SIXTH EDITION

DARBY AND WALSH
DENTAL HYGIENE

THEORY (AND) PRACTICE

Jennifer A. Pieren, RDH, BSAS, MS
Adjunct Faculty
Department of Health Professions
Dental Hygiene
Youngstown State University
Youngstown, Ohio

Cynthia C. Gadbury-Amyot, MSDH, Ed.D
Professor Emeritus
Dental Hygiene
University of Missouri-Kansas City
Kansas City, Missouri

ELSEVIER

Elsevier
3251 Riverport Lane
St. Louis, Missouri 63043

Notice

Practitioners and researchers must always rely on their own experience and knowledge in evaluating and
using any information, methods, compounds or experiments described herein. Because of rapid advances
in the medical sciences, in particular, independent verification of diagnoses and drug dosages should be
made. To the fullest extent of the law, no responsibility is assumed by Elsevier, authors, editors or contributors for any injury and/or damage to persons or property as a matter of products liability, negligence or
otherwise, or from any use or operation of any methods, products, instructions, or ideas contained in the
material herein.

Previous editions copyrighted 2020, 2015, 2010, 2003, and 1995 by Saunders, an imprint of Elsevier, Inc.

Publishing Director, Education Content: Kristin Wilhelm
Director, Content Development: Ellen Wurm-Cutter
Senior Content Strategist: Kelly Skelton
Senior Content Development Specialist: Kathleen Nahm
Publishing Services Manager: Julie Eddy
Senior Project Manager: Cindy Thoms
Senior Book Designer: Margaret Reid

Printed in India

Last digit is the print number: 9 8 7 6 5 4 3 2

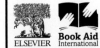

For Michele, Peggy, and Denise. This book's legacy is built on the reputation of giants. We aspire to continue your work in every edition and move closer to fulfilling your vision for the dental hygiene profession. Also, for everyone else who helped build and foster this book, current and past editions, you are an inspiration to the dental hygiene profession.

For my entire family, especially Steve, and Riley; Cynthia C. Gadbury-Amyot, my co-editor, mentor, and friend, who deserves special thanks for joining me on this journey, Diane P. Kandray, my mentor and friend, and Nikki Fillman, who is always there for me. You are my incredible support system, who have been instrumental in making this edition a reality. Your unwavering love, understanding, and encouragement have been the driving force in my success and wellness. I would not be who I am without you. Also, for my niece Lauren – you have demonstrated remarkable dedication, perseverance, and resilience in pursuing your dreams. I am so proud of you.

Jennifer A. Pieren

For my husband of 47 years who has never failed to support my crazy endeavors – thank you Bernie; to my children, Megan and Caleb, of whom I am immensely proud of the adults they have become; to my co-editor, Jennifer Pieren, who has taken me on this journey of co-editorship and between her depth and breadth of knowledge has also made the process fun! For my colleagues at the University of Missouri-Kansas City School of Dentistry who have always pushed and supported me in my 30+ years at the university to be "all that I could be". And last but by far not least, to my parents who raised me to believe that I could do and be anything I wanted. I use my maiden name of "Gadbury" to honor them for my academic endeavors.

Cynthia C. Gadbury-Amyot

CONTRIBUTORS

Diana Aboytes, RDH, MS
Associate Professor
Division of Dental Hygiene
Department of Dental Medicine
University of New Mexico
Albuquerque, New Mexico

Melanie Aley, BOH, BHSc(Hons), MEd, PhD
Associate Professor
Sydney Dental School
The University of Sydney,
    Camperdown
NSW
Australia

Joanna Asadoorian, AAS(DH), BSc, MSc, PhD
Professor/Coordinator
School of Dental Health
George Brown College, Toronto
Ontario
Canada

Curtis Aumiller, PhD, RRT-ACCS, RRT-NPS, RPFT
Professor, Program Director of Respiratory
    Therapy
Health Sciences
Harrisburg Area Community College
Harrisburg, Pennsylvania

Kylie J. Austin, RDH, MS
Consultant
School of Dentistry
University of Missouri-Kansas City
Kansas City, Missouri

Marleen Azzam, DHSc, RDH
Assistant Professor
Dental Hygiene
Farmingdale State College
Farmingdale, New York

Katelyn Bartone, RDH, BS, MPH
Clinic Coordinator
Dental Hygiene
University of New Haven
West Haven, Connecticut

Kimberly Bastin, CDA, EFDA, CRDH, MS
Director
Dental Hygiene
State College of Florida
Bradenton, Florida

Katy Battani, RDH, MS
Project Manager
National Maternal and Child Oral Health
    Resource Center
Georgetown University
Washington, DC

Helene Sharon Bednarsh, BS, RDH, MPH
Dental Director New England AIDS Education
    and Training Center
Department of Family Medicine and Community
    Health
UMASS Chan Medical School
Sharon, Massachusetts

Kathryn Bell, EdD, RDH
Associate Professor and Director
Doctor of Science Program
Associate Dean for Interprofessional Education
Pacific University
Hillsboro, Oregon

Laurie V. Bercasio, RDH, BS, MSDH
Dental Hygiene Instructor
Dental Hygiene
Chabot College
Hayward, California

Mary Bertone, BSc(DH), MPH, DSc(c)
Director and Associate Professor
School of Dental Hygiene
University of Manitoba
Winnipeg, Manitoba
Canada

Leciel Bono, RDH-ER, MS
Graduate Program Director, Associate Professor
Dental Hygiene
Idaho State University
Pocatello, Idaho

Joaquin Borrego Jr., PhD, MA, BA
Professor and Associate Dean for Faculty Devel-
    opment and Student Success
School of Graduate Psychology, College of Health
    Professions
Pacific University
Portland, Oregon

Dani Botbyl, RDH
Professional Education and Research
Clinical Affairs
Dentsply Sirona
Toronto, Ontario
Canada

Kimberly S. Bray, PhD, RDH
Professor
School of Dentistry
University of Missouri-Kansas City
Kansas City, Missouri

Ann M. Bruhn, BSDH, MS, RDH
Associate Professor and Chair
School of Dental Hygiene
Old Dominion University
Norfolk, Virginia

Ann Brunick, MSDH
Professor Emeritus
Department of Dental Hygiene
University of South Dakota
Vermillion, South Dakota

Ruth Lynn Bushby, RDH, MEd, BScDH, dip DH
Professor
Oral Health Programs
Confederation College
Thunder Bay, Ontario
Canada

Susan Camardese, RDH, MS
Co-Founder for Mid-Atlantic Prevent Abuse and
    Neglect (PANDA)
Columbia, Maryland

Dina Marie Canasi, DHSc, MSDH, CRDH
Professor
Dental Hygiene
Hillsborough Community College
Tampa, Florida

Anthony S. Carroccia, DDS, MAGD, DDOCS, MaCSD, FICD, FACD, FPFA, ABGD
St. Bethlehem Dental Care
Clarksville, Tennessee

Denise M. Claiborne, MS, PhD
Assistant Professor
Graduate Program Director
Dental Hygiene
Old Dominion University
Norfolk, Virginia

Matt Crespin, MPH, RDH
Executive Director
Children's Health Alliance of Wisconsin
Children's Wisconsin
Milwaukee, Wisconsin

Eve Cuny, BA, MS
Executive Associate Dean
Administration
Professor
Diagnostic Sciences
University of the Pacific Arthur A. Dugoni School
    of Dentistry
San Francisco, California

Sandra D'Amato-Palumbo, RDH, MPS, EdD
Professor
Allied Health
University of New Haven
West Haven, Connecticut

Tracee Sokolik Dahm, MS, BSDH
Adjunct Faculty
Clinic
North Idaho College
Coeur d'Alene, Idaho

Diane M. Daubert, RDH, MS, PhD
Associate Teaching Professor
Periodontics
University of Washington
Seattle, Washington

Joan M. Davis, RDH, PhD
Professor, Assistant Dean of Research
Missouri School of Dentistry and Oral Health
A. T. Still University
St. Louis, Missouri

Lauren C. DeSantis, RDH, MDH, EFDA
Part Time Faulty
Department of Health Professions
Youngstown State University
Youngstown, Ohio

Haley Dollins, BSDH, MSDH Ed
President and Dental Hygiene Clinician
Dental Experts, LLC
Minneapolis, Minnesota

Leeann Donnelly, Dip DH, BDSc(DH), MSc, PhD
Associate Professor
Oral Biological and Medical Sciences
University of British Columbia
Vancouver, British Columbia
Canada

Catherine Kelly Draper, MS, RDH
Adjunct Faculty
Biological and Health Sciences
Foothill College
San Jose, California
Managing Editor
Journal of Dental Hygiene
American Dental Hygienists' Association
Chicago, Illinois

Nadia Dubreuil, HD, cert EFPT
Professor
Dental Hygiene
Cégep Garneau
President of Group For Research and Education in Dental Hygiene
Québec City, Québec
Canada

Kathy J. Eklund, RDH, MHP
Sr. Director of Occupational Health and Safety
Administration
The Forsyth Institute
Cambridge, Massachusetts
Adjunct Faculty
Dental Hygiene
Regis College
Westin, Massachusetts

John D. Featherstone, MSc, PhD
Professor Emeritus and Dean Emeritus
Preventive and Restorative Dental Sciences
University of California San Francisco
San Francisco, California

Margaret J. Fehrenbach, RDH, MS
Oral Biologist and Dental Hygienist
Educational Consultant and Oral Biology Writer
Past Adjunct Faculty
Dental Hygiene Program
Seattle Central College
Seattle, Washington

Jane L. Forrest, EdD, MS, BSDH
Professor Emerita
Dental Public Health and Pediatric Dentistry
Ostrow School of Dentistry
University of Southern California
Los Angeles, California
Director, National Center for Dental Hygiene
   Research & Practice, Inc.
Cave Creek, Arizona

Cynthia C. Gadbury-Amyot, MSDH, EdD
Professor Emeritus
Division of Dental Hygiene
University of Missouri-Kansas City
Kansas City, Missouri

Marie D. George, RDH, MS
Adjunct Faculty
Dental Hygiene
West Liberty University
West Liberty, West Virginia
Clinical Instructor
Dental Hygiene
Westmoreland County Community College
Youngwood, Pennsylvania

Lorraine Frances Glassford, BA, Dip DH, MA (IS)
Senior Instructor
School of Dental Hygiene
University of Manitoba
Winnipeg, Manitoba
Canada

Joan I. Gluch, PhD, RDH, PHDHP
Associate Dean, Division Chief and
   Professor, Community Oral Health
Preventive and Restorative Sciences
University of Pennsylvania School of Dental Medicine
Philadelphia, Pennsylvania

Matthew Greaves, DDS, MS
Assistant Professor
Missouri School of Dentistry & Oral Health
A.T. Still University
St. Louis, Missouri

Gwen Grosso, RDH, MS
Assistant Professor
Dental Hygiene
University of New Haven
West Haven, Connecticut

Adrien Gupton, DNP, FNP, CNM
Associate Clinical Professor
School of Nursing
Northern Arizona University
Flagstaff, Arizona

Lesley A. Harbison, RDH, EPDH, MS
Assistant Professor
School of Dental Hygiene Studies
Pacific University
Hillsboro, Oregon

Joanna Harris-Worelds, EdD, MSDH, RDH
Assistant Professor
Dental Hygiene
Georgia State University
Perimeter College
Dunwoody, Georgia

Harold Henson, BS, RDH, MEd, PhD
Professor
Periodontics and Dental Hygiene
The University of Texas at Houston School of
   Dentistry
Houston, Texas

Kathleen Olivia Hodges, RDH, MS
Professor Emerita
Dental Hygiene
Idaho State University
Pocatello, Idaho

Lorie Holt, AS, BS, MS, PhD
Associate Professor
Division of Dental Hygiene
Director RDH to BSDH Degree Program
Division of Dental Hygiene
Cafe Pillar Lead
Center for Advancing Faculty Excellence
University of Missouri-Kansas City
Kansas City, Missouri

Alice M. Horowitz, RDH, MA, PhD
Research Professor
Behavioral and Community Health
School of Public Health, UMD
College Park, Maryland

Amber W. Hunt, BSDH, MS, RDH
Clinical Assistant Professor
Junior Clinic Coordinator
Gene W. Hirschfeld School of Dental Hygiene
Old Dominion University
Norfolk, Virginia

Russell Johnson, DDS, MS
Affiliate Assistant Professor
Restorative Dentistry
University of Washington
Seattle, Washington

Beth Jordan, RDH, MS
Scientific Relations Manager
Portland, Maine

Jessica Lopez Jorquera, BS, RDH, RDHAP
Manager, Infection Prevention and Control
Environmental Health and Safety
Clinical Assistant Professor
Diagnostic Sciences
University of the Pacific, Arthur A. Dugoni School
    of Dentistry
San Francisco, California

Mark Kacerik, RDH, MS
Chair, Associate Professor
Allied Health
University of New Haven
West Haven, Connecticut

Diane P. Kandray, EdD, RDH
Professor
Health Professions, Dental Hygiene Program
Youngstown State University
Youngstown, Ohio

Juliana J. Kim, PhD, MBA
Adjunct Assistant Professor
School of Dental Hygiene
Old Dominion University
Norfolk, Virginia
Vice President
Business Development, Pharma
Univision Communications
New York, New York

Mina C. Kim, DDS
Practice Manager
Dental
Bryant Park Dental Associates
New York, New York

Elizabeth C. Kornegay, MS, RDH
Assistant Professor
Comprehensive Oral Health
University of North Carolina at Chapel Hill
Chapel Hill, North Carolina

Gwen Lang, RDH, MS
Professor
Dental Hygiene
Diablo Valley College
Pleasant Hill, California

**France Lavoie, DH, BA, MA, DIU
Posturology**
Independent Practice
Dental Hygiene
Coop HD Quebec
Trois-Rivieres, Quebec
Research
Group of Research and Education in Dental
    Hygiene (GREDH)
Quebec, Quebec
Canada

Jennifer Leicht, RDH, RDHAP, MS Ed
Full Time Tenure Track Faculty
Dental Hygiene
Foothill College
Los Altos Hills, California

Margaret Lemaster, MS, BSDH, RDH
Adjunct Professor
School of Dentistry
Virginia Commonwealth University
Richmond, Virginia

**Laura L. MacDonald, DipDH, BScD(DH),
MEd, PhD**
Associate Professor
School of Dental Hygiene, College of Dentistry
Member, College of Dentistry
Office of Interprofessional Collaboration
Rady Faculty of Health Sciences
University of Manitoba
Winnipeg, Manitoba
Canada

L. Lynda McKeown, RDH, HBA, MA
Dental Hygienist
Palliative Dental Hygiene Oral Care Mobile
    Practice
Oral Health Programs
Confederation College
Thunder Bay, Ontario
Canada

L. Teal Mercer, RDH, BS, MPH
Assistant Professor
Dental Hygiene
Montgomery County Community College
Blue Bell, Pennsylvania

Elizabeth Michaud-Jobin, RDH, BS
Professor
Dental Hygiene
Cégep Garneau
Quebec, Quebec
Canada

Syrene A. Miller, MSW
Project Manager
National Center for Dental Hygiene Research
Cave Creek, Arizona

Tanya Villalpando Mitchell, RDH, MS
Professor and Chair
Division of Dental Hygiene
University of Missouri-Kansas City School of
    Dentistry
Kansas City, Missouri

**Cara Michiko Miyasaki, CDA, RDA,
RDHEF, MS**
Program Director
Dental Assisting Department
Instructor
Dental Hygiene Program
Foothill College
Los Altos Hills, California

Tracye A. Moore, RDH, MS, EdD
Department Chair
Department of Dental Hygiene
Northern Arizona University
Flagstaff, Arizona

Ann Kim Mora, RDH, BASDH
Registered Dental Hygienist
Dental Hygiene
Andrew Kapust, DDS
Olympia, Washington

Antonio Moretti, DDS, MS
Professor
Periodontology
University of North Carolina School of Dentistry
Chapel Hill, North Carolina

Laura Mueller-Joseph, BSDH, MS, EdD
Vice President for Academic Affairs and
    Professor
Department of Dental Hygiene
Farmingdale State College
Farmingdale, New York

Christine N. Nathe, RDH, MS
Professor and Director
Dental Hygiene
University of New Mexico
Albuquerque, New Mexico

**Caroline Tram Nguyen, DMD, MS, FACP,
FRCD(C)**
Director of Examinations
The National Dental Examining Board of Canada
Maxillofacial Prosthodontist
Dentistry
The Ottawa Hospital-Civic Campus
Ottawa, Ontario
Canada

**Michaela Trang-Thu Nguyen,
RDH, MS**
Clinical Assistant Professor
Infection Control, Diagnostic Sciences and
    Periodontology
Ostrow School of Dentistry of University of
    Southern California
Los Angeles, California

Sheila Kensmoe Norton, BS, RDH
Retired Restorative Lead
Dental Hygiene
Pierce College
Lakewood, Washington

Danette Ocegueda, RDH, MS
Professional Education, Manager-West
Dental Professional
Philips Oral Healthcare
Stanford, Connecticut

Uhlee Oh, MS, RDH
Assistant Professor
Forsyth School of Dental Hygiene
Massachusetts College of Pharmacy and Health
    Sciences
Boston, Massachusetts

Sarah O. Ostrander, RDH, DHSc
Senior Manager, Dental Licensure and Education
Education and Professional Affairs
American Dental Association
Chicago, Illinois

Ruth Palich, RDH, MHHS, CHES
Assistant Professor
Dental Hygiene
Youngstown State University
Youngstown, Ohio

Karen M. Palleschi, AS, BSDH, MS
Professor Emeritis - retired
Dental Hygiene
Hudson Valley Community College
Troy, New York

Victoria Patrounova, RDH, MHA
Associate Professor
Periodontics and Dental Hygiene
The University of Texas
Bellaire, Texas

Jennifer A. Pieren, RDH, BSAS, MS, FADHA
Adjunct Faculty
Department of Health Professions
Dental Hygiene
Youngstown State University
Youngstown, Ohio
Adjunct Professor
Allied Health
University of New Haven
West Haven, Connecticut

Susan Raynak, Diploma
Professor/ Coordinator - Retired
Oral Health Programmes
Confederation College
Thunder Bay, Ontario
Canada

David Alan Reznik, DDS
Chief, Dental Medicine
Medical Staff
Executive Director
Oral Health Center/Infectious Disease Program
Grady Health System
Atlanta, Georgia

Melanie Simmer-Beck, PhD, RDH
Chair and Professor
Dental Public Health and Behavioral Science
University of Missouri-Kansas City
Kansas City, Missouri

Suzanne Smith, RDH, MEd
Associate Professor
Health Professions
Youngstown State University
Youngstown, Ohio

Phyllis Anne Spragge, RDH, MA
Professor
Dental Hygiene
Foothill College
Los Altos Hills, California

Herve Sroussi, DMD, PhD
Surgery
Brigham and Women's Hospital
Harvard School of Dental Medicine
Boston, Massachusetts

Joyce Y. Sumi, RDH, BSDH, MSDH
Associate Professor
Dental Public Health and Community Outreach
Director
Community Oral Health Certificate Program
Infection Control Safety Specialist
Herman Ostrow School of Dentistry of
University of Southern California
Los Angeles, California

Sheryl L. Syme, RDH, MS
Associate Professor
Advanced Oral Sciences and Therapeutics
Periodontics Division
University of Maryland School of Dentistry
Baltimore, Maryland

Bryn K. Taylor, BSDH, MHHS, RDH, EFDA
Interim Program Administrator
Department of Health Professions
Youngstown State University
Youngstown, Ohio

Thomas Viola, RPh, CCP, CDE, CPMP
Adjunct Instructor
College of Dentistry
New York University
New York, New York

Carolyn Weiss, RDH
Registered Independent Dental Hygienist
Dental Hygiene
Carolyn Weiss Dental Hygiene Mobile Services
Thunder Bay, Ontario
Canada

Meghan Wendland, DDS, MPH
Assistant Professor
Dental Public Health and Behavioral Sciences
University of Missouri-Kansas City School of
Dentistry
Kansas City, Missouri

Rebecca Wilder, RDH, MS
Distinguished Professor and
Associate Dean for Professional Development and
Faculty Affairs
Adams School of Dentistry
University of North Carolina at
Chapel Hill
Chapel Hill, North Carolina

Rachelle Williams, BS, MS
Assistant Professor
Dental Hygiene Sciences
Idaho State University
Pocatello, Idaho

Heather Woodbeck, BScN, MHSA
Long Term Care Best Practice Coordinator
International Affairs and Best Practice Guidelines
Centre
Registered Nurses' Association of Ontario
Thunder Bay, Ontario
Canada

Kathy Yerex, BSc, RDH, MS
Professor
School of Dental Hygiene
University of Manitoba
Winnipeg, Manitoba
Canada

Pamela Zarkowski, JD, MPH
Provost and Vice President for Academic Affairs
Academic Affairs
Professor
Practice Essentials and Interprofessional Education
University of Detroit Mercy School of Dentistry
Detroit, Michigan

REVIEWERS

Aicha Sid Ahmed, DDS
Clinical Tutor of Periodontics
Lecturer of Periodontics
Sharjah University
College of Dental Medicine
Sharjah, United Arab Emirates

Chukwuemeka Anyikwa, BDS
University of Nigeria Teaching Hospital
Enugu, Enugu State
Nigeria

Maureen Archer-Festa, RDH, DDS
Chairperson of the Dental Hygiene Department
New York City College of Technology
Dental Hygiene Department
Brooklyn, New York

Barbara Bennett, RDH, MS
Director of Medical Education and Curriculum
    Management
University of Illinois Urbana-Champaign
College of Medicine
Urbana, Illinois

Peg Boyce, RDH, MA
Professor
Parkland College
Champaign, Illinois

Kristin H. Calley, RDH, MS
Associate Professor
Idaho State University
Department of Dental Hygiene
Pocatello, Idaho

Lezlie M. Cantrell, RDH, PhD
Dental Hygiene Educator
Freelance Writer, Healthcare Content
Missouri Southern State University
Joplin, Missouri

Tammy S. Clossen, RDH, PHDHP, PhD
Assistant Professor
Dental Hygiene
Pennsylvania College of Technology
Williamsport, Pennsylvania

Lorinda L. Coan, MS, RDH
Associate Professor
University of Southern Indiana
College of Nursing and Health Professions
Evansville, Indiana

**JoAnn Gurenlian, RDH, MS, PhD,
AAFAAOM, FADHA**
Director, Education, Research & Advocacy
American Dental Hygienists' Association
Chicago, Illinois

Julie Collette, RDH, BSc
Registered Dental Hygienist
University of Alberta
Edmonton, Alberta
Canada

Sharon M. Compton, BSc, MA(Ed), PhD, RDH
Professor
University of Alberta
Edmonton, Alberta
Canada

**Satyawan Damle, MDS, MBA, PhD, FAMS,
FIAMS**
Ex-Dean, Professor and Head Pediatric and
    Preventive
Nair Hospital Dental College, Mumbai,
Ex-Vice Chancellor
Maharishi Markandeshwar University, Mullana,
Nair Hospital Dental College Mumbai
Bombay University
Mumbai, Maharashtra
Ambala, Haryana
India

Stephanie Eisner, RDH, BS, MEd
Dental Hygiene Instructor
Wallace State Community College
Hanceville, Alabama

Gwen Essex, RDH, RDHAP, MS, EdD
Clinical Professor
University of California, San Francisco,
School of Dentistry
Department of Preventive and Restorative Dental
    Sciences
San Francisco, California

Tabitha Fair, RDH, PhD
Assistant Professor/Dental Hygiene Program
    Director
East Tennessee State University
Johnson City, Tennessee

Christine Fambely, RDH, BA, MEd
Theoretical and Clinical Instructor
John Abbott College
Ste-Anne-de-Bellevue, Quebec
Canada

Shokoufeh Shahrabi Farahani, DDS, MS, DMSc
Associate Professor and Director
University of Tennessee Health Science Center
College of Dentistry
Memphis, Tennessee

Varinder Goyal
Professor and Chair, Pediatric Dentistry
Guru Nanak Dev Dental College and Research
    Institute
Sunam
India

Tawnya Guthrie, RDH
University of Missouri-Kansas City School of
    Dentistry
Division of Dental Hygiene
Kansas City, Missouri
Class of 2023

Rosemary Menta Herman, RDH, MEd
Assistant Professor
First Year Dental Hygiene Coordinator
Montgomery County Community College
Blue Bell, Pennsylvania

Laura Hettinger, MSDH
Associate Professor
Parkland College
Champaign, Illinois

Sarah Jackson, RDH, MSDH
Professor of Dental Hygiene
Eastern Washington University
Spokane, Washington

Pravesh Jhingta
Professor
HP Government Dental College and
    Hospital-Shimla
Shimla, Himachal Pradesh
India

Deborah L. Johnson, RDH, EA/EP, MS
Professor
Eastern Washington University
Spokane, Washington,
University of Bridgeport
Bridgeport, Connecticut
Lone Star College
Porter, Texas

Terri Johnson, RDH, BS
Clinical Coordinator
Southern University at Shreveport
Shreveport, Louisiana

Merri L. Jones, RDH, MSDH
Associate Professor
Eastern Washington University
Spokane, Washington

Zohaib Khurshid
Doctor
Department of Prosthodontics and Dental
    Implantology
College of Dentistry
King Faisal University, KSA
Hofuf, Saudi Arabia

Venkata Sandeep Kumar
Assistant Professor
Narayana Dental College
Nellore, Andhra Pradesh
India

Crystal Kanderis Lane, RDH, MSDH
Assistant Professor
Idaho State University
Pocatello, Idaho

Lory Laughter, RDH, MS
Assistant Professor/Program Director, Dental
  Hygiene
University of the Pacific, Arthur A. Dugoni School
  of Dentistry
San Francisco, California

**Gabriele Eva Maycher, BSc, PID, Dip DH,
RDH (Alberta,
British Columbia)**
Private Consultant
CEO, Founder
GEM Dental Experts Inc.
Vancouver, British Columbia
Canada

Tanya Villalpando Mitchell, RDH, MS
Professor and Chair-Division of Dental Hygiene
University of Missouri-Kansas City School of
  Dentistry
Kansas City, Missouri

Christine Nielsen Nathe, RDH, MS
Professor and Program Director
University of New Mexico
Division of Dental Hygiene
Albuquerque, New Mexico

Elizabeth Ann North, RDH, BSc, PID
Registered Dental Hygienist
Vancouver College of Dental Hygiene
New Westminster, British Columbia
Canada

Veerinder Pannu, BDS, MS
Assistant Professor
The Dental College of Georgia
Augusta University
Augusta, Georgia

Alfredo Torres Parra, DDS, MSc
Dental surgeon
Universidad San Sebastián
Concepción, Chile

**Brian B. Partido, PhD, MSDH, RDH,
RDA, CDA**
Executive Director, Dental Programs
Seattle Central College
Seattle, Washington

Anna Matsuishi Pattison, RDH, MS
Associate Professor Emeritus
Co-Director
University of Southern California
Ostrow School of Dentistry
Pattison Institute
Los Angeles, California

Suprabha Rathee
Professor
IP Dental College and Hospital
Uttar Pradesh, India

Samantha Reidenbach, RDH, BSDH, MA
Dental Hygiene Faculty
Kalamazoo Valley Community College
Kalamazoo, Michigan

Arvind Babu Rajendra Santhosh, BDS, MDS
Doctor
School of Dentistry
Faculty of Medical Sciences
The University of the West Indies
Mona Campus, Kingston
Jamaica

Cynthia Seaman, BS, MBA, MS, PhD
Team Leader/Registered Dental Hygienist
College of Southern Idaho
Twin Falls, Idaho

Kylie J. Siruta-Austin, RDH, MS, ECP-III
Consultant and Course Director
University of Missouri-Kansas City
Kansas City, Missouri

**Laura J. Sleeper, DHSc, RDH, NYS, AAS, BS,
MA, DHSc**
Dean, School of Dental Sciences
Plaza College
Forest Hills, New York

Dawn R. Smith, BSDH, MS
Associate Professor
Howard University
Washington, DC

Lorie Speer, RDH, MSDH
Associate Professor
Eastern Washington University
Spokane Campus
Spokane, Washington

Jill L. Stoltenberg, RDH, MS, RF
Associate Professor
University of Minnesota
Minneapolis, Minnesota

Mary E. Terkoski, DDS
Supervising Dentist and Adjunct Faculty
Dental Hygiene Program
Middlesex Community College
Bedford, Massachusetts

Michelle W. Terry, BS, RDH
Registered Dental Hygienist
Southern Jersey Family Medical Centers
Hammonton, New Jersey

Terri Tilliss, RDH, BS, MS, MA, PhD
Professor
University of Colorado School of Dental Medicine
Aurora, Colorado

Kelly Turner, BA (Kin), RDH, PME (c. 2021)
Professor of Dental Hygiene
Fanshawe College
London, Ontario
Canada

Lancette VanGuilder, BS, RDH, PHEDH
Professional Educator
Speaker and Public Health Dental Hygienist
Hygienist for Health
Community Dental Connections
Reno, Nevada

**Laura J. Webb, MSHSA, RDH, FAADH,
CDA-emeritus**
Allied Dental Education Consultant and Speaker
TMCC Dental Hygiene Program
Faculty Emerita
Truckee Meadows Community College
Reno, Nevada

I-Tsen Weng
University of Michigan School of Dentistry
Ann Arbor, Michigan

Rebecca S. Wilder, RDH, BS, MS, ICF-ACC
Professor and Associate Dean for Professional
  Development and Faculty Affairs
University of North Carolina-Chapel Hill
Adams School of Dentistry
Chapel Hill, North Carolina

Stefania Moglia Willis, RDH, MA, DMH
Clinical Associate Professor
New York University College of Dentistry
New York City, New York

**Sharman Woynarski, RDH, RDA, BDSc,
MAEd**
Academic Chair Dental Programs
Saskatchewan Polytechnic
Regina, Saskatchewan
Canada

Simith Yadav, BDS, MDS
Doctor
Community Health Centre, DADHA
Greater Noida, Uttar Pradesh
India

PREFACE

Darby and Walsh Dental Hygiene: Theory and Practice, sixth edition, continues the legacy of Michele Darby and Margaret "Peggy" Walsh while continuing the enhancement of their seminal work that was started in the fifth edition. The focus of enhancements both for the fifth and now sixth edition is to create a book that (1) heightens its focus on the expanding opportunities for dental hygienists as primary care providers, (2) is aware of the changing public health needs following an unprecedented public health emergency; (3) is visually appealing and easy to use, and (4) is suitable for the needs of modern learners.

The book provides a strong foundation in critical thinking, evidence-based practice, related theory, and safe clinical care in all settings. One of the greatest challenges for educators is to connect course content to the current culture while making learning outcomes and activities relevant to these students' goals and interests. Addressing these learning preferences is a continued objective in this edition and its accompanying online resources.

Dental hygiene is changing as dental hygienists practice in an ever-evolving variety of settings. Dental hygienists are primary care providers who work interprofessionally and intraprofessionally with other health care providers. Critical thinking in health care improves the quality of services delivered and patient outcomes. We want to provide dental hygiene students, faculty, and practitioners opportunities to understand and experience this enhanced vision of our profession.

As educators, clinicians, and editors, we realize that the exclusive use of the word *client* versus *patient* is not universal in our discipline nor in other disciplines. Our compromise is to use the term *patient* when referring to clinical procedures provided for individuals and the term *client* when referring to educational or motivational interactions requiring a cotherapy or collaborative approach and when dental hygienists work with clients other than those seen in the clinical practice setting.

Our philosophy continues to be one of embracing the Dental Hygiene Paradigm concepts developed by Darby and Walsh and adopted by the American Dental Hygienists' Association (ADHA): client (potential or actual recipients of dental hygiene care including individuals, families, groups, and communities), health (wellness-illness continuum), environment (factors other than dental hygiene actions that affect the client's attainment of optimal oral health), and dental hygiene actions (preventive and therapeutic oral health services requiring cognitive, affective, and psychomotor skills, including the dental hygiene process of care). We also embrace the Dental Hygiene Human Needs Conceptual Model developed by Darby and Walsh. As with the last edition, this text will present other validated health and behavioral theories and other dental hygiene conceptual models such as the Oral Health-Related Quality of Life Conceptual Model.

CHAPTER FORMAT

The book and chapters are organized as follows.

Opening Features
Professional Opportunities

Each chapter begins with a brief statement explaining why this information is important for the dental hygienist's growth and future opportunities in the discipline or in interaction with patients.

Competencies

Competencies, or learning outcomes, are included for each chapter. The learning competencies reflect higher levels of learning domains that the student will acquire from studying the chapter and completing related activities.

Evolve Instructor Resources

Content and curriculum experts have developed a comprehensive listing of specific objectives, presentation content, learning strategies, and lesson plans for our complementary online instructor section on the Evolve site.

PROFESSIONAL OPPORTUNITIES

Dental hygienists have the responsibility to both understand and provide quality care to patients with disabilities. No one is alike. People with disabilities are not handicapped; they are genuinely special. That is why disabilities are special needs. Dental hygienists can improve the quality of life of these individuals by caring for their oral health needs and helping them prevent dental disease requiring treatment that is more complex.

COMPETENCIES

By the end of this chapter, the reader will be able to:
1. Define "disability" and acquire knowledge about major developments or circumstances affecting patients with disabilities.
2. Distinguish different classifications for patients with disabilities.
3. Consider and recommend means to address healthcare barriers, assistive devices, and oral self-care devices for patients with disabilities. Provide oral self-care education to patients with disabilities and their caregivers.
4. Explain how to use protective stabilization and patient-positioning techniques throughout the delivery of professional care.
5. Care for patients in wheelchairs and recommend opportunities to advocate for patients with disabilities.

▶ EVOLVE VIDEO RESOURCES

View two videos on one-person and two-person wheelchair transfer procedures and technique demonstrations on Evolve (http://evolve.elsevier.com/Pieren/hygiene/).

Body of Chapter

Many of the descriptions, basic concepts, key trends, and discoveries, as well as some of the conclusions, are presented in figures or boxes. Tables are also used to succinctly and clearly present the bulk of the detailed information in each chapter for the learner.

- Procedure Boxes: Up-to-date, evidence-based procedures tables outline functions and tasks that require succinct, systematic, step-by-step instructions. Elements of legal documentation are included for procedures performed.
  - Fifty-five instructional videos accompany the procedure tables. These online resources are complimentary for any faculty member adopting the textbook for their students' use.
- Client or Patient Education Tips: Key points to teach the client or patient in order to decrease risk of disease and promote health are listed in boxes.
- Legal, Ethical, and Safety Issues: Legal or ethical responsibilities of the dental hygienist are listed or presented using brief scenarios that require application of these requirements, principles, or issues.

- Key Concepts: At the conclusion of each chapter, the key "take-home messages" discussed in the chapter are summarized.
- Critical Thinking Scenarios: New scenarios, such as challenging case studies, can be used by learners and educators to apply key concepts. These scenarios allow the learner to do one or more of the following:
  - Apply research-based evidence in practice
  - Make evidence-based clinical decisions
  - Exercise professional judgment and self-assessment skills
  - Evaluate significant information
  - Collaborate with others on the health care team or interprofessionally
- Key Terms: Key terms are bolded in black where they are defined in the chapter.
- References: Current citations using the highest level of evidence or current health policy are included.

PROCEDURE 59.1 Proper Use of Mouth Prop and Establishing a Double Fulcrum

Steps

1. Hold the mouth prop using the hand opposite to the half of the mouth receiving treatment. For example, if the dental hygienist intends to provide treatment on the right half of the mouth, then hold the mouth prop with the left hand and vice versa.
2. Gently pull the patient's lower lip forward using the index finger and thumb of the available hand. This step is essential in preventing the patient from inadvertently biting the lip when the mouth prop is inserted into the mouth.
3. Gently insert the smaller end of the mouth prop horizontally into the patient's mouth while continuing to protect the lower lip from biting trauma.

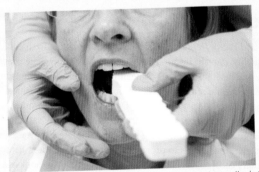

Gently insert smaller end of the mouth prop horizontally into the patient's mouth while continuing to protect the lower lip from a biting trauma. (Courtesy Faizan Kabani and Kathleen Muzzin, Texas A&M College of Dentistry, Caruth School of Dental Hygiene, Dallas, TX)

4. Carefully turn the mouth prop from a horizontal to a vertical position to help open the patient's mouth. Be sure to use the mouth prop only between the patient's posterior teeth, which are built to withstand biting pressure.
5. Place the ring finger of the hand holding the mouth prop on the gingiva buccal to the mandibular anterior sextant. The ring finger establishes the first fulcrum and prevents the lower lip from biting trauma.
6. Place the pinky finger of the hand that is holding the mouth prop on the patient's chin. The pinky finger establishes the second fulcrum and assists in stabilizing the mouth prop (see Fig. 59.6).

BOX 20.7 Client Education Tips

- Explain the purpose of both the comprehensive periodontal examination and risk factor assessment.
- Show the clinical appearance of healthy gingiva, periodontal pocket readings, bleeding on probing, and other signs of disease; use a mirror and the patient's radiographic images for teaching.
- Engage the patient as a team member, self-monitor clinical signs of oral disease, and perform self-examination.
- Explain the significance of the risk factors so that the patient understands the personal degree of risk for periodontal disease, the disease progression, and the importance of an effective oral self-care program and regular professional treatments.

BOX 20.9 Legal, Ethical, and Safety Issues

- Information gained from the periodontal assessment and shared with the patient provides the basis for patient autonomy and informed consent.
- Communication about the assessment, proposed procedures, risks of procedures, and alternatives to care (including refusal) must be in the terminology and language that the patient understands.
- The patient must be given information about current risks, periodontal disease status, prognosis, and the risks involved in treatment.
- Documentation of the assessment objective and subjective findings and patient communication are legal documents that must be accurate and complete.
- Importantly, clinicians should encourage and give the patient opportunities to ask questions, and then document both the question and the corresponding response.

CRITICAL THINKING EXERCISE ON DESIGNING ORAL SELF-CARE ASSISTIVE DEVICES

Design oral self-care devices for the following patient conditions:
- Inability to grasp and hold,
- Inability to raise the arm and hand, and/or
- Inability to move the forearm in a back-and-forth motion.

PROTECTIVE STABILIZATION AND PATIENT POSITIONING

Understanding Protective Stabilization

Patients with disabilities, from subtle

KEY CONCEPTS

- Risk factor assessment is important for appropriate targeted care planning that focuses on prevention and treatment, specific risk factors, and reparative therapies.
- The origin of periodontal disease is strongly linked to periodontal pathogens (e.g., *Aggregatibacter actinomycetemcomitans*, *Tannerella forsythia*, and *Porphyromonas gingivalis*). Clinical observations of inflammation and probing depths, the determination of clinical attachment levels, and radiographic images provide primary information for determining periodontal health, diagnosing periodontal conditions, and planning dental hygiene therapy. Dental biofilm–induced gingivitis is a reversible inflammatory periodontal disease without attachment loss and is characterized by any or all of the following tissue changes: redness, edema, enlargement, spongy consistency, and BOP.
- Gingival bleeding is the key clinical characteristic of dental biofilm–induced gingivitis.
- Periodontitis is an inflammation of the periodontium characterized by clinical attachment loss, resulting from the destruction of the periodontal ligament and alveolar bone. It can exhibit periods of exacerbation (i.e., disease activity) and quiescence (i.e., inactivity). Other forms of periodontitis include necrotizing periodontitis and periodontitis as a manifestation of systemic disease.
- Periimplant diseases include periimplant mucositis and periimplantitis.
- The host's immunoinflammatory and immunologic responses to bacteria in oral biofilm is responsible for tissue destruction in periodontal disease.
- Gingival bleeding occurring at sequential continued care visits is associated with an increased risk for periodontal destruction.
- Periodontitis cannot be determined by the appearance of the gingiva, which can appear pale and firm with slight bleeding on probing or fiery red, and boggy, with heavy bleeding. Periodontal pockets can vary from site to site, from tooth to tooth, and even from site to site on the same tooth.
- Radiographic images reveal the amount of alveolar bone present, the pattern, and the extent of bone loss.
- Radiographic images must be used in conjunction with a thorough clinical assessment.
- Vertical bitewing radiographic images are recommended instead of horizontal bitewing exposures for evaluation of periodontitis.
- Continued attachment loss over time, not current clinical attachment loss, indicates a progression of periodontal disease.
- Documentation of periodontal assessment findings at every visit is essential for accurate diagnosis, periodontal disease management, and risk management.
- Individual immune response and susceptibility to periodontal disease varies widely.
- Periodontal risk factors modulate periodontal disease susceptibility and influence the onset, progression, and severity of the disease.
- The most significant periodontal risk factors are smoking, poor oral hygiene, genetics, stress, diabetes, and obesity.

EVOLVE CONTENT

In addition to all of these learning resources, faculty who adopt this book and students who purchase it will have access to a multitude of instructional resources at the online Evolve site. Faculty can download the materials on their own course management site or use them from the Evolve site. These are some of the exciting features accompany the textbook whether in print or as an ebook.

Instructor Resources

Test Bank

2000+ NBDHE-style questions include answers, rationales for correct and incorrect responses, cognitive leveling, and mapping to chapter objectives and to National Board Dental Hygiene Examination (NBDHE) test blueprint.

TEACH Instructor Resources

- TEACH Lesson Plans
- TEACH PowerPoint Slides
- TEACH Student Handouts
- Image Collection
- Competency Evaluation Forms
- Case-Based Assessments

Student Online Resources (PIN code protected)

- Practice Quizzes for self-assessment with approximately 1000 questions
- Fifty-five Dental Hygiene Procedure Videos
- Expanded Searchable Glossary

CONCLUSION

Darby and Walsh Dental Hygiene: Theory and Practice, sixth edition, offers high-quality, current information regarding dental hygiene practice, preventive oral health interventions, health education and promotion, and the link between oral and systemic health while addressing critical thinking skills and ethical decision making. Dental hygiene encompasses autonomous, intraprofessional, and interprofessional collaboration for shared knowledge and decision making with other oral health professionals and healthcare professionals to provide comprehensive patient-centered care. As primary care providers, dental hygienists can use this book as a resource to enhance delivery of clinical oral health services to individual patients using the process of dental hygiene care: assessment, dental hygiene diagnosis, implementation, evaluation, and documentation.

Jennifer A. Pieren
Cynthia C. Gadbury-Amyot

ACKNOWLEDGMENTS

We would like to express our sincere appreciation to all the contributors who helped make *Darby and Walsh Dental Hygiene: Theory and Practice,* sixth edition, a reality, including all contributors to earlier editions.

We acknowledge the authors and publishers who granted permission to use concepts, quotes, photographs, figures, and tables. Several individuals who contributed content reviews of selected chapters also are appreciated.

Our special thanks to our Elsevier supporters: our team for the current edition – Kelly Skelton, Senior Content Strategist, who provided critical leadership to ensure that the ideas for what this edition could be were realized. Kathleen Nahm, Senior Content Development Specialist, Cindy Thoms, Senior Project Manager, and Margaret Reid, Senior Book Designer, for their incredible work, commitment, enthusiastic support, and encouragement as they shepherded the manuscript throughout the publication process making it as smooth as possible. Other supporters who we wish to recognize include Kristin Wilhelm, Publishing Director, Education Content, who has been an advocate for this project and its editors from the beginning and Joslyn Dumas, Inclusion and Diversity Program Manager, who has been long committed to the success of this book.

As with any new edition of a textbook, we are grateful to readers who have shared their suggestions for additions or revisions with us. This edition reflects our ever-evolving profession of dental hygiene, the state of the science and current evidence, and responses to feedback provided by our dental hygiene community.

Jennifer A. Pieren
Cynthia C. Gadbury Amyot

CONTENTS

1

The Dental Hygiene Profession

Jennifer A. Pieren and Cynthia C. Gadbury-Amyot

PROFESSIONAL OPPORTUNITIES

Dental hygienists are licensed professionals who focus on oral health, prevention of oral diseases, and health promotion. Dental hygiene encompasses autonomous intra- and interprofessional collaboration for shared knowledge and decision making with other oral health professionals and healthcare professionals to provide comprehensive person-centered care. The profession serves clients such as individuals, families, groups, and communities. As primary care providers, dental hygienists deliver clinical oral health services to individual patients using the process of dental hygiene care: assessment, dental hygiene diagnosis, planning, implementation, evaluation, and documentation (ADPIE). Aims of the **dental hygiene profession** include promoting health and improving access to oral healthcare, oral health literacy, and health outcomes for the populations it serves.

COMPETENCIES

1. Apply knowledge of the discipline of dental hygiene, the role of the dental hygienist, and the dental hygiene process of care to succinctly elucidate the primary focus of dental hygiene and approaches taken by dental hygienists to prevent oral diseases and foster overall wellness.
2. Relate the concepts in the metaparadigm for the discipline of dental hygiene to differences in clients and environment.
3. Consider the professional roles of the dental hygienist to determine if more than one of them might appeal to you and why.
4. Compare and contrast the different workforce models for dental hygienists and how they are affected by professional regulation in the United States and Canada.
5. Contemplate the role and importance of various professional dental hygiene associations, highlight why participation is important for professionals, and select at least two of interest.

THE DENTAL HYGIENE PROFESSION

Since its inception, the basis of the profession of dental hygiene has been oral hygiene, oral health education, and preventive oral healthcare. In 1913, Dr. Alfred Civilion Fones opened the first dental hygiene school in Bridgeport, Connecticut, United States. The curriculum was designed to prepare dental hygienists to educate children in self-care and provide preventive oral health services. In other words, dental hygiene was

conceptually conceived on the idea of prevention and health. The first licensed dental hygienist was Irene Newman (cousin of Dr. Fones) in 1917, and by 1952, all 50 states in the United States had licensed dental hygienists. Today, the profession builds upon this foundation of expertise by expanding its scope to include the promotion of health and wellness as oral health is now known to be integral to overall health. The American Dental Hygienists' Association (ADHA), established in 1923, defines the discipline of **dental hygiene** as "the art and science of preventive oral healthcare, including the management of behaviors to prevent oral disease and to promote health."[1] ADHA's vision "calls for the integration of dental hygienists into the healthcare delivery system as essential primary care providers to expand access to oral health care."[2] Established in 1963, the Canadian Dental Hygienists Association's (CDHA's) vision to inspire the profession and communicate the essence and value of who dental hygienists are and what they do, states, "I am a dental hygienist. I educate and empower Canadians to embrace their oral health for better overall health and well-being."[3] The vision of the International Federation of Dental Hygienists (IFDH), established in 1986, states that IFDH "is dedicated to enhancing the recognition of the dental hygienists as being the key provider of preventive oral health care worldwide, and ensuring that oral health is integrated as a key aspect of overall health."[4] While dental hygiene was started in the United States, dental hygiene is currently recognized in over 30 countries, all of which are members of the IFDH. It is important to note that not all of these countries have licensing boards or exams, as required in the United States and Canada, for example.

The art of dental hygiene encompasses caring, ethics, professional judgment, critical thinking, and reflections to enhance patient-provider interactions and outcomes in healthcare settings and the community. The science of dental hygiene involves the integration of biological, psychological, and social science knowledge, precise practice skills, and use of current evidence-based practices to deliver the highest quality of dental hygiene care. One hallmark of a profession is to accept responsibility for the quality of care provided to the public.[5]

THE DENTAL HYGIENIST

Dental hygienists are primary oral healthcare professionals. So what does it mean to be part of a profession? As stated above, in most instances, the dental hygienist is licensed and has graduated from an accredited dental hygiene program in an institution of higher education.[5] They have the knowledge, skills, and professional responsibility to provide oral health promotion and health protection strategies for clients, including individuals/patients, families, groups, and communities of all ages, genders, educational backgrounds, and sociocultural and economic states. As licensed professionals, they are accountable, both legally and ethically, for the care and services they provide.[1,5]

Dental hygiene students who are reading this chapter have chosen to become a dental hygienist, which means they have chosen to enter a licensed healthcare profession. Being licensed is unique in the work world. The individual is held accountable through licensing boards, where determination of qualification for licensure to practice and ensuring high standards of professional competence and ethical conduct among members of the profession are a few of the functions carried out. The people of our states/provinces/countries entrust us through the legislative processes to practice ethical standards, follow practice regulations, and autonomously provide services to the highest standards set by the profession. Being a licensed practitioner demands responsibility for one's own practice of dental hygiene. In the Standard Occupational Classification, dental hygienists are recognized by the US Bureau of Labor Statistics as healthcare diagnosing or treating practitioners, like dentists.[6] And similar to dentists, licensed dental hygienists are expected to take ownership of their portion of the practice, regardless of where they work, for example, private dental practice, community health center, etc.

Through these services, dental hygienists promote and maintain oral wellness and thereby contribute to overall health and quality of life. If an individual's oral health changes, the dental hygienist, within the scope of dental hygiene practice, provides the highest quality of dental hygiene care to guide the person back to oral wellness. If oral wellness cannot be achieved, dental hygiene care helps to attain and maintain the best possible level of oral health. In addition, the dental hygienist interconnects care with other oral healthcare providers and healthcare professionals and assists individuals in seeking other healthcare services as needed.

THE DENTAL HYGIENE PROCESS OF CARE

The **dental hygiene process of care** is the foundation of professional dental hygiene practice and provides a framework for delivering high-quality dental hygiene care to all types of clients in any environment or professional role. This process requires decision making and assumes that dental hygienists are responsible for supporting positive health behaviors and both identifying and resolving client problems and needs within the scope of dental hygiene practice.

The dental hygiene process of care involves six key behaviors,[5] or steps, namely assessment, dental hygiene diagnosis, planning, implementation, evaluation, and documentation. Fig. 1.1 illustrates these six steps of the dental hygiene process. During **assessment**, the dental hygienist collects and analyzes oral health data collected through a systematic, comprehensive individualized assessment of the client (individual/patient, group, community, population) who may have or be at risk for oral disease or complications.[5] In a clinical setting, patient assessment includes the health history; examinations of extraoral, intraoral, periodontal, and hard tissue (dental charting); and risk assessments. The **dental hygiene diagnosis**[5,7] involves identifying an individual's health behaviors, attitudes, and oral healthcare needs within the scope of services the dental hygienist is licensed and educated to provide. The dental hygiene diagnosis uses critical analysis of all assessment findings to reach conclusions about the patient's treatment needs. Multiple dental hygiene diagnoses can be made, and the need for referrals within dentistry or to other healthcare providers is determined. The first two steps in the process of care provide the basis for the care plan. The first is **planning** for realistic overall patient goals for behavioral outcomes, oral health, and overall health while planning dental hygiene interventions to move

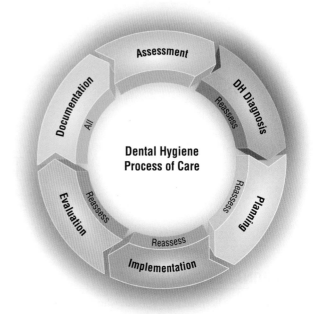

Fig. 1.1 The dental hygiene process of care.

the client toward oral health.[5] The care plan involves the patient and the provider, ultimately leading to informed consent for dental hygiene care. It lays the groundwork for evaluating the effectiveness of care and documenting all related information. **Implementation** is the actual process of completing the plan and engaging the patient as a cotherapist. **Evaluation** involves assessment of oral and health conditions and patient behaviors by collecting and interpreting data using measurable outcomes. It occurs throughout the process of care, and the care plan or treatment implemented is modified as needed. **Documentation** also occurs throughout the process of dental hygiene care by accurately recording all assessment findings, leading to a dental hygiene diagnosis, treatment planned and delivered, patient communication, treatment outcomes, and recommendations. It is intended to provide for continuity of care and communication between providers, and as an accurate, legal document to minimize risk of malpractice claims.[5] Throughout the dental hygiene process of care, the dental hygienist takes into account any individual and environmental factors that may impact the patient's oral health needs, including but not limited to age, gender, culture, lifestyle, oral health literacy, health beliefs, socioeconomic status, and physical abilities.

The process of dental hygiene care described in the ADHA Standards for Clinical Practice is universally applied to other settings where dental hygienists provide services to promote wellness and oral health, provide oral health education, and help the public attain oral health and wellness. For example, dental hygienists working in public health programs assess the needs of the group they are serving, diagnose needs of that group, plan preventive programs to address those needs, and evaluate the outcomes in terms of oral health or health behaviors. A dental hygienist might be engaged in a program targeting tobacco cessation in a group of preteens and teens. The program might include educational efforts, early screenings for oral cancer, and health promotion activities in favor of laws to limit tobacco use and advertising. Dental hygienists identifying community needs based on high dental caries rates in underserved young children might plan, implement, and evaluate a school-based fluoride varnish and sealant program in area elementary schools. Thus the dental hygiene process of care is universal in the discipline (see Fig. 1.1; Box 1.1).

BOX 1.1 Steps of the Dental Hygiene Process of Care[1]

Steps	Definition
Assessment	The systematic collection of data to identify oral and general health status based on client problems, needs, and strengths (includes health history, clinical assessment, and risk assessments)
Dental hygiene diagnosis	The use of critical decision-making skills to reach and communicate conclusions about the client's dental hygiene needs based on all available assessment data and evidence in the literature (includes referrals to a dentist or other medical professionals)[3]
Planning	The establishment, in collaboration with the client, of realistic goals and outcomes based on client needs, expectations, values, and current scientific evidence to obtain informed consent and plan dental hygiene interventions to facilitate optimal oral health (includes collaboration with a dentist or other medical professionals)
Implementation	Delivery of dental hygiene services based on the dental hygiene care plan, including any required modifications, while minimizing risk and optimizing oral health, as well as any needed patient education following treatment for self-care, followup, continuing care, or maintenance
Evaluation	Use measurable outcomes to review and assess the outcomes of delivered dental hygiene care (and collaboration with a dentist or other medical professionals)
Documentation	Complete and accurate recording of all collected data, interventions planned and provided, recommendations, interactions with the client, and other information relevant to client care and treatment while complying with any record-keeping requirements and ensuring client confidentiality[2]

DENTAL HYGIENE'S PARADIGM

A **paradigm** is a widely accepted worldview of a discipline that shapes the direction and methods of its practitioners, educators, administrators, and researchers.[8] It specifies the unique perspective of each discipline; it is the first level of distinction between disciplines and defines the profession's major concepts as its central ideas.[7] These major concepts are known as paradigm concepts. The four major paradigm concepts for the discipline of dental hygiene as defined by the ADHA[1] include the *client*, the *environment*, *health and oral health*, and *dental hygiene actions* (Fig. 1.2). Definitions of these paradigm concepts and their interrelationship are discussed in detail in Chapter 2.

Dental hygienists serve many clients—individuals/patients, families, groups, and communities—in different settings, always with a focus on wellness rather than illness and with an active dental hygienist–client relationship. In clinical practice, the term *patient* is most commonly used to describe individual recipients of dental hygiene care, as it is by many healthcare professionals based on the biomedical model. The term *patient* is narrower than client, however, and it

is not used for recipients of dental hygiene interventions in public health programs, schools, and community settings, for example. Thus the term *client* was chosen for the metaparadigm. This selection of the broader term for the metaparadigm providing a worldview of the profession does not discount our relation with patients when we are providing person-centered clinical dental hygiene services and engaging them as cotherapists. Regardless of the word used or the setting in which dental hygienists interact with the public, our aim is wellness and active participation of the recipients of our services, our clients. Recognizing this distinction, one approach is to use the term *client* when referring to dental hygienists' interactions with clients in health promotion, oral health education, or motivational activities and to use the term *patient* when referring to clinical care interactions.

The paradigm concept of *environment* refers to the different settings where dental hygienists interact with various clients. Factors that affect a client's or patient's attainment of optimal oral health include, for example, economic, psychologic, cultural, physical, legal, educational, ethical, and geographic variables. The environment impacts *dental hygiene actions*, the interventions provided by a dental hygienist for the benefit of and in collaboration with the client to promote oral and overall wellness and prevent oral disease. The paradigm concept, *health/oral health*, refers to the client's state of well-being, which fluctuates over time. Dental hygienists provide services and care to prevent disease that might affect health and wellness or to restore health/oral health when disease is present.

These four paradigm concepts are central to the discipline of dental hygiene (see Fig. 1.2). They are defined further and expanded in numerous ways by the development of conceptual models of dental hygiene (see Chapter 2).

PROFESSIONAL ROLES OF DENTAL HYGIENISTS

Dental hygienists learn not only to provide clinical dental hygiene care but also to be administrators, communicators, collaborators, critical thinkers, researchers, advocates, and coordinators of health as part of their education.[5,9] Dental hygienists are involved in providing patient education as well as diagnostic and preventive treatment to position patients to take control of their own oral health, intervene early in the disease process, and increase the overall oral health of the various populations they serve, including vulnerable and underserved ones (see Box 1.2).

Contemporary dental hygiene practice requires that dental hygienists possess a range of knowledge and skills in a variety of areas. In the past, the principal services of dental hygienists were oral health education and professional removal of calculus, biofilm, and other exogenous accretions from the tooth surface. Changes in healthcare knowledge and practice have expanded the scope of dental hygiene to include the professional roles of clinician, corporate executive, public health professional, researcher, educator, administrator, and entrepreneur (Fig. 1.3, Table 1.1; see also Chapter 63).[10] Dental hygienists in these roles share a common goal of improved oral health for society. Although many dental hygienists are clinical practitioners, others have pursued nonclinical careers by going into business for themselves (e.g., dental staff placement agencies, private continuing education companies, consulting firms, or independent oral healthcare providers in long-term care facilities) or working in public health, private industry, public schools, or academia, or with government agencies.

Regardless of the roles selected by a dental hygienist during the span of a professional career, dental hygienists are a vital part of the healthcare workforce, focusing on prevention of oral disease and promoting oral wellness by working in collaboration with others involved in healthcare in a variety of settings for all populations.

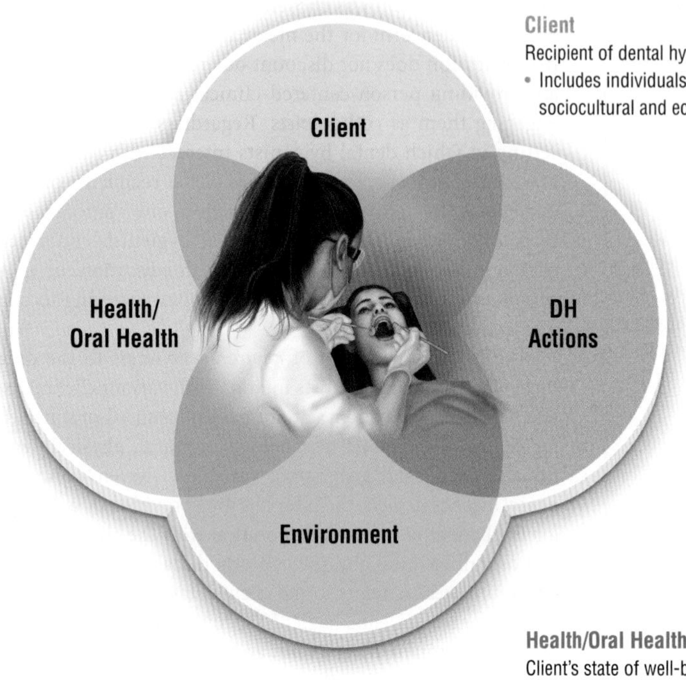

Dental Hygiene (DH) Metaparadigm and Concepts

Client

Recipient of dental hygiene care.

- Includes individuals/patients, families, groups and communities of all ages, genders, and sociocultural and economic states.

DH Actions

Involve cognitive, affective, and psychomotor performances including assessing, DH diagnosis, planning, implementing, evaluating, and documenting (DH process of care) preventive oral health care.

- May be provided independently, interdependently, and/or collaboratively with the client and healthcare team members.
- Also incorporate leadership, research, and behavioral principles in the management of the client's health/oral health status on the wellness/illness continuum.
- Reflect and affirm dental hygiene's unique commitment to preventive oral healthcare.

Environment

Factors other than dental hygiene actions that affect the client's attainment of optimal oral health.

- Includes economic, psychologic, cultural, physical, legal, educational, ethical, and geographic.
- Some factors may be more related to the client; others may be more related to the provider.

Health/Oral Health

Client's state of well-being, which exists on a continuum from optimal wellness to illness and fluctuates over time as a result of biologic, psychologic, spiritual, and developmental factors.

- Oral health and overall health are interrelated; each influences the other.
- Preventive oral health care maintains or improves the client's health/oral health position on the continuum; thus maintains or improves the client's quality of life.

Fig. 1.2 The dental hygiene metaparadigm.

BOX 1.2 Critical Thinking Scenario A

"Going to the Dentist"

You just met a former high school classmate at the grocery store. As you were catching up, you mentioned that you are enrolled at a university and taking classes to become a dental hygienist.

Your friend: "Oh that reminds me. I have to go to the dentist next week."

You: "What are you having done?"

Your friend: "Just a cleaning; no big deal."

You: "Does your dentist usually clean your teeth?"

Your friend: "No, I think somebody else, the dental assistant or hygienist, maybe?"

Consider what it means to the profession and the advancement of the profession when your friend innocently indicates he is seeing the dentist, not the dental hygienist, for services his hygienist is providing. The word *dentist* is used as a placeholder, much the same as the word *Coke* is used when referring to cola. Regardless, most people know the difference between Coca-Cola (Coke) and other types of cola beverages. Discuss the long- and short-term effects when your patients and the public are uninformed of your education and the value of your preventive/therapeutic treatment and care. How does the word "cleaning" minimize our preventive/therapeutic treatment and care?

DENTAL HYGIENE WORKFORCE MODELS

Dental hygienists deliver preventive services to address the oral healthcare needs of the public. In Canada, hygienists can work as independent practitioners without dental or other employers. In the United States, several different practice models provide opportunities for dental hygienists to serve vulnerable and underserved populations (either independently or under the supervision of a dentist), and dental hygienists are working to improve access to preventive oral health.

Midlevel Oral Health Practitioner

Historically, in the United States, dental healthcare access has been limited by the lack of dentists practicing in rural or inner-city areas and serving citizens faced with educational, economic, cultural, and health status disadvantages. Because of these barriers, some people suffer from pain or delay preventive care and treatment until the oral condition is severe and expensive to correct. When dental problems reach a crisis, some people seek dental care from hospital emergency rooms, where healthcare providers may alleviate pain temporarily without treating dental disease, or in safety net clinics with limited services.

In response to this access crisis identified more than a decade ago, the ADHA, with the support of various policy and professional interest organizations, has been advocating for new dental hygiene–based workforce models to extend oral healthcare delivery systems and improve oral health access to underserved populations. One of these systems is based on the creation of a midlevel oral health practitioner. The ADHA defines a **midlevel oral health practitioner** as a licensed dental hygienist and graduate from an accredited dental hygiene program who is a primary oral healthcare provider of dental hygiene services directly to patients. Midlevel oral health practitioners have an expanded scope of care, as set forth by the appropriate licensing agency or regulatory authority.[1]

As of 2023, 42 states provide legal avenues for dental hygienists to provide patient care outside the private dental office without the physical presence of a dentist.[11] The models are designed to extend the reach of the existing oral healthcare system to underserved populations.

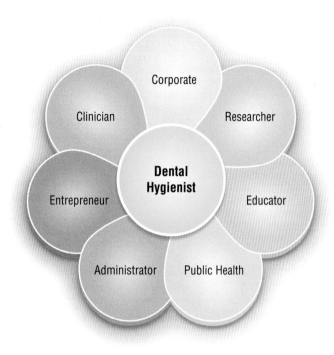

Fig. 1.3 Seven professional roles of the dental hygienist identified by the American Dental Hygienists' Association.[5]

Examples of states that have specifically enacted a midlevel oral healthcare workforce model include:
- Minnesota—Advanced Dental Therapist (may be dually licensed as a dental hygienist)
- Maine—Dental Hygiene Therapist (may be dually licensed as a dental hygienist)
- Vermont—Dental Therapist (must be dually licensed as a dental hygienist)

Many additional states are pursuing midlevel oral healthcare workforce models.[12]

Dental hygienists prepared as midlevel providers and providing direct access to dental hygiene services help the professions of dentistry and dental hygiene meet the oral healthcare needs of the community. The development of these midlevel oral healthcare workforce models should result in cost-effective, quality primary dental care and healthier citizens in the United States.

Other Practice Models for Direct Access to Dental Hygiene Care

The ADHA defines **direct access** as "the ability of a dental hygienist to initiate treatment based on their assessment of a patient's needs without the specific authorization of a dentist, treat the patient without the presence of a dentist, and maintain a provider-patient relationship."[1] Although midlevel provider models and independent dental hygiene practice are two means of providing direct access to dental hygiene care, many other models exist. Other states have the Registered Dental Hygienist Alternative Practice (RDHAP), extended care permits (ECPs), extended access endorsements, and limited access permits (LAPs) or other provisions for public health dental hygienists to provide direct access to care.[11,13]

Laws and regulations in various states, provinces, and countries determine the level of supervision required by a dentist, if any. These requirements are changing as more jurisdictions adopt newly evolving practice models to improve access to oral healthcare. Dental hygienists can check the ADHA or applicable state regulatory agency websites for supervision requirements and dental hygienists' involvement in regulation in the United States, and the CDHA's website for practice regulation authority in Canada. Given the lack of access to oral healthcare within all dental practice populations and settings (due in part to disparities in the healthcare delivery system), direct access models can play a key role in providing greater access to quality oral healthcare for all individuals (Box 1.3).

Collaborative Practice Model and Agreements

Collaboration occurs when individuals with differing strengths work together as equal partners to achieve better results than each could achieve working alone. According to the **collaborative practice model**[14] created nearly 25 years ago and commonly embraced today, dentists and dental hygienists work together as colleagues, each offering professional expertise for the goal of providing optimum oral healthcare to the public. Although both professions can and should work together to improve the oral health status of the public, each has a specific role that complements and enhances the effectiveness of the other.

The collaborative practice model emphasizes the distinct roles of dental hygienist and dentist and their ability to enter into a collegial relationship as healthcare providers. In this model, the dentist and the dental hygienist are in a cotherapist relationship. In a collaborative practice, dental hygienists are viewed as experts in their field, are consulted about appropriate dental hygiene interventions, are expected

TABLE 1.1 Seven Roles of the Professional Dental Hygienist[10]

Roles	Sample Settings	Sample Responsibilities
Clinician	Clinical practice in any public or private dental treatment setting Managed-care programs Extended-care facilities School-based programs	Use dental hygiene process of care to control oral diseases and partner with clients to promote health Provide care to clients based on evidence-based decision making and skill Collaborate with and refer to other healthcare professionals as needed
Corporate	Oral healthcare industry Medical industry Product research Publishing	Apply educational and practice expertise as sales representatives, product researchers, educators, and administrators to support various oral healthcare and related industries in providing quality products, services, and information
Public Health/ Interprofessional	Public health clinics Native American Health Services Head Start Programs Public health departments Medical settings (colocating)	Address unmet needs of underserved or groups with special needs Deliver care in school- or community-based settings Plan, conduct, and evaluate community and public oral health programs
Researcher	Research institutions Educational institutions Governmental institutions Oral healthcare industry	Conduct original qualitative or quantitative research Develop and implement evidence-based plan to address problems with budgets, expected outcomes, and evaluation procedures Interpret and evaluate research findings and apply findings to practice
Educator	University faculty member Continuing education instructor Public health programs Public school programs Oral healthcare industry	Apply educational theory and the teaching-learning process Design and produce instructional materials and media
Administrator	Community-based health programs Professional organizations Educational institutions Dental health programs Oral healthcare industry	Identify and manage resources Participate in strategic planning Formulate policies and procedures Apply organizational skills and solve problems Evaluate and modify programs based on evaluation outcomes
Entrepreneur	Oral healthcare industry Product development and sales industry Independent clinical practices Employment and staffing services Continuing education businesses Consulting businesses Nonprofit organizations	Initiate or finance new commercial enterprises Initiate or finance new commercial enterprises to address needs of consumers and providers Bring available resources together to resolve problems or deliver professional services Develop business opportunities to provide state-of-the-art knowledge, technology, skills, and procedures

BOX 1.3 Client or Patient Education and Professional Awareness

Educating the public and individual clients or patients about the dental hygiene profession and the value of dental hygiene services is critical to promoting health and also awareness of the profession. While the scope of dental hygiene practice continues to evolve and expand, ensuring adequate oral healthcare for all individuals remains a challenge. Some jurisdictions provide avenues for direct access to dental hygiene care, whereas others have laws and regulations prohibiting it and requiring dental supervision as requisite to dental hygiene care. The dental hygiene profession advocates for access to care for vulnerable and underserved populations not served by other oral healthcare providers. Each contact with clients and patients is an opportunity to explain the value of the dental hygiene practice. It is important not to minimize the services provided (i.e., refer to comprehensive dental hygiene care as "a cleaning" or to describing what dental hygienists do as "cleaning teeth") but rather to explain how professional dental hygiene services improve their oral and systemic health. The more the public views dental hygienists as essential primary care providers, the more likely it is that the laws and regulations will support efforts of dental hygienists to carry out their fullest potential.

to make clinical dental hygiene decisions, and are given freedom in planning, implementing, and evaluating the dental hygiene component of the overall care plan.

Many states have provisions for collaborative practice agreements within the laws and regulations governing dental hygiene. This delivery model encourages more dental hygienists to participate in direct access to their care in specified settings, especially where the public has significant barriers to accessing oral healthcare. Examples include schools, public health programs, and long-term care facilities—locations that are convenient and accessible to the public. A collaborative practice agreement is an option specified in the laws and regulations governing dental hygiene in several jurisdictions. The contractual agreement provides a legal means to remove dental supervision barriers while retaining the legally defined scope of dental hygiene practice. The agreement clarifies details regarding a referral system for followup care by a dentist. A collaborative practice agreement generally includes the following:

- A legally defined protocol setting out the circumstances in which the dental hygienist can initiate treatment
- Description of the scope of dental hygiene services
- Practice protocols

- Responsibilities of the collaborating dentist regarding consultation with the dental hygienist
- Maintenance of the dental record
- Emergency management plan
- Referral methods[13,14]

Other examples of collaboration can be found in the 2021 *Oral Health in America: Advances and Challenges* report, where multiple models of medical-dental integrated care can be found.[15] The integration of oral and general healthcare delivery is based on evidence that shows how oral and general health conditions are related and coordinating treatment between medical and dental providers is important to maintain overall health.

Integrating dental hygienists into medical teams in primary care practices is one strategy that is being used to address lack of access to oral healthcare services. Colorado has been active in this arena, with the colocation of direct-access dental hygienists into medical practices.[16] It is an exciting time to be entering the profession of dental hygiene as expanded scopes of practice are emerging.

Independent Practitioner

Independent dental hygiene practitioners own their own businesses, or independent practices, and provide preventive oral healthcare services to the public as primary care providers where permitted by law. Under the laws and regulations of a jurisdiction adopting this model, dental supervision is not required, and dental hygienists have provisions for owning a dental hygiene practice. Thus independent dental hygiene practice is also called unsupervised practice.

A few states, such as Maine and Colorado, have provisions for independent dental hygiene practice in the United States. In Canada, more than 1000 dental hygienists are independent dental hygiene practitioners.[17] The CDHA has an Independent Practice Network to provide support, resources, and training for independent dental hygiene practitioners. The network provides information about business plans, insurance reimbursement protocols and carriers, service codes, marketing, financing, partnerships, and incorporation.

Some dental hygienists who own their own businesses offer dental hygiene services to vulnerable and underserved populations while having legal arrangements for dentist collaboration or general supervision. Although these practices are independently owned, they are not independent dental hygiene practices.

THE DENTAL HYGIENIST IN INTERPROFESSIONAL PRACTICE

Improving access to affordable preventive oral healthcare is important for healthy development and healthy aging, but it is unlikely to be an adequate approach for reducing the burden of oral disease.[18] Dental caries is the most common chronic disease in children, and a significant number of adults have untreated caries and chronic periodontal disease. To effectively combat oral disease, we need to expand the oral disease prevention workforce and intervene earlier in the course of disease. Oral healthcare services provided in primary care settings present an opportunity to expand access to care and a structure for improving referrals for dental care beyond the scope of dental hygiene practice. This model also provides/facilitates the delivery of preventive oral healthcare as a part of overall wellness (Fig. 1.4).[19]

Interprofessional collaboration, also known as **interprofessional practice** in healthcare, is shared responsibility and collaboration among healthcare professionals in patient-centered healthcare delivery systems to attain optimal health outcomes for populations with, or at risk for, oral diseases. An interprofessional approach is important for improving patient outcomes beyond what could be achieved by delivering care within one discipline because each profession brings complementary knowledge, skills, values, and attitudes to each client case.[18] Interprofessional education for all healthcare professionals and students is common throughout the world to prepare the healthcare workforce for interprofessional practice.

Dental hygienists work in interprofessional practice in a variety of settings with healthcare workers from multiple backgrounds. For example, dental hygienists work in community clinics and medical practices with pediatricians, family physicians, nurse practitioners, nurses, and

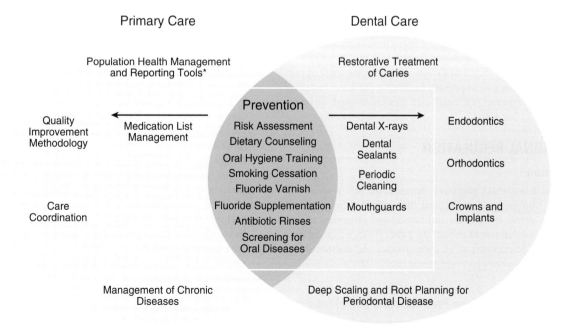

*Including structured EHR data and diagnostic codes, disease registries, and other tools

Fig. 1.4 An interprofessional practice model of partnering to expand prevention. (From Hummel K, Phillips KE, Holt B, et al. Oral health: an essential component of primary care. Seattle. *Qualis Health*, June 2015.)

BOX 1.4 Interprofessional Practice

Interprofessional Practice
Dental hygienists can collaborate interprofessionally in many roles and settings, most often as clinicians and educators. Consider the following examples:

Company Wellness Programs
Many companies are implementing wellness programs to improve the health of their employees and promote healthy habits. Many of these programs include offering a wide variety of online resources, free screenings, and educational services to their participants. Consider the impact dental hygienists have when they are part of these programs. They can manage the educational resources available to patients, screen and counsel patients on their needs, facilitate referrals, and consult with other disciplines to ensure optimal overall health.

Obstetrics Practice Settings
Hormonal changes during pregnancy can increase the potential for inflammation of periodontal tissues. Preventive oral healthcare is essential and recommended during pregnancy to avoid oral infections such as periodontal disease, which has been linked to preterm birth. Consider the impact of a dental hygienist colocated in an obstetrician's office. Women who schedule appointments with their obstetricians early in their pregnancy are usually seen more frequently by these practices than other healthcare professionals during pregnancy. The availability of a dental hygienist in these practices could result in early and consistent intervention, potentially improving patient outcomes. The dental hygienist could provide preventive/therapeutic care as needed in these settings, assess for other oral health concerns and infections, provide patient-centered education and resources on finding a dental care provider or dental home for the mother's child, and facilitate necessary referrals. A dental hygienist could also reinforce the importance of the human papillomavirus (HPV) vaccine for protection from cervical and oral cancer.

Pediatric Practice Settings
The high caries rate in children and guidelines by pediatric professional associations' recommendations for regular oral examinations, caries risk assessments, and fluoride varnish applications in pediatric primary care provide interprofessional opportunities for dental hygienists. The dental hygienist can partner with registered dieticians to educate families about meal planning to reduce sugar intake, offer anticipatory guidance, and manage sugar addiction. Pediatricians are developing preventive oral care programs within their practice settings, and dental hygienists are valued for their expertise and ability to save time and collaborate with the medical care professionals and staff. In community clinic systems providing care for vulnerable and underserved children, dental hygienists are employed to coordinate preventive oral care services with the primary healthcare and facilitate referrals between dental and medical providers.

Urgent Care and Emergency Departments
Patients without a dental care provider often go to the emergency department when they have dental pain or problems. Imagine if a dental hygienist were available in every emergency/urgent care department to triage patients who had suspected infections. They could identify current concerns and unmet dental needs, educate patients, expose dental radiographs as needed, and work with the emergency department professionals to facilitate referrals and followup for definitive dental care.

Identify Opportunities in Your Community
Reflect on the characteristics of the communities in which you have lived or worked and consider how dental hygienists can affect the unique needs of those communities. Identify other settings where hygienists can improve access to oral care or improve oral healthcare. What different roles can they assume within these settings? What services can they provide and what populations can they help?

physician assistants, completing pediatric oral assessments, applying fluoride varnish, and teaching parents about oral healthcare practices important to their child's oral health. Dental hygienists in long-term care facilities work with nurses' aides and registered nurses to monitor residents' oral health, care for dentures, provide preventive oral healthcare, and make dental care referrals. The opportunities are expanding, and dental hygienists are being trained to work with healthcare providers in many disciplines. Dental hygienists are embracing these opportunities as well as their role as primary healthcare providers to deliver comprehensive preventive oral healthcare services through interprofessional practice (Box 1.4).

PROFESSIONAL REGULATION

Accreditation

Accreditation is a formal, voluntary nongovernmental process that establishes a minimum set of national standards that promote and ensure quality across educational institutions and programs, as well as serving as a mechanism to protect the public.[20] Accreditation documents include descriptions of all competencies and abilities that a beginning dental hygiene practitioner must consistently perform accurately and efficiently.

Dental and Dental Hygiene Practice Acts and Licensure

Dental and dental hygiene practice acts are laws established in each applicable jurisdiction—that is, states (United States) or provinces (Canada)—to regulate the practice of dental hygiene. In some jurisdictions, dental hygienists are self-regulated; in others, dental hygienists

participate with consumers in regulation of the profession as a part of the dental practice act, and dentists are largely in control of the regulation of dental hygiene practice. Although the laws that regulate dental hygiene practice vary with each licensing jurisdiction, they have common elements. In general, the practice act does the following:

- Establishes criteria for dental hygiene education, licensure, and relicensure
- Defines the legal scope of dental hygiene practice
- Protects the public by making illegal the practice of dental hygiene by uncredentialed and unlicensed persons
- Creates a board empowered with legal authority to oversee the policies and procedures affecting the dental hygiene practice in that jurisdiction

Dental hygiene is a self-regulated profession in most Canadian provinces, so registration is a provincial responsibility. A certificate of registration to practice is issued only to those who meet established standards of qualification and practice established by the profession of dental hygiene in each province.

In the United States, virtually every state requires certain measures before a license is granted:

- Graduation from an accredited dental hygiene program
- Successful completion of the written National Board Dental Hygiene Examination
- Successful completion of a regional or state clinical board examination, although a national clinical examination has been proposed.

The board in each state is given legal authority to design and administer licensing examinations to graduates of approved schools of dental hygiene or to accept standardized examinations offered by testing

<table>
</table>

BOX 1.5 Legal, Ethical, and Safety Issues

- Dental hygienists must be licensed in the jurisdiction in which they practice and adhere to the laws, rules, and regulations governing the practice of dental hygiene.
- Dental hygienists are obligated to provide the highest quality of care for clients/patients they serve.
- A code of ethics for dental hygiene establishes ethical principles and responsibilities for dental hygienists across all practice areas including clinical care, education, research, administration, and any other roles in which dental hygienists serve (see ADHA Code of Ethics and CDHA Codes of Ethics).
- Standards for Clinical Dental Hygiene set forth guidelines for clinical practice of dental hygienists.
- Health professionals must use the best current evidence to support decisions about healthcare services they provide for the public.
- As professionals, dental hygienists should become involved in professional associations representing the profession and their professional interest areas.
- Oral health professionals need to branch out from traditional roles and settings to collaborate with other healthcare professionals in interprofessional practice.

agencies. Individuals who pass the licensing examination earn a license to practice dental hygiene as it is defined in that state. The license can be denied, revoked, or suspended for a variety of reasons, such as incompetence, negligence, chemical dependency, illegal practice, and criminal misconduct. Realizing the limitation of single states requiring repeat licensing examinations for dental hygienists who are relocating, some state boards have established licensing by credential as an alternative. Licensing by credentials recognizes the dental hygiene license received in other states when appropriate. Documents are provided for the board's approval in meeting licensure requirements so the dental hygienist does not have to repeat a licensure examination after relocating. Due to the issues associated with portability of licenses within the United States, there are currently ongoing discussions regarding a new interstate compact to increase the ease of license portability, which will ultimately improve access to oral healthcare.[21] See Box 1.5.

The Dental Hygiene National Board

To be eligible for regional and/or state licensure examinations, after graduation from an accredited dental hygiene program, dental hygienists must also pass the written National Board Dental Hygiene Examination administered by the American Dental Association Joint Commission on National Dental Examinations. The purpose of the national examination is to assist state boards in determining qualifications of dental hygiene licensure applicants by assessing their ability to recall important information from basic biomedical, dental, and dental hygiene sciences, as well as their ability to apply such information in problem-solving situations. A case-based segment of the examination focuses on the ability to use knowledge related to clinical dental hygiene and the dental sciences in solving client problems and addressing client needs.

STANDARDS FOR DENTAL HYGIENE PRACTICE AND COMPETENCIES FOR ENTRY INTO THE PROFESSION

Standards in the United States

The ADHA *Standards for Clinical Dental Hygiene Practice* define and guide professional dental hygiene practice.[5] The primary purpose of

the *Standards* is to offer guidance to dental hygienists and the public at large about the expected practice behavior for dental hygiene practitioners seeking to provide client-centered and evidence-based clinical care. In addition, dental hygienists functioning as educators, researchers, and administrators can use the *Standards* to guide implementation of collaborative, client-centered care in multidisciplinary teams of health professionals. Such collaborations occur in community-based settings such as community and public health centers, hospitals, schools, and long-term care programs. Although dental hygienists are individually accountable to the *Standards* set by the discipline, these *Standards* do not substitute for professional judgment. However, they do provide a framework that describes a competent level of dental hygiene care based on the dental hygiene process of care. These *Standards* are likely to be continuously evaluated and modified as necessary as new scientific evidence, and federal and state regulations develop to ensure optimal, comprehensive client care.[5]

In addition to the ADHA *Standards for Clinical Dental Hygiene Practice,* the American Dental Education Association (ADEA) has developed *ADEA Competencies for Entry into the Allied Dental Professions,* to supplement existing competencies for the profession of dental hygiene.[22] These competency documents describe the abilities needed by a dental hygienist entering the dental hygiene profession to be able to perform independently and inform dental hygiene accreditation bodies. The standards for clinical practice, along with the competencies for entry-level dental hygienists, serve the profession and society in the following ways:

- Define the activities of dental hygienists unique to dental hygiene
- Provide consumers, employers, and colleagues with guidelines as to what constitutes high-quality dental hygiene care
- Provide guidelines for establishing goals for clinical dental hygiene education
- Serve as the foundation to ensure competence and for continued professional development.

Standards in Canada

The current standards for dental hygiene practice in Canada, *Practice Competencies and Standards for Canadian Dental Hygienists,* was a collaborative project involving many stakeholders.[9] This document defines a national perspective on the knowledge and abilities dental hygienists require to practice competently and responsibly.

The CDHA combined competency statements and practice standards in the same document to be considered as a whole. The practice competencies are intended for use primarily by educators in curriculum development to define the outcomes of entry-level professional education. The practice standards specify a level to which entry-level dental hygienists must practice as outlined by the Federation of Dental Hygiene Regulatory Authorities. These standards also include the CDHA definition of dental hygiene and scope of practice. Some provincial professional associations have developed additional standards for practicing dental hygienists.

PROFESSIONAL ASSOCIATIONS FOR DENTAL HYGIENISTS

Professional associations collectively represent the views of a profession or professional special interest group and influence resolution of issues relevant to education, practice, and research. Professional organizations have an enormous effect on dental hygiene because they address issues of professional growth, education, access to care, research and theory development, quality assurance, manpower, legislation, and collaboration with other professionals. Although many professional associations exist, only the major organizations are discussed in this chapter.

American Dental Hygienists' Association

The **American Dental Hygienists' Association (ADHA)** is a national organization of dental hygienists. The ADHA advocates for dental hygienists to be valued and integrated into the comprehensive healthcare delivery system in order to improve oral and overall health.[23] ADHA works to support dental hygienists throughout their careers and advance the dental hygiene profession by developing new career avenues, expanding opportunities for care, and providing the latest training and information.

The ADHA has a trilevel structure by which individual members are automatically part of local (component), state (constituent), and national levels of its associated organizations. A few states have options for membership in independent dental hygiene professional associations. The official publication of the ADHA is the *Journal of Dental Hygiene*. Its legislative body is the House of Delegates, which is composed of voting members who proportionately represent each constituent. The Board of Directors, presided over by the organization's elected president, consists of voting members (president, president-elect, vice president, treasurer, immediate past president, and 12 district trustees) and nonvoting, ex officio members (executive director and speaker of the House of Delegates). The ADHA plays a major role in issues that deal with legislation, access to care, education, practice, research, public relations, and health policy. The ADHA offers a variety of tangible and intangible benefits. Membership and support by professional and student dental hygienists in the United States is important.

National Dental Hygienists' Association

In 1932, the **National Dental Hygienists' Association (NDHA)** was founded by African American dental hygienists to address the needs and special challenges of minority dental hygienists. The mission of the NDHA is to do the following:[24]

- "Promote the highest standards of education and ethics for dental hygienists; create specific position statements on issues impacting the dental hygiene profession.
- Enhance recruitment efforts for communities of minority students in need.
- Assist in access to oral care for underserved communities in the United States.
- Improve the Association's visibility via public service.
- Provide a professional foundation for minority dental hygienists.
- Increase the number of minority dental hygienists."

The NDHA executive board includes five officers, and the Board of Trustees includes the immediate past president and five trustees elected by the growing general membership body. It holds an annual convention in conjunction with the National Dental Association.

Canadian Dental Hygienists Association

The **Canadian Dental Hygienists Association (CDHA)**, officially founded in 1965, is the national association for registered dental hygienists in Canada. The CDHA's purpose is to enable its members to provide quality preventive and therapeutic oral healthcare as well as health promotion for all members of the Canadian public.[25] As the collective voice of dental hygiene in Canada, the CDHA contributes to the health of the public by leading the development of national positions and encouraging standards related to dental hygiene practice, education, research, and regulation.

The CDHA Board's actions are directed toward its members with specific measurable outcomes, including the following:[25]

- **Public Policy Environment**—favorable to dental hygienists' ability to practice as primary healthcare providers.
- **Public Recognition**—dental hygienists' value is recognized by the Canadian public.
- **Professional Practice**—standards, competencies, and resources for dental hygienists to work independently and interprofessionally as an integral part of the healthcare team.
- **Professional Knowledge**—means for dental hygienists to create, contribute to, and utilize a growing body of professional knowledge and research.
- **Leadership**—dental hygienists' potential for professional leadership is developed.

With a structure similar to that of the ADHA, the CDHA has provincial organizations supported by local components. The CDHA publishes *The Canadian Journal of Dental Hygiene* as its official journal and has played a prominent role in developing continuing education, formal dental hygiene education, portability of licensure, and dental hygiene research and theory. The ADHA and CDHA have worked together to achieve many common goals.

International Federation of Dental Hygienists

The **International Federation of Dental Hygienists (IFDH)** is an international organization, free from any political, racial, or religious ties, formed to unite dental hygiene associations worldwide in their common goal of promoting oral health. The IFDH's purposes are as follows:[26]

- "Safeguard and defend the interests of the profession of dental hygiene, represent and advance the profession of dental hygiene.
- Promote professional alliances with its association members as well as with other interdisciplinary associations, federations, and organizations whose objectives are similar.
- Promote and coordinate the exchange of knowledge and information about the profession, its education, evidence-based research, and best practice.
- Promote access to quality preventive oral health services and foster social responsibility programmes to enhance oral health.
- Increase public awareness that oral disease can be prevented through proven regimens and can have significant impact on general health.
- Provide an international scientific forum for education and networking the understanding and discussion of issues pertaining to dental hygiene."

The IFDH provides a formal network by which dental hygienists worldwide can promote collegiality among nations, commitment to maintaining universal standards of dental hygiene care and education, and access to high-quality oral healthcare. The IFDH is governed by its House of Delegates, which has two delegates from each member country's association. Normally, this governing body meets every 2 years, in conjunction with the International Symposium on Dental Hygiene, hosted and organized by a selected member country. An executive council (president, president-elect, vice president, and treasurer) is elected by the House of Delegates to execute the goals established by the House of Delegates every 2 years.[26]

Other Professional Associations of Interest to Dental Hygienists

In addition to membership in national and local organizations that primarily represent the interests of the dental hygiene profession, for example, the ADHA, CDHA, etc., dental hygienists can consider other professional associations that exist in dental hygienists' areas of interest. A few examples of such organizations follow:

- American Dental Education Association (ADEA)—The only national organization representing academic dentistry, thus the voice of dental education. Members include educators, corporations, and institutions from general dentistry, specialties, dental hygiene, dental assisting, and dental laboratory technology. http://www.adea.org
- Special Care Dentistry Association (SCDA)—The Special Care Dentistry Association is a resource for all oral healthcare professionals who have an interest in patients with special needs; it provides education and networking to increase access to oral healthcare for these patients. http://www.scdaonline.org
- National Center for Interprofessional Practice and Education (NEXUSIPE)—This organization provides resources, guidance, and leadership in this area, and avenues for interprofessional practice and education professionals to connect with colleagues, researchers, practitioners, educators, and consultants with NEXUS, an integrated learning system to transform education and care, summits, and their online directory. https://nexusipe.org
- International Association for Dental Research (IADR)—IADR supports the advancement of research and knowledge to improve oral health, represents the oral health research community, and enables communication of research findings. While dental hygiene researchers belong to many groups within IADR, the oral health research group was created by the efforts of a dental hygiene researcher and many choose that group for participation. http://www.iadr.org
- American Public Health Association (APHA)—The APHA brings together members from all public health fields, including dental hygiene. It advocates for the health of all people and communities to strengthen the public health profession by addressing public health issues and policies backed by science. https://www.apha.org
- American Academy of Oral Medicine (AAOM)—The AAOM's vision is to integrate medicine and dentistry to promote optimal health. Their mission is to advance excellence in patient care, education, and research and to promote access to quality affordable oral medicine care while increasing professional and public awareness of oral medicine. https://www.aaom.com/
- American Association of Dental Office Management (AADOM)—AADOM provides resources, education, and networking for office administrators. https://www.dentalmanagers.com
- The Dental Trade Alliance (DTA)—DTA is an association of companies that provide dental equipment, supplies, materials, and services to dentists and other oral care professionals, serving as a strong voice for the industry and promoting market growth. https://www.dentaltradealliance.org

ACKNOWLEDGMENT

The authors acknowledge and honor the original authors of this chapter, Margaret M. Walsh, Michele L. Darby, and Denise Bowen.

EVOLVE RESOURCES

Please visit http://evolve.elsevier.com/Pieren/hygiene/ for additional practice and study support tools.

KEY CONCEPTS

- Dental hygiene is the study of preventive oral healthcare, including the management of behaviors to prevent oral disease and promote health.
- Dental hygienists are licensed, primary oral healthcare professionals with knowledge, skills, and responsibility to provide oral health promotion, education, and clinical services to clients including individuals/patients, families, groups, and communities of all ages, genders, educational backgrounds, and sociocultural and economic states.
- The dental hygienist is a licensed oral healthcare professional with career paths available including the professional roles of clinician, corporate, researcher, educator, public health, administrator, and entrepreneur to support total health through the prevention of oral disease and the promotion of health.
- The dental hygiene process of care includes assessment, diagnosis, planning, implementation, evaluation, and documentation. It is the foundation of professional dental hygiene practice and provides a model for organizing and providing dental hygiene care in a variety of settings.
- A metaparadigm specifies the unique perspective of each discipline and is the first level of distinction between disciplines.
- The metaparadigm for the discipline of dental hygiene consists of the following four major paradigm concepts: client, environment, health and oral health, and dental hygiene actions.
- The collaborative practice model assumes that dentists and dental hygienists work together as colleagues, each offering professional expertise for the goal of providing optimum oral healthcare to the public.
- The dental hygiene clinician provides preventive, therapeutic, and educational services and makes decisions independently or in collaboration with the client and family, the dentist, or other healthcare professionals.
- Several dental hygiene workforce models have been developed to increase access to preventive oral healthcare for vulnerable and underserved populations.
- A midlevel oral health practitioner, as a licensed dental hygienist who is a primary oral healthcare provider of dental hygiene services directly to patients, has an expanded scope of care as defined by the appropriate regulatory agency.
- Independent dental hygiene practitioners own their own businesses or independent practices and provide preventive oral healthcare services to the public as primary care providers where permitted by law.
- Interprofessional collaboration or practice is an approach to providing comprehensive healthcare through the teamwork of healthcare workers from more than one discipline.
- Standards of practice provide consumers, employers, and colleagues with guidelines as to what constitutes high-quality dental hygiene care.
- Licensure and registration are processes by which a government agency certifies that individuals are minimally qualified to practice in its jurisdiction.
- Professional organizations represent collectively the views of a profession or special interest group and influence resolution of relevant issues.

REFERENCES

1. American Dental Hygienists' Association. *Policy Manual*. Adopted 2022. Available at: https://www.adha.org/wp-content/uploads/2023/01/ADHA_Policy-_Manual_FY22.pdf. Accessed February 25, 2023.
2. Battrell A, Lynch A, Steinbach P. The American Dental Hygienists' Association leads the profession into 21st century workforce opportunities. *J Evid Based Dent Pract*. 2016;16(suppl):4–10.

3. Canadian Dental Hygienists Association. *Our Professional Identity – In Search of Our Identity*. Available at: http://www.cdha.ca/cdha/ The_Profession_folder/Professional_Identity/CDHA/The_Profession/ The_Profession.aspx?hkey=0d786b25-f9e4-4551-8ad8-869b0b4b5e64. Accessed February 25, 2023.

4. International Federation of Dental Hygienists. *History of the IFDH*. Available at: https://www.ifdh.org/about-ifdh/history/. Accessed February 25, 2023.

5. American Dental Hygienists' Association. *Standards of Care for Clinical Dental Hygiene Practice*. 2016. Available at: https://www.adha.org/ education-resources/professional-resources/clinical-practice-resources/. Accessed on February 23, 2023.

6. U.S. Bureau of Labor Statistics, U.S. Office of Management and Budget. *2018 SOC Definitions*. Jan 2018. Available at: https://www.bls.gov/ soc/2018/soc_2018_definitions.pdf. Accessed February 26, 2023.

7. American Dental Hygienists' Association. *Dental Hygiene Diagnosis*. Revised September 2015. Available at: https://www.adha.org/advocacy/ scope-of-practice/dental-hygiene-diagnosis/. Accessed on February 23, 2023.

8. Walsh MM, Ortega E, Heckman B. The dental hygiene scholarly identity and roadblocks to achieving it. *J Dent Hyg*. 2016;2:79–87.

9. Canadian Dental Hygienists' Association. Entry-to-Practice Competencies and Standards for Dental Hygienists. A collaborative project of the Canadian Dental Hygienists Association (CDHA), Federation of Dental Hygiene Regulatory Authorities (FDHRA), Commission on Dental Accreditation of Canada (CDAC), National Dental Hygiene Certification Board (NDHCB) and dental hygiene educators. 2021. Available at: https:// www.cdho.org/docs/default-source/pdfs/standards-of-practice/epccodh_ fdhrc_november_2021.pdf. Accessed on February 25, 2023.

10. American Dental Hygienists' Association. *Career Paths*. Available at: https://www.adha.org/membership/students/student-resources/career-paths/. Accessed February 25, 2023.

11. American Dental Hygienists' Association. *Direct Access States*. Revised December 2017. Available at: https://www.adha.org/advocacy/scope-of-practice/direct-access/. Accessed February 25, 2023.

12. American Dental Hygienists' Association. *Dental Therapy Authorized by State*. Available at: https://www.adha.org/wp-content/uploads/2022/12/ Dental_Therapy_Authorized_by_State_Law.pdf. Accessed February 26, 2023.

13. American Dental Hygienists' Association. *Direct Access States*. Revised August 2022. Available at: https://www.adha.org/wp-content/ uploads/2023/01/ADHA_Direct_Access_Chart_2022-08.pdf. Accessed February 25, 2023.

14. Darby M. Collaborative practice model: the future of dental hygiene. *J Dent Educ*. 1983;47:589.

15. National Institutes of Health. *Oral Health in America: Advances and Challenges [Internet]*. National Institute of Dental and Craniofacial Research; 2021. [cited Oct 25, 2022]. Available at: https://www.nidcr.nih. gov/oralhealthinamerica. Accessed February 27, 2023.

16. Braun PA, Budzyn SE, Chavez C, Barnard JG. Integrating Dental Hygienists into Medical Care Teams: Practitioner and patient perspectives. *American Dental Hygienists' Association*. 2021;95(3):6–17.

17. Canadian Dental Hygienists Association. *Independent Practice. Welcome to the Independent Practice Network*. Available at: http://www.cdha.ca/ cdha/The_Profession_folder/Independent_Practice_folder/CDHA/The_ Profession/Independent_Practice/Introducing_Independent_Practice_ Network.aspx?hkey=6baa1969-bb7a-45db-8596-b2a498f678f5. Accessed February 23, 2023.

18. National Network for Oral Health Access. *A User's Guide for Implementation of Interprofessional Oral Health Core Clinical Competencies: Results of a Pilot Project*; 2015. Available at: https://www. hrsa.gov/sites/default/files/hrsa/oral-health/ipohccc-users-guide-2015. pdf. Accessed February 25, 2023.

19. Qualis Health. *Oral Health: An Essential Component of Primary Care: Executive Summary*. June 2015. Available at: www.qualishealth.org/sites/ default/files/Executive-Summary-Oral-Health-Integration.pdf. Accessed February 25, 2023.

20. Commission on Dental Accreditation. *Accreditation Standards for Dental Hygiene Education Programs*. Revised 2022. Available at: https://coda.ada. org/-/media/project/ada-organization/ada/coda/files/dental_hygiene_ standards.pdf?rev=aa609ad18b504e9f9cc63f0b3715a5fd&hash= 67CB76127017AD98CF8D62088168EA58. Accessed February 25, 2023.

21. American Dental Hygienists' Association. *License Portability*. Available at: https://www.adha.org/advocacy/license-portability/. Accessed on February 26, 2023.

22. American Dental Education Association. ADEA competencies for entry into the allied dental professions. *J Dent Educ*. 2011;75(7):949.

23. American Dental Hygienists' Association. *ADHA website*. Available at: www.adha.org. Accessed February 25, 2023.

24. National Dental Hygienists' Association. *NDHA website*. Available at: http://www.ndhaonline.org. Accessed February 25, 2023.

25. Canadian Dental Hygienists Association. *CDHA website*. Available at: www.cdha.ca. Accessed February 25, 2023.

26. International Federation of Dental Hygienists. *IFDH website*. Available at: http://www.ifdh.org/about.html. Accessed February 25, 2023.

2

Dental Hygiene Metaparadigm Concepts and Conceptual Models Applied to Practice

Laura L. MacDonald and Katherine E. Yerex

PROFESSIONAL OPPORTUNITY

Dental hygienists provide client-centered preventive and therapeutic clinical services, and foster health promotion and disease prevention. How a dental hygienist does this depends on how the dental hygienist views or thinks about the needs of the client and the dental hygienist's role in facilitating the client's health, and how they conceptualize those needs and their role. Disciplines have distinct ideas, views, ways of looking at things, or thought patterns impacting their actions and fortifying values, that is, epistemological perspectives (beliefs about knowledge and how knowledge is constructed). The set of concepts and how these are arrived is called a paradigm. The discipline embodies the concepts, shapes conceptual models, theorizes and engages in research exploring the concepts and models, and thus informs practice and education within the profession and its discipline.

COMPETENCIES

1. Discuss the dental hygiene metaparadigm and its four paradigm concepts.
2. Define conceptual model.
3. Discuss the key features of the Dental Hygiene Human Needs Conceptual Model, illustrate how the model enables the dental hygienist to diagnose patient needs based on assessment and/or formulate a plan of action to help meet the need, and apply the model to two fictional patient cases.
4. Discuss the key features of the Oral Health-Related Quality of Life Model, a conceptual model, illustrate how the model enables the dental hygienist to diagnose patient needs based on assessment and/or formulate a plan of action to help meet the need, and apply the model to two fictional patient cases.
5. Discuss the key features of the Client Self-Care Commitment Model, a conceptual model, illustrate how the model enables the dental hygienist to diagnose patient needs based on assessment and/or formulate a plan of action to help meet the need, and apply the model to two fictional patient cases.

THE DENTAL HYGIENE METAPARADIGM AND PARADIGM CONCEPTS

Most disciplines have a metaparadigm, a widely accepted view of the discipline that includes paradigm concepts defined by the discipline as its unique perspective. The concepts defined for each discipline help differentiate the discipline from others. Fig. 2.1 illustrates the dental hygiene metaparadigm and its four paradigm concepts.[1] Dental hygienists need to consider how the four paradigm concepts of the dental hygiene discipline interrelate: client, environment, health and oral health, and dental hygiene actions. These grand concepts fundamentally shape different dental hygiene conceptual practice models which inspire theories and ultimately inform practice, education, and research within the profession. They are grand concepts because they are overarching, no matter the dental hygienist's practice setting.

Even before reflecting on the paradigm concepts, dental hygienists are invited to explore on their positionality with respect to how they view health, in general, given dental hygienists are healthcare professionals. Indeed, dental hygienists are reminded that "health is created and lived by people within the settings of their everyday life; where they learn, work, play, and love."[2] Salutogenesis is health creation.[3] Pathogenesis is about the origins of disease and disease. Dental hygienists perceiving the profession as one focused on health creation and the promotion of health would be salutogenic agents. Consider the difference between the dental hygienist positioning their practice from a salutogenic perspective vs a pathogenic one. Should the dental hygienist's perspective be informed from a pathogenic viewpoint, they would likely focus practice on prevention and treatment of disease and disease with little or no consideration regarding salutogenesis. Whereas should the dental hygienist's frame of reference be that of salutogenesis, they would expand their view from that of pathogenesis and embrace a role in health creation and understanding the determinants of health. The perspective matters as it informs thought and thought processes, and fortifies attitudes, values, and assumptions within each of the dental hygiene paradigm concepts and metaparadigm.

Dental Hygiene's Paradigm Concepts

A discipline's paradigm concepts are defined very broadly, or globally, so conceptual models can be developed about the concepts.[4] Dental hygienists need to be prudent regarding their understanding of the four paradigm concepts: client, health/oral health, environment, and dental hygiene actions. Fig. 2.1 illustrates the interrelationship and unity of the concepts. Given the dental hygiene profession is person-centered, the first concept to be described is the client. Moving counterclockwise around Fig. 2.1, descriptions of the oral/health and environment concepts follow, with the concept of dental hygiene actions described last as the other three concepts inform the actions (the ways of knowing).

The client concept includes persons, families, groups, and communities of all ages, genders, sociocultural, and economic backgrounds, and importantly, whether they accessed or would benefit from dental hygiene care.[1,4,5] The term *client*, rather than *patient*, was selected as a paradigm concept because the term *client* is broad, suggests wellness rather than illness, and represents an active rather than passive relationship with the dental hygienist.[4] Still, people receiving treatment and prevention focused dental hygiene care are often referred to as patients, and thus client and patient are used, depending on the dental hygienist engagement with the person(s). The use of both terms is seen in the 2021 policy manual of the American Dental Hygienists

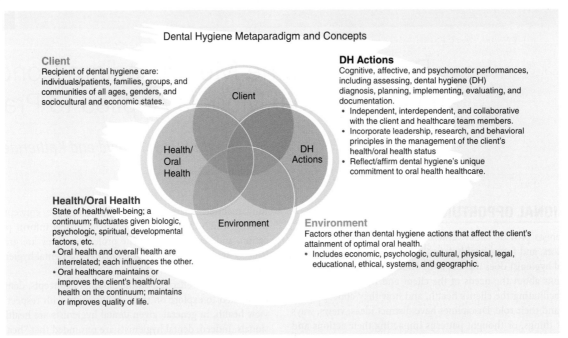

Fig. 2.1 The Dental Hygiene Discipline's Metaparadigm and Paradigm Concepts.

Association (ADHA).[5] The paradigm concept of client has a broader definition than that of patient. Importantly, dental hygienists value and practice person-centered care.

The concept of health/oral health is defined as the client's state of well-being on a continuum from maximum wellness to maximum illness (see Fig. 2.1).[1,4] Oral health and overall health are interrelated because each influences the other. For example, there is a bidirectional relationship between diabetes and periodontal disease. Poorly controlled diabetes is a risk factor for periodontal disease, and periodontal disease is a risk factor for diabetes, whereas clients with well-controlled diabetes can enjoy good periodontal health. A healthy diet is required for oral health, for example an eating disorder may result in systemic health issues as well as oral diseases such as dental caries and enamel erosion. The dental hygienist needs to explore the determinants of health and not only the associations and causation of disease and disease, and further, do so knowing the intricate relationship between the health/oral health concept with the other three dental hygiene paradigm concepts. For example, consider the relationship between health/oral health and an environmental culture of racism, a known public health crisis, and how it must be addressed and dismantled at all structural and systems levels to ensure health equity,[6] including oral health equity.[7]

The concept of the environment is defined as the surroundings in which the client and dental hygienist are interacting (see Fig. 2.1).[1,4] This concept includes, for example, social, ethno-cultural, financial, political, and educational factors that can be barriers or facilitators to health, oral health, and dental hygiene actions. The environment affects the client and the dental hygienist, and the client and the dental hygienist also influence the environment. A few examples follow. Notably, attention is given to the social determinants of health (e.g., access to care, education, geographical location) which are inherent within the environment concept, but also intertwined with and between the other three paradigm concepts. A dental hygienist providing clinical care to patients in a dental or dental hygiene practice would be influenced by a practice environment different, for example, from a practice setting in a school or a primary healthcare clinic. Clients, culture, and the environment in a rural area may differ from clients, culture, and the environment in an urban area. Elderly clients in long-term

care facilities would uniquely affect dental hygiene actions. The dental hygienist needs to know the system, policies, and protocols within the facility, and further, the legislation and regulation within their practice jurisdiction. Dental hygienists serving a client community with low oral health literacy would need to ensure that resources exist so they can facilitate the client's understanding of their oral conditions, recommended treatment, and self-care instructions. Importantly, the dental hygienist needs to stay abreast of the ongoing global calls for better health that influence the environment concept such as global health; interprofessional collaboration; pandemic awareness and practice management; social determinants of health; anti-racism; deconstructing colonial ideologies informing practice and systems; patient safety and quality assurance; and healthy policy and healthy decision-making processes at organizational, institutional, and societal levels.

The concept of dental hygiene actions is defined as the interventions provided by a dental hygienist for the benefit of, and in collaboration with, the client to promote wellness and oral wellness and prevent oral disease (see Fig. 2.1).[1,4] Importantly, dental hygiene actions embrace interprofessional collaboration. Dental hygiene actions occur throughout the dental hygiene process of care in any setting, role, or environment. For example, the actions of a dental hygienist employed in a public health setting might include planning, implementation, and screenings for oral cancer in a high school or facilitating an oral health education program for a group of caregivers. Over the past several decades, dental hygiene actions have evolved and/or emerged resulting in changes and scope of practice. For example, pandemics impacted dental hygiene actions with respect to infection control and prevention. For many dental hygienists, regulation is such that their scope of practice includes local anesthetic and for some, the ability to prescribe medications or administer vaccinations.

The above examples begin to illuminate the interaction among the four paradigm concepts as the clients differ, for example, in age, culture, socioeconomic groups, education, and health/oral health status; the environment where dental hygienists serve the client differs; and, accordingly, dental hygiene actions must vary to address the health/oral health needs of these various clients in their unique environments. Thus, the metaparadigm represents the discipline of dental hygiene,

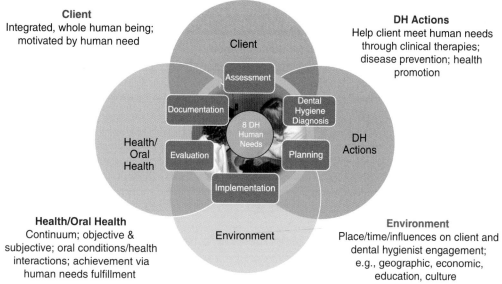

Client
Integrated, whole human being;
motivated by human need

DH Actions
Help client meet human needs
through clinical therapies;
disease prevention; health
promotion

Health/Oral Health
Continuum; objective &
subjective; oral conditions/health
interactions; achievement via
human needs fulfillment

Environment
Place/time/influences on client and
dental hygienist engagement;
e.g., geographic, economic,
education, culture

Fig. 2.2 Dental hygiene's paradigm concepts are explained in terms of human needs theory in the Human Needs Conceptual Model.

and the paradigm concepts apply to all situations in which dental hygienists provide oral healthcare services, oral health education, and oral health/health promotion and creation.

DENTAL HYGIENE CONCEPTUAL MODELS

A conceptual model represents concepts and relationships between them. Conceptual models are like schools of thought. Most disciplines have several conceptual models from which to guide professional practice, develop and evolve disciplinary science, and inform the profession's education process and outcome. Although the dental hygiene discipline draws on many theories, in this chapter, conceptual models that draw on the dental hygiene discipline's paradigm concepts are presented and applied to clinically based dental hygiene practice settings. Each describes a unique process of care that is distinct for dental hygiene. Sometimes, authors of models use the term conceptual in the title, and sometimes it is implied.

The Dental Hygiene Human Needs Conceptual Model was developed by two dental hygiene scholars, Michelle Darby and Margaret Walsh, building on nursing theory and applying it specifically to dental hygiene.[8,9] The model is based on the premise that human behavior is motivated by fulfillment of human needs, and it defines the paradigm concepts in terms of human need theory (Fig. 2.2). The model explicitly draws upon the four dental hygiene disciplinary concepts to develop an understanding of client human needs throughout the dental hygiene process of care. It is a theoretically sound dental hygiene model.[10] The way the model relates the paradigm concepts to the steps of the dental hygiene process as per the American Dental Hygienist Association standards of practice is explained in Table 2.1. Box 2.1 outlines the eight dental hygiene human needs. The dental hygienist identifies deficits in these needs with the client during the assessment and diagnosis phases of the dental hygiene care process of care and then, in collaboration with others, plans, implements, evaluates, and documents interventions to resolve and meet the client needs.

The two fictional cases, Edward Gilly (Box 2.2) and Pia Tran (Box 2.3), provide scenarios to apply to the dental hygiene theoretical model. Keep in mind that the Dental Hygiene Human Needs Conceptual Model is about knowing the needs of the client through assessment, dental hygiene diagnosis, and the resulting dental hygiene care plan.

Chapter 22 on the dental hygiene diagnosis and Chapter 23 on dental hygiene care planning, evaluation, and documentation further illustrate the application of the model and others to dental hygiene practice.

The Oral Health–Related Quality of Life Model, a conceptual model developed by dental hygiene educator-researchers at the University of Missouri—Kansas City, is a framework for looking at the complex interrelationship between wellness, disease, characteristics of the individual or population, and general quality of life (Fig. 2.3).[11,12] It is based on the premise that oral health, comfort, and function is an integral element of general health. It builds on three previous models, with wellness and disease being on a dynamic continuum that encompasses health, preclinical disease, biological and physiological variables, symptom status, functional status, oral health perceptions, and general quality of life.[11,12] Sociocultural, environmental, and economic characteristics influence and modify each domain. Importantly, the model emphasizes the biopsychosocial perspectives, and thus affiliates well with the practitioner's attention to the social determinants of health. Additionally, the model was designed to aid dental hygienists knowing patient-centered care, that is, the dental hygiene care plan emerges from and is driven by the patient's perceptions of and reactions to their own oral health status as it relates to their quality of life, and not just the diagnosis of disease.

The Client Self-Care Commitment Model, a conceptual model developed by dental hygiene educators at Idaho State University, draws on several previous models from different disciplines to provide a unique, specific application to dental hygiene (Fig. 2.4).[13] The model is based on the premise of clients as co-therapists in their oral health decisions to enhance motivation, commitment, and compliance with oral self-care. A primary role of the dental hygienist is as an oral health educator and practitioner with a pivotal role in establishing trusting client-provider relationships to provide oral health-promoting information, and preventive and therapeutic care. The model recognizes that relationship and proposes five interrelated domains to encourage active client self-involvement in oral health maintenance and empower clients to make decisions to enhance their own health through commitment and compliance.

All three models apply to the dental hygiene process of care (assessment, dental hygiene diagnosis, planning, implementation, evaluation, and documentation). The concepts of client, environment, health/

TABLE 2.1   Comparison of Dental Hygiene Process of Care Between ADHA Standards for Clinical Dental Hygiene Practice and Human Needs Conceptual Model

Steps	ADHA Definition and Standards for Clinical Dental Hygiene Practice[15]	Human Needs Conceptual Model[8,9]
Assessment	Systematic collection and analysis of systematic and oral health data to identify client needs.	Systematic data collection and evaluation of eight human needs as being met or unmet based on all available assessment data.
Dental hygiene diagnosis	Identification of an individual's health behaviors, attitudes, and oral healthcare needs for which a dental hygienist is educationally qualified and licensed to provide.	Identification of unmet human needs among the eight related to dental hygiene care (i.e., human need deficit) and of the cause as evidenced by signs and symptoms.
Planning	The establishment of realistic goals and selection of dental hygiene interventions that can move the client closer to optimal oral health.	Establishment of goals for client behavior with time deadlines to meet identified unmet human needs.
Implementation	The act of carrying out the dental hygiene plan of care.	The process of carrying out planned interventions targeting causes of unmet needs.
Evaluation	Measurement of the extent to which the client has achieved the goals specified in the dental hygiene care plan.	The outcome measurement of whether client goals have been met, partially met, or unmet.
Documentation	The complete and accurate recording of all collected data, treatment planned and provided, recommendations (both oral and written), referrals, prescriptions, patient/client comments and related communication, treatment outcomes and patient satisfaction, and other information relevant to patient care and treatment.	The complete and accurate recording of human need deficits related to the client's eight human needs, and dental hygiene diagnoses, goals, interventions, and evaluations based on human need theory.

ADHA, American Dental Hygienists Association.

BOX 2.1   Eight Human Needs Related to Dental Hygiene Care[8,9]

Protection from health risks
Freedom from fear and stress
Freedom from pain
Wholesome facial image
Skin and mucous membrane integrity of the head and neck
Biologically sound and functional dentition
Conceptualization and problem solving
Responsibility for oral health

BOX 2.2   Critical Thinking Scenario A

Fictional Client (Edward Gilly) and Dental Hygienist (Siobhan McNicol)

Edward Gilly, an 84-year-old government administrator, presents for his annual appointment with his long-term dental hygienist, Siobhan McNicol. Health history findings include normal vitals, history of hypertension, high cholesterol, asthma, allergy to codeine, and former tobacco use with a resolved desire to remain tobacco-free. He reports compliance with antihypertensive, blood-thinning, cholesterol-lowering, and bronchodilation medications, and regular visits to his primary healthcare team. This year, Mr. Gilly had coronary bypass surgery. He is proud of his quick, full recovery and current good health due to regular exercise with his personal trainer.

Examination findings reveal numerous restorations, well-fitting lower and upper partial dentures, root caries, and dry mouth. Mr. Gilly has localized Stage III Grade B periodontitis in the posterior teeth, 4- to 6-mm probing depths, 6- to 7-mm clinical attachment loss, bleeding upon probing, class I and II furcations, and radiographic evidence of horizontal bone loss extending to the middle third of roots of posterior teeth, localized light subgingival calculus, and moderate supragingival calculus on the lingual of mandibular anterior teeth, generalized marginal and interdental dental plaque, and a coated tongue.

Mr. Gilly uses a manual toothbrush and fluoridated dentifrice twice a day, an interdental brush twice a week, and cleans and soaks his partial dentures nightly. He manages his dry mouth from medications with sugarless chewing gum and drinking sweetened iced tea, and he snacks frequently on cookies that his loving wife of 50 years bakes for him.

---

oral health, and dental hygiene action remain the main elements of the discipline's metaparadigm, regardless of the conceptual model. The worldview or paradigm concepts and the dental hygiene process of care influences the dental hygienist's approach or experience depending on the conceptual model.

The Paradigm Concepts Viewed Through the Dental Hygiene Human Needs Conceptual Model

In the Dental Hygiene Human Needs Conceptual Model, the client is defined as a biological, psychological, spiritual, social, cultural, and intellectual human being who is an integrated, organized whole and whose behavior is motivated by human need fulfillment (see Fig. 2.2). Human need fulfillment restores a sense of wholeness as a human being. The client is viewed as having eight human needs especially related to dental hygiene care (see Box 2.1). For fictional client Edward Gilly (see Box 2.2), dental hygienist Siobhan McNicol would likely diagnose the following human need deficits (meaning possible unfilled needs): protection from health risks given his health history; biologically sound and functional dentition given active root caries; skin and mucous membrane integrity of the head and neck given periodontal disease condition, tongue coating, and dry mouth; and responsibility for oral health related to his diet and active root caries.

In the Dental Hygiene Human Needs Conceptual Model, the environment influences the manner, mode, and level of human need fulfillment for the person, family, and community (see Fig. 2.2). To illustrate this concept, fictional client Pia Tran (see Box 2.3) informs dental hygienist Emery Sinclair that she is a married mother of two children. Pia and her husband do not support fluoride use. From a human need perspective, Emery, wanting to help fulfill Pia's human

Fictional Client (Pia Tran) and Dental Hygienist (Emery Sinclair)

Pia Tran, a 40-year-old, married, full-time salesperson with two children, presents for the first time to dental hygienist Emery Sinclair. Pia's health history includes normal vitals, long-term pharmacologically managed depression, regular physician visits, and an active lifestyle. Pia reports being busy with daily family activities and a resulting diet of fast food, energy bars, and protein/fruit shakes or store-bought prepared meals.

During the extraoral examination, Emery notes a herpetic lesion in the crusting healing phase after 1 week of over-the-counter medication. Intraoral findings include several crowns, anterior interproximal resin restorations, rolled and red gingival margins around the crowns, white spot lesions on the buccal of the second maxillary molars, normal probing depths, and normal clinical attachment levels. There is light supragingival calculus on the lower anterior teeth; coffee stains that motivated her to see Emery; light, localized dental plaque; light tongue coating; and a low salivary flow. Pia drinks water frequently and does not report dry mouth symptoms.

Pia brushes twice daily using a power-driven toothbrush with a nonfluoridated toothpaste and an antimicrobial rinse, but no flossing. She and her husband do not believe in fluoride. Pia does not brush her tongue because of a gag reflex. Mid-appointment with Emery, Pia mentions that neither of her elementary-school children have seen a dentist or dental hygienist. She thinks both might have a couple of cavities as they have "black spots" on some posterior teeth.

need, would likely begin to engage Pia in conceptualization and problem-solving as well as responsibility for oral health with respect to her children's dentition given the presence of potential carious lesions and Pia's concern about them. The environment in which the children are growing up has multiple influences, including client beliefs, that impact health and oral health and resulting dental hygiene actions within the dental hygiene care plan. At this point, note that the paradigm concepts are interrelated and that one does not exist without the other.

The concept of health and oral health exists on a continuum from maximal wellness to maximal illness. Along the health and oral health continuum, degrees of wellness and illness are associated with varying levels of human need fulfillment (see Fig. 2.2). Fictional client Edward Gilly (see Box 2.2) presents himself as a person who perceives himself as healthy because he defines health as being all you can be, realizing aspirations, and adapting to life. His dental hygienist, Siobhan McNicol, would likely employ motivational interviewing (see Chapter 5) to identify how Edward knows himself this way and how she can help him facilitate this perspective while adapting and managing health risks such as high cholesterol, asthma, and related oral-health impacts resulting from the medications. Edward has access to healthcare that enables him to manage his health condition, and he appears health literate. These factors and his clinical findings illustrate the paradigm concepts of environment, oral health/health, and client, respectively. Siobhan used her assessment of Edward's human needs and dental hygiene diagnosis based on human needs within the process of dental hygiene care to understand this about Edward.

Dental hygiene actions are behaviors of the dental hygienist aimed at assisting clients in meeting their eight human needs related to optimal oral wellness and quality of life throughout the life cycle. The process of dental hygiene care is inherent in the concept of dental hygiene actions (see Table 2.1). After initial collection of client histories and completing all assessments, including identifying client needs, findings

are evaluated to determine whether the eight human needs related to dental hygiene care are met. These eight human needs relate, for example, to physical, emotional, intellectual, social, and cultural dimensions of the client and the environment that are related to dental hygiene care. Findings from the assessment of these human needs ensure a comprehensive and humanistic approach to care. Dental hygienists use these findings to make dental hygiene diagnoses based on unmet human needs (i.e., human need deficits) and then plan (i.e., set goals, sequence appointments, select interventions), implement, evaluate, and document outcomes of dental hygiene care (i.e., goals met, partially met, or unmet). Fictional client Pia Tran's health history reveals management of depression with the use of medications, regular appointments with her physician, and lifestyle modifications (see Box 2.3). Dental hygienist Emery Sinclair will engage in dental hygiene actions such as interprofessional collaboration and recommending strategies to minimize the oral implications of having low salivary flow, a challenge to her human need for soft tissue integrity and sound dentition.

The Dental Hygiene Human Needs Conceptual Model's Eight Human Needs in Clinical Care

The dental hygienist seeks to understand a client/patient's (hereafter referred to as patient given clinical-based care) dental hygiene human needs via the assessment and diagnostic phases of the dental hygiene process of care, plans with the patient how to address deficit needs, implements the dental hygiene care plan, and evaluates it, documenting throughout the process. Hence, this model is client/patient centered. The dental hygienist comes to know the client/patient's needs by using effective communication strategies and developing a practitioner-client/patient therapeutic relationship. In this way, the dental hygienist learns from the client/patient about their needs, and the client/patient learns from the dental hygienist about oral/systemic health, thus promoting oral/health literacy. Each of the eight human needs is described and examples are provided to illustrate how the dental hygienist assesses the client/patient's needs and implications of deficit or unmet needs on the dental hygiene care plan. A comprehensive dental hygiene care plan is thus developed with and for the client/patient. Description of the eight human needs represented as the inner circle of the Dental Hygiene Human Needs Conceptual Model (see Fig. 2.2) follows.

Protection From Health Risks

Protection from health risks is the need to avoid medical contraindications related to dental hygiene care and to be free from harm or danger. This human need includes a patient's need to be in a state of good general health through efficient functioning of body organs and systems, or under the active care of a physician or other primary healthcare provider to be in a controlled state of general health.

During the assessment, indications that the patient's need for protection from health risks is *unmet* include but are not limited to the following:

- Evidence from the patient's health history of the need for immediate referral to or consultation with a primary care provider regarding uncontrolled disease (e.g., blood pressure reading or blood glucose level outside of normal limits).
- Evidence of lifestyle practices that place the patient at risk for oral injury (e.g., inconsistent use of an athletic mouthguard) or for oral disease (e.g., a tobacco user).

When dental hygienists need specific information about the status of a patient's general health to complete a care plan, they consult and collaborate with the patient's other healthcare providers, such as the primary care provider, medical specialist, or pharmacist, to ensure safe dental hygiene care. Generally, patients with no healthcare provider are referred to one for examination. Obtaining initial information related

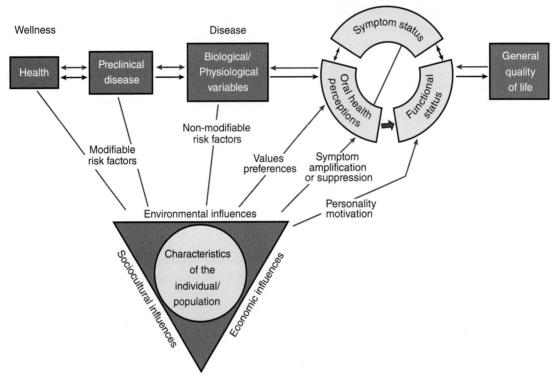

Fig. 2.3 The Oral Health–Related Quality of Life Model. (Redrawn from Williams KB, Gadbury-Amyot CC, Bray KK, et al. Oral health–related quality of life: a model for dental hygiene. *J Dent Hyg.* 1998a;72(2):19–26.)

to a patient's general and oral health and updating it at each dental hygiene care appointment are essential steps to ensure that the patient's need for protection from health risks is met or fulfilled.

In the case of Edward Gilly, this need is met by the dental hygienist monitoring his vitals and updating his health history at each appointment for safety purposes (see Box 2.2). Dental hygienist Siobhan will want to ensure that the blood thinners are not a concern with respect to bleeding associated with any dental hygiene action, such as periodontal debridement; she will also want to monitor his cardiovascular health, knowing the potential for oral systemic health connections (see Chapter 21).

Freedom From Fear and Stress

Freedom from fear and stress is the need to feel safe and to be free from emotional discomfort in the oral healthcare environment and to receive appreciation, attention, and respect from others. People often state they fear needles, do not like having to deal with dental issues, or dislike the feeling of having their teeth "scraped." The dental hygienist must fulfill the patient's need to be free from fear and stress while the patient is in their care. During assessment, indications that the patient's need for freedom from fear and stress is unmet may include previous negative experiences, triggering situations reminding the dental hygienist of the need for trauma-informed care, cost of care, and signs of stress such as clenched hands or perspiration (see Chapter 11). To some patients, the dental hygiene appointment itself may signal threat or danger and may trigger fear and stress. Being confronted with strangers, use of objects in their mouth (e.g., dental hygiene instruments), loss of parental protection (for children), and the fear of contracting an infectious or life-threatening disease such as hepatitis C, coronavirus disease (COVID-19), or acquired immunodeficiency syndrome (AIDS) are threats to the need for freedom from fear and stress.

If fear and stress are apparent at the beginning of, during, or following the dental hygiene appointment, the dental hygienist initiates

fear- or stress-control interventions. Such interventions include, for example, reassuring the patient that every effort will be made to provide care in as comfortable and safe a manner as possible, communicating with empathy, discussing culturally associated behaviors, answering all questions as completely as possible, and using pharmacologic agents such as nitrous oxide sedation and local anesthesia. Neither patient Edward Gilly nor patient Pia Tran appear to be expressing a human need for freedom from fear and stress; however, as the dental hygienist continually develops and attends to the patient-clinician therapeutic relationship (see Chapter 5), such need may be disclosed, with the dental hygienist responding to it accordingly.

Freedom From Pain

The human need of freedom from pain is the patient's need to be exempt from physical discomfort not only in the head and neck area but also in general. During the assessment, indications that the patient's need for freedom from pain is unmet include but are not limited to patient self-report and signs of discomfort or pain during dental hygiene care, such as wincing or squinting of the eyes or continual repositioning in the chair, seeking a comfortable position.

The patient must be relieved of pain—this is the highest priority. If pain is apparent, the dental hygienist initiates pain control interventions immediately and if outside of the scope of practice, collaborates with appropriate others, for example, a dentist. Given that fictional patient Edward Gilly (see Box 2.2) has root caries and localized Stage III Grade B periodontitis, he may experience or anticipate pain with periodontal debridement; hence, his dental hygienist, Siobhan, would recommend pain management such as a local anesthetic (see Chapter 43).

Wholesome Facial Image

Wholesome facial image is the need to feel satisfied with one's own oral-facial features and breath. Facial image is influenced by normal

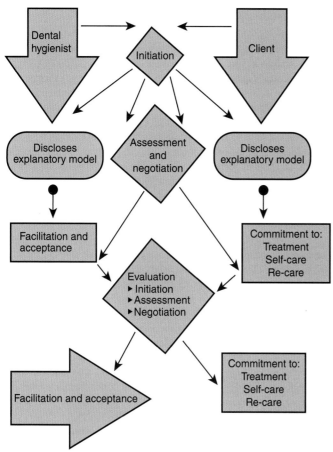

Fig. 2.4 The Client Self-Care Commitment Model. (Redrawn from Calley KH, Rogo E, Miller DL, et al. A proposed client self-care commitment model. *J Dent Hyg.* 2000;74(1):24–35.)

and abnormal physical changes, and for example, by cultural and societal attitudes and values. During assessment, dental hygienists look for indications that the patient's need for a wholesome facial image is unmet and listen for patients' concern about appearance or breath. Personal perceptions matter. For example, someone who associates possession of natural teeth with femininity or masculinity would view loss of teeth as a significant alteration. Similarly, patients with dentures, a cleft lip, or facial disfigurement after surgical treatment of oral cancer may reduce social contacts out of fear of people's reactions to them. An indication that the patient's need for a wholesome facial image is fulfilled might be the patient expressing satisfaction with his or her appearance. To facilitate identification of the wholesome facial image need, the dental hygienist engages in effective communication strategies (see Chapter 5) and aside from closed-ended questions asks open-ended questions such as, "I am wondering how you feel about your teeth and mouth?" Such questions may elicit responses indicating dissatisfaction with tooth stain, calculus, receding gums, a discolored restoration, tooth loss, maligned teeth, or disfigurement from facial trauma. For example, fictional patient Pia Tran presents for her dental hygiene appointment expressing dissatisfaction with tooth discoloration from coffee stains (see Box 2.3). Dental hygienist Emery Sinclair would suggest meeting her need by including stain management and removal strategies (see Chapter 32). Importantly, the dental hygienist listens to patient needs and discusses treatment outcomes related to wholesome facial image needs while providing information, reassurance, and referrals. The dental hygienist also may collaborate with others to help fulfill the patient's need.

Skin and Mucous Membrane Integrity of the Head and Neck

Skin and mucous membrane integrity of the head and neck is the need for an intact and functioning covering of the person's head and neck area, including the oral mucous membranes and periodontium. These intact tissues defend against harmful microbes, provide sensory information, resist injurious substances and trauma, and reflect adequate nutrition. During the assessment, indications this human need is unmet include but are not limited to extraoral and intraoral lesions, tenderness, or swelling; periodontal disease; and nutritional deficiency manifestations.

The dental hygienist examines all skin and mucous membranes in and about the oral cavity, including the periodontium, and documents findings. The examination informs the dental hygiene care plan, the patient's dentist and primary healthcare provider, and the patient about evidence of abnormal tissue changes and/or disease. Recognition, treatment, and followup of specific lesions may be of great significance to the general and oral health of the patient. Routine extraoral and intraoral examination of patients at the initial appointment and at each continued care appointment provides an excellent opportunity to control oral disease by early recognition and treatment. For example, patients must be screened regularly to detect potentially cancerous lesions. Moreover, a current appointment may be postponed because of a patient's need for urgent medical consultation, a positive screening outcome for COVID-19, or because of evidence of infectious lesions, such as herpes labialis. Dental hygienist Emery Sinclair, after performing an extraoral examination on fictional patient Pia Tran, decided along with Pia to continue with the intraoral examination, given that the herpetic lesion on Pia's lip was in the crusting-over healing phase, and the intraoral examination was not contraindicated at this time.

Biologically Sound and Functional Dentition

Biologically sound and functional dentition refers to the need for intact teeth and/or dental prosthetic appliances and dental restorations that defend against harmful microbes and provide adequate functioning and esthetics. During the assessment, indications that the patient's need for a biologically sound dentition is unmet include but are not limited to dental caries; teeth with calculus, oral biofilm, or stain; sound or failing restorations; occlusal alignment; dentinal sensitivity; and missing teeth and prosthetic appliances.

The dental hygienist identifies and documents existing conditions of the teeth, including all teeth with signs of disease and/or functional problems that require care within and beyond the dental hygienist's scope of practice. There are numerous dental hygiene actions to help a patient fulfill this human need—for example, providing fluoride therapy, pit and fissure sealants, dietary counseling, and, in some jurisdictions, restorative care. Both fictional patients, Edward Gilly and Pia Tran would benefit from preventive interventions (see Boxes 2.2 and 2.3). Edward has exposed roots that are susceptible to root caries and biofilm and calculus deposits, consumes cariogenic foods daily, and has medication-induced dry mouth. He also has numerous repaired teeth and wears well-fitting partial dentures; thus, his dental hygienist would likely reinforce denture care and fluoride therapy. Pia also has numerous repaired teeth, plaque biofilm and calculus deposits, possible salivary flow issues, and dietary habits that may be concerns, and she does not use fluoride. She, too, would benefit from dental hygiene actions.

Conceptualization and Problem Solving

Conceptualization and problem solving involve the need to understand ideas and abstractions to make sound judgments about one's oral health. This need is met if the patient understands the rationale for recommended oral healthcare interventions; participates in setting goals for dental hygiene care; has no questions about professional dental hygiene care or dental treatment; and has no questions about the cause of the oral problem, its relationship to overall health, and the importance of the solution suggested to solve the problem.

During the assessment, the dental hygienist assesses this need by listening to a patient's questions and responses to the dental hygienist's answers and observing nonverbal responses. Oral health literacy is assessed, as it strongly influences a client's ability to process and understand the basic health/oral health information and services to make appropriate health decisions. Oral examination findings indicating this human need include the observation that the patient's conditions are incongruent with the patient's expressed beliefs, attitude, and knowledge and professed behaviors. Evidence that the patient has questions, misconceptions, or a lack of knowledge indicates this need is unmet. Examples of information critical to a client's decision making and participation as a co-therapist in their own oral healthcare include providing informed consent for recommended dental hygiene care, understanding oral-systemic health connections, and selecting and performing daily effective preventive self-care practices.

During patient education, dental hygienists present the rationale and details of recommended self-care methods and ensure the patient understands. They use educational materials including the demonstration of oral hygiene device(s), clarify patient understanding, and evaluate ability to use the device or tool. For example, to help a patient conceptualize dental biofilm and gingivitis, the dental hygienist may show the patient signs of gingival inflammation, use a disclosing agent, and demonstrate how selected oral hygiene techniques effectively remove the biofilm. To illustrate this human need, dental hygienist Emery Sinclair will help patient Pia Tran problem solve her gag reflex, which has inhibited her willingness to perform daily tongue hygiene.

Responsibility for Oral Health

Responsibility for oral health refers to the need for accountability for one's oral health given interaction between one's motivation, physical and cognitive capability, and social environment. During the assessment, indications this need is unmet include but are not limited to inadequate oral self-care, lengthy time periods between oral examinations, and statements such as "My mother had bad teeth and so I have bad teeth."

The dental hygienist assesses the patient's oral health behaviors and suggests behaviors to the patient (or to the parent/healthcare decision maker or proxy) that could be initiated to obtain and maintain oral health and wellness. The dental hygienist encourages the patient to participate in setting goals for dental hygiene care, offers choices, and facilitates and reinforces patient decision making. In addition, the dental hygienist addresses deficits in the patient's psychomotor skills and recommends strategies to enhance proper manipulation of the toothbrush, floss, or other oral self-care aids (e.g., use of a power toothbrush to facilitate biofilm removal).

A primary role of the dental hygienist is to motivate and empower patients to adopt and maintain positive oral health behaviors. Dental hygienist Siobhan McNicol will engage patient Edward Gilly in conversation about his dry mouth, habit of drinking sweetened tea throughout the day, periodontal disease, and root caries (see Box 2.2). Knowing he has been successful in the past in quitting tobacco use is a good starting point for Siobhan to begin to help Edward consider goals related to improving his oral health. Goals must be related realistically to the patient's individual needs, values, and ability level.

Simultaneously Meeting Needs

Identification of the eight human needs related to dental hygiene care is a way for dental hygienists to evaluate and understand the needs of all patients and to achieve a patient-centered practice. In Chapter 22 on Dental Hygiene Diagnosis, Fig. 22.2 provides an example of a clinical form for use in assessing the eight human needs and making dental hygiene diagnoses which together inform the plan (dental hygiene actions), implementation and evaluation of the plan, and also documentation as it relates to meeting the patient's needs. Fig. 22.3 provides an example of the form in use. The Dental Hygiene Human Needs Conceptual Model provides a holistic and humanistic perspective for dental hygiene care. The model addresses the client's needs in the physical, psychologic, emotional, intellectual, spiritual, and social dimensions, and informs the practice of client-centered dental hygiene in any role or setting.

After identifying a client's unmet human needs, the dental hygienist, in collaboration with the client, sets goals and establishes priorities for providing care to fulfill these needs. Setting goals and establishing priorities, however, does not mean that the dental hygienist provides care for only one need at a time. For example, when providing care for a patient with painful gingivitis whose human needs for skin and mucous membrane integrity of the head and neck and for freedom from pain require immediate attention, the dental hygienist also takes into consideration the patient's need for freedom from stress and wholesome facial image. It is not unusual that one needs to take priority. The dental hygienist must be concerned first with the highest-priority need (such as helping the patient cope with a fear of pain). However, frequently, the dental hygienist simultaneously addresses needs such as assisting a patient in meeting the need for responsibility for oral health while also helping the patient achieve freedom from pain. Applying this model when interacting with clients, whether the client is an individual, a family, or a community, enhances the dental hygienist's relationship with the client and promotes the client's adoption of and adherence to the dental hygienist's professional recommendations.

For additional examples of how to apply the Dental Hygiene Human Needs Conceptual Model, please refer to Chapters 22 and 23, where cases and case scenarios are used to walk the reader through the application of this model.

ORAL HEALTH–RELATED QUALITY OF LIFE MODEL

The conceptual model, the Oral Health–Related Quality of Life Model, focuses on how the individual or population defines its own satisfactory level of oral health, comfort, and function. Inherent to the model is a recognition that the oral cavity is a primary source of sensory perception and a key means of social interaction and functioning.[11,12] This model provides a framework that allows the dental hygienist to view and approach patient care while placing emphasis on the multidimensional nature of oral problems and considering an individual patient's or population group's preferences for health outcomes (see Fig. 2.3). The model encourages the dental hygienist to investigate and understand each patient's perceptions of their oral health and to allow the patient to express their desires for oral health and overall health. The dental hygienist questions the patient about any symptoms or signs of oral disease or conditions needing dental hygiene care and addresses a patient's functional status based upon their physical, social, and psychological function. Similar to the Dental Hygiene Human Needs Conceptual Model, yet with a different lens, this model emphasizes respecting a patient's individuality and perceptions of their lived experience as important to help patients achieve their desired health outcomes and oral health-related quality of life.

During the assessment, the dental hygienist has a dialogue with patients to identify their oral-health quality of life. In Chapter 22, Dental Hygiene Diagnosis, Figs. 22.6 and 22.7 provide examples of clinical forms with patient information assessing the domains and key elements of the Oral Health–Related Quality of Life Conceptual Model.[12] Figs. 22.4 and 22.5 are the OHRQL Questionnaire forms that are used to solicit patient perceptions of their general and oral health quality of life. This information is integrated with clinical assessment findings to develop a comprehensive dental hygiene care plan. This approach allows dental hygienists to identify issues of importance to the patient that might not be priorities of the dental hygienist and areas of important health or clinical findings that the patient is unaware of. For example, the patient may perceive they have halitosis that is not detected by the clinician. Conversely, the dental hygienist might detect an asymptomatic abnormal oral lesion that the patient does not know is present.

Domains and Key Elements of the Oral Health–Related Quality of Life Model

A domain is a specific area or sphere of knowledge. The Oral Health–Related Quality of Life Model includes six domains, each with key elements related to dental hygiene care (see Fig. 2.3).

Health and Preclinical Disease Domain

In the Oral Health–Related Quality of Life Model, health is defined by an individual as their ideal level of well-being, including physical, psychological, social, and emotional health. Preclinical disease frequently is preceded by changes that are not observable, yet these changes can be influenced by health promotion and prevention, key defining components of the discipline of dental hygiene. Dental hygienists focus on helping individuals, families, groups, and communities prevent oral disease and provide interventions and programs specifically designed to foster oral and general health. Clinical or community dental hygiene interventions such as fluoride therapy and pit and fissure sealants are preventive in nature, whereas oral health education and tobacco cessation efforts promote health.

In the fictional case of Edward Gilly (see Box 2.2), dental hygienist Siobhan McNicol recognizes Edward's self-perceived good health and quality of life (despite his complex medical history, dry mouth, and age of 84 years), while also identifying signs of inflammation associated with his biofilm and calculus deposits, periodontal disease, and bleeding upon probing. She will reinforce his daily measures to maintain good health such as exercise, twice-daily brushing with a fluoride toothpaste, and use of sugarless gum or mints for his dry mouth, and discuss the need for daily interdental oral hygiene and less frequent sugary snacks as important means of prevention and health promotion.

Biological and Physical Clinical Variables

The Oral Health–Related Quality of Life Model also includes biological and physical clinical variables (see Fig. 2.3). This area encompasses clinical assessment findings indicating oral and systemic disease—for example, history of diabetes, dental caries, clinical attachment loss, and gingival inflammation. In the dental hygiene process of care, assessment findings are used to formulate a dental hygiene diagnosis. The dental hygienist then centers on implementing interventions to address the clinical disease and evaluating resultant changes.

In the case of Edward Gilly (see Box 2.2), his dental hygienist, Siobhan, will provide fluoride varnish therapy and periodontal debridement, and suggest more frequent periodontal maintenance visits as a means of addressing his periodontal disease and decreasing inflammation as a potential factor in preventing or reducing future coronary heart disease events. She will then evaluate the outcomes of care in combination with improved oral hygiene practices to determine the need for additional dental hygiene care, modifications in the care plan, or success allowing for no further treatment until the continuing care periodontal maintenance appointment when the dental hygiene process of care begins again. Siobhan will collaborate with a dentist regarding the presence of root caries.

Symptom Status Domain

The domains of symptom status, functional status, and health perception include the interrelated concepts that define quality of life (see Fig. 2.3). These aspects of the model assist the dental hygienist in recognizing the complex relationships between the concepts of the client (individual or population) and environment and determining dental hygiene actions. In the symptom status domain, the focus of the dental hygienist is redirected from clinical assessment findings to the client's subjective feelings about their state of well-being.

In the fictional case of Pia Tran (see Box 2.3), dental hygienist Emery Sinclair knows that Pia perceives her depression as controlled and believes her coffee stain is unappealing. This oral symptom served as a motivating factor for Pia to seek preventive oral health-care. She experiences no symptoms associated with her low salivary flow, incipient dental caries, and gingivitis, and she treated her herpes symptoms with over-the-counter medications. Conversely, Edward Gilly reports dry mouth and measures he takes to address the symptoms. The dental hygienist would want to determine the effectiveness of his frequent use of sugarless gum and consider the need to augment it with sugarless gum containing xylitol, oral moisturizers, or salivary substitutes.

Functional Status Domain

The functional status domain includes the client's ability to perform specific physical oral functions such as chewing food, speaking, and swallowing. These oral functions relate to important daily living activities and life tasks. Symptoms can influence oral function and vice versa. Oral conditions affecting the appearance of the mouth also can affect psychological well-being and functioning as they may reduce self-esteem or affect social interactions. Certainly, oral disease resulting in pain would affect an individual's functional status. Neither of the fictional patients, Edward Gilly or Pia Tran, report concerns regarding functional status.

Health Perceptions Domain

The domain of health perceptions is defined as the individual's subjective opinion of oral and general health and well-being, including its impact on physical, psychological, and social aspects of quality of life (see Fig. 2.3). Oral health perceptions combined with oral health beliefs about susceptibility, significance, and self-efficacy will influence oral health–related quality of life. For example, one individual could believe that losing all their natural teeth and getting full-mouth dentures would not be all that significant and there is nothing a person can do about it, whereas another individual might perceive a natural dentition as critical to aesthetics, sensuality, and oral functions. These health perceptions would influence dental hygiene actions and communication with the patient, for example, regarding existing periodontitis.

The case of Pia Tran (see Box 2.3) illustrates this domain. Pia is concerned about her children's likelihood of active dental caries, but she and her husband do not believe in fluoride therapy. The dental hygienist will need to determine why the parents have this belief and, if appropriate based on that information, discuss the importance and effectiveness of fluoride therapy or discuss other approaches to caries prevention. In either event, the dental hygienist would stress the importance of regular dental and dental hygiene care and dietary factors related to dental caries risk.

General Quality of Life Domain

The domain of general quality of life encompasses the client's overall satisfaction with life. The impact of oral and systemic health and disease on an individual's perceptions of overall quality of life can vary considerably. One individual might accept their health challenges as a part of life, ignore them, and enjoy a good quality of life, especially if symptoms and functional status are not significantly impacted. Another individual might perceive a poor general quality of life due to constantly feeling tired or not being athletic despite being free of oral and systemic disease. Environment—for example, living conditions, economic status, and peer groups—also affects general quality of life. Fictional patient Edward Gilly illustrates this. Edward (see Box 2.2) is satisfied with his general quality of life at age 84. His heart disease, recent major surgery, and periodontal disease are not major factors impacting how he perceives his life, yet his regular exercise and loving wife are factors that positively influence his satisfaction with life.

For examples of how to apply the Oral Health–Related Quality of Life Conceptual Model, please refer to Chapters 22 and 23, where cases and case scenarios are used to walk the reader through the application of this model.

THE CLIENT SELF-CARE COMMITMENT MODEL

The Client Self-Care Commitment Model, a conceptual model, focuses on client self-care.[13,14] The Client Self-Care Commitment Model uses components of three other models to create a new one. Those three models are the Dental Hygiene Human Needs Model, Client Empowerment Model, and Explanatory Model. The model proposes that interaction between the dental hygienist and client encourages sharing of explanatory models and self-care perspectives, active client participation, and negotiation of self-care behaviors (see Fig. 2.4). The dental hygienist empowers clients to commit to selected self-care behaviors, rather than proposing what the client "should" do and expecting compliance. The model includes five domains.

Initiation Domain

Each patient presenting for clinical dental hygiene care has pre-existing beliefs and values, a unique understanding of health and disease, and existing self-care methods, be they minimal or maximal. The Client Self-Care Commitment Model proposes that the dental hygienist assesses these client perceptions during the assessment phase of the dental hygiene process of care. The dental hygienist's role is to remain open, elicit these views from the patient, and accept them without judgment.

Fictional patient Pia Tran (see Box 2.3) says she and her husband do not believe in fluoride, while also expressing concern about her children's probable dental caries, and she has not brought them to the dentist prior to enrollment in elementary school. Pia's dental hygienist, Emery Sinclair, likely supports fluoride therapy and finding a dental home by the age of 1 year, and Emery might be disheartened by the fact that their apparent active decay was not prevented or treated. Regardless of these differences in beliefs and perspectives, the dental hygienist has the responsibility to accept these differences and Pia's explanatory model and to create an environment of collaboration.

Assessment Domain

During assessment, the dental hygienist assesses the patient's self-care practices and symptoms with open-ended questions and sincere,

respectful, and attentive listening. The clinician recognizes the individuality of each client and asks one or more questions without trying to control the patient's responses. The dental hygienist shares their explanatory model of disease and its prevention while accepting the patient's view, knowing people may assimilate new information from healthcare providers if it fits their own beliefs or if they see the new information as more useful than their existing thoughts. When the patient does not accept the dental hygienist's explanation, the patient's priorities become the dental hygienist's priorities.

Again, referring to fictional patient Pia Tran (see Box 2.3), the possibility exists that her beliefs about fluoride are strong, and an explanation of its safety and benefits would not change her mind about fluoride therapy for herself and her children. Accepting this health belief, the dental hygienist might suggest diligent oral hygiene, dietary counseling to reduce sugar exposures throughout the day, immediate restoration of the active caries lesions to reduce *Streptococcus mutans* (bacteria identified as causing dental decay), and use of remineralizing agents—while also explaining the effectiveness of fluoride, but these actions will potentially help reduce caries risk.

Negotiation Domain

Once the dental hygienist and the patient share their explanatory models, they become co-therapists who can negotiate self-care practices and other elements of the care plan, including treatment interventions and frequency of regular oral health visits. It is important that the dental hygienist does not lead the patient to decisions and that negotiation is honest and open. The patient may want to explore alternatives as described in the example provided for the assessment phase, or other options they propose based on their knowledge and beliefs. Patients will make judgments about these options and potential outcomes before making a commitment.

Commitment Domain

After negotiation, the client is able to commit to self-selected goals for self-care, and the dental hygienist can facilitate decisions on treatment and continuing care intervals, or dental hygiene actions. The client makes the decision; the dental hygienist supports choices made and helps the patient achieve their goals. The client's commitment and goals are documented in the dental record.

In the case of Edward Gilly, the dental hygienist will explain the rationale for more frequent periodontal maintenance appointments and daily use of the interdental brush given the inflammation, periodontitis, probing depths, and attachment loss (see Box 2.2). If Mr. Gilly wants to commit to daily interdental cleaning but begin with 6-month or 4-month (rather than annual) appointments and "see how it goes," the dental hygienist will accept that commitment and reassess these conditions at the next maintenance appointment. In this way, the client learns from daily living and personal results, rather than solely from information provided by the dental hygienist. Depending on findings shared with the patient, the interval between appointments is discussed again, and the patient is empowered to make a new commitment or a decision to stay with the current interval for reasons in accordance with their own beliefs and needs. The patient and the dental hygienist evolve as co-therapists.

Evaluation Domain

In this last phase of the Client Self-Care Commitment Model, the patient self-reports actual self-care practices performed and progress toward achieving their goals. The dental hygienist shares clinical assessment findings, and the process of client interaction continues through the subsequent phases of the client-provider process described by the domains of the Client Commitment Model.

KEY CONCEPTS

- Dental hygienists come to understand, process, envision, and validate the client need with respect to oral and health client issues, environment, and subsequent formulation of dental hygiene actions as per the process of dental hygiene care and planning.
- From a clinical dental hygiene perspective, the four dental hygiene paradigm concepts of client, oral health/health, environment, and dental hygiene actions weave together and form practice model(s), assumptions, processes, and principles.
- There are many theories, models, principles, and assumptions from which the dental hygienist might draw for practice and/or aspects of practice. Three examples of conceptual models are as follows: the Dental Hygiene Human Needs Conceptual Model, the Oral Health–Related Quality of Life Model, and the Client Self-Care Commitment Model.
- The Dental Hygiene Human Needs Conceptual Model is about enabling, mediating, and advocating for client-centered, human need fulfillment. Identification of the eight human needs related to dental hygiene care is a way for dental hygienists to provide a holistic and humanistic perspective for dental hygiene care.
- The Oral Health–Related Quality of Life Conceptual Model provides a framework that allows the dental hygienist to look at the complex interrelationship between health and disease, and its biologic, psychologic, and social consequences, based on the premise that a satisfactory level of oral health, comfort, and function is an integral element of general health.
- The Client Self-Care Commitment Conceptual Model considers human needs, client empowerment, and explanatory models of the client and dental hygienist. Client-provider interaction recognizes the client's perspective as central to a client's commitment to self-care, treatment interventions, and continuing care intervals.

CONCLUSION

Regardless of one's conceptual model, it is the responsibility of the dental hygienist to ensure that practice is accountable to the client and the dental hygiene profession. The paradigm concepts of client, environment, health/oral heath, and dental hygiene actions provide the disciplinary frame of reference for the profession. Within these concepts, dental hygienists must be evidence based and informed in applying their practice model(s); respect the dental hygiene profession and other professions' knowledge, expertise, and contributions to healthcare; employ the dental hygiene process of care guided by the regulatory and professional standards of care; and self-assess with respect to quality care and practice model(s). These obligations require the dental hygienist to think in a systematic and methodologic way with respect to quality oral healthcare. Each step along the way means applying a theoretical model, principles, or processes informing practice—for example, the evidence–decision making model (see Chapter 3); the Guidance-Cooperation Model and the Transtheoretical Model (see Chapter 5); the Diversity Continuum in Communication Model (see Chapter 6); the Infection Control Model (see Chapter 10); the Hydrodynamic Theory with respect to dentinal sensitivity (see Chapter 42); and the HIV Continuous Care Model (see Chapter 51). Each of these models can be interpreted through the four dental hygiene concepts: client, environment, health/oral health, and dental hygiene actions. To illustrate this, consider infection control. The processes involved uphold the culture of safety (environment) for all (client) by applying universal precautions (dental hygiene actions) to minimize risk to health and well-being (oral health/health). Most of the time, the dental hygiene paradigm concepts are implicit within

practice; however, a prudent dental hygienist would make explicit how the concepts are ever-present in their thinking as they are foundational to knowing them self distinctly as a dental hygienist. A review of the Oral Health Related Quality of Life Model conducted eighteen years after the development of this model found that it was being used minimally in education, research, and practice.[16] For the health and development of the discipline and profession, it is critical to continually explore and create theoretical models for the dental hygiene profession.[17,18]

EVOLVE RESOURCES

Please visit http://evolve.elsevier.com/Pieren/hygiene/ for additional practice and study support tools.

REFERENCES

1. American Dental Hygienists Association. *ADHA Framework for Theory Development*; 1993. Available at: https://www.dropbox.com/s/lpp75i3qnl9it9r/ADHA%20Framework%20for%20Theory%20Development%20Archived.docx?dl=0. Accessed August 2022.
2. WHO. *Ottawa Charter for Health Promotion [Internet]*. Geneva: Ottawa Charter for Health Promotion; 1986. Available from: http://www.who.int/healthpromotion/conferences/previous/ottawa/en/.
3. Antonovsky A. *Unraveling the Mystery of Health. How People Manage Stress and Stay Well*. London: Jossey-Bass Publishers; 1987.
4. Walsh MM, Ortega E, Heckman B. The dental hygiene scholarly identity and roadblocks to achieving it. *J Dent Hyg*. 2016;90(2):79–87.
5. American Dental Hygienists' Association. *ADHA Policy Manual*; 2021. Available at: https://www.adha.org/sites/default/files/ADHA_Policy_Manual.pdf. Accessed August 2022.
6. American Public Health Association. *Racism is a Public Health Crisis*. Available at: https://www.apha.org/topics-and-issues/health-equity/racism-and-health/racism-declarations . Accessed August 2022.
7. Fleming E, Burgette J, Lee HH, Buscemi J, Smith PD. Oral health equity cannot be achieved without racial equity. *Health Affairs Forefront*. 2022. https://doi.org/10.1377/forefront.20220420.398180.
8. Darby ML, Walsh MM. A human needs conceptual model for dental hygiene, Part I. *J Dent Hyg*. 1993;67:326–334.
9. Walsh MM, Darby ML. Application of the human needs conceptual model to the role of the clinician: Part II. *J Dent Hyg*. 1993;67:335–346.
10. MacDonald L, Bowen D. Theory analysis of the dental hygiene human needs conceptual model. *Int J Dent Hyg*. 2017;15:e163–e172.
11. Williams KB, Gadbury-Amyot CC, Bray KK, et al. Oral health-related quality of life: a model for dental hygiene. *J Dent Hyg*. 1998;72(2):19–26.
12. Kesekyak NT, Gadbury-Amyot CC. Application of an oral health-related quality of life model to the dental hygiene curriculum. *J Dent Educ*. 2001;65(3):253–261.
13. Calley KH, Rogo E, Miller DL, et al. A proposed client self-care commitment model. *J Dent Hyg*. 2000;74(1):24–35.
14. Miles SS, Rogo EJ, Calley KH, Hill NR. Integration of the client self–care commitment model in a dental hygiene curriculum. *Int J Dent Hyg*. 2014;12(4):305–314.
15. American Dental Hygienists' Association (ADHA). *ADHA Standards for Clinical Dental Hygiene Practice*. Revised 2016. Available at: https://www.adha.org/practice. Accessed August 2022.
16. Gadbury–Amyot, Austin K, Simmer–Beck M. A review of the oral health–related quality of life (OHRQL) model for dental hygiene: eighteen years later. *Int J Dent Hyg*. 2018;16(2):267–278. https://doi.org/10.1111/idh.12277.
17. Gurenlian JR, Rogo EJ, Spolarich AE. The doctoral degree in dental hygiene: Creating new oral healthcare paradigms. *J Evid Based Dent Pract*. 2016;16:144–149.
18. Palmer, Rogo EJ, Gurenlian JR. (2021). Exploration of the scholarship of doctoral prepared dental hygienists. *J Dent Hyg*. 2021;95(6):63–72.

3

Evidence-Based Decision Making

Jane L. Forrest and Syrene A. Miller

PROFESSIONAL OPPORTUNITIES

As a dental hygienist, you need to know how to address clinical questions and make the most appropriate decisions for your patients' care based on the highest levels of evidence. However, keeping current, answering patient questions, and finding relevant clinical evidence when needed is nearly impossible with the increase in the number of published articles, new devices, products, and drugs. One approach to help bridge the gap between current research evidence and your practice is through evidence-based decision making (EBDM).[1]

COMPETENCIES

1. Define EBDM, list the two fundamental principles of EBDM, and discuss evidence sources and levels of evidence.
2. Ask a good PICO question; identify the specific problem, intervention, comparison, and clinical outcome; and conduct a PubMed clinical query to determine if the PICO question efficiently generates relevant, high-quality sources to address the PICO question.
3. Apply the EBDM process and skills to access different sources of evidence, critically appraise and apply it when appropriate, and communicate findings as it relates to providing evidence-based patient care.

How would you respond to a patient who saw on social media how an oral cancer screening is performed using different adjunctive devices and then questions you about how thorough you were in performing one because you did not use one of the devices? Or, what would you say to patients who refuse to have radiographs taken because of a report on the evening news associating dental x-rays with brain tumors (meningiomas)? Would you know how to find the most current scientific information on these topics to locate the most current evidence and determine if the evidence supports the procedure you performed, or what they saw on social media? Would you understand the level of evidence that was obtained in the study and how to present this to your clients?

These two examples reinforce the importance of EBDM, which requires becoming a good consumer of the scientific literature. It is important that you understand what you are reading, the level of evidence it represents, and how much confidence you can put into the findings. In this regard, EBDM is patient-centered and supplements the traditional decision-making process by incorporating the most relevant scientific information.

WHAT IS EVIDENCE-BASED DECISION MAKING?

Evidence-based decision making (EBDM) is defined as "the integration of best research evidence with our clinical expertise and our patient's unique values and circumstances."[2] Thus, optimal decisions are made when all components are considered (Fig. 3.1). To practice EBDM, online searching and evaluation skills are needed along with

an understanding of research design. These skills and knowledge allow clinicians to efficiently access and critically appraise scientific articles to see if they are relevant to guiding their decision making or answering specific patient questions. EBDM is not unique to medicine or any specific health discipline, which is why it is referred to here as EBDM rather than evidence-based dentistry or evidence-based dental hygiene.

PRINCIPLES OF EVIDENCE-BASED DECISION MAKING

The use of an evidence-based approach in clinical practice is intended to close the gap between what is known (research) and what is practiced. EBDM is about solving clinical problems, whether patient care issues, the patient's clinical condition, or questions based on personal interest. In solving these problems, there are two **fundamental principles of EBDM**[3]:

1. Evidence alone is never sufficient to make a clinical decision: that is, clinical research is only one key component of the decision-making process and does not tell a practitioner what to do (see Fig. 3.1).
2. **Levels of evidence** exist: a hierarchy of evidence is available to guide clinical decision making. As the term *hierarchy* implies, not all evidence is equal.
   - As you move up the hierarchy, the research designs allow more control so that intervention or treatment outcome differences are not due to chance.
   - As you move up the hierarchy, the number of published studies decreases, and yet these are more clinically relevant studies (Fig. 3.2).[4]

Evidence Sources and Levels of Evidence

There are two categories of evidence sources: primary and secondary research. Understanding the distinction between these two helps with the search for evidence and critical analysis of it.

Primary Research

Primary research includes original research studies. These studies can be divided into two categories: experimental studies and nonexperimental, or observational, studies (see Fig. 3.2).

1. In **experimental research**, the researcher is testing a hypothesis, most likely to establish cause and effect. To accomplish this goal:
   - The researcher controls or manipulates the variables under investigation, such as in testing the effectiveness of a treatment.
   - The researcher uses complex study designs that include randomized controlled trials (RCTs) and controlled clinical trials.

   The **randomized controlled trial (RCT)** provides the strongest evidence for demonstrating cause and effect: that is, the treatment has caused the effect, rather than it occurring by chance.
2. **Nonexperimental, or observational, research** includes studies in which the researcher *does not give a treatment, intervention, or*

provide an exposure; that is, data are gathered without intervening to control variables. This type of research includes cohort studies and case-control studies.

- **Cohort studies** and **case-control studies** are used to describe and interpret conditions or relationships that already exist. These studies are used when the possibility exists that testing a treatment or intervention has the potential to cause harm. For example,
  - In a **cohort study** the investigator could not give tobacco to subjects to test if tobacco causes cancer but instead would recruit subjects who already are exposed to the risk (tobacco) and then follow them to see who develops cancer.
  - In a **case-control study**, subjects who already have cancer would be recruited and the investigator would examine what could have caused the cancer, i.e., tobacco.

Secondary Research

Secondary research includes pre-appraised or filtered research—that is, research on already-conducted individual studies. This category includes the following:

- Meta-analyses (MAs) of systematic reviews
- Systematic reviews (SRs)
- Critical summaries

In Fig. 3.2, the hierarchy of evidence is shown. Sources regarded as providing level 1 evidence, the highest level of evidence, are within the category of secondary research. An individual RCT is also considered level 1 evidence. This highest level of evidence is followed by cohort studies (level 2), and case-control studies (level 3), respectively. Case reports, narrative reviews, and editorials (levels 4 and 5 evidence) do not involve a research design. Although animal and laboratory research studies are extremely important, they are at the bottom of the hierarchy because they do not involve human subjects, and evidence-based practice is all about how it works in people. An excellent short, graphic review of each of these research methods and designs can be found at the SUNY Downstate Medical Center, Evidence-Based Medicine Course, "Guide to Research Methods—The Evidence Pyramid,"[5] which can be accessed at https://guides.upstate.edu/ebp/pyramid.

Fig. 3.3 illustrates the relationship between primary research, which includes individual studies (RCTs, cohort, and case-control studies), and secondary research, which is the synthesis of the findings from individual research studies that answer the same question (e.g., treatment, products, procedures, techniques, materials). A **systematic review (SR)**

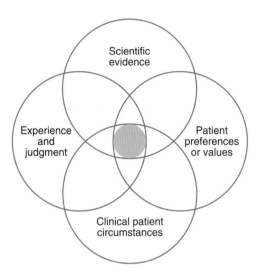

Fig. 3.1 Evidence-based decision making. (Adapted from Forrest JL, Miller SA: Evidence-based decision making in dental hygiene education, practice, and research. *J Dent Hyg.* 2001;75:50.)

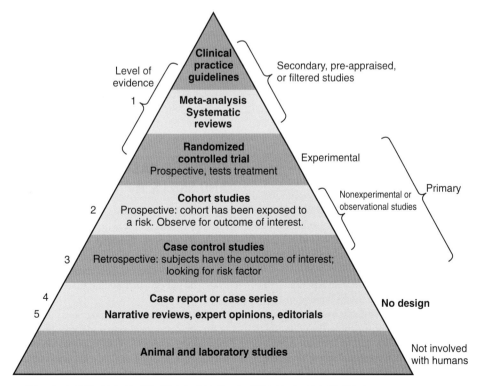

Based on ability to control for bias and to demonstrate cause and effect in humans

Fig. 3.2 Hierarchy of research designs and levels of scientific evidence. (Reprinted with permission. Copyright 2012 JL Forrest, NCDHRP, National Center for Dental Hygiene Research and Practice.)

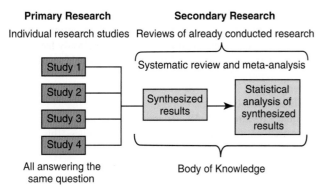

Primary Research

Individual research studies

Secondary Research

Reviews of already conducted research

Study 1
Study 2
Study 3
Study 4

All answering the same question

Systematic review and meta-analysis

Synthesized results → Statistical analysis of synthesized results

Body of Knowledge

Fig. 3.3 Primary versus secondary research. (Reprinted with permission. ©2020, JL Forrest & SA Miller, EBDM in ACTION: Developing Competence in EB Practice, 2nd ed.)

is the synthesis of the findings from individual studies on the same topic. When data from the individual studies that make up the SR can be combined, an analysis conducted of this pooled data is known as a **meta-analysis (MA)**. The benefits of pooling the data are that the sample size and power usually increase and the combined effect can increase the precision of estimates of treatment effects and exposure risks.[6]

At the top of the hierarchy are **clinical practice guidelines (CPGs)**. A clinical practice guideline does not have a research design per se but is a secondary source of evidence in that it incorporates the best available scientific evidence to support a clinical practice. SRs and MAs support the process of developing clinical practice guidelines by putting together all the evidence known about a topic in an objective manner. This evidence then is analyzed by a panel of experts who make specific recommendations based on the level and quality of evidence. Clinical practice guidelines are intended to translate the research into practical applications.

Clinical practice guidelines change over time as the evidence evolves, underscoring the importance of keeping current with the scientific literature. One example of this evolving nature of evidence is the change in the American Heart Association Guidelines for the Prevention of Infective Endocarditis related to the need for premedication before dental and dental hygiene procedures.[7] In the 2007 update, the rationale for revising the 1997 document was provided. Excerpts from their rationale include the following (notice the references to types of studies, use of evidence, and experts in updating the guidelines):

The rationale for prophylaxis was based largely on expert opinion and what seemed to be a rational and prudent attempt to prevent a life-threatening infection. … Accordingly, the basis for recommendations for Infective Endocarditis (IE) prophylaxis was not well established, and the quality of evidence was limited to a few case-control studies or was based on expert opinion, clinical experience, and descriptive studies that utilized surrogate measures of risk. … The present revised document was not based on the results of a single study but rather on the collective body of evidence published in numerous studies over the past two decades … and would represent the conclusions of published studies and the collective wisdom of many experts on IE and relevant national and international societies.[8]

Other currently updated evidence-based clinical practice guidelines that support dental hygiene practice include the Evaluation of Potentially Malignant Disorders in the Oral Cavity; the Systematic Review on Nonsurgical Treatment of Patients with Chronic Periodontitis by Means of Scaling and Root Planing (SRP) with or Without Adjuncts; and the Management of Patients with Prosthetic Joints Undergoing Dental Procedures Clinical Practice Guideline. Each of these clinical practice guidelines can be found on the ADA's Center for Evidence-Based Dentistry website: http://ebd.ada.org.

Other sources of clinical practice guidelines, clinical recommendations, parameters of care, position papers, or academy statements related to clinical dental hygiene practice can be found in professional journals such as the *International Journal of Dental Hygiene, the Canadian Journal of Dental Hygiene,* and specialty journals, and on the websites of professional organizations, such as the following:

- *American Academy of Pediatric Dentistry:* Under Definitions, Oral Health Policies, and Clinical Guidelines (http://www.aapd.org/policies/)
- *American Academy of Periodontology:* Under AAP Clinical and Scientific Papers (https://www.perio.org/resources-products/clinical-scientific-papers.html)
- *American Dental Association:* Science & Research Institute website (http://ada.org/sri) provides links to SRs and critical summaries; clinical recommendations on fluorides, sealants, oral cancer screening along with chairside guides on many of these topics; and links to a variety of external resources, including PubMed and Cochrane.
- *Centers for Disease Control and Prevention:* Under Guidelines and Recommendations (https://www.cdc.gov/oralhealth/infectioncontrol/guidelines/index.htm)
- ***Cochrane Collaboration:*** The Cochrane Collaboration is an international, independent, not-for-profit organization comprising more than 28,000 contributors from more than 100 countries dedicated to producing SRs as a reliable and relevant source of evidence about the effects of healthcare for making informed decisions. Their work is recognized as the gold standard for SRs. The Cochrane Oral Health Group is but one of 52 groups. All Cochrane Review groups have an obligation to update the review every 2 to 4 years to account for new evidence (http://www.cochrane.org [Oral Health Group, http://oralhealth.cochrane.org]).

Ideally, dental hygienists want to be able to quickly access new research that is valid, is easy to read, and has been pre-appraised. If a clinical practice guideline does not exist, another source of pre-appraised evidence includes **critical summaries**. These are 1- to 2-page reviews of the original research and include an expert commentary on the strengths and weaknesses of how the study was conducted, the strength of the evidence, and the clinical application. Critical summaries can be found as part of the ADA's Center for Evidence-Based Dentistry, and in the journals of the ADA (*JADA*) and two evidence-based dentistry journals: *Evidence-Based Dentistry* (http://www.nature.com/ebd/index.html) and the *Journal of Evidence-Based Dental Practice* (http://www.jebdp.com).

EVIDENCE-BASED DECISION-MAKING PROCESS AND SKILLS: A PRACTICAL APPLICATION

The growth of "evidence-based" practice has been made possible through two factors. The first is the development of online scientific databases, such as **PubMed** and the Cochrane Library. The second factor is having access to computers and/or hand-held devices that provide Internet access. This combination allows quick location of relevant clinical evidence so that there is no excuse for not doing so (see Box 3.1).

EBDM requires developing new skills. These **EBDM skills** consist of the ability to formulate a specific clinical question, then find, critically appraise, and correctly apply current relevant evidence to clinical decisions so that the evidence known is reflected in the care provided. Following the application of evidence is the evaluation of the outcomes. Translating these skills into action include the five steps outlined in Box 3.2.

BOX 3.2   Skills Needed to Apply the Evidence-Based Decision Making Process

1. **ASK**: Convert information needs/problems into clinical questions so that they can be answered.
2. **ACCESS**: Conduct a computerized search with maximum efficiency for finding the best external evidence with which to answer the question.
3. **APPRAISE**: Critically appraise the evidence for its validity and usefulness (clinical applicability).
4. **APPLY**: Apply the results of the appraisal, or evidence, in clinical practice.
5. **ASSESS**: Evaluate the process and your performance.

From Straus SE, Glasziou P, Richardson WS, et al. Evidence-based medicine: how to practice and teach it. 4th ed. London, England: Churchill Livingstone Elsevier; 2011.

BOX 3.3   Critical Thinking Scenario A

Mrs. Sanchez is a 58-year-old woman who is concerned about her risk of developing root caries. She knows her children have received fluoride treatments to prevent cavities on their teeth and asks you if she should be getting professionally applied fluoride treatments, and what she should be doing at home.

Having recently read an article on the role of chlorhexidine varnish (CHX-V) for the prevention of root caries, you want to reread it and double-check to see if CHX-V would be more effective than fluoride varnish. Because Mrs. Sanchez has a second appointment with you next week, you tell her you would like to look up the most current scientific information and discuss the findings with her at that appointment. Apply the principles of EBDM, PubMed search strategy learned, and critical appraisal to find the best evidence and answer her question.

These EBDM skills provide a structured process and, just as in learning technical clinical skills, these too require practice. Staying current is not an option but a requirement for all professionals because the body of evidence is constantly evolving over time as individual research studies are conducted. What is learned in school during the first year may not be current by the time of graduation. Only by devoting time to this never-ending process of updating current knowledge and skills will the dental hygienist be prepared to give clients the best evidence-based care.

How Is EBDM Used in Everyday Practice?

The following clinical scenario is provided to illustrate the five steps and skills necessary to practice EBDM (Box 3.3).

Step 1. Asking Good Questions: the PICO Process

Asking a good clinical question is a difficult skill to learn, but it is fundamental to EBDM. To help meet this challenge, the **PICO** process has been formulated.[2] The PICO process almost always begins with a client's question or problem.

A "well-built" PICO question includes four parts, beginning with the patient problem or population (P); the intervention (I); the comparison (C), a second intervention and often the gold standard; and the outcome(s) (O). Once these four components are identified clearly, the following format is used to structure the PICO question:

"For a client with _____ (P), will _____ (I) as compared to _____ (C) increase/decrease/provide better/be more effective/be as effective in doing _____ (O)?"

The formality of using PICO to frame the question facilitates the online search by identifying key terms to use. Based on Mrs. Sanchez's clinical case, the PICO question would be,

"For a client concerned about developing root caries," will chlorhexidine varnish (I) as compared to fluoride varnish (C) be more effective in preventing root caries (O)?[a]

Step 2. Conduct an Efficient Online Search

The second step in using EBDM is to conduct an online search to find the best external evidence for answering the question. Finding relevant evidence requires conducting a focused search of the peer-reviewed professional literature based on the appropriate research methodology.

PubMed is used to demonstrate finding the evidence because it provides free access to MEDLINE, the largest scientific database (PubMed, http://www.ncbi.nlm.nih.gov/pubmed/ or just pubmed.gov; Fig. 3.4). Also, starting with PubMed may save time because many references found on other databases, including the ADA's Center for Evidence-Based Dentistry, directly link to PubMed.

Although it takes time to develop searching skills, the PubMed features, such as Article Type, can be used immediately once you start limiting the citations you find (Fig. 3.5). The features provide specialized searches using evidence-based filters to retrieve articles. The built-in algorithms streamline the process of searching for clinically relevant articles, making it one of the most valuable features for busy professionals and students. Being able to search electronically across hundreds of journals at the same time for specific answers to client questions also overcomes the challenges of knowing which journals to subscribe to and to finding relevant clinical evidence when it is needed to help make well-informed decisions.

To use PubMed, begin by typing in the search box the primary terms identified in the PICO question, the *Intervention* and *Comparison* (Fluoride varnish and Chlorhexidine varnish). Next, click on Search (Fig. 3.6). Ideally, these two components retrieve citations that compare the two and quickly assist in answering the question. By clicking on Search, you will be brought to the PubMed search page, with the limitation features listed down the left side of the page (see Fig. 3.5). Next, scroll down to **Article Type** to limit the 157 citations (Fig. 3.7) to the highest level of evidence by clicking on **Meta-analysis (MA)**. The citations go from 157 to 7 (Fig. 3.8), a much more reasonable number to scan through. If none of the seven answer the question, then uncheck MA and click on the next highest level of evidence, **Systematic Review (SR)**. In this case, 12 citations are found (Fig. 3.9). Again, if there are none or if none answer the question, the next option is to select the next level of evidence, Randomized Controlled Trial, under Article Type.

If the I and C are used or applied for other purposes, then run the search including the P (problem), *root caries*. This narrowed the 157 results to 30 studies that focused on the caries-preventive effectiveness of chlorhexidine (CHX) rather than comparing the two treatments.[9] Results reported in these abstracts indicated the evidence on using

[a]For an in-depth review on EBDM and PICO, complete the course *Evidence-Based Decision Making: Introduction and Formulating Good Clinical Questions* on Dentalcare.com under the Course Listings Topic of Electives, http://www.dentalcare.com.

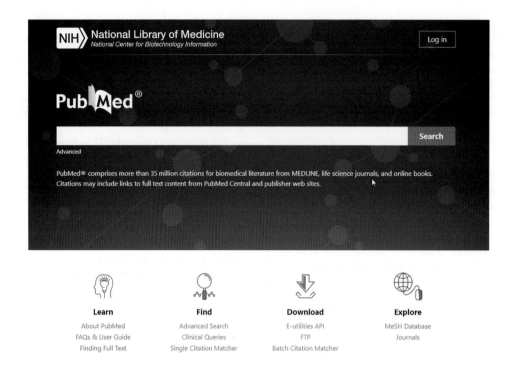

Fig. 3.4 PubMed homepage with search box. (*From https://pubmed.ncbi.nlm.nih.gov/.*)

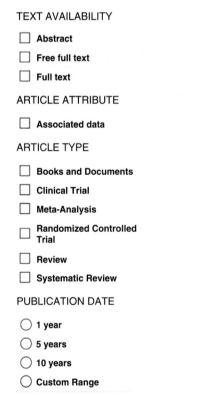

Fig. 3.5 PubMed features. (*From https://pubmed.ncbi.nlm.nih.gov/.*)

NaF pastes/gels and 5% NaF varnishes were *moderately effective in higher-risk adults*. Because Mrs. Sanchez is at *low risk* but still interested in what she could do at home to prevent root caries development, the ADA clinical recommendations on topical fluoride for caries prevention was identified.[12,13] The strength of their fluoride guidelines runs from "Strong—evidence strongly supports the intervention" to "Against—evidence does not support and discontinue using the intervention." Root caries prevention falls under the recommendation "Expert Opinion For" because of the lack or inconclusiveness of the evidence. For those at risk, both professionally applied fluoride treatments and homecare recommendations are provided.

Without knowing about the PubMed features or combining the Intervention and Comparison, the most common way of beginning a search is to type in the main search term in the search box on the homepage. Typing in "fluoride varnish" garnered 1890 citations (Fig 3.11). Someone not familiar with the PubMed filters feature or levels of evidence would spend considerable time reviewing the 1890 titles and abstracts to determine which ones might be useful or, more likely, would become discouraged after reviewing the first 10 or 20 and stop.[b]

> **BOX 3.4   Key Tips for Learning How to Search Using PubMed**
>
> - Keep the search simple.
> - Limit the search terms to the key terms identified in the PICO question.
> - Begin your search using the PubMed Clinical Queries feature.
> - Complete the PubMed Tutorial to learn how to take full advantage of PubMed.
> - Complete the courses on Dentalcare.com that are tailored to EBDM and Searching PubMed.

CHX varies from being weak at best[8] to inconclusive[9] or not recommending CHX at all.[10]

Subsequently, a second search was run for fluoride varnish and root caries (Fig. 3.10). Of the 101 results, 5 were identified as MA; however many included silver diamine fluoride, which were not of interest. Conclusions of an SR "Supplemental fluoride use for moderate and high caries risk adults: a systematic review"[11] found that 1.1%

---

[b]For a comprehensive, step-by-step guide on how to conduct a search, complete the course *Strategies for Searching the Literature Using PubMed* on Dentalcare.com, under the Course Listings Topic of Electives, http://www.dentalcare.com.

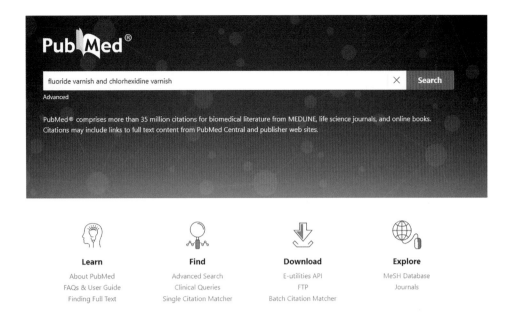

Fig. 3.6 Intervention and comparison typed into search box. (*From https://pubmed.ncbi.nlm.nih.gov/.*)

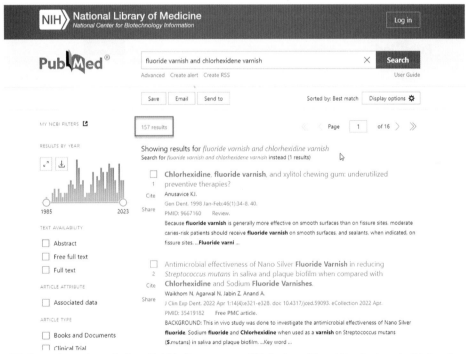

Fig. 3.7 General search results from PubMed homepage – 157 citations. (*From https://pubmed.ncbi.nlm.nih.gov/.*)

Key tips to keep in mind when beginning to learn how to search using PubMed are outlined in Box 3.4.

Step 3. Critically Appraise the Evidence for Its Validity and Usefulness (Clinical Applicability)

Once the most current evidence is located, the next step in the EBDM process is to understand it and its relevance to the client's problem and answering the PICO question. Three key questions guide the critical analysis process[2]:

1. Are the results of the study valid?
2. What are the results?
3. Will the results help in caring for my client?

1. Are the results of the study valid? The first question focuses the analysis on the research design, methods, and way the study was conducted. This focus on results reinforces the importance of understanding research design and the corresponding level of evidence it provides. Little confidence can be placed in the results if the study was not conducted appropriately. Therefore, answering the first

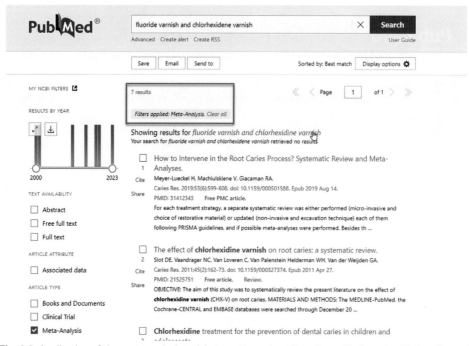

Fig. 3.8 Application of the meta-analysis article type, 7 results. (*From https://pubmed.ncbi.nlm.nih.gov/.*)

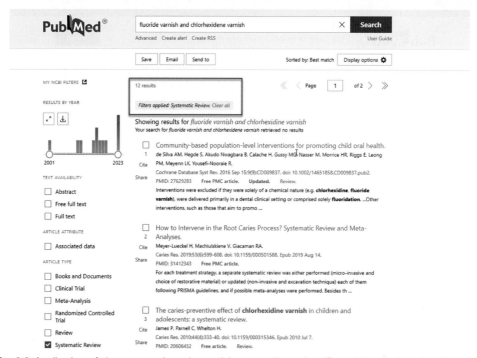

Fig. 3.9 Application of the systematic review article type, 12 results. (*From https://pubmed.ncbi.nlm.nih. gov/.*)

question can help determine whether to continue reading the study or go on to the next article. Fortunately, to assist with this process, several evidence-based groups provide **critical appraisal** checklists of questions that can be downloaded to use.[14] These tools consist of a structured series of questions that help determine the study's validity by exploring the strengths and weaknesses of how a study was conducted, or of how information was collected, and how useful and applicable the evidence is to the specific patient problem or question being asked.

*2. **What are the results?*** Once it has been determined that the results are valid, the next step is to determine if the results or

potential benefits (or harms) are important, and then whether to apply the evidence to patient care. The researchers' conclusions are specifically helpful as they discuss the implications for practice and research.

Statistical vs. clinical significance. Another consideration in appraising the evidence is understanding the difference between statistical significance and clinical significance. **Statistical significance** refers to the likelihood that the results were unlikely to have occurred by chance at a specified probability level and that the differences would still exist each time the experiment was repeated. Therefore statistical

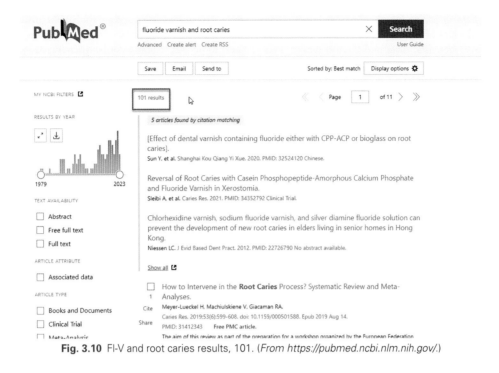

Fig. 3.10 Fl-V and root caries results, 101. (*From https://pubmed.ncbi.nlm.nih.gov/.*)

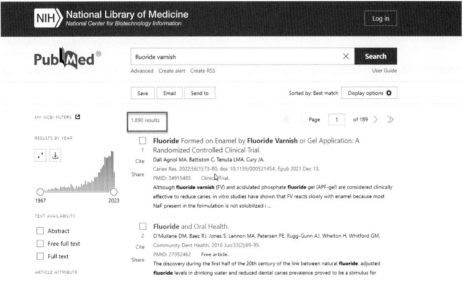

Fig. 3.11 Fl-V general search results, 1890. (*From https://pubmed.ncbi.nlm.nih.gov/.*)

significance is reported as the probability related to chance, or "p" level. Levels of statistical significance are set at thresholds at the point where the null hypothesis (the statement of no difference between groups) will be rejected, such as at $P <.05$, which means that the probability is less than 5 in 100 that the difference occurred by chance.

Clinical significance is used to distinguish the importance and meaning of the results reported in a study and is not based on a comparison of numbers, as is statistical significance. A study can have statistical significance without being clinically significant and vice versa. Statistical significance does not determine the practical or clinical implications of the data. For example, small differences may be statistically significant, a difference of 0.05 to 1.0 mm in levels of attachment; however, this difference may not be clinically significant because this small a difference could be due to measurement error and/or chance.

On the other hand, analysis of the results of a study may find no statistically significant difference between two treatments, which may mean that a new treatment was as effective as (no better or no worse than) the gold standard treatment. This finding could be clinically significant, especially if the new treatment is easier to apply/less technique sensitive, takes less time/fewer visits, and/or is less costly.

As previously mentioned, the results related to CHX-V were inconclusive, having either weak or insufficient evidence to recommend CHX-V for root caries prevention. It appears that the results of the SR and studies demonstrate statistical and clinical significance for providing a fluoride treatment, especially for those at high risk or with incipient lesions.[11] In reviewing the ADA's clinical recommendations, "patients at low risk of developing caries may not need additional topical fluorides other than over-the-counter fluoridated toothpaste and fluoridated water."[13]

3. Will the results help in caring for my client? It is critical to review the results from the lens of the client and consider the client's values, preferences, costs, benefits, risks and circumstances. It is helpful to recognize how closely the studied population describes your specific client. For example, had all the fluoride studies had been conducted with children and adolescents, then the results would have to be extrapolated by the clinician to decide if the results would be helpful in caring for the patient. This situation would refer to the first fundamental principle of EBDM: the evidence alone is never sufficient to make a clinical decision, and the clinician determines whether the level and quality of the evidence is useful and how much confidence can be placed in the findings. This principle helps dental hygienists decide which, if any, of the scientific evidence to incorporate with their experience and judgment, along with the clinical circumstances and patient preferences or values. Also, it allows hygienists to educate their patients about changes based on new research. See Box 3.5.

BOX 3.5   Client or Patient Education Tip

- Evidence-based decision making allows the clinician to discuss the rationale for new therapies and new approaches based on the evolving science so that patients can participate in making informed decisions.
- Evidence-based decision making allows the clinician to discuss the rationale for changing or eliminating previous procedures that now, through sound research, have been found not to be effective.

Step 4. Apply the Results of the Appraisal, or Evidence, in Clinical Practice

After completing the review of the evidence, the next step is to discuss findings with Mrs. Sanchez. You share the scientific evidence, review her caries risk assessment, and share your experience and judgment and allow Mrs. Sanchez to make an informed decision that includes her preferences and values and specific clinical circumstances. Consequently, Mrs. Sanchez decided to continue her homecare routine of brushing with a fluoridated toothpaste but opted for a professionally applied fluoride varnish treatment at her maintenance appointments. A client with similar risk may choose to continue homecare with over-the-counter fluoridated toothpaste and fluoridated water only. Both would be evidence-based choices.

Step 5. Evaluate the Process and Your Performance

The final step in EBDM is evaluation of the effectiveness of the process. This step includes evaluating two aspects: the outcomes of the care

provided and the application of the EBDM process. Mastering the skills of EBDM takes time, practice, and reflection, and a clinician who is new to the steps should not be discouraged by early difficulties. Self-evaluation of developing skills is a most critical aspect in mastery of EBDM. Following the five skills/steps in the EBDM process, questions that can be used to evaluate performance are outlined in Box 3.6.

BOX 3.6   Questions for Evaluating the Evidence-Based Decision-Making Process

- Were my questions focused and answerable?
- Did I use the PICO components to find high levels of evidence quickly and efficiently?
- Did I appraise the evidence effectively?
- Was I able to integrate the appraisal with my own expertise and the unique features of the situation to present the findings in an unbiased and understandable manner to my client?
- Did I evaluate the outcome of care provided to my client?

The path for development of expertise in any skill involves learning the basic steps followed by practice in applying the skills; however, practice without reflection on how to improve is trial-and-error learning rather than following a systematic process. Reflective practitioners are continually self-assessing results of their actions to enhance their abilities and development of expertise. This self-assessment also is the case with development of skills in EBDM. The practitioner who makes time to apply *and* evaluate the results of EBDM develops expertise and quickly and conveniently stays current with scientific findings on topics that are important to practice.

CONCLUSION

EBDM provides a strategy for improving the efficiency of integrating new evidence into patient care decisions. Being able to search electronically across hundreds of journals at the same time for specific answers to clinical problems and patient questions overcomes the challenge of finding relevant clinical evidence when it is needed to help make well-informed decisions. As EBDM becomes standard practice, dental hygienists must be knowledgeable about what constitutes the evidence and how it is reported. Understanding research designs and levels of evidence allows you to better judge the validity and relevance of reported findings. By integrating good science with clinical judgment and patient preferences, you enhance your decision-making ability and maximize the potential for successful patient care outcomes.

KEY CONCEPTS

- The desire to improve the oral health of patients must start with the hygienist's commitment to keeping current with important and useful scientific knowledge. Although the increase in the number of published articles, new devices, products, and drugs has made it nearly impossible to keep up to date, dental hygienists have an ethical responsibility to provide the most appropriate care to their clients.
- Evidence-based decision-making skills and knowledge allow clinicians to efficiently access and critically appraise scientific articles to see if they are relevant to guiding their decision making or answering specific client questions.
- Evidence alone is never sufficient to make a clinical decision: that is, clinical research is only one key component of the decision-making process and does not tell a practitioner what to do.
- A hierarchy of evidence exists to guide clinical decision making and, as a hierarchy implies, not all evidence is equal.

- There are two categories of evidence sources: primary and secondary research. Understanding the distinction between these two helps in searching for evidence and critically analyzing it.
- Evidence changes over time as more and more research is conducted, underscoring the importance of keeping current with the scientific literature.
- Multiple sources provide clinical practice guidelines, clinical recommendations, parameters of care, position papers, or academy statements that support clinical dental hygiene practice.
- Evidence-based decision making requires developing new skills, such as the abilities to find, critically appraise, and correctly apply current evidence from relevant research to decisions made in practice so that what is known is reflected in the care provided.
- Being able to search electronically across hundreds of journals at the same time for specific answers to client questions overcomes the challenges of knowing which journals to subscribe to and to finding relevant clinical evidence when it is needed to help make well-informed decisions.

CRITICAL THINKING EXERCISE

Kevin is a 27-year-old bartender who has used chewing tobacco for 13 years. He is a frequent user who chews almost 5 hours a day. He has just learned from his oral healthcare provider that he has developed precancerous lesions in the vestibular area where he holds the tobacco plug. This new information has motivated him to quit.

Kevin knows he cannot quit by will power alone because he has tried in the past. He wants to know if Zyban, a nonnicotine aid, or the nicotine patch is more effective in helping chewing tobacco users permanently quit.

1. Identify the PICO components and write out the PICO question.
2. Once you have the PICO question, conduct a PubMed search.
3. After finding citations, analyze them critically to determine which are helpful in answering your question.
4. Discuss how you would incorporate the evidence into your clinical decision making, including how you would discuss your findings with Kevin.
5. Evaluate your strengths and weaknesses in using the EBDM process.
6. Explain why evidence alone is never sufficient to make a clinical decision.
7. Explain why an RCT is not always the appropriate research design to use.
8. Discuss how EBDM influences dental hygiene practice today.
9. Once you have completed the EBDM process, discuss how you can use these skills to provide better care for your patients.

EVOLVE RESOURCES

Please visit *http://evolve.elsevier.com/Pieren/hygiene/* for additional practice and study support tools.

REFERENCES

1. Committee on Quality of Health Care in America, IOM. *Crossing the Quality Chasm: A New Health System for the 21st Century*. Washington, DC: The National Academy of Sciences; 2000.
2. Straus SE, Glasziou P, Richardson WS, et al. In: *Evidence-Based Medicine: How to Practice and Teach it*. 4th ed. London, England: Churchill Livingstone Elsevier; 2011.
3. Evidence-Based Medicine Working Group. In: *Users' Guides to the Medical Literature, A Manual for EB Clinical Practice*. 2nd ed. Chicago: AMA; 2008.
4. McKibbon A, Eady A, Marks S. *PDQ, Evidence-Based Principles and Practice*. Hamilton, Ontario: B.C. Decker; 1999.
5. SUNY Downstate Medical Center. Evidence Based Medicine Course, Guide to Research Methods - the Evidence Pyramid. Available at: https://guides.upstate.edu/ebp/pyramid. Accessed May 15, 2022.
6. Mulrow C. Rationale for systematic reviews. In: Chalmers I, Altman DG, eds. *Systematic Reviews*. London, England: BMJ Publishing Group; 1995:1.
7. Wilson W, Taubert KA, Gewitz M, et al. Prevention of Infective Endocarditis, Guidelines from the American Heart Association: A Guideline from the American Heart Association Rheumatic Fever, Endocarditis, and Kawasaki Disease Committee, Council on Cardiovascular Disease in the Young, and the Council on Clinical Cardiology, Council on Cardiovascular Surgery and Anesthesia, and the Quality of Care and Outcomes Research Interdisciplinary Working Group. *Circulation*. 2007:1736–1754. Available at: http://circ.ahajournals.org/content/116/15/1736.full.pdf+html?sid=ada268bd-1f10-4496-bae4-b91806aaf341. Accessed May 15, 2022.
8. Wilson W, Taubert KA, Gewitz M, et al. Prevention of infective endocarditis. *Circulation*. 2007;116:1736.
9. Slot DE, Vaandrager NC, Van Loveren C, et al. The effect of chlorhexidine varnish on root caries: a systematic review. *Caries Res*. 2011;45(2):162.
10. Autio-Gold J. The role of chlorhexidine in caries prevention. *Oper Dent*. 2008;33(6):710.
11. Gibson G, Jurasic MM, Wehler CH, et al. Supplemental fluoride use for moderate and high caries risk adults: a systematic review. *J Public Health Dent*. 2011;71(3):171.
12. Maguire A. ADA clinical recommendations on topical fluoride for caries prevention. *Evid Based Dent*. 2014;15(2):38.
13. Weyant RJ, Tracy SL, Anselmo TT, et al. Topical fluoride for caries prevention: executive summary of the updated clinical recommendations and supporting systematic review. *J Am Dent Assoc*. 2013;144(11):1279. Available at: https://pubmed.ncbi.nlm.nih.gov/24177407/. Accessed May 15, 2022.
14. Critical Appraisal Skills Programme: Making Sense of the Evidence. CASP Critical Appraisal Checklists. Available at: http://www.casp-uk.net and https://casp-uk.net/casp-tools-checklists/. Accessed May 15, 2022.

4

Community Health

Mary Bertone and Laura L. MacDonald

PROFESSIONAL OPPORTUNITIES

The dental hygienist is a primary healthcare provider. Dental hygienists collaborate with others to facilitate clients (persons, families, groups, and communities) in meeting their needs and promoting quality of life through oral disease treatment, oral disease prevention, and oral health promotion across the healthcare continuum. Dental hygienists, no matter their practice site, can engage in each of these activities and thereby be client advocates, educators, and oral health promoters. Doing so requires dental hygienists to think of their clients as part of the community from which they came, susceptible to and influenced by forces much bigger than the individual or group—that is, dental hygienists must "think" **community health**.

COMPETENCIES

1. Describe the healthcare continuum of dental hygiene care and discuss related critical thinking scenarios.
2. Define "health" and discuss healthcare promotion. Understand that dental hygiene practice, no matter the setting, impacts the client at the individual/family, group, community, and advocacy/policy level.
3. Discuss the concept of the healthcare continuum and that dental hygienists practice along a continuum of care, promoting health and well-being in terms of disease treatment, disease prevention (primary, secondary, and tertiary), and health promotion.
4. Take action and apply health promotion strategies to facilitate client and/or community oral health.

DENTAL HYGIENE AND THE HEALTHCARE CONTINUUM

The dental hygienist engages with the client along the continuum of healthcare (Fig. 4.1) based on the client's needs. They do so no matter the practice setting in which they encounter or seek out their client. Thus, the term *client* is used to refer to individuals in the context of their communities, or to families, or to communities or populations in a larger context. If the client's entry point of care is disease treatment, then the dental hygienist helps manage the disease, thus facilitating the client's movement along the continuum toward health and wellness. If a client or community is known to be at risk of an oral condition detrimental to health, the dental hygienist would suggest a preventive intervention—for example, an educational program on cannabis use and health/oral health for high school students known to be susceptible to experimentation with substances (see Chapter 56). Moving along the continuum toward health, the dental hygienist promotes oral health by engaging in health promotion activities that enable, mediate, and advocate for health for all—for example, ensuring access to dental hygiene care for those who are underserved, given that access to healthcare is

a social determinant of health. Though dental hygienists practice in many settings, the philosophic approach to health and health promotion is about addressing the determinants of health, for example, access to healthcare and healthy childhood development and, importantly, quality of life.

Consider Boxes 4.1 to 4.3, where the dental hygienists are thinking about their patients' oral health in relation to their overall state of well-being. The practice settings differ in the scenarios, but the dental hygiene approach remains the same. The dental hygienists are considering the interrelationship, for example, of the individual's life events, diagnosed disease, healthcare access, and personal lifestyle. At the foreground of the dental hygienists' thinking are these questions: What constitutes being healthy? How does a patient achieve health and maintain it? The dental hygiene care plan for the patient in the three scenarios will take into consideration each patient's respective needs.

In Box 4.1, George's dental hygienist shares her expertise with George's support group, thus advocating not only for George but for others within his support community. In Box 4.2, Jennifer, the dental hygienist, understands that social support networks may be a determinant of health for Sophia. Thus she discusses with Sophia support within the community that would enable Sophia to meet her needs. In Box 4.3, Adi critically thinks about the needs of the Abdul children, knowing the care plan must be culturally responsive, there may be a need for language interpretation, and she can help connect the family with not only oral health resources but also other community resources such English as a Second Language (ESL) courses and job reentry. She knows she needs to review current evidence regarding the recommended interprofessional multiagency approach to helping people after a traumatic experience. In addition, she knows how to engage in advocacy/policy activity to facilitate better government benefits coverage for immigrants. The dental hygienists in all three scenarios are embracing a full continuum of care from treatment to health promotion.

HEALTH

What is health? The World Health Organization (WHO) in 1948 defined health as "a state of complete physical, social and mental well-being, and not merely the absence of disease or infirmity."[1] Over the decades, the concept of health has come to encompass much more. It is about being able to realize aspirations and satisfy needs, as well as being able to change and cope with an ever-changing environment; health is an investment in and resource for living.[2] This broader conceptualization of health evoked a perspective on achieving health that recognizes personal lifestyles as just one determinant of health and that other factors, such as where an individual/community lives, educational levels, and social supports, are broader determinants, with significant impact on individual and community or population health. Health promotion is the process of enabling people to increase control over

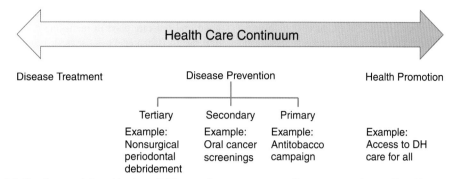

Fig. 4.1 Continuum of dental hygiene (DH) care: disease treatment, disease prevention, and health promotion.

BOX 4.1 Critical Thinking Scenario A

George Fountaine is attending his dental hygiene appointment with Phyllis at the Starlight Dental Clinic. During the health history interview, George informs Phyllis that he is a self-employed graphic designer. George leads an active lifestyle. He has been diagnosed with multiple sclerosis and is beginning to work with an occupational therapist who is helping him adapt his lifestyle and enjoy a better quality of life. He tells Phyllis he has begun to attend a support group, and he has learned a lot from the various speakers. Phyllis tells George she could speak on oral health/health. He thinks that is a great idea. Phyllis connects with the support group and provides an oral health/health education session. After the session, a participant asked if she could present a similar session to another support group. Phyllis becomes a regular speaker for support groups for persons with multiple sclerosis.

BOX 4.2 Critical Thinking Scenario B

Sophia Perez, 28 years old, and her husband moved 2 years ago to the town of Riverview. They have two sons who are doing very well in school and their extracurricular activities. Since the move, Sophia has not found employment in her field. During a dental hygiene appointment, she tells Jennifer, the dental hygienist, that although she has been busy with the family, she is distraught about not furthering her career. Sophia recognizes she is short-tempered, tired, and uninterested in activities she formerly found fun. Jennifer asks Sophia if she has a good support network, and Sophia replies, "Not really. I have been so busy getting the family settled, I haven't thought about making friends." Jennifer knows that having a social support network is important to health, so she suggests that Sophia visit the local community center that offers programs at a reasonable price for people to meet and share similar interests. Wondering if Sophia may benefit from counseling, Jennifer asks Sophia if she wants to connect with one. Sophia thanked Jennifer for her attentive listening as they continued with the dental hygiene care plan.

BOX 4.3 Critical Thinking Scenario C

Adi Klein, a dental hygienist, has worked in public health for many years. As an independent contractor, she has provided dental hygiene services and educational programming for clients of the community health safety net clinic. It is here that she meets the Abdul family, who emigrated under distress from Syria 2 months ago. The family consists of partners Paula and Paolo, and their children, 9-year-old Hassan and 7-year-old Adnan. The family has come to the clinic because the children were identified by the healthy child school screening program as having tooth decay. The family has an interim publicly provided health benefit program for temporary coverage of basic dental and dental hygiene needs, but Adi has seen many new immigrants at the safety net clinic and knows that the temporary coverage will be insufficient to meet all their needs. Adi cochairs the local ad hoc committee on publicly funded oral health benefits program with a family physician.

---

and to improve their health.[1] All people have the right to be healthy. Actions, decisions, and policies at all levels are held accountable for their effects on health. Worldwide, the call for action involves not only health professionals but also government and communities. All are called to make a difference with respect to the determinants of health. This means action is taken at the individual, family, group, community, and advocacy/policy levels to enable health creation, with health not merely being known as the absence of disease. Chapter 2 describes the difference between a health creation (salutogenic perspective) and a pathogenic one. Perspectives always matter.

Oral health is viewed as a resource for being able to live a good quality of life. This connection is seen in both the Dental Hygiene Human Needs Model and the Oral Health-Related Quality of Life Model, for example:

- Viewed from the human needs perspective, having a sound dentition and oral soft tissue integrity indicates good oral health, which enables a person to enjoy a variety of foods, which support good nutrition, thus enabling the body to build and repair tissue. A person must have access to foods that enrich and fortify the body. Dental hygienists need to keep food security needs at the forefront. High costs of nutritious food, knowing what food is nutritious, and having readily available foods all play a role in food security. Good nutrition is part of being able to be healthy and hence a human need. Similarly, the quality-of-life model would recognize food security as an environmental influence on a client's ability to enjoy quality of life.
- Viewed from a quality-of-life perspective, consider a community with limited access to dental hygiene or dental care. Many children experience early childhood caries (ECC). Children with severe, long-standing ECC may live with the condition for many years and be placed on long surgical waitlists requiring general anesthesia. For this, the child may be treated at a location far from home and spend time in a potentially frightening environment away from family and support. This scenario illustrates one of the goals emphasized in the Oral Health-Related Quality of Life Model of Care, that is, to promote quality of life, health development, and health behaviors across all life stages. Note that the human needs approach would capture this severe early childhood caries problem and see it as a deficit in sound dentition, necessitating protection of the child from health risks.
- Since the entry of e-cigarettes into the marketplace, previous nontobacco users have chosen to engage in e-cigarette use. This expanded use includes youth. Position statements are being provided by health professional associations to provide the healthcare provider with the best available evidence for health education. In

addition, at a public policy level, e-cigarette use is prohibited in public places, and in some places, the sale of e-cigarettes to minors is illegal. From a human needs viewpoint, this approach appeals to a client's responsibility for oral health. From a quality-of-life perspective, both the environmental influence (mass marketing of e-cigarettes) and the individual's own decision making would be recognized as impacting and enabling quality of life.

Importantly, the dental hygienist knows that health is determined by more than access to healthcare. This means that all dental hygienists—whether offering care one-to-one within a private clinical practice, a community clinic, or within a dental public health program, serving in a broader public health position, or working interprofessionally with other healthcare providers—do their part to promote health for all, by all.

HEALTHCARE CONTINUUM

Dental hygienists practice along a continuum of care promoting health and well-being:
- Disease treatment
- Disease prevention
- Health promotion

Fig. 4.1 illustrates the continuum of dental hygiene practice and provides examples of dental hygiene actions in each approach. Dental hygiene actions occur along the continuum at the individual, family, group, community, and advocacy/policy levels of client engagement.

Disease Treatment

Disease treatment is about treating a disease or condition. When the dental hygienist works in a clinical capacity providing dental hygiene treatment or preventive interventions, the client may be identified as a patient, given that the person is seeking the dental hygienist's clinical expertise. When disease, disability, or adversity challenges health, this condition is treated so the patient's health is reestablished or in some way improved as a result of the treatment or intervention. Disease treatment is critical on the continuum of dental hygiene care and is likely how the patient most strongly identifies the clinical dental hygienist in terms of patient–dental hygienist encounters. Dental hygienists recognize, however, that confining their practice to disease treatment ignores the synergy of care that results when disease is not only treated but prevented and health is promoted. For example, in the case of Sophia Perez in Box 4.2, the dental hygienist, at an individual level of intervention, knows that this patient's emotional stress as a result of unemployment has the potential to affect her oral health/ health. Box 4.3 demonstrates individual and policy levels of disease treatment. The Abdul family needs therapeutic interventions and can access treatment because of financial support offered to newcomers; however, that funding is insufficient to meet their needs. Access to healthcare for the treatment of disease is a determinant of health.

Disease Prevention: Primary, Secondary, and Tertiary Prevention

Disease prevention focuses on avoiding or eliminating the disease's causative agent(s) to prevent the disease from recurring or progressing. Several examples follow. For example, the dental hygienist in clinical practice would consider the effect the oral biofilm has on the dentition and periodontium (Chapter 19—Dental Caries Management by Risk Assessment and Chapter 20—Periodontal Assessment and Charting). Further, they would consider the relationship between health conditions and or medications and oral health (Chapter 15—Pharmacologic History and Chapter 21—Oral-Systemic Health Connection). The dental hygienists working with a diabetes education resource center would

facilitate collaboratively delivered educational sessions about the role good oral self-care plays in managing diabetes as well as maintaining oral health (Chapter 49—Diabetes). From a community perspective, the dental hygienist knows that local governments, along with the people whom they serve, decide whether to fluoridate the community water supply. Thus the dental hygienist advocates and engages with policy decision makers regarding community health needs, wants, and demands. The client-centered need informs the dental hygienist's action and level of prevention on the continuum of care. The levels of disease prevention are as follows: primary, secondary, and tertiary (Table 4.1).
- **Primary prevention** consists of interventions to prevent the onset of disease or injury. Examples of such dental hygiene actions include advocating for community water fluoridation, implementing sealant programs for caries-free school-aged children, dietary counseling for the prevention of dental caries, and setting up a dental hygiene mouthguard clinic at the local sports arena. Importantly, by engaging with the client at this level of prevention, the dental hygienist has already assessed that a disease or adverse condition is not present but that the client is at risk of such.
- **Secondary prevention** consists of early identification of disease and interventions designed to stop or minimize the progression of early disease. The disease or condition is present. Examples of dental hygiene actions include oral cancer screenings, fluoride varnish programs for children with incipient (beginning stage) decay, and needs assessments for people residing in long-term care facilities using an oral health assessment tool. There is a gray area between primary and secondary prevention, which may be best differentiated via the purpose for implementation of the dental hygiene action. For example, the dental hygienist in a K–6 school dental/hygiene clinic observes that 55% of the students over the past 2 years have incipient carious lesions. This early identification prompts a school fluoride varnish program. Thus the dental hygienist is implementing a secondary prevention measure. However, at the same time, the dental hygienist begins an investigation as to why this high prevalence of caries is occurring and finds out that this group of students is from a surrounding community without water fluoridation. The dental hygienist wanting to prevent dental caries connects with the municipality and begins an advocacy campaign about the benefits of water fluoridation, a primary prevention intervention.
- **Tertiary prevention** consists of intervening with the progress of an existing established disease or condition and preventing further

TABLE 4.1 Modes of Oral Health Intervention for the Three Levels of Prevention

Level	Focus	Activity
Primary	No disease, condition, or injury; prevent it from occurring	Daily mouth care Tobacco-use abstinence Athletic mouth protectors Water fluoridation Fluoridated dentifrice Pit and fissure sealants
Secondary	Early detection and prompt intervention	Oral cancer screening Tobacco-use cessation Fluoride varnish school-age program
Tertiary	Treatment and rehabilitation	Periodontal therapy Fluoride therapy for person with perimylolosis

disability by improving or restoring function, thus preventing further deterioration. Examples of dental hygiene tertiary prevention actions are nonsurgical periodontal therapy and interim therapeutic restorations or arresting caries using silver diamine fluoride. This level of prevention also is about treatment of disease; hence treatment is viewed as part of prevention of disease.

Health Promotion

Health promotion is the process of enabling people to increase control over and improve their current and future health.[1,2] Everyone and every entity (e.g., individuals, healthcare organizations, and governments) is seen as responsible for the creation of environments that predispose and enable people as individuals and communities to achieve health and realize their own aspirations. There are known **social determinants of health**, or conditions in the environment where people live, work, and play, that affect health, functioning, and quality of life, given as follows:[2,3] income and socioeconomic status; social support networks; education and literacy; employment and working conditions; social environment; physical environment; personal health practices and coping skills; healthy child development; biology and genetic endowment; health services; and gender and culture. The determinants of health require a **population health** approach, that is, knowing that health is more than individual decision making; the individual exists within a community, and thus community health is integral to individual health.

Box 4.4 illustrates the determinants of health for Meaghan Woo, a healthy, active teen residing in a small city. Several social and psychological determinants have impacted Meghan's health in her short lifetime. These determinants are seen in both the Dental Hygiene Human Needs Model and the Oral Health-Related Quality of Life Model. For example, from a human needs perspective, education and lifestyle have helped Meghan and her parents conceptualize her oral health conditions and use problem solving to make informed health decisions. From an oral health quality of life viewpoint, the ability to pay for oral healthcare has been an economic determinant of health by improving access to care. Importantly, Healthy People 2030, published online by the Office of Disease Prevention and Health Promotion, describes and emphasizes the importance of focusing on the determinants of health.[4] Tools for taking action to address the social determinants of health are available through the Centers for Disease Control and Prevention—for example, guides, webinars, and other interactive tools and evidence-based resources.[5]

Lines may be blurred between disease prevention and health promotion. For clarity, the fundamental difference between the two is the primary purpose or intent. Consider asking, "What makes the client healthy?" This is not the same as asking, "What makes the client sick?" or "Why does this community experience high rates of tooth loss?" The focus on health is the aim of health promotion. It is directed toward the determinants of health. Whether working with individual clients or patients one on one or with community clients, dental hygienists approach health promotion from a population health perspective. For example, the dental hygienist seeks to understand the client's lifestyle and personal health practices, health literacy, access to healthcare, and the client's childhood growth and development.

Just as the Dental Hygiene Human Needs Model and the Oral Health-Related Quality of Life Model are practice models, the Population Health and Health Promotion Model presents a way of understanding client need and dental hygiene actions. The health promotion approach is illustrated in the line of inquiry regarding why the young boy named Jason, with extensive and long-standing ECC, is in the hospital (Box 4.5).[3]

Similarly, the scenario could be layered to understand why Jason has severe early childhood caries or why the Abdul family in Box 4.3 needs further healthcare coverage. Seeking to understand client need, the dental hygienist asks questions such as what determines oral health disparities, why some populations are at risk for disease while others are not, and why some people are healthy and others not. The population health approach aims at promoting health for all by focusing on specific challenges, identifying mechanisms, and implementing health promotion strategies to meet these challenges. The goal of health promotion is to lessen inequities by addressing the determinants of health and work to strengthen those so that people are more likely to be healthy than to develop disease.

The World Health Organization (WHO) principles for taking action with respect to the social determinants of health are outlined in Table 4.2. The WHO speaks to a holistic view of the social determinants of health and health equity from a social justice lens, with the determinants being affected by the global economic and political environment.[6] For example, being poor is a determinant of health associated with other determinants such as income, education, and working conditions, not just access to health and other services. The unequal distribution of health globally and locally is a result of poor policies, programs, economic arrangements, and politics that impact the creation of healthy living settings.[6] Figure 4.2 presents the global health promotion effort to enable, mediate, and

---

BOX 4.4 Critical Thinking Scenario D

Meghan Woo, a 17-year-old Canadian citizen, was raised with two younger siblings in a middle-class-income household in a small city with active community programs and clean air and water. Meghan sees her family's healthcare team regularly for preventive healthcare, immunizations, and benchmarks of growth and development. Meghan had one 3-day hospital stay for an appendectomy. This hospitalization was completely covered by Canada's national healthcare plan. At the age of 13, Meghan's parents took her to the orthodontist because her teeth needed to be straightened. Meghan wore orthodontic appliances for 2 years, like most of her friends. Fortunately, the cost of care was covered by her parent's health insurance plans as benefits of their employment. The family enjoys "quality time" together and regularly participates in community activities. Meghan plays soccer and belongs to a church youth group. She is a good team player, mindful of her actions affecting others and the environment. Meghan has never had a toothache, has a strong stance against using tobacco and other substances, eats a good breakfast every day, and wears a custom-made mouthguard when playing sports. She knows herself as healthy.

BOX 4.5 Determinants of Health

- Why is Jason in the hospital?
  - Because he has a bad infection in his leg.
- But why does he have an infection?
  - Because he has a cut on his leg and it got infected.
- But why does he have a cut on his leg?
  - Because he was playing in the junkyard next to his apartment building and there was some sharp, jagged steel there that he fell on.
- But why was he playing in a junkyard?
  - Because his neighborhood is kind of run down; a lot of kids play there, and there is no one to supervise them.
- But why does he live in that neighborhood?
  - Because his parents can't afford a nicer place to live.
- But why can't his parents afford a nicer place to live?
  - Because his dad is unemployed and his mom is sick.
- But why is his dad unemployed?
  - Because he doesn't have much education and he can't find a job.
- But why? …

From *Toward a Healthy Future*. Public Health Agency of Canada. Published September 1999. Available at: http://publications.gc.ca/collections/Collection/H39-468-1999E.pdf. Accessed August 2022.

TABLE 4.2	Three Principles of Action With Respect to the Social Determinants of Health		
Principle of Action	**Meaning**	**Elaboration**	**Example**
Improve conditions of daily life	People are born, grow, live, work, and age in a variety of circumstances that determine their health	Equity from the start: policy, programming, and education that ensures all children have a healthy start to life Healthy places, healthy people: quality housing, clean water, and sanitation Fair employment and decent work Social protection throughout life Universal healthcare	Born into poverty, live in substandard housing in high-crime neighborhood, work at an early age to bring in household income, drop out of school, sustain workplace injury, no disability insurance, no long-term income for elder years
Tackle inequitable distribution of power, money, and resources	Power, money, and resources at all levels (globally, nationally, and locally) determine daily life existence	Address social norms, policies, and practices that enable and promote unfair distribution of and access to power, wealth, and other necessary social resources	Gender equity in the workplace; shared decision making; access to resources (e.g., food, education)
Measure the problem, evaluate action, expand knowledge base, train a workforce to address social determinants of health, and create public awareness of them	Assess, plan, implement, and evaluate actions to reduce the inequities and enable all to enjoy quality of life	Shared and accountable global, national, local, private, and interagency efforts to assess determinants of health with effective strategies based on quality decision making	Collaboration; person- and community-centered focus; evidence-based best practice; health literacy; healthy public policy

Adapted from Commission on Social Determinants of Health (CSDH). *Closing the Gap in a Generation: Health Equity Through Action on the Social Determinants of Health. Final Report of the Commission on Social Determinants of Health.* World Health Organization; 2008. Available at: http://www.who.int/social_determinants/thecommission/finalreport/en/. Accessed October 2022. Permission to adapt granted from WHO Press, October 2017.

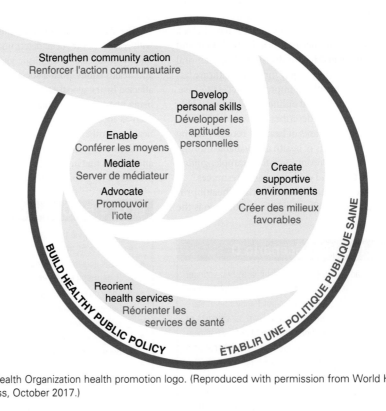

Fig. 4.2 World Health Organization health promotion logo. (Reproduced with permission from World Health Organization Press, October 2017.)

advocate for health for all by creating supportive environments, facilitating the development of personal skills, strengthening community action, and reorienting health services. From an oral health perspective, this effort is seen in the 2021 *Oral Health in America: Opportunities and Challenges* report,[7] and the World Health Organization.[8] The efforts promote understanding of the interaction between oral health and general health and well-being through the life span and call for action on the evidence that oral health is more than an outcome of individual lifestyle and behaviors. Indeed, access to oral health is a matter of health inequities, with social and commercial determinants impacting oral health.[9] Thus global oral health aims to eliminate inequities through health promotion, disease prevention, and importantly, approaches that address the determinants of oral health.[10]

The population health approach positions the health professional in an interprofessional collaborative leadership role. Whether working in a clinical environment or with a public health agency, the dental hygienist advocates for the understanding that oral health is integral to overall health and well-being, and the taking of action. People are healthy because they have the knowledge base to engage in healthy behaviors. They have the knowledge base because they are educated. They are educated because they live in a country where the law states that all people have the right to receive an education. Though the dental hygienist is well positioned for leadership in oral health promotion, the health promotion movement calls to more than the health professional. It calls to all levels of influence—individuals, communities, institutions, and governments.

The call is to take action by building public policy that honors health; strengthens community action by empowering communities to assume ownership and control of their own destinies; reorients health services to be health promotion focused; creates supportive environments; and, on an individual level, facilitates the development of personal skills. Thus dental hygienists, being health professionals with a body of knowledge and expertise, are ethically obligated to integrate oral health promotion within practice, even if that practice setting is focused on disease prevention (primary, secondary, and tertiary) and disease treatment. Dental hygienists commit to health promotion and hence to the full continuum of healthcare.

Some may argue that the health promotion movement is the responsibility of the public health dental hygienist and that the clinical dental hygienist in a private practice setting is not integral to the movement. Health promotion, however, is about the individual client who is part of a community of people who are influenced by and who influence their environment and other communities. It is also about policies developed by communities for support of healthy environments and services for the individual client and the community. Box 4.3 about the Abdul family is an example of a health-promoting policy whereby financial support is provided to immigrants so that they can access basic oral healthcare. Another example is Wren Marks (Box 4.6). This scenario demonstrates health promotion thinking at all levels. On an intrapersonal level, the client, Wren, is challenged to quit smoking. She encounters the dental hygienist, Fayez, who is offering a smoking cessation program along with her colleagues at a local community clinic. The program, on a personal level, is about enhancing participants' health literacy with respect to tobacco use. By participating, Wren will learn that her dependency on tobacco reflects physical and psychological addiction, and that nicotine replacement therapy

is now more inclusive of a variety of options than in the past. On an interpersonal level, she will gain support given the social networking built into the program. At the community level, the policy is in effect that prevents her from smoking in public places. Indeed, Wren's drive to quit smoking may be coming from social forces at the public policy level—thus broader than her own personal level.

HEALTH PROMOTION: TAKING ACTION

One of the social determinants of health is access to health services. Health professionals are health-promoting resources and agents and are not merely focused on the treatment of and prevention of disease and/or infirmity. Health professionals can take action by employing strategies of health promotion such as social marketing of the concept of oral health, offering health education, collaborating with others, using mass and or social media, and focusing on community organization, advocacy, and legislation (Fig. 4.3).

Social Marketing of Oral Health as a Concept

When a concept is marketed, such as oral health, it is referred to as **social marketing**. With social marketing, the intent is to impact behavior like active living versus marketing or selling a product like a certain brand of dentifrice. Still, the social marketing process draws upon marketing strategies employed to attract people to want a product, but in the case of social marketing, the aim would be to promote people wanting good oral health, as an example. Unlike marketing a tangible product, such as a specific over-the-counter tooth-whitening agent or an antibacterial mouth rinse, marketing oral health is intangible. Herein lies the difference—making the intangible product a tangible one. The promotion of oral health behaviors and health-promoting environments requires the dental hygienist to market a concept that, if accepted, results in a product, that being oral health. To help understand this strategy, consider the social marketing campaigns against spouse, child, and elder abuse; drinking and driving; tobacco and substance abuse; and promoting breastfeeding. An example of a dental hygienist employing social marketing is Karen in Box 4.7. She is marketing oral health to the surrounding community in response to the call for health services.

Social marketing is essential for promoting oral health. It persuades people, through exposure, awareness, reinforcement, and provision of knowledge and skills, to accept responsibility for their health and that of their community. The Surgeon General's report on oral health states that to reduce oral health disparities and promote oral health for all, there is a need to increase understanding of the health–oral health connection by the public, practitioners, and policymakers. Social marketing emphasizes the need to define the product (make the intangible tangible) and to identify how the product will be promoted, where it will be promoted, and the price of that promotion. Consider the healthy tooth development campaign called "Smile," aimed at parents and caregivers of babies and young children and outlined in Table 4.3. If the campaign reaches the public through media outlets but the

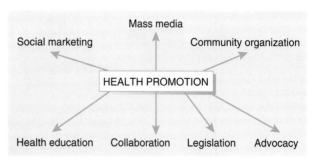

Fig. 4.3 Health promotion strategies.

practitioner does not reinforce it at the individual level, the importance or value of the message misses a critical one-on-one interface among the credible health professional, the caregiver, and the message itself.

Health Education

Health education is "any combination of learning experiences designed to help individuals and communities improve their health, by increasing their knowledge or influencing their attitudes."[1] Education is a social determinant of health. The dental hygienist engages in health education at chairside with their clients but as well, has the responsibility, given their knowledge and expertise, to help others learn about oral health/health in places where people live, learn, play, and work. Health education may be provided at the individual level, at the community level, and at the level of legislation and advocacy.

BOX 4.7 Critical Thinking Scenario F

Karen Fraser recently became a licensed dental hygienist. She was enjoying her practice in a large downtown shopping center. Soon enough, Karen realized that she was reaching only those individuals who came to her practice for dental hygiene care. She knew that accessing oral health services was a determinant of health and, as an advocate for social justice and health equity, she felt responsible for ensuring that the community knew about the value and evidence base regarding professional oral health services for oral and systemic health. This responsibility and other legal and ethical issues are outlined in Box 4.8. Karen developed a website on evidence-based oral-systemic-health connections and invited people in the community to contact her with their concerns and questions. In no time, she realized the impact she had on raising awareness of the importance of professional care because many of the people who visited her site sought out her professional care.

TABLE 4.3 Marketing Applied to Oral Health

Marketing	Oral Health Example
Product	Oral health as part of total health
	Name of campaign, e.g., "Smile"
	Make "Smile" a tangible product, e.g., with photographs
Promotion	Social media platform messages
	National dental hygiene campaign
	Interactive webpage on oral health
Place	Workplace and public school locations
	Booth display at local mall
	Social media (apps)
Price	Time and effort
	Resource costs

Table 4.4 provides examples of health education offered at these three levels. The individualistic approach enhances self-help; for example, the dental hygienist discusses with the client that health is an investment in and resource for living, or explores with the client the role oral health plays in their ability to achieve aspirations and realize goals. The community level identifies with people helping people. A dental hygienist who designs and delivers oral health education sessions for caregivers of persons living in long-term care facilities is an example of the community level of engagement of health education. Importantly, the dental hygienist collaborates with the community to identify their needs and then develops educational programs to meet those needs, for example, a hands-on workshop on how to provide daily oral hygiene for persons requiring assistance with daily living activity skills. The legislative/advocacy approach considers the creation of healthy public policy and programming. The dental hygienist serves as a client advocate, enabling the client to access interventions that promote enablement and decision making by and for the client. An example would be offering educational sessions for decision makers regarding the value of good oral health for residents of long-term care facilities. The intention of such education is to incorporate daily oral hygiene/oral health programming and to inform policy directed at residents' oral health.

Interprofessional Collaboration

Interprofessional collaboration is an important element of healthcare. In the spirit of collaboration, health professionals provide clients with information on health-promoting resources and programs in the community, such as smoking-cessation programs, cardiovascular fitness programs, cooking programs, and various support groups. In addition, collaboration also must occur among decision makers and society outside of the healthcare arena to create healthy environments. An illustration of this collaboration is mandating elder abuse as a reportable condition. Another is the creation of practice guidelines for healthcare providers of adult survivors of childhood sexual abuse. Society does not tolerate abuse, and healthcare professionals are in a position to detect abuse. Government bodies (on behalf of the people) require action to be taken to help abuse victims. The expression "It takes a community" is fundamental to health promotion.

Boxes 4.9 and 4.10 illustrate scenarios where health professionals who collaborate interprofessionally provide better quality care and

BOX 4.8 Legal, Ethical, and Safety Issues

- Health is a fundamental right of all people.
- Oral health is part of overall health and wellness.
- Access to dental hygiene care enables disease treatment, disease prevention, and health promotion.
- Health promotion is everyone's responsibility.

TABLE 4.4 Health Education Examples

Approach	Health Promotion Strategy	Health Education Example
Individual	Develop personal skills	• One-to-one oral health education on relationship between diabetes and periodontal disease • Basic oral hygiene skills education • Tobacco-use cessation counseling
Community	Strengthening community action	• Holding informational town hall meeting on community water fluoridation • Creating "Basic Oral Hygiene" certification program for caregivers of persons requiring assistance with daily living skills
Legislative/advocacy	• Reorient health services • Create supportive environments • Build healthy public policy	• Letters to legislators or members of parliament regarding universal oral healthcare • Lobbying for self-regulation of dental hygiene practice

BOX 4.9 Critical Thinking Scenario G

While completing a routine blood pressure screening for Mr. Smith, his dental hygienist, Harriet Bezu, finds that his blood pressure is higher than normal, despite his medication to control hypertension. With Mr. Smith's permission, she calls his physician, and the physician's office schedules an appointment in 1 week. The physician asks Harriet about Mr. Smith's salivary flow or any other oral changes resulting from the medication. During Harriet's dental hygiene dietary assessment, Mr. Smith says he detests cooking and has relied on toast and soup as his mainstay meal since his wife passed away. Harriet provides information about an agency that delivers prepared hot meals every day. He thinks that would be marvelous; in fact, the social worker at the community center suggested this, and he just hadn't followed through. Harriet demonstrates interprofessional healthcare collaboration by being aware of a client's holistic health to enhance the person's capacity to adopt preventive, self-care, and health promotional practices.

BOX 4.10 Critical Thinking Scenario H

Jean Schnarr, a dental hygienist in a rural community with a primary healthcare center, became involved in a health promotion initiative. The local public health nurses approached them about babies' first oral health visits. Recently, nurses worked interprofessionally with dental therapists to offer baby visits promoting healthy child development, but these services were eliminated. The nurses invited them to join them as an oral health promotion consultant. They met with parents community health workers, health directors, and other key individuals/groups for guidance regarding how the team could foster healthy early childhood development for all children in the community. All team members were residents of the community, thus promoting strengthened community action. Jean contributed their expertise about what to include in an oral health kit to distribute to parents, including oral health education literature and how to access dental products. The kits were assembled according to the developmental needs of the child and included a message for parental oral health.

BOX 4.11 Critical Thinking Scenario I

Dental hygienist Roland Pantel is employed in a dental practice in a neighborhood where only about half of the 5-year-olds have had an oral health screening, referral, and followup. The families in the neighborhood are of low income, with no private or publicly funded oral health insurance or coverage. Roland observes that children he sees in his practice have a high caries rate and knows that they would benefit from a fluoride varnish. He thinks that along with a screening program, the community would benefit from a school-based fluoride varnish program. Roland takes the initiative to find dental hygienists to perform oral health screenings in the community school. He confers with his dental hygiene colleagues, the mayor, and the school's parent council, all of whom collaborate to apply for a grant for funding and other resources. Roland continues to advocate for regulatory changes for his profession, given that the settings in which he can provide dental hygiene care are limited due to scope of practice regulation dating back 50 years. Knowing that the regulations restrict or limit access to care by the 5-year-old children in need of oral healthcare in his community, Roland becomes actively involved in his professional association's legislative committee.

health outcomes for those they serve. Dental hygienist Harriet Bezu, in Box 4.9, illustrates interprofessional collaborative practice promoting the health and well-being of her patient, Mr. Smith. Another example is when a healthcare team invited a dental hygienist to join them because they value the knowledge base the dental hygienist brings to the resource center regarding the oral health–diabetes bidirectional relationship. In Box 4.10, dental hygienist Jean Schnarr collaborates with nurses to ensure healthy childhood development for children of a remote northern community.

Mass and/or Social Media

Mass and/or social media allows many people to receive a message at one time, thus creating awareness of a concept or engaging people in thinking and talking about the message. Mass and/or social media offer some means of social marketing the concept of oral health and engaging in health education as well. There are many forms of mass and/or social media, and each has pros and cons. Not everyone accesses the Internet, nor does everyone read the newspaper, so use of the Internet and/or newspaper announcements only reaches some people. Importantly, whatever the form of mass or social media, the reader's literacy must be considered. Examples of dental hygiene actions for marketing oral health are as follows:
- Mass media
  - Holding press conferences during local, state, or national dental hygiene gatherings
  - Performing radio and television spots
  - Serving as contributing health editors to household magazines

- Social media
  - Creating a blog on oral systemic health on a social media platform
  - Sharing a Facebook page
  - Posting key messages on YouTube

Community-Centered Organization: Building Capacity

Community-centered organization aims at developing the skills and abilities of groups of people for the purpose of self-led improvement. It focuses on building capacity from within the community for sustainability and longevity of the change. It creates supportive environments and strengthens community action. School-based breakfast programs exemplify community-centered initiatives. It is well known that hunger is a disabler for learning. Parents, teachers, and administrators have reached out to school communities and set up breakfast programs so that all children have a healthy start to their day. Another example of strengthening community is a group of veterinarians who used the "One Health" concept. They reached out and collaborated with agencies, industry, and other health professionals, including dental hygienists, to engage street youth as pet owners to learn about pet and human health education and care. "One Health" respects the connections among people, animals, and the environment.

Fundamental to community centeredness is that the community identifies and clarifies its needs and wants—community members best know what these are and how to strategize to meet them. This community engagement is illustrated in Box 4.11, when dental hygienist Roland Pantel collaborates with the school parent council, local mayor, and dental hygiene colleagues to provide better access to dental hygiene care for the community children.

Advocacy, Legislation, and Public Policy

Advocacy, legislation, and public policy are essential tools for achieving health for all, the mission of health promotion. All the scenarios in this chapter address aspects of advocacy, legislation, and public policy. Thus the scenarios illustrate that these health promotion efforts may be between the dental hygienist and the individual patient accessing better healthcare or at a public policy level, with the dental hygienist involved to promote environments enabling health for all. Advocacy and legislation are intertwined; advocacy is generally the precursor to legislation. Advocacy, in this context, is the education of decision makers to provide the essential political support for changes, whereas legislation makes these behaviors mandatory. Examples of public policy for health

---

BOX 4.12   Critical Thinking Scenario J

Bruce Front had been practicing dental hygiene for 5 years when legislative change occurred, enabling dental hygienists to offer direct access to the full scope of practice for all people. Further, long-term care policy mandated the inclusion of oral health assessment on an annual basis for all residents. In response, Bruce established a mobile dental hygiene service and now provides oral health assessments and dental hygiene care to residents in more than 15 long-term care facilities. Bruce was hired by the facilities to provide monthly and refresher mouthcare training sessions for the caregivers—mouthcare became a valued part of overall daily hygiene and health.

---

instigated through advocacy and legislation include smoke-free public spaces, age limits on the legal purchase of tobacco products, and immunization programs for school-age children. Dental hygienist Roland Pantel, in Box 4.11, illustrates a dental hygienist engaging in advocacy, legislative change, and public policy. Taking action to enable access to dental hygiene care for all people is part of the creation of a healthy public policy. Another example is dental hygienist Bruce Front in Box 4.12, who took action as a result of new public policy and legislation.

KEY CONCEPTS

- Health is the extent to which an individual or group is able to realize and satisfy its needs and to change and cope with the environment.
- Dental hygienists engage with the client along the continuum of healthcare based on the client's needs.
- Dental hygienists have an important role to play in promoting oral health as integral to overall health, preventing oral disease, and reducing inequities among population groups.
- Three levels of disease prevention are primary, secondary, and tertiary.
- Primary prevention focuses on preventing the existence of disease, conditions, or injury. The dental hygienist has roles and responsibilities in all areas of prevention.
- Secondary prevention identifies early signs and symptoms of disease, conditions, or injury and aims at prompt intervention and lessening of disability.
- Tertiary prevention treats existing disease, conditions, or injury and rehabilitates a person to recovery of health.
- Health promotion enhances health by enabling, mediating, and advocating for healthy public policy; creating supportive environments; strengthening community action; developing personal skills; and reorienting health services.
- Strategies for health promotion include marketing, health education, interprofessional collaboration, mass media use, community organization, and advocacy/legislation/policy.
- Dental hygienists collaborate with individuals, groups, and other health professionals to prevent oral disease and promote health.
- Dental hygiene, like all health professions, is called to facilitate the worldwide mission to achieve health (oral health) for all.

EVOLVE RESOURCES

Please visit http://evolve.elsevier.com/Pieren/hygiene/ for additional practice and study support tools

REFERENCES

1. World Health Organization. *Health Promotion Glossary of Terms 2021.* World Health Organization; 2021. License: CC BY-NC-SA 3.0IGO. Available at: https://www.who.int/publications/i/item/9789240038349. Accessed September 2022.
2. World Health Organization (WHO). *Ottawa Charter for Health Promotion*; 1986. Available at: https://www.who.int/publications/i/item/ottawa-charter-for-health-promotion. Accessed September 2022.
3. Public Health Agency of Canada, Population Health. *Population Health Approach: An Integrated Model of Population Health and Health Promotion.* Available at: https://www.canada.ca/en/public-health/services/health-promotion/population-health.html. Accessed September 2022.
4. United States Department of Health and Human Services. Office of Disease Prevention and Health Promotion. *Healthy People 2030 Framework.* Available at: Healthy People 2030. Accessed September 2022.
5. Centers for Disease Control and Prevention. *Social Determinants of Health: Know What Affects Health.* Available at: https://www.cdc.gov/socialdeterminants/. Accessed September 2022.
6. Commission on Social Determinants of Health (CSDH):. *Closing the Gap in a Generation: Health Equity Through Action on the Social Determinants of Health. Final Report of the Commission on Social Determinants of Health.* World Health Organization; 2008. Available at: http://www.who.int/social_determinants/thecommission/finalreport/en/. Accessed October 2022.
7. National Institutes of Health. *Oral Health in America: Advances and Challenges. Surgeon General Report 2021.* US Department of Health and Human Services, National Institutes of Health, National Institute of Dental and Craniofacial Research; 2021. https://www.nidcr.nih.gov/sites/default/files/2021-12/Oral-Health-in-America-Advances-and-Challenges.pdf, Accessed from https://www.nidcr.nih.gov/research/oralhealthinamerica.
8. World Health Organization. *Oral Health*; 2022. Available at: https://www.who.int/health-topics/oral-health#tab=tab_1.
9. Peres Macpherson LMD, Weyant RJ, Daly B, et al. Oral diseases: a global public health challenge. *The Lancet (British Edition).* 2019;394(10194):249–260. https://doi.org/10.1016/S0140-6736(19)31146-8.
10. Seymour B, James Z, Shroff Karhade D, et al. A definition of global oral health: an expert consensus approach by the Consortium of Universities for Global Health's Global Oral Health Interest Group. *Glob Health Action.* 2020;13:1. https://doi.org/10.1080/16549716.2020.1814001.

5

Sustainable Health Behavior Change

Kimberly Krust Bray

PROFESSIONAL OPPORTUNITIES

The dynamics of health behavior change are among the most frustrating and rewarding for dental hygienists. Understanding sources of motivation and promoting autonomy are keys to facilitating oral health education. These strategies of client-centered communication not only are applicable to clients but may also facilitate intraoffice communications.

COMPETENCIES

1. Discuss extrinsic and intrinsic motivation.
2. Examine motivational interviewing as a client-centered approach to addressing behavior change.
3. List and describe the four core motivational interviewing communication skills.
4. Discuss various communication styles between a client and a healthcare provider, including guiding, following, and directing.
5. Describe professional dental hygiene relationships, including the PACE principles.
6. Describe factors that inhibit behavior change.
7. Discuss communication with clients throughout the life span.

Effective client communication is essential for providing optimal dental hygiene care. For example, during the assessment phase of the dental hygiene process of care, the dental hygienist communicates effectively with the client to obtain and validate information concerning medical, dental, personal, and social histories and oral health status and behaviors. Dental hygienists' communication skills also influence client adherence to preventive and therapeutic recommendations. In an environment of autonomy, support, competence, and relatedness, a client is more likely to share confidential information and to follow specific oral healthcare recommendations. If dental hygienists possess technical skills and knowledge but are unable to communicate effectively, they may fail to engage clients. This chapter presents foundational concepts about communication and highlights motivational interviewing (MI),[1] a recommended approach to resolving client issues that inhibit positive behavior change. MI actively engages the client in the communication process.

Health professionals encounter and are often frustrated by the dynamics of behavior change—particularly why people don't change. An individual's behavior best predicts health-related outcomes. As such, a number of theories and strategies have been developed to regulate motivation and thus modify behavior. The relationships between types of motivation and associated regulation are illustrated in Fig. 5.1.

EXTRINSIC MOTIVATION

In a reciprocal form, the environment acts on a person and influences decisions about behavior change. The person acts on the environment, and the environment changes.[2] **Extrinsic motivation** is action initiated from an environmental source. This action is not based on a desire, reason, ability, or need to make a change; it is based on contingencies in the environment. Extrinsic motivation is based on three key concepts of incentives, consequences, and rewards. Incentives occur prior to the target behavior and entice or deter action. Consequences follow the target behavior and increase or decrease the strength of the behavior. Rewards are given in exchange for a person's service, effort, or achievement. These forms of external regulation of behavior can weaken the quality of performance, diminish long-term capacity for autonomous self-regulation, and interfere with learning when they are expected and tangible. These can be offset by using unexpected and/or verbal (i.e., praise) rewards.

INTRINSIC MOTIVATION

Intrinsic motivation is an inherent inclination toward exploration, spontaneous interest, and environmental mastery emerging from inherent strivings for personal growth and from the experience of need satisfaction. Autonomy, competence, and relatedness are three distinct types of regulation supported by the environment and one's relationships associated with intrinsic motivation. Individuals perceive autonomy when experiencing an internal perceived locus of causality (control), volition (feeling free), and perceived choice over one's actions. Competence is the psychologic need to be effective in interactions with the environment and reflects the desire to pursue and master optimal and developmentally appropriate challenges.[2] The fulfillment of the psychologic need for competence is satisfaction and enjoyment. Relatedness is the psychologic need to establish close emotional bonds and attachments with other people and reflects an innate desire to be emotionally connected to and interpersonally involved in warm relationships.[3] This need for relatedness causes us to gravitate toward people whom we trust will care for our well-being.

MOTIVATIONAL INTERVIEWING

In the communication process, a dental hygienist is striving constantly to influence the client's motivations to perform recommended oral health behaviors. **Motivational interviewing** (MI) is a client-centered, directive method for enhancing intrinsic motivation to change by exploring and resolving ambivalence through active engagement.[4] MI is a form of client-centered communication to help clients get "unstuck from the ambivalence that prevents a specific behavioral change." It is a philosophic approach to client-centered education that emphasizes the following:

- Collaboration, not persuasion
- Eliciting information, not imparting information
- Client's autonomy, not authority of the expert

In this approach to behavioral change, the client does most of the talking, with the dental hygienist listening carefully. The goal

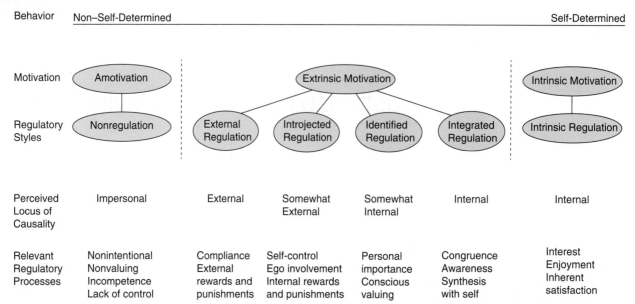

Fig. 5.1 Types of motivation and associated regulatory style. (From Ryan RM, Deci EL. Self-determination theory and the facilitation of intrinsic motivation, social determination and well-being. *Am Psychol* 2000;55(1):68.)

of MI is to have the client voice the arguments for positive change, which is called "**change talk**." Examples of change talk would be reasons for concern about their current behavior or talking about the good things to be gained if they made the recommended behavior change. An example of change talk would be a client saying, "I know I need to floss more because I am really concerned that I have bad breath." Another example of change talk would be a client saying, "I know if I brushed and flossed more, my gums would not bleed so much. My mother had to have a denture because she had gum disease. I do not want that to happen to me." Thus any time a client voices an advantage of desired change, the dental hygienist affirms the client's comment by saying something such as, "I can tell this is something you want to do. What is the next step?"

MI "engages" clients to help them resolve ambivalence so that they can make a decision to perform the recommended behavior. Ambivalence is feeling two ways or having contradictory thoughts about making a behavior change. It is a natural part of the behavior change process. In this client interaction, the dental hygienist explores both sides of the ambivalence by asking clients, for example, the benefit of flossing and then asking if they have any concerns about not flossing. The dental hygienist should never argue with the client. Raising only one side of the argument causes an ambivalent person to defend the opposite point of view, which may cause what is known as the paradoxical effect. The **paradoxical effect** occurs when the client becomes more committed to refraining from doing the recommended desired behavior. In psychology, there is a saying: "As I hear myself talk, I learn what I believe." Therefore it is important to explore *both* sides of the ambivalence and to resist the "yes, but …" syndrome when the client voices what is good about not flossing (or whatever the undesirable behavior may be). When the dental hygienist tries to persuade ambivalent clients to adopt the dental hygienist's point of view, it causes these clients to defend the opposite point of view, which often results in a behavioral outcome that is the opposite behavior to the one the dental hygienist intended to promote.

Therefore if a client refuses to follow the dental hygienist's oral health recommendation, it is important to support the client's decision by doing the following:

- Stating that the dental hygienist understands the client is not ready to engage in the recommended behavior now

- Offering some written information on the benefits of engaging in the recommended behavior, perhaps for clients to read at their leisure
- Informing clients that the hygienist is ready to help when and if they become ready to make the recommended behavioral change
- Asking clients' permission to revisit the issue in the future to assess where they are in their decision-making process
- Noting in the client's electronic record to ask again about the issue at the next visit

Becoming comfortable with MI as a client behavior change tool enhances client communication and positive outcomes in terms of compliance with recommendations to promote oral health. MI is empirically supported as a treatment for substance abuse as well as other health issues including diabetes, HIV, hypertension, and smoking. Many of these health issues are risk factors for caries and periodontal disease as well. MI is associated with sustained adoption of brushing frequency and thoroughness, resulting in lower plaque accumulation and reduced bleeding on probing.[5] The effects of MI on reducing caries or periodontal disease are mixed, some showing positive outcomes while others show no difference from controls. These mixed results may be due in part to the multifactorial nature of these diseases.

CORE MOTIVATIONAL INTERVIEWING COMMUNICATION SKILLS

The four core MI communication skills are easily remembered using the pneumonic OARS: Open-Ended Questions, Affirmations, Reflective Listening, and Summarizing.

Open-Ended Questions

One of the most critical and valuable tools in the dental hygienists' arsenal of communication skills is the art of questioning. Among the many types of questions, there are only two basic forms: closed-ended questions, which are directive, and open-ended questions, which are nondirective.

Closed-Ended Questions

Closed-ended questions require narrow answers to specific queries. The answer to these questions is usually "yes" or "no" or some other brief answer. An example is, "Do you want to bleach your teeth?"

Open-Ended Questions

Open-ended questions generally are used to elicit a wide range of responses on a broad topic. Open-ended questions usually have the following characteristics:

- Cannot be answered with a single word or a simple "yes" or "no."
- Begin with *what, how,* or *why.*
- Do not lead the client in a specific direction.
- Encourage dialogue by drawing out the client's feelings or opinions.

Open-ended questions are usually more effective than questions that require a simple "yes" or "no" answer. Open-ended questioning allows clients to elaborate and show their genuine feelings by bringing up whatever they think is important (Box 5.1). Skillful questioning by the dental hygienist promotes communication.

Affirmations

Validate, confirm, or state positively the patient's interests or efforts. Affirmations support engagement, foster the client to further explore the change process, and build confidence (Fig. 5.2). To form an affirmation, the dental hygienist finds an effort the client is making or an observed strength and reflects it back to them. Affirmations can be short such as, "Good job making sure you brush twice a day," or more content specific such as, "You know a lot about gum disease."

Reflective Listening

Caring involves an interpersonal interaction that is much more than two persons talking back and forth. In a caring relationship, the dental hygienist establishes trust, opens lines of communication, and listens to what the client has to say. Listening attentively is key because it conveys to clients that they have the hygienist's full attention and interest. Listening to the meaning of what a client says helps create a mutual relationship.

The dental hygienist indicates interest by appearing natural and relaxed and facing the client with good eye contact (Fig. 5.3). Whatever the services being rendered, the client should remain the center of attention, with the hygienist's ears available to evaluate and respond. Interpersonal attending skills shown in Table 5.1 facilitate active listening and communication.

Paraphrasing

Paraphrasing is one of the simplest forms of reflection. It means restating or summarizing what the client has just said. Through paraphrasing, the client receives a signal that their message was received and understood and is prompted to continue a communication effort by providing further information. The client may say, "I don't understand how I could have periodontal disease. My teeth and gums feel fine. I have absolutely no pain." The hygienist could paraphrase the statement by saying, "You're not convinced you have periodontal disease or any gum problems because you have no discomfort?" The client may respond, "Right, I just can't believe anything is wrong with my mouth." By actively listening and paraphrasing, the dental hygienist's response allows further analysis of the problem and opens the conversation for communication and problem solving.

The dental hygienist actively listens and analyzes messages received, however, so that the paraphrase is an accurate account not only of what the client actually says but also of what the client feels. For example, if a client sends verbal or nonverbal messages of anger or frustration about being told to floss more, the dental hygienist could say, "It sounds like this situation has really upset you and that you are frustrated with me for not recognizing your efforts." This response encourages clients to

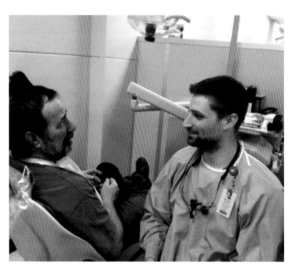

Fig. 5.3 Dental hygienist using eye contact to communicate reassurance.

BOX 5.1 Examples of Open-Ended Questions

How do you feel about your oral health?
What are you currently doing each day to care for your mouth?
Why do you feel you will never be able to floss regularly?
What are you currently doing to prevent caries?

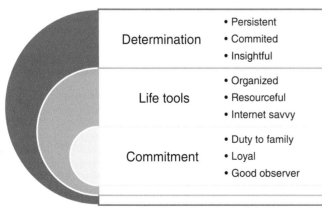

Determination
- Persistent
- Commited
- Insightful

Life tools
- Organized
- Resourceful
- Internet savvy

Commitment
- Duty to family
- Loyal
- Good observer

Fig. 5.2 Positive characteristics to support change.

TABLE 5.1 Checklist of Interpersonal Attending

Skill Area	Criterion
Eye contact	Listener consistently focuses on the face and eyes of the speaker
Body orientation	Listener orients shoulders and legs toward the speaker
Posture	Listener maintains slight forward lean, arms maintained in a relaxed position
Listening	Listener avoids interrupting the speaker and uses periods of silence to facilitate communication
Following cues	Listener uses verbal and nonverbal cues to facilitate communication and indicate interest and attention
Distance	Listener maintains distance of 3 to 4 feet from speaker
Distractions	Listener avoids distracting behaviors such as pencil tapping, looking at a clock, and extraneous movements

Adapted from Geboy MJ. *Communications and Behavior Management in Dentistry.* Williams and Wilkins; 1985.

communicate further about health problems. Passive listening or silence on the part of the dental hygienist, with no attempt to decode the message, could result in an uncomfortable impasse in the communication process.

Clarifying

At times, the message sent by the client may be vague. When clarification is needed, the discussion should be stopped temporarily until confusing or conflicting statements have been understood. For example, consider Communication Scenario 5.1, in which a client has come to the oral care environment for an oral prophylaxis.

In responding this way, the hygienist is trying to get clarification. The client's rush of words seems to be related to her own problems, but the hygienist cannot be sure until the client states it clearly. Table 5.2 provides subcategories of open-ended questions that enhance communication. In addition, the hygienist should be aware that statements made to the client may need clarification. To fulfill their human need for conceptualization and problem solving, clients need to understand why they are asked to comply with a specific homecare regimen. In Communication Scenario 5.2, the dental hygienist has completed nonsurgical periodontal therapy on the mandibular left quadrant, which has been anesthetized. The more specific the hygienist can be, the clearer the message to the client.

Focusing

Sometimes when clients discuss health-related issues, the messages become redundant or rambling. Important information may not surface because the client is off on a tangent. Dental hygienists ask questions to clarify when the client is unclear or confused. When focusing, however, the hygienist knows what the client is talking about. Instead, the hygienist is having trouble keeping the client on the subject so that data gathering and assessment can be completed. In such cases, the

---

> ### COMMUNICATION SCENARIO 5.1
>
> Client: My mother had pyorrhea and lost all her teeth at a young age. I'm sure it's hereditary. I can only hope to stall it.
> Hygienist: Sounds like you are a little concerned about tooth loss.

TABLE 5.2   Subcategories of Open-Ended Questions That Enhance Communication

Type	Purpose	Example
Clarifying questions	To seek verification of the content and/or feeling of the client's message	If I am hearing correctly, your major concerns are _____. Is that so? From what you are telling me, I get the impression you are frustrated, or am I misreading your feelings?
Developmental questions	To draw out a broad response on a narrow topic	Can you tell me more about that? Can you give me an example of what you mean by that?
Directive questions	To change the conversation from one topic to another	Can you tell me about the other issue you wanted to discuss with me?
Testing questions	To assess a client's level of agreement or disagreement about a specific issue	How does that strike you? What would living with that be like for you?

---

dental hygienist encourages verbalization but steers the discussion back on track as a technique to improve communication. Rather than a question, a gentle command may be appropriate, such as, "Please point to the tooth that seems to be causing your discomfort," or "Show me exactly what you do when you floss your back teeth" (see Table 5.2).

Reflective Observations

Clients may be unaware of the nonverbal messages they are sending. When a client is asked, "How are you, Mrs. Jones?" as a friendly greeting, she may respond, "Oh, just fine." Her appearance, gait, and mannerisms may indicate something different. She may look slightly disheveled, walk with a slow shuffle, and display generally unenthusiastic gestures and facial expressions. When nonverbal cues conflict with the verbal message, stating a simple straightforward observation may open the lines of communication. The hygienist may say, "You appear worn out, Mrs. Jones." This is likely to cause the person to volunteer more information about how she feels without need for further questioning, focusing, or clarifying. It is important to note that if you try reflecting feelings or emotions and do not get it right, the client will correct you, and you can redirect with the new clarified information.

To promote positive communication, however, the dental hygienist uses respectful language. The client may feel sensitive about how observations are worded. Saying a person looks "tired" is different from saying they look "haggard," which could embarrass or anger them Other observations that can soften a client's response are stating that teeth are "crowded" rather than "crooked," that a troublesome tongue is "muscular" and not "fat," and that gingiva is "pigmented" and not "discolored." See Table 5.3 on Levels of Reflection.

Summarizing

Summarizing points discussed at a regularly scheduled appointment focuses attention on the major points of the communicative interaction. For example, the dental hygienist may conclude the appointment with, "Today, we discussed the purpose of nonsurgical periodontal therapy and the periodontal disease process. We also practiced flossing technique. Remember, you decided to floss daily and to try to slip the floss carefully down below the gum line." If the client is coming in for multiple appointments to receive quadrant or sextant nonsurgical periodontal therapy, the discussion from the previous appointment is summarized before new information is given. Documentation in the client's chart at each appointment reflects topics discussed at the appointment as related to the client's goals.

The summary serves as a review of the key aspects of the information presented so that the client can ask for clarification. Adding new information in the summary may confuse the client; however, a comment about what will be discussed at the next appointment is appropriate. Such a statement may be, "At your next appointment, we will talk about use of the Perio-Aid and continue discussion of the periodontal disease process." See Box 5.2.

> ### COMMUNICATION SCENARIO 5.2
>
> Hygienist: Mr. Johnson, after you leave, try not to chew on your left side for a while.
> Client: Do you mean today or for several days?
> Hygienist: Oh no, I just mean for a few hours.
> Client: What might happen if I do chew on that side? Will it hurt my teeth or gums?
> Hygienist: Oh no, I was referring to your anesthesia. I'm afraid you might bite your cheeks or tongue if you chew on that side, because everything is numb. The numbness should be completely gone by about 5:00 PM.

TABLE 5.3	Levels of Reflection		
Repeat	Direct restatement of what the person said		You brush twice every day but do not always floss.
Rephrase	Saying the same thing in slightly different words		You do a good job flossing right after your visit, but that wears off over time and you go back to just brushing again.
Paraphrase	Making a guess about meaning; continuing the paragraph; usually adds information.		Flossing is just too difficult. If there were something easier you could do to reduce the gum inflammation besides flossing, you would do it.
Other Types of Reflection			
Double-sided reflection	Captures both sides of the ambivalence (… AND …)		So on the one hand, you know it is better if you quit smoking, but it is hard to quit when so many of your friends at work smoke on breaks.
Amplified reflection	Overstates what the person says		You are NEVER going to floss, even if you lose a few teeth because of it.

BOX 5.2 Critical Thinking Scenario A

Considering yourself personally, identify an unhealthy behavioral practice of your own. Engage in motivational interviewing with a student-partner to consider why you continue the unhealthy behavior.

BOX 5.3 Provide Explanatory Rationales

Provide clients with the value, worth, meaning, utility, or importance of engaging in behaviors to support well-being. Communicating value means using informational language to offer clients an explanatory rationale in a tolerant manner that supports autonomy. Expressions of negative affect need to be acknowledged and accepted as okay.

COMMUNICATION STYLES

Communication styles are an approach of sending and receiving messages between a client and a healthcare provider to help the client make decisions and reach goals related to comfort and health. No single communication technique works with all clients. A skillful practitioner can shift flexibly between the three different communication styles (directing, following, and guiding) as appropriate to the client and situation,

Dental hygienists typically learn and approach patient encounters in a persuasive authoritative manner, offering knowledge and prescriptive strategies to lead the patient in making required behavior change. Conversely, improved adherence has been demonstrated when a more behavioral than cognitive focus is used. A relatively simple shift in style can positively change the encounter. One individual may be encouraged to express feelings when the dental hygienist is silent, whereas another may need coaxing with active questioning. Practice and experience, based on a strong theoretical foundation, are required for choosing communication techniques to use in different situations. The three communication styles discussed here are often used in different circumstances, based on which fits and works best.[4]

Guiding

The **guiding** style is a combination of approaches in which the dental hygienist listens actively and empathetically to understand a client's problems or concerns. Ask about various options the client is considering and explore together the pros and cons of each. Offer information and alternatives that were helpful to others in similar circumstances, all the while acknowledging that it is ultimately the client's decision. If a decision emerges, assist the client in setting a plan consistent in moving in the chosen direction.

Following

In the **following** style, listening predominates. This requires clinicians to set aside their internal dialogues, with no agreeing or disagreeing, persuading or advising, warning or analyzing. This can be difficult for healthcare providers, who often believe that they know what will help others. Based on what is known about autonomous regulation, dental hygienists must suspend their role as experts in order to see the situation through

the client's eyes. This can be especially helpful at the beginning of a consultation, when a brief period of just listening helps to understand the client's symptoms and how these fit into the bigger picture of their life and well-being.

Directing

The **directing** communication style is useful for helping those who are stuck and unable to make a decision or for whom a specific direction is critical to their well-being. Some patients prefer and even depend on their providers to make the decision for them. It should, however, be conveyed that the directives are being offered with the client's best interest at heart. Exercise care not to revert to this often-learned style in all circumstances. From a coaching standpoint, however, directing should not play a significant part. There may be times when delivering concrete information the dental hygienist happens to have that could be of use to a client may be appropriate, with permission, but that should be a very small percentage of the time of a health coaching session. Many circumstances are effectively handled by a balanced mix of the aforementioned styles of communication. In order to overcome the tendency to rely on the directing style that many healthcare providers learned and continue to use, it is recommended to guide and follow before reverting to a directing style (Box 5.3).

PROFESSIONAL DENTAL HYGIENE RELATIONSHIPS

Having a philosophy based on caring and respect for others helps dental hygienists to establish relationships with clients. PACE is a simple mnemonic, or memory-assisting technique, to identify a philosophy important to establishing effective dental hygienist–client helping relationships (Fig. 5.4). The spirit of MI is the foundation for all interactions.

Partnership

A key aspect of establishing a **partnership** (*P* in the mnemonic) with the client is using language and nonverbal cues that are supportive rather than persuasive. This can be difficult in a relationship that

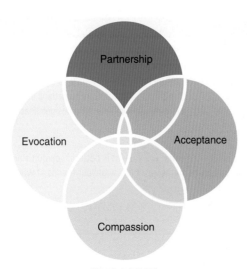

Fig. 5.4 PACE.

already has a socially normed hierarchy. As such, the clinician actively attempts to diminish their expert role. It is necessary to collaborate because the patient, not the clinician, is viewed as the expert on their life and the challenges of the behavior change in question. This does not mean the practitioner agrees with the client's entire perspective on the nature of the problem or changes that need to be addressed. It is simply about mutual understanding.

Acceptance

Acceptance (*A* in the mnemonic) refers to the dental hygienist's ability to accept clients as the people they are without allowing any judgment of clients' attitudes or feelings to interfere with communication. For example, a client may appear unwilling to assume responsibility for their health and may be critical or untrusting. The client's poor oral health may seem self-imposed and related to an unhealthy lifestyle. But the client's appearance and attitudes may have deep cultural roots that are unfamiliar to the hygienist. The dental hygienist must develop an attitude of acceptance toward individuals whose values and sociocultural backgrounds seem unusual or foreign (see Chapter 6).

Conveying acceptance requires a tolerant, nonjudgmental attitude toward clients. An open, accepting approach is needed to foster a helping relationship between hygienist and client. Care is taken to avoid nonverbal behavior that may be offensive or that may prevent free-flowing communication. Gestures such as frowning, rolling eyes upward, or shaking the head may communicate disagreement or disapproval to the client. The dental hygienist shows willingness to listen to the client's viewpoint and provide feedback that indicates understanding and acceptance of the person.

Empathy is another means of conveying acceptance. Empathy means perceiving clients as they see themselves, sensing their hurt or pleasure as they sense it, accepting their feelings, and communicating this understanding of their reality.[4] It results when we place ourselves in another's shoes. In expressing empathy, the dental hygienist communicates an understanding of the importance of the feelings behind a client's statements. Empathy statements are neutral and nonjudgmental. They can be used to establish trust in difficult situations. For example, the dental hygienist may say to an angry client who has lost mobility after a stroke, "It must be very frustrating to know what you want and not be able to do it." This perception of clients' viewpoints helps the dental hygienist to better understand them, their reaction to dental hygiene care, and their capabilities for taking responsibility for their own health.

Compassion

Compassion (*C* in the mnemonic) refers to the hygienist's ability to deal with the welfare of clients, to be aware of the client's physical and emotional response during dental hygiene care, and to provide verbal support to a client who fears oral healthcare procedures. Aspects of dental hygiene practice related to client compassion include clients' inability to seek oral healthcare because of financial difficulties, fear of injections, and discomfort from having their personal space "invaded" during care.

Evocation

Evocation (*E* in the mnemonic) or responsiveness in a healthcare provider is the ability to reply to messages at the moment they are sent. It requires sensitive alertness to cues that something more must be said. When a client arrives for a dental hygiene appointment and mentions oral discomfort, the comment should be pursued immediately. Nonsurgical periodontal therapy may have been scheduled, but other problems may be an immediate priority and supersede the planned care. Box 5.4 includes some techniques that can be applied by the dental hygienist.[2] See Box 5.5 for a discussion of client rights.

FACTORS THAT INHIBIT COMMUNICATION

The dental hygienist unintentionally may impede communication. **Nontherapeutic communication** is a process of sending and receiving messages that does not help clients make decisions or reach goals related to their comfort and health (Box 5.6). The dental hygienist should avoid these nontherapeutic communication techniques because they inhibit communication.[2]

Prescriptive Directives

Autonomy support fosters clients' ability to make their own decisions about health. A hygienist may be tempted to offer directives to persuade others to behave in a prescribed manner, which likely weakens the clients' autonomy and jeopardizes their need for responsibility for oral health. Clients may volunteer personal information about themselves and may ask for the hygienist's opinion. It is best in such a situation to acknowledge the individual's feelings but to avoid the transfer of decision making from client to hygienist. Communication Scenario 5.3 is a hypothetical situation presenting two possible responses by the dental hygienist in an interaction with a client.

The first response by the dental hygienist could make the client feel worse by confirming a doubt she has about her daughter. The latter response recognizes the client's feelings without expressing an opinion that could make the client feel worse.

Offering False Reassurance

Hygienists may at times offer reassurance when it is not well grounded. It is natural to want to alleviate the client's anxiety and fear, but reassurance may promise something that cannot occur. For example, the dental hygienist should not promise clients that they will experience no discomfort during an anticipated dental treatment. Although the dental hygienist may feel confident that the oral surgeon or periodontist is competent and kind, discomfort may be unavoidable. In addition, when clients are distraught about having periodontal disease it is best not to say, "There's nothing to worry about. You'll be fine." Indeed, depending on the amount of bone loss present and the client's disease susceptibility, the periodontist may not be able to control the disease, even with extensive therapy. Communication Scenario 5.4 illustrates how the dental hygienist can listen to and acknowledge a client's feelings without offering false assurance that the problem is a simple one.

BOX 5.4   Contextual Factors Influencing Communication

Psychophysiologic Context

The internal factors influencing communication are as follows:

- Physiologic status (e.g., pain, hunger)
- Emotional status (e.g., anxiety, anger)
- Growth and development status (e.g., age)
- Unmet needs (e.g., emotional stress, physical pain)
- Attitudes, values, and beliefs (e.g., meaning of oral health)
- Perceptions and personality (e.g., optimist or pessimist, introvert or extrovert)
- Self-concept and self-esteem (e.g., positive or negative)

Situation Context

Reasons for the communication include the following:

- Information exchange
- Goal achievement
- Problem resolution
- Expression of feelings

Relation Context

The nature of the relationship between the participants involves the following:

- Social, helping, or working relationship
- Level of trust between participants
- Level of self-disclosure between participants
- Shared history of participants
- Balance of power and control

Environmental Context

The physical surroundings in which communication takes place involve the following:

- Privacy level
- Noise level
- Comfort and safety level
- Distraction level

Cultural Context

The sociocultural elements that affect the interaction are as follows:

- Educational level of participants
- Language and self-expression patterns
- Customs and expectations

Adapted from Potter PA, Perry AG. *Fundamentals of Nursing.* 7th ed. Mosby; 2009.

BOX 5.5   Legal, Ethical, and Safety Issues

- Clients have the right to accept or reject the dental hygiene care plan and still retain the respect of the dental hygienist.
- It is important to meet the client's need for conceptualization and understanding of health information to promote health literacy and informed oral healthcare decisions.
- The client has the right to personalized, up-to-date, evidence-based recommendations and care from the dental hygienist.

Being Defensive

When clients criticize services or personnel, it is easy for the hygienist to become defensive. A defensive posture may threaten the relationship between dental hygienist and client by communicating to clients that they do not have a right to express their opinions. Instead, it is better

BOX 5.6   Factors That Inhibit Communication

Giving an opinion
Offering false reassurance
Being defensive
Showing approval or disapproval
Asking why
Changing the subject inappropriately

COMMUNICATION SCENARIO 5.3

Hygienist: Mrs. Smith, you look troubled today.
Client: Well, actually, I'm feeling quite down in the dumps. Yesterday was my birthday and I didn't hear a word from my daughter. I'm sure you wouldn't do such a thing to your mother!
Hygienist: (Response #1) Heavens, no! How terribly inconsiderate of her.
  The hygienist may have answered differently:
Hygienist: (Response #2) You seem really disappointed. I'm sorry you're so upset.

COMMUNICATION SCENARIO 5.4

Mrs. Frank, a 75-year-old woman, has been told by the dentist that her remaining teeth are hopeless and must be extracted for a full denture placement. The hygienist enters the room as the dentist leaves.
  Mrs. Frank: I can't believe this is happening to me. I don't deserve it. I've tried to take good care of my teeth. I'm so upset. Oh, I'm sorry, I know you don't want to hear about my problems.
  Hygienist: You are frustrated to hear you need extractions after doing everything you could to take care of your teeth. Is it okay if I share some information about tooth loss with you? There are many risk factors besides daily care that can lead to tooth loss, so I am glad to hear you did what you could.

COMMUNICATION SCENARIO 5.5

Client: I hope I don't have to see Dr. Herman today.
Hygienist: You sound upset. Can you tell me more about it?
Client: I just don't think he should have sent me to that oral surgeon.
Hygienist: You think the visit there was unnecessary?
Client: Yes. I didn't mind the biopsy, the results were negative, but first I got lost trying to find the place, then I couldn't find a parking place, then they made me wait for 2 hours, and finally they charged me a fortune for the procedure. Actually, I didn't mind the cost as much as the inconvenience.
Hygienist: Sounds frustrating.

for the hygienist to use the therapeutic communication techniques of active listening to verify what clients have to say and to learn why they are upset or angry. Active listening does not mean the dental hygienist needs to agree with what is being said but rather, conveys that the negative affect is acknowledged, accepted, and okay. This latter approach is illustrated in Communication Scenario 5.5.

Some care in listening led to discovery of the source of the client's anger, which was the inconvenience of a particular oral surgeon's location, parking, and office procedures. By avoiding defensiveness and applying active listening and paraphrasing, the hygienist allowed the client to vent his anger. Therefore communication was facilitated, not blocked.

Showing Approval or Disapproval

Showing either approval or disapproval in certain situations can be detrimental to the communication process. Excessive praise may imply to the client that the hygienist thinks the behavior being praised is the only acceptable one. Often clients may reveal information about themselves because they are seeking a way to express their feelings; they are not necessarily looking for approval or disapproval from the dental hygienist. In Communication Scenario 5.6, the hygienist's response cannot be interpreted as neutral.

The discussion in Communication Scenario 5.6 is likely to stop with the dental hygienist's statements. The client probably sees the hygienist's viewpoint as supportive of her daughter. Perhaps the woman is better off having her daughter drive her. It is also possible that she is capable of walking, likes the exercise, and enjoys the independence of getting to her own appointments. The dental hygienist's strong statements of approval may inhibit further communication.

In addition, behaviors that communicate disapproval cause clients to feel rejected and their desire to interact further with the dental hygienist may be weakened. Disapproving statements may be issued by a dental hygienist who is not thinking carefully about how the client may react. Communication Scenario 5.7 exemplifies a dental hygienist's response that communicates hasty disapproval.

Instead of this response, the dental hygienist may have said, "You're making progress. Tell me more about your activities on those 3 days when you weren't able to floss. Perhaps together we could find a better way of integrating flossing into your lifestyle."

Asking Why

When people are puzzled by another's behavior, the natural reaction is to ask, "Why?" When dental hygienists discover that clients have not been following recommendations, they may feel a natural inclination to ask why this has occurred. Clients may interpret such a question as an accusation. They may feel resentment, leading to withdrawal and a lack of **motivation** to communicate further with the dental hygienist.

Efforts to search for reasons why the client has not practiced the oral healthcare behaviors as recommended can be facilitated by simply rephrasing a probing "why" question. For example, rather than saying, "Why haven't you used the oral irrigator?" the hygienist may say, "You said you haven't used the oral irrigator. Tell me more about that." For anxious clients, rather than asking, "Why are you upset?" the hygienist may say, "You seem upset—what are some aspects you are not so happy about?"

Changing the Subject Inappropriately

Changing the subject abruptly shows a lack of empathy and could be interpreted as rude. In addition, it prevents the client from discussing an issue that may have important implications for care. Communication Scenario 5.8 is a sample client–dental hygienist interaction.

The dental hygienist's response shows insensitivity and an unwillingness to discuss the client's complaint. It is possible that the client has a periodontal or periapical abscess or some other serious problem. The dental hygienist is remiss in ignoring the client's attempt to communicate a problem. Communication has been stalled and the client's oral health jeopardized. The client should be given an opportunity to elaborate on the message she is trying to send. See Box 5.7.

COMMUNICATIONS WITH CLIENTS THROUGH THE LIFE SPAN

Effective communication can be further impacted by the age of the target audience. The purpose of this section is to address considerations for communication with clients through the life span. Table 5.4 summarizes the key developmental characteristics at different age levels over the life span and those communication techniques that are appropriate at each level.[6]

Preschool and Younger School-Age Children

Communicating with children requires an understanding of the influence of growth and development on language, thought processes, and motor skills. Children begin development with simple, concrete language and thinking and move toward the more complex and abstract. Communication techniques and teaching methods also can increase in complexity as the child grows older.

Nonverbal communication is more important with preschoolers than it is with the school-age child, whose communication is better developed. The preschooler learns through play and enjoys a gamelike atmosphere. Therefore dentists often call the dental engine their "whistle" or the "buzzy bee," and hygienists often refer to their polishing cup as the "whirly bird" and the saliva ejector as "Mr. Thirsty." Imaginary names help lighten the healthcare experience for small children. Oral health professionals are advised to use simple, short sentences, familiar words, and concrete explanations.

COMMUNICATION SCENARIO 5.6

Client: I've been walking to my dental appointments for years. My daughter offered to drive me today and I accepted. She feels that the walk has become too much for me.

Hygienist: I'm so glad you didn't walk over. You definitely made the right decision. Your daughter should drive you to your appointments from now on.

COMMUNICATION SCENARIO 5.7

Client: I've been working so hard at flossing! I only missed 2 or 3 days last week.

Hygienist: Two or 3 days without flossing! You'll have to do better than that. Your inflammation will not improve at that rate.

COMMUNICATION SCENARIO 5.8

Hygienist: Hello, Mrs. Johnson. How are you today?
Client: Not too well. My gums are really sore.
Hygienist: Well, let's get you going. We have a lot to do today.

BOX 5.7   Critical Thinking Scenario B

Identify therapeutic and nontherapeutic communication techniques by name as two people role-play the following client–oral healthcare educator sessions.

- In the first session, the "client" should improvise a story of frustration with their current oral hygiene regimen by explaining that a heavy workload, family responsibilities, or other interference that makes it difficult to maintain a good homecare regimen. While glancing at a list of the possible responses as a prompt, the "dental hygienist" tries to respond with only therapeutic comments. Classroom listeners should try to determine which specific categories of therapeutic communication fit the educator's comments.
- In the second session, the "dental hygienist" glances at the list of possible responses and answers with mostly nontherapeutic responses. Classroom listeners should try to determine which specific categories of nontherapeutic communication fit the dental hygienist's comments.

TABLE 5.4	Techniques for Communicating With Clients Through the Life Span	
Level	**Developmental Characteristics**	**Communication Techniques**
Preschoolers	Beginning use of symbols and language; egocentric, focused on self; concrete in thinking and language	Allow child to use their five senses to explore oral healthcare environment (handle a mirror, feel a prophy cup, taste and smell fluoride, etc.) Use simple language and concrete, thorough explanations of exactly what is going to happen Let child see and feel cup "going around" or compressed air before putting in their mouth
School-age children	Less egocentric; shift to abstract thought emerges but much thought still concrete	Demonstrate equipment, allow child to question, give simple explanations of procedures
Adolescents	Concrete thinking evolves to more complex abstraction; can formulate alternative hypotheses in problem solving; may revert to childish manner at times; usually enjoy adult attention	Allow self-expression and avoid being judgmental Give thorough, detailed answers to questions Be attentive
Adults	Broad individual differences in values, experiences, and attitudes; self-directed and independent in comparison with children; have assumed certain family and social roles; periods of stability and change	Appropriately applied therapeutic communication techniques: maintaining silence, listening attentively, conveying acceptance, asking related questions, paraphrasing, clarifying, focusing, stating observations, offering information, summarizing, reflective responding
Older adults	May have sensory loss of hearing, vision; may have high level of anxiety; may be willing to comply with recommendations but forgetful	Approach with respect, speak clearly and slowly Give time for client to formulate answers to questions and to elaborate Be attentive to nonverbal communication

Adapted from Potter PA, Perry AG. *Fundamentals of Nursing: Concepts, Process, and Practice.* 3rd ed. Mosby; 1993.

Preschool and school-age children are eager to learn and explore but may have fears about the oral healthcare environment, personnel, and treatment. Studies have shown that dental fears begin in childhood, and making early oral care a positive experience is necessary if the dental hygienist is interested in the client's long-term attitude toward oral health.[3] Rapport must be established as a foundation for cooperation and trust. The best teaching approaches for younger children follow behavioral rather than cognitive theory. Positive reinforcement used as immediate feedback, short instructional segments with simplified language and content that is concrete rather than abstract, close monitoring of progress, and encouragement for independence in the practice of oral hygiene skills are indicated.

The Guidance-Cooperation Model

Five principles for communicating with young children are suggested in the Guidance-Cooperation Model.[7] Because the model is neither permissive nor coercive, it is ideally suited for the preschool or young school-age child. According to this model, health professionals are placed in a parental role whereby the child is expected to respect and cooperate with them. The principles inherent to the Guidance-Cooperation Model follow.

Tell the child the ground rules before and during treatment. Let the child know exactly what is expected. A comment such as, "You must do exactly as I ask, and please keep your hands in your lap like my other helpers," prepares the child to meet expectations. Structuring time so that the child also knows what to expect may be useful. For fluoride treatments, a timer should be set and made visible so that the child knows how long it will be before the trays will come out of their mouth.

Praise all cooperative behavior. When children respond to a directive such as, "Open wide," praise them with, "That's good! Thank you!" When children sit quietly, remember to praise them for cooperation. It is a mistake to ignore behavior until it is a problem.

Keep your cool. Ignore negative behavior such as whining if it is not interfering with the healthcare. Showing anger only makes matters

worse. Showing displeasure and using a calm voice for statements such as, "I get upset [or unhappy, etc.] when you ..." is likely to communicate the point more successfully.

Use voice control. A sudden change in volume can gain attention from a child who is being uncooperative. Modulate voice tone and volume as soon as the child begins to respond.

Allow the child to play a role. Let the child make some structured choices. For example, ask, "Would you like strawberry- or grape-flavored fluoride today?" Most younger children enjoy the role of "helper" and are happy to hold mirrors, papers, and pencils and to receive praise for their good work.

Avoid attempting to talk a child into cooperation. Do not give lengthy rationales for the necessity of procedures. Rather, acknowledge the child's feelings by making statements such as, "I understand that you don't like the fluoride treatment; however, we must do it to make your teeth stronger. I understand that you would rather be outside playing, but we need to polish your teeth now." Then firmly request the child's attention and cooperation and proceed with the service.

Older School-Age Children and Adolescents

Adolescence is not a single stage of development. The rate at which children progress through adolescence and the psychologic states that accompany the changes can vary considerably from one child to another.[8] In early adolescence (about 13 to 15 years old), children may rather suddenly demonstrate an ambivalence toward parents and other adults manifested by questioning of adult values and authority. By late adolescence (18 years and older), much of the ambivalence is gone, and values that characterize the adult years have emerged. Friendship patterns in early and middle adolescence are usually intense as the child begins to explore companionship outside the family and become established as an independent person (Fig. 5.5).

Some common complaints from the adolescent's point of view can sensitize health professionals for positive interactions with this group of young people. First, a frequently voiced complaint of adolescents is that

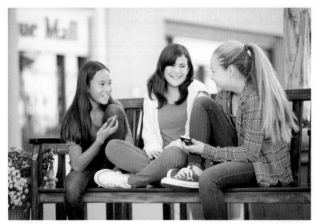

Fig. 5.5 Interacting with peers helps to establish independence. (Copyright iStock/bowdenimages.)

adults do not listen to them. They seem to feel that adults are in too much of a hurry, appear to be looking for certain answers, or listen only to what they want to hear. A second complaint is that, too often, a conversation turns into unsolicited advice or a mini-lecture. A young person, asked to describe specific experiences in dentistry, related, "My dentist bugged me a lot. He would become angry if I felt pain. He pushed my hair around and lectured constantly about young people and their hair."[7] Other less-common complaints from adolescents are that they are patronized, that they do not understand questions being asked, and that adults lack humor.

Dental hygienists should carefully consider these complaints and practice behaviors that enhance communication with adolescents. Being attentive and allowing the adolescent time to talk enhance rapport and communication. Some rapport-building questions at the beginning of the appointment may relate to family, school, personal interests, or career intentions. It is useful to have some knowledge of the contemporary interests of adolescents, which may include trends in music, sports, and fashion. They want a sense of being understood and do not want to be judged or lectured.

Adolescents have a strong human need for responsibility. An astute dental hygienist can use these unfulfilled needs to motivate the adolescent client to adopt oral self-care behaviors. This educational approach, based on human needs theory, can enhance adolescents' sense of personal responsibility toward the care of their mouths. To prevent adolescents from feeling singled out, a dental hygienist may say, "We encourage all of our adult clients to floss daily. This is because we know it works. We've seen the results." Teenagers do not feel patronized or confused if questions and advice are offered in a sincere, straightforward manner.

Adults

Havinghurst delineated three developmental stages for adults and listed common adult concerns at each stage.[6] Although communication techniques may not differ greatly for the adult stages, knowledge of general differences in characteristics among age groups can enlighten the hygienist about typical concerns of clients at different periods of adulthood. An awareness of how priorities in life change for adults as they develop can help the hygienist identify learning needs and "teachable moments" for different clients. The Havinghurst adult stages are summarized in Box 5.8 according to early adulthood, middle age, and late maturity. The dental hygienist should be aware, without asking personal questions, that young adults may be trying to institute oral self-care behaviors while adjusting to major life stresses such as bringing up young children, managing a home, or starting a demanding career. Adults in the middle years may be more settled in careers and have less responsibility for childcare but may be involved heavily in social responsibilities, adjusting to their personal physical changes, or

---

BOX 5.8 Havinghurst's Description of the Adult Developmental Stages

Early Adulthood
Selecting a mate
Learning to live with a marriage partner
Starting a family
Bringing up young children
Managing a home
Getting started in an occupation
Taking on civic responsibilities
Finding a congenial social group

Middle Age
Achieving adulthood and social responsibilities
Establishing and maintaining an economic standard of living
Assisting one's children to become adults
Developing durable leisure-time activities
Relating to one's marriage partner as a person
Accepting and adjusting to physical change
Adjusting to one's aging parent

Late Maturity
Adjusting to decreasing physical strength and to death
Adjusting to retirement and to reduced income
Adjusting to death of one's marriage partner
Establishing an explicit affiliation with one's age group
Meeting social and civic obligations
Establishing satisfactory physical living arrangements in light of physical infirmities

Adapted from Darkenwald GG, Merriam SB. *Adult Education: Foundations of Practice.* Harper & Row; 1982.

the demands of caring for aging parents. Older adults may be adjusting to decreasing physical strength, a chronic health problem, retirement, or death of a spouse. The elderly population is a highly diversified group. The wide variations in health and psychologic states dictate the necessity of careful assessment of each individual (see Chapter 47).

Health Behavior Theories

Communication approaches appropriate for adults are the therapeutic communication techniques discussed previously in this chapter. In using the techniques, the dental hygienist must be familiar with the adult developmental stages and aware of what demands may be preventing adults in the different stages from easily making oral healthcare behavioral changes. Modern adult learning theory has been supported by some basic assumptions. Keeping these assumptions in mind facilitates communication with adults who become "learners" as dental hygienists become "teachers" in the healthcare setting. These assumptions can enhance communication and the dental hygiene educator's approach to teaching adults.

Reviews of research on changing a variety of health behaviors show that interventions based on psychosocial theory or theoretical constructs are more effective than are those not using theory. However, the mechanisms that explain the larger effects have not been studied.[5] The most often used theories of health behavior are self-determination theory (SDT), social cognitive theory (SCT), the transtheoretical model (TTM)/stages of change, the health belief model (HBM), and the theory of planned behavior (TPB).[9]

Self-Determination Theory

SDT is a contemporary theory referring to an individual's ability to make choices and manage their life. People are motivated to grow

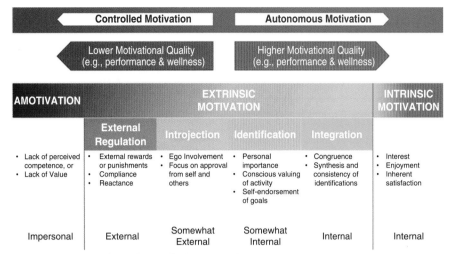

From Ryan & Deci (2000); © 2017 Center for Self-Determination Theory

Fig. 5.6 Self-Determination Theory. (Copyright © 2000, American Psychological Association. Ryan, RM, Deci, EL (2000). Self-determination theory and the facilitation of intrinsic motivation, social development, and well-being. *Am Psychol*, 55(1) ,68-78.)

and change by three innate and universal psychological needs: autonomy, competence, and relatedness. The links between SDT and MI are extensive and include similar assumptions about individuals and psychological health and growth. They both posit that individuals have an innate tendency for personal growth toward psychological integration. SDT examines experimentally how the processes and structures of rewards, directives, feedback, praise, positive regard, and other change-related factors enhance or diminish self-motivation and outcomes. SDT proposes that all behaviors can be described as lying along a continuum of relative autonomy, reflecting the extent to which the person fully endorses and is committed to what they are doing (Fig. 5.6).

At the more controlled end of this continuum is behavior that is motivated by external regulations, such as the rewards and punishments that others might control. Controlled motivation consists of both external regulation, in which one's behavior is a function of external contingencies of reward or punishment, and introjected regulation, in which the regulation of action has been partially internalized and is energized by factors such as an approval motive, avoidance of shame, contingent self-esteem, and ego involvements.[10] An example of external regulation is a client engaging in a behavior because they were pressured or mandated to do so by a dental hygienist.

The more autonomous end of this continuum reflects motives for engaging in behavior for the inherent interest and satisfaction derived from engaging in the action itself. Autonomous motivation is relevant to both intrinsic motivation and extrinsic motivation, which refers to activities that are not inherently rewarding (such as health behaviors or schoolwork). According to SDT, extrinsic motivations also have the potential to be autonomous if the individual has identified with the activity's value and ideally integrated it into their sense of self. SDT differentiates types of extrinsic motivation in terms of the degree to which it has been internalized, suggesting that the more fully it is internalized and integrated with one's self, the more autonomously regulated the behavior is said to be.

The transtheoretical model (TTM)/stages of change. One theory that has gained wide acceptance in recent years is the simple notion that behavior change is a process, not an event.[9] TTM recognizes stages of readiness and cognitive decisions to take action. Even individuals with the best of intentions to adopt a lifestyle change struggle with relapse. TTM implicitly addresses this phenomenon.[11]

Social determination theory (SDT). Sustaining behavior change focuses on establishing new behavior patterns that emphasize autonomy, environmental management, and improved self-efficacy. These strategies are an eclectic mix drawn from SCT.[12]

Theory of planned behavior (TPB). TTM distinguishes between the stages of contemplation and preparation and overt action.[13] A further application of this distinction comes from TPB, which proposes that intentions are the best predictors of behavior. Implementation intentions are even more closely related and may be better predictors of behavior and behavior change.[11] The most empirical applications of health behavior theory are part of public health intervention programs. Such programs have demonstrated only modest impact, which is due in part to weaknesses in application of available theoretical models.[14]

KEY CONCEPTS

- Communication during the dental hygiene process of care is a dynamic interaction between the dental hygienist and the client that involves verbal and nonverbal components.
- Factors that may affect the communication process include internal factors of the client and the dental hygienist (e.g., perceptions, values, emotions, and knowledge), the nature of their relationship, the situation prompting communication, and the environment.
- Some communication approaches are therapeutic and helpful in assisting clients to make decisions and attain goals related to their comfort and health. Other approaches are nontherapeutic and unsuccessful in helping clients make decisions and attain goals related to their comfort and health.
- Communication techniques used by the dental hygiene clinician must be flexible to relate to the full range of client ages through the life span.
- MI is an approach designed to facilitate resolution of client issues that inhibit positive behavior by actively engaging the client in the communication process.
- MI emphasizes collaboration, eliciting information from the client, and respecting client autonomy.
- The goal of MI is to have the client voice the arguments for positive change, which is called "change talk."
- The tools of MI are open-ended questions, affirming change talk, reflective responding, and summarizing the results of the dialogue.
- MI can be useful in addressing behavioral problems dental hygienists face every day.

ACKNOWLEDGMENT

The author acknowledges Margaret M. Walsh, Sandra K. Rich, and Hope Oliver for their past contributions to this chapter.

REFERENCES

1. Miller W, Rollnick S. *Motivational Interviewing: Preparing People for Change*. 2nd ed. Guilford Press; 2002.

2. Deci EL, Ryan RM. *Intrinsic Motivation and Self-Determination in Human Behavior*. Plenum; 1985.

3. Carvallo M, Gabriel S. No man is an island: the need to belong and dismissing avoidant attachment style. *Pers Soc Sycholl Bull*. 2006;32(5):697–709.

4. Rollnick S, Miller WR, Butler CC. *Motivational Interviewing in Health Care: Helping Patients Change Behavior*. Guilford Press; 2008.

5. Cascaes AM, Bielemann RM, Clark VL, et al. Effectiveness of motivational interviewing at improving oral health: a systematic review. *Rev Saude Publica*. 2014;48(1):142–153.

6. Havinghurst RJ. *Developmental Tasks and Education*. McKay; 1952.

7. Weinstein P, Getz T, Milgrom P. *Oral Self-Care: Strategies for Preventive Dentistry*. 3rd ed. University of Washington Continuing Dental Education; 1991.

8. Ryan RM, Deci EL. Self-determination theory and the facilitation of intrinsic motivation, social determination and well-being. *Am Psychol*. 2000;55:68–78.

9. Glanz K, Bishop DB. The role of behavioral science theory in development and implementation of public health interventions. *Annu Rev Public Health*. 2010;31:399–418.

10. Ryan RM, Deci EL, Vansteenkiste M, Soenens B. Building a science of motivated persons: self-determination theory's empirical approach to human experience and the regulation of behavior. *Mot Sci*. 2021;7(2):97.

11. Prochaska JO, Redding CA, Evers KE. The transtheoretical model and stages of change. In: Glanz K, Lewis FM, Rimer B, eds. *Health Behavior and Health Education: Theory, Research, and Practice*. Jossey Bass Publishers; 2008:97–121.

12. Deci EL, Ryan RM. A motivational approach to self-integration in personality. In: Diensibier D, ed. *Perspectives on Motivation. Nebraska Symposium on Motivation*. Vol. 38. University of Nebraska Press; 1991:237–288.

13. Ajzen I. The theory of planned behavior. *Org Behav Hum Decis Proc*. 1991;50:179–211.

14. Gollwitzer PM. Implementation intentions: strong effects of simple plans. *Am Psychol*. 1999;54:493–503.

6

Inclusive Practices in Healthcare

Danette Ocegueda and Lorie Holt

PROFESSIONAL OPPORTUNITIES

On a daily basis, healthcare providers encounter people from diverse backgrounds with differing values, beliefs, and lifestyles. Therefore, it is imperative that healthcare providers develop the necessary knowledge and skills to interact and communicate with patients and other healthcare professionals in a culturally diverse world.

COMPETENCIES

1. Discuss the relationship between culture and health, and work toward developing cultural sensitivity through self-awareness and exploration of cultural self-identify and identity of others.
2. Understand the relationships among cultural competence, cultural humility, and patient-centered care.
3. Describe healthcare literacy and value the importance of cultural values, health beliefs, and cultural sensitivity.
4. Value the importance of verbal, nonverbal, and written communication utilizing Motivational Interviewing techniques and LEARN frameworks to communicate with patients in inclusive encounters.
5. Discuss the importance of cultural sensitivity when making shared decisions in the healthcare environment.
6. Discuss the process of care in patient-centered environments.

DIVERSITY, EQUITY, AND INCLUSION DYNAMICS

The study of Diversity, Equity, and Inclusion (DEI) is very fluid, with shifts in pedagogy and terminology occurring regularly. In previous versions of this text, this chapter has been titled "Cultural Competency in Healthcare." In recent years, researchers have recognized the shortcomings of cultural competence alone and have emphasized the need for elevating cultural humility pedagogy. Critics of cultural competence pedagogy dispute the idea that individuals can learn a defined set of attitudes, behaviors, and skills that would allow them to work within the cultural context of the patient and that there is an end point to this learning.[1] Instead, cultural humility is seen as an alternative approach to cultural competence and is seen as a dynamic and lifelong process that focuses on self-exploration and self-critique combined with a willingness to learn from others. Many in the healthcare community recognize that the concepts of cultural competence and cultural humility are not in contrast to each other, but both are pieces to the same puzzle. The lens of this current chapter will reflect that shift in pedagogy and terminology.

HEALTHCARE FOR A DIVERSE POPULATION

The changing cultural landscape and increasing globalization have led to increasingly culturally diverse societies. According to data from the US Census Bureau, ethnic minorities account for one-third of the current US population and are expected to make up nearly 60% of the total US population by 2060.[2] Regularly, healthcare professionals encounter patients with different backgrounds, belief systems, values, attitudes, norms, traditions, and languages. Cultural differences can lead to patient and clinician dissatisfaction, decreased trust, poor adherence to recommendations, and adverse health outcomes.

Many events in society highlight the need to increase diversity and inclusion in healthcare. For example, the COVID-19 pandemic's disproportionate impact on Black, Latino, Native American, and other underserved communities is well documented and cause for concern. It was another example in a long history of **health inequities** and **health disparities** affecting underserved individuals and communities in our society.

Therefore, there is an essential need for a healthcare workforce that can interact and communicate effectively with patients and other healthcare providers in an inclusive, **patient-centered** environment. This concept is articulated in the *Healthy People 2030* document published by the US Department of Health and Human Services (HHS). The HHS developed an action plan outlining the need for a workforce and healthcare system able to identify racial and ethnic health disparities and to develop sensitivity for culture differences.[3] The HHS has also established standards for healthcare organizations to advance health equity, improve quality, and help eliminate healthcare disparities in its publication "National Standards for Culturally and Linguistically Appropriate Services (CLAS) in Health and Health Care."[4] The Principal Standard is that healthcare must "provide effective, equitable, understandable and respectful quality care and services that are responsive to diverse cultural health beliefs and practices, preferred languages, health literacy and other communication needs."[4]

The American Dental Hygienists' Association (ADHA) and the Canadian Dental Hygienists Association (CDHA) have established minimum standards and competencies for dental hygienists related to treating a diverse patient population.[5,6] In addition, the Commission on Dental Accreditation (CODA) current accreditation standards speak to the need for dental hygiene graduates to achieve competence in **interprofessional** collaborations that impact the delivery of health services to a diverse patient population.[7] See Box 6.1 for a Critical Thinking activity.

HEALTH INEQUITY AND LITERACY

There is exhaustive evidence to support that social factors, including education, employment status, income level, gender, and ethnicity, have an influence on a person's health. For example, the lower an individual's socioeconomic status, the higher the risk of poor health and difficulty verbalizing health concerns, asserting needs, determining the level of participation in care, and seeking second opinions. The World Health Organization notes that **health inequities** are often the result of systematic differences in health status or the distribution of health determinants between different population groups.[8] Health inequities are the result of complex interactions among environmental, biological, social, and economic factors. Race or ethnicity, sex, gender identity, age, disability, socioeconomic status, geographic location, lifestyle, and other factors all contribute to an individual's ability to achieve optimal health, which can look different for different people and cultures. Knowledge of health inequities is essential to understanding the different **determinants of health**. See Fig. 6.1 and Box 6.2.

These barriers can lead to lower levels of **healthcare literacy**. Healthcare professionals play a role in assuming responsibility for their patient's healthcare literacy and must take action to help rectify health inequities caused by social determinants of health such as poverty. Health equity requires focused and ongoing societal efforts to address historical and contemporary injustices; overcome economic, social, and other obstacles to health and healthcare; and eliminate preventable health disparities. Employing cultural humility in patient care is often seen as a foundational pillar for reducing disparities through culturally sensitive and unbiased quality care by respecting diversity in the patient population and cultural factors that can affect health and health outcomes.

CULTURAL HUMILITY/CULTURAL COMPETENCE

As the world becomes increasingly diverse, developing cultural humility and cultural competence is a growing imperative. To be effective healthcare providers, individuals at all levels need to develop and deepen their capacities to work across differences and create environments that are welcoming, equitable, and inclusive. Whether it is treating patients, working in healthcare teams, or engaging with community members, individuals need to cultivate their personal cultural humility by developing an awareness of self to help inform how they see others.

Cultural competence is characterized as a skill that can be taught or achieved and is often seen as necessary for working effectively with diverse patients. The underlying assumption of cultural competence is that the greater the knowledge one has about another culture, the greater the competence in practice. Cultural competence suggests an outcome—a tangible and achievable end goal, and **cultural humility** is the mindset that fuels that journey toward achieving that goal.[9]

At its core, cultural humility requires opening a conversation in a way that genuinely attempts to understand a person's identities related to race and ethnicity, gender, sexual orientation, socioeconomic status, education, social needs, and others. Developing cultural humility is often seen as a fluid and ongoing learning process that involves continual self-awareness. The ability to recognize possible biases and develop a nonjudgmental stance about what they hear, recognizing an

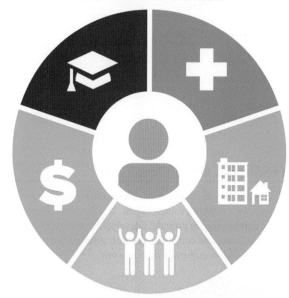

Social Determinants of Health

Fig. 6.1 Social Determinants of Health. (From https://health.gov/healthypeople/priority-areas/social-determinants-health)

inherent status of privilege as a provider, and developing the capacity to be taught by their patients are inherent traits of cultural humility. It involves entering a relationship with another person with the intention of honoring their beliefs, customs, and values.

A recent paradigm of thought regarding the relationship between cultural competence and cultural humility is **cultural competemility**, which infuses the principles of cultural humility with that of cultural competence. Cultural competemility suggests that healthcare professionals maintain both an attitude and a lens of cultural competence and cultural humility as they engage in cultural encounters, obtain cultural knowledge, demonstrate the cultural skills of both their own biases and the presence of "ism" (e.g., racism, sexism, ableism, classism, ageism, anti-Semitism, heterosexism, colorism, ethnocentrism).[1] Reframing cultural competence as an ongoing process is critical in pursuing cultural competemility.

"To become different from what we are, we must have some awareness of what we are."

Eric Hoffer

CULTURE AND HEALTH

Culture is a fluid concept, continually changing and adapting to different developments and environments. **Culture** is often seen as a set of guidelines that one can inherit as a member of a particular group or society. It can influence the way a member of that society or group views the world. Culture is inclusive of but not limited to race, ethnicity, gender identity, sexual orientation, faith, age, socioeconomic status, disability, or profession. It is important to note that not all individuals who are born and raised within one culture embrace its normative values and attitudes reconfirming the notion that "even in sameness there is difference." See Boxes 6.3 and 6.4.

Cultural beliefs and practices can influence an individual's health status, such as an appreciation for the important preventive measures or therapeutic interventions can play in establishing good oral health. However, being part of any cultural group does not automatically lead

BOX 6.2 Social Determinants of Health: 5 Domains

Neighborhood and Built Environment
- Access to foods that support healthy eating patterns
- Quality of housing
- Crime and violence
- Environmental conditions

Healthcare Access and Quality
- Access to healthcare
- Access to primary care
- Health literacy

Social and Community Context
- Social cohesion
- Civil participation
- Discrimination
- Incarceration

Education Access and Quality
- High school graduation
- Enrollment in higher education
- Language and literacy
- Early childhood education and development

Economic Stability
- Poverty
- Employment
- Food insecurity
- Housing instability

Adapted from HHS ODPHP *Healthy People 2030* https://health.gov/healthypeople/priority-areas/social-determinants-health.

BOX 6.3 Cultural Humility

"Cultural humility involves understanding the complexity of identities — that even in sameness there is difference — and that a clinician will never be fully competent about the evolving and dynamic nature of a patient's experiences."

From Cultural Humility vs. Cultural Competence, available at https://healthcity.bmc.org/policy-and-industry/cultural-humility-vs-cultural-competence-providers-need-both.

BOX 6.4 Cultural Awareness Exercise

Describe your own culture(s). Think in terms of your race(s), ethnic background(s), profession, gender, sexual orientation, faith, or even your age. Reflect on traditions, family, and/or social influences that have played a role in the way you view yourself, others, and the world in general. Synthesize how you see or react to individuals from cultures different than your own. Reflect on your personal cultural identity and consider how it affects your view of healthcare. Contemplate how and from whom you seek healthcare advice or services.

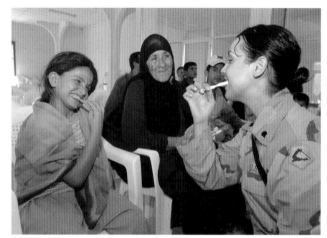

Fig. 6.2 A United States Army Specialist teaching an Iraqi girl proper tooth brushing techniques. (From https://commons.wikimedia.org/wiki/File:Toothbrush_teaching_1.jpg)

a person to have poor oral or overall health. Within all cultural groups are substantial differences in beliefs and behaviors. Cultural norms contribute to how members of a specific group determine health expectations and explanations for health, disease, or illness. Cultural norms may also determine where and from whom the patient may seek health advice, guidance, and treatment if they become ill. This inevitably leads to varying degrees of health.[10,11] Health and illness are not only physical conditions but are also based on perceptual judgments. The way a person understands illness—oral or systemic—can largely be culturally determined. These beliefs and practices can facilitate or act as barriers to accessing healthcare services.

Health professionals must realize that patients within any cultural group have individual variability in their perceptions of health, sometimes having sociocultural health beliefs that do not match the clinician's perspective (Fig. 6.2). It is imperative that all healthcare professionals be aware of their own biases and ethnocentric behaviors, and avoid stereotyping others. **Ethnocentric** beliefs and **stereotyping** an individual based solely on culture context decreases trust and communication between the patient and provider and makes forming a patient/provider relationship difficult, which often leads to less than ideal healthcare outcomes.

DEVELOPING A CULTURALLY INCLUSIVE FRAMEWORK

Cultural differences often exist in any clinical encounter and must be assessed conscientiously. A major challenge for healthcare providers lies in trying to develop a personal culturally inclusive pedagogy. Since culture is a fluid concept, changing and adapting to different developments and environments, cultural humility must also be a dynamic process entailing an ongoing process of self-exploration, self-awareness, and critique by acknowledging one's own biases. It recognizes the shifting nature of intersecting identities.

Awareness of self is central to the notion of cultural humility—who a person is informs how they see others. Developing cultural humility is critical to the development of cultural competence, which focuses on the ability to engage knowledgeably with people across cultures. Cultural competence suggests that having knowledge and understanding of another person's culture allows one to better adapt interventions and approaches to healthcare specific to the culture of the patient, family, and social group. The development of cultural humility and cultural competence can be seen as a continuum and an ongoing learning process (Fig. 6.3).[11,12]

A framework was developed in 2011 for incorporating cultural awareness into the delivery of healthcare services.[1] Within this model, constructs such as **cultural awareness, cultural knowledge, cultural skills, cultural encounters, and cultural desire** were central to its use. The Process of

Cultural Competence in the Delivery of Health Care Services model (Fig. 6.4) is one that has been widely adopted and used in healthcare education and practice.[11] This framework for providing culturally competent healthcare is represented by a Venn diagram showing the interrelation of the five constructs that must be present to move toward becoming a culturally inclusive individual and healthcare provider.

Going beyond traditional approaches to cultural competence and cultural humility that tend to focus solely on self-awareness, the appreciation of cultural differences, and interpersonal skills, the framework of Cultural Competency for Equity and Inclusion (CCEI) (Fig. 6.5) integrates an intersectional perspective and social justice concepts such as issues of power, privilege, oppression, and systemic change that are often seen with health inequities.[13] The unique characteristic of the CCEI model is the commitment to equity and inclusion. Similarities with other models of cultural competence can be seen in the CCEI model as well.

The five core constructs in this model are: self-awareness, understanding and valuing others, knowledge of societal inequities, interpersonal skills to effectively engage across differences in different contexts, and skills to foster transformation toward equity and inclusion.

Self-awareness entails the ability to understand who we are and how our race, ethnicity, religion/spirituality, socioeconomic class, sexual orientation, gender identity, ability, national origin, age, and other social identities affect our worldviews, relationships, perspective, experiences, and behaviors. The result of self-awareness is the knowledge of appreciation for and valuing others' social identities, cultures, and perspectives and understanding their biases.

Like self-awareness, knowledge of others' cultures and social identity groups and how they intersect is important. Understanding how other's socialization, life experiences, and cultural background shape who they are, their worldviews, beliefs, and values is important to

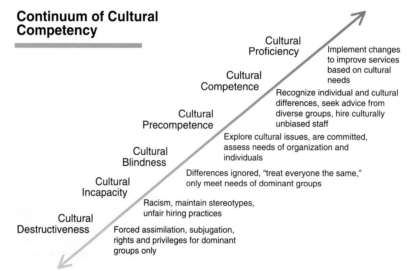

Fig. 6.3 Cultural Competency Continuum. (Adapted from Cross TL, Bazron B, Dennis K, Isaacs M. *Towards a Culturally Competent System of Care: A Monograph of Effective Service for Minority Children Who Are Severely Emotionally Disturbed.* Included with permission of the Georgetown University Center for Child & Human Development, Georgetown University Medical Center.)

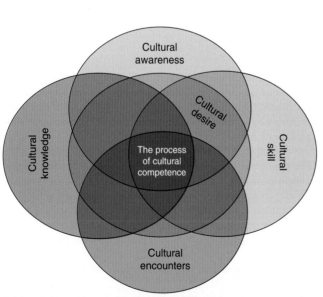

Fig. 6.4 The Process of Cultural Competence in the Delivery of Healthcare Services Model. (Redrawn from Campinha-Bacote J. Process of cultural competence in the delivery of healthcare services: a model of care. *Journal of Transcultural Nursing.* 2002;13(3):181.)

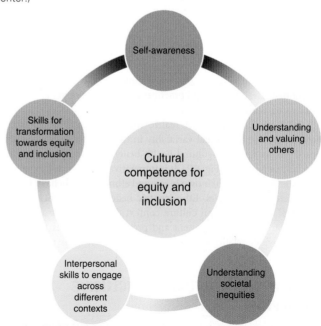

Fig. 6.5 CCEI. (Redrawn from Goodman DJ. Cultural competence for equity and inclusion. *Understanding and Dismantling Privilege.* 2020;10(1):41–60.)

developing cultural humility and competence. In addition to understanding self, others, and society, the ability to adapt to and work collaboratively with a diverse group of people in a range of situations impacts an individual's ability to reconsider personal assumptions and find ways to embrace a wide range of cultural encounters.

CCEI entails more than interpersonal skills and an understanding of the impact of structural inequities. It requires being able to identify and address inequities and choose appropriate interventions to create environments and practices that foster diversity, equity, inclusion, and social justice. For cultural inclusive critical thinking activities, see Boxes 6.5 and 6.6.

INCLUSIVE COMMUNICATION

Openness, caring, and mutual respect are essential to building relationships and maximizing effective communication. Inclusive communication emphasizes the importance of addressing all people with respect.[14] In interactions with patients, the healthcare provider can follow actions outlined in the LEARN Model[15] (Box 6.7) for inclusive communication. This model highlights the act of active listening, sharing of perspectives, acknowledging the differences and similarities in each perspective, and negotiating a mutually agreed upon course of treatment. See Box 6.8 for a role play activity using the LEARN model.

Inclusive communication can be divided into three subcategories: verbal communication, nonverbal communication, and written communication. Cultural sensitivity should be used in all forms of provider/patient communication. For inclusive communication in healthcare settings, the Centers for Disease Control and Prevention encourage healthcare providers to consider the following concepts:[14]

1. Avoid jargon or complex terms; use active verbs and plain language to convey information.
2. Recognize that not all patients/colleagues have the same ability to interpret and understand information shared.
3. Acknowledge that many people with English as a secondary language may be highly literate in a non-English language.
4. Acknowledge that some people may not be literate in their primary language and may not understand written information when translated into their primary language.
5. Recognize that while people may not be literate, they possess other skills to understand and comprehend information.
   For written communication pieces:
1. Offer multiple forms of written communication.
2. Recognize some people may lack digital access and/or literacy.

Verbal and Nonverbal Communication

Cultural perspective needs to be considered in verbal communications. To have inclusive dialogs in culturally sensitive interactions, healthcare providers might employ **motivational interviewing** techniques (see Chapter 5) and communication methods outlined in the LEARN model[15] for inclusive communication. Utilizing these skills can allow the patient and provider to reach a mutually agreeable treatment plan for optimal health outcomes. The provider needs to be able to recognize the potential for communication difficulties and find solutions to overcome any real or perceived barriers. For example, when language is a barrier, it is most appropriate to use a trained medical interpreter.

Interpreting is the process of understanding and analyzing a spoken or signed message and reexpressing that message accurately and objectively in another language. The inability to communicate with a care provider can undermine trust and decrease appropriate followup, and may cause diagnostic errors and inappropriate treatment. Therefore

---

BOX 6.5   Critical Thinking Scenario A

You, as a dental hygienist, have been treating a 22-year-old college student for the past 16 years. She is from an affluent family whom you have known socially for years. She has always presented with good health and fair oral hygiene. In the past, she has been compliant with all treatment recommendations and oral hygiene instructions. Today, she comes in on a break from college for routine prophylaxis services. She seems a little different. She shares that she fasts daily and consume only plant-based foods because of religious practices that may be new to her. She appears very pale and presents with glossitis, angular cheilitis, and aphthous ulcers, which she state she gets frequently. She refuse any fluoride products and to have her teeth polished. Can you relate to the scenario in terms of the patient's healthcare beliefs or values that may have changed? Are they different or the same as yours? Do you have any biases that could play into your treatment recommendations for this patient? How might you learn from this scenario to develop your cultural humility? Your cultural competence? How will you reach mutually agreeable treatment options? What model(s) for cross-cultural communication could be used to provide nutritional counseling to this patient?

BOX 6.6   Critical Thinking Scenario B

Your new patient today is an 8-year-old male. He comes back to the treatment area by himself; a woman, who you assume is his mother, escorts him to the office but remains in the waiting area during treatment. Upon reviewing his medical/dental/social history form, you see that his mother is listed but the line for his father is left blank. When inquiring about his oral hygiene habits, you ask him who assists him with his brushing, and he replies, "Mom and mommy." You ask if his father also helps him brush his teeth. He does not respond to your question. Later, you go out to the waiting room to share his oral findings with his mother. Two women get up and accompany you back to the treatment room.

What strategies could you use in this scenario in an effort to provide this family with culturally sensitive care? Is the medical, dental, and social history form culturally appropriate? Why or why not? What, if any, are the potential legal implications in this scenario?

BOX 6.7   LEARN Model

L Listen to the patient's perspective.
E Explain and share one's own perspective.
A Acknowledge differences and similarities between these two perspectives.
R Recommend a treatment plan.
N Negotiate a mutually agreed-on treatment plan.

BOX 6.8   Role Play Activity: Communicating With Patients Using the LEARN Cultural Communication Model

With a partner or small group, take turns playing the role of the patient with moderate periodontitis and extensive restorative needs, the dental hygienist, and an observer. Use the LEARN model to communicate in a culturally inclusive environment. Use different cultural environments, such as a newcomer to the United States with health beliefs different from your own as a healthcare provider, or maybe a patient from the same geographical area and cultural background as you but who is opposed to suggested treatment options because of faith-based or lifestyle beliefs and behaviors.

How will you practice culturally sensitive or culturally inclusive care and still reach mutually agreeable treatment outcomes?

it is the responsibility of the healthcare provider to ensure effective communication via a trained medical interpreter.[10] To communicate efficiently and effectively with a patient, the healthcare provider must determine when a trained medical interpreter is needed. A healthcare provider should consider the following questions and/or statements when evaluating whether a trained medical interpreter is required:

- What is the patient's primary language?
- Is the healthcare provider fluent in that language?
- Does the patient have a hearing or other impairment that may require an interpreter for healthcare services?
- Assess the patient's language and English proficiency skills by asking open-ended questions.
- Assess the patient's healthcare literacy. A patient may be fluent in a language but lack understanding of medical and dental terminology.
- If possible, avoid the use of family members, especially minor children, as interpreters.

If a healthcare provider does not have access to a trained medical interpreter, the healthcare provider will be challenged to find suitable alternatives to communicate with the patient. If possible, try to avoid family members, especially young children. A healthcare provider might find the use of electronic translating applications and devices as an effective means for communication. If available, a colleague who is fluent in the patient's native language might be able to serve as an interpreter. Boxes 6.9 and 6.10 provide tips for working with a trained medical interpreter and legal considerations of using an unqualified interpreter.

Culture can also play an important role in determining the meaning and interpretation of nonverbal communication. Behavioral etiquette, eye contact, facial expressions, body gestures, and physical contact all may be determined by cultural norms and background.[16] Even the way in which individuals use space to communicate nonverbally, often called proxemics, can vary by culture.[17] Table 6.1 lists some behavioral considerations for working with patients. In any interaction, the use of one's hands or other parts of the body in nonverbal communication can be a source of misunderstanding. Healthcare providers should be cognizant of nonverbal communication, such as facial expressions and eye contact, as culture context often dictates the appropriate amount that is desired or acceptable for both the healthcare provider and patient.

Physical contact or touch is divided into two categories: necessary touch and nonnecessary touch. An intraoral examination is an example of necessary touch; holding a patient's hand while explaining a procedure is an example of nonnecessary touch. Physical contact or touching can often be misinterpreted. In the clinical healthcare setting, the patient's personal space is often invaded out of necessity by the healthcare provider. When personal space is invaded, patients may communicate their discomfort nonverbally through hesitation or attempting to readjust to a more comfortable distance. A patient may even request a provider of a specific gender for religious, cultural, or personal reasons. Such requests should be honored and not seen as a slight against a particular provider. When in doubt, ask permission to touch a patient prior to making any physical contact and limit your contact to necessary touching only.

Written Communication

As with verbal and nonverbal communication, healthcare providers might contemplate cultural factors when formulating and disseminating written/electronic materials. Written/electronic materials may include, but are not limited to, medical, dental, and social history forms, as well as other educational or postoperative materials/instructions. Healthcare providers should be familiar with the written or electronic materials disseminated to patients and/or their family members. Healthcare providers need to be aware of word choices and images in these materials. Use media materials that are equitable and inclusive, avoid stereotypes, and consider the gender, ability, and race or ethnicity of the people in images.

In the United States and many other countries, the law requires patients to give informed consent, signing a form indicating full understanding of the information provided in relation to their health and disease, and their agreement with a proposed treatment plan. For some patients, this concept of choice may conflict with cultural values and specific life circumstances. Illiteracy, lack of familiarity with the healthcare system, and financial concerns also may impair patient autonomy and participation in shared decision making.

THE PROCESS OF PATIENT-CENTERED CARE

Practicing culturally sensitive healthcare is the effective integration of patients' diverse cultural backgrounds into the **patient-centered process of care** (Chapter 23). As health professionals, caring for individuals who have similar traits and beliefs, e.g., gender identity, religious beliefs, skin tone, etc., may not present the same challenges as caring for individuals with different traits and beliefs. This process may require additional effort and may be time consuming. Healthcare providers may need to take the time and effort to learn about different cultures, subcultures, and health practices of the individuals they are treating. Additional time may need to be scheduled to accommodate the need for learning about an individual's culture context, beliefs, and health traditions. Extra time may also be needed for translation, repetition, clarification, and socialization to the healthcare care setting.[10] See Box 6.11 for Patient-Centered Care strategies.

TABLE 6.1 Behavioral Considerations for Working With Patients*

Category	Types of Behavior	Range of Behavior	Category	Types of Behavior	Range of Behavior
Communication (verbal and nonverbal)	Voice quality	Soft, strong	Basic beliefs and concepts	Belief in supernatural forces	Yes / No
	Pronunciation and enunciation	Clear, slurred / Dialect		Belief in extent of control over environment/health	Internal control / External control (fatalism, luck, etc.)
	Use of silence	Infrequent, often / Length of silence (brief to long)		Individual responsible for treatment/advice related to illness	Traditional medical professional / Nontraditional medical professional / Spiritual advisor / Culturally specific individuals / Combination of approaches
	Use of nonverbal	Hands / Eyes / Body / Expressions / Gestures / Posture		Perception of treatment/advice	Authoritarian / Recommendations
	Touch	Avoids touch / Accepts touch readily / Touches others readily		Treatment of illness	Traditional medicine / Holistic medicine / Nontraditional medicine / Spiritual treatment / Culturally specific treatments / Combination of approaches
	Eye contact	Direct / Avoided / Frequency / Infrequent / Often / Intermittent		Perception of health	Freedom from illness or disease / Stable condition / Harmony/disharmony with nature, mind, body or spirit / Punishment from spiritual being / Other
	Formality of address	Values formality / Doesn't value formality / Formal until directed otherwise		Perception of medical/ dental professionals	Respect for authority/professionals / Trusted / Distrusted / Other
Personal space	Comfort	Moves/doesn't move when personal space is compromised	Social organization (collectivistic vs. individualistic)	Identification of family unit/group	Nuclear family / Extended family / Community / Others
	Normal speaking distance	0 to 18 inches / 18 inches to 3 feet / More than 3 feet		Level of involvement of family/social groups in decision making	Involved—immediate or extended family / Involved—others / Not involved
	Formal/informal	Personal space is closer with family/friends than others			

*Many ethnic, cultural, and/or religious practices may shape values, behaviors, health, and illness beliefs of a particular group. Not all people from a given cultural group act in a standard manner. Great variability exists within cultural groups based on socioeconomic status, level of education, and overall life experiences. This list is by no means exhaustive or extensive but merely serves as an overview of the range of potential beliefs and behaviors exhibited by some individuals.
Adapted from Giger JN. *Transcultural Nursing: Assessment and Intervention.* 7th ed. Elsevier; 2017.0.

BOX 6.11 Strategies for Patient-Centered Care

- Approach each patient as a valued, unique individual.
- Reflect on your culture, personal characteristics, values, and life experiences. Identify potential biases and prejudices that can impact your effectiveness as a healthcare provider, educator, administrator, manager, researcher, and advocate.
- Become a lifelong student of cultures and diversity in general. In all encounters, strive to move toward cultural humility.
- Demonstrate knowledge and recognition of the patient's cultural practices throughout each interaction. Encourage patients to continue cultural health practices that can bring no harm.
- Display an accepting, nonjudgmental demeanor when presented with diversity.
- Consider dietary practices. Provide nutritional counseling within the framework of the patient's cultural values and norms.
- Develop collegial relationships with healthcare providers from diverse cultural groups.
- Promote cultural exchanges that contribute to patient-centered care.

To provide culturally sensitive care, the healthcare provider must understand the patient's view or cultural context for making healthcare decisions. In some cultures, decisions are not made independently but as a group. In a **collectivistic** environment, the group is viewed as the fundamental unit of society and healthcare decisions are made by the group. In contrast, a patient from an **individualistic** culture is often viewed as the single unit with autonomy and self-determination, and healthcare decisions are made by the individual. A clear understanding of both the collectivistic and individualistic viewpoints is essential to negotiate a mutually acceptable care plan with the patient. Characteristics of collectivistic and individualistic cultures are described in Table 6.2.

Assessment

The cultural assessment is an important part of the overall dental hygiene assessment of the patient. Table 6.3 outlines culturally relevant considerations that healthcare providers might encounter when treating patients. Through the utilization of motivational interviewing

TABLE 6.2   Characteristics of Collectivistic and Individualistic Cultures

Characteristic	Collectivistic	Individualistic
Goals	Emphasis is on group goals over individual goals	Emphasis on individual goals over group goals
Responsibility	Tend to belong to groups that look after one another	Tend to assume responsibility only for themselves and their immediate family
Self-actualization	Involves cooperation and solidarity with fellow members of one's group	More self-centered
Identity	Tend to identify self within the group they are part of	Clearly see themselves as an individual
Social life	Work and social life intertwined	Personal privacy is protected
Work values	Harmony and loyalty within company is important	Emphasize success in job or private wealth
Communication	Do not disagree with someone in public, avoid confrontation	Prefer clarity and being direct; to the point
Decision making	Family and friends are involved in decision-making patterns; group often will determine who will be responsible for healthcare decisions	The individual tends to make the final decision, based on their own expectations and values, in general and in relation to healthcare decisions

TABLE 6.3   Cultural Assessment

Culturally Relevant Considerations	Key Questions or Considerations
Ethnic origin	Ethnic identification of the patient? Place of birth? Place of childhood?
Racial identification	Racial background?
Gender identification	Gender preference? Preferred pronouns?
Domicile history	Where the patient lived and where the patient now lives? Years in this country?
Valued habits, customs, and behaviors	Behaviors, customs, values, and beliefs about health, healthcare providers, and the healthcare system? How the patient values courtesy, family, work, and gender roles? How the patient expresses emotion, stress, pain, spirituality, fear?
Communications	Communication style, e.g., manner of speaking, language spoken, need for interpreter, reading skills, methods of showing respect or deference, eye contact, personal space?
Health beliefs and practices	Healing systems and nontraditional practices used by the patient? Explanation of disease and illness (fatalism, punishment from higher being(s), germ theory, spirits, etc.)? How the patient determines seriousness of a health problem; when to seek care and from whom?
Nutritional factors	Culturally or religiously determined food preferences or restrictions? Foods used to treat illness or to achieve a desired characteristic?
Sociologic factors	Impact of socioeconomic status and environment on health and disease, living conditions, lifestyle, access to healthcare? Family's (or significant other's) role in healthcare? Key people or institutions that influence patient's health behavior (family, school, mosque, church, synagogue, tribal council or organization, etc.)
Psychologic factors	Patient's response to the healthcare system (e.g., anxiety, hope, distrust, fear, avoidance)? Patient's relationship to people, institutions, and environments from other cultures?
Physical characteristics	Normal limits for individuals within this ethnic group (e.g., skin color, gingival color, and facial characteristics)? Growth and development pattern variations within the cultural groups? Disease risk factors prevalent within patient's cultural, racial, or ethnic group?

BOX 6.12 Patient Education Tips

- Use models and educational materials that are culturally inclusive.
- Assess and verify patient's beliefs and practices. Be familiar with common healthcare beliefs and practices in the patient's culture as a starting point without stereotyping.
- Integrate self-care and professional care therapies for oral disease management with the patient's culture in mind; conventional and nonconventional approaches may be encouraged if not harmful.
- Provide nutritional counseling within the context of the patient's culture values and beliefs.

techniques, the healthcare provider can gain valuable insights into a patient's values, beliefs, and attitudes pertaining to their oral and overall health.

Dental Hygiene Diagnosis and Care Planning

The dental hygiene diagnosis should identify the patient's unmet human needs or any other factors affecting the patient's quality of life (see Chapters 2 and 22). Using a nonjudgmental, nonethnocentric approach as outlined in the LEARN model for inclusive communication, an individualized, patient-centered care plan can be developed and appropriate interventions proposed. This can allow the patient to have informed interactions with their healthcare provider, which helps to establish an inclusive encounter. Such encounters help build a pathway for a mutually beneficial two-way relationship where trust and rapport can flourish so that culturally appropriate care plans with mutually agreeable self-care aids and treatment options can be negotiated for optimal health outcomes. See Box 6.12 for patient education tips.

Implementation

Interventions should be culturally acceptable for ideal adherence. Oral health therapy and promotion strategies, including the planning of interventions and the implementation of the care plan, must be delivered in relation to the cultural environment of the patient. Patient values and needs guide the selection of interventions. Health interventions, whether educational, technical, or interpersonal in nature, are most effective when the intervention is congruent with the patient's personal values (Fig. 6.6).

Evaluation

In all clinical encounters, it is important to gain insight into the patient's perspectives of success, level of understanding, psychomotor skill development, and self-care practices. Evaluation determines whether the health services are meeting the patient's needs. Inviting patients to talk about their health practices can help with improving culturally inclusive communication.

Documentation

Documentation relates to all components of the dental hygiene process of care. It is critical to record completely and accurately all collected data, planned and provided treatment(s), interventions recommended, and all information relevant to patient care, including but not limited to any

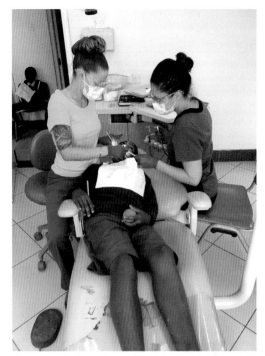

Fig. 6.6 Dental hygienists Jimmie McClain, RDH, BS, and Sarah Pea, RDH, BS, performing dental hygiene services on a Kenyan child. (Courtesy of Jimmie McClain, RDH, BS.)

BOX 6.13 Legal and Ethical Considerations

- Investigate the patient's expectations and beliefs; one can minimize risk of patients apportioning blame by establishing a trusting relationship.
- Provide care that is patient centered and respectful.
- Barriers to access and participation in care must be identified and addressed.
- Investigate culturally based treatment options and therapies to ensure safety and efficacy of treatment.
- Patients have a right to an interpreter. When language is a barrier, an interpreter enhances and authenticates communication.
- Document patient's use of culturally based therapies and patient's response to professional care, instructions, and recommendations, as well as the level at which the patient (or patient's social group) wants to be involved in the decision-making process.

personal beliefs and practices affecting any phase of care. It is important to recognize the legal and ethical responsibilities of documentation (Box 6.13), including compliance with state regulations and statutes and the federal Health Insurance Portability and Accountability Act (HIPAA). See Box 6.14 for a vignette of traditional care versus culturally sensitive care.

"If we are open and we prepare for promoting dialogue and love, and a better understanding of each other, and tolerance and so forth, that's what the world will become, a more tolerant, loving place."

Russell Simmons

BOX 6.14   Vignette of Traditional Care Versus Culturally Inclusive Care

Original Scenario—Cursed

A dental hygienist has an encounter with a young girl and her mother who recently arrived in the United States. The young child presents with poor oral health. The mother refuses to accept standard oral hygiene recommendations such as toothbrushing or flossing. The dental hygienist assumes that the mother sees little value in her child's primary teeth. Seeing no other option, the dental hygienist instructs the mother to bring the child back for prophylaxis services in 3 months, which the mother agrees to do. The family returns in 3 months for an evaluation, and not much has changed. The dental hygienist documents her findings in the chart.

Culturally Inclusive Approach—Cursed

A dental hygienist has an encounter with a young girl and her mother who recently arrived in the United States. The young child presents with poor oral health. The mother refuses to accept standard oral hygiene recommendations such as toothbrushing or flossing. On further questioning, the dental hygienist learns that the girl's family believes that child is cursed and that any items placed in her mouth will become a danger to family members who may touch them. Understanding their cultural context, the dental hygienist realizes that the only acceptable intervention is to allow the girl to use her own finger and commercial antimicrobial mouth rinse, which the family readily accepts. The family returns in 6 months for an evaluation, and the girl's oral hygiene has improved greatly. The dental hygienist documents her finding in the chart, including the family's cultural beliefs.

KEY CONCEPTS

- Culture is the set of behaviors learned for a person to adapt successfully to life within a particular group; it includes beliefs, traditions, experiences, customs, rituals, and language.
- Culture can be integral in oral care because an individual's conception of oral health, disease, and illness can be determined culturally.
- Culture can influence how people view their health and the healthcare services they receive. Clinicians should be aware of these potential differences and respect them. The parameters are set by the patient's values and beliefs, and clinicians have to work within them.
- Focusing on characteristics of cultural groups as the basis for culturally appropriate action can lead to stereotypes and risk of misunderstanding. Clinicians should strive to understand cultural practices of diverse groups by asking questions and avoiding assumptions.
- Cultural humility and competence are essential for the delivery of healthcare to achieve desired health outcomes.
- The clinician must respect differences in other people, including customs, thoughts, behaviors, communication styles, values, traditions, and institutions.

- Cultural humility starts with the clinician exploring his or her own beliefs and attitudes before assessing the individual patient. Clinicians must recognize their own cultural values and be able to identify biases, prejudices, and stereotypes that can prevent them from communicating effectively with patients from different cultural backgrounds.
- A culturally sensitive oral health professional regards all patients as unique and is aware of the fact that the patient's experiences, beliefs, values, and language can affect the perception of the clinical service delivery, diagnosis, and adherence.
- Many nonverbal behaviors associated with respect, genuine interest, and openness are appropriate for most patients regardless of their cultural background, even when a clinician's cultural knowledge is limited.
- Social determinants of health impact one's general and oral health status.
- The oral health professional has a responsibility to reduce barriers to improve access to care.

ACKNOWLEDGMENT

The authors wish to acknowledge Michele L. Darby, Devan L. Darby, and Ron J. M. Knevel for their past contributions to this chapter.

REFERENCES

1. Campinha-Bacote J. Cultural competemility: a paradigm shift in the cultural competence versus cultural humility debate—Part I. *Online J Issues Nurs.* 2019;24(1). Available at: http://ojin.nursingworld.org/MainMenuCategories/ANAMarketplace/ANAPeriodicals/OJIN/TableofContents/Vol-24-2019/No1-Jan-2019/Articles-Previous-Topics/Cultural-Competemility-A-Paradigm-Shift.html. Accessed August 30, 2022.
2. Vespa J, Median L, Armstrong D. *Demographic Turning Points for the United States: Population Projections for 2020 to 2060. [Internet]*; 2020. Available at: https://www.census.gov/content/dam/Census/library/publications/2020/demo/p25-1144.pdf. Accessed August 22, 2022.
3. U.S. Department of Health and Human Services. *HHS Action Plan to Reduce Racial and Ethnic Disparities: A Nation Free of Disparities in Health and Health Care.* U.S. Department of Health and Human Services, Office of Minority Health [Internet]; 2011. Updated 2020 Available at: https://www.minorityhealth.hhs.gov/assets/PDF/Update_HHS_Disparities_Dept-FY2020.pdf. Accessed September 6, 2022.
4. National Standards for Culturally and Linguistically Appropriate Services (CLAS) in Health and Health Care. U.S. Department of Health and Human Services Office of Minority Health Website. Available at: https://thinkculturalhealth.hhs.gov/CLAS/. Accessed August 28, 2022
5. Standards for Dental Hygiene Practice. *American Dental Hygienists Association Website*; 2017. Available at: www.adha.org/resources-docs/2016-Revised-Standards-for-Clinical-Dental-Hygiene-Practice.pdf. Accessed August 28, 2022.
6. Entry-to-Practice Canadian Competencies for Dental Hygienists. *Canadian Dental Hygienists Association*; 2021. Available at: https://www.cdho.org/docs/default-source/pdfs/standards-of-practice/epccodh_fdhrc_november_2021.pdf. Accessed August 28, 2022.
7. Accreditation Standards for Dental Hygiene Education Programs. *Commission on Dental Accreditation*; 2022. Available at: https://coda.ada.org/~/media/CODA/Files/dental_hygiene_standards.pdf?la=en.
8. *Health Inequality and Inequity Definition.* World Health Organization website; 2017. Available at: https://www.who.int/news-room/facts-in-pictures/detail/health-inequities-and-their-causes. Accessed August 28, 2022.
9. Stubbe DE. Practicing cultural competence and cultural humility in the care of diverse patients. *Focus.* 2020;18(1):49–51.
10. Cultural Competency Program for Oral Health Providers. U.S. Department of Health and Human Services Office of Minority Health Website. Available at: https://oralhealth.thinkculturalhealth.hhs.gov/. Accessed September 6, 2022.
11. Campinha-Bacote J. The process of cultural competence in the delivery of healthcare services: a model of care. *J Transcult Nurs.* 2002;13(3):181–184.
12. Cross TL, Bazron BJ, Dennis KW, Isaacs MR. *Toward a culturally competent system of care. Volume One: A Monograph of Effective Service for Minority Children Who Are Severely Emotionally Disturbed. CASSP Technical Assistance Center.* Georgetown University Child Development Center; 1989.

13. Goodman DJ. Cultural competence for equity and inclusion. *Understanding and Dismantling Privilege.* 2020;10(1):41–60.

14. Centers for Disease Control and Prevention website. Using a Health Equity Lens [Internet]. Available at: https://www.cdc.gov/healthcommunication/Health_Equity_Lens.html. Accessed September 6, 2022.

15. Berlin E, Fowkes WA. A teaching framework for cross-cultural health care. *West J Med.* 1983;139:934–938.

16. Riggio RE, Feldman RS. Introduction to Applications of Nonverbal Communication. *Applications of Nonverbal Communication;* 2005.

17. Prabhu T. Proxemics: some challenges and strategies in nonverbal communication. *IUP Journal of Soft Skills.* 2010;4(3).

7

Legal and Ethical Decision Making

Pamela Zarkowski

PROFESSIONAL OPPORTUNITIES

Understanding legal and ethical obligations in patient care and professional interactions provides a framework for written and oral communication, decision making, and record keeping and contributes to risk management. Dental hygienists who know the legal protections they are afforded as employees and employers will better understand their rights and responsibilities in an employment setting.

COMPETENCIES

1. Demonstrate an understanding of the dental hygiene codes of ethics and key ethical principles given ethical scenarios.
2. Apply the ethical decision-making framework to resolve ethical dilemmas encountered in practice.
3. Explain the ethical challenges of the dental hygienist-patient relationship, the dental hygienist-dental hygienist relationship, and the employer-employee relationship. Also, discuss the usage of a dental ethics committee.
4. Discuss and describe the basic legal concepts, contract and tort principles, and risk management strategies that affect oral health professionals.
5. Explain legal concepts in the dental hygienist-patient relationship, the dental hygienist-dentist relationship, and employer-employee relationship.
6. Suggest risk management strategies to reduce legal risks and liabilities of dental hygienists engaged in various roles.
7. Describe ethical dilemmas, legal issues, and roles of the dental hygienist as a dependent and independent clinical practitioner, independent contractor, administrator or manager, educator, consumer advocate, and public health professional.

FOUNDATIONS OF ETHICAL DECISION MAKING

Ethics Defined

Ethics is a branch of philosophy that deals with thinking about morality, moral problems, and moral judgments. Ethics is a concern for everyone because it forces the question of what people should do and why. A discussion of professional ethics relates to what is professionally right or conforms to professional standards of conduct. This definition reflects the traditional view of a profession as a group that determines its standards, writes its code of ethics, and regulates and disciplines its members. This traditional view is changing to include a broader perspective that argues professional ethics involves not merely what practitioners regard as custom but rather what the profession and society agree are appropriate rules of conduct. For example, the American Dental Hygienists' Association (ADHA) Code of Ethics[1] points out that a dental hygienist should not discuss a patient's medical condition with anyone without the individual's authorization. Another example found within the ADHA Code of Ethics is a statement that the dental hygienist should inform the patient of proposed care and allow the person to become involved in treatment decisions.

A code of ethics recognizes the following three relationships:

- Professional and client
- Professional and professional
- Professional and society

In dental hygiene, ethics focuses on the moral duties and obligations of the professional to patients, colleagues, and society.

Historically, society respected health professionals because they believed they followed codes of ethics and monitored their members. However, recurring charges of malpractice, impropriety, and fraud have projected the health professions into the arena of public concern and criticism. Consumers aware of inappropriate or perceived unethical behaviors contact professional organizations and licensing or regulatory agencies to express their concerns. Recognizing its importance, professional conferences and publications address professionalism, ethics, ethical decision making, and peer review issues. State boards of dentistry require continuing education courses in ethics and jurisprudence for licensure. Health profession associations regularly review their codes of ethics and professionalism policies to appropriately update them based on societal changes and provide guidance on emerging issues. Examples include social media use, cultural competence, and sustainability.

Legal obligations and ethical obligations are distinct. Promulgated by state or federal statutes, rules of conduct are obligatory customs or practices of a community (legal obligation). A dental hygienist must follow legal obligations or face the consequences. For example, a hygienist is obligated by both federal and state statutes not to discriminate against individuals belonging to certain classes or to sexually or ethnically harass another person. Such behaviors may result in legal action against the dental hygienist. Consequences for violating statutory laws include fines or imprisonment, depending on the severity of the violation.

Rules of conduct promulgated by the ADHA or the Canadian Dental Hygienists Association (CDHA)[2] serve as guidelines for conduct or ethical obligations. Both documents refer to the client in the broad sense as defined in the dental hygiene paradigm. The term *client* may refer to a patient undergoing patient care, a client-cotherapist relationship, a family, a community, or a population. A professional who violates an ethical code may frustrate a client or lose the respect of professional colleagues. Still, there may or may not be legal consequences. For example, the dental hygienist who refuses to provide care to individuals on Medicaid violates the ethical standard that suggests a provider should not discriminate, but there are no legal consequences.

Accountability and Responsibility

Accountability refers to people's ability to answer for their actions. Dental hygienists provide patient care and are accountable for their actions to themselves, their patients, the profession, employers, and society.

BOX 7.1 How to Maintain Professional Accountability

Self
- Report any conduct or conditions that endanger patients.
- Seek lifelong learning opportunities, stay informed, and practice current dental hygiene theory.
- Make judgments and evaluate based on evidence.
- Maintain current licensure and continuing education requirements

Client or Individual Patient
- Provide clients with thorough and accurate information about care.
- Conduct dental hygiene care in a manner that ensures client safety and well-being.
- Encourage respectful communication within a professional client–provider relationship.
- Be knowledgeable of state and federal laws protecting patients.

Profession
- Maintain ethical standards in practice.
- Encourage professional colleagues to follow the same ethical standards.
- Report colleagues' unethical behavior to appropriate peer review entities.

Employment Situation
- Remain current regarding state rules and regulations governing dental and dental hygiene practice.
- Follow employment setting policy and procedures.

Society
- Maintain ethical conduct in the care of all clients in all settings.
- Integrate sensitivity to diversity and cultural competency in patient care.

The purposes of professional accountability are as follows:
- Evaluate new professional practices and reassess existing ones
- Maintain standards of care
- Facilitate personal reflection, ethical thought, and personal growth on the part of health professionals
- Provide a basis for ethical decision making
- Demonstrate qualities important to professional status

Dental hygienists are accountable for dental hygiene care and do not rely on others to assume this responsibility (Box 7.1).

Fundamental Ethical Principles

The ethical principles that underlie healthcare are:
- Autonomy
- Beneficence
- Nonmaleficence
- Justice
- Veracity
- Fidelity

Autonomy is based on the principle of respect for persons. It is the belief that others should not constrain an individual's independent actions and choices. Individuals have a right to self-determination, that is, the freedom to make judgments based on their evaluations. Recognizing autonomy occurs when the dental hygienist involves the patient in decision making about their oral healthcare and obtains informed consent. A dental hygienist should provide all clients with understandable information about their oral health status and treatment options. To meet this obligation, a dental hygienist uses communication appropriate for the client's comprehension and competence level.

Beneficence is the provision of benefit, preventing evil or harm, removing evil or harm, or promoting good. A professional has a duty to help others by doing what is best for them. Acting on this principle, a professional is responsible for contributing to the health and welfare of others. Examples of benevolent actions include taking only necessary radiographs and maintaining equipment to prevent patient injury, such as replacing worn instruments, so that instrument tips do not break in a patient's mouth. A dental hygienist participating in a community-based oral cancer screening and referral program is another example of promoting good.

Nonmaleficence is summarized as "above all, do no harm." A dental hygienist seeks never to harm a client. An example of potential harm is when a dental hygienist is asked to provide treatment that they are not qualified to perform. A dental office allows the dental hygiene staff to offer tooth-bleaching treatments to patients. A dental hygienist, although not appropriately trained, provides the treatment. Due to a lack of expertise, the action may inflict harm and violate the principle of nonmaleficence.

Justice relies on fairness and equality. A person is treated justly when given what they are due, owed, deserve, or can legitimately claim. All clients receiving care should be treated equally. A dental hygienist who provides substandard care to persons in a nursing home because they are institutionalized is not treating all clients equally.

Veracity, truth telling or integrity, is critical to meaningful communication and relationships between individuals. Dental hygienists are obligated to be truthful with clients and associates. For example, a dental hygienist fails to tell a patient that during sealant application to tooth 19, the primary tooth anterior to tooth 19 fractured. A dental hygienist on a commission-based salary erroneously codes a procedure for insurance reimbursement to receive higher financial payment. The dishonest behavior is apparent in these situations.

Fidelity is the obligation to keep implied or explicit promises. A dental hygienist who says they will call the patient with additional information about dental implants and then follows through with that promise demonstrates fidelity.

Other core principles suggested in ethics forums warrant a brief review. *Societal trust* is a perception of the honesty, integrity, and reliability of others. Societal trust obligates the provider to follow a health profession's highest ideals and standards. *Confidentiality* requires a provider not to reveal information to a third party. *Integrity* is consistency in actions, values, methods, expectations, and outcomes.

Ethical principles are the foundation of legal obligations as well. Ethical principles and legal obligations discussed in this chapter will provide the dental hygienist with resources to provide ethically based care while meeting their professional duties (Box 7.2).

Codes of Ethics

The ADHA Code of Ethics[1] and the CDHA Code of Ethics[2] assist dental hygienists in achieving high ethical consciousness, decision making, and practice. The Codes describe the fundamental beliefs on the importance of oral health and the role of dental hygienists in preventing and treating oral diseases. The ADHA Code contains categories of Standards of Professional Responsibilities, a key section of the code. The categories begin by explaining the dental hygienist's responsibility to maintain personal health and well-being, competence, and a collaborative and safe work environment. Also highlighted are responsibilities to clients, colleagues, employees and employers, the dental hygiene profession, the community, society, and scientific investigation. The responsibilities within each category reflect themes, including professional obligations to contribute to society and the profession, communication with clients and colleagues, professional collaboration, and participation in advancing the profession. The responsibilities under each category provide a framework for reflection and guide the identification of a potential ethical concern or resolution of an ethical

Ethical principles provide the foundation for legal obligations.

Ethical Principle	Legal Obligation
<u>Autonomy:</u> respect for a client and their right to make informed decisions about their healthcare	• Duty to obtain informed consent • Duty to obtain informed refusal
<u>Beneficence:</u> preventing harm or removing harm; promoting good	• Following OSHA requirements for sterilization and disinfection
<u>Nonmaleficence:</u> acting to do no harm	• Practicing within the defined scope of practice and following the rules of the dental practice act in one's state or province
<u>Justice:</u> treating clients with equality and fairness	• Not discriminating in employment or patient care services; not harassing
<u>Veracity:</u> truth telling and demonstrating integrity	• Appropriately coding or not committing insurance fraud when billing for dental services
<u>Fidelity:</u> keeping promises	• Contractual arrangements are respected and not breached

OSHA, Occupational Safety and Health Administration.

dilemma. The CDHA Code outlines ethical principles and describes specific responsibilities. The CDHA Code describes ethical distress, ethical dilemmas, and ethical violations, and provides a framework for ethical decision making and guidelines for reporting ethical violations. Codes of ethics serve as an element of the self-policing responsibility of a profession. Code of ethics documents can be obtained from the ADHA[1] and the CDHA[2] websites.

ETHICAL PROBLEMS IN DENTAL HYGIENE

Ethical, moral, and legal issues interweave among the many dilemmas faced by dental hygienists. An **ethical dilemma** is a situation in which two ethical principles conflict, making it challenging to make a choice. Regardless of the dental hygienist's decision or actions, an ethical principle will be violated. Both ethical and legal issues may be encountered in a dilemma. The CDHA Code also addresses ethical distress. Ethical distress occurs when dental hygienists know or believe they know the right thing to do in a particular situation. However, they do not or cannot take the right actions or prevent particular harm for various reasons. For example, a dental hygienist observes signs of child abuse. The dental hygienist's employer forbids them from contacting the appropriate agency. This directive causes ethical distress. Because they are legally and ethically obligated, the dental hygienist reports the abuse, choosing ethical courage. Before a discussion about frequently encountered ethical dilemmas in different career situations, an ethical decision-making framework is introduced to assist dental hygienists in resolving dilemmas.

ETHICAL DECISION-MAKING FRAMEWORK

A dental hygienist may face various ethical dilemmas in the employment setting. Dilemmas occur in patient care situations or between an employee and employer. Ethical dilemmas occur in other professional settings including dental hygiene education, professional organizations, research, and community outreach settings. A provider must be prepared with a framework for resolving ethical dilemmas.[3] A six-step decision-making model is a valuable tool in providing guidance.

DEFINE THE CONFLICT OR DILEMMA

It is advisable to define precisely the problem or conflict creating the dilemma. Ethical or legal standards or a combination of ethical and legal principles may define the problem. Personal criteria may also determine the problem, moral code, or differences in philosophy, management style, or professional priorities. It is important to consider what ethical principles conflict. For example, it is vague to state that a conflict has arisen because of different educational backgrounds. It is more precise to identify the conflict as a lack of consistency in referring for biopsy or patient assessment techniques. An office does not refer suspicious lesions for biopsy. In that situation, they are not being truthful to the patient (veracity) and putting the patient in a potentially harmful situation by not doing something that benefits the patient (beneficence). Ethical dilemmas can be complex and involve legal obligations.

IDENTIFY THE ETHICAL ISSUES

What are the issues? Can one major issue be defined? For example, when a conflict exists between the dental hygienist's suggestion to refer to a specialist versus the dentist's refusal to support the request, the dilemma occurs between a professional obligation to follow the dentist's diagnosis and the dental hygienist's obligation to assess the patient's needs and provide high-quality care. From the patient's point of view, the referral may satisfy the patient's need for a specialist's evaluation and possible treatment. Suppose the dental hygienist's recommendation is incorrect. In that case, the second opinion creates an additional expense in time and money for the patient, resulting in conflict within the employment setting and a frustrated patient.

GATHER RELEVANT INFORMATION

When faced with an ethical dilemma, the dental hygienist must gather all relevant information (e.g., family status, age, lifestyle, habits, medical and dental facts, and patient values). Subjective and objective information is included to evaluate the evidence-based and human-based elements. As part of information gathering, the dental hygienist may want to reevaluate a patient's condition, research the evidence, investigate a diagnosis, or obtain a third opinion. If the dilemma is focused on an office protocol or policy, the dental hygienist may want to contact other healthcare providers, a lawyer, or a professional association representative to verify standard practices.

IDENTIFY THE ETHICAL ALTERNATIVES

A dental hygienist should consider more than one course of action. For example, in one situation, alternatives may include resigning from a position, confronting an employer, or calling the patient to express a concern or suggest a course of action. Each alternative may carry serious personal, financial, and professional implications for the dental hygienist and the patient.

In most situations, the list of alternatives considers the parties involved: the client, employer, supervising dentist, dental hygienist, and coworkers. When listing the alternatives, consider the following:
- Obligation(s) to the client (legal, professional, and ethical)
- Obligation(s) to others involved (patient's family, employer, colleagues)
- Personal beliefs and values
- Client's culturally based health beliefs and practices
- Client's or patient's legal rights, responsibilities, values, and interests
- Alternatives that protect the client's best interests
- Alternatives that protect the professional's best interests

- Alternatives that do the least amount of harm
- Practical constraints
- Professional judgment

ESTABLISH AN ETHICAL POSITION AND PRIORITIZE THE ALTERNATIVES

Each alternative requires evaluation using ethical and legal principles, personal and professional factors, and anticipated outcomes. For example, a patient at high risk of an adverse outcome from infective endocarditis refuses to premedicate with an antibiotic before an appointment. If the dental hygienist chooses an alternative that honors the patient's request, the ethical principle of autonomy is followed; however, ethically, the dental hygienist who treats a patient without appropriate premedication would potentially cause harm, violating nonmaleficence. In selecting the course of action, you may weigh which action promotes the best balance between the negative and positive aspects of the situation. The dental hygienist may also be at legal risk for an allegation of negligence and violating the standard of care.

Or you may evaluate the alternatives and choose the least negative alternative. For example, a dental hygienist chooses to balance their recommendations versus the dentist's decision not to refer a patient for a lesion biopsy, to schedule a follow-up appointment in 2 weeks, and reevaluate the lesion. The consequences may include a harmonious working relationship, an opportunity to study the pathology further, and the ability to keep open the possibility that in 2 weeks, both the dental hygienist and dentist can conduct a more informed assessment. The conflict may be internal with the parties involved, such as the dentist-employer. If you are resolved that the ethical choice is the correct one, however, identifying the consequences assists you in anticipating and preparing for implementing or acting on the choice.

SELECT, JUSTIFY, AND DEFEND THE PROVIDER'S CHOSEN ALTERNATIVE

Once you have evaluated the consequences of a choice and before you act on the choice, you should review the decision. What are the supporting ethical principles? Does the ADHA or CDHA Code address the issue or offer guidance? What might be a strong argument against the position? Identifying an argument, aside from an ethical position, which supports the decision is helpful. Evaluation at this stage assists the decision maker before the choice is implemented or acted upon. Individuals need to evaluate their decisions. It may be that the consequences are so harmful that another alternative or compromise might need to be considered.

ACT ON THE ETHICAL CHOICE

The dental hygienist takes the appropriate step to implement the chosen alternative to resolve the conflict or dilemma. Codes of ethics, dental practice acts, and state or provincial laws serve as guideposts for decision making and final choice (Box 7.3).

Clinical Practice

Dental hygienists may encounter ethical issues and dilemmas, including substandard care, unnecessary dental treatment; dental team members practicing outside the legal scope of practice; insurance fraud; violation of patient confidentiality; impaired professional colleagues; sexual, gender, or ethnic harassment; failure to report suspected abuse; incomplete health assessment; delegation to unqualified personnel; and substandard care. A dental hygienist may have a daily production quota, expecting a certain number of patients treated in a specific workday. A schedule with short appointments results in an inability to assess the patient and provide patient education appropriately and may result in poor quality care. The ethical principles of justice, beneficence, and fidelity are violated.

Failure to refer a patient to a periodontist occurs in dental hygiene care situations. For example, the dental hygienist responsible for patient assessment observes a deteriorating periodontal status. The dental hygienist's employer, a general dentist, chooses not to refer; however, the dental hygienist recognizes that the office staff's skill level cannot meet the patient's periodontal needs. The failure to inform the patient of the need for a periodontal referral depending on the facts may constitute an ethical dilemma and malpractice. The ADHA Code of Ethics speaks specifically to the responsibility to refer clients to other healthcare providers when the client's needs are beyond the dental hygienist's ability or scope of practice. Another ethical obligation is to advocate for clients' welfare; however, in some states, the dental hygienist cannot legally refer. Alternatives for solving the dilemma may include working to change office policy, educating colleagues about current referring guidelines, informing clients of their need to seek care in another office, or seeking another position. Each solution carries consequences such as upsetting the employer, frightening the client, performing an activity outside the scope of dental hygiene practice, or losing a valued position.

Consider the scenario when the dental hygienist-dentist team fails to detect dental disease. Perhaps a thorough assessment does not occur. The dental hygienist has the skills to assess the patient and record findings but is not given adequate time to fulfill those responsibilities. The dentist conducts a cursory dental caries examination, but other conditions such as periodontal disease, cancer, malocclusion, or temporomandibular joint dysfunction are ignored. Violation of the Code includes failing to provide optimal oral healthcare, compromising the public's confidence in members of the dental health profession, and failing to educate clients about quality oral healthcare.

The legal obligations include completing appropriate clinical examinations and following consistent referral protocols. Legal terminology generally uses the term *patient* rather than *client* in the healthcare provider-patient relationship. It is suggested that dental offices have a standard protocol for patients with medical and dental conditions that require evaluation and treatment beyond the scope of dental practice. Adherence to the protocol may protect the practitioner from malpractice. The office protocol should comply with the Americans with Disabilities Act, ensure that the patient is counseled and referred to an appropriate healthcare agency or provider, and ensure that consultations and referrals are documented in the services rendered section of the dental chart. The protocol should be used consistently with all patients (Box 7.4).

The use of social media may result in a violation of patient confidentiality. A dental hygienist discusses a patient's case on social media and seeks input from other colleagues about the management of the case. The information provided by the dental hygienist makes the patient easily identifiable. Patient confidentiality is compromised. Dental offices should have clear policies for staff regarding social media use pertaining to the office, colleagues, and patient care (Box 7.5). The policy should guide staff postings focusing on patients to prevent HIPAA or other privacy violations.

Public Health

Public health hygienists frequently face ethical problems because their decisions concern allocating limited resources and maximizing benefits for a large population. A dental hygienist must implement a dental sealant program for elementary school children. Funding is limited and therefore not all students can participate. How are the recipients selected? Should children receive the benefits of water fluoridation and also have the benefit of a dental sealant program? Or should children without access to water fluoridation or other fluoride therapies participate in the sealant program? With the knowledge that sealants are useful in preventing occlusal caries, children without the benefit of fluoridation are at a higher risk for developing smooth-surface dental

BOX 7.3 Example of the Ethical Decision-Making Process

Scenario

The dental hygienist works late one evening a week with a dentist. The dental hygienist notices that throughout the evening, the dentist steps into the laboratory and drinks from a small flask hidden in the laboratory, followed by using mouthwash and returning to treating patients. His care of patients does not appear compromised. He meets all the requests of the dental hygienist and the evening office hours run smoothly; however, the dental hygienist notes that the dentist's drinking behavior is repeated weekly. The dental hygienist questions the staff about the drinking. The staff indicates that they find him a great dentist, the office environment is good, they really like their jobs, and they don't want to lose them. They imply that they hope the dental hygienist will ignore the situation so everything will remain the same. Using the ethical decision-making framework, how would the dental hygienist use the model to assist in evaluating the decision?

Define the Conflict or Dilemma

The dental hygienist may find it personally offensive that a person is drinking on the job and providing patient care. The dental hygienist may feel that the quality of care the dentist provides is compromised by the drinking, thus violating the ethical mandate of providing the most comprehensive care available. There may be legal issues, such as negligent care provided by the dentist. There are also interpersonal issues with the staff members ignoring the situation and pressuring the dental hygienist to do the same. The problem is that the dentist drinks, provides patient care, and compromises patient safety and staff interaction. The dental hygienist's dilemma is whether or not to do something about the situation. Using the ethical decision-making model, the following should be considered.

Identify the Ethical Issues

A professional is responsible for protecting patients' well-being (nonmaleficence, beneficence). A dental hygienist must prioritize their responsibilities to the patient versus the staff's wishes to ignore the situation. Working with someone in an alcoholic state may affect patient care, decision making, and problem solving by the dentist (confidentiality, veracity).

Gather Relevant Information

Information gathering includes getting the following questions answered:
- Are other staff members witnessing the behavior?
- How long has the pattern existed?
- Does the drinking occur throughout the whole day?
- Have any untoward incidents been identified with the dentist's care or patient management? Has or is the dentist currently participating in alcohol rehabilitation?
- Is there a personal crisis in the dentist's life?

The dental hygienist should document their observations and those of others. The dental hygienist may want to investigate the types of services available to professionals with substance abuse problems. Perhaps a protocol is in place within the state dental society to work with the dentist to overcome this problem and maintain his professional status, or Alcoholics Anonymous may have information about programs. The dental hygienist may want to research alcoholism and the characteristics of an alcoholic to assist in confirming that a problem exists.

Identify the Ethical Alternatives

In this situation, alternatives may include the following:
- Discussing observations with the dentist involved
- Discussing and confirming observations with coworkers
- Confronting a single staff member to get additional support
- Discussing observations with others
- Ignoring the situation
- Contacting appropriate agencies, such as the dental association or state board
- Quitting the employment situation
- Refusing to work with the dentist
- Contacting the local dental hygiene or dental component for guidelines or advice
- Talking to peers to get ideas or solutions
- Consulting the Code of Ethics and the state statutes that govern practice

The Code requires the dental hygienist to follow the rules and regulations governing dental hygiene practice. Thus if a mandate requires the dental hygienist to report situations when patient care may be compromised, the alternative of choice is delineated. In most dilemmas, the ethical code helps generate alternatives for consideration.

Establish an Ethical Position and Prioritize the Alternatives

The dental hygienist should evaluate each alternative and weigh the ethical principles that impact each alternative and the personal and professional implications of choosing one alternative. As each alternative is identified, its advantages, disadvantages, and consequences are reviewed. The mental exercise of justifying and defending assists the dental hygienist in decision making and helps generate additional alternatives. The dental hygienist goes through a "what if" process and finishes the sentence. For example, seeking help from the local or state dental society may allow for intervention by a dentist colleague. Confronting the dentist may result in the dentist taking steps to address the problem or firing the dental hygienist. The consequences of each alternative must be considered and the alternative prioritized in rank order.

For this situation, the dental hygienist chooses to confront the dentist and offer information about counseling services available to persons with a drinking problem.

Select, Justify, and Defend the Chosen Alternative

The hygienist considers the decision in light of supporting ethical principles. In this case, the principles include beneficence, nonmaleficence, veracity, and confidentiality. The hygienist may also consider a strong argument against the position, such as the dentist's possible denial, or a consequence such as the dentist terminating the dental hygienist's employment rather than admitting a substance abuse problem. Evaluation of the alternatives is an ongoing part of the process.

Act on the Ethical Choice

The most difficult part is acting on the choice. In the best scenario, the dentist welcomes the identification of a problem and seeks counseling to overcome it. The worst scenario may be denial and an effort on the part of the dentist to dismiss the dental hygienist; however, the guiding ethical principle of nonmaleficence, the ADHA Code of Ethics, and genuine concern for fellow employees should strengthen the dental hygienist, whatever the consequences.

---

caries. Does socioeconomic status play a role in access to dental services? In this situation, the ethical standard of providing optimal oral healthcare using sound professional judgment to meet the oral health needs of the public guide decision making. Another ethical responsibility is access to oral health services for all, supporting justice and fairness in distributing healthcare resources. The dental hygienist may choose to maximize the preventive potential by using the funding for a sealant program in the fluoridated community. One outcome may reduce the incidence of caries in children living in the fluoridated community. Another outcome may be that the children at risk for caries without access to fluoride or dental sealants continue to be at risk.

Consider the situation of a dental hygienist employed by the state department of public health. The position's responsibilities include monitoring the quality and quantity of oral health services provided by different public health clinics throughout the state. State law prohibits dental hygienists from practicing unless a dentist is on the premises. The dental hygienist responsible is aware that dental hygienists treat patients in settings where a dentist is not always present. However, they are also aware that high-quality care within the dental hygienist's scope of practice is being offered to individuals in need. A legal and ethical dilemma exists. Should the dental hygienist at the local clinic continue care? Is it fair to discontinue services in specific communities because a

- Nondental personnel making treatment decisions
- Compromising or alternating patient care or populations served due to local or state politics

local clinic cannot afford to employ a dentist full time? To whom is the dental hygienist ethically responsible—the citizens of the state, the profession, or the state board? From a legal perspective, the dental hygienist is violating the law. The standard to advocate for the provision of care and prevention of dental disease can be used to argue that the dental hygienist is ethically meeting the obligation; however, ethical codes also direct dental hygienists to uphold the laws and regulations governing the profession. This dilemma is difficult. Unethical and illegal behavior cannot be justified. The dental hygienist coordinating the clinics should seek to remedy the situation legislatively or through creative strategies such as staffing alternatives and affiliation agreements with local dentists or clinics.

In another situation, the dental hygienist travels with a mobile dental clinic program throughout a metropolitan area, providing oral health education and preventive services to city residents. The program receives state funding to provide care for underserved populations. The dental hygienist has been a strong advocate of the program, a pilot project, as a model for other regions. The dental hygienist begins receiving telephone calls reporting that the dentist staffing the mobile clinic, deluged by many patients, is providing substandard care. The dental hygienist knows that reporting the dentist may discontinue services to a population in need. The dental hygienist could begin by discussing the complaint with the dentist and deciding how the situation might be rectified immediately. At the same time, the dental hygienist is obligated to document and report inadequate or substandard care. Ultimately, the dental hygienist must protect the patients and stop inadequate care. Suppose patient care cannot be improved immediately by intraprofessional collaboration between the dentist and the dental hygienist care coordinator. In that case, solutions to the dilemma may include working with a local dental society or dental school to assist in staffing the clinic until a replacement dentist is identified.

Other examples of ethical problems in public health may include the following:
- Misuse of funds supporting items other than patient care

Administration and Management

Administrators, whether in educational or business-based organizations, face ethical dilemmas. A patient visits a dental hygiene clinic for care. The patient refuses to be treated by a specific student and makes unpleasant comments about the student's ethnic background. The administrator is obligated to protect the student and provide a harassment-free and safe learning environment. At the same time, the reputation of the dental hygiene program to willingly treat all persons in the community must be maintained. The administrator may educate the patient about their rights and responsibilities or dismiss the patient and refer them to another provider. In some instances, institutional protocol guides the administrator in choosing a particular option, or the institution may seek the advice of institutional legal counsel.

In another example, dental hygiene students are assigned to provide nonsurgical periodontal therapy at an urban hospital-based clinic. The patients treated at the clinic are at high risk for acquired immunodeficiency syndrome (AIDS). The dental hygiene program director is aware that there is always the possibility of a puncture wound occurring, with the result that a contaminated instrument may injure a dental hygiene student. Does the director choose not to have students assigned to the clinic? Should the students be informed of the risk? The situation may create a dilemma in some settings, but using the principle that all individuals should be treated without discrimination and the knowledge that students are using the appropriate standard of care, all students should be assigned.

An administrator also deals with ethical problems among colleagues. The administrator is asked to evaluate the faculty for merit salary raises. Not all faculty members contribute equally to the department. One tenured faculty member fulfills the minimum responsibilities; however, if that faculty person's raise is not comparable to others' raises, they may contribute even less and accuse the administrator of discrimination. Some less-productive faculty members may decide to quit, leaving those remaining with the burden of heavier workloads. Does the administrator recognize all the faculty members as equally meritorious? Is there an obligation to report weaker faculty contributions to the administration? What obligation exists to those who are most productive? The administrator must identify the problem and evaluate the alternatives with the questions raised. One solution is to suggest a merit raise for the weak faculty person, then structure that faculty member's obligations to improve their productivity. The consequences include other faculty members' lowered morale when all faculty members receive merit raises, although not all are justified.

Research

Informal research occurs in practice when a dental hygienist surveys patients' attitudes, evaluate their acceptance of products and procedures, or compiles salary survey data. Dental hygienists are also involved in research conducted at educational institutions or with an oral health product manufacturer.

Perhaps a dental hygienist is conducting research to evaluate the effectiveness of a chemotherapeutic agent on selective pathogenic and nonpathogenic microorganisms. The manufacturer is providing funding for the research. The dental hygienist discovers that although the research design is valid, the coinvestigator allows personal bias to influence observations and interpretations. Both are aware that if the research establishes the chemotherapeutic agent as effective, the pharmaceutical company that produces the agent will provide generous funding in the future. Should the dental hygienist confront the coinvestigator? Should the dental hygienist ignore the unethical and illegal behavior of the coinvestigator? Knowing that research is replicated, should the dental hygienist ignore what has occurred and assume that followup research will reveal the flaws of the current research?

Other examples of ethical problems in research include:
- Individuals who steal another's idea or concept
- Individuals who take credit for a colleague's success in research
- Manipulation of data
- Intentional bias in sampling and failure to report research that does not support or confirm a hypothesis
- Misuse of funds or resources

COLLEAGUE RELATIONSHIP ETHICAL CHALLENGES

Dental Hygienist–Dentist-Patient Relationships

The dental employment setting involves numerous relationships that present ethical dilemmas. One of the most challenging and frequent problems is when the dental hygienist and dentist disagree on the oral healthcare required by a patient. A dental hygienist observes signs of cancerlike soft tissue changes during the patient's assessment. The dental hygienist suggests that the lesion be biopsied. The dentist disagrees. The dental hygienist feels a responsibility to the patient that conflicts with that of the dentist. Does the dental hygienist express concern to the patient? Should the dental hygienist identify another dentist in the office for a second opinion? Should the dentist's decision stand? The dental hygienist considers all the alternatives and chooses one that supports ethical principles. If the dental hygienist seeks another dentist in the office to evaluate the patient, the dental hygienist may be satisfied with a second opinion. The consequences can include an unhappy dentist and a frightened patient; however, if a biopsy is performed, the personal and professional satisfaction gained by the dental hygienist and the outcome of the biopsy on the patient's health outweighs the other consequences. Conflicts between the dental hygienist and dentist are not easily solved.

Dental hygienists are subject to the employer's policies and procedures. When policies and procedures dictate that the dental hygienist is allowed 45 minutes for all patient appointments, that care must be completed in one appointment, or that everyone gets a "routine oral prophylaxis," the dental hygienist is forced to provide substandard care. Should the dental hygienist work within the policies, ignoring the quality of care standard? Does the dental hygienist leave the position? It may be difficult to quit because of location, salary, and benefits. Does the dental hygienist inform the patient that care is limited and recommend referral for a second opinion? Or does the dental hygienist attempt to provide optimal care and work more diligently? The preemployment process should address issues about patient care, length of time allotted for care, referral protocols, and other work expectations. If issues arise after employment, the dental hygienist may resolve the concerns by scheduling an appointment with the employer or as part of an employee evaluation process, whichever occurs earliest.

Conflicts arise when a patient refuses specific treatment, decides to ignore a referral, or continues an unhealthy practice. What ethical obligations does the dental hygienist have to the patient and the employer?

A patient decides based on information. Some ethical dilemmas created by patient actions or failure to act could be eliminated if the patient were given an appropriate amount of information. With overly brief appointments, ill-informed or uncommunicative staff members cannot adequately educate clients. Education and service should remain priorities and should guide office practice and policies.

Other examples of ethical problems in dental hygienist–dentist-patient relationships may include:
- Ethnic, gender, gender identity, or racial harassment of staff, vendors, or clients
- Office staff practicing outside the defined scope of practice
- Inappropriate use of social media
- Violation of appropriate business practices (i.e., denying a patient a copy of their dental records)
- Bullying by dental suppliers, staff, supervisors, and patients
- Patient requests to commit insurance fraud

Dental Hygienist-Dental Hygienist Relationships

Working in an environment where a colleague's care is below the acceptable standard is challenging. For example, the dental hygienist colleague may be compromising patient care by not thoroughly assessing the patient or may be performing services beyond the scope of dental hygiene care. Situations affecting the patient's care or health status create an immediate dilemma. Do you report the activity to the employer, regulatory boards, or the ethics board of the professional association? Do you attempt to educate or update the colleague? Or do you ignore the situation, assuming it is the employer's responsibility?

Talking with the dental hygienist in question may be the best alternative. The dental hygienist may be unaware of the quality of care issues or illegal activities. Respectfully confronting individuals while offering solutions to the problem is a step toward resolution. Other solutions may include a staff in-service session reviewing the dental practice act, attending a continuing education class, or developing a dental hygiene office manual outlining specific roles and responsibilities.

Employer-Employee Relationships

Various professional, personal, and business relationships coexist in a dental or dental hygiene practice or other work environments. An employment situation may present dilemmas for the dental hygienist. As an employee, you may suspect that an employer is sexually harassing a colleague, that insurance fraud occurs during billing procedures, or that a colleague has a substance abuse problem. Is it the dental hygienist's responsibility to act, or the dentist owner of the practice? Should the dental hygienist be concerned about ethical and legal violations? Do you address the issue with the offending practitioner? What if after the problem is addressed, no change occurs? It is especially frustrating when you recognize that the dental hygienist is expected to practice within the ADHA or CDHA Code of Ethics but is not in control of the work environment.

The ADHA Code of Ethics says to participate in the development and advancement of the profession. Many dental hygienists are not members of their professional association. Are dental hygienists not members of the association aware of the Code of Ethics? Is it the ethical obligation of a dental hygienist who is a member to encourage nonmembers to join the professional association? As a professional association member, a dental hygienist has access to scientific literature, continuing education courses, and other resources. Should these items be shared with nonmember dental hygiene colleagues? Each question raises multiple ethical dilemmas. The Code of Ethics encourages a work environment that promotes individual growth and development. Educating nonmember dental hygienists about the association or sharing new knowledge or expertise supports the professional development philosophy.

Dental Ethics Committee

Dental professionals must use ethical principles and codes to resolve an ethical dilemma. Establishing a dental ethics committee (DEC) for the office is one action to facilitate ethical decision making.[4] The DEC could identify dilemmas, use the ethical decision-making model and existing codes of ethics for dental hygienists and dentists for in-service and discussion to address concerns, and create a team approach to resolve difficult issues. Guidelines could be developed for the DEC, outlining its purposes, functions, and membership. Staff meetings could periodically include the DEC as one of the agenda items. A committee approach assists in raising issues of concern to all office members and educates staff members about ethical decision making. This approach encourages an ethics-based office philosophy.

LEGAL CONCEPTS

Oral Health Professionals at Risk

Patients have become sophisticated consumers of high-quality healthcare that is accessible and reasonably priced. Therefore an individual dissatisfied with oral healthcare frequently looks to the legal system for assistance. Malpractice suits against dental professionals have consistently become more prevalent (Box 7.6).

Common malpractice litigation includes accusations of the following:
- Violation of standard of care, negligence
- Failure to treat problems related to temporomandibular joint disease
- Failure to diagnose, refer, or treat periodontal disease
- Failure to detect oral pathology
- Failure to obtain informed consent
- Use of defective products
- Abandonment of the patient
- Failure to identify and protect a person with a medically compromising condition, such as a heart murmur or drug allergy
- Failure to maintain proper records
- Incorrect medical or dental history taking; medical history not updated
- Failure to meet the standard of care, administering improper treatment

Oral health professionals are governed by statutory laws enacted by legislators, administrative laws (regulations) promulgated by regulatory boards, and common law or case law determined by judicial decisions in court cases (Fig. 7.1). Each governing body affects the practice of dental hygiene. Sanctions for violations exist, and a practitioner who

---

BOX 7.6 Are You Contributing to Potential Malpractice Situations or Illegal Dental Hygiene Practice?

It is not my responsibility to report violators of the dental practice act. I assume that it is someone else's responsibility.

I sometimes treat patients with severe periodontal disease for years rather than refer them.

If I run late on my schedule, I may not update a patient's health history.

There is probably a procedure or two that a dental assistant performs in my office that is not allowed under state law.

Before treating a patient, I rarely explain the reason for the procedure or the risks involved because it takes too much time.

If a patient insists, we do not always premedicate an individual who should have appropriate antibiotics before treatment.

I sometimes talk about my patients on Facebook after a bad day at work.

If a dentist asks me to do something that I know is illegal, I should do it because the dentist will get sued, not me.

I may eliminate the name from my continued-care list if I dislike a patient.

If you checked any of these statements, you or your patients are at risk.

---

violates a particular rule may be adjudicated under multiple governing bodies. The professional is presumed to know all the rules and regulations influencing practice and cannot claim ignorance of the law.

For example, a dental hygienist who administers nitrous oxide–oxygen analgesia in a state that restricts dental hygiene to traditional practice has violated the rules and regulations outlined by the state regulatory board and may, based on a review by the board, have their license revoked or suspended. If harm results, the individual may be charged with a civil violation, such as negligence. In addition, there may be allegations of a criminal violation, specifically administering drugs without a license, depending on state and local statutes, resulting in court action or fines. A dental hygienist must know the rules and regulations governing dental hygiene practice in the jurisdiction where licensing is maintained.

Basic Legal Concepts

The **law** is divided into civil and criminal categories. Although these categories are separate, a person can be accused of both a civil and a criminal violation simultaneously.
- **Civil law** includes offenses for violating private or contractual rights or, in simpler terms, a breach of legal duty against a person. A violation against a person is purported to have occurred in a civil lawsuit. The remedy that a person seeks is to be "whole" because some damage has occurred, and how the person is made whole is to receive monetary damages.
- **Criminal law** is established to prevent harm to society and describes a criminal act and the appropriate punishment. In a criminal lawsuit, the individual found guilty is punished based on society's rules and regulations. Fines, prison terms, or other penalties are based on the specific criminal violation.

Two distinctly different levels of proof are used to determine innocence or guilt:
- The level of proof required for a criminal act is beyond a reasonable doubt. To meet the level of proof, a jury or judge must be convinced that the criminal act occurred to establish guilt. If they are not absolutely convinced, an individual must be found innocent.
- A civil action requires a less strict level of proof, called a **preponderance of evidence.** Based on the evidence presented, this level requires the jury or judge to be 51% certain that someone is guilty or innocent. For example, a dental hygienist committed an error during patient care. If the jury or judge is 51% sure that the error caused harm, the dental hygienist will be liable.

The requirement of a preponderance of evidence to prove guilt or innocence is weaker than a requirement of proof beyond a reasonable doubt. Professional malpractice suits filed against oral health professionals are usually in the civil arena; therefore the level of proof required is a preponderance of evidence. Understanding the proof required for civil lawsuits assists in explaining how dental hygienists or dentists are found guilty or innocent when charges are filed against them.

Parties in a lawsuit include the plaintiff(s) and the defendant(s). In a legal dispute, the **plaintiff** is the person who brings the action or files the suit; the **defendant** is the person denying the action charged.

Contract Principles and Relationships

Malpractice lawsuits are civil. A common concept of liability used in dental malpractice lawsuits is **breach of contract** (i.e., failure to perform a promise). Business transactions come to mind when people think of a contract violation rather than oral healthcare. Applications of the breach of contract concept were initially limited to business transactions; however, society has become more consumer oriented, and the courts now recognize the dentist-patient relationship as a contract.

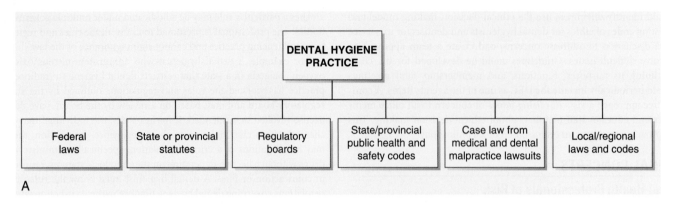

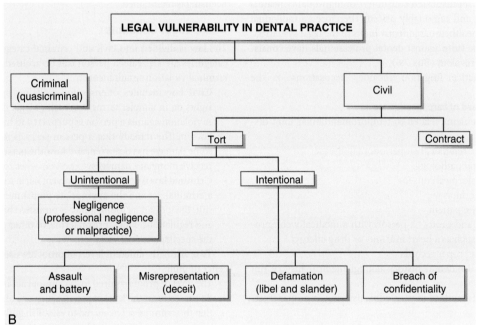

Fig. 7.1 (A) Diagram of governing bodies affecting the practice of dental hygiene. (B) Diagram of legal vulnerability in dental practice. (B, Redrawn from Pollack B. *Risk Management Manual*, Fort Lauderdale, Fla, 1986, National Society of Dental Practitioners.)

A legal definition states that a contract is an agreement between two or more consenting and competent parties to do or not to do a legal act for which there is sufficient consideration. **Consideration** is exchanging something of value, such as money, between two people.[5] The contractual relationship between the oral health practitioner and the patient is one of the following two types:

- An **implied contract** can begin in several situations, including the performance of a professional act, such as taking radiographs or expressing a professional opinion. Although there is no written document of agreement in an implied contract, a contractual relationship exists.
- An **express contract** is one in which the terms are expressed and includes either a verbal or a written agreement.

The **contract**, whether written or oral, may outline specific conditions or obligations that must be satisfied by the patient or oral healthcare provider, such as fees, method of payment, or type of services to be provided. In addition, both parties require certain warranties or duties based on the contractual relationship. The word **duty** in legal vernacular means obligatory conduct or service or conducting oneself in a particular manner. Professionals in the legal system evaluate medical malpractice case law to determine the contractual rights and duties shared between the practitioner and the patient based on the

contractual relationship. Based on that contractual relationship, in accepting the patient for care, the oral healthcare provider promises to do the following:[6]

- Be properly licensed and registered and meet all other legal requirements to engage in the practice of dentistry or dental hygiene
- Use reasonable care in providing services as measured against acceptable standards set by other practitioners with similar training
- Never exceed the scope of practice
- Not use experimental procedures or medications
- Complete care within a reasonable time frame or arrange other sources of treatment when appropriate to complete treatment
- Never abandon the patient by abruptly stopping oral healthcare
- Obtain informed consent from the individual or the party responsible (i.e., guardian) before examination or treatment
- Arrange care for the patient during an absence and ensure that care is available in emergencies
- Make appropriate referrals and request necessary consultations
- Maintain patient privacy and confidentiality of information
- Maintain a level of knowledge in keeping with current advances in the profession
- Keep patients informed of their treatment progress and health status
- Inform the patient of unanticipated occurrences

- Never permit any person acting under another's direction to engage in unlawful acts
- Keep accurate records of the care provided to the patient
- Comply with all laws regulating the practice of dentistry and dental hygiene
- Practice in a manner consistent with the code of ethics of the profession
- Charge a reasonable fee for services based on community standards
- Not attempt a procedure for which the practitioner is unqualified

The duties or warranties listed are enforceable, although not written or stated in any document given to the patient. Legal obligations can intersect with ethical obligations. A dental hygienist who uses experimental periodontal therapy rather than evidence-based procedures may be violating a contractual responsibility to use only standard procedures. A dental hygienist who casually discusses confidential information during the health history interview violates a contractual obligation, ignoring the principle of fidelity and committing a breach of confidentiality. A dental hygienist practicing outdated techniques also violates a duty to remain current and ignores the principle of beneficence.

The patient has contractual duties, including cooperating in care, providing accurate information, paying fees, and keeping appointments. Practitioners encounter patients who do not pay fees. Collection procedures may result from the patient's failure to meet the contractual obligation. Failing to cooperate in care, such as missing appointments or refusing to take premedication, does not necessarily result in a lawsuit filed by the dentist. Rather than filing a lawsuit, the practitioner may choose to dismiss the patient from the practice.

If a breach of contract occurs, the patient can use the contract concept to remedy the situation and obtain damages. Perhaps a patient discovers that a dental assistant, not a dental hygienist, is providing root planing, which only a licensed dental hygienist can perform. The assistant did not harm the patient; however, the dentist warranted, based on the contractual relationship between the dentist and patient, that employees within the office were properly licensed and that the staff would never exceed the scope of practice. In this example, three violations occurred and a breach of contract exists. At the same time, if the patient has not met obligations, such as keeping an appointment, that patient has breached the contract. Although the practitioner would probably not seek damages in this situation, the failure of the patient to meet their responsibilities (**contributory negligence**) may be a reason to end the practitioner-patient relationship.

Terminating the Practitioner-Patient Relationship

Termination of the practitioner-patient relationship frequently occurs in practice; however, the practitioner must be cautioned never to abandon the patient. **Abandonment** is a relinquishment of all connection with the patient. The relationship between professional and patient may end without charges of abandonment if the following conditions are met:

- Both parties agree to end it.
- The death of the patient or oral health practitioner occurs.
- The patient ends the relationship by act or statement.
- The patient is cured or treatment is completed, as with a specialist.
- The practitioner unilaterally decides to terminate care.

If the practitioner seeks to end the relationship, the following specific steps are necessary:

- The patient should receive written notification of termination and the reasons (e.g., lack of payment for services rendered or nonadherence to recommended care).
- The reason for termination should be provided in objective language. If a patient is terminated because of harassing behaviors,

the letter does not have to describe the specific behaviors. Instead, the letter can indicate that the dentist is terminating the relationship because of "disrespectful attitudes and behaviors toward staff." Another reason may be noncompliance impacting the prognosis.
- The letter should state that the individual will remain a patient of the practice for a certain length of time, the date services will be terminated, and that if necessary, emergency care will be provided for a designated period.
- The letter must suggest that the patient seek another dental care provider and state that copies of the patient's records will be forwarded to the new provider. Indicate if a fee is associated with acquiring a copy of the patient's records. It is advisable to include a permission slip to transfer records that the patient can sign and return to expedite the process (Fig. 7.2).
- The termination process is done carefully to ensure continuity of care and diminish the possibility of charges of abandonment. The letter should be sent by certified or registered mail with the return receipt requested. A copy of the termination letter and return receipt should be kept in the patient's file.

Avoiding charges of abandonment becomes an issue in dental hygiene care when patients of record do not respond to a continued-care notice. Although office procedures may not require that an individual receive notification that they are no longer a patient of record, actions such as written notification should be taken.

Another example of a situation that may require termination of the practitioner-patient relationship is when the patient refuses necessary oral radiographs or prophylactic antibiotic premedication to prevent infective endocarditis. Rather than jeopardize the quality of care, the dental hygienist may dismiss the patient of record from the practice. Again, written notification of termination is necessary to protect the dental hygienist and the employer from abandonment charges.

Related Responsibilities

A practitioner may refuse to treat a patient. The justification for refusal may include that the provider does not feel competent to provide the care. A dental office may refer patients for prosthodontic care to another office. However, an office cannot deny treatment to a patient if the reason is based on race, creed, color, national origin, or certain conditions such as a disability. For example, a practice specializing in prosthodontic care may refuse to accept children as patients. As long as there is no discriminatory reason such as ethnic origin, not accepting children as patients is legal. An office that fails to schedule individuals with Hispanic-sounding surnames, however, is discriminating based on national origin.

Dental hygienists should obtain information about the rules and regulations governing the care of patients within their state to avoid charges of discrimination. Different jurisdictions (states, commonwealths, provinces) have defined special groups with specific statutory implications relating to civil rights and discrimination. For example, in some states, statutes pertaining to the rights of the disabled protect persons with human immunodeficiency virus (HIV) infection. Other states offer protection based on marital status, height, weight, or gender identity.

A practitioner can refuse to treat a patient of record and not violate a contract obligation. A practitioner should refuse to treat a patient if they are not competent to provide the appropriate standard of care. Without the necessary skills, the practitioner is expected to refer the patient to the appropriate oral health provider. If a certain skill level is required to provide the appropriate treatment (e.g., root planing and periodontal surgery) and those skills are not present in the personnel of that practice, the practitioner has failed to meet the obligation to refer. Lawsuits have resulted from practitioners attempting to provide

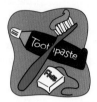

Fisher Lake Dental Group

1952 Glen

Lakeshore, MI 48111

September 27, 2022

Mr. Daniel Powers
12214 Yale Rd.
Point Park, MI 48000

Dear Mr. Powers:

Our records indicate that you have filed to respond to six notices for periodontal maintenance care. Notices have been forwarded from this office for 4 years from 2018-2022, requesting that you schedule an appointment for an examination and oral maintenance. Your lack of responses to both the mail and telephone messages suggests that you disagree with our preventive philosophy. Effective October 27, 2022, your relationship with this office will be terminated. Dr. Jones will be available to treat any emergency you have for the next 30 days, provided that you call the office and schedule an appointment.

I encourage you to seek regular care from another dentist and dental hygienist. The office will forward a copy of your records once that practitioner is identified. Enclosed is a permission slip to transfer your records. Please return the signed and dated copy to the office to allow for the release of your records to your new provider.

Thank you.

Mary L. Mesial, RDH, BS, MSDH

cc: Patient record

Fig. 7.2 Letter of protection, terminating dental hygienist-patient relationship.

care beyond the practitioner's level of competence. Perhaps a dental hygienist evaluates the patient's periodontal health and, although referral is indicated by the condition presented, the dentist chooses to provide treatment. The referral is not viewed as discriminatory but is the appropriate action under contract principles.

Tort Principles

The negligence principle is the legal basis most commonly used by patients to file a lawsuit against healthcare providers. Negligence falls within the category of law known as *torts*. A **tort** interferes with another's right to enjoy person, property, or privacy.[5] Categories of torts are as follows:
- Intentional torts
- Unintentional torts

Intentional Torts

Intentional torts are committed with intent on the part of the person. Intentional torts include battery, assault, false imprisonment, mental

distress, breach of confidentiality, interference with property (e.g., trespassing on private property), and misrepresentation or deceit. Professional liability insurance frequently covers only the unintentional tort of negligence. Intentional torts require that the person accused of the tort intended the harm that occurred. An intentional tort is a serious offense. Some intentional torts of interest to dental hygienists are discussed in the following paragraphs.

An **assault**[5] occurs when someone intends to cause apprehension in another person without touching them. An example of an assault may be threatening someone with a raised hand. A practitioner who threatens to harm someone or causes fear may be guilty of assault, as in the example, "If you do not sit still, I am going to stick you with the needle."

A **battery**[5] is harmful or offensive contact with someone—touching someone without their permission (e.g., restraining a child without parental permission). A **technical battery**[7] is when a dental hygienist, in the course of treatment, exceeds the consent given by the patient. It is described as intentional touching without permission. The person bringing the charges, the plaintiff, does not have to prove that the provider intended any harm. Examples of technical battery include placing dental sealants on teeth or giving a fluoride treatment to a child without the parent's consent. In such cases, the plaintiff argues that the contact was offensive, and the dental hygienist (defendant) could be charged with technical assault and battery. Assault and battery are considered intentional torts, and professional liability insurance may not provide coverage for charges filed under these categories. The dental hygienist should obtain informed consent to prevent accusations of assault and battery. (Informed consent is discussed later in the section.)

Deceit or **misrepresentation** can occur in the provision of oral healthcare. An example of deceit is a failure to inform a patient that an instrument tip has broken and is lodged in the sulcus. A practitioner must always educate patients on their oral healthcare status and not misrepresent the services rendered. If a dental hygienist is ill and a dental assistant substitutes, there is an intent to misrepresent the dental assistant as a dental hygienist, and the employer is guilty of an intentional tort.

Another tort that could be classified as intentional is a **breach of confidentiality**. A dental hygienist who violates the confidential relationship between the dental hygienist and the patient is committing a tort. Discussing a patient's history over lunch with a friend violates confidentiality between the practitioner and the patient. The confidential relationship is violated if a dental hygienist responds to a request for patient information without obtaining the patient's permission.

Unintentional Torts and Negligence

Unintentional torts are not intended by the person accused of committing the tort. Negligence and dental malpractice are used synonymously. **Negligence**[5] is a failure of a person who owes a duty to another to do what a reasonable and prudent person would ordinarily have done under the circumstances. The defining characteristics of negligence are the following:

- A duty or standard exists (e.g., health history taking, determining blood pressure levels, assessing periodontal health, recording oral health status, referral).
- A breach or failure to exercise requisite care occurs (e.g., failing to assess and/or treat the patient, failing to meet the standard of care for dental hygiene practice, incorrectly using anesthesia).
- A harm results (e.g., medical emergency, periodontal status declines, paresthesia develops).
- The breach of duty directly causes harm.

The plaintiff's responsibility is to prove that the defendant was negligent. The plaintiff must prove all of the elements listed previously by a preponderance of the evidence. For example, a dental hygienist places dental sealants on a child's teeth. The treatment area is typical, with the operator's supplies on the dental bracket tray. The supplies include a receptacle with acid etch material. The dental hygienist is etching the teeth while holding the acid etch–filled container. The child suddenly moves, the acid etch spills on the child, and a chemical burn occurs on the side of the child's face. Has negligent behavior occurred? You would need to evaluate the elements of negligence to answer the question. The dental hygienist did not intend to burn the child; however, a duty existed to be careful while applying the acid etch solution. For the most part, the dental hygienist was practicing cautiously; however, evidence may indicate that keeping the acid etch solution away from the child is recommended to avoid spilling. The dental hygienist failed to use certain precautionary measures (reasonably prudent person rule), and harm resulted. The dental hygienist's actions proximately caused the harm, and thus the hygienist is found negligent by a judge or a jury. The jury or judge must be only 51% sure (weight of the evidence) that the dental hygienist's actions caused the harm. The jury or judge may

recognize that the child's actions influenced what occurred but may still find the dental hygienist negligent.

Another example of negligent behavior is if a dental hygienist leaves infection control chemical (like those used to clean suction units) in a cup on a counter. If, when the dental hygienist is away from the treatment room, a patient mistakes the liquid for water or mouthrinse and drinks it, harm occurs, although there was no intent to harm the client.

Standard of Care

Standard of care[5] is the degree of care a reasonably prudent professional would exercise under the same or similar circumstances. The standard of care is not defined by the courts but rather, is determined by members of the profession. In negligence actions, expert witnesses are called to testify to explain the standard of care and determine if the defendant is guilty or innocent. (A lawyer may seek information from a professional association, such as the ADHA or CDHA, professional literature, or a nationally recognized group, such as the Centers for Disease Control and Prevention, as a source of acceptable standards.)

Lawyers for both the plaintiff and defendant may call expert witnesses who best satisfy their arguments in court. An expert witness is a member of the defendant's professional group with a similar background (e.g., in a periodontal malpractice lawsuit, a dental hygienist working in a periodontal practice). Therefore the dental hygienist, who may be defending specific actions, may identify an expert witness to support the standard of care demonstrated by that dental hygienist's practices. The plaintiff also has an expert witness testify that the dental hygienist did not meet the acceptable standard of care. The decision of liability rests with the jurors and judge using the preponderance of evidence as the standard of proof.

After listening to the expert witnesses' testimony, jurors decide whether the plaintiff was negligent. If there is a failure to meet that standard as determined by the jurors or a judge, the dental hygienist may be found negligent. For example, a dental hygienist fails to monitor and record a patient's blood pressure before care. During treatment, the patient experiences a cardiac arrest related to high blood pressure. The standard of care for dental hygiene includes taking and recording blood pressure as part of patient assessment. The dental hygienist failed to meet the standard.

The failure to meet the standard of care can include the following:
- An act of omission (i.e., not doing something)
- An act of commission (i.e., performing an act inappropriately)

Omitting a procedure or step because you are unaware that it is the current standard is not an acceptable excuse in a court of law.

Dental hygienists must practice the concepts and techniques currently accepted (i.e., to meet the standard of care). Although in most jurisdictions, the dentist is ultimately responsible for the actions of the dental hygienist, the dental hygienist still may be found negligent in a court of law if a required duty is not met. Dental practitioners may be negligent when harm is caused to the patient due to failure to stay current. It is difficult for any dental professional to accept a verdict of negligence because there is no intent on the professional's part to provide inadequate care; however, members of the legal system attempt to evaluate the facts objectively. They evaluate the actions of the practitioners and then assess the impact of those actions on the patient. If harm occurs, the legal system decides who is at fault and awards damages, if appropriate.

Informed Consent

Another legal argument that falls within the negligence theory used in lawsuits against practitioners is the lack of informed consent. **Informed consent** is a person's agreement to allow something to happen based on full disclosure of facts required to make an intelligent decision; consent is the individual's right to self-determination. As part of the consent process, patients must be informed of the material risks involved in care. Obtaining informed consent cannot be delegated to an assistant; it is the professional's responsibility to obtain consent.

A material risk is one that a "reasonable person" would consider in determining whether to proceed with the proposed treatment. Court decisions have determined that the patient has the final say in their care, the patient must be of sound mind when giving consent, and the consent must be informed to be valid.[5]

To achieve informed consent, clients must be told, in a language that they understand, the following information:

- Diagnosis of the condition
- Recommended procedure
- Nature and reasons for the procedure
- Benefits of the procedure
- Material risks in performing the procedure
- Prognosis if the procedure is performed or not performed
- Alternatives to the recommended procedure
- Risks and benefits of the alternative procedures
- Potential consequences if the patient does not choose the recommended procedure (Fig. 7.3)

In lawsuits that focus on violating the duty to obtain informed consent, specific issues arise. A patient claims a lack of understanding of the risks involved in the care or that treatment alternatives were not presented. The dental hygienist should explain technical terms and ensure that the patient comprehends the information; a linguistic interpreter may be necessary. Consent must be obtained for minors from parents or guardians. It is important to obtain consent from the parent(s) legally allowed to provide consent for medical and dental treatment. Issues of consent for minors with divorced or separated parents must be carefully monitored so that legal consent is obtained. A minor may be able to give consent if they are an emancipated minor. An emancipated minor is a child considered an adult because of a specific circumstance or court order. The minor is not under the parent's control and can make their own health-related decisions. Individual states define an emancipated minor differently. In some states, a minor who has a child is considered emancipated or a financially independent individual. Other states require a court order. If a patient is legally incompetent or lacks decision-making capacity, consent must be obtained from a guardian or surrogate. Consent can be documented using a standardized form that allows portions to be completed on a case-by-case basis (see Chapter 23).

Patients should sign the consent form. If care is modified or additional invasive procedures are performed, consent should be obtained again. Dental hygienists must take the time to obtain informed consent and allow the patient an opportunity to ask questions. This opportunity to ask questions and have them answered also must be documented in the patient's record. Informed consent should be obtained for all surgical and invasive procedures, fluoride therapy, radiographs, and similar services. It is suggested that office policy be developed so that informed consent is obtained consistently from all patients.

Informed Refusal

The risk of a lawsuit occurs when the patient refuses to follow the advice of the treating dentist or dental hygienist. A lawsuit may arise if a patient experiences serious injury or consequences after refusing care and claims they did not fully understand the effects of refusing a recommendation or treatment. A basic rule to follow when a patient refuses advice is to inform the patient of possible consequences and obtain an **informed refusal** (Fig. 7.4; see Chapter 23). The rules for informed refusal follow those for obtaining informed consent to care. They include that the patient is told in understandable language the following information:

- The diagnosis and recommendation for treatment or referral
- The reasons for the recommendation
- Risks and possible consequences to the patient's oral and general health

There must be discussion about the refusal and the effects and an opportunity to discuss the recommendation. During the discussion, if it appears that the patient refused care because of a lack of understanding, the dental hygienist should again explain the recommendation. The patient's refusal can be documented on an informed refusal form that includes the following:

- Recommendation
- List of the consequences of refusal
- Documentation that the patient understood the risks of refusing care
- The date
- Signatures of the dentist, patient, and a witness

If the patient refuses to sign the informed refusal, this should be noted and the form signed by the provider and the witness. A copy of the form should be given to the patient and another copy kept in the chart. An informed refusal form may also be called a declination of treatment.

Statute of Limitations

The **statute of limitations** is the length of time an aggrieved person has to enter lawsuits against another for an alleged injury.[5] A statute of limitations places a time limit on a contract or tort action. Once the period has ended, the lawsuit cannot be filed. For example, the statute of limitations for a contract action may be 6 years and for a tort action 3 years. In some states, the statute of limitations starts either when an injury occurs or when the plaintiff discovers the injury or reasonably should have discovered the injury. This ability to sue when an injury is discovered expands the length of time someone can file a lawsuit. Perhaps a patient is diagnosed with severe periodontal disease 5 years after ending a patient-provider relationship. The patient may still be allowed to file a lawsuit. Risk constantly exists for a lawsuit to be filed. Practitioners must be aware of the statute of limitations and rules within their state to assist in planning for record keeping and record storage.

Legal Concepts and the Dental Hygienist-Patient Relationship
Confidentiality

The dental hygienist-patient relationship raises additional areas of concern that extend the legal duties and obligations outlined. The practitioner must maintain the confidentiality of information in all settings and take steps to protect patient privacy and confidentiality. Confidentiality means that information about a patient's care is not to be shared without the patient's permission. To release confidential information without the patient's permission is an invasion of privacy. Invasion of privacy includes releasing patient information to an unauthorized person, such as a spouse, or discussing a patient's health history outside the scope of treatment. In large, open clinics, discussions with patients may appear less private.

A person can waive confidentiality through words or actions. For example, an individual who is referred to a specialist waives confidentiality. The referring practitioner is expected to inform the specialist of the patient's status. Confidentiality can be waived by action of law, such as a requirement to report specific communicable diseases or the suspicion of child abuse to a state or provincial agency. A patient's waiver of confidentiality should be documented in a progress note or separate form titled Waiver of Confidentiality.

Defamation

Defamation is a communication that injures an individual's reputation. Defamation may be:

Great Smiles Dental Office
1234 Wade Street
Seaview, CA 90000

Informed Consent Form
Procedure: Root Planing and Scaling

Please initial and date each section after you have
read and had all your questions answered.

What is scaling and root planing, and what are its benefits?

Scaling and root planing, also called periodontal therapy or deep cleaning, is used to treat the beginning stages of periodontal or gum disease. This condition is usually indicated by deeper pocket depths than normal, bleeding gums, tartar accumulation below the gum line, and x-ray evidence of bone loss. The goal of periodontal therapy is to reduce these pocket depths, remove unhealthy tissue, and thoroughly clean the root surfaces of the teeth. These efforts are done to help a patient retain their teeth and improve periodontal health. There is not a cure for periodontal disease, only treatment.

Patient/Guardian Initials: _____

What are the risks?

The following may be risks to the root planing and scaling procedure:

- The treatment will not be effective and the gum disease will progress, requiring more invasive procedures (e.g., surgery).
- The treatment will not be effective and the gum disease will progress, requiring extractions.
- Pain, soreness, and sensitivity to hot and cold stimuli.
- The gums may shrink (recession), exposing more tooth surface, which may result in sensitivity or create aesthetic (appearance) or cosmetic changes.
- Increased mobility (looseness) for teeth during the healing period or after.
- There may be an infection.

Patient/Guardian Initials: _____

The following may be risks to the use of anesthesia during the root planing and scaling procedure:

- The injection may cause and is not limited to swelling, bruising, soreness, elevated blood pressure or pulse, or allergic reaction.
- Numbness may occur after the dental appointment and, in rare cases, may extend for a period or time or be permanent.

Patient/Guardian Initials: _____

What are my alternatives and risks to the alternatives?

- Treatment that only includes a prophy (dental cleaning) that is a treatment for gum disease because the roots cannot be appropriately treated
- No treatment that will permit the gum disease to progress and may result in loss of teeth.

Patient/Guardian Initials: _____

INFORMED CONSENT: I have been given the opportunity to ask any questions regarding the nature and purpose of the proposed treatment and have received satisfactory answers. I do voluntarily assume any and all possible risks.

By signing this form, I am freely giving my consent to authorize treatment.

Patient's name (please print):

Signature of patient/legal guardian:

Witness:

Date:

Fig. 7.3 Sample informed consent for root planing and scaling.

Informed Refusal

Date: 11-5-22

Progress Notes

Care plan suggests periodontal surgery. Explained justification for surgery, risks, and alternative of three-month maintenance care, with reevaluation of need for surgery; client opted for three-month maintenance care. Client states that she understands three-month regimen must be strictly followed. Explained limitations of maintenance care versus surgery. Client asked questions about procedures at maintenance appointment.

I, Monica Gooten, refuse periodontal surgery as recommended by Tameka Simpson. I opt to cooperate in a three-month maintenance care appointment program for a nine-month period. The risks, benefits, and reasons for both treatment alternatives have been adequately explained, and my questions answered.

Patient's Signature   _____

Operator Signature   _____

Fig. 7.4 Informed refusal.

- **Libel** (written defamation)
- **Slander** (verbal defamation)

To be libelous or slanderous, the defamatory comment must be false. If the defamatory comment does not harm an individual's reputation, there is no libel or slander. Malice (intent to inflict an injury) must be shown in certain defamation cases. If a lawsuit is filed, the plaintiff must show actual damages to property, business, trade, profession, or occupation or diminish the esteem, respect, or confidence held by the person. Thus an informal comment to one person about an "incompetent dentist" by a recently fired dental hygienist would not be considered slander. The dentist's reputation was not harmed and those listening would consider the source and not necessarily believe the comment. Repeated comments by a dental hygienist in a periodontal practice stating that one periodontist is more skilled than another may result in a lawsuit if the comments harm the dentist's reputation or influence patients' return to the practice.

Legal Concepts and the Dental Hygienist–Dentist Relationship
Discrimination in Employment
In seeking employment, an individual is protected against unlawful discriminatory practices. Federal and state labor laws exist to protect both employers and employees. State laws protecting against discrimination may be more inclusive than federal laws. Employees who believe they have been the subject of discrimination are advised to consult with an attorney familiar with state law. A federal statute, Title VII of the Civil Rights Act of 1964, prohibits discrimination based on race, color, religion, gender, or national origin relating to hiring, firing, and terms, conditions, or privileges of employment. Gender discrimination includes discrimination based on pregnancy, childbirth, and related medical conditions such as gynecologic or gender-related problems. Title VII applies to employers with 15 or more employees; however, human rights acts in almost all states outlaw the same discriminatory activity and may affect employers with as few as one employee. State laws may also expand the types of discrimination banned (e.g., discrimination based on marital status, physical handicap, sexual orientation, or gender identity). The Age Discrimination in Employment Act of 1967 (ADEA) is a federal law that affects employers with 20 or more

employees. The act prohibits discrimination based on age between 40 and 70 years.

The Equal Employment Opportunity Commission (EEOC) deals with discrimination on federally prohibited grounds. The EEOC assists by investigating or advising on appropriate agencies to contact. There are strict guidelines on the timeliness of the complaint, such as a requirement to bring a complaint within 180 days. If the EEOC cannot obtain a solution, an individual may have the right to file a lawsuit. The EEOC has local offices that will answer questions or direct individuals to appropriate sources to resolve issues. Federal laws prohibiting employment discrimination are available on the EEOC website. Dental hygienists who believe they have been discriminated against in employment should contact their state civil rights agency. Discrimination can occur in a dental office. If an employer learns about an employee's religious or ethnic background and fires that employee based on the information or if an older dental hygienist is terminated and replaced by a younger, recent graduate, this may be discrimination. If employees believe they have been the subject of discrimination, they should contact their EEOC office in their state or region.

Americans With Disabilities Act

The Americans with Disabilities Act (ADA) prohibits employment discrimination against qualified individuals with disabilities. The law applies to employers with 15 or more employees. Individuals qualify for protection under this act if they have a physical or mental impairment that substantially limits one or more major life activities. Major life activities include but are not limited to caring for oneself, performing manual tasks, seeing, hearing, eating, sleeping, walking, standing, lifting, bending, speaking, breathing, learning, reading, concentrating, thinking, communicating, and working. If an individual satisfies the position requirements, the employer must provide reasonable accommodations such as modifying equipment, facilities, schedules, or job routine. For example, an office receptionist with a hearing impairment may require telephone amplification to meet the job requirements.

Equal Pay Act

The Equal Pay Act of 1963 protects men and women who perform substantially equal work in the same establishment from gender-based wage discrimination. The law would not allow an employer to reduce the wages of either a man or a woman to equalize inequities in pay.

Pregnancy and Employment Status

A significant percentage of dental hygienists are female; therefore discrimination based on pregnancy is an important issue. Federal law prohibits an employer from terminating or refusing to hire or promote a woman because of childbirth, pregnancy, or related medical conditions, such as abortion. The EEOC is the agency that administers Title VII provisions. Guidelines distributed by the EEOC state that disabilities caused by or contributed to pregnancy or childbirth must be treated like any other disability. Mandatory leave arbitrarily set at a specific time for pregnant women without regard to their ability to work is also prohibited, as well as a policy that prohibits an employee from returning to work for a predetermined length of time after childbirth. Pregnancy benefits cannot be limited to married women only. To be informed and to assist their employers, dental hygienists should obtain information from a local human rights department if maternity leave is anticipated.

Employer-Employee Relationships

Seeking employment is a common occurrence. An employment application can include the following:
- Identification of the applicant (e.g., name, address, telephone number)
- Applicant's interests (jobs, salary levels)
- Summary of applicant's background, including education, employment history, and skills
  Unlawful preemployment inquiries include the following:
- Applicant's maiden or birth name
- Birthplace of applicant
- Religious denomination or affiliation
- Complexion or skin color
- Disability status
- Requirement of a photograph
- Height, weight
- Marital status or children
- Arrest record
- National origin, ancestry, or descent
- Society or club memberships or affiliations

Applicants need not provide information that falls within the unlawful category. During the interview, if an applicant is asked a question considered illegal, they must respond tactfully and indicate they need not answer the question. Often, the applicant can redirect the interviewer by asking a question about the position or office and simply not answering the illegal question. If the interviewer insists on an answer, the applicant can respond by indicating the question is unlawful and does not need a response.

Individual states have legislation that regulates employment. An excellent resource is a state civil rights department or a related agency.

Unlike some employer-employee relationships, dental hygienists rarely have a written employment contract. The contract is written documentation that clearly outlines the rights and responsibilities of the parties involved (see Chapter 64). Traditionally, employment responsibilities, financial arrangements, benefits, and length of employment are verbally agreed on. The lack of a written agreement may leave the dental hygienist in a precarious situation. The ADHA provides a reference guide for members that includes suggestions for résumé writing, interviewing, and additional strategies for seeking and getting a job at https://mymembership.adha.org/images/pdf/2016_ADHA_Employment_Guide.pdf

The CDHA has a template for an Employment Contract at https://www.cdha.ca/pdfs/Career/students_sec.pdf

A dental hygienist-employee needs to assist an employer so that a complete and fair contract is drafted, addressing the following issues:
- Position title and responsibilities
- Scheduled days and hours of the week
- Salary (remuneration):
  - Amount
  - Pay period schedule
  - Benefits to be deducted
  - How the salary will be calculated—commission, hourly, daily
- Schedules of employee review or evaluation:
  - Influence on salary
  - Method of evaluation: formal or informal
- Fringe benefits, e.g., health insurance, continuing education support, retirement, payment of dues for professional association membership
- Notification requirements for contract severance by the dental hygienist or employer
- Specific expectations, e.g., evening or weekend hours

In most jurisdictions, the dental hygienist works as an employee of the dentist. The law views this as a fundamental employer-employee relationship where there is direct control and supervision of the employee by the employer. The doctrine governing the relationship is **respondeat superior**,[5] Latin for "let the superior [master] answer." Based on the traditional structure of most state dental practice acts, the dentist-employer answers for the actions of the dental hygienist. The dental hygienist is legally accountable and can be sued as a licensed professional. Because of the doctrine of respondeat superior, however, dentists are also named in lawsuits filed against dental hygienists. Including the dentist as one of the parties of a lawsuit reflects the "deep pocket" theory. The monetary damages sought can be increased because of the dentist-employer's more significant malpractice insurance coverage.

Another business relationship with the dentist-employer that may exist for the dental hygienist is that of an independent contractor. The general rule is that an individual is an independent contractor if the payer has the right to control or direct only the result of the work and not what will be done and how it will be done. If you are an independent contractor, then you are self-employed. If a dental hygienist is offered an opportunity to be an independent contractor, they should seek legal advice or research the requirements. The IRS instructs businesses to consider three categories of "facts that provide evidence of the degree of control and independence" in the relationship.

The three categories are:
1. Behavioral: Does the company control or have the right to control what the worker does and how the worker does their job?
2. Financial: Are the business aspects of the worker's job controlled by the payer? (These include how the worker is paid, whether expenses are reimbursed, who provides tools/supplies, etc.)
3. Type of Relationship: Are there written contracts or employee-type benefits (i.e., pension plan, insurance, vacation pay, etc.)? Will the relationship continue and is the work performed a key aspect of the business?

A dental office and the dental hygienist must apply the factors listed and determine whether the hygienist is an employee or an independent contractor. The two parties must consider and evaluate the entire relationship and determine the degree of control based on the circumstances of the relationship. If it is unclear, the recommendation is to complete a Form SS-8, Determination of Worker Status for Purposes of Employment Taxes and Income Tax Withholding, to allow the IRS to decide. See https://www.irs.gov/forms-pubs/about-form-ss-8[8]

If the dental hygienist is classified as an independent contractor, the hygienist is considered to be self-employed. With the increased freedom of independent contracting, there is also an increased liability and total responsibility for income and Social Security taxes. Individuals interested in achieving an independent relationship should seek legal and tax advice to protect themselves.

Sexual Harassment

Federal guidelines classify sexual harassment as a form of sexual discrimination. **Sexual harassment** is defined as sexual discrimination because it forces a female or male to work under adverse employment conditions. Harassment does not have to be of a sexual nature, however, and can include offensive remarks about a person's sex. For example, it is illegal to harass a woman by making lewd comments about women in general.

The victim and the harasser can be either female or male, and the victim and harasser can be of the same sex. The EEOC defines sexual harassment as follows:

Unwelcome sexual advances, requests for sexual favors, and other verbal or physical conduct of a sexual nature when submission to or rejection of this conduct is made either explicitly or implicitly a term or condition of an individual's employment; submission to or rejection of such conduct by an individual is used as the basis for employment decisions affecting the individual; or such conduct has the purpose or effect of unreasonably interfering with an individual's work performance or creating an intimidating, hostile, or offensive working environment.[7]

Two types of sexual harassment occur, as follows:

- **Quid pro quo**, which means something for something, involves a superior-subordinate relationship in which the offender controls the victim's working conditions. Examples of sexual harassment include demands for sexual favors in exchange for better working conditions or reviews, raises, or promotions.
- **A hostile environment** includes unwelcome, demeaning verbal or physical conduct of a sexual nature that creates a hostile, intimidating, or offensive work environment. Behaviors that may create a hostile work environment include a conversation with sexual content, telling sexually explicit jokes, displaying sexually suggestive objects or pictures, sending inappropriate texts or email messages, and using names such as "honey," "sweetie," or "blondie." The environment may interfere with the ability of the harassed employee to do the job; however, no tangible employment loss is evident. Supervisors, coworkers, or nonemployees may be involved.

Sexual harassment occurs in the dental environment. A dental hygienist reported that whenever they asked for a dentist "to check" a patient after a dental hygiene appointment, the dentist asked the dental hygienist to perform a sexual act. The dental hygienist, flustered and embarrassed, did not want to work alone with the dentist. Although the request for sexual favors was not related to salary or employee evaluation, it quickly could have developed into that situation. The dentist's actions constitute sexual harassment.

A second example may be a patient who makes inappropriate remarks or gestures of a sexual nature. Patients, considered nonemployees, influence the environment in which a dental hygienist is employed. A dental hygienist should report the behavior of the patient to the employer. The employer is obligated to make the working environment nonthreatening.

An employer must maintain a professional, businesslike relationship among employees and prevent or stop all situations considered harassment in the workplace. Prevention is the best strategy. Employers should communicate to all employees that sexual harassment will not be tolerated. If an individual has been the victim of sexual harassment, immediate action is necessary. An employee's response to either

physical or verbal harassment must be prompt, serious, specific, and assertive. If faced with sexual harassment, you should do the following:

- Directly inform the harasser that the conduct is unwelcome, and specifically identify the conduct.
- Directly inform the harasser that the conduct is to stop.
- Review office policies and protocol and/or notify an employer or supervisor of the incident.
- Talk to coworkers; determine whether others have shared similar experiences or if others have witnessed harassing behaviors.
- If a refusal may affect the job, report the incident to practice coowner or appropriate supervisory personnel.
- Document the harassment and keep accurate notes of what was said and done, the date, the time, the place, and the names of any witnesses.

If the situation is not remedied, options exist. In settings that employ 15 or more employees, the district office of the EEOC is contacted. The EEOC will guide an individual through filing a complaint against the harasser. If there are fewer than 15 employees, assistance may be available from a state agency such as the state department of civil rights. Although hiring a lawyer may not be necessary, legal representation is helpful to guide the victim and represent the victim if the case progresses. The district EEOC office is a resource (Box 7.7).

Termination of Employment

Dental hygienists are frequently at-will employees. At will allows the dentist to terminate the employment for little or no reason. The small business atmosphere of dental practice allows "at-will termination" by either party to exist. Some states have developed legal remedies for individuals wrongfully terminated. Some jurisdictions, for example, have laws that allow employers to terminate employees for good cause (i.e., someone can lose their position with a documented cause, such as failure to meet performance standards). A dental hygienist should be familiar with the state's policy on termination. Various states have developed criteria that must be met to prove either appropriate or inappropriate employer behavior if an employee is terminated. The termination process can also be outlined in a contract (e.g., termination requiring 2-week written notice). Given the "at-will" termination process, notice of termination is a courtesy but not a requirement to end employment.

BOX 7.7 Critical Thinking Scenario B

An assistant, your pregnant best friend, is employed in the office where you practice dental hygiene. The dentist has been very understanding about her condition; however, she is scheduling her physician visits during the workday. Your employer "gently" asks her to schedule the doctor appointments toward the end of the day, when the office is closed. She becomes very offended and quits. She calls you the evening she quits and tells you that she plans to call the state OSHA office and report violations she observed in the dental office. You think this is unfair because the office is complying, and she is creating issues where none exist. She also starts saying unkind things about the employer and suggests that she is also considering contacting the EEOC concerning possible sexual harassment.

1. Accusations of sexually harassing behaviors are serious. Discuss the types of sexual harassment that can occur in a dental office. If the dentist had been sexually harassing the assistant, what steps should she have taken?
2. If the employer had not been supportive of the pregnant assistant, what steps could the assistant have taken to resolve the conflict?
3. Use the ethical decision-making model to resolve the dilemmas presented.
4. What aspects of the ADHA or CDHA Code of Ethics apply to this situation?

RISK MANAGEMENT

A risk management program is recommended to identify potential risks in the delivery of oral care.[6] After risk is identified and measured, the office staff can make efforts to minimize or eliminate the risk. Potential areas of risk exposure include the following:

- Liability associated with professional actions of employers or employees
- General liability exposures for injuries to patients, vendors, and others
- Property and casualty exposures related to the office, building, or surrounding area (e.g., parking lot)
- Exposure to defamation actions among staff, office managers, and other personnel
- Exposure to financial losses such as fraud, embezzlement, or theft
- Exposure to contracts, warranties, and similar entities associated with the purchase and use of goods and services
- Fraud and abuse exposure associated with federal and state third-party reimbursement programs
- Exposure to losses related to staff hiring, promotions, and termination practices
- Inappropriate or incorrect use of dental equipment or dental materials
- Violation of privacy or confidentiality requirements

Box 7.8 provides sample questions that can be considered when assessing the potential risks in an employment setting.

Communication as a Risk Management Tool
Employment Setting Considerations

Communication plays a vital role in an employment setting. Professional and respectful interpersonal interactions are expected among colleagues, patients, and clients in the educational, research, and industry environment. Today's educational and employment setting has seen an increase in unprofessional and disruptive behaviors, including incivility and bullying. Such behaviors violate the ethical principles and, in some instances, legal obligations that professionals aspire to follow. Incivility and bullying can also impact productivity, patient safety, and staff morale, resulting in employee illness or health issues. Bullying is the deliberate misuse of power to target another individual with repeated, unwanted words or actions, hurting them physically and/or emotionally. An example in private practice could be repeated name calling of a dental assistant by the dentist's employer. Incivility is low-intensity deviant behavior with ambiguous intent to harm the target. Examples of incivility in the workplace include verbal outbursts, sarcastic comments, ignoring someone, and sarcastic comments.

Dental Hygienist-Client/Patient

Client or patient education is the dental hygienist's primary ethical and legal responsibility (Box 7.9). Open communication between the dental hygienist and all clients also minimizes misunderstandings, reducing the likelihood of lawsuits and allowing for immediate, timely resolution of problems. A dental hygienist who spends 45 to 60 minutes in a one-on-one relationship with a patient can reduce the potential for negligent actions. The one-on-one relationship allows the dental hygienist to explain the care that will occur and answer questions. Concepts must be presented clearly, with appropriate use of professional jargon. A patient who senses professional interest and expertise on the part of the dental hygienist may not be as prone to file a lawsuit if a procedure is unsuccessful. A diverse clientele may require an office to employ bilingual staff to improve communication.

Dental Hygienist-Employer

The dental hygienist is essential in educating employers about potential liabilities for dental hygienists and their prevention. Written standards

---

BOX 7.8 Sample Checklist for Assessing Litigation Risk in a Dental Employment Setting

Is the staff properly licensed and practicing within the appropriate scope of practice?

Is the dental equipment adequately maintained and monitored?

Are there procedures for educating and updating staff concerning the components of the dental record and the electronic record software?

Do the staff members use appropriate verbal and nonverbal communication techniques?

Are the health and dental histories updated at every appointment?

Are appropriate intraoral and extraoral data collected and recorded?

Do the staff members comprehensively document crucial data or conversations?

Are referrals (to dentists, physicians, or other healthcare providers) documented?

Is informed consent or informed refusal documented?

Does the office have a medical emergency protocol and has the procedure been rehearsed?

Are the staff qualified for cardiopulmonary resuscitation (CPR) and first aid?

Is a medical emergency kit available and are its drugs kept current? Is someone in the office capable of administering the medications in the emergency kit?

Is there an office manual outlining protocols for patient care, referral, and termination?

Is office protocol or documentation available to all staff outlining roles, responsibilities, and important policies, such as sexual/ethnic harassment prevention guidelines?

Are there social media guidelines for staff?

According to Occupational Safety and Health Administration (OSHA) and Centers for Disease Control and Prevention (CDC) guidelines, are the staff members practicing the latest infection control procedures?

Are the staff members familiar with the uses of major equipment in the office (e.g., digital radiography equipment, ultrasonic devices, dental handpieces, sedation equipment, and autoclaves)?

Are broken toys or sharp objects removed promptly from the reception area?

Are the sidewalks, parking lots, and driveways clear of debris (e.g., nails, glass, ice)?

Are the handicapped ramps operable?

Is signage clear and understandable?

BOX 7.9 Client or Patient Education Tips

- Educate the client about the legal justification for particular activities (e.g., questions about the use of protective barriers can result in a discussion about Occupational Safety and Health Administration [OSHA] regulations).
- Explain issues of standards of care, the scope of practice, and duty to the client. Help the patient understand the different members of the dental team or interprofessional education team and their legal roles and responsibilities in providing care.
- As the operator records information, such as periodontal assessment data, the need to keep accurate records to assist in clinical care and protection from health risks can be described.
- If an individual refuses a particular recommendation for treatment, the ethical principles of autonomy, beneficence, and nonmaleficence can be discussed.
- If a professional is concerned about treating particular clients, such as those with infectious diseases, the legal issues of discrimination and the ethical principle of justice can be discussed.

for office protocol can be developed and coordinated by the dental hygienist in conjunction with the employer. A resource library that includes updated website addresses, literature, textbooks, and other related material, such as a current copy of the rules and regulations outlining the rights and responsibilities of licensed office staff, provides a quick resource if questions arise. The dental hygiene staff can assist in developing an employee handbook available to all staff. The handbook can summarize employee expectations, dress code, social media use guidelines, benefits, and important office policies. Policies can address sexual and gender harassment, bullying, and incivility. Web-based resources allow an extensive array of resources to be available quickly to respond to inquiries, clarify information, or identify potential risks. If a risk management philosophy is practiced and reinforced by the employees and the employer, legal risks are reduced for the entire staff.

Dental Hygienist-Colleagues

The personnel within the employment setting are the best resources for developing a risk management philosophy. Persons in similar roles should meet for a risk management day to identify potential risk areas and develop mechanisms to reduce that risk. Consistent criteria for record keeping and referral can be developed; specific evidence-based literature to support particular treatment modalities can be shared, and office protocols and handbooks can be developed. Each activity contributes to improved practice habits. Suggested activities are the following:

- Brainstorm to identify risks, including treatment techniques, patient management, record keeping, communication, and preventive practices.
- Have each person review the plan of care for a patient; write down the key steps followed.
- Sample patient records and review record-keeping styles, abbreviations, charting records, informed consent and refusal, and other written aspects of care.
- Discuss risky practices that have become apparent.
- Develop a consensus that focuses on reducing risky behaviors that all employees consistently follow (e.g., procedures for patient care, charting techniques, abbreviations, referral guidelines, periodontal and other preventive therapies).
- Develop a dental hygiene office manual, which can be separate or incorporated as a component of a larger manual. It can focus on the dental hygiene staff; patient assessment, treatment, and evaluation insurance information; risk management suggestions; record-keeping protocol; standardized periodontal assessment and charting guidelines; and premedication information. Once consensus occurs, chapters can be delegated and written. The manual serves as a guidebook to assist current and future employees. The manual is also helpful to other office staff and dentists.
- Propose and/or conduct a similar risk management workshop for the dentists and assistants on staff.

Patient Record

The patient record can be a provider's best defense or worst enemy in a malpractice action. Every member of the dental team must recognize their responsibility for recording patient information. The record provides the following information:

- Complete description of the health and dental status at the time of the initial examination, including the pharmacologic and fluoride history and subsequent updates
- Comprehensive and chronologic documentation of treatment provided
- Communication mechanism among health professionals involved in the patient's care
- Identification of specific providers by name

- Potential legal document on the patient's behalf (e.g., use in corpse identification or insurance claims or fraud)
- Legal document for the defense of litigious claims against a dental practitioner
- Records as required in some states as part of the laws regulating professional practice
- Tool for quality assessment and assurance

State dental practice acts outline required elements of a patient record. Documentation begins with the initial contact and continues throughout the relationship between the provider and the patient, including reasons for termination of the relationship, if that occurs. It is advisable to regularly review the law to determine the specific information required in a patient record. For example, a state recently modified its law to require written informed consent for all procedures.

Patient Identification Data

Patient identification data are standard information such as name, address, telephone numbers, e.g., cell, work, the best time to call, emergency contact person(s), legal guardian or surrogate, physician of record, and insurance-related information such as a Social Security number. Practices have grown, patient numbers have increased, and patient populations reflect multicultural backgrounds. Inaccurate patient data make it difficult to identify a record that may be critical in a lawsuit. Photographs for treatment, payment, or healthcare operations purposes do not require patients' written authorization. However, obtaining written consent for the photograph is advised.

Information about a patient may change frequently, so periodic updating should be routine. Updated material should be dated.

Health and Dental History

All health and dental history information should be pursued and answered. If an item on the history form is inappropriate, it should be indicated "NA" (not applicable) (see Chapter 13). A notation such as "WNL" (within normal limits) is appropriate if the condition is normal. The oral healthcare provider should review the history to ensure every question has been answered. Patient history should be obtained at every visit. After a review is complete, notations should be made and dated in the progress notes or on the health history, noting changes.

Documenting the individuals involved in each step of the history-taking process is necessary. For example, the names of those who completed the health history or reviewed the history with the patient (if not the dentist or dental hygienist) and dates and signatures for each step should be recorded.

Assessment data should be recorded consistently. For example, a patient initially comes to the office with moderate periodontitis. If the condition does not improve, the practitioner has a record of the condition from when care begins. Therefore the dentist or dental hygienist cannot be accused of contributing to the patient's condition.

Clinical Assessment and Diagnosis

A protocol should be established for the initial clinical assessment and subsequent visits. A diagnosis should be documented to justify treatment. The plaintiff's attorney frequently suggests that malpractice occurred because there was no clear diagnosis documented in the dental chart that would guide treatment.

Treatment Information

Concise, accurate, clear, and comprehensive records of care should include the following:

- Nature of the care or treatments provided
- Area in the mouth where care is provided
- Use of special dental equipment, such as an ultrasonic scaler
- Type and dose of anesthetic agent and/or analgesia used

- Details about conditions presented, gingival health, oral hygiene status, specific areas of change
- Language that is specific (e.g., a notation such as "some deep pockets in the posterior" provides little definitive information)
- Details of conditions noted during or as the result of treatment, such as hematomas or excessive bleeding
- Specific recommendations for postoperative instructions and whether written postoperative instructions were provided to the patient
- Medication prescribed or administered and dosages
- Unexpected occurrences or reactions, such as fractured restorations
- Patient education was conducted, and the patient's response
- Continued-care interval or maintenance schedule

All procedures must be documented. Each patient has one dental hygienist and remembers each visit. Each dental hygienist has a large clientele and needs to record information that may be required in future litigation. Cancellations, late arrivals, changes of appointments, and conversations with front desk personnel are documented.

A record must be maintained professionally. The record should reflect objective information; subjective information is included only if it affects patient care (e.g., writing "Patient was very apprehensive and asked many questions during the procedure," rather than "Patient was a bother and questioned everything"). It is advisable not to comment on patient or guardian personalities or characteristics, such as "Parent is very protective."

The record assists in the defense against a charge of breach of contract, negligence, or lack of informed consent. The lawyer for the plaintiff who reviews a thorough, complete record may determine that there is no reason to pursue a lawsuit (Box 7.10). The record may clearly indicate that the practitioner met all obligations and caused no harm. An incomplete or inaccurate record under scrutiny provides multiple opportunities for the plaintiff's lawyer to prove inadequate or negligent care. Poor documentation reflects on the oral healthcare provider. There may be an assumption that sloppy records reflect sloppy care.

LEGAL ISSUES AND ROLES OF THE DENTAL HYGIENIST

Dependent Practitioner

The status of a dependent practitioner may be somewhat misleading. An individual is dependent as a result of the licensing and regulation laws of the state; however, the individual is not dependent on the employer to assume legal responsibility for their actions. The dependent practitioner is providing patient care. Based on the educational background and licensed status, the dental hygienist has professional obligations and legal duties that must be fulfilled. Failure to fulfill specific legal duties may result in negligence (malpractice) charges.

A dental hygienist may be charged with **negligence** if a breach of duty occurs and harm results. A practitioner can omit a service, such as assessing a patient's blood pressure, resulting in negligence. A practitioner can also commit a negligent act, such as harming a patient with incorrect instrumentation. In any situation, the duty or standard of care expected is evaluated. A conflict arises when the dental hygienist cannot provide care at an acceptable standard. For example, an individual has a periodontal condition that requires four 1-hour appointments to adequately root plane and scale, followed by an appointment for reevaluation. The care planning philosophy of the dentist is to allow two appointments. The dental hygienist may fail to adequately treat the patient in two appointments, contributing to a declining periodontal status. The issue of the standard of care for the dental hygienist is addressed during a lawsuit. Thus the dental hygienist is liable for professional actions taken or omitted.

BOX 7.10 Suggestions for Managing Dental Records

A dental hygienist may use an electronic record or paper record. The following guidelines apply to both:

- All members of the dental team are responsible for accurate and factual records.
- When there is more than one person making entries, entries should identify the provider.
- Errors must be corrected.
- A record should never be altered once there is some indication that legal action is contemplated by the patient.
- Standard abbreviations should be used consistently.
- Financial information should not be kept on the treatment record.
- All cancellations, late arrivals, and changes of appointments are recorded.
- Consents are documented, including all risks and alternative treatments presented to the patient and remarks made by the patient.
- The patient was informed of any adverse occurrences or untoward events that take place during the course of care.
- All requests for consultations and responses are recorded.
- All conversations held with other health practitioners relating to the care of the patient are documented.
- All dental records should be retained for at least the period of the statute of limitations equal to that of contract actions. In most jurisdictions, it is 6 years; however, it can be longer. In the case of minors, it is until the person reaches the age of 24 years. However, a case of alleged negligence involving a very young patient may arise 16 to 18 years after treatment. Check for special laws in your local jurisdiction. A dental office may consider additional record retention options that may include record storage facilities, microfilm, and/or imaging to allow retrieval at a later date. If at all possible, keep records forever.
- No subjective evaluations, such as an opinion about the patient's mental health, should be recorded on the treatment record unless the writer is qualified and licensed to make such evaluations.
- Confidentiality of information contained on the record should be guarded and HIPAA guidelines followed.
- The original record should not be surrendered to anyone except by court order. A patient has a right to a copy of the record and can be charged a reasonable fee for duplication.
- Staff are instructed that they must retain the records of patients and comply with any written request for a copy.

Electronic Records
- Electronic records should never be altered. There should be a standardized protocol that includes daily backup of records and weekly transfer of records. Software programs allow transfer of information. Security measures may be integral to the system. HIPAA security regulations should be followed.

Paper Records
- Entries should be legible, written in black ink or ballpoint pen.
- All terms, procedures, and dental materials should be spelled correctly.
- When errors occur, they should not be blocked out so that they cannot be read. Instead, a single line should be drawn through the entry and a note made above it, stating, "error in entry, see correction below." The correction should be dated at the time it is made.
- Entries should be uniformly spaced on the form. There should be no unusual or irregular blank spaces.

Independent Practitioner

In many states, defined circumstances allow a qualified dental hygienist to treat patients with limited or no contemporaneous supervision from a dentist. In such a manner, the hygienist directly interacts with a patient.

These "direct access" situations are established under state law and typically monitored by the respective state boards of dentistry. The rules that permit such a practice are specific, vary by state, and must be adhered to carefully. Accordingly, a hygienist interested in practicing in a direct patient access situation must assume a greater level of competency in areas in addition to those required of a dependent practitioner.

As an independent practitioner, a hygienist is responsible for all the legal principles influencing patient care, including negligence, referral, abandonment, informed refusal, and informed consent. The independent practitioner can also be an employer responsible for knowledge of labor and employment laws, discrimination issues, tax laws, and related business obligations. Assessing and minimizing those risks contributes to long-term success in practice as an independent practitioner.

Accordingly, an independent practitioner is advised to seek legal and business assistance for some of the following items. Contracts and other related agreements are necessary if the independent practitioner is a business owner and must be drafted, negotiated, and signed. Suppose the independent practitioner is the owner of an independent business. In that case, that role requires managerial skills outside the realm of patient care (e.g., building and equipment maintenance, material and human resources management, and strategic planning). State and federal laws affect many aspects of the business, including hiring, firing, and evaluating personnel. Other laws affect the physical plant, such as incorporating barrier-free access or selecting and maintaining equipment according to Occupational Safety and Health Administration (OSHA) guidelines.

An independent practitioner is responsible for policies and procedures, quality of care provided, documentation, and the actions of any employees. Given the litigious environment affecting dentistry and dental hygiene, the independent practitioner may be scrutinized by those seeking to find errors or illegalities. A clear understanding of the laws governing practice is imperative. The financial commitment required to be an independent practitioner may be significant. If the independent practitioner establishes a business, it is essential to protect personal assets and keep personal and professional expenses separate. Separate accounts are advisable for ease of bookkeeping. In addition, the separation of personal and professional assets is important, so personal assets cannot be taken if the business is affected by either financial or legal problems.

Independent Contractor

A dental hygienist performing services as an independent contractor must recognize the increased responsibilities inherent in business matters and as an independent professional practice. The independent contractor dental hygienist is contracting to provide services to another party. Both parties in the relationship, the dental hygienist and the contracting party, have specific rights and responsibilities. For example, the dental hygienist assumes that the contracting party will compensate the hygienist for services rendered and provide certain facilities and possibly support staff. Failure of either party to fulfill specific obligations of a contract is considered a breach of contract.

Dental hygienists should seek legal counsel before any commitment to practice as an independent contractor. Business issues such as labor laws, income tax, Social Security taxes, and liability issues are additional and important considerations. The independent contractor and the other contracting party must also remain aware of the legal issues affecting patient care, such as negligence, informed consent, referral, abandonment, and record keeping.

The dental hygienist, as an independent contractor, must approach practicing with a strong risk management philosophy. A dental hygienist should not be put at risk because of the poor quality of care provided by someone else. Therefore during the engagement process and before establishing a contractual relationship, the dental hygienist should evaluate the hosting party in terms of potentially negligent activities, referral philosophies, infection control, and record keeping, to name a few considerations. Reviewing dental records (with an understanding of HIPAA regulations) to observe how patient care is managed may assist a dental hygienist in deciding whether to contract with a specific care provider. Appropriate malpractice insurance coverage should be considered. Both parties' respective rights and responsibilities must be clearly outlined to define and understand the working relationship. The reasons and methods for ending the relationship, such as justification, if any, and notice requirements, are matters to be identified. Both contracting parties must review and agree on postterm concerns such as record retention.

In summary, practicing as an independent contracting hygienist requires understanding and scrutiny of various tax, business, and professional issues that an employed hygienist may not need to address. Accordingly, it is recommended that legal counsel be consulted before committing to an independent contractor relationship.

Educator

An educator has contact with both colleagues and students. Confidentiality—an obligation not to violate confidences shared—is one aspect of the relationships developed in an educational setting. In today's society, issues that must remain confidential have become more difficult to define. Educators are grappling with issues such as the student who confides in a high-risk lifestyle for contracting a sexually transmitted disease or a colleague who has had a positive HIV test result. Higher education institutions have developed policies to address such situations, but state and local laws may also address topics such as student rights and health issues.

Some states have general policies concerning issues such as the infected healthcare worker that institutions can use to guide their activities. Discrimination may also be an issue. Educators must be certain that decisions affecting admission, hiring, clinical assignments, workload, promotion, and evaluation are not influenced by actions that are considered discriminatory. Clearly outlined policies for personnel hiring and management and student admission and continuance assist in decreasing potentially discriminatory practices. Informal comments previously made about an individual or group of individuals may resurface if allegations of discrimination occur.

Educators are responsible for participating in professional development that will assist them in fulfilling their roles and responsibilities. Mandates for Title IX protections for students related to sexual assault and sexual harassment require an educational institution to educate faculty and staff about their obligation to report incidents of sexual misconduct as reported to them by a student. Professional development assists educators in learning about the institutional personnel and resources available to help them in areas such as disability services and support, diversity and inclusivity, student protections, and campus safety.

The educator who serves as a clinical instructor must recognize that the legal principles apply to clinical education. Informed consent, the standard of care, confidentiality, referral policies, and contract and tort duties must be purposefully applied. Clinical faculty members are ultimately liable for a student's actions. Therefore patient interactions and care should be carefully monitored. Patient information written by a student and cosigned by a faculty member should be read critically to ensure accuracy and completeness. Student-faculty interactions in a clinical setting must be free of bias or discriminatory practices. Similar issues apply to the educator, who also may provide clinical care as part of in-house faculty practice. Policies to prevent charges of abandonment must be developed and implemented. Careful documentation of patient care, referral, and dismissal with standardized language ensures consistency within the institution.

An educator may be involved in the supervision of clerical and clinical staff. Legal issues involve employee rights, contractual responsibilities, personnel evaluations, and dismissals. The educator must consider written documentation, discriminatory practices, civil rights issues, and issues within the areas of labor law and employer-employee relationships. Some institutions have unionized employees and a supervisor must consider the contract requirements. Educators should seek legal guidance for assistance when appropriate.

The educator also works with administrators. Issues such as the educator's contractual rights, civil rights, and related topics should be understood, and legal counsel may be sought if an issue arises. Failure on the part of an institution to recognize specific rights may lead to legal challenges by an employee. Promotion and tenure decisions, salary and equity issues, and job descriptions and responsibilities also have a legal component.

Administrator or Manager

The administrator or manager is involved in hiring, evaluating, and possibly dismissing students, colleagues, or employees. Knowledge of federal and state laws affecting civil rights and sexual harassment and protecting those rights are important to know and follow. Administrators must recognize that specific questions cannot be asked during an employment interview. Evaluation of an employee should be completed carefully and documented. Sometimes dismissal of an employee or student can occur only after a series of evaluations, warnings, and required counseling is completed. Again, colleagues who make discriminatory remarks, exhibit sexual misconduct, or conduct themselves inappropriately reflect on the administrator's ability to manage effectively.

Contracts are a common part of an administrator's or manager's life. A **contract**, the agreement between two consenting parties, reflects certain rights and responsibilities. All parties involved require a clear understanding of the rights and responsibilities delineated in the contract. Failure to understand the contract may lead to charges of a **breach of contract** based on the failure to fulfill a responsibility. For example, if a breach of contract occurs, there may be financial ramifications. If an employee is inappropriately dismissed without due process of law, the court may require that the employer be responsible for fulfilling the salary terms of the contract. The employer is still obligated to pay salary and benefits under the law.

The administrator or manager may be responsible for ensuring the safety of an employee from the tortious acts of another (e.g., a responsibility to protect an employee from a patient or student who may commit an assault or battery). In addition, an obligation exists to prevent negligence in the maintenance of the physical plant, such as faulty steps, icy or wet entrances, or other dangerous situations. The administrator or manager may be responsible for following federal or state mandates in areas such as employment or safety. The manager may be responsible for adhering to workplace laws, rules, and regulations.

Labor laws and related legal concepts may dictate what documentation is essential and appropriate. Employees have access to their employment files, so an administrator or manager must be objective and thorough in documenting events and personal interactions. State and federal laws seek to protect the rights of involved individuals.

Consumer Advocate

The consumer rights advocate should be aware of legislation on legal issues, civil rights, healthcare, labor issues in the employment of the disabled, geriatrics, and issues regarding children and adolescents. Advocates should focus on areas that best meet personal needs and the needs of the population group(s) they represent. Understanding the political system, enacting laws, and lobbying techniques help the advocate to keep updated by pursuing information and getting on mailing lists. Working with professional groups with similar interests also provides a valuable resource for information or to respond to a situation, such as through a letter-writing campaign.

The legal implications of contracts and torts are applicable in many situations. Did a group promise to provide services, fail to meet its obligation, and breach its contract? Did an agency violate the terms of its contract? Was an individual negligent in their responsibilities in fulfilling the contract? Was informed consent obtained? Is there a duty to an individual or group of individuals based on an interpretation of the law? Can it be argued that some have misrepresented themselves or an issue? In most instances, a lawyer can assist in defining the legal principles that apply. The code of ethics for lawyers suggests that they perform some legal work pro bono (for free). Therefore an individual working as a consumer advocate may find legal assistance from someone willing to work pro bono and obtain valuable advice and guidance from the legal perspective.

Researcher

Researchers should be familiar with issues such as institutional review boards, confidentiality, rights of human and animal subjects, informed consent, record keeping, data management, and abandonment. For instance, researchers must also consider legal issues not addressed in this chapter, such as product liability, fund management, and tax issues.

KEY CONCEPTS

- Ethics focuses on the moral duties and obligations of the oral healthcare provider to self, the profession, clients, colleagues, employees, employers, family, friends, the community, scientific investigations, and society.
- Dental hygienists are guided by the core ethical principles of autonomy, veracity, justice, beneficence, nonmaleficence, and fidelity.
- Dental hygienists are accountable to clients, colleagues, employers, and society.
- A code of ethics is characteristic of a profession and assists in raising ethical sensitivity and providing a guiding framework for decision making.
- An ethical decision-making model includes identifying the conflict and the ethical principles involved and gathering relevant information to identify a list of alternatives from which a dental hygienist can choose one ethically based alternative on which to act.
- Civil law is that branch of law that includes offenses violating private or contractual rights.
- Dental hygienists can have a contractual relationship with a patient that requires the dental hygienist to fulfill specific obligations.
- Abandonment results if a relationship between a practitioner and patient is severed without appropriate notification and documentation.
- Technical battery occurs if a practitioner performs a procedure on a patient without informed consent.
- Negligence is a professional's failure to fulfill a specific duty to a patient that results in injury or harm.
- A dental hygienist must meet the standard of care for the profession (i.e., the degree of care a reasonably prudent professional would exercise under the same or similar circumstances).
- Informed consent allows a patient to agree to permit something to happen based on full disclosure of information and is based on the ethical principle of autonomy and recognition of an individual's right to self-determination.
- Informed refusal allows a patient to decline dental advice; the refusal should be documented to protect the practitioner.
- Confidentiality is an important responsibility that protects a patient's privacy.
- Federal and state laws protect dental hygienists from employment discrimination in hiring, firing, compensation, and promotion decisions.
- Dental hygienists may be subject to sexually or ethnically based harassing behaviors and should be familiar with steps to stop or prevent the behavior.
- Risk management involves identifying risks and implementing strategies to reduce or eliminate risks.
- Record keeping is important to protect the practitioner and the patient and to assist in patient care.

CRITICAL THINKING EXERCISES

1. Obtain a current document from the ADHA (Dental Hygiene Practice Act Overview: Permitted Functions and Supervision Levels by State, available at https://www.adha.org/resources-docs/7511_Permitted_Services_Supervision_Levels_by_State.pdf or CDHA that provides a synopsis of the supervision requirements for services provided by dental hygienists by state or province. How is the legal doctrine of respondeat superior affected by this variability in supervision requirements in the various legal jurisdictions?
2. Obtain the current Code of Ethics from both the ADHA and the CDHA. Read both. How are they similar? How do they differ? Was there a statement that was unexpected?
3. Reflect on current social media. Draft guidelines for social media use in private practice that could be included in an employee handbook and provide guidance to staff to prevent unprofessional conduct, e.g., bullying or patient privacy violations.
4. Answer the questions in the Ethical and Legal Decision-Making Scenarios 7.1 to 7.4 for analysis and discussion.

ETHICAL AND LEGAL DECISION-MAKING SCENARIO 7.1

Ivy Smith has been a licensed dental hygienist for 8 years. She is not active in the dental hygiene professional association and looks to her employer, Dr. Albert Brady, to keep her "updated." She relies on Dr. Brady to tell her what is "legal" or "illegal" in dental hygiene. She rarely attends professional meetings or reads scientific publications. Her employer has told her that she can perform some expanded duties under his direction. Based on his direction, she has cemented some crowns and used nitrous oxide–oxygen analgesia during patient care activities (both of which are illegal for dental hygienists in the state/province). Dr. Brady also told her not to spend time reviewing health or dental histories or using other patient assessment methods, such as evaluating periodontal disease status, to save time. According to Dr. Brady, when it comes to history review and assessment, "once is enough," and her job is to "clean teeth." She has raised a concern to you about potential malpractice liability, but Dr. Brady told her not to worry because he is responsible under the doctrine of respondeat superior.

1. Which sections of the ADHA or CDHA Code of Ethics apply to this case?
2. Is Ivy Smith meeting the standard of care for dental hygiene?
3. What strategies would you use to encourage Ivy to join the dental hygiene professional association?
4. Does the concept of respondeat superior excuse Ivy Smith from her legal and ethical responsibilities?
5. Assume Ivy Smith schedules a meeting to discuss her concerns with Dr. Brady. What legal and ethical issues should she raise with her employer?

ETHICAL AND LEGAL DECISION-MAKING SCENARIO 7.2

You have worked in practice for 3 years and have developed a close friendship with Alice Gunn. Alice moved from Georgia 3 years ago, is a single parent, and is a technically proficient dental hygienist. Her dental hygiene and communication skills with patients and staff impressed you. One night after work, you and Alice go out for dinner, and she confides in you that she is not licensed in the state. Alice admits that because of the employment opportunity, the great health benefits, the hours, and the employer and employees, she could not wait to get a license and take the job. Your employer never asked for proof of licensure, so she never had to admit or deny that she wasn't licensed. She asks you not to mention the situation because she can't afford to stop practicing until she gets a license. She also does not want to be exposed because she is active in the local dental hygiene association, which would be embarrassing. She promises to try to get a license but doesn't want anyone to know that she isn't currently licensed.

1. Use the ethical decision-making model to resolve the dilemma presented.
2. How would a copy of the dental practice act assist the dental hygienist?
3. How could the employer have prevented this situation?
4. What aspects of the ADHA or CDHA Code of Ethics apply to this situation?

ETHICAL AND LEGAL DECISION-MAKING SCENARIO 7.3

Andrew Pierce is a second-year dental hygiene student who has been described as patient centered. Andrew works diligently and carefully to ensure that his patients receive outstanding dental hygiene care. Many of the patients who visit the dental hygiene clinic are on limited incomes and do not have dental insurance. Andrew knows the importance of fluoride therapy for his child and adult patients. He tries to give fluoride treatments, when appropriate, to all patients. He knows that preventive therapies are important and feels he is serving the needs of the patients; however, he knows that some of his patients cannot afford the fluoride fee and would decline the treatment if given a choice. Andrew gives a fluoride treatment to patients who cannot afford the treatment or do not have insurance coverage. For them not to be charged, he does not record the fluoride treatment in the progress notes and does not indicate the fluoride treatment on the charge slip given to the cashier. The dental hygiene faculty members often do not notice that the fluoride treatment is not documented because they are busy with many students.

1. Which ethical principles apply to this case?
2. Identify some risks to the client, student, faculty, and dental hygiene program.
3. Take the part of the dental hygiene program director. What steps would you take with the student and dental hygiene faculty to address the problem?
4. Take the role of a student colleague of Andrew Pierce who is aware of the situation. What would you do based on your program's academic and professional decorum policies?

ETHICAL AND LEGAL DECISION-MAKING SCENARIO 7.4

The new dental associate in the office likes to make it known that they are "in charge." The associate recently graduated from dental school and has repeatedly reminded the staff that they have a significant student loan balance to pay off. The new associate frequently checks your patients after you have completed dental hygiene care. The dentist receives a percentage of the fee for every patient with a treatment plan, including a root planing and scaling appointment. You begin noticing that they appear to be overtreating and overdiagnosing patients. Examples of these behaviors include convincing patients to agree to extensive restorative work, advocating cosmetic procedures, and classifying patients as needing root planing and scaling when it is evident from their condition that it is not necessary. Privately, you have asked them about some of these treatment plans. They firmly inform you that they are the licensed dentist in the office and you are the registered dental hygienist.

1. Use the ethical decision-making model to resolve the dilemma(s) presented. What resources would you draw on?
2. Which legal principle or principles are involved in this scenario?
3. Does your state or province have a dental society peer review process?

REFERENCES

1. American Dental Hygienists' Association. *American Dental Hygienists Code of Ethics*; 2019. Available at: https://www.adha.org/resources-docs/ADHA_Code_of_Ethics.pdf. Accessed November 9, 2022.
2. Canadian Dental Hygienists Association. *Code of Ethics*; 2012. Available at: https://www.cdha.ca/pdfs/Profession/Resources/Code_of_Ethics_EN_web.pdf. Accessed June 15, 2022.
3. Beemsterboer PL. Ethical decision making in dental hygiene and dentistry. In: Beemsterboer PL, ed. *Ethics and the Law*. 3rd ed. Elsevier; 2017.
4. Homenko DF. *Dentist Offices Prepare for Ethical Dilemmas through the Formation of an Office Committee*; 1999. https://www.rdhmag.com/patient-care/radiology/article/16404631/a-committees-morals. Accessed November 9, 2022.
5. Garner BA. *Black's Law Dictionary*. 11th ed. Thomson Reuters; 2019.
6. Pollack BR. Risk management in the dental office. *Dent Clin North Am*. 1985;29(3):557–580.
7. Equal Employment Opportunity Commission. Sexual Harassment Defined. Available at: https://www.eeoc.gov/harassment. Accessed November 9, 2022.
8. Internal Revenue Service (IRS). Independent Contractor (Self-Employed) or Employee? Available at: https://www.irs.gov/businesses/small-businesses-self-employed/independent-contractor-self-employed-or-employee. Accessed November 9, 2022.

8

Professional e-Portfolios

Phyllis Spragge and Catherine Kelly Draper

PROFESSIONAL OPPORTUNITIES

Building a professional portfolio usually begins during the student years; however, portfolios have far-reaching applications, including the demonstration of ongoing competencies required for licensure renewal, providing a means to display skills and experiences as part of an employment interview, or as a way to take one's dental hygiene career in a brand-new direction.

COMPETENCIES

1. Differentiate between the various types and formats of portfolios and their uses.
2. Describe the process for creating a student portfolio and identify artifacts or projects that demonstrate competency.
3. Examine the role of reflection within the portfolio.
4. Discuss the role that ethics plays in portfolio authorship.
5. Describe how the student portfolio can be transitioned for use throughout the career of the dental hygienist.

Portfolios are becoming an integral part of the dental hygiene education and career process. Beginning as a way to assess and showcase student work while in the dental hygiene program, the professional portfolio demonstrates the growth and achievements throughout the career of the dental hygienist. Portfolios also help students document their progress while in the dental hygiene program by providing a place to archive, reflect on, and share their best work with faculty members. Portfolios can also serve as evidence of a student's competency in many of the educational standards required by the Commission on Dental Accreditation. In addition, portfolios provide a much deeper level of insight into a student's learning and accomplishments and may be a requirement for scholarship, degree completion, and graduate program review committees. Maintaining a professional portfolio is also a critical component of the employment process for the new graduate as well as the seasoned professional. A portfolio can provide the potential employer with evidence of a candidate's range of skills and experiences extending far beyond the traditional résumé. Portfolios are also considered by some states and Canadian provinces for licensure as well as a requirement for the demonstration of ongoing competency throughout the licensed professional's career.

WHAT IS A PROFESSIONAL PORTFOLIO?

A **professional portfolio** is defined as an organized collection of **artifacts,** the term commonly used for the physical evidence or items included in a portfolio, which have been selected carefully to document an individual's competency, growth, and accomplishments over time. Portfolios include a reflection component, providing an opportunity for an individual to thoughtfully comment or reflect on their artifacts, ongoing personal growth, and professional goals. Reflection also plays

a key role in self-assessment, evaluation of one's competencies, and one's ability to think critically. Historically, portfolios have been used by students in fields ranging from art and photography to journalism and education as a means to visually display actual examples of their work as part of the application process for admission into specialty or graduate degree programs. Today, portfolios are being used by a wide range of healthcare professionals, including physicians, nurses, pharmacists, dietitians, dentists, and dental hygienists in the United States as well as internationally as a way to demonstrate ongoing competency and document professional growth.[1]

TYPES OF PORTFOLIOS

Academic or Learning

Various forms of academic or learning portfolios are being used in more than half of all colleges and universities in the United States. Student portfolios have been used in dental and dental hygiene education programs since 1998 as a means to demonstrate competency or the skills, knowledge, and values of an individual ready to enter independent practice.[2] The student portfolio is a compilation of academic work or other artifacts that have been organized to demonstrate learning progress, academic achievement, and evidence of meeting institutional standards or course requirements. Student portfolios may also include formative feedback from faculty and student reflection on academic and clinical performance and competency evaluations. Academic portfolios may also be used for summative capstone or final projects designed to demonstrate content mastery as a requirement for graduation.[3]

Employment

Looking beyond academia, professional portfolios are being used by individuals seeking employment in a variety of disciplines as a way to expand beyond the one-page résumé by providing a more complete visual record of the candidate's abilities and accomplishments. The professional portfolio also can be used as a marketing tool to potential employers, illustrating the applicant's knowledge, skills, and relevant experiences. The process of updating the student portfolio in preparation for an employment interview can instill renewed confidence in the applicant as they reflect on all they have accomplished during their education.[4] A portfolio can also serve as a visual prompt in the interview process, highlighting an experience or area of expertise that may go unnoticed or forgotten during the verbal interview.

Demonstration of Ongoing Competency for Licensure

Healthcare professionals are also turning to the professional portfolio as a means to document competency and professional development throughout their careers. Competency, as it relates to a healthcare professional, means that one is able to provide safe and reliable care on a consistent basis over time. Graduating from an accredited healthcare education program and passing written and clinical boards are no longer being accepted as adequate evidence of preparedness for a lifetime of practice, especially considering the rapidly changing science and technology required for patient care in the 21st century. Registered nurses are among the healthcare providers currently using professional portfolios for documenting continued competency within their specific area of expertise as well as for seeking new positions and career ladder promotions. Some nursing boards in the United States also have joined their international counterparts in requiring the submission of a portfolio for licensure renewal.[4]

Pathway to Initial Clinical Licensure

The professional portfolio also is being used to measure clinical competency in dentistry and dental hygiene. The California legislature approved the hybrid portfolio as a pathway for initial licensure for general dentists applying for licensure by the Dental Board of California. Dental students have the option to apply for licensure based on a portfolio of completed clinical experiences and competency examinations in seven subject areas that are evaluated over the final year of dental school. Once all the clinical experiences and assessments have been completed to the satisfaction of calibrated faculty members, students must submit their completed portfolio to the Dental Board of California for final review before becoming eligible to apply for a license to practice dentistry. Since the approval of the California hybrid portfolio in 2014, Colorado and Iowa also accept the hybrid portfolio as a means to demonstrate clinical competency for initial licensure in dentistry.[5]

Professional Development Requirement

Although initial licensure by portfolio is not an option for dental hygienists in the United States at this time, the state of Minnesota currently requires all dental professionals to maintain a **professional development** portfolio to record, monitor, and document both fundamental continuing education courses and elective professional development activities. Fundamental courses include a mandatory infection control course, ethics, patient communication, medical emergencies, diagnosis and treatment planning, record keeping, and the Health Insurance Portability and Accountability Act (HIPAA). Elective activities can include attendance at professional conferences, community service, and scholarly work, including professional presentations. Dentists, dental therapists, dental hygienists, and dental assistants must maintain documentation of their professional development activities (continuing education course details, logs of activities, etc.) in a portfolio for both the current and previous renewal cycles. Actual portfolio submission is not required as part of the licensure renewal process; however, licensed

professionals may be randomly audited and required to submit their portfolio to the Minnesota Board of Dentistry for review.[6]

The majority of the dental hygienists licensed in Canada are required to maintain a professional development portfolio as a requirement for quality assurance and licensure renewal. The required contents of the portfolio vary depending on the province; however, the licensed professional's self-assessment of their knowledge and skills and the setting of learning goals for ongoing professional development courses are common elements to the Canadian portfolios. For example, dental hygienists licensed in Ontario must complete detailed learning portfolio and practice worksheets, and dental hygienists may be audited as part of their provincial quality assurance program requirements.[7] Much further abroad, dental hygienists in New Zealand are also using professional portfolios for licensure renewal.[8]

In summary, the student portfolio lays the foundation for the future dental hygiene professional. It can serve as an effective tool for the new graduate in seeking entry-level employment or as part of the application process for a degree completion or postgraduate program. More important, maintaining a professional portfolio is becoming a requirement for licensure and specialty certification boards across a wide range of disciplines in healthcare. Developing the necessary skills to demonstrate competency via a professional portfolio begins early in the dental hygiene education process.

PORTFOLIO FORMATS

Portfolio formats can range from very simple templates for professional development or student competency requirements to the more complex multimedia versions often used by visual artists. The most common types of portfolios used in education and beyond are electronic versions or **e-portfolios**, while the traditional paper-based formats may still be used for some purposes.

Paper Formats

The paper-based portfolio typically is organized in a binder or folders. This method is relatively easy and inexpensive initially; however, a paper portfolio is limited to exclusively print-based artifacts and projects and cannot be easily shared with multiple viewers or regulatory agencies for licensure renewal.

Electronic Formats

Electronic or e-portfolios are either Web- or computer-based (Fig. 8.1). Electronic formats have the advantage of communicating an

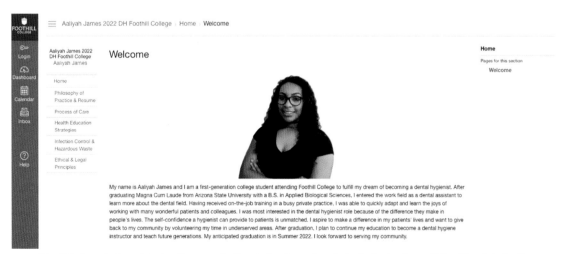

Fig. 8.1 Sample template for the organizational structure of a student electronic portfolio. (Reprinted with permission from Foothill College Dental Hygiene Program, Los Altos Hills, California.)

individual's work and accomplishments not only through written text but also by allowing for the incorporation of graphic, audio, and video formats. An individual's work then can be stored electronically and shared on a website or on a personal computer. Creating a computer-based e-portfolio may require purchasing additional software and a scanner. Printed portfolio contents can be scanned and saved as electronic files. Once the computer-based e-portfolio is completed, it can be stored virtually in the cloud or electronically shared with others. Although there are no recurring setup or maintenance fees with this type of portfolio, a computer-based e-portfolio is not as easily accessible as a Web version. Web-based e-portfolios are created on dedicated websites, often with the help of design templates and user-friendly software for uploading files. Annual user fees for accessing the Web domain are common for this type of e-portfolio. Institutional or academic portfolios may also be created on a designated site within the learning management system. Examples of e-portfolio websites can be found in Box 8.1. Many Web-based e-portfolios can be linked to the user's email signature, social media accounts, or professional networking sites, such as LinkedIn, and can create advantages for future employment opportunities. This chapter focuses on the creation of a dental hygiene student portfolio with specific examples adaptable for electronic formats.

CREATING THE STUDENT PORTFOLIO

Selecting the contents for a dental hygiene portfolio depends on a number of factors, in particular the purpose of the portfolio. Student projects or experiences included in a portfolio are often based on the guidelines, learning outcomes, and competencies developed by the specific dental hygiene program, college, or university, demonstrating how the graduate has met the educational standards required by the Commission on Dental Accreditation (Table 8.1).[9]

General examples of the elements common to any student portfolio include biographic data, examples of core clinical competencies, student research projects and presentations, summaries of patient/client experiences, professional activities, community service experiences, interprofessional learning, and related projects and experiences outside of the classroom. A strong portfolio should be built with the key projects or assignments that demonstrate achievement of the dental hygiene program competencies as well as examples of the student's critical thinking and problem-solving skills. The portfolio is meant to be a dynamic documentation of growth and development. Web-based e-portfolios often have an interactive feedback box where faculty or other site visitors, such as other healthcare professionals, can provide comments to the portfolio owner. Based on the feedback provided, the student may choose to change or enhance the portfolio content. Examples of best work chosen at the beginning of the dental hygiene program will change over time and should be updated regularly as the

BOX 8.1   Selected e-Portfolio Website Resources

foliotek: https://www.foliotek.com
LiveText: https://www.livetext.com
PebblePad: https://www.pebblepad.co.uk
Weebly: www.weebly.com
FolioSpaces: https://www.foliospaces.org/
Canvas Learning Management System: https://www.instructure.com/higher-education
Moodle Learning Management System: https://moodle.org/
Blackboard Learning Management System: www.blackboard.com

student progresses toward graduation. Portfolios created for the purpose of documenting professional development or ongoing continuing education should include a comprehensive record of all relevant coursework, conferences, workshops, and related activities.

The first step in the portfolio process is to begin to collect the contents or artifacts (Fig. 8.2). Regardless of whether the e-portfolio is Web or computer based, it is important to choose an organizational structure or template to effectively display the artifacts to fit the portfolio's purpose. The design and accompanying photographs and images should always project the image of a healthcare professional. It is important to remember that a portfolio is not a digital scrapbook, photo album, or social media page. Although the specific organizational requirements for a student portfolio may vary depending on the school and the dental hygiene program, the elements listed in Box 8.2 can be used to help guide the organizational process of building an e-portfolio template. Examples of specific artifacts that could demonstrate competency in various sections of the e-portfolio are shown in Table 8.2. See Box 8.3.

Reflection and the Professional Portfolio

Reflection is a key component of any portfolio, adding depth extending beyond the description of the project or activity. Without meaningful reflection, the portfolio is little more than a filing system of projects and activities. At its simplest level, reflection means to look back and consider or think about something. However, when considering reflection within the context of providing healthcare, it is a process that can create a greater understanding of one's self and any given situation or event, particularly as it relates to the delivery of patient care. The ability to think deeply and critically has been defined as a desirable attribute in the competent healthcare professional. Portfolios provide students the opportunity to select artifacts such as a clinical case study and reflect on the critical thinking skills, problem solving, and self-directed learning that led to their competence in patient care.

Reflection and critical thinking also play a major role in the self-assessment process that should guide lifelong learning and professional growth.[10,11] The ability assess gaps in knowledge, skills, and attributes starts in school. Regular formative feedback from faculty members plays an important role in helping students to identify the gaps and develop the strategies to acquire new knowledge and clinical skills. Students who develop reflective learning skills have demonstrated that they are more proactive in their learning and are better able to identify the areas where they need more self-improvement and skill development. Rather than simply focusing on learning rote information and clinical skills, the reflective student and future healthcare professional are more focused on critical thinking, problem solving, and self-motivated change.[10,11]

Reflecting on experiences both in and outside of the dental hygiene clinic is challenging for any beginning student, but it is a process that can be developed with guidance from dental hygiene faculty members and mentors. It is important to remember that the project or artifact in a student portfolio is not the evidence of the learning; it is the reflection that demonstrates the transfer of knowledge learned in the classroom or elsewhere to the clinical experience or situation.[10]

Putting one's thoughts into written reflection statements can be difficult for seasoned professionals as well as students but again, it is a skill that can be developed with practice. A reflection statement should not be a detailed summary of the activity or assignment. Meaningful reflection comes by moving past the activity to a deeper level of thinking, with a focus on one's feelings, values, or assumptions surrounding the activity or event.[12] It can be helpful to spend some time thinking first before rushing to write a reflection statement on the selected assignment or activity.

TABLE 8.1 Mapping Commission on Dental Accreditation (CODA) Standards to e-Portfolio Artifacts

CODA Standards	e-Portfolio Artifact Samples
2-12 Graduates must be competent in providing dental hygiene care for child, adolescent, adult, geriatric, and special needs patients. 2-13 Graduates must be competent in providing the dental hygiene process of care including: • Comprehensive collection of patient data • Analysis of assessment findings to address the patient's dental hygiene treatment needs • Establishment of a dental hygiene care plan • Provision of comprehensive patient-centered treatment • Measurement of achievement of the dental hygiene care plan • Accurate documentation of patient care	• Research on dental hygiene care for patients/clients across the lifespan • Case studies • Clinical competency evaluations • Patient care logs and statistics • Reflections on the challenges and successes in the delivery of patient/client care
2-14 Graduates must be competent in providing dental hygiene care for all types of classifications of periodontal disease, including patients who exhibit moderate to severe periodontal disease.	• Periodontal research papers/projects • Periodontal competency evaluations • Experiences with periodontal disease staging and grading • Periodontal patient care logs and statistics • Reflections on periodontal patient/client experiences
2-15 Graduates must be competent in communicating and collaborating with other members of the healthcare team to support comprehensive patient care.	• Interprofessional education activities/projects • Examples of collaborative care strategies for patients with special healthcare needs • Community oral health projects • Professional meeting and community service logs • Reflections on interprofessional education/collaboration activities; community outreach activities; collaborations with other oral healthcare providers
2-16 Graduates must demonstrate competence in: • Assessing the oral health needs of community-based programs • Planning an oral health program to include health promotion and disease prevention activities • Implementing the program • Evaluating the effectiveness of the program	• Community oral health project; research, literature review, planning documents, data analysis, and presentations • Reflections on the challenges and outcomes of the implementation of a community oral health program
2-19 Graduates must be competent in the application of the principles of ethical reasoning, ethical decision making, and professional responsibility as they pertain to the academic environment, research, patient care, and practice management. 2-20 Graduates must be competent in applying legal and regulatory concepts to the provision and/or support of oral healthcare services.	• Law and ethics research project and/or case studies • Infection and hazard control research project • Reflections on ethical dilemmas as a student dental hygienist
2-21 Graduates must be competent in the application of self-assessment skills to prepare them for lifelong learning.	• Professional development logs • Self-assessment of dental hygiene process of care skills and patient competencies • Feedback and reflections on patient/client care • Reflections on program competencies and strategies for growth
2-22 Graduates must be competent in the evaluation of current scientific literature.	• Research projects and abstracts • Reviews of the literature • Case studies • PICO questions for evidence-based practice decisions • Reflections on professional responsibilities of evaluating scientific literature and the impact of misinformation and disinformation

Consider the scenario of a second-semester, first-year dental hygiene student caring for a 5-year-old pediatric patient in the school clinic. The parent and child are late for their appointment and when they finally arrive, the child is frightened by the big clinic and is uncooperative for the kindergarten screening and oral prophylaxis. The screening reveals visible caries in all the primary molars and although the prophylaxis was eventually completed, the overall experience was stressful for the child, parent, and student dental hygienist. Immediately following the clinic session, the student may have been initially focused on their own needs, such as their clinic grade or competency requirement. However, deeper reflection on this scenario could include consideration of the student's false assumptions regarding the patient's oral health status, access to care issues, and oral health literacy levels, as well as any necessary advance preparation that was needed for this child and parent. Reflective thinking would include considering the underlying factors that contributed to this less-than-positive outcome and what can be done in the future for an improved experience for the patient, the parent, and the healthcare provider. The process of critical reflection includes analyzing, questioning, and reframing an experience to make an assessment of either the learning or ways to improve clinical practice.[13] Student learners can be guided by their instructors in developing the skills needed to

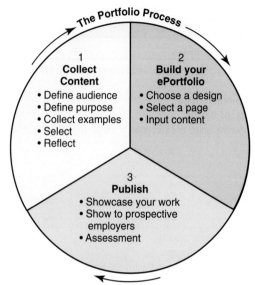

Fig. 8.2 The portfolio process: from content collection to publication. (Reprinted with permission from San Francisco State University, http://eportfolio.sfsu.edu.)

BOX 8.2   Portfolio Development Guidelines

- Best work versus professional development/competency or combination
- Portfolio audience
- Dental hygiene faculty versus potential employers
- College or university guidelines
- Institutional required elements
- Dental hygiene program requirements
- Demonstration of program competencies

TABLE 8.2   Portfolio Sample Template

Tabs for the e-Portfolio	Content Under Each Section Tab
Home Page	• Introduction and photograph • Résumé • Philosophy of practice statement
Process of Care	• Reflection/introduction • Patient care log and statistics • Patient competencies and research papers
Health Education Strategies	• Reflection/introduction • Oral health research project • Community service • Professional development • Community dental health project
Infection and Hazard Control	• Reflection/introduction • Infection control research project
Ethical and Legal Principles	• Reflection/introduction • Law and Ethics research project

Reproduced with permission from Foothill College Dental Hygiene Program, Los Altos Hills, CA.

BOX 8.3   Critical Thinking Scenario A

Using the competencies of your dental hygiene program, create a working template for your student portfolio. Review the accreditation standards in Table 8.1 and consider the various artifacts that could be used to demonstrate mastery of each competency at your school. Explain why you chose these artifacts as examples of the specific competency you are highlighting.

BOX 8.4   Example of Student Journal Log Versus a Reflection

Journal Log Entry

I cared for a young adult patient with albinism and who was legally blind. I learned a lot about working with a visually impaired patient and I can use this experience for my special needs competency requirement.

Reflective Entry

This semester I had the experience of working with a 20-year-old patient who was legally blind due to albinism, a genetic disorder. I didn't know anything about this condition prior to their appointment. Working with this patient required me to reconsider everything I did automatically in clinic—from the simple task of escorting the patient to my cubicle to taking x-rays and giving oral hygiene instructions. I had to put myself in their shoes and think how I would want to be cared for. I discovered that the best approach was to just ask my patient what sort of guidance worked best with their limited vision rather than make assumptions about their needs. This was especially helpful when discussing self-care strategies. I was able to make some helpful suggestions on toothbrush placement and ways to recognize proper placement by the sense of touch. I found that by taking a few minutes to get to know my patient as a person, rather than someone with impaired vision, that we were able to develop effective strategies together for maintaining oral health. I also did some research on albinism following the appointment and found that in addition to skin and vision problems, people with albinism may experience social and emotional challenges due to their condition. Knowing more about the impact of this genetic condition made me realize the role that trust and empathy plays in patient care.

---

be able to describe a clinical experience, to analyze the situation, and ultimately develop a new perspective for future practice through regular formative feedback.[14]

Journal writing allows students a more private opportunity to critique their clinical practice activities and allows for reflection on any assumptions and values underlying the experiences. The differences between a nonreflective, factual journal entry as compared with a thoughtful reflection of the same activity are illustrated in Box 8.4. Although there are a number of prompts for triggering critical reflection, the four "Rs" of revisit, react, relate, and respond, as outlined in Box 8.5, provide helpful guidelines for reflective thinking and writing a reflection statement.[13] A reflection statement based on the experiences of the dental hygiene student and the pediatric patient described previously is shown in Box 8.6. Again, feedback from faculty members on how to move past simply reporting on an experience to thinking more deeply on what was actually learned and how the experience will impact future behavior plays an important role in developing the ability to reflect, think critically, problem solve, and self-assess.[15]

Reflection statements can be inserted in a variety of places depending on the specific purpose of the portfolio. Student reflections are often part of each competency section and should be updated at the end of each academic term to demonstrate one's personal growth as a future healthcare provider. Reflections should also be included as part of an introduction to an artifact, giving more depth regarding the deeper

BOX 8.5 Formulating Reflection Statements[13]

Revisit

Briefly describe the activity or situation

React

How did the activity or situation make you feel?

What actions did you take?

What choices did you make?

Relate

What was the impact of your actions or choices?

How did your actions challenge your value system?

Respond

What did you learn from this activity or situation?

How can you prepare to improve your ability to respond in similar circumstances in the future?

Tsang AK, Walsh LK. Oral health students' perceptions of clinical reflective learning relevance to their development as evolving professionals. *Eur J Dent Educ.* 2010;14:99–105.

BOX 8.6 Reflection on Pediatric Patient

One of my most memorable pediatric patient experiences was caring for a 5-year-old male who presented with his mother for a kindergarten screening and oral prophylaxis appointment. I realized that I had not adequately prepared for their visit when they arrived 20 minutes late. More importantly, I did not know in advance that this was the child's first dental visit and that he would need extra time to become comfortable with the clinic. My initial concerns were that I would not be able to complete this requirement and the impact this clinic session might have on my daily grade. I felt stressed and anxious because I was not able to deal with the child's fears with the shortened appointment time. Given that the examination revealed significant decay and this patient would need dental care as soon as possible, I should have been better prepared with referral sources for the patient's mother. Working with this patient gave me a new perspective on the need to establish a dental home, the importance of oral health education for parents of young children, and the many challenges parents face just getting their children to dental appointments. It made me realize that I have been focusing on periodontal disease management and have overlooked the importance of pediatric oral healthcare in the bigger picture of disease prevention.

BOX 8.7 Critical Thinking Scenario B

Reflective writing takes thought and practice. Think back to caring for your very first patient in clinic. In what ways have you grown as a student dental hygienist? Are there new ways you are providing patient care and making recommendations based on scientific evidence and the needs of the individual patient? In what ways have you grown in your communication skills you're your patients as well as your instructors? Write a one- to two-paragraph statement on the ways you have changed and the challenges you still face as a student dental hygienist.

Introductions to dental hygiene student portfolios often include a brief description of why the student chose dental hygiene as a profession and their personal career goals. This page undoubtedly will change as the student progresses through the dental hygiene program (Fig. 8.3 and Box 8.8).

A philosophy of practice statement is a personal written statement, unique to the individual students, and reflects their values, commitment to the dental hygiene profession, and short-term and long-term career goals as future oral healthcare providers. The perfect time to write a philosophy of practice statement is as the student nears graduation. The process of reflecting and writing this statement helps dental hygiene graduates identify their professional values and communicate to potential employers their unique skills and abilities (Fig. 8.4). Guidelines for writing a philosophy of practice statement can be found in Box 8.9. See Box 8.10.

The biographic data section is the ideal place to keep a current résumé and curriculum vitae. A **résumé** should be a brief document succinctly summarizing an individual's education, employment history, and experiences relevant to a specific employment position. The purpose of a résumé combined with a cover letter is to get an interview. Résumés should be written in a concise style, using bulleted lists rather than sentences or paragraphs, and are designed to fit on a single page. It is advisable to maintain a general résumé on file and then tailor it with the most relevant professional experiences that meet the specific requirements of the potential employment position. Additional information on résumé writing can be found in Chapter 63. The **curriculum vitae** (CV), or course of life as the Latin term implies, is an overview of a person's lifetime of professional activities. The CV should be an ongoing documentation of one's employment, education, teaching, publications, honors, and volunteer activities. Educators in all disciplines are required to maintain a current CV as part of the institution's accreditation process. In the United States, a CV is usually necessary when applying for academic appointments, grants, fellowships, and scholarships. Outside the United States, almost all employers expect a CV as part of the application process. The résumé and the CV should be part of the professional portfolio and must be updated regularly to remain current. The CV can also provide potential artifacts for a portfolio depending on how the portfolio will be used, such as selected research projects or presentations given.

Portfolio Artifacts

An artifact for an e-portfolio may be an electronic file of a student-created brochure, research paper, community service project, or any other document that demonstrates a particular competency.[15] Documents and artifacts must be selected carefully and organized to support the portfolio purpose. Remember, the portfolio should not be a display of every assignment or class project but rather, a well-documented, selective collection of evidence designed to illustrate a particular competency (Figs. 8.5 and 8.6). Each artifact must be accompanied by a label or caption clearly explaining its significance in relationship to the competency or skill, the title of the artifact, the author(s), and the

meaning and significance of the project or activity rather than a detailed explanation of what was done. If the portfolio is used as evidence of competency for the licensed oral healthcare professional, reflection is an integral part of the clinician's self-assessment of competency and guides the planning of future continuing education and professional development activities. An example of this would be the practicing clinician's self-identification of the need to improve their technique for panoramic radiographs. This requires the clinician to first recognize the suboptimal diagnostic quality of their panoramic images and develop a plan for improvement. In this case, the clinician might seek out resources such as a hands-on radiography course at a dental hygiene conference or a continuing education course as ways to meet their self-identified learning goal of improved panoramic images. See Box 8.7.

Introduction and Biographic Data

The portfolio should begin with a brief introduction designed to orient the reader, followed by biographic information on the portfolio's owner.

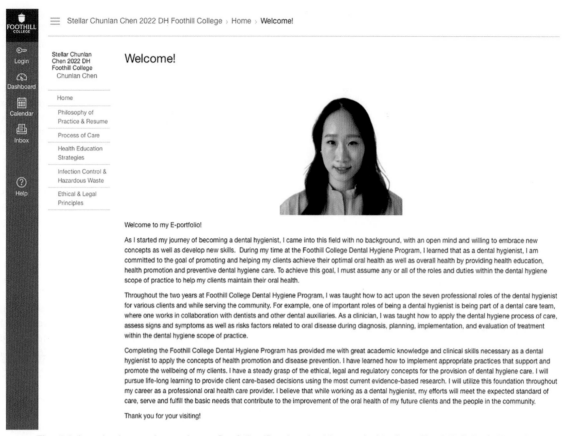

Fig. 8.3 Introduction to the student e-Portfolio. (Reprinted with permission from Foothill College Dental Hygiene Program, Los Altos Hills, California.)

BOX 8.8   Critical Thinking Scenario C

Think about how you would orient a member of the dental hygiene faculty to your portfolio. Consider the key factors and experiences that have been part of your education and personal journey. Write a one-paragraph introduction to your portfolio. Include some brief information about your background and your future dental hygiene career goals. Trade your statement with a peer in your dental hygiene program and give each other feedback on the overall impression you have after reading the introduction.

---

date it was completed. Reflective statements in the form of sentences or short paragraphs should also be included in the descriptive label. Patient care experiences can also be included as an artifact in the student portfolio (Fig. 8.7A). A graphic summary of the various types of patients treated by a dental hygiene student can later serve to demonstrate competency as a new graduate (see Fig. 8.7B). Artifacts demonstrating interprofessional learning or collaborative experiences can be useful for both students and new graduates (Box 8.11).

References and Citations

All documents and artifacts used in the professional portfolio must have appropriate referencing and attribution. If another person's work or research contributed to the project, the work must be appropriately cited. As stated in the *Chicago Manual of Style,* "ethics, copyright laws, and courtesy to readers require authors to identify the sources of direct quotations and of any facts or opinions not generally known or easily checked."[16] Citations not only give credit to others for their work but also allow the reader to further explore the topic by providing the information to locate the original resource. Multiple references also add evidence and credibility to support the project or artifact.

The particular system for listing references and the specific citation style guidelines for student projects depends on the individual school, department, or dental hygiene program; however, there are numerous ways to reference resources. Many medical or biomedical publications require authors to use the American Medical Association (AMA) or the National Library of Medicine (NLM) style, whereas nursing publications frequently use the American Psychological Association (APA) style guidelines. *Citing Medicine,* complete with comprehensive examples of all types of NLM citations, is available free of charge on the National Library of Medicine website, https://www.ncbi.nlm.nih.gov/books/NBK7256/.

Confidentiality and Permissions

One of the core values in the American Dental Hygienists' Association (ADHA) Code of Ethics is **confidentiality,** the responsibility to keep patient information private. Applying this concept to a portfolio means that there must not be any identifiable patient information used in the portfolio. Eliminating names or any identifying information by substitution with initials or pseudonyms can protect the privacy of the individual and institution. Images used in portfolio artifacts can present challenges with patient privacy. Photographs of actual patients must be used with caution. Written permission in the form of a model or photograph release must be obtained to use original photographs, videos, or any other media in which the individuals depicted can be identified. Care must be taken in the selection of artifacts, particularly in online Web-based portfolios, to preserve confidentiality of the patients, faculty, fellow students, and clinical sites that may be described in the artifacts or reflections.

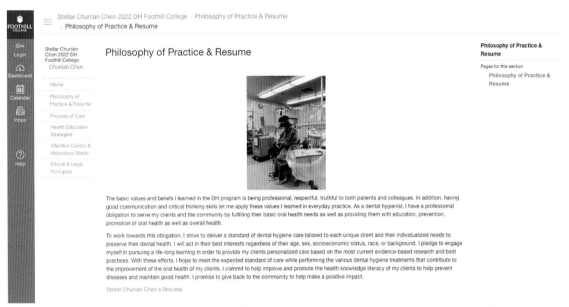

Fig. 8.4 Philosophy of Practice Statement. (Reprinted with permission from Foothill College Dental Hygiene Program, Los Altos Hills, California.)

BOX 8.9 Writing a Healthcare Philosophy of Practice Statement

A healthcare philosophy of practice statement should be a succinctly written paragraph or bulleted highlights that serve as the foundation for one's professional beliefs. Reflection on the following topics can guide the philosophy statement:

- Definition of personal objectives
- Career goals: short term and long term
- Healthcare values
- Interprofessional and intraprofessional collaboration
- Ethical considerations of practice
- Commitment to cultural diversity, special needs, and vulnerable populations
- Definition of excellence
- Vision for the future

BOX 8.10 Critical Thinking Scenario D

You are preparing to graduate and look for your first position as a clinician in private practice. Reflect on your professional values and future career goals and write your philosophy of practice statement to include as part of your portfolio.

BOX 8.11 Critical Thinking Scenario E

It can be challenging to select appropriate content and artifacts for a student portfolio. Discuss with your classmates the differences between a portfolio and professional information posted on social media sites such as Facebook and LinkedIn.

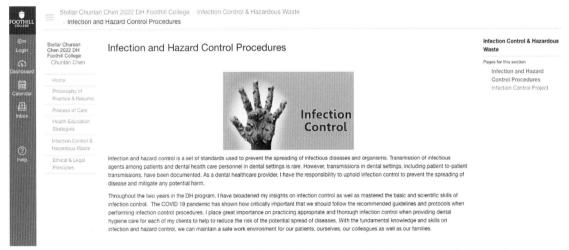

Fig. 8.5 Infection and Hazard Control Introduction. (Reprinted with permission from Foothill College Dental Hygiene Program, Los Altos Hills, California.)

Copyright and Fair Use

Copyright is a widely enacted legal concept which in the simplest of terms means "right to copy." Copyright protects the authors and creators of all types of original work, including writing, composing, graphic and visual arts, and architectural and industrial designs, from others copying their work. It also grants the creator of the work, or copyright holder, the right to be credited for their work and to determine who may adapt or use the work and who may benefit financially from the work. Although copyright does not protect facts, ideas, systems, or methods of operation, it may protect the way these concepts are used or expressed. Copyright protection is available to published and unpublished work and lasts the lifetime of the creator plus a specified number of years.

Copyright does not always prohibit all forms of replication or copying. The **fair use** doctrine in the United States permits some copying and distribution without asking direct permission of the copyright holder. Under certain conditions, fair use can grant educators and students instructional rights to use copyrighted materials while still preserving the rights of the creator and not financially benefiting the user. Although there are no limits to the number of words, images, text, or sounds that can be used safely without prior permission under fair use, it is still best to obtain permission before using copyrighted material when possible. The guidelines defining fair use for educational purposes can be found in Box 8.12. In general, students and professionals creating a portfolio post their own original work in the portfolio. However, there may be occasions in which the portfolio author may want to use an image, link to a website, or quote from a source of literature. It is best to get written permission from the owner of the image and always use the appropriate attribution and reference.[17]

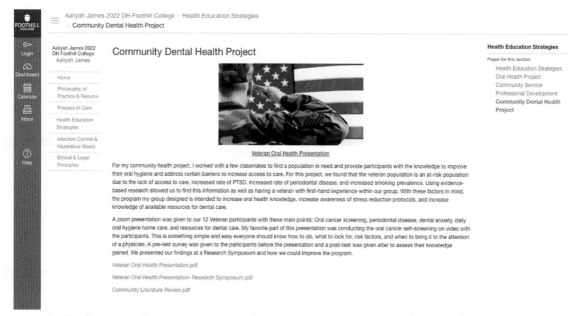

Fig. 8.6 Community Oral Health Project Description. (Reprinted with permission from Foothill College Dental Hygiene Program, Los Altos Hills, California.)

Patient care log

Pt.	ASA	Calculus class and AAP type	Age/ethnicity/ gender	Special needs	Summary of treatment and learning outcomes
1	I	Light calculus/ AAP I: periodontium healthy	3/Asian/F	Pediatric	Pediatric competency. In addition to the regular assessments. I completed a caries risk assessment, plaque index, dmft, and a nutritional assessment. I performed a FM toothbrush prophylaxis and coronal polishing. RS presented with good hygiene but she was in the unaware stage of the learning ladder. Both RS and her mother were receptive to my suggestions and recommendations. It took me one visit to complete care.
2	II	Light calculus/ AAP II: Gingivitis on intact periodontium	30/Caucasian/M	Asthma: Inhaler on counter TMJ: Frequent breaks due to TMJ soreness.	I performed FM scaling with the USS and hand instruments as well as applied 5% fluoride varnish. Patient has good hygiene home care and presented with light calculus, so I was able to complete his treatment while getting comfortable with the process of seeing patients. It took me two visits to complete care.
3	II	Light calculus/ Light calculus/ AAP III: Periodontitis, stage 1, grade A	35/Asian/F	Hypertension: monitor vitals, stress-reduction protocols hypersensitivity	The first patient that I saw this quarter, I performed FM scaling with the USS and hand instruments, selective coronal polishing, and applied 5% fluoride varnish. She presented with generalized slight horizontal bone loss so the oral hygiene instructions focused on products to reduce hypersensitivity and continuing to perform good oral hygiene care at home to maintain the health of her oral status. It took me three visits to complete care.

A

Fig. 8.7 (A) Patient Care Log.

FHDHC Patient Experience Charts

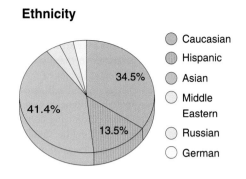

Ethnicity

- Caucasian
- Hispanic
- Asian
- Middle Eastern
- Russian
- German

41.4% 34.5% 13.5%

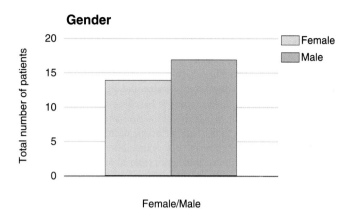

Gender

- Female
- Male

Female/Male

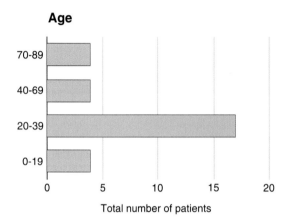

Age

Total number of patients

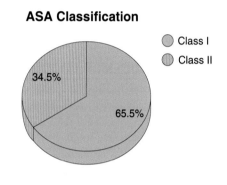

ASA Classification

- Class I
- Class II

34.5% 65.5%

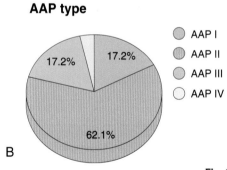

AAP type

- AAP I
- AAP II
- AAP III
- AAP IV

17.2% 17.2% 62.1%

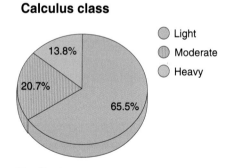

Calculus class

- Light
- Moderate
- Heavy

13.8% 20.7% 65.5%

B

Fig. 8.7, cont'd (B) Patient Demographics Charts.

BOX 8.12 General Guidelines for Fair Use in Education[18]

Fair Use	Not Fair Use
Teaching, scholarship, education	Commercial purposes, profit
Nonfiction based, factual information	Creative work (art, music, films, plays, books)
Commentary or criticism	Entertainment
Small sample of work used	Large part of work is used
Limited or restricted access	Open access on Internet or a public forum

Bylaws and Code of Ethics June 2021. American Dental Hygienists Association. Available at: http://www.adha.org/resources-docs/7611_Bylaws_and_Code_of_Ethics.pdf. Accessed July 8, 2022.

A number of resources for photos and other images without copyright protection are available. Creative Commons, a nonprofit organization, has developed a standardized licensing approach for individuals wishing to make their creative works available for public use via the Internet. Images licensed through Creative Commons can be found through a number of search engines including Google, Yahoo, Flickr, and Unsplash. Appropriate credit must still be given for images and content licensed by Creative Commons.

PORTFOLIO AUTHORSHIP AND ETHICAL PRINCIPLES

The ethical principles of **veracity, beneficence, autonomy,** and **confidentiality** apply to the creation of a professional portfolio and the artifacts presented (Box 8.13). Veracity is defined as the adherence to the truth or conformity to factual evidence. The student dental hygienist or professional is bound by the ADHA Code of Ethics to present artifacts or documents that are the work or accomplishments of the portfolio owner.[18] Work done by others, such as images and outside research, must always be attributed and properly cited. Beneficence is the provision of benefit, preventing harm, or promoting good as a profession. Dental hygiene e-portfolios often include examples of participating in community service and health screenings, an example of beneficence. Autonomy is based on the concept that individuals have the right to self-determination and decision making. Autonomy is related to the legal principle of informed consent. Patients should be asked for consent before including artifacts related to them. Confidentiality protects a client's right to privacy; therefore any client data must be deidentified, which relates to HIPAA regulations. Digital ethics is a growing field that is universal in the ever-increasing digital world. Digital ethics include the use of respectful and appropriate language, gaining consent for the use of information, and the ethical values associated with an online presence in a variety of technologies in safe, responsible, and legal ways. A dental hygiene e-portfolio should be created and maintained with this in mind.[19]

TRANSITIONING THE STUDENT PORTFOLIO

Initially, the student portfolio can be used for entry-level employment interviews, degree completion programs, and postgraduate study. Over time, the portfolio can be transitioned to fulfill a variety of purposes. The student portfolio can become a "working portfolio," serving as a repository for organizing and storing artifacts acquired during one's professional life. Looking back to the core competency areas for the student dental hygienist related to infection control, patient care, health education, and legal and ethical principles, the licensed oral healthcare professional could choose to continue to organize artifacts or evidence of ongoing competencies in these same key areas. The ADHA's "Standards for Clinical Dental Hygiene Practice" also can be used as a guideline for demonstration and self-assessment of clinical competencies.[20] Professional development should be ongoing, even for the recent graduate. Logs chronicling courses, workshops, in-services, and other activities, including the date, presenter, and a short summary/reflection on the activity, should be created for this section. Once the templates for the professional development log have been created, adding the content becomes an easy task (Fig. 8.8). Many state boards of dentistry, as well as the Dental Hygiene Board of California, conduct random audits of the continuing education courses and professional development activities required for licensure renewal. It is the responsibility of the licensed professional to maintain accurate records of their required courses and documentation of attendance.

The portfolio introduction and biographic data section is another area that should be customized to fit the specific purpose of the portfolio. This is the ideal area to state the portfolio owner's philosophy of practice or career goals. Writing a philosophy of practice takes thought and reflection and will most likely change over time and with experience. A philosophy of practice will also vary, depending on the purpose of the portfolio. A portfolio used to interview for a clinical position in private practice differs from one used for a position in education or the corporate world; the philosophy should be written according to the specific purpose. A well-written introduction and philosophy of practice should catch the interest of the reader to review the portfolio more deeply in addition to leaving a professional impression.

Transitioning the student portfolio is an excellent way to showcase the new professional's strengths and experiences in addition to validating clinical competency, ongoing professional development, and self-reflection. Consider Box 8.14. Further information on ethics and ethical decision making can be found in Chapter 7.

BOX 8.13   Legal, Ethical, and Safety Issues

- Apply the core principles of the ADHA Code of Ethics when creating a portfolio.
- Honesty and accuracy are key elements of a student or professional portfolio.
- Consider digital ethics and best practices when creating and sharing e-portfolios.
- Confidentiality, privacy, and consent are important legal/ethical concepts in development of a portfolio.

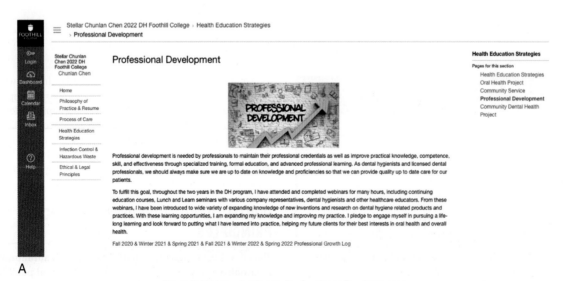

Fig. 8.8 (A) Introduction to Professional Development.

Spring 2022 Professional Growth/CE Activities Log

Date/Course/Meeting	Speaker/Topic	Hours	Summary
4/20/22	Akta Amin – *HuFriedy*	1	In this Zoom meeting, Akta Amin introduces us some of the popular products from HuFriedy, including the PPE and different kinds of instruments with detailed information on their characteristics and usage. Akta Amin then briefly talks about the history of HuFriedy and HuFriedy Group. What's more, Akta Amin also offers us good price for trade-in instruments or new instruments.
4/20/22	Jennifer Lomanto RDH, BSDH - *"Beyond Gut Health: Applications for Use of Probiotics in Dentistry"* ; Dana Yumul RDHEF II, BSDH - *"Music Therapy to Reduce Dental Anxiety"*	2	"Beyond Gut Health: Applications for Use of Probiotics in Dentistry" presented by Jennifer Lomanto, RDH, BSDH covers a brief review of bacteria, chronic oral health conditions, beneficial bacteria, probiotics and their use in dentistry. "Music Therapy to Reduce Dental Anxiety" presented by Dana Yumul, RDHEF II, BSDH introduces the benefits of music therapy and dental anxiety among dental patients.
4/27/22	Sunita Rai – *Pacific Dental Services*	1	In this Zoom meeting, Sunita Rai from Pacific Dental Services briefly explains how the company works as well as what she expects from us if we work as temp RDHs through her company. Rai also provides a lot of practical and useful tips for various aspects of being a dental hygienist. This helps broaden my eyes in the job market of dental hygienist.
5/4/22	Melissa Calhoun – *Arm & Hammer*	1	In this Zoom meeting, Melissa from Arm & Hammer introduces us some of their dental hygiene care products, such as different types of toothpaste. I am so glad that I can learn about the new dental hygiene care products from this company. I will recommend

B

Fig. 8.8, cont'd (B) Professional Development Log.

KEY CONCEPTS

- Portfolios are becoming an integral part of the dental hygiene education and development of the healthcare professional. The foundation begins as student dental hygienist with a learning portfolio and should transition to a professional portfolio, reflecting the growth and achievements throughout the career of the dental hygienist.
- Healthcare professionals must be able to provide ongoing evidence of competency throughout their careers. Maintaining a professional portfolio with artifacts documenting professional development activities is a requirement for license renewal for dental professionals in some states, Canadian provinces, and internationally. Licensure by portfolio is an alternative for the live patient exam for dental students in California, Colorado, and Iowa and may be considered in the future by other states as well.
- Reflective thinking supports critical thinking, problem solving, and self-directed learning, key characteristics of a healthcare professional. Reflection statements should be integrated into the professional portfolio to support each artifact, competency, or section of the portfolio and to direct self-assessment and the lifelong learning process of the healthcare professional.
- A professional portfolio can serve as a visual tool to guide or support the interview process. A well-organized portfolio can assist the practitioner in articulating their philosophy of practice, experiences, education, and ongoing professional growth.
- The professional portfolio must be an honest representation of the individual. Artifacts must have appropriate attribution and follow ethical and legal guidelines.

BOX 8.14 Critical Thinking Scenario F

You are a newly licensed dental hygienist and are getting ready for your first interview for a position in private practice. Practice for the interview by role playing with a peer using artifacts to support your range of clinical experiences from your portfolio.

REFERENCES

1. Siddiqui ZS, Fisher MB, Slade C, et al. Twelve tips for introducing e-Portfolios in health professions education. *Med Teach.* 2022:1–6.
2. Gadbury-Amyot C, Bray KK, Austin KJ. Fifteen years of portfolio assessment of dental hygiene student competency: lessons learned. *J Dent Hyg.* 2014;88(5):267–274.
3. Douglas ME, Peecksen S, Rogers J, Simmons M. College students' motivation and confidence for e-portfolio use. *Int J EPortfolio.* 2019;9(1):1–6.
4. Chamblee TB, Dale JC, Drews B, Spahis J, Hardin T. Implementation of a professional portfolio: a tool to demonstrate professional development for advanced practice. *J Pediatr Health Care.* 2015;29(1):113–117.
5. Dental Licensure and CE Requirements Maps. American Dental Association. Updated May 27, 2022. Available at: https://www.ada.org/resources/licensure/dental-licensure-by-state-map. Accessed July 7, 2022.
6. Minnesota Administrative Rules. Minnesota Legislature. Available at: https://www.revisor.mn.gov/rules/3100.5100/administrativerules. Accessed July 7, 2022.
7. Requirements of the Quality Assurance Program and Guidelines for Continuing Competency. College of Dental Hygienists of Ontario. Updated January 2021. Available at: https://www.cdho.org/docs/default-

source/pdfs/quality-assurance/qaprogram_guidelines.pdf. Accessed July 7, 2022.

8. Kardos RL, Cook JM, Buston RJ, et al. The development of an e-portfolio for life-long reflective learning and auditable professional certification. *Eur J Dent Educ.* 2009;13(3):135–141.

9. Accreditation Standards for Dental Hygiene Programs July 2022. Commission on Dental Accreditation. Available at: https://coda.ada.org/~/media/CODA/Files/dental_hygiene_standards.pdf?la=en. Accessed July 7, 2022.

10. Gwozdek AE, Springfield EC, Kerschbaum WE. Eportfolio: developing a catalyst for critical self-assessment and evaluation of learning outcomes. *J Allied Health.* 2013;42(1):11–17.

11. Woldt JL, Nenad MW. Reflective writing in dental education to improve critical thinking and learning: a systematic review. *J Dent Educ.* 2021;85(6):778–785.

12. Asadoorian J, Schoenwetter DJ, Lavigne SE. Developing reflective health care practitioners: learning from experience in dental education. *J Dent Educ.* 2011;75(4):472–484.

13. Tsang AK, Walsh LK. Oral health students' perceptions of clinical reflective learning relevance to their development as evolving professionals. *Eur J Dent Educ.* 2010;14:99–105.

14. Heeneman S, Driessen E, Durning SJ, et al. Use of an e-portfolio mapping tool: connecting experiences, analysis and action by learners. *Perspect Med Educ.* 2019;8(3):197–200.

15. Gadbury-Amyot CC, Godley LW, Nelson Jr JW. Measuring the level of reflective ability of predoctoral dental students: early outcomes in an e-portfolio reflection. *J Dent Educ.* 2019;83(3):275–280.

16. University of Chicago Press Staff. *Chicago Manual of Style.* 17th ed. University of Chicago Press; 2017:1174.

17. Copyright law of the United States of America. Copyright.gov. Available at: https://www.copyright.gov/title17/. Accessed July 8, 2022.

18. Bylaws and Code of Ethics June 2021. American Dental Hygienists Association. Available at: http://www.adha.org/resources-docs/7611_Bylaws_and_Code_of_Ethics.pdf. Accessed July 8, 2022.

19. Wilson CB, Slade C, Kirby MK, et al. Digital ethics and the use of eportfolio: a scoping review of the literature. *Int J EPortfolio.* 2018;8(2):115–125.

20. Standards for Clinical Dental Hygiene Practice. American Dental Hygienists Association. Available at: https://www.adha.org/resources-docs/2016-Revised-Standards-for-Clinical-Dental-Hygiene-Practice.pdf. Accessed July 8, 2022.

9

Dental Hygiene Patient Care Settings

Tracee Sokolik Dahm

PROFESSIONAL OPPORTUNITIES

Dental hygienists deliver preventive and therapeutic oral healthcare services in many different practice settings. Being aware of the various practice environments enables a dental hygienist to adapt to differing equipment and situations for patient care.

COMPETENCIES

1. Discuss the equipment and areas included in a patient treatment area in a dental/dental hygiene office or clinic.
2. Compare and contrast the dental hygiene care environment in a dental office, college or university, and correctional facility to include the components of the dental hygiene treatment area.
3. Apply knowledge of the dental hygiene care environment unique to a correctional facility and an institutionalized setting and delivery of patient care services in that setting.
4. Explain the adjustments that a dental hygiene care provider must consider when delivering services in a school-based oral health prevention program, mobile dental facility, or outreach setting using teledentistry. Also, describe the influence of patient setting on the dental hygiene care environment.

DENTAL HYGIENE CARE ENVIRONMENT

The **dental hygiene care environment** is the physical setting that contains equipment and instruments where the dental hygienist delivers professional oral care. This chapter identifies the structural components of a conventional **treatment area** (formerly called an operatory) in a dental or dental hygiene practice setting, as well as community locations that include higher education, hospital, correctional facility, and outreach settings using teledentistry and mobile dental equipment. In addition, this chapter describes dental equipment the dental hygienist uses and maintains and discusses the legal, ethical, and safety issues associated with the dental hygiene care environment (Box 9.1). Dental hygienists deliver preventive and therapeutic clinical services in various settings. In some states, dental hygienists provide direct access to oral healthcare as they initiate treatment based on their assessment of a patient's needs without the specific authorization of a dentist, treat a patient without a dentist, and maintain healthcare provider-patient relationships.[1] An oral healthcare practice or clinic in the private, corporate, and public sectors commonly includes treatment areas for dental units, general structural fixtures, radiographic equipment, a radiographic processing area, an instrument processing area, a

laboratory, supply storage, reception and clerical areas, and a restroom. Some practices and clinics also have staff areas for breaks and private consultation rooms for patient care.

Dental or Dental Hygiene Offices or Clinics

In a dental or dental hygiene practice setting, multiple rooms make up the dental office. Dental hygienists often work in a separate treatment area. The reception area is the first room a patient enters and confirms their appointment (Fig. 9.1). Décor, lighting, temperature, sound, and smell influence the environment in a dental office. These factors also leave a lasting impression on patients and set the tone for the visit. Décor in a general practice should be calm and relaxing, with no overwhelming color schemes. The lighting should be adequate for reading, and appropriate reading material should be available for patients. Soft sounds, such as a water fountain bubbling or classical music, may also help the patient to relax before the appointment. The clerical area is located adjacent to the reception area and contains computer terminals, telephones, and intraoffice communication systems, in addition to an area for printed patient-related dental records and office supplies. The clerical area should remain private because of the exchange of patient information in accordance with the Health Insurance Portability and Accountability Act (HIPAA) (see Chapter 64). The complexity of this area depends on the size and needs of the practice. The dentist has an office to consult the patient's medical records and to converse privately with other staff members and/or patients. Private dental offices often provide a break room or kitchen for employees to eat their food throughout the workday.[2]

Dental Hygiene or Dental Treatment Area
Stools and Chairs

The dental treatment area, where the dental hygienist provides professional oral care, contains stools, dental chair, dental unit, and equipment (Fig. 9.2). The **operator stool** adjusts for seat height and back support with controls located under the seat cushion (Fig. 9.3). It should provide ergonomic support, especially in the lumbar region of the back, and allow for the operator's feet to be flat on the floor to maintain proper circulation in the lower extremity. Stool designs range from saddle stools with no back or armrests to traditional stools with back and low armrests. The stools are lightweight, portable, and easily adjustable to solve a multitude of ergonomic problems. A **saddle stool** adjusts easily with one lever and lends itself to multiple users (Fig. 9.4). The saddle stool helps correct poor ergonomics and body positions by placing the dental hygienist halfway between standing and sitting, increasing the hip angle up to 135°, thus allowing for lower positioning

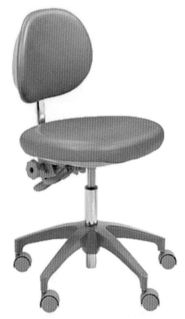

Fig. 9.3 Operator stool. (Courtesy A-dec, Inc., Newberg, OR.)

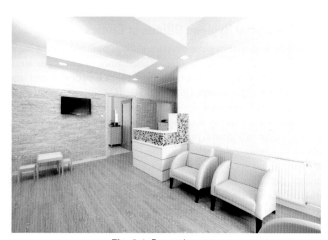

Fig. 9.1 Reception area.

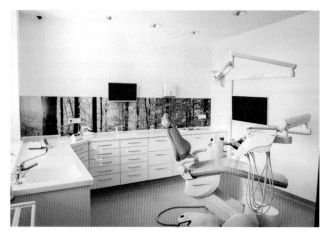

Fig. 9.2 Treatment area.

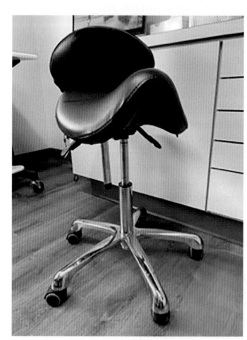

Fig. 9.4 Saddle stool. (Courtesy Tracee Dahm, Coeur d'Alene Dental Center, Coeur d'Alene, Idaho.)

of the patient and a more relaxed shoulder posture for the clinician. Regardless of the stool chosen, properly adjusting the stool for the clinician's body stature is important to prevent musculoskeletal disorders. The **dental assistant stool**, taller than an operator stool, differs in function and usually has a bar to support the feet and a torso support bar to allow the dental assistant to lean forward over the patient while assisting the operator (Fig. 9.5). The **dental chair**, a reclining elongated lounge, has arm supports and is adjustable by switch, touch pad, or foot control for height, headrest, swivel, and tilt. Coverings on dental stools and chairs vary and are durable and easily disinfected. The dental chair is adjustable and should be comfortable for the patient during the dental hygiene process of care. It also is an ideal place to provide patient education and teach self-care practices such as the correct use of oral hygiene aids (Box 9.2).[3]

The Dental Unit

The **dental unit** contains the **delivery system** and a dental light (Fig. 9.6). The delivery system, attached to a bracket table, movable arm, or mobile cart, typically contains the air-water syringe, the high-speed

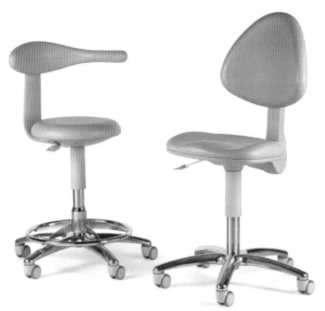

Fig. 9.5 Options for the dental assistant stool are available with or without a torso support bar.

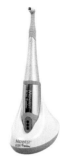

Fig. 9.7 Wireless handpiece.

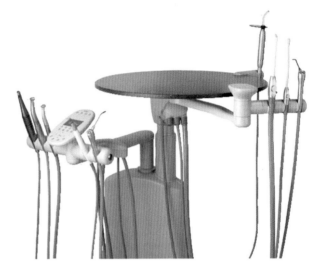

Fig. 9.8 Two dental delivery system. (Courtesy A-dec, Inc., Newberg, OR.)

BOX 9.2   Client or Patient Education Tips

The dental hygiene chair and treatment is the best place for dental hygienists to educate their patient on proper oral hygiene instruction. Coupled with today's technology, dental hygienists have numerous tools, both visual and hands, to help teach patients how to care for their oral cavity. The dental chair, in an upright position, is an excellent place because it keeps both the hygienist and patient at the same eye level for constructive criticism when it comes to oral hygiene instruction. Most dental hygienists start by handing their patients a soft manual toothbrush or interdental aid and asking them to demonstrate normal use. The dental hygienist holds a handheld mirror so that patients can see what they are doing. A dental hygienist can show patients why they are missing specific areas of the mouth, leaving behind bacterial biofilm, and demonstrate how to adapt the oral hygiene device(s) in the oral cavity. If equipment is available and time permits, then the dental hygienist can show patient education videos to introduce or reinforce oral hygiene instruction. In addition, an intraoral camera (IOC), available in many operatories, is an effective educational tool to demonstrate missed areas of bacterial biofilm.[2]

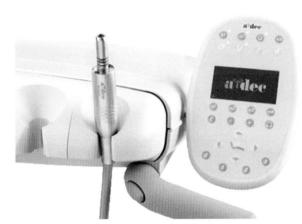

Fig. 9.9 Dental unit touch pad. (Courtesy A-dec, Inc., Newberg, OR.)

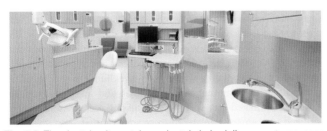

Fig. 9.6 The dental unit contains a dental chair, delivery systems, monitor, rheostat, and light.

and low-speed handpiece tubing, and the handpiece prophy angle. Dental handpieces and other equipment can have wired and wireless settings. Wireless handpieces allow for their use outside of the traditional dental setting and help to maintain better ergonomics for the dental professional (Fig. 9.7). The dental light can be mounted on a ceiling track or on a pole attached to the dental unit. Some clinicians also choose to wear wireless light-emitting diode (LED) headlights. A

switch or rheostat (foot control) controls electrical power, light, and water; most units have separate power and water switches independent of each other. Some delivery systems have touch pads mounted on the bracket or instrument table that operate components of the system (Figs. 9.8 and 9.9). Many variations in design are available for a bracket or instrument table, which can hold instruments and the components of the delivery system for oral healthcare providers. Additional mounted tubing on the delivery system arm may include an ultrasonic, piezoelectric, or sonic scaler; an air polishing handpiece or unit; a fiberoptic light; a composite curing light; and a laser, all of which may be activated by switch or rheostat. Mounted on the delivery arm could be a monitor for a computer to display electronic dental records. This equipment can be mounted either in front of the clinician for a 9 o'clock seating position or behind the patient's head for a 12 o'clock delivery system with a seating position for the clinician behind the patient's head (Fig. 9.10). High-volume evacuation (HVE) and low-volume evacuation (LVE) tubing or suction lines facilitate patient rinsing and maintain visibility and a dry field during care. Adapters and devices are available for suction lines that accommodate narrow and wide suction tip inserts and saliva ejectors. The evacuation system has a trap to catch debris evacuated from the oral cavity, and it requires daily cleaning and replacement after cleaning. Dental units have a separate water bottle supply (closed water system) for the unit (Fig. 9.11) or a facility-wide water treatment system. The Centers for Disease Control and Prevention (CDC) has established recommendations for all dental devices (e.g., handpieces, ultrasonic scalers, air-water syringe) connected to the water system.[4] Water used for routine dental treatment should meet the nationally recognized standards set by the U.S. Environmental Protection Agency (EPA) for drinking water (<500 CFU/mL for heterotrophic plate count). Dental units and their various equipment use distilled water according to manufacturers' instructions. Daily treatments such as iodine tablets for water bottles or suction line chemical treatments are necessary to prevent biofilm formation in the water tubing or lines. Most contemporary dental units have antiretraction valves

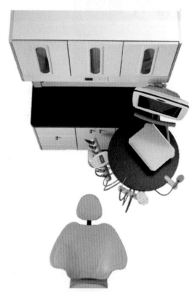

Fig. 9.10 A 12 o'clock dental delivery system. (Courtesy A-dec, Inc., Newberg, OR.)

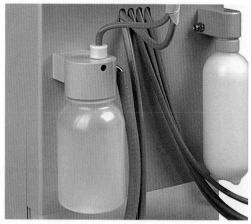

Fig. 9.11 Dental water bottle.

on the water lines to prevent the backflow of contaminated water into the water lines of the unit. The CDC recommends that dental professionals advise their patients not to close their mouths tightly on suction tips to prevent a possible backflow of liquids.[4] Water line disinfection products are available (see Chapter 10). Dental hygienists need to follow dental equipment suppliers' published information on the use and maintenance of these products. If these documents are not available in the treatment area, then most manufacturers publish maintenance information on their websites.[5]

Structural Fixtures

Most treatment areas have storage cabinets, a sink, paper towel dispensers, and alcohol hand rub and antibacterial soap dispensers with manual (often with foot or laser) controls. Infection control standards mandate an emergency eyewash station attached to the faucet of a sink in the facility. A biohazard sharps container to collect contaminated needles and sharp objects is in the treatment area to help prevent needlestick exposures during disposal. The EPA asks dental offices to keep a disposal container for anesthetic carpules that are not fully used. The counter in a treatment area holds material referenced during patient care (e.g., paperwork, educational or study models, patient education materials). The walls and flooring in the treatment area are functional, easily cleaned, and sturdy. Draperies, carpeting, and delicate furnishings are not appropriate in treatment areas because they hold contaminants and are difficult to disinfect.

A compressor provides compressed air to run the dental units and delivery systems. Because of its size and noise production, the compressor is usually housed in a mechanical room with other devices such as circuit breakers, fuse box, central suction, water heater, and heating and air conditioning units.[6]

Other Areas Found in a Dental Facility or a Dental Hygiene Office or Clinic
Instrument Recirculation Area

Contaminated instruments are sterilized or processed for reuse (see Chapter 10 on Infection Control) in the instrument recirculation area or sterilization area. Contaminated instruments are carried to this area in a covered container or cassette by a clinician wearing full personal protective equipment (PPE). The area should have a clearly demarcated entrance point to bring in contaminated instruments and an exit point for the sterile instruments. Demarcated areas prevent the accidental exposure of sterile instruments and people to blood and bodily fluids from contaminated instruments. This well-ventilated area contains ultrasonic instrument cleaning device(s) and one or more methods to sterilize the various instruments: dry heat, steam pressure or chemical pressure, and/or flash sterilizer(s). The contaminated area provides storage for products used in preparing instruments for sterilization and in cleaning and disinfection supplies, as well as a container with a high-level liquid chemical instrument disinfectant. Another biohazard trash and sharps container is in the contaminated section of the processing area or isolated area. Sterilized instruments are stored in wrapped preset trays, cassettes, or pouches, away from the contaminated processing area, and handled according to CDC guidelines (see Chapter 10).[3] Following manufacturers' directions for all equipment is necessary to ensure that all procedures are consistently implemented for optimal performance of the equipment.[2–6]

Radiographic equipment. Radiographic equipment used by the dental hygienist varies because radiographs are either film or digital and are taken at chairside, in a designated or separate area, or with wireless equipment. The radiographic equipment can consist of a wall-mounted control panel with an on-off switch, an indicator light, exposure settings, an x-ray tube mounted on a long movable arm with an open cylinder or rectangular position indicating device (PID) at the end, and a wall-mounted exposure button (Fig. 9.12). Wireless radiographic equipment is operated as a handheld radiography device (Fig. 9.13). The lead apron with a thyroid collar is required for patient protection.

Digital radiographic technology uses the same x-ray tube as conventional methods; however, a charged photoreceptor sensor, the size of 0, 1, or 2 film, is used in lieu of a conventional film packet (Fig. 9.14). Images appear almost instantaneously on the computer monitor after exposure. Digital radiographic images can be viewed on a computer screen, stored, transmitted electronically, or printed.[7]

Panoramic radiography produces a film or digital image of the maxillary and mandibular jaws. A digital panoramic image appears on the computer monitor while exposure is in progress. The image can be saved to the computer software, transmitted electronically, or printed. Large treatment areas can house the panoramic x-ray machine; some facilities have separate rooms for this machine (Fig. 9.15).[7]

Intraoral cameras (IOCs) were first used in dentistry in 1987. Since then, IOCs have evolved from oversized mobile units to pocket-sized, lightweight wands. The IOC magnifies teeth to 40 to 60 times their original size, which allows for the identification of defects within the oral cavity. Operators use IOCs for chairside patient education, oral examinations, comparisons, and specialist referrals (Fig. 9.16).[7]

Radiographic Processing Area

A **radiographic processing area** or darkroom houses automatic dental radiographic film processing units that provide standardized processing of films using premixed solutions, automated time and temperature exposure, and rinsing and drying of films. Safe lights located in the processing area should be 4 feet away from the processors. Automatic

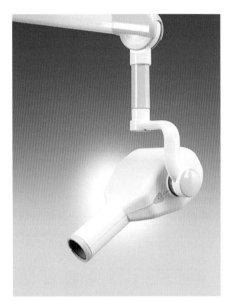

Fig. 9.12 Radiographic tube head.

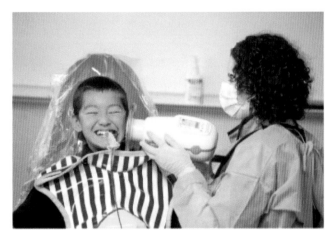

Fig. 9.13 Nomad wireless x-ray unit. (Photo by Jeff Gritchen/Digital First Media/Orange County Register via Getty Images.)

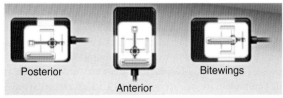

Fig. 9.14 Digital radiographic sensors. (Courtesy DENTSPLY Rinn, a division of DENTSPLY International, Elgin, IL.)

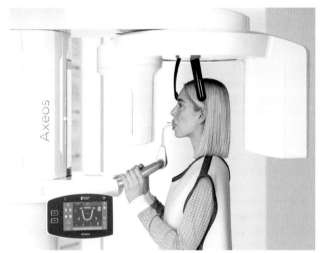

Fig. 9.15 Panoramic radiography. (Courtesy DENTSPLY Sirona, York, PA.)

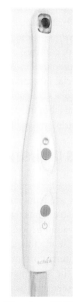

Fig. 9.16 Intraoral camera. (Courtesy Old Dominion University, Norfolk, VA.)

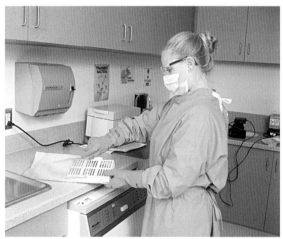

Fig. 9.17 A dental laboratory. (From Bird DL, Robinson DS. *Modern Dental Assisting.* 4th ed. Saunders; 2018.)

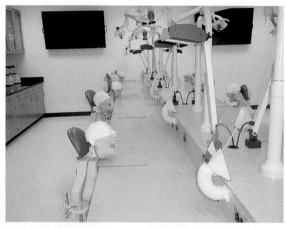

Fig. 9.18 Educational setting patient simulator. (Thomas Nelson Community College, Williamsburg, VA.)

processors with a daylight loader do not require a darkroom. In addition to overhead lighting in the darkroom, an outside warning light prevents accidental entry into the darkroom while films are being processed. Dental offices or clinics using digital or wireless radiographic settings do not have a radiographic processing area.[7]

Dental Laboratory

Although most extensive dental laboratory work, such as construction of crowns and bridges or implants, is sent to a separate dental laboratory employing dental laboratory technicians, many dental offices have small areas for minor laboratory work to support patient care. The dental laboratory within the dental facility is a well-ventilated area for dental work not directly performed with the patient. PPE is required while working in the laboratory. Examples of minor laboratory work include construction of study models, adjustment of dental appliances, and fabrication of mouth guards and custom fluoride or whitening trays. To accomplish these tasks, the laboratory has various equipment such as a model articulator, dental lathe, lathe hood, a vacuum machine to shape acrylic, shears and nippers, and a dental engine with a laboratory handpiece. In addition, air and gas outlets, a gas torch, alcohol or Bunsen burners, casting ovens, and waxing units may be in the laboratory. Commonly found dental materials in the dental laboratory include impression trays, rubber bowls, alginate, spatulas, dental plaster, dental stone, tray formers, a model vibrator, and a model trimmer. A sink and water source with temperature controls are standard dental laboratory features. In some facilities, preparation of impressions or prostheses for transmittal to a commercial laboratory takes place in the laboratory. Dust, byproducts, and noises are usually present in the laboratory. Whenever possible, the dental laboratory is accessible to the treatment areas but out of sight and hearing range of patients (Fig. 9.17).[2,3,6]

ACADEMIC SETTINGS IN INSTITUTIONS OF HIGHER EDUCATION

In academia, dental hygiene students encounter most of the structural fixtures, equipment, instruments, radiology, and dental laboratories similar to those in private practice. The school setting differs in that dental hygiene schools use mannequin simulation for preclinical teaching (Fig. 9.18). With mannequin simulation or typodont mounts, instructors can safely teach the students to work with the public by engaging them in real-life scenarios without jeopardizing anyone's health. A simulation laboratory is an asset in some academic dental hygiene settings.

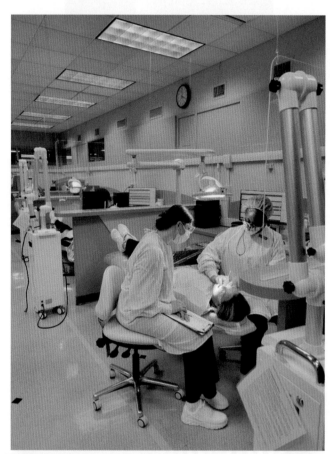

Fig. 9.19 Academic setting. (Courtesy Jennifer Pieren, Youngstown State University, Youngstown, OH.)

Some are media equipped and used to view and record instruction from professors. As the students become more confident with mannequin instruction, they can then move on to treating patients. The design of the clinic's floor plan and academic treatment areas typically promotes opportunities for teaching and learning, offering faculty members the opportunity to work with multiple students in different yet clustered areas (Fig. 9.19). Central areas may accommodate radiographic equipment, storage areas, and sterilization areas that are accessible to all students. Faculty offices may also be available for clinical faculty supervising students' patient care.[8]

DENTAL HYGIENISTS IN SETTINGS BEYOND TRADITIONAL PRIVATE PRACTICE

The release of the 2021 *Oral Health in America: Advances and Challenges* report discussed how the current oral health system in the United States delivers predominantly office-based care that, while convenient for providers, is not accessible for many, including older adults, persons with disabilities, and others.[9] Dental hygienists have experienced an increase in access to care legislation in the past 20 years that has resulted in hygienists working in settings where care is taken to the patient, rather than the patient coming to a dentist's office. The impact of these modules of care can be seen in the 2021 report. Following are examples of how dental hygienists have expanded their practice settings to include community-based centers, schools, nursing homes, and beyond.

CORRECTIONAL FACILITY SETTING

The care environment for the registered dental hygienist who works in a correctional facility (prison) is very different. Although the facility typically houses one or more treatment areas, similar to those mentioned in previous settings, the setup should be altered to protect both the dental professional and the patient (Fig. 9.20). As a result of patient circumstances and the disciplinary environment, the patients who are being treated are under strict 24-hour monitoring and are only allowed certain "freedoms," depending on the facility's regulations. The dental hygiene care environment in the correctional facility has only instruments and equipment deemed necessary for treatment. Treatment areas contain the dental chair, bracket table, operator stool, and possibly a dental assistant stool, if needed. A small desk for note taking and either a digital or paper chart may be found in the treatment area. Supplies and equipment are counted and monitored to ensure that they are not left alone with the patient. Inventory, sterilization, and storage of instruments are locked and out of sight of the treatment area because sharp edges or chemicals could cause bodily harm to prisoners if not safely guarded.[10]

INSTITUTIONALIZED SETTING

As part of a specialized oral healthcare team, dental hygienists provide therapeutic services to medically complex individuals. These individuals are often too ill to provide care to themselves because of various diseases or ailments and the natural process of aging. The institutionalized setting is a hospital, mental health facility, long-term care facility, or nursing home that provides housing for individuals unable to live without assistance. In both acute and chronic care settings, dental hygienists may provide bedside care to clients too ill to be transported or may work in a traditional treatment area. Some institutionalized settings have additional dental hygiene care environments, including a radiographic processing area. The dental hygiene environment can be improvised because care for persons who are homebound, bedridden, or wheelchair bound requires the clinician to use portable or hand-activated methods of instrumentation and/or portable dental equipment, and to work in unique areas such as a hospital room and an operating room (Figs. 9.21 and 9.22). Some patients in wheelchairs may be able to be transported to a traditional dental operatory, while others may elect to have the dental hygienist treat them while sitting in their wheelchairs. The portable dental equipment used in the institutionalized setting may be equipped with other medical equipment to help provide dental care. For example, a dental hygienist may use the hospital wall suction to help keep the oral cavity dry during treatment.[10]

School-Based Oral Health Prevention Programs

Dental hygienists deliver preventive oral health services in school-based oral health programs that provide fluoride varnish and dental sealants to children. In school-based programs, dental hygienists provide screenings, fluoride varnish, dental sealants, and oral health education to students and, if needed, refer patients to local dentists for dental care. In school-based sealant programs, dental hygienists

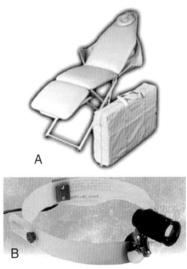

Fig. 9.21 (A) Portable dental chair. (B) Headband light. (Courtesy DNTL-works Equipment Corporation, Centennial, CO.)

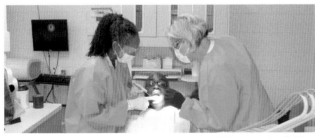

Fig. 9.20 Correctional facility. (Federal Bureau of Prisons). Available at: www.bop.gov/jobs/positions/index.jsp?p=Dental%20Hygienist

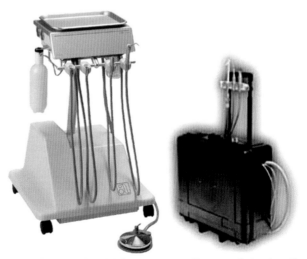

Fig. 9.22 Portable dental delivery systems. (Courtesy A-dec, Inc., Newberg, OR.)

provide pit and fissure sealants to children in a school setting. These programs generally target vulnerable populations of children who are at greater risk for developing dental caries and are less likely to receive preventive care. These programs may have a room converted into a dental treatment area. More commonly, mobile dental equipment is used by dental hygienists visiting different schools in a school district.[10]

Mobile Dental Facility Setting

Mobile dental facilities are entirely structured on the basis of space, supplies, and need. Dental hygienists can travel; therefore the dental hygiene care setting is comprised of easily portable equipment. These facilities are unique and not structured as typical dental hygiene care environments; there is no defined radiographic, laboratory, or clerical area. Some community health agencies and private foundations own fully equipped mobile dental vans for providing preventive and therapeutic services to underserved populations (Fig. 9.23). Fully equipped train cars travel on existing rail systems (e.g., the Smile Train) or in large motor home–type vehicles, bringing high-quality oral care to underserved areas.

Some dental hygienists also have mobile equipment carts or trailers that are used to travel from one facility to another to provide care to people lacking access to preventive and therapeutic dental and dental hygiene services. Dental hygienists also provide direct access to patient care for individuals in long-term care facilities, in areas with no available dental professionals, and in assisted living facilities.[10]

Outreach Settings Using Teledentistry

Telehealth dentistry (teledentistry) originated in 1924. The idea was to reach out to underserved, remote populations and to provide oral

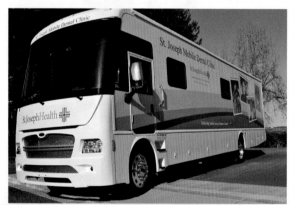

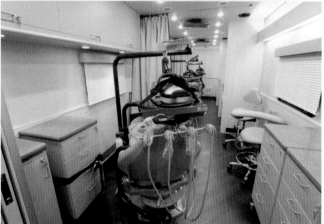

Fig. 9.23 Mobile dentistry. (Courtesy St. Joseph Health, Sonoma County, CA.)

care through the help of an oral professional coupled with technologic advancements. Teledentistry became increasingly popular during the COVID-19 pandemic in 2020.[11] A registered dental hygienist working in telehealth could work in a dental hygiene environment such as those previously mentioned (see Chapter 65 on Teledentistry). Teledentistry occurs in remote areas; therefore the facility size, number of clinicians, operatories, supplies, and equipment vary. Dental hygienists may be in an environment where they work with advanced technology that includes wireless equipment or find themselves using portable equipment such as that described for mobile dentistry settings. Electronic telehealth dentistry depends on electronic communication, both visual and verbal, between the dental hygienist treating the patient and the supervising or collaborating dentist. A dental hygienist may discuss a patient's care and health status over the telephone or via the computer. The telehealth dental hygiene care environment has access to these types of communication devices, either directly in the treatment area or in a clerical office, as long as each patient's case is kept confidential.[10]

INFLUENCE OF PRACTICE SETTING ON THE DENTAL HYGIENE CARE ENVIRONMENT

The dental hygiene care environment often is influenced by the practice setting. Within the private or corporate dental office settings, the facilities are similar; however, the availability of instruments, equipment, technology, and spaces differ from one practice to another. When changing work settings or substituting in various practices, dental hygienists must adapt to varying environments for patient care. Dental hygienists practicing in settings other than the private or corporate settings, such as a college or university, correctional facility, mobile, or teledentistry setting, experience additional differences in the patient care environment (see Critical Thinking Exercise).

CRITICAL THINKING EXERCISE

Visit the different facilities and/or contact dental hygienists who work in the following settings: dental office, college or university, school, and prison. Compare the practice environments and the components of the dental hygiene treatment areas.

KEY CONCEPTS

- A dental hygiene care environment is the physical setting in which professional care is delivered; defined areas are designed for the delivery and support of professional care. The environment may be stationary or mobilized to place-bound or underserved populations.
- Additional space for instrument and radiographic processing is in separate rooms or in clearly designated areas.
- High-quality professional care may be delivered in private practices, academic and research facilities, hospitals, community clinics, mobile vehicles, long-term care facilities, and correctional facilities.
- The dental hygienist is responsible for learning effective, safe practices for using and maintaining equipment, supplies, and instruments used in the delivery of care.
- Inadequate equipment and supplies undermine the quality of services rendered and jeopardize the health and welfare of clinicians and patients.
- Practitioners and dental facility administrators are responsible for injuries or damages resulting from inadequate equipment or negligent maintenance procedures.

ACKNOWLEDGMENT

The author acknowledges Denise M. Claiborne for her past contributions to this chapter.

REFERENCES

1. American Dental Hygienists' Association. ADHA Policy Manual, 13–15. Updated June 2020. Available at: https://www.adha.org/resources-docs/7614_Policy_Manual.pdf. Accessed November 8, 2022.
2. Bird DL, Robinson DS. *Modern Dental Assisting*. 13th ed. Saunders; 2021.
3. Gaylor LJ. *The Administrative Dental Assistant*. 5th ed. Elsevier; 2019.
4. Centers for Disease Control and Prevention. Medical and dental equipment. Updated October 11, 2016. Available at: https://www.cdc.gov/healthywater/other/medical/med_dental.html. Accessed November 8, 2022.
5. Centers for Disease Control and Prevention. Saliva ejector & backflow. Updated March 3, 2016. Available at: https://www.cdc.gov/oralhealth/infectioncontrol/faqs/saliva.html. Accessed November 8, 2022.
6. Finkbeiner B, Finkbeiner C. *Practice Management for the Dental Team*. 9th ed. Mosby; 2020.
7. Thomson E, Johnson O. *Essentials of Dental Radiography for Dental Assistants and Hygienists*. 10th ed. Pearson; 2018.
8. Allaire JL. Assessing critical thinking outcomes of dental hygiene students utilizing virtual patient simulation: a mixed methods study. *J Dent Educ.* 2015;79(9):1082–1092.
9. National Institutes of Health (NIH). *Oral Health in America: Advances and Challenges*; 2021. Available at: https://www.nidcr.nih.gov/oralhealthinamerica. Accessed November 9, 2022.
10. Beatty CF. *Community Oral Health Practice for the Dental Hygienist*. 5th ed. Elsevier; 2021.
11. Abbas B, Wajahat M, Saleem Z, et al. Role of teledentistry in COVID-19 pandemic: a nationwide comparative analysis among dental professionals. *Eur J Dent.* 2020;14(S 01):S116–S122. https://doi.org/10.1055/s-0040-1722107. Epub December 31, 2020. PMID: 33383589; PMCID: PMC7775233.

Infection Prevention and Control

Eve Cuny, Kathy Eklund, and Jessica Jorquera

PROFESSIONAL OPPORTUNITIES

Infection prevention and control (IPC) is an essential part of every clinical practice. Patients and dental hygiene professionals may be exposed to infectious agents during the course of dental treatment. The risk of infectious disease transmission can be greatly reduced, even eliminated, through the strict adherence to evidence-based infection prevention practices. Dental hygienists with strong infection-control skills and knowledge can take a leadership role within the dental setting to educate and guide the rest of the dental team.

COMPETENCIES

1. Discuss basic infection prevention and control concepts.
2. Explain the similarities and differences between the infection-control model and the model of dental hygiene care.
3. Identify the government agencies that play key roles in regulation of infection-control standards.
4. Discuss the standard of care, including assessment of risk of disease transmission in oral healthcare and planning of appropriate control measures.
5. Explain, in detail, the four principles of IPC, including:
   - Select appropriate protective attire for dental hygiene patient care.
   - Prepare the dental environment before and after patient care.
6. Discuss strategies to prevent disease transmission and actions healthcare personnel can take to stay healthy.

BASIC INFECTION PREVENTION AND CONTROL CONCEPTS

IPC is a critical component of safe dental care.[1] In healthcare settings, including dental healthcare settings, the primary objective is to prevent: (1) healthcare-associated infections (HAIs) in patients, and (2) occupational injuries and illnesses in personnel.[1–3] Although transmission of infectious agents among patients and dental healthcare personnel (DHCP) in dental settings is rare, transmission of infectious diseases has been documented in dental care settings. Noncompliance with infection prevention procedures increases the likelihood for transmission to occur.[1,4–6]

Infection prevention and control refers to a comprehensive, systematic program that when applied, reduces the risk of transmission of infectious agents among persons who are in direct or indirect contact with the healthcare environment. The goal of IPC is to create and maintain a safe clinical environment to eliminate or significantly reduce the potential for disease transmission from clinician to patient, patient to clinician, or patient to patient.[2,4] The risk of infectious disease transmission occurs when an infectious agent has a viable portal of entry to a susceptible host. This can occur when a dental hygienist has an accidental puncture with a contaminated instrument or when inadequately reprocessed instruments are used on subsequent patients.

Although IPC practices cannot reduce unintended harm from the care itself, they can prevent unintended harm to the dental hygienist, patient, and other staff members. The hygienist uses patient assessment findings to make decisions about appropriate interventions. With infection-control practices, the hygienist considers procedures and behaviors indicated to reduce risk of disease transmission.

Infection prevention begins with an assessment of the healthcare delivery environment to determine the site-specific IPC measures that are indicated. There are steps to take to prevent exposure to potential infectious hazards. Dental hygienists conduct an infection-control assessment based on the care plan as follows:
1. What procedures will be performed?
2. What exposure risks are associated with those procedures?
3. What IPC measures are indicated (Box 10.1)?

INFECTION PREVENTION AND CONTROL MODEL

A **model of IPC** parallels the model of dental hygiene care. For example, patients must understand the selection and use of IPC procedures and the protective outcomes. However, the infection-control model differs from the traditional patient care model in that it focuses on tasks and procedures to protect both the patient and the provider.

Scrutinizing each individual health history does not determine the degree of risk for disease transmission, which is a primary rationale for the use of standard precautions. Patients may be unknowingly infected with an infectious microorganism and display no symptoms. However, many infectious organisms can be contagious before an infected person has detectable clinical symptoms. Examples include the common cold, influenza, COVID-19, and other highly contagious infectious diseases. Individuals infected with the hepatitis B virus (HBV) or the hepatitis C virus (HCV) may have no symptoms, yet they may have the virus circulating in their blood and other body fluids. Dental procedures generate widely variant amounts of body fluids, and the dental instruments used vary in their tendency to release body fluids. Therefore, IPC is procedurally based, not patient based. Cognitive goals in the infection-control model relate to the explanation of IPC, the protective intent of IPC, and its benchmark status as a standard of care. Effective goals in the infection-control model are designed to change a patient's attitude in a positive manner and reduce fear or anxiety associated with dental hygiene care. The patient must see IPC as protective, not punitive.

GOVERNMENT AGENCIES AND INFECTION PREVENTION AND CONTROL

Four agencies of the United States government play key roles in IPC. Guidelines and regulations developed by these four agencies have established national standards for IPC related to patient care, patient care equipment and materials, and the environment. In addition to federal agencies, many state, county, and city government agencies have

Summary of Infection Prevention Practices in Dental Settings: Basic Expectations for Safe Care. https://www.cdc.gov/oralhealth/infectioncontrol/pdf/safe-care2.pdf

Infection Prevention Checklist for Dental Settings: Basic Expectations for Safe Care (Print Friendly). https://www.cdc.gov/oralhealth/infectioncontrol/pdf/safe-care-checklist.pdf

Infection Prevention Checklist for Dental Settings: Basic Expectations for Safe Care (Fillable Form). https://www.cdc.gov/oralhealth/infectioncontrol/pdf/dentaleditable_tag508.pdf

Recommendations from the Guidelines for Infection Control in Dental Health-Care Settings—2003. https://www.cdc.gov/oralhealth/infectioncontrol/pdf/recommendations-excerpt.pdf

Guidelines for Infection Control in Dental Health-Care Settings—2003. *MMWR*, December 19, 2003:52(RR-17). https://www.cdc.gov/mmwr/PDF/rr/rr5217.pdf

Screening and Evaluating Safer Dental Devices. https://www.cdc.gov/oralhealth/infectioncontrol/forms.htm

[a] https://www.cdc.gov/oralhealth/infectioncontrol/guidelines/
CDC, Centers for Disease Control and Prevention.

regulations that apply to IPC. These include state boards of licensure, state health departments, and city and county health departments, among others (Table 10.1).

The **Centers for Disease Control and Prevention (CDC)** is one of eight federal public health agencies within the US Department of Health and Human Services (HHS). Its mission is to promote health and quality of life by preventing and controlling disease, injury, and disability. The CDC develops guidelines and recommendations; among these are infection-control recommendations for healthcare settings. The CDC is not a regulatory agency and does not enforce the guidelines it develops. (See Boxes 10.1 and 10.2 for relevant CDC guidance documents and resources.)

The **Occupational Safety and Health Administration (OSHA)**, within the US Department of Labor, protects persons by ensuring a safe and healthy workplace. OSHA enforces workplace safety regulations, including those for IPC in healthcare settings. In approximately half of the states, there are state-administered OSHA agencies. The remainder of the states are exclusively regulated by the federal OSHA. Where there is a state plan, if it is more stringent than the federal plan, then the state plan must be followed. See Box 10.3 for relevant OSHA documents and resources.

The **US Food and Drug Administration (FDA)** and the **US Environmental Protection Agency (EPA)** also provide regulatory oversight in the area of products used in the application of infection-control procedures. The FDA regulatory mission is to do the following:

TABLE 10.1   Federal Agencies and Organizations

Agency/ Organization	Website	US Federal Agency	Standard Setting Organization	Regulatory Authority (Yes/No)	Key Document or Activity That Impacts Infection Prevention and Control in Dentistry
Centers for Disease Control and Prevention (CDC)	http://www.cdc.gov/	US Department of Health and Human Services www.hhs.gov		No Develops evidence-based guidelines Develops and applies disease prevention and control, environmental health, health promotion, and health education	CDC Guidelines for Infection Control in Dental Healthcare Settings—2003 Other CDC guidelines and guidance for healthcare settings and personnel
National Institute for Occupational Safety and Health (NIOSH)	http://www.cdc.gov/niosh/	US Department of Health and Human Services www.hhs.gov CDC www.cdc.gov		No Conducts research and makes recommendations to prevent DHCP injury and illness	Personal Protective Equipment http://www.cdc.gov/niosh/topics/PTD/ Eye safety Respirators Protective clothing Selecting sharps containers http://www.cdc.gov/niosh/docs/97-111/ Sharps injury prevention http://www.cdc.gov/niosh/topics/bbp/safer/step1b.html
Occupational Safety and Health Administration (OSHA)	www.osha.gov	US Department of Labor www.dol.gov		Yes Employers in the private sector are responsible for the health and safety of employees.	OSHA Bloodborne Pathogens Standard Hazards Communication Standards
US Environmental Protection Agency (EPA)	www.epa.gov	US Environmental Protection Agency		Yes A variety of public and private sector regulations are provided.	Hospital antimicrobial disinfectant registrations Hazardous waste regulations (RCRA)

Continued

TABLE 10.1   Federal Agencies and Organizations—cont'd

Agency/ Organization	Website	US Federal Agency	Standard Setting Organization	Regulatory Authority (Yes/No)	Key Document or Activity That Impacts Infection Prevention and Control in Dentistry
US Food and Drug Administration (FDA)	www.fda.gov	US Department of Health and Human Services www.hhs.gov		Yes Regulates through premarket clearance for safety and efficacy	Medical device clearance Medical product clearance Medical device safety and reporting (MAUDE)
American National Standards Institute (ANSI)	www.ansi.org		Yes	No	Standards for protective clothing and eyewear, and other items
Association for the Advancement of Medical Instrumentation (AAMI)	www.aami.org		Yes	No	ST79, Updated Steam Sterilization Standard for Healthcare Facilities
International Organization for Standardization (ISO)	http://www.iso.org/ iso/home.html		Yes	No	ISO 9000 series Quality Management
American Dental Association (ADA) Standards Committee	http://www. ada.org/en/ science-research/ dental-standards/ us-tag-for-iso-tc-106-dentistry		Yes	No	Sub-TAG 3: Dental Terminology Sub-TAG 4: Dental Instruments Sub-TAG 6: Dental Equipment
Organization for Safety, Asepsis and Prevention (OSAP)	www.osap.org		No	No	Credible resources and tools for infection prevention and control in dentistry

DHCP, Dental healthcare personnel; *MAUDE,* Manufacturer and User Facility Device Experience; *RCRA,* Resource Conservation and Recovery Act.

- Promote and protect the public health by helping safe and effective products reach the market in a timely way.
- Monitor products for continued safety after they are in use.
- Help the public obtain accurate, science-based information needed to improve health.

The FDA's regulatory approaches are as varied as the products it regulates. The FDA regulates all medical devices, from simple items such as tongue depressors and thermometers to complex technologies such as heart pacemakers and dialysis machines. Different levels of approval are required, based on the complexity and use of products or devices. These differences are dictated by the laws enforced and the relative risks that the products pose to consumers. Some products, such as new drugs and complex medical devices, must be proven safe and effective before companies sell them or otherwise make them available to consumers. Other products, such as x-ray machines and medical sterilizers, must meet performance standards.

Since 1970, the EPA's regulatory mission has been to protect human health and the environment. Areas of the EPA's regulatory authority that affect IPC include regulation of chemical germicides used in healthcare and regulation of biohazardous and chemical waste.

STANDARD OF CARE

The standard of care is the level of care that a reasonably prudent practitioner would exercise. It is not a maximum standard; rather, it is the minimum level acceptable in all aspects of patient care.

Infection-control regulations, evidence-based guidelines, government agencies, licensing boards, other dental practitioners, and expert opinion determine the standard of care for appropriate infection-control practices in dentistry. The standard of care provides a basis from which to promote excellence and encourage performance improvement to develop and implement best practices.

The goal of IPC is to prevent HAIs among patients, as well as injuries and illnesses in DHCP.[1,4] Dental patients and DHCP can be exposed to pathogenic (disease-producing) microorganisms.[1,4] Human pathogens include cytomegalovirus (CMV), HBV, HCV, herpes simplex virus types 1 and 2, human immunodeficiency virus (HIV), *Mycobacterium tuberculosis* (TB), staphylococci, streptococci, influenza, coronavirus, and other viruses and bacteria that colonize or infect the oral cavity and respiratory tract. These organisms can be transmitted in dental healthcare settings by the following means:[2–4,7]

- Direct contact with blood, oral fluids, or other patient materials
- Indirect contact with contaminated objects (e.g., instruments, equipment, environmental surfaces)
- Contact of conjunctiva, nasal membranes, or oral mucosa with droplets (e.g., spatter) that contain microorganisms generated from an infected person and propelled a short distance by coughing, sneezing, or talking
- Inhalation of airborne microorganisms that can remain suspended in the air for long periods

Infection through any of these routes requires that all of the following conditions be present:

BOX 10.2 Additional CDC Infection Prevention and Control Guidelines

General Infection Prevention Guidelines 2007—Guideline for Isolation Precautions: Preventing Transmission of Infectious Agents in Healthcare Settings. www.cdc.gov/hicpac/pdf/isolation/Isolation2007.pdf

Guideline for Disinfection and Sterilization in Healthcare Facilities, 2008 (Updated 2019). https://www.cdc.gov/infectioncontrol/pdf/guidelines/disinfection-guidelines-H.pdf

Guideline for Hand Hygiene in Health-Care Settings, 2002. https://www.cdc.gov/mmwr/PDF/rr/rr5116.pdf

Guideline for Infection Control in Healthcare Personnel, 1998. www.cdc.gov/hicpac/pdf/InfectControl98.pdf

Guidelines for Environmental Infection Control in Health-Care Facilities, updated 2019. https://www.cdc.gov/infectioncontrol/pdf/guidelines/environmental-guidelines-P.pdf

Guidelines for Preventing the Transmission of *Mycobacterium Tuberculosis* in Health-Care Settings, 2005. www.cdc.gov/mmwr/pdf/rr/rr5417.pdf

Immunization of Health-Care Personnel: Recommendations of the Advisory Committee on Immunization Practices (ACIP), 2011. www.cdc.gov/mmwr/pdf/rr/rr6007.pdf

Management of Multidrug-Resistant Organisms in Healthcare Settings, 2006. https://www.cdc.gov/mrsa/pdf/mdroGuideline2006.pdf

Key Links for Additional Information
CDC Division of Oral Health. www.cdc.gov/oralhealth
CDC/Healthcare Infection Control Practices Advisory Committee (HICPAC). https://www.cdc.gov/hicpac/index.html
CDC website on Hand Hygiene. www.cdc.gov/handwashing
CDC website on Influenza (flu). www.cdc.gov/flu
CDC website on Injection Safety. www.cdc.gov/injectionsafety

CDC, Centers for Disease Control and Prevention.

BOX 10.3 OSHA Resources: Blood-Borne Pathogens and Needle Stick Prevention

OSHA's Bloodborne Pathogens Standard (29 CFR 1910.1030). https://www.osha.gov/pls/oshaweb/owadisp.show_document?p_id=10051&p_table=STANDARDS

OSHA Fact Sheet OSHA's Bloodborne Pathogens Standard. OSHA Fact Sheet, (January 2011). https://www.osha.gov/OshDoc/data_BloodborneFacts/bbfact01.pdf

National Occupational Research Agenda (NORA), Stop Sticks Campaign. (2019) https://www.cdc.gov/nora/councils/hcsa/stopsticks/safersharps-devices.html

Occupational Exposure to Bloodborne Pathogens; Needlestick and Other Sharps Injuries; Final Rule (PDF). OSHA Federal Register Final Rules 66:5317–5325, (January 18, 2011). OSHA revised the Bloodborne Pathogens standard in conformance with the requirements of the Needlestick Safety and Prevention Act. https://www.osha.gov/pls/oshaweb/owadisp.show_document?p_table=FEDERAL_REGISTER&p_id=16265

Bloodborne Pathogens and Needlestick Prevention. https://www.osha.gov/SLTC/bloodbornepathogens/index.html

Most Frequently Asked Questions Concerning the Bloodborne Pathogens Standard. OSHA Standard Interpretation, (February 1, 1993; updated November 1, 2011). Responses to common questions about the blood-borne pathogens standard. https://www.osha.gov/laws-regs/standardinterpretations/1993-02-01-0

Quick Reference Guide to the Bloodborne Pathogens Standard. OSHA, (2011). Provides answers to frequently asked questions regarding blood-borne pathogen hazards. https://www.osha.gov/SLTC/bloodbornepathogens/bloodborne_quickref.html

Reducing bloodborne pathogens exposure in dentistry: an update. http://www.dir.ca.gov/DOSH/REU/bloodborne/REU_BBPdent1.html

OSHA, Occupational Safety and Health Administration.

management of work-related illness, postexposure management, counseling, work restrictions, and immunization.[1,4]

- A pathogenic organism of sufficient virulence and in adequate numbers to cause disease
- A reservoir or source (e.g., blood) that allows the pathogen to survive and multiply
- A mode of transmission from the source to the host
- A portal of entry through which the pathogen can enter the host
- A susceptible host (i.e., one who is not immune)

These conditions constitute a **chain of infection** by which disease transmission may occur. Effective infection-control strategies prevent disease transmission by interrupting one or more links in the chain.[4]

FOUR PRINCIPLES OF INFECTION CONTROL AND PREVENTION

The CDC identifies four principles of IPC that help protect the health of all individuals in the dental environment.[8]

Principle 1: Take Action to Stay Healthy

All persons must take positive steps to maintain their own health, which is especially true for those working in any healthcare setting, including DHCP. A basic strategy for **healthcare personnel (HCP)** to take action to stay healthy is to develop a personnel health program based on the CDC 2003 Dental Infection-Control Guidelines and the 2016 Summary of Infection Prevention Practices in Dental Settings: Basic Expectations for Safe Care. The recommended program includes hand hygiene, medical evaluation, health safety education and training,

Immunizations for Vaccine-Preventable Diseases

Immunization is one of the most effective means of preventing disease transmission. Once a person has acquired immunity through vaccination, the disease no longer poses a threat to that person. In addition to standard childhood immunizations, hygienists should obtain immunizations specifically recommended for HCP. The CDC's **Advisory Council on Immunization Practices (ACIP)** routinely reviews, updates, and revises immunization recommendations. Therefore the most current ACIP recommendations should be used when making immunization decisions (Table 10.2).[1,4,9]

HCP in specific geographic locations or with underlying medical conditions may need immunizations in addition to those currently recommended by the CDC.[9,10] It is important for HCP to consult with their physicians to determine which immunizations are appropriate, based on disease risk in the specific location. All children in the United States and most other countries receive immunization for diphtheria, pertussis, and tetanus (DPT) as a combined vaccine. Adults should receive the tetanus-diphtheria (Td) booster every 10 years, more often if recommended or indicated because of exposure. In addition, a tetanus, diphtheria, and acellular pertussis (Tdap) vaccine is recommended for all adolescents and adults. It is a one-time booster given in place of the Td booster.[9,11] After receiving the one-time Tdap, individuals should resume the schedule of Td boosters. Additional vaccines recommended for all HCP include HBV, annual influenza, measles, mumps, rubella, and varicella, unless the DHCP has naturally acquired immunity

TABLE 10.2   CDC Recommended Immunizations for Healthcare Personnel, Including Dental Healthcare Personnel

Hepatitis B virus	If a healthcare worker does not have documented evidence of a complete hepB vaccine series or if they do not have an up-to-date blood test that shows an immunity to hepatitis B (i.e., no serologic evidence of immunity or prior vaccination), then they should get the following: • Three-dose series (dose 1 now, dose 2 in 1 month, and dose 3 approximately 5 months after dose 2); and • Anti-HBs serologic tested 1 to 2 months after dose 3.
Influenza (flu)	Get 1 dose of influenza vaccine annually.
Measles, mumps, and rubella (MMR)	If a healthcare worker was born in 1957 or later and has not had the MMR vaccine or if they do not have an up-to-date blood test that shows an immunity to measles or mumps (i.e., no serologic evidence of immunity or prior vaccination), then they should get two doses of MMR (dose 1 now and dose 2 at least 28 days later).
Varicella (chickenpox)	If a healthcare worker has not had chickenpox (varicella) and has not received the varicella vaccine or does not have an up-to-date blood test that shows an immunity to varicella (i.e., no serologic evidence of immunity or prior vaccination), then they should get two doses of varicella vaccine, 4 weeks apart.
Tetanus, diphtheria, and pertussis (Tdap)	Get a one-time Tdap vaccination as soon as possible if any healthcare worker has not previously received the Tdap vaccine, regardless of when a previous dose was received. They should get Tdap booster vaccinations every 10 years thereafter. Healthcare workers who are pregnant need to get a Tdap vaccination during each pregnancy.

To learn more about these diseases and the benefits and potential risks associated with the vaccines, read the Vaccine Information Statements (VISs). For Healthcare Personnel Vaccination Recommendations, visit http://www.immunize.org/catg.d/p2017.pdf.
Source: Centers for Disease Control and Prevention (CDC): Vaccine Information for Adults: https://www.cdc.gov/vaccines/adults/rec-vac/hcw.html
Adapted from CDC. Immunizations of Health-Care Personnel. Recommendations of the Advisory Committee on Immunization Practices (ACIP), *MMWR* 2011;60(7).

stemming from a past infection. In addition, the CDC recommends pneumococcal vaccine for all adults age 65 or older.[9,11] Additional vaccines may be indicated during public health emergencies due to significant outbreaks, such as the Severe Acute Respiratory Syndrome Coronavirus 2 (SARS-CoV-2) pandemic and the monkeypox outbreak.

OSHA requires employers to offer all personnel at risk of exposure to blood and other potentially infectious materials (OPIM) the HBV vaccination unless they have verification of previous HBV immunization or naturally acquired immunity.[12] If the employee declines immunization, they must sign a specific OSHA-designated declination waiver.[12] Before declination, the employer must provide information on the safety and efficacy of the vaccine, the benefits to receiving the vaccine, and the risks associated with not receiving vaccination.[12] If the employee initially declines HBV vaccination but at a later date, decides to accept the vaccination, the employer must make HBV vaccination available at that time.[12]

OSHA states that the administration of the vaccination be provided according to recommendations of the current US Public Health Service at the time these evaluations and procedures take place.[12] The vaccination is currently administered in a three-part series, with postvaccine testing for hepatitis B surface antibodies (anti-HBs) 1 to 2 months after the third dose of the vaccine.[11,13] Persons who fail to respond should consult their healthcare professional. Either an additional single dose or a second three-dose series may be offered. When any additional dose(s) are completed, an anti-HBs titer should be completed to check antibody response. Those who fail to develop detectable anti-HBs after additional doses should be considered nonresponders and tested for hepatitis B surface antigen (HBsAg), which indicates active infection or carrier status. If the result of this test is negative, the individual is considered susceptible to HBV infection and counseled on precautions to avoid exposure and appropriate postexposure management.[11,13]

Work Restrictions

DHCP should be aware of their personal health and take action to stay healthy. Within a written infection-control plan, discussing the conditions that require a restriction or exclusion from direct patient care

is necessary. The US Public Health Service recommends work restrictions for HCP with specific infections and following exposure to some diseases. Many of these infections are preventable with vaccines. The following precautions help protect HCP and patients:[1,2,4,9,10]

- HCP diagnosed with diphtheria should refrain from working until the illness resolves.
- HCP with mumps or measles should refrain from working during the acute illness phase as well as after exposure and during the incubation phase if not immunized.
- HCP diagnosed with hepatitis A should refrain from direct patient contact and avoid handling food others will eat.
- HCP with an upper-respiratory infection should avoid contact with medically compromised persons as defined by the ACIP for complications from influenza.
- HCP with active herpes zoster (shingles) may continue to work unrestricted but should cover lesions to protect against exposure of nonintact skin to blood and body fluids.
- In 2012, the CDC published *Updated CDC Recommendations for the Management of Hepatitis B Virus–Infected Health-Care Providers and Students.*[14] Because of the lack of documented infected DHCP-to-patient transmission of HBV after the adoption of universal precautions and more recently of standard precautions, the CDC recommends no restrictions for practitioners performing dental procedures, with the exception of major oral or maxillofacial surgery.[14]
- HCP with HIV are not specifically restricted, but some modifications may be necessary for certain procedures. An expert review panel and physician should be consulted.[14]

It is important to consult current CDC recommendations for HCP and specific and applicable state laws or recommendations for additional information about applicable workplace restrictions.

Principle 2: Avoid Contact With Blood and Other Infectious Body Substances

Avoid contact with blood and other potentially infectious body fluids by using a combination of safe-work practices and behaviors, and

engineering controls. Infection-prevention and infection-control measures include the following:
- Effective use of personal protective equipment (PPE) (e.g., gloves, face masks, protective eyewear, protective gowns) (Fig. 10.1)
- Safe handling of sharp instruments and objects
- Use of high-speed evacuation and rubber dams to reduce the amount of spray from dental devices

Core Infection and Prevention Practices

In 2014, the Healthcare Infection Control and Prevention Advisory Committee (HICPAC), an advisory group to the CDC, voted to adopt the *Core Infection Prevention and Control Practices for Safe Healthcare Delivery in All Settings*. These core practices represent widely agreed upon IPC practices that are elements of care that are not expected to change based on additional research, either because of an overwhelming preponderance of evidence (e.g., hand hygiene requirements) or, in some cases, due to ethical concerns (e.g., randomizing patients to procedures performed by trained versus untrained personnel) Table 10.3.[15]

Standard Precautions

Standard precautions are the IPC practices by which HCP follow the same protocols for all patients, regardless of infectious status or health history. When consistently used, standard precautions ensure the safe delivery of oral healthcare. Health history alone will not reliably identify all persons with HIV infection, HBV infection, or other blood-borne diseases. In fact, standard precautions do not depend on the health, dental, and pharmacologic histories since some infected individuals are unaware of their status and others may choose not to disclose their disease status on the health history. Certain precautions prevent the transmission of these viruses when applied during patient care. These precautions protect the HCP and the patient from disease transmission.[1-4]

Standard precautions are a synthesis of the major features of universal precautions and body substance isolation precautions and apply to the following:
- Blood
- Other bodily fluids, secretions, and excretions except sweat, regardless of whether they contain visible blood
- Nonintact skin
- Mucous membranes

Therefore standard precautions apply to all body fluids, excretions, and secretions, with the exception of sweat and tears.[2,3]

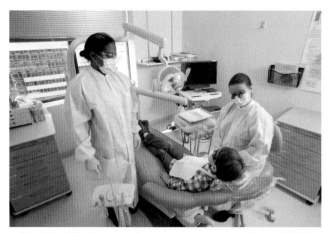

Fig. 10.1 Effective use of personal protective equipment (PPE).

Transmission-Based Precautions

Certain diseases require measures in addition to standard precautions, based on the route of transmission. Expanded or **transmission-based precautions** may be necessary to prevent potential spread of certain diseases (e.g., TB, influenza, varicella, measles, COVID-19) that are airborne or transmitted by droplet or contact (e.g., sneezing, coughing, contact with skin). Acutely ill persons with these diseases do not usually seek routine dental care and should not be treated in a typical dental outpatient setting while they are infectious. Nonetheless, a general understanding of precautions for diseases transmitted by all routes is critical for the following reasons:[2,3]
- Some DHCP are based in hospitals or work part-time in hospital settings.
- Persons infected with these diseases may seek urgent treatment at outpatient dental offices.
- DHCP may become infected with these diseases.

Necessary transmission-based precautions may include patient placement (isolation), adequate room ventilation, respiratory protection (N95 masks) for DHCP, or postponement of nonemergency dental procedures.

The CDC has identified the following three categories of transmission-based precautions:[2-4]
- Contact
- Droplet
- Airborne

Transmission-based precautions are used when the routes of transmission are not interrupted completely using standard precautions alone. For some diseases that have multiple routes of transmission (e.g., measles), more than one transmission-based precaution category may be used. Whether transmission-based precautions are used singly or in combination, standard precautions always apply as well.[2-4]

In the case of clinically active TB, the level of protection afforded by standard precautions is not sufficient to prevent transmission.[2-4] Risk of TB transmission is reduced by a hierarchy of measures that include administrative controls, environmental controls, and personal respiratory protection. For patients known or suspected to have active TB, the CDC recommends the following:
- Evaluate the patient away from other patients and DHCP. When not being evaluated, the patient should wear a surgical mask or cover mouth and nose when coughing or sneezing.
- Defer elective dental treatment until the person is noninfectious.
- Refer patients requiring urgent dental treatment to a previously identified facility with TB engineering controls and a respiratory protection program.

Health History

The health history is an important tool for the following:
- Understanding the patient's overall health
- Assisting in making appropriate care and referral decisions

DHCP should be aware of signs and symptoms of infectious diseases and mindful of the steps required to minimize risk of transmission. This is particularly important if a patient has active TB, signs and symptoms of which may include coughing, chest pain, sweating, weight loss, night sweats, and fever. Box 10.4 provides additional information that DHCP should consider regarding TB.

Engineering Controls

OSHA considers engineering controls to be the most effective in reducing the risk of workplace injury, followed by work practice controls and, finally, by administrative controls. Employers should always ensure the highest-level type of control available is implemented to prevent injury.

TABLE 10.3 **Core Infection Prevention and Control Practices for Safe Healthcare Delivery in All Settings—Recommendations of the HICPAC**

Core Practice Category	Comments
Leadership support	To be successful, infection prevention programs require visible and tangible support from all levels of the healthcare facility's leadership.
Education and training of healthcare personnel on infection prevention	Training should be adapted to reflect the diversity of the workforce and the type of facility and tailored to meet the needs of each category of healthcare personnel being trained.
Patient, family, and caregiver education	Include information about how infections are spread, how they can be prevented, and what signs or symptoms should prompt reevaluation and notification of the patient's healthcare provider. Instructional materials and delivery should address varied levels of education, language comprehension, and cultural diversity.
Performance monitoring and feedback	Performance measures should be tailored to the care activities and the population served.
Standard precautions	Standard Precautions are the basic practices that apply to all patient care, regardless of the patient's suspected or confirmed infectious state, and apply to all settings where care is delivered. These practices protect healthcare personnel and prevent healthcare personnel or the environment from transmitting infections to other patients.
Hand hygiene	Unless hands are visibly soiled, an alcohol-based hand rub is preferred over soap and water in most clinical situations due to evidence of better compliance compared to soap and water. Hand rubs are generally less irritating to hands and are effective in the absence of a sink.
Environmental cleaning and disinfection	When information from manufacturers is limited regarding selection and use of agents for specific microorganisms, environmental surfaces, or equipment, facility policies regarding cleaning and disinfecting should be guided by the best available evidence and careful consideration of the risks and benefits of the available options.
Infection and medication safety	Refer to "Guideline for Isolation Precautions: Preventing Transmission of Infectious Agents in Healthcare Settings, 2007" for details.
Risk assessment and appropriate use of personal protective equipment	PPE, e.g., gloves, gowns, face masks, respirators, goggles, and face shields, can be effective barriers to transmission of infections but are secondary to the more effective measures such as administrative and engineering controls.
Minimizing potential exposures	Refer to "Guideline for Isolation Precautions: Preventing Transmission of Infectious Agents in Healthcare Settings, 2007" for details.
Reprocessing reusable medical equipment	Manufacturer's instructions for reprocessing reusable medical equipment should be readily available and used to establish clear operating procedures and training content for the facility. Instructions should be posted at the site where equipment reprocessing is performed. Reprocessing personnel should have training in the reprocessing steps and the correct use of PPE necessary for the task. Competencies of those personnel should be documented initially upon assignment of their duties, whenever new equipment is introduced, and periodically (e.g., annually).
Transmission-based precautions	Implementation of transmission-based precautions may differ depending on the patient care settings (e.g., inpatient, outpatient, long-term care), the facility design characteristics, and the type of patient interaction, and should be adapted to the specific healthcare setting.
Temporary invasive medical devices for clinical management (generally not applicable to most dental settings)	Early and prompt removal of invasive devices should be part of the plan of care and included in regular assessment. Healthcare personnel should be knowledgeable regarding risks of the device and infection prevention interventions associated with the individual device and should advocate for the patient by working toward removal of the device as soon as possible.
Occupational health	It is the professional responsibility of all healthcare organizations and individual personnel to ensure adherence to federal, state, and local requirements concerning immunizations, work policies that support safety of healthcare personnel, timely reporting of illness by employees to employers when that illness may represent a risk to patients and other healthcare personnel, and notification to public health authorities when the illness has public health implications or is required to be reported.

Adapted from Healthcare Infection Control Practices Advisory Committee. Core Infection Prevention and Control Practices for Safe Healthcare Delivery in All Settings–Recommendations of the Healthcare Infection Control Practices Advisory Committee (HICPAC), 2017.

Engineering controls are devices or equipment that reduce or eliminate a hazard.[4,12] In the context of oral healthcare, these include the following:
- Devices that contain or remove sharp items
- Anesthetic syringes that contain retractable needles, shielding, or encapsulation mechanisms
- Anesthetic needles that contain shielding mechanisms (Fig. 10.2)
- Disposable scalpels that do not require removal of a used blade
- Scalpel handles with retractable blades or blade guards

- Safety intravenous (IV) needles and needle-free ports for adding medications to IV lines

Consider the use of engineering controls when it is reasonable to believe that the control measure will reduce the potential for exposure to a patient's blood or body fluids.[4,12] OSHA requires the use of sharps with engineered injury protection when available and when found to both provide superior protection compared with the standard devices and not interfere with the delivery of patient care.[4,12]

BOX 10.4 Tuberculosis Considerations for Dental Healthcare Personnel

Coughing, especially if persistent and if blood is present, is a key indicator of infection. A patient with active tuberculosis (TB) or suspected of having active TB should be isolated from other patients, asked to wear a face mask, and encouraged to contact their physician of record for definitive medical diagnosis (e.g., presence or absence of TB).[4,16,17]

The tuberculin skin test (TST), previously known as the Mantoux test, is the most common screening test for TB. The CDC recommends the TST, which involves an intradermal injection of purified protein derivative (PPD) into the skin of the forearm. The area is observed for 48 to 72 hours after the injection for development of a wheal, which is an area of skin that is temporarily raised, typically red, and measures at least 10 mm across.[16,17] If it has been several years since the last time a person had a TB skin test, the physician may recommend repeating the test to rule out the potential for a false-negative result.[16,17] For HIV-infected individuals, a 5-mm wheal is an indication of infection owing to the tendency of immunocompromised individuals to develop a lesser reaction.[17] A positive TST result is an indication of infection with the bacterium but is not an indication of active disease. In fact, the majority of individuals with a positive TST result do not have active TB.[17] About 10% of infected individuals develop active TB in their lifetime. About 5% develop the active disease shortly after exposure and 5% develop active disease later in life, usually owing to a compromised immune system.[16,17]

Occasionally, a person may have a positive TST because they previously received a TB vaccine called bacillus Calmette-Guérin (BCG).[16,17] BCG is often given to people born and living in countries with a high prevalence of TB to help prevent childhood TB meningitis. For these individuals, a positive TST may indicate either an infection or a false-positive reaction due to the BCG vaccine. A blood test, called an interferon-gamma release assay (IGRA) may be used to test for TB infection.[17] It is useful in ruling out false-positive tests in those who were previously vaccinated with BCG.[17]

Most people who experience a positive TST result receive preventive chemotherapy for 6 months. The standard drug for prevention of active infection is isoniazid (INH). To treat an active infection (i.e., in a symptomatic person), physicians use INH in combination with other medications such as rifampin and pyrazinamide.[16,17] Rare cases of TB do not respond to traditional therapy. These cases, referred to as drug-resistant TB, are more likely to result in death of the infected individual.[16,17]

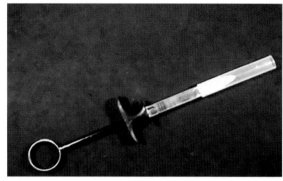

Fig. 10.2 Anesthetic syringe with an engineering control.

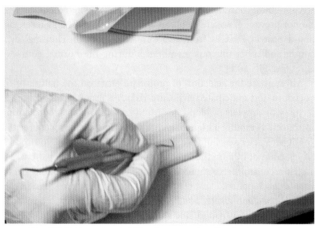

Fig. 10.3 Use of a stabilized sponge to wipe instruments.

Work Practice Controls

Work practice controls are precautionary measures that reduce the likelihood of exposure to bloodborne pathogens by altering the way a task or procedure is performed.[4,12] The use of a stabilized sponge or cotton rolls to wipe instruments rather than wrapping cotton gauze around a finger to debride helps protect the hygienist's fingers from accidental scrapes or punctures with a sharp instrument (Fig. 10.3). Proper patient positioning that allows a 14- to 18-inch focal distance may reduce the hygienist's exposure to contaminated droplets generated during certain procedures. The use of magnifying loupes may assist in achieving optimal focal distance. Proper patient and operator positioning also increases visibility and access to the mouth, further decreasing the risk for accidental injury. Using a high-speed evacuator while spraying a patient's mouth with air and water reduces the amount of droplet splash compared with the use of low-speed suction or no suction.[4] Using an ultrasonic cleaner, washer, or washer/disinfector to decontaminate used dental instruments before sterilization is another example of work practice controls. Using automated instrument cleaning reduces the need for the DHCP to handle contaminated instruments. A one-handed scoop technique to recap used anesthetic needles is also

an example of a work practice control. In this case, if a suitable engineering control is also available, it should be implemented as an engineering control instead of resorting to the lower-level work practice control.

Several risk reduction protocols center on the need to prevent percutaneous injuries by using both engineering and work-practice controls:

- Use medical devices with engineered safety features designed to prevent injuries and/or use safer techniques.
- Never recap needles by hand.
- Never disengage needles from a single-use syringe.
- Use a holding device to remove needles from reusable syringes.
- Dispose of needles and sharps in appropriate sharps disposal containers.
- Avoid hand contact with sharps.
- Never wipe instruments on gauze in a hand or wrapped around a finger; instead, use a single-hand technique, such as a commercial safe wipe or sponge device.
- Announce instrument passes to warn others of sharps and exposure potential.
- Create a neutral zone for sharps to avoid passing directly between DHCP.
- Use appropriate cleanup procedures to minimize hand contact with sharps.

Work-practice controls have some of the greatest impact on preventing blood-borne disease transmission. Given the types of exposures found in dental settings, more than 90% are associated with needles or other sharp devices. The CDC determined that most transmissions occur outside of the mouth and on the hands and fingers of the DHCP. Many of these transmissions are preventable with proper caution and with the use of safer devices.

Administrative Controls

Administrative controls are actions that are taken to reduce or eliminate a hazard. While engineering controls relate to devices and work practice controls relate to the way a person performs duties, administrative controls rely on actions such as rotating duties, taking breaks, and other similar measures. These types of controls are normally used in combination with other controls that more directly prevent or control exposure to the hazard.[18]

Personal Protective Equipment

The term **personal protective equipment (PPE)** refers to protective clothing, eye protection, airway protection, and other attire worn with the intent to protect the DHCP from blood and body fluid exposure.[1,4,12] Work practice controls and engineering controls are the preferred methods of protection.[4,12] PPE is indicated when those controls will not prevent exposure to blood and body fluids. The PPE selected should protect DHCPs from exposure to their skin, clothing, eyes, mouth, and other mucous membranes during the normal course of duties (see Fig. 10.1).[4,12]

Always base the selection of protective attire on the nature of the procedure and anticipated exposure risks.[4,12] Procedures that generate spray or droplets of blood or saliva (e.g., scaling and root planing, air polishing) require a higher level of protection than procedures that do not produce body fluids (e.g., x-ray examinations).[4,12] Do not base the selection of PPE on the infectious disease status of the patient. The infection-control precautions for any given procedure should be the same for each patient.

Eye and face protection. Appropriate eye protection includes goggles, glasses with solid side shields, or a face shield that protects the eyes from exposure to infectious, chemical, and physical hazards (Fig. 10.4).[4,12] The CDC recommends and OSHA regulates that protective eyewear meet standards for spatter protection.[4,12] HCP who wear prescription eyeglasses should consult an eyecare professional to ensure that the style and materials of the eyewear meet standards for protective eyewear or whether they should use goggles or face shields that fit over the prescription eyewear.[4,12]

When laser technologies are used, additional eye protection may be required. Every pair of safety goggles or safety glasses intended for use with laser beams must bear a label with the following information:[4]

- Laser wavelengths in use
- Optical density of those wavelengths
- Visible light transmission

Follow recommended manufacturer instructions for cleaning and disinfecting of protective eyewear.[19]

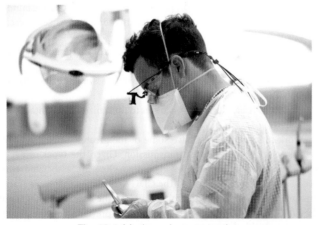

Fig. 10.4 Masks and eye protection.

Masks. A surgical mask protects the mucous membranes of the nose and mouth from exposure to spatter generated under a variety of dental procedures. Wear masks under the same circumstances that warrant the use of eye protection (see Fig. 10.4).[4] Base the selection of masks on comfort, how well the periphery of the mask conforms to the contours of the face, and the level of filtration the mask provides.[4] Surgical face masks are divided into performance classes based on their fluid resistance, bacterial filtration efficiency, submicron particle filtration efficiency, and flame spread potential.[4,20]

The FDA provides specific guidance to manufacturers for clearing surgical masks for the market.[20] The American Society for Testing and Materials (ASTM) rating designation recognized by the FDA includes levels 1, 2, and 3.[21] Level 1 has the lowest barrier performance and level 3 carries the highest. Procedures with no or minimal potential for blood splatter could be performed using a level 1 mask. Since most dental hygiene procedures are likely to produce some level of splatter, excess moisture, visible blood, and higher velocity (e.g., prophy angles, ultrasonic instrumentation), the clinician should consider using a level 2 or level 3 mask.

Respirators and respiratory protection. During the COVID-19 pandemic, interim IPC guidelines were regularly issued by the CDC. One area that was new to dentistry was the use of respirators in place of face masks for protection against airborne transmission. A respirator provides greater protection for the respiratory system. Commonly used dental equipment and procedures are known to create aerosols and airborne contamination, including ultrasonic scalers, high-speed dental handpieces, air/water syringes, air polishing, and air abrasion units. Therefore respiratory protection should be used when performing aerosol-generating procedures on patients, particularly on patients who are suspected or confirmed to have infections that are transmitted through aerosols, including SARS-CoV-2. When presented with such a patient, the DHCP should correctly wear recommended PPE (including National Institute of Occupational Health and Safety [NIOSH]-approved N95 equivalents or higher-level respirators in counties with substantial or high levels of transmission) and use other appropriate mitigation methods designed to minimize droplet spatter and aerosols, including four-handed dentistry, high evacuation suction, and dental dams.

Respirator fit testing, medical evaluation, education, and training are important elements of a comprehensive respiratory protection program. OSHA's Respiratory Protection Standard (29 CFR1910.134 and 29 CFR 1926.139) defines the specific regulations to develop, implement, and manage a respiratory protection program. OSHA also provides a number of resources including training videos, guidance documents, and online tools related to respiratory protection. Additionally, the NIOSH approves respirators, including particulate filtering facepiece respirators (e.g., N95 respirators).

Protective clothing. Protective clothing (e.g., reusable or disposable gown, laboratory coat, uniform) should cover personal clothing and skin (e.g., forearms).[4,12] The protective clothing provides a barrier to protect work clothes (i.e., scrubs) or street clothes from exposure to spray or spatter generated during dental procedures.[4] In most dental settings, a long-sleeved lab coat that falls at or below the knees is adequate. However, during exposure-prone procedures, such as surgical procedures, the DHCP may need a more fluid-resistant material.[4] Protective clothing is removed before leaving the work area, including during breaks or going into nonclinical areas of the facility.[4,12] Scrubs alone are not protective attire and should be worn in combination with a long-sleeved gown or lab coat. The gown or lab coat is the protective attire. OSHA regulations require the employer to arrange for laundering reusable protective attire.[12]

Gloves. Gloves used for dental and dental hygiene procedures fall into the following three categories:

1. Medical examination gloves are nonsterile gloves that are available in a variety of sizes and materials and are either ambidextrous or right- or left-hand specific.[4] Medical exam gloves are appropriate for all nonsurgical dental procedures.
2. Sterile surgeon's gloves (indicated for oral surgical procedures) are sterile gloves individually packaged in sized pairs. To maintain sterility of gloves, do not open the package until ready to use for surgical procedures.[4]
3. Heavy-duty utility gloves are puncture-resistant gloves (Fig. 10.5) used when handling contaminated sharps to reduce risk of accidental puncture injury.[4,12]

The CDC recommends that DHCP:[1,4]
- Wear medical gloves when a potential exists for contacting blood, saliva, OPIM, or mucous membranes.
- Wear sterile surgical gloves in connection with surgical procedures.
- Wear a new pair of medical gloves for each patient.
- Promptly remove the gloves after use and immediately perform hand hygiene to avoid transfer of microorganisms to other patients or environments.
- Remove gloves that are torn, cut, or punctured, and wash hands before regloving.[1,4]

Medical gloves and sterile surgeon's gloves are regulated by the FDA. The FDA provides resources for healthcare professionals.[22]

Dermatitis or allergic reactions may arise from exposure to materials used in the manufacture of gloves. HCP may experience allergic dermatitis of the hands. Many of these reactions are the result of contact with chemicals used in the manufacture of gloves. However, a small percentage involve a potentially serious allergic reaction to the proteins found in natural rubber latex.[4] Today, most medical examination gloves are made of nitrile rubber, not latex. When experiencing dermal problems related to the use of medical gloves, it is important to consult with a qualified healthcare professional (e.g., physician specializing in dermatitis and allergies) for accurate diagnosis and treatment.[4]

Hand Hygiene

Hand hygiene is the most important behavior in the prevention of disease transmission.[1,4,23]

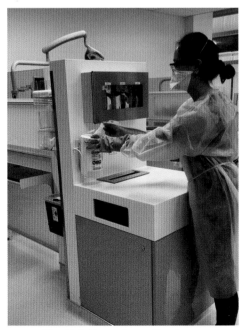

Fig. 10.5 Heavy-duty utility gloves.

The preferred method for hand hygiene depends on the type of procedure, the degree of contamination, and the desired persistence of antimicrobial action on the skin (Table 10.4). Remove transient microbial flora and disease by cleaning the hands with detergent and water. The presence of colonized or resident flora on the hands requires the use of antiseptic agents. For routine dental procedures (e.g., screening, examination, nonsurgical procedures), wash hands with either plain or antimicrobial soap and water. If the hands are not visibly soiled, an alcohol-based hand rub is adequate.[1,4,23] Hand hygiene for surgical procedures (e.g., periodontal surgery, surgical extraction of teeth, biopsy) requires surgical hand antisepsis to eliminate transient flora and reduce resident flora.[1,4,23]

Rings and hand jewelry should be removed before performing hand hygiene. Some studies have shown that skin underneath rings contains more germs than comparable areas of skin on fingers without rings.[23] Rings may also make donning gloves more difficult.[4,23]

The CDC recommends keeping fingernails short, with smooth, filed edges to allow thorough cleaning and prevent glove tears.[4,23] The CDC further recommends healthcare personnel not wear artificial fingernails or extenders when having direct contact with patients due to the difficulty to adequately clean the artificial nail material and its potential to harbor microorganisms.[4,23]

Dermatitis may arise from the effects of frequent use of hand hygiene products and exposure to water.[4,23] There are several strategies that may help maintain good skin integrity in spite of the need for frequent hand hygiene procedures:[4]
- Thoroughly dry hands after washing with soap and water and before donning gloves.
- Use powder-free gloves.
- Frequently use appropriate lubricating hand lotions throughout the day.
- Use cool water when washing hands.
- Protect hands from chapping and drying during cold weather.
- Protect hands from cuts and scratches when performing household chores.

The CDC provides many hand hygiene resources for HCP, including when and how long to perform hand hygiene and hand health, at https://www.cdc.gov/handhygiene/.[24]

Principle 3: Make Patient Care Items (Dental Instruments, Devices, and Equipment) Safe for Use

Instruments, devices, and equipment used to provide direct patient care become contaminated. Appropriate infection-control measures must be taken to prevent transmission of infectious agents from patient to patient through these contaminated items. Patient care items are either single-use disposable items or reusable items that require sterilization between uses. Methods of appropriate infection-control measures include the following:
- Cleaning, sterilization, or disinfection of reusable patient care items
- Appropriate containment and disposal of all single-use items

Sterilization is the destruction of all living organisms, including highly resistant bacterial spores.[25] Properly performed cleaning and sterilization procedures offer the highest level of assurance that no pathogenic organisms remain on instruments and devices. The intent of instrument and equipment sterilization is not to establish a sterile-care environment. Indeed, such an environment would be impossible to establish because the mouth is not a sterile environment. Rather, the sterilization process ensures the destruction of all organisms transferred to an item during use on a patient before reuse of the item on a subsequent patient.[4,26]

Instrument Classification

Dental instruments fall into three broad categories for determining the minimal level of management between patients (Table 10.5):[1,4]

TABLE 10.4   Types of Hand Hygiene

Methods	Agent	Purpose	Area	Duration (Minimum)
Routine handwash	Water and nonantimicrobial soap (i.e., plain soap[a])	To remove soil and transient microorganisms[b]	All surfaces of hands and fingers	15 seconds[c]
Antiseptic handwash	Water and antimicrobial soap (i.e., FDA-cleared antiseptic handwash agent for healthcare settings)	To remove or destroy transient microorganisms and to reduce resident flora[d] (persistent activity[e])	All surfaces of hands and fingers	15 seconds[c]
Antiseptic handrub	Alcohol-based handrub[f]	To remove or destroy transient microorganisms and to reduce resident flora[d] (persistent activity[e])	All surfaces of hands and fingers	Until hands are dry
Surgical antisepsis	Water and antimicrobial soap (i.e., FDA-cleared antiseptic handwash agent for healthcare settings) using a surgical handscrub technique	To remove or destroy transient microorganisms, and to reduce resident flora[d] (persistent activity[e])	Hands and forearms[g]	2 to 6 minutes
	Water and nonantimicrobial soap, followed by an alcohol-based surgical handscrub product with persistent activity following a surgical handscrub technique		Hands and forearms	Follow manufacturer's instructions for surgical handscrub product with persistent activity[h]

[a]Pathogenic organisms have been found on or around bar soap during and after use. Using a liquid soap with hands-free controls for dispensing is preferable.

[b]Transient microorganisms are often acquired by healthcare personnel during direct contact with patients or contaminated environmental surfaces. Transient microorganisms are most frequently associated with healthcare-associated infections and are more amenable to removal by routine hand washing than resident flora.

[c]This minimum time is reported as effective in removing most transient flora from the skin. For most procedures, a vigorous and brief (at least 15 seconds) rubbing together of all surfaces of premoistened, lathered hands and fingers, followed by rinsing under a stream of cool or tepid water, is recommended. Hands should always be thoroughly dried before gloves are donned.

[d]Resident flora are species of microorganisms that are always present on or in the body, not easily removed by mechanical friction, and less likely to be associated with healthcare-associated infections.

[e]Persistent activity is prolonged or extended activity that prevents or inhibits proliferation or survival of microorganisms after application of a product. Previously, this term was sometimes referred to as *residual activity*.

[f]Waterless products (e.g., alcohol-based hand rubs) are especially useful when water facilities are unavailable (e.g., during dental screenings in schools, during boil-water advisories). Alcohol-based hand rubs should not be used in the presence of visible soil or organic material.

[g]Removal of all jewelry, washing the hands and forearms, holding the hands above the elbows during final rinsing, and drying the hands with sterile towels.

[h]Before beginning surgical hand scrub, remove all arm jewelry and any hand jewelry that may make donning gloves more difficult, cause gloves to tear more readily, or interfere with glove usage (e.g., ability to wear the correct-sized glove or altered glove integrity).

From Centers for Disease Control and Prevention (CDC). Frequently asked questions. Hand hygiene. Available at: https://www.cdc.gov/oralhealth/infectioncontrol/faqs/hand-hygiene.html. Accessed August 1, 2017.

TABLE 10.5   Infection-Control Management of Instruments and Devices Based on Classification

Category	Definition	Process	Examples
Critical	Penetrate soft tissue or bone	Sterilization	Surgical instruments, periodontal scalers, surgical dental burs
Semicritical	Contact mucous membranes or nonintact skin	Sterilization or high-level disinfection	Dental mouth mirrors, amalgam condensers, dental handpieces, most hand instruments
Noncritical	Contact intact skin	Low- to intermediate-level disinfection	X-ray head or cone, blood-pressure cuff, facebow

1. **Critical instruments** are instruments that penetrate soft tissue or bone. Critical instruments must be heat sterilized between each use or discarded if disposable. Examples of critical instruments and devices include periodontal probes, explorers, scaling and root planing instruments, and the tip insert of an ultrasonic scaling unit.

2. **Semicritical instruments** are not intended to penetrate soft tissue or bone but contact oral fluids. Examples include mouth mirrors, ultrasonic scaling handpieces, impression trays, and oral photography retractors. These instruments also should be heat sterilized between each use. The use of high-level disinfectants is indicated for semicritical instruments that cannot be heat sterilized. These germicides are chemical disinfectants that provide sterilization under certain conditions. Chemical germicides are not as reliable as heat sterilization methods and raise DHCP safety concerns; therefore

heat-stable or disposable alternatives are preferred. Some semicritical items cannot be either heat sterilized or subjected to high-level disinfectants. These items include digital x-ray sensors and intraoral imaging devices such as digital scanners, among others. These items should be barrier-protected at a minimum, with a new barrier used for each patient. If the underlying surfaces may have been exposed to contaminants, they should be cleaned and disinfected with an appropriate intermediate-level disinfectant before reuse.

3. **Noncritical instruments and devices** are those items that come into contact only with intact skin. Examples include an x-ray head, light handles, high- and low-volume evacuator handles, tubing for handpieces, instrument trays, countertops, and chair surfaces. Use surface barriers or clean and disinfect these items with an EPA-registered low- to intermediate-level disinfectant.

Sterilization Process

The processing of instruments for reuse on patients requires attention to very specific steps that must be completed in the same sequence each time the process is performed. A sterilization area separate from patient treatment rooms will help reduce the risk of cross-contamination in the patient-care environment. Sterilization areas should be arranged to minimize the potential for errors that could result in the release of unsterilized items into the patient care areas. Use a workflow that encourages a one-directional flow of the instruments during the entire process, which includes receiving, cleaning, inspection and packaging, sterilization, and storage.[1,4,26]

Instrument transportation. Used instruments should be transferred from the patient care area to the sterilization area in a container that is solid on the sides and bottom and is labeled with the universal biohazard symbol (Fig. 10.6).[12] Soiled instruments and equipment should be placed in a designated area that will not allow the items to be mixed with sterile items.[1,4,26]

Cleaning. If instruments are heavily soiled or will not be immediately cleaned, the use of a presoak or prespray may help ensure more thorough cleaning of the instruments.[4,27] For items heavily soiled with blood or other organic material, a product that contains an enzyme may be useful. Always follow the manufacturer's instructions for safe use of the product.[4,26,27]

The most effective means of cleaning instruments before sterilization are automated devices specifically intended for this purpose.[4,27] Ultrasonic cleaning baths and instrument washers or washer/disinfectors have been shown to provide superior cleaning to hand scrubbing. Heavy-duty gloves, face protection such as a face shield or goggles with a face mask, in addition to a gown or lab coat, should be worn

throughout the instrument processing procedures until removal of sterile packs from the sterilizer.[4]

After cleaning, instruments should be inspected for residual debris and carefully cleaned with a solvent, brush, soap, or by other suitable means. After drying, instruments should be either placed in sterilization pouches or placed on trays intended for the sterilization process being used and wrapped with an appropriate sterilization wrap. Instrument cassettes should be packaged according to the manufacturer's instructions. Instrument packs should be placed in either a single layer or loosely on their sides.[27] Packs should not overlap as this may prevent the penetration of the sterilizing agent (e.g., steam, heat) to the center of the load. When using paper/plastic pouches, pouches should be placed on their sides, with paper facing plastic of the adjacent pouch.[27] Upon removal from the sterilizer, instrument packs should be stored in a dry area away from contamination and should remain packaged until they are needed for patient care.[4,26,27]

Heat methods of sterilization. Heat-based sterilization methods are more time efficient and reliable than chemical germicides. It is important to determine the method of sterilization that provides a safe and effective outcome for the type of devices.

DHCP must use an FDA-approved sterilization device and follow the manufacturer's instructions for cycle time, temperature, and other parameters necessary to achieving sterilization.[4,26,27] For satisfactory results, thoroughly clean instruments before placing them into appropriate packaging and sterilizing them. Three major types of heat sterilization are available:

- Steam autoclave, the most common method of heat sterilization in the dental office, uses steam in a pressurized chamber to sterilize heat-stable instruments and devices. The user places distilled water into a chamber that dispenses the amount needed to provide steam for the process. Most steam autoclaves require several minutes to achieve the temperature necessary to begin the sterilization process. Additional time at the end of the sterilization cycle allows depressurization of the chamber and drying of instrument packs. Two methods of air evacuation are available in autoclaves: (1) dynamic air removal and (2) gravity displacement.

- A **dynamic air removal sterilizer** usually consists of a sterilization chamber surrounded by a secondary jacket. When the sterilization cycle is initiated, the air is pumped out of the chamber, creating a vacuum into which steam is injected. Some devices accomplish this by drawing a vacuum and then injecting steam, while others use a steam flush–pressure pulse process. This more efficient way of air removal results in a shorter sterilization cycle and better penetration of steam into devices that contain a lumen (hollow inside), such as air-driven dental handpieces. Once the chamber reaches the desired temperature and pressure, the sterilization process begins. In many dynamic air removal sterilizers, the actual sterilization time is 4 to 5 minutes, followed by a 20-minute drying cycle. When using a dynamic air removal sterilizer, follow the manufacturer's instructions to conduct an air removal test; one such test is the Bowie-Dick test (Fig. 10.7). Many sterilizers require the test at the beginning of each day to ensure the process removes all air from the chamber. Pockets of air remaining after the air removal may result in incomplete sterilization of the contents.

- **Gravity displacement sterilization** relies on gravity to evacuate the air from the sterilizer chamber. Pressurization of the autoclave relies on the effective removal of all air. As steam enters the gravity displacement sterilizer, gravity forces the air out through ventilation ports in the chamber. Gravity displacement is less efficient than dynamic air removal, resulting in a typically longer process to achieve sterilization.

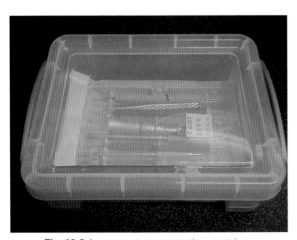

Fig. 10.6 Instrument transportation container.

- An **unsaturated chemical vapor sterilizer** uses a process similar to that of the autoclave; however, in place of steam, a chemical vapor enters the pressurized sterilization chamber. The use of chemical vapor instead of steam reduces the humidity of the sterilization process, reducing the risk of instrument rust and corrosion, primarily in carbon steel instruments. These sterilizers should be ventilated according to the manufacturer's instructions.
- **Dry-heat sterilization** uses high heat for a specific amount of time to achieve sterile results. Temperatures often reach 350° F; therefore dry heat is likely to damage heat-sensitive items such as dental handpieces and some plastics.

Chemical disinfectants and sterilants. Several classes of chemical agents are available that provide high-level disinfection and sterilization under given conditions. Varying degrees of corrosion and damage to certain materials occur if instruments or devices are in prolonged contact with the chemical agent. In addition, the CDC discourages the use of these chemicals because of their toxic properties.[4]

Sterility assurance. To ensure effectiveness of sterilization, several levels of sterility assurance are available, and a combination approach is best.

- **Chemical indicators** allow the operator to determine the presence of certain necessary parameters such as heat or steam. These indicators often appear as arrows or color-change indicators on pouches used to package instruments during sterilization (Fig. 10.8). They

are also available as tape embedded with stripes that change color or indicator strips. There are six types of chemical indicators.[27] Use chemical indicators on the inside of every packet of instruments as a signal to the user that the particular packet completed a heat sterilization process. If the indicator cannot be seen from the outside of the pouch, an additional chemical indicator should be used on the outside of the pack.[4,23] Many of the commercially available pouches have chemical indicators built into the paper. The indicator is not an indication of effectiveness of the sterilization process itself because many factors may interfere with adequate sterilization.

- **Biologic indicators (BIs)**, also called **spore tests**, are the highest level of sterility assurance (Fig. 10.9). BIs use nonpathogenic spores that are especially resistant to the sterilization process. The spores are embedded on a strip or in a solution that is placed in the sterilizer with a load of instruments. Incubation of the spore test confirms the destruction of the spores, which indicates a successful sterilization process.[27]

The following spores are commonly used as BIs:
- *Geobacillus stearothermophilus* is a standard organism for testing steam and chemical vapor sterilization.
- *Bacillus pumilus* spores are the organisms most resistant to dry heat sterilization.
- For monitoring a combination of sterilization methods, dual species biologic indicators (containing both types of spores) would be an appropriate choice.

Destruction of spores that are resistant to specific sterilization methods indicates the elimination of all of the organisms of concern. Spore test at least weekly and with each implantable device to verify the proper functioning and operation of the sterilizer.[4] Maintain records of spore testing and the results in the dental office. Many states require biologic monitoring/spore testing and specify the length of time to maintain the test result records.

Dental Water Quality

Water is essential to the practice of dentistry. Water is used to irrigate surgical sites, cool dental devices such as handpieces and ultrasonic scalers, and irrigate restorative sites for better visibility; water is used in nearly every modern dental practice (Box 10.5).

Nonsurgical procedures. Standards for safe drinking water quality are established by the EPA, the American Public Health Association (APHA), and the American Water Works Association (AWWA).[28] The standards set limits for heterotrophic bacteria of ≤500 CFU/mL (colony-forming units per milliliter) of drinking water. Thus the

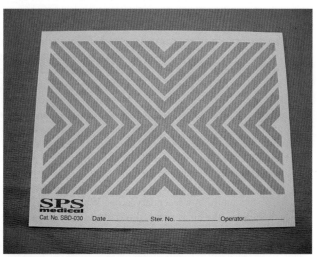

Fig. 10.7 Bowie-Dick Air Removal Test.

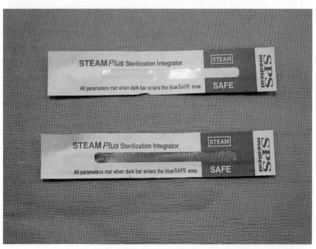

Fig. 10.8 Chemical indicator strips.

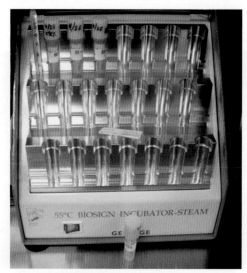

Fig. 10.9 Biologic indicators.

number of bacteria in water used as a coolant/irrigant for nonsurgical dental procedures should be as low as reasonably achievable and, at a minimum, ≤500 CFU/mL, the regulatory standard for safe drinking water established by the EPA and APHA/AWWA.

Since 2003, the CDC has recommended that all dental units use systems that provide output treatment water that meets drinking water standards (i.e., ≤500 CFU/ mL of heterotrophic water bacteria) for nonsurgical procedures.[1,4] These systems include:

- Self-contained water systems (e.g., independent water reservoir), combined with chemical treatment (e.g., periodic or continuous chemical germicide treatment protocols or purifying filters that replace uptake straws in the reservoir bottles).
- Systems designed for single-chair or entire-practice water lines that purify or treat incoming water to remove or inactivate microorganisms.

Most new dental units in the United States now have a separate water reservoir. Using a separate water reservoir system enables the use of water other than the local municipal water supply. In addition to having better control over the quality of the source water used in patient care, it eliminates interruptions in dental care when boil-water notices are issued by local health authorities. The separate water reservoir, even when using distilled or sterile water, does not prevent biofilm development in the dental unit water lines. To achieve the CDC's recommended water quality for nonsurgical dental procedures, separate water reservoirs must be combined with another approach, such as periodic or continuous chemical treatments or filters or a centralized water treatment system.[1,4,29]

The CDC has further clarified that independent reservoirs—or water-bottle systems—alone are not sufficient and should be combined with commercial products and devices that can improve the quality of water used in routine (i.e., nonsurgical) dental treatment. The CDC recommends consulting the dental unit manufacturer as well as the product or device being used to control the biofilm, for appropriate water quality maintenance methods, and for recommendations for monitoring dental water quality.

Chemical products remove, inactivate, or prevent formation of biofilm. Chemical treatments are either continuously infused into or intermittently added to the dental unit water. It may be necessary to remove biofilm in the dental unit water lines using a shock treatment before initial use of a chemical treatment product. Beyond initial shocking of the dental unit water lines the specific chemical treatment

product manufacturer should provide instructions for routine or periodic shocking of the lines.

Two types of treatment systems are available: (1) treatment cartridges that release an active ingredient that disinfects and (2) filter devices that remove solid particles from water. The treatment cartridge is connected to the dental unit's existing water bottle pickup tube. Treatment cartridges need to be replaced at regular intervals, according to the product-specific manufacturer's instructions for use (IFU). Filter devices are installed in the water line, between the dental unit water line and the dental instrument (e.g., dental handpiece, air/water syringe). The filter does not affect biofilm in water lines but removes microorganisms as the water exits the water line through the filter to the dental instrument. Filters must be periodically replaced, with the frequency depending on the amount of biofilm in the water lines and the manufacturer's instructions. The filters may or may not remove endotoxin.

Consult the dental unit manufacturer to determine the compatible methods, products, and devices that are needed to maintain the quality of dental water for the specific dental unit. For other dental devices, such as ultrasonic scalers with independent water reservoirs, consult the manufacturer of each device that uses water for instructions and recommended products to control biofilm in the water lines.

Critical elements of a successful dental unit water line treatment approach include training of DHCP in site-specific dental unit water line treatment protocols and monitoring compliance. DHCP should follow the manufacturer-specific directions and IFU for all commercial products and devices used. Personnel responsible for maintenance of independent reservoir bottles must handle the bottles with clean gloves and follow the manufacturer's instructions for cleaning and aseptically managing the bottles. The CDC 2016 Summary of Infection Prevention Practices in Dental Settings contains a two-part checklist to assess compliance with the CDC's 2003 Recommendations for Dental Healthcare Settings.

Dental unit water line treatment products and devices are regulated by either the FDA or the EPA. Continuous chemical treatment products, systems, and filters designed for dental unit water line treatment are regulated by the FDA. Intermittent chemical treatment products are registered with the EPA as cleaners or disinfectants for dental unit water line treatment.

Surgical procedures. During surgical procedures, the CDC recommends the use of only sterile solutions as coolants and irrigants in an appropriate delivery device, such as a sterile bulb syringe, sterile tubing that bypasses dental unit water lines or sterile single-use devices.[1,4] The Guidelines for Infection Control in Dental Health-Care Settings—2003 define an Oral Surgical Procedure as "the incision, excision, or reflection of tissue that exposes the normally sterile areas of the oral cavity. Examples include biopsy, periodontal surgery, apical surgery, implant surgery, and surgical extractions of teeth (e.g., removal of erupted or nonerupted tooth requiring elevation of mucoperiosteal flap, removal of bone or section of tooth, and suturing if needed)."

Principle 4: Limit the Spread of Blood and Other Infectious Body Substances

Although environmental surfaces and waste products are less likely to provide an efficient mechanism for transmission of infectious agents, they are subject to contamination in oral healthcare settings. Examples of infection-control measures to limit the spread of contamination include:

- Protective surface covers or barriers (Fig. 10.10)
- Use of high-volume evacuation
- Cleaning and surface disinfection
- Limiting touching of objects and surfaces while wearing medical gloves
- Management of medical waste (sharps and soft wastes)

Environmental Surface Disinfection

Surfaces in the dental treatment room are a potential source of infectious agents, either from the spray and spatter generated by dental devices or by contact with contaminated gloves during and after the procedure. Surfaces and equipment that cannot be disassembled for sterilization should be cleaned and **disinfected** between each patient.

The CDC designates environmental surfaces in the oral healthcare setting into two categories:

1. **Housekeeping surfaces** are surfaces such as floors, walls, and sinks. These surfaces may become contaminated during patient care but carry less risk of disease transmission than clinical contact surfaces. These surfaces can be cleaned with soap and water. If they become visibly contaminated with blood or OPIM, they should be cleaned and disinfected.

2. **Clinical contact surfaces** are surfaces that become contaminated from spray or droplets of oral fluids or by touching with gloved hands during the procedure. Some clinical contact surfaces may be difficult or impossible to clean, including switches, knobs, hoses, and brackets. Protect these surfaces by covering them with fluid-impervious barriers (see Fig. 10.10). Always change barriers between patients.[4,30] Clean and disinfect or barrier-protect clinical contact surfaces, including the following:

   - Touch areas on the dental chair
   - Touch areas on the operator chair
   - Dental unit
   - Dental light handle(s)
   - X-ray unit touch areas
   - Countertops that are contacted by contaminated items
   - Air and water syringe handle and tubing
   - Pencils, pens
   - Keyboards, pointing devices, monitors
   - Mirror for patient education
   - Dental unit suction controls and disposable-tip connection tubing
   - Saliva ejector holder and tubing
   - Bracket tables and bracket tray
   - Portable equipment (e.g., ultrasonic cleaner and scaler, airpolisher, curing light, vitalometer, laser)[4,30]

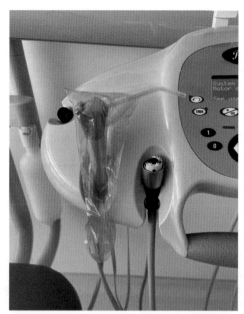

Fig. 10.10 Protective surface covers or barriers.

In the absence of barriers, clean and disinfect surfaces and equipment between patients with an EPA-registered hospital disinfectant (low-level disinfectant) or an EPA-registered hospital disinfectant with a tuberculocidal claim (intermediate-level disinfectant). Use intermediate-level disinfectant for surfaces with visible blood or OPIM.[4,30]

Follow the manufacturer's directions for the handling, use, and storage of all disinfectant and cleaning products. Manufacturers of dental devices and equipment should provide information regarding material compatibility with liquid chemical germicides, precautions regarding immersion of devices for cleaning, and how to decontaminate the item if servicing is required. DHCP who perform environmental cleaning and disinfection should wear gloves and other PPE to prevent occupational exposure to infectious agents and hazardous chemicals. Chemical- and puncture-resistant utility gloves offer more protection than latex examination gloves when chemicals such as disinfectants are used (Fig. 10.5).

EXPOSURE MANAGEMENT

As previously discussed, risk reduction strategies include the use of safer work practices, safer devices, PPE, proper policies and procedures, awareness of personal health status, attention to standard precautions, and a program of ongoing education. The majority of exposures are preventable, but exposures can occur. The risk of infection with a blood-borne disease after an occupational exposure to blood or other body fluids in dental settings appears to be low.[5] However, every exposure to blood and body fluids carries some risk for transmission of blood-borne pathogens (Box 10.6). Every dental facility must have a postexposure management program for occupational exposures.[12] The written program should identify the specific steps to follow after an exposure incident and include training and education

---

> ### BOX 10.6   Epidemic and Pandemic Outbreaks
>
> Epidemics occur when an infectious disease rapidly spreads and affects a greater number of people than generally expected within a given population. When an epidemic spreads worldwide, it is referred to as a pandemic. Often, epidemics start as outbreaks, during which the spread of disease is limited to a specific area. An example is the Ebola outbreak in 2014 that started in the West African nation of Sierra Leone but spread to multiple countries and remained an uncontained epidemic for 2 years. Another example was the severe acute respiratory syndrome (SARS) epidemic of 2003 that spread from Asia to North America, South America, and Europe and sickened more than 8000 people. The H1N1 influenza virus, which began in Mexico in 2008 and spread to multiple continents well beyond the usual time frame of influenza season, led the World Health Organization to issue the highest pandemic alert level in 2009. More recently, the SARS-CoV-2 pandemic in 2019 is still, at the publication of this chapter, impacting countries across the globe.
>
> Many of the diseases involved in epidemics and pandemics are spread via infectious droplets or respiratory secretions and may require transmission-based precautions. During pandemics or local epidemics, all DHCP should be aware of and follow public health department guidelines. Being aware of the symptoms of a specific illness is important. Patients should be asked about symptoms suggestive of infection when confirming appointments and instructed to reschedule if they show signs of the illness. DHCP should remain home when symptomatic to prevent spreading the infection to patients and other DHCP. The spread of influenza can also be reduced by good hand-hygiene practices and cough etiquette, including covering the mouth with a tissue when coughing and immediately discarding the tissue, or coughing or sneezing into the inside of the arm at the elbow.

concerning the types of exposure that place DHCP at risk and procedures for prompt reporting and evaluation, including counseling, testing, and followup, according to the most current US Public Health Service (USPHS) guidelines. These policies should be in compliance with the OSHA bloodborne pathogen standard and with any state or local laws or regulations.

Exposure and Exposure Risk

The CDC defines an occupational exposure as a percutaneous injury or contact of mucous membrane or nonintact skin with blood, saliva, tissue, or other body fluids that are potentially infectious.[4] Exposure incidents may pose a risk of HBV, HCV, or HIV infection and are a matter of medical urgency. Exposure risk varies with the amount of blood to which the HCP has been exposed, the titer of virus in the patient, the depth of the injury with the contaminated device or instrument, type of exposure (e.g., percutaneous, mucous membrane, nonintact skin), and the immune status of the HCP.[4]

Postexposure Management

When an injury occurs, the goal is to contain the injury as soon as possible to reduce the risk of transmission. If an exposure occurs, offer the exposed DHCP immediate postexposure management in accordance with the most recent USPHS guidelines. Selecting a **qualified healthcare provider (QHCP)** trained to evaluate and treat infectious diseases, including HIV infection, is critical.[12] For the QHCP to provide appropriate treatment and assess the need for followup, they must receive specific information regarding the exposure incident. This information includes the circumstances, devices, degree, and severity of exposure. If the source patient consents, the QHCP determines the source patient's infectious disease status through testing. Basic steps of postexposure management are as follows:

Step 1

If an injury occurs, there are basic first aid measures to apply immediately, such as washing an area of percutaneous exposure or flushing the nose, mouth, eyes, or skin with clean water, saline, or sterile irrigants. No scientific evidence indicates that the use of antiseptics for wound care or bleeding the wound reduces the risk of transmission of a bloodborne pathogen. The exposed DHCP should not use caustic agents such as bleach or attempt to "milk" the wound, which would serve to further irritate the area.[4]

Step 2

Report the incident to a designated individual. That individual must complete an incident report form, which includes the source patient's name and the nature of the exposure. The completion of a report should not cause a delay or defer treatment.

Step 3

A designated individual should discuss the incident with the source patient, if identified.

Step 4

Initiate immediate referral to a QHCP who is capable of treating an exposed individual.

Step 5

Begin medical evaluation and followup in accordance with the most recent USPHS guidelines. Medical followup should include counseling and testing as indicated and determined by the infection potential of the exposure. Testing may be for HIV, HBV, or HCV; the QHCP may need to repeat testing at certain intervals. A rapid test for HIV and HCV

is available in many settings. The QHCP must have access to this test. Results from a rapid test are available in less than 30 minutes rather than in days. Use of rapid testing results can assist in decision-making for medical management. Postexposure management begun within the first 1 to 2 hours with antiretroviral drugs may reduce the risk of infection by approximately 80% but will not prevent all cases of infection.[31] Postexposure management may fail because of a resistant virus, an increased titer of virus, an increased dose of blood, or host factors. Postexposure prophylaxis (PEP) may not be effective unless promptly initiated.

Exposure Followup Guidelines

Followup also involves counseling regarding signs and symptoms of infection, the importance of measures to avoid infecting others, and the importance of seeking advice if illness occurs:

- HBV: Followup of occupational exposure to HBV depends on the HBsAg status of the source patient and the vaccination and anti-HBs response of the exposed DHCP.[13] If the exposed DHCP is unvaccinated for HBV, it is likely that the vaccination series will be initiated. A prevaccination titer test is not necessary. If the source individual has a history of HBV infection, administration of hepatitis B immune globulin will likely be part of the management protocol. Treatment should begin as soon as possible, preferably within 24 hours and in less than 1 week. If the exposed DHCP has been vaccinated and is a known responder, no action is necessary because the HBV vaccine has strong immunologic memory. However, if the immune status is unknown or the individual is a known nonresponder to the vaccine, other actions must be taken.
- HCV: There is neither preexposure vaccination nor PEP for occupational exposure to HCV. The most current recommendation for followup of occupational exposure to HCV is to test the source patient for HCV RNA. No additional testing is required if the source patient is HCV-negative. If the source individual is HCV-positive or unknown, the CDC provides a recommended algorithm for followup of the exposed DHCP (https://www.cdc.gov/hepatitis/pdfs/testing-followup-exposed-hc-personnel-3d.pdf). Testing is recommended for the source patient at baseline and at ≥3 weeks for the exposed healthcare worker if the source is positive or unknown. Monitoring liver function may be necessary and the DHCP should be tested for HCV RNA at 3 weeks or later. Should transmission occur, early identification of the HCV infection and a referral of the exposed individual to a specialist are important. Limited data suggest that antiviral treatment initiated early in the course of infection may be beneficial.
- HIV: Recommendations for HIV PEP are based on situations in which there has been an occupational exposure to a source patient who either has or is considered likely to have an HIV infection. Baseline testing is part of the standard protocol, and repeat testing may be indicated at 6 weeks, 12 weeks, and 6 months. If indicated, the DHCP should begin postexposure treatment as soon as possible (within 2 hours). If the patient is known to be HIV positive, the course of treatment usually involves a 4-week regimen of 2 or more antiretroviral drugs, depending on the nature of the exposure and the medications being taken by the source patient. The DHCP may require drug toxicity tests.[32]

Postexposure management is an area of rapidly changing recommendations. As new antiretroviral agents become available, some are replacing drugs previously used. Seeking the advice and care of an appropriate provider who is familiar with the most current USPHS recommendations for testing and PEP is important. Counseling as to the potential side effects and reporting of illness are essential to the appropriate medical management of an occupational exposure to HIV.

The CDC recommends counseling regarding risks and benefits for the pregnant DHCP and extensive followup. Pregnancy may affect the selection of antiretroviral drugs because some of these are contraindicated during pregnancy.

Risk of Infection

Most exposures do not lead to infection and the risk of seroconversion may vary, depending on the agent, the type of exposure, the amount of blood involved, and the amount of circulating virus in the source patient. When assessing an occupational exposure and determining the management and followup, QHCP review the following:

- Type of exposure (percutaneous, mucous membrane, nonintact skin, or bite)
- Type and amount of fluid (blood versus fluids containing blood)
- Infectious status of the source (presence of HBsAg, presence of HCV antibody, and/or presence of HIV antibody)
- Susceptibility of the exposed person with consideration to the HBV vaccine response status and the HBV, HCV, and/or HIV status

For HBV, the risk of infection ranges from 6% to 30% in persons not protected by vaccination or previous infection.[4,13] Source individuals who are hepatitis e-antigen–positive are potentially more infectious and more likely to transmit disease. The best protection is vaccination against HBV.

For HCV, the risk is about 1.8% on average for percutaneous exposures.[4] There are no exact estimates of the number of DHCPs occupationally infected with HCV, but the risk to a DHCP is no higher than the average community risk.[4]

For HIV, average risk after a percutaneous exposure is about 0.3%. The risk after exposure to eyes, nose, or mouth is about 0.1% and the risk to skin is estimated to be less than that unless the skin is damaged or compromised, in which case the risk would be higher.[4,32]

Understanding the risk and taking action to prevent exposure is the appropriate approach, not selectively referring patients elsewhere based on infectious disease status. To refuse treatment to a patient of record because that person has an infectious disease or to refuse to treat a person based on the presence of an infectious disease is unethical and illegal. Consider the critical thinking scenario in Box 10.7.

Infection Prevention and Control Program Evaluation

A successful and compliant IPC program requires ongoing monitoring and evaluation. Tools for evaluating and monitoring compliance with CDC recommendations include the CDC Summary of Infection Prevention Practices in Dental Settings: Basic Expectations for Safe Care and the companion two-part compliance Infection Prevention Checklist for Dental Settings (http://www.cdc.gov/oralhealth/infectioncontrol/guidelines/index.htm). Additional resources for program evaluation are in Box 10.8.[1]

Each dental healthcare setting should have a designated infection prevention and safety coordinator to facilitate effective and efficient implementation of the written infection program.[1,33] In a small facility, it may be one individual; in a larger facility, it may be a shared activity by a committee of designated personnel. The infection prevention coordinator should ensure that equipment and supplies (e.g., hand hygiene products, safer devices to reduce percutaneous injuries, PPE) are available and maintain communication with all staff members to address specific issues or concerns related to infection prevention.[1] The Organization for Safety, Asepsis and Prevention (OSAP) has many resources and tools for infection prevention and safety, including information about the roles and responsibilities of the infection prevention coordinator (www.osap.org).

Developing a true culture of safety requires the commitment to IPC by all personnel as demonstrated by day-to-day infection prevention practices. Ways in which the safety culture may be demonstrated include ensuring that patients are part of the care team in making informed decisions about their care, explaining the infection prevention practices in place for their safety, and eliciting questions from patients (Box 10.9). The dental hygienist must ensure infection prevention practices are firmly based on evidence and must be vigilant in ensuring new information is evaluated and, when appropriate, implemented into clinical practice (Box 10.9).

BOX 10.7 Critical Thinking Scenario

You have been hired by one of the most reputable dental practices in the community. On the second day of employment, while treating your patient, you accidentally insert a used hypodermic needle percutaneously into your thumb after administering a local anesthetic agent. Because your patient is a high-profile state legislator and you do not want to appear incompetent to your new employer or the patient, you say nothing about the exposure incident. After 3 days of thinking about the situation, you report the incident to the office manager. Use the principles of postexposure management to determine the following:

1. What should the office manager do to protect the health and safety of the new dental hygienist?
2. What errors in judgment were made by the dental hygienist?
3. What steps of the postexposure management protocol should the dental hygienist have taken?
4. What tertiary preventive strategies must be initiated by the office manager for the practice to ensure that a similar exposure incident does not occur again?

An exposure response resource is available at The Clinician Consultation Center at the University of California, San Francisco. The Center provides expert advice on managing occupational exposure incidents to HIV, HBV, and HCV and has the most up-to-date information on this subject. The Center is available on the Web (http://nccc.ucsf.edu/) or by toll-free telephone (1-888-448-4911) between 9:00 AM and 9:00 PM EST, 7 days a week. Access the online PEP Quick Guide for Occupational Exposures at http://nccc.ucsf.edu/clinical-resources/pep-resources/pep-quick-guide/.

BOX 10.8 Resources for Monitoring and Evaluating an Infection Prevention and Control Program

CDC: Summary of Infection Prevention Practices in Dental Settings: Basic Expectations for Safe Care. Centers for Disease Control and Prevention, US Dept. of Health and Human Services; October 2016. https://www.cdc.gov/oralhealth/infectioncontrol/pdf/safe-care2.pdf.
Infection Prevention Checklist for Dental Settings: Basic Expectations for Safe Care (Fillable Form). https://www.cdc.gov/oralhealth/infectioncontrol/pdf/dentaleditable_tag508.pdf.
OSAP: Portable and Mobile Dentistry: Site assessment and checklist. https://www.osap.org/portable-mobile.
Joint Commission Resources: Infection Prevention and Control Workbook: The APIC/JCR Infection Prevention and Control Workbook, 4th ed. https://store.jcrinc.com/the-apic-jcr-infection-prevention-and-control-workbook-4th-edition/.

BOX 10.9 Client or Patient Education Tips

There must be evidence of the use of sound and appropriate infection-control practices and there must be an explanation of rationales before care is delivered. Patients need to realize that their safety is paramount; this instills the belief that subsequent care is most appropriate as well.

KEY CONCEPTS

- Heat sterilization is the most effective means for reprocessing semicritical and critical patient care items and equipment.
- Clinical contact surfaces should be cleaned and disinfected or covered with impervious barriers.
- Hand washing is a key strategy in the prevention of infection and disease transmission.
- The Centers for Disease Control and Prevention recommendations for standard precautions indicate that healthcare personnel use personal protective equipment when exposure to body fluids is likely.
- The basic tenet of standard precautions is that all body fluids, except sweat and tears, should be considered potentially infectious.
- Healthcare practitioners should adhere to standard precautions to reduce the risk of infection for themselves, their families, and their patients.

ACKNOWLEDGMENT

The authors wish to acknowledge Helene Bednarsh for her past contributions to this chapter.

REFERENCES

1. Centers for Disease Control and Prevention. Summary of Infection Prevention Practices in Dental Settings Basic Expectations for Safe Care; March 29, 2016. Available at: http://www.cdc.gov/oralhealth/infectioncontrol/guidelines/index.htm. Accessed June 6, 2017.
2. Siegel JD, Rhinehart E, Jackson M, et al. 2007 Guideline for Isolation Precautions: preventing transmission of infectious agents in healthcare settings. *Am J Infect Control.* 2007;35(10 suppl 2):S65–S164. Available at: www.cdc.gov/hicpac/dhqp/pdf/isolation2007.pdf. https://www.cdc.gov/infectioncontrol/pdf/guidelines/isolation-guidelines.pdf. https://www.cdc.gov/infectioncontrol/guidelines/isolation/index.html Accessed June 21, 2017.
3. Harte JA. Standard and transmission-based precautions: an update for dentistry. *J Am Dent Assoc.* 2010;141(5):572–581. Available at: http://jada.ada.org/article/S0002-8177(14)61533-6/abstract.
4. Centers for Disease Control and Prevention. Guidelines for infection control in dental health-care settings—2003. *MMWR Recomm Rep (Morb Mortal Wkly Rep).* 2003;52(RR-17):1–61. Available at: https://www.cdc.gov/mmwr/PDF/rr/rr5217.pdf. Accessed June 21, 2017.
5. Cleveland JL, Gray SK, Harte JA, et al. Transmission of blood-borne pathogens in US dental health care settings: 2016 update. *J Am Dent Assoc.* 2016;147(9):729–738. Available at: http://www.cdc.gov/OralHealth/publications/articles/index.htm#infection. Accessed June 27, 2017.
6. Centers for Disease Control and Prevention. Viral Hepatitis > Outbreaks. Healthcare-Associated Hepatitis B and C Outbreaks Reported to the Centers for Disease Control and Prevention (CDC) 2008–2015. Available at: http://www.cdc.gov/hepatitis/outbreaks/healthcarehepoutbreaktable.htm. Accessed June 21, 2017.
7. Garner JS. Guideline for isolation precautions in hospitals. The hospital infection control practices advisory committee. *Infect Control Hosp Epidemiol.* 1996;17:53–80.
8. Summers CJ, Gooch BF, Marianos DW, et al. Practical infection control in oral health surveys and screenings. *J Am Dent Assoc.* 1994;125:1213–1217.
9. Centers for Disease Control and Prevention. Recommended Vaccines for Healthcare DHCPs. Healthcare Personnel Vaccination Recommendations. Available at: http://www.immunize.org/catg.d/p2017.pdf. CDC Vaccine Information for Adults. Available at: https://www.cdc.gov/vaccines/adults/rec-vac/hcw.html. Accessed June 21, 2017.
10. Bolyard EA, Tablan OC, Williams WW, et al. Guideline for infection control in healthcare personnel, 1998. Hospital infection control practices advisory committee. *Infect Control Hosp Epidemiol.* 1998;19(6):407–463.
11. Centers for Disease Control and Prevention. Immunization of health-care personnel: recommendations of the advisory committee on immunization practices (ACIP). *MMWR Recomm Rep (Morb Mortal Wkly Rep).* 2011;60(RR–07):1–45.
12. US Department of Labor. Occupational Safety and Health Administration. 29 CFR part 1910.1030. Occupational exposure to bloodborne pathogens; needlesticks and other sharps injuries; final rule. *Federal Regist.* 2001;66:5317–5325. As amended from and includes 29 CFR part 1910.1030. Occupational exposure to bloodborne pathogens; final rule. *Fed Regist.* 1991;56:64174–64182. Available at: http://www.osha.gov/SLTC/dentistry/index.html.
13. Centers for Disease Control and Prevention. CDC guidance for evaluating health-care personnel for hepatitis B virus protection and for administering postexposure management. *MMWR Recomm Rep (Morb Mortal Wkly Rep).* 2013;62(RR10):1–19. Available at: http://www.cdc.gov/mmwr/preview/mmwrhtml/rr6210a1.htm. Accessed June 21, 2017.
14. Centers for Disease Control and Prevention (CDC). Updated CDC recommendations for the management of hepatitis B virus-infected health-care providers and students. *MMWR Recomm Rep (Morb Mortal Wkly Rep).* 2012;61(RR–3):1. Erratum in: *MMWR Recomm Rep.* 2012;61(28):542.
15. Healthcare Infection Control Practices Advisory Committee. Core Infection Prevention and Control Practices for Safe Healthcare Delivery in All Settings—Recommendations of the Healthcare Infection Control Practices Advisory Committee. (HICPAC); 2017.
16. Centers for Disease Control and Prevention. Guidelines for preventing the transmission of *Mycobacterium tuberculosis* in health-care settings, 2005. *MMWR Recomm Rep (Morb Mortal Wkly Rep).* 2005;54(RR–17):1–141. Available at: http://www.cdc.gov/mmwr/preview/mmwrhtml/rr5417a1.htm?s_cid=rr5417a1_e. Accessed June 21, 2017.
17. Tuberculosis (TB) Centers for Disease Control and Prevention. Testing Health Care DHCPs. http://www.cdc.gov/tb/topic/testing/healthcareDHCPs.htm. Accessed June 21, 2017.
18. Occupational Safety and Health Administration (OSHA). Hazard Prevention and Control. fy11_sh-22318-11_Mod_3_HazardPrevention.pdf (osha.gov).
19. Centers for Disease Control and Prevention. Strategies for Optimizing the Supply of Eye Protection. Available at: https://www.cdc.gov/coronavirus/2019-ncov/hcp/ppe-strategy/eye-protection.html.
20. FDA Resource for Health Professionals: Surgical Masks. Available at: https://www.fda.gov/MedicalDevices/ProductsandMedicalProcedures/GeneralHospitalDevicesandSupplies/PersonalProtectiveEquipment/ucm055977.htm#s2. Accessed July 21, 2017.
21. ASTM. Standard Specification for Performance of Materials Used in Medical Face Masks. F2100-11 (2018). Available at: https://www.astm.org/Standards/F2100.htm. Accessed January 22, 2018.
22. FDA Resource for Health Professionals: Medical Gloves. Available at: https://www.fda.gov/MedicalDevices/ProductsandMedicalProcedures/GeneralHospitalDevicesandSupplies/PersonalProtectiveEquipment/ucm056077.htm. Accessed July 21, 2017.
23. Boyce JM, Pittet D, Healthcare Infection Control Practices Advisory Committee. Society for Healthcare Epidemiology of America; Association for Professionals in Infection Control; Infectious Diseases Society of America; Hand Hygiene Task Force. Guideline for hand hygiene in health-care settings: recommendation of the healthcare infection control practices advisory committee and the HICPAC/SHEA/APIC/IDSA hand hygiene task force. *Infect Control Hosp Epidemiol.* 2002;12(suppl):S3–S40. Available at: www.cdc.gov/mmwr/PDF/rr/rr5116.pdf.
24. Centers for Disease Control and Prevention. Hand Hygiene in Healthcare Settings. Available at: https://www.cdc.gov/handhygiene/. Accessed June 17, 2017.
25. Block SS. *Disinfection, Sterilization, and Preservation.* 5th ed. Lippincott Williams & Wilkins; 2001.
26. Rutala WA, Weber DJ. Healthcare infection control practices advisory committee. Guideline for disinfection and sterilization in healthcare facilities, 2008. *Am J Infect Control.* 2013;41(5 suppl):S67–S71. Available at: www.cdc.gov/hicpac/pdf/guidelines/Disinfection_Nov_2008.pdf. https://www.cdc.gov/infectioncontrol/pdf/guidelines/

disinfectionguidelines.pdf. https://www.cdc.gov/infectioncontrol/ guidelines/disinfection/index.html. Accessed June 17, 2017.

27. American National Standard/Association for the Advancement of Medical Instrumentation ANSI/AAMI ST79 Comprehensive guide to steam sterilization and sterility assurance in health care facilities 2017. Available at: http://my.aami.org/store/detail.aspx?id=ST79.

28. US Environmental Protection Agency. *National Primary Drinking Water Regulations, 1999: List of Contaminants.* US Environmental Protection Agency; 1999. Available at: https://www.epa.gov/safewater/mcl.html. Accessed January 17, 2017.

29. Centers for Disease Control and Prevention. Questions and Answers on Dental Unit Water Quality. Available at: https://www.cdc.gov/oralhealth/ infectioncontrol/questions/dental-unit-water-quality.html. Accessed January 27, 2017.

30. Sehulster L, Chin RY. Healthcare Infection Control Practices Advisory Committee. Guidelines for environmental infection control in health-care facilities. Recommendations of CDC and the healthcare infection control practices advisory committee. *MMWR Recomm Rep (Morb Mortal Wkly Rep).* 2003;52(RR–10):1–42. Available at: https://www.cdc.gov/ infectioncontrol/pdf/guidelines/environmental-guidelines.pdf.

31. Cardo DM, Culver DH, Ciesielski CA, et al. A case-control study of HIV seroconversion in health care workers after percutaneous exposure. *N Engl J Med.* 1997;337:1485–1490.

32. U.S. Public Health Service Working Group on Occupational Postexposure Prophylaxis, Kuhar DT, Henderson DK, et al. *Updated U.S. Public Health Service Guidelines for the Management of Occupational Exposures to HIV and Recommendations for Postexposure Prophylaxis;* 2013. Available at: https://stacks.cdc.gov/view/cdc/20711.

33. Centers for Disease Control and Prevention. Healthcare Infection Control Practices Advisory Committee. Core infection prevention and control practices for safe healthcare delivery in all settings— recommendations of the Healthcare Infection Control Practices Advisory Committee (HICPAC) 2017. Available at: https://www.cdc.gov/hicpac/ recommendations/index.html.

11

Preventing and Managing Medical Emergencies

Jennifer A. Pieren and Diane P. Kandray

PROFESSIONAL OPPORTUNITIES

Dental hygienists work in a variety of settings, including dental offices, public health settings, schools, and other nontraditional settings, which enables them to work in the absence of a dentist. The dental hygienist is responsible for completing and updating the patient's health history at each appointment and for identifying patients with risk factors that may increase the likelihood of a medical emergency. Appropriate knowledge and preparation will allow dental hygienists to effectively recognize, prevent, and manage medical emergencies.

COMPETENCIES

1. Prepare the dental hygienist to recognize, prevent and manage a medical emergency.
2. Discuss the importance of documentation in relation to medical emergencies.
3. Understand the role of anxiety in dental treatment and emergencies.
4. Describe responses to and management of medical emergencies.
5. Recognize necessary legal considerations for medical emergencies.

PREVENTING MEDICAL EMERGENCIES

Life-threatening emergencies may occur in the oral healthcare setting. Although these emergencies are infrequent, the following factors increase the likelihood of such incidents:
- Increased number of medically compromised individuals seeking care;
- Medical advances in drug therapy;
- Increased number of invasive procedures and longer appointments; and
- Increased use of drugs, such as local anesthetics, sedatives, and analgesics in the oral healthcare setting.

Fortunately, prevention can minimize life-threatening incidents. Prevention begins with a comprehensive health history and risk assessment, with special attention paid to medication usage, vital signs, and anxiety recognition and management. Prevention also includes treatment modifications and stress reduction protocols to minimize medical risks. All assessment findings should be documented in the patient's record and updated at each subsequent visit.

Dental personnel must be prepared to assist in the recognition and management of any potential emergency situation. Updated and complete patient-related information, well-trained dental personnel, and availability of appropriate emergency equipment are vital to ensure the best possible outcome.

PREPARING THE DENTAL TEAM AND ENVIRONMENT

Preparing both dental personnel and the dental environment is critical to prevent and manage a medical emergency.

Training

Training and current certification in **Basic Life Support** (BLS), practice sessions in emergency simulations, and updated knowledge or completion of a refresher course in emergency management are necessary should a medical emergency arise.

Basic Life Support

BLS is the level of care or intervention used for those with life-threatening illnesses or injuries until they can be given full medical care at a healthcare facility. Emergency medical personnel should be notified at the onset of a medical emergency. **Cardiopulmonary resuscitation** (CPR) is an emergency procedure performed to manually preserve brain function until further actions are taken to restore spontaneous blood circulation and breathing in a person who is not breathing, not breathing normally (only gasping), and/or has no pulse.[1] Dental professionals should have current certification in BLS, including CPR and automated external defibrillator (AED) training. See the American Heart Association (AHA) or the International Liaison Committee on Resuscitation for BLS/CPR Guidelines (Box 11.1). Various levels of BLS training are available from organizations such as the AHA and the American Red Cross. Healthcare professionals should maintain appropriate certifications based on licensure requirements, type of practice, and environment. All oral healthcare personnel should be currently certified at the level of BLS appropriate for their practice.

CRITICAL THINKING EXERCISE

Use the Internet to locate a Quick Reference Card for Basic Life Support. Discuss how the information on the card could be used during training or an actual medical emergency.

In the event of an emergency, the AHA chain of survival includes recognition that a medical emergency is occurring, activation of an emergency response system, and initiation of CPR and defibrillation, if needed, until emergency personnel arrive on the scene. These BLS procedures are applied until recovery, until the person can be stabilized and transported to an emergency care facility, or until advanced life support is available. Emergency cardiac care, including CPR and the use of an AED, is part of BLS for healthcare providers.

Healthcare providers often work together in the management of medical emergencies. Coworkers should be trained together at appropriate intervals to maintain proficiency so that they may effectively respond as a team when medical emergencies arise. A plan should be in place to ensure that all members of the dental team work efficiently in managing a medical emergency.

DENTAL ENVIRONMENT PREPARATION

The dental environment must be supplied with the proper drugs and equipment to manage a potential medical emergency. Emergency contact information should be readily available if an emergency arises. The emergency assistance numbers and the emergency drug kit and equipment such as oxygen and an AED should be readily available. Local police, fire, and poison control center telephone numbers should be visibly posted next to the telephones and updated annually. The address of the facility and room number should also be posted to ensure emergency personnel are directed to the appropriate location.

Every dental setting should have a medical emergency plan. Each member of the oral care team should have a specific role to play in the event of an emergency. These roles should be periodically reviewed and practiced. Protocols for managing a medical emergency should be reviewed no less than annually and provided to all new employees. An annual refresher course in medical emergency management is highly recommended. Practice emergency simulations should be used to prepare the dental personnel for the implementation of protocols and the use of emergency equipment. These simulations should routinely occur to ensure that all staff members are prepared to deal with emergency situations that may arise.

Emergency Equipment

The dental emergency kit should contain all drugs, equipment, and supplies needed to handle a medical emergency in the oral healthcare setting. Dental facilities should have a first aid kit, an emergency drug kit, a portable oxygen tank, and an AED available (Fig. 11.1).

Drugs

The emergency kit should contain the basic drugs and items listed in Table 11.1. At a minimum, it should include epinephrine, histamine blocker, nitroglycerin, bronchodilator, oxygen, pulse oximeter, aspirin, and oral glucose.

The emergency kit should contain only drugs that the dentist or dental hygienist is trained to administer. For example, if intravenous medications that are used for advanced life support are in an emergency drug kit, the dentist or professional staff members would need training to ensure they can be competently administered (e.g., in an oral surgery office with an anesthetist). These medications, however, may not be used in a dental or dental hygiene practice setting without advanced training in sedation and anesthesia.

Dental settings where opioids or benzodiazepines are administered should include reversal drugs in their emergency kit. Naloxone (Narcan) can reverse an opioid overdose by blocking the effects of an opioid, and flumazenil (Romazicon) reverses the effects of a benzodiazepine that is typically used for anesthesia or conscious sedation. Maintaining medications

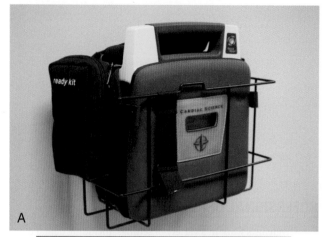

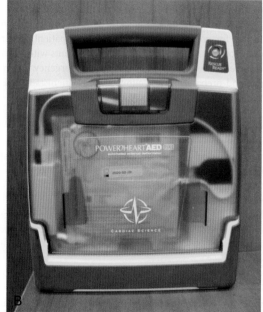

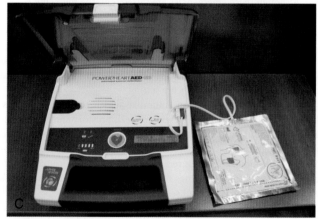

Fig. 11.1 (A) Wall-mounted automated external defibrillator (AED). (B) AED in a case. (C) AED opened. (Courtesy of Jennifer A. Pieren.)

in the dental emergency kit without the training to administer them could subject the dental hygienist or dentist to liability claims (Box 11.2).[2]

Oxygen

Oxygen (O_2) is an essential drug in an emergency kit. In the dental setting, oxygen is generally provided by a portable oxygen tank. Portable oxygen tanks are green in the United States but may also be found

TABLE 11.1 Contents of the Basic Dental Emergency Kit

Drugs,* Equipment, and Supplies	Administration Route and Use†	Action	Indications
Epinephrine pen	Subcutaneous or intramuscular	Acts as a cardiac stimulant and bronchodilator	Acute allergic reaction (anaphylaxis), acute bronchospasm (asthma)
Nitroglycerin	Sublingual	Relaxes smooth muscle and dilates coronary arteries	Angina pectoris
Bronchodilator (albuterol)	Inhaled	Dilates bronchi	Bronchospasm, asthma
Antihistamine (diphenhydramine)	Oral	Decreases the allergic response by blocking the action of histamine	Mild or localized allergic reaction
Aspirin (81-mg chewable tablets)	Oral	Provides a fibrinolysis effect to reduce clotting	Myocardial infarction
Pulse oximeter	Patient's finger	Monitors oxygen saturation of hemoglobin in arterial blood	To monitor oxygen saturations to determine whether oxygen should be administered
Automatic external defibrillator (AED)	Appropriate placement of electrical pads	Provides a shock to the heart to allow for the correction of an irregular, ineffective rhythm of heartbeat	Unresponsive patient, cardiac arrest
Oxygen tank, mask, and cannula	Nasal	Delivers free-flowing oxygen to a person with inadequate oxygen saturation	Oxygen saturation below target peripheral capillary oxygen saturation (SpO$_2$)
Pocket mask (optional: bag-valve-mask)	Mouth and nose	Provides a barrier for safety during rescue breathing	Basic Life Support
Blood pressure cuff and stethoscope	Appropriate sites	Monitors blood pressure	Before dental hygiene care, before and after the administration of drugs, as indicated during an emergency, and after stabilization in an emergency
Glucose (e.g., sugar cubes, orange juice, nondiet soft drink)	Oral	Elevates blood sugar	Hypoglycemia in a conscious patient
Injectable glucose (e.g., glucagon)	Intramuscular or subcutaneous	Elevates blood sugar	Hypoglycemia for an unconscious patient or conscious patient at risk for choking (i.e., seizures or convulsions)

*Other medications may be included for use in advanced cardiac life support, but advanced training is needed to administer them.
†If patients are conscious and aware as their medical situations are occurring, then they should be encouraged to administer their own medications whenever possible, which may include nitroglycerin, albuterol inhalers, EpiPens, and diabetic medications.

BOX 11.2 Ammonium Inhalants: Evidence-Based Update

The use of ammonia inhalants to prevent or treat syncope has long been the most common protocol in medical emergency management. However, evidence against the use of ammonia for an unconscious patient is increasing. Their use as a respiratory stimulant is not only nonspecific to the cause of syncope but may even be harmful to a patient with respiratory distress or compromised airway.

The violent physical response to the noxious smell, including wild and forceful motions of the extremities, may pose a challenge to the safety of the patient and to the dental professional. In addition, the use of ammonia is contraindicated in patients with a head injury or intracranial bleeding. Ammonia use may also produce coughing, nausea, and vomiting, which may exacerbate the risk of aspiration in a patient with an impaired gag reflex.

The use of ammonia inhalants for unconscious individuals is no longer recommended by emergency medical services (EMS) workers because of the complications that may arise. For example, the state of Michigan no longer recommends their use by EMS personnel.[3] Similarly, their use in the dental setting is also being reevaluated.[4]

in white tanks in other countries that have adopted the recommended standards for international color coding for medical gas (Fig. 11.2). However, not all countries have adopted standardized colors for oxygen tanks, so dental professionals should check the label before administering oxygen.[5] Most dental settings use a size E cylinder, which will supply approximately 30 minutes of oxygen. Oxygen delivery is measured in liters per minute (L/min). The flow rate is determined by patient characteristics and the type of emergency situation that is being treated.[2,6]

In the past, oxygen was commonly recommended for use in nearly every emergency except hyperventilation. Recent research has indicated that routine use of supplemental oxygen without appropriate titration may be associated with adverse outcomes. Therefore, **oxygen saturation**, the proportion of oxygen-saturated hemoglobin to overall hemoglobin in the blood, should be determined with a **pulse oximeter** before administering (Fig. 11.3). If a patient appears to be stable with a peripheral capillary oxygen saturation (SpO$_2$) of 90% to 94%, then they may not require further oxygen supplementation.[7] However, a patient who is acutely ill, having difficulty breathing, or showing obvious signs of heart failure or hypoxemia should have a target SpO$_2$ of 94% to 98%.[8]

Oxygen is delivered in several ways: nasal cannula (Fig. 11.4), a simple face mask, or a nonrebreather mask. When initiating oxygen therapy, the lowest concentration should be used via a nasal cannula

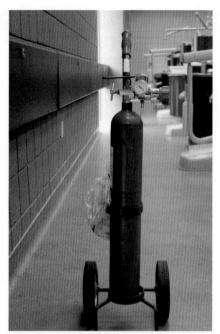

Fig. 11.2 Portable oxygen tank. (Courtesy of Jennifer A. Pieren.)

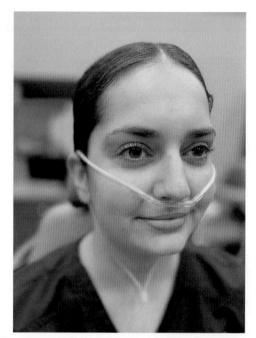

Fig. 11.4 Nasal cannula. (Courtesy of Jennifer A. Pieren.)

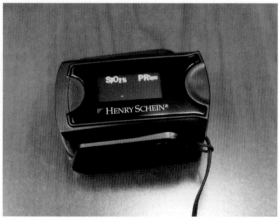

Fig. 11.3 Pulse oximeter. (Courtesy of Jennifer A. Pieren.)

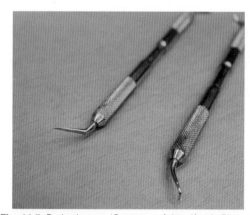

Fig. 11.5 Periotrievers. (Courtesy of Jennifer A. Pieren.)

at a 2 L/min flow rate. The liter flow should be titrated up if necessary to achieve an SpO$_2$ of 94% or greater without exceeding the maximum of 6 L/min. If sufficient oxygenation is not achieved, use a simple face mask and then a nonrebreather mask, if needed, to achieve target oxygen saturation.[8] Special attention should be paid to minimizing oxygen therapy in patients with potential reperfusion conditions such as acute coronary syndrome and acute ischemic stroke.[1,9]

Additional Items

Additional items in an emergency kit may include a pocket mask, syringes for delivery of intramuscular (IM) and subcutaneous (SC) drugs, sugar packets, a blanket, thermometer, emesis basin, and Magill forceps. Magnetized instruments, such as periotrievers, may also be beneficial to retrieve broken instrument tips (Fig. 11.5). However, magnetized retrieval instruments may not work on all types of instrument metals. It is recommended that dental hygienists have their own resuscitation masks in their treatment area to ensure that a mask is always available during patient care in the event of an emergency requiring CPR (Fig. 11.6). An individual in the dental setting should be designated to monitor contents regularly and to resupply and update the dental emergency kit at least quarterly and after every emergency.

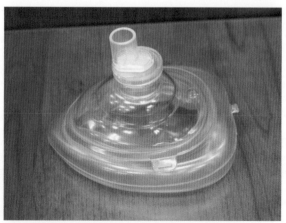

Fig. 11.6 Pocket mask. (Courtesy of Jennifer A. Pieren.)

CRITICAL THINKING EXERCISE: EMERGENCY MEDICAL KIT

Visit a local facility where dental hygiene care is delivered. Locate the dental emergency kit in the healthcare facility. Identify all equipment, supplies, and drugs in the kit, and describe their intended use. Check the expiration dates on all items. How is the dental emergency kit systematically updated to ensure currency of all items? How are the staff members trained to ensure that all of the contents of the emergency kit can be used when necessary? What is the emergency protocol in the healthcare facility? Does each member of the healthcare team have a clear role to play in the event of an emergency? Define these roles.

DOCUMENTATION

Dental hygienists are required to document all procedures performed during a dental visit, including those that occur during a medical emergency. Emergency medical report forms should be available to record the time of onset, treatment or drugs administered, and vital signs. A copy of the report should be kept on file and given to emergency medical services (EMS) personnel upon arrival and accompany the patient to the emergency department (Fig. 11.7).

Comprehensive Patient History

Dental hygienists should evaluate information from the comprehensive health history and risk assessment to create a care plan that will reduce the likelihood of a medical complication. If a patient is

---

MEDICAL EMERGENCY REPORT

Patient's Name _____Jane Smith_____   Today's Date _____1-5-18_____

Description of Incident:

Patient was standing in the panoramic machine and said she was feeling "light-headed and warm."
She was immediately placed on the floor and feet were elevated.
The patient's vital signs were monitored, and she remained responsive.
However, patient continued feeling uneasy and reported this was her first time she felt light-headed; no apparent
cause was determined. Patient consented to activation of EMS.

Time of Onset	Time EMS Summoned	Time EMS Arrived
9:30 am	9:39 am	9:45 am

Time Patient Released	
10:00 am	Patient Released to: EMS with a copy of this report.

	Finding	Time	Finding	Time	Finding	Time
Blood Pressure	114/76	9:32 am	108/68	9:38 am		
Pulse	82		68			
Respirations	14		18			
Oxygen Saturation	98% SpO2		98% SpO2			

Cessation of Breathing	Cessation of Pulse	CPR Initiated
Time: N/A	Time: N/A	Time: N/A

Drugs Administered	Route	Dosage	Time
N/A			

Fig. 11.7 Medical emergency report. (Adapted from Youngstown State University.)

BOX 11.3 Interprofessional Collaboration Opportunity

Interprofessional collaboration among healthcare providers can lead to a better understanding of a patient's needs. Consultation between a dental hygienist and a patient's primary healthcare provider regarding a health issue may lead to modifications in the care plan to prevent a medical emergency from occurring. Encouraging a collaborative approach among all healthcare disciplines can improve and enhance patient outcomes.

BOX 11.4 Client or Patient Education Tips

- Explain the importance of having an accurate health, dental, and pharmacologic history to prevent medical emergencies.
- Explain the importance of taking prescribed medications to prevent medical emergencies.
- Teach stress reduction strategies.
- Explain that complying with medication schedules, seeking regular preventive care, and immediately reporting unusual symptoms to a healthcare professional can prevent medical emergencies.

BOX 11.5 Signs of Dental Anxiety

- Cold, sweaty palms
- High blood pressure and pulse rate
- History of canceled appointments for nonemergency treatments
- History of emergency dental care only
- Muscle tightness
- Nervous conversations with others in the reception area
- Nervous play with tissue or hands
- Perspiration on forehead and hands
- Questioning the receptionist regarding injections or the use of sedation
- Quick answers
- Restlessness
- Unnaturally stiff posture
- White-knuckle syndrome

found to be at high risk, the dentist and/or the patient's physician are consulted as needed (see Chapter 13). Medical consultation should be obtained before intraoral invasive treatment is initiated. The dental professional should be prepared to provide the physician with detailed information about the proposed oral healthcare plan and any anticipated problems. Based on this consultation, an appropriate care plan and/or medications can be used to reduce the risk of emergencies (Box 11.3).

Managing and reducing stress by careful appointment planning, good communication, and patient rapport are essential. When indicated, the administration of conscious sedation or antianxiety premedication may also improve clinical outcomes. The purpose of the patient assessment process is to establish the patient's physical and psychologic risk and management during proposed treatment.[2,6,10]

American Society of Anesthesiologists Classifications

The American Society of Anesthesiologists (ASA) physical status classification may be used as a medical assessment framework to determine a patient's physical status (Table 11.2).[11] The acronym ASA and Roman numerals I through VI are used to classify physical status based on existing conditions, functional limitations, and blood pressure readings, with physical status becoming progressively worse as the ASA classification increases.

The ASA I category represents a "green light" for elective dental treatment. An ASA II or III represents a "yellow light" for elective dental treatment, which requires caution before proceeding. Dental hygienists will commonly see patients classified as ASA I, II, and III. A "red light" represents categories ASA IV, V, and VI. Although an ASA IV patient may present for dental hygiene treatment, these patients should only receive conservative emergency dental treatments until their condition stabilizes or improves to at least an ASA III category. Patients categorized as ASA V and VI are hospitalized or moribund and are not likely to receive dental treatment outside of the hospital environment.[2,11]

Vital Signs

Monitoring vital signs is an important aspect of assessing a patient's overall health status. Baseline vital signs are recorded to enable the healthcare provider to determine the health status of the patient and compare normal readings with readings that occur during a medical emergency (see Chapter 14).

Vital signs recorded outside the normal ranges may indicate underlying medical issues. Discussing vital signs with a patient is an important aspect of treatment (Box 11.4). A physician consultation may be needed to determine whether modifications or a delay in treatment is necessary.

ANXIETY RECOGNITION AND MANAGEMENT

Heightened anxiety and fear of dental care can lead to hyperventilation and **syncope** or an acute exacerbation of conditions such as heart attack, stroke, angina, seizures, and asthma. One of the goals of patient assessment is to determine whether a patient is psychologically capable of tolerating the stress associated with the planned care. Recognizing anxiety can be as simple as asking the patient about fear, anxiety, and past traumatic or painful dental experiences during the comprehensive health history and interview. Many patients underestimate or do not want to acknowledge dental anxiety; therefore, direct observation of signs and symptoms is an important component of assessing anxiety (Box 11.5). The use of dental anxiety scales and questionnaires may be helpful to assess dental anxiety in patients.[10]

CRITICAL THINKING EXERCISE: SYNCOPE

Syncope is one of the most common medical emergencies occurring in the dental setting. Discuss steps to prevent an episode of syncope. Review the signs and symptoms of syncope and the management of this condition.

Direct Observation

Careful observation may identify anxious individuals. Severely anxious individuals may be recognized by the following:
- Increased blood pressure and heart rate
- Trembling
- Excessive perspiration
- Dilated pupils
- Overall appearance of extreme uneasiness

Stress Reduction Protocols

Many medical emergencies are associated with stress. The **stress-reduction protocols**, or steps taken to reduce dental anxiety and fear, are listed in Box 11.6. Prevention or reduction of stress should start before the dental appointment, continue throughout treatment, and follow through into the postoperative period, if necessary (Box 11.7).[2,6,10]

TABLE 11.2 American Society of Anesthesiologists (ASA)

ASA Classification	Definition	Functional Limitations	Examples
ASA I	Normal health	• Able to walk up one flight of stairs or two level city blocks without distress • Can withstand whatever stress is associated with planned dental treatment without added risk of serious complications	Adult: Healthy, no or minimal alcohol use, no smoking Pediatric: Healthy (no acute or chronic disease), normal BMI percentile for age
ASA II	Mild stable systemic disease without substantive functional limitations or extreme anxiety and fear in the dental environment	• Able to walk up one flight of stairs or two level city blocks before needing to stop	Adult: Obesity (BMI between 30 and 40), well-controlled diabetes mellitus (DM) and hypertension (HTN), mild lung disease, social alcohol drinker, current smoker Pediatric: Asthma without exacerbation, cancer state in remission, abnormal BMI for age, well-controlled epilepsy, noninsulin-dependent diabetes mellitus Obstetric: Normal pregnancy, well-controlled gestational HTN, controlled preeclampsia, diet-controlled gestational DM
ASA III	Severe systemic disease, one or more moderate to severe diseases or substantive functional limitations	• Able to climb one flight of stairs or walk two city blocks but must stop and rest before completing because of the distress	Adult: Morbid obesity (BMI ≥40), poorly controlled DM or HTN, alcohol dependence or abuse, history (>3 months) of myocardial infarction (MI), cerebrovascular accident (CVA), transient ischemic attack (TIA), coronary artery disease (CAD) or stents, active hepatitis, end-stage renal disease (ESRD) with regularly scheduled dialysis, chronic obstructive pulmonary disease (COPD), implanted pacemaker Pediatric: Asthma with exacerbation, poorly controlled epilepsy, insulin-dependent DM, morbid obesity Obstetric: Severe preeclampsia, gestational DM with complications
ASA IV	Severe systemic disease that constantly threatens life	• Cannot climb a flight of stairs or walk two-level city blocks because of shortness of breath or fatigue	Adult: Recent (<3 months) MI, CVA, TIA, CAD or stents, ongoing cardiac ischemia or severe valve dysfunction, ESRD without regularly scheduled dialysis, acute respiratory distress, sepsis, disseminated intravascular coagulation Pediatric: Symptomatic or unstable cardiac disease, severe respiratory distress, advanced cancer state Obstetric: Severe preeclampsia
ASA V	Near death and not expected to survive without medical intervention		Significant cardiac pathologic conditions, ruptured abdominal or thoracic aneurysm, intracranial bleeding with mass effect, massive trauma, ischemic bowel, multiple organ or system dysfunction
ASA VI	Declared brain dead; organs are being removed for donor purposes		

Adapted from Malamed SF. *Medical Emergencies in the Dental Office*. 8th ed. Elsevier; 2023; and Appukuttan DP. Strategies to manage patients with dental anxiety and dental phobia: literature review. *Clin Cosmet Investig Dent*. 2016;8:35–50.
American Society of Anesthesiologists. *ASA Physical Status Classification System*. Updated: December 13, 2020. Available at: https://www.asahq.org/standards-and-guidelines/asa-physical-status-classification-system. Accessed February 24, 2023.
Böhmer A, Defosse J, Geldner G, et al. The updated SA classification. *Anästh Intensivmed* 2021;62:223–227. https://doi.org/10.19224/ai2021.223. Available at: https://www.ai-online.info/images/ai-ausgabe/2021/05-2021/AI_05-2021_Sonderbeitrag_Boehmer_englisch.pdf.

BOX 11.6   Stress-Reduction Protocols

General:
- Build patient rapport to evaluate and relieve anxiety.
- Maintain communication with the patient about fears and anxiety.
- Minimize waiting time.
- Schedule short, preferably morning, appointments.

Pharmacologic options as needed:
- Use adequate pain control medications during and after the procedure.
- Prescribe preappointment sedation (e.g., a short-acting benzodiazepine drug).
- Offer sedation during the appointment (e.g., nitrous oxide sedation).
- Administer profound local anesthesia.
- Follow up with the patient after treatment.

BOX 11.7   Management Techniques for Dental Anxiety

- Acupuncture
- Biofeedback
- Cognitive therapy
- Distraction
- Guided imagery
- Hypnotherapy
- Positive reinforcement
- Relaxation techniques (e.g., deep breathing, muscle relaxation)
- Systematic desensitization or exposure therapy
- Tell-show-do
- Conscious sedation
- Pharmacologic management

BOX 11.8   Informed Consent for Emergency Medical Treatment

If a patient is conscious, they are and consent is expressly obtained before providing any assistance. If a patient is unconscious, permission can be assumed and emergency assistance can begin immediately.

RESPONSE TO MEDICAL EMERGENCIES

Recognition of Unresponsiveness

Unresponsiveness, also called unconsciousness, must be quickly recognized and effectively managed. The unresponsive (unconscious) person does not respond to sensory stimulation such as gently shaking and shouting, "Are you all right?" Lack of response to this stimulation indicates that the person is unconscious. When an apparently unconscious person is discovered, the health professional checks for responsiveness and breathing. If the patient is unresponsive, not breathing, or breathing abnormally (only gasping), BLS is immediately activated (Box 11.8).

Terminate Dental Hygiene Care, Summon Assistance, and Position the Patient

As soon as unresponsiveness is recognized, the hygienist terminates dental hygiene procedures and activates EMS (e.g., 911 in the United States and Canada; 000 in Australia; 119 in Japan; 112 or 999 in the United Kingdom; and 112 in most of Europe; is standard on Global System for Mobile Communications [GSM] mobile phones). Box 11.9 lists information to be given to the EMS dispatcher.

BOX 11.9   Information Given to the Emergency Medical Services Dispatcher

- Your name
- Location of the emergency (with names of cross streets, if possible)
- Telephone number from which the call is made
- What has happened (e.g., heart attack, seizure)
- Condition of the patient
- Aid being given to the patient
- Any other information requested

Note: The caller should hang up only when told to do so.

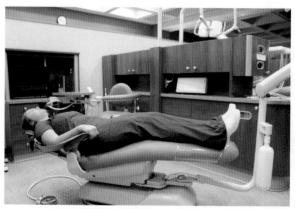

Fig. 11.8 Supine position. (Courtesy of Jennifer A. Pieren.)

The unconscious person is placed into the supine (horizontal) position (Fig. 11.8). In the supine position, the brain is at the same level as the body positioned on a flat plane. A major objective in the management of unconsciousness is the delivery of oxygenated blood to the brain. The horizontal position helps the heart accomplish this task and prepares the patient for CPR if needed. Any extra head supports, such as pillows, must be removed from the headrest of the dental chair when the patient loses consciousness to ensure that the body is in the supine position.

The next step is to begin life support by delivering high-quality CPR. When office personnel are available to assist, they can be directed to notify EMS while CPR is started and to obtain the AED for the rescuer. Assisting personnel can also obtain other items from the medical emergency kit (e.g., oxygen, bag-valve-mask (Fig. 11.9), aspirin) as needed.[1]

Effective Emergency Response

To effectively respond to life-threatening emergencies outside of the hospital setting, understanding the importance of the chain of survival is helpful (Fig. 11.10).

The six links in the chain are as follows:
- *Early recognition of the emergency and early access to EMS.* The sooner the local emergency number is called, the sooner advanced EMS personnel will arrive and take over.
- *Early CPR.* CPR helps supply oxygen to the brain and other vital organs to keep the individual alive until an AED is used or advanced medical care is given.
- *Early defibrillation.* An electrical shock called defibrillation may restore a normal heart rhythm. Each minute of delayed defibrillation reduces the patient's chance of survival by approximately 10%.

- *Basic and advanced medical care.* EMS personnel provide more advanced medical care and transport the patient to the hospital.
- *Advanced life support and postcardiac arrest care.* Comprehensive multidisciplinary care is provided by hospital personnel.
- *Recovery.* Emphasis on additional treatment, observation, rehabilitation, and any other needed support for recovery.[1,12]

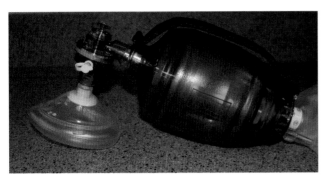

Fig. 11.9 Bag-valve-mask. (Courtesy of Jennifer A. Pieren.)

MANAGEMENT OF SPECIFIC MEDICAL EMERGENCIES

Recognition of medical emergencies is essential for early intervention and appropriate treatment. When a medical emergency arises, the patient's symptoms and vital signs must be rapidly assessed. Guided by symptoms and vital signs, an assessment of the patient's state of consciousness and neurologic, respiratory, or cardiac status is performed. From this information, the type of emergency is identified and treatment is rendered. Signs and symptoms of various conditions and the treatments for specific medical emergencies are listed in Table 11.3. In all cases, the hygienist begins by assessing the patient's responsiveness, breathing, and pulse. If the patient is unresponsive, is not breathing, or has no pulse, the BLS sequence should be followed.

CRITICAL THINKING EXERCISE

A patient complains of squeezing chest pain and shortness of breath and exhibits significant diaphoresis. What condition(s) should you suspect? Discuss appropriate management for this patient's condition. What steps could have been taken to reduce the risk of this medical emergency occurring?

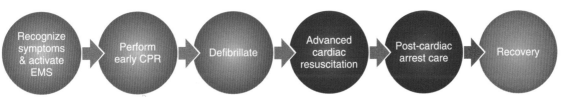

Fig. 11.10 Chain of Survival image. (Modified from Kaji A, Pedigo RA. Emergency Medicine Board Review E-Book. Elsevier Health Sciences; 2021.)

TABLE 11.3   Management of Specific Medical Emergencies

Condition and Overview	Signs and Symptoms	Management
In all medical emergencies, terminate dental treatment upon onset, activate facility emergency procedures, and monitor vital signs and peripheral capillary oxygen saturation (SpO_2). If the patient becomes unconscious or is unresponsive, then begin the Basic Life Support (BLS) sequence.		
Adrenal crisis: cortisol deficiency	<ul><li>Confusion</li><li>Weakness</li><li>Lethargy</li><li>Respiratory depression</li><li>Headache</li><li>Shocklike symptoms</li><li>Weak, rapid pulse</li><li>Low blood pressure</li><li>Abdominal or leg pain</li><li>Possible loss of consciousness</li></ul>	If responsive:<ul><li>Place the patient in the supine position with feet slightly elevated.</li><li>Assess SpO_2; administer oxygen if needed.</li><li>Ask the patient to self-administer a stress dose of their own corticosteroid medication. Initiate BLS and activate emergency medical services (EMS), if needed.</li></ul>If unresponsive:<ul><li>Place the patient in the supine position with feet slightly elevated.</li><li>Activate EMS.</li><li>Initiate BLS as needed.</li></ul>
Partial (mild) airway obstruction: partial blockage of the airway with adequate oxygen exchange	<ul><li>Effective coughing</li><li>Choking</li><li>Wheezing</li><li>Grasping throat with hands</li><li>Able to speak</li><li>Possible cyanosis</li></ul>	<ul><li>Evaluate air exchange.</li><li>If adequate, encourage the patient to continue coughing to dislodge the object and clear the airway.</li><li>If inadequate, cough becomes silent, or the patient is unable to speak, treat as severe airway obstruction.</li></ul>
Complete (severe) airway obstruction: severe or complete blockage of the airway with inadequate oxygen exchange	<ul><li>Silent cough</li><li>Choking</li><li>Possible high-pitched noise</li><li>Grasping throat with hands</li><li>Unable to speak</li><li>Cyanosis</li></ul>	<ul><li>Begin abdominal thrusts (Heimlich maneuver) until the object is dislodged; if the patient is pregnant or obese, use chest compressions until the object is dislodged.</li><li>If the patient becomes unresponsive, activate EMS and begin BLS.</li></ul>

Continued

TABLE 11.3   Management of Specific Medical Emergencies—cont'd

Condition and Overview	Signs and Symptoms	Management
Angina pectoris: chest pain due to inadequate blood and oxygen supply to the heart muscle	• Crushing, burning, or squeezing chest pain, radiating to left shoulder, arms, neck, or mandible (lasting less than 15 minutes) • Shortness of breath • Perspiration	In a patient with a history of stable angina: • Place the patient in a comfortable position, usually upright. • Assess SpO$_2$; administer oxygen as needed. • Administer nitroglycerin 0.4 mg sublingually (preferably self-administered) every 5 minutes, with a maximum of three doses, until pain is relieved. • Reassure the patient. • If the pain is not relieved, activate EMS and treat as a myocardial infarction. In a patient with no history of angina or if pain is more intense than normal: • Activate EMS.
Asthma attack: narrowing of the bronchial airways due to bronchospasm, excessive mucus, or inflammation	• Nonproductive cough • Wheezing • Increased respiratory efforts • Shortness of breath • Perspiration • Pallor • Anxiety • Possible cyanosis • Increased pulse rate	• Position the patient to facilitate breathing (upright is usually best). • Administer bronchodilator (preferably self-administered). • Assess and maintain airway. • Assess SpO$_2$; administer oxygen as needed. • If the patient recovers, care can be continued if appropriate. • If not, terminate dental hygiene services, have the patient self-medicate one more time with the inhaler, administer oxygen, activate EMS, and initiate BLS as needed. • If the patient becomes unresponsive, administer epinephrine 0.3 mg of 1:1000.
Cardiac arrest: sudden cessation of heart function	• Ashen, gray, and/or cold, clammy skin • Cyanosis • Dilated pupils • Absence of a pulse • Absence of heart sounds • Absence of respirations • Unconsciousness	• Place the patient in a supine position. • Activate EMS. • Initiate BLS.
Cerebrovascular accident (CVA) or stroke: occlusion or hemorrhage of cerebral blood vessel, resulting in ischemia	• Sudden weakness of one side • Severe headache • Difficulty speaking or loss of speech • Vision changes • Dizziness • Nausea • Convulsions	• Place the patient in a semisupine position. • Activate EMS. • Assess SpO2; administer oxygen as needed. • Monitor and maintain airway; suction if needed. • Keep the patient quiet and still. • Initiate BLS as needed.
Eye injury: trauma, exposure or introduction of a foreign body or substance[13]	• Tearing • Blinking • Pain • Change in eye movement • Changes to vision • Redness or bleeding • Unusual pupil size, shape, or orientation	For all eye injuries: • Do not touch, rub, or apply medicine or pressure to the eye. • Do not try to remove the object. • Seek either advanced medical care or facilitate emergency care. For an eye puncture or cut: • Activate EMS. • Place a shield over the eye. • Do not rinse with water. For a particle or foreign material in the eye: • Wash your hands and apply clean gloves. • Examine the eye by gently pulling down the lower eyelid; ask the patient to look up while holding the upper lid open. • If debris is visible, rinse the surface of the eye mesially to distally to remove the object, or advise the patient to lift the upper eyelid over the lashes of the lower lid and blink. • If the particle remains, advise the patient to keep eyes closed and immediately seek medical attention. For a chemical burn: • Immediately flush the surface of the eye mesially to distally with clean water or saline for 15 minutes. • Activate EMS.
Hemorrhage: profuse bleeding	• Arterial blood is red in color and spurts. • Venous blood is darker in color and oozes.	• Apply compression over the hemorrhage, usually with gauze. For bleeding from a dental extraction or surgical site: • Pack the area with gauze and have the patient bite down until the bleeding stops, or pack the site with absorbable material (if trained). For nosebleeds: • Apply pressure to the bleeding side or pack the bleeding nostril with gauze. For severe bleeding: • Watch for signs of shock and activate EMS if bleeding continues.

TABLE 11.3 Management of Specific Medical Emergencies—cont'd

Condition and Overview	Signs and Symptoms	Management
Hypertensive crisis (hypertensive urgency): severe blood pressure elevation in an otherwise stable patient, without acute or impending target organ damage or dysfunction Hypertensive emergency: severe blood pressure elevation with evidence of target organ damage[14]	Urgency and emergency: • Systolic blood pressure >180 mm Hg and/or • Diastolic blood pressure >120 mm Hg Emergency: • Evidence of target organ damage	Urgency: • Advise patient to seek advanced medical assessment and care immediately. Emergency: • Requires immediate reduction of blood pressure to limit further target organ damage. • Activate EMS or facilitate transfer to an advanced care setting.
Hyperventilation: respiratory alkalosis resulting from an excessive loss of carbon dioxide	• Rapid or shallow respirations • Lightheadedness • Dizziness • Confusion • Tingling in extremities and/or perioral numbness • Tightness in chest • Fast pulse • Panic-stricken appearance • Carpopedal tetany • Cold hands	• Place the patient in an upright position. • Explain what is happening. • Remove the source of anxiety. • Remove objects from the oral cavity. • Reassure the patient, using a quiet voice to calm. • Encourage slow, normal breathing; have the patient breathe through pursed lips or into cupped hands. • Do not administer oxygen.
Myocardial infarction (heart attack): necrosis of the myocardium due to total or partial occlusion of an artery	• Chest pain, usually more severe than angina • Pain in the left arm, jaw, and possibly teeth; not relieved by rest and nitroglycerin • Cold and/or clammy skin • Nausea • Anxiety or impending sense of doom • Shortness of breath • Weakness • Perspiration • Burning feeling of indigestion	• Place the patient in a comfortable position, usually semisupine or upright. • Activate EMS. • If possible, have the patient chew 162 to 325 mg of chewable, nonenteric-coated aspirin or two to four 81 mg baby aspirin tablets. • Assess SpO2; administer oxygen if needed. • Calm and reassure the patient. • If the patient becomes unconscious, begin BLS.
Pulmonary edema (acute): impairment of the heart muscle from left ventricular failure, resulting in fluid accumulation in the lungs	• Shortness of breath • Difficulty breathing • Possible cyanosis • Weakness • Feeling of suffocation • Swelling of lower extremities • Perspiration • Pink, frothy sputum • Distention of jugular vein when upright	• Place the patient in an upright position. • Activate EMS. • Calm and reassure the patient. • Assess and maintain the airway. • Assess SpO_2; administer oxygen as needed. • Administer 0.8 to 1.2 mg (2 to 3 tablets or sprays) of nitroglycerine every 5 to 10 minutes. • Initiate BLS as needed.
Psychogenic shock: cerebral hypoxia (treated the same as syncope) Other forms of shock: type will depend on etiology[15]	• Hypotension • Pale, clammy skin • Change in mental status • Fainting • Dizziness • Rapid weak pulse • Rapid shallow respirations • Eventual unconsciousness if untreated	• Place the patient in a supine position with elevated feet. • Activate EMS. • Assess and maintain airway responsiveness and pulse. • Assess SpO2 and administer oxygen as needed. • Administer BLS as needed.
Syncope: sudden transient loss of consciousness (fainting)	• Pallor • Nausea • Fast pulse (early), followed by slow pulse (late) • Perspiration • Pupil dilation • Dimming of vision • Yawning • Eventual loss of consciousness	• Place the patient in a supine position with legs slightly elevated; for a pregnant patient, roll her on to the left side. • Loosen binding clothes. • Assess and maintain airway. • Assess SpO2 and administer oxygen as needed. • Allow the patient to recover. • If hypoglycemia is suspected, administer oral glucose during postsyncopal recovery. • If the patient does not rapidly regain consciousness after proper positioning and treatment, activate EMS.

Continued

TABLE 11.3   Management of Specific Medical Emergencies—cont'd

Condition and Overview	Signs and Symptoms	Management
Seizure Disorders		
Generalized tonic-clonic (grand mal) seizure: generalized electronic abnormality in the brain with a loss of consciousness	• Aura (change in taste, smell, or sight preceding seizure) • Loss of consciousness • Sudden cry • Involuntary tonic-clonic muscle contractions • Altered breathing • Possible involuntary defecation or urination	• Place patient in supine position. • Lower dental chair and protect patient from personal injury. • Clear area of all sharp and dangerous objects. • Do not attempt to restrain the person. • After convulsion, assess and monitor airway. • Assess SpO2; administer oxygen as needed. • If unresolved (status epilepticus), activate EMS. • If stable, allow patient to rest, arrange for medical followup, and arrange for transportation assistance.
Nonconvulsive (petit mal) seizure: generalized electronic abnormality in the brain without a loss of consciousness	• Sudden momentary loss of awareness without loss of postural tone • Blank stare • Muscle twitches • Duration of several to 90 seconds	• Place the patient in a supine position. • Observe closely. • Clear area of sharp objects to ensure patient safety. • Provide supportive care. • Request a physician evaluation if needed.
Diabetic Emergencies		
Hyperglycemia (ketoacidosis): excess glucose and insufficient insulin levels	• Excessive thirst • Excessive urination • Excessive hunger • Labored respirations • Nausea • Dry, flushed skin • Low blood pressure • Weak, rapid pulse • Fruity smell to the breath • Blurred vision • Headache • Unconsciousness	• Place the patient in a supine position. • Activate EMS. • Assess SpO2 and administer oxygen as needed. • Provide BLS as needed. If responsive: • Ask when the patient ate last, whether insulin has been taken, and whether insulin is available. • Retrieve the patient's insulin. • If able, the patient should self-administer the insulin.
Hypoglycemia (hyperinsulinism or insulin shock): insufficient glucose levels	• Mood changes • Hunger • Headache • Perspiration • Nausea • Confusion • Irritation • Dizziness • Weakness • Increased anxiety • Possible unconsciousness	If responsive: • Place the patient in an upright position. • Give concentrated form of oral sugar (e.g., sugar packet, cake icing, concentrated orange juice, apple juice, sugar-containing soda). • If symptoms worsen or do not resolve within 10 minutes, emergency services should be activated. If unresponsive: • Place the patient in a supine position. • Activate EMS. • Assess SpO_2, and administer oxygen as needed. • If available and trained, administer intramuscular or subcutaneous glucagon (1 mg).
Allergic Reactions		
Anaphylaxis: an allergic reaction with immediate hypersensitivity	• Rapid and severe hives • Itchy skin • Swelling of mucous membranes such as lips, tongue, larynx, and pharynx • Respiratory distress • Wheezing • Weak pulse • Low blood pressure • May progress to unconsciousness and cardiovascular collapse	If unresponsive: • Place the patient in the supine position. • Activate EMS. If responsive: • Place the patient in a comfortable position, usually upright. • Administer epinephrine (0.15 mg for individuals up to 30 kg; 0.3 to 0.5 mg for individuals greater than 30 kg); if ineffective, a repeat dose can be considered if advanced care will not arrive within 5 to 10 minutes. For both: • Assess and maintain the airway. • Assess SpO2 and administer oxygen as needed. • Initiate BLS as needed.

TABLE 11.3   Management of Specific Medical Emergencies—cont'd

Condition and Overview	Signs and Symptoms	Management
Localized skin response: hypersensitivity to an allergen	Slow onset of: • Mild itching • Mild skin rash • Hives	• Place the patient in a comfortable position, usually upright. • Call for assistance. • Administer diphenhydramine, 1 mg/kg for children, not to exceed 25 mg; 25 mg to 50 mg for adults. • Discontinue exposure to the allergen if known. • Assess vital signs. • Be prepared to administer BLS if needed. • Have the patient consult their physician about a repeat dose every 6 hours for 2 days after reaction if needed.
Reactions to local anesthesia: sensitivity to an ingredient in a local anesthetic (see Chapter 43 for more information)	Toxicity from local anesthesia: • Light headedness • Blurred vision • Slurred speech • Confusion • Drowsiness • Anxiety • Tinnitus • Slow pulse rate • Fast respirations Toxicity from vasopressor or vasoconstrictor: • Anxiety • Fast pulse rate • Fast respirations • Chest pain • Dysrhythmias • Cardiac arrest	If unresponsive: • Place the patient in the supine position. • Activate EMS. If responsive: • Place the patient in a comfortable position, usually upright. • Assess vital signs. • Assess SpO$_2$ and administer oxygen as needed. • Activate EMS as needed. • Initiate BLS as needed.
Other Emergencies		
Tooth avulsion		• Immediately reimplant the tooth. • If reimplantation is not possible, store the tooth in Hanks' balanced salt solution or wrap the tooth in cling film until tooth can be reimplanted by a dental professional. • Storage in tap water is not recommended.

Available at First Aid Medical Emergencies, American Heart Association/Red Cross https://cpr.heart.org/en/resuscitation-science/first-aid-guidelines/first-aid Pellegrino JL, Charlton NP, Carlson JN, et al. 2020 American Heart Association and American Red Cross focused update for first aid. *Circulation.* Oct 27, 2020;142(17):e287–303. Available at: https://www.ahajournals.org/doi/epub/10.1161/CIR.0000000000000269. Accessed February 21, 2023; Malamed SF. *Medical Emergencies in the Dental Office.* 8th ed. Mosby; 2023; Little JW, Miller CS, Rhodus NL. *Little and Falace's Dental Management of the Medically Compromised Patient.* Elsevier; 2018; National Association of State EMS Officials. *National Model EMS Clinical Guidelines.* March 2022. Available at: https://nasemso.org/wp-content/uploads/National-Model-EMS-Clinical-Guidelines_2022.pdf. Access February 21, 2023.

CRITICAL THINKING EXERCISE

During periodontal debridement, the tip of your instrument breaks off and your patient aspirates it. What is the appropriate response to this situation? What steps could have been taken to prevent this incident?

CRITICAL THINKING EXERCISE

Role play these emergency situations: stroke, cardiac arrest, insulin shock, diabetic coma, seizure, reaction to the local anesthetic agent, anaphylactic shock, obstructed airway, and syncope.

Documentation

Proper documentation of an emergency is required. The medical emergency incident report form (see Fig. 11.7 for an example) can be used for this purpose. A member of the oral care team should be assigned the responsibility of recording information on the medical incident report form during the emergency situation. The form is kept in the patient's record. In the event that the patient is transferred to a hospital, a copy of the incident report and health history forms should accompany the patient.[2]

LEGAL CONSIDERATIONS FOR MEDICAL EMERGENCIES: GOOD SAMARITAN STATUTES

A **Good Samaritan** is a legal term that refers to someone who renders aid in an emergency to an injured person on a voluntary basis. Usually, if a volunteer comes to the aid of an injured or ill person who is a stranger, the person providing the aid owes the stranger a duty of being reasonably careful. Good Samaritan statutes generally provide immunity from civil liability for those rendering care in emergency situations in certain circumstances. Under these statutes, a health professional providing care in an emergency would not be liable for any civil damages as a result of acts or omissions in rendering first aid or emergency care, nor is the person liable for any civil damages as a result of any act or failure to act to provide or arrange for further medical treatment or care for the injured person. Certain stipulations apply:

- Emergency care is provided at the scene of the emergency.
- The healthcare professional has proper training for the care provided.
- The volunteer acts gratuitously and in good faith but without remuneration or the expectation of remuneration.

These statutes were enacted so that healthcare professionals and volunteers can render care to persons in emergencies and be protected from lawsuits for negligent harm. These laws vary from state to state, but gross negligence or willful misconduct is not covered in most jurisdictions. Gross negligence is the intentional failure to perform a task, with reckless disregard for the consequences that affect the life of another or a conscious act or omission that may result in grave injury.

In addition, under Good Samaritan statutes, emergency care cannot be denied if providing such care is part of a person's job responsibilities. Dental hygienists have a duty to deliver emergency services within the scope of their training. All dental professionals also have a duty to remain competent through training, retraining, certification, and practice so that they can manage a medical emergency in the practice setting.

KEY CONCEPTS

- Completing an assessment of the patient, including health, dental, and pharmacologic history and vital signs, is essential in the prevention of medical emergencies.
- Assessing the potential for a medical emergency includes consideration of the risk level of the patient, the procedure planned, and the anxiety level of the patient.
- Use stress reduction protocols to prevent anxiety-related emergencies.
- If a patient is found to be at risk, consult the patient's physician and adjust the care plan and appointment schedule to avoid possible emergency situations.
- Dental professionals must be competent in using the medical emergency kit, including all drugs and equipment, and should practice medical emergency drills using a variety of scenarios.
- When a medical emergency arises, conduct a rapid and thorough assessment of the patient. Document any details related to the emergency situation, including onset, treatment, and outcome.
- Include a completed medical emergency incident report in the patient's record as documentation of the event.

ACKNOWLEDGMENTS

The authors acknowledge Lynn Utecht and Denise Bowen for their past contributions to this chapter. The authors also appreciate the time and expertise contributed to this chapter by Joseph J. Mistovich.

REFERENCES

1. American Heart Association. *2020 American Heart Association Guidelines for Cardiopulmonary Resuscitation and Emergency Cardiovascular Care.* Available at: https://cpr.heart.org/en/resuscitation-science/cpr-and-ecc-guidelines/executive-summary.
2. Malamed SF. *Medical Emergencies in the Dental Office.* 8th ed. Mosby; 2023.
3. Wahl K. *Ammonia Inhalants. State of Michigan.* Department of Health and Human Services; 2016.
4. Goodchild JH, Donaldson M. Is it time to omit ammonia inhalants from dental emergency kits? *Gen Dent.* 2022;70(4):6–9.
5. Whitaker DK, Wilkinson DJ. *Anesthesia Patient Safety Foundation. Medical Gases: Time to Adopt the Global Standard?* June 2014. Available at: https://www.apsf.org/newsletters/html/2014/June/06_medicalgases.htm.
6. Little JW, Miller CS, Rhodus NL. *Little and Falace's Dental Management of the Medically Compromised Patient.* Elsevier, Inc.; 2018.
7. Cornet AD, Kooter AJ, Peters MJ, et al. The potential harm of oxygen therapy in medical emergencies. *Crit Care.* 2013;17:313.
8. National Association of State EMS Officials. *National Model EMS Clinical Guidelines*; 2022. Available at: https://nasemso.org/wp-content/uploads/National-Model-EMS-Clinical-Guidelines_2022.pdf. Accessed February 21, 2023.
9. O'Connor RE, Al Ali AS, Brady WJ, et al. Part 9: acute coronary syndromes: 2015 American Heart Association guidelines update for cardiopulmonary resuscitation and emergency cardiovascular care. *Circulation.* 2015;132(suppl 2):S483–S500.
10. Appukuttan DP. Strategies to manage patients with dental anxiety and dental phobia: literature review. *Clin Cosmet Investig Dent.* 2016;8:35–50.
11. American Society of Anesthesiologists. *ASA Physical Status Classification System.* Updated: December 13, 2020. Available at: https://www.asahq.org/standards-and-guidelines/asa-physical-status-classification-system. Accessed February 24, 2023.
12. American Heart Association. 2020 AHA guidelines for CPR and ECC. https://cpr.heart.org/en/resuscitation-science/cpr-and-ecc-guidelines. Accessed February 21, 2023.
13. American Academy of Ophthalmology. Recognizing and Treating Eye Injuries. Updated March 4, 2021. Available at: https://www.aao.org/eye-health/tips-prevention/injuries Accessed February 21, 2023.
14. American College of Cardiology/American Heart Association Task Force on Clinical Practice Guidelines. *American Heart Association. Detailed Summary from the 2017 Guideline for the Prevention, Detection, Evaluation and Management of High Blood Pressure in Adults*; 2017.
15. National Library of Medicine. Medline Plus. *Shock.* Updated 2020. Available at: https://medlineplus.gov/ency/article/000039.htm. Accessed February 21, 2023.

12

Ergonomics and Work-Related Musculoskeletal Disorders

Melanie J. Aley

PROFESSIONAL OPPORTUNITIES

Work-related musculoskeletal disorders (MSDs) are a significant occupational health issue in dentistry. By applying ergonomic principles and undertaking regular physical activity, these disorders are preventable, improving the likelihood of career satisfaction and longevity.

COMPETENCIES

1. Apply ergonomic principles in dental hygiene practice, considering environmental, equipment, positioning, performance, and person-level factors.
2. Demonstrate strengthening and chairside stretching exercises. Also discuss the importance of a regular exercise regimen.
3. Compare and contrast common **repetitive strain injuries (RSIs)** in terms of signs, symptoms, and risk factors. Also practice chairside measures for prevention of RSIs and other musculoskeletal disorders (MSDs) that a dental hygienist should take before, during, and after patient care appointments.
4. Demonstrate exercises recommended for reducing the risk of injury.

PRINCIPLES OF ERGONOMICS

Ergonomics is the study of human performance and workplace design. Dental hygienists are at risk for work-related injuries and disorders involving the tendons, tendon sheaths, muscles, and nerves of hands, wrists, arms, elbows, shoulders, neck, and back. RSIs describe a range of painful injuries to areas of the body that are caused by overuse or repetitive tasks. MSDs more broadly refer to injuries that affect movement and the body's musculoskeletal system, including RSIs. When ergonomic principles are applied (Fig. 12.1), a dental hygienist can comfortably practice and avert disability. When clinicians ignore ergonomic principles, an RSI may occur. Minimizing occupational risks increases the likelihood of long-range health and wellness for the practitioner.

Environmental Factors

Environmental factors within the dental clinic, such as the room temperature and noise levels, affect the musculoskeletal health of dental hygienists. Flexibility of muscles and tendons, which is important for reducing the occurrence of an RSI, develops through physical exercise and comfortable room temperatures. Cold room temperatures relate to less relaxed and less flexible muscles and tendons. Stress and strain of stiff muscles and tendons lead to RSIs. Relaxed atmospheres with minimal background noise contribute to a positive psychologic state for both clinicians and patients. Dental hygienists working in clinical settings other than the dental hygiene or dental office, such as long-term

care facilities, may need to consider additional factors associated with the lifting or transferring of patients.

Equipment Factors

Equipment within the dental clinic, including the dental unit, clinician's chair, gloves, and instruments, can affect musculoskeletal health and ergonomics.

Dental Unit

The treatment area consists of the dental unit and chair, including the dental light. The dental chair supports the patient's head, torso, and feet. The dental chair also provides for easy maneuvering of the patient via an articulating headrest and foot and side power controls. The dental light transmits illumination to maximize the clinician's view of the patient's oral cavity. The dental unit contains essential treatment equipment such as the handpiece lines, water lines, a self-contained water source, an air and water syringe, evacuation lines, and instrument tray(s). Correct positioning of the clinician and patient in a particular place or way and the arrangement of controls, light, and equipment are prerequisites to the prevention of RSIs and MSDs.

Clinician's Chair

The clinician's chair is one of the most important pieces of equipment for the delivery of care. It should have a broad, heavy base and be readily mobile to maneuver around the patient's head during delivery of care. The chair seat should allow for adequate body support and be easily adjusted for the proper height to ensure that the clinician's feet are flat on the floor with the knees positioned slightly below the hips (105° to 125° hip angle). New, ergonomically designed chairs put the clinician in the proper position and lend total body support to reduce the strain on the spine, lower back, shoulders, and arms (Fig. 12.2). In addition to a traditional clinician chair, other available designs include the saddle stool and Ghopec chair. Too high of a chair position causes the spine, back, and shoulders to support the body weight. Too low of a position causes the clinician to slump and sit with a curved spine.

Gloves

Wearing properly fitting gloves during the delivery of dental care reduces RSIs. Each glove should fit the hand and fingers snugly but be neither too tight nor too loose from the fingers to the forearm. Tight gloves compromise proper circulation to the clinician's hands and fingers and place pressure on the carpal tunnel across the wrist. Loose gloves cause the clinician to grasp the instrument handle more tightly to compensate for the feeling of a lack of control. Excess glove material at the fingertips hinders the clinician's ability to roll the instrument adequately in the fingers to adapt around line angles. The clinician compensates by twisting the wrist or by flexing and hyperextending the wrist.

1. Environmental Factors
- ✔ Comfortable temperature
- ✔ Comfortable noise level

2. Equipment Factors
- ✔ Properly designed clinician chair with freedom of movement
- ✔ Properly designed dental chair
- ✔ Bracket tray and dental light within reach
- ✔ Properly maintain cutting edge
- ✔ Use ergonomic handles
- ✔ Variations in handle diameter and shape
- ✔ Use balanced instruments
- ✔ Use ultrasonic and sonic instruments
- ✔ Avoid curly or retracting cords on motor-driven instruments and air/water syringes
- ✔ Limit the use of instruments that cause vibrations

3. Positioning Factors
- ✔ Proper clinician positioning
- ✔ Proper client positioning

4. Performance Factors
- ✔ Proper grasp and fulcrum
- ✔ Maintained neutral wrist, elbow, and shoulder position
- ✔ Maintained neck and back support
- ✔ Proper wrist motion; limited digital motion and wrist extension and flexion
- ✔ Appointment management

5. Person-Level Factors
- ✔ Limit psychosocial stressors in the workplace
- ✔ Be aware of any nonoccupational risk factors such as age and gender

6. Exercises
- ✔ Strengthening exercises
- ✔ Chairside stretching exercises

Fig. 12.1 Ergonomic checklist for dental hygienists.

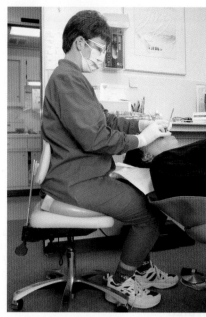

Fig. 12.2 Neutral position of clinician. Note shoulders are level and held in a relaxed position, with the elbows close to body and forearms in same plane as wrists, hands, and patient's mouth. (Valachi B. Evidence-based strategies for dental hygienists—and those who travel. *ADHA Access.* July 2012:14–18.)

Instruments

Hand instrument cutting-edge sharpness. Sharp instruments are essential to the elimination of fatigue and stress on the clinician's hand, wrist, arm, and shoulders that cause RSIs. Therefore any instrument with a cutting edge should be kept sharp during the entire procedure. Dull instruments that deviate from their original design cause the clinician to apply additional force, resulting in increased lateral pressure applied, excess stroke repetitions, and a tightened grasp. Fatigue and RSIs can ensue.

Ergonomic instrument handles. Ergonomic instrument handles are large in diameter and light in weight.[1] Using instrument handles with a variety of ergonomic adaptations (e.g., weight, diameter, padding) can modify muscle activity throughout the day to reduce RSIs for dental hygienists.[1] Large-diameter handles open the grasp just enough to dissipate the mechanical forces over a large area of muscles. Instrument setups that contain several styles of handle give the clinician the opportunity to rest different muscle groups while completing care, thereby decreasing the occurrence of RSIs. Another ergonomic design feature to consider is the use of instruments with padded, gripped, or silicone handles (Fig. 12.3). Padded instrument handles cushion the fingertips while grasping the handle. (See the section on parts and characteristics of dental instruments in Chapter 28, including Fig. 28.2.)

Mechanized and vibrating instruments. The use of ultrasonic and sonic instruments significantly reduces repetitive hand-wrist-forearm motions (see Chapter 29). Supragingival and subgingival debridement requires numerous repetitive strokes and significant lateral pressure when using hand-activated instrumentation techniques.

Instruments causing vibrations, such as the ultrasonic scaler and motor-driven handpieces, may cause fatigue and hand, arm, and shoulder muscle strain. Applying the principles of selective scaling and polishing limits the time during which the clinician uses a hand or vibrating instrument. There appears to be an association between greater use of ultrasonic handpieces and a diagnosis of sensorineural dysfunction.[2] A common RSI caused by vibratory instruments is Raynaud syndrome, which results in blanching and often painful fingers. Mechanized instruments also expose dental hygienists to the risk of noise-induced hearing loss. Prolonged exposure to high-frequency noise–emitting devices such as ultrasonic scalers may result in symptoms such as muffled hearing and tinnitus. Dental hygienists may consider wearing hearing protection such as earmuffs, foam earplugs, ear canal plugs, or active sound control devices.[3]

Dental mirrors. The mouth mirror is held in the nondominant hand. Practitioners focus on the hand, wrist, and arm position of the dominant hand during instrumentation with limited regard for the nondominant hand. Ergonomic adaptations in mouth mirror handles have been associated with increases and decreases in muscle activity. The clinical impact of this increase or decrease in muscle activity amplifies as force is exerted. When comparing the function of the dominant and nondominant hands during dental hygiene procedures, the difference between the techniques of the scaling hand and the hand holding the mirror is significant. The nondominant hand holding the mirror functions to increase access and visualization by retracting the tongue and cheeks. Unlike the multitasking dominant hand, the static nondominant hand often requires a forceful grip, retracting the tongue and cheek throughout delivery of care. This continuous static position of the nondominant hand decreases blood flow to the hand and fingers, increasing the risk of RSIs. Similar to other hand instruments, mirror handles have ergonomic adaptations in weight, diameter, and padding to vary muscle activity throughout the day to reduce the risk of RSIs for dental hygienists.

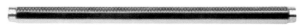

 # 2 HANDLE
The #2 handle features a .25-inch diameter, octagonal handle shape
for stability, with a patented diamond knurl design that provides
enhanced grip.

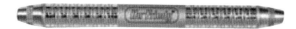

 # 6 HANDLE SATIN STEEL®
Satin Steel instruments are all about comfort, control, and efficiency.
The exclusive comfort zone is an extra-wide, gradual taper that reduces
pressure points for increased comfort all day long.

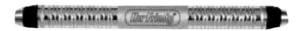

 # 7 HANDLE SATIN STEEL COLORS®
A large diameter handle, balanced weight, sharp blades, and soft
silicone grips provide great tactile sensitivity and rotational control.
Black grips are standard.

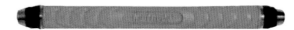

 # 8 RESIN EIGHT™ HANDLE
Large, lightweight handle for comfortable grasp. Textured-wave knurl
design increases rotational control. Comfort cone zone allows handle
transition, which reduces pressure points. Black signature series grips
with built-in color-coding capabilities.

 # 8 RESIN EIGHT™ COLORS HANDLE
Lightweight resin handle with large diameter and textured design for a
comfortable and secure grip. Color options assist clinicians in quick
and easy instrument selection.

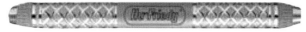

 # 9 EVEREDGE™ HANDLE
The EverEdge handle employs state-of-the-art technology for less hand
fatigue and greater comfort throughout the day.

Fig. 12.3 Variety of instrument handles. (Image courtesy of Hu-Friedy Mfg Co., LLC, Chicago.)

POSITIONING FACTORS

The concept of neutral positioning is important in the prevention of musculoskeletal injuries in dental hygiene practice. A neutral position is achieved through proper joint alignment and muscle balance and should be complemented by ergonomically designed equipment as described in the previous sections under Equipment Factors.

Patient-Clinician Positioning

The following are commonly used patient positions:
- **Upright.** For interviewing and educating patients
- **Semiupright.** For treating patients with cardiovascular and respiratory diseases
- **Supine.** For treating most patients
- **Trendelenburg.** For treating patients who experience syncope

In the supine position, the patient's mouth should be approximately at the height of the seated clinician's elbow. The headrest is adjustable for maxillary or mandibular arch visibility. During treatment of the maxillary teeth, the maxilla should be perpendicular to the floor; during treatment of the mandibular teeth, the mandible should be parallel to the floor.

The face of a clock best represents clinician-patient positioning (Fig. 12.4):
- Patient's head is the center of the clock.
- Clinician moves around the face of clock and is between the 9 o'clock and the 3 o'clock positions.
- Right-handed clinicians use the 9 o'clock to 2 o'clock range.
- Left-handed clinicians predominantly work in the 10 o'clock to 3 o'clock range.
- Working from the 8 o'clock position (4 o'clock for left-handed clinicians) is not recommended; this position requires challenging physical demands of the lower back.[4]

A variety of patient positions can be used during delivery of dental hygiene care (Fig. 12.5).

Box 12.1 provides tips for educating patients on patient-clinician positioning.

Position of the Clinician

Clinician comfort and safety cannot be sacrificed for the patient. Repetitive use of incorrect clinician positioning causes stress and fatigue. Therefore patient positioning should allow the hygienist to perform

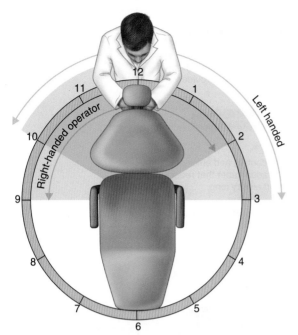

Fig. 12.4 Possible clinician positions around the patient. Right-handed clinician: 9 to 2 o'clock. Left-handed clinician: 3 to 10 o'clock. (From Levi PA, Jeong YN, Rudy RJ, Coleman DK. Patient examination and assessment. In: *Non-Surgical Control of Periodontal Diseases*. Springer; 2016.)

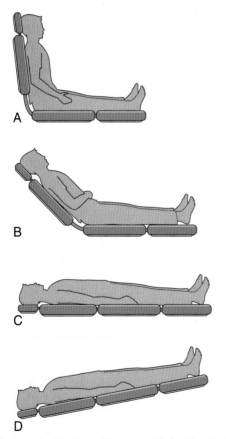

Fig. 12.5 Basic patient body positions used during the dental hygiene process of care. (A) Basic upright position; patient is seated at an 80° to 90° angle. (B) Semiupright position; patient is seated at a 45° angle. (C) Supine position has been modified for mandibular instrumentation. (D) Supine position has been modified for maxillary insertion.

TABLE 12.1   Correct Clinician Positioning

Body Region	Correct Positioning
Neck	Centered with minimal bending of the neck (front to back, side to side), and minimal rotation of neck (<20°)
Shoulders	Relaxed and in a neutral position, parallel to the floor
Elbows	Relaxed, close to body (elevated <20°)
Wrists	Aligned with hand and forearm, and minimal flexion or extension (<15°)
Back	Natural curvature of spine, minimal bending (front to back, side to side), and minimal rotation of torso (<20°)
Hips	Level on clinician's chair
Knees	105° to 125° angle from hips and shoulder-width apart
Feet	Flat on the floor and shoulder-width apart

intraoral procedures without increasing the risk of RSIs.[5] Table 12.1 lists the correct positioning of the clinician's arms, shoulders, legs, feet, back, head, and eyes during delivery of care.

Wrist, Arm, Elbow, and Shoulder Positions

Maintaining a neutral position of the wrist, arm, elbow, and shoulder reduces clinician fatigue and injury during delivery of care. Neutral positions are basic to the prevention of occupational pain and risks related to RSIs and other MSDs.

Neutral positions include the following (see Fig. 12.2):

- **Shoulders.** Are level and held in their lowest, most relaxed position
- **Elbow.** Is held close to the clinician's body at a 90° angle
- **Forearm.** Is held in the same plane as the wrist and hand
- **Wrist.** Is never bent but is held straight

Back and Neck Support

Adequate back and neck support reduces the occurrence of MSDs to the spine. Intervertebral disks in the spine resemble a jelly donut. When uneven pressure is placed on an intervertebral disk, the effect is the same as if one side of a jelly donut is pushed down; the contents of the disk (jelly donut) are pushed out. Poor posture of the clinician results in uneven support of the spine and rupture of an intervertebral disk. Maintaining a straight back, straight neck, and erect head, with the feet flat on the floor and knees positioned slightly below the hips at a 105° to 125° hip angle, properly supports the spine.

Eye loupes (telescopes) are magnification devices that are worn instead of traditional eyeglasses to improve the clinician's operative field of vision, visual accuracy, and posture during delivery of patient care (Fig. 12.6). The use of multilens telescopic loupes in the 2× to 2.5× magnification range offers the necessary depth of field and ensures a specific physical distance between the dental hygienist and patient. These loupes keep the dental hygienist's back and spine straight, preventing occupational pain caused by cumulative trauma.[6] If the clinician is too close to or too far away from the patient, the visual field seen

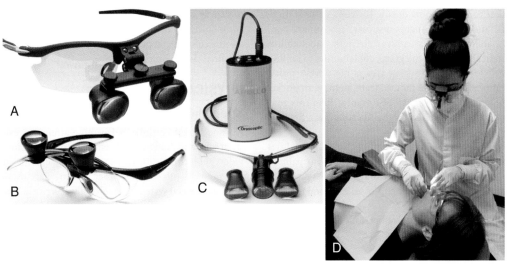

Fig. 12.6 (A) Flip-up loupe on a black Rudy sport frame. (B) Revolution through-the-flip loupe with insert; is available with prescription. (C) Rudy loupe with Apollo light-emitting diode (LED) bulb. (D) Correct clinician position when using loupes. (A to C, Courtesy Orascoptic, Middleton, Wisconsin.)

through the magnification device is blurred. Once back into the proper position, the clinician's field of vision is clear. Ensuring correct fitting of loupes by a trained manufacturer's representative is essential to avoid eyestrain and headaches. Clinicians may also consider the addition of a headlight attachment to their loupes, which provides optimal illumination of the oral cavity and prevents the continual need to adjust the overhead light during treatments. The following Critical Thinking Exercise box focuses on patient or client positioning.

CRITICAL THINKING EXERCISE

Practice positioning a patient or classmate in the dental chair. The clinician must be positioned for access to and visibility of the patient's mouth without compromising personal health and comfort.
1. Position yourself in the clinician's chair according to ergonomic principles. Position the patient in a semisupine position in preparation for debridement of quadrant 4. Prepare to begin treatment sitting at the 10 o'clock position. If no adjustments are made to the clinician's position, what aspects of body dynamics are compromised? How can the clinician reposition and still follow the ergonomic principles? How might you reposition the patient?
2. Position yourself in the clinician's chair according to ergonomic principles. Position a small child patient in the dental chair in a supine position in preparation for placing a fissure sealant on the upper first molars. Prepare to begin treatment sitting at the 10 o'clock position. If no adjustments are made to the position of the clinician, what aspects of body health are compromised? How can the clinician reposition self, patient, and chair to follow ergonomic principles? How might you reposition the patient?

PERFORMANCE FACTORS

Five Categories of Motion

Motions and movements can be stressful to the physical well-being of dental clinicians. Stresses caused by movement can harm the back, neck, arms, and wrists. There are five categories of motion, based on the amount of movement and the bone and muscle support needed to carry out the movement (Table 12.2). Dental clinicians should limit their movements to Classes I, II, and III.

Grasp and Fulcrum

The fundamentals of grasp include firmly holding the instrument, maintaining a secure grip, and maintaining control of the instrument

TABLE 12.2	**Five Categories of Motion**
Classification	**Motion**
Class I	Using fingers only
Class II	Using fingers and wrist
Class III	Moving fingers, wrist, and arm
Class IV	Moving entire arm and shoulder
Class V	Moving arm and twisting body

without causing undue strain or fatigue to the clinician's hand, arms, and shoulders. The modified pen grasp is a three-finger grasp using the thumb, index finger, and middle finger. A space must be maintained between the index finger and thumb to facilitate freedom of movement when rolling the instrument into interproximal spaces and around line angles of the teeth during instrumentation. Rolling the instrument between the index finger, middle finger, and thumb eliminates turning and twisting of the wrist, which can lead to an RSI such as **carpal tunnel syndrome** (CTS). CTS is a painful condition of the hands and fingers caused by nerve compression where the nerve passes over the carpal bones through a channel at the front of the wrist, adjacent to the flexor tendons of the hand.

Holding the instrument with all four fingers securely wrapped around the handle is the palm grasp. The modified pen grasp and palm grasp may be firm or light, depending on the procedure performed. (See Chapters 28 and 29 for a thorough discussion of instrumentation principles.)

Fulcrum and Hand Stabilization

The fulcrum is the area on which the finger rests and against which it pushes while instrumentation is performed. The fulcrum provides a basis for steadiness and control during stroke activation. Proper fulcrum and hand stabilization reduces RSIs.

The intraoral fulcrum is established by resting the pad of the fulcrum (ring) finger inside the mouth against a tooth surface. The fulcrum finger must remain locked during instrument activation. A locked fulcrum allows the clinician to pivot on and gain strength from the fulcrum finger. Pivoting on the fulcrum finger helps maintain a firm grasp, stability, and proper wrist motion. Middle and fulcrum fingers work together to add support during instrument activation. Splitting the middle and fulcrum fingers decreases instrument control, strength, and stability. With less control, strength, and stability, the clinician automatically tightens the grasp, contributing to an RSI. Placing the fulcrum close to the working area is not always possible owing to space limitations in the mouth, teeth alignment, pocket depth, or the angle of access. A variety of intraoral fulcrums may be necessary. (See Chapter 28, section on the fulcrum, for a detailed explanation.)

The extraoral fulcrum can also be used during clinical procedures and is accomplished by placing the broad side of the clinician's palm or back of the hand against an outside structure of the patient's face such as the chin or cheek (see Chapter 28). Benefits of an extraoral fulcrum are as follows:

- Easier, less strenuous accessibility to deep periodontal pockets and difficult access areas
- Stability and control
- Less twisting of the wrist during activation of maxillary posterior areas
- Decreased chance of RSIs to the nerves, tendons, and ligaments in the clinician's wrist and elbow (e.g., action of the activation or pulling stroke is transmitted to the arm and shoulder and away from the wrist)

When no fulcrum is used, lateral pressure on the instrument during activation causes the instrument to slip in the hand. To stabilize and control the instrument, the clinician automatically tightens the grasp. Tightening the grasp places stress on hand and arm muscles, tendons, and ligaments, leading to an increased occurrence of RSIs.

Wrist Motion During Instrument Activation

Wrist motion and the fulcrum are interdependent. Safe wrist motion is vital to the health of the clinician's hand, wrist, and forearm muscles, tendons, and ligaments. Pivoting on the fulcrum causes the hand, wrist, and forearm to move in one unified motion. Failing to handle instruments using the unified motion causes the clinician to extend or flex the wrist. Continued flexion or extension of the wrist contributes to a variety of RSIs.

Digital motion during instrument activation is also a factor that contributes to RSIs. Digital motion is the push-and-pull motion of the instrument using only fingers. Muscle fatigue quickly results from digital motion, and a decrease in instrument power and stability occurs.

Appointment Management

Control of appointment procedures and time may reduce the possibility of RSIs. The dental hygienist should achieve the following:

- Alternate new patients with continued-care patients.
- Alternate root debridement and therapeutic scaling with maintenance appointments.
- Alternate difficult appointments with less taxing ones.
- Shorten continued-care intervals.
- Ensure planning of adequate breaks in the daily schedule.

PERSON-LEVEL FACTORS

Psychosocial stress appears to be a risk factor for work-related MSDs. Research indicates that satisfaction with wage, work-life balance, and involvement in practice decisions can impact the prevalence of MSDs.[7] Eliminating or limiting workplace stress is important for maintaining health and well-being.

A number of nonoccupational factors are risk factors for MSDs. It is widely acknowledged that increasing age and female gender correlate

positively with MSDs, as well as hereditary traits and systemic illness.[8] Although such risks cannot be eliminated, knowledge of their effects on musculoskeletal health can ensure that clinicians are aware of their personal risks of injury.

PHYSICAL EXERCISE

Strengthening Exercises

No one would consider performing strenuous exercise without first stretching and doing strengthening maneuvers. However, oral care providers subject their muscles to strenuous activities daily without properly preparing their bodies for the workplace. Maintaining a healthy musculoskeletal system through daily exercise has the following results:

- Improves strength and flexibility
- Improves lumbar spine, neck muscle, and lower back health
- Stretches and extends back muscles
- Strengthens abdominal muscles
- Strengthens finger, hand, and arm muscles

Regular performance of strengthening exercises repairs and maintains a healthy musculoskeletal system (Box 12.2).

Chairside Stretching Exercises

Stretching and warm-up **exercises**[9] reduce muscle and joint soreness and injury and psychologically prepare the individual for activities requiring skill and dexterity. Before work and throughout the day, dental hygienists should perform the following **tendon-gliding exercise** (TGE) (Fig. 12.7), which diffuses synovial fluid, the lubricant around the hand and finger tendons:

1. Hold hand and fingers straight, pointing upward.
2. Bend fingers into a 90° angle from the hand.
3. Close fingers into the hand.
4. Arch hand back toward the top of the wrist.
5. Further arch fingers in the same direction.
6. Briefly hold position, and then release.
7. Repeat this exercise four times.

Regular Exercise Regimen

Regular aerobic exercise improves blood flow to tissues, reduces blood pressure and body fat, and has recognized psychologic benefits. Yoga and physical activity appear to reduce the incidence of MSDs among dental professionals.[10] Core strength will help the body support a neutral position and stabilize the spine and pelvis. A systematic review of yoga interventions for health professionals and health profession students reported that the physical benefits of yoga included reduced MSD, specifically pain in the lower back, neck, and wrist.[11]

REPETITIVE STRAIN INJURIES

RSIs are common MSDs in dentistry. The most frequently reported RSIs, their signs and symptoms, risk factors, and chairside preventive measures are outlined in this section.[12]

Hand, Wrist, and Finger Injuries
Carpal Tunnel Syndrome

Carpal tunnel syndrome (CTS) is defined earlier in this chapter and has the following causes:

- Congenital: anatomic structure and development
- Self-limiting conditions: pregnancy
- Systemic conditions: edema or arthritis
- Nonmedical: occupational or work-related reasons

Up to one-quarter of dental hygienists report symptoms of CTS,[7] which occurs when the median nerve becomes compressed within

BOX 12.2 Strengthening Exercises

Pelvic Tilt: Strengthens the Lumbar Spine
1. Ideally, lie on your back or, if at work, stand flat against the wall.
2. Keep knees slightly bent.
3. Flatten and press back into floor (or wall).
4. Briefly hold this position.
5. Repeat this exercise.

Hyperextension: Safeguards the Lumbar Curve
1. Lie on your stomach.
2. Arch your body backward in an upward direction.
3. Briefly hold this position.
4. Repeat this exercise.

Knee-to-Chest: Stretches the Lumbar Spine
1. Lie on your back.
2. Bring both knees to your chest.
3. Briefly hold this position.
4. Return to original position; avoid straightening legs.
5. Repeat this exercise.

Sit-Ups: Strengthen the Abdominal Muscles
1. Lie on your back.
2. Bend both knees.
3. Support neck.
4. Gently raise shoulders toward knees.
5. Briefly hold this position, and then return to original position.
6. Repeat this exercise.

Suspend From a Bar: Relieves Lower Back Pain
1. Firmly grasp bar.
2. Suspend your body from bar; slowly lift feet.
3. Hold this position for a short time.
4. Repeat this exercise.

Doorway Stretch: Reverses Poor Posture
1. Stand in front of an open doorway.
2. Place your hands on either side of doorframe.
3. Gently allow your body to lean forward through doorway.
4. Hold this position and return to original position.
5. Repeat this exercise.

Neck Isometric: Stretches the Cervical Spine and Relieves Neck Muscle Strain
1. Grasp your hands behind head.
2. Gently press your head back.
3. Do not allow any backward movement.
4. Briefly hold this position.
5. Repeat this exercise.

Rubber Ball Squeeze: Strengthens the Hand and Finger Muscles
1. Firmly grasp a rubber ball in your hand.
2. Gently squeeze.
3. Briefly hold this position.
4. Repeat this exercise.

Rubber Band Stretch: Strengthens the Hand and Finger Muscles
1. Extend a rubber band between fingers of your hand.
2. Gently stretch the rubber band until you feel resistance.
3. Briefly hold this position.
4. Release the rubber band.
5. Repeat this exercise.

the carpal tunnel (Fig. 12.8). The median nerve has both sensory and motor functions and supplies:

- Sensation to the thumb, index finger, middle finger, and one-half of the ring finger; and
- A branch to the thumb (thenar) muscles.

Repetitive force and motion to the wrist result in tendon inflammation and swelling within the carpal tunnel. The enlarged tendons and lack of space in the carpal tunnel place undue pressure on the median nerve, causing pain. Once the nerve is compressed, CTS begins. Repeated wrist flexion and hyperextension during instrumentation aggravate the tendons and cause further swelling.

Signs and symptoms. Signs and symptoms of CTS are the following:
- Numbness in the areas supplied by the median nerve (earliest sign)
- Pain in the hand, wrist, shoulder, neck, and lower back
- Nocturnal pain in hand(s) and forearm(s)
- Pain in hand(s) while working
- Morning and/or daytime stiffness and numbness
- Loss of strength in hand(s) and a weakened grasp
- Cold fingers
- Increased fatigue in fingers, hand, wrist, forearm, and shoulders
- Nerve dysfunction

Risk factors. Repetition is the foremost risk factor causing CTS. Tightly holding the instruments places excessive force on the wrist and hand. Vibrating instruments, including low-speed handpieces and ultrasonic scalers, have been identified as risk factors for CTS.[2] Cold temperatures in the dental treatment area decrease flexibility of the clinician's fingers, hand, arm, shoulder, neck, and back muscles. This inflexibility causes

stiffness, making workplace performance stressful. In addition, wearing gloves that are too tight can pinch the median nerve at the wrist.

Chairside preventive measures. The following measures can prevent CTS:

- Maintain good operator posture. The patient's mouth should be even with the clinician's elbow, and the elbow should be in the neutral position (90° angle created by the upper arm and forearm).
- Maintain proper position to support the clinician's body. The knees should be positioned slightly below the hips at a 105° to 125° hip angle, with feet flat on floor.
- Maintain a neutral forearm and wrist position. Avoid pinching the median nerve in the carpal tunnel.
- Keep shoulders relaxed.
- Use a unified motion. A unified motion of wrist, hand, and forearm should be used during scaling and polishing. Avoid flexing and extending the wrist.
- Avoid extremes in temperatures.
- Avoid or limit exposure to vibrating instruments.
- Avoid forceful pinching and gripping of instrument handles.
- Wear properly fitting gloves.
- Alternate clinician positions.
- Perform TGEs.

Thoracic Outlet Compression

Thoracic outlet compression (TOC) is an RSI resulting in compression of the brachial artery and plexus nerve trunk at the thoracic outlet (Fig 12.9). TOC affects the hand, wrist, arm, and shoulder. Compression of

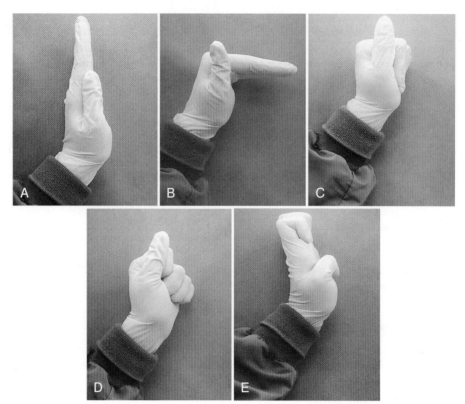

Fig. 12.7 Tendon-gliding exercises. (A) Hand and fingers are straight, pointing upward. (B) Fingers are bent to an L position at a 90° angle from hand. (C) Fingers are closed into palm. (D) Hand in a fist is arched back toward the top of wrist. (E) Knuckles are bent so that tips of fingers touch palm and hand is arched back.

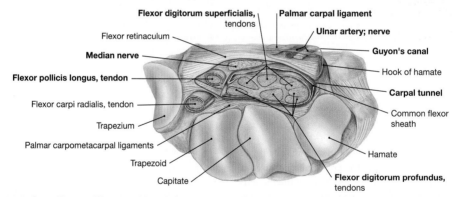

Fig. 12.8 Carpal bones. The carpal bones form a trough through which the flexor tendons and median nerve traverse into the hand. (From Hombach-Klonisch S, Klonisch T, Peeler J. *Clinical Atlas of Human Anatomy.* Elsevier; 2019.)

the neurovascular bundle (i.e., brachial plexus, subclavian artery, subclavian vein) results in decreased blood flow to the nerve functions of the arm. The compression occurs at the neck, where the scalene muscles create an outlet or tunnel. The nerves and blood vessels run from the neck into the arm and hand.

Symptoms. Symptoms of TOC are the following:
- Numbness and tingling along the sides of arms and hands
- Neck and shoulder muscle spasms
- Weakness and clumsiness in hand and fingers
- Cold extremities
- Absence of a radial pulse

Risk factors. Poor posture is the primary cause. Tilting the head too much, hunching the shoulders, and positioning the dental chair too high are risk factors for TOC.

Chairside preventive measures. The following measures can prevent TOC:
- Maintain proper clinician position with head erect, back straight, and shoulders in a neutral position.
- Maintain proper height of the dental chair and proper patient positioning.

Guyon Canal Syndrome

Guyon canal syndrome (GCS), caused by ulnar nerve entrapment at the wrist, differs from CTS in that the ulnar nerve does not pass through the carpal tunnel. Rather, the ulnar nerve passes through a tunnel formed by the pisiform and hamate bones and the ligaments that connect them (Fig. 12.8).

Symptoms. Symptoms of GCS are the following:

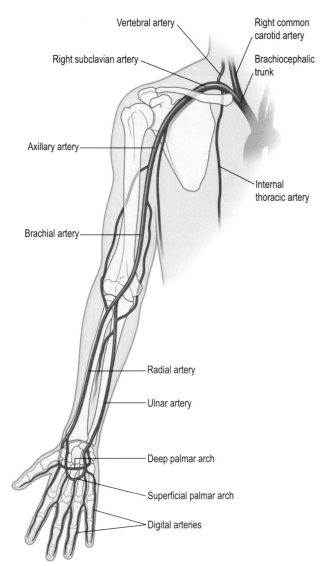

Fig. 12.9 The main arteries of the right arm. (Copyright © 2023 by Elsevier Ltd, All rights reserved.)

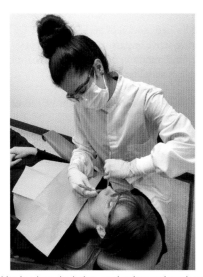

Fig. 12.10 Wrist in ulnar deviation, and spine and neck are out of alignment.

- Numbness and tingling in the little finger and right side of fulcrum (ring) finger
- Loss of strength in lower forearm
- Loss of movement of small muscles in hand
- Clumsiness of hand

Risk factors. During instrumentation, holding the little finger close to the fulcrum finger for stability and control is important. Maintaining this position of the two fingers avoids an RSI. Holding the little finger a full span away from the hand and fulcrum finger causes nerve entrapment and symptoms of GCS.

Chairside preventive measures. Attention placed on hand and finger position during instrumentation reduces the risk of GCS and includes the following:

- Repositioning the little finger during scaling and extrinsic stain removal
- Performing periodic hand stretches

De Quervain Syndrome

De Quervain syndrome is an inflammation of the tendons and tendon sheaths at the base of the thumb (the *anatomic snuffbox*). This condition occurs from repetitive motion combining hand twisting and forceful gripping, along with prolonged work with the wrist held in ulnar deviation (Fig. 12.10). Symptoms occur when the pollicis longus and extensor pollicis longus tendons are unable to glide through the tunnel on the side of the wrist.

Symptoms. Symptoms of De Quervain syndrome are the following:
- Aching and weakness of thumb (along the base)
- Pain migrating into forearm

Risk factors. Repetitive ulnar deviation of the wrist while reaching for instruments or during instrumentation is the biggest risk factor causing De Quervain syndrome. Twisting and bending the wrist in an ulnar direction (toward the little finger) and using a forceful grip on instrument handles are also risk factors.

Chairside preventive measures. The following measures can prevent De Quervain syndrome:
- Avoid ulnar wrist deviation during instrumentation.
- Avoid twisting wrist when reaching for dental instruments.
- Maintain a neutral wrist position and unified motion during dental care.

Elbow and Forearm Injuries
Lateral Epicondylitis

Lateral epicondylitis (LE) is a degenerative elbow disorder caused by inflammation of the wrist extensor tendons on the lateral epicondyle of the elbow.

Symptoms. Symptoms of LE are the following:
- Aching or pain in the elbow
- Sharp, shooting pain during elbow extension

Risk factors. Repetitive and constant use of a forceful grip or grasp, forceful wrist and elbow movement, and extension of wrist during dental care all increase the risk of LE.

Chairside preventive measures. The following measures can prevent LE:
- Avoid wrist extension during dental care.
- Maintain proper neutral wrist position during instrumentation.
- Use proper clinician positions, allowing maintenance of neutral body positions.

Radial Tunnel Syndrome

Radial tunnel syndrome (RTS) is a condition affecting the radial nerve entrapped in the radial tunnel. The radial nerve starts at the side of the neck and travels through the armpit and down the arm to the hands and fingers; the nerve passes in front of the elbow through the radial tunnel and allows the hand to turn in a clockwise direction.

Symptoms. Increased tenderness and pain at the lateral side of the elbow when the arm and elbow are used may indicate RTS.

Chairside preventive measures. As with LE, maintaining proper wrist position and motion during care is important.

Cubital Tunnel Syndrome

Cubital tunnel syndrome is a condition affecting the ulnar nerve as it crosses behind the elbow through the cubital tunnel (Fig. 12.8). The ulnar nerve controls the muscles in the right half of the ring finger and little finger of the hand. When the elbow is bent, the nerve is raised between bones, causing compression and entrapment of the ulnar nerve. Nerve compression slows impulses.

Symptoms. Symptoms of cubital tunnel syndrome are the following:
- Pain and numbness on the outer side of ring and little fingers
- Pain that is sometimes relieved when straightening the elbow

Risk factors. The clinician should avoid all prolonged gripping or grasping of instruments in the palm of the hand and holding the elbow in a flexed position during procedures.

Chairside preventive measures. The following measures can prevent cubital tunnel syndrome:
- Maintain a neutral elbow position during procedures.
- Alter instrument grasps and avoid prolonged use of palm grasp.
- Avoid repetitive crossing of arms across the chest.
- Avoid leaning on the elbow when sitting at a table.

Shoulder Injuries
Rotator Cuff Injuries

Rotator cuff injuries (RCIs) include rotator cuff tendonitis and rotator cuff tears. Both injuries affect the connective tissue in the shoulder and cause common shoulder pain. The supraspinatus tendon is most often affected. RCIs are associated with repetitive motion and excessive and forceful exertion of shoulder and arm.

Symptoms. Symptoms of RCIs are the following:
- Pain when lifting the arm 60° to 90°
- Functional impairment

Risk factors. Static loading on the shoulder muscles and improper body support lead to RCIs.

Chairside preventive measures. The following measures prevent RCIs:
- Avoid repetitive twisting and reaching.
- Maintain neutral shoulder and arm positions.
- Use proper clinician positions during dental care.

Adhesive Capsulitis

Adhesive capsulitis (AC), also known as *frozen shoulder,* results from immobility of the shoulder because of severe shoulder injury or repeated occurrences of rotator cuff tendonitis.

Symptoms. Symptoms are similar to those of RCIs:
- Pain in shoulder
- Limited range of shoulder motion

Risk factors. Static loading and improper strain placed on shoulder joint owing to static loading increase the risk for AC.

Chairside preventive measures. The following measures can prevent AC:
- Avoid repetitive twisting and reaching.
- Maintain proper shoulder and arm positions; that is, maintain neutral positions.

- Use proper clinician positions and movement during instrumentation. The following Critical Thinking Exercise focuses on shoulder pain.

Neck and Back Injuries
Tension Neck Syndrome

Tension neck syndrome (TNS), also called *tension myalgia,* involves the cervical muscles of the trapezius muscle.

Signs and symptoms. Signs and symptoms of TNS are the following:
- Pain or stiffness around cervical spine (neck)
- Pain between the shoulder blades that may radiate down the arms
- Muscle tightness and tenderness in neck
- Palpable hardness in neck
- Limited neck movement

Risk factors. Risks include improper positioning of the clinician's head and neck during delivery of dental care. The head must be held erect; bending the neck places tremendous pressure and stress on the cervical spine.

Chairside preventive measures. The following measures prevent TNS:
- Maintain proper clinician head and neck position to support the neck and spine.
- Maintain proper height of the dental chair and patient position.
- Support the weight of the head over the entire spine, not only over the cervical portion of the spine.
- Keep the back straight during dental care.
- Take periodic breaks and perform stretching exercises.

Cervical Spondylolysis and Cervical Disk Disease

Cervical spondylolysis (CS) and cervical disk disease (CDD) lead to degeneration of the cervical spine. These RSIs affect the neck, scapula, shoulders, and arms, causing osteoarthritis of the cervical spine, disk degeneration, and herniation.

Signs and symptoms. Signs and symptoms of CS and CDD are the following:
- Stiffness and limited motion of neck
- Crepitus during active or passive neck movements
- Pain in upper and middle cervical regions of the spine
- Pain in scapula of shoulder regions
- Muscle spasms

Risk factors. Repeated stress and strain placed on the neck and cervical spine are risk factors.

Chairside preventive measures. The following measures can prevent CS and CDD:
- Maintain proper position of the clinician's head and neck to support the neck and spine.
- Position patients for easy access to the mouth.

Assessing symptoms. Signs and symptoms of CS and CDD include but are not limited to pain, tingling sensations, coldness, loss of strength, reduced range of motion, and numbness. A medical practitioner should assess all such symptoms.

Treatment. Clinicians should seek expert medical advice for any symptoms they are experiencing to ensure an accurate diagnosis and treatment plan. Treatment may include but is not limited to rest, antiinflammatory medications, corticosteroidal agents, physical therapy, compression, wearing an immobilization splint, or, in severe cases, surgery.

To Change or Not to Change

Recognition of RSIs in dentistry was reported as early as 1946 and yet, as recently as 2010, between 60% and 93% of dental hygienists were still reporting MSDs.[7] In addition, dental hygiene students report MSDs beginning during their education and training. The combination of learning new clinical skills with increased use of the computer and desk-based study appears to place students at an increased risk for developing MSDs.

Recognition of unsound ergonomic practices helps stop the cycle of occupational pain for dental workers. Research has demonstrated that education on clinician and patient positioning and the use of loupes has a protective effect against injury.[6] Compliance with ergonomic principles is the foundation for a long, successful career in practice. Clinicians should consider the legal, ethical, and safety issues that occupational injuries have on their own health and on patient care (Box 12.3).

BOX 12.3 Legal, Ethical, and Safety Issues

- Dental hygienists have an ethical obligation to prevent disability and disease in themselves.
- Working while experiencing an untreated physical disability and pain may have ethical and legal implications if a poor level of quality care is the outcome.
- To improve their own safety, dental hygienists should use proper ergonomics, take chairside preventive measures, and regularly perform strengthening exercises to prevent RSIs and MSDs.

KEY CONCEPTS

- Applying ergonomic principles in the workplace reduces the risk of developing RSIs and MSDs.
- Regular strengthening and stretching exercises increase the flexibility and strength of muscles and tendons, reducing the risk of RSIs in the clinician.
- If signs and symptoms of an RSI occur, assessment of the environment and workplace practices should be conducted, and prompt medical attention should be sought.

ACKNOWLEDGMENT

The author acknowledges Lori Drummer for her past contributions to this chapter.

REFERENCES

1. Simmer-Beck M, Branson BG. An evidence-based review of ergonomic features of dental hygiene instruments. *Work*. 2010;35(4):477–485.
2. Cherniack M, Brammer AJ, Nilsson T, et al. Nerve conduction and sensorineural function in dental hygienists using high frequency ultrasound handpieces. *Am J Ind Med*. 2006;49(5):313–326.
3. Henneberry K, Hilland S, Haslam SK. Are dental hygienists at risk for noise-induced hearing loss? A literature review. *Canadian J Den Hyg*. 2021;55(2):110.
4. Howarth SJ, Grondin DE, La Delfa NJ, et al. Working position influences the biomechanical demands on the lower back during dental hygiene. *Ergonomics*. 2016;59(4):545–555.
5. Pîrvu C, Pătraşcu I, Pîrvu D, et al. The dentist's operating posture–ergonomic aspects. *J Med Life*. 2014;7(2):177.
6. Hayes MJ, Osmotherly PG, Taylor JA, et al. The effect of wearing loupes on upper extremity musculoskeletal disorders among dental hygienists. *Int J Dent Hyg*. 2014;12(3):174–179.
7. Hayes MJ, Taylor JA, Smith DR. Predictors of work-related musculoskeletal disorders among dental hygienists. *Int J Dent Hyg*. 2012;10(4):265–269.
8. Hayes MJ, Smith DR, Cockrell D. An international review of musculoskeletal disorders in the dental hygiene profession. *Int Dent J*. 2010;60(5):343–352.
9. Kumar DK, Rathan N, Mohan S, et al. Exercise prescriptions to prevent musculoskeletal disorders in dentists. *J Clin Diagn Res*. 2014;8(7):ZE13.
10. Koneru S, Tanikonda R. Role of yoga and physical activity in work-related musculoskeletal disorders among dentists. *J Int Soc Prev Community Dent*. 2015;5(3):199.
11. Ciezar-Andersen SD, Hayden KA, King-Shier KM. A systematic review of yoga interventions for helping health professionals and students. *Complementary Ther Med*. 2021;58:102704.
12. Chopra A. Musculoskeletal disorders in dentistry—a review. *JSM Dent*. 2014;2(3):1032.

13

Personal, Dental, and Health Histories

Dina M. Canasi

PROFESSIONAL OPPORTUNITIES

Personal, dental, and health histories can influence decision making, guide the selection of appropriate dental care, and affect patient outcomes. The collection of accurate health history data is therefore vital for proper patient assessment and treatment planning.

COMPETENCIES

1. Explain the purpose of recording personal, dental, and health histories.
2. Discuss a health history assessment, the data collection process, and documentation by utilizing patient-centered interviewing techniques.
3. Describe the legal and ethical issues related to collecting and documenting health history information.
4. Discuss the process of decision-making after obtaining the health history to include the interpretation of patient data, understanding the indications and rationale for prophylactic antibiotic premedication, and identifying the need for collaboration with other healthcare professionals for medical risk assessment to establish an individual dental-hygiene care plan.

PURPOSE OF PERSONAL, DENTAL, AND HEALTH HISTORIES

Collecting and recording personal, dental, and health histories will provide information that the dental hygienist needs to assess risks and contraindications that may influence treatment planning and determine the need for supportive medical consultation. The collection of this data facilitates complete and accurate assessment to ensure a client is never treated as a stranger. The personal, dental, and health histories are legal documents that enable the dental hygienist to:

- Understand patient concerns, attitudes, and goals for the dental visit
- Establish patient rapport
- Document baseline information regarding a patient's complete health status
- Identify key risk factors that affect the provision of dental hygiene care
- Determine the need for consultation with other healthcare professionals
- Prepare preoperative and postoperative care plans for the prevention of medical emergencies

- Facilitate medical and dental diagnoses of various symptoms and conditions
- Recognize special physiologic states such as pregnancy or menopause
- Identify patient's social determinants of health
- Manage risks to minimize potential litigation.

Using a culturally sensitive, patient-centered approach is recommended as the dental hygienist creates a dialog to establish a therapeutic relationship with the patient that will promote quality care. The personal history can uncover patient perceptions, motivations, and value of dental care. The dental history provides information relating to past experiences, recognizes chief complaints, and guides treatment modalities. The health history identifies existing medical conditions that may influence clinical procedures and outcomes or identify the need for prophylactic antibiotic premedication. During the psychologic, systemic wellness, and oral evaluations, the foundation for clinical decision making develops. Fig. 13.1 identifies the dimensions of the health history assessment from the physical, personal, societal, cognitive, emotional, and spiritual perspectives.

HEALTH HISTORY ASSESSMENT

Health status is dynamic, and the health history requires constant monitoring for changes at each dental appointment. A complete health history includes documentation, building rapport through patient-centered interviewing, and verifying key elements to guide care planning. In most practice settings, the patient completes the health history questionnaire at annual visits before initiating professional services.

Numerous formats for the written or electronic health history questionnaires are available. A preferable design includes a clearly demarcated area, usually at the top of the form, to identify critical medical information. This section is reserved for preevaluation of high-risk medical alerts and conditions, such as antibiotic allergies, cardiovascular diseases, and prophylactic antibiotic premedication before initiating dental care. Fig. 13.2 provides examples of the various sections of the health history.

Patient-Centered Health History Interview

The patient-centered health history interview is the first step toward establishing rapport and trust with a patient (see Chapter 22—Human Needs Assessment Form and OHRQL Questionnaire). One of the primary objectives of the health history interview is to form a constructive **dental hygienist–patient partnership**. The dental hygienist–patient partnership maintains a mutual goal—the patient's overall well-being. Patients respond more completely to a friendly, caring, nonjudgmental

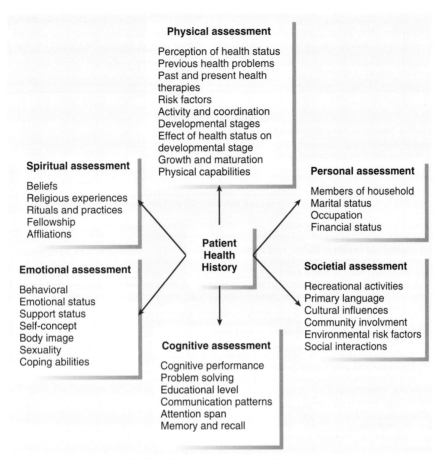

Physical assessment

Perception of health status
Previous health problems
Past and present health
therapies
Risk factors
Activity and coordination
Developmental stages
Effect of health status on
developmental stage
Growth and maturation
Physical capabilities

Spiritual assessment

Beliefs
Religious experiences
Rituals and practices
Fellowship
Affliations

Emotional assessment

Behavioral
Emotional status
Support status
Self-concept
Body image
Sexuality
Coping abilities

**Patient
Health
History**

Personal assessment

Members of household
Marital status
Occupation
Financial status

Societial assessment

Recreational activities
Primary language
Cultural influences
Community involvment
Environmental risk factors
Social interactions

Cognitive assessment

Cognitive performance
Problem solving
Educational level
Communication patterns
Attention span
Memory and recall

Fig. 13.1 Dimensions of the health history.

interviewer. Therefore, the practitioner must demonstrate verbal and nonverbal acceptance and respect for the patient's values. If a positive relationship has been established, the patient will feel more comfortable asking questions about treatments and will trust the practitioner's recommendations.[1] Evidence-based interventions can then follow as determined by the health assessment.

A patient-generated health information survey should be clarified and validated during the interview. The dental hygienist should identify potential barriers to effective communication. Such barriers may include language or cultural differences, the presence of a physical or mental challenge (e.g., hearing loss, dementia), or a low level of health literacy. Patients experiencing poor **health literacy**—basic reading and numerical skills that allow a person to function in the healthcare environment—or reading comprehension require verbal confirmation for information accuracy. Most healthcare materials are written at a 10th-grade level, but most adults read at an 8th-grade level.[2]

During the interview process, the practitioner may also identify risk factors such as smoking, work stress, or poor living conditions. These are considered **social determinants of health** and can affect a patient's willingness or ability to seek dental care. Early recognition of barriers and social determinants of health can influence treatment planning and approach to patient care.

Patient-Centered Interview Process

Patient-centered interviewing is a process that elicits the patient's emotions and personal health agenda to allow for a better understanding of the psychosocial context for disease. In contrast to solely gathering disease- and symptom-related data during the traditional clinician-centered interview, the patient-centered approach shifts the focus to patient concerns, anxieties, and perceptions of the individual's disease in

a humanistic and scientific manner.[3] The five steps in patient-centered interviewing are: (1) establishing a private setting; (2) eliciting the patient's chief concerns and setting the agenda for the appointment; (3) using open-ended questioning to help the patient express themselves; (4) using active listening and response techniques; and (5) briefly summarizing the interview for accuracy, clarification, and confirmation.[4]

Interview Setting

The dental professional should understand the importance of the physical environment when collecting health information for care planning. The health history interview should be conducted in a setting that ensures privacy and discretion. The interview should occur in private unless the patient is a minor, in which case the parent or legal guardian is present, or when an interpreter is needed. Allowing patients to identify their concerns during the office visit by asking, "What has brought you in today?" is the primary theme in patient-centered interviewing (see Chapter 5).

Patient-Centered Interview

Patient-centered interviewing enables the clinician to obtain a deeper understanding of the patient's concerns, improves the therapeutic relationship, and increases patient and provider satisfaction.[5] Using **motivational interviewing techniques** to modify patient behavior during the interview process promotes better communication and elicits **change-talk**, a technique that encourages patients to discuss their desires, abilities, reasons, and need for change in their dental care.[3] During the health history interview, the dental hygienist should observe the patient's use of eye contact, nonverbal communication, and body language as part of the patient assessment process. Highly anxious patients may not express fear, although their behavior may provide clues concerning their mental state. Patients experiencing stress, fear, and anxiety during the dental visit may be at risk for medical emergencies such as vasovagal syncope (a common cause of fainting), cardiac arrhythmia (irregular heartbeat), or hyperventilation (rapid breathing or overbreathing). Stress and fear reduction techniques and protocols should be part of the interview process and incorporated into the **dental hygiene care plan** as a strategy to avoid a medical emergency (see Chapter 11).

The patient-centered interview is an opportunity for the dental hygienist to apply effective verbal and nonverbal communication skills

---

MEDICAL HISTORY

*Please write **YES** or **NO** in answering the following questions:*

1. Are you in good health? _____
2. Has there been any change in your general health in the past year? _____If answer is yes, what was the change?_____
   _____
3. Are you having pain or discomfort at this time? _____If yes, where?_____
4. When was your last physical exam? _____
5. Are you now under the care of a physician? _____If answer is yes, what condition is being treated? _____
   _____
6. Have you had any serious illness or operation? _____ Have you ever been hospitalized? _____
   If answer is yes, for what problem? _____
7. Do you have or have you had any of the following diseases or problems?
   a. Rheumatic fever or rheumatic heart disease:_____
   b. Congenital heart lesions or scarlet fever:_____
   c. Cardiovascular disease (heart trouble, heart attack or heart attack within the last 6 months, coronary artery insufficiency, coronary occlusion, high blood pressure, arteriosclerosis, stroke, heart murmur, congestive heart failure, mitral valve prolapse, or angina pectoris) _____
      1. Do you have chest pains upon exertion? . _____
      2. Do you have shortness of breath after mild exercise? _____
      3. Do your ankles swell? _____
      4. Do you get short of breath when you lie down, or do you require extra pillows when you sleep? _____
      5. Do you have a cardiac pacemaker, implanted defibrillator? _____
      6. Do you have artificial joints/valves/implants/transplanted organ? _____
   d. Allergy (e.g., iodine, latex) _____
   e. Sinusitis/hayfever/seasonal allergy: _____
   f. Asthma:_____
   g. Hives or a skin rash: _____
   h. Fainting spells or seizures such as epilepsy
   i. Diabetes _____
      1. Do you have to urinate more than 6 times a day?. _____
      2. Are you thirsty much of the time? _____
      3. Does your mouth frequently become dry? _____
   j. Hepatitis, jaundice or liver disease: _____
   k. Arthritis: _____
   l. Inflammatory rheumatism (painful swollen joints) : _____
   m. Low blood pressure: _____
   n. High blood pressure: _____
   o. Herpes virus (cold sores) _____
   p. Stomach ulcers: _____
   q. Kidney trouble: _____
   r. Tuberculosis: _____
   s. Venereal Disease:_____
   t. Acquired Immune Deficiency Syndrome/HIV Infection: _____
   u. Hyperactive thyroid gland (unexplained weight loss):_____
   v. Underactive thyroid gland (unexplained weight gain): _____
   w. Cholinesterase deficiency:_____
   x. Pain in jaw joints:_____
   y. Psychiatric treatment:_____
8. Do you have a history of drug/alcohol dependency? _____
9. Have you had abnormal bleeding assoicated with previous extractions, surgery or trauma? _____
10. Do you have any blood disorder, such as anemia, hemophilia, or bruise easily? _____
11. Have you had surgery or x-ray treatment for a tumor, growth or other condition of your head or neck? _____
12. Have you ever had a blood transfusion? _____If so, explain:_____
    _____
13. Have you ever had or are you currently having kidney dialysis? _____ If so, explain:_____
    _____
14. Are you taking any of the following now or within the past two years?
    a. Antibiotics or sulfa drugs:_____
    b. Anticoagulants (blood thinners): _____
    c. High blood pressure medication: _____
    d. Cortisone (steroids): _____
    e. Tranquilizers:_____

Fig. 13.2 Sample medical history and dental history questionnaire, as well as an informed consent agreement. (Courtesy of and adapted from Youngstown State University, Youngstown, Ohio.)

f. Aspirin:_____

g. Insulin, Tolbutamide (Orinase), or similar drug:_____

h. Digitalis or drugs for heart trouble:_____

i. Nitroglycerin:_____

j. Antihistamine: _____

k. Oral contraceptive or other hormonal therapy:_____

l. Fosamax or similar bisphosphonates: _____

15. Are you taking any other drug, medication, or vitamin/herbal supplements? _____ If so, specify:_____
_____

16. Are you allergic or have you reacted adversely to any of the following?

a. Local anesthetics: _____

b. Penicillin or other antibiotics:_____

c. Sulfa drugs: _____

d. Barbiturates, sedatives, or sleeping pills:_____

e. Aspirin:_____

f. Codeine or other narcotics:_____

g. Other _____

17. Are you wearing contact lenses? _____

18. WOMEN: Are you pregnant? _____

19. Have you ever had a bad experience in the dental office? _____If so, please explain:_____
_____
_____

20. Do you have any other disease, condition, or problem that is not listed above? _____If so, please explain:_____
_____
_____

DENTAL HISTORY

1. What is your chief complaint or what brings you to this office? _____

2. Who referred you to this office? _____

3. In general, do you feel uncomfortable or nervous receiving dental treatment? _____

4. When did you last visit the dentist? _____

5. When was the last time you had your teeth cleaned?_____

6. How often do you brush your teeth? _____How often do you floss your teeth? _____

7. Do your gums bleed when you brush or floss? _____

8. Have you ever had periodontal surgery or orthodontic treatment? _____

9. Do you smoke? _____If yes, how much?_____

10. Do you use snuff or smokeless tobacco? _____If yes, what kind, how often, and where?_____

11. Do you have any mouth habits? _____What kind?_____

12. Do you snack between meals? _____What kind?_____

13. Do you participate in sports?_____ Which sports? _____

INFORMED CONSENT AGREEMENT

Having been informed of the procedures and given an opportunity to ask questions, I consent to the following with my initials:

_____ oral prophylaxis (scaling and polishing)

_____ local anesthesia

_____ fluoride

_____ sealants

_____ radiographs

_____ ultrasonic scaling

_____ oral irrigation

_____ obtaining and/or use of photographs, radiographs, tape recordings, video recordings or drawings for the purpose of education, including publication in professional journals and books or for professional presentations.

_____ placement of restorations

_____ study models

_____ diabetes screening

_____ plaque smear

_____ dietary management

_____ cleaning removable appliances

_____ other, specify _____

Patient Signature _____Date_____

Fig. 13.2, cont'd

while adhering to two ethical obligations: (1) honest listening without prejudgment and (2) honest responses without bias. The response technique of **back channeling** uses words, including "I see," and gestures, such as nodding with an attentive gaze, to demonstrate active listening. This technique allows for the dental professional to express empathy and agreement or request more information or clarification. The use of **open-ended questions** requires the patient to offer more than a yes or no response. For example, the dental hygienist may say, "Tell me more about the discomfort you are feeling." This technique leads to a discussion during which the patient describes the issue in greater detail for better assessment. Other strategies that support effective communication skills include initiating and encouraging interaction, helping patients identify with their feelings, and ensuring mutual understanding without inhibiting communication.[3] Box 13.1 contains additional information on key concepts used in the patient-centered interview process.

Completing a Comprehensive Health History

The dental hygienist must review the patient's responses, assess their significance, determine their implications for professional dental care, and refer the patient to a dental specialist or physician of record if necessary. A comprehensive health history should contain demographic information; the patient's chief complaint; and the personal, dental, and medical or health histories.

Demographic information is necessary for the business aspects of the dental practice to establish familiarity with new patients and facilitate followup care. This information may also include the patient's **social history** regarding marital and family status, occupation, living situation, cultural practices, social determinants of health, or other identifiable barriers that interfere with the patient seeking or acquiring healthcare. Table 13.1 provides examples of a patient's personal history,

including demographic information and social history, which can be found in the patient record.

The **chief complaint** is the patient's primary reason for seeking oral healthcare services and is recorded in the patient's own words. Inquiring about the reason for the appointment clarifies the dental needs and identifies potential topics. This information may lead to patient education or identify community resources to meet the chief complaint. The patient's primary concern should be addressed early in the care plan to facilitate patient satisfaction, build trust, and elicit cooperation. The **dental history** identifies preexisting conditions that are relevant for diagnosing and care planning:

- Previous dental treatments, frequency of dental visits, and any unpleasant experiences
- Complications from adverse effects of local anesthetic agents or dental procedures
- Current symptoms and concerns (e.g., fear of dental care, bleeding gums, loose teeth, oral malodor, toothache, tenderness, swelling, unpleasant appearance, pain)
- Current oral habits (e.g., bruxism, nail biting, thumb sucking, cheek biting, tobacco use)
- Oral self-care practices (e.g., products or home remedies, methods, frequency, duration of use)
- Fluoride history (e.g., professional applications; fluoridated community water; home water filtration; bottled water; fluoride toothpaste, rinses, drops, or tablets)
- Use of prescribed or over-the-counter oral care products (e.g., antimicrobial mouthrinse, moisturizing mouthrinse, saliva substitute, amorphous calcium phosphate, xylitol gum, mints)
- Type of diet and snacking habits
- Beliefs and values related to oral health, noting family history of periodontitis or dentures

A separate dental history form may be used to collect this information on a patient's prior dental experiences. Table 13.2 provides examples of interview questions regarding the patient's dental history and chief complaints.

The **medical history** documents the patient's overall medical health and identifies the need for medical consultations. The medical history includes diagnosed medical conditions, current symptoms suggestive of undiagnosed conditions, use of prescription and over-the-counter medications (see Chapter 15), alcohol and illicit drug use, types of allergies, drug reactions, and the need for **prophylactic antibiotic premedication**. The extent and severity of medical conditions must be explored for better treatment planning and care. To determine a patient's health status, a comprehensive survey of medical questions, including rationales for professional care, is provided in Table 13.3.

BOX 13.1 Patient-Centered Interview Process

- *Initialize and encourage conversation* by providing information for the patient to reflect on by using open-ended questions for in-depth responses and by focusing questions on topics of concern to evoke a deeper understanding of the patient's condition. Rationale: Creates a rapport with the patient, builds trust, and develops a knowledge base.
- *Identify and express feelings* by sharing observations, paraphrasing the patient's comments, and focusing comments to reflect feelings. Rationale: Promotes the patient's awareness, clarifies meaning, and encourages communication.
- *Ensure mutual understanding* by seeking clarification through summarizing and validating the patient's comments. Rationale: Confirms your interpretation of the patient's concerns and maintains focus.
- *Avoid inhibiting communication* with false reassurances, giving advice, stereotyping responses, or providing a defensive response to a patient's comment. Rationale: Diminishes patient–clinician rapport and decreases patient's willingness to communicate.

Adapted from Saleeby JR. Communication and collaboration. In: Perry AG, Potter PA, Ostendorf W, eds. *Nursing Intervention and Clinical Skills*. 6th ed. Elsevier; 2016.

TABLE 13.1 Patient Personal History (Demographic and Social Status)

Items	Implication for Use
Name, contact information, gender, date of birth, emergency contact, completion date on form	Identifies the patient, contains the facility's correspondence, establishes emergency contact, and determines legal obligation for consent of care.
Marital status, occupation, children or dependents, living situation, cultural practices	Identifies barriers or social determinants related to health and disease.
Insurance information	Determines financial obligations and identifies primary and secondary payers for dental services.
Previous dental providers and contact information	Facilitates acquisition of previous dental records, radiographs, and consultation with dental care providers for comparison or monitoring of oral conditions.
Physician's name and contact information	Identifies the physician to facilitate assistance in consultation and management of medical conditions and emergencies.
Referral source	Identifies who should receive acknowledgment for the patient referral.

TABLE 13.2 Patient Dental History and Chief Complaint

Item	Relevant Questions	Implications for Professional Care
1. Chief complaint	What brings you in today? Are you experiencing any oral problems or concerns?	Identify purpose for the appointment, address the chief complaint, create patient autonomy, and build patient rapport.
2. Prior dental care	When was your last dental visit? What treatment was provided? Were there any problems with your prior dental care? Have you ever had any type of specialized dental care? Do you feel anxious during dental appointments?	Establish prior dental care, identify specific needs, and determine the patient's anxiety or fear, which may require the use of stress-reduction protocols.
3. Radiation history	When was the last time you received dental x-rays? How many images were taken? Have you had recent medical radiographs taken? If so, what type?	Request prior oral radiographs from the former dentist, limit radiographic exposure to only necessary images, and determine medical radiation exposure.
4. Dental complications	Have you experienced any dental-related complications? Do you have allergies to any medicines or other substances? If so, what type of reaction occurs?	Avoid dental complications, such as allergic reactions and adverse events from local anesthetics or dental products.
5. Patient anxiety	What causes you to fear dental treatment? Have you ever taken medication to reduce your anxiety? How can I help make this a more pleasant experience for you?	Evaluate patient anxiety, determine need for stress-reduction protocols, and prepare for medical emergencies (e.g., syncope, hyperventilation). Be empathetic and establish confidence and trust.
6. Patient perception	What do you know about oral health and entire body health? Do you know it is possible to keep your teeth for the rest of your life?	Evaluate medical conditions affecting oral health, such as diabetes, infective endocarditis, and autoimmune diseases, as well as the patient's overall health status.
7. Adverse events	Are you experiencing pain? When did it occur and where? What aggravates the pain? What improves the pain?	Conduct an oral examination with a focus on complications. Provide recommendations for self-care and oral products to relieve discomfort.
8. Chewing ability	Do you have difficulty chewing or swallowing? Can you describe the experience? Is it painful? Do you wear dentures? How do they fit?	Identify any difficulty chewing or swallowing that is related to ill-fitting dentures, oral appliances, missing teeth, or extensive decay. Consider nutritional counseling and refer the patient to the dentist.
9. Periodontal health	Can you describe your oral hygiene habits? Do your gums bleed when you brush or floss? Do you have loose teeth, bad breath, or receding gums? How long have you experienced these conditions? Do you understand why these situations are occurring?	Assess periodontium for systemic-related health concerns. Assess the patient's oral health literacy and determine an education plan. Complete a periodontal assessment for biofilm control and gingival architecture to establish oral hygiene instruction. Determine an appropriate treatment schedule.
10. Oral lesions	Where are the sores located? How long have they been present? Do you have any idea of their cause?	Determine the differential diagnosis or implement precautions for infectious lesions by identifying the cause (e.g., trauma, herpes virus, aphthae, leukemia, blood dyscrasia, syphilis, malignancy, medical disorders). Determine appropriate referrals. Assess the patient's oral health literacy and determine an education plan.
11. Oral habits	Do you clench or grind your teeth? Does your child use a pacifier or suck his or her thumb? Do you know what is causing this problem?	Determine the impact and appropriate counseling of oral habits. Assess the patient's oral health literacy and determine an education plan.
12. Patient satisfaction	What causes dissatisfaction? Have you considered treatment to improve the situation?	Identify conditions relating to dissatisfaction (e.g., periodontal disease, lack of regular dental care, medical problems, and developmental issues). Determine alternative treatment options and schedules.
13. Facial or oral injuries	Have you experienced any injury to your mouth or face? Do you have jaw trouble or pain when opening your mouth?	Identify temporomandibular joint (TMJ) dysfunction or previous injuries. Determine appropriate care scheduling and use of mouth props for patient comfort.
14. Oral biofilm control	What type of toothpaste, toothbrush, and floss do you use? What type of oral rinses do you use? Can you tell me about your oral hygiene habits?	Determine the patient's oral health habits and need for product recommendations. Assess the patient's oral health literacy and determine an education plan.
15. Fluorides and sealants	Do you use fluoride products or have fluoridated water? Do you want a topical fluoride treatment today? Have you had sealants placed on teeth?	Assess the patient's need for caries prevention products and treatment.
16. Carcinogenic diet	How often do you drink sugar-sweetened beverages, coffee, or tea? How about sugar-free drinks and bottled water? How often do you snack between meals or eat sweets?	Assess the patient's carcinogenic diet and determine the need for nutritional counseling.
17. Beliefs and values regarding oral health	How important is your oral health? Did you know it is possible to keep your teeth for your entire life?	Assess motivational strategies and an education plan to improve the patient's oral health beliefs and values.

TABLE 13.3   Patient Health History

Item	Relevant Questions	Purpose and Implications for Professional Care
General Health		
1. Determination of general health	How is your health?	Determine whether conflicting data in the health history exist. Investigate the patient's misunderstandings of health status for accurate documentation and treatment planning.
2. Change in general health	Has there been any recent change in your health? What has happened?	Determine whether medical consultation is warranted.
3. Last physical examination	When was your last physical examination? What were the results? Who performed the examination?	Determine the patient's previous health history and compliance with regular medical care.
4. Currently under medical care and the reason	Do you see a physician for any ongoing illness? What type of treatment are you undergoing? Are you experiencing any complications?	Determine the patient's current health status, chronic health problems, risk for medical emergencies, and the need for medical consultation before initiating oral care, as well as the need for modifications to treatment planning.
5. Serious illness or hospitalization within the past 5 years	Have you experienced any hospitalizations or surgeries in the last 5 years? Did you experience any complications? Do you take any medications because of the illness or hospitalization?	Identify recent surgeries or hospitalizations and potential for antibiotic prophylaxis (e.g., cardiac valve replacement). Determine risk of pharmacologic effect, interactions with local anesthetics, or prescribed medications.
6. Medical radiation or x-ray examination within the past 5 years	Have you undergone any x-ray examinations in the last 5 years? Was it diagnostic or treatment radiation? Did you experience any complications from radiation therapy? If so, please describe them.	Determine the patient's current health status, based on the reason for radiation therapy. Determine the need for oral care product recommendations, based on oral needs. Although digital oral radiographs have lower ionizing radiation exposure compared to traditional x-rays, only take images that are necessary for diagnosis. Identify cancer therapy or any other medical problem, such as hyperthyroidism. **Alert:** Limit oral radiographic exposure.
7. Medications, including nonprescription agents and herbs	Are you taking any medications, including nonprescription drugs or herbs? Why are you taking each drug or herb, and what is the dose and frequency for each? Have you noticed any side effects from each drug or herb? (Consult a drug reference for potential side effects relevant to oral procedures.)	Identify prescriptions to investigate in a drug reference. Identify drug effects or side effects that may influence patient management (e.g., xerostomia, bleeding, drug-influenced gingival enlargement, vital sign changes). Consider medical conditions being pharmacologically managed and their effect on oral care (e.g., interaction with local anesthesia). Identify current drug or herbal effects relevant to oral care. Consider effects of each drug or herb and potential side effects relevant to oral care.
8. Allergies and reactions	Did you experience hives, rash, or itching or become short of breath? Did you report all reactions to your physician?	True allergic reactions usually involve rash, itching, or anaphylaxis (e.g., facial swelling, bronchial constriction, hypotension, shock). Use the appropriate antibiotic from a different class. If the patient is allergic to penicillin, select azithromycin or cephalexin. Avoid the offending drug and drug class when an allergy exists. Identify any allergy to drugs and substances used in dental hygiene care. Differentiate between a true allergic reaction and a side effect.
Medical Conditions		
9(a). Cardiovascular disease, artificial heart valves or prosthetic material for cardiac valve repair, prior infective endocarditis, unrepaired cyanotic congenital heart disease, repaired congenital heart disease with prosthetic material within 6 months of the procedure, valvular disease in a cardiac transplant	Do you have any medical problems with your heart? Tell me about the cardiac condition and when it developed. Has your physician told you to take antibiotics before dental treatment? Did you take your antibiotic? What did you take? What dose, and how long ago did you take it?	Investigate the patient's cardiac condition and current outcome (may need medical consultation). If applicable, record the antibiotic agent, dose, and time it was administered in the patient record. Current regimen suggests taking an appropriate antibiotic 1 hour before the appointment; if inadvertently forgotten, it can be administered at the dental appointment or within 2 hours of the appointment. Advise the patient to notify the dentist if fever develops within 2 weeks of the appointment, as this is a sign of endocarditis. Antibiotic prophylaxis may be indicated before any dental hygiene procedure for these cardiac conditions. **Alert:** Medical consultation may be necessary.

TABLE 13.3　Patient Health History—cont'd

Item	Relevant Questions	Purpose and Implications for Professional Care
9(b). Vascular disease (heart trouble, heart attack, coronary artery disease, chest pain [angina], hypertension, arteriosclerosis, stroke, cardiac bypass, cardiac surgery)	Have you experienced any medical problems with your heart or blood vessels? When? What was the outcome? Is the condition controlled? Do you take any medications for it? Did you have complications from the condition or the medical therapy? Has your physician warned you about receiving dental care?	Monitor patient vital signs and functional capacity to assess cardiovascular recovery.[5] Determine the time since the cardiovascular event and the physician's recommendations regarding dental care. A recent event may require physician consultation. A prior myocardial infarction (MI) requires 1 month for convalescence and a prior stroke requires 6 months' convalescence before dental hygiene care can be provided. Identify specific cardiac diseases. Determine functional capacity and extent of damage to cardiac muscle.
9(b) 1. Do you have chest pain on exertion?	Tell me more about your chest pain. When does it occur? What do you do for it? What makes the pain lessen? What makes it increase? Do you have a recent prescription for nitroglycerin? When was your last attack of chest pain? What were you doing? Has it occurred at a dental appointment?	Determine the risk for an anginal attack during the appointment. Identify nitroglycerin therapy. Ensure that nitroglycerin is brought to all appointments by the nitrate-dependent patient and that the date on bottle shows the prescription to be current. If angina occurs, administer a sublingual tablet every 5 minutes with a maximum of 3 doses. Ensure that the patient is lying down or safely seated since hypotension and syncope can occur. Monitor the patient's blood pressure every 5 minutes during angina management. Record management procedure in the patient record. Identify coronary arteriosclerosis and reduced blood flow to cardiac muscle. **Alert:** There is an increased risk for unstable angina or heart attack.
9(b) 2. Are you ever short of breath after mild exercise or when lying down? Can you walk up a flight of stairs without stopping to rest?	What does your physician say about your shortness of breath or your problem walking up a flight of stairs? Let me know if you begin to feel any problem as I provide treatment.	Cardiologists report that for patients with a history of an MI or heart failure, the degree of functional capacity relates to their ability to receive noncardiac procedures.[5] Adequate functional capacity to receive dental procedures includes the ability to walk a block at a moderate speed or the ability to climb a flight of stairs without stopping.[5] A contraindication to dental care exists if an MI occurred less than 1 month earlier. Determine the patient's functional capacity.
9(b) 3. How many pillows do you need to sleep?	Have you always used that number of pillows to sleep? Why do you need to be upright to sleep? Have you been evaluated for heart failure?	Since the inability to sleep in a supine position may be a sign of congestive heart failure, determine the reason for needing to be in an upright position to sleep. Investigate whether a medical evaluation has been completed and, if so, the results of that evaluation. Stress can exacerbate heart failure. Consider medical consultation and implementing stress-reduction protocol. **Alert:** Identify uncontrolled congestive heart disease.
9(b) 4. Do your ankles swell?	Do you know why your ankles swell? Have you seen your physician about it? Is there any pain associated with the swelling?	Determine the reason for swelling. Pain is not a feature of swelling in extremities associated with heart failure. Determine whether the condition has been medically evaluated. Identify initial signs of heart failure. Leg and ankle swelling may also relate to noncardiac reasons such as venous varicosities or pregnancy.
9(b) 5. Do you have an implanted cardiac pacemaker or defibrillator?	When was your last pacemaker implanted? Have you experienced any complications since the procedure?	Medtronic, St. Jude, or Guidant brands of pacemakers are not disrupted by an electromagnetic ultrasonic scaler or unit. Monitor the patient's pulse rate for regularity and qualities. Antibiotic prophylaxis is not indicated. An implanted cardiac pacemaker or defibrillator indicates a cardiac disorder but not the need for antibiotic prophylaxis. An ultrasonic scaler is not contraindicated for shielded pacemakers.

Continued

TABLE 13.3   Patient Health History—cont'd

Item	Relevant Questions	Purpose and Implications for Professional Care
9(b) 6. Have you recently had severe headaches?	Have you seen your physician to learn the cause of your headaches? Have you ruled out sinus issues and migraine?	Try to identify the cause of the severe headaches. Medical consultation may be indicated. **Alert:** Identify signs of prestroke condition. **Alert:** Monitor the patient's blood pressure; severe hypertension increases the risk of stroke.
10(a). Allergy, hives, skin rash	Do you have any allergies? What reaction do you have? How do you treat it?	Avoid using a product to which the patient is allergic. Monitor vital signs, patient appearance, and respiration characteristics. **Alert:** Identify dental-related allergens.
10(b). Sinus trouble, hay fever, cold	Do you have any cold symptoms? Do you have any trouble with your sinuses? Have you had any postnasal drainage today?	Consider the need for semisupine chair position. Determine risk for the spread of infection and airway constriction.
11. Respiratory problems (emphysema, bronchitis, chronic obstructive pulmonary disease [COPD], asthma)	How do you control signs and symptoms of your breathing disease? What makes your respiratory disease worse? What makes it better? Do you carry a rescue inhaler? When were you diagnosed? What are your asthma triggers? Can you tolerate being placed in a supine position?	Monitor the patient's respiration rate. Determine the need for semisupine positioning. Continuous oxygen ventilation by nasal cannula may be needed. Avoid aerosol production. Avoid nitrous oxide for analgesia. A bronchodilator must be present at every appointment. **Alert:** Stress may cause an acute attack. **Alert:** Identify risk for a constricted airway. **Alert:** Identify the patient who cannot tolerate supine position for care. **Alert:** Nitrous oxide–oxygen analgesia may be contraindicated in the patient with COPD.
12. Fainting spells	What causes you to faint? When was the last time it occurred? Have you fainted during a dental appointment?	Determine the cause of the fainting and prevent its reoccurrence. Fainting can be associated with some cardiac and neurologic disorders. Identify risk for an emergency involving loss of consciousness.
13. Epilepsy or other neurologic disorders	Do you have a history of a seizure disorder or any problems with your nervous system? Are you taking antiseizure medication? Did you take it today? What type of seizure disorder do you have? Do you know when a seizure is about to happen? When was your last seizure? Have you ever had to go to the hospital because of a prolonged seizure?	Determine risk for a seizure during the oral care appointment. Avoid flashing overhead light in the patient's eyes and use of any device that may precipitate a seizure. Plan for seizure management and watch the patient for signs of seizure (e.g., loss of consciousness, abnormal movements, stiffness, fluttering eyelids, blank stare). Move dental equipment to ensure that the patient is not injured during a seizure and immediately notify medical personnel. Investigate side effects of seizure pharmacotherapy (e.g., drug-influenced gingival enlargement, bleeding). **Alert:** A recent attack is a heightened risk factor for an emergency situation. **Alert:** The patient's failure to take antiseizure medication is a risk factor for recurrent seizures.
14. Low blood pressure	Have you ever lost consciousness after lying down or rising from a chair? Have you consulted a physician about it?	Low blood pressure may be normal for individuals with good physical stamina and may represent "normal limits" for a given patient. Consider collecting supine, sitting, and standing blood pressures. Determine risk for postural hypotension and follow the protocol to prevent it at end of the appointment. **Alert:** Risk for postural (orthostatic) hypotension and syncope is increased.
15. Bowel and bladder problems	Do you have any problems with your bowel or bladder function? Which condition? How do you manage the condition? Do you need to go to the restroom before we begin? Let me know if we need to stop during the appointment.	Determine the cause of the problem and appropriately and respectfully manage care. Assess the need for a bathroom break during the appointment. Identify the need for planning restroom breaks. Symptoms of bowel and bladder problems can be associated with a variety of disorders (e.g., urinary tract infection, neurologic disease, acquired immunodeficiency syndrome [AIDS], malignancy, bowel disorders, febrile illness).

TABLE 13.3   Patient Health History—cont'd

Item	Relevant Questions	Purpose and Implications for Professional Care
16. Diabetes mellitus (DM)	Have you been diagnosed with diabetes or prediabetes? When were you diagnosed? When was your last medical evaluation for diabetes? What was your last hemoglobin A_{1c} value? How do you manage your diabetes—by diet, exercise, and/or medication? Do you have low blood sugar (hypoglycemic) episodes? Do you use a glucose meter? What was your reading this morning? Did you eat before coming in today?	Controlled DM is characterized by a recent hemoglobin A_{1c} test result of <7%. Blood sugar is usually monitored in the evening and morning by pricking the finger and placing blood on a test strip to be inserted in the blood glucose meter. A morning score of 70–130 mg/dL is the goal for treatment. Levels >200 mg/dL should be referred for medical evaluation. Determine risk for hypoglycemia (glucose <70 mg/dL) and keep sugar available to reverse hypoglycemia should it develop (see Chapter 49). An appointment is scheduled for morning hours after a meal is consumed. **Alert:** Determine risk for a hypoglycemic emergency. Patients with controlled diabetes are treated the same as normal healthy patients. Uncontrolled DM may cause reduced healing and greater periodontal destruction. Prophylactic antibiotics are not indicated.
16(a). Do you have to urinate (pass water) more than six times a day? More than three times during the night? 16(b). Are you thirsty much of the time? 16(c). Have you had a recent weight change of more than 10 pounds? 16(d). Are you slow to heal or do you get frequent infections?	Have you ever been checked for diabetes? Does anyone in your family have diabetes? I recommend that you be checked for diabetes. Do you have high blood pressure?	If the cause for symptoms cannot be determined, the patient should be referred for medical evaluation. The patient may need to have medical evaluation before treatment. Examine oral tissues for signs of uncontrolled DM (e.g., periodontal abscess, extensive attachment loss, fruity breath odor, candidiasis). Monitor vital signs; hypertension and atherosclerosis are associated with DM, especially uncontrolled disease. Cardiovascular disease may be present. In case of emergency, call 911. **Alert:** These are signs and symptoms of undiagnosed or uncontrolled DM. **Alert:** Risk for a hyperglycemic event (diabetic coma or ketoacidosis) is increased.
17. Thyroid problems	Are you aware of any problems with your thyroid gland? Have you been diagnosed with hypothyroidism or hyperthyroidism? Are you currently being treated for a thyroid disorder? Are there any drugs that you cannot tolerate?	Uncontrolled hyperthyroidism is characterized by an increased pulse rate and increased body temperature. Monitor vital signs during each appointment. Uncontrolled hypothyroidism is characterized by edema, enlarged tongue, bradycardia, and hypotension. **Alert:** Uncontrolled thyroid disease poses an increased risk for a medical emergency. **Alert:** A thyroid storm is associated with uncontrolled hyperthyroidism; monitor the patient's pulse rate and body temperature.
18. Arthritis, rheumatism, or painful swollen joints	Do you have any problems with your joints? How does this affect your ability to perform oral self-care such as brushing and flossing? What medications do you take? What did you take today? Are you able to lie down without discomfort? When is the best time for your appointment—midmorning or afternoon? Is your jaw (temporomandibular joint [TMJ]) affected?	Evaluate effects of each drug taken before the appointment. Monitor for clotting during care and use digital pressure to achieve hemostasis during oral procedures. Upper extremity impairments may necessitate oral hygiene modifications (e.g., large-handle toothbrush, floss aid). Determine the best time for an appointment around daily pattern of symptoms. The patient may have difficulty opening the mouth widely if the TMJ is affected. Identify the patient who may have disabilities of the hands or fingers and who may not tolerate supine positioning. Identify pharmacologic therapy with side effects that may complicate oral care such as immunosuppression and increased bleeding.

Continued

TABLE 13.3   Patient Health History—cont'd

Item	Relevant Questions	Purpose and Implications for Professional Care
19. Problems of the immune system or organ transplant	Do you have any condition that weakens your immune system or increases your risk for infections? What is the cause of the condition? Has your physician told you to take antibiotics before a dental appointment? What medicines are you taking for your condition?	Determine the potential complications associated with oral care such as poor healing and infection. Investigate drug therapy and possible drug-influenced gingival enlargement with cyclosporine. Identify the immunocompromised patient who is susceptible to infection and may have a reduced healing response. Determine the need for physician consultation regarding antibiotic prophylaxis.
20. Stomach ulcers or hyperacidity or gastroesophageal reflux disorder	Do you have problems with your stomach or esophagus? Does lying flat cause a reflux problem? Are your teeth sensitive?	Hyperacid conditions are sometimes associated with reflux of stomach acid into the mouth, leading to erosion and caries. Examine dentition for erosion, caries, and chipped teeth. Acetaminophen is the indicated analgesic for oral pain. Consider semisupine chair position. Identify the patient who is predisposed to erosion. Note the contraindication for aspirin and nonsteroidal antiinflammatory drugs with peptic ulcer disease. Identify positioning modifications.
21. Kidney disease	Do you have any problem with your kidneys? How are you being treated?	Some renal disorders, such as glomerulonephritis, may require medical consultation before oral care is initiated. If the patient is on hemodialysis, take the blood pressure reading in the arm without a fistula or graft. Antibiotic prophylaxis is not generally indicated for shunts and catheters in hemodialysis. Evaluate each patient individually for need based on risk factors (see Chapter 54). Reveal the risk for hypertension and the inability to excrete drugs normally.
22. Tuberculosis ([TB]; positive purified protein derivative test result, or chest x-ray image)	Have you been tested for TB infection? What was the result? If the test was positive, do you have symptoms such as cough, fever, or weight loss? Was a chest x-ray image performed? Are you or did you ever receive antibiotics? For how long? Have you had sputum tests?	Medical consultation must be completed to ensure the absence of active infection. Anti-TB drugs taken for >2 weeks should render the patient noninfectious. Be alert to side effects of anti-TB drugs (e.g., rifampin may cause a red-orange discoloration of saliva and tears). **Alert:** Patients with active TB should not receive oral treatment.
23. Persistent cough or cough that produces blood	Have you sought medical evaluation? What was the medical diagnosis? Are you currently in treatment? Do you know if you are infectious to others?	Medical consultation is needed to rule out infectious TB. If a non-TB lung infection is suspected, wash your hands and wear gloves and a surgical mask to prevent cross contamination. **Alert:** Identify the patient with infectious lung disease, such as TB.
24. Sexually transmitted diseases ([STDs], e.g., syphilis, gonorrhea, chlamydia)	Have you ever been diagnosed with a sexually transmitted infection? When were you diagnosed? Are you currently in treatment? When will you finish your antibiotics? Are you infectious to others?	Ensure that adequate barrier protection is maintained. If an oral STD infection is suspected, defer oral care until medical consultation verifies that the patient is noninfectious. Medical consultation is needed to verify diagnosis and current medical therapy. Identify the patient with an untreated STD who may have oral infectious lesions.
25. Acquired immunodeficiency syndrome (AIDS) or human immunodeficiency viral (HIV) infection	Have you ever been tested for an HIV infection? When? What was the result? Are you currently taking medications? What was your most recent CD4 cell count?	Consultation with the referring physician may be required when considering antibiotic prophylaxis. Opportunistic infections are more likely at CD4 counts <200 cells/μL. Anticipate oral and/or esophageal candidiasis. Investigate all drugs for side effects relevant to oral care. **Alert:** Identify the immunocompromised patient. Maintain standard precautions.
26. Oral herpes (cold sores, fever blisters)	Do you have an oral lesion today? What usually causes an outbreak? How do you treat the lesion?	Inform the patient that a lesion is communicable, so the appointment will be rescheduled. Recommend using a new toothbrush after the lesion resolves to reduce reinfection. Acyclovir or over-the-counter products can be advised. **Alert:** Oral treatment is contraindicated when labial lesions are present and the risk of cross infection is high.

TABLE 13.3 Patient Health History—cont'd

Item	Relevant Questions	Purpose and Implications for Professional Care
27. Blood disorder (e.g., anemia, bruising, leukemia) 27(a). Do you have abnormal bleeding? 27(b). Have you required a blood transfusion? If yes, when?	Do you easily bruise or bleed? When was the condition diagnosed? Are you receiving medical therapy for the condition? What do you do to stop bleeding?	Monitor for increased bleeding and reduced healing. Determine the cause of the condition and manage as needed. Reveal the blood disorder that may complicate healing during oral care. Identify risk for increased bleeding or hemorrhage.
28. Mental health problems	Have you sought help from a mental health professional in the past? Are you currently being treated for any condition? What medications are you taking?	Show concern and try to encourage self-interest in a healthy oral cavity. Identify the need to initiate stress-reduction protocols. Investigate medication side effects; xerostomia is common. Identify emotional issues that may complicate oral care and patient self-care.
29. Cancer, tumors, growths, or persistent swollen glands	Have you ever been diagnosed with cancer? What type of cancer? What treatments have you been receiving? What is your current white blood cell count?	Chemotherapy often reduces the number of white blood cells; medical consultation is needed to establish the time when the patient can receive oral care while undergoing chemotherapy. For oral malignancy, monitor tissues during every maintenance appointment for a new lesion or recurrence. Investigate drug therapy for relevant side effects (e.g., mucositis, ulceration, xerostomia). Identify any malignant disease and the need for an examination for recurrence at maintenance appointments.
30. Tumor or growth	What type of tumor did you have? What treatment did you receive (e.g., surgery, radiation, chemotherapy)? What was the outcome? Did you develop oral complications? Describe them.	Determine the cause and treatment success and manage as needed. For radiation-induced xerostomia, consider salivary substitutes or oral lubricating products. Monitor for oral effects, depending on the therapy received. Identify the patient with a history of malignancy or neoplastic disease.
31. Liver disease	Do you know of any problems with your liver? If hepatitis B virus (HBV): Are you being treated with antiviral agents? Are you contagious? Do you bleed for a long time after a cut?	Determine etiology Liver disease may increase bleeding risk. All practitioners should have immunity to HBV from a vaccine that is verified by a blood test to determine adequate antibody formation. Take care to avoid an injury that may compromise the standard precaution of gloves. If a puncture occurs, immediately seek medical evaluation for recommended therapy. Determine whether blood-borne transmission of a viral condition exists. Determine whether increased bleeding is probable.
32. Allergic reactions to the following: • Local anesthetics • Penicillin or antibiotics • Sulfa drugs • Barbiturates, sedatives, or sleeping pills • Aspirin • Iodine • Codeine or narcotics • Latex • Metals (silver, mercury) • Other	What type of reaction did you have? Describe it. What antibiotic can you take?	New legislation gives some prescribing abilities to dental hygienists. Medications or over-the-counter products to which an allergy has occurred should not be recommended or provided to the patient. Determine whether a reaction was a hypersensitivity reaction or a side effect. Latex: Select nonlatex gloves, prophy cup, or other product; cover the arm with a barrier before placing the blood pressure cuff. Identify the allergies relevant to products used in dentistry. Indicate the medications that should not be prescribed or products that should not be used in oral care.
33. Serious event associated with a previous dental treatment	Have you had a serious event associated with a previous dental treatment? What happened? How can it be prevented today?	Investigate the event and institute procedures to prevent it. For anxious patients, talking about their interests to keep the current treatment "off their mind" may reduce anxiety. Identify the patient who may be at increased risk for syncope or other emergencies.
34. Disease, condition, or problem not previously listed that is important	Do you have a disease, condition, or problem not previously listed that is important? What is the condition? Have you received medical treatment? What was the outcome?	Determine the cause of the condition and manage as needed. Identify any condition not included on the history form.

Continued

TABLE 13.3 Patient Health History—cont'd

Item	Relevant Questions	Purpose and Implications for Professional Care
35. Contact lenses	Are you wearing contact lenses? Do you want to take your contact lenses out before treatment?	Consider the possibility of introducing an aerosol irritant to the eyes. Wearing protective eyewear is the standard of care, but prophylaxis paste spatter may cause irritation in some cases. Identify special considerations, remove lenses, and provide protective eyewear.
36. Tobacco use	Do you use or have you ever used tobacco? If so, what type? For how many years? How much tobacco did you use each day? If you stopped, how long ago did you stop? Follow up responses as indicated. How do you feel about stopping smoking? If you are contemplating or are ready to quit, would you like information on local tobacco cessation programs?	Offer information on local counseling programs for tobacco cessation. Counsel that nicotine replacement drugs may be available from physicians or from dentists in some practices. Regardless of the interest in quitting, encourage tobacco cessation to avoid lung, cardiovascular, and oral cancer conditions. Identify the issues for tobacco cessation programs.
37. Alcohol and substance use and abuse	How often do you drink alcohol? How much do you drink? Has your drinking ever been a problem? Do you have any problems with your liver? When was your last drink? Do you use recreational drugs? Do you use cocaine? How do you use it and when was your last use?	Do not recommend mouthrinse with alcohol to a patient who is a recovering alcoholic. Withdrawal of alcohol in an alcohol-dependent patient can precipitate a seizure. Vasoconstrictors (epinephrine) are contraindicated when cocaine has been used within the past 24 hours. Cocaine use increases the risk for stroke and cardiac arrhythmias. Identify the alcohol or substance abusing patient. **Alert:** Identify cocaine interaction with a vasoconstrictor.
38. X-rays or ionizing radiation	Are you employed in a facility that regularly exposes you to x-rays or ionizing radiation? Do you have regular assessments to determine your level of ionizing radiation exposure? Can we take dental x-rays if they are necessary?	Consider whether there is a need to avoid or limit dental x-ray exposure. Identify the need for reducing patient exposure to ionizing radiation.
For women only: 39. Pregnancy	Are you pregnant? If yes, when is your due date?	Radiographs can be taken during pregnancy using standard precautions. The second trimester is the preferred time for elective oral care. During the third trimester, to avoid supine hypotension, place a pillow under the right hip and rotate the abdomen to the left to avoid compression of the vena cava. Identify the time for an appointment plan.
40. Menstruation	Do you have problems with menstrual periods? If yes, what are the problems? What do you do about them?	Determine the cause and manage as needed. Identify hormone imbalance.
41. Nursing	Are you nursing? Can we schedule your appointment after your nursing time?	Schedule an appointment as directed by the patient. Identify an appointment planning schedule.
42. Birth control	Are you taking birth control pills? Do your gums bleed more since you started taking them? Are you experiencing any side effects?	Monitor patient blood pressure: there is a risk for increased values when hormones are taken. Avoid antibiotics or use an additional birth control method when taking antibiotics. Strict biofilm control is useful. Identify potential side effects relevant to oral care.
43. Hormone replacement therapy	Do you have hot flashes or signs of menopause? Are you taking hormone replacement therapy? Have you had a bone density test? If so, what was the result?	Monitor the patient's vital signs and identify the increased risk for cardiovascular complications. Identify issues involving hormone replacement therapy.
44. Risk for osteonecrosis	Have you had a bone density test? Have you been diagnosed with osteopenia or osteoporosis? How long have you taken antiresorptive agents? Which agent were or are you taking? Have you ever taken bisphosphonates or denosumab? Was it taken orally or intravenously?	Provide patient information on the small risk of osteonecrosis of the jaw when oral agents are taken for 3 or more years or with intravenous bisphosphonates taken for 10 months or longer. Examine oral cavity for signs of osteonecrosis affecting the bone of the jaws. Identify the patient at risk for osteonecrosis of the jaw.

Legal and Ethical Issues Related to the Health History

Both the American Dental Hygienists' Association (ADHA) and Canadian Dental Hygienists' Association (CDHA) publish codes of ethics that are governed by public health statutes, rules, and regulations associated with the practice of dental hygiene in their legal jurisdictions. Public health statutes may identify responsibilities such as mandatory reporting of abuse and neglect, domestic violence, and infectious diseases. Confidentiality relating to the patient's health history is protected by the Health Insurance Portability and Accountability Act (HIPAA). HIPAA requires that all "individually identifiable" personal health information or health-related information, such as name, birth date, address, or Social Security number, remain private and unavailable to others without the written approval of the patient or patient's guardian.[4] One exception to the HIPAA guidelines is an emergency situation, during which disclosing protected health information is in the best interest of the patient. Dental hygienists are expected to exercise the utmost professionalism necessary to uphold the HIPAA guidelines, including refraining from discussing patient care with third parties and keeping protected health information in secure areas.

Health history data can be collected using paper or electronic medical records. Paper medical records must be completed in permanent ink. Recording errors are to be lined out neatly, initialed, and dated. Verification and accuracy of health information is affirmed by the patient's signature (electronic or written) and dating of the health history form at the time of completion. Written comments and modifications to the health history should be initialed by the patient to verify accuracy. If the patient is younger than 18 years of age, a parent or legal guardian must sign and date the health history form. A separate consent form (Fig. 13.3) can be used to verify permission for services rendered during appointments.

The importance of patient education regarding the accuracy of health information helps protect against legal justification of dental-related activities. It is important to provide an explanation for standards of care, provisions in the scope of practice, and duties of the patient to aid in keeping accurate records and to protect against health risks. Additional suggestions for the management of patient records to protect against litigation are included in Box 13.2.

DECISION MAKING AFTER THE HEALTH HISTORY IS OBTAINED

Interpretation of Patient Data and Degree of Medical Risk

American Society of Anesthesiologists' Physical Status Classification System

A physical status classification system was developed by the American Society of Anesthesiologists (ASA) to categorize medical risk on six levels, based on disease or disorder for patients receiving local or general anesthesia (see Chapter 11).[5]

Oral health professionals use the ASA classification system to decide whether treatment is safe for patients with certain medical conditions. A patient classified as ASA IV or higher should not receive elective dental treatment. Treatment can resume when conditions improve, and the status is downgraded. For example, a patient with uncontrolled diabetes or angina at rest (ASA IV) should be referred for a medical evaluation before dental hygiene care can be performed. If a patient with an ASA IV status needs emergency oral care, then a hospital environment should be used in case a life-threatening emergency occurs. Only palliative care is recommended for a patient with an ASA V status.

1. I consent to the recommended procedure or treatment _____

to be completed by Dr./Ms./Mr._____.
2. The procedure(s) or treatment(s) have been described to me.
3. I have been informed of the purpose of the procedure or treatment.
4. I have been informed of the alternatives to the procedure or treatment.
5. I understand that the following risk(s) may result from the procedure or treatment:

_____
_____
_____

6. I understand that the following risk(s) may occur if the procedure or treatment is not completed:

_____
_____
_____

7. I do—do not—consent to the administration of anesthetic.
   a. I understand that the following risks are involved in administering anesthesia:

   _____
   _____
   _____

   b. The following alternatives to anesthesia were described: _____

   _____
   _____

All my questions have been satisfactorily answered.

Signature: _____
            Date

Representative: _____
            Date

Signature of Witness: _____
            Date

Fig. 13.3 Sample consent form.

Assessment of Functional Capacity

Increases in medical risk may exist for certain conditions that involve cardiovascular dysfunction, respiratory impairment, or acute and chronic diseases. A patient who can walk up a flight of stairs or walk two level city blocks without symptomatic limitations has reached a safe level of functional capacity to undergo dental procedures. The American College of Cardiology and the American Heart Association (ACC/AHA) have determined that the first month following a myocardial infarction is the period with the highest degree of medical risk. After the first month, functional capacity decides the level of recovery and risk.[6]

Use of Drug References

Before providing professional care, the dental hygienist must investigate and document all medications taken by the patient. Medications can create adverse reactions, affect outcomes, and alter clinical treatment. These situations may necessitate change to the dental care plan or require a medical consultation before initiating treatment. Several print and electronic medical references are available and provide valuable information on drugs and diseases applicable to dental care. These references include the *Prescriber's Digital Reference (PDR), Mosby's Dental Drug Reference,* the *Drug Information Handbook for Dentistry,* and the *Merck Manual of Diagnosis and Therapy.*[7-10] Fig. 13.4 illustrates

BOX 13.2   Suggestions for Managing Patient Records

Procedures required of all types of record keeping:
- Financial information should not be noted on the treatment record.
- All referrals, consultations, and conversations to or with other health practitioners are to be documented, dated, and signed by personnel, including the reason for the referral, consultation, or conversation; contact information of other practitioner's office and personnel; details of any conversations; and specifics relating to medical issues affecting the delivery of oral healthcare. A copy of this information should be sent to the physician.
- All cancelations, late arrivals, and changes of appointments are to be recorded.
- Informed consents are documented, including all risks and alternative treatment options presented to the patient and comments made by the patient; for minors, a parent's or legal guardian's consent is documented.
- All health history questions are to be answered, or a "not applicable" (NA) response is to be documented.
- No subjective evaluations, such as an opinion about the patient's mental health, should be recorded on the treatment record unless the writer is qualified and licensed to make such evaluations.
- Completion of the health history is performed by the patient and jointly amended by the patient and healthcare practitioner.
- A patient record should never be altered.
- The current physician's name and contact information should be readily available in the event of a medical emergency.
- Documentation identifying medical alerts is clearly placed on health history form to capture the reader's attention for the prevention of medical emergencies.
- All patient records should be retained for at least the period of the statute of limitations applicable to contract actions, which is usually no more than 7 years. In the case of a minor, the applicable statute of limitations is 3 years after the patient becomes of age under state law (typically 18 years of age) or 7 years after the last date of treatment, whichever is longer. Check for special or different laws in your location. A dental office may consider additional record retention options that may include record storage facilities, microfilm, and/or scanning to electronic records. If possible, keep records indefinitely.
- The patient record should not be surrendered to anyone other than the patient, except by order of a court or as otherwise required by law or regulation; ensure Health Insurance Portability and Accountability Act (HIPAA) compliance and confidentiality of patient's health information.
- Heirs are instructed that they must retain the records of patients and comply with any written request for a copy.

Procedures specific to paper documentation:
- Entries are to be legible and written in black ink; all health information is recorded in permanent ink. Changes and additions are reviewed with the patient, and the patient signs or initials the documented information to verify its accuracy.
- All entries are to be signed or initialed.
- Entry errors are to be drawn through using a single line, accompanied by a notation stating, "Error in entry, see correction below," initialed by the person correcting the error, and dated at time of correction.
- Entries are to be uniformly spaced on the form (i.e., no unusual or irregular blank spaces).

Procedures specific to electronic documentation:
- Entry errors are to be accompanied by a notation stating, "Error in entry, see correction below," initialed by the person correcting the error, and dated at time of correction.
- A standardized protocol that includes daily backup of records and weekly transfer of records to an encrypted electronic database is to be used to ensure patient records are not altered.

Adapted from Saleeby JR. Communication and collaboration. In: Perry AG, Potter PA, Ostendorf W, eds. *Nursing Intervention and Clinical Skills.* 6th ed. Elsevier; 2016:12–34.

---

carvedilol (CAR-veh-DILL-ole)

Coreg

■♦■ **Dilatrend**

Drug Class: Alpha-adrenergic blocker; Beta-adrenergic blocker

PHARMACOLOGY

Action
Blocks alpha$_1$-receptors and nonselective beta-receptors to decrease BP.

Uses
Management of essential hypertension; treatment of mild to severe heart failure of ischemic or cardiomyopathic origin. Reduce cardiovascular mortality in clinically stable patients who have survived the acute phase of MI and have a left ventricular ejection fraction of 40% or less.

Unlabeled Uses
Angina pectoris.

➡◀ DRUG INTERACTIONS RELATED TO DENTAL THERAPEUTICS

COX-1 inhibitors: Decreased antihypertensive effect (decreased prostaglandin synthesis)
- Monitor blood pressure.

Sympathomimetic amines: Decreased antihypertensive effect (pharmacological antagonism)
- Use local anesthetic agents containing a vasoconstrictor with caution.
- Monitor blood pressure.

ADVERSE EFFECTS

⚠ **ORAL:** Periodontitis (1% to 3%); dry mouth.
CNS: Dizziness (32%); fatigue (24%); headache (8%); lung edema (for treatment of left ventricular dysfunction following MI [>3%]); somnolence, vertigo, hypesthesia, paresthesia, depression, insomnia (1% to 3%).
CVS: Bradycardia, postural hypotension, edema (2%).
GI: Diarrhea (12%); nausea (9%); vomiting (6%); melena, GI pain (1% to 3%).
RESP: Upper respiratory tract infection (18%); increased cough (8%); sinusitis, bronchitis (5%); rales (4%); dyspnea (for treatment of LVD following MI [>3%]).
MISC: Asthenia (11%); pain (9%); edema generalized, arthralgia (6%); edema dependent (4%); allergy, malaise, hypovolemia, fever, leg edema, infection, viral infection, back pain muscle cramps, arthritis, hypotonia, flu-like syndrome, peripheral vascular disorder (1% to 3%).

CLINICAL IMPLICATIONS

General
- Determine why drug is being taken. Consider implications of condition on dental treatment.
- Monitor vital signs (e.g., BP, pulse pressure, rate, and rhythm) at each appointment to assess disease control. Do not provide elective dental treatment when BP is ≥180/110 or in the presence of other high-risk CV conditions. Refer to the section entitled "The Patient Taking Cardiovascular Drugs" in Chapter 6: *Clinical Medicine.*
- Evaluate respiratory function.
- Use local anesthetic agents with vasoconstrictor with caution based on functional capacity of the patient and use aspirating technique to prevent intravascular injection.
- Beta blockers may mask epinephrine-induced signs and symptoms of hypoglycemia in patients with diabetes.
- Determine ability to adapt to stress of dental treatment. Consider short appointments.
- *Postural hypotension:* Monitor BP at the beginning and end of each appointment; anticipate syncope. Have patient sit upright for several min at the end of the dental appointment before dismissing.
- If GI or respiratory side effects occur, consider semisupine chair position.
- Chronic dry mouth is possible; anticipate increased caries, candidiasis, and lichenoid mucositis.

Oral Health Education
- If chronic dry mouth occurs, recommend home fluoride therapy and use of nonalcoholic oral health care products.
- Encourage daily plaque control procedures for effective self-care in patients at risk for cardiovascular disease.

Fig. 13.4 Illustration of information in dental drug reference with clinical implications. (From Pickett FA, Terezhalmy GT. *Lippincott Williams and Wilkins' Dental Drug Reference With Clinical Implications.* 2nd ed. Lippincott Williams and Wilkins; 2009.)

drug information including generic and brand names, drug action, indication for use, interactions with dental therapeutics, adverse effects, and clinical implications.

Prophylactic Antibiotic Premedication for the Prevention of Infective Endocarditis

Routine dental procedures such as professional prophylaxis and the administration of local anesthetics in areas of infection can introduce bacteremia into the bloodstream that can allow microorganisms to lodge on damaged or abnormal areas of the heart valves and underlying connective tissue. Infective endocarditis (IE) is a life-threatening infection of the tissue lining the heart.

Dental procedures for which antibiotic premedication may be beneficial for patients at highest risk include the manipulation of gingival and periapical tissues and the perforation of oral mucosa.

The AHA guidelines recommend prophylactic antibiotic premedication before such dental procedures for patients with the following: prosthetic cardiac valves or prosthetic material used for cardiac valve repair with device including annuloplasty, rings, chords, or clips; previous, relapse, or recurrent IE; unrepaired cyanotic congenital heart disease, including palliative shunts and conduits; congenital heart defects that have been completely repaired with prosthetic material or a device within the last 6 months (endothelialization of prosthetic material requires 6 months); repaired congenital heart disease with residual defects at or adjacent to the site of a prosthetic patch or prosthetic device; and recipients of cardiac transplantation who develop cardiac valvulopathy.[11]

Preventive measures are taken to avoid bacteremia and infection by administering prophylactic antibiotic premedication one-half to 1 hour before dental procedures. If the dose of antibiotic is inadvertently not administered before the procedure, the dose may be administered up to 2 hours after the procedure.[12] For this reason, some facilities keep a supply of antibiotics available to ensure that oral procedures can be provided with no delay when indicated. The theoretical rationale for administering prophylactic antibiotic premedication to prevent transient bacteremia from developing into IE is controversial.[12] Bacteremia is detectible after dental procedures and through common daily activities such as tooth brushing and chewing. Although a strong emphasis on prevention exists, the risk for contracting IE from dental procedures versus routine oral activities is unknown.

The standard prophylactic antibiotic premedication regimen for IE prevention recommended by the AHA is referenced in Table 13.4.[11] Individuals who are currently taking an antibiotic regimen should receive an antibiotic from a different class. For example, for a patient with a history of IE who would normally take amoxicillin for prophylactic antibiotic premedication but who is currently taking amoxicillin for another medical reason, azithromycin, doxycycline, or cephalexin can be administered. An alternate suggestion is to delay the dental procedure for 10 days after the completion of amoxicillin antibiotic therapy and administer a one-time dose of amoxicillin before the dental procedures. This 10-day period may allow for the usual oral flora to reestablish.

Current American Dental Association (ADA) guidelines no longer recommend the antibiotic clindamycin for dental prophylaxis or therapeutic use for patients with a history of penicillin allergies. This antibiotic is known to provoke more frequent and serious adverse reactions when compared to other prophylactic alternatives. Clindamycin

can cause *Clostridioides difficile* or *C. difficile*, a bacterial infection that induces diarrhea and colitis (an inflammation of the colon). Premedication guidelines are continuously being reviewed and updates can be found on the ADA Premedication webpage: https://www.ada.org/resources/research/science-and-research-institute/oral-health-topics/antibiotic-prophylaxis.

A complete assessment of the patient's drug history should be recorded in the patient's chart to include the identification of prescribed antibiotics, recommended doses, and times of administration to ensure that the antibiotic is taken within 2 hours of the appointment. The importance of patient education regarding the need for prophylactic antibiotic premedication for certain medical conditions before the initiation of dental hygiene procedures becomes a conscious effort on the part of the patient and clinician. Table 13.5 provides a summary of considerations for prescribing prophylactic antibiotic premedication.

TABLE 13.4 Prophylactic Antibiotic Premedication for a Dental Procedure (Single Dose 30 to 60 Minutes Before the Procedure)

Situation	Agent	Adults	Children
Oral	amoxicillin	2 g	50 mg/kg
Unable to take an oral medication	ampicillin or	2 g IV/IM	50 mg/kg IV/IM
	cefazolin or ceftriaxone	1 g IV/IM	50 mg/kg IV/IM
Allergic to penicillin or ampicillin and able to take an oral medication	cephalexin*†	2 g	50 mg/kg
	azithromycin or clarithromycin	500 mg	15 mg/kg
Allergic to penicillin or ampicillin and unable to take an oral medication	cefazolin or ceftriaxone†	1 g IM or IV	50 mg/kg IV/IM

*Or other first- or second-generation oral cephalosporin in equivalent adult or pediatric dose.
†Cephalosporins should not be taken by a person with a history of anaphylaxis, angioedema, or urticaria with penicillin or ampicillin.
IM, Intramuscular; *IV,* intravenous.
Data from Prevention of infective endocarditis: guidelines from the American Heart Association.[11]

TABLE 13.5 Considerations for Prescribing a Prophylactic Antibiotic Premedication

Management of Individuals Who Are at High Risk	Management Rationale
Use prophylactic antibiotics during the perioperative period (30 minutes to 1 hour before treatment) or within 2 hours after the appointment.	Use these measures to prevent infective endocarditis.
Establish and maintain optimal oral health.	Use these measures to prevent infective endocarditis and to improve the patient's oral health literacy.
Schedule appointments 10 days apart for procedures requiring antibiotic prophylaxis.	Reduce the emergence of resistant microorganisms. Allow for the repopulation of antibiotic-susceptible flora.
Administer an alternative prophylactic antibiotic therapy when: (a) Procedures are less than 9 days apart; or (b) The patient is currently taking antibiotics for another reason.	Reduce the emergence of resistant microorganisms.
Combine prophylaxis with other dental procedures during premedicated time frames.	Reduce the emergence of resistant microorganisms by reducing the number of premedicated dental visits.
Encourage full or partial denture wearers to have periodic oral examinations and return to their provider if discomfort develops.	Ill-fitting removable oral prostheses can cause tissue ulceration with concomitant bacteremia of oral origin.

Data from American Dental Association: 2017 Oral Health Topics: Antibiotic prophylaxis prior to dental procedures.[12]

BOX 13.3   Critical Thinking Scenario

Patient Profile: Mrs. Smith is a 52-year-old woman who has been referred for a periodontal evaluation.

Chief Complaint: "Facial swelling and gingival pain in the lower right quadrant"

Dental History: Mrs. Smith has avoided dental care for over 15 years until she recently developed facial swelling, pain, and a low-grade fever, which caused her to visit the emergency department over the weekend. The attending physician prescribed antibiotic therapy and pain medication for 1 week and referred Mrs. Smith to a general dentist for a complete periodontal evaluation. Mrs. Smith has rescheduled her initial evaluation appointment with the general dentist and dental hygienist several times because of work-related conflicts and her reluctance to seek dental care. It has been 1 month since her visit to the emergency department, and she arrives today with apprehension as the pain and swelling are gradually returning.

Health History: Mrs. Smith has a history of depression, hypertension, and type 2 diabetes. She manages her depression with Zoloft (sertraline hydrochloride, 25 mg once daily) and Accupril, an angiotensin-converting enzyme inhibitor that controls her hypertension and slows the progression of kidney damage associated with diabetes mellitus. Mrs. Smith's type 2 diabetes is controlled by daily insulin and diet. She is compliant in taking her medications as prescribed and sees her physician on a regular basis. She cannot recall her most recent hemoglobin A_{1c} (HbA_{1c}) test level or if she has experienced any hypoglycemic episodes. Her vital signs are within normal limits. In her health history questionnaire, she notes unpleasant experiences in the dental office—a probable cause for her dental anxiety.

Social History: Mrs. Smith is married with two grown children. She has worked for many years as an executive secretary.

Extraoral Examination: All findings are within normal limits.

Supplemental Notes: The patient arrives 30 minutes late for her 4:00 PM appointment. At 4:35 PM, the dental hygienist escorts her to the treatment room to review her health and dental history. The dental hygienist notices that Mrs. Smith appears anxious since she is clutching her purse and speaking very rapidly. The health history is reviewed, vital signs are measured, and no changes to the health history are recorded in the patient record. Consider the following questions when assessing Mrs. Smith:

1. What are Mrs. Smith's concerns for the dental visit? How would you prioritize her concerns with her dental needs?
2. What behavior modifications for the management of dental anxiety are warranted?
3. What questions should the dental hygienist ask Mrs. Smith regarding her medical conditions and medications to prevent a medical emergency?
4. What is Mrs. Smith's American Society of Anesthesiologists (ASA) classification and the protocol associated with this classification?
5. Does Mrs. Smith require prophylactic antibiotic premedication?
6. Due to Mrs. Smith's medical conditions, is a physician's consultation necessary before initiating treatment?
7. How would Mrs. Smith's medical conditions or medications alter the scheduling of her dental appointments and procedures (e.g., appointment time, meals)?
8. Due to Mrs. Smith's medical conditions, are any modifications to the selection or dose of the local anesthetic agent necessary (e.g., type of local anesthetic agent, cardiac dose)?

Treatments and Conditions Not Requiring Prophylactic Antibiotic Premedication

Prophylactic antibiotic premedication is not recommended when exposing dental radiographs, before initiating fluoride treatments, when placing removable prosthodontic appliances, before operative restorative dentistry (with or without a retraction cord, placement of rubber dams, postoperative suture removal, and taking of impressions), before adjusting or placing orthodontic appliances and brackets, before shedding of primary teeth, or when bleeding from trauma to the lips or oral mucosa is present.[11] The awareness of adverse events associated with the misuse and overuse of antibiotics, such as allergic reactions and increases in antibiotic-resistant microorganisms that exist worldwide, promotes careful consideration when prescribing prophylactic antibiotic premedication.

The American Academy of Orthopaedic Surgeons (AAOS) and the ADA do not recommend prophylactic antibiotic premedication, regardless of the procedure, for patients with prosthetic joint implants. The AHA and the ACC agree that maintaining good oral hygiene is an important precaution for all patients with prosthetic joints.[12] The evidence suggests that antibiotic prophylaxis is unwarranted in patients who have undergone a variety of surgical interventions such as stem cell transplant, organ transplant, ventriculoarterial and ventriculoperitoneal shunts, nonvascular devices including indwelling vascular catheters (e.g., central lines), cardiovascular implantable electronic devices (CIEDs), breast augmentation, and penile implants unless the person is predisposed to infection, in which case consulting the treating physician to prescribe the antibiotics may be appropriate. This guidance is also observed for patients with the following conditions: immunocompromised, immunosuppressed, inflammatory arthropathies (e.g., rheumatoid arthritis, systemic lupus erythematosus), drug-induced immunosuppression, radiation-induced immunosuppression, and comorbidities (e.g., previous prosthetic joint infections, malnourishment, hemophilia, HIV infection, type 1 diabetes, and malignancy). See Box 13.3.

Physician Consultation and Referral

The physician of record is consulted if the patient reveals a condition that may jeopardize safety during dental care. Medical consultations are initiated for the following:

- Conditions that may need prophylactic antibiotic premedication
- Suspicion of an undiagnosed or uncontrolled medical condition
- Abnormal vital signs (see Chapter 14)
- Precautionary treatment modifications (e.g., local anesthetics with reduced levels of vasoconstrictor (see Chapter 43)
- Person taking anticoagulant or blood-thinning medication (e.g., warfarin [Coumadin]).

Patients are referred for medical evaluation when a nonurgent but potentially undiagnosed condition is suspected (e.g., presence of hypertension or diabetes) or when needed laboratory test results are not available (e.g., blood test to determine the risk for excessive bleeding when warfarin is taken) (see Chapter 15). Urgent consultation with the referring physician is indicated if the client reveals a condition that precludes dental hygiene care or needs prompt dental or medical attention. Consultations should be documented in the patient's dental record and followed with a written consultation form (Fig. 13.5). To expedite the receipt of information, a request for the physician to send information electronically is recommended.

When requesting additional medical information from a patient's referring physician, the dental hygienist must obtain consent for information release from the patient before the request per HIPAA regulations. An entry in the treatment record should document to whom the medical request was sent and the reason for the request. Information

PHYSICIAN'S CONSULTATION FORM
Facility Name, Address, Phone and Fax Number

Date: _____

Patient's Name: _____ Birth Date: _____ Phone #: _____

Address: _____
Street   City   State   Zip

Physician's Name: _____ Phone #: _____ FAX #: _____

Address: _____
Street   City   State   Zip

I hereby authorize the release of medical information as requested. _____
Patient's Signature   Date

The above named patient is seeking dental care in our office. In order to provide the best care possible, it is necessary that we know the following information. The patient indicates a history of:

___ adrenal insufficiency or steroid therapy ___ chemotherapy/radiation therapy ___ leukemia ___ prescription diet drug (_____)
___ anemia ___ diabetes (type_____) ___ liver disease ___ pulmonary disease
___ anticoagulant therapy ___ heart murmur ___ Marfan's syndrome ___ renal dialysis with shunts
___ artificial prosthesis ___ hepatitis (type_____) ___ mitral valve prolapse ___ renal disease
(valvular, orthopedic, etc.) ___ HIV ___ myocardial infarction ___ rheumatic heart disease
___ by-pass surgery ___ hypertension ___ organ transplant ___ systemic lupus erythematosus
___ blood disorder ___ immunodeficiency ___ systemic pulmonary artery shunt
___ cardiovascular accident ___ pacemaker (type_____) ___ other:_____

Comments: _____

Treatment was postponed until an appropriate medical clearance, medical treatment and/or pre-medication could be obtained. The client has rescheduled an appointment for dental treatment on (Date) _____

SECTION 1 – MEDICAL HISTORY VERIFICATION
1. Do your records agree to what the patient has indicated? ☐ yes ☐ no
2. If not specify and comment: _____
3. ASA Status ☐ I ☐ II ☐ III ☐ IV
4. Diabetic – Acceptable Serum Glucose Range: _____
5. Hypertension – Acceptable Reading: _____
6. Hepatitis – Antigen/Antibody Status: _____
7. Other: _____

SECTION 2 – ANTIBIOTIC PRE-MEDICATION
1. Should this patient be pre-medicated with antibiotics prior to dental treatment? ☐ yes ☐ no
If yes, do you recommend the regimen of the American Heart Association or an alternative?
☐ AHA Regimen – Standard General Prophylaxis (amoxicillin 2.0 gm 1 hour before dental treatment)
☐ AHA Regimen – Penicillin Allergic Patient (clindamycin 600 mg 1 hour before dental treatment)
☐ Other, specify: _____
Comments: _____

SECTION 3 – MEDICAL RELEASE
1. ☐ This patient may receive dental hygiene care without limitations.
2. ☐ This patient may receive dental hygiene care with limitations.
Specify limitations: _____
3. ☐ This patient may not receive dental hygiene care at this time.

Physician's Signature _____ Date_____

Fig. 13.5 Sample physician's consultation form. (Adapted from and courtesy of Youngstown State University, Youngstown, Ohio.)

BOX 13.4 Patient or Client Education Tips

Educate patients regarding the following:
- Predispositions for medical emergencies occurring in the dental setting from information obtained in the patients' health history (e.g., counseling patients with diabetes mellitus to eat after taking medication before their dental appointment).
- Need for medical consultation before initiating dental procedures to avoid risks and emergency situations.
- Administration of prophylactic antibiotic premedication for certain medical conditions before initiating dental hygiene procedures.
- Importance of regular oral examinations to reduce the severity of oral disease and decrease the costs of oral care.
- Legal justification for dental-related activities, including an explanation of the issues of standards of care, scope of practice, and duty to the patient.
- Need to maintain accurate records of patient care to protect against health risks.

obtained from the patient's physician should be placed in the patient's dental record. A formal written request for medical consultation is the preferred procedure for medical-legal documentation. Consent may also be needed for a medical clearance before initiating dental care.

Referral

Initiating patient referrals for medical evaluations of an undiagnosed condition (e.g., presence of signs and symptoms of diabetes mellitus), for reassessment of a condition (e.g., high blood pressure), or for laboratory tests to determine health status before treatment (e.g., blood test to eliminate risks of excessive bleeding due to medications, chemotherapy, risk of infection) may be necessary in the delivery of dental care. Patients must understand the importance of maintaining communication between medical and dental providers to reduce risks and avoid emergency situations in the dental office. Box 13.4 provides additional information for patient education.

ACKNOWLEDGMENTS

The author acknowledges Frieda Atherton Pickett and Cara Miyaski for their past contributions to this chapter, as well as Dr. Devan Darby for her previous review.

KEY CONCEPTS

- The health history is a legal document containing protected information regarding the patient's health status.
- The dental hygienist–patient partnership is a patient-centered relationship based on trust and dedicated to the patient's overall well-being.
- The patient completes the written health history questionnaire during the first visit. The dental hygienist reviews, discusses, and verifies the information during the patient interview. At subsequent appointments, the health history is updated, and changes are investigated and documented in writing or electronically.
- The dental hygienist builds rapport during the health history interview by applying patient-centered interviewing techniques such as open-ended questioning, active listening and responding, and excellent verbal and nonverbal communication skills.
- The ASA physical status classification system categorizes patients who are medically *"at risk"* and determines the probability of medical emergencies in the dental setting. Only patients in the ASA I through III classifications should receive elective oral care.
- Stress reduction protocols can minimize the risk of medical emergencies and create a satisfactory experience for the anxious patient.
- Medical references, such as the *Physician's Desk Reference* (*PDR*), *Mosby's Dental Drug Reference,* the *Drug Information Handbook for Dentistry,* and the *Merck Manual of Diagnosis and Therapy*, are available to identify drug actions, interactions, contraindications, adverse reactions, oral health implication, and information on diseases.
- Infective endocarditis (IE) can be a life-threatening condition. Routine dental procedures including prophylaxis and administration of local anesthesia may place patients with certain heart conditions at risk for IE. Only patients at the highest risk for complications from IE should receive prophylactic antibiotic premedication before dental hygiene procedures.
- Patients with prosthetic joints or orthopedic implants do not require prophylactic antibiotics before dental procedures.
- The selection of prophylactic antibiotics is based on recommended guidelines, concurrently prescribed antibiotic agents, and patient tolerance of the medication.
- A patient may have an undiagnosed disease that can be recognized by a comprehensive health history review and observation of signs and reported symptoms. The health history review and physical assessment are monitors of a patient's health and risk status.

REFERENCES

1. Greene J, Ramos C. A mixed method examination of health care provider behaviors that build patients' trust. *Patient Ed Couns*. 2021;104(5):1222–1228.
2. Health Literacy. Updated October 1, 2021. Available at: https://www.cdc.gov/healthliteracy/. Accessed April 16, 2022.
3. Saleeby JR. Communication and collaboration. In: Perry AG, Potter PA, Ostendorf W, eds. *Nursing Intervention and Clinical Skills*. 6th ed. Elsevier, Inc.; 2016:12–34.
4. Summary of the HIPAA Privacy Rule. US Department of Health and Human Services, Office for Civil Rights. Updated March 31, 2022. Available at: https://www.hhs.gov/hipaa/for-professionals/privacy/laws-regulations. Accessed April 16, 2022.
5. American Society of Anesthesiologists (ASA). Physical status classification system. Updated December 13, 2020. Available at: https://www.asahq.org/resources/clinical-information/asa-physical-status-classification-system. Accessed April 16, 2022.
6. Heidenreich PA, Bozkurt, B, Aguilar, D., et al. 2022 ACC/AHA/HFSA guideline for the management of heart failure: Executive summary: A report of the American College of Cardiology/American Heart Association Joint Committee on Clinical Practice Guidelines. *Circulation*. 2022. Available at: https://www.ahajournals.org/doi/10.1161/CIR.0000000000001062. Accessed April 16, 2022.
7. *Physicians' Desk Reference*. 71st ed. PDR Network; 2017.
8. *Mosby's Dental Drug Reference*. 13th ed. Elsevier; 2022.
9. Wynn RL, Meiller TF, Crossley HL. *Drug Information Handbook for Dentistry*. 27th ed. LexiComp Wolters Kluwer; 2020.
10. Porter RS. *The Merck Manual of Diagnosis and Therapy*. 20th ed. Merck and Company; 2018.
11. American Heart Association Scientific Statement. *Prevention of Viridans Group Streptococcal Infective Endocarditis*; 2021. Available at: https://www.ahajournals.org/doi/pdf/10.1161/CIR.0000000000000969. Accessed April 16, 2022.
12. Sollecito TP, Abt E, Lockhart PB, et al. The use of prophylactic antibiotics prior to dental procedures in patients with prosthetic joints. *JADA*. 2015;146(1):11–16.

14

Vital Signs

Cara M. Miyasaki and Jennifer R. Leicht

PROFESSIONAL OPPORTUNITIES

Vital signs are often an indication of a patient's cardiovascular and overall health. A dental hygienist must be able to assess vital signs accurately as part of a comprehensive dental hygiene treatment. Patients may exhibit abnormal vital signs due to a variety of causes, including pathologic conditions and other external factors that may be unrelated to health. Patients may have dental appointments more frequently than medical appointments, which presents opportunities to screen patients for asymptomatic deviations in their vital signs. Therefore it is important to establish a baseline and monitor patients accordingly.

COMPETENCIES

1. Discuss vital signs and the importance of minimizing the risk of a medical emergency via vital signs assessment.
2. Discuss the significance of body temperature, assess and record body temperature, and make decisions based on observed body temperature.
3. Discuss the significance of pulse rate, assess and record pulse rate, and make decisions based on observed pulse rate.
4. Discuss the significance of respiration rate, assess and record respiration rate, and make decisions based on observed respiration rate.
5. Discuss the significance of blood pressure, assess and record blood pressure, and make decisions based on observed blood pressure.

VITAL SIGNS

Body temperature, pulse rate, respiration rate, and blood pressure are indicators of health status and are referred to as **vital signs**. Inspection, palpation, and **auscultation** (i.e., listening either directly or with a stethoscope for sounds produced in the body) are techniques used to determine vital signs. At the initial patient appointment, vital signs help identify undiagnosed medical conditions or establish baseline measurements for comparison at future appointments (Box 14.1). Box 14.2 lists appropriate occasions for the dental hygienist to measure and record the patient's vital signs.

Vital signs outside an acceptable range may indicate health problems or undiagnosed conditions, which could lead to the need for a referral to a physician or the need to postpone dental hygiene care. In addition, other factors can influence vital signs, such as illness, age, gender, medications, the temperature of the environment, altitude, body position, physical exertion, diet, stress, improperly used equipment, and unreliable equipment. Vital signs are analyzed to interpret their significance and make clinical decisions. If abnormal readings are obtained, the dental hygienist questions the patient about possible causes and repeats the measurement. When readings that have exceeded normal limits are validated, the dental hygienist communicates the findings to the patient, dentist, and physician of record (Box 14.3).

The following practice guidelines assist the dental hygienist in obtaining accurate vital signs:

- Use properly functioning and appropriate equipment that is designed for the size and age of the patient (e.g., an adult-size blood pressure cuff should not be used for a child or for a patient who is obese).
- Be familiar with the patient's baseline measurements, health status, and pharmacologic history. Some illnesses, treatments, behaviors, and medications can affect vital signs.
- Minimize environmental factors that may affect vital signs (e.g., allow patients to sit quietly for at least 5 minutes before taking blood pressure readings).
- Use a systematic approach for each procedure.
- Approach the patient in a calm, caring manner while demonstrating competence in measuring vital signs.
- Use critical thinking skills to determine when the dentist should be notified and whether a medical consultation is needed (Boxes 14.4 and 14.5).

BODY TEMPERATURE

Body **temperature** is regulated by the brain's hypothalamic area, which acts as the body's thermostat. The hypothalamus senses changes in temperature and sends impulses out to the body to correct them. On a hot day, the hypothalamus detects a rise in body temperature and signals the body to lower the body temperature (e.g., skin to perspire). In cold weather, the hypothalamus detects a lowering of the body's temperature and signals the body to increase the body temperature (e.g., to shiver). No single temperature is normal for all people. The normal range for body temperature is 97°F to 99.6°F (or 36.1°C to 37.5°C).

Maintaining body temperature requires a balance between heat loss and heat production. With aging, the normal temperature range gradually narrows because the mechanisms that control thermoregulation start to deteriorate.

Body Temperature Measurement Sites

Five sites are used to measure body temperature: oral, ear, rectal, axilla, and forehead. The infrared contact-free device, used to scan across the forehead, is generally accurate and easy to use since it is noninvasive. Digital oral devices are also accurate; however, caution should be taken to prevent inaccurate readings if hot or cold foods have been ingested (wait 20 to 30 minutes) or if the patient has been smoking. Alternative sites such as the tympanic membrane (ear) or axilla (armpit) should be used when the patient's safety is a consideration. For example, unconscious patients, infants, small children, or patients who are cognitively challenged may have difficulty with the oral thermometer under the tongue or may bite the thermometer and break it.

175

BOX 14.1   Vital Signs: Acceptable Ranges for Adults

Body Temperature[1]
Range: 97°F to 99.6°F (or 36.1°C to 37.5°C).

Pulse[2]
60 to 100 beats per minute

Respirations[2]
12 to 20 respirations per minute

Blood Pressure[2]
<120/<80 mm Hg

Adapted from Potter PA, Perry AG, Stockert P, Hall A. *Fundamentals of Nursing.* 11th ed. Elsevier Health Sciences (US); 2023.
Adapted from Malamed SF. *Medical Emergencies in the Dental Office.* 8th ed. Mosby; 2023.

BOX 14.2   When to Take Vital Signs

- At the initial appointment
- At every continued-care appointment (3-month, 4-month, 6-month, 12-month recall appointments) for a patient whose vital signs are within normal limits
- Whenever a significant change occurs in the patient's health history
- At each appointment for a patient with readings that fall outside the normal limits but who is being monitored by a physician
- When a patient is taking a medication that can affect blood pressure and/or when a patient has a condition that indicates a need for monitoring blood pressure (e.g., a pregnant woman)
- Before the administration of a local anesthetic agent, nitrous oxide–oxygen analgesia, or any other medication that could affect cardiovascular and respiratory regulation and after administering nitrous oxide
- Before, during, and after surgical procedures
- When the patient makes statements about feeling physically ill
- If the patient reports symptoms that indicate a potential emergency situation or when a medical emergency is in progress

BOX 14.3   Legal, Ethical, and Safety Issues

When abnormal vital signs are detected, the patient should be informed of the actual reading; however, the dental hygienist should refrain from diagnosing systemic conditions based solely on vital signs taken in the clinical setting. Ensure that the patient is referred to a primary healthcare provider of record for medical consultation when vital signs exceed normal ranges. Include copies of the referral letter in the patient's chart for access and confirmation.

BOX 14.4   Client or Patient Education Tips

- Inform the patient when abnormal vital signs are present; ensure that the patient is referred to a primary healthcare provider physician referral when appropriate.
- Encourage compliance with recommended primary healthcare provider referrals and prescriptive medications to control abnormal vital signs.
- Explain risk factors for abnormal vital signs (e.g., patients with high blood pressure may have no overt symptoms yet be at increased risk for cardiac arrest and stroke).

Thermometers

Many types of **thermometers** are available for measuring body temperature. The **mercury-in-glass thermometer** is no longer the standard of care and is no longer recommended because of the environmental hazard of mercury. Digital thermometers are commonly used at home and in professional practice.

Digital thermometers consist of a probe or infrared scanner attached to an electronic display (Figs. 14.1 and 14.2) to measure oral, axillary, tympanic membrane, and superficial temporal (forehead)

BOX 14.5   Legal, Ethical, and Safety Issues

- The dental hygienist is following the ethical principles of integrity and nonmaleficence (do no harm) by ensuring vital signs are taken when necessary. By properly using the equipment and following standard procedures, the dental hygienist is following the ethical principle of competence and professionalism.
- The dental hygienist must be sensitive to diverse patient cultures, beliefs, and preferred gender identities (see Chapter 6). Describe the procedure to the patient before performing it, especially when there will be physical contact. Some cultures prefer a same-sex care provider, and a language barrier may necessitate a family member's presence for moral support and translation assistance.

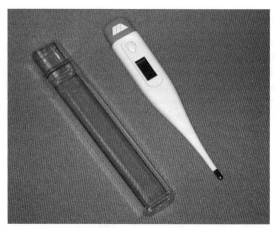

Fig. 14.1 Electronic (digital) thermometer. (Courtesy Sedation Resource, Lone Oak, TX. www.sedationresource.com.)

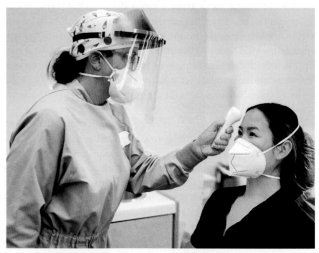

Fig. 14.2 Infrared contact-free digital thermometer measuring temperature on forehead.

artery temperatures. When an oral thermometer is placed in the mouth, a disposable plastic sheath is used over the oral probe as a protective barrier for infection control. A pacifier thermometer, a type of digital thermometer, obtains a reasonably accurate reading in young children within 3 minutes. Axillary digital thermometers have a short reading time (8 to 30 seconds) and are easy to use in young children. Tympanic membrane thermometers are easy to use, are less invasive, and achieve a reading within seconds, but they may not be as reliable as other assessment devices. Oral, axillary, and superficial temporal artery thermometers can indicate a patient's body temperature within seconds. Disposable single-use thermometers are primarily used for oral temperature screening. The body temperature is recorded in degrees Fahrenheit.

Decision Making Based on Observed Body Temperature

A thermometer should be available in case there is a need to take a patient's temperature. Usually, an elevated body temperature (known as fever or pyrexia) indicates that the body is fighting an infection. For elective dental treatment, the patient should be rescheduled if a fever is suspected. If the infection is not dentally related, then a referral for medical evaluation by the patient's primary healthcare provider may be indicated. If the fever is due to a dental infection, then immediate dental treatment and antibiotic therapy may be indicated.

PULSE

The **pulse**, an indicator of the integrity of the cardiovascular system, is the intermittent beat of the heart felt through the walls of an artery. **Tachycardia** (above 100 beats per minute [bpm]) is an abnormally elevated heart rate; however, it is a normal response to stress or physical exercise. **Bradycardia** (below 60 bpm) is an abnormally slow heart rate (Table 14.1). Athletes may be bradycardic at rest as a result of physical conditioning. Table 14.2 describes factors that influence pulse rate.

Pulse Rate Measurement Sites

Pulse points are body sites where the rhythmic beats of an artery can be felt. The most common site for assessing the **radial pulse** is on the thumb side of the inner wrist, where the radial artery can be felt (Fig. 14.3 and Procedure 14.1 and the corresponding Competency Form). The clinician's fingertips of the first two fingers are used to feel for the pulse (a throbbing sensation). (*Note:* Never use the thumb to feel for the pulse because it has a pulse of its own that can be mistaken for

the patient's pulse.) If the radial pulse cannot be felt, the carotid pulse, located on the side of the neck over the carotid artery, is an alternative site. In emergency situations, the carotid pulse should be palpated because the body delivers blood to the brain for as long as possible, whereas peripheral blood supply can decline. The pulse is recorded in beats per minute. Heart rhythm (regular or irregular) and pulse quality (thready, strong, bounding, or weak) also are assessed when the pulse is measured (Box 14.6).

Decision Making Based on Observed Pulse Rate

If the adult patient's heart rate falls below 60 bpm or rises above 100 bpm, the patient should be evaluated for causative factors or conditions. If no cause can be determined, a medical consultation with the patient's physician should be conducted. A medical consultation is recommended in the following circumstances:

- Occasional **premature ventricular contractions** (PVCs), defined as a break in the rhythm of the beats, are common and can be caused by smoking, fatigue, certain medications, stress, caffeine, and alcohol. Occasional PVCs in an otherwise healthy person are not usually a concern; however, if the patient experiences frequent symptoms, a medical referral should be initiated.
- **Pulsus alternans**, defined as alternating strong and weak heartbeats, may indicate ventricular failure.
  See Box 14.7.

RESPIRATION RATE

Respiration rate is assessed by counting the rise and fall (i.e., inspiration and expiration) of the patient's chest and is recorded as respirations

TABLE 14.1 Acceptable Ranges of Heart (Pulse) Rate	
Age	**Heart Rate (Beats per Minute)**
Infant	120–160
Toddler	90–140
Preschooler	80–110
School-age child	75–100
Adolescent	60–90
Adult	60–100

Adapted from Potter PA, Perry AG, Stockert P, Hall A. *Fundamentals of Nursing.* 11th ed. Elsevier Health Sciences (US); 2023.

TABLE 14.2 Factors That Influence Pulse (Heart) Rate		
Factor	**Increases Pulse Rate**	**Decreases Pulse Rate**
Exercise	Short-term exercise	A heart conditioned by long-term exercise, resulting in a lower heart rate at rest and a quicker return to resting level after exercise
Temperature	Fever and heat	Hypothermia
Emotions	Acute pain and anxiety increase sympathetic stimulation, affecting heart rate	Effect of chronic pain on heart rate varies; unrelieved severe pain increases parasympathetic stimulation, decreasing heart rate
Medications	Positive chronotropic drugs (e.g., epinephrine)	Negative chronotropic drugs (e.g., digitalis, beta-blockers, calcium blockers)
Hemorrhage	Loss of blood increases sympathetic stimulation	
Postural changes	Standing or sitting	Lying down
Pulmonary conditions	Diseases causing poor oxygenation such as asthma, chronic obstructive pulmonary disease (COPD)	

From Potter PA, Perry AG, Stockert P, Hall A. *Fundamentals of Nursing.* 11th ed. Elsevier Health Sciences (US); 2023.

per minute (rpm). The dental hygienist makes this assessment without the patient's awareness to prevent the patient from changing breathing patterns.

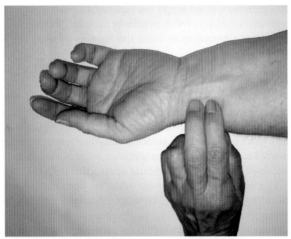

Fig. 14.3 Position of the fingers in measuring the radial pulse.

Respiration Rate Measurement Site

Respiration rate may be measured before or after the patient's pulse rate is assessed. The dental hygienist's hand remains on the patient's radial pulse while the hygienist inconspicuously counts the rise and fall of the patient's chest.

The normal adult range is 12 to 20 rpm. Children have a more rapid respiratory rate (20 to 30 rpm) than adults. Infants and young children also tend to have a less regular breathing cycle. Advancing age produces variations in the respiration rate. Steps for measuring respirations are shown in Procedure 14.2 and the corresponding Competency Form.

Decision Making Based on Observed Respiration Rate

Alterations in the rate, depth, or rhythm should be noted. If an abnormal respiratory rate is detected, the dental hygienist refers the patient

---

BOX 14.6   Legal, Ethical, and Safety Issues

Always record the patient's vital signs on the treatment record and refer to the patient's baseline readings for comparison. These should be routinely performed at continued care appointments and at each appointment when indicated by the patient's health and pharmacologic history.

BOX 14.7   Critical Thinking Scenario A

The dental hygienist takes the patient's pulse several times. The patient reports an increase in the frequency of fluttering or flip-flops in the chest. The findings are discussed with the patient, and the patient is resistant to seeing a physician concerning the problem. Role play with a partner to demonstrate how to manage this situation effectively.

PROCEDURE 14.1   Measuring the Radial Pulse

Equipment
Timer with a seconds display
Pen
Patient record
Vital signs chart

Steps
1. Use a timer with a seconds display.
2. Perform hand hygiene.
3. Explain the purpose and method of the procedure to the patient. Advise the patient to relax and not to speak.
4. Ask the patient to assume a sitting position, bend the patient's elbow 90°, and support the patient's lower arm on the armrest of the chair. Extend the wrist with the palm up.
5. Place the first two fingers of your hand along the patient's radial artery (thumb side of wrist), and lightly compress (Fig. 14.3).
6. Obliterate the pulse initially, then relax the pressure so that the pulse is easily palpable.
7. Determine the rhythm and quality of the pulse—regular, irregular, full and strong, weak and thready.
8. When the pulse can be regularly felt, use the timer and begin to count the rate, starting with 0 and then 1, and so on.
9. If the pulse is regular, count for 30 seconds and multiply the total by 2.
10. If the pulse is irregular, count for 1 full minute.
11. Record heart rate (beats per minute [bpm]), rhythm of the heart (regular or irregular), quality of the pulse (thready, strong, weak, bounding), and the date in the chart. Pulse rates outside the normal range should be evaluated by the patient's physician.
12. Document completion of this service in the patient's record under "Services Rendered." Record heart rate (bpm), rhythm of the heart (regular, regularly irregular, or irregularly irregular), the quality of the pulse (thready and weak [not easily felt], strong and full [easily felt]), and the date in the record. For example: "The patient's pulse taken on 08/01/2024 has a regular rhythm and strong quality with rate of 65 bpm."

Data from Potter PA, Perry AG, Stockert P, Hall A. *Fundamentals of Nursing.* 11th ed. Elsevier Health Sciences (US); 2023.

PROCEDURE 14.2   Measuring Respirations

Equipment
Timer with a seconds display
Pen
Patient record
Vital signs chart

Steps
1. Use a timer with a seconds display.
2. Place a hand along the patient's radial artery and inconspicuously observe the patient's chest before or after taking the patient's pulse rate.
3. Observe the rise and fall of the patient's chest. Count complete respiratory cycles (one inspiration and one expiration).
4. For an adult, count the number of respirations in 30 seconds and multiply that number by 2. For a young child, count respirations for a full minute.
5. If an adult has respirations with an irregular rhythm or if respirations are abnormally slow or fast (<12 or >20 respirations per minute [rpm]), count for a full minute.
6. While counting, note whether depth is shallow, normal, or deep, and whether rhythm is normal or one of the altered patterns.
7. Document in the patient record the completion of this service under "Services Rendered." Record the date and the patient's respiration rate in the record, for example: "The patient's respiration rate taken on 08/01/2024 has a regular rhythm with rate of 18 rpm." A respiration rate with an irregular pattern or that is outside of the normal range should be evaluated by the physician.

Data from Potter PA, Perry AG, Stockert P, Hall A. *Fundamentals of Nursing.* 11th ed. Elsevier Health Sciences (US); 2023.

to the physician of record for a medical evaluation. Table 14.3 provides acceptable ranges of respiratory rates by age. **Tachypnea** (rapid breathing) greater than 20 rpm may indicate restrictive lung disease or inflammation of the lungs. An increase in breathing rate and depth could be associated with physical exercise, anxiety, or metabolic acidosis. A deep and labored breathing pattern is associated with diabetic ketoacidosis (Kussmaul respirations). Obstructed breathing from narrowed airways may occur with asthma, chronic bronchitis, congestive heart disease, and chronic obstructive pulmonary disease.

BLOOD PRESSURE

Blood pressure, the force exerted by the blood against the arterial walls when the heart contracts, is an important indicator of current cardiovascular function and a risk indicator of future cardiovascular morbidity and mortality. Chronic **hypertension** causes thickening and loss of elasticity in the arterial walls, which can lead to myocardial infarction (heart attack), heart failure, stroke, and kidney disease. **Hypotension** (low blood pressure) is not dangerous unless the patient has noticeable chronic signs and symptoms, or if the patient is in a state of shock or is affected by a disorder or condition that lowers the blood pressure. In fact, the lower the blood pressure, the better the long-term prognosis for cardiovascular health. An acute change in blood pressure can indicate an emergency situation, such as shock or rapid hemorrhaging (Box 14.8).[1,2]

Blood pressure is measured in millimeters of mercury (mm Hg). The two measurements taken for blood pressure are systolic blood pressure and diastolic blood pressure:

- **Systolic blood pressure** measures the maximum pressure occurring in the blood vessels during cardiac ventricular contraction (systole) and is the number on the **sphygmomanometer** (blood pressure cuff) when the first heart sound is heard.[1,2]
- **Diastolic blood pressure** measures the minimum pressure occurring against the arterial walls as a result of cardiac ventricular relaxation (diastole) and is the number on the sphygmomanometer when the last heart sound is heard.[1,2]

When documenting blood pressure, the dental hygienist records the date and arm used. Blood pressure is recorded as a fraction. The optimal systolic and diastolic measurements for adults 18 years of age and older are less than 120 and less than 80 mm Hg, respectively. The first reading of a given blood pressure is the systolic measurement, and the second reading is the diastolic measurement. Multiple consistent readings need to be taken in order to demonstrate the patient's blood pressure. The blood pressure is considered to be elevated if the systolic blood pressure is 120 to 129 mm Hg and the diastolic blood pressure is less than 80 mm Hg. A patient is considered hypertensive stage 1 if the systolic blood pressure is 130 to 139 mm Hg or the diastolic blood pressure is 80 to 89 mm Hg. A patient is considered hypertensive stage 2 if the systolic blood pressure is equal to or greater than 140 mm Hg or the diastolic blood pressure is equal to or greater than 90 mm Hg. A **hypertensive crisis** is a systolic blood pressure greater than 180 mm Hg and/or a diastolic blood pressure greater than 120 mm Hg (consult a medical doctor immediately).[3] Children and adolescents should be screened for hypertension as well. Table 14.4 lists blood pressures for different ages of children and adolescents that require further evaluation. Table 14.5 describes factors that influence blood pressure.[1,4]

Decision Making Based on Observed Blood Pressure

Hypertension is the major cause of stroke and is a contributing factor to myocardial infarction (Table 14.6).[5] An elevated blood pressure (systolic of 120 to 129 mm Hg or diastolic of lower than 80 mm Hg) identifies patients who are likely to develop high blood pressure unless steps are taken to control it, such as adopting a healthier lifestyle and being reassessed in 3 to 6 months. Patients who have elevated blood pressure are usually not candidates for drug therapy unless risk factors for hypertension (e.g., diabetes and kidney disease) are present and only

---

TABLE 14.3 Acceptable Ranges of Respiratory Rate According to Age

Age	Rate (Respirations per Minute)
Newborn	30–60
Infant (6 months)	30–50
Toddler (2 years)	25–32
Child	20–30
Adolescent	16–20
Adult	12–20

Adapted from Potter PA, Perry AG, Stockert P, Hall A. *Fundamentals of Nursing.* 11th ed. Elsevier Health Sciences (US); 2023.

BOX 14.8 Critical Thinking Scenario B

The dental hygienist takes the patient's blood pressure and obtains a reading of 126/90 mm Hg in the right arm. The dental hygienist measures the blood pressure again in 5 minutes, and the blood pressure is 110/70 mm Hg in the right arm. What circumstances could have caused the differences observed in the two readings? Discuss how the problem could be prevented in the future.

TABLE 14.4 Normal Vital Sign Ranges at Various Ages

Age	Heart Rate (Beats/Min)	Blood Pressure (mm Hg)	Respiratory Rate (Breaths/Min)
Premature	120–170	55–75/35–45	40–70
0–3 months	100–150	65–85/45–55	35–55
3–6 months	90–120	70–90/50–65	30–45
6–12 months	80–120	80–100/55–65	25–40
1–3 years	70–110	90–105/55–70	20–30
3–6 years	65–110	95–110/60–75	20–25
6–12 years	60–95	100–120/60–75	14–22
12+ years	55–85	110–135/65–85	12–20

Modified from: Malamed SF. *Medical Emergencies in the Dental Office.* 8th ed. Mosby; 2023.

TABLE 14.5 Factors Influencing Blood Pressure

Factors	Effects
Age	Blood pressure rises with age. Newborns have the lowest mean systolic blood pressure (65 to 115/42 to 80 mm Hg). As people age, elasticity in the arteries declines, producing an increase in blood pressure (>55 years for men and >65 years for women).
Race	The prevalence of hypertension in African, Hispanic, or Native Americans is considerably higher than in the White population, and hypertension tends to appear earlier in life in these groups.
Weight	Blood pressure tends to be elevated in individuals who are overweight and obese. Oversized blood pressure cuffs are necessary for accurate readings.
Gender	Hormonal variation causes women to have lower blood pressure after puberty than men; however, postmenopausal women tend to have higher blood pressure than men of similar age. Preeclampsia is abnormal hypertension experienced by some women during pregnancy.
Emotional stress	Stress stimulates the sympathetic nervous system which, in turn, increases cardiac output and vasoconstriction. The outcome is elevated blood pressure.
Severe pain	Pain decreases blood pressure and, if severe, can cause shock.
Oral contraceptives	These agents can increase blood pressure by a small but detectable amount. If not within normal limits, blood pressure should be monitored on a regular basis.
Exercise	After exercise, blood pressure is increased for the first 30 minutes, followed by a decrease.
Eating	A decrease of 5 to 10 mm Hg in blood pressure can occur in older adults 1 hour after eating.
Medications	Medications vary in their ability to increase and decrease blood pressure. Medications must be reviewed at each appointment to determine their effects on blood pressure.
Diurnal variation	Blood pressure varies with metabolic rate. Pressure is lowest in the morning, then rises and peaks in the late afternoon or early evening.
Chronic disease	Diseases that affect cardiac output, blood volume, blood viscosity, or arterial elasticity, which will increase blood pressure.
Tobacco, alcohol, and caffeine use	Elevates blood pressure.
High fat and saturated fat intake	High blood cholesterol, especially high low-density lipoprotein (LDL) cholesterol, and high triglycerides cause atherosclerosis which, in turn, can cause an increase in blood pressure.
Dehydration	Accompanied by sudden changes in posture (lying to standing) can cause orthostatic or postural hypotension.
White-coat hypertension (isolated office hypertension)	Approximately 15% to 30% of patients with stage 1 hypertension may have elevated blood pressure in the presence of a healthcare worker, especially a physician.[4] Consistent measurements require annual blood pressure monitoring with a physician or home blood pressure monitoring for means of comparison.

Muntner P, Shimbo D, Carey RM, et al. Measurement of blood pressure in humans: a scientific statement from the American Heart Association. *Hypertension.* 2019;73(5):e35–e66. https://doi.org/10.1161/HYP.0000000000000087.
Adapted from Potter PA, Perry AG, Stockert P, Hall A. *Fundamentals of Nursing.* 11th ed. Elsevier Health Sciences (US); 2023.

TABLE 14.6 Healthy and Unhealthy Blood Pressure Readings

Blood Pressure Classification	Systolic Blood Pressure (mm Hg)	and/or	Diastolic Blood Pressure (mm Hg)
Normal	Less than 120	and	Less than 80
Elevated	120–129	and	Less than 80
Stage 1 hypertension	130–139	or	80–89
Stage 2 hypertension	140 or Higher	or	90 or Higher
Hypertensive crisis (urgency and emergency)	Higher than 180	and/or	Higher than 120

American Heart Association. Understand Symptoms and Risk of High Blood Pressure. Available at: https://www.heart.org/en/health-topics/high-blood-pressure/understanding-blood-pressure-readings. Accessed July 2022.

after lifestyle modifications have failed to reduce the blood pressure to normal levels. A medical consultation is indicated for persons with abnormal blood pressure (Table 14.7) before administering dental or dental hygiene care (Box 14.9).[3,5]

If the patient's blood pressure is unknown, a baseline blood pressure should be obtained by using the auscultatory method for aneroid manometers (see the text under Sphygmomanometer [Blood Pressure Cuff]). Patients in hypertension-prone groups or those who are taking medications that affect blood pressure should have their blood pressure measured at each dental or dental hygiene appointment. The use of epinephrine for hypertensive patients has minimal effect; however, caution should be taken with uncontrolled hypertensive patients before any surgical procedure (see Chapter 43).

Blood Pressure Equipment and Measurement
Sphygmomanometer (Blood Pressure Cuff)
The **sphygmomanometer** consists of a pressure-measuring device called a *manometer* and an inflatable cuff that wraps around the arm or leg. Portable and lightweight, the **aneroid manometer** is used to assess blood pressure; it has a glass-enclosed circular gauge containing a needle that registers millimeter calibrations. Aneroid manometers require periodic biomedical calibration to ensure their accuracy. The **mercury manometer** is an upright tube containing mercury and was considered the standard for blood pressure measurement. However, the mercury in the manometer poses a health hazard and is no longer

TABLE 14.7   Guidelines for Blood Pressure for Adults for Use in the Dental Hygiene Process of Care

Systolic Blood Pressure (mm Hg)		Diastolic Blood Pressure (mm Hg)	Dental Hygiene Therapy Considerations
<120	and	<80	Routine dental treatment is permitted No unusual precautions related to patient management based on BP readings are needed
120–139	and/or	80–89	Recheck in 5 minutes Routine dental treatment is permitted Implement stress-reduction protocols
140–180	and/or	90–120	Recheck in 5 minutes If still elevated, medical consultation needed prior to dental treatment
≥180	and/or	≥120	Refer to hospital if immediate dental therapy indicated

Adapted from Malamed SF. *Medical Emergencies in the Dental Office.* 8th ed. Mosby; 2023.

BOX 14.9   Critical Thinking Scenario C

Ethics

A patient has arrived for his first office visit and his blood pressure is above normal treatment limits. You have taken his vital signs several times and have determined that no extraneous factors could be affecting the patient's blood pressure. The Physical Status Classification System developed by the American Society of Anesthesiologists (ASA) categorizes a patient with this elevated level of blood pressure as an ASA IV, which indicates the need for a medical consultation before elective dental treatment. You consult the dentist and inform the patient of the need for medical clearance before treatment. The patient states that his blood pressure is always elevated, and his physician considers the readings "normal" for him. The patient insists on continuing with treatment. What emergency is most likely to happen with high blood pressure? What are the ethical implications of continuing with treatment?

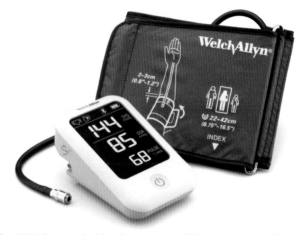

Fig. 14.5 Automatic blood pressure cuff for home use. (Courtesy Welch Allyn, Inc., Skaneateles, NY.)

BOX 14.10   Patient Conditions Not Appropriate for Electronic Blood Pressure Measurement

- Irregular heart rate
- Peripheral vascular obstruction (e.g., clots, narrowed vessels)
- Shivering
- Seizures
- Excessive tremors
- Inability to cooperate

From Potter PA, Perry AG, Stockert P, Hall A. *Fundamentals of Nursing.* 11th ed. Elsevier Health Sciences (US); 2023.

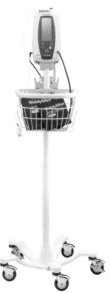

Fig. 14.4 Hospital-grade mobile aneroid blood pressure unit. (Courtesy Welch Allyn, Inc., Skaneateles, NY.)

recommended. An **electronic hospital-grade blood pressure device** (Fig. 14.4) is accurate and can also provide pulse rate and oxygen saturation levels.

The **electronic over-the-counter-type manometer** for home use automatically determines blood pressure (Fig. 14.5) without the use of a stethoscope. Electronic devices are sensitive to outside interference such as patient movement or noise. Such factors interfere with the manometer's sensor signal. An electronic over-the-counter manometer can easily become inaccurate and should be recalibrated more than once a year. This manometer is not appropriate for patients with certain conditions (Box 14.10). Regardless of whether the equipment is aneroid or electronic, the equipment should be recalibrated for accuracy every 1 to 2 years. Recalibration can be accomplished by comparing blood pressure readings with a calibrated model.

Parts of a manometer are similar, regardless of the type, and include an occlusive cloth cuff that encloses an inflatable rubber bladder and a pressure bulb with a release valve that inflates the bladder. Large adult cuffs, thigh cuffs, and pediatric sizes are also available. Proper cuff size is necessary for accurate blood pressure readings. The cuff size selected is proportional to the circumference of the upper arm being assessed. The recommended cuff width should be 20% more than the upper arm diameter.

In an adult, the bladder within the cuff should encircle at least 80% of the arm, and it should circle the entire arm of a child (Fig. 14.6). Patients with muscular arms who have prominent biceps or obese individuals require the use of a large adult cuff. Using a cuff on the forearm of a large adult is not recommended as it can lead to a higher systolic reading of up to 20 mm Hg.[6] Although cuffs may be labeled newborn, infant, child, small adult, and large adult, the practitioner should not rely on patient age as the basis for cuff selection. False readings can occur with faulty equipment and poor techniques (Tables 14.8 and 14.9).

Stethoscope

The **stethoscope**, an instrument used to amplify sound, consists of two earpieces, binaurals, plastic or rubber tubing, and a chestpiece. The

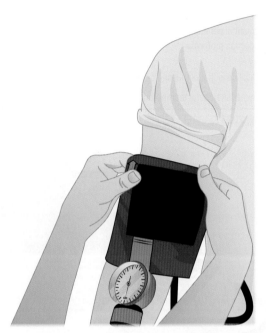

Fig. 14.6 In an adult, the bladder within the cuff should encircle at least 80% of the arm. (From Bonewit-West. *Clinical Procedures for Medical Assistants.* 11th ed. St Louis: Elsevier, Inc.; 2024.)

TABLE 14.8   Primary Types of Manometers Used in Blood Pressure Measurement

Name	Advantages	Disadvantages
Hospital-grade mobile aneroid blood pressure unit	Can be used on most patients Good reliability	Cost
Aneroid sphygmomanometer	Lightweight Portable Compact	Must be recalibrated Requires clinical skill
Electronic sphygmomanometer	Easy to use Stethoscope not required	Must be recalibrated Sensitive to outside interference Susceptible to error

Adapted from Medicines and Healthcare Products Regulatory Agency (MHRA): Blood Pressure Measurement Devices, 2019. https://assets.publishing.service.gov.uk/government/uploads/system/uploads/attachment_data/file/841944/BP_monitoring_2019_v2.2.pdf. Accessed June 2020.

TABLE 14.9   Common Mistakes in Blood Pressure Assessment

Effect	Error
False high readings	Bladder or cuff is too small, too narrow, or too short. Cuff is wrapped too loosely or unevenly. Cuff is deflated too slowly (produces a false high diastolic reading). Arm is below the heart level. Arm is not supported and should not be held by patient. Cuff is inflated too slowly. Assessments are repeated too quickly (produces a false high systolic reading). Bladder not fully deflated before beginning measurement. Patient is talking. Back and feet are unsupported. Legs are crossed. Patient is not resting quietly for 3–5 minutes before assessment.
False low readings	Failure to identify the auscultatory gap. Bladder or cuff is too wide. Arm is above the heart level. Stethoscope is pressed too firmly (produces a false low diastolic reading). Inflation level is inadequate (produces a false low systolic reading).
False high or false low readings	Multiple examiners use different Korotkoff sounds (produces a false high systolic reading and a false low diastolic reading). Stethoscope fits poorly or the examiner's hearing impairment causes the sounds to be muffled (produces a false low systolic reading and a false high diastolic reading). Cuff is deflated too quickly (produces a false low systolic reading and a false high diastolic reading). Cuff is over clothing.

Adapted from Muntner P, Shimbo D, Carey RM, et al. Measurement of blood pressure in humans: a scientific statement from the American Heart Association. *Hypertension.* 2019;73(5):e35–e66. https://doi.org/10.1161/HYP.0000000000000087.

chestpiece has two sides, the bell and the diaphragm (Fig. 14.7; Box 14.11).

When the bladder within the occluding cuff is deflated, the blood begins to flow intermittently through the brachial artery (Fig. 14.8),

producing rhythmic, knocking sounds. These sounds are referred to as **Korotkoff** (ko-rot-kof) **sounds**. As the cuff is deflated further, the Korotkoff sounds become less audible, and the pulse eventually disappears. See Fig. 14.9 for the five Korotkoff sounds described in phases.

An **auscultatory gap**, a period of abnormal silence that occurs between the Korotkoff phases, can occur when measuring blood pressure in older patients with a wide pulse pressure. This gap usually appears between the first and second systolic sounds. Failure to recognize the auscultatory gap results in an underestimation of the systolic pressure. Therefore it is important that the dental hygienist use palpation to assess the point at which the pulse is obliterated (the systolic reading) while increasing the pressure in the bladder before taking the blood pressure by auscultation. Moreover, the clinician should increase the bladder pressure 30 mm Hg higher than the point at which the pulse is obliterated when measuring blood pressure (Procedure 14.3 and the corresponding Competency Form). Once taken, blood pressure should be documented in writing and dated in the patient's chart under services rendered (e.g., "8/1/2024—Blood pressure in right arm, 160/90 mm Hg with auscultatory gap between 160 and 120 mm Hg") (Boxes 14.12 and 14.13).

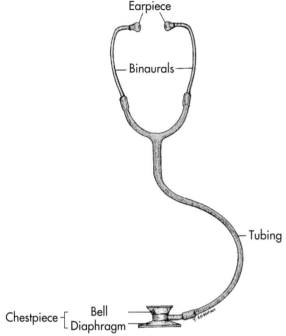

Fig. 14.7 Parts of a stethoscope. (From Potter PA, Griffin AG, Stockert P, et al. *Fundamentals of Nursing.* 9th ed. Mosby; 2017.)

BOX 14.11 Legal, Ethical, and Safety Issues

Disinfect the earpiece of the stethoscope before and after its use to avoid disease transmission.

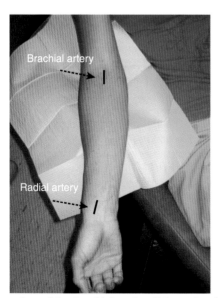

Fig. 14.8 Location of the brachial and radial arteries. The brachial artery is located on the medial half of the antecubital fossa, whereas the radial artery is on the lateral volar aspect of the wrist. (From Malamed SF. *Medical Emergencies in the Dental Office.* 7th ed. Mosby; 2015.)

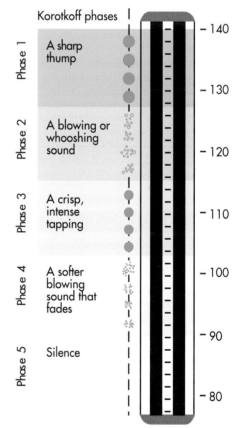

Fig. 14.9 The sounds auscultated during blood pressure measurement can be differentiated into five Korotkoff phases. In this example, blood pressure is 140/90 mm Hg. A scale ranging from 80 to 140 shows five Korotkoff phases as follows:

Phase 1: A sharp thump between 127 and 140.
Phase 2: A blowing or whooshing sound between 115 and 127.
Phase 3: A crisp, intense tapping between 103 and 115.
Phase 4: A softer blowing sound that fades between 90 and 103.
Phase 5: Silence between 80 and 90.

Note: Data is approximate.

(From Potter PA, Perry AG, Stockert P, Hall A. *Fundamentals of Nursing.* 11th ed. Elsevier Health Sciences (US); 2023.)

PROCEDURE 14.3 Assessing Blood Pressure by Auscultation

Equipment
Blood pressure cuff or sphygmomanometer
Stethoscope
Pen
Patient record
Vital signs chart

Steps
1. Allow the patient to sit quietly for at least 5 minutes with their back and feet supported (legs uncrossed).
2. Ask the patient about recent activities that could alter the patient's normal blood pressure. Avoid assessing blood pressure if the patient has ingested caffeine, smoked or used other nicotine products, or exercised within the last 30 minutes.
3. Determine the proper cuff size. Inspect the parts of the release valve and the pressure bulb. The valve should be clean and freely movable in either direction.
4. Perform hand hygiene.
5. Explain the purpose of the procedure, but avoid talking to patient for at least a minute before taking the patient's blood pressure.
6. Assist the patient into a comfortable sitting position, with their arm slightly flexed and forearm supported at heart level.
7. Fully expose the upper arm.
8. Palpate the brachial artery. Position the cuff approximately 1 inch above the antecubital space.
9. Ensure that the cuff is fully deflated. Wrap the cuff evenly and snugly around the upper arm.
10. Center the arrow on the cuff over the artery. If there is no arrow, then estimate the center of the bladder and place over the artery.
11. Ensure that the manometer is positioned for easy reading.
12. If the patient's normal systolic pressure is unknown, palpate the radial artery and rapidly inflate cuff to a pressure 30 mm Hg above the point above which the radial pulsation disappears. Deflate the cuff and wait 30 seconds.

13. Place the stethoscope earpieces in ears and ensure that the sounds are clear, not muffled.
14. Place the diaphragm (or bell) of the stethoscope over the brachial artery in the antecubital fossa. The antecubital fossa is the depression in the underside of the arm at the bend of the elbow. Avoid contact with the blood pressure cuff or clothing.
15. Close the valve of the pressure bulb clockwise until tight.
16. Inflate the cuff to 30 mm Hg above the patient's normal systolic level.
17. Slowly release the valve, allowing the needle of the aneroid gauge to fall at a rate of 2 mm Hg per second.
18. Note the point on the manometer at which the first clear sound is heard.
19. Continue cuff deflation, noting the point on the manometer at which the sound muffles (phase IV) and disappears (phase V). Listen for 10 to 20 mm Hg after last sound.
20. Rapidly deflate the cuff. To determine an average blood pressure and ensure a correct reading, wait 2 minutes, then repeat the procedure for the same arm. Calculate the average of the two readings.
21. Remove the cuff from the patient's arm. Assist the patient into a comfortable position, and cover the upper arm.
22. Disinfect the earpieces of the stethoscope, fold the cuff, and properly store the stethoscope in a cool, dry place.
23. Disclose the findings to the patient.
24. Document the completion of this service in patient's record under "Services Rendered." Record the systolic pressure reading over the diastolic blood pressure reading in mm Hg and include the date of services, the cuff size (if it was an atypical size), and the arm used for measurement in the patient's record. For example: "The patient's blood pressure, taken on 08/01/2024 and measured with adult size cuff, is 110/75 mm Hg, right arm sitting."

Initiate proper physician referral when appropriate.

Data from Potter PA, Perry AG, Stockert P, Hall A. *Fundamentals of Nursing.* 11th ed. Elsevier Health Sciences (US); 2023.

BOX 14.12 Legal, Ethical, and Safety Issues

Never provide dental hygiene care to a patient with a consistent blood pressure reading of ≥180 and/or ≥120.

BOX 14.13 Critical Thinking Scenario D

The patient, a 40-year-old medical resident who works in a hospital emergency department, has a history of missing several dental appointments, making numerous cancellations, and rescheduling appointments. She is 10 minutes late for her appointment and, on arrival, is still dressed in scrubs. On inquiry, she wearily states that she has had approximately 20 hours of sleep during the last week because of her residency assignment. Her health and pharmacologic history reveals migraine headaches, depression, a prosthetic heart valve, and petit mal and grand mal (tonic-clonic) epileptic seizures. She is currently taking a nonsteroidal antiinflammatory agent for her migraines when needed, a tricyclic antidepressant for depression, and Depakote (an anticonvulsant medication) for her epilepsy. She takes her antidepressant and anticonvulsant on a regular basis and states that she has taken the medications on the day of the appointment. She also must take amoxicillin for a prosthetic heart valve and reports an allergy to aspirin products, which has been confirmed by her physician. Her vital signs are pulse 70 bpm, respirations 16 rpm, and blood pressure 120/90 mm Hg.

A. Before initiating dental hygiene care, what should the dental hygienist do?
B. The dental hygienist administers 2% lidocaine with 1:100,000 epinephrine for the posterior superior alveolar (PSA) injection, giving a total of three-fourths of the total cartridge with no complications. Proper local anesthetic technique was observed during administration, including aspiration that was negative. The patient unexpectedly has a petit mal seizure. What is the most likely cause of the seizure?
C. After the seizure, the patient admits that she forgot to take her prophylactic amoxicillin premedication for a prosthetic heart valve. The dental hygienist reschedules the patient for treatment, and no treatment other than the administration of the local anesthesia was given. What recommendation concerning the premedication is indicated before the patient is dismissed?
D. The patient calls the next day and reports difficulty with mouth opening and soreness of her jaw. What is the most likely cause of the problem?

KEY CONCEPTS

- Abnormal vital signs can be attributed to patient conditions, equipment failure, or operator error. The dental hygienist must accurately take the vital signs and control factors that contribute to errors.
- Baseline blood pressure, pulse, and respiration measurements should be taken as a comparison for subsequent appointments.
- A thermometer should be available in case there is a need to take a patient's temperature.
- Pulse rate is recorded in bpm. The pulse in the radial or carotid artery is often measured using the first two fingers of the clinician's hand.
- Normal pulse rate for an adult at rest can range from 60 to 100 bpm. Children usually have a more rapid pulse rate than adults.
- If the patient is experiencing frequent PVCs per minute, a medical consultation should be considered.
- Respiration rate is determined by observing the rise and fall of the patient's chest and is recorded as rpm.
- Normal adult range for respiration rate is 12 to 20 rpm. Children have a more rapid respiratory rate than adults (e.g., 20 to 30 rpm for a 6-year-old child).
- Two measurements taken for blood pressure are systolic blood pressure and diastolic blood pressure.
- Optimal systolic and diastolic measurements for adults 18 years of age and older are lower than 120/80 mm Hg.
- Lifestyle changes are recommended for patients with blood pressure classified as elevated with the goal of reducing and/or preventing hypertension.
- Treatment is recommended for stages 1 and 2 hypertension with the goal of reducing the blood pressure to a healthy range.
- Rhythmic, knocking sounds heard via the stethoscope when measuring blood pressure are referred to as Korotkoff sounds.

REFERENCES

1. Potter PA, Perry AG, Stockert P, Hall A. In: *Fundamentals of Nursing*. 11th ed. Elsevier Health Sciences (US); 2023.
2. Malamed SF. In: *Medical Emergencies in the Dental Office*. 8th ed. Mosby; 2023.
3. Whelton PK, Carey RM, Aronow WS, et al. 2018 ACC/AHA/AAPA/ABC/ACPM/AGS/APha/ASH/ASPC/NMA/PCNA guideline for the prevention, detection, evaluation, and management of high blood pressure in adults. *J Am Coll Cardiol*. 2018;19:71.
4. Muntner P, Shimbo D, Carey RM, et al. Measurement of blood pressure in humans: a scientific statement from the American Heart Association. *Hypertension*. 2019;73(5):e35–e66. https://doi.org/10.1161/HYP.0000000000000087.
5. American Heart Association. *Understand Symptoms and Risk of High Blood Pressure*. Available at: http://www.heart.org/HEARTORG/Conditions/HighBloodPressure/High-Blood-Pressure_UCM_002020_SubHomePage.jsp. Accessed July 2022.
6. Brown RJ, Rich K, Treat-Jacobson D. Considerations for accurate blood pressure measurement in clinical care and research. *J Vasc Nurs*. 2019;37(4):274–276.
7. Medicines and Healthcare Products Regulatory Agency (MHRA). *Blood Pressure Measurement Devices*; 2019. https://assets.publishing.service.gov.uk/government/uploads/system/uploads/attachment_data/file/841944/BP_monitoring_2019_v2.2.pdf. Accessed June 2020.

15

Pharmacologic History

Thomas Viola

PROFESSIONAL OPPORTUNITIES

The ability to successfully gather and interpret a patient's pharmacologic, or medication, history is an essential skill necessary to formulate a patient's comprehensive overall health history. Dental patients have never been more medically complex. They are living longer with chronic diseases, and advances in the treatment of those diseases have led to the development of wide variety of new medications. In addition, managing those chronic diseases requires patients to be under the care of multiple healthcare providers, all of whom may be prescribing more medications.

Thus dental patients are at high risk for adverse medication effects and drug interactions that may increase health risks and negatively impact their quality of life. Dental hygienists play a vital role in monitoring for the appropriate use of medications by their patients and by employing patient management strategies aimed at successfully reducing medication-induced oral complications.

COMPETENCIES

1. Discuss the importance of formulating and interpreting a comprehensive medication history.
2. Identify fundamental questions to collect a comprehensive medication history and accomplish the following:
    a. Describe adverse medication events, including side effects, drug toxicity, and drug hypersensitivity reactions
    b. Describe common side effects caused by medication use
    c. Discuss strategies to improve patient compliance with medication use
    d. Discuss dental hygiene interventions to manage the oral complications of medication use.

INTRODUCTION

Initial patient assessment includes collecting a comprehensive **medication history** or pharmacologic history, which provides information regarding a patient's past and present medication use and offers clues about a patient's current health status and behaviors. Often, patients do not consider information about their systemic health conditions or the medications they are taking for the treatment of those conditions to be within the scope of dental hygiene care, and therefore patients may not include this information on their dental hygiene health history questionnaire.

Omission of information about medical conditions or medications may be intentional if the patient knows that divulging the information to the dental hygienist may require that the course of dental hygiene treatment be altered or postponed, or that additional testing or medical treatment will be required before dental hygiene treatment may proceed. For example, this situation may be encountered with patients who dislike having to take prophylactic antibiotic premedication or to undergo monthly testing required to monitor the efficacy of their medications, such as warfarin.

Omission of information about medical conditions or medications may also be intentional if the patient fears discrimination because of a violation of confidentiality. Thus sensitive issues, such as the patient's use of medications for human immunodeficiency virus (HIV) infection, sexually transmitted diseases, mental illness, substance addiction, or gender affirmation, must be appropriately managed to ensure patient privacy and respect.

Conversely, a conscientious patient may forget to report over-the-counter (OTC) medications, dietary supplements, or substances such as cannabis simply because the patient does not view these as "medications." This assumption is often the case with oral contraceptives, antacids, dietary supplements, and aspirin. Because many OTC medications, dietary supplements, and substances interact with medications used in dentistry and/or produce side effects, including oral complications, they may also have the potential to compromise patient safety and function.

Thus obtaining a complete and accurate medication history enables the dental hygienist to assess risks associated with treating patients who are taking all types of medications, supplements, and substances and employ treatment strategies necessary for reducing those risks.

COMPREHENSIVE PHARMACOLOGIC HISTORY

Medication List

The first step in obtaining a complete and accurate medication history is to compile a list of all medications, both prescription and nonprescription, as well as any herbal and dietary supplements that the patient is currently taking. This list should include the name of each medication or supplement and the **dose** (the specific amount taken) and the **dosage schedule** (frequency of taking that dose), as well as any special instructions for its use. With the patient's informed consent, a consultation with the patient's physician, pharmacy, legal guardian, or caregiver may be necessary to verify this information.[1]

Patients are asked about their own perceptions regarding their medication use to assess their knowledge about their medications. Some people take drugs without understanding why they have been prescribed or knowing the expected outcome of medication therapy (Box 15.1).

Patients should be encouraged to keep their medication list, including dosage schedules and the name of the prescribing physician, with them at all times. This is helpful to all health professionals treating the patient and may be especially useful during an emergency situation. The dental hygienist can help the patient develop this record as a health promotion activity and update it at each appointment (Box 15.2).

The medication list is also helpful for assessing the patient's attitude toward health and wellness. For example, patients using OTC vitamins and dietary supplements may be more interested in nutritional counseling or may seek complementary and alternative medicine services.

In addition, it is important to have a candid conversation with the patient about their use of alcohol and substances, such as cannabis, and even misuse of medications. At times, unhealthy behaviors and attitudes may be determined by a patient's drug misuse, such as abusing OTC stimulants for weight loss or recreationally using illegal drugs and alcohol. **Medication misuse** is defined as using a medication for a purpose that is not consistent with legal or medical guidelines, such as abusing OTC stimulants for weight loss (see Chapter 56). Box 15.3 lists the drug references that are used to access current medication information to support clinical decision making at chairside.

Eight Fundamental Assessment Questions
See Table 15.1.

Question 1: Why Is the Patient Taking Medication?
The dental hygienist assesses the reason the patient is taking medication. Generally, medications are taken for the following purposes:

BOX 15.1 Patient or Client Education Tip

The "teach back" method should be used whenever a patient is given a prescription or recommendation for a new medication. After receiving instructions from the provider, the patient should be able to identify the name and indication for use of each medication and instruct the healthcare provider about how the medication is to be used. This method helps ensure that the patient has received adequate instructions and understands how to use the medication safely. The "teach back" method helps prevent medication errors. Consent must be obtained to request this information from either the patient or the patient's legal guardian.

BOX 15.2 Legal, Ethical, and Safety Issues

The medication list should be updated at every visit, verified, and entered into the patient dental record. If a copy of the list has been obtained from another healthcare provider, such as from a head nurse at a long-term care facility or a pharmacist, the original document should be date stamped on receipt, scanned, and electronically uploaded into the patient dental record. A note should be included in the treatment notes that the medication list was requested and obtained from the named source and has been scanned into the patient's permanent record.

BOX 15.3 Chairside Drug References

Lexicomp Online for Dentistry. Available at: http://www.wolterskluwercdi.com/online-for-dentistry/
Epocrates. Athenahealth Inc. Available at: https://www.epocrates.com/
ADA/PDR Dental Therapeutics Online. Available at: http://www.ada.org/en/publications/ada-news/2014-archive/february/subscribe-to-ada-pdr-dental-therapeutics-online
Prescribers Digital Reference (PDR). ConnectiveRx. Available at: http://www.pdr.net/
Mosby's Dental Drug Reference. Jeske A, ed. 13th ed. Mosby/Elsevier; 2021.
U.S. Food and Drug Administration. Available at: www.fda.gov
Herbs at a Glance. National Institute for Complementary and Integrative Health. Available at: https://nccih.nih.gov/health/herbsataglance.htm
RxList. Available at: www.rxlist.com
Drugs.com Available at: www.drugs.com

- *To treat an acute systemic condition.* Medications that are taken to treat acute conditions (e.g., cough and cold preparations, antibiotic medications, antifungal medications, antidiarrheal agents, pain relievers) are generally recommended or prescribed for a defined time frame, usually of short duration, to manage the symptoms of an acute condition or to eliminate an infection. The assumption is that when the medication is gone, so too will be the cause of the symptoms or the condition being treated.
- *To treat a chronic systemic condition.* Medications that are taken to treat chronic conditions are prescribed for a longer duration or for extended periods throughout the lifetime (e.g., oral hypoglycemic medications, allergy medications, antihypertensive agents).
- *To prevent a condition from occurring.* Medications may be indicated for the prevention of a disease or condition (e.g., oral contraceptives to prevent pregnancy).
- *To prevent a recurrence of an existing condition.* Medications may be preventively used to ward off the recurrence of a chronic problem (e.g., inhaled steroids for asthma, anticonvulsants to prevent seizures).
- *To satisfy a habit, with no clinical indication or need.* Substances may be consumed even though there is no clinical indication to justify their usage. This might include alcohol, caffeine, nicotine, and, of course, illegal substances. However, it may also include medications, such as aspirin, and vitamin and dietary supplements which are habitually taken because of a perceived health benefit that may or may not truly exist (Box 15.4).

TABLE 15.1 Eight Fundamental Questions of the Pharmacologic History

Question	Dental Hygiene Process of Care
1. Why is the patient taking the medication(s)? 2. What are the adverse effects of this medication? 3. Are there potential drug interactions? 4. Is there a problem with the medication dosage? 5. How is the patient managing their medications?	Assessment
6. Will any oral side effects of this medication require intervention? 7. Are the patient's symptoms caused by a known or unknown condition, or are the symptoms possible medication side effects?	Diagnosis
8. Given the pharmacologic history and other assessment data, what are the risks of treating this patient?	Planning

---

BOX 15.4 Legal, Ethical, and Safety Issues

A 63-year-old male patient includes marijuana on his list of medications on the written health history form. The dental hygienist is unsure whether to write notes about the patient's disclosure in the pharmacologic history or in the section about the social history of the patient. Upon further questioning, the patient states that he recently developed an allergy to several prescription eye drops; consequently, his ophthalmologist prescribed marijuana as an adjunctive treatment for his glaucoma. In this instance, cannabis has been prescribed for approved medical use. The use of medical marijuana documented under the pharmacologic history is not to be confused with recreational marijuana use. The legalized use of cannabis products for medical and recreational use varies at state and federal levels.

Question 2: What Are the Adverse Effects of This Medication?

All medications have the potential to cause harm. When a medication is selected to treat a condition, the potential risks of the use of that medication must be carefully weighed against the benefits of its use. In the United States, medications are extensively tested and regulated by the Food and Drug Administration (FDA) to ensure safety and efficacy. The FDA requires medication manufacturers to report known adverse effects listed in the medication's monograph, which can be accessed using reference databases or from the FDA website (see Box 15.3). This information also appears on the package insert of all FDA-approved medications. Common side effects are listed in Box 15.5.

Medications interact with their target tissues to produce a desired effect, also known as their **therapeutic effect**. However, medications also may interact with nontarget tissues, resulting in effects that differ from their intended therapeutic effects. These effects, which are typically undesirable, are also known as medication **side effects**, the severity of which may be dose related. For example, a patient takes an angiotensin-converting enzyme (ACE) inhibitor to treat hypertension and although it is effective in lowering the patient's blood pressure, it also produces a persistent dry cough. All medications produce side effects, but most are tolerable and usually disappear when the medication is discontinued. The FDA requires the reporting of all known side effects, which are organized by body system and the percentage of population affected.

Drug toxicity refers to toxin-induced cell damage and/or cell death from a medication. Typically, the medication itself does not produce damage directly to the cell. Rather, the damage is usually caused by a **metabolite** formed during metabolic breakdown of the medication by the liver or kidneys. Metabolites may cause biochemical damage to cellular components, resulting in altered metabolism of the affected cell, cell mutation, or even cell death. Unlike side effects, toxicity reactions usually cannot be tolerated and cause permanent tissue damage on either the microscopic or macroscopic level. This is especially dangerous if major organ systems are involved. Medications that produce these types of reactions may be labeled as hepatotoxic (causing liver damage), nephrotoxic (causing kidney damage), neurotoxic (causing nerve damage), or cardiotoxic (causing heart damage). Drug toxicity often occurs when the dose of the medication administered exceeds the established therapeutic level (drug overdose).

Drug hypersensitivity, or allergy, occurs when either the medication and/or its metabolites act as immunogens, triggering the immune response. Signs of a true allergic reaction include skin rash, itching, hives, bronchospasm, and rhinitis. Life-threatening allergic reactions include anaphylaxis, hemolysis, and bone marrow suppression. Allergic reactions are managed with epinephrine, antihistamines, and corticosteroids, as well as assistance from emergency support personnel. Allergic reactions are dangerous because they are not predictable and are not related to the prescribed dose. Patients with a history of an allergy to a medication in a specific class of medications may be allergic to all of the medications in that same class. In addition, some medications, such as penicillins and cephalosporins, show cross sensitivity to medications in other classes with similar chemical structures. The dental hygienist must recognize the warning signs of an allergic reaction to ensure that appropriate treatment interventions can be promptly administered (see Chapter 11).

Other adverse medication effects include negative effects on fetal development, or **teratogenicity**. Many medications cross the placenta and are secreted in breast milk; therefore, medications are typically not tested in pregnant and lactating women. The FDA recently adopted the Pregnancy and Lactation Labeling (Drugs) Rule, changing the way that medications are labeled according to risk.[2] The new labeling requirements replace the former pregnancy risk factors (A, B, C, D, X) and allow healthcare providers to weigh risk versus benefit for pregnant women who need to take medication (see Chapter 46).

Occasionally, a patient experiences a side effect from a medication that is completely unexpected or qualitatively different from any other known published side effects. This unique response to a medication is called a **drug idiosyncrasy**. Idiosyncratic drug reactions are usually related to a genetic variant. Patients may also report **drug tolerance**, which manifests as the need to take increased doses of the medication to produce the same response as that produced in other patients. This is often due to rapid medication metabolism.

To answer Question 2, the dental hygienist assesses the following:
- What are the known published side effects of the medication(s)?
- Could the symptoms reported by the patient be side effects of the medication(s)?
- Are reported symptoms indicative of a medication allergy?

BOX 15.5 Common Side Effects of Medications

Central Nervous System Effects
Hyperexcitability
Dizziness
Insomnia
Drowsiness

Cardiac Effects
Hypertension
Hypotension
Orthostatic hypotension or fainting
Edema
Cardiac arrhythmias

Hematologic Effects
Changes in bleeding time
Blood dyscrasias

Gastrointestinal Effects
Weight changes
Appetite changes
Nausea
Vomiting
Diarrhea
Constipation
Xerostomia

Genitourinary Effects
Urinary changes
Sexual dysfunction

Dermatologic Effects
Photosensitivity
Skin disorders

Respiratory Effects
Dyspnea
Coughing

Effects on Special Senses
Blurred vision
Visual disturbances
Taste alteration
Acoustic and balance disorders

Other Common Side Effects
Opportunistic infections (e.g., yeasts, fungal)

Question 3: Are There Potential Drug Interactions?

Adverse medication effects can also be caused by **drug interactions**, the negative effects that can occur when two or more medications are taken simultaneously. Drug interactions range in severity from mild alterations in medication efficacy to life-threatening conditions in the patient (e.g., major alterations in medication efficacy, toxicity reactions, and other dangerous reactions such as hypertensive crisis, extended bleeding time, and respiratory depression). Medications also may interact with foods and dietary and herbal supplements.

Drug interactions are prevented by knowing medication relationships. Dental hygienists must keep apprised of drug interactions by routinely reviewing lists of known interactions in standard medication reference sources and scientific publications. Drug interactions arise from a variety of mechanisms and may result in either a decreased or an increased effect of one or more medications. The greater the number of medications taken, the greater the likelihood that the patient will experience an interaction. Medication compatibility must always be confirmed before prescribing any medication to a patient.

To assess whether the patient is experiencing a drug interaction, the dental hygienist and dentist may reference a current medication database and assesses the following:

- Are there any known drug interactions for this medication?
- Could the patient's symptoms be indicative of a drug interaction?

Question 4: Do These Findings Suggest a Problem With Medication Dosage?

Standard medication dosage schedules may be too strong for pediatric and older adult patients, and doses may have to be altered to prevent adverse medication effects. The need to alter doses in these populations is directly related to a medication's **pharmacokinetics**, which refers to how the medication is absorbed, distributed, metabolized, and excreted from the body. For example, children may more readily and more quickly absorb and metabolize medications than their adult counterparts. Pediatric doses are typically based on the weight of the child. (Boxes 15.6 and 15.7).

In older adult patients, normal physiologic changes of aging may also dictate the need for a reduction in a dosage. Altered stomach acidity may affect medication absorption into circulation. Normally, the liver converts lipid-soluble medications to water-soluble metabolites, thus inactivating the medication and allowing for filtration and elimination by the kidney. However, liver and kidney function declines with age and, therefore more medication may stay active after passing through the liver. The portion of the medication that remains lipid soluble is scavenged by the kidneys and either recirculated or stored in body fat. The production of plasma proteins and the binding sites for medications in circulation also decline with age. The portion of the medication that is unbound in the circulation is the active medication. The amount of active medication in circulation increases when the patient takes multiple medications, all of which are competing for fewer binding sites. These physiologic changes manifest as an increased medication effect in the patient and contribute to unwanted side effects. As with pediatric patients, doses for older adult patients may also have to be reduced. Liver and kidney function also must be considered when determining the proper dose, especially in patients with hepatic and renal disease.

To assess the potential for complications caused by the medication dose, the dental hygienist considers the following:

- Have the patient's age and weight been considered when determining the medication dose?
- Could the symptoms be attributed to altered medication pharmacokinetics caused by normal physiologic changes of aging?
- Could the symptoms be attributed to altered medication pharmacokinetics caused by hepatic and renal disease?

Question 5: How Is the Patient Managing Medications?

Most patients take multiple medications and are treated by many different healthcare providers. The lack of communication among these providers, all of whom may be prescribing medications, results in an increased risk for adverse medication reactions, drug interactions, and duplication of therapy. As an advocate for the patient, the dental hygienist encourages compliance and works with the patient to assess risks associated with medication use.

The patient's ability to manage their medications is confounded by several variables. First, the patient may be self-medicating with OTC medications, prescription medications, or supplements. Patients are usually unaware of potential adverse medication effects and drug interactions that may occur as a result of mixing medications, altering recommended dosage schedules, or mixing medications with supplements, alcohol, or certain foods. Second, patients may not read the warning labels on the medication packaging or may not understand what they are reading. Misunderstanding is especially prevalent when the label warns against using certain classes of medications or warns against using the medication because of a preexisting condition. Patients may not be aware that they have a preexisting condition such as an enlarged prostate, hypertension, or thyroid disease. Other patients simply choose to ignore the warnings and take the medication anyway. In fact, the small type size on many labels may pose yet another challenge for older adult patients and the visually impaired.

Lack of compliance with medication use, intentionally or unintentionally, must be discerned by the dental hygienist. The dental hygienist should never assume that the patient intuitively understands the prescribed regimen or reads the instructions from the pharmacy. Whenever a medication is dispensed or prescribed from the dental office, the dental hygienist and dentist provide detailed instructions. Even patients who are normally compliant are given instructions and an opportunity to ask questions to reinforce adherence to the prescribed regimen (Box 15.8).

BOX 15.6 Legal, Ethical, and Safety Issues

All dental hygienists should know how to calculate safe medication doses. The American Heart Association has formulas for calculating pediatric doses for antibiotic prophylaxis. Doses of local anesthetic agents and vasoconstrictors are determined according to a patient's weight.

BOX 15.7 Critical Thinking Scenario A

Calculating a Medication Dose

An 8-year-old female patient weighing 64 pounds requires antibacterial prophylaxis before receiving dental hygiene treatment. According to the American Heart Association, the pediatric dose is based on a milligram of medication per kilogram of body weight (mg/kg), with a total dose not to exceed the adult dose. How much antibacterial premedication should be prescribed for this child for a single dose of premedication for amoxicillin (50 mg/kg)? Azithromycin (15 mg/kg)?

BOX 15.8 Health Literacy

When assessing patient compliance, the dental hygienist should also assess the level of health literacy. Clinicians should not assume that patients make decisions about medication compliance based solely on their ability to read and understand label instructions. Compliance may also be affected by cultural and social norms within the individual's family or community (see Chapter 6).

Familiarity with a routine can breed laziness in compliance. Just as patients learn proper dosage schedules, they may also learn to give the "right answer" to inquiries about taking their medications. In these instances, the dental hygienist may rely on the patient's physical presentation as well as personal intuition to discern whether the patient truly is following instructions. A patient's compliance with medication use can reflect the patient's willingness to comply with other professional recommendations, including self-care instructions and referrals.

Dental hygienists may also facilitate the transfer of information between the patient and other healthcare professionals. By simply placing a call to the patient's physician, dental hygienists may clarify discrepancies in the patient's understanding of their medications and may confirm that it is safe to provide treatment. Conversations between the dental hygienist and other practitioners should be documented in the patient record.

When assessing patient compliance with medications, the dental hygienist focuses on the following:

- How many medications is the patient taking?
- How many providers are prescribing medication for the patient?
- When was the patient last seen by a physician?
- When did the patient last see the physician who prescribed the medication?
- What is the prescribed regimen for the medication?
- How long is the patient to remain on the medication?
- Does the patient understand why the medication was prescribed?
- Have patient instructions been provided for taking the medication? If so, by whom?
- Does the patient understand the instructions for using the medication?
- Is the patient self-medicating, undermedicating, or overmedicating?
- How many refills are there for the medication?
- Has the medication expired?

Question 6: Will Any Oral Side Effects of This Medication Require Intervention?

Management of oral side effects is an ongoing challenge (Box 15.9). Oral side effects negatively affect oral health–related quality of life. Patients frequently experience discomfort and difficulty with chewing, swallowing, and digesting food. Some oral side effects place the patient at risk for oral trauma, and others lead to infection, pain, and possible tooth loss. Dental hygienists may recognize these oral conditions in a timely manner and recommend appropriate treatment interventions. Professional intervention is often necessary to improve patient comfort and function. More than 500 medications cause dry mouth, making it the most commonly reported oral side effect, especially among older adult clients (Box 15.10).[3,4]

Medication-induced dry mouth is a combination of reduced salivary flow rate (**hyposalivation**) and a change in the nature and quality of the residual saliva. Residual saliva is more mucinous and viscous, facilitating food and oral biofilm adherence to tooth surfaces, appliances, dentures, and oral tissues. The patient retains more food in the buccal vestibule after eating as a result of the loss of natural salivary cleansing. The pH of the mouth becomes more acidic because of the reduction of natural physiologic buffers which, when combined with oral biofilm and food accumulation, places the client at increased risk for dental caries. Dental caries are evident along the gingival margin on exposed buccal and lingual root surfaces, at and underneath crown margins, on incisal edges and cusp tips with dentinal exposure from attrition, and in root furcations.

Dental caries can lead to extensive tooth destruction and tooth loss, which is particularly significant for teeth that serve as anchors for dental prostheses. Increased biofilm acidity also contributes to dentinal hypersensitivity. Patients with hyposalivation should be placed on supplemental daily fluoride with consideration for use of remineralization therapies to reduce caries and dentinal hypersensitivity risks (see Chapter 19 and Chapter 42). Incorporating daily therapeutic doses of xylitol-containing products also may be recommended to reduce *Streptococcus mutans* and stimulate saliva production.

The subjective perception of **xerostomia**, or dry mouth, requires symptomatic relief with artificial salivary substitutes and other products that lubricate the oral tissues. More serious cases of objective dryness, or true **salivary gland hypofunction**, may be treated with the prescription medications pilocarpine (Salagen) or cevimeline (Evoxac), which stimulate serous salivary flow. Compatibility must be confirmed

---

BOX 15.9   Common Oral Side Effects of Medications

Xerostomia
Dental caries
Change in taste
Difficulty with mastication
Difficulty wearing appliances
Oral ulcerations
Atrophic mucosa
Hairy tongue
Infection
Mucositis or stomatitis
Burning mouth or tongue
Difficulty with speech
Difficulty with swallowing
Increased periodontal disease progression
Opportunistic infections (e.g., candidiasis)
Bleeding
Gingival enlargement

BOX 15.10   Classes of Medications That Cause Xerostomia

Anorexiants
Antiacne agents
Antianxiety agents
Anticholinergics
Anticonvulsants
Antidepressants
Antidiarrheals
Antiemetics
Antihistamines
Antihypertensives
Antiinflammatory analgesics
Antinauseants
Antiparkinsonian agents
Antipsychotics
Antispasmodics
Bronchodilators
Decongestants
Diuretics
Muscle relaxants
Opiate analgesics
Sedatives

with the patient's existing health status and concurrent medication use before these systemic medications are prescribed.

Under normal conditions, saliva maintains the balance of the oral ecosystem with immunologic and antibacterial processes that regulate the population of oral flora. When the ecosystem becomes unbalanced, the proportions of pathogenic and opportunistic organisms increase. Therefore patients with dry mouth are at greater risk for oral infections, including gingivitis, periodontitis, and viral and fungal infections. People with dry mouth greatly benefit from the use of daily antimicrobial therapy at home. Chlorhexidine and essential oil mouthrinses have demonstrated efficacy against a broad spectrum of oral pathogens and seven species of *Candida* organisms (see Chapter 27). Fungal infections are associated with use of antibiotics, immunosuppressants, and underlying systemic diseases such as diabetes mellitus. Prescription antifungal medications, such as nystatin, are indicated and often repeated in patients with xerostomia who develop recurrent fungal infections. Fungal infections may present as white plaques overlying red oral mucosa, burning mouth syndrome, symptomatic geographic tongue, and angular cheilitis.

Salivary mucins lubricate the oral mucous membranes, protect against ulceration and penetration of toxins, and assist with wound healing and repair. Patients with xerostomia have friable mucous membranes, which are highly susceptible to trauma from toothbrushing, mastication, and rubbing against appliances and dentures. Numerous OTC products are available for topical pain control associated with aphthous ulcerations and oral mucositis; most contain benzocaine to improve comfort. Viscous lidocaine oral solution may also be used as a rinse for pain relief.

Salivary mucins also play a role in initiating the breakdown of food in preparation for swallowing and digestion. Often, patients with xerostomia experience gastrointestinal disorders related to their inability to digest food adequately. These problems are further compounded in patients who are taking medications that cause taste alterations as a side effect. More than 250 medications alter taste and smell. Saliva is needed to help carry tastants (chemicals that produce taste sensations by activating taste receptor cells) to the taste buds, which is diminished in patients with xerostomia. Medications may also be excreted into saliva and gingival crevicular fluid or may concentrate electrolytes in the saliva. These adverse effects may lead patients to make poor food choices or stop eating because of discomfort, disinterest, or chewing difficulties. Patients may experience weight loss, which alters the fit and comfort of dentures and appliances, leading to a cycle that requires intervention. Weight loss and poor nutritional status are of great concern in those with serious medical conditions or those undergoing cancer therapy (see Chapter 50).

Anticonvulsant medications (e.g., phenytoin), antirejection medications (e.g., cyclosporine), and calcium channel blockers (e.g., amlodipine) may cause medication-induced gingival enlargement as a side effect. Black, hairy tongue is typically associated with antibacterial agents. Other medication-induced oral side effects include glossitis, erythema multiforme, lichenoid medication reaction, and taste alteration. The dental hygienist should consult a medication reference to verify the potential for a medication to produce these adverse effects. For a list of strategies to manage oral side effects associated with medication use, see Box 15.11.

To determine the need for intervention, the dental hygienist must consider the following:

- Is the patient having difficulty speaking, chewing, swallowing, or wearing dental appliances?
- Is the patient taking medications that could be contributing to these problems?
- Has the patient reported changes in weight that could be attributed to a change in nutritional status?
- Are oral assessment findings consistent with known side effects of the medications that the patient is taking?

BOX 15.11 Dental Hygiene Interventions to Manage the Oral Side Effects of Medications

Dental Caries Preventive and Dentinal Hypersensitivity Therapies
Prescription fluorides: dentifrices, gels, and rinses
Professional in-office application of topical fluorides
Amorphous calcium phosphate (ACP), licensed from the ADA
Arginine
Calcium sodium phosphosilicate (NovaMin)
Tricalcium phosphate
Milk casein phosphopeptide (CPP) complexed with ACP (CPP-ACP) (Recaldent)
OTC dentinal hypersensitivity protection dentifrices
Xylitol

Salivary Replacement Therapy
Artificial saliva
Water

Salivary Stimulation
Pilocarpine (Salagen)
Cevimeline (Evoxac)
Sonic toothbrushing

Daily Antimicrobial Therapy
Chlorhexidine mouthrinse (0.12%)
Essential oil mouthrinse
Cetylpyridinium chloride mouthrinse (0.07%)

Antifungal Therapy
Prescription medications: topical ointments, liquids, powders, and troches (e.g., nystatin [Mycostatin]); systemic medications (e.g., fluconazole [Diflucan])
Daily antimicrobial therapy with 0.12% chlorhexidine or essential oil mouthrinse

Antiviral Therapy
Prescription topical ointments, systemic medications (e.g., acyclovir [Zovirax], penciclovir [Denavir], valacyclovir [Valtrex], famciclovir [Famvir])
OTC topical ointments (e.g., docosanol 10% [Abreva])
OTC topical benzocaine ointments for pain control

Topical Pain Control for Ulcerations or Mucositis
OTC benzocaine or tetracaine ointments
OTC liquid Benadryl mixed with coating agent
Viscous lidocaine oral rinse (prescribed by a dentist)
Amlexanox (Aphthasol) ointment (prescribed by a dentist)

Oral Hygiene Devices
Power toothbrush
Power flosser
Oral irrigator
Interdental cleaning aids

ADA, American Dental Association; *OTC,* over-the-counter.

Question 7: Are Symptoms Reported During the Patient's Health History Interview Caused by a Medical Condition or Are They Medication Side Effects?

Answering this question may be a challenge; therefore dental hygienists should pay close attention to findings from the health history interview. The dental hygienist attempts to match the physical findings or symptoms reported by the patient with existing medical or dental conditions. Medications that the patient is taking should be suitable for the medical and dental conditions for which the patient is being treated. Consider that a physician may prescribe a medication for an off-label use. When symptoms do not correlate with known conditions, the dental hygienist must then discern whether the patient's medications may be contributing to the problem or whether an undiagnosed condition may be present, either of which could explain the patient's symptoms.

The following questions facilitate problem solving:

- Does the patient have a known systemic condition?
- What are the symptoms reported by the patient?
- Do these symptoms correlate with the patient's known systemic condition?
- Do the reported symptoms indicate the presence of an undiagnosed condition?
- What are the indications for the medications being taken?
- Could the medications be causing or contributing to the symptoms in question?

Question 8: Given the Pharmacologic History and Other Assessment Data, What Are the Risks of Treating This Patient?

Assessing the risk of proceeding with treatment is the final and most important determination made. Treatment risks associated with medication use vary in nature and severity and are not always obvious. Life-threatening risks may be associated with conditions for which the patient is taking medication or with medication-related side effects (Box 15.12).

To assess risk, the following questions must be considered:

- If treatment is initiated, will the patient be placed in a situation that is potentially dangerous or life-threatening?
- Will the planned treatment temporarily or permanently compromise the patient's health or ability to function?
- Will the treatment compromise the patient's safety or comfort?
- Will the treatment compromise the provider's safety or comfort?

Patients who are immunocompromised from cancer chemotherapy or immunomodulatory medications, organ transplant antirejection therapy, or acquired immunodeficiency syndrome (AIDS) are at greater risk for developing infections from poor oral hygiene or invasive dental hygiene procedures (see Chapters 47, 50, 51, 53, and 54). Good oral self-care practices, preprocedural antimicrobial rinsing, and prophylactic antibiotic premedication are strategies to minimize the risk for infection. Antibiotic therapy associated with professional care is determined in consultation with the dentist or physician on a case-by-case basis (see Chapter 13).

Given global concerns about antimicrobial resistance and risk for life-threatening infections caused by resistant organisms, antibacterial agents (antibiotics) must be used judiciously, avoiding unnecessary use. Risks associated with antibacterial agent use must be carefully weighed against potential benefits, and patients must be informed of these risks and participate in the decision about whether antibacterial premedication is desired. There is no evidence that antibiotic premedication changes the risk for either infective endocarditis or prosthetic joint infection.[5,6] Dental hygienists should follow published clinical practice guidelines and the appropriate use criteria from the American Dental Association, the American Heart Association, and the American

Academy of Orthopedic Surgeons to determine the need for antibiotic premedication before treatment.[6-9]

The risk for hypertensive crisis and stroke has been associated with the use of vasoconstrictors, and the dental hygienist must verify the compatibility of administering epinephrine with all medications taken by the patient before giving an injection (see Chapter 43). The use of substances such as cocaine, methamphetamine, and cannabis sensitizes patients to the effects of epinephrine, posing an even greater risk for hypertensive crisis, myocardial infarction, and stroke in the oral care environment. In addition, myocardial infarction, stroke, and anaphylaxis as a result of an unexpected allergic reaction are perhaps the most dangerous risks. Insulin shock, aspiration, and seizures are mostly preventable with proper patient assessment and use of safety precautions.

All dental hygienists must be currently certified in cardiopulmonary resuscitation (CPR) and managing medical emergencies in the dental office. The dental hygienist can help establish a safety plan that includes monitoring oxygen tanks to ensure the availability of adequate levels, the expiration dates on emergency medications, and the use of medications dispensed from the office (see Chapter 11).

Dental hygienists should use laboratory test results, medical records, and information obtained from the dentist, physician, and pharmacist to assist with clinical decision making. Maintaining a patient's systemic health always takes priority over dental hygiene care needs, and treatment should never be initiated when the patient's safety is a concern (see Chapter 13). The patient and the dental hygienist must know about any medication risks associated with treatment, and these risks should be thoroughly explained and documented in the treatment record.

The dental hygienist is exposed to personal health risks when treating patients with medications. Inhalation risks are associated with general anesthetics and nitrous oxide–oxygen systems with inadequate scavenging systems (see Chapter 44). For example, pregnant

---

BOX 15.12   Legal, Ethical, and Safety Issues

The dental hygienist seats a 73-year-old female for the first of four scheduled visits for quadrant nonsurgical periodontal therapy. After hearing about the planned procedures for the day, the patient asks whether she will receive a prescription for a "painkiller" since she is worried that she will be uncomfortable later that evening after the local anesthesia wears off. She states, "Since I had my hip replaced last year, I have found that I do so much better with Percocet than with ibuprofen for anything that might cause me pain. I want to be able to sleep comfortably tonight. Please ask the dentist to give me a prescription to get me through all of this dental work." The dental hygienist consults with the dentist and shares concerns about the patient's request.

Addiction to opioid medications is a common occurrence, especially among older adults who are susceptible to this medication risk after opioid use for a legitimate invasive medical procedure. Using the sedative side effect of opiates for other reasons, such as a sleep aid or for anxiety, is a warning sign of drug misuse and dependency. Requesting specific opioids, as in this case, is also a warning sign. Healthcare professionals should be aware that drug dependency affects individuals of all ages. The patient is unaware that neither the oxycodone nor acetaminophen contained in Percocet is effective at reducing the inflammation associated with periodontitis and nonsurgical periodontal therapy; thus its use is not an appropriate medication for this clinical situation. The dentist discusses concerns with the patient and obtains further information about the patient's frequency of opioid use. The patient is referred to a pain management specialist for further evaluation. The dentist recommends the use of a nonsteroidal antiinflammatory analgesic for anticipated minor postoperative pain. The dental hygienist and dentist document the conversation and referral in the patient's treatment record.

practitioners should exercise caution when in the presence of nitrous oxide, a medication that may cause spontaneous abortion as a teratogenic effect (i.e., capable of producing genetic mutations). However, use of a proper scavenging system significantly minimizes this inhalation risk. Topically applied agents have the potential to come in contact with the skin, mucous membranes, and eyes of the dental hygienist, requiring the use of personal protective equipment (see Chapter 10). The dental hygienist also must assess the treatment environment for potential hazards to protect themselves and the patient in case the patient falls or has a seizure. The risk for falls increases with patients who take medications that cause orthostatic hypotension or central nervous system side effects that alter equilibrium.

KEY CONCEPTS

- The pharmacologic history provides clues regarding a patient's general health status and health behaviors and protects the patient's health and safety.
- Using a logical, systematic approach to history taking helps the dental hygienist formulate questions and evaluate patient responses to safely provide care.
- Interpreting data obtained from the eight fundamental questions of the medication history enables the dental hygienist to assess the risks of treating patients taking medications.
- All medications have the potential to cause adverse effects.
- Drug interactions range in severity from mild alterations in drug action to life-threatening conditions in the patient.
- Standard medication doses are too strong for children, older adults, and those with hepatic and renal disease and therefore may need to be altered to prevent adverse effects.
- The dental hygienist is a patient advocate who facilitates patient compliance and education on use of medications.
- Patients may fail to comply with medication use for several reasons, including multiple providers prescribing multiple medications, self-medication, cost, and failure to adhere to prescribed dosage regimens.
- Oral side effects of medications negatively affect oral health–related quality of life.

ACKNOWLEDGMENTS

The author acknowledges Ann Eshenaur Spolarich for her past contributions to this chapter.

REFERENCES

1. Choi HJ, Stewart AL, Tu C. Medication discrepancies in the dental record and impact of pharmacist-led intervention. *Int Dent J*. 2017;67(5):318–325.
2. United States Department of Health and Human Services. Food and Drug Administration. Pregnancy and Lactation Labeling Final Rule (PLLR). 21 CFR Part 201. June 30, 2015. Available at: https://s3.amazonaws.com/public-inspection.federalregister.gov/2014-28241.pdf.
3. Han P, Suarez-Durall P, Mulligan R. Dry mouth: a critical topic for older adult patients. *J Prosthodont Res*. 2015;59(1):6–19. Epub Dec 9, 2014. Review.
4. Wolff A, Joshi RK, Ekström J, et al. A guide to medications inducing salivary gland dysfunction, xerostomia, and subjective sialorrhea: a systematic review sponsored by the World Workshop on Oral Medicine VI. *Drugs R*. 2017;17(1):1–28.
5. Oliver R, Roberts GJ, Hooper L, et al. Antibiotics for the prophylaxis of bacterial endocarditis in dentistry. *Cochrane Database Syst Rev*. 2008;4:CD003813.
6. Sollecito TP, Abt E, Lockhart PB, et al. The use of prophylactic antibiotics prior to dental procedures in patients with prosthetic joints: evidence-based clinical practice guideline for dental practitioners – a report of the American Dental Association Council on Scientific Affairs. *J Am Dent Assoc*. 2015;146(1):11–16.
7. American Dental Association–Appointed Members of the Expert writing and Voting Panels contributing to the development of American Academy of Orthopedic Surgeons Appropriate Use criteria. American Dental Association guidance for utilizing appropriate use criteria in the management of the care of patients with orthopedic implants undergoing dental procedures. *J Am Dent Assoc*. 2017;148(2):57–59.
8. American Academy of Orthopedic Surgeons. Ortho guidelines. Appropriate use criteria. Management of patients with orthopaedic implants undergoing dental procedures. Available at: http://www.orthoguidelines.org/go/auc/default.cfm?auc_id=224995&actionxm=Terms. Accessed July 21, 2022.
9. American Heart Association Scientific Statement. *Prevention of Viridans Group Streptococcal Infective Endocarditis*; 2021. Available at: https://www.ahajournals.org/doi/pdf/10.1161/CIR.0000000000000969. Accessed December 27, 2022.

16

Assessment of Head and Neck Examination

Margaret J. Fehrenbach

PROFESSIONAL OPPORTUNITIES

The dental hygienist must provide a comprehensive collection of patient findings relating to the head and neck to identify their general and oral health status. This includes being able to perform a thorough examination of the head and neck as well as the oral cavity, along with careful overall patient evaluation. This is followed by an assessment of examination findings using critical thinking along with evidence-based decision making (EBDM) to address the patient's dental hygiene treatment needs. This is an essential part of planning and providing optimal dental hygiene care.

COMPETENCIES

1. Apply knowledge of head and neck anatomic structures during extraoral and intraoral examination to recognize lesions.
2. Perform an extraoral and intraoral examination with overall patient evaluation using correct methods and sequence while involving the patient in basic self-examination techniques as well as giving related oral health information.
3. Assess the examination findings using critical thinking along with EBDM to determine if any lesions discovered are an atypical or abnormal finding.
4. Describe and document significant findings in the patient's record using precise descriptive terminology to form a dental hygiene diagnosis and then inform the patient's dentist when abnormal findings are present to allow for differential diagnosis formation as well as documenting referrals.
5. Describe common types of head and neck cancer (HNC) and understand how it affects the patient while being aware of the current cancer detection methods.

ASSESSMENT OF EXAMINATION FINDINGS

The status of the head and neck is considered an indicator of one's general health as well as oral health. To meet the challenge of performing a head and neck examination and then being able to assess the examination findings so as to recognize any status changes, the dental hygienist must be thoroughly familiar with the anatomy of head and neck structures. Thus any change from a characteristic **typical finding** in the head and neck structures or what some clinicians call *normal* discovery must be noted.

A **lesion** indicates this change in structure of an organ or part, which can be attributable to injury, pathologic condition, or developmental disturbance. The lesion may also be the first indication of systemic pathologic processes. For example, certain systemic pathologic conditions that may first present in the oral cavity as localized lesions include diabetes, human immunodeficiency virus (HIV) infection, leukemia, and nutritional deficiency.

Lesions are common within the head and neck as well as the oral cavity of the adult population.[1] An estimated 10% of dental patients have a lesion. Most of these lesions fall into the category of an **atypical finding,** a discovery that some clinicians call a *variation from normal.*

However, the lesion could instead be an **abnormal finding,** a discovery that is not only not typical but is serious pathologic condition, and possibly can even prove fatal, such as with cancer. First, one must understand the general use of *tumor,* or now more specifically called **neoplasm,** when discussing cancer, which is an abnormal mass of tissue that forms when cells grow and divide more than usual or never die off. One classification is *cancer* or **malignant neoplasm,** which can invade nearby tissue and later can undergo **metastasis,** which means that cancer has spread to a different body part or region from where it started.

In contrast, a *noncancerous* or **benign neoplasm** does not invade nearby tissue but stays at its primary location and does not undergo metastasis. However, a benign neoplasm can still have a serious impact on health if they are considered aggressive in growth or prevent body function.[2]

When performed, cancer screening as part of overall patient examination is most frequently accomplished by the dental hygienist in the dental office and not usually by the dentist since the patient is more regularly seen for preventive care.[1] However, research shows that currently less than an estimated 15% to 25% of those who regularly visit a dental office report having had a cancer screening.

Thus as a dental professional, it is the dental hygienist's responsibility to recognize any lesions as either atypical or abnormal findings during the head and neck examination and to inform the patient's dentist of any abnormal findings (Box 16.1). Imaging may also be indicated to assert the baseline status of the findings, possibly along with other clinical procedures to assess cancer risk.

Taking such appropriate action after recognizing an abnormal finding is absolutely necessary for promoting health and, in the case of cancer, possibly preventing premature death. In addition, informing the patient of the need for regular self-examination allows them to assume some responsibility for the care and control of their own oral and associated systemic health.

Lesion Diagnosis

By definition, a **diagnosis** is the identification of the lesion by assessment of the symptoms and signs after examination. After assessing any atypical or abnormal findings during the examination, the dental hygienist accurately describes and documents them in the patient record to form the **dental hygiene diagnosis** for the patient. This level of diagnosis of the patient by the dental hygienist includes clinical findings, radiographic findings, oral homecare needs, and future oral care needs. This level of diagnosis of a possible lesion can include "like" or "related to" or "due to" and "evidenced by" if consistent with a known

TABLE 16.1 Extraoral and Intraoral Examination Skills

Skills	Application Examples
Observation: surveillance of patient to detect atypical or abnormal findings	Noting patient movement; body structure and symmetry; skin and mucous membrane color, surface texture, contour, and form; patient knowledge, attitude, behavior
Palpation: using touch to detect atypical or abnormal findings; see Table 16.2 for examination methods	Noting tenderness, surface texture, consistency, temperature
Olfaction: sensing odors to detect atypical or abnormal findings	Noting alcohol breath with recent consumption and possible alcohol abuse; smoker's breath with nicotine use; halitosis or bad breath associated with dental caries and periodontal disease or gastrointestinal difficulties, which is especially strong with necrotizing periodontitis; sweet, fruity acetone breath with ketosis from diabetic acidosis

lesion type. The dental hygiene diagnosis provides the basis for the dental hygiene care plan; see Chapters 22 and 23.

The dental hygiene diagnosis will then support the dentist in forming an accurate differential diagnosis, using both signs and symptoms noted during further examination or any additional testing. A **differential diagnosis** or *clinical diagnosis* is the identification of a lesion by differentiating between pathologic processes that may produce lesions with similar signs and symptoms.

The **definitive diagnosis** or *surgical diagnosis* formed by the patient's dentist or referred specialist is achieved after forming a clinical picture and receiving test results, such as biopsies, that are performed to determine whether a certain pathologic condition is present. Further referrals to a dental specialist or other healthcare professionals are also made as needed by the dentist.

The dental hygiene diagnosis, as with any type of later diagnosis, also serves as a baseline for subsequent examination and future treatment planning in the dental setting, as well as a legal record in case of a claim or patient identification after an accident or disaster.

OVERALL PATIENT EVALUATION

Initially, the patient is observed while seated during reception and as they enter the treatment room to be seated. The clinician notes any physical characteristics and impairments that may require special dental care modification or further consultation. This overall evaluation includes any differing aspects of speech and hearing; the functional level of hands, arms, and legs; and personal hygiene status.

For example, an overall evaluation may suggest an oropharyngeal cancer (OPC), with its hoarse speech. A history of stroke may be indicated with slurred speech or aphasia, from traumatic brain injury with its difficulty when forming words. That type of difference in speech may also be present with the use of prescribed medications or drug abuse. Breathing difficulties may be attributable to respiratory or emotional condition, and the clicking of dentures may indicate a possible poor fit.

Hearing loss, possibly with extra-loud speech, may be the result of developmental disturbance, aging, or injury. Compromised hearing when exchanging greetings may be a result of medications or an infection. A history of loss of blood supply to the brain area that controls speech as a result of stroke, high blood pressure, or diabetes could also be involved.

Functional loss of the arms and legs may indicate a history of injury as well as presence of a pathologic condition or developmental disturbance. Compromised hand and arm function may indicate the need to modify future oral homecare. There may also be a need to modify the patient's seating arrangements during treatment and there may be difficulty attending future dental appointments. Personal hygiene status may reflect the patient's overall concern about health and care given to the oral cavity as well as their oral health literacy (OHL).

EXAMINATION PROCEDURE

Before performing extraoral and intraoral examinations, the dental hygienist reviews the patient's medical and dental history, as well as imaging history and other procedural tests, and explains the examination procedure to the patient. Screening questions are also asked before the examinations to establish the risk for cancer, such as nicotine use, alcohol abuse, and history of human papillomavirus (HPV) infection or related cancer. Establishing an examination sequence and systematically following it reduces the possibility of overlooking an area.[3,4]

The skills of **observation**, **palpation**, and **olfaction** are basic to examination of a lesion (Table 16.1).[5,6] Palpation examination methods that are used to examine a lesion include **digital palpation**, **bidigital palpation**, **manual palpation**, **bimanual palpation**, **bilateral palpation**, and **circular palpation** (Table 16.2).[3]

The clinician must always observe the lesion first and only then palpate it using the correct method to avoid possibly altering the lesion before fully observing it. To obtain maximum information about a lesion, the clinician always palpates against a firm or bony structure, such as a muscle or bone, as well as other fingers. In addition, nearby lymph nodes, salivary glands, temporomandibular joints (TMJs), and thyroid gland are then palpated to establish any possible associated involvement.[6]

EXTRAORAL EXAMINATION

An extraoral examination includes a thorough examination of the structures of the head and neck. Procedure 16.1 for head regions examination and Procedure 16.2 for neck regions examination detail the steps for examining the structures along with examples of typical findings.[3] Importantly, Table 16.3 for head regions and Table 16.4 for neck regions suggest possible atypical findings and abnormal findings.

TABLE 16.2 Palpation Examination Methods

Methods	Application Examples
Digital palpation: compressing and moving along using the index finger(s)	Used for oral vestibules, floor of the mouth, lingual border of mandible 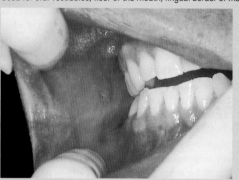
Bidigital palpation: compressing and rolling along using the fingers and thumbs	Used for lips, labial and buccal mucosa, tongue 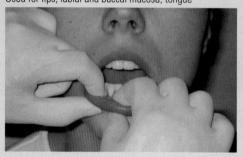
Manual palpation: compressing and moving along simultaneously using the fingers of one hand	Used for lymph nodes, thyroid gland 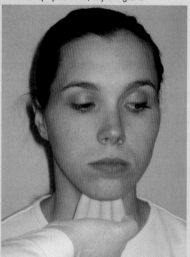
Bimanual palpation: compressing and moving along using the index finger of one hand and fingers of the other hand simultaneously on opposite sides	Used for the floor of the mouth 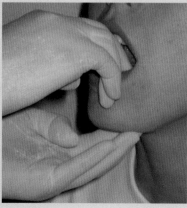

TABLE 16.2 Palpation Examination Methods—cont'd

Methods	Application Examples
Bilateral palpation: compressing and moving along using a finger or the fingers of both hands simultaneously on contralateral sides	Used for general palpation to allow for bilateral comparison 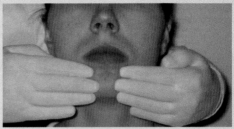
Circular palpation: compressing and rotating around the fingertips of one hand	Used for suspected lesion 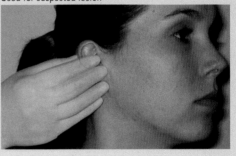

Figures courtesy of Margaret J. Fehrenbach, RDH, MS, and from Fehrenbach MJ, Herring SW. *Illustrated Anatomy of the Head and Neck*. 6th ed. Saunders; 2021.

PROCEDURE 16.1 Performing Extraoral Examination: Head Regions

Equipment
Personal protective equipment
Mouth mirror instrument
Patient hand mirror

Extraoral Head Regions	Steps	Typical Findings
Overall evaluation, including skin 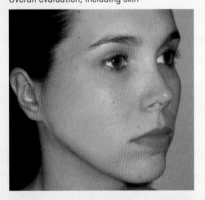	Observe symmetry and skin coloration of face and neck with patient sitting upright and relaxed; allow patient to observe in handheld mirror	Face and head symmetric; skin is firm with coloration similar to rest of body, possibly with physiologic pigmentation
Frontal region, including forehead and frontal sinuses 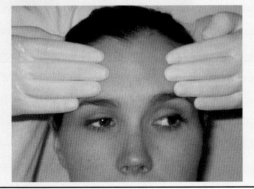	Observe and bilaterally palpate forehead, including frontal sinuses	Area firm and smooth, without tenderness

Continued

PROCEDURE 16.1   Performing Extraoral Examination: Head Regions—cont'd

Extraoral Head Regions	Steps	Typical Findings
Parietal and occipital regions, including scalp, hair, occipital nodes	Observe entire scalp by moving hair, especially around hairline, starting from one ear and proceeding to the other ear and bilaterally palpate occipital nodes on each side of the base of the head while asking the patient to lean the head forward	Scalp firm and continuous and without changes; hair free of debris; nodes not clinically palpable or visible

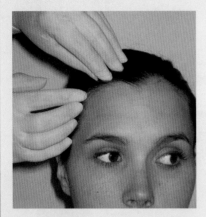

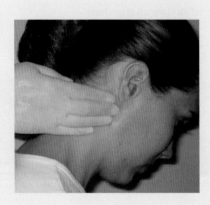

Temporal and auricular regions, including scalp, ears, auricular nodes	Observe and bilaterally palpate external ears as well as scalp, face, and auricular nodes around each ear	Nodes not clinically palpable or visible; ears without discharge or inner canal redness or darkness

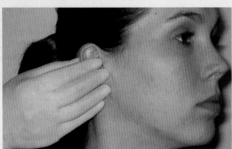

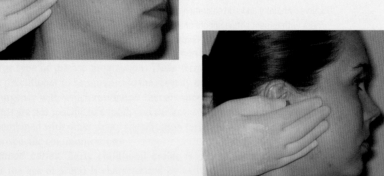

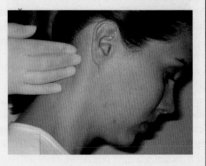

PROCEDURE 16.1 Performing Extraoral Examination: Head Regions—cont'd

Extraoral Head Regions	Steps	Typical Findings
Orbital regions, including eyes 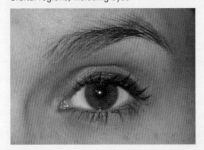	Observe movements and responses of eyes to light and action	Each iris clear and exhibiting response to light via the pupil; sclera is white; no swelling, bruising, and/or drainage; can open and close eyes
Nasal region, including nose 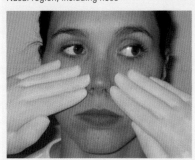	Observe and bilaterally palpate external nose starting at the root and proceeding to the apex	Nose symmetric and no signs of discharge, redness or darkness, as well as overlying skin ulceration
Infraorbital and zygomatic regions, including the muscles of facial expression, facial nodes, maxillae, maxillary sinuses, and temporomandibular joints 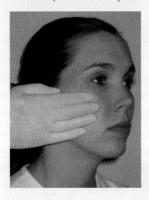 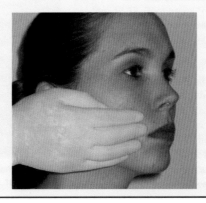	Observe areas inferior to orbits, noting use of muscles of facial expression; observe and bilaterally palpate each side of face and facial nodes, moving from infraorbital region to labial commissure and then to surface of mandible; observe and bilaterally palpate maxillary sinuses Ask patient to open and close the mouth several times; ask patient to move opened jaw left, then right, then forward; then ask whether pain or tenderness is experienced and note sounds made by either joint. To further access joints, gently place a finger into the outer parts of each external acoustic meatus during these movements.	Can use of muscles of facial expression on both sides of face; joint movement is smooth, continuous, and silent; both sides of the joint function similarly; both the joint and associated musculature are free of pain

Continued

PROCEDURE 16.1   Performing Extraoral Examination: Head Regions—cont'd

Extraoral Head Regions	Steps	Typical Findings

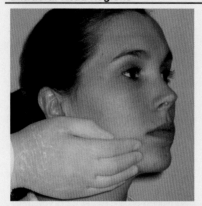
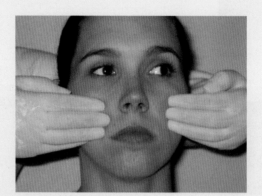
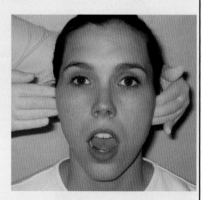
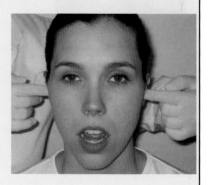

PROCEDURE 16.1   Performing Extraoral Examination: Head Regions—cont'd

Extraoral Head Regions	Steps	Typical Findings
Buccal regions, including masseter muscle, parotid salivary glands, superficial parotid nodes, and mandible 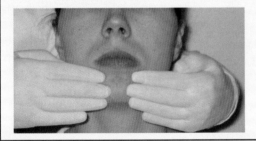	Observe and bilaterally palpate masseter muscle and parotid salivary glands by starting in front of each ear, moving to zygomatic arch and inferior to angle of the mandible; then place the fingers of each hand over the masseter muscle and then ask patient to clench teeth together several times as best they can	Area is firm and smooth, without tenderness or increased size or density
Mental region, including chin	Observe and bilaterally palpate the chin	Area is firm and smooth, without tenderness

Figures courtesy of Margaret J. Fehrenbach, RDH, MS, and from Fehrenbach MJ, Herring SW. *Illustrated Anatomy of the Head and Neck.* 6th ed. Saunders; 2021.

After performing the extraoral examination, the clinician proceeds with the intraoral examination (discussed later).

Lymph Node Examination

Lymph nodes are bean-shaped structures grouped in clusters along the connecting lymphatic vessels, positioned to filter toxic products from the lymph to prevent their entry into the blood (Fig. 16.1).[4] The nodes can be superficially located along with the superficial veins or found deeper within the tissue with the associated deeper blood vessels. All head and neck nodes are paired and usually drain either the right or the left tissues, structures, or organs in the area, depending on their location; one exception is for the midline submental nodes, which bilaterally drain the tissue in the region.

In healthy patients, the nodes are usually small, soft, and free or mobile in the surrounding tissue and thus cannot be observed or palpated within their usual location during an extraoral examination of the head and neck. Palpable and possibly observed nodes during extraoral examination are those that have undergone **lymphadenopathy**, with its associated enlargement resulting from an increase in size and a change in consistency of the lymphoid tissue.[3] Changed node consistency can range from firm to hard.

Lymph nodes also can become attached or fixed to the surrounding tissue as the pathologic process progresses. Nodes also can be tender or even painful to the patient when palpated because of the pressure an enlarged node can place on the area nerves. However, most deeper enlarged nodes cannot be observed or even palpated due to

PROCEDURE 16.2 Performing Extraoral Examination: Neck Regions

Equipment
Personal protective equipment
Patient hand mirror

Extraoral Neck Regions	Procedural Steps	Typical Findings
Submandibular and submental triangles, including submandibular and sublingual salivary glands and associated nodes 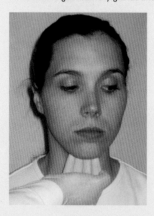 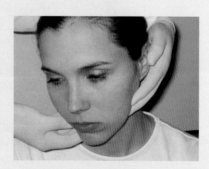	While asking to lower chin, manually palpate submandibular and sublingual glands and associated nodes directly underneath the chin and on the inferior border of mandible; then push tissue in area over bony inferior border of mandible on each side, where it is grasped and rolled	Mandible is symmetric, with continuous borders; nodes not clinically palpable or visible
Anterior and posterior cervical triangles, including sternocleidomastoid muscles and associated nodes 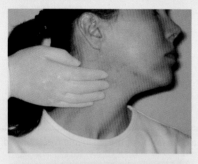 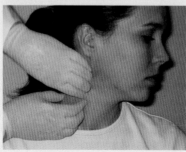	With patient looking straight ahead, observe and then use both hands to manually palpate the superficial cervical nodes on either side of the neck, starting inferior to the ears and continuing the length of the sternocleidomastoid muscles surface to clavicles Next, ask patient to tilt the head to each side to palpate superior deep cervical nodes on underside of anterior and posterior aspects. Then ask patient to raise shoulders up and forward to palpate inferior deep cervical, accessory, and supraclavicular nodes over each trapezius muscle surface.	Nodes not clinically palpable or visible

PROCEDURE 16.2 Performing Extraoral Examination: Neck Regions—cont'd

Extraoral Neck Regions	Procedural Steps	Typical Findings
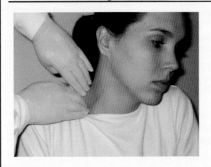 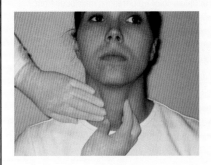 Anterior midline cervical region, including hyoid bone, thyroid cartilage, thyroid gland, larynx	Locate thyroid cartilage and pass fingers up and down thyroid gland, examining for abnormal masses and assessing overall size; then place one hand on each side of the trachea and gently displace the thyroid gland tissue to contralateral side of neck while the other hand manually palpates displaced tissue. Compare the two thyroid lobes for size and texture, using observation and bimanual palpation. Ask the patient to swallow, possibly with water, to check for gland mobility by observing while it moves superiorly and then back inferiorly. Finally, bidigitally palpate both the hyoid bone and larynx, deliberately and gently moving each one.	Thyroid gland is not enlarged, tender, or with abnormal consistency and moves during swallowing; larynx is without tenderness and freely movable when deliberately moved and palpated

Figures courtesy of Margaret J. Fehrenbach, RDH, MS, and from Fehrenbach MJ, Herring SW. *Illustrated Anatomy of the Head and Neck*. 6th ed. Saunders; 2021.

their hidden position, even when there is a change in consistency or attachment.

Palpable lymph nodes may help determine where a pathologic process such as infection or cancer is active and may help establish whether it has become widespread.[2] Documentation of palpable nodes assists in the diagnosis, treatment, and prognosis of a pathologic condition. Thus understanding the relationship between the node location and its drainage patterns is important.[1] Furthermore, it is important to keep in mind that the head and neck nodes drain not only intraoral structures such as the teeth but also the eyes, ears, nasal cavity, and deeper areas of the pharynx (Box 16.2).

Head and Neck Regions

The clinician begins by performing an overall evaluation of the head and neck, including the surrounding skin, before moving on to each specific region of the head and neck. The head and neck are generally symmetric and the skin is continuous and firm, possibly with **physiologic pigmentation**.[4] This typical variation in coloration results from melanin increase and can range from light brown to almost black tones in specific areas or throughout the region; it is more common with darker skin tones. It can happen anywhere on the skin as well as oral cavity but is mainly found intraorally within the attached gingiva.

Next, the clinician divides the head and neck into specific regions to observe and bilaterally palpate each region in sequence, moving from the superior to the inferior regions using observation first and then

palpation as discussed earlier (Fig. 16.2).[3] The patient is seated, if possible, in an upright, relaxed position. Adequate lighting and exposure of the area being evaluated are essential, including removal of any neck-related clothing or glasses as well as contact lenses for comfort.

Frontal Region

The frontal region includes the forehead and the area superior to the eyes. The paired frontal sinuses are located in the frontal bone just superior to the nasal cavity, and each communicates with and drains into the nasal cavity (Fig. 16.3).

Parietal and Occipital Regions

The parietal and occipital regions are covered by the scalp, which overlies the skull. The occipital nodes are bilaterally located on the posterior base of the head in the occipital region and drain this part of the scalp (see Fig. 16.1). The occipital nodes then empty into the deep cervical nodes in the neck.

Temporal and Auricular Regions

Within the temporal and auricular regions is the external ear, which is comprised of an auricle, the larger flap of the ear, and its external acoustic meatus, an inner tube through which sound waves are transmitted to the middle ear within the skull.

The anterior and posterior auricular nodes are located anterior and posterior to each ear (see Fig. 16.1). These nodes drain the external

TABLE 16.3 Atypical and Abnormal Findings for Extraoral Regions: Head Regions

Extraoral Head Regions	Atypical Findings	Abnormal Findings
Overall evaluation, including skin	Moles, freckles, scarring, cosmetic facial piercings, tattoos	Needle marks from drug use; trauma from domestic abuse; cosmetic facial piercing or tattoo infections
Frontal region, including forehead and frontal sinuses	Tenderness from sinusitis	Redder or darker red as well as ulcerous and abnormal pigmentation with skin cancer
Parietal and occipital regions, including scalp, hair, occipital nodes	Debris found on scalp or hair; palpable nontender node with scarring from past chronic infection	Scalp lesions under hair such as redder or darker red as well as ulcerous and abnormal pigmentation with skin cancer; soft, tender, enlarged, and freely movable nodes with acute infection; hard, nontender, and fixed nodes with chronic infection or cancer; hair loss or patches or thinning from alopecia, chemotherapy, eating disorder, or hormonal and nutritional disorder
Temporal and auricular regions, including scalp, ears, auricular nodes	Discharge or inner canal redder or darker red; cosmetic ear piercings	Soft, tender, enlarged, and freely movable nodes with acute infection; hard, nontender, and fixed nodes with chronic infection, cancer, or trauma from domestic abuse; redder or darker red as well as ulcerous and abnormal pigmentation with skin cancer, especially on sun-exposed auricles; cosmetic piercing infection
Orbital regions, including eyes	Tearing and eye redness from emotional distress or respiratory condition; eyeglasses or contact lenses; cosmetic eyebrow piercings	Yellow sclerae with jaundice or bluish color from trauma; iris cloudy from pathologic process or pinpoint from drug intake; yellowish discharge with infection; excessive tearing and redness from drug or alcohol intake or obstructing mass in maxillary sinus, nose, or facial soft tissue; traumatic swelling and bruising from domestic abuse; swelling from cancer in palate or maxillary and ethmoidal sinuses; inability to close eye on affected side with facial paralysis from Bell palsy or stroke; cosmetic piercing infection
Nasal region, including nose	Nasal discharge with skin redness or darkness from respiratory conditions from allergies and infections; loss of symmetry with deviated septum or broken nose; cosmetic nose piercings	Inflammation, infection, and necrosis of tissue, nasal septum perforation, saddle nose deformity from cocaine snorting; redder or darker red as well as ulcerous and abnormal pigmentation from skin cancer; traumatic swelling and bruising from domestic abuse; cosmetic piercing infection
Infraorbital and zygomatic regions, including muscles of facial expression, facial nodes, maxillae, maxillary sinuses, temporomandibular joints	Tenderness with maxillary sinusitis; joint sounds or deviation of mandible upon opening	Facial paralysis from Bell palsy or stroke; joint disorder with jaw movement limitations, subluxation, pain
Buccal regions, including masseter muscle, parotid salivary glands, mandible	Overdeveloped masseter muscle with parafunctional habits	Soft, tender, enlarged, and freely movable nodes from acute infection; hard, nontender, and fixed nodes with chronic infection or cancer; constant glandular pain with cancer; redder or darker red as well as ulcerous and abnormal pigmentation with skin cancer; odontogenic infection signs
Mental region, including chin	Dimple or slight cleft at mandibular symphysis	Traumatic swelling and bruising from domestic abuse or scarring from accidents; odontogenic infection signs

TABLE 16.4 Atypical and Abnormal Findings for Extraoral Regions: Neck Regions

Extraoral Neck Regions	Atypical Findings	Abnormal Findings
Submandibular and submental triangles, including submandibular and sublingual salivary glands and associated nodes	Palpable nontender node with scarring from previous chronic infection	Blocked duct from stone or trauma; excessive salivary flow or xerostomia; soft, tender, enlarged, and freely movable nodes with acute infection; hard, nontender, and fixed nodes with chronic infection or cancer; odontogenic infection signs
Anterior and posterior cervical triangles, including sternocleidomastoid muscles and associated nodes	Palpable nontender node with scarring from previous chronic infection; palpable jugulodigastric or tonsillar node from inflamed palatine tonsils and/or pharynx	Soft, tender, enlarged, and freely movable nodes with acute infection; hard, nontender, and fixed nodes with chronic infection or cancer, especially with breast cancer history
Anterior midline cervical region, including hyoid bone, thyroid cartilage, thyroid gland, larynx		Thyroid enlargement with goiter; thyroid tender with rubbery or hard masses from cyst or cancer; thyroid lack from surgery; thyroid lacking movement during swallowing; not freely movable larynx with stiffness and/or tenderness; also voice and speech changes

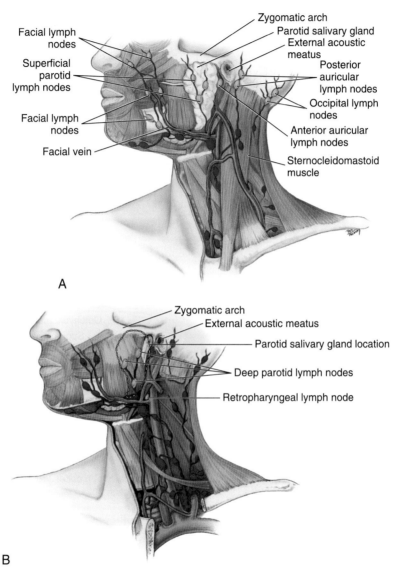

A

B

Fig. 16.1 Diagram of lymphatic drainage system of the head and neck. (A) Superficial lymph nodes of the head; (B) deep lymph nodes of the head.

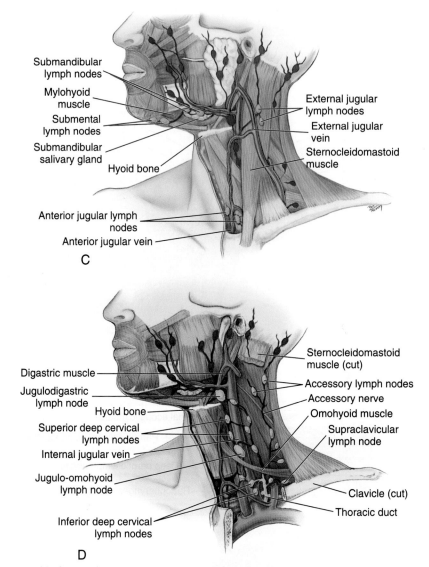

Fig. 16.1, cont'd (C) superficial cervical lymph nodes; (D) deep cervical lymph nodes.From Fehrenbach MJ, Herring SW. *Illustrated Anatomy of the Head and Neck*. 6th ed. Saunders; 2021.)

ear, the lacrimal or tear gland superior to the eye, and the surrounding regions of the scalp and face, and then empty into the deep cervical nodes.

Orbital Region

In the orbital region, the eyeball and all its supporting structures are contained in the bony socket, the orbit. The white area, or sclera, with its central area of coloration, the circular iris, is located on the eyeball. The opening in the center of the iris is the pupil, which appears black and changes size as the iris responds to changing light conditions. The conjunctiva is the delicate and thin membrane lining the inside of the eyelids and the front of the eyeball. The outer corner where the upper and lower eyelids meet is the outer canthus; the inner corner is the inner canthus.

Nasal Region

The external nose is the main feature in the nasal region. Inferior to the apex on both sides of the nose are the nostrils or nares (singular, naris).

The nares are separated internally by the midline nasal septum. The nares are laterally bounded on each side by a winglike cartilaginous structure(s), the ala (plural, alae) of the nose. The tip of the nose is flexible when palpated.

Infraorbital and Zygomatic Regions

The infraorbital and zygomatic regions are both located on the face (see Fig. 16.2). The infraorbital region is located inferior to the orbital region and lateral to the nasal region. Farther laterally is the zygomatic region, which is comprised of the zygomatic arch that forms the cheekbone. The zygomatic arch extends from just inferior to the eye's lateral margin toward the middle part of the ear.

Facial lymph nodes are superficially positioned along the length of the facial vein and are usually small and variable in number and further categorized according to their location (see Fig. 16.1). Each facial node group drains the skin and mucous membranes where they are located and finally drains into the deep cervical nodes by way of the submandibular nodes. The paired maxillary sinuses are each located

The patient of record is a 75-year-old male retired chess player who had bypass surgery over a year ago. He has what appears to be a lesion on the mandibular alveolar process anterior to his mandibular right third molar. He is taking a diuretic medication and an angiotensin-converting enzyme. He says he is always very thirsty but likes soft drinks rather than water.

- What conditions may be noted during the intraoral examination that are attributable to being thirsty?
- To obtain information pertinent to the health of his dentition during the intraoral examination, which procedures related to his salivary glands will be important?
- How should the lesion on the mandibular alveolar process anterior to his mandibular right third molar be assessed by the clinician?
- What lymph nodes are related to the draining of his mandibular right third molar?
- How might the involved lymph nodes have reacted to the recent change in his oral health?

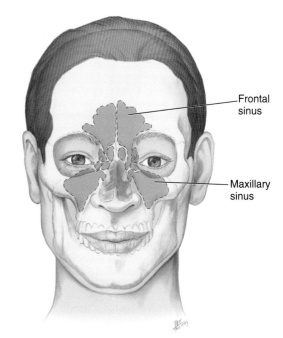

Fig. 16.3 **Diagram of anterior view of the skull and the palpable paranasal sinuses.** Note that the ethmoidal sinus is not included since it is not palpable. (Adapted from Fehrenbach MJ, Herring SW. *Illustrated Anatomy of the Head and Neck.* 6th ed. Saunders; 2021.)

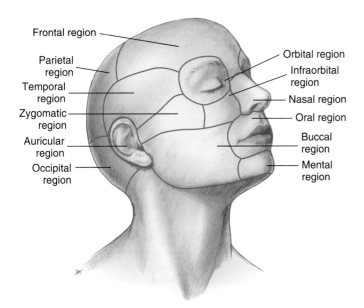

Fig. 16.2 Diagram of regions of the head for examination. (From Fehrenbach MJ, Herring SW. *Illustrated Anatomy of the Head and Neck.* 6th ed. Saunders; 2021.)

in the body of each maxilla, superior to the maxillary canine and premolars, and drain into the nasal cavity (see Fig. 16.3). For the maxillary and mandibular arch anatomy, see Chapter 17.

Inferior to the zygomatic arch and just anterior to the ear is the TMJ, which is where the upper skull forms a joint with the lower jaw. The joint on each side of the head involves the temporal bone of the maxilla and the condyle of the mandible. Joint movements during the examination are observed and palpated when opening or closing the mouth or when moving the lower jaw to the right, left, or forward and also gently placing a finger into the outer part of external acoustic meatus when opening and closing the jaw. Listening to any joint sounds during movement may also be noted in the patient's record; this can be considered using *auscultation*.

Buccal Region

The buccal region is located laterally on the face with its cheek, mainly formed by a fat and muscle mass (see Fig. 16.2). This includes the

strong masseter muscle, which is felt when a patient clenches the teeth. The sharp outer part of lower jaw that is inferior to the earlobe is the angle of the mandible. The parotid salivary gland is also within this region since it occupies the area anterior and inferior to each ear as well as posterior to the mandibular ramus (Fig. 16.4). The superficial parotid nodes are located just on the surface of each gland; under each are the deep parotid nodes.

Mental Region and Submandibular and Submental Triangles

The chin is the mental region's major feature. Inferiorly, the neck presents with a large strap muscle, the sternocleidomastoid (SCM) muscle, which diagonally divides each side of the neck into two cervical regions (Fig. 16.5). The SCM muscle originates from the clavicle and sternum and passes posteriorly and superiorly to insert onto the temporal bone, just posterior and inferior to the ear. When the patient's head is tilted to the side for observation and palpation, the SCM muscle is more prominent.

The anterior neck region corresponds to the two anterior cervical triangles, which are separated by a midline. The lateral neck region posterior to each SCM muscle forms the posterior cervical triangles on each side. There are many superficial cervical nodes in this region, such as the external jugular nodes, which are located along the external jugular vein and are superficial to the SCM muscle and serve as secondary nodes for the more superior nodes that then empty into the deep cervical nodes (see Fig. 16.1). Another regional group is the anterior jugular nodes located on each side of the neck along the length of the anterior jugular vein, anterior to the larynx, trachea, and superficial to the SCM muscle, which drain the infrahyoid region of the neck and then empty into the deep cervical nodes.

The neck's anterior cervical triangle can be further subdivided into smaller triangular regions by parts of neck muscles and the mandible. The submandibular region is the superior part of the anterior cervical triangle on each side of the neck. The paired submandibular salivary glands are located in this region posterior to the paired sublingual glands (see Fig. 16.4).

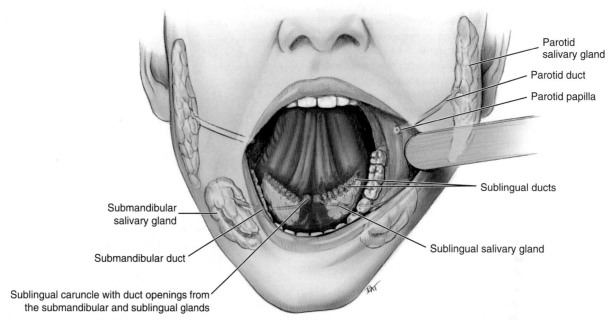

Fig. 16.4 Diagram of major salivary glands and associated structures. (From Fehrenbach MJ, Herring SW. *Illustrated Anatomy of the Head and Neck.* 6th ed. Saunders; 2021.)

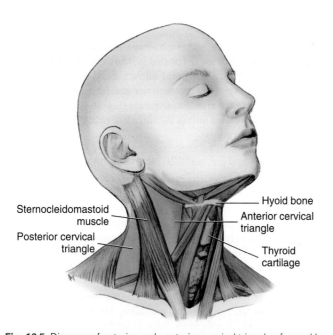

Fig. 16.5 Diagram of anterior and posterior cervical triangles formed by the sternocleidomastoid muscle. (From Fehrenbach MJ, Herring SW. *Illustrated Anatomy of the Head and Neck.* 6th ed. Saunders; 2021.)

The submandibular nodes are located at the inferior border of the ramus of the mandible, just superficial to the submandibular gland (see Fig. 16.1). They drain the cheeks, upper lip, body of the tongue, anterior hard palate, sublingual and submandibular salivary glands, and all the dentition and associated tissue except the mandibular incisors and maxillary third molars. The submandibular nodes then empty into the deep cervical nodes.

Near the midline of the anterior cervical triangle is the submental region, where both the sublingual salivary glands are located (see Fig. 16.4). The sublingual and submental nodes are located inferior to the chin in this region (see Fig. 16.1). These nodes drain both sides of the chin, the lower lip, the floor of the mouth, the apex of the tongue, and the mandibular incisors and associated tissue. They then empty into the submandibular nodes or directly into the deep cervical nodes.

Anterior and Posterior Cervical Triangles

The inferior and superior deep cervical nodes are also bilaterally located along the neck's length, deep to the SCM muscle (see Fig. 16.1). These nodes drain the nasal cavity, posterior hard palate, soft palate, base of the tongue, maxillary third molars, esophagus, trachea, and thyroid gland. These inferior nodes may be involved with breast cancer since they also communicate with the axillary nodes under the arms which drains that tissue.

In addition to the deep cervical nodes in the neck's most inferior area are the supraclavicular nodes that are located along the clavicle and drain the anterior cervical triangles (see Fig. 16.1). The supraclavicular nodes then empty into one of the jugular trunks or directly into the right lymphatic duct or thoracic duct. Thus these nodes are the final endpoint of lymphatic drainage from the entire body; for instance, cancer starting from the lungs, esophagus, and stomach may exist in these nodes. Posterior to the supraclavicular nodes are the accessory nodes, which drain the posterior scalp and neck regions and then drain into the supraclavicular nodes.

Anterior Midline Cervical Region

Within the anterior midline cervical region is the hyoid bone, which has various muscle groups attached to it and which controls the position of the base of the tongue (Fig. 16.6). The hyoid bone can be effectively palpated inferior and medial to both angles of the mandible because it is suspended in the neck without any bony connection. When palpating the neck, the clinician should not confuse the hyoid bone with the more inferiorly placed thyroid cartilage, which also is found within the anterior midline. The thyroid cartilage is the prominence of the voice box or larynx (see Fig. 16.6). The thyroid cartilage's anterior part is visible as the "Adam's apple," which is especially prominent in adult males. The vocal cords or ligaments of the larynx are posteriorly attached to the thyroid cartilage.

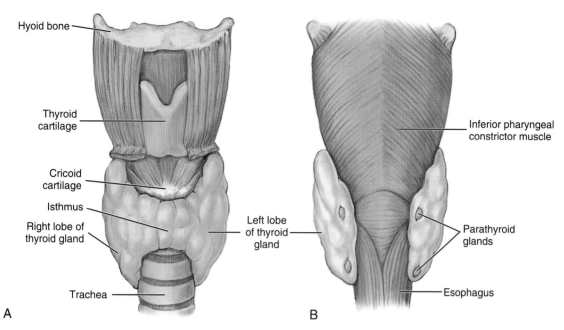

Fig. 16.6 Diagram of (A) anterior and (B) posterior view of the thyroid cartilage, thyroid gland, and associated structures. (From Fehrenbach MJ, Herring SW. *Illustrated Anatomy of the Head and Neck.* 6th ed. Saunders; 2021.)

The thyroid gland also is located in this region inferior to the thyroid cartilage and at the junction of the larynx and the trachea. The gland has two lobes on either side of the neck, anteriorly connected by an isthmus.

INTRAORAL EXAMINATION

The intraoral examination includes evaluation of the oral cavity and associated structures such as the palate, pharynx, tongue, and floor of the mouth. The patient is seated in a relaxed, supine position and will need to remove any dentures or oral appliances. A nonpetroleum lubricant applied to the lip areas makes patients more comfortable.

After an overall intraoral evaluation with a mouth mirror, the clinician next divides the oral cavity into specific regions to examine each in sequence using observation first and then palpation, as discussed earlier. During the evaluation of mucosal surfaces, gently drying these surfaces with a gauze or an air syringe is important to ensure that color and surface texture changes will become more obvious. Patients are encouraged to inform the clinician of any discomfort during the evaluation, possibly by raising one hand to allow discussion.

Procedure 16.3 details the steps for examining structures during an intraoral clinical evaluation with examples of typical findings.[3] Importantly, Table 16.5 suggests both possible atypical and abnormal findings for the oral cavity. After performing the intraoral examination, dentition examination is performed along with caries and periodontal disease risk assessment; see Chapters 17 through 20.

Oral Region

The oral region contains the lips and oral cavity. The lips are outlined from the surrounding skin by a transition, the mucocutaneous junction at the vermilion border (Fig. 16.7). Each lip's vermilion zone has an appearance of being redder or darker in those with darker skin tones than the surrounding skin, possibly with localized physiologic pigmentation. On the upper lip midline extending downward from the nasal septum is a vertical groove, the philtrum, which terminates in a thicker area or tubercle. The upper and lower lips meet at each corner of the mouth, the labial commissure.

The oral cavity is the inner part of the mouth. The anatomic landmarks in the oral cavity can be used as a general point of reference during an intraoral examination (Fig. 16.8). The oral cavity is lined by oral mucosa (Fig. 16.9). The lip inner area consists of labial mucosa. The labial mucosa is continuous with buccal mucosa that lines the inner cheek. The buccal mucosa covers a dense inner tissue pad, the buccal fat pad. On the buccal mucosa just opposite the maxillary second molar is a small, raised tissue mass, the parotid papilla, which contains the parotid gland ductal opening (see Figs. 16.4 and 16.9).

The upper and lower spaces between the cheeks and lips and the gingival tissue are the maxillary and mandibular oral vestibules. Deep within each vestibule, the thicker labial or buccal mucosa that is pink to darker pink in those with darker skin tones meets the thinner redder or darker red alveolar mucosa at the mucobuccal fold, possibly with localized physiologic pigmentation (see Fig. 16.9). The labial frenum is a fold of tissue located at the midline between the labial mucosa and the alveolar mucosa on each jaw.

The dentition is located in the upper and lower jaws, the maxilla and mandible. Just posterior to the most distal maxillary tooth position is a rounded, raised area, the maxillary tuberosity. Just posterior to the most distal mandibular tooth is a dense tissue pad, the retromolar pad (see Fig. 16.8). Surrounding the teeth is the attached gingiva with its free or marginal gingiva that is also pink to darker pink in those with darker skin tones, possibly with localized physiologic pigmentation. The interdental gingiva with its interdental papillae occupies the interdental space coronal to the alveolar crest; clinically, it fills the embrasure space, possibly having a higher pigmentation level (see Fig. 16.10).

Palate and Pharynx

The roof of the mouth has both a firmer anterior part, the hard palate, and a looser posterior part, the soft palate (Fig. 16.11; see also Fig. 16.8). The midline ridge of the tissue on the hard palate is the median

PROCEDURE 16.3   Performing Intraoral Examination

Equipment
Personal protective equipment
Mouth mirror instrument
Patient hand mirror
Gauze

Intraoral Regions	Procedural Steps	Typical Findings
Oral cavity, including lips, labial commissures, buccal mucosa and labial mucosa, parotid salivary glands and ducts, alveolar processes, and attached gingiva	Allow patient to observe in handheld mirror. Observe lips at rest. Then ask the patient to smile and then to open the mouth slightly; bidigitally palpate as well as observe lower and upper lips from one commissure to the other.	Lips and oral mucosa have redder or darker red coloration than skin, possibly with physiologic pigmentation, firm in texture, free of lesions, and moist; parotid papilla is visible, same color as surrounding mucosa, and can produce saliva. Buccal and labial mucosa are generally smooth but with pebbly texture due to minor salivary glands. Attached gingiva has stippling in varying degrees with firm consistency, and is tightly anchored to teeth and underlying alveolar process.

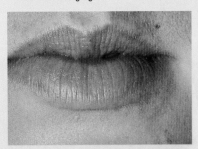

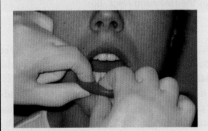

Then gently pull lower and upper lip away from the teeth to observe labial mucosa and then bidigitally palpate inner lips. Gently pull buccal mucosa slightly away from the teeth to bidigitally palpate inner cheeks on each side using circular palpation. Dry area and observe salivary flow of each parotid duct near parotid papillae.

Retract buccal mucosa and labial mucosa to observe vestibular area and gingival tissue, including maxillary tuberosity and retromolar pad on each side. Then bidigitally palpate these inner areas using circular palpation.

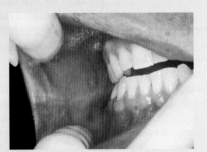

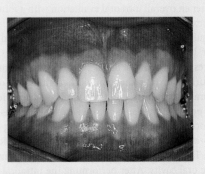

PROCEDURE 16.3 Performing Intraoral Examination—cont'd

Intraoral Regions	Procedural Steps	Typical Findings
Palate and pharynx, including median palatine raphe, incisive papilla, faucial pillars, palatine tonsils, uvula, and visible parts of oropharynx and nasopharynx 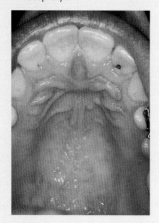	Ask the patient to tilt the head back slightly and extend the tongue to observe palatal and pharyngeal regions while using a mouth mirror to intensify light source. Gently place a mouth mirror with mirror side down on middle of dorsal surface of the tongue and ask the patient to say "ah" without sticking out the tongue. Now observe soft palate with uvula and fauces with palatine tonsils as well visible parts of the pharynx. Palpate the hard palate with first or second finger of one hand, avoiding palpation of soft palate to prevent gag reflex. 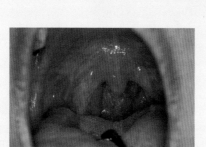	Coloration similar to other oral mucosa, with yellowish hue in soft palate area; tissue is well hydrated and free of lesions and free of lesions
Tongue, including lingual papillae, sulcus terminalis, foramen cecum, lingual tonsil 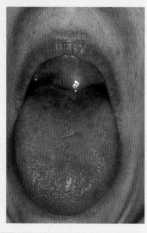	Ask the patient to extend the tongue. Wrap gauze around anterior third to obtain firm grasp to observe, and then digitally palpate dorsal surface, making sure not to force patient to extend the tongue too far and trigger gag reflex. Then slightly turn the tongue on its side to observe its base and lateral borders and bidigitally palpate lateral surfaces. Ask the patient to lift the tongue to observe and digitally palpate the ventral surface. Ask the patient to swallow; observe swallowing pattern while holding the lips apart, possibly giving water to swallow.	Bilaterally symmetric, extremely vascular, admoist, with coloration similar to other oral mucosa, possibly with physiologic pigmentation; full range of movement noted

Continued

PROCEDURE 16.3 Performing Intraoral Examination—cont'd

Intraoral Regions	Procedural Steps	Typical Findings

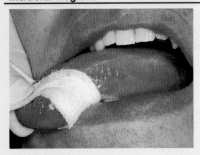

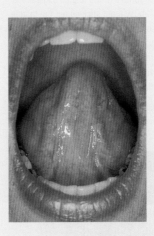

Floor of the mouth, including lingual frenum, sublingual caruncle, and submandibular and sublingual salivary glands and ducts

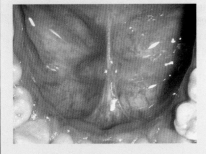

Ask the patient to touch the tongue to the palate. Using a mouth mirror to intensify light source, observe mucosa of floor of the mouth and check lingual frenum. Dry each sublingual caruncle and observe saliva flow from the ducts.

Then bimanually palpate the sublingual region by intraorally placing one index finger intraorally behind each mandibular canine and the other index finger extraorally under the chin.

Bilaterally symmetric, extremely vascular, coloration similar to other oral mucosa, and moist; sublingual caruncle is as firm as the surrounding mucosa and can produce saliva

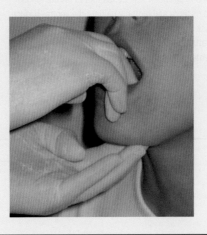

Figures courtesy of Margaret J. Fehrenbach, RDH, MS, and from Fehrenbach MJ, Herring SW. *Illustrated Anatomy of the Head and Neck.* 6th ed. Saunders; 2021.

TABLE 16.5   Atypical and Abnormal Findings: Intraoral Regions

Intraoral Regions	Atypical Findings	Abnormal Findings
Lips, including labial mucosa and oral vestibules	Lip dryness or cracks with xerostomia; ulcerations, irritation, and scarring with parafunctional habits of biting and chewing lips; inflamed labial commissures with angular cheilitis from parafunctional habits of licking lips or local and systemic infections; surrounding ulcerations or vesicles from herpetic infection; cosmetic lip piercings	Vermilion zone loss; redder, darker red, or whiter as well as ulcerous and abnormal pigmentation from cancer or erosive dermatologic pathologic condition; sagging lips on affected side from facial paralysis with Bell palsy or stroke; odontogenic infection signs; cosmetic piercing infections
Oral cavity, including buccal mucosa and fat pads, ducts at parotid papillae, alveolar mucosa, labial frenum, mucogingival junction, alveolar process of maxillae and mandible, dentition, gingiva, maxillary tuberosity, retromolar pad	Inflamed facial gingival tissue from mouth breathing; ulcerations and scarring from traumatic lesions; whitened areas with spit tobacco; bony projections or exostoses on alveolar ridges; amalgam tattoo from restorative treatment; third-molar surgery scarring	Redder, darker red, or whiter as well as ulcerous and abnormal pigmentation with cancer or erosive dermatologic pathologic condition; whiter with candidiasis or lichen planus; excessive salivary flow or xerostomia; odontogenic infection signs; ulceration and scarring with parafunctional habits; trauma with domestic abuse; stone or trauma with blocked duct
Palate, including median palatine raphe and incisive papilla, faucial pillars, palatine tonsils, uvula, visible parts of oropharynx and nasopharynx	Palatal torus; food burns; red or dark petechiae on whiter background with nicotinic stomatitis; bifid uvula; inflamed tonsillar tissue; third-molar surgery scarring; redness and soft palate swelling from postnasal drip	Denture stomatitis; redder, darker red, or whiter as well as ulcerous with cancer; trauma from child abuse; sagging palatal tissue from facial paralysis with stroke; asymmetry, ulceration, or masses on tonsils or pillars with cancer
Tongue, including lingual papillae, sulcus terminalis, foramen cecum, lingual tonsil	Dorsal surface clefting with fissured tongue; dorsal white and red patches from geographic tongue; dorsal raised or flat redder or darker red central area with central papillary atrophy; lingual varicosities; dorsal surface coated or stained; large with macroglossia; thrusting movements during swallowing; lateral scalloped or scarred from parafunctional habits of chewing or clenching; cosmetic piercing	Hairy leukoplakia with human immunodeficiency virus infection; papillae loss, soreness, or burning with nutritional disorders; limited movement, enlargement, or induration with cancer; trauma with child abuse; cosmetic piercing infection; difficulty swallowing with dysphagia or deviation from nerve disorders or oropharyngeal cancers
Floor of the mouth, including lingual frenum and submandibular and sublingual salivary glands and ducts	Mandibular torus or tori; cosmetic frenum piercings	Blocked or traumatized duct from stone with mucocele or ranula; limited movement of the lingual frenum from ankyloglossia; excessive salivary flow or xerostomia; soreness; enlargement or induration; redder, darker red, or whiter as well as ulcerous and abnormal pigmentation from cancer; trauma from child abuse; cosmetic piercing infections

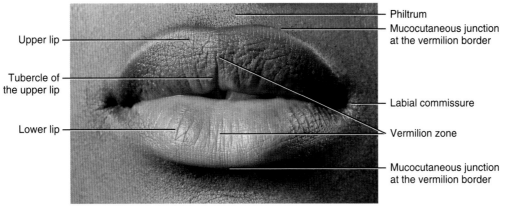

Fig. 16.7 Frontal view of the lips and related anatomic landmarks. (From Kindel Media, Los Angeles, 2022 with adaption from Fehrenbach MJ, Herring SW. *Illustrated Anatomy of the Head and Neck.* 6th ed. Saunders; 2021.)

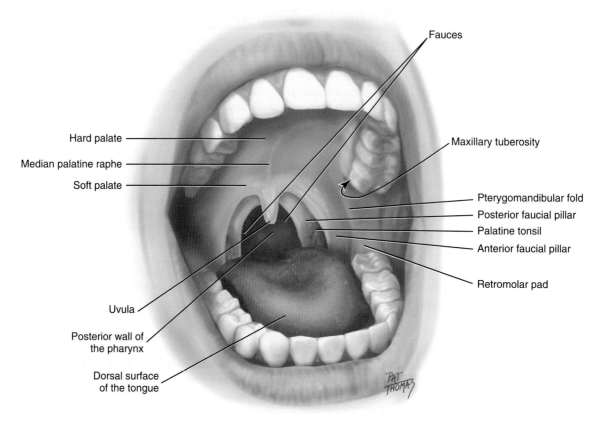

Fig. 16.8 Diagram of anatomic landmarks in the oral cavity. (From Fehrenbach MJ, Herring SW. *Illustrated Anatomy of the Head and Neck.* 6th ed. Saunders; 2021.)

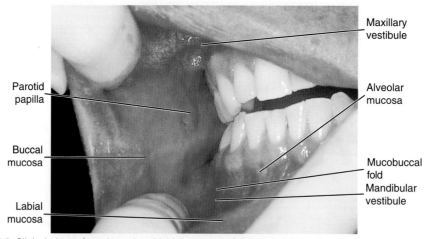

Fig. 16.9 Clinical view of the buccal and labial mucosa of the oral cavity, with anatomic landmarks noted. (Courtesy of Margaret J. Fehrenbach, RDH, MS, and from Fehrenbach MJ, Herring SW. *Illustrated Anatomy of the Head and Neck.* 6th ed. Saunders; 2021.)

palatine raphe. A small bulge of tissue at the most anterior part, palatal to the anterior teeth, is the incisive papilla. The palatine rugae, firm irregular ridges of tissue, are directly posterior to this.

A midline muscular structure, the uvula, hangs from the posterior margin of the soft palate. The pterygomandibular fold is a fold of tissue that extends from the junction of the hard and soft palates down to the mandible, just behind the retromolar pad. This fold stretches when a patient opens the mouth wide, separating the buccal mucosa from the pharynx (see Fig. 16.8).

The oral cavity also provides the entrance into the pharynx or throat, a muscular tube that serves both the respiratory and digestive systems. Parts of the nasopharynx and oropharynx are observable; the laryngopharynx is inferior to these two structures and is not observable. The part of the pharynx that is superior to the level of the soft palate is the nasopharynx, which is continuous with the nasal cavity.

The oropharynx is the part of the pharynx that is between the soft palate and the opening of the larynx. The opening from the oral cavity into the oropharynx is the fauces, laterally formed by two folds of tissue consisting of both the anterior and posterior faucial pillars. The palatine tonsils are masses of lymphoid tissue located between these two pillars (see Fig. 16.8). The tonsils, similar to lymph nodes, contain lymphocytes that remove toxic products. The atypical finding of

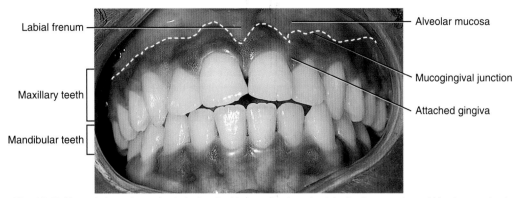

Fig. 16.10 Frontal view of attached gingiva, in this case having physiologic pigmentation within the attached gingiva. (Courtesy of Margaret J. Fehrenbach, RDH, MS, and from Fehrenbach MJ, Herring SW. *Illustrated Anatomy of the Head and Neck.* 6th ed. Saunders; 2021.)

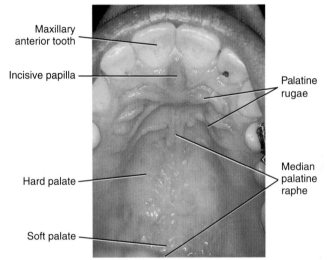

Fig. 16.11 View of the palate, with its anatomic landmarks noted. (Courtesy of Margaret J. Fehrenbach, RDH, MS, and from Fehrenbach MJ, Herring SW. *Illustrated Anatomy of the Head and Neck.* 6th ed. Saunders; 2021.)

lymphadenopathy also can occur in the palatine tonsils (see earlier discussion).

Tongue

Parts of the tongue can be important potential lesion sites and must be carefully examined (Fig. 16.12). The posterior one-third of the tongue is its base, which attaches to the floor of the mouth. The base of the tongue does not lie within the oral cavity, but it is located within the oropharynx. The anterior two-thirds of the tongue is its body, which lies within the oral cavity. The dorsal surface or top of the tongue has a midline depression, the median lingual sulcus.

The dorsal surface is pink to darker pink in those with darker skin tones (see Fig. 16.12). This top tongue surface also has raised small structures of specialized mucosa, the lingual papillae of various types. The slender, whitish, threadlike filiform lingual papillae give the dorsal surface its velvety texture. The less-numerous, mushroom-shaped, fungiform lingual papillae are redder or darker red in those with darker skin tone, possibly with localized physiologic pigmentation at the tops. Because of lingual papillae, the dorsal surface of the tongue is not exceptionally smooth.

Farther posteriorly on the tongue's dorsal surface and more difficult to observe clinically is a V-shaped groove, the sulcus terminalis (see Fig. 16.12).

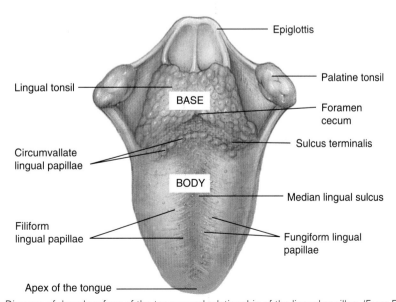

Fig. 16.12 Diagram of dorsal surface of the tongue and relationship of the lingual papillae. (From Fehrenbach MJ, Popowics, T. *Illustrated Dental Embryology, Histology, and Anatomy.* 6th ed. Saunders; 2020.)

The sulcus terminalis separates the base from the body of the tongue and has a small pitlike midline depression, the foramen cecum, and together, they point toward the pharynx.

The circumvallate lingual papillae are 10 to 14 in number, lining up along the anterior side of the sulcus terminalis on the body of the tongue. These lingual papillae are larger red or darker red and mushroom shaped. Farther posteriorly on the dorsal surface of the tongue base is an irregular mass of the lingual tonsil, which is clinically more difficult to see. The side or lateral surface of the tongue has vertical ridges, which are the foliate lingual papilla.

The ventral surface or undersurface is noted for its visible large blood vessels, the deep lingual veins, that run close to the surface on either side (Fig. 16.13). Lateral to each deep lingual vein is the plica fimbriata, a bilateral fold of tissue.

Floor of the Mouth

The floor of the mouth is inferior to the ventral surface of the tongue (Fig. 16.14). The lingual frenum is a midline fold of tissue between the tongue's ventral surface and the mouth floor. There is also a tissue ridge on each side of the mouth, the sublingual folds, that together form a V-shaped configuration from the lingual frenum to the base of the tongue. The sublingual folds contain duct openings from the sublingual salivary gland. The sublingual caruncle at the anterior end of each sublingual fold contains the submandibular and sublingual duct openings from the submandibular and the sublingual salivary glands.

LESION DESCRIPTION

An overall descriptive terminology for lesions includes atrophy, bulla, macule, nodule, papule, plaque, pustule, ulcer, and vesicle (Table 16.6).[4] In addition, there are other more specific related findings that need to be considered such as location and distribution, size and shape, color changes, surface texture and consistency, attachment, depth, and mobility, as well as related symptoms and signs.

Location and Distribution

When documenting the location of a lesion or area of concern, the dental hygienist must be as accurate as possible so that a precise followup examination by the patient's dentist may occur, even when the lesion may have subsequently healed and no longer remains.

This location is also key because some lesions characteristically occur in specific regions or within specific tissue types; this can further support the formation of the dentist's differential diagnosis. For example, hairy leukoplakia with an HIV infection, with its thick white plaque having long fingerlike papillary projections, mainly occurs bilaterally on the lateral borders of the tongue.

When describing this location at this level of specificity, the clinician identifies the region discussed earlier and the nearest anatomic landmark (e.g., upper lip, labial mucosa, tongue surface, or specific teeth). The clinician then notes the location and the lesion's anatomic relationship to the structure, such as whether it is anterior or posterior, medial or lateral, inferior or superior.

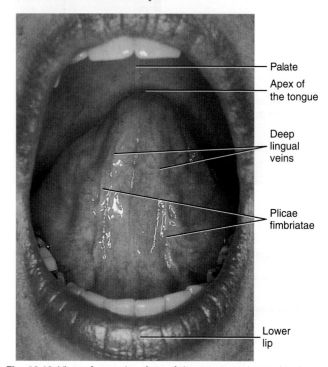

Fig. 16.13 View of ventral surface of the tongue and associated structures. (Courtesy of Margaret J. Fehrenbach, RDH, MS, and from Fehrenbach MJ, Herring SW. *Illustrated Anatomy of the Head and Neck.* 6th ed. Saunders; 2021.)

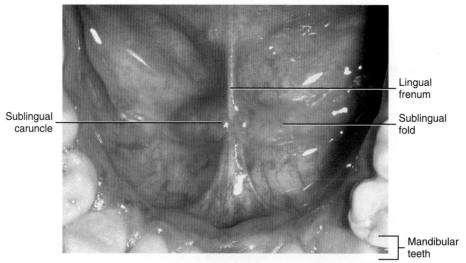

Fig. 16.14 View of the floor of the mouth and associated structures. (Courtesy of Margaret J. Fehrenbach, RDH, MS, and from Fehrenbach MJ, Herring SW. *Illustrated Anatomy of the Head and Neck.* 6th ed. Saunders; 2021.)

TABLE 16.6 Descriptive Lesion Terminology

Terms With Application Examples*	Associated Dental Hygiene Patient Record Notes†
Atrophy: surface tissue thinning; size varies 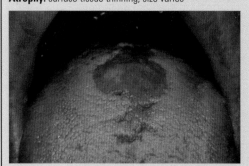	Long-term, large (2 cm × 4 cm), painless, smooth, well-defined, single, darker red, and rhomboidal-shaped patch on posterior midline dorsal surface of tongue that slightly burns with spicy food like central papillary atrophy.
Bulla: large, and well-defined blister containing clear serum and/or blood; >1 cm 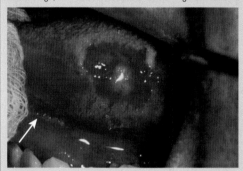	Unilateral, single, short-term, large (10 cm × 10 cm), painful, poorly-defined, and superficial bulla with clear fluid and surrounded with multiple ulcerations on left lateral tongue border; past history of similar lesions throughout mouth that easily break and heal with crusting but without scarring like pemphigus vulgaris.
Macule: well-defined, and small, flat patch, with different coloration from surrounding area; <1 cm 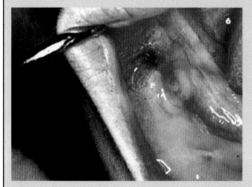	Unilateral, bluish, long-term, flat, small (1 cm × 1 cm), well-defined, single, painless, and rounded macule on edentulous right alveolar ridge; had been previously associated with extracted second molarlike amalgam tattoo.
Nodule: well-defined, and raised, hard mass; 0.5 to 2 cm 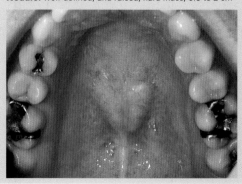	Long-term, moderate-sized (2 cm × 1.5 cm), painless, well-defined, multiple, hard, unsymmetrical, connected, and raised nodules with same coloration as surrounding area on midline hard palate like palatal torus.

(continued)

TABLE 16.6   Descriptive Lesion Terminology—cont'd

Terms With Application Examples*	Associated Dental Hygiene Patient Record Notes†
Papule: well-defined, raised, and firm mass; <0.5 cm 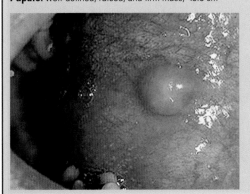	Long-term, painless, unilateral, slightly raised, small (1 cm × 1 cm), round, firm, and sessile papule with same coloration as surrounding area on right buccal mucosa like oral traumatic fibroma.
Plaque: well-defined, and slightly raised area, with surface texture or coloration different from surrounding area; >0.5 cm 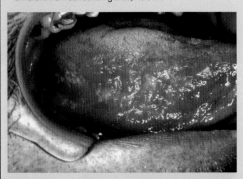	*Painless, long-term, bilateral, well-defined, large (1 cm × 10 cm), thick, and whiter plaque on tongue lateral borders that does not wipe off like HIV-associated hairy leukoplakia associated with HIV-positive diagnosis.*
Pustule: well-defined, and blisterlike but filled with pus; size varies 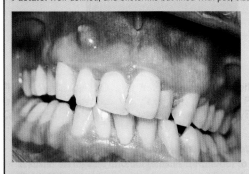	*Unilateral painful, short-term, large, (2 cm × 2 cm), rounded, and raised pustule on attached gingiva superior to both maxillary right lateral incisor and canine having deep periodontal pocketing but unable to determine exact source clinically like periodontal abscess.*
Ulcer: depressed and erythematous area with loss of epithelial layer; size varies 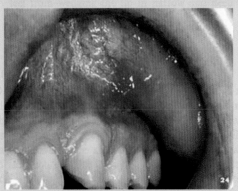	*Unilateral, painful, short-term, multiple, large (around 2 cm × 4 cm), depressed, and shallow ulcers surrounded by erythematous halos on labial mucosa superior to maxillary left premolars with past history of similar lesions throughout that heal without scarring like recurrent aphthous stomatitis.*

TABLE 16.6 Descriptive Lesion Terminology—cont'd

Terms With Application Examples*	Associated Dental Hygiene Patient Record Notes[†]
Vesicle: well-defined and small blister filled with clear fluid; <0.5 cm 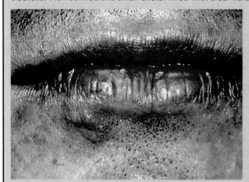	Short-term, painful, multiple, well-defined, small (less than 0.5 mm × 0.5 mm), and itchy vesicles with clear fluid coalesced at vermilion border of lower lip with past history of similar lesions in same location that do not easily break but leave ulcerations and heal with crusting but without scarring like herpes labialis.

*Figures courtesy of Margaret J. Fehrenbach, RDH, MS.
[†]Patient Record notes of dental hygiene diagnosis should include *"To be followed by differential diagnosis upon evaluation by dentist"*.

This description of the location must also use terminology in relation to the larger region of the head or neck.[4] This includes whether the lesion is **unilateral**, which means that it is located on either the right side or the left side, or whether it is **bilateral**, which means it is located on both sides. In addition, the location of the lesion must consider whether it is **contralateral**, which means it is located on the opposite side of a specific structure, or whether it is **ipsilateral**, which means it is located on the same side as a specific structure.

Bilateral structures are usually anatomic structures and thus a unilateral finding may indicate a higher probability of it being a lesion. Thus it is important to compare the right and left sides of the head and neck using bilateral palpation to obtain this vital information when indicated. In contrast, some lesions may be located in the midline that divides the body into right and left halves.

In addition to location, the distribution of the lesion must be described and that can be either single or multiple in its spread over an area. For example, a mucocele, which is a raised lesion caused by an accumulation of saliva from a blocked duct, is a single lesion. In contrast, a herpes simplex virus infection evident on the attached gingiva or skin around the lips often produces multiple lesions in the area.

Multiple lesions may be described as either separate or coalescing.[4] Multiple lesions that are distinct and do not run together are considered **separate** by having **well-defined borders** or being *well circumscribed*. In contrast, lesions that seem to merge are **coalescing** by having **poorly defined borders**.

A lesion with borders that are poorly defined can make it impossible to detect the exact parameters of the lesion, which may make treatment more difficult and, depending on the biopsy results, *radical* surgery may have to be implemented. Such is the case with a malignant neoplasm or even an aggressive benign neoplasm, with the surgical removal having to include a wide band of healthy tissue.

In addition, multiple lesions may be localized or generalized.[4] **Localized** lesions are limited to a single area (e.g. aphthous ulcer); in contrast, **generalized** lesions involve more than one area, possibly indicating a systemic dermatologic pathologic condition (e.g., lichen planus).

Size and Shape

Lesion size is determined by using a periodontal probe or small metric ruler to measure the legion's length, width, and height from the surrounding surface. The size of lesions varies, but generally a lesion is not apparent to the patient when it is smaller than 1 to 2 cm. In addition, this description needs to note whether the lesion is a papule, which is raised, or a macule, which is flat.

The contour of the lesion's borders related to its shape also must be described by documenting the lesion's border as being either well defined or poorly defined, as discussed earlier (see Table 16.6). Generally, noncancerous or benign neoplasms have well-defined borders and are usually round or ovoid shaped. In contrast, cancerous or malignant neoplasms have poorly defined borders and thus have an irregular shape. These poorly defined borders are usually from the invasion of the cancer into the surrounding region, resulting in tissue inflammation and fibrosis. This invasion can continue until the neoplasm has further undergone metastasis, as discussed earlier.[2]

Color Changes

Abnormal color changes in the tissue may signal an abnormal finding. Common lesion colors are redder, as in having *erythema*, or darker red in those with darker skin tones, as well as whiter, with white lesions predominating overall. Other, less common colors include blue, purple, yellow, black, and gray. However, lesions can also exhibit the same color as the surrounding tissue, differing only in other notable ways.

Redder or darker red lesions may be the result of increased vascularity in the subepithelial tissue, thinning of the superficial epithelium, or a dissolution of connective tissue. White lesions that cannot be removed with a gauze may be the result of opacity in similar tissue layers from decreased vascularity, excess keratin, or fibrosis, with its increased fibers.

Brown, blue, or black lesions indicate a tissue deposit of melanin, blood, or even heavy metal such as amalgam particles with an amalgam tattoo. In addition, fluid-filled lesions or lesions with increased or enlarged blood vessels can appear bluish to translucent, depending on the skin tone beneath. Importantly, all localized brown, blue, or black lesions should be immediately discussed with the patient's dentist, who will quickly refer them to a dental or medical specialist because of the high risk of being metastatic cancer such as with oral malignant melanoma (OMM), as discussed later.[7]

Yellow lesions usually contain sebaceous glands or adipose tissue or the presence of purulent suppuration or pus from infection.

TABLE 16.7 Lesion Surface Texture Terminology

Terms	Descriptions
Corrugated	Wrinkled, with parallel and alternating ridges and grooves
Cratered	Central depression surrounded by raised margin
Crusted	Hard brittle covering of dried serum, blood, or pus, or combination
Fissured	Ridges and irregularities forming craterlike areas
Indurated	Hardness from increased number of surrounding epithelial cells
Papillary	Roughness having small raised fingerlike projections
Pseudomembranous	Inflammatory exudate layer
Reticular	Lacelike textured pattern on tissue surface
Smooth	Tissue surface without texture
Velvety	Soft, smooth, and thick layer on tissue surface
Verrucous	Rough and wartlike, with multiple irregular folds

TABLE 16.8 Lesion Consistency Comparisons

Lesion Consistency	Tissue Consistency Comparisons
Soft: mainly comprised of cells without much intervening dense fibrous connective tissue; completely flexible during palpation	Adipose tissue, loose connective tissue, glandular tissue
Firm or Rubbery: denser than surrounding softer oral mucosa or skin, indicating presence of increased fibrous connective tissue; more flexible during palpation than bone	Cartilage
Hard: harder than soft tissue and even harder than firm or rubbery tissue, indicating presence of bone or other calcified material; without any flexibility during palpation	Bone or enamel

Sometimes, multiple colors can be present at the same time within the lesion area, as discussed later with melanoma. In addition, if the lesion is spontaneously hemorrhaging, with abnormal bleeding or easy bleeding when palpated, then that condition requires documentation.

Surface Texture and Consistency

The **surface texture** of a lesion can involve being **corrugated, cratered, crusted, fissured, indurated, papillary, pseudomembranous, reticular, smooth, velvety,** or **verrucous** (Table 16.7).[4] Surface texture is an important consideration when establishing a list of possible differential diagnoses since most of the oral cavity has a relatively smooth surface texture except the palatal rugae, attached gingiva stippling, and lingual papilla. Superficial epithelial tissue lesions frequently have a rougher surface, whereas deeper ones involving connective tissue as well as muscle and bone continue to have a smoother surface.

The tissue **consistency of a lesion** refers to the degree of firmness or density. Categorization of the firmness of the lesion is therefore accomplished by first palpating the lesion and then secondarily comparing its degree of consistency with the typical consistency of nearby

healthy tissue types that when palpated are soft, firm or rubbery, and hard (Table 16.8).

Soft lesions more than 1 cm in diameter also should be tested for **fluctuance** by placing the fingers of one hand on one side of the lesion and gently pressing on the lesion with the fingers of the other hand. If the fingers can detect a wave passing through the lesion, then the lesion is fluctuant. The lesion also should be checked for **emptiability**, which is the temporary loss of fluctuance caused by the brief evacuation of the lesion fluid into the surrounding tissue.

Attachment, Depth, and Mobility

If a lesion has a broad base of attachment to the surface as wide as the lesion itself, then its attachment is **sessile**. In contrast, **pedunculated** lesions have a narrow pedicle or stalklike base of attachment to the surface. Lesions can also be superficial, which means located toward the surface, or they can be deep, which means located inward and away from the surface. Lesion depth is determined with palpation of the area of concern after initial observation.

During palpation, it is important to note if a lesion has either mobility or has undergone fixation. **Mobility** refers to the lesion being freely movable from the surrounding tissue with palpation. When the lesion has undergone **fixation**, it cannot freely move in relationship to the surrounding tissue with palpation.

Evaluation by palpation for either mobility or fixation occurs first by stabilizing the lesion with the fingers of one hand while moving the superficial tissue over the lesion with the other hand to see if it is fixed, or attached, to its overlying tissue. Then the clinician attempts to move the lesion independently from its underlying structures or tissue to demonstrate if the lesion is freely movable in all directions. However, certain regions of the oral mucosa usually do not allow movement of the oral mucosa separate from the deeper structures such as the attached gingiva, median palatine raphe, or hard palate.

Generally, the following considerations of mobility or fixation with palpation can help support a differential diagnosis of the unknown lesion. If freely movable in all directions, then the lesion is encapsulated or likely not a cancer. If fixed to overlying skin or oral mucosa only, then the lesion originates from the overlying tissue. If fixed to underlying structures only, then the lesion originates from the underlying tissue. If fixed to both overlying and underlying tissue or structures, then the lesion involves either fibrosis or invasion into deeper structures from cancerous growth.

Symptomatology

By asking questions of the patient, symptoms are discovered related to the finding. A **symptom** is a subjective condition reported by the patient (Box 16.3). In contrast, a **sign** is an objective condition that can be directly observed by both the patient and clinician. In this regard, there are certain considerations about their symptoms to be documented in the patient record (Box 16.4).

HEAD AND NECK CANCER

The incidence of HNC accounts for 6% of all cancers, with diagnoses of around 68,000 annually in the United States. Cancer appearance can vary in type and with individuals. Thus the associated signs and symptoms of these cancers must be kept in mind during the examination, which can be further divided into either early and late presentations (Table 16.9). However, most of the patient population is not aware of these signs and symptoms associated with HNC or even risk factors. In a recent NIH study, only 25% of surveyed adults could identify even one sign or symptom of HNC.[1]

The largest risk factors for HNCs are nicotine use (cigarettes, cigars, and chewing tobacco) and alcohol abuse, especially when combined. In fact, 70% to 80% of HNCs are linked to nicotine use; importantly, continued nicotine use may also affect a cancer's prognosis due to slowing recovery.[7]

Other risk factors include prolonged exposure to occupational, dietary, or pharmacologic toxins or sunlight, HPV and other infections, and gastroesophageal reflux disease (GERD), as well as previous HNC history. In addition, secondhand/thirdhand smoke or marijuana use may increase a person's risk. Risks with carcinogenic air pollution exposure and electronic cigarette use remain unknown and will only be evident in the coming decades. For information on dental hygiene care for persons with cancer, see Chapter 50.

SKIN CANCER

Skin cancer is the most common form in the United States and is generally classified as either nonmelanoma skin cancer (NMSC) or melanoma.[8] There has been an increasing incidence of both over the past several decades. The most common forms of NMSC are basal cell carcinoma (BCC) and squamous cell carcinomas (SCCs). Importantly, more than 90% of HNCs are head and neck squamous cell carcinomas (HNSCCs).

Approximately 85% of skin cancers are located on the skin of the head and neck because of excessive ultraviolet (UV) exposure from sunlight. Sunlight generates DNA damage that leads to mutation formation and also reduces the host immune system's ability to recognize and remove malignant cells. Most NMSCs are from cumulative UV exposure; specifically, melanoma is highly correlated to adolescent exposure. All patients, even those with darker skin tones with lower skin cancer rates, should be encouraged by the dental hygienist to use sunscreen or sun coverage. However, when skin cancer develops in skin with darker tones, it can occur in areas not exposed to sunlight and color changes are not reliable, so it is often in a late stage when diagnosed.

Usually, NMSCs start as small pearly or pale papules on the skin (with BCCs); other forms are redder or darker red in those with darker skin tones such as appearing as a scaly, flat patch or plaque on the skin (with SCCs). Although NMSCs types usually do not spread or undergo metastasis, if not completely removed, they frequently invade and destroy the local skin, muscle, and nerves in their path. Fortunately, these skin cancers usually are recognized in their early stages because of their slow growth; therefore they generally have a better prognosis than more fatal forms of skin cancer.

A less common type and possibly fatal form of skin cancer is melanoma, especially if the initial lesion is detected at an advanced stage.[9] In the affected area, multiple colors are present within the lesion, with streaks of tan, brown, or black, and sometimes white, blue, and red, always darker in those with darker skin tones. This coloration is not just from increased melanocytic activity like physiologic pigmentation but rather, increased numbers of abnormal melanocytes. Thus this abnormal color mixture is one of the more important presenting signs, as well as rapid irregular growth, abnormal shape, and possible bleeding at the site.

BOX 16.3 Critical Thinking Scenario B

A 35-year-old emergency female patient who is 7 months pregnant has been referred by another dental office. In addition, because the referred dentist's schedule is full, the dental hygienist sees the patient first. The patient says she has pain in the jaw area when she opens or even closes her mouth and has frequent bouts of vomiting. She has slight inflammation of her marginal gingival tissue throughout her mouth but has only one restoration that was placed at her last regular 6-month appointment; her palatal tissue seems moderately inflamed. She recently told her obstetrician about the jaw pain and reported there were no overriding concerns, except that her right cheek area seems larger than the left.

- What techniques should be used to initially examine the jaw and its joint during an extraoral examination?
- What condition might be involved in her larger cheek area on one side and how should its examination be performed by the clinician?
- What modification in seating during the appointment might be warranted during the extraoral examination for this patient?
- Why might her marginal tissue and palatal tissue be inflamed at this time?
- How would the dental hygienist's extraoral and intraoral examination findings be entered into the patient record?

BOX 16.4 Symptomology Considerations for Patient Record Documentation

- If the lesion is known to the patient, then how long has it been present? Have changes in its size and appearance occurred over time?
- Has the patient experienced related neurologic symptoms with the lesion, such as pain, tingling, burning, or paresthesia with its numbness? If so, it must first be determined whether the pain is present with or without palpation. Generally, painful lesions are caused by inflammation but in some cases, can also involve cancerous growth near the area nerves.
- If procedural tests such as laboratory findings or imaging have been performed, then these reports must be documented in the patient record, including evaluations made by the patient's other healthcare providers.

TABLE 16.9 Associated Oral and Oropharyngeal Cancer Signs and Symptoms

ASSOCIATED ORAL AND OROPHARYNGEAL CANCER SIGNS AND SYMPTOMS

Early Presentations	Late Presentations
Abnormal surface changes	Indurated area with surrounding hardness with palpation
Nonhealing ulcerous area	Paresthesia with numbness and dysesthesia with abnormal sensation of tongue or lips
Persistent redder/darker red and/or whiter patch and abnormal pigmentation	Altered vision
Progressive enlargement or swelling with palpation	Chronic serous otitis media with ear infection or otalgia with ear pain
Sudden tooth mobility without apparent cause	Trismus with difficulty opening mouth or dysphagia with difficulty swallowing
Abnormal tissue bleeding	Cervical lymphadenopathy with palpation
Epistaxis with nose bleeding	Persistent or referred pain
Prolonged hoarseness and feeling of persistent lump in throat	Airway obstruction

Melanomas frequently develop from or near an existing nevus or mole but can be found anywhere on the skin as well as on the scalp and in the eye. Melanomas can also metastasize to the oral cavity as an OMM. Risk factors for melanoma are the same as for the other NMSCs, as well as having close relatives with history.

ORAL AND OROPHARYNGEAL CANCER

It is estimated that more than 75% of HNCs originate in the oral cavity and oropharynx. More than 54,000 Americans will be diagnosed yearly with oral and oropharyngeal cancer (OC/OPC).[10,11] As one of the most serious conditions that can occur in the oral cavity and oropharynx, this cancer is an especially devastating pathologic condition when detected in its later stages. Late-stage treatment usually involves radical surgery, radiation, and chemotherapy.

Current reports show that OC/OPCs cause more than 11,000 deaths per year, or around 2% of all cancer deaths in the United States, mainly because these cancers are routinely discovered late. Even with the death rates for these cancers decreasing over the last 30 years, the rate for these cancers is still higher than for cancers having public awareness such as cervical or ovarian cancer; Hodgkin lymphoma; leukemia; cancer of the brain, liver, testes, or kidney; and a serious skin cancer such as melanoma.

Important to note is that OC/OPCs are more than twice as common in males as they are in females; they are about equally common in various races. The average age of most people diagnosed with these cancers is 62 years, but they can occur in younger persons. These cancers are rare in children, but around 20% now occur in those younger than 55 years of age. In the United States, cancers of the oral cavity and oropharynx are strongly associated with same risk factors as NMSCs. However, extraoral lesions on the lower lip are mainly attributable to prolonged sun exposure.

Oral Squamous Cell Carcinoma

Oral squamous cell carcinoma (OSCC) makes up around 90% of OC/OPCs and develops from the mucosal epithelium in the oral cavity, oropharynx and larynx.[10] One type of OSCC is verrucous carcinoma (VC), which is a rare, nonmetastasizing, well-differentiated variant. The remainder of OC/OPCs include salivary gland neoplasms, lymphoma, and sarcoma. Importantly, OSCC has a higher mortality rate compared with other carcinomas (discussed later).

The risk of cancerous transformation in ulcerous, redder, or darker red areas in those with darker skin tones is higher than in more commonly found white patches, although the latter can often prove to be cancerous. The earliest form of OSCC is *carcinoma in situ*, meaning that the cancer cells are present only in the outer layers; this presentation is different from *invasive* OSCC, in which the cancer cells have invaded the deep layers of the oral cavity or oropharynx.

Although cancer may arise at any site in the oral cavity, the most common sites for OSCC in the United States (in order) are as follows: lower lip; lateral border of the tongue; floor of the mouth; and oropharynx, including the posterior soft palate, uvula, and faucial arches.[1]

However, as discussed in the next section, newer reports related to the rise of HPV infection within populations may indicate that these trends for common sites are changing, with cancers of the palatine and lingual tonsils, tonsillar pillar and crypt, base of the tongue, and oropharynx now having rapidly higher incidence rates.[1,10,11]

Human Papillomavirus–Related Cancer

In recent years, the overall rate of new cases of OC/OPCs has been stable in males and slightly dropping in females, as noted earlier. However, there has been a recent rise in cases of HPV-related OPCs linked to specific types.

This mainly involves nonusers of nicotine and alcohol products and White males under the age of 55 years. It now comprises the fastest-growing OPC segment, approximately one-third of the total cases as diagnosed via genetic testing.[10] Importantly, this cancer often takes years, even decades, to develop after a person undergoes HPV infection.

Additionally, most people with HPV infections of the oral cavity and oropharynx have no initial symptoms or signs to support an early diagnosis, but on the positive side, only a small percentage of those with an HPV infection develop cancer. In fact, these cancers that contain HPV genetic material tend to have a better prognosis than those without the HPV.

Both nicotine- and alcohol-related lesions are located mostly in the regions of the oral cavity, larynx, and hypopharynx, with symptoms possible. In contrast, HPV-related OPCs are located mainly in the regions of the palatine and lingual tonsils of the oropharynx, again without the typical cancer symptoms or signs in the oral mucosa. Instead, skin lesions such as warts and sores can identify HPV infection as well as genital lesion history. Thus palpation during an extraoral examination for hard and painless fixed lymph nodes is an important diagnostic feature for HPV-related OPCs.[10]

The increased rate of HPV-related OPCs is thought to be due to changes in sexual practices in recent decades and number of sex partners. Over the next 20 years, it is estimated that these cancers will represent the majority of HNCs in the United States.

To combat HPV infections, vaccines that reduce the risk of infection with certain types of HPV have become available in recent years. Thus the dental hygienist needs to encourage vaccination according to the latest recommendations by the Centers for Disease Control and Prevention (CDC).[12] Dental offices can also offer screening using a salivary DNA oral rinse test to check for an oral HPV mucosal infection history. However, recent research after a large group sample size now questions the advisability of routine HPV screening in dentistry.[13]

Recent research has also found a possible association of OC with cases of severe periodontal disease but still having coexisting lifestyle risk factors: further research is needed to make a direct correlation.[14] It is thought that an accumulation of dental biofilm results in a chronic inflammatory process, possibly creating an environment promoting cancer development. If it is conclusively found to be correlated, then preserving periodontal health may minimize this serious risk.

ORAL AND OROPHARYNGEAL CANCER PROGRESSION

Unlike traumatic or infective lesions in the same region that are short term, OC/OPCs are persistent since they do not show healing and resolution after a 2-week window of time, nor do they respond to treatment (see Table 16.9). Thus the patient may be asked to return after a 2-week period for further examination. Examples of the most common atypical lesions that mimic OC/OPC initially but instead show healing and resolution over this 14-day time period are traumatic aphthous ulcerations or infective herpetic simplex ulcerations. In contrast, the OC/OPC starts to develop abnormal changes in color, shape, and size during this long-term presence, as discussed earlier.

More extensive cancer-related terminology relating to this long-term presence as well as these noted abnormal changes includes **chronicity, erosion, erythroplakia, erythrolcukoplakia, fixation, leukoplakia,** or **lymphadenopathy** (See Table 16.10).[3] Also associated with cancer are some of the descriptive terminologies already discussed, such as being fissured from abnormal cell growth, indurated from inflammatory infiltrate, and ulcerated from cell maturation discrepancy, intercellular attachment loss, and basement membrane.

When the malignant lesion is biopsied, the cells show severe abnormalities or *anaplasia*. In some cases, a lesion when biopsied is noted to have only slight abnormalities or *dysplasia*, which may signify a

TABLE 16.10 Cancer-Related Terminology

Terms

Chronicity: Long-term presence due to failure of healing and resolution during A 2-week time period such as with persistent red/dark and/or white patch or nonhealing ulcer

Erosion: Surface layer(s) thinning resulting from epithelial integrity destruction due to cell maturation discrepancy, intercellular attachments loss, basement membrane disruption

Erythroplakia: Redder/darker red patch that is granular (rough) or velvety (smooth) that cannot be diagnosed as any other lesion without biopsy

Erythroleukoplakia: Abnormal "speckled" patch with *both* redder or darker red and whiter areas; see also erythroplakia and leukoplakia in this table

Fixation: Immobility with palpation in contrast to mobile surrounding tissue resulting from abnormally dividing cells invading deep areas such as muscle and bone

Leukoplakia: Whiter patch that cannot be wiped off and cannot be diagnosed as any other lesion without biopsy

Lymphadenopathy: Involvement of regional lymph nodes and/or tonsils, resulting in painful, firm, or rubbery or even hard enlarged nodes with palpation; possibly fixed and painless

BOX 16.5 Critical Thinking Scenario C

A 34-year-old female social worker in a rural township has had a recent history of OPC. Her involvement with the human papillomavirus (HPV-related OPC) was caught early, but she is still smoking cigarettes. She still has many questions and wonders how she can reduce her risk of further involvement. She states that her life is full of stress attributable to her work, in addition to a personal life with a blended family situation. She states that she really needs to smoke during her breaks and right after work to relax. She has four preteen children and is considering having them receive the related vaccine.
- How could this patient reduce the risk of further OPC?
- What methods of tobacco cessation could work for this patient?
- Why would the related vaccine possibly prevent OPC in the patient's children?
- How could the patient integrate self-examination into her schedule?
- Which methods of cancer detection in the dental setting could be considered for this patient?

stage preceding the development of cancer and thus the presence of a **premalignant neoplasm**. This can also occur with evolving of certain benign neoplasms into a malignant neoplasm. The neoplasm then progresses through various stages that are categorized within the traditional **TNM Staging System**, which includes specific findings under "T" for neoplasm size, "N" for lymph node involvement, and "M" for metastasis. Although lymph node metastasis is not an early event, as many as 21% of OC/OPC present at diagnosis with nodal metastasis.[1]

Once the malignancy is categorized, then the prognosis or outlook is determined by staging, which is one of the most important factors in choosing the treatment for the patient. However, recent acceptance of a more complex staging system than TNM staging now involves depth of invasion and nodal staging revisions as well as a novel staging system for HPV-related cancers.[12]

Around 400,000 people are living with OC/OPCs in the United States. In addition, some patients successfully treated may experience recurrent or relapsed cancer when it returns. There also may be development of another type of cancer later in the oral cavity, oropharynx, or other nearby regions as well as in the associated lymph nodes. For this reason, these patients always must have semiannual followup dental examinations.

Patients with a history of OC/OPCs will also need to avoid using nicotine and alcohol products to decrease the risk of recurrence. One of the most important predictors for the recurrence of cancer may be the onset of area pain that is increased during oral function. The dental hygienist is again in an important position to provide information about the early symptoms and signs and to assist the patient in eliminating high-risk behaviors such as with tobacco cessation; see Chapter 37.

ORAL AND OROPHARYNGEAL CANCER DETECTION

The increased mortality rate for OC/OPC is mainly a result of late detection of the pathologic condition. The **mortality rate** is the incidence of deaths in a given population during a defined time period. The overall 5-year survival rate for this cancer is 66%. However, if the cancer is diagnosed at an early stage, the overall 5-year survival rate for all people is 85%. Only around 29% of these are diagnosed at this early stage.

In contrast, if this cancer has spread to surrounding tissue or organs and/or the regional lymph nodes by metastasis, the overall 5-year

survival rate is 67%. Sadly, almost half of cases are diagnosed at this late stage. If this cancer has spread to a distant part of the body, the overall 5-year survival rate is 40%.[10,11]

Public awareness of OC/OPC, as compared with other cancers, continues to be low, and this contributes to delays in diagnosis, followed by delays in obtaining treatment, especially in underserved populations.[1,15] In addition, many early cancerous lesions seem to only be an atypical finding such as a traumatic lesion, and determining with certainty which lesions are cancerous is not possible without performing a biopsy.[1] Because a biopsy often seems extreme to the patient for what appears to be a harmless lesion, many early OC/OPCs remain undiagnosed; consequently, they progress to a more advanced stage.

Dental hygienists have a unique opportunity during an extraoral and intraoral examination to detect these OC/OPCs while they are still unsuspected by the patient. As discussed earlier, cancer screening should be performed annually for those older than 18 years of age and twice a year for those with a high-risk history. It is also important to assure patients that performing these examinations does not necessarily mean that the clinician thinks they have cancer.

Patient Self-Examination

The patient-dental hygienist interaction is an opportunity to inform the patient about the need for regular self-examination. This need can be supported by having them observe basic examination techniques during professional examinations. This information and resultant action will empower them with the skills to see any changes themselves. In addition, this discussion with patients further supports a review of their OC/OPC risk and then modification of any high-risk behaviors if indicated. Thus the dental hygienist will need to inform the patient, as noted in Table 16.9, about its signs and symptoms as well as its risks as noted (Box 16.5). Patient education about OC/OPC is truly one of the most important services a dental hygienist can render (Box 16.6).

Biopsy

As discussed, the definitive diagnosis formed by the patient's dentist or referred specialist is achieved after forming a clinical picture and receiving test results, such as biopsies, that are performed to determine whether a certain pathologic condition is present. **Biopsy** is the surgical removal of a section of tissue or other material by a dentist or referred specialist that undergoes histopathologic assessment for the purposes of diagnosing, estimating the prognosis, and monitoring the course of the pathologic condition.[4] It is considered the gold standard for forming a definitive diagnosis

- When informing the patient about the need for self-examination for early detection of OC/OPC and then allowing them to observe a dental professional's examination to obtain the basic technique, make sure to slow down and take time during the examination to adjust the information shared to the patient's needs as well as their OHL.
- When informing the patient about the early signs and symptoms of OC/OPC, counsel the patient about the need to have them shared if present as soon as possible with dental professionals since anxiety and denial concerning cancer may allow a delay in this. Thus it is important not to make the discussion negative and fear based but instead, positive and health based.
- Be careful when suggesting the elimination of high-risk behaviors that predispose a patient to OC/OPC, especially in those with an OC/OPC history. Make sure not to judge the patient but to enter into a facilitating relationship so as to work together on a change plan. Use critical thinking to establish the best possible ways for this patient to move forward to oral health by listening carefully to lifestyle clues. Small steps to reduce the risk of cancer are a good way to approach change, so focus on one risk factor at a time.

When the entire lesion with borders is removed for assessment it is considered an **excisional biopsy**. In contrast, only representative tissue samples are obtained by excising a wedge of tissue during **incisional biopsy**.

After the specimen is obtained and packaged for transport, it is sent to a laboratory. A report of the findings is issued by the pathologist, who assesses the histopathologic appearance of the suspected lesion in conjunction with the stated differential diagnosis by the patient's dentist. This report is then sent to the dentist, who determines any further action.

Oral and Oropharyngeal Cancer Diagnostic Adjuncts

Several adjunctive techniques have been suggested for early evaluation of lesions to determine whether they show cellular changes and may be a *potentially malignant disorder* (PMD) and need a biopsy.[16] These include cytology, vital staining, and light-based adjuncts.

To understand and compare the efficacy of each method, it is important to understand the overall structure of epithelial tissue such as the oral mucosa that lines the oral cavity.[17] Epithelium consists of three layers: the basal cell layer, the intermediate layers, and the superficial layers. Cell division occurs in the basal cell layer, near the basement membrane. Cells then move through the intermediate layers to the superficial layers to be shed. An important feature of a reliable method designed for early detection is that it evaluates a full thickness of the epithelium to note cellular changes.

However, clinical guidelines developed by the American Dental Association Council on Scientific Affairs and the Center for Evidence-Based Dentistry state that for patients with suspicious lesions, the patient's dentist needs to immediately perform a biopsy of the lesion or refer the patient to a specialist.[18]

The Council at this time does not recommend the use of any adjuncts in the diagnosis of a PMD since they feel that stronger evidence is needed to support their use. In addition, the Council suggests that for adult patients with no clinically evident lesions or symptoms, no further action is necessary at that time. Dental settings can offer adjuncts but not without explanations as to their lack of evidence at this time in forming a diagnosis. Instead, the Council emphasizes the need for counseling because patients may delay diagnosis due to of anxiety and denial (see Box 16.6).

Cytology

Cytology is a procedure that involves the scraping of tissue from a suspected lesion so that it can undergo histopathologic assessment.[16] Dental settings now use **transepithelial cytology**, which uses a specially designed brush to remove sample cells from lesions that may not otherwise be subjected to biopsy because they have only an atypical appearance.[1] The brush captures cells from a full thickness of epithelium because the brush penetrates the basement membrane so as to determine whether a lesion should be submitted for biopsy; see related video on Evolve.

In the case of atypical or what is considered a positive result with transepithelial cytology, the laboratory recommends biopsy of the lesion, since these test results are limited to reporting the presence or absence of cellular abnormalities and do not provide a definitive diagnosis. Although this adjunct method makes the diagnostic process more effective, it is possible for the patient's dentist to reach a comprehensive differential diagnosis through only observation and palpation.[1] At this time, the Council believes cytology can be helpful only if a patient refuses a biopsy to confirm the need for it for definitive diagnosis or lives in a rural area with limited access to care.

Vital Staining

Toluidine blue (ToB) **dye** has been used as a vital stain for many years for the screening of cancerous cells such as those occurring in the oral cavity and pharynx since it differentially discolors the cells.[16] The dye is selectively taken up by these abnormal cells due to their accumulation of abundant nuclear material from increased mitoses and poor cell-to-cell adhesion, which is the premise for its use to confirm clinical impressions of abnormal cellular changes that happen with cancer. A drawback to using the dye on the surface of a lesion to detect cellular changes is that inflammatory cells are often present with a benign neoplasm and also take up the dye stain, making interpretation of the test difficult; thus it is not considered a truly diagnostic procedure.

It is important to note that only the darkest royal blue staining attributable to nuclear staining by ToB dye should be regarded as positive; benign neoplasms have no nuclear staining and are more often a paler blue in color. However, the ToB dye can be used with a higher level of certainty during biopsy to define the margins of the lesions and to discover secondary lesions.

Light-Based Adjuncts

Another detection method involves the surface tissue's reactions to light sources.[19] **Tissue reflectance** includes either a disposable handheld light or a reusable battery-powered light that provides a similar blue-white illumination, and a flavored acetic acid mouth rinse before use of a respective light source. Healthy epithelium absorbs the device's illumination and appears darker, whereas abnormal epithelium reflects it and appears bright white.

A kit that combines tissue reflectance and ToB dye is also available; however, these tests have not been shown by research to be effective in early detection. Rather, they detect dysplasia, a condition that may or may not be precancerous.

A handheld device is also available that provides the direct observation of **autofluorescence** (or narrow emission) and the changes in fluorescence that can occur when abnormalities are present. The unit emits a cone of blue light into the oral cavity, creating different fluorescence responses, depending on the health of the tissue being screened. Healthy epithelium appears pale green under the light, whereas lesions considered abnormal look dark green to black. However, at this time, the loss of fluorescence is not strictly limited to epithelial abnormalities and can be seen with prominent surface vascularity, including areas of inflammation and melanin.

Another testing procedure, **autofluorescence spectroscopy**, combines the technologies of tissue reflectance and autofluorescence with a conventional white light source. It can help identify oral epithelial abnormalities attributable to even minor alterations of the oral mucosa that otherwise may not be apparent, as well as help discern the superficial tissue vascularity; spectrograph analysis is performed in an objective manner by computer. However, the small probe size that is presently used is only useful on smaller localized lesions and only on those initially noted by observation; therefore its value is questionable or limited.

Future Cancer Diagnostic Adjuncts

It is understood that there is a need to identify head and neck cancerous lesions as early as possible to reduce the need for aggressive treatment and avoid high mortality rates. However, at the time of diagnosis, more than 50% of patients with OSCC had advanced pathologic conditions, indicating the lack of availability of early specific biomarkers as for other cancers. A **biomarker** is a measurable indicator of change in biologic state or condition.[20]

Biomarkers can be carbohydrates, DNA, mRNAs, proteins, or small molecules like metabolites and other cellular molecules. *A predictive biomarker* leads to detection of the causes for the abnormalities, while a *diagnostic biomarker* narrows down a diagnosis that is significantly more specific to individual patients. Additionally, a *prognostic biomarker* and genetic drivers help in predicting therapy response and prognosis of the patient.[20,21]

When considering genetic drivers for other body cancers, finding mutated oncogenes by using polymerase chain reaction (PCR) allows amplification of even tiny amounts of genetic material from noninvasive simple sampling and yields information on the genetic status of cancerous lesion.[16] One specific area showing a strong possibility within the head and neck is in genetic material isolation from HPV-related OPCs, which could serve in determining successful therapy and thus bettering the prognosis.

EVOLVE RESOURCES

Please visit http://evolve.elsevier.com/Pieren/hygiene for additional practice and study support tools.

REFERENCES

1. Oral Cancer Foundation. Available at: oralcancerfoundation.org/dental/role-dental-medical-professionals/ and oralcancerfoundation.org/cdc/early-detection-diagnosis-staging/. Accessed October 2023.
2. Patel A. Benign vs malignant tumors. *JAMA Oncol.* 2020;6(9):1488. Available at: https://jamanetwork.com/journals/jamaoncology/fullarticle/2768634. Accessed October 2023.
3. Fehrenbach MJ, Herring SW. In: *Illustrated Anatomy of the Head and Neck.* Saunders; 2021.
4. Fehrenbach MJ (editor-in-chief), et al. In: *Mosby's Dental Dictionary.* Mosby; 2019.
5. Ball JW, Dains JE, Flynn JA, et al. In: *Seidel's Physical Examination Handbook: An Interprofessional Approach.* Elsevier; 2023.
6. Evaluation of the Dental Patient. *Merck Manual;* 2021. Available at: www.merckmanuals.com/professional/dental-disorders/approach-to-the-dental-patient/evaluation-of-the-dental-patient. Accessed October 2023.
7. Smith RA, Andrews KS, Brooks D, et al. Cancer screening in the United States, 2019: a review of current American Cancer Society guidelines and current issues in cancer screening. *CA, Cancer J Clin.* 2019. Available at: acsjournals.onlinelibrary.wiley.com/doi/10.3322/caac.21557. Accessed October 2023.
8. National Center for Biotechnology Information, National Library of Medicine. *StatPearls: Skin cancer.* Available at: www.ncbi.nlm.nih.gov/books/NBK441949/. Accessed October 2023.
9. National Center for Biotechnology Information, National Library of medicine. *StatPearls: Malignant melanoma.* Available at: www.ncbi.nlm.nih.gov/books/NBK470409/. Accessed October 2023.
10. American Cancer Society. *Oral Cavity and Oropharyngeal Cancer, Key Statistics.* Available at: www.cancer.org/cancer/oral-cavity-and-oropharyngeal-cancer/about/key-statistics.html. Accessed October 2023.
11. Johnson DE, Burtness B, Leemans CR, et al. Head and neck squamous cell carcinoma. *Nat Rev Dis Primers.* 2021;6(1):92. Available at: www.ncbi.nlm.nih.gov/pmc/articles/PMC7944998/. Accessed October 2023.
12. Centers for Disease Control and Prevention. *Human Papillomavirus (HPV) Vaccine.* Available at: www.cdc.gov/hpv/parents/vaccine.html. Accessed October 2023.
13. Rindal DB, Gilbert GH, Carcelén C, et al. Feasibility and acceptance of oral HPV detection in the dental office: results from the National Dental PBRN. *JADA.* 2019;150(2):130–139. e4. Available at: www.ncbi.nlm.nih.gov/pmc/articles/PMC6800070/. Accessed October 2023.
14. Komlós G, Csurgay K, Horváth F, et al. Periodontitis as a risk for oral cancer: a case–control study. *BMC Oral Health.* 2021:640. https://doi.org/10.1186/s12903-021-01998-y. Accessed October 2023.
15. Ge S, Lu H, Li Q, et al. Classification tree analysis of factors associated with oral cancer exam. *Am J Health Behav.* 2019;43(3):635–647.
16. Chaurasia A, Alam SI, Singh N. Oral cancer diagnostics: an overview. *Natl J Maxillofac Surg.* 2021;12(3):324–332. Available at: www.ncbi.nlm.nih.gov/pmc/articles/PMC8820315/. Accessed October 2023.
17. Fehrenbach MJ, Popowics T. In: *Illustrated Dental Embryology, Histology, and Anatomy.* Saunders; 2020.
18. American Dental Association. *Evaluation of Potentially Malignant Disorders in the Oral Cavity Clinical Practice Guideline;* 2017. Available at: www.ada.org/resources/research/science-and-research-institute/evidence-based-dental-research/oral-cancer-guideline. www.ada.org/-/media/

KEY CONCEPTS

- Structures of the head and neck as well as the oral cavity provide an indication of general systemic health status; any changes discovered may be the first indication of a systemic pathologic condition.
- Performing a careful overall evaluation and a thorough examination of the head and neck as well as the oral cavity are essential to planning and providing optimal dental hygiene care.
- The dental hygienist must establish a sequence and systematically follow it during the examination, incorporating the examination skills of observation, palpation, and olfaction and using palpation examination methods.
- During the examination, the dental hygienist carefully checks for palpable regional lymph nodes and documents them, if present, since they may pinpoint where a pathologic process is active, which assists in the diagnosis and treatment of the pathologic condition.
- After the assessment of findings from observation and palpation of atypical or abnormal findings, the dental hygienist accurately describes and documents them in the patient record as a dental hygiene diagnosis.
- The ability to describe a lesion is critical to the examination process; precise descriptive terminology enables the dental hygienist to communicate with the patient's dentist.
- Because many patients are more regularly seen for preventive dental care, dental hygienists have a unique opportunity during an examination to detect cancer in its early presentation.
- After recognizing atypical or abnormal findings, the dental hygienist is responsible for informing the patient's dentist to support formation of a differential diagnosis by the dentist.
- Only cytology is a recommended diagnostic adjunct for determining a potentially malignant disorder and only in certain cases. However, after examination, a biopsy followed by histopathologic assessment of suspicious lesions is still required for formation of a definitive diagnosis by the patient's dentist.

project/ada-organization/ada/ada-org/files/resources/research/10870a_
chairside_guide_oralcancer_final.pdf?rev=74b8c9f18ce54fab955e4aface43
2df8&hash=55B1C9403FCD62F2B10DCB27BCE354BE. Accessed
October 2023.

19. Schorn L, Rana M, Madry A, et al. Does autofluorescence help detect
recurrent squamous cell carcinoma? A prospective clinical study. *Oral
Surg Oral Med Oral Pathol Oral Radiol.* 2020;130(3):258–263.

20. Pillai J, Chincholkar T, Dixit R, Pandey M. A systematic review of
proteomic biomarkers in oral squamous cell cancer. *World J Surg Onc.*
2021:315. https://doi.org/10.1186/s12957-021-02423-y. Accessed October
2023.

21. Li Q, Ouyang X, Chen J, Zhang P, Feng Y. A review on salivary
proteomics for oral cancer screening. *Curr Issues Mol Biol.* 2020;37:47–56.
Available at: www.caister.com/cimb/v/v37/47.pdf. Accessed October 2023.

17

Hard Tissue Assessment and Dental Charting

L. Teal Mercer, Gwen Grosso, and Katelyn Bartone

PROFESSIONAL OPPORTUNITIES

Proper documentation allows the dental team to function as a cohesive unit. A full understanding of how to accurately detect and describe clinical findings is vital to the development of a clear, comprehensive treatment plan.

COMPETENCIES

1. Apply the proper methods of documentation required to fulfill dental hygiene responsibilities.
2. Demonstrate the use of different tooth numbering systems and the proper application of charting symbols.
3. Discuss the classification of dental caries and restorations.
4. Recognize hard tissue assessment methods, including identification of signs and symptoms of dental caries, tooth damage, and clinically evident developmental anomalies.
5. Compare different malocclusion classifications.
6. Discuss common problems of occlusion.
7. Integrate tooth assessment and documentation into the dental hygiene process of care.

INTRODUCTION

Hard tissue assessment is used to determine whether the patient's dentition is biologically sound and functional. Assessment is also used to assist the clinician in appropriately developing a treatment plan that will ultimately enhance the patient's well-being. Hard tissue assessment and documentation initially occur during the assessment phase of the dental hygiene process of care and are updated during the implementation, evaluation, and maintenance phases of dental hygiene care. The goal of hard tissue assessment is to recognize and document signs of dental caries, acquired tooth damage, and developmental anomalies to optimize patient care. An accurate and complete hard tissue documentation of findings will:

- Visually describe the patient's current dental status for use in planning patient care
- Enhance communication with the patient, other members of the oral healthcare team, and third-party payers, such as insurance companies and health maintenance organizations
- Provide a legal document of the actual care provided that is admissible evidence in a court of law
- Assist in verifying oral healthcare services provided during financial audits
- Contain a detailed history of the patient's clinical examination findings, dental diagnosis, treatment plan, and rendered treatment for quality-assurance audits
- Assist in forensically identifying unknown victims of criminal incidents and mass casualties.

See Box 17.1 for the American Dental Hygienists' Association (ADHA) definition of assessment.

DOCUMENTATION

Dental charting is the graphic representation of the condition of the patient's teeth on a specific date. The recorded data are based on clinical and radiographic assessments and the patient's reported symptoms. The exact location and condition of all teeth and restorations, including normal and abnormal findings, are documented on an odontogram as part of the patient's permanent record.

An ideal dental charting system, whether electronic or paper based, must be easy to interpret and contain sufficient space for the complete recording of data (Box 17.2). To facilitate continuity, sequencing, and ongoing documentation of care, the odontogram should be available for reference and amendment during subsequent appointments.

Electronic Charting

Paper charting has been used for years; however, many offices have recently begun to replace paper charts with **electronic charting** systems. Although the changeover to electronic formats continues to expand, some dental offices still use paper systems.

Many electronic charting programs are available. Similar to paper charts, electronic charts generally provide a two-dimensional anatomic representation. However, as electronic technologies advance, three-dimensional (3D) chart software systems are now available. 3D charting programs provide a more accurate representation of the patient's current condition (Fig. 17.1). Data collected for electronic systems are digitally stored. A completed charting form can be printed when a hard (paper) copy is needed.

Electronic charting systems can save office space and are readily retrievable chairside. They also allow for the incorporation of digital clinical data, intraoral photography, and radiographic images into the patient record. However, implementing an electronic-based system is not without its challenges. These systems are expensive to implement, and the learning curve may be steep while practitioners become familiar with electronic procedures. In addition, the risk of documentation errors is increased during the learning process. Input methods must be closely monitored to ensure infection control protocols are being maintained (Procedure 17.1; see also Chapter 10).

BOX 17.1 Definition of Assessment

The American Dental Hygienists' Association (ADHA) defines assessment as the systematic collection and analysis of systemic and oral health data to identify patient needs. In its code of ethics, the ADHA further states that patients must be kept informed of their treatment progress and health status. To provide documentation of their needs and treatment, it is essential that accurate records are kept and that confidentiality of this information is maintained.

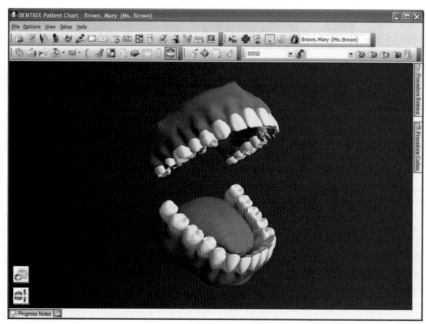

Fig. 17.1 An example of a three-dimensional Dentrix Clinical Chart. (Courtesy Dentrix.com. Available at https://www.dentrix.com/solutions/clinical-efficiency.)

PROCEDURE 17.1   Dentrix Patient Chart

Using the Dentrix Patient Chart Window

The Dentrix Patient Chart is divided into the following areas: panels, toolbars, graphic chart, procedure codes and buttons, status buttons, progress notes, and progress notes control buttons.

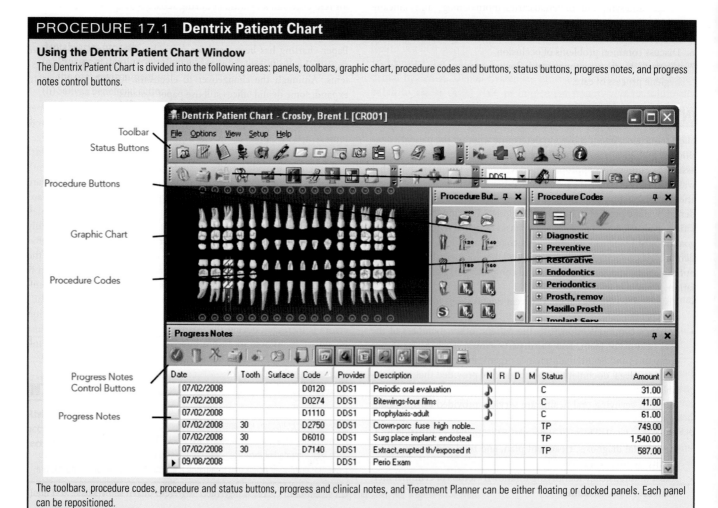

The toolbars, procedure codes, procedure and status buttons, progress and clinical notes, and Treatment Planner can be either floating or docked panels. Each panel can be repositioned.

PROCEDURE 17.1 Dentrix Patient Chart—cont'd

Using the Dentrix Procedure Buttons

The procedure buttons collectively represent the most common procedures performed. Each user-definable button represents a single procedure code, multicode, or condition. For a more complete explanation of the procedure buttons, see "Setting Up Procedure Buttons" and related topics in Dentrix Help.

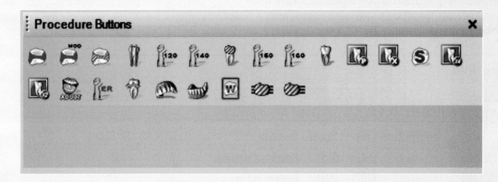

Using the Dentrix Procedure Codes

Procedure codes can be used to enter the treatment. Each procedure code category expands to display specific procedure codes that correspond to a category title. For example, the prophylaxis codes can be accessed from the Preventative list since they are preventative procedures.

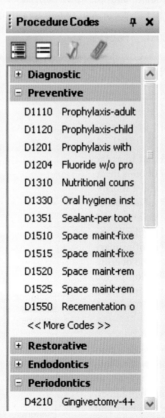

Note: Procedure code categories can be customized in the Office Manager. For more information, see "Customizing Procedure Code Categories" in Dentrix Help.

Using the Dentrix Status Buttons

The status buttons and lists indicate the type of treatment that can be entered in the progress notes.

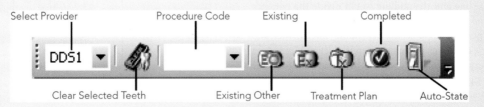

Continued

PROCEDURE 17.1   Dentrix Patient Chart—cont'd

Using Dentrix Progress Notes

The progress notes panel centralizes documentation and examination information, making it easy to review a patient's history. Each time a procedure, examination, condition, treatment plan, referral, or clinical note is entered in the Patient Chart, Dentrix adds a line to the progress notes. For each item recorded in the progress notes, the date the treatment was entered, treatment areas (if applicable), procedure code, provider, treatment description, treatment status, and dollar amount associated with the procedure are all recorded. The "N" column represents progress notes. A musical note symbol in the "N" column indicates that a procedure note is available for that item. The "R" column represents referrals. The "D" column represents diagnostic codes. The "M" column represents medical cross-codes.

Progress Notes

Date	Tooth	Surface	Code	Provider	Description	N	R	D	M	Status	Amount
07/02/2008			D0120	DDS1	Periodic oral evaluation	♪				C	31.00
07/02/2008			D0274	DDS1	Bitewings-four films	♪				C	41.00
07/02/2008			D1110	DDS1	Prophylaxis-adult	♪				C	61.00
07/02/2008	30		D2750	DDS1	Crown-porc fuse high noble...					TP	749.00
07/02/2008	30		D6010	DDS1	Surg place implant: endosteal					TP	1,540.00
07/02/2008	30		D7140	DDS1	Extract,erupted th/exposed rt					TP	587.00
09/08/2008				DDS1	Perio Exam						

For an explanation of each toolbar button on the Progress Notes panel and its function for working with the listed treatment, see "Using Progress Notes Toolbar Buttons" in the Dentrix Help.

From Dentrix G4 User's Guide, Copyright Henry Schein Practice Solutions.

Tooth Classification

Humans have two sets of natural teeth, commonly referred to as the primary and the permanent dentitions. The primary dentition is made up of 20 teeth, 5 in each quadrant: 2 incisors, 1 canine, and 2 molars. The permanent or secondary dentition contains 32 teeth. Each quadrant is made up of 8 teeth: 2 incisors, 1 canine, 2 premolars, and 3 molars. The functions of the individual tooth types are similar in the primary and the permanent dentitions. The classifications of primary and permanent teeth, along with the expected age at the time of eruption, are provided in Figs. 17.2 and 17.3. The mixed dentition period generally occurs between 6 and 12 years of age, when both primary and permanent teeth are present. See Box 17.3 for identification tips.

Quadrant and Sextant Classification

To clearly describe dentition areas and individual teeth, the dentition is divided into quadrants and sextants, and each tooth is divided into specific surfaces.

Quadrant classification. If an imaginary vertical (longitudinal) line divided the patient's face into two equal halves, the maxillary and mandibular arches of the mouth would be divided into two mirror images or halves. This imaginary vertical line that bisects the patient's face is referred to as the **midline**. If a horizontal imaginary line divided the maxillary arch from the mandibular arch, the combination of this imaginary horizontal line and the midline would divide the patient's mouth into four equal sections termed **quadrants** (Q). Each quadrant contains between five and eight teeth, depending on whether the patient has a primary, mixed, or permanent dentition (Fig. 17.4A).

Sextant classification. Another way to designate sections of dentition is by drawing imaginary lines to create divisions between the anterior and the posterior teeth. Dividing the dentition in this manner creates six areas called **sextants** (S). Each anterior sextant contains

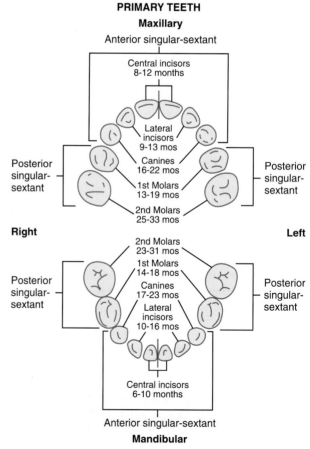

PRIMARY TEETH

Maxillary

Anterior singular-sextant

Central incisors
8–12 months

Lateral incisors
9–13 mos

Canines
16–22 mos

1st Molars
13–19 mos

2nd Molars
25–33 mos

Posterior singular-sextant

Posterior singular-sextant

Right   **Left**

2nd Molars
23–31 mos

1st Molars
14–18 mos

Canines
17–23 mos

Lateral incisors
10–16 mos

Posterior singular-sextant

Posterior singular-sextant

Central incisors
6–10 months

Anterior singular-sextant

Mandibular

Fig. 17.2 Classifications of primary teeth with ages of eruption.

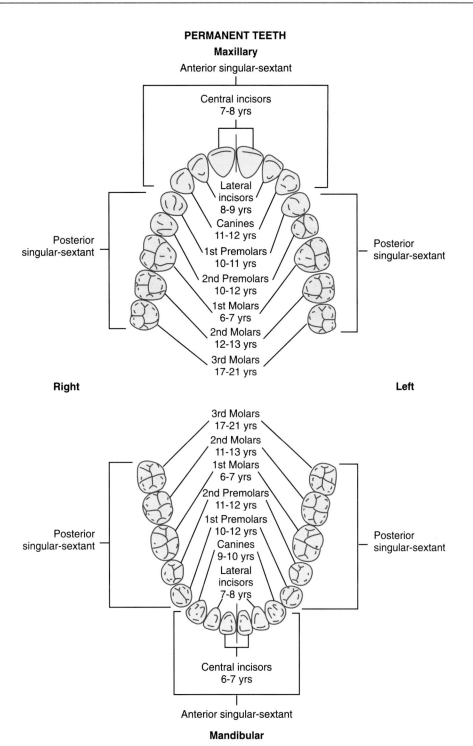

PERMANENT TEETH

Maxillary

Anterior singular-sextant

Central incisors
7-8 yrs

Lateral
incisors
8-9 yrs

Canines
11-12 yrs

1st Premolars
10-11 yrs

2nd Premolars
10-12 yrs

1st Molars
6-7 yrs

2nd Molars
12-13 yrs

3rd Molars
17-21 yrs

Posterior
singular-sextant

Posterior
singular-sextant

Right

Left

3rd Molars
17-21 yrs

2nd Molars
11-13 yrs

1st Molars
6-7 yrs

2nd Premolars
11-12 yrs

1st Premolars
10-12 yrs

Canines
9-10 yrs

Lateral
incisors
7-8 yrs

Posterior
singular-sextant

Posterior
singular-sextant

Central incisors
6-7 yrs

Anterior singular-sextant

Mandibular

Fig. 17.3 Classifications of permanent teeth with ages of eruption.

incisors and canines, and each of the posterior sextants contains premolars and molars. Fig. 17.4B illustrates sextants.

Tooth Surface Classification. The differentiation of tooth surfaces provides a means of pinpointing specific areas of the tooth for accurate assessment, charting, treatment, and evaluation (see Chapter 39).

- **Mesial** (M). Refers to the tooth surfaces closest to the midline.
- **Distal** (D). Refers to the tooth surfaces farthest from the midline.
- **Facial** (F). Includes the buccal and labial surfaces of teeth and refers to the front of each tooth that is most visible when retracting the lips and cheeks.
- **Lingual** (L). Includes the palatal surfaces of teeth and refers to the surfaces closest to the palate or tongue.
- **Occlusal** (O). Refers to the chewing surfaces of premolars and molars.
- **Incisal** (I). Refers to the cutting edges of incisors and canines.
  Fig. 17.5 identifies the classification of tooth surfaces.

Tooth divisions into thirds. The tooth crown and root can each be divided into imaginary thirds (Fig. 17.6). The root can be divided horizontally into the **apical third** (the area involving the root apex), the **middle third**, and the **cervical third** (the area that borders the cementoenamel junction [CEJ]). The tooth crown can also be divided into horizontal thirds: the **gingival third** (the area that borders the CEJ), the **middle third,** and the **incisal** or **occlusal third**. Vertically, the crown of the tooth can be divided from the facial view, to

---

BOX 17.3   Tooth Identification Tips

When learning to chart types of teeth that are present, think through the following factors:
- How old is the patient?
- Is mixed dentition likely?
- How many teeth are in the quadrant?
- Teeth usually erupt in pairs. How big is the tooth? How white is it?

---

include the mesial, middle, and distal thirds. The mesial and distal views can be divided into labial (facial), middle, and lingual views for the anterior teeth and buccal (facial), middle, and lingual for the posterior teeth.

Tooth Numbering Systems

Tooth numbering systems were developed to simplify the task of identifying individual teeth. Tooth numbering systems are essential for charting and recording procedures. The three most common systems are the Universal Numbering System, the International Numbering System, and the Palmer System.

Universal Numbering System

The **Universal Numbering System** provides a standard sequential numbering system (1 through 32) for all permanent teeth. Primary teeth are identified by capital letters A to T. Maxillary primary numbering starts at the right second molar (tooth A) and proceeds clockwise to the maxillary left second molar (tooth J). The mandibular primary numbering continues clockwise from the left mandibular (tooth K) to the mandibular right second molar (tooth T) (see Fig. 17.7A). Maxillary permanent numbering starts at right maxillary third molar (tooth 1) and proceeds clockwise to left maxillary third molar (tooth 16). The mandibular permanent numbering continues clockwise from left mandibular third molar (tooth 17) to right mandibular third molar (tooth 32) (see Fig. 17.7B).

International Numbering System (Fédération Dentaire Internationale)

The **International Numbering System** uses two digits to identify each tooth (see Fig. 17.7). The first digit indicates the quadrant in which the tooth is located and the second digit identifies the specific tooth. For quadrant designation numbers 1 through 4 are used to specify permanent quadrant and numbers 5 through 8 to designate primary quadrants. The second digit identifies the specific tooth within the quadrant: the numbers 1 through 8 are used for permanent teeth and

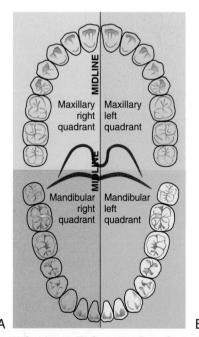
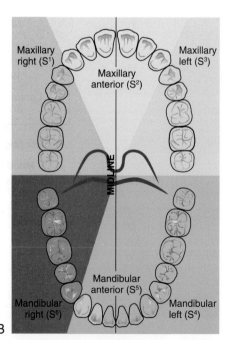

Fig. 17.4 (A) Quadrants. (B) Sextants. (From Gaylor LJ. *The Administrative Dental Assistant.* Elsevier; 2017.)

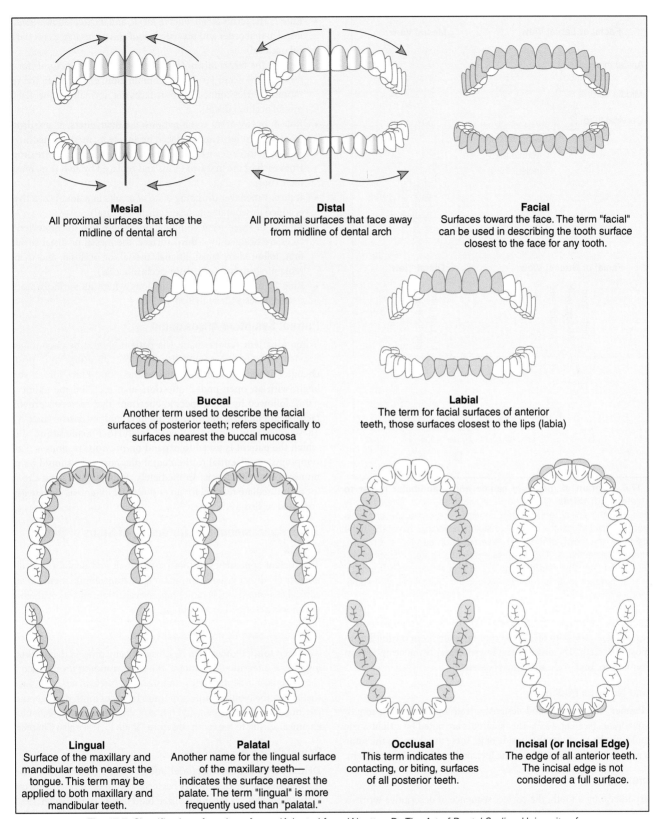

Mesial
All proximal surfaces that face the midline of dental arch

Distal
All proximal surfaces that face away from midline of dental arch

Facial
Surfaces toward the face. The term "facial" can be used in describing the tooth surface closest to the face for any tooth.

Buccal
Another term used to describe the facial surfaces of posterior teeth; refers specifically to surfaces nearest the buccal mucosa

Labial
The term for facial surfaces of anterior teeth, those surfaces closest to the lips (labia)

Lingual
Surface of the maxillary and mandibular teeth nearest the tongue. This term may be applied to both maxillary and mandibular teeth.

Palatal
Another name for the lingual surface of the maxillary teeth—indicates the surface nearest the palate. The term "lingual" is more frequently used than "palatal."

Occlusal
This term indicates the contacting, or biting, surfaces of all posterior teeth.

Incisal (or Incisal Edge)
The edge of all anterior teeth. The incisal edge is not considered a full surface.

Fig. 17.5 Classification of tooth surfaces. (Adapted from Wootton D. *The Art of Dental Scaling.* University of Vermont; 1991.)

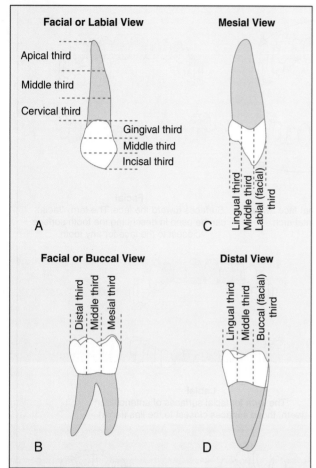

Fig. 17.6 Diagram of maxillary canine and mandibular molar to illustrate tooth thirds. (A) In the labial view, the root is horizontally divided into the apical, middle, and cervical thirds, and the crown is horizontally divided into the gingival, middle, and incisal thirds. (B) In the buccal view, the crown of the tooth is vertically divided into the mesial, middle, and distal thirds. (C) The mesial view of an anterior tooth is vertically divided into labial (facial), middle, and lingual thirds. (D) The distal view of an anterior tooth is vertically divided into buccal (facial), middle, and lingual thirds.

the numbers 1 through 5 for primary teeth. In each dentition, tooth 1 is the central incisor, with the numbers progressing from the midline to the posterior teeth. The order of the International Numbering System is pronounced "one, six," rather than "sixteen."

Palmer Notation Method

The **Palmer Notation Method** designates teeth by dividing the mouth into quadrants (see Fig. 17.7). The quadrants are noted by a right angle symbol with the tooth number inside of it. These numbers are the same ones used for tooth designation in the International Numbering System.

Nomenclature

When describing a tooth, the correct sequence of descriptive terms is based on a **D-A-Q-T System**. **D** is for *dentition*, **A** is for *arch*, **Q** is for *quadrant*, and **T** is for *tooth*. An example would be: permanent mandibular right second molar. In describing a cavity or a restoration, specific nomenclature is used that involves the combination of anatomic terms. Basic rules for nomenclature used to describe a cavity or restoration are as follows.

- Rule 1: The terms *mesial* and *distal* precede all other terms, with *mesial* taking precedence (e.g., mesial occlusal).

- Rule 2: The terms *labial, buccal, facial,* and *lingual* follow *mesial* and *distal* in that order and precede *incisal* and *occlusal* (e.g., mesial buccal occlusal).
- Rule 3: The terms *incisal* (for anterior teeth) and *occlusal* (for posterior teeth) occur last in any combination, except when the restoration or caries connects two surfaces not normally connected (e.g., mesial occlusal distal).
- Rule 4: In two-term combinations, the final letters, *al*, are dropped from the first term and replaced by an *o* (e.g., mesiolingual).
- Rule 5: In three-term combinations, the final letters, *al*, are dropped from each of the first two terms and replaced by an *o* (e.g., mesiolabioincisal).
- Rule 6: Whenever dropping of an *al* results in a double *o*, a hyphen is added to separate them (e.g., disto-occlusal).
- Rule 7: In three-term combinations where two unconnected surfaces are bridged by a third surface, the mesial or distal surface is first, followed by facial, lingual, incisal, or occlusal, and then the remaining surface (e.g., disto-occlusobuccal).
- Rule 8: In three-term combinations where all surfaces are connected, rules 1 through 3 apply.

Patient Symptom Assessment

When a patient reports pain, the patient should be encouraged to provide information about the location, duration, and postural changes, as well as characteristics of the pain.[1] Questioning should begin with an open-ended question such as, "Tell me about your pain," followed by more specific questions that focus on provoking factors, attenuating factors, frequency, and intensity (Box 17.4). These questions can be followed by further exploration, during which the patient is asked to expand on previous responses. Patient symptoms are essential to the dental diagnosis and should be communicated to the dentist immediately. Factors indicating the need for an immediate referral for an endodontic diagnosis and treatment are listed in Box 17.5.

Tooth Assessment and Detection of Signs of Dental Caries

The current approaches to tooth assessment and dental caries detection are (1) direct visual examination, (2) transillumination, (3) tactile clinical examination, (4) radiographic evaluation, and (5) evaluation of symptoms described by the patient.

Acquired Tooth Damage Assessment

Acquired tooth damage can be caused by any process that results in a loss of the integrity of the tooth. The most common form of acquired tooth damage is dental caries, an infectious disease caused by bacteria that live in the biofilm. Other common forms of tooth damage, such as attrition, abrasion, erosion, and fracture, are the result of mechanical or chemical assault to the tooth structure (Table 17.1; see also Chapter 39).

Dental Caries Assessment

Dental caries is a multifactorial infectious and transmissible disease, the primary factor of which is bacterial action on fermentable carbohydrates that affects the mineralized hard tissues (see Chapter 19). Susceptible sites that favor biofilm retention and are particularly prone to caries include the following:
- Pits and fissures on occlusal, buccal, and lingual surfaces
- Interproximal contacts
- Free gingival margin
- Areas of recession where root surfaces are exposed
- Deficient or defective margins of restorations
- Surfaces that are adjacent to bridges and dentures

BOX 17.4 Questions to Determine Quality of Pain

- General: "Tell me about your pain."
- Provoking factors: "Can you describe what causes your pain? Does temperature change, such as hot or cold, initiate the pain? Does chewing or biting hurt?"
- Attenuating factors: "Does anything relieve the pain?"
- Intensity: "When you have pain, is it mild, moderate, or severe?"
- Location: "Please point to the tooth or area that hurts."
- Duration: "How long does the pain last?"
- Postural: "Do you have any pain when you lie down? Bend over?"
- Quality: "What is the nature of the pain? Sharp? Dull? Stabbing? Throbbing?"

BOX 17.5 Considerations for Referral to Endodontic Diagnosis and Treatment

- Sharp, severe, intermittent pain that may be hard to localize
  - Pain when biting or chewing
  - Sensitivity to hot and cold
- Clinical and/or radiographic evidence of tooth damage such as caries, tooth fracture, or defective restorations
- Observation of soft tissue redness or swelling and presence of a fistula (sinus tract drainage)
- Rounded radiolucency at the apex of the tooth
- Pulpal vitality test results
- Facial asymmetry caused by swelling
- Skin lesions (occasionally, facial lesions may be traced to a tooth source, for example, sinus tract drainage.)

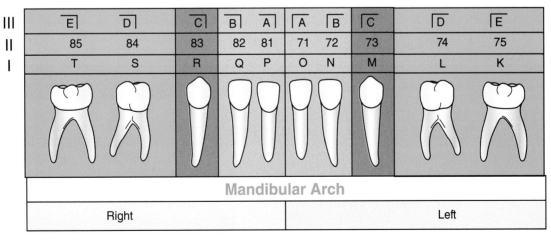

- I   Universal Numbering System
- II International Numbering System
- III Palmer Notation Method

A

Fig. 17.7 Tooth designation systems including the Universal Numbering System, the International Numbering System, and the Palmer Notation Method. (A) Primary dentition. (From Fehrenbach M, Popowics T. *Illustrated Dental Embryology, Histology, and Anatomy.* 5th ed. Saunders/Elsevier; 2021.)

	Molars			Premolars		Canine	Incisors				Canine	Premolars		Molars		

Maxillary Arch

	Molars			Premolars		Canine	Incisors				Canine	Premolars		Molars		
I	1	2	3	4	5	6	7	8	9	10	11	12	13	14	15	16
II	18	17	16	15	14	13	12	11	21	22	23	24	25	26	27	28
III	8⌋	7⌋	6⌋	5⌋	4⌋	3⌋	2⌋	1⌋	⌊1	⌊2	⌊3	⌊4	⌊5	⌊6	⌊7	⌊8

III	8⌉	7⌉	6⌉	5⌉	4⌉	3⌉	2⌉	1⌉	⌈1	⌈2	⌈3	⌈4	⌈5	⌈6	⌈7	⌈8
II	48	47	46	45	44	43	42	41	31	32	33	34	35	36	37	38
I	32	31	30	29	28	27	26	25	24	23	22	21	20	19	18	17

Mandibular Arch

Right	Left

I   Universal Numbering System

II International Numbering System

III Palmer Notation Method

B

Fig. 17.7, cont'd

TABLE 17.1 Acquired Tooth Damage

Name	Description	Clinical Appearance	Image
Attrition[*,†]	Tooth-to-tooth wear of the dentition is pathologic in nature and may be caused by bruxism, grinding, or clenching.	Appears as excessive wear to the occlusal and incisal surfaces. Restoration of a tooth with excessive attrition may include complete tooth coverage by a crown.	

TABLE 17.1 Acquired Tooth Damage—cont'd

Name	Description	Clinical Appearance	Image
Dental abrasion**	Pathologic tooth wear may be caused by a foreign substance, commonly seen as a result of traumatic toothbrushing.	Appears as a notch *(arrow)* worn into the teeth near the gingival margin.	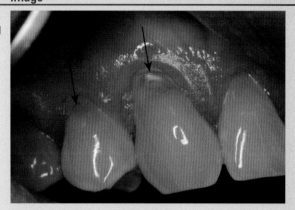
Dental erosion††,***,†††	Loss of tooth surface may occur as a result of chemical agents from acid reflux disease, excessive vomiting with morning sickness, anorexia, and bulimia. Tooth erosion may also result from habits such as sucking on lemons and holding mouth fresheners, cough drops, or candies in the mucobuccal fold. The erosive action of these chemicals causes local destruction of tooth enamel.	Enamel will appear very smooth. As the enamel thins, the dentin may be evident under the enamel *(arrows)*.	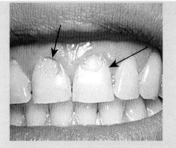 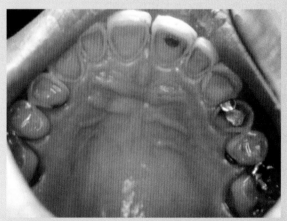 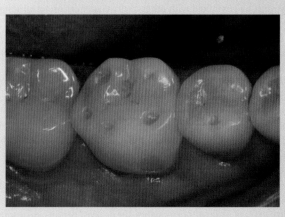

Continued

TABLE 17.1   Acquired Tooth Damage—cont'd

Name	Description	Clinical Appearance	Image
Noncarious cervical lesions****	Noncarious cervical lesions (NCCLs) defects are caused by biomechanical forces on teeth that result in tooth flexure and a wedge- or V-shaped loss of tooth structure at the cementoenamel junction (CEJ); the tooth is more susceptible to toothbrush abrasion.	Cervical stress lesion that exhibits a V- or wedge-shaped defect at the CEJ.	
Tooth fracture††††	Tooth fractures may range from small chips of the enamel to breaks that penetrate deeply into the tooth.	Minor enamel fractures often require nothing more than polishing of rough surfaces. More severe fractures require various levels of restoration. Some fractured teeth may not be restorable and, as a result, require removal.	

*Figure courtesy of Gary Nack, DDS, FAGD.
†Figure courtesy Margaret J. Fehrenbach, RDH, MS. In: Bird DL, Robinson DS, eds. *Modern Dental Assisting*. 12th ed. Saunders; 2018.
**Figure courtesy of Gary Nack, DDS, FAGD.
††Figure courtesy of Margaret Walsh, University of California–San Francisco.
***Figure from Sapp JP, Eversole LR, Wysocki GW. *Contemporary Oral and Maxillofacial Pathology*. 2nd ed. Mosby; 2004.
†††Figure courtesy of Gary Nack, DDS, FAGD.
****Figure courtesy Dr. Geoffrey Sperber, University of Alberta, Canada.
††††Figure courtesy of Margaret Walsh, University of California–San Francisco.

Types of Dental Caries

The classification of dental caries is intended to describe the rate, direction, and/or type of disease progression. These terms allow the oral healthcare practitioner to communicate the severity or rapidity of attack and the urgency with which restorative therapy should be delivered. These terms are not specific to a tooth and surface; consequently, they must be combined with other cavity classification terminology to permit location-specific communication.

Early childhood caries. **Early childhood caries** is observed in children under the age of 5 and is characterized by early onset and rapid progression of the disease (see Chapter 45).

Rampant caries. **Rampant caries** describes sudden, rapid destruction of many teeth and requires urgent intervention (Figs. 17.8 and 17.9). Rampant caries is often associated with early childhood caries in infants, in teens who frequently consume cariogenic snacks and beverages, and in persons of any age with an emotional disturbance or with reduced saliva flow resulting from, for example, head and neck cancer radiation therapy.[2]

Chronic caries. **Chronic caries** describes a slow, progressive decay process that requires intervention. The carious dentin is firm and often brown to black. In large, open cavities, the decayed dentin can be scooped out in large segments and has the consistency of firm leather (Fig. 17.10).

Arrested caries. Dental caries is not a continuous demineralization process. Evidence supports a continuous demineralization-remineralization process that can be tipped out of balance by changes in diet and oral environment (see Chapter 19). **Arrested caries** exhibit recalcified lesions resulting from remineralization that occurs when the caries process halts. It is noted by its dark staining without further breakdown of tooth tissues. Arrested lesions are characterized by their light or brown color and firm and glasslike surface when evaluated.

Recurrent caries. **Recurrent caries** describes new caries that occurs under or around a restoration or its margins. These lesions pose a unique threat because they may be difficult to detect and can invade the tissue beneath the restoration.

Types of Carious Lesions by Location

Carious lesions are often referred to by their specific location on a tooth. This descriptive mechanism may assist when describing the dental problem to the patient. The location description may include anatomic representations such as pit and fissure caries, smooth surface caries, and root caries. Another method of describing the carious lesion location is to identify the specific tooth surface(s) with the lesion. It is not uncommon for noncarious tooth surfaces to become involved in the restoration process because of the need for access or restoration design. For example, a tooth with a carious lesion on the distal surface may require the involvement of the occlusal or disto-occlusal surface for preparation and placement of the final restoration.

Pit and fissure caries. **Pit and fissure caries** is most frequently found in the grooves and crevices of the occlusal surfaces of premolars and molars (Fig. 17.11). They may also be found in maxillary incisor

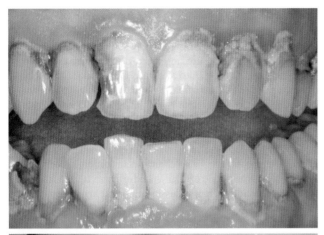

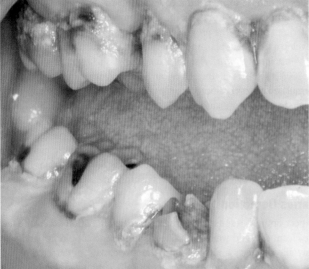

Fig. 17.8 Rampant caries. (From Ritter AV, Boushell LW, Walter R. *Sturdevant's Art and Science of Operative Dentistry.* 7th ed. Elsevier; 2019.)

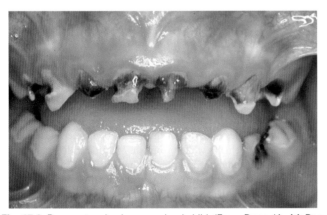

Fig. 17.9 Rampant caries in a preschool child. (From Dean JA. *McDonald and Avery's Dentistry for the Child and Adolescent.* 10th ed. Elsevier; 2016.)

lingual pits, mandibular molar buccal pits, and maxillary molar lingual grooves. Pits and fissures are particularly susceptible to a carious attack because of the protected bacterial niche provided by the coalesced developmental lobes of enamel.

Proximal caries. Dental caries between teeth at the point of their **proximal contact** (i.e., the contact between teeth that stabilizes their

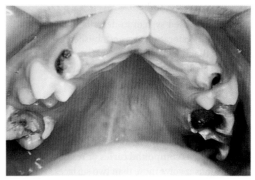

Fig. 17.10 Chronic caries.

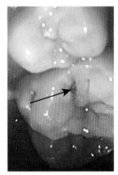

Fig. 17.11 Pit and fissure caries *(arrow).*

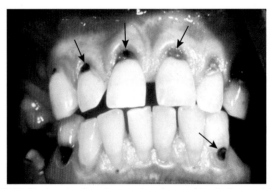

Fig. 17.12 Root caries found on root surfaces of teeth *(arrows).* (Courtesy Dr. John D. B. Featherstone, School of Dentistry, University of California San Francisco.)

position in the dental arch and prevents food impaction between the teeth) is called **proximal caries**.

Smooth surface caries. **Smooth surface caries** is found on the facial, buccal, lingual, mesial, and distal surfaces of the dentition. The proximal smooth surfaces are the most susceptible to dental caries because of the shelter these surfaces provide for biofilm development. The gingival third of the facial, buccal, and lingual surfaces is also more susceptible to caries because this area is often neglected while brushing.

Root caries. **Root caries** is dental caries that involves the tooth root, cementum, or cervical area of the tooth. Root caries is most frequently found in the older adult population in whom root exposure is common because of gingival recession (Fig. 17.12). Root caries can be exacerbated because of xerostomia.

Classification of Dental Caries and Restorations

Dental caries and dental restorations are commonly classified by either Black Classification System or the Complexity Classification System.

Black Classification System

The most commonly used system to describe the types and locations of dental caries and restorations was established by G. V. Black in the early 1900s. The **Black Classification System** is a descriptive system consisting of six classifications (Table 17.2).

Complexity Classification System

The **Complexity Classification System** identifies dental caries and restorations by the number of surfaces they involve. **Simple caries** or restorations are those involving only one tooth surface. Those that involve two surfaces are classified as **compound caries** or restorations, and **complex caries** or restorations involve more than two surfaces. The usual practice is to refer to the caries or restoration using the abbreviation of the surfaces affected, such as *O* for occlusal, *DO* for disto-occlusal, and *MOD* for mesio-occlusodistal. When using abbreviations, the letters are pronounced separately, such as a D-O caries or an M-O-D restoration.

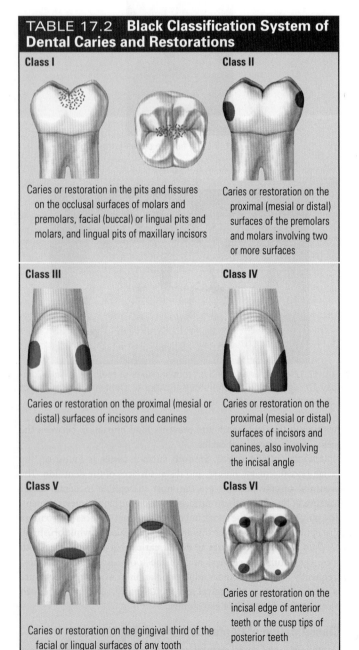

TABLE 17.2   Black Classification System of Dental Caries and Restorations

Class I

Caries or restoration in the pits and fissures on the occlusal surfaces of molars and premolars, facial (buccal) or lingual pits and molars, and lingual pits of maxillary incisors

Class II

Caries or restoration on the proximal (mesial or distal) surfaces of the premolars and molars involving two or more surfaces

Class III

Caries or restoration on the proximal (mesial or distal) surfaces of incisors and canines

Class IV

Caries or restoration on the proximal (mesial or distal) surfaces of incisors and canines, also involving the incisal angle

Class V

Caries or restoration on the gingival third of the facial or lingual surfaces of any tooth

Class VI

Caries or restoration on the incisal edge of anterior teeth or the cusp tips of posterior teeth

Figures adapted from Bird DL, Robinson DS. *Modern Dental Assisting.* 10th ed. Saunders/Elsevier; 2012.

Other Caries Classification Systems

The American Dental Association Caries Classification System (ADACCS) incorporates the International Caries Detection and Assessment System (ICDAS). These systems are used together to determine the extent of caries.

International Caries Detection and Assessment System and International Caries Classification and Management System. The **International Caries Detection and Assessment System** (ICDAS) is a method of assigning caries detection codes by combining patient risk assessment and clinical assessment of the tooth surface to assist clinicians in developing a plan that is focused and uses a preventive treatment approach. The visual clinical examination is performed on clean, dry teeth with the aid of a ball-ended explorer. ICDAS is associated with the **International Caries Classification and Management System** (ICCMS). The ICCMS focuses on prevention and long-term health maintenance. Those using the ICCMS may use all six ICDAS caries codes or choose to merge the codes to include fewer steps. Regardless of the number of codes used, the clinician will be using clearly defined criteria to monitor the progression or remission of the caries process to develop a treatment plan and establish a method to monitor outcomes.[3]

American Dental Association Caries Classification System. In 2008, members of the American Dental Association (ADA) met to formulate a caries classification system that would allow clinicians to classify tooth structure from sound, unaffected tooth structure to tooth structure that is fully cavitated. This group developed the ADA Caries Classification System (CCS), which allows clinicians to identify the current tooth classification and then determine what clinical treatments and/or therapeutic measures are appropriate. Fig. 17.13 illustrates the ADA CCS. See Box 17.6 for factors to consider when determining a patient's risk for caries.

Caries Detection

Expect optimal results from a hard tissue examination when the teeth are clean, dry, and well illuminated. The presence of biofilm and saliva may allow defects and signs of disease to remain undetected. A hard tissue examination should be systematically conducted, beginning, for example, with the most distal tooth in the maxillary right quadrant. The examination continues across the arch and through the last tooth in the maxillary left quadrant. Then the mandible is examined in reverse order, beginning with the most distal tooth in the mandibular left quadrant and ending with the last tooth in the mandibular right quadrant.

Visual Assessment

An evaluation of location, color, and surface texture all add to the clinician's ability to determine the presence of a carious lesion. Utilizing the ICDAS, the clinician visually assesses the appearance of occlusal surfaces and assigns a number from 0 to 6. Fig. 17.13 illustrates the occlusal images/rating scale. Caries is found where biofilm is allowed to accumulate. Caries can increase the opacity of enamel and may also change color to a chalky white or brown. Marginal ridges, especially in anterior teeth, should be examined under a well-directed light. The careful use of an intraoral mirror for transillumination may show signs of decay (Box 17.7). All of these findings need to be noted and included in the dental hygiene diagnosis.

Radiographic Assessment

Bitewing radiographs are standard diagnostic tools for detecting interproximal caries and periodontal bone loss in posterior teeth. Because of the contrast between the oral tissues and the restorative materials, radiographs readily illustrate the fit and contours of restorations. Carious lesions appear as radiolucent (black) images on radiographs because dental caries cause localized demineralization and loss of tooth tissue (Fig. 17.14). Depending on their density, restorative materials produce relatively radiopaque (white) images.

American Dental Association Caries Classification System.

	AMERICAN DENTAL ASSOCIATION CARIES CLASSIFICATION SYSTEM			
	Sound	**Initial**	**Moderate**	**Advanced**
Clinical Presentation	No clinically detectable lesion. Dental hard tissue appears normal in color, translucency, and gloss.	Earliest clinically detectable lesion compatible with mild demineralization. Lesion limited to enamel or to shallow demineralization of cementum/dentin. Mildest forms are detectable only after drying. When established and active, lesions may be white or brown and enamel has lost its normal gloss.	Visible signs of enamel breakdown or signs the dentin is moderately demineralized.	Enamel is fully cavitated and dentin is exposed. Dentin lesion is deeply/severely demineralized.
Other Labels	No surface change or adequately restored	Visually noncavitated	Established, early cavitated, shallow cavitation, microcavitation	Spread/disseminated, late cavitated, deep cavitation
Infected Dentin	None	Unlikely	Possible	Present
Appearance of Occlusal Surfaces (Pit and Fissure)*,†	ICDAS 0	ICDAS 1 ICDAS 2	ICDAS 3 ICDAS 4	ICDAS 5 ICDAS 6
Accessible Smooth Surfaces, Including Cervical and Root‡				
Radiographic Presentation of the Approximal Surface§	E0¶ or R0# No radiolucency	E1¶ or RA1# E2¶ or RA2# D1¶ or RA3# Radiolucency may extend to the dentinoenamel junction or outer one-third of the dentin. Note: radiographs are not reliable for mild occlusal lesions.	D2¶ or RB4# Radiolucency extends into the middle one-third of the dentin	D3¶ or RC5# Radiolucency extends into the inner one-third of the dentin

* Photographs of extracted teeth illustrate examples of pit-and-fissure caries.
† The ICDAS notation system links the clinical visual appearance of occlusal caries lesions with the histologically determined degree of dentinal penetration using the evidence collated and published by the ICDAS Foundation over the last decade; ICDAS also has a menu of options, including 3 levels of caries lesion classification, radiographic scoring and an integrated, risk-based caries management system ICCMS. (Pitts NB, Ekstrand KR. International Caries Detection and Assessment System [ICDAS] and its International Caries Classification and Management System [ICCMS]: Methods for staging of the caries process and enabling dentists to manage caries. *Community Dent Oral Epidemiol* 2013;41[1]:e41-e52. Pitts NB, Ismail AI, Martignon S, Ekstrand K, Douglas GAV, Longbottom C. ICCMS Guide for Practitioners and Educators. Available at: https://www.icdas.org/uploads/ICCMS-Guide_Full_Guide_US.pdf. Accessed April 13, 2015.)
‡ "Cervical and root" includes any smooth surface lesion above or below the anatomical crown that is accessible through direct visual/tactile examination.
§ Simulated radiographic images.
¶ E0-E2, D1-D3 notation system.[33]
# R0, RA1-RA3, RB4, and RC5-RC6 ICCMS radiographic scoring system (RC6 = into pulp). (Pitts NB, Ismail AI, Martignon S, Ekstrand K, Douglas GAV, Longbottom C. ICCMS Guide for Practitioners and Educators. Available at: https://www.icdas.org/uploads/ICCMS-Guide_Full_Guide_US.pdf. Accessed April 13, 2015.)

Fig. 17.13 The American Dental Association Caries Classification System. (From Young DA, Nový BB, Zeller GG, et al. The American Dental Association Caries Classification System for clinical practice: a report of the American Dental Association Council on Scientific Affairs. *J Am Dent Assoc.* 2015;146(2):79–86.)

BOX 17.6 Critical Thinking Scenario

Patient Caries Risk

Patients depend on the expertise of the dental hygienist to interpret and discuss all clinical findings. The dental hygienist should put together a plan that is clinically sound, evidence based, and individualized to the unique needs of the patient.

Dental caries is a multifactorial disease. Discuss the daily habits of patients. What is their daily sugar intake? How frequently does the patient ingest any sugar? How often do they brush? Are children properly assisted or supervised while brushing their teeth? Do they have an increased risk for xerostomia?

What are possible treatment considerations for an initial lesion (Fig. 17.13)? What oral hygiene aid can help prevent approximal (proximal) surface decay indicated on E1, E2, RA1, or RA2 lesions (Fig.17.13)?

BOX 17.7 Caries Detection

When conducting a visual assessment for caries, consider turning off the overhead lights in the treatment area. Use the light from an intraoral camera to transilluminate the anterior teeth. Closely look for shade changes as the light passes behind the anterior teeth and shines through the enamel and dentin.

As an example, clinicians can verify suspected overhanging margins of fillings by referring to radiographs (Fig. 17.15).

The ADACCS relies on the radiographic presentation of the approximal surfaces. The goal is to determine the depth of a radiolucency using the following scoring systems, E0-E2 (enamel involvement), D1-D3 (dentin involvement), and R0-R6 (pulpal involvement). Fig 17.13 illustrates the radiographic images.

Periapical radiographs, which are radiographs that include the root apex, may be used to examine anterior and posterior teeth if they are determined to be necessary during the clinical examination (Fig. 17.16). In addition, periapical radiographs are required of any tooth in which the health of the pulp is in question (see Chapter 39). Box 17.8 lists tips that enhance the effective use of radiographs.

Explorer Assessment

Conducting a hard tissue examination and evaluating for caries using an explorer is no longer recommended when suspected carious lesions are visually observed.[4,5] Historically, clinicians used an explorer to probe the tooth surface to detect caries since the surface of the caries may feel rough to an explorer passing over it. If the explorer stuck or felt tacky, then the area was determined to be positive for caries. This approach is no longer recommended because the explorer may:

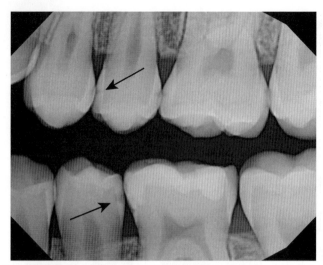

Fig. 17.14 Radiographic image of interproximal caries *(arrows)*. (Courtesy of Gary Nack, DDS, FAGD.)

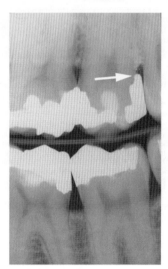

Fig. 17.15 Radiographic image of restoration; an overhang is revealed *(arrow)*. (From Newman MG, Takei HH, Klokkevoid PR, Carranza FA. *Carranza's Clinical Periodontology.* 13th ed. Saunders/Elsevier; 2019.)

- Disrupt the tooth surface and inhibit remineralization
- Transfer cariogenic microorganisms from tooth to tooth[6]
- Give a false-positive assessment attributable to the sticky or tacky feel from wedging the tip in narrow and deep pits and fissures rather than caries
- Fail to show improved detection of pit and fissure caries over visual inspection alone.[6]

Emerging Technologies

Developing new technologies complement traditional methods of caries diagnosis. The aim of new technologies is to provide objective information about the presence and severity of a carious lesion. It has been well established that by the time dental caries is observed visually or radiographically, it is often deeper and larger than it appears and may not be receptive to remineralization strategies.[7] Using new caries detection devices as an adjunctive technique along with traditional methods to diagnosis caries enables the implementation of preventive strategies to promote remineralization. These adjunctive techniques also help monitor the effectiveness of the interventions by assessing the state of the lesion over time.[7] Table 17.3 presents a few technologies currently available to clinicians.

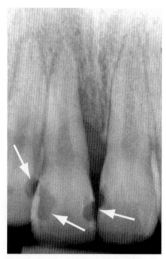

Fig. 17.16 Maxillary anterior periapical radiograph reveals signs of dental caries *(arrows)*. (From Newman MG, Takei HH, Klokkevoid PR, Carranza FA. *Carranza's Clinical Periodontology.* 11th ed. Saunders/Elsevier; 2012.)

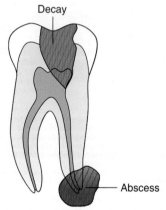

Decay

Abscess

Fig. 17.17 Illustration shows extensive decay into the pulp and formation of a periapical abscess. (From Bird DL, Robinson DS. *Modern Dental Assisting.* 11th ed. Saunders/Elsevier; 2015.)

BOX 17.8 Enhancing Digital Radiographs

When using digital radiographs, optimize the tools available. These are generally found along the software tool bar. Magnify the image to see calculus most clearly. Use contrast features to make caries more visible.

Intraoral cameras (IOCs) are used to document current conditions in the mouth. IOCs are shaped similarly to a small wand that enables a digital image to be magnified onto a computer screen. By enabling the patient to visualize a condition clearly, a treatment plan can be easily explained and understood. Research has shown that the use of IOCs has positively influenced patient compliance regarding home-care methods. These cameras do have a learning curve for the clinician, and their cost should be considered.

Pulpal Damage

The most common causes of pulpal nerve damage are bacterial infection and trauma. Bacterial infection is caused most often by extensive caries. If bacteria reach the nerves and blood vessels, the infection results in an abscess (Fig. 17.17). Endodontics is the specialty of dentistry that manages the prevention, diagnosis, and treatment of the dental pulp and the periradicular tissues that surround the root of the tooth. Endodontic treatment, or root canal therapy, provides

TABLE 17.3	Technologies Available for Dental Caries Detection			
Technology	**Description**	**Mechanism of Action**	**Advantages**	**Disadvantages**
Fiberoptic transillumination (FOTI)	An intense light is transmitted through the tissue of the tooth via a fiberoptic cable.	As light passes through the tooth structure, demineralized areas will produce a dark shadow.	The light source used is readily available in dental offices and can enhance detection of caries by a well-trained clinician.[8]	The risk of missing a carious lesion is high.
Digital imaging fiberoptic transillumination (DIFOTI)	Is a computerized version of FOTI; is a computer system with a monitor, mirror, and light source.[8]	Shines a concentrated beam of visible light on the tooth and, via a mirror, the computer system captures an image on the other side of the tooth that is seen on the computer monitor. Allows for the detection of optical changes at or near the surfaces such as cracks.	Is a useful adjunct to radiographic assessment and clinical decision making. The computer stores the images so they can be compared with future images.	Measures only optical changes near the tooth surface. Does not quantify the images; therefore the examiner makes a subjective analysis, based on the appearance of the stored images.[9]
Quantitative light-induced fluorescence (QLF)	Fluorescent-filtered images are transmitted from an intraoral camera to the computer screen.	An enamel lesion has increased porosity, causing a decrease in the emitted fluorescence. This difference can be quantitative.	Can be used for the early detection of carious lesions and for monitoring demineralization and remineralization of white spots by quantifying the mineral loss and the size of smooth surface lesions.	The outcome may be influenced by the presence of biofilm, calculus, surrounding light, or vitality of the tooth. QLF is also limited in its ability to measure interproximal caries.
Laser fluorescence (LF)	The LF device, with its solid-state diode laser, detects and measures changes in tooth structure.[8]	The actual mechanism is not fully understood; two theories exist: 1. When the red incident light connects with the increased porosity of a demineralized tooth, it stimulates the fluorescent light of a different wavelength and this fluorescent light is analyzed. 2. Metabolites of cariogenic bacteria emit fluorescence. The LF device measures the level of cariogenic bacterial activity and works on the assumption that if a high level of bacteria is present, the probability of having decalcified enamel is high.[8]	Is a useful adjunct to conventional visual and tactile detection methods for lesions on the occlusal surface. The reading gives a guideline on when to intervene with preventive measures, and the lesions can be monitored at subsequent recall appointments.[8]	There are many substances that can cause fluorescence, including stains, biofilm, calculus, prophy paste, and food. Some cariogenic bacteria do not produce fluorescence.[8] Therefore, in the aforementioned order, LF can give false-positive or false-negative results.
Electrical caries monitor (ECM)	An ECM is a battery-powered device with a low-frequency output of 21 Hz. The ECM probe is directly applied to the tooth, typically on an occlusal fissure, and the site is measured.	This technology is based on the differences in electrical conductivity between demineralized and sound enamel. Demineralized enamel has greater porosity, and the electrical conductivity increases.	ECM has the potential to monitor lesion progression in the depth and mineral content of the enamel. It has good sensitivity in detecting occlusal caries.[9]	This technology is time consuming to use and may not be feasible during a standard dental examination appointment.[8] In addition, a number of other factors can affect results, such as tooth temperature, thickness of enamel and tissue, and hydration or dryness of the teeth.[9]

From Heyman HD, Swift EJ Jr, Ritter AV. *Sturdevant's Art and Science of Operative Dentistry.* 6th ed. Mosby; 2013.

an effective means of saving a tooth that otherwise may have to be extracted. Although patients may experience symptoms differently, Box 17.5 provides a list of the most common signs and symptoms of pulpal nerve damage.

Although thermal testing using hot or cold appliances is used to detect vital pulp tissue, electric pulp testers are considered more reliable. Electric pulp testing is based on electric stimulation that causes the patient to react if the pulp is vital.

Developmental Anomalies

A tooth anomaly is a developmental disorder that is usually the result of a congenital or hereditary defect or an environmental disturbance. The extent of the dental anomaly depends on the stage of dental development when the disruption occurs. **Developmental anomalies** may include deviations from the usual number of teeth or irregularities within specific tooth tissue.

Tables 17.4 through 17.9 describe the more frequently noted dental anomalies.

TABLE 17.4   Anomalies of Number of Teeth

Name	Description	Clinical Appearance	Image
Hyperdontia[*,†]	Extra teeth, beyond the normal complement, are referred to as *supernumerary* or *supplemental* teeth.	Supernumerary teeth are extra teeth of abnormal shape. Supplemental teeth are extra teeth of normal shape.	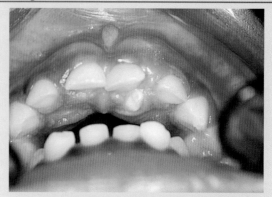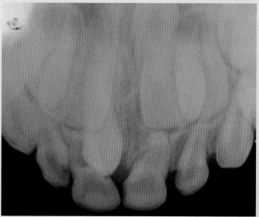
Mesiodens[**,††]	These supernumerary teeth are usually misshapen, small, and peglike.	Mesiodens may be seen as an extra tooth at the midline between the maxillary anterior incisors.	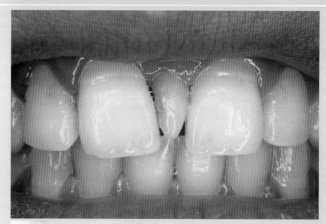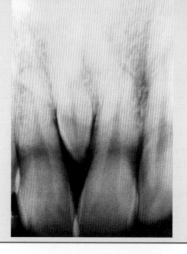

TABLE 17.4 Anomalies of Number of Teeth—cont'd

Name	Description	Clinical Appearance	Image
Hypodontia***,††† (also called *anodontia*)	One or more teeth are absent. Complete anodontia is failure of all teeth to develop and is a rare condition. Partial anodontia is the absence of one or several teeth.	Most frequently, congenitally missing teeth are the following: • Third molars • Maxillary lateral incisors • Mandibular premolars Teeth least frequently absent are the first permanent molars.	
Fusion****	The dentin and enamel of two or more teeth join together during development.	Fusion will reduce the number of teeth found in an arch.	

*Figure from Zitelli B, Nowalk A, McIntire S. *Zitelli and Davis' Atlas of Pediatric Physical Diagnosis*. 8th ed. Elsevier; 2021.
†Figure courtesy Wikimedia Commons, commons.wikimedia.org/.
**Figure from Chi A, Neville B, Allen C, Damm D. *Oral and Maxillofacial Pathology*. 4th ed. Saunders; 2016.
††Figure from Sciubba J, Regezi J, Jordan J. *Oral Pathology: Clinical Pathologic Correlations*. 7th ed. Saunders; 2017.
***Figure from Zitelli BJ, Davis HW. *Atlas of Pediatric Physical Diagnosis*. 8th ed. Saunders; 2023.
†††Figure from Regezi JA, Sciubba JJ, Jordan RCK. *Oral Pathology: Clinical Pathologic Correlations*. 7th ed. Elsevier; 2017.
****Figure from Regezi JA, Sciubba JJ, Jordan RCK. *Oral Pathology: Clinical Pathologic Correlations*. 7th ed. Elsevier; 2017.
Figures adapted from Darby ML, Walsh MM. *Dental Hygiene: Theory and Practice*. 4th ed. Saunders/Elsevier; 2015.

TABLE 17.5 Anomalies of the Whole Tooth

Name	Description	Clinical Appearance	Image
Macrodontia*	Is defined as larger than normal teeth.	May be larger in width, length, or height *(arrow)*.	
Microdontia†	Many supernumerary teeth are small and can be classified as microdonts. *Peg-lateral* is a term used to describe a type of microdont that can stem from a variety of causes.	Microdonts are teeth that are smaller than normal. It may be one tooth *(arrow)*, several teeth, or all teeth in the dentition. Are seen as conical lateral incisors.	
Gemination**	Is defined as a large tooth, resulting from the splitting of a single tooth germ that attempts to form two teeth.	Usually results in a partially or completely divided crown that is attached to a single root with one canal.	
Dens in dente††,***	Is defined as a tooth within a tooth *(arrow)*, which is caused by invagination of the enamel organ during development.	Is most frequently observed on the lingual aspect of the maxillary lateral incisors.	

TABLE 17.5	Anomalies of the Whole Tooth—cont'd		
Name	**Description**	**Clinical Appearance**	**Image**
Dilaceration[†††]	Is defined as an abnormal distortion of a crown or root caused by trauma during tooth formation. It is usually observed as a severely angulated root.	The root angulation may create extraction challenges for the dentist.[2]	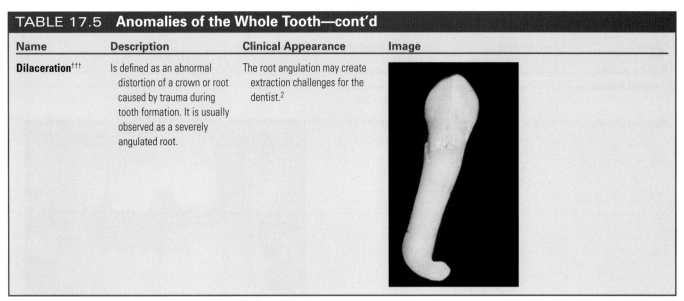

*Figure courtesy Steven R. Singer, Rutgers School of Dental Medicine.
[†]From Berkovitz B, Holland G, Moxham B. *Oral anatomy, histology, and embryology*. ed 4. Edinburgh: Mosby; 2009. Courtesy Dr. M. Cobourne.
**Figure from Bouquot J, Neville B, Allen C, Damm D. *Oral and Maxillofacial Pathology*. 3rd ed. Saunders; 2009.
[††]Figure from Rajendran A, Sivapathasundharam B, eds. *Shafer's Textbook of Oral Pathology*. 7th ed. Elsevier India; 2012.
***Figure from Bird D, Robinson D. *Modern Dental Assisting*. 12th ed. Saunders; 2018.
[†††]Figure courtesy Oral Pathology University of Alberta, Canada.
Figures adapted from Darby ML, Walsh MM. *Dental Hygiene: Theory and Practice*. 4th ed. Saunders/Elsevier; 2015.

TABLE 17.6	Anomalies of Enamel Formation: Enamel Dysplasia		
Name	**Description**	**Clinical Appearance**	**Image**
Enamel hypoplasia*	Is the result of a disturbance of the ameloblasts during matrix formation.	Enamel surface is pitted or rough and striated.	
Types of Enamel Hypoplasia			
Dental fluorosis[†]	Excessive amounts of systemic fluoride may be responsible for enamel hypoplasia or enamel hypocalcification.	Ranges from mild fluorosis, with white flecking, to severe conditions, with teeth that are deeply pitted or that have brown stains.	

Continued

TABLE 17.6 Anomalies of Enamel Formation: Enamel Dysplasia—cont'd

Name	Description	Clinical Appearance	Image
Syphilis-related enamel hypoplasia	Congenital syphilis is a rare cause of enamel hypoplasia.	Nodular enamel growths appear on the cusp surfaces of the permanent molars.	
Hutchinson incisors[**]	This term is used to describe the appearance of syphilitic incisor teeth, which is a sign of congenital syphilis.	Permanent incisor teeth are narrow and notched.	
Mulberry molars[††]	This term is used to describe molar anomalies associated with congenital syphilis.[6]	Rounded cusps, mottled mulberry-shaped molars.	
Peg lateral teeth[***]	May be associated with syphilitic conditions; however, as discussed in Table 17.5, microdontia can arise from several causes.	Are seen as conical lateral incisors.	
Enamel hypocalcification[†††]	This defect occurs in the enamel as the result of a disturbance during mineralization.	Exhibits white spotting of the enamel surface, which is generally smooth in texture.	

Name	Description	Clinical Appearance	Image
Amelogenesis imperfecta****	Is a form of enamel dysplasia as a result of many inheritance patterns such as autosomal dominant, recessive, or X-linked gene.	Exhibits partial or total malformation of enamel. The dentin and pulp develop normally, but the enamel is easily chipped or worn away.	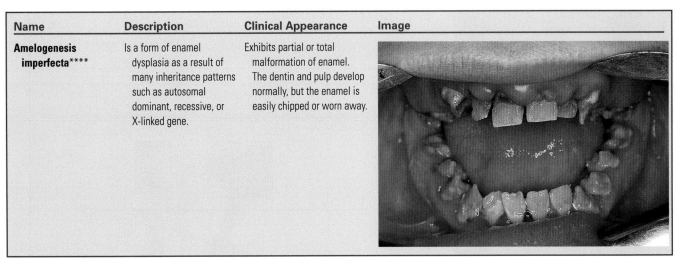

*Figure from Regezi JA, Sciubba JJ, Jordan RCK. *Oral Pathology: Clinical Pathologic Correlations*. 7th ed. Saunders; 2017.

†Figure from Daniel SJ, Harfst SA, Wilder R: *Mosby's Dental Hygiene: Concepts, Cases, and Competencies*. 2nd ed. St. Louis, 2008, Mosby; courtesy Dr. George Taybos, Jackson, Mississippi.

**Figure from Halstead CL, Blozis GG, Drinnan AJ, et al. *Physical Evaluation of the Dental Patient*. Mosby; 1982.

††Figure from Darby ML. *Mosby's Comprehensive Review of Dental Hygiene*. 7th ed. Mosby; 2012.

***Figure courtesy of Dr. Gururaj N, CSI Dental College, Madurai, Tamil Nadu. In: Rajendran A, Sivapathasundharam B, eds. *Shafer's Textbook of Oral Pathology*. 7th ed. Elsevier India; 2012.

†††Figure from Heymann HO, Swift EJ, Ritter AV. *Sturdevant's Art and Science of Operative Dentistry*. 6th ed. Mosby; 2013.

****Figure from Regezi JA, Sciubba JJ, Jordan RCK. *Oral Pathology: Clinical Pathologic Correlations*. 7th ed. Elsevier; 2017.

Figures adapted from Darby ML, Walsh MM. *Dental Hygiene: Theory and Practice*. 4th ed. Saunders/Elsevier; 2015.

TABLE 17.7 Enamel Anomalies Not Classified as Enamel Dysplasia

Name	Description	Clinical Appearance
Dens evaginatus*	Is also referred to as *tuberculated cusp*. This rare developmental anomaly is caused by a proliferation of enamel epithelium that forms an accessory cusp found on the occlusal surface. It is believed to form from an outpouching (evagination) of the enamel epithelium during the early stages of odontogenesis. The tissue mass contains normal pulp and is subject to occlusal wear.	Exhibits a small mass of enamel or accessory cusp, projecting on the occlusal surface of molars and premolars *(arrow)*.
Talon cusp†	The lingual cusp of anterior teeth is reported to resemble an eagle's talon and was named accordingly. The talon cusp has well-developed enamel and dentin and contains a pulp horn.[2]	Exhibits one or more well-delineated cusps on the lingual surfaces of maxillary *(arrows)* and mandibular anterior teeth.

*Figure courtesy of Margot Van Dis.

†Figure courtesy of Geoffrey Speber, University of Alberta, Canada.

Figures adapted from Darby ML, Walsh MM. *Dental Hygiene: Theory and Practice*. 4th ed. Saunders/Elsevier; 2015.

TABLE 17.8 Anomalies of Dentin Formation

Name	Description	Clinical Appearance	Image
Dentinogenesis imperfecta[*][†][**]	Is associated with a dominant inherited disorder and is characterized by faulty formation of connective tissues. Enamel formation occurs normally, but the enamel easily breaks or chips away, resulting in tooth attrition and dentinal hypersensitivity. Irregular formation or an absence of dentinal development is exhibited.	Displays a softer than normal consistency as a result of increased water and organic content. Teeth display a larger than normal width, length, or height. Dental treatment usually includes placement of crowns to preserve an existing crown.	
Dentin dysplasia[††]	Dentin dysplasia has two subdivisions: type I (radicular dentin dysplasia) and type II (coronal dentin dysplasia). Dentin dysplasia type I is an autosomal-dominant inheritance pattern characterized by teeth with normal crowns and abnormal roots. The defect is connected to a disturbance in the Hertwig epithelial root sheath, which guides the formation of the root. Dentin dysplasia type II has an autosomal dominant inheritance pattern. A mutation in the gene dentin sialophosphoprotein (*DSPP*) has occurred. Dentinogenesis imperfecta and dentin dysplasia type II share the *DSPP* mutation.[6]	Type I exhibits a total or partial lack of pulp chambers and root canals on radiographic images. Primary and secondary dentitions are equally affected. Because the roots are short, the teeth are easily affected by any trauma, even minor, and the teeth are generally lost prematurely. Type II exhibits an obliterated and partial lack of coronal pulp chambers and small root canals.[6]	

*,†Figures courtesy Dr. Edward V Zegarelli.

**Figure from Dean J, Avery DR, McDonald RE. *McDonald and Avery's Dentistry for the Child and Adolescent.* 10th ed. Elsevier; 2016.

††Figure courtesy Carl J Witkop.

TABLE 17.9 Anomalies of Pulp Formation

Name	Description	Clinical Appearance	Image
Taurodontism	The term *taurodontism* means bull-like teeth and is an inherited phenomenon that is genetically determined.	The crowns of these teeth develop normally; however, the pulp chambers are significantly enlarged *(arrow)* at the expense of the dentinal walls.[2]	

Figure adapted from Darby ML, Walsh MM. *Dental Hygiene: Theory and Practice.* 4th ed. Saunders/Elsevier; 2015. Courtesy Dr. George Blozis.

Dentition Charting

Charting tooth assessment data is conducted at the patient's initial assessment appointment and updated at each subsequent appointment. Although no set sequence is required for charting, a systematic approach avoids omitting important information. For common charting symbols and examples, see Appendix A at the end of this book. Examples from Dentrix **dental software** program are shown in Procedure 17.1 (Dentrix example).

Occlusion

Hard tissue assessment includes classifying occlusion and documenting the relationships present among the teeth. **Occlusion** is defined as the contact relationship between all teeth when the maxilla and mandible are in a fully closed position. As the primary teeth erupt, occlusion is influenced by the development of facial muscles and neuromuscular patterns.

Centric Occlusion

Centric occlusion is a term used to describe the spatial relationship between the maxillary and mandibular teeth when the teeth come in contact with one another. This spatial relationship optimizes the occlusal surface contact areas. Ideally, it exists when the patient closes naturally. When the teeth of a normal occlusion are in centric occlusion, each tooth of one arch contacts two teeth in the opposite arch, except for the mandibular central incisors and the maxillary third molars. This positioning of the teeth equally distributes the forces of occlusion. Because of this arrangement, the alignment of the opposing jaw is not disturbed immediately if a tooth is lost. If, however, restorative treatment is not performed for a period of time, the neighboring teeth may begin to drift mesially. The teeth may tilt, and the opposing teeth may supererupt. Thus the loss of one tooth can change the occlusal relationship of the entire dentition. When teeth do not occlude properly, unnatural stress is placed on them that may lead to pain and/or occlusal trauma. Although occlusal trauma does not cause periodontal disease directly, it may be an adverse factor in an already diseased periodontium. Box 17.9 discusses considerations that address the dental care needs of patients with occlusal trauma to reduce the risk of periodontal disease.

Centric Relation

Centric relation is the relation of the mandible to the maxilla when the condyles are in their most posterior and superior positions in the

BOX 17.9 Dental Care Considerations for Occlusal Trauma

Malocclusion can create unique patient needs. A variety of oral hygiene options should be addressed to meet these needs: floss, interdental brushes, power toothbrushes, end tuft brushes, and oral mouthwashes, among others.

The possibility of pain and/or occlusal trauma attributable to changes in the occlusion highlights the importance of maintaining proper or normal occlusion when placing dental restorations or sealants. All restorations and sealants must be checked with articulating paper to ensure health is being maintained.

mandibular fossae. Ideally, the mandible is in centric relation when the dentition is in centric occlusion. Usually, the teeth slide about 1 mm when patients shift their occlusion from centric relation to centric occlusion.[9]

Overjet

When teeth come together in centric occlusion, there is often a horizontal projection of the maxillary teeth beyond the mandibular teeth. This is termed **overjet** (Fig. 17.18). To measure overjet, have the patient close in centric occlusion. Measure the distance between the labial surface of the mandibular incisor and the incisal edge of the maxillary incisor while the probe is held at a right angle to the labial surface of the mandibular incisor.[7]

Overbite

In centric occlusion, the maxillary incisors generally overlap the mandibular incisors vertically, a position called **overbite**. Vertical overlap allows maximum contact between the posterior teeth during mastication. Overbite is classified as normal, moderate, or severe, based on the depth of the overlap. When the maxillary incisors overlap within the incisal third of the mandibular incisors, the patient has a normal overbite. Moderate overbite occurs when the maxillary incisors overlap with the middle third of the mandibular incisors, and severe overbite occurs when the incisal edges of the maxillary teeth reach the gingival third of the mandibular incisors (Fig. 17.19A–C).

To measure overbite, the tip of the periodontal probe is placed at the incisal edge of the maxillary incisor at right angles to the mandibular incisor, when the patient is in centric occlusion. As the patient opens

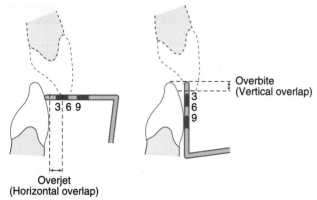

Overbite
(Vertical overlap)

3
6
9

Overjet
(Horizontal overlap)

Fig. 17.18 Overjet and overbite. (From Fehrenbach M, Popowics T. *Illustrated Dental Embryology, Histology, and Anatomy.* 4th ed. St Louis: Saunders/Elsevier; 2016.)

slowly, the clinician can observe which third of the mandibular incisor the probe is contacting.

Contact Area

In an ideal dental arch, contact areas are where the teeth touch their proximal neighbors. These contact areas protect the interdental papilla and stabilize each tooth within the dental arch. When there is an open contact area between teeth, food can be trapped, resulting in gingival inflammation. The use of floss is an effective tool, along with radiographs, to assess the status of a contact area. Open contacts must be called to the attention of the dentist for evaluation and possible treatment (Box 17.10).[9]

Normal Occlusion

In the late 1800s, Dr. Edward H. Angle established a system of classification of occlusion, Angle's Classification of Malocclusion. Because of their stability within the dental arch, the permanent first molars, and later the canines, were used to assess the relationship between the maxillary and the mandibular arches. In a normal molar relationship, the mesiobuccal cusp of the maxillary permanent first molar occludes with the mesiobuccal groove of the mandibular permanent first molar. In a normal canine relationship, the maxillary permanent canine occludes with the distal half of the mandibular permanent canine and the mesial half of the mandibular first premolar.

Malocclusion

Malocclusion is a deviation from the normal relationship between the maxilla and mandible while in centric occlusion. Malocclusion may increase the risk of occlusal trauma. In addition, malocclusion negatively impacts the patient's ability to maintain effective oral hygiene. Therefore individuals with malocclusion are at increased risk for periodontal disease attributable to the high levels of biofilm retention. Malocclusion may also contribute to temporomandibular joint pain. As part of the dental hygiene assessment, occlusion is classified on both the right and left sides of the dentition. Malocclusion and temporomandibular joint dysfunctions, such as pain or popping on opening and closing of the mandible, are referred to the dentist for further evaluation (see Chapter 40 for detailed discussion of malocclusion and orthodontic treatment).

In Angle's classification system, there are three types of malocclusion in the permanent dentition: Class I, Class II, and Class III. Class II malocclusion is further divided into divisions 1 and 2 (Fig. 17.20).

Class I malocclusion. Angle defined **Class I malocclusion** as occurring when an individual tooth or groups of teeth are not ideally positioned, even though the canine and first molars are in normal

BOX 17.10   Notes on Open Contacts

A thin floss that easily glides can assist with the determination of open contacts. Open contacts need to be kept free of plaque. Although floss is effective, patients may need to be instructed to use a wide floss or dental tape. Interproximal brushes are also effective in cleaning these areas and maintaining optimal health. Open contacts may also indicate the need for a restoration to be recontoured or replaced.

occlusion. For example, there may be problems with crowding, causing the teeth to be out of line within the dental arch. Some patients with Class I malocclusion have slight, moderate, or severe overbites, or an open bite in which some teeth do not occlude. Some patients have an **end-to-end bite** (sometimes referred to as edge-to-edge bite) in the anterior sextant, in which the teeth occlude without the maxillary teeth overlapping the mandibular teeth, or a **crossbite**, in which the maxillary teeth are positioned lingual to the mandibular teeth (Fig. 17.19D–F, Fig. 17.21A–B).

Class II malocclusion. In **Class II malocclusion**, the molar relationship is such that the mesiobuccal cusp of the permanent maxillary first molar is situated mesial to the mesiobuccal groove of the permanent mandibular first molar by at least the width of a premolar, whereas the maxillary permanent canine is mesial to the mandibular permanent canine by at least the width of a premolar. If the distance is less than the width of a premolar, it is classified as having a "tendency toward Class II." An individual with a Class II malocclusion usually has a retrognathic facial profile.

Two subdivisions of the Class II malocclusion are used to indicate the relationship of the maxillary and mandibular anterior teeth. In Class II division 1, the maxillary incisors facially protrude from the mandibular incisors. As a result, the incisors may supererupt, causing a severe overbite. In Class II division 2, one or more of the maxillary central incisors are lingually inclined or retruded (see Fig. 17.20). The maxillary lateral incisors may overlap the central incisors. Overbite is often severe.[9]

Class III malocclusion. In **Class III malocclusion**, the mandible is relatively large compared with the maxilla; thus a prognathic profile results (see Fig. 17.20). The molar relationship is such that the mesiobuccal cusp of the permanent maxillary first molar is situated distal to the mesial buccal groove of the permanent mandibular first molar by at least the width of a premolar, whereas the maxillary permanent canine is distal to the distal surface of the mandibular permanent canine by at least the width of a premolar. Similar to the case with the Class II malocclusion, if the distance of movement in the molars or canine is less than the width of a premolar, the classification of occlusion is labeled as having a "tendency toward Class III."[9]

Primary Occlusion

Similar to the permanent dentition, an ideal relationship exists when the primary maxillary canine occludes with the distal half of the mandibular canine. The **terminal plane** is the ideal molar relationship when the primary teeth are in centric occlusion. There are two ways this can occur. The first is the **flush terminal plane**, in which the primary maxillary and mandibular second molars occlude in an end-to-end relationship. The second is the **mesial step**, which occurs when the primary mandibular second molar is mesial to the primary maxillary second molar.

A distal step relationship occurs when the primary mandibular molar occludes distal to the primary maxillary second molar, which is not an ideal molar relationship (Fig. 17.22).[2]

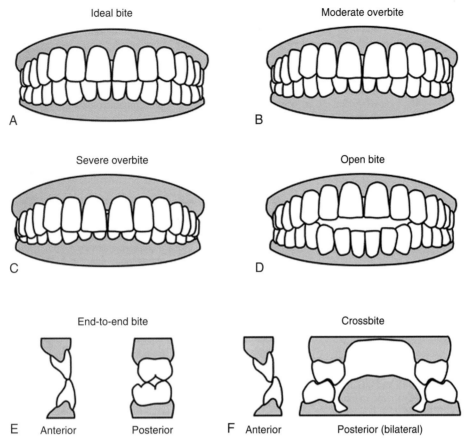

Fig. 17.19 Malrelationships of individual teeth or groups of teeth. (A) Ideal bite. (B) Moderate overbite. (C) Severe overbite. (D) Open bite. Abnormal vertical spaces between the mandibular and maxillary teeth are most frequently observed in the anterior teeth; however, open bite may occur in the posterior areas. (E) End-to-end bite. The teeth occlude without the maxillary teeth overlapping the mandibular teeth. An end-to-end bite can occur anteriorly and posteriorly and unilaterally or bilaterally. (F) Crossbite. The maxillary teeth are lingually positioned to the mandibular teeth and may occur unilaterally or bilaterally. (From Fehrenbach M, Popowics T. *Illustrated Dental Embryology, Histology, and Anatomy,* ed 5, Saunders, Elsevier; 2021.)

Parafunctional Habits

Parafunctional habits are movements of the mandible, such as clenching and bruxism, which are considered outside or beyond the functions of eating, speech, or respiration. These parafunctional habits often subconsciously occur during sleep or while deeply concentrating on something.

Clenching occurs when the teeth occlude for a long period while in centric occlusion without giving the mandible a rest. People who clench their teeth may have enlarged masseter muscles and may consider it normal to feel muscle tension in the facial and masticatory muscles. Directed relaxing of these muscles may help in some cases. Clenching may be attributable to stress or the way an individual processes neurologic impulses (Box 17.11).[9]

Bruxism is the forceful grinding of opposing occlusal surfaces, often making an audible noise. Bruxism causes attrition and wear facets of the incisal or occlusal surfaces of the teeth, especially of the canine cusp tips. People who clench or grind their teeth should be referred to a dentist for an occlusal guard, which is an oral appliance that covers the dentition. An occlusal guard can be worn during waking hours and/or when sleeping. It protects the teeth from further attrition and helps spread the occlusal force generated throughout the dentition.

Thumb or finger sucking. Sucking the thumb or fingers usually occurs in infancy and early childhood. If this behavior persists into childhood, it can cause malocclusion, a high, arched palate, a callused thumb or finger, or improper swallowing patterns (see Chapter 45).[2]

Trauma from occlusion. Two types of trauma from occlusion can result—primary and secondary. **Primary trauma from occlusion** is an injury that occurs from excessive occlusal forces on a periodontium that have not been altered by disease. There is no attachment loss, apical migration of the junctional epithelium, or loss of connective tissue. Primary trauma from occlusion is caused by high restorations, improperly fitting removable partial dentures or bridges, malaligned teeth, clenching, or bruxism and is reversible if the trauma is removed or altered, usually by occlusal adjustment. Signs of primary trauma include widened periodontal ligament space, tooth mobility, and pain.

Secondary trauma from occlusion is an injury that occurs from normal or excessive occlusal forces placed on a weakened periodontium. It occurs when the surrounding periodontium has been weakened by periodontal disease with evidence of apical migration of the junctional epithelium and loss of connective tissue. With secondary occlusal trauma, the clinician may observe rapid bone loss and pocket formation in the patient. The patient

Occlusal Relationships in Centric Occlusion	Molar Relationships	Canine Relationships	Anterior Relationships	Face Profile
Normal occlusion 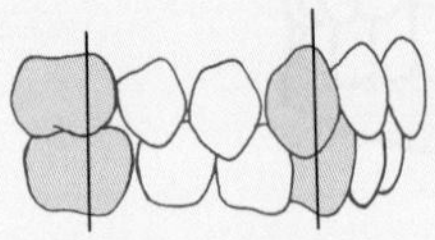	MB cusp of the maxillary first molar occludes with the MB groove of the mandibular first molar	Maxillary canine occludes with the distal half of the mandibular canine and the mesial half of the mandibular first premolar	No dental malalignments present, such as crowding or spacing	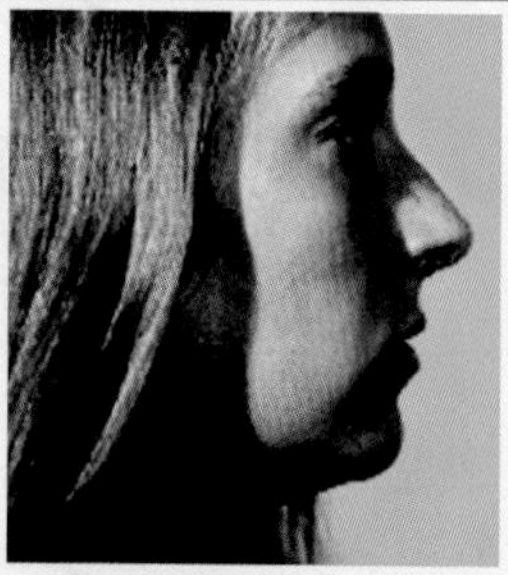 Mesognathic profile
Class I malocclusion 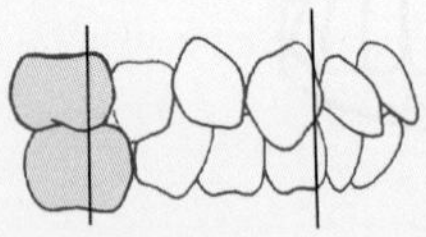	Same as above but malpositions of individual or groups of teeth may occur	Same as above but malpositions of individual or groups of teeth may occur	Dental malalignments present, such as crowding or spacing	Same as above
Class II Distal I malocclusion 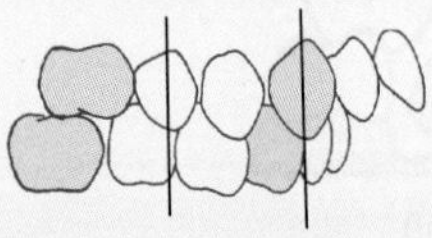	MB cusp of the maxillary first molar occludes (by more than the width of a premolar) mesial to the MB groove of the mandibular first molar	Distal surface of the mandibular canine is distal to the mesial surface of the maxillary canine by at least the width of a premolar	Maxillary anteriors protrude facially from the mandibular anteriors, with deep overbite	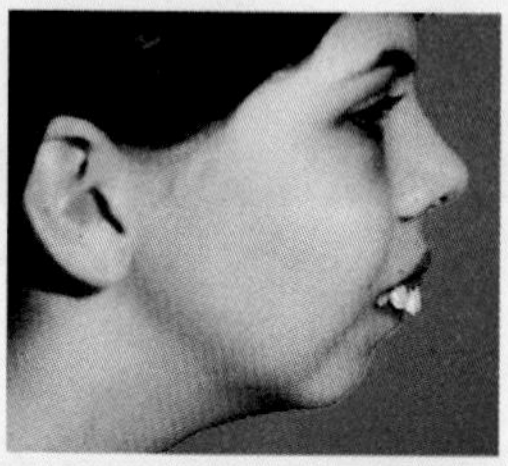 Retrognathic profile with lip incompetence
Class II Division II malocclusion 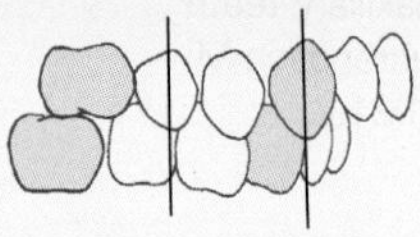	Same as Class II division 1	Same as Class II division 1	Maxillary central incisors are upright or retruded, and lateral incisors are tipped labially or overlap the central incisors with deep overbite	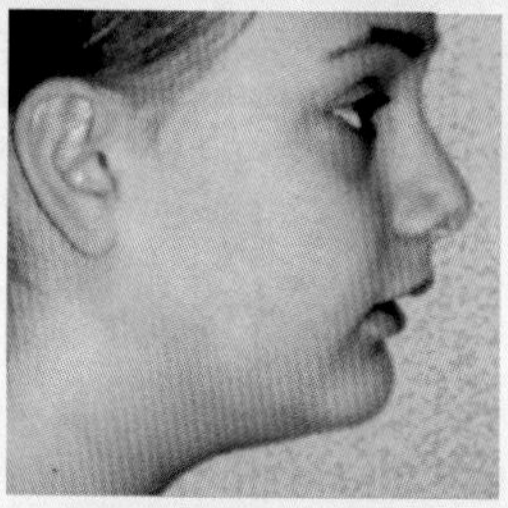 Retrognathic profile
Class III malocclusion 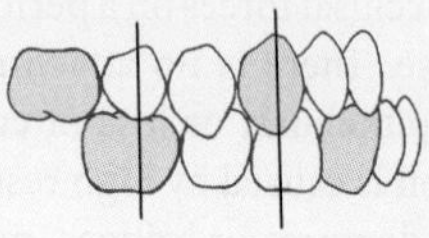	MB cusp of the maxillary first molar occludes (by more than the width of a premolar) distal to the MB groove of the mandibular first molar	Distal surface of the mandibular canine is mesial to the mesial surface of the maxillary canine by at least the width of a premolar	Mandibular incisors in complete crossbite	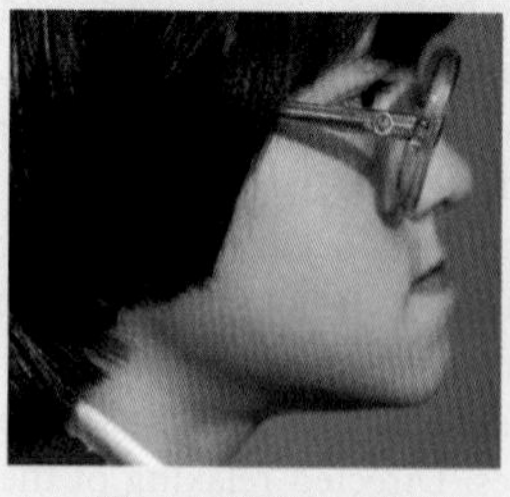 Prognathic profile

Fig. 17.20 Classification of malocclusion. *MB,* Mesiobuccal. (Adapted from Bath-Balogh MB, Fehrenbach, MJ. *Illustrated Dental Embryology, Histology, and Anatomy.* 3rd ed. Saunders/Elsevier; 2006. Photographs from Proffit WR, Fields HW, Sarver DM. *Contemporary Orthodontics.* 5th ed. Mosby/Elsevier; 2013.)

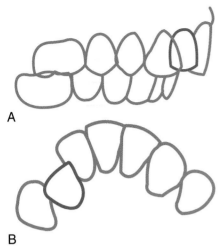

Fig. 17.21 Labioversion and linguoversion. (A) Labioversion. A tooth is labially or facially positioned to its normal position. (B) Linguoversion. A tooth lingually positioned to its normal position. (A–B, Adapted from Popowics, Margaret Fehrenbach, T. *Illustrated Dental Embryology, Histology, and Anatomy*. 4th ed. Elsevier Health Sciences (US), 2016. Available from: VitalSource Bookshelf.)

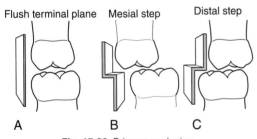

Fig. 17.22 Primary occlusion.

BOX 17.11   Patient or Client Education Tips

- Share information concerning acquired tooth damage and provide caries preventive strategies based on the caries risk (see Chapter 19).
- Interpret and discuss the charted findings with the patient.
- Report the factors—local (e.g., trauma), systemic (e.g., diseases, nutritional deficiencies, excess systemic fluoride), hereditary, and idiopathic (unknown)—that may cause anomalies in enamel formation.
- Discuss the importance of tooth replacement to prevent occlusal disharmonies.
- Educate the patient about the need for treating open contacts that trap food, which may result in gingival inflammation and periodontal breakdown.
- Teach strategies to the patient to treat parafunctional habits.

should be referred to the dentist or periodontist for further evaluation and treatment.

KEY CONCEPTS

- Documentation of tooth assessments is important for care planning, communication, legal documentation, and quality assurance.
- Dental charting is the graphic representation of the condition of the patient's teeth observed on a specific date. The data recorded are based on clinical and radiographic assessments and the patient's report of symptoms.
- The dental chart is part of the permanent patient record and must be accessible for reference during all appointments, thus facilitating continuity, treatment planning, and ongoing documentation of care.
- The goal of tooth assessment for the dental hygienist is to recognize signs of disease, defective restorations, developmental anomalies, and acquired tooth damage.
- Collaboration with other healthcare professionals will optimize patient care.
- Consistent use of terms, symbols, and nomenclature will facilitate accurate transfer of knowledge between providers.
- Direct examination can be effectively performed only if the teeth are clean, dry, and illuminated with good light. Care should be exercised to avoid exploring early carious lesions and known sensitive areas.
- The dental hygienist must use a well-organized and thorough clinical assessment of signs, symptoms, radiographs, and any available additional information to assist in making a dental hygiene diagnosis.
- Thorough dentition assessment includes classifying occlusion and documenting tooth malrelationships, as well as assessing parafunctional habits.

ACKNOWLEDGMENTS

The author acknowledges Janice F. L. Pimlott, Joan D. Leakey, Cheryl Cameron, and Glen E. Gordon for their past contributions to this chapter.

REFERENCES

1. Araújo M-R, Alvarez M-J, Godinho CA, et al. Psychological, behavioral, and clinical effects of intra-oral camera: a randomized control trial on adults with gingivitis. *Community Dent Oral Epidemiol.* 2016;44:523–530.
2. Dean J. *McDonald and Avery's Dentistry for the Child and Adolescent.* 10th ed. Elsevier; 2016.
3. Pitts NB, Ekstrand KR. On behalf of the ICDAS Foundation: International Caries Detection and Assessment System (ICDAS) and its International Caries Classification and Management System (ICCMS)—methods for staging of the caries process and enabling dentists to manage caries. *Community Dent Oral Epidemiol.* 2013;41:e41–e52.
4. Featherstone JDB. The science and practice of caries prevention. *J Am Dent Assoc.* 2000;131:887.
5. Featherstone JDB, O'Reilly MM, Shariati M, et al. Enhancement of remineralization in vitro and in vivo. In: Leach SA, ed. *Factors Relating to Demineralization and Remineralization of the Teeth.* IRL Press; 1986.
6. Loesche WJ, Svanberg ML, Pape HL. Intraoral transmission of streptococcus mutans by a dental explorer. *J Dent Res.* 1979;58:765.
7. Amaechi BT. Emerging technologies for diagnosis of dental caries: the road so far. *J Appl Phys.* 2009;105:102047.
8. Cohen S. Diagnostic procedures. In: Cohen S, Burns RC, eds. *Pathways of the Pulp.* 10th ed. Mosby; 2011.
9. Fehrenbach M, Popowics T. *Illustrated Dental Embryology, Histology, and Anatomy.* 4th ed. Elsevier; 2016.

18

Assessment of Dental Deposits and Stain

Mark G. Kacerik

PROFESSIONAL OPPORTUNITIES

A dental hygienist must be competent in the assessment of dental deposits to provide quality dental hygiene treatment. Dental deposits contribute to destructive dental diseases. The prevention of such diseases begins with the ability to accurately assess deposits, develop an appropriate treatment plan, and educate the patient on oral self-care practices.

COMPETENCIES

1. Compare and contrast the different types of oral deposits and stains.
2. Apply appropriate techniques for the assessment of dental deposits.
3. Discuss with patients the impact of dental deposits on oral health.
4. Utilize oral hygiene indices for patient assessment and education.
5. Explain the significance of record keeping and documentation as it relates to the assessment of dental deposits and stains.

DENTAL DEPOSITS

Dental deposits include soft and hard deposits and dental stains.

Dental Deposits: Soft
Oral Biofilm
A **biofilm** is a complex, highly organized, three-dimensional community of microorganisms that adhere to a surface where moisture and nutrients are available. Unlike **planktonic** (free-floating) bacteria, bacteria in a biofilm community are able to maximize nutrients, keep their community clean, protect the community when under attack, and relocate to start new biofilm communities. As a host-associated biofilm, **oral biofilm** (also known as microbial plaque, dental plaque, dental plaque biofilm, or bacterial plaque biofilm) is a dense, transparent, nonmineralized mass of bacterial colonies in an extracellular matrix, sometimes called glycocalyx or referred to as a slime layer, that is attached to a moist environmental surface.

Oral biofilm lends other protective properties to the associated bacteria, including resistance to antibacterial agents such as chlorhexidine gluconate, essential oils, cetylpyridinium chloride, systemic antibiotics, and host defense mechanisms (e.g., immune system, inflammation). Hypotheses regarding the factors that protect biofilm include an extracellular slime layer, cell variations that protect bacteria in the oral biofilm from antibiotics, slow penetration of antibiotics into the biofilm, and an altered chemical microenvironment within the biofilm.[1]

Bacteria within the oral biofilm adhere to one another, tooth surfaces, dental appliances, restorations, and oral mucosa. The structure of the oral biofilm includes channels that use the motion of saliva within the oral cavity or gingival crevicular fluid for bacterial colonization, nutrition, and transportation of bacterial wastes. Loosely attached and unattached microbes are found at the surface of the oral biofilm (Fig. 18.1).[1–3]

Oral biofilm consists of hundreds of different microorganisms that establish **microbiomes** (a collection of microorganisms in a particular environment). Many different microbiomes exist within and on the human body, including the skin, respiratory tract, digestive tract, and oral cavity. Organisms in a microbiome adapt to the body over time and can play an important role in maintaining health. When there is dysbiosis, a change in the balance or quantity of organisms in a particular microbiome, the host is at increased risk of infection and disease. In regard to oral biofilm, this imbalance in the microbiome contributes to dental caries and periodontal disease.[2]

Mutans streptococci and lactobacilli bacteria within the oral biofilm metabolize sugars and produce lactic acid. The prolonged exposure to lactic acid is responsible for the demineralization observed in dental caries. A shift in the microbiome that favors these bacteria places the host at an increased risk for dental caries. Because of the protective and self-sustaining properties of oral biofilm, associated bacteria are likely to survive within the mouth, and oral diseases may become chronic. Recognition of the self-sustaining nature of the oral biofilm community helps explain why caries and periodontal disease is difficult to control and why pathogens resist antimicrobial agents, antibiotic therapies, and host defense mechanisms. The specific mechanisms that contribute to dysbiosis within the microbiome are still under investigation; a better understanding of the complex nature of how microorganisms interact with each other may provide new ways to manage oral disease.

Microorganisms Within Oral Biofilm
Supragingival microorganisms. In a healthy mouth, oral biofilm is primarily supragingival and confined to enamel surfaces and oral mucosa. Typically, the bacteria associated with supragingival oral biofilm include gram-positive aerobic rods and cocci with very few motile species. The bacterial species associated with periodontal health include *Streptococcus mitis, Streptococcus sanguinis, Streptococcus gordonii,* and *Streptococcus oralis*; however, these species may also be present with disease. As undisturbed oral biofilm matures, the bacterial population shifts to increasing numbers of gram-negative anaerobic flora; this change in bacterial species brings signs of oral infection and inflammation.[3,4]

Subgingival microorganisms. In dental plaque (oral biofilm)–induced gingival disease, the type and quantity of bacteria that are present shifts. As supragingival oral biofilm grows undisturbed, it extends below the gingival margins. Bacterial species associated with dental plaque–induced gingival disease include gram-negative spirochetes and motile rods, such as *Fusobacterium nucleatum,* species of *Prevotella* and *Treponema,* and *Campylobacter rectus.* In advancing periodontal disease, a zone of gram-positive organisms is present on the tooth surface and a loosely adherent zone of gram-negative species is adjacent to the pocket wall. Bacteria associated with periodontitis are predominantly anaerobic and include but are not limited to

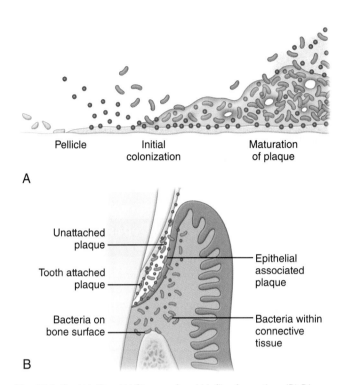

Fig. 18.1 Oral biofilm. (A) Stages of oral biofilm formation. (B) Diagram depicting oral biofilm bacteria associated with tooth surface and periodontal tissues.

Porphyromonas gingivalis, *Prevotella intermedia*, *Tannerella forsythia*, and *Aggregatibacter actinomycetemcomitans*.

Although a correlation exists between certain bacteria and periodontal disease, research is still ongoing to determine the extent to which these bacteria are responsible, rather than the oral biofilm community in which they live, and the host response.[2,5]

Stages of Oral Biofilm Formation

Oral biofilm formation occurs in stages that include pellicle formation, colonization, bacterial growth and maturation, and dispersion.

Pellicle formation. The first stage is the deposition of the **acquired pellicle**, a tenacious, unstructured, acellular film comprised of glycoproteins found in saliva. The acquired pellicle forms on tooth surfaces, restorations, and calculus. Although the pellicle performs a protective function, acting as a barrier to acids, it also serves as a medium for the attachment of planktonic bacteria, beginning the first stage of oral biofilm development. Salivary proteins and peptides promote bacterial adhesion to oral surfaces. Immediately after cleansing the tooth, the pellicle begins to reform.[3,4]

Colonization. During the next stage of oral biofilm formation, planktonic microorganisms attach to the acquired pellicle and begin to form sessile (fixed) colonies. Gram-positive cocci are the first microorganisms to colonize the teeth. Initial colonizers consist primarily of aerobic gram-positive cocci such as *Streptococcus mutans* and *S. sanguinis*. Due to the nature of bacterial attachment, the complete removal of oral biofilm requires mechanical action, such as toothbrushing, flossing, or the use of other oral hygiene adjuncts. As the planktonic bacteria become sessile, bacterial growth lags and colonization continues in stratified layers against the tooth surface. If left undisturbed, filamentous forms of bacteria grow on the surface of the coccal colonies and begin to infiltrate the sessile colonies, replacing the cocci.[3,4]

Bacterial growth and maturation. During the growth and maturation stage of oral biofilm formation, adherent bacteria secrete extracellular polysaccharides (carbohydrates) to form an extracellular matrix. The organic component of the matrix is comprised of polysaccharides, glycoproteins (protein-carbohydrate compounds) from saliva, and lipids (fatty acids) of host and bacterial origins. The matrix is sticky and therefore further facilitates microbial adhesion. A patient may experience this phenomenon as a "fuzzy" or "filmy" feeling on the teeth. In addition to providing a method of adherence for the bacterial colonies, the matrix and its polysaccharides trap other nutrients, provide a food source for the bacteria, and contribute to the protective functions of oral biofilm.

Within 1 to 2 weeks, the load of gram-negative anaerobic species and pathogenic spirochetes increases. At approximately 2 weeks, clinical signs of inflammation can be observed.[3,4]

Dispersion. The growth of the biofilm continues as it derives nutrients from the gingival crevicular fluid, saliva, and the microbial matrix. Ultimately, bacteria within the oral biofilm slow their growth or become static, while other bacteria detach or disperse and relocate to form new oral biofilm colonies.[6]

These changes in the bacterial composition of oral biofilm as it ages along with the host response are what leads to a change from a state of health to one that favors disease.

The formation and destructive nature of oral biofilm highlight the need for its daily removal by mechanical means. The longer the oral biofilm remains undisturbed, the greater its pathogenic or disease-producing potential for the host. The host's immune response is activated and eventually overresponds, causing the connective tissue and bone destruction in periodontal disease (see Chapter 20).[7]

Materia Alba and Food Debris

Materia alba (white material) is a loosely attached collection of oral debris, desquamated epithelial cells, leukocytes, salivary proteins and lipids, and microorganisms that may appear as a white, yellow, or grayish mass (Fig. 18.2). Typically, materia alba resembles small curds of cottage cheese, is less adherent than oral biofilm, and can be found in areas of poor oral hygiene.

Food debris is comprised of unstructured particles that remain in the mouth after eating. Rinsing, use of an oral irrigator, and the self-cleansing action of the tongue and saliva can remove materia alba and food debris unless it is impacted between the teeth (Fig. 18.3). If present in great amounts, materia alba and food debris accumulations can impede the dental hygienist's ability to accurately assess the level of oral biofilm and calculus. The presence of soft deposits may indicate inadequate oral hygiene knowledge and skill, infrequent oral self-care, poor manual dexterity, or a low motivational level. The bacteria in materia alba and food debris contribute to oral disease and supply nutrients to the oral biofilm; therefore both need to be regularly removed.

Skill, Motivation, and Compliance

The dental hygienist must assess the patient's ability to manage oral self-care practices. Assessment occurs through the following:
- Questioning the patient and/or caregiver about oral care practices
- Direct observation of oral self-care techniques used by the patient and/or caregiver
- Evaluation of the patient's oral hygiene status and dental history (Procedure 18.1 and the corresponding Competency Form)

Patient assessment includes assessing the patient's readiness to change behavior. The dental hygienist utilizes all relevant information to educate and motivate the patient and/or caregiver using small steps to encourage change that will support oral and systemic health.

As part of professional care, discussing the characteristics of oral deposits can serve as a useful motivator for patients who are having difficulty controlling oral biofilm. Patient knowledge of oral biofilm provides a rationale for frequent professional subgingival debridement because oral biofilm in deep periodontal pockets cannot be reached by toothbrushes, interdental cleaners, and mouthrinses. Educating the patient about the resistant nature of oral biofilm and the importance of daily disruption and removal of oral biofilm via mechanical and chemical measures remains the most effective means for its control (Box 18.1) (see Chapters 24–27). Motivational interviewing techniques may improve acceptance of behavior change (see Chapter 5).

Clinical Assessment of Oral Biofilm

Clinically, oral biofilm appears as a transparent film that begins to form within minutes after removal. The extent and quantity of biofilm present will influence the methods needed for assessment. When particularly heavy amounts of oral biofilm are present, these can be assessed by direct observation or by passing an explorer over the tooth surface near the gingival margin. In most cases, assessment is best when done with the use of a disclosing agent.

Disclosing Agents

Disclosing agents, also known as disclosants, are used to make oral biofilm clinically visible (Fig. 18.4). Available in liquid, gel, or tablet form, disclosants contain ingredients that temporarily stain oral biofilm, making it visible and measurable. Traditional disclosants contain erythrosine dye, which stains oral biofilm red. Two-tone disclosing agents stain older oral biofilm blue and new oral biofilm red. Three-tone disclosing gels are also available, which identify new, mature, and

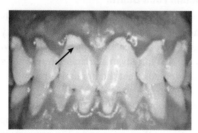

Fig. 18.2 Materia alba generalized throughout the mouth with the heaviest accumulation near the gingiva. Note the presence of plaque-induced gingivitis (arrow).

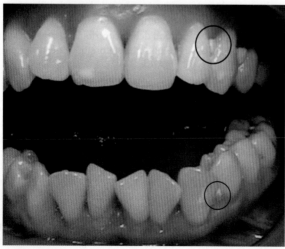

Fig. 18.3 Localized food debris found in interdental spaces (circles).

acid-producing oral biofilms in red to pink, blue to purple and light blue, respectively (Fig. 18.5).

Application of disclosing agents occurs after oral and periodontal assessment because they can camouflage clinical signs of disease. When signs of disease are present, it is the dental hygienist's responsibility to make the patient aware of its presence. The use of a disclosant is a critical tool in helping the patient understand the correlation between oral hygiene and oral disease (see Chapters 19 and 20).

The application of disclosant varies depending on the type of product used:

- Solutions may be applied without dilution using a cotton swab or diluted with water in a cup for the patient to use as an oral rinse.
- Tablets are chewed, swished in the mouth, and expectorated.

PROCEDURE 18.1   Oral Deposit Assessment

Equipment

Personal protective equipment
Antimicrobial mouthrinse
Mouth mirror
Periodontal explorer
Gauze
Disclosing solution
Cotton tip applicators
Compressed air
Intraoral light source
Patient hand mirror
Oral hygiene assessment form, including a dental index

Steps

1. Place the patient in supine position; position the light source to illuminate the patient's mouth.
2. Using compressed air, dry the supragingival tooth surfaces a sextant at a time. Using a mouth mirror and direct and indirect vision, examine for supragingival calculus deposits.
3. Identify surfaces with supragingival calculus and stain. Record these areas in the patient record.
4. Apply a disclosing agent.
5. Examine tooth surfaces with a mouth mirror for areas of stained oral biofilm. Ask the patient to observe using a hand mirror.
6. Record oral biofilm in the patient record, including documentation of biofilm present on soft tissues and appliances.
7. Using a periodontal explorer and mouth mirror, explore subgingival tooth surfaces for calculus deposits.
8. Record subgingival calculus deposits in the patient record.
9. Communicate findings to the patient.
10. Record services rendered in the patient record.

BOX 18.1   Critical Thinking Scenario A

Olivia arrives for her recare appointment. She is typically diligent with her oral self-care regime and her maintenance appointments. An update in her medical history reveals a recent diagnosis of arthritis. During the assessment of dental deposits, you note interproximal food debris, as well as an overall decline in Olivia's oral hygiene.

1. When comparing Olivia's previous oral hygiene assessment with today's findings, what might be the cause of the decline in her oral hygiene effectiveness?
2. Considering this patient's particular needs, what oral hygiene adjuncts should you recommend?

- Gels are applied with a swab, microbrush, or cotton pellet; the mouth is then rinsed with water.

Depending on the method used for application of the disclosant, the patient will expectorate after rinsing, or the dental hygienist will suction to remove excess disclosant from the mouth. Following the application of the disclosant, the patient is provided a mirror, and the dental hygienist reviews the location of the deposits with the patient or caregiver.

Deposit-free surfaces do not absorb the dye unless roughness is present (e.g., demineralization, hypocalcification, restorations, cementum). Acquired pellicle, oral biofilm, debris, and calculus absorb the disclosing agent.

The dental hygienist assists the patient in identifying deposits and correlates the findings with areas of gingivitis, periodontitis, and dental caries. The hygienist and patient can then discuss oral self-care options. The dental hygienist introduces mechanical and chemotherapeutic oral biofilm control techniques based on patient need and with the goal of improving oral health. Following this introduction, the dental hygienist will provide the patient an opportunity to perform the techniques while the dental hygienist observes. The dental hygienist will use this opportunity to ensure that the patient's oral biofilm removal is safe and effective. Disclosants should be included for at-home self-evaluation following oral hygiene instruction. Seeing, feeling, and smelling the oral biofilm deposits teaches and motivates individuals to improve and monitor their self-care effectiveness.

Assessment

Oral biofilm is classified by its *location* (supragingival and/or subgingival), *amount* (e.g., no oral biofilm present or light, moderate, or heavy oral biofilm present), and *extent* (e.g., localized or generalized presence of biofilm).

The assessment of oral biofilm begins with its location:
- Supragingival, coronal to the free gingival margin, and subgingival, apical to the margin of the free gingiva
- Subgingival oral biofilm accumulates in the sulcus or periodontal pocket
- Supragingival oral biofilm can form on any exposed surface in the oral cavity including soft tissues such as the gingiva, oral mucosa, and specialized mucosa (tongue)

The hygienist will then determine the amount of oral biofilm present (e.g., no oral biofilm present or light, moderate, or heavy biofilm present). The extent is an assessment of whether the oral biofilm is generalized, present throughout the dentition, or localized, present on less than 30% of the dentition. Oral hygiene assessment includes the host (patient) immune response to the oral biofilm. In a healthy mouth, there is a balance between the oral biofilm and the host, where irreversible damage does not occur. If the oral biofilm contributes to tissue destruction that exceeds the reparative ability of the host, then disease occurs. The quality of oral biofilm and the host immune response to that bacterial challenge assist with treatment planning. For example, a patient with a high oral biofilm score on the lingual surfaces of the teeth but with oral biofilm-free facial tooth surfaces and healthy gingival tissue requires instructions targeting the lingual areas while reinforcing effective techniques in the facial area. A patient with a small quantity of oral biofilm accumulation but with severe gingival bleeding requires a different approach to care, perhaps considering systemic factors or appointments that are more frequent. The patient's oral contributing factors influence the growth, retention, and removal of oral biofilm:
- Tight lingual frenum interferes with the natural self-cleansing action of the tongue.

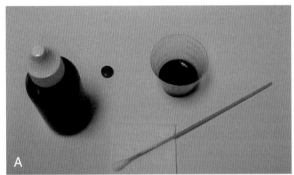
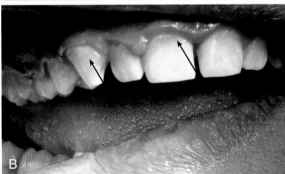

Fig. 18.4 Application of disclosing agents used to identify oral biofilm. (A) Examples of traditional oral biofilm disclosants. (B) Clinical photograph of disclosed oral biofilm *(arrows)*.

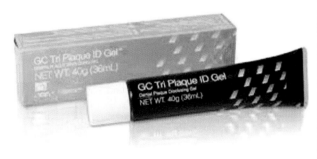
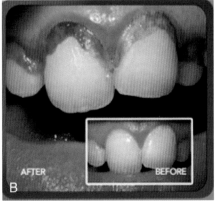

Fig. 18.5 Three-tone disclosant. (A) Example of three-tone gel disclosant. (B) Clinical photograph identifying new, mature, and acid-producing oral biofilm. (Courtesy of GC America, Inc.)

- Papillae on the tongue are conducive to oral biofilm growth (coated tongue).
- Faulty restorations with open or overhanging margins or poorly contoured surfaces readily harbor oral biofilm.
- Missing teeth contribute to oral biofilm retention and inhibit the self-cleaning effectiveness of occlusal surfaces during mastication.
- Malocclusions result in crowding and tipping of teeth, which can make oral biofilm removal difficult and/or can lead to a greater accumulation of oral biofilm.
- Mouth breathing, with its drying effects on oral tissues, favors growth of oral biofilm in the absence of the bactericidal action of saliva. Ropey, viscous saliva is less self-cleansing than watery saliva.
- The rough, porous surface of calculus provides an area where bacteria reside.
- Extrinsic tooth stain provides a rough surface for bacteria to colonize.

All of these factors influence retention and can make oral biofilm control challenging (Box 18.2).

Dental Deposits: Hard

Dental calculus, commonly referred to as *tartar*, is mineralized oral biofilm. The source of minerals is primarily calcium and phosphate derived from saliva or gingival crevicular fluid. Although calculus is not the causative factor in periodontal infections, it facilitates the attachment and retention of oral biofilm; therefore, professional calculus removal is necessary. The dental hygienist removes calculus to ensure that the teeth exhibit a biologically acceptable surface. Similar to oral biofilm, the classification of dental calculus includes location, amount, and extent.

Calculus Formation

Because calculus is mineralized oral biofilm, its formation follows the stages of oral biofilm formation. Calculus forms and grows by

the apposition of new layers of oral biofilm. Mineralization occurs in the intermicrobial matrix of the oral biofilm. The mineral source for supragingival calculus is primarily saliva. The sources for subgingival calculus are gingival crevicular fluid and inflammatory exudate. Crystals of hydroxyapatite, octacalcium phosphate, whitlockite, and brushite form in the intercellular matrix. Approximately 10 days (rapid calculus formers) to 20 days (slow calculus formers) are required for undisrupted oral biofilm to change to mineralized calculus, although the mineralization process can begin within 24 to 48 hours.[4,8] Heavy calculus formers have higher salivary concentrations of calcium and phosphate than light calculus formers. In contrast, light calculus formers have higher levels of pyrophosphate, a known inhibitor of calcification used in an anticalculus dentifrice (see Chapter 26).[8]

Calculus composition. Calculus composition is similar in supragingival and subgingival deposits:

- Inorganic components include calcium, phosphorus, carbonate, sodium, magnesium, and potassium.[8]
- Organic components include nonvital microorganisms, desquamated epithelial cells, leukocytes, salivary mucins, phospholipids, fatty acids, sugars, carbohydrates, proteins, and amino acids.[4]

Supragingival calculus. Supragingival calculus is mineralized oral biofilm formed above the free gingival margin. Although supragingival calculus can form in any location (Fig. 18.6), it is most commonly located on surfaces adjacent to the sublingual and parotid salivary gland ducts, resulting in mineralized deposits on the mandibular anterior lingual surfaces and maxillary posterior buccal surfaces of teeth. The most efficient method of identifying supragingival calculus is visual observation in conjunction with compressed air. Generally, calculus deposits are yellow-white, but they may take on surface stains and appear dark yellow to brown (Fig. 18.7). Drying the teeth with compressed air allows for a more accurate assessment; as the calculus is dried, it takes on a chalky-white appearance, making it easier to see.

Subgingival calculus. Subgingival calculus is mineralized oral biofilm formed below the free gingival margin. Unlike supragingival calculus, subgingival calculus is more likely to have a dark color due to the absorption of blood pigments from the gingival sulcus or diseased periodontal pocket. These deposits may be hard and tenacious and are occasionally visible within the sulcus or pocket by deflecting the gingival margin with compressed air or are visible through thin gingival tissues. The most accurate method of detecting subgingival calculus is with the use of a periodontal explorer. However, the dental hygienist may also feel calculus during periodontal probing.

With transillumination, calculus appears as a dark, opaque, shadowlike area against the translucent enamel. Heavy deposits of calculus may be visible on radiographic images (Fig. 18.8).

BOX 18.2 Critical Thinking Scenario B

During Jackson's initial appointment, disclosing agents were used during oral hygiene instruction. He arrives today for a recare appointment.

1. What process would you use when discussing this patient's oral self-care techniques?
2. How might this process differ in comparison with the initial oral hygiene education provided to Jackson?

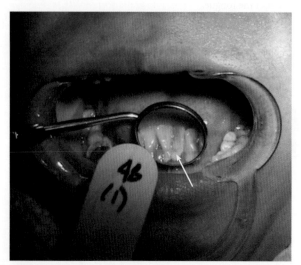

Fig. 18.6 Supragingival calculus adjacent to the sublingual salivary duct.

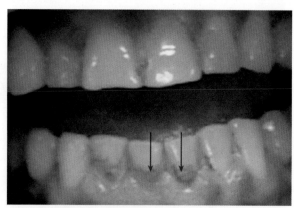

Fig. 18.7 Calculus superimposed with brown stain *(arrows)*.

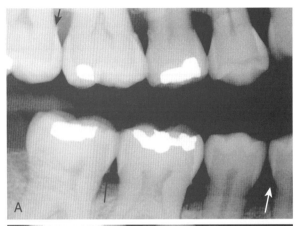

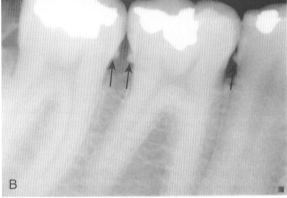

Fig. 18.8 Radiographic images depicting subgingival calculus deposits. (A) Interproximal calculus visible on a horizontal bitewing radiograph *(arrows)*. (B) Mandibular periapical showing calculus deposits as interproximal spurs *(arrows)*.

Subgingival calculus frequently occurs in interproximal spaces because these areas are difficult for a patient to clean. Subgingival calculus may take several forms, including granular deposits, thin layers, and spurs or rings that extend around several surfaces of the root. The dental hygienist feels for this change in tooth surface texture and dimension when assessing for subgingival calculus with an explorer. Calculus may feel like a nodule, a ledge, or a ring around a tooth, or it may be smooth when it is in thin layers.

Dental Deposits: Tooth Stains

Tooth stain is a discolored deposit or area on a tooth that is in contrast with the rest of the tooth color (Fig. 18.9). The classification of stains depends on their source and location. The terms exogenous and endogenous refer to the stain's source, while the terms extrinsic and intrinsic refer to the stain's location. The dental hygienist must be able to identify the source and location of stains to develop an appropriate treatment plan for the patient (Table 18.1).

Exogenous stains originate from sources outside of the tooth such as food, beverages, tobacco products, or **chromogenic bacteria** (color-producing bacteria). **Endogenous stains** originate from within the tooth; examples include tetracycline, pulpal trauma, and developmental conditions such as dentinogenesis and amelogenesis imperfecta.

Intrinsic stains occur within the tooth structure. Scaling and polishing are not effective in removing the stain, but alternative methods are available to reduce intrinsic stains (see Chapter 32). Such stains can result from alterations during tooth development and are associated with antibiotic use, fever, trauma, infection, and ingestion of high amounts of systemic fluoride. Examples include dental fluorosis (mottled, opaque, or brownish discoloration) and tetracycline stain (brown

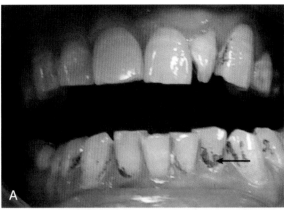

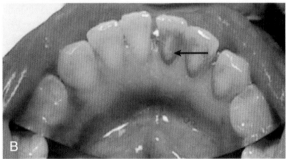

Fig. 18.9 Tooth stains. (A) Dark brown exogenous extrinsic stain on facial surfaces *(arrow)*. (B) Brown exogenous extrinsic stain on mandibular lingual surfaces *(arrow)*. Image depicts before and after removal of stains.

or grayish brown within the substance of the tooth) from the use of tetracycline during tooth development (Fig. 18.10).

Extrinsic stains occur on the tooth surface. Removal of the stain is by mechanical means and includes scaling with manual or ultrasonic instruments and polishing (see Chapter 32). Extrinsic stains develop due to the presence of chromogenic bacteria and substances such as tobacco, red wine, tea, coffee, soda, blueberries, certain drugs, and exposure to metallic compounds. Over time, extrinsic stains may become intrinsic (Fig. 18.11).

To identify the source of the stain, the dental hygienist takes into account the location and color of the stain and questions the patient about diet, work environment, and oral habits. Identification of the stain and its source assists in developing a specific care plan that facilitates stain control and a more aesthetic appearance for patients. The patient can often reduce stain formation with improved oral hygiene practices and appropriate product selection (e.g., whitening products, power toothbrushes) (Box 18.3).

DENTAL DEPOSIT ASSESSMENT

Assessment of dental deposits and stains is essential for effective care planning and the prevention of oral disease. Assessment of deposits occurs during the initial visit to establish a baseline and at subsequent visits to monitor the progress toward reaching treatment goals (see Procedure 18.1).

Deposit Assessment Armamentarium

The following armamentarium assists in the comprehensive assessment of deposits.
- *Light:* increases visual detection.
- *Compressed air:* aids in the detection of supragingival and subgingival soft and hard deposits.
- *Mouth mirror:* provides indirect vision, illumination, transillumination, and retraction.

TABLE 18.1   Tooth Stains

Type	Source(s)	Clinical Approach
Extrinsic Stains		
Green	Chromogenic bacteria and fungi (*Penicillium* and *Aspergillus* species) from poor oral hygiene and often seen in children with enamel irregularities	Potential for underlying demineralized enamel. Have the patient remove stains during toothbrush instruction or by lightly polishing; may use hydrogen peroxide to help with bleaching and removal.
Black stain	Iron in saliva, iron-containing oral solutions, *Actinomyces* species, industrial exposure to iron, manganese, and silver	Scale/ultrasonic because of its calculus-like nature, and selectively polish for complete removal.
Black-line stain	Thin band approximately 1 mm wide and slightly coronal to the gingival margin; associated with bacteria and iron in the saliva, most common in middle-aged women with good oral hygiene	Scale/ultrasonic and polish selectively.
Orange stain	Chromogenic bacteria (*Serratia marcescens* and *Flavobacterium lutescens*) from poor oral hygiene	Scale and polish selectively.
Brown stain	Tobacco; tars from smoking, chewing, hookah, and dipping tobacco; food and beverage pigments and tannins	Scale/ultrasonic and polish selectively.
Brown stain (chemotherapeutic agents)	Stannous fluoride, chlorhexidine, or cetylpyridinium chloride mouthrinses	Scale/ultrasonic and polish selectively.
Gray/brown-green stain	Marijuana	Scale/ultrasonic and polish selectively.
Yellow stain	Oral biofilm	Have the patient remove stains during toothbrush instruction.
Blue-green stain	Mercury and lead dust	Scale/ultrasonic and polish selectively.
Red-black stain	Chewing betel nut, betel leaf; found in Western Pacific and South Asian cultures	Scale/ultrasonic and polish selectively.
Intrinsic Stains		
Dental fluorosis (white-spotted to brown-pitted enamel)	Excessive fluoride ingestion during enamel development	Scaling and polishing are not effective. Consider tooth-whitening procedures.
Hypocalcification (white spots on enamel)	High fever during enamel formation	Scaling and polishing are not effective. Consider tooth-whitening procedures.
Demineralization (white or brown spots on enamel, may be smooth or rough)	Acid erosion of enamel caused by oral biofilm	Cannot be removed by scaling or polishing. Recommend daily 0.05% sodium fluoride rinses for remineralization.
Tetracycline (grayish-brown discoloration)	Use of tetracyclines during tooth development	Scaling and polishing are not effective. Consider tooth-whitening procedures.

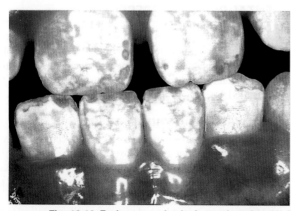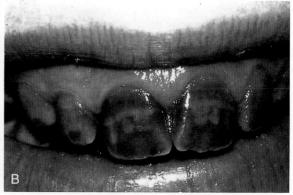

Fig. 18.10 Endogenous intrinsic tooth stains. (A) Dental fluorosis. (B) Tetracycline stain. (Berkovitz BKB, Holland GR, Moxham BJ. *Oral Anatomy, Histology and Embryology*. 4th ed. Mosby/Elsevier; 2009.)

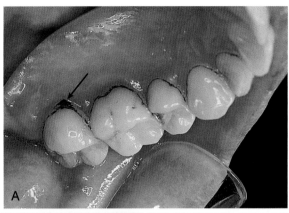

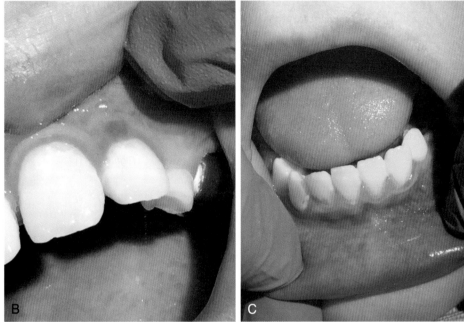

Fig. 18.11 Exogenous extrinsic tooth stains. (A) Black-line stain *(arrow)*. (B) Orange stain in a patient with poor oral hygiene, severe periodontal disease, and rampant caries. (C) Green stain. ([A] Courtesy Dr. George Taybos, Jackson, MS. From Daniel SJ, Harfst SA, Wilder RS. *Mosby's Dental Hygiene: Concepts, Cases, and Competencies*. 2nd ed. Mosby/Elsevier; 2008.)

BOX 18.3 **Critical Thinking Scenario C**

During patient assessment, you observe a moderate amount of brown stain on Jude's teeth. Jude indicates that he is concerned about the appearance of his smile. What is the most effective way of exploring the nature of the stains and assisting Jude in maintaining a more aesthetic appearance between professional care visits?

- *Periodontal explorer (e.g., ODU 11/12 and EXTU 17):* allows subgingival access for accurate assessment of calculus and optimal tactile sensitivity.
- *Gauze:* maintains a clean instrument tip to prevent translocating soft deposits from one site to another.
- *Disclosing solution:* enhances visual assessment of supragingival oral biofilm.

Concepts for Oral Hygiene Assessment

Documentation of dental deposits includes the following.
- *Location:* identify if deposits are supragingival and/or subgingival.

- *Amount:* identify if deposits are light, moderate, or heavy, or if no deposits are present.
- *Extent:* identify if deposits are generalized (present throughout the dentition), involving more than 30% of the dentition; or localized (present on a single tooth or select areas of the dentition), involving less than 30% of the dentition.

Assessment also involves evaluating the patient's knowledge, skill, attitude, and motivation related to oral self-care habits. Oral biofilm is an etiologic agent for dental caries, periodontal diseases, certain stains, and oral malodor. Stain and calculus have aesthetic implications and are risk factors for oral disease because they promote the retention of oral biofilm on teeth, dental appliances, and adjacent periodontal structures. The location, amount, and extent of oral biofilm, stain, calculus, materia alba, and food debris are important variables to measure and record during baseline assessment and at continued-care intervals. The dental hygienist must inform patients regarding the presence of dental deposits and stains and encourage daily oral self-care for the prevention of oral and systemic disease.

Oral hygiene assessment allows the dental hygienist to determine unmet human needs, educate patients to improve the quality of their oral health, and instruct them in effective self-care behaviors (Box 18.4). Individualizing oral hygiene instruction based on patient need is important; no one plan is appropriate for all patients.

ORAL HYGIENE INDICES

Indices provide a way to monitor oral hygiene of an individual or group over time. Dental indices provide a quantitative measure of oral status (see Chapter 20 for periodontal indices). A **dental index** is a data collection instrument that allows the practitioner (or researcher) to convert specific clinical observations into numeric values that can be quantified, summarized, analyzed, and interpreted. Oral hygiene indices measure levels of oral hygiene to accomplish the following:

- Establish a baseline, monitor an individual's oral self-care progress, and motivate the patient to achieve higher levels of oral wellness
- Survey the oral hygiene status within a population as is accomplished in an epidemiologic research study
- Establish a baseline and monitor the oral health status of a target population to evaluate the effectiveness of a community-based program or intervention
- Evaluate an intervention, drug, or device as is found in a clinical trial. The index used must meet criteria for validity, reliability, and usability (Boxes 18.5 and 18.6).

BOX 18.4 Client or Patient Education Tips

- Explain the role of oral biofilm and host response in the development and control of gingival inflammation and the progression of periodontal disease.
- Use disclosing agents, bleeding points, and the patient's concerns to identify areas that need self-care interventions.
- Explain contributory factors in oral deposit accumulation.
- Explain the relationship between oral hygiene index scores and the patient's current oral health status.
- Discuss how and where calculus forms and review methods of calculus management (e.g., anticalculus dentifrices and mouthrinses).
- Educate the patient on individualized and effective product selection.

BOX 18.5 Criteria for an Effective Dental Index

- Simple to use
- Minimal discomfort to patient
- Time efficient
- Cost effective
- Statistically valid (measures what it is intended to measure) and reliable (reproducible)
- Translates clinical descriptions to numeric values on a graduated scale

---

BOX 18.6 Critical Thinking Scenario D

While working with a patient, you notice a decrease in the amount of oral biofilm on the posterior lingual surfaces of the mandibular teeth from the last time an oral hygiene index was performed. By reviewing the chart, you note that at the last dental hygiene care visit, particular attention was paid to these areas during oral hygiene instruction. What are the best means of conveying this information to your patient to maximize positive reinforcement?

Indices Used for Assessing Oral Deposits

Use of a standardized method of assessment can be valuable for motivating a patient and documenting progress. The ability to show improvement is a positive reinforcement technique that can help a patient follow oral self-care recommendations. An index can illustrate repeated neglect of a specific area of the mouth and thus guide a patient in adhering to a self-care regimen. For maximum effectiveness, an index performed with an individual should evaluate the entire dentition rather than a specific sample of teeth. Indices originally designed to measure a sample of teeth in a research subject's mouth can be adapted to measure all teeth present in the dentition.

A long-standing and commonly used index is the Simplified Oral Hygiene Index (OHI-S), which can assess the degree of both oral biofilm and calculus. The Simplified Debris Index (DI-S) assesses oral biofilm and the Simplified Calculus Index (CI-S) assesses calculus. For efficiency, the OHI-S includes only six teeth, the buccal surfaces of the maxillary first molars, the lingual surfaces for the mandibular first molars, and the facial surfaces of incisors 8 and 24 (Fig. 18.12). If a first molar is missing, the second or third molar in the quadrant can serve as a substitute; if a central incisor is missing, the adjacent incisor can serve as a substitute. To obtain the oral debris score, run the side of an explorer along the surface of the tooth to determine the amount of debris present. To determine the calculus score, use an explorer or

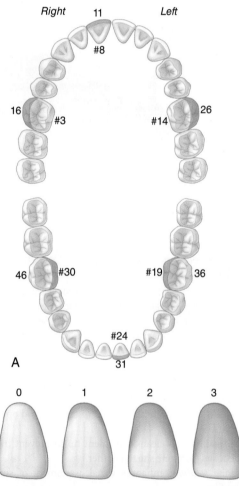

Fig. 18.12 Tooth selection. (A) Tooth selection for completing the Simplified Oral Hygiene Index (OHI-S). Teeth are numbered by the FDI Numbering System on the outside of the arch and by the Universal Numbering System on the inside of the arch. (B) Example of the Simplified Debris Index (DI-S) scoring the degree of soft deposits.

periodontal probe. Table 18.2 lists the criteria for scoring debris and calculus. To calculate the DI-S and CI-S scores, divide the score by the number of teeth assessed. To determine the OHI-S, add the DI-S and the CI-S scores.[9]

Example:
DI-S: 9/6 = 1.5
CI-S: 4/6 = 0.66
OHI-S: 1.5 + 0.66 = 2.16

Table 18.3 provides an interpretation of the numeric scores that may be more meaningful to the patient. Using an index allows patients to monitor their own progress and therefore facilitates patient motivation to improve oral self-care behaviors. If available, an intraoral camera can also capture and provide a point-in-time reference of health and disease of soft and hard tissue. Table 18.4 provides additional oral hygiene indices (Box 18.7).

RECORD KEEPING AND DOCUMENTATION

Maintaining a record of a patient's oral hygiene status is part of the assessment phase of care. Records provide a baseline reference for

TABLE 18.2 Oral Debris and Calculus Scoring Criteria[9]

Oral Debris Index (DI-S)

Score	Criteria
0	No debris or stain is present.
1	Soft debris covers one-third or less of the tooth surface being examined, or extrinsic stains without debris are present, regardless of surface area covered.
2	Soft debris covers more than one-third of the area being examined but not more than two-thirds of the exposed tooth surface.
3	Soft debris covers more than two-thirds of the exposed tooth surface.

Calculus Index (CI-S)

Score	Criteria
0	No calculus is present.
1	Supragingival calculus covers one-third or less of the exposed tooth surface being examined.
2	Supragingival calculus covers more than one-third but not more than two-thirds of the exposed tooth surface, or individual flecks of subgingival calculus are around the cervical portion of the tooth.
3	Supragingival calculus covers more than two-thirds of the exposed tooth surface, or a continuous heavy band of subgingival calculus is present around the cervical portion of the tooth.

TABLE 18.3 Interpretation of Simplified Oral Hygiene Index Scores

Interpretation of DI-S and CI-S Scores
0.0 = Excellent
0.1–0.6 = Good oral hygiene
0.7–1.8 = Fair oral hygiene
1.9–3.0 = Poor oral hygiene

Interpretation of OHI-S Scores
0.0 = Excellent
0.1–1.2 = Good oral hygiene
1.3–3.0 = Fair oral hygiene
3.1–6.0 = Poor oral hygiene

TABLE 18.4 Oral Hygiene Indices

Index and Purpose	Procedure for Use	Interpretation
Plaque Control Record[10] *Purpose:* Records the presence of plaque on all individual tooth surfaces, enabling the patient to monitor progress over time.	This procedure is best suited for use with an individual patient for oral biofilm identification and oral hygiene motivation. All teeth are included in the assessment. Oral biofilm that is present on four tooth surfaces is recorded: facial-buccal, lingual, mesial, and distal. Apply disclosing agent, and rinse the mouth. Examine the gingival margin for oral biofilm, and record each surface with plaque with a slash. Multiply the number of teeth present by 4 (number of surfaces examined), count the number of surfaces with oral biofilm, and multiply by 100. Divide this number by the total number of available tooth surfaces to obtain the percentage of tooth surface with oral biofilm.	This procedure is scored as a percentage of tooth surfaces with oral biofilm. An emphasis on the oral biofilm–free status can be a positive approach with many patients.
Plaque-Free Score[11] *Purpose:* Measures the location, number, and percentage of plaque-free surfaces in the entire mouth.	This procedure is best suited for use with an individual patient for oral biofilm identification and positive reinforcement of oral biofilm control behaviors. All teeth are included in the assessment. Four tooth surfaces are evaluated for the absence of oral biofilm: facial-buccal, lingual, mesial, and distal. Apply disclosing agent, and rinse the mouth. Surfaces with oral biofilm are recorded. Add the total number of teeth present and the number of surfaces with oral biofilm. Multiply the total number of teeth by four, and subtract the number of surfaces with plaque to obtain the number of oral biofilm–free surfaces. Multiply this number by 100 for the percentage of oral biofilm–free surfaces.	This procedure is scored as a percentage of plaque-free surfaces; the ideal is 100% oral biofilm free. An emphasis on oral biofilm–free areas can be a positive approach with many patients.

Continued

TABLE 18.4   Oral Hygiene Indices—cont'd

Index and Purpose	Procedure for Use	Interpretation
Plaque Index (PI)[12] *Purpose:* Assesses the thickness of oral biofilm at the gingival area and general oral biofilm accumulation.	This procedure is useful for either an individual patient who has significant oral biofilm accumulation or a population-based assessment. Four gingival scoring units (mesial, distal, facial-buccal, and lingual) are examined on the following teeth: 3, 9, 12, 19, 25, and 28. Missing teeth are not substituted. A mouth mirror, dental explorer, and air are used to score the above tooth surfaces for oral biofilm using the following criteria: 0 = No oral biofilm 1 = Oral biofilm adhering to the free gingival margin and adjacent area of the tooth. Oral biofilm may be recognized only after applying a disclosing agent or by running the explorer across the tooth surface. 2 = Moderate accumulation of soft deposits within the gingival pocket can be seen with the naked eye or on the tooth and gingival margin. 3 = Abundance of soft matter is present within the gingival crevice and/or the tooth and gingival margin. For individual patients, the PI is obtained by totaling the four oral biofilm scores per examined tooth and dividing by 4. Obtain a PI score within a group by adding the PI scores per tooth and dividing by the number of teeth examined. A PI may be obtained for a segment or group of teeth.	A PI is scored as follows: 0.0 = Excellent oral hygiene 0.1–0.9 = Good oral hygiene 1.0–1.9 = Fair oral hygiene 2.0–3.0 = Poor oral hygiene
Patient Hygiene Performance (PHP)[13] *Purpose:* Assesses the extent of oral biofilm and debris over a tooth surface as an indication of oral cleanliness.	This procedure is most useful with individual patients who have significant oral biofilm accumulation. Apply disclosing solution to the following teeth: 3, 8, 14, 19, 24, and 30. Divide each tooth into five areas: three longitudinal thirds—distal, middle, and mesial; the middle third is subdivided horizontally into incisal, middle, and gingival thirds. An individual patient score is obtained by totaling the five subdivision scores per tooth surface and dividing that total by the number of tooth surfaces examined.	The PHP is scored as follows: 0.0 = Excellent 0.1–1.7 = Good 1.8–3.4 = Fair 3.5–5.0 = Poor

---

BOX 18.7   Critical Thinking Scenario E

Select an appropriate oral hygiene assessment index for a patient whom you are currently treating and provide the rationale for its selection.

BOX 18.8   Legal, Ethical, and Safety Issues: Treatment Considerations

- **Prophylactic antibiotic premedication:** Prophylactic antibiotic premedication may be indicated for patients considered at high risk of adverse outcomes resulting from infective endocarditis during invasive dental procedures (see Chapter 13).
- **Record keeping and documentation:** Dental hygienists have a responsibility to document oral hygiene assessment data over time and patient compliance with oral hygiene recommendations in the treatment record. Noncompliance may be viewed as contributory negligence in malpractice suits. Documenting a lack of compliance is a risk management strategy and may establish, if necessary, contributory negligence on the part of the patient.

subsequent visits and a basis for making professional care and product recommendations. Documenting oral hygiene products used and previous instructions discussed with the patient provides continuity of care and ensures that educational interventions are appropriate.

Documentation of assessment scores allows the clinician to expand the patient's oral health knowledge, reinforce instructions, and encourage effective use of techniques and products. Patients expect a continuing conversation about their success with recommended oral products and devices; an index that documents this information supports such interaction (Box 18.8).

KEY CONCEPTS

- Oral hygiene assessment provides the clinician with an accurate understanding of the patient's oral hygiene status. The interpretation of oral hygiene assessment data includes the host response.
- Oral hygiene assessment yields information that can motivate the patient to achieve or maintain oral health.
- Assessment of soft and hard deposits, their origins, and locations is essential for dental hygiene diagnosis and care planning.
- Many factors contribute to the retention of oral biofilm, including stains, calculus, oral factors, specialized mucosa of the tongue, and saliva.
- Oral biofilms are resistant to traditional chemotherapeutic and antibiotic treatments.
- Oral biofilm can form on any surface in the oral cavity.
- Mechanical removal is the most effective method to control oral biofilm.
- Although dental calculus and extrinsic tooth stains are not causative agents in gingival inflammation, they contribute by providing an environment for oral biofilm attachment.
- Tracking indices over time provides an objective measure of a patient's progress with oral self-care activities.

ACKNOWLEDGMENTS

The author acknowledges Michele Darby, Margaret Walsh, Gwen Essex, Donna Eastabrooks, and Renee Garcia-Prajer for their past contributions to this chapter.

REFERENCES

1. Sharma D, Misba L, Khan AU. Antibiotics versus biofilm: an emerging battleground in microbial communities. *Antimicrob Resist Infect Control.* 2019;8:76.
2. Valm AM. The structure of dental plaque microbial communities in the transition from health to dental caries and periodontal disease. *J Mol Biol.* 2019;431(16):2957–2969.
3. Seneviratne CJ, Zhang CF, Samaranayake LP. Dental plaque biofilm in oral health and disease. *Chin J Dent Res.* 2011;14(2):87–94.
4. Newman MG, Takei HH, Klokkevold PR, Carranza Fermín A. *Newman and Carranza's Clinical Periodontology.* Elsevier, Inc; 2019.
5. Perez-Chaparro PJ, Goncalves C, Figueiredo LC, et al. Newly identified pathogens associated with periodontitis: a systematic review. *J Dent Res.* 2014;93:846–858.
6. Berger D, Rakhamimova A, Pollack A, Loewy Z. Oral biofilms: development, control, and analysis. *High Throughput.* 2018;7(3):24.
7. Hajishengallis G. Periodontitis from microbial immune subversion to systemic inflammation. *Nat Rev Immunol.* 2015;15(1):30–44.
8. Aghanashini S, Puvvalla B, Mundinamane DB, et al. A comprehensive review on dental calculus. *J Health Sci Res.* 2016;7(2):42–50.
9. Greene JC, Vermillion JR. The simplified oral hygiene index. *J Am Dent Assoc.* 1964;8:7–13.
10. O'Leary TJ, Drake RB, Naylor JE. The plaque control record. *J Periodontol.* 1972;43(1):38.
11. Grant DQ, Stern IB, Everett FG. *Periodontics.* 5th ed. Mosby; 1979:529–531.
12. Löe H. The gingival index, the plaque index and the retention index systems. *J Periodontol.* 1967;38(6 suppl):610–616.
13. Podshadley AG, Haley JV. A method for evaluating oral hygiene performance. *Public Health Rep.* 1968;83(3):259–264.

19

Dental Caries Management by Risk Assessment

John D.B. Featherstone*

PROFESSIONAL OPPORTUNITIES

Dental hygienists provide preventive oral healthcare services for patients that are based, in part, on knowing how to identify patients at risk for dental caries, by using a caries risk assessment form, and being able to advise patients regarding behavior modification, dietary lifestyle choices, and/or the use of therapeutic agents to prevent and reverse caries lesions. Providing the tools to reduce the risk for dental caries to patients and parents is an important component of dental hygiene care.

COMPETENCIES

1. Explain the team approach and primary purpose in integrating caries management by risk assessment (**CAMBRA®**) into an oral healthcare practice.
2. Describe the caries process and relate each of the following to the dental caries process:
   (a) Process of demineralization and remineralization that occurs in the oral environment
   (b) Saliva's beneficial actions
   (c) Dental caries balance
3. Assess risk of dental caries for patients 6 years of age through adult, including the following:
   (a) Caries disease indicators
   (b) Caries risk factors
   (c) Caries protective factors
   (d) Use the caries risk assessment form and test salivary flow rate.
4. Assess level of dental caries in children from birth to 5 years of age, including the caries risk factors and the caries protective factors. Also, explain the parent/caregiver recommendations for caries prevention.
5. Use clinical guidelines for dental caries management.
6. Relate the risk level of dental caries to the indications for the several types of fluoride therapies.
7. Relate dental caries risk level to indications for evidence-based nonfluoride caries-preventive agents.
8. Discuss legal, ethical, and safety issues related to caries management, as well as future possibilities for caries management products.

INTRODUCTION

Risk assessment is an estimation of the likelihood that an event will occur in the future.[1,2] For more than two decades, medical science has recommended that physicians identify and treat patients based on their risk status, rather than treating all patients as if they were the same. Although individual factors that contribute to risk of dental caries have been identified for more than two decades, only recently have combinations been put together in validated procedures for application to everyday clinical practice.[2,3] Caries risk assessment is the first step in CAMBRA (**Ca**ries **M**anagement **b**y **R**isk **A**ssessment), which is an evidence-based disease caries management protocol. With the CAMBRA methodology, the clinician first assesses an individual's risk for caries by assessing disease indicators, risk factors, and protective factors. Consideration of these factors (according to the caries balance concept) then determines the caries risk level as low, moderate, high, or extreme. Based on the caries risk level, an evidence-based care plan is developed that includes specific behavioral, chemical, and minimally invasive preventive and therapeutic procedures to manage the individual's dental caries disease.[1] A well-trained dental professional who correctly assesses the caries risk and coaches patients to improve their oral health is a first step in successful management of dental caries.

Many of the CAMBRA procedures fall within the purview of the dental hygienist. Dental hygienists must be knowledgeable and prepared to assess caries risk, to implement noninvasive or minimally invasive procedures according to state or province practice acts, and to promote an interdependent clinician-patient partnership to achieve best outcomes for patients. In addition, the dental hygienist can provide leadership in promoting synergistic relationships with other team members to create an environment of evidence-based excellent patient care. Every member of the dental team is essential to establish a CAMBRA prevention–focused practice and to achieve successful patient outcomes.[4] Compliance of the patient with the home-use regimens is paramount to success in caries management. The dental hygienist plays a key role in this aspect.

This chapter reviews the dental caries disease process and the background, rationale, and step-by-step procedures for the CAMBRA approach. It also provides an overview of topical fluoride use and other chemical (nonfluoride) interventions to manage the disease of dental caries based on the level of caries risk.

DENTAL CARIES: A CONTINUING HEALTH ISSUE

Dental caries is a multifactorial disease caused by a prolonged acid imbalance in the mouth, primarily facilitated by bacterial biofilm (dental plaque). Dental caries is considered a transmissible bacterial infection that can be prevented, arrested, and, in some cases, even reversed (remineralized). Dental caries is also the most common dental disease affecting children and adults in the United States and Canada, and

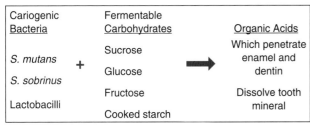

Fig. 19.1 Demineralization: Step 1.

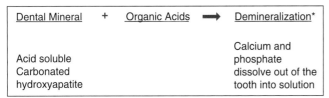

*If fluoride is present in the solution between the crystals, it inhibits mineral loss.

Fig. 19.2 Demineralization: Step 2.

it remains a significant worldwide disease and public health issue.[5] Largely a preventable disease, dental caries can be reduced by changing lifestyle and dietary habits, applying therapeutic products, and improving home care.

REVIEW OF THE DENTAL CARIES PROCESS

pH: Measure of Alkalinity or Acidity

pH values range from 0 (acidic) to 14 (alkaline). The lower the number on the pH scale, the more acidic the oral environment; the higher on the pH scale, the more alkaline. A pH of 7 is neutral; the pH of pure water, for example, is close to 7. Demineralization is a net loss of mineral from the tooth surface that occurs around pH 5.5 and below.

Demineralization

Dental caries is caused by several groups of acid-producing bacteria such as mutans streptococci (e.g., *Streptococcus mutans*, *Streptococcus sobrinus* species) and *Lactobacillus* species, and numerous other so-called acidogenic species, that live in the plaque biofilm attached to teeth. These bacteria metabolize dietary fermentable carbohydrates (e.g., sugars, cooked starch) and produce acids as a by-product. These acids cause a substantial change in the pH level of **plaque biofilm**. At rest, the pH of plaque biofilm is typically neutral (pH 7). When fermentable carbohydrates are ingested, the plaque biofilm pH rapidly drops (below pH 5.5); consequently, then, biofilm fluid in contact with the tooth surface is acidic. The acids diffuse into the tooth and dissolve calcium and phosphate from the so-called carbonated hydroxyapatite mineral of the enamel and dentin. This process is called **demineralization** (Figs. 19.1 and 19.2).[5–7]

Remineralization

After the ingestion of fermentable carbohydrates stops, the pH level gradually returns to neutral in 30 to 60 minutes, provided that saliva flow is adequate. A variety of factors mediate the return to a neutral pH. Saliva plays a key role in that it neutralizes acids and provides minerals and proteins that protect the teeth (Box 19.1). Once calcium and phosphate are lost from the tooth structure and the pH in the adjacent environment returns to neutral, the area experiences remineralization. Minerals in the saliva and minerals dissolved out of the tooth are available to redeposit onto existing

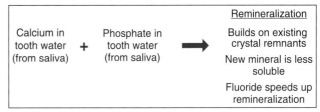

Fig. 19.3 Remineralization and tooth repair.

crystal remnants inside the noncavitated, partially demineralized, carious lesion. This deposition of minerals into demineralized areas of tooth structure is called **remineralization**, which repairs the initial carious lesion (Fig. 19.3). This ongoing process of destruction (demineralization) and repair (remineralization) occurs with each carbohydrate challenge. Remineralization is the natural repair mechanism of the precavitated carious lesion and anything that we can do to encourage this is beneficial because it can stave off cavitation, which is not reversible.

Whether an initial carious lesion progresses and develops into a frank carious lesion (i.e., hole or cavitation) depends on a variety of factors. To prevent the lesion from progressing, there must be enough deposition of salivary minerals to repair and strengthen the area and to provide support for the enamel surface and subsurface. Minerals in the saliva initially enable the host to repair demineralized areas. However, if the flow of saliva is low, the level of acid-producing bacteria is high, and if the frequency of eating and/or drinking fermentable carbohydrates is high, the tooth mineral lost by acid attacks is too great for repair by natural salivary remineralization. This oral imbalance leads to the start of dental caries, evidenced clinically first as a white spot lesion (Fig. 19.4). However, fluoride plays a very important role in the remineralization repair process and the overall prevention of carious lesions. Fluoride works primarily via topical surface mechanisms to inhibit demineralization, enhance remineralization, and inhibit (at high concentrations) plaque biofilm bacteria.[8]

White Spot Lesion

Demineralization results in the greatest loss of calcium and phosphate minerals in the subsurface zone of the enamel and the formation of a **white spot lesion**. The enamel surface of the white spot typically remains intact, but the demineralized area appears white, which is caused by the net loss of mineral in the subsurface zone of the enamel (see Fig. 19.4) and thus results in a change of light

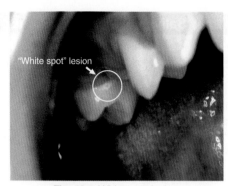

Fig. 19.4 White spot lesion.

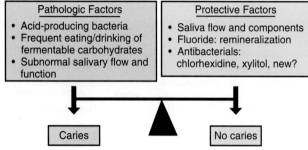

Fig. 19.5 The caries balance. (Redrawn from Featherstone JDB. The caries balance: contributing factors and early detection. *J Calif Dent Assoc.* 2003;31:129.)

refraction. By comparison, the enamel surrounding the white spot appears sound and translucent.[8] Thus a white spot lesion is a demineralized area of enamel that usually has an intact surface remaining over the body of the demineralized early carious lesion. It is partially reversible with appropriate topical fluoride intervention. The white spot lesion, which is noncavitated, is a signal to consider an intervention to avoid the development of a frank carious lesion or cavity. Nevertheless, the activity of the white spot lesion needs to be checked. Because of the change in refraction, completely remineralized white spots, which do not have active demineralization happening, typically still appear white. In any case, a white spot lesion is not a signal to perform a surgical intervention (e.g., drill and fill, place a restoration).[8] The demineralization process for cementum and dentin is similar to that for enamel, except that the process typically does not result in an intact surface remaining over the body of the carious lesion.

CARIES BALANCE OR IMBALANCE

Dental caries is a result of an imbalance between caries pathological factors and protective factors in the oral cavity. Pathologic factors include (1) **acidogenic bacteria** (acid-producing bacteria), including mutans streptococci, *Lactobacillus* species, and several other acid-producing species; (2) frequent eating and/or drinking of fermentable carbohydrates; and (3) subnormal salivary flow and function. Protective factors include (1) calcium, phosphate, proteins, and fluoride in the saliva; (2) normal salivary flow; and (3) antibacterial agents, if needed (Fig. 19.5).[8,9] The goal of caries management is to restore and maintain a balance, known as the **caries balance**, between protective factors and pathologic factors, to remineralize early carious lesions and/or to prevent future caries or the progression of existing carious lesions.[1,5]

DENTAL CARIES RISK ASSESSMENT FOR PATIENTS AGES 6 THROUGH ADULT

There are many published caries risk assessment forms and procedures but there are only two in the world that are clinically validated.[2] These are the CAMBRA developed at the University of California-San Francisco (UCSF)[1] and the Cariogram system developed in Sweden.[2,10] The CAMBRA methodology for caries risk assessment and caries management is described in detail in this chapter. Performing a **caries risk assessment** is the first step in the CAMBRA philosophy. A group of experts from across the United States convened at a consensus conference in 2002 and produced a caries risk assessment procedure and form for patients 6 years of age through adults that was subsequently validated in two large cohort studies and a clinical trial.[3,11] Several iterations have followed over a period of 20 years as more evidence has become available, with the latest update being published in 2021.[1] Fig. 19.6 part 1 presents the refined and updated version of the caries risk assessment form for this patient age group.[1] This updated version of the assessment form is comprised of a hierarchy of disease indicators, risk factors, and protective factors (Fig. 19.6) that are based on scientific evidence and clinical outcomes studies on thousands of patients.[12] Use of this caries risk assessment form as the basis for caries management is discussed later in this chapter.

The goal of caries risk assessment for patients 6 years old and older is to assign a patient's caries risk level for development of future caries as the first step in managing the caries disease process. This assessment occurs in two phases. First, the clinician assesses the individual's caries disease indicators, risk factors, and protective factors. Second, the clinician then determines the level of caries risk (e.g., low, moderate, high, extreme), based on the presence of caries disease indicators and the balance between pathologic and protective factors.[1]

Caries Disease Indicators

Caries disease indicators are four clinical observations from the clinical examination that indicate caries history and past activity.[1] The four caries disease indicators are listed in Box 19.2. Clinicians mark the presence of each of these caries disease indicators by checking a positive response (i.e., "yes") on the caries risk assessment form (Fig. 19.6 Part 1). Usually, one or more disease indicators coincide with assessment as **high caries risk** for a new patient, depending on other additional factors identified during the caries risk assessment process. If this is a patient of record with whom therapeutic measures are in place and the disease indicators have not progressed since the last visit, the caries risk level will be determined by the balance between caries risk factors and caries protective factors according to the procedure documented in Fig. 19.6 part 1. The presence of any one of these caries disease indicators in the presence of inadequate salivary flow usually indicates **extreme caries risk**.[1]

Caries Risk Factors

Caries risk factors are biologic or environmental influences that contribute to the level of risk for developing new carious lesions in the future or to the progress of existing lesions.[1,3,12] Some risk factors can be avoided or modified by the clinician or patient. The following eight risk factors are listed on the caries risk assessment form (see Fig. 19.6 part 1):[1]

1. Frequent (more than three times daily) snacking between meals.
2. Hyposalivatory medications (medications that markedly reduce salivary flow).
3. Recreational drug use.
4. Visible heavy plaque biofilm on teeth.
5. Inadequate salivary flow by observation or measurement (e.g., caused by medications, head and/or neck radiation, systemic condition). See below for measuring procedure.
6. Deep pits and fissures.
7. Exposed roots.

Figure 19.6 (Part 1). CAMBRA Caries Risk Assessment form[#] for ages 6 year through adult.[##]
Refer to the second page (part 2) for instructions for use as guidelines for caries risk assessment.

Patient Name: Reference Number:
Provider Name: Date:

Caries risk assessment component	Column 1 Score: -1	Column 2 Score: +2	Column 3 Score: +3
Protective factors – Question items	**Check if Yes***		
1. Fluoridated water			
2. F toothpaste at least once a day			
3. F toothpaste 2X daily or more			
4. 5000 ppm F toothpaste			
5. F varnish last 6 months			
6. 0.05% sodium fluoride mouthrinse daily			
7. 0.12% chlorhexidine gluconate mouthrinse daily 7 days monthly			
8. Normal salivary function			
Biological or environmental risk factors Question items		**Check if Yes***	
1. Frequent snacking (>3 times daily)			
2. Hyposalivatory medications			
3. Recreational drug use			
Biological risk factors – Clinical Exam			
4. Heavy plaque on the teeth			
5. Reduced salivary function (measured low flow rate) **			
6. Deep pits and fissures			
7. Exposed tooth roots			
8. Orthodontic appliances			
Disease Indicators – Clinical exam			**Check if Yes***
1. New cavities or lesion(s) into dentin (radiographically)			
2. New white spot lesions on smooth surfaces			
3. New non-cavitated lesion(s) in enamel (radiographically)			
4. Existing restorations in last 3 years (new patient) or the last year (patient of record)			
Column total score (Columns 2 + 3 -1):	Column 1 Total:	Column 2 Total:	Column 3 Total:
Yes in column 3 likely indicates high or extreme risk Yes's in columns 1 and 2: use the caries balance-below **Hyposalivation plus high risk factors = extreme risk			
Final Overall Caries Risk Assessment Category (check) determined as per guidelines below			
LOW ☐ MODERATE ☐ HIGH ☐ EXTREME ☐			

***Check the yes answers in the appropriate column. Shading indicates which column to place the appropriate yes. Assess the caries risk as per instructions in Fig.19.6 (part 2) below.**

[#] Reproduced with permission from Featherstone et al., *Front Oral Health.*, 2021 doi.org/10.3389/froh.2021.657518).
[##] This material may be used free of charge for the purposes of patient care, education, academic works, research, health promotion, health policy and related activities. However, permission must be obtained before this material is used for commercial purposes. Copyright © 2003, 2007,2010, 2011, 2019, 2020, 2021 The Regents of The University of California. CAMBRA® is a trademark of the Regents of The University of California. Except where otherwise noted, this content is licensed under a Creative Commons 4.0 International license (CC BY-NC-ND 4.0).

Fig. 19.6 (part 1 and part 2). CAMBRA caries risk assessment form for patients 6 years through adult. (Reproduced with permission from Featherstone et al. *Front Oral Health.* April 2021. https://doi.org/10.3389/froh.2021.657518.)

Figure 19.6 (Part 2). Caries Risk Assessment Guidelines for ages 6 years through adult. Assessing the caries risk as low, moderate, high or extreme.

The dental caregiver has the responsibility of making a caries risk assessment and then deciding on a caries management plan for the patient that leads from the risk assessment and a personalized assessment of the needs of the individual patient. These guidelines can assist in the process.

Determining the caries risk as low, moderate, high or extreme - guiding principles

1. *Low risk.* If there are no disease indicators, very few or no risk factors, and the protective factors prevail, the patient is most likely at low risk. Usually this is obvious.
2. *Moderate risk.* If the patient is not obviously at high, or extreme risk and there is doubt about low risk, then the patient should be allocated to moderate risk and followed carefully, with additional chemical therapy added. An example would be a patient who had a root canal as a result of caries 4 years ago and has no new clinical caries lesions but has exposed tooth roots and only uses a fluoride toothpaste once a day.
3. *High and extreme risk.* One or more disease indicators most likely signals at least high risk. If there is also hyposalivation, the patient is likely at extreme risk. Even if there are no positive disease indicators, the patient can still be at high risk if the risk factors definitively outweigh the protective factors. Think of the caries balance: visualize the balance diagram as illustrated below.

Any items checked "yes" should also be used as topics to modify behavior or determine additional therapy.

<u>Use the following modified caries balance</u> to visualize the overall result and determine the risk level. It may be helpful to allocate scores for each "yes" checked on the risk assessment form with a score of -1 for each yes in column 1 and +2 and +3 respectively each yes in columns 2 and 3. The final total will help guide the risk level decision. **Low** = -8 to -2; **Moderate** = -1 to +2; **High** = +3 to +17; **Extreme** = +18 to +30 and/or is a high risk level plus measured or observed hyposalivation. Use the caries balance to visualize the overall result and determine the risk level for the individual patient.

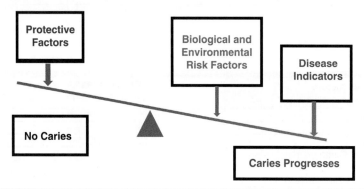

Additional caries-related components for caries management and caregiver/patient counseling.
Record in patient chart at each visit.

Dietary counseling to reduce frequency and amount of fermentable carbohydrates. Record number and type of daily snacks, drinks and juices used.
Oral hygiene and fluoride(F) toothpaste use. At each visit note frequency and amount used.
Record all recommended therapy such as F toothpaste, F varnish, chlorhexidine and usage by patient.
Record medications at each visit and check for changes.
Record participation in assistance programs such as "school lunches," "Head Start," appropriate to the state or country.
Child or adult has developmental problems or special care needs (CHSCN).
Inadequate saliva flow and related medications, medical conditions, or illnesses.
Discuss self-management goals with caregiver/patient and set two goals together at each visit. Provide in writing.

Fig. 19.6, cont'd

8. Oral appliances (e.g., orthodontic appliances, removable partial dentures, night guards).

These risk factors also help clinicians understand the reason behind an ongoing caries problem. If no clinical signs of caries disease indicators are present, the caries risk status (e.g., low, moderate, high, extreme) is determined by the balance between the caries risk factors and protective factors described in the following section (see Fig 19.6, part 1 and calculation method described in Fig. 19.6, part 2).

Caries Protective Factors

Caries protective factors are biologic or therapeutic influences that can collectively offset the challenge presented by the caries risk factors.[1] The more severe the risk factors, the more protective factors

that are needed to keep the patient in balance or to reverse the caries process.

Currently, the following eight protective factors are included on the caries risk assessment form (see Fig. 19.6 part 1)[1]:

1. Lives, works, or attends school in a fluoridated water community.
2. Uses fluoride toothpaste at least once daily.
3. Uses fluoride toothpaste at least two times daily (implies an additional benefit over and above once a day or less tooth brushing with toothpaste).
4. Uses 5000 parts per million (ppm) fluoride toothpaste (prescription only) daily.
5. Has had fluoride varnish applied in the last 6 months.
6. Uses fluoride mouth rinse (0.05% sodium fluoride [NaF]) daily.

7. Has used prescribed 0.12% chlorhexidine gluconate (CHX) (or other proven caries antibacterial agent) daily for 1 week in each of the last 6 months.
8. Has adequate salivary flow (>1 mL/min stimulated).

Use of the Caries Risk Assessment Form for Ages 6 Years Through Adult

Procedure 19.1, together with Part 2 of Fig. 19.6, describes how to use the caries risk assessment form and how to assess caries risk as low, moderate, high, or extreme for this age group. Fig. 19.6 part 2 lists the criteria for each of these four caries risk levels, including the use of the "caries imbalance" illustrated in that figure.

As presented in this chapter, the CAMBRA caries risk assessment (CRA) tool for use with children ages 6 and older as well as adults allows easy recording of disease indicators and pathologic and protective factors in everyday practice. The procedure to use the form is straightforward and follows the dental history and clinical examination. A 2011 study was conducted to evaluate the validity of this CRA procedure as it related to existing caries and to determine its predictive value for future caries. Data were collected retrospectively from electronic and paper charts by a systematic process of chart reviews for 12,954 records over a 6-year period. Findings provided convincing evidence that the CAMBRA CRA tool is valid in an adult population seeking care and demonstrated that the CAMBRA CRA form can be implemented successfully and used in everyday clinical dental practice. The CAMBRA CRA form accurately identified patients at high risk and extreme risk levels.[3] Low-risk patients were also adequately identified.

Salivary Flow Rate Test

If visually inadequate salivary flow is noted or if the patient reports having a dry mouth, a salivary flow rate test should be conducted (Procedure 19.2). Saliva neutralizes acids and provides minerals and proteins that protect the teeth from dental caries. Therefore, a salivary flow rate test is essential for assisting in the assessment of extreme caries risk.

The reason for any low salivary flow rate must be determined to plan for caries management. The patient should be informed of the results and their implications for dental caries.

Caries Bacteria Testing

Ideally, all patients should be screened for cariogenic bacteria levels, which would enhance the caries risk categorization procedure. However, at the time of this writing, no validated chairside caries bacteria test system is commercially available, nor is it likely to be in the near future. The best currently available measure is "heavy plaque on the teeth," which has been validated as a statistically significant caries risk factor in clinical outcomes studies in thousands of patients.[3]

CARIES MANAGEMENT FOR AGES 6 YEARS THROUGH ADULT

Based on the level of caries risk as described above, an evidence-based care plan is developed that includes specific behavioral, chemical, and minimally invasive preventive and therapeutic procedures to manage the individual's dental caries disease (see Chapter 5 for motivation for behavior change). Caries management is aimed at restoring and maintaining a balance between protective factors and pathological/risk factors (see Figs. 19.5 and 19.6 part 2). Caries management involves the following (see also Box 19.3):
- Reducing bacteria that cause the bacterial-based disease
- Remineralizing early noncavitated carious lesions by enhancing salivary flow, using fluoride products, and possibly using calcium and

---

PROCEDURE 19.1 Use of the Caries Risk Assessment Forms (Figs. 19.6 part 1 and 19.8 part 1)

Step 1
Based on data obtained from the health histories, clinical examination, and answers to the questions, check the *Yes* categories in the three columns on the caries risk assessment form (see Fig. 19.6 part 1; Fig. 19.8 part 1).

Step 2
Make notations regarding the number of carious lesions present, the oral hygiene status, the brand of fluorides used, the type of snacks eaten, and the names of medications or drugs causing dry mouth.

Step 3
Allocate a score of −1 for each yes in column 1, +2 for each yes in column 2, and +3 for each yes in column 3. Add these up for each column and enter the totals at the bottom of the caries risk assessment form (Fig 19.6 part 1; Fig. 19.8 part 1). Calculate the overall numerical score by adding the scores for columns 2 and 3 and subtracting the total from column 1. Refer to Fig. 19.6 part 2; Fig. 19.8 part 2; and step 4 below for further instructions.

Step 4
Make an overall judgment as to whether the patient is at low, moderate, high, or extreme risk levels, depending on the balance between the disease indicators or risk factors and the protective factors, using the caries balance concept and the numerical score as calculated above. Fig. 19.6 and Fig. 19.8 part 2 provide a modified caries balance and a table of ranges for the numerical values related to each risk level, together with further details of the procedure and additional information.

PROCEDURE 19.2 Measuring Stimulated Salivary Flow Rate

Equipment
Paraffin pellets or sugar-free chewing gum
Measuring cup (10 mL)
Personal protective barriers

Steps to Measure Saliva Flow Rate
- Ask the patient to chew a paraffin pellet or sugar-free gum for 3 to 5 minutes (timed) and spit all saliva generated into a measuring cup.
- At the end of the 3 to 5 minutes, measure the amount of saliva in milliliters (mL) and divide that amount by the time to determine the mL per minute (mL/min) of stimulated salivary flow.
- A flow rate of 1 mL/min or higher is considered normal; a level of 0.7 mL/min is low; and any rate at 0.5 mL/min or less is considered dry, indicating severe salivary gland hypofunction.
- Investigate the reason (e.g., medication, radiation, systemic condition) for the flow rate if 0.7 mL/min or less.

BOX 19.3 Guiding Principles for Caries Management for High-Risk Individuals

- Reducing bacterial challenge through antibacterial therapy. This therapy is essential because placing restorations fixes defects, cavities, etc., in the specific tooth but does not reduce the bacterial challenge in the remainder of the mouth.
- Using fluoride at an increased concentration for enhanced remineralization and to inhibit demineralization
- Reducing pathologic (caries risk) factors, such as the frequent ingestion of fermentable carbohydrates, to be at least balanced with protective factors

phosphate paste products, and sodium bicarbonate to influence the pH level, especially if the patient is at the extreme caries risk level (e.g., low salivary flow)

- Preventing demineralization by using fluorides
- Protecting tooth surfaces by using sealants
- Decreasing the frequency of ingesting fermentable carbohydrates (sugars and cooked starches)
- Surgically removing carious lesions that are beyond hope of remineralization and restoring the teeth with minimally invasive techniques and materials[13]

Decreasing caries risk factors and increasing protective factors involve strategies such as patient education, oral hygiene instruction, a reduction of the intake of fermentable carbohydrates, and addition of the use of CHX rinse.[1] Box 19.3 summarizes guiding principles for caries management for individuals at high or extreme risk for caries.

When the caries risk assessment described above has been is completed a treatment plan that includes in-office and home-use chemical therapy appropriate to the caries risk level of the patient is prepared. Details are provided in Table 19.1. The treatment plan also includes appropriate in-office preventive and restorative work. Patients with one (or more) cavitated lesion(s) are at high risk for caries. Patients with one (or more) cavitated lesion(s) and severe hyposalivation are usually at extreme risk for continuing caries.

All restorative work should be performed with the minimally invasive philosophy in mind. Obviously, cavitated lesions require restoration as part of the treatment plan. The use of glass ionomer restorations is recommended where considered appropriate. Composite resin restorations should be used where appropriate. Composite resins with sustained antibacterial properties are now on the market in the United States and should be used if possible.[14] Existing smooth surface lesions that do not penetrate the dentin-enamel junction and are not cavitated should be chemically, not surgically, treated. Fluoride varnish in-office and home-use high-concentration fluoride (5000 ppm F) toothpaste are very important for high and extreme caries risk patients in this age group (Table 19.1).

The chemical therapy and restorative work for each of the four caries risk levels is summarized in Table 19.1. Details of the chemical therapy and preventive measures are described later in this chapter. The treatment plan is discussed with the patient and with the parent if the patient is a child. It is very important that the patient (and parent) understand the rationale for the treatment plan and that they especially buy into the home care plan. Motivational interviewing should be used and the patient/parent guided to decide on their goals and what they think they can achieve prior to the next visit (see Chapter 5 to learn more about motivational interviewing). For all risk levels, patients must maintain good oral hygiene and a diet low in frequent ingestion of fermentable carbohydrates. Where patients have indicated frequent snacking during the risk assessment, dietary counseling is important. See Box 19.4 for educational tips when working with parents, caregivers, or patients.

TABLE 19.1	Chemical Therapy by Caries Risk Level for the Age Group 6 Years Through Adult		
Caries Risk Level	Chemical Therapy Diet Control	Recall Frequency	In-Office Preventive or Restorative Dentistry
Low	OTC fluoride toothpaste 2× daily. Keep doing what you are doing.	12 months	Not applicable
Moderate	Option 1: OTC fluoride toothpaste 2× daily. OTC 0.05% NaF mouth rinse 2× daily. Reduce frequency of snacking on carbohydrates. Option 2: 5000 ppm F toothpaste 2× daily. Reduce frequency of snacking on carbohydrates.	6 months	Sealants for deep pits and fissures. If noncavitated lesions are present, fluoride varnish is appropriate. Do not drill and fill.[†]
High	5000 ppm F toothpaste 2× daily. Fluoride varnish in office at each recall visit. Chlorhexidine gluconate 0.12% rinse once daily for one week every mont Reduce frequency of snacking on carbohydrates*	3 to 4 months	Sealants for deep pits and fissures. If noncavitated lesions are present, do not drill and fill.[†] Restore cavitated lesions with minimal intervention dentistry using glass ionomer or composite, as appropriate.[†] Use antibacterial composite, if possible.
Extreme	5000 ppm F toothpaste 2× daily. Fluoride varnish in office at each recall visit. Chlorhexidine gluconate 0.12% rinse once daily for one week every month. Baking soda rinse daily ad libitum (2 teaspoons baking soda in 250 mL water, made fresh daily). Reduce frequency of snacking on carbohydrates.*	3 months	Sealants for deep pits and fissures. If noncavitated lesions are present, do not drill and fill.[†] Restore cavitated lesions with minimal intervention dentistry using glass ionomer or composite, as appropriate.[†] Use antibacterial composite, if possible.

*For all risk levels: Patients must maintain good oral hygiene and a diet low in frequent ingestion of fermentable carbohydrates.
[†]Patients with one (or more) cavitated lesion(s) are at high risk for caries. Patients with one (or more) cavitated lesion(s) and severe hyposalivation are at extreme risk for caries.
All restorative work should be performed with the minimally invasive philosophy in mind. Existing smooth surface lesions that do not penetrate the dentin-enamel junction and are not cavitated should be chemically, not surgically, treated.
Note that in-office fluoride therapy is appropriate for high- and extreme-risk patients of all ages in this category, for adults as well as children.
Adapted from Featherstone et al. *Front Oral Health.* 2021. https://doi.org/10.3389/froh.2021.657518

It is useful to provide the patient with educational material about the caries process (see http://www.cdafoundation.org for a patient information sheet on tooth decay) to help them in their desire to comply with the recommended home care plan. The patient's compliance with recommendations is assessed at the next recall visit. Recommendations should be modified or reinforced, based on patient compliance and reevaluations.[1] Compliance with the home care regimen is critical. The hygienist can play a pivotal role in this important aspect of caries management (Box 19.4).

DENTAL CARIES RISK ASSESSMENT FOR CHILDREN FROM BIRTH TO 5 YEARS OF AGE

Early childhood caries (ECC) is an infectious disease that affects children from birth to 5 years of age and rapidly destroys newly erupted teeth.[15] Initially, ECC appears as bands of demineralized areas usually first observed on the primary maxillary incisors. These areas of demineralization quickly become yellow or brown cavitated areas (Fig. 19.7).

The causes of ECC are complex. The primary cause of demineralization in infants and toddlers basically involves cariogenic bacteria and a diet high in fermentable carbohydrates. Parents, caregivers, siblings, and other children transmit mutans streptococci and other cariogenic bacteria to infants and young children. Additional causes are frequent or prolonged feeding with bottled milk, formula, human breast milk, fruit juice, or sugared drinks. Box 19.5 lists high-risk factors for caries in children ages birth to 5 years and Box 19.6 lists protective factors for this same age group.[15]

Dental Visit and Caries Risk Assessment

The American Dental Association (ADA), the American Academy of Pediatric Dentistry (AAPD), and the American Association of Public Health Dentistry recommend that all children have their first preventive dental visit before reaching 1 year of age. Fig. 19.8 presents the CAMBRA CRA form for children from birth to 5 years of age.[1] The protocol for a comprehensive CAMBRA visit includes the following components:

- Parent interview; initial parts of CRA form
- Examination of the child; next sections of the CRA form

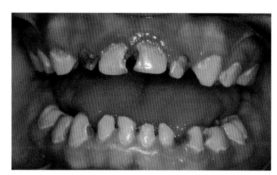

Fig. 19.7 Early childhood caries. (Courtesy Dr. Frank Hodges.)

> ### BOX 19.4   Patient or Parent/Caregiver Education Tips*
>
> Dental hygienists engage the patient, parent, or caregiver in cotherapy for the prevention and management of dental caries.
> - Explain the disease of dental caries, including carbohydrate frequency and acid-producing bacteria.
> - Explain that the conventional restorative approach alone does not eliminate the disease of caries.
> - Explain the dental caries balance.
> - Explain the importance of (1) promoting oral flora to favor health, (2) reducing or eliminating risk factors, (3) enhancing salivary function where needed, (4) enhancing the caries repair process by remineralization, and (5) using a minimally invasive approach when restorative treatment is needed.
> - Explain that dental caries infections can be prevented and controlled with the help of the patient, and explain preventive and therapeutic choices.
> - Present products and services that are available to prevent and control future caries.
> - Inform patients of their current caries risk status and provide an evidence-based care plan based on their level of risk as determined by the balance or imbalance between the pathologic factors and protective factors of each patient.
> - Explain that caries is an infection that can be transmitted from parent to child or from person to person.
> - Emphasize the frequent use of low-dose fluoride-containing products (e.g., dentifrices, oral rinses) to repair demineralized areas.
> - Describe how a reduced salivary flow can increase dental caries risk. Recommend products that will help counteract xerostomia symptoms and combat caries.
> - Explain that dental caries management is a lifelong issue.
> - Teach parents and caregivers that they are critical partners in management of dental caries in children under 6 years of age.
> - Explain that fluoride is an effective agent in management of caries and that it must be safely used and stored.
> - Explain that when well water is the primary water source, it should be tested to determine its fluoride level.

*For further details please go to http://www.cdafoundation.org for a patient information sheet that will be helpful. Scroll down to the lower part of this page to locate the Patient Fact Sheet.

> ### BOX 19.5   Factors for High Caries Risk: Patients Ages Birth to 5 Years
>
> - Parent or primary caregiver has had active dental decay in the last 12 months.
> - Sleeps with a bottle or nurses on an ad lib basis.
> - Bottle contains fluids other than milk or water.
> - Cavities, white spots, or obvious decalcification are visible.
> - Recent (less than 2 years) dental restorations have been provided.
> - Bleeding gums or heavy plaque on teeth is revealed.
> - Between-meal snacks of sugars or cooked starch are frequently eaten (more than three times daily).
> - Appliances (e.g., space maintainers, obturators) are present.
> - Salivary flow is visually inadequate.
> - One or both of the following saliva-reducing factors are revealed:
>   - Medications, such as for asthma or hyperactivity
>   - Medical reasons (cancer treatment) or genetic predisposition

---

> ### BOX 19.6   Protective Factors: Patients Ages Birth to 5 Years
>
> - Patient is a resident in a community with fluoridated water.
> - Parent or caregiver cleans child's teeth twice a day with fluoride toothpaste (small amount).
> - Dental examination is combined with oral hygiene instruction for parent or caregiver.
> - Salivary flow is visibly adequate.
> - Parent or caregiver has no caries activity.

- Completion of the caries risk assessment form
- Assignment of caries risk level
- Treatment plan including restorative work if needed, in-office therapy, and home care (see below for care paths for this age group)
- Motivational interview with parent or caregiver

A motivational interview with parent or caregiver for caries control includes the following topics:

- Individualized treatment based on risk level
- Individualized homecare recommendations
- Setting of self-management goals with parent or caregiver and child
- Anticipatory guidance according to a specific age category

- Determination of the interval for recall and periodic oral examinations
- Collaboration with other healthcare professionals[15]

Parent Interview

A parent interview is conducted before the child is examined to identify protective factors already in place, potential caries risk factors, and related environmental factors (Fig. 19.8 part 1). If the parent and/or caregiver has active decay, this potentially places the child at high risk because of the high likelihood of bacterial transmission from parent or caregiver to child.[15]

Fig. 19.8 (Part 1). CAMBRA Caries Risk Assessment form[#] for ages 0-6 years.[##] Refer to the second page of this form (part 2) for instructions for use as guidelines for caries risk assessment.

Patient Name: Reference Number:
Provider Name: Date:

Caries risk assessment component	Column 1 Score: -1	Column 2 Score: +2	Column 3 Score: +3
Biological or environmental risk factors* **Question items**		**Check if Yes****	
1. Frequent snacking (more than 3 times daily)			
2. Uses bottle/nonspill cup containing other than water or milk			
3. Parent/primary caregiver or sibling has current decay or a recent history of decay (see high risk description below)			
4. Family has low socioeconomic and/or low health literacy status			
5. Medications that induce hyposalivation			
Protective factors - Question items	**Check if Yes****		
1. Lives in a fluoridated drinking water area			
2. Drinks fluoridated water			
3. Uses fluoride (F)-containing toothpaste at least two times daily-a smear for ages 0-2 years and pea size for ages 3-6 years of 1000 ppm F.			
4. Has had fluoride varnish applied in the last 6 months			
Biological risk factors - Clinical exam*		**Check if Yes****	
1. Heavy plaque on the teeth			
Disease indicators – Clinical exam			**Check if Yes****
1. Evident tooth decay or white spots			
2. Recent restorations in last 2 years (new patient) or the last year (patient of record)			
Column total score (Columns 2 + 3 -1):	Column 1 Total:	Column 2 Total:	Column 3 Total:
Yes's in columns 1 and 2 only: use the caries balance-below Yes or yes's in column 3 likely indicates high or very high risk			
Final Overall Caries Risk Assessment Category (check) determined as per guidelines below			

LOW ☐   MODERATE ☐   HIGH ☐   VERY HIGH ☐

***Biological and environmental risk factors are split into a) question items, b) clinical exam**
****Check the yes answers in the appropriate column. Shading indicates which column to place the appropriate yes. Assess the caries risk as per instructions in Fig 19.8 (part 2) below.**

[#] (Reproduced with permission from Featherstone et al., Front Oral Health, 2021 doi.org/10.3389/froh.2021.657518).
[##] This material may be used free of charge for the purposes of patient care, education, academic works, research, health promotion, health policy and related activities. However, permission must be obtained before this material is used for commercial purposes

Fig. 19.8 (part 1 and part 2). CAMBRA caries risk assessment form for children, from birth to 5 years of age. (Reproduced with permission from Featherstone et al. *Front Oral Health*. April 2021. https://doi.org/10.3389/froh.2021.657518.)

Fig. 19.8 (Part 2). Caries Risk Assessment Guidelines 0-6 years.
Assessing the caries risk as low,moderate, high or very high.

The dental caregiver has the responsibility of making a caries risk assessment and then deciding on a caries management plan for the patient that leads from the risk assessment and a personalized assessment of the needs of the individual patient. These guidelines can assist in the process.

1. *Low risk.* If there are protective factors, very few or no risk factors, no disease indicators, and the protective factors prevail, the patient is at low risk.
2. *Moderate risk.* If there are no disease indicators and the risk factors and protective factors appear to be balanced, then a moderate caries risk determination is appropriate. If in doubt, move the moderate to a high classification.
3. *High risk.* If there is a "YES" in column 3 (one or both disease indicators) the patient is very likely at high risk. Even if there are no "yes" disease indicators, the patient can still be at high risk if the risk factors definitively outweigh the protective factors. Parent or caregiver with current or recent dental decay most likely indicates high caries risk for the child
4. *Very high risk.* If the above process indicates high risk and the existing or recent decay is severe and/or extensive, a designation of "very high" caries risk is appropriate and will guide a more aggressive caries management plan.

Any items checked "yes" should also be used as topics to modify behavior or determine additional therapy.

Use the following modified caries balance to visualize the overall result and determine the risk level. It may be helpful to allocate scores for each "yes" checked on the risk assessment form with a score of -1 for each yes column 1, and +2 and +3 respectively for each yes in columns 2 and 3. The final total will help guide the risk level decision. **Low** = -4 to -1; **Moderate** = 0 to +3; **High** = +4 to +13; **Very high** = +14 to +18 and/or is a high risk level plus extensive and/or severe recent or existing decay.

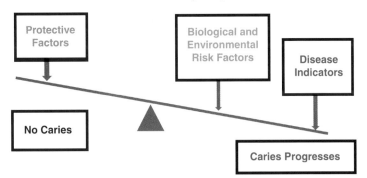

Additional caries-related components for caries management and caregiver/patient counseling. Record in patient chart at each visit.
Dietary counseling to reduce frequency and amount of fermentable carbohydrates, especially sucrose, fructose (high fructose corn syrup) and continual fruit juice (e.g. apple juice). Record number and type of daily snacks, drinks and juices used.
Bottle used continually, bottle used in bed or nursing on demand. Record details provided.
Fluoride (F) toothpaste use. Note frequency and amount used at each visit.
Record all recommended therapy such as F toothpaste, F varnish, use of silver diamine fluoride in appropriate cases. Record usage provided by parent/caregiver.
Record medications at each visit and check for changes.
Record participation in assistance programs such as "school lunches," "Head Start," appropriate to the state or country.
Child has developmental problems/child has special care needs (CHSCN).
Inadequate saliva flow and related medications, medical conditions, or illnesses.
Discuss self-management goals with parent/caregiver and set two goals together at each visit. Provide in writing.

Fig. 19.8, cont;d

Examination of the Child

The examination of the child completes the disease indicator–risk factor list (Fig 19.8 part 1). If the child has obvious decalcification (e.g., active white spot lesions) or cavities, this factor places the child at high risk for future caries.[1,15]

Assignment of Caries Risk Level for Ages Birth Through 5 Years

The CAMBRA CRA for this age group is presented in Fig. 19.8 part 1. Each of the items on the form with a yes is checked in the appropriate column as the parent interview and clinical exam proceed. Once the disease indicators and risk and protective factors have been checked,

the provider assigns a caries risk level (low, moderate, high, or very high) based on the balance between caries risk factors and protective factors and the contribution of the disease indicators.

Procedure 19.1, together with Part 2 of Fig. 19.8, describes how to use the caries risk assessment form and how to assess caries risk as low, moderate, high, or very high for this age group. Fig. 19.8 Part 2 lists the criteria for each of the caries risk levels including the use of the "caries imbalance" illustrated in that figure. The procedure for using the form is straightforward and follows the parent interview, the dental history, and clinical examination. Fig. 19.8 part 2 also includes a list of topics for discussion with the parent that will aid in the development of a risk-based treatment plan specific to that child.

Individualized Caries Management and Home Care Recommendations for Ages Birth Through 5 Years Based Upon the Caries Risk Level

Once the caries risk level is determined, the provider develops an individualized treatment plan, customizes homecare recommendations, engages the parent or caregiver in the process by conducting a motivational interview,[16] involves the parent or caregiver in setting self-management goals, educates the parent or caregiver about age-specific interventions for prevention (anticipatory guidance), and determines the interval for recall and periodic reevaluations. Informed consent from the parent and assent from the child is required before implementing individual therapies.

Table 19.2 presents the recommended care pathways, including home care and caries prevention measures for parent or caregiver of children from birth to 5 years of age.[1] Details of each of the therapies are provided below. Based upon the caries risk level and the recommendations in Table 19.2, a detailed individualized treatment plan is prepared, including restorative work if needed. This treatment plan is discussed with the parent or caregiver and implemented with their cooperation and consent (Box 19.7 and Table 19.2). Education of the parent and/or caregiver and motivational interviewing is critical for success (Box 19.4).

CARIES MANAGEMENT THERAPIES FOR ALL AGES

Fluoride Therapies

Fluoride is a natural-occurring element present in many minerals, water supplies, and foods. Fluoride delivered from water, foods, beverages, and fluoride products to the tooth surface and the plaque biofilm can have a dramatic caries preventive and reparative effect if delivered at the right concentrations and at the right time.

Primary Mechanisms of Fluoride Action

Fluoride primarily and most effectively works via topical (surface) mechanisms (whether delivered in drinking water, foods, beverages, or products) to inhibit demineralization, enhance remineralization, and inhibit plaque bacteria.[5,8]

BOX 19.7   Parent or Caregiver Recommendations for Caries Prevention: Patients Ages Birth to 5 Years (Use in Conjunction With Table 19.2)

Daily Oral Hygiene
- Small amount of fluoride-containing toothpaste applied with a cloth or brush at least twice daily. Use a smear for ages 0 to 2 years and a pea size for ages 3 to 5 years.
- Selective daily flossing

Diet
- Elimination of bottles containing sugared fluids or juices
- Limited between-meal snacks and sodas, with the substitution of non-caries-causing snacks

---

TABLE 19.2   Care Pathways (Preventive/Restorative Therapy/Dentistry) by Caries Risk Level for the Age Group Birth Through 5 Years*

Caries Risk Level	Fluoride Diet Control	Recall Exam		In-Office Preventive or Restorative Dentistry
		Radiographs		
Low	OTC fluoride toothpaste 2× daily.[†] Maintain diet control.**	Recall 6 to 12 months Radiographs 12 to 24 months		Not applicable
Moderate	OTC fluoride toothpaste 2× daily.[†] F varnish every 6 months. Reduce frequency of snacking on fermentable carbohydrates.**	Recall 6 months Radiographs 6 to 12 months		Sealants on enamel defects and pits and fissures at risk. If noncavitated lesions are present, do not drill and fill. Use fluoride treatment.[††]
High	OTC fluoride toothpaste 2× daily.[†] Brush and spit, do not rinse. F varnish every 3 months. Reduce frequency of snacking on carbohydrates.**	Recall 3 months Radiographs 6 months		Sealants for pits and fissures at risk. If noncavitated lesions are present, remineralize with fluoride.[††] Restore cavitated lesions with minimal intervention dentistry using glass ionomer or composite, as appropriate.[††] Use antibacterial composite, if available. Use nonsurgical management with ITR or SDF as appropriate.
Very high, with extensive existing disease	OTC fluoride toothpaste 3× daily.[†] Brush and spit, do not rinse. F varnish every 1 to 3 months. Reduce frequency of snacking on carbohydrates.** Consider additional therapies.***	Recall every month Radiographs 6 months		Sealants for all pits and fissures. If noncavitated lesions are present, remineralize with fluoride.[††] Consider caries arrest with SDF prior to restoration. Use nonsurgical management with ITR or SDF as appropriate. Restore cavitated lesions with minimal intervention dentistry using glass ionomer or composite, as appropriate.[††] Use antibacterial composite, if available.

*Adapted with permission from Featherstone et al. *Front Oral Health*, 2021. https://doi.org/10.3389/froh.2021.657518
[†]Smear of 1000 ppm fluoride toothpaste for 0- to 2-year-olds, pea size of fluoride toothpaste for 3- to 6-year-olds (or equivalent for specific area).
**For all risk levels: Patients must maintain good oral hygiene and a diet low in frequent ingestion of fermentable carbohydrates.
[††]Patients with one (or more) cavitated lesion(s) are at high risk for caries. All restorative work should be performed with the minimally invasive philosophy in mind. Existing smooth surface lesions that do not penetrate the dentin-enamel junction and are not cavitated should be chemically, not surgically, treated.
***Possible additional therapy for very high risk: wipe teeth with baking soda/xylitol, use casein phosphopeptide–amorphous calcium phosphate (ACP/CPP) paste.

Fluoride can be very effectively delivered via drinking water and/or fluoride products, which include toothpaste, mouth rinses, tablets, varnishes, and gels.

Inhibition of Demineralization

Fluoride present on the tooth surface and in plaque fluid from any of the sources previously listed inhibits acid demineralization by reducing the solubility of the tooth mineral.[5,8]

Enhancement of Remineralization

Fluoride accelerates the remineralization process by adsorbing to mineral crystals within the tooth, especially in a partially demineralized carious lesion, attracting calcium and phosphate ions, and building new crystal surfaces. Therefore fluoride ions incorporate into the remineralizing tooth structure, resulting in the development of fluorapatite-like surfaces on the individual crystals. These crystals are less soluble than the original enamel mineral and make remineralized lesions less susceptible to future demineralization.[5,17] Fluoride levels in the mouth from fluoridated water are sufficient to enhance remineralization. Primarily, fluoridated water has a topical effect.

Inhibition of Plaque Bacteria

Fluoride that is present in plaque biofilm is taken up by acid-producing bacteria and interferes with acid production.[5,6]

COMMUNITY WATER FLUORIDATION AND ANTIFLUORIDATIONISTS

Evidence supports community water fluoridation as a safe and effective public health intervention for the prevention of dental caries (Chapter 45). Although the benefits of community water fluoridation are well documented, some individuals continue to oppose this public health measure and actively seek and have succeeded in preventing or reversing water fluoridation programs.[18]

The opposition acknowledges that fluoride is beneficial in fighting decay but questions whether it is safe for consumption. Some associate fluoride ingestion with an increased risk for certain systemic diseases and conditions (e.g., congenital anomalies, bone fractures, Alzheimer's disease, cancer, skeletal fluorosis, intellectual disabilities). Antifluoridationists also cite cost, freedom of choice, and a violation of individual and religious rights as reasons for their stance against adding fluoride to community water supplies.

FLUORIDE IN FOOD AND BEVERAGES

Community water fluoridation has a more than 70-year history of success in reducing caries incidence and prevalence. However, the public is currently exposed to a variety of fluoride-containing food, beverages, and additives that have become part of everyone's overall exposure to topical and systemic fluoride. Consequently, considerable variation in the amount of fluoride exists in products routinely ingested. It might be of interest, especially to young patients, to calculate their daily source of fluoride intake.

Infants primarily ingest breast milk, cow's milk, or milk- and soy-based formulas. Fluoride levels are generally low in human breast milk (<0.01 ppm) and cow's milk (0.05 ppm). When the formula and infant food industry recognized that milk-based formula may be reconstituted with fluoridated water, many voluntarily reduced the fluoride content in powdered formula. Formula packaging should be consulted to determine fluoride levels in prepared powders; for example, soy-based formulas contain more fluoride than milk-based products.[7]

Beverages prepared from natural ingredients can be a systemic and topical source of fluoride. Raw tea leaves and tea tree oils are high in fluoride content. Children may be at risk for dental fluorosis (i.e., chronic excessive fluoride) in some areas (e.g., England, Australia, India, parts of Asia) where it is customary to drink tea regularly at a young age during tooth development.[7]

The fluoride level in processed beverages and bottled waters varies considerably. For example, fluoride content in fruit juices and carbonated beverages ranges from less than 0.1 to 6.7 ppm. Differences in fluoride content in processed beverages are attributed to the variations in the fluoride levels of the water used to prepare these products. Although the fluoride content in bottled waters (e.g., distilled, drinking, mineral, natural spring) varies, these beverages generally have low fluoride concentrations. Given that consumption of tap water among children in the United States has declined and consumption of other beverages, especially bottled water, has grown, assessing a patient's fluoride exposure by fluid intake is becoming increasingly difficult.

PRESCRIPTION FLUORIDE SUPPLEMENTS[19]

Fluoride supplements in the form of drops, syrups, lozenges, and tablets can provide topical fluoride if a lozenge or tablet is sucked or chewed for 2 minutes or preferably longer by children residing in communities without water fluoridation or where well water has low or undetectable levels of fluoride (Chapter 45).[19] The goal of supplementation is to offer children in nonfluoridated communities a caries-reduction advantage, similar to children living in fluoridated communities.

Fluoride supplementation recommendations are based on an assessment of whether a patient resides in a community without water fluoridation, patient's age, and all other sources of fluoride derived from diet (Chapter 45). Fluoride supplementation remains a dilemma because numerous other sources provide children with fluoride. Dental hygienists can play an important role in analyzing patients' intake and consulting with pediatricians, primary medical care providers, and pediatric dentists. Consultation prevents duplicate prescriptions for supplements and thus reduces the risk of chronic fluoride toxicity.

In 2010, the ADA Council on Scientific Affairs issued a statement saying that only children at high risk of developing caries along with a deficient primary water supply should receive supplements as follows: ages 6 months to 3 years, 0.25 mg per day; ages 3 to 6 years, 0.25 to 0.5 mg per day; and ages 6 to 16 years, 0.5 to 1.0 mg per day (depending on fluoride content in drinking water) (see the ADA Fluoride Supplements Dosage Schedule in Chapter 45).[19]

TOPICAL FLUORIDE

Beyond the fluoride in drinking water and some beverages, **topical fluorides** are taken into the oral cavity in three primary forms:

1. Self-applied by patients in the form of nonprescription products available over the counter (OTC)
2. Self-applied by patients in the form of prescription products
3. Professionally applied prescription products[20]

The myriad of product types and concentrations offered by OTC and prescription products can be confusing. Focusing on the fluoride concentration (parts per million) and patient's risk level is important when choosing and recommending products for a patient.[20] Typically, the topical self-applied fluoride agents available for at-home use are lower in fluoride concentration than those that are applied professionally.

FLUORIDE THAT IS SELF-APPLIED BY PATIENTS

Self-Applied Dentifrices (Toothpastes)

Other than the fluoride consumed in drinking water, dentifrices (commonly referred to as toothpaste) are the most widely used fluoride preparations. ADA-approved fluoride dentifrices for caries prevention provide a sufficiently high concentration of fluoride to facilitate enamel remineralization (Fig. 19.9).[21,22] The majority of OTC commercial dentifrices available in the United States contain around 1000 to 1100 ppm fluoride. In many other parts of the world, the standard concentration in OTC toothpastes is 1450 ppm fluoride. Most OTC dentifrices marketed in the United States contain one of the following:

- Sodium fluoride (NaF) formulated with a highly compatible, hydrated silica abrasive
- Sodium monofluorophosphate (NaMFP)
- Stannous fluoride (SnF$_2$)

Brushing twice daily with a fluoride-containing dentifrice is effective for preventing dental decay and is much more effective than brushing once a day.[21,23,24] The patient should be taught to expectorate (spit) completely after brushing *but not to rinse* afterward; otherwise, the beneficial fluoride will be immediately washed away from the oral cavity. Numerous clinical trials reported a reduction of approximately 30% in caries incidence with fluoride dentifrice containing 1000 to 2800 ppm fluoride.[21] Curnow and colleagues[23,24] reported a 56% reduction with supervised brushing twice daily compared with unsupervised brushing.

High-fluoride concentration prescription products such as 5000 ppm fluoride toothpaste are more effective than 1100 ppm fluoride toothpaste in high-risk individuals and are also proven effective for root caries prevention.[25,26] Fig. 19.10 shows examples of high-concentration prescription fluoride products for individuals at high risk for caries. Such high fluoride concentration dentifrices require a prescription from a dentist and are usually available in the dental office. Baysan and colleagues[26] reported that 5000 ppm fluoride toothpaste gave a statistically significant extra reduction in root carie compared with 1100 ppm fluoride toothpaste. Nordstrom and Birkhed[25] demonstrated a 40% reduction in caries in teenagers using 5000 ppm F toothpaste versus 1450 ppm F toothpaste. Caries progression still occurred, however, in many subjects in both studies. Thus a very high bacterial challenge

in high-caries-risk individuals overcomes the therapeutic effect of fluoride and requires use of additional antibacterial chemical agents to improve the protective factors. A combination of a fluoride dentifrice, varnish professionally applied quarterly, and the use of antimicrobial agents[1] such as CHX or silver diamine fluoride is recommended.[1,27]

Self-Applied Daily Fluoride Mouth Rinses and Gels

Low-concentration fluoride rinses are available as OTC products. For example, 0.05% NaF rinses have a fluoride concentration of approximately 220 ppm. These products are used as an adjunct to brushing with a fluoride dentifrice. OTC fluoride rinses (0.05% NaF) (Fig. 19.11) are effective when used once or twice daily for 1 minute, along with a fluoride-containing dentifrice.[28] Individuals are taught to use the metered dose of the rinse from the bottle, to swish the rinse in the mouth vigorously, and then to expectorate thoroughly. Because young children may swallow fluoride rinses, these products are not recommended for children under 6 years of age. For the same reason, fluoride rinses should be stored out of the reach of young children.[15]

Self-applied fluoride gels also may be used in addition to a fluoride-containing dentifrice to help manage dental caries. Similar to the

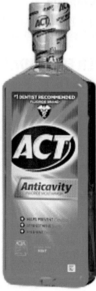

Fig. 19.11 Sample of over-the-counter 0.05% NaF rinse that has the American Dental Association Seal of Acceptance for dental caries prevention. (Courtesy Colgate Oral Pharmaceuticals, New York; and Chattem, Inc., Chattanooga, Tennessee.)

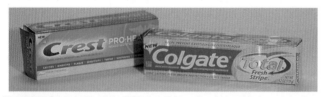

Fig. 19.9 Sample fluoride OTC dentifrices that have the American Dental Association Seal of Acceptance for dental caries prevention. (Courtesy Dr. Mark Dillenges.)

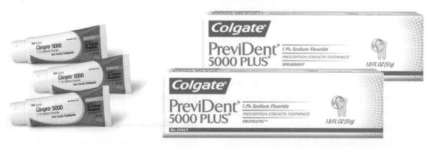

High-concentration 5000 ppm fluoride toothpaste/gel for caries high-risk clients from age 6 years and older

Fig. 19.10 Sample prescription fluoride products. (Courtesy Dr. Mark Dillenges.)

rinses, a majority of the gels have a low- to mid-range concentration of fluoride and, as such, are administered with higher frequency. The scientific literature indicates that low-potency fluoride rinses and gels reduce caries by 30% to 35%.[5,8]

Fluoride gels are marketed as SnF_2 products at 1000 ppm, neutral (NaF), and acidulated phosphate fluoride (APF) products at 5000 ppm. These products are designed for daily use and are typically brushed on the teeth after toothbrushing with a conventional fluoride dentifrice.[5] When increased duration of contact with the teeth is desired, the 5000 ppm products can be used in custom trays. Because of the risk for young children to swallow fluoride gels, these products are not recommended for children under 6 years of age.

Although few studies document their efficacy, the ADA Council on Scientific Affairs approved SnF_2 gels. In addition, the U.S. Food and Drug Administration (FDA) approved OTC SnF_2 gels for sale because they contain the same fluoride concentration as conventional SnF_2 dentifrices. SnF_2 gels do not contain abrasives and should not be substituted for dentifrices that achieve good oral hygiene and stain removal; therefore SnF_2 dentifrices that have the same concentration of SnF_2 would be preferable over the gel.

Self-applied, prescription-strength neutral fluoride gels (5000 ppm) may be used for individuals at extreme risk for caries such as that resulting from the administration of radiation for head and neck cancers, those with systemic medical conditions, and those who routinely use medications that reduce salivary flow. For example, extreme-risk patients who are not responding to the regime shown in Box 19.4 could have a home-use gel of 5000 ppm added for use in trays. These products are available as gels without abrasives and as gels with abrasives (marketed as prescription dentifrices). Although the 5000 ppm gels lack approval from the ADA Council on Scientific Affairs for caries prevention, an evidence-based clinical practice guideline developed by an expert panel of the ADA recommends use of 5000 ppm fluoride (1.1% NaF) once a day for cavitated or noncavitated root caries lesions.[29] These products have gained widespread use for individuals with special needs. Careful education is required when these products are recommended for unsupervised home use. Fluoride gels should be used as directed in a custom tray or brushed on the teeth and kept in the oral cavity for 1 minute and then expectorated. Patients should be reminded that these products are available by prescription because of their high levels of fluoride; therefore they should be carefully stored out of the reach of children.[11]

PROFESSIONALLY APPLIED FLUORIDE (IN-OFFICE ADMINISTRATION)

Fluoride treatments are one of the last procedures performed in the appointment sequence and are administered solely by licensed or certified dental professionals.

Forms of professionally applied topical fluoride supported by evidence of clinical effectiveness for caries prevention include the following:[20]
- Gel
- Varnish (Fig. 19.12)

Evidence-based general clinical recommendations are listed in Box 19.4.[1,20]

Although fluoride foams (not ADA endorsed) and in-office rinses (not FDA approved) also are available, few data support their efficacy. More research is needed before foams and rinses can be used with the same confidence as gels and varnishes.

Gels

Clinical practice guidelines developed by the ADA recommended 2.26% fluoride varnish or 1.23% APF gel for caries risk.[20] Care must be

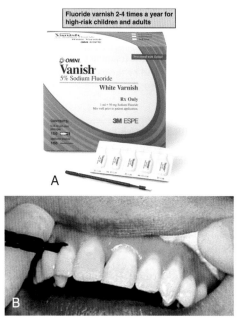

Fig. 19.12 (A) Fluoride varnish. (B) Fluoride varnish can be colored for visibility during application (*yellow*), although most products are white to satisfy patient preference. ([A] Courtesy 3M ESPE, St. Paul, Minnesota.)

taken by the clinician to explain the need to avoid swallowing during the procedure, especially with children, as ingesting the gel can result in nausea or vomiting. See Chapter 45 and Procedure 45.1 for a discussion of professionally applied fluoride gel using CAMBRA with a 5-year-old child.

Varnishes

Fluoride varnish is a concentrated topical fluoride with a resin or synthetic base that is painted on the teeth to prolong fluoride exposure. It can be used for risk categories as shown in Tables 19.1 and 19.2. Evidence from systematic reviews of randomized controlled trials by the ADA Council on Scientific Affairs and the Cochrane Oral Health Group has shown that fluoride varnish applied two to four times a year has a substantial caries-inhibiting effect in both primary and permanent teeth in children and adolescents and in high-risk populations.[30,31]

Fluoride-containing varnishes typically contain 5% NaF, which is equivalent to 2.26% or 22,600 ppm fluoride ion. Only 2.26% varnish is recommended for children.[31,32] Some fluoride varnish products also contain additional remineralization agents. Fluoride varnish applications take less time, create less patient discomfort, and achieve greater patient acceptability than fluoride gel, especially in preschool-aged children as well as infants and toddlers.[15] Fluoride varnish dispensed in unit doses has a lower potential for harm (i.e., nausea, vomiting) than other forms of high-concentration topical fluoride agents because the amount of fluoride that is placed in the mouth by using a fluoride varnish is approximately one-tenth that of other professionally applied products.[30]

Varnish hardens on the tooth upon contact with saliva. The varnish system offers patients a prolonged (1 to 7 days) temporary exposure to a high concentration of fluoride. Varnish holds fluoride in close proximity to teeth surfaces for longer periods than other concentrated fluoride products.[4] Teeth are dried with gauze a quadrant at a time, and a thin coat of the varnish is applied with a tiny brush (see Chapter 45, Procedure 45.2). Patients should be instructed to avoid drinking for 1 hour and to avoid ingesting hot, hard, or crunchy foods and brushing and flossing for 4 to 6 hours after placement.

In addition, fluoride varnishes contain a smaller total quantity of fluoride, compared with the formerly used fluoride gels. Therefore use of a fluoride varnish reduces the risk of inadvertent ingestion in children younger than 6 years.[30] The frequency of application for a fluoride varnish should be determined by the patient's level of risk for developing caries (Tables 19.1 and 19.2).

Patient Selection

Based on the CAMBRA approach to care, professional application of fluoride gel or fluoride varnish at 3- to 6-month intervals is recommended for individuals with a high or extreme caries risk (Tables 19.1 and 19.2).

Product Selection

Once it is determined that a patient will benefit from a professionally applied topical fluoride treatment, the dental hygienist, in conjunction with the dentist, decides which fluoride varnish product will be used.

Safety of Fluoride Varnish

No incidents of acute or chronic fluoride toxicity as a result of using a fluoride varnish have been documented. The rapid setting characteristic of fluoride varnishes seems to prevent ingestion, minimizing the risk for a toxic dose, which is especially important for children, older adults, and intellectually challenged individuals. The varnish breaks down over a period of several days; consequently, ingestion slowly occurs over time, reducing the likelihood of acute fluoride toxicity. Because some varnishes contain rosin, it should not be used on individuals with a known sensitivity to this material or with patients with ulcerative gingivitis, stomatitis, or large, open lesions.[4]

ACUTE AND CHRONIC FLUORIDE TOXICITY

Fluoride is a toxic element if ingested in high amounts.[33–35] Subtoxic levels can lead to fluorosis and other symptoms. Ingestion of approximately 5 mg fluoride per kilogram of body weight can lead to death (Chapter 45).

SILVER DIAMINE FLUORIDE

Silver diamine fluoride (SDF) is a noninvasive dental caries treatment that has been shown to arrest and remineralize caries lesions.[27,36,37] The silver ion is antibacterial and the fluoride is in a high concentration to aid in remineralization. The FDA approved SDF for dentinal sensitivity in 2014; however, until late 2016, its use in the United States as a caries-preventing or caries-arresting agent was off-label. At that time, the FDA granted breakthrough therapy designation to 38% SDF as a product to arrest and prevent tooth decay in children and adults. It is available in unit dose ampules or an 8-ounce bottle as Advantage Arrest. It has been in use for some time in Japan, Australia, China, Portugal, and Spain.

Several literature reviews have been published. One review by Crystal and Niederman[36] combined the results of previous systematic reviews and came to the following conclusions: "By arresting and preventing caries, silver diamine fluoride (SDF) offers an alternate care path for patients for whom traditional restorative treatment is not immediately available. Current data from controlled clinical trials encompassing more than 3900 children indicate that biannual application of SDF reduces progression of current caries and risk of subsequent caries."

SDF is applied directly to the affected (decayed) area of the tooth dropwise, according to manufacturer's instructions. However, the biggest side effect is that demineralized enamel, dentin, softened areas of the tooth, and organic matter are stained black. This esthetically unpleasing appearance can pose major problems. Crystal studied parental attitudes to this issue[37] and came to the following conclusions: "Staining on posterior teeth was more acceptable than staining on anterior teeth. Although staining on anterior teeth was undesirable, most parents preferred this option to advanced behavioral techniques such as sedation or general anesthesia. Clinicians need to understand parental sensitivities regarding the staining effect of SDF to plan adequately for the use of SDF as a method of caries management in pediatric patients."

The AAPD recently published revised guidelines for the use of SDF in children.[27] The SDF panel supports the use of 38% SDF for the arrest of cavitated caries lesions in children, adolescents, or individuals with special healthcare needs as part of a comprehensive caries management program consistent with the goals of a dental home.

NONRESTORATIVE TREATMENTS FOR CARIOUS LESIONS

A 2018 evidence-based clinical practice guideline was developed by an expert panel of the ADA. It included the following recommendations to arrest or reverse cavitated or noncavitated lesions:[29]

- Use sealants plus 5% NaF varnish on occlusal surfaces, 5% NaF varnish on approximal surfaces, and 1.23% APF gel or 5% NaF varnish alone on facial or lingual surfaces.
- Prioritize the use of 5000 ppm fluoride (1.1% NaF) toothpaste or gel to arrest or reverse lesions on root surfaces of permanent teeth.
- Use 38% silver diamine fluoride biannually to arrest or reverse advanced cavitated or noncavitated caries on occlusal surfaces of primary teeth, and follow the same protocol on permanent teeth with advanced lesions (based on extrapolated data from primary teeth).

These recommendations and others are supported by evidence and discussed in the published clinical guideline. Each of these treatments falls within the dental hygienist's scope of practice in most states and provinces and is particularly important for populations without access to oral healthcare. The nonrestorative treatments for caries offer expanded evidence-based options for provisions of comprehensive dental hygiene care for patients with caries.

NONFLUORIDE CARIES-PREVENTIVE AGENTS

Although the use of fluoride therapy alone is highly effective for low and moderate risk levels for caries, additional therapy and behavior modifications are needed to control the disease in individuals at high and extreme risk. Nonfluoride options include antibacterial therapy; however, clinical evidence is limited. Based on the caries balance concept previously described, nonfluoride therapy alone is unlikely to control caries more effectively than fluoride therapy alone. Hence combined therapy is essential for individuals at high and extreme risk levels for caries. The following agents can be used in conjunction with fluoride as described earlier in this chapter for effective management of caries.[1]

Antibacterial Therapy
Bacterial Culture

Ideally, a chairside cariogenic bacterial assessment would be made, but there is currently no validated system commercially available. The use of antibacterial therapy is therefore decided by the caries risk level. Antibacterial therapy is essential for high- and extreme-risk patients in the 6-year-old through adult category, or the caries progression will not be controlled. For younger children the care pathways shown in Table 19.2 are recommended. These pathways include additional fluoride therapy for high-risk and very-high-risk infants and toddlers.

Chlorhexidine as an Antibacterial Component of Dental Caries Management

CHX gluconate is a broad-spectrum antibacterial agent that works by opening up the cell membranes of the bacteria. It has immediate bactericidal action and prolonged bacteriostatic action (**substantivity**, or period of action, is 8 to 12 hours) resulting from adsorption onto pellicle-coated enamel surfaces. CHX is administered in the United States by prescription and is available only as a 0.12% CHX gluconate antibacterial mouth rinse for the management of dental caries and periodontal diseases (Fig. 19.13). For individuals at high and extreme caries risk levels, use of 0.12% CHX gluconate rinse for 1 minute daily for 1 week each month is recommended to reduce mutans streptococci and lactobacilli levels in the plaque biofilm[1,38] (see Table 19.1). This regimen, in conjunction with an OTC fluoride dentifrice, was shown in a 3-year clinical trial to reduce caries incidence by 24% in individuals at high-risk level for caries, as compared with a conventional treatment control group.[38]

Noting the CHX regimen is very important, because this was developed during the abovementioned clinical trial and shown to be effective compared with other less-frequent doses that have been proposed by previous authors and were mostly not effective for caries control. CHX therapy reduces the bacterial challenge but must be used in conjunction with fluoride remineralization therapy as previously described in detail. Rinsing once daily for 1 week significantly reduces the levels of mutans streptococci, but they begin to return quickly. Hence, repeating the regimen each month is needed, thereby driving the bacterial levels down to safe regions over a period of 6 months.[38]

In a recent practice-based clinical trial by Rechmann and coworkers,[39,40] in older children and adults, the current CAMBRA approach was employed where 5000 ppm F toothpaste was used twice daily and CHX rinse was used daily for 1 week each month. A 70% reduction in the number of high-caries-risk patients was observed within 18 months, commensurate with a 68% reduction in dental caries in the initially high-risk patient group.

In individuals with a high bacterial challenge, this therapy must be continued for approximately 1 year. However, problems are associated with long-term use of this compound; it can alter taste; cause staining of oral tissues; and increase calculus formation, resulting in a need for more frequent recare appointments, and compliance is often poor.[1] Nevertheless, at the time of writing, CHX therapy is one of the best options available that has clinical proof of efficacy as part of a caries management protocol. No problems with the abovementioned side effects were reported in either of the clinical trials described above,[38,39] where the CHX was only used for one week each month.

In regard to the practical use of the CHX rinse, it should be used at least 1 hour after using a fluoride dentifrice to allow time for the fluoride to work; otherwise, rinsing washes away the fluoride. Conversely, brushing with fluoride toothpaste should not occur within an hour after the CHX rinse. One possible regimen is to brush with a fluoride toothpaste after the evening meal and then administer the CHX rinse before bed, enabling it to act overnight to control the bacteria.

Remineralization Products

Products are available to deliver additional calcium and phosphate for remineralization. Although calcium and phosphate levels are sufficient for remineralization in healthy saliva, such products might be beneficial to patients with inadequate salivary flow. Additional evidence of effectiveness in this population is needed.

Casein Phosphopeptide–Amorphous Calcium Phosphate

Decades of research have led to a product that combines amorphous calcium phosphate (ACP) with casein phosphopeptides (CPPs). ACP has the same calcium and phosphate levels as tooth mineral but is not crystalline. ACP is significantly more soluble and can enhance remineralization. However, it binds fluoride and is difficult to use alone. The combined CPP-ACP compound has greater affinity for bacterial biofilm because the presence of CPP stabilizes ACP and allows calcium and phosphate ions to be slowly released for remineralization.[41,42] CPP is an ingredient derived from **casein**, part of the protein found in cow's milk; therefore it is contraindicated in people with milk protein allergies.

CPP-ACP products (e.g., RECALDENT, GC America) help maintain calcium and phosphate in a soluble form that may bind to tooth structure. This compound is also found in Trident Xtra Care Gum (Cadbury Adams USA) and prescription-only MI Paste, MI Paste Plus with fluoride (GC America), and MI Varnish with fluoride. Per the manufacturer's directions, MI Paste or MI Paste Plus should be applied directly to the teeth using the fingers rather than a brush. It can also be used in disposable applicator trays. After applying, patients use the tongue to spread saliva over the paste to initiate the release of ACP (saliva enzymes break open the protein component CPP). Similar to products with only ACP, CPP-ACP–containing products are not a substitute for fluoride therapy. Additional long-term clinical trials are

Antibacterial Therapy: Age 6 Years and Older

Chlorhexidine gluconate 0.12% has not been studied in children under 18 years old; however, it is not contraindicated. CAMBRA recommends:
- Rinse 10 mL daily for 1 week
- Repeat every month for 6 months and reassess
- Continue until caries is controlled
- Must be used together with fluoride therapy

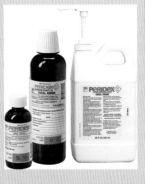

Fig. 19.13 Chlorhexidine mouth rinse. (Courtesy 3M ESPE, St Paul, Minnesota.)

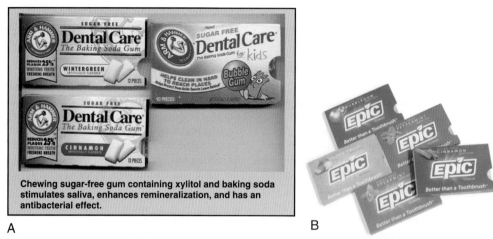

Chewing sugar-free gum containing xylitol and baking soda stimulates saliva, enhances remineralization, and has an antibacterial effect.

A   B

Fig. 19.14 Sample xylitol products. (A) Spry gum. (B) Epic Dental. ([A] Copyright Xlear, Inc. All rights reserved. [B] Epic Dental LLC. All rights reserved.)

needed to document its effectiveness in caries reduction. An evidence-based clinical practice guideline developed by an expert panel of the ADA recommended against using CPP-ACP to arrest or reverse cavitated or noncavitated caries lesions on occlusal surfaces of permanent or primary teeth.[29]

Tricalcium Phosphate

Tricalcium phosphate (TCP) is another calcium phosphate technology on the market. It is used as an ingredient in fluoride products to enhance calcium availability and remineralization. Once TCP is exposed to saliva on the tooth surface and in the plaque, calcium, phosphate, and fluoride ions are released. TCP is an ingredient in Clinpro 5000 toothpaste and Omni varnish. Additional evidence is needed to support effectiveness.

Xylitol

Xylitol is a naturally occurring 5-carbon sugar alcohol, a sweetener that looks and tastes like sucrose (Fig. 19.14). Xylitol is not a source of energy for cariogenic bacteria nor is it fermented by them. Therefore it is an excellent sucrose or fructose substitute to avoid frequent ingestion of fermentable carbohydrates between meals. Early laboratory studies and clinical trials indicated that xylitol has antibacterial properties and that it may reduce caries in humans, but this early promise has not been upheld. However, chewing on xylitol gum stimulates saliva, thereby enhancing remineralization as well as being a substitute for sugar-containing snacks.

Sodium Bicarbonate

Sodium bicarbonate (baking soda) neutralizes acids produced by acidogenic bacteria and has antibacterial properties. It can be delivered to patients at extreme risk for caries (e.g., those at high risk plus dry mouth or special needs) in a solution for individuals with low salivary flow[1] (see Chapter 52; Table 52.1). Sugar-free gum with sodium bicarbonate and fluoride dentifrices with sodium bicarbonate are available with significantly lower quantities of the ingredient than the rinse (Fig. 19.15). Some examples include Arm & Hammer Dental Care Sugar Free Gum and Arm & Hammer Complete Care.

Arginine

Arginine-containing toothpastes are available in some countries but not in the United States. Arginine is processed by some

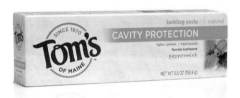

Fig. 19.15 Example of sodium bicarbonate toothpaste. Tom's of Maine. (Copyright Colgate-Palmolive.)

oral bacteria to neutralize acid that is produced by the cariogenic bacteria. Clinical trials and supporting science have shown these products to be effective as part of a caries management regimen, especially when fluoride and arginine are combined in the same product. However, additional studies are needed to make a conclusive recommendation.[29]

Probiotics

Use of probiotics to replace and displace cariogenic bacteria with noncariogenic bacteria has shown promising preliminary results; however, evidence regarding its effectiveness in reducing incidence of caries is lacking. This approach to caries control creates a balance between beneficial and pathogenic bacteria in the oral cavity. Probiotics are live microorganisms which, when administered in adequate amounts, are supposed to award a health benefit to the host. Research has focused on identifying which bacteria prevent the development of pathogenic oral biofilms. The effectiveness of probiotics is still under investigation. Current evidence is insufficient for recommending probiotics for the management of dental caries.[43] No proven anticaries probiotics are available in the United States.

LEGAL, ETHICAL, AND SAFETY ISSUES

Dental hygienists are responsible for providing the highest quality care using the best evidence. Safety and efficacy of all products used professionally or at home should be discussed with the patient or parent, and informed consent should be obtained before providing any clinical service (Boxes 19.8 and 19.9). Box 19.9 provides a summary of legal, ethical, and safety considerations related to management of caries.

BOX 19.8 Critical Thinking Scenario

Sue works as a dental hygienist in a large group practice that employs a total of three full-time dental hygienists. This general practice is located in a town that has had community water fluoridation for the past 30 years; nearly all of the patients treated in the office reside in the town. Sue is providing a preventive appointment for a 5-year-old patient. The patient is new to the practice; her mother is waiting for her in the reception area. The patient has the following dental history:

- Mixed dentition
- A healthy diet; infrequently ingestion of snacks containing fermentable carbohydrates
- Twice-daily brushing with a fluoridated toothpaste (The mother monitors toothbrushing at bedtime.)
- Fair-to-good oral hygiene
- Apparently normal salivary flow
- No clinical evidence of demineralization
- No restorations

The office policy is that professionally applied fluorides (tray technique) are administered to all children (3 to 16 years of age) two times annually. As Sue nears the end of her appointment, she explains to the patient that she is going to administer a fluoride treatment; the patient has never had this procedure before. Sue asks the patient what flavor fluoride she would prefer—tutti-frutti, strawberry, or double chocolate. The patient says that she loves chocolate, so she selects the double chocolate flavor.

Sue explains the 4-minute tray application to the patient, the use of the saliva ejector, and the need to avoid swallowing the fluoride during the treatment. Sue selects a small, hinged fluoride tray and fills it two-thirds full with 1.23% APF. Sue then dries the teeth, concurrently inserts both trays, inserts the saliva ejector, and begins timing the treatment for 4 minutes. Sue remains chairside during the treatment and distracts the patient by talking about her favorite sport.

As Sue removes the fluoride trays, the patient immediately begins talking about how much she liked the taste of the double chocolate fluoride. Sue says that she is glad that the patient enjoyed her first fluoride treatment and hopes she will look forward to the next appointment in 6 months.

Sue prepares to dismiss the patient and return with her to the reception area to talk with the patient's mother. As Sue and the patient entered the reception area, the patient reports to her mother that her stomach "does not feel good" and that she thinks she might "be sick."

1. What aspects of the patient assessment did Sue take into consideration when she decided to administer a professional fluoride application to this patient?
2. Did Sue's administration technique affect the risk for a fluoride reaction?
3. Is Sue professionally and ethically bound to carry out the office policy regarding professionally applied fluoride applications? Are there any potential legal issues involved?
4. Is the office policy consistent with the evidence in the literature regarding professionally applied fluorides?
5. What should Sue and the mother do to assist the child?
6. How should this appointment be documented in the dental record?

APF, Acidulated phosphate fluoride.

BOX 19.9 Legal, Ethical, and Safety Issues

The dental hygienist is responsible for the following considerations related to the management of caries:
- Carefully assess disease indicators and risk factors to determine risk level for dental caries.
- Inform patients of their current risk status for dental caries.
- Carefully analyze patient's overall fluoride exposure, and take a fluoride history.
- Make recommendations based on risk status for dental caries of the individual as determined by the balance or imbalance between the pathologic factors and the protective factors, and document recommendations and findings in the patient's chart.
- Explain the risks, benefits, and after-treatment instructions that pertain to fluoride and nonfluoride agents to patient.
- Never insist that a patient accept fluoride therapy if it is refused.
- Emphasize the safe use of self-applied products, especially with children younger than 6 years of age.

- Document recommendations regarding self-applied products in the patient record, including information regarding type of product, frequency of its use, its safe use, and its storage.
- Thoroughly document the administration of in-office products in the dental record.
- Safely store and manage professional-strength fluoride products in the dental treatment setting and at home.
- Have a clear understanding of the amount of professional-strength fluoride that should be administered and how it relates to a certainly lethal dose and a safely tolerated dose.
- Work in collaboration with other oral care professionals to develop a response plan in the event of an acute fluoride overdose in the dental treatment setting.
- Regularly consult the professional literature for current information and clinical evidence regarding strategies for managing dental caries.

FUTURE POSSIBILITIES FOR CARIES MANAGEMENT PRODUCTS

Several avenues, which may come to fruition as products or procedures are approved for use at some point in the future, are being explored by scientists around the world. Several additional approaches are being taken for the development of antibacterial products. Novel compounds that can alter the acid-base balance within the biofilm show promise. Genetic exploration of key biofilm components may lead to procedures that beneficially alter the biofilm. The area of probiotics, as previously mentioned, has shown great potential and is being actively explored clinically in Europe. Novel peptides that enhance subsurface remineralization are in clinical trials in Europe. Biomaterials that incorporate antibacterial agents in microparticles are an exciting development. One such range of products was cleared by the FDA for marketing in the United States in 2022 and has the potential to reduce markedly the incidence of secondary caries around restorations if widely used and if successful over time.[14]

The future is bright for new and more effective agents to supplement the dental hygienist's ability to manage dental caries.

KEY CONCEPTS

- Caries management is aimed at restoring and maintaining a balance between pathologic and protective factors.
- The team approach is essential for a successful caries management program, and the role of the dental hygienist can be critical in the overall management of the CAMBRA program.
- Caries is defined as an infectious, transmissible disease process in which a complex cariogenic biofilm, in the presence of an oral environmental status that is more pathologic than protective, leads to the demineralization and eventual cavitation of dental hard tissues.
- Pathologic factors include cariogenic bacteria (*Streptococcus mutans, Streptococcus sobrinus, Lactobacillus* species and numerous other species), frequent ingestion of fermentable carbohydrates (sugars and starches), and salivary dysfunction.
- Protective factors include but are not limited to adequate saliva and its caries-preventive components, fluoride therapy, and antibacterial therapy.
- Saliva plays a key role in that it neutralizes acids and provides minerals and proteins that protect the teeth.
- To determine caries risk, the dental hygienist evaluates disease indicators, risk factors, and protective factors.
- Risk factors are biologic, behavioral, or socioeconomic contributors to the caries disease process that can be modified as part of the care plan.
- The overall aim of the caries management care plan is to reduce the bacterial challenge, reduce or eliminate other risk factors, enhance salivary function where needed, enhance the repair process by remineralization, and use a minimally invasive approach when restorative treatment is needed.
- Individuals at high and extreme risk levels for caries require antimicrobial therapy, reduction of identified risk factors, and agents for arrest of cavitated or noncavitated caries lesions (e.g., SDF). Individuals at an extreme risk level with severe salivary dysfunction require additional therapy, such as the use of buffering agents.
- Individuals at moderate risk level for caries require improved remineralization therapy and a reduction of other risk factors, which may include antimicrobial therapy.
- Management of caries includes treating the bacterial infection that causes dental caries rather than simply treating the carious lesion.
- Caries management involves suppressing bacteria that cause the infection; remineralizing early noncavitated carious lesions by enhancing salivary flow and using fluorides; protecting tooth surfaces by using sealants and fluorides; decreasing the frequency of sugar intake, especially between meals; and referring patients to the dentist for surgical removal of carious lesions that are beyond hope of remineralization and for restoration of teeth with minimally invasive techniques and materials.
- CHX is used as a mouth rinse (10 mL once daily for a 1-week period every month). In individuals with high bacterial challenge, this therapy must be continued for at least 1 year depending on change in caries risk status. Use of the CHX rinse, separated by at least 1 hour from fluoride use, continued for a full week, and repeated every month, is critical for success in high- and extreme-risk patients.[1,39] Less frequent use is ineffective as shown by several studies.
- Demineralization and remineralization occur in the oral cavity on a daily basis.
- Saliva and fluoride are instrumental in the remineralization process.
- Demineralization is an issue from the time the primary dentition erupts into the oral cavity until death or the permanent teeth are prematurely lost.
- Topical fluoride delivery systems play key preventive roles.
- Community water fluoridation is an important delivery system.
- Fluoridated dentifrices play a key role in delivery of fluoride for the prevention and control of caries.
- Various self-applied dentifrices, rinses, and gels are available, and the market continues to expand in this area.
- Use of professionally applied fluoride gels depends on caries risk level.
- Use of fluoride varnish is a key strategy for the management of dental caries.
- It is the dental hygienist's ethical responsibility to document thoroughly the use of and recommendations made regarding chemotherapeutic agents for the management of dental caries.
- Dental hygienists should pay special attention to oral hygiene instructions and product recommendations for patients with xerostomia; risk for caries is usually higher in these patients.
- Dental hygienists are ethically responsible for reading the scientific literature and using it to provide the evidence to substantiate professional decisions.

ACKNOWLEDGMENTS

The author acknowledges Peter Rechmann and Ivy H. Zellmer for their major contributions to this chapter in the previous edition. The author also acknowledges Michele Darby, Jeanne Maloney, Anne Miller, and Denise Bowen for their past contributions to this chapter in prior editions. The author would also like to acknowledge the many people who contributed to the development and updates to the CAMBRA caries management system, especially my coauthors on the update published in 2021 in *Frontiers in Oral Health* that has formed the basis of the updates to the present chapter. Those coauthors to be acknowledged are Drs. Pamela Alston, Benjamin Chaffee, Yasmi Crystal, Sophie Domejean, Francisco Ramos-Gomez, Peter Rechmann, and Ling Zhan.

REFERENCES

1. Featherstone JDB, Crystal YO, Alston P, et al. Evidence-based caries management for all ages-practical guidelines. *Front Oral Health*. 2021;2(14). https://doi.org/10.3389/froh.2021.657518.
2. Featherstone JDB, Crystal YO, Alston P, et al. A comparison of four caries risk assessment methods. *Front Oral Health*. 2021;2(15). https://doi.org/10.3389/froh.2021.656558.
3. Domejean S, White JM, Featherstone JD. Validation of the CDA CAMBRA caries risk assessment–a six-year retrospective study. *J Calif Dent Assoc*. 2011;39(10):709–715.
4. Gutkowski S, Gerger D, Creasey J, Nelson A, Young DA. The role of dental hygienists, assistants, and office staff in CAMBRA. *J Calif Dent Assoc*. 2007;35(11):786–789. 92–93.
5. Featherstone JD. The science and practice of caries prevention. *J Am Dent Assoc*. 2000;131(7):887–899.
6. Featherstone JD. Dental caries: a dynamic disease process. *Aust Dent J*. 2008;53(3):286–291.
7. Selwitz RH, Ismail AI, Pitts NB. Dental caries. *Lancet*. 2007;369(9555):51–59.
8. Featherstone JD. Prevention and reversal of dental caries: role of low level fluoride. *Community Dent Oral Epidemiol*. 1999;27(1):31–40.
9. Featherstone JD. The caries balance: contributing factors and early detection. *J Calif Dent Assoc*. 2003;31(2):129–133.
10. Bratthall D, Hansel Petersson G. Cariogram–a multifactorial risk assessment model for a multifactorial disease. *Community Dent Oral Epidemiol*. 2005;33(4):256–264.
11. Chaffee BW, Cheng J, Featherstone JD. Baseline caries risk assessment as a predictor of caries incidence. *J Dent*. 2015;43(5):518–524.
12. Featherstone JDB, Chaffee BW. The evidence for caries management by risk assessment (CAMBRA(R)). *Adv Dent Res*. 2018;29(1):9–14.

13. Domejean S, Banerjee A, Featherstone JDB. Caries risk/susceptibility assessment: its value in minimum intervention oral healthcare. *Br Dent J*. 2017;223(3):191–197.

14. Featherstone JDB. Dental restorative materials containing quaternary ammonium compounds have sustained antibacterial action. *J Am Dent Assoc*. 2022;153(12):1114–1120.

15. Ramos-Gomez FJ, Crall J, Gansky SA, Slayton RL, Featherstone JD. Caries risk assessment appropriate for the age 1 visit (infants and toddlers). *J Calif Dent Assoc*. 2007;35(10):687–702.

16. Borrelli B, Tooley EM, Scott-Sheldon LA. Motivational interviewing for parent-child health interventions: a systematic review and meta-analysis. *Pediatr Dent*. 2015;37(3):254–265.

17. Featherstone JD, Domejean S. The role of remineralizing and anticaries agents in caries management. *Adv Dent Res*. 2012;24(2):28–31.

18. Spencer AJ, Do LG. Caution needed in altering the "optimum" fluoride concentration in drinking water. *Community Dent Oral Epidemiol*. 2016;44(2):101–108.

19. Rozier RG, Adair S, Graham F, et al. Evidence-based clinical recommendations on the prescription of dietary fluoride supplements for caries prevention: a report of the American Dental Association Council on Scientific Affairs. *J Am Dent Assoc*. 2010;141(12):1480–1489.

20. Weyant RJ, Tracy SL, Anselmo TT, et al. Topical fluoride for caries prevention: executive summary of the updated clinical recommendations and supporting systematic review. *J Am Dent Assoc*. 2013;144(11):1279–1291.

21. Wong MC, Clarkson J, Glenny AM, et al. Cochrane reviews on the benefits/risks of fluoride toothpastes. *J Dent Res*. 2011;90(5):573–579.

22. Marinho VC. Cochrane reviews of randomized trials of fluoride therapies for preventing dental caries. *Eur Arch Paediatr Dent*. 2009;10(3):183–191.

23. Curnow MM, Pine CM, Burnside G, et al. A randomised controlled trial of the efficacy of supervised toothbrushing in high-caries-risk children. *Caries Res*. 2002;36(4):294–300.

24. Pine CM, Curnow MM, Burnside G, Nicholson JA, Roberts AJ. Caries prevalence four years after the end of a randomised controlled trial. *Caries Res*. 2007;41(6):431–436.

25. Nordstrom A, Birkhed D. Preventive effect of high-fluoride dentifrice (5,000 ppm) in caries-active adolescents: a 2-year clinical trial. *Caries Res*. 2010;44(3):323–331.

26. Baysan A, Lynch E, Ellwood R, et al. Reversal of primary root caries using dentifrices containing 5,000 and 1,100 ppm fluoride. *Caries Res*. 2001;35(1):41–46.

27. Crystal YO, Marghalani AA, Ureles SD, et al. Use of silver diamine fluoride for dental caries management in children and adolescents, including those with special health care needs. *Pediatr Dent*. 2017;39(5):135–145.

28. Marinho VC, Chong LY, Worthington HV, Walsh T. Fluoride mouthrinses for preventing dental caries in children and adolescents. *Cochrane Database Syst Rev*. 2016;7:CD002284.

29. Slayton RL, Urquhart O, Araujo MWB, et al. Evidence-based clinical practice guideline on nonrestorative treatments for carious lesions: a report from the American Dental Association. *J Am Dent Assoc*. 2018;149(10):837–849.e19.

30. Marinho VC, Worthington HV, Walsh T, Clarkson JE. Fluoride varnishes for preventing dental caries in children and adolescents. *Cochrane Database Syst Rev*. 2013;7:CD002279.

31. Bonetti D, Clarkson JE. Fluoride varnish for caries prevention: efficacy and implementation. *Caries Res*. 2016;50(suppl 1):45–49.

32. Weintraub JA, Ramos-Gomez F, Jue B, et al. Fluoride varnish efficacy in preventing early childhood caries. *J Dent Res*. 2006;85(2):172–176.

33. Ekstrand J, Fomon SJ, Ziegler EE, Nelson SE. Fluoride pharmacokinetics in infancy. *Pediatr Res*. 1994;35(2):157–163.

34. Fomon SJ, Ekstrand J. Fluoride intake by infants. *J Public Health Dent*. 1999;59(4):229–234.

35. Fomon SJ, Ekstrand J, Ziegler EE. Fluoride intake and prevalence of dental fluorosis: trends in fluoride intake with special attention to infants. *J Public Health Dent*. 2000;60(3):131–139.

36. Crystal YO, Niederman R. Silver diamine fluoride treatment considerations in children's caries management. *Pediatr Dent*. 2016;38(7):466–471.

37. Crystal YO, Janal MN, Hamilton DS, Niederman R. Parental perceptions and acceptance of silver diamine fluoride staining. *J Am Dent Assoc*. 2017;148(7):510–518.e4.

38. Featherstone JD, White JM, Hoover CI, et al. A randomized clinical trial of anticaries therapies targeted according to risk assessment (caries management by risk assessment). *Caries Res*. 2012;46(2):118–129.

39. Rechmann P, Chaffee BW, Rechmann BMT, Featherstone JDB. Changes in caries risk in a practice-based randomized controlled trial. *Adv Dent Res*. 2018;29(1):15–23.

40. Rechmann P, Chaffee BW, Rechmann BMT, Featherstone JDB. Caries management by risk assessment: results from a practice-based research network study. *J Calif Dent Assoc*. 2019;47:15–24.

41. Su N, Marek CL, Ching V, Grushka M. Caries prevention for patients with dry mouth. *J Can Dent Assoc*. 2011;77:b85.

42. Zhao J, Liu Y, Sun WB, Zhang H. Amorphous calcium phosphate and its application in dentistry. *Chem Cent J*. 2011;5:40.

43. Gruner D, Paris S, Schwendicke F. Probiotics for managing caries and periodontitis: systematic review and meta-analysis. *J Dent*. 2016;48:16–25.

20

Periodontal Assessment and Charting

Diana Aboytes and Christine N. Nathe

PROFESSIONAL OPPORTUNITIES

An important part of each patient's evaluation is the periodontal assessment, which is critical to an accurate dental hygiene diagnosis and care plan. Once a dental hygienist accurately assesses periodontal health or disease and records the information, the next step is to communicate the findings, identify a dental hygiene diagnosis, develop a self-care program for the patient, and recommend treatments to the patient and to other dental or healthcare professionals.

COMPETENCIES

1. Relate periodontal assessment and its significance to the dental hygiene process of care.
2. Discuss the four physical units of a healthy periodontium, as well as the clinical signs and histologic characteristics of a healthy and diseased periodontium.
3. Discuss periodontal diseases, including characteristics/signs, types, and causes. Also, classify periodontal diseases using the classification systems of the American Academy of Periodontology (AAP) and the European Federation of Periodontology (EFP).
4. Perform thorough and accurate periodontal assessment of the periodontium and implants.
5. Discuss risk factors for periodontal diseases and their relationship stages and grades of periodontitis and dental hygiene care planning.
6. Explain proper documentation and record keeping for periodontal assessment and treatment.

PERIODONTAL ASSESSMENT

The American Dental Hygienists' Association (ADHA) defines assessment as a collection and analysis of oral health data to establish patient needs[1] This is the first step in the process of providing dental hygiene care (Fig. 20.1). Assessing a patient's risk for periodontal disease is important because conditions associated with specific diseases may affect treatment, disease management, and prognosis. Risk factors are characteristics of an individual that increase the likelihood of developing a disease or injury and thus influence one's susceptibility to periodontitis.[1,2] In addition, assessment provides the framework to develop treatment plans targeting risk factors and for creating opportunities for enhanced treatment outcomes.

Components of the Periodontium

A healthy periodontium consists of four physical units: gingiva, periodontal ligament (PDL), alveolar process (supporting bone), and cementum.

Gingiva

Gingiva is masticatory oral mucosa that covers the alveolar process and surrounds the cervical portion of the teeth. Histologically, the gingiva has a protective layer of stratified squamous epithelium covering a dense, fibrous connective tissue. Gingiva is divided into four anatomic areas: (1) free or unattached gingiva; (2) gingival sulcus; (3) attached gingiva; and (4) interdental gingiva or interdental papilla (Fig. 20.2).

Free or unattached gingival sulcus. Gingival tissue closest to the crown is the free or unattached gingiva. Free gingiva does not directly attach to the underlying alveolar bone. In healthy adult dentitions, the free gingiva is located on the tooth enamel 0.5 to 2 mm coronal to the cementoenamel junction (CEJ) and fits tightly around each tooth. The edge of the free gingiva nearest the incisal or occlusal area of the tooth is the gingival margin or the gingival crest. The gingival margin marks the opening of the gingival sulcus.

Gingival sulcus. The space between the free gingiva and the tooth is the **gingival sulcus** or gingival crevice. A healthy gingival sulcus generally measures 0.5 to 3 mm from the gingival margin to the base of the sulcus. Boundaries of the gingival sulcus are the

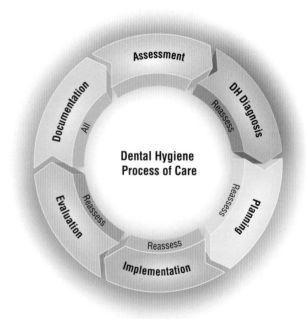

Fig. 20.1 The dental hygiene process of care begins with assessment. Thorough and accurate documentation of each process component is essential.

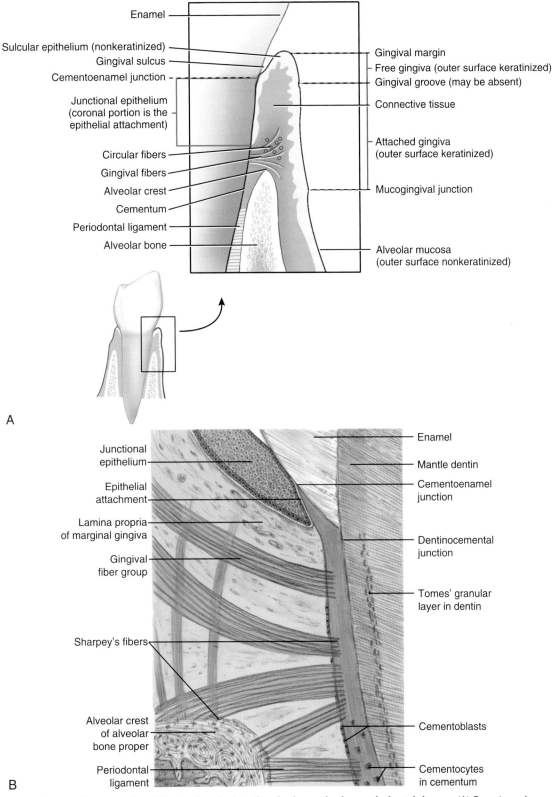

Fig. 20.2 Cross-sectional illustration depicts the gingiva and other periodontal tissues. (A) Overview of tissues. (B) Enlargement and details of area marked with box in A.

sulcular epithelium and the tooth. The **sulcular epithelium** is the nonkeratinized continuation of the keratinized epithelium covering the marginal gingiva. The sulcular epithelium is clinically significant in that it is a semipermeable membrane, allowing bacterial endotoxins from the plaque biofilm to penetrate the underlying tissue.

Attached gingiva. Free gingiva connects with the alveolar gingiva at the gingival groove. The alveolar or **attached gingiva**, continuous with the free gingiva, is covered with stratified squamous epithelium. The free marginal gingiva joins to the attached gingiva at the gingival groove. This shallow groove is clinically visible in less than one-half of the population. Attached gingiva covers the crestal portion of the alveolar bone on the facial and lingual surfaces and the roof of the mouth. It is firmly attached to the alveolar bone, unlike the marginal gingiva, which has no attachment fibers. The mandibular facial and lingual attached gingiva and the maxillary facial attached gingiva are demarcated from the alveolar mucosa by the mucogingival junction (MGJ); the width of alveolar gingiva varies throughout the mouth (from 1 mm to 9 mm). The facial aspect of the maxillary anterior teeth has the widest attached gingiva. In general, at least 1 mm of attached gingiva is adequate for gingival health. This 1 mm minimum width measurement has significance for planning educational and therapeutic interventions for persons with periodontal disease.

Gingival papilla. An **interdental** or **gingival papilla** is located in the interdental space between two adjacent teeth. The tip and lateral borders of the interdental papilla are continuous with the marginal gingiva, and the center is comprised of attached gingiva at the base. The shape of the interdental papilla varies with the space or distance between two adjacent teeth. Given a wide space, the papilla is flat or saddle shaped. If the interdental space is narrow, then the papilla is pointed or pyramidal. When two teeth are in contact, the facial and lingual aspects of the papilla are connected by the **col**, a nonkeratinized area of interdental gingiva. Because the col is not keratinized, it is highly susceptible to disease (Fig. 20.3).

Alveolar Mucosa

Alveolar mucosa is movable tissue loosely attached to underlying alveolar bone. Its surface appears smooth and shiny and is comprised of thin, nonkeratinized epithelium. The alveolar mucosa is separated from the alveolar gingiva at the MGJ. The alveolar mucosa blends into the palatal gingiva in the maxilla; consequently, no MGJ is distinguishable there. Alveolar mucosa is a darker shade of red than gingiva because of its vascularity.

Junctional Epithelium

Inside the gingival sulcus, the sulcular epithelium attaches to the tooth at the coronal portion of the junctional epithelium (JE). The JE is a cuff-like band of squamous epithelium that completely encircles the tooth and is attached to the tooth. The base of the sulcus is formed by the JE (see Fig. 20.2). The epithelial attachment is the innermost part of the JE that attaches to the tooth by hemidesmosomes and the basal lamina. A hemidesmosome is one-half of a dense plate near the cell surface that forms a site of attachment between the JE and the surface of the tooth. The basal lamina is a thin layer of delicate, noncellular material underlying the epithelium, with the principal component being collagen.

Gingival crevicular fluid (GCF) is a serum-like fluid secreted from the underlying connective tissue into the sulcular space. Little or no fluid is found in the healthy gingival sulcus, but GCF has been found to flow after 1 day without oral biofilm control and increases with gingival inflammation. The GCF, part of the body's defense mechanism, transports antibodies and can also transport certain systemically administered drugs used in the treatment of periodontal disease.

Clinical Appearance of Gingiva

In both a healthy and diseased periodontium, gingiva has a distinctive color, consistency, surface texture, contour, and size (Fig. 20.4 and Table 20.1).

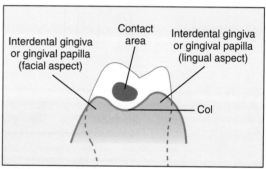

Fig. 20.3 The col is significant because it is anatomically predisposed to the growth of oral biofilm and hence susceptible to inflammation and disease progression.

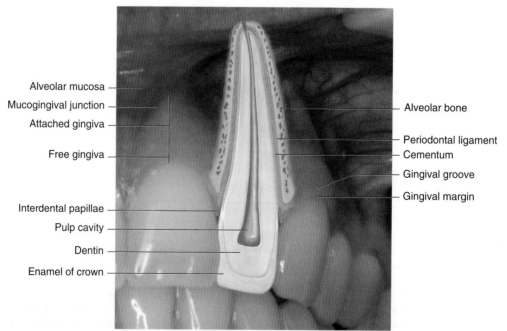

Fig. 20.4 Anatomic relationship of normal gingiva. The gingival tissues are alveolar mucosa, mucogingival junction, attached gingiva, free gingiva, and interdental papillae.

TABLE 20.1 Clinical Characteristics in Healthy and Inflamed Gingiva in Dental Biofilm–Induced Gingivitis

Characteristic	Healthy	Inflamed
Color	Is uniformly pale pink, with or without generalized dark brown pigmentation.	Is red. Is bluish, blue-red. Is pink if fibrotic.
Consistency	Is firm and resilient.	Is soft and spongy. Easily dents when pressed with a probe.
Bleeding	Exhibits ≤10% bleeding sites.	Exhibits ≥10% bleeding sites.
Surface texture	Free gingiva is smooth. Attached gingiva is stippled.	Loss of stippling occurs; is shiny. Is fibrotic with stippling; is nodular and hyperkeratotic.
Contour	Gingival margin is 1 mm above CEJ in fully erupted teeth. Marginal gingiva is knife edged; flat; follows a curved line around the tooth; and fits snugly around the tooth. Papilla is pointed and pyramidal; fills interproximal spaces.	Margins are irregular from edema, fibrosis, clefting, and/or festooning. May be rounded, rolled, or bulbous; thus is more coronal to the CEJ. Is bulbous, flattened, blunted, and cratered.
Size	Free marginal gingiva is near the CEJ and closely adheres to the tooth.	Is enlarged from excess extracellular fluid in the tissues or fibrotic from the formation of scar tissue within the connective tissue. Free marginal gingiva may be highly retractable with air.
Probing depth	Depth is usually 1 to 3 mm, with no apical migration of the JE or CAL in an intact periodontium. In a reduced periodontium, CAL may be present.	Depth is 4 mm, with apical migration of the gingiva or JE below the CEJ in an intact periodontium and apical migration of the gingiva and/or JE.

CAL, Clinical attachment loss; *CEJ,* cementoenamel junction; *JE,* junctional epithelium.

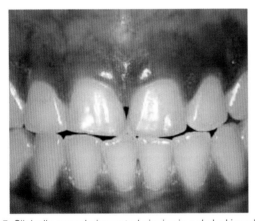

Fig. 20.5 Clinically normal pigmented gingiva in a dark-skinned individual.

Gingival color varies according to degree of vascularity, amount of melanin pigmentation, degree of epithelial keratinization, and thickness of the epithelium. Pigment-containing cells in the basal layer of the epithelium are commonly present in persons of color (Fig. 20.5). Therefore some individuals naturally have brown melanin pigmentation throughout the gingiva. Healthy attached gingiva is resilient, firm, and tightly bound to the underlying bone by gingival fibers running between the connective tissue and the periosteum of the alveolar bone.

Healthy gingiva, when visually examined, air dried, and probed, does not bleed or exude fluids. Healthy attached gingiva may have a stippled (orange peel) texture that varies with individuals and areas of the mouth. A healthy gingival margin is located 1 to 2 mm coronal to the CEJ, and the gingival contour follows the contour of the teeth. In addition, the contour, size, and shape of the gingiva depend on location, tooth size, and tooth alignment.

Cementum, a mineralized bone-like substance, covers the roots of the teeth and provides attachment and anchorage for periodontal fibers. Cementum is usually a very thin cellular layer, not as hard as dentin, and lacks blood vessels and nerves. In a healthy periodontium, apical to the epithelial attachment, the PDL protects the cementum and has no exposure to the oral cavity.

Periodontal Ligament

The PDL is the fibrous connective tissue that surrounds and attaches the tooth roots to the alveolar bone. The width of the PDL, seen in radiographic images as only a black (radiolucent) space, depends on the age of the individual, stage of eruption, function of the tooth, and angle of the exposure. Collagen fibers of the ligament insert into the cementum and prevent tooth mobility by anchoring the tooth into its alveolar socket. The PDL connects to the cementum and bone by collagen fibers called Sharpey fibers. Functions of the PDL also include the formation and maintenance of fibrous and calcified tissue, nutrient transport, and the sensory functions of pain and pressure.

Alveolar Bone

Alveolar bone is comprised of compact or cortical bone and of spongy bone marked by trabecular spaces as visualized on radiographic images. Compact bone is the outside wall of the alveolar bone, where the PDL fibers are anchored and the rich vascular supply penetrates. Spongy bone is the interior of the alveolar bone. It increases and decreases in response to physical pressure, function, bacterial infection, and inflammation. The alveolar crest—the portion of the alveolar bone located between the teeth—varies in size and shape, depending on tooth position.

Periodontal Assessment Instruments

The basic instruments needed to assess clinical parameters include a good source of light, compressed air to dry the tissues, a mouth mirror, an explorer, a periodontal probe, and a current full-mouth radiographic series.

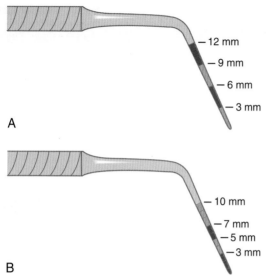

Fig. 20.6 (A) Marquis probe calibrated with color bands to indicate 3-, 6-, 9-, and 12-mm levels of penetration. (B) Williams probe calibrated in 3-, 5-, 7-, and 10-mm increments.

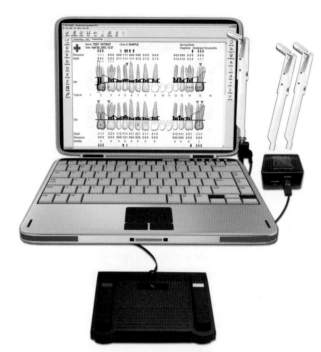

Fig. 20.7 Computer-assisted probing device and setup. (Courtesy Florida Probe Corporation, Gainesville, Florida.)

Many kinds of periodontal probes are available. All probes use millimeters for assessing the health of the periodontium and may be made of plastic or metal. Fig. 20.6A shows the Marquis probe with its colored bands, which indicate different measurement levels of 3-, 6-, 9-, and 12-mm markings, and the Williams probe (Fig. 20.6B), which is calibrated with 3-, 5-, 7-, and 10-mm markings. When a probe is inserted into the space between the tooth and the gingiva, the calibrations show the depth of the space in millimeters. Probing depths are used to monitor periodontal health and disease.

Computer-assisted, pressure-sensitive, and voice-activated probes are options to manual probing. Probing depths are entered using a computer keyboard and software (Fig. 20.7). In addition to probing depths, most computerized systems store and reveal information on attachment levels, recession, mobility, and furcation involvement. The clinician operates the probe by gently probing around the tooth. A foot pedal is used in conjunction with the probe handpiece to select from a list of periodontal data to be entered. The resulting computer-generated chart (Fig. 20.8) aids periodontal assessment, may save time over traditional methods, and provides a visual tool for educating patients. Pressure-sensitive probes, primarily used in research, have the advantage of maintaining a standard probing force, typically 15 g, improving accuracy (Fig. 20.9).

A technologic advance in periodontal assessment and treatment is the **periodontal endoscope**, an illuminated fiberoptic instrument that provides high magnification views (24× to 48×) of the gingival sulcus or periodontal pocket. The instrument consists of a miniature camera attached to a tiny diagnostic explorer or probe. Images of the actual subgingival conditions are exhibited on a monitor. The probe is placed subgingivally, a water irrigation sheath flushes the pocket, and subgingival images—periodontal pocket, root surface, bone, and furcation areas—are immediately displayed on a chairside color screen. This technology assists in visualizing and assessing the extent of the patient's periodontal disease (see Chapter 28).

CLASSIFICATIONS OF PERIODONTAL AND PERI-IMPLANT DISEASES AND CONDITIONS

The AAP-EFP jointly developed the new system for classifying periodontal and peri-implant diseases and conditions in 2017 (Table 20.2).[3] These changes and associated papers describing these diseases and conditions were published in 2018. The former classification of periodontal diseases and conditions had been used since 1999 (Boxes 20.1 and 20.2). As of 2019, practitioners and insurance companies have adapted to the new system. To classify periodontal disease, the practitioner must decide whether health, biofilm-induced gingivitis, nongingival disease, periodontitis, other periodontal conditions, or peri-implant diseases are present.

Periodontal Health, Gingival Diseases and Conditions
Periodontal and Gingival Health

Gingival health can exist in an intact or a reduced periodontium after successful treatment. Periodontal health in a reduced periodontium requires lifelong supportive periodontal therapy, also known as periodontal maintenance.[4]

Dental Biofilm–Induced Gingivitis

Understanding the characteristics of the healthy periodontium provides a foundation on which to recognize the signs of disease and to make evidence-based decisions regarding care. The term *periodontal disease* includes many types of diseases and conditions affecting the periodontium. The 2017 gingival diseases have two classifications: (1) dental biofilm–induced gingivitis and (2) nondental biofilm (nonplaque)-induced gingival diseases (Box 20.3), whereas the 1999 classification had many (see Box 20.1).[5] **Dental biofilm–induced gingivitis**, also referred to as **gingivitis**, is inflammation of the gingival tissue and a reversible bacterial infection confined to the gingiva. It can occur in an intact or reduced periodontium that has been successfully treated. Among all the periodontal diseases gingivitis is considered to be the commonest. In gingivitis, the free gingiva shows signs of inflammation, but no apical migration of the JE has occurred beyond the CEJ or no bone loss is evident. It has the following characteristics:
- Presence of gingival inflammation
- Presence of a bacterial burden posed by dental biofilm
- Bleeding on probing (BOP) score (%)
  - Intact periodontium with a BOP score ≥10%
    - Localized (BOP score ≥10% and ≤30%)
    - Generalized (BOP score ≥30%)

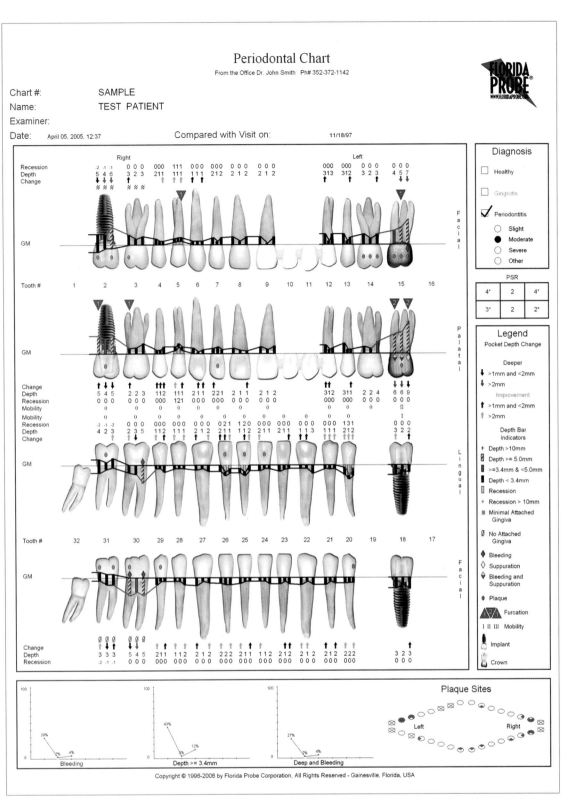

Fig. 20.8 Computer-generated periodontal chart. (Courtesy Florida Probe Corporation, Gainesville, Florida.)

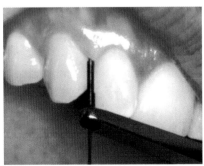

Fig. 20.9 Pressure-sensitive periodontal probe. (Courtesy Florida Probe Corporation, Gainesville, Florida.)

TABLE 20.2 Classification of Periodontal and Peri-implant Diseases, 2017

PERIODONTAL DISEASES AND CONDITIONS

Periodontal Health, Gingival Diseases and Conditions			Periodontitis			Other Conditions Affecting the Periodontium				
Chapple et al.: 2018 Consensus Report Trombelli et al.: 2018 Case Definitions			Papapanou et al.: 2018 Consensus Report Jepsen et al.: 2018 Consensus Report Tonetti, Greenwell, Kornman: 2018 Case Definitions			Jepsen et al.: 2018 Consensus Report Papapanou et al.: 2018 Consensus Report				
Periodontal health and gingival health	Gingivitis: dental biofilm–induced	Gingival diseases: nondental biofilm–induced	Necrotizing periodontal diseases	Periodontitis	Periodontitis as a manifestation of systemic disease	Systemic diseases or conditions affecting the periodontal-supporting tissues	Periodontal abscesses and endodontic-periodontal lesions	Mucogingival deformities and conditions	Traumatic occlusal forces	Tooth- and prosthesis-related factors

PERI-IMPLANT DISEASES AND CONDITIONS

Berglundh et al.: 2018 Consensus Report

Peri-implant health	Peri-implant mucositis	Peri-implantitis	Peri-implant soft and hard tissue deficiencies

BOX 20.1 1999 Classification of Gingival Diseases

Dental Plaque–Induced Gingival Lesions*
1. Gingivitis associated with dental plaque only
   a. Without other local contributing factors
   b. With local contributing factors
2. Gingival diseases modified by systemic factors
   a. Associated with the endocrine system
      1) Puberty-associated gingivitis
      2) Menstrual cycle–associated gingivitis
      3) Pregnancy-associated gingivitis
         a) Gingivitis
         b) Pyogenic granuloma
      4) DM-associated gingivitis
   b. Associated with blood dyscrasias
      1) Leukemia-associated gingivitis
      2) Other
3. Gingival diseases modified by medications
   a. Drug-influenced gingival enlargements
   b. Drug-influenced gingivitis
      1) Oral contraceptive–associated gingivitis
      2) Other
4. Gingival diseases modified by malnutrition
   a. Ascorbic acid–deficiency gingivitis
   b. Other

Nondental Plaque–Induced Gingival Lesions
1. Gingival diseases of specific bacterial origin
   a. Neisseria gonorrhoeae–associated lesions
   b. Treponema pallidum–associated lesions
   c. Streptococcal species–associated lesions
   d. Other
2. Gingival diseases of viral origin
   a. Herpesvirus infections
      1) Primary herpetic gingivostomatitis
      2) Recurrent oral herpes
      3) Varicella-zoster infection
   b. Other

3. Gingival diseases of fungal origin
   a. Candida species infections
   b. Generalized gingival candidiasis
   c. Linear gingival erythema
   d. Histoplasmosis
   e. Other
4. Gingival lesions of genetic origin
   a. Hereditary gingival fibromatosis
   b. Other
5. Gingival manifestations of systemic conditions
   a. Mucocutaneous disorders
      1) Lichen planus
      2) Pemphigoid
      3) Pemphigus vulgaris
      4) Erythema multiforme
      5) Lupus erythematosus
      6) Drug-induced disorders
      7) Other
   b. Allergic reactions
      1) Dental restorative materials
         a) Mercury
         b) Nickel
         c) Acrylic
         d) Other
      2) Reactions attributable to
         a) Toothpastes or dentifrices
         b) Mouthrinses or mouthwashes
         c) Chewing gum additives
         d) Foods and additives
      3) Other
6. Traumatic lesions (factitious, iatrogenic, accidental)
   a. Chemical injury
   b. Physical injury
   c. Thermal injury
7. Foreign body reactions
8. Not otherwise specified (NOS)

*Can occur on a periodontium with no attachment loss or on a periodontium with attachment loss that is not progressing (reduced periodontium with inflammation).
Adapted from Armitage GC. Development of a classification system for periodontal diseases and conditions. *Ann Periodontol.* 1999;4(1):1–6.

BOX 20.2 1999 Classification of Periodontal Diseases and Conditions—Periodontitis

I. Chronic periodontitis*
  A. Localized
  B. Generalized
II. Aggressive periodontitis*
  A. Localized
  B. Generalized
III. Periodontitis as a manifestation of systemic diseases
  A. Associated with hematologic disorders
    1. Acquired neutropenia
    2. Leukemias
    3. Other
  B. Associated with genetic disorders
    1. Familial and cyclic neutropenia
    2. Down syndrome
    3. Leukocyte adhesion–deficiency syndromes
    4. Papillon-Lefèvre syndrome
    5. Chédiak-Higashi syndrome
    6. Histiocytosis syndromes
    7. Glycogen storage disease
    8. Infantile genetic agranulocytosis
    9. Cohen syndrome
    10. Ehlers-Danlos syndrome
    11. Hypophosphatasia
    12. Other
  C. Not otherwise specified (NOS)
IV. Necrotizing periodontal diseases
  A. Necrotizing ulcerative gingivitis (NUG)
  B. Necrotizing ulcerative periodontitis (NUP)
V. Abscesses of the periodontium
  A. Gingival abscess
  B. Periodontal abscess
  C. Periocoronal abscess
VI. Periodontitis associated with endodontic lesions
VII. Combined periodontic-endodontic lesions
VIII. Developmental or acquired deformities and conditions
  A. Localized tooth-related factors that modify or predispose to plaque-induced gingival diseases and periodontitis
    1. Tooth anatomic factors
    2. Dental restorations and appliances
    3. Root fractures
    4. Cervical root resorption and cemental tears
  B. Mucogingival deformities and conditions around teeth
    1. Gingival soft tissue recession
      a. Facial or lingual surfaces
      b. Interproximal (papillary)
    2. Lack of keratinized gingiva
    3. Decreased vestibular depth
    4. Aberrant frenum or muscle position
    5. Gingival excess
      a. Pseudopocket
      b. Inconsistent gingival margin
      c. Excessive gingival display
      d. Gingival enlargement
    6. Abnormal color
  C. Mucogingival deformities and conditions on edentulous ridges
    1. Vertical and/or horizontal ridge deficiency
    2. Lack of gingiva or keratinized tissue
    3. Gingival soft tissue enlargement
    4. Aberrant frenum or muscle position
    5. Decreased vestibular depth
    6. Abnormal color
  D. Occlusal trauma
    1. Primary occlusal trauma
    2. Secondary occlusal trauma

* Can be further classified on the basis of extent and severity based on 1999 criteria.
Adapted from Armitage GC. Development of a classification system for periodontal diseases and conditions. *Ann Periodontol.* 1999;4(1):1–6. In 2017, the American Academy of Periodontology and the European Federation of Periodontology revised and updated this classification system.

BOX 20.3 2017 Classification of Periodontal Diseases and Conditions—Gingival Diseases

Dental Biofilm–Induced Gingivitis and Modifying Factors
A. Associated with bacterial dental biofilm only
B. Potential modifying factors of biofilm-induced gingivitis:
  1. Systemic conditions
    a. Sex steroid hormones
      i. Puberty
      ii. Menstrual cycle
      iii. Pregnancy
      iv. Oral contraceptives
  2. Hyperglycemia
  3. Leukemia
  4. Smoking
  5. Malnutrition
  6. Oral factors enhancing plaque accumulation
    a. Prominent subgingival restoration margins
    b. Hyposalivation
C. Drug-influenced gingival enlargements

Nondental Biofilm–Induced Gingival Diseases
- Genetic and developmental—hereditary gingival fibromatosis
- Specific infections—bacterial, viral, and fungal
  - Bacterial—gonorrhea, syphilis, tuberculosis, and streptococcal gingivitis
  - Viral—coxsackie virus (hand, foot, and mouth disease), herpes simplex, and herpes zoster
  - Human papilloma virus (HPV)
  - Fungal—candidiasis and other mycoses
- Inflammatory and immune conditions—hypersensitivity (allergy) reactions; autoimmune diseases of skin and mucous membrane, such as pemphigus vulgaris, pemphigoid, lichen planus, and lupus erythematosus; granulomatous inflammatory conditions, including Crohn disease and sarcoidosis; endocrine, nutritional (vitamin deficiencies), and metabolic diseases
- Reactive processes—epulides (tumorlike enlargements in the alveolar mucosa or gingiva) and neoplasms (cancerous lesions)
- Endocrine, nutritional, and metabolic diseases
- Traumatic lesions—physical and/or mechanical, chemical (toxic), and thermal (burns)
- Gingival pigmentation

Adapted from Murakami S, Mealey BL, Mariotti A, et al. Dental plaque-induced gingival conditions. *J Clin Periodontol.* 2018;45(suppl 20):S17–S27.

- Reduced periodontium with an attachment loss and a BOP score ≥10%; but
  - Without BOP in any site probing ≥4 mm in depth.
- Reversible with the removal or disruption of biofilm
- Systemic modifying factors (e.g., hormones, systemic disorders, drugs), which can affect the severity of inflammation
- Stable attachment levels on an intact periodontium or a successfully treated case of periodontitis with reduced attachment levels.[5]

Dental biofilm–induced gingivitis is associated with bacterial dental biofilm only, although it can be mediated or modified by systemic or local factors. These factors include the following:

- Systemic conditions exacerbating periodontal destruction
  - Sex steroidal hormones—puberty, menstruation, pregnancy, oral contraceptives
  - Hyperglycemia (undiagnosed or poorly controlled diabetes)
    - Leukemia
    - Smoking
    - Malnutrition
  - Oral factors enhancing plaque accumulation
    - Prominent subgingival restoration margins
    - Hyposalivation
    - Drug-influenced gingival enlargements[5]

Nondental biofilm–induced gingival conditions are organized by their causes into the following categories:

- Genetic and/or developmental—hereditary gingival fibromatosis
- Specific infections—bacterial, viral, and fungal

- Inflammatory and immune conditions—hypersensitivity (allergy) reactions; autoimmune diseases of skin and mucous membrane; granulomatous inflammatory conditions; and endocrine, nutritional, and metabolic diseases
- Reactive processes—epulides and neoplasms
- Endocrine, nutritional, and metabolic diseases
- Traumatic lesions
- Gingival pigmentation[6]

Nondental Biofilm–Induced Gingival Diseases

This category of periodontal diseases includes conditions that are not as common as gingivitis, but they can have significance for patients.[6] These oral lesions are often manifestations of a systemic disease; consequently, their classification is related to their cause. A diagnosis would be specified using the medical disease classification codes developed by the World Health Organization (WHO). Nondental biofilm–induced gingival conditions are less common than gingivitis and are categorized by their cause (see Box 20.3.)[6]

Periodontitis

The 2017 AAP-EFP classification includes the following three distinct categories of periodontitis (see Table 20.2)[7]:

- Periodontitis (previously chronic or aggressive periodontitis)
  - New staging and grading system (Tables 20.3 and 20.4)
  - Radiographic evidence of **clinical attachment lost** (CAL), bone loss

TABLE 20.3   Classification of Periodontitis Based on Stages Defined by Severity (According to the Level of Interdental Clinical Attachment Loss, Radiographic Bone Loss and Tooth Loss), Complexity, and Extent and Distribution

Periodontitis Stage		Stage I	Stage II	Stage III	Stage IV
Severity	Interdental CAL at site of greatest loss	1 to 2 mm	3 to 4 mm	≥5 mm	≥5 mm
	Radiographic bone loss	Coronal third (<15%)	Coronal third (<15% to 33%)	Extending to middle or apical third of the root	Extending to middle or apical third of the root
	Tooth loss	No tooth loss due to periodontitis		Tooth loss due to periodontitis of ≤4 teeth	Tooth loss due to periodontitis of ≥5 teeth
Complexity	Local	Maximum probing depth ≤4 mm Mostly horizontal bone loss	Maximum probing depth ≤5 mm Mostly horizontal bone loss	In addition to stage II complexity: Probing depth ≥6 mm Vertical bone loss ≥3 mm Furcation involvement Class II or III Moderate ridge defect	In addition to stage III complexity: Need for complex rehabilitation due to: Masticatory dysfunction Secondary occlusal trauma (tooth mobility degree ≥2) Severe ridge defect Bite collapse, drifting, flaring Fewer than 20 remaining teeth (10 opposing pairs)
Extent and distribution	Add to stage as descriptor	For each stage, describe extent as localized (<30% of teeth involved), generalized, or molar/incisor pattern			

The initial stage should be determined using clinical attachment loss (CAL); if not available, then radiographic bone loss (RBL) should be used. Information on tooth loss that can be attributed primarily to periodontitis—if available—may modify stage definition. This is the case even in the absence of complexity factors. Complexity factors may shift the stage to a higher level; for example, furcation II or III would shift to either stage III or IV, irrespective of CAL. The distinction between stage III and stage IV is primarily based on complexity factors. For example, a high level of tooth mobility and/or posterior bite collapse would indicate a stage IV diagnosis. For any given case, only some, not all, complexity factors may be present; however, in general, it only takes one complexity factor to shift the diagnosis to a higher stage. It should be emphasized that these case definitions are guidelines that should be applied using sound clinical judgment to arrive at the most appropriate clinical diagnosis.

For posttreatment patients, CAL and RBL are still the primary stage determinants. If a stage-shifting complexity factor(s) is eliminated by treatment, the stage should not retrogress to a lower stage since the original stage complexity factor should always be considered in maintenance phase management.

TABLE 20.4 **Classification of Periodontitis Based on Grades That Reflect Biologic Features of the Disease Including Evidence of, or Risk for, Rapid Progression, Anticipated Treatment Response, and Effects on Systemic Health**

Periodontitis Grade			Grade A: Slow Rate of Progression	Grade B: Moderate Rate of Progression	Grade C: Rapid Rate of Progression
Primary criteria	Direct evidence of progression	Longitudinal data (radiographic bone loss or CAL)	Evidence of no loss over 5 years	<2 mm over 5 years	≥2 mm over 5 years
	Indirect evidence of progression	% bone loss/age	<0.25	0.25 to 1.0	>1.0
		Case phenotype	Heavy biofilm deposits with low levels of destruction	Destruction commensurate with biofilm deposits	Destruction exceeds expectation given biofilm deposits; specific clinical patterns suggestive of periods of rapid progression and/or early onset disease (e.g., molar/incisor pattern; lack of expected response to standard bacterial control therapies)
Grade modifiers	Risk factors	Smoking	Nonsmoker	Smoker < 10 cigarettes/day	Smoker ≥ 10 cigarettes/day
		Diabetes	Normoglycemic/no diagnosis of diabetes	HbA1c < 7.0% in patients with diabetes	HbA1c ≥ 7.0% in patients with diabetes

Grade should be used as an indicator of the rate of periodontitis progression. The primary criteria are either direct or indirect evidence of progression. Whenever available, direct evidence is used; in its absence, indirect estimation is made, using bone loss as a function of age at the most affected tooth or case presentation (radiographic bone loss expressed as percentage of root length divided by the age of the subject, RBL/age). Clinicians should initially assume grade B disease and seek specific evidence to shift towards grade A or C, if available. Once grade is established based on evidence of progression, it can be modified based on the presence of risk factors. *CAL,* Clinical attachment loss; *HbA1c,* glycated hemoglobin A1c; *RBL,* radiographic bone loss.

- Necrotizing periodontal diseases—necrotizing ulcerative gingivitis (NUG), necrotizing ulcerative periodontitis (NUP), necrotizing stomatitis (NS)
- Other conditions affecting the periodontium
  - Systemic diseases, periodontal and/or endodontic abscesses, mucogingival deformities and conditions (recession), traumatic occlusal forces (not CAL), tooth- and prostheses-related factors (recession)
  - Conditions independent of biofilm (periodontal abscesses may or may not be associated with periodontitis and biofilm and should be classified by etiology)

Periodontitis (Previously Chronic or Aggressive Periodontitis)

Periodontitis is a group of chronic, multifactorial disease classifications associated with dysbiotic (causing gut imbalance associated with disease) plaque accumulation. Evidence suggests that lipopolysaccharide (LPS), which is an endotoxin found on the outer membrane of Gram-negative bacteria, is absorbed by intestinal tissue. Periodontitis is a bacterial infection with inflammation extending from the gingival epithelium into the connective tissue and alveolar bone that supports the teeth. In periodontitis, apical migration of the JE occurs with an associated loss of attachment and irreversible destruction of alveolar bone (Fig. 20.10).

The 1999 classification of periodontitis included chronic and aggressive forms (see Box 20.2). This division was revised in the new classification scheme (see Table 20.2) because evidence no longer supported the differentiation of these two diseases into distinct categories. Periodontitis for individual patients under the current system is further classified into stages, grades, and extent of distribution.[7]

The four stages are based on severity according to the level of CAL, amount and percentage of radiographic bone loss, probing depths,

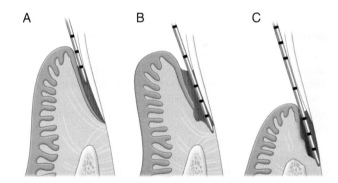

Fig. 20.10 Parameters of probing in health, in gingivitis, and in periodontitis. (A) Probing a normal sulcus with a long junctional epithelium (JE), the probe penetrates approximately one-third to one-half the length of the JE. (B) In gingivitis, enlarged gingiva and probe penetration beyond the apical end of the JE results in 4-mm gingival pockets. (C) In periodontitis, the probe penetrates through the JE and into the connective tissues; the loss of bone and periodontal fibers result in greater probing depths.

presence of furcation involvement, and mobility, as well as the number of teeth lost due to periodontitis, complexity, and extent of distribution (see Table 20.3).[7] Stage I is initial, stage II is moderate, and stages III and IV are severe with increasing complexity.

Grade indicates the rate of progression and is based on risk factors affecting progression, general health status, and other considerations such as smoking or the level of control of diabetes (see Table 20.4). Grades include three levels: grade A indicates low risk, grade

B indicates moderate risk, and grade C indicates high risk for progression.[7] The rate of progression varies considerably for individual patients with periodontitis; however, evidence does not support the separate classification of aggressive periodontitis. The localized form of this rapidly progressive form of periodontitis continues to have the characteristics of a healthy patient, young age of onset, and a pattern of initial CAL and alveolar bone loss in the anterior teeth and first molars.

Describing the extent (localized or generalized) of the affected sites can further define periodontal conditions:

- Localized—Fewer than 30% of the sites in the mouth are affected.
- Generalized—More than 30% of the sites in the mouth are affected. A dental hygiene diagnosis of periodontitis for an individual patient requires recognition of the history and clinical signs of the disease, followed by staging and grading. A patient with generalized periodontitis would exhibit one of the following:
  - ≥2 mm CAL in interdental areas of nonadjacent teeth, or
  - ≥2 or 3 mm CAL with ≥3 mm probing depths in buccal or oral surfaces of two teeth when the CAL cannot be attributed to a nonperiodontitis cause, such as gingival recession from trauma, cervical dental caries, malposed or extracted third molars, an endodontic lesion, and a vertical root fracture.[7]

Clinical descriptions usually include localized or generalized BOP, as well as the proportion of sites with periodontal pockets ≥4 mm and ≥6 mm or CAL ≥3 mm and ≥5 mm.

Periodontitis is most prevalent in adults, affecting more than 50% of the adult population, with its severe forms affecting 11% of adults.[8] The rate of attachment loss per year varies considerably. Periodontitis is cyclic in nature, with variable rates of progression. There may be bursts of periodontal destruction or inactivity, although activity and remission episodes are hard to measure clinically. Loss of connective tissue attachment during the active stage can vary from minor changes to extensive tissue loss. An increase in probing depth and CAL is considered to be a cumulative effect.

Necrotizing Periodontal Diseases

This AAP-EFP classification of periodontitis includes necrotizing gingivitis (NG), necrotizing periodontitis (NP), and necrotizing stomatitis (NS) because they are unique in their initial presentation and development. These **necrotizing periodontal diseases** have three key clinical features—papillary necrosis, bleeding, and pain, usually with rapid onset.[7] In NG, necrosis is limited to the gingiva; in NP, it affects the periodontal attachment and bone, and in NS, it affects the oral mucosa. NG rarely progresses to NP. Both are associated with a compromised host immune response—for example, in patients with the human immunodeficiency virus (HIV) or acquired immunodeficiency syndrome (AIDS) with CD4 counts <200 cells per cubic millimeter of blood (cells/mm^3) and measurable viral loads, other conditions causing immunosuppression, severe malnutrition, severe viral infections, uncontrolled stress or smoking, or previous episodes of necrotizing periodontal diseases.[7]

Periodontitis as a Manifestation of Systemic Diseases

This type of periodontitis is also listed under the next category, *Other Conditions Affecting the Periodontium*. At times, periodontitis as a manifestation of systemic diseases meets the criteria for periodontitis (CAL and bone loss); at other times, it will have developmental or acquired deficiencies affecting the teeth or gingiva. Thus it is discussed in the next section.

Other Conditions Affecting the Periodontium

Various systemic diseases affect the course of periodontitis or have a negative effect on the periodontal tissues.[9] Gingival recessions are common and can lead to mucogingival deformities, sensitivity, and dental caries. Periodontal abscesses and endodontic-periodontic lesions are caused by infection in the periodontal ligament that affects the periodontal apparatus. Occlusal forces can result in damage to the teeth and periodontium. Other developmental or acquired conditions associated with the dentition or prosthetic restorations and appliances may also be predisposing factors to periodontal diseases.[9]

Systemic Diseases Affecting the Periodontium

Some systemic diseases influence the course of periodontitis, whereas some affect the periodontium, independent of dental biofilm–induced inflammation. These systemic diseases include rare disorders (e.g., Papillon-Lefèvre syndrome, Down syndrome, cyclic neutropenia, leukocyte adhesion deficiency, hypophosphatasia) that have a major impact on the age of onset and severity of periodontitis.[9] Other rare conditions, such as oral cancer, can affect the periodontium, independent of dental-plaque biofilm. Clinical changes mimic the characteristics of periodontitis. This category also includes common systemic diseases affecting the course of periodontal disease but that do not affect the magnitude of the systemic disease, such as diabetes and osteoporosis.

Mucogingival Deformities and Conditions

Gingival recession is the apical migration of the margin of the gingiva, causing root exposure. It is associated with CAL and mucogingival changes. Recession can occur on all tooth surfaces—mesial, distal, and buccal, which causes esthetic concerns, hypersensitivity, root caries, and noncarious cervical lesions adjacent to defective prostheses. Gingival recession may be related to the periodontal phenotype of thin gingival tissue, environmental risk factors, and a genetic predisposition.[9] Orthodontic treatment can result in gingival recession, but this effect is not universal. Recession of the gingival tissues into the attached gingiva result in mucogingival deformities, such as scanty or no attached gingiva. Mucogingival conditions or defects can also occur without gingival recession and may be attributed to tooth position, frenum pulling on the attached gingiva, or a lack of adequate vestibular depth.

Traumatic Occlusal Force

Traumatic occlusal force is defined as any occlusal force that damages the teeth and/or periodontal attachment tissues.[9] **Occlusal trauma** is the injury to the periodontium (Box 20.4). There is no evidence that traumatic occlusal force causes CAL, and limited evidence suggests that it results in inflammation. Occlusal trauma is associated with the severity of periodontitis, but it does not influence the rate of progression

---

BOX 20.4   Signs of Occlusal Trauma

Clinical Signs

- Tooth pain or discomfort on chewing or percussion
- Tooth migration
- Wear facets exceeding expected levels
- Fremitus
- Chipped enamel
- Tooth mobility
- Root fracture

Radiographic Signs

- Widening of the periodontal ligament space
- Loss of lamina dura
- Radiolucencies at tooth apices in a vital tooth
- Root resorption

of periodontitis. Traumatic occlusal force does not cause noncarious cervical lesions or abfractions (i.e., wedge-shaped defects at the CEJ of an affected tooth) or gingival recession.

Tooth- and Prosthesis-Related Factors

Supracrestal attached tissues (formerly the biologic width) are the JE and connective tissues that attach the gingiva to the alveolar bone above the crest of the bone. Infringement by a tooth or prosthesis-related factor, such as nonoptimal fixed or partial dentures or rough or overhanging margins of restorations, can cause periodontal inflammation and CAL. Less commonly, tooth anomalies, such as enamel pearls, close root proximity, abnormal root fractures, and tooth position in the arch, can result in loss of the periodontal apparatus.

Abscesses and Endodontic-Periodontal Lesions

Although not specified in the new classifications of periodontal diseases, periodontal abscesses and acute endodontic-periodontal lesions are characterized by rapid onset and rapid destruction of the periodontium and pain or discomfort. These characteristics often lead to a patient seeking urgent care.[3] **Periodontal abscesses** are localized periodontal infections that result in inflammation and can ultimately lead to the formation of **purulent exudate** (containing pus). They are caused by bacterial or foreign body invasion of the periodontal tissues surrounding the sulcus or periodontal pocket. The exudate must be drained to prevent growth of the abscess. Periodontal abscesses can occur in patients with untreated periodontitis or after periodontal instrumentation when residual calculus remains, or they can develop in a healthy patient with an impaction (e.g., toothpick tip subgingivally broken during self-care) or who has unhealthy habits that cause injury to the tissues.[7]

Peri-implant Diseases and Conditions

Osseointegrated dental implants are artificial replacement teeth surgically inserted into the alveolar bone replacing a single tooth, multiple teeth, or multiple implanted support dentures of edentulous patients (Fig. 20.11). As with natural teeth, assessment of dental implant

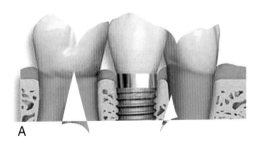
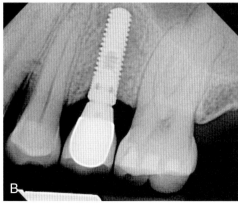

Fig. 20.11 (A) Illustration of an integrated implant. (B) Radiographic image of a dental implant.

periodontal health is important because of the similar risks of bacterial plaque–biofilm infection and inflammatory response. Implants are monitored for peri-implant health, peri-implant mucositis, peri-implantitis, or peri-implant soft and hard tissue deficiencies.[10]

Peri-implant Health

Peri-implant health is defined as an absence of redness (erythema), swelling (edema), bleeding, and suppuration of the tissue surrounding a dental implant. A probing depth range is not defined; some reduction in bone support that is not progressing and without signs of inflammation may accompany peri-implant health.[10]

Peri-implant Mucositis

Peri-implant mucositis is inflamed gingival tissue surrounding a dental implant and is characterized by erythema, bleeding, swelling, and/or suppuration.[10] Slight deepening of probing depths is possible, due to tissue enlargement and inflammation rather than from loss of bone around the implant. There is no bone loss other than that caused by initial bone remodeling. Dental plaque–biofilm is believed to be the primary cause. Host response to the bacterial irritation can be modified by smoking and systemic diseases. Peri-implant mucositis can progress to peri-implantitis without regular oral hygiene and peri-implant maintenance appointments.

Peri-implantitis

Peri-implantitis is also a dental biofilm–induced disease; however, it can also be caused by placement of the implant or surgical trauma. It is characterized by the same inflammatory signs in the gingival tissue as peri-implant mucositis, as well as progressing alveolar bone loss around the implant (≥3 mm around the most coronal portion of the intraosseous part of the implant). Thus deeper probing depths than at the previous examination (or ≥6 mm if no prior probing depth for comparison) and/or recession of the gingiva can be present in peri-implantitis. Smoking, poor plaque control, and irregular implant maintenance appointments are risk factors for peri-implantitis.[10]

Peri-implant Soft and Hard Tissue Deficiencies

Peri-implant soft and hard tissue deficiencies are reduced dimensions of the alveolar bone or ridge that occur during the healing process after tooth loss. Greater deficiencies may occur at sites affected by the following factors: loss of periodontal support, endodontic lesions, root fractures, placement of the implant in the bone, and extraction of additional teeth for other reasons.[10]

IMMUNOPATHOLOGIC RESPONSES IN DENTAL BIOFILM–INDUCED GINGIVITIS AND PERIODONTITIS

Diseased Periodontium

The histopathologic changes of **periodontal disease** progress in four stages (Table 20.5).[11,12] Three of the stages describe a sequence of events resulting in gingivitis, and the last stage describes events resulting in periodontitis. The progression of periodontal disease involves the destruction of connective tissue attachment at the most apical portion of a periodontal pocket. Associated with this attachment loss are the apical growth of the subgingival flora, apical migration of the JE, and alveolar bone resorption.

The following two distinct causative components cause periodontal destruction:

- A complex pathogenic microbiota in the subgingival biofilm, including endogenous Gram-negative bacteria *Porphyromonas*

TABLE 20.5 Histopathologic Changes of Periodontal Disease Page and Schroeder Model of Inflammation

Stage	Histopathologic Changes	Time	Clinical Signs
Initial lesion	Vasoconstriction, followed by migration and infiltration of PMNs into JE and gingival sulcus Alteration of the most coronal part of the JE Increase in gingival crevicular fluid flow Loss of perivascular collagen	2 to 4 days of bacterial irritation from oral biofilm accumulation	None Subclinical infection
Early lesion	Accentuation of the initial lesion features Chronic inflammatory cells, such as the accumulation of lymphocytes in the connective tissue Junctional epithelium forms rete pegs 70% loss of collagen fibers	7 to 14 days of oral biofilm accumulation growing thicker	Acute signs of inflammation Redness Edema Loss of tissue tone Bleeding on provocation
Established lesion	Persistence of acute inflammation manifestations Plasma cells predominating in the connective tissue Increased collagen loss with loss of connective tissue fiber support • JE and oral epithelium continue to proliferate with areas of ulceration; epithelium is more permeable. • JE moves apically with connective tissue destruction; no bone loss.	2 weeks or more Varies, may never progress beyond this stage; depends on host response	Chronic signs of inflammation Continuation of changes from early lesion; may become more severe Chronic changes such as fibrosis occur over time Reversible condition
Advanced lesion	Continuation of features in established lesion Extension of the pocket epithelium deep into connective tissue Extensive destruction of collagen and gingival fibers Extension of irritants into the alveolar bone and PDL, resulting in bone loss Periodontal pockets Conversion of bone marrow distant from the lesion into connective tissue Periods of quiescence and exacerbation	Varies and depends on risk factors, control of etiologic factors, and host response	Signs of periodontitis Attachment loss Crestal bone resorption Periodontal pockets Irreversible condition

JE, Junctional epithelium; *PDL,* periodontal ligament; *PMNs,* polymorphonuclear neutrophilic leukocytes.

gingivalis, Tannerella forsythia (both red complex bacteria), Aggregatibacter actinomycetemcomitans, and Treponema denticola, trigger a response in a susceptible host. Importantly, recent evidence indicates periodontal disease is initiated by a synergistic and dysbiotic bacterial community versus individual bacteria.

- Innate inflammatory and immune responses to the periodontal pathogens and adaptive immunity cells and characteristic cytokines initiate periodontal destruction.[13]

When bacterial plaque biofilm is not adequately removed, it accumulates at the gingival margin; over several days, biofilm bacteria shift from Gram-positive to Gram-negative and induce an initial innate response of polymorphonuclear (PMN) leukocytes and the production of cytokines, specifically, interleukin-1β and tumor necrosis factor-α. Periodontal inflammation caused by proinflammatory cytokines can release destructive enzymes. These responses result in capillary permeability and chemotaxis of neutrophils into the JE and gingival sulcus. The subsequent adaptive response of proinflammatory cytokines, inflammatory mediators, and T4 helper cells has the potential to promote alveolar bone loss and collagen destruction by means of matrix metalloproteinases (MMPs), which are a group of degrading enzymes or proteases.[13] Over time, if this process continues, it can result in connective tissue destruction, attachment loss, and periodontitis (Fig. 20.12).

Periodontal diseases are inflammatory processes characterized by an accumulation of immune cells including PMN leukocytes and T cells (lymphocytes), which are important in regulating B lymphocytes, as well as plasma cells, mast cells, and macrophages. An interaction between the host immune system and the periodontal pathogens is responsible for the pathogenetic development of periodontitis. The cytokines and inflammatory mediators can act alone or together to stimulate a breakdown of connective tissue, BOP, and eventually alveolar bone resorption, which are the clinical manifestations of periodontal diseases. Mechanisms involved in the role of the host as protective versus destructive continue to be studied.[12,13]

Signs of Dental Biofilm–Induced Gingivitis

Clinical signs of inflammation (gingivitis). Inflammation begins in the epithelium of the col and the marginal gingiva as a result of bacterial invasion or endotoxins.[2] Endotoxins and enzymes from Gram-negative periodontal pathogens break down epithelial intercellular substances, causing sulcular epithelium ulceration. This ulceration permits enzymes and toxins to penetrate further into the underlying connective tissue and allows for gingival bleeding to occur with inflammation. Connective tissue inflammation results in dilation of capillaries, which can result in redness for the gingiva with inflammation and increased permeability of capillaries, fostering extracellular fluid accumulation in the tissues known as edema. In summary, these changes result in the following four characteristic signs of gingival or periodontal inflammation:

1. Changes in color—dilated capillaries
2. BOP—ulceration of the JE and sulcular epithelium
3. Swelling or edema—inflammatory and immune cellular infiltrate
4. Presence of exudate from the gingival sulcus—increased gingival crevicular fluid (GCF)

Oral tissues are assessed for these signs after they have been dried with compressed air or gauze if a patient's teeth are sensitive to air.

Changes in color. During assessment, the first characteristic noted is gingival tissue color. **Erythema** (reddened gingiva), common in

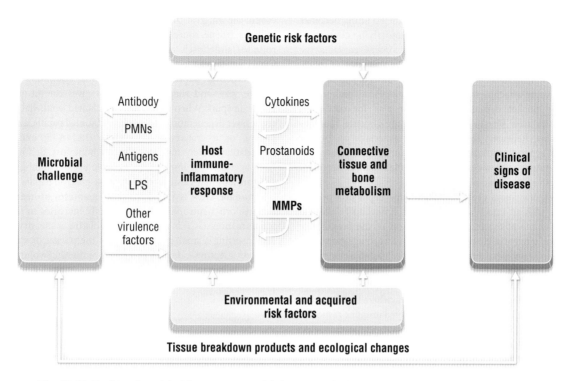

Fig. 20.12 Traditional model of host response, risk factors, and microbial challenge in periodontal disease. *LPS,* Lipopolysaccharide; *MMPs,* matrix metalloproteinases; *PMNs,* polymorphonuclear leukocytes. (Adapted from Kornman KS. Host modulation as a therapeutic strategy in the treatment of periodontal disease. *Clin Infect Dis.* 1999;28:520.)

TABLE 20.6	Terminology Used to Describe Observations Associated With Clinical Assessment of Gingiva		
Characteristic	**Terminology**	**Description**	**Example**
Gingival color	Location	Generalized or localized	Localized, with slight marginal redness in the lingual aspects of teeth 18, 20, 30, 31; all other areas are coral pink and uniform in color
	Distribution	Diffuse, marginal, or papillary	
	Severity	Slight, moderate, or severe	
	Quality	Pink, red, bright red, cyanotic	
Gingival contour	Location	Generalized or localized	Localized, with moderately cratered papilla of teeth 6 to 11 and 22 to 27; all other areas are within normal limits
	Distribution	Diffuse, marginal, or papillary	
	Severity	Slight, moderate, or severe	
	Quality	Bulbous, flattened, punched out, cratered	
Consistency of gingiva	Location	Generalized or localized	Generalized, with moderate marginal sponginess more severe on facial aspect of teeth 8, 9; all other areas are coral pink with moderate, generalized melanin pigmentation
	Distribution	Diffuse, marginal, or papillary	
	Severity	Slight, moderate, or severe	
	Quality	Firm (fibrotic), spongy (edematous)	
Surface texture of gingiva	Location	Generalized or localized	Localized, with smooth gingiva on the facial aspect of teeth 7, 8; all other areas with generalized stippling
	Distribution	Diffuse, marginal, or papillary	
	Quality	Smooth, shiny, eroded, stippling	

inflammation, indicates an increase in the vascular supply attributable to the body's effort to defend itself against bacterial invasion or trauma (e.g., oral biofilm, calculus) or foreign objects (e.g., a popcorn shell). Bright red gingival color indicates acute gingival inflammation; blue or purple gingival color indicates venous congestion (cyanosis) in the connective tissue from long duration and chronic inflammation.

Dental hygienists monitor and record changes in gingival color, contour, consistency, and texture, noting the location, distribution, severity, and quality of such changes (Table 20.6). Patients are informed of the clinical findings and are taught to monitor their gingival health. Using a hand mirror and/or an intraoral camera, the dental hygienist points out gingival characteristics to the patient and compares an inflamed gingival area of the mouth with an area that is healthy while teaching the patient about his or her periodontal status.

Bleeding on probing. Healthy gingival epithelium acts as a barrier to the bacterial plaque biofilm and irritants. As a result of the inflammatory processes, the sulcus' gingival epithelial lining becomes ulcerated. Consequently, capillary beds in the underlying connective tissue are exposed. During probing, the instrument contacts the ulcerated epithelium, which causes bleeding. As a predictor of future periodontal breakdown, BOP alone has minimal value. Bleeding is not a predictor of future attachment loss; however, BOP, in combination with increasing pocket depths, increases the risk for continued periodontal destruction. Bleeding is the key feature of dental biofilm–induced gingivitis. Repeated absence of BOP, especially on two or more occasions, generally indicates good periodontal health. Cessation of bleeding correlates with reduced gingival inflammation, repair of gingival connective tissue, and pocket reduction.

The use of a periodontal probe to measure the depth of a healthy sulcus (i.e., one with an intact layer of sulcular epithelium) yields no bleeding. BOP is one of the earliest clinical signs of the presence of inflammation and gingivitis. However, false-positive readings may occur if a clinician uses heavy force during probing, resulting in a punctured JE. This instrumentation error could result in bleeding from healthy gingival tissues. In most cases, the more severe the inflammation, the more severe the bleeding, except in tobacco users, where bleeding may be reduced by associated vasoconstriction and altered immune response.

- BOP predicts attachment loss approximately 30% of the time. Furthermore, fibrotic tissue resulting from long-term, chronic inflammation may bleed little or not at all.
- Gingival bleeding occurring at several sequential continued-care visits is associated with an increased risk for loss of attachment.
- Bleeding can be minimized or masked in tobacco users.
- Absence of bleeding is associated with a lack of disease progression; however, the mere presence or absence of bleeding does not predict periodontal breakdown.
- BOP sites are recorded in the patient record and monitored at each appointment.

The dental hygienist explains to the patient that bleeding when conducting periodontal probing indicates the existence of inflammation. Infection is what causes the inflammation. The hygienist can point out that bleeding, when brushing, flossing, or using interdental cleaning aids, is a sign that infection and inflammation are present. This information gives the individual a self-test for monitoring gingival health status at home.

Swelling or edema. Microorganisms in oral biofilm produce harmful toxins, and enzymes increase permeability of the blood vessels in the connective tissue underlying the gingival epithelium. Increased blood vessel permeability allows lymphocytes, plasma cells, and extracellular fluid to accumulate in gingival connective tissue, known as a cellular infiltrate. This accumulation results in enlarged, edematous tissue. When no apical migration of the JE has occurred, the sulcus deepens from gingival tissue edema, producing a gingival pocket, also called an *artificially deepened sulcus* or a **pseudopocket**, because the marginal gingiva has moved coronally, not apically. Deeper periodontal structures are not involved, and no migration of the JE has occurred.

A gingival pocket can be reversed to a healthy gingival sulcus by the patient's daily plaque control regimen supplemented by professional mechanical therapy. When oral bacterial plaque biofilm is controlled and calculus is removed, inflammation subsides and gingival enlargement decreases with a resultant decrease in gingival pocket depth.

Changes in texture and contour. Swelling or edema produces gingival texture and contour changes. In gingivitis, gingival texture becomes shiny and smooth (i.e., loss of stippling) from an increase in fluids, resulting in edema. Swelling from edema causes gingival contour changes attributable to enlargement. With severe enlargement, the coronal position of the gingival margin partially or almost covers the enamel and anatomic crown; however, enlargement more commonly

covers the gingival third of the tooth. Marginal gingiva can become bulbous, friable, rounded, or rolled, rather than knife-edged or slightly rounded and closely adapted to the tooth. In chronic inflammation, gingival surfaces may become nodular or fibrotic (Fig. 20.13).

Interdental papillae changes. While examining gingival color, texture, size, and shape, the clinician gives careful attention to the gingival papilla. When the col area is inflamed, epithelial and connective tissue layer degeneration can result in a blunted papilla, a split interdental papilla, or a cratered papilla (Figs. 20.14A–E; and 20.15). Such degradation usually indicates alveolar bone loss. Self-induced trauma from aggressive or improper use of dental floss, toothpicks, and other self-care aids may cause laceration of the gingival papilla.

Exudate. GCF is found in small quantities in healthy gingiva as it transports neutrophils. It significantly increases in the presence of inflammation. GCF is measured by isolating a site, drying it with air, and inserting a small paper strip into the pocket or sulcus for 3 to 5 seconds. Electronic devices can measure the GCF volume of the paper strip, although the clinical value of such a test renders it less relevant to practitioners than to researchers.

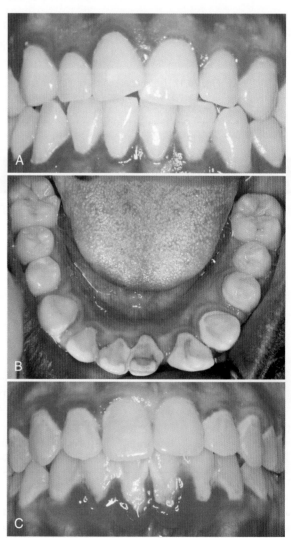

Fig. 20.13 (A) In edema, note the loss of stippling and erythema associated with plaque-induced gingivitis. (B) A type of lifesaver enlargement of the gingival margins exhibits changes in color, contour, and consistency. Note the large amount of supragingival calculus. (C) Diffuse enlargement and redness in the mandibular anterior, affecting the free and attached gingiva.

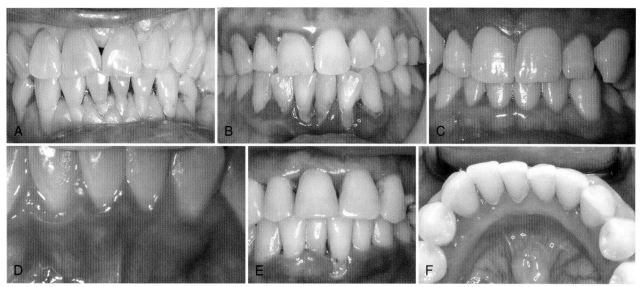

Fig. 20.14 (A) Significant recession of varying degrees is displayed throughout the mouth. Note composite restorations at the cervical areas on the teeth, along with the tobacco stain in the mandibular interproximal areas. (B) Severe inflammation is demonstrated in the mandibular anterior tissues. Note the blue color. Moderate erythema, edema, and loss of stippling are evident throughout. Note the significant recession caused by the calculus and oral biofilm in the mandibular anterior. (C) Generalized marginal erythema with shiny, smooth, enlarged gingival tissues is demonstrated. (D) Plaque-induced gingivitis is present, and interdental papillae have lost their knifelike shape and display puffy, rolled borders with erythematous tissues. (E) The loss of interdental papillae is evident in the anterior areas with significant recession on tooth 25. Note the pigmented gingival tissues. (F) Slight calculus in the mandibular anterior is displayed, with slight inflammation of the gingival tissues.

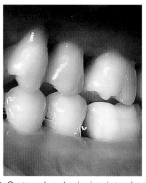

Fig. 20.15 Cratered and missing interdental papilla.

GCF is called *suppuration* when it is a clear, serous liquid and *purulent exudate* when it contains living and dead polymorphonuclear neutrophilic leukocytes (PMNs), bacteria, necrotic tissue, and enzymes. The increase of GCF volume in inflammation is known as an inflammatory exudate; however, it is not purulent because it does not contain pus. When **purulent exudate** is present, pus escapes the pocket during probing. Applying pressure to the base of a pocket with one's finger while moving coronally can express exudate. Although purulent exudate is a dramatic sign of inflammation, it does not indicate the severity of inflammation or pocket depth. Although some shallow and some deep pockets have suppuration, some do not. The presence of pus is, however, an indicator of active periodontal destruction. Suppuration correlates with specific attachment loss 2% to 30% of the time; therefore it is not a reliable indicator of active periodontal destruction. When suppuration or purulent exudate is observed, it is recorded for each area found and reassessed at subsequent visits.[5]

Documentation of the clinical gingival assessment. When assessing the gingiva (see Table 20.1), the clinician describes changes in gingival color, consistency, surface texture, contour, and size with regard to the following:

- Location (generalized throughout or localized to a specific area)
- Distribution (diffuse, marginal, or papillary)
- Severity (slight, moderate, or severe)
- Quality

The phrase, healthy periodontium with reduced support, is appropriate for sites that are disease free but have attachment loss and/or recession, resulting from previous episodes of periodontitis. For example, successfully treated sites fall into this category. When successfully treated periodontitis sites show signs of gingival inflammation in areas with ≤3 mm at subsequent appointments, the condition is termed dental biofilm–induced gingivitis on a reduced periodontium.[5]

Signs of Disease Progression (Periodontitis)

Periodontal pocket. **Probing depth** is the distance from the gingival margin to the base of the sulcus or pocket, as measured by the periodontal probe (Fig. 20.16). Unlike a gingival pocket or pseudopocket (Fig. 20.17B), a **periodontal pocket** is a pathologically deepened sulcus caused by the host, that is, the patient's inflammatory response to a biofilm-induced bacterial infection. It is characterized by a loss of connective tissue and alveolar bone supporting the tooth. When the coronal end of the JE (the surface that forms the actual sulcus or pocket bottom) contacts oral biofilm, it detaches from the tooth. At the same time, the apical end of the JE apically migrates, thus deepening the sulcus into a periodontal pocket. As the inflammatory process causes apical migration of the JE, it also causes gradual alveolar bone resorption, reducing bone support for the tooth (Fig. 20.16). Periodontal pockets are classified as follows:

- **Suprabony periodontal pocket** occurs when the JE has migrated below the CEJ but remains above the crest of the alveolar bone. Suprabony pockets are most commonly associated with horizontal bone loss (see Fig. 20.17C).

- **Intrabony periodontal pocket**, also known as infrabony pocket, occurs when the JE has migrated below the crest of the alveolar bone. Intrabony pockets are associated with vertical bone loss (see Fig. 20.17D).

Periodontal pockets may be present without obvious clinical signs of gingival inflammation or apparent in radiographic images. Therefore clinical probing is the only accurate way to assess the gingiva for the presence of periodontal pockets. The probe is gently "walked" in 1-mm increments along the epithelial attachment at the bottom of the pocket, keeping the tip in contact with the tooth (Fig. 20.18). Because periodontal pockets can develop at any point around a tooth, the probe must be gently inserted and the entire circumference of the tooth must be measured (Fig. 20.19). The clinician should record the deepest measurement for each of the six tooth surfaces on the patient's periodontal charting form. If calculus impedes insertion of the probe to the base of the pocket, then the probe is teased over the calculus, or the calculus is removed to allow insertion of the probe to the bottom of the pocket (Fig. 20.20).

Interproximal areas are the most difficult areas for patients to clean and, consequently, are the areas where periodontal pockets tend to form. To probe the interproximal area just apical to the contact, the probe is placed up against the interdental contact and mesially or distally tilted as appropriate to keep the tip touching the tooth (Fig. 20.21). Failure to tilt the probe enough to keep its tip in contact with the tooth surface is a common error and causes inaccurate interproximal probing readings (Fig. 20.22). The interproximal tooth surfaces should be probed from the facial and lingual sides of each tooth, as loss of attachment may differ at each site (Fig. 20.23).

Gingival recession. The causes of gingival recession are not clearly defined by current evidence. Once gingival recession exposes the root surface, the connective tissue cannot reattach because collagen breaks

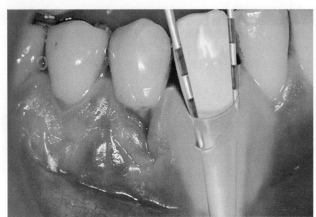

Fig. 20.16 Probing depth and attachment loss are measured on same tooth using the Marquis probe. Note that the probe on the left reveals a probe depth of 4 mm and a clinical attachment loss reading of 5 mm. The probe on the right reveals a probe reading within normal limits of 2 mm with no clinical attachment loss. Tooth 28 shows a good example of a gingival cleft. (Adapted from Newman MG, Takei HH, Klokkevold PR, Carranza F, eds. *Carranza's Clinical Periodontology*. 11th ed. Saunders; 2012.)

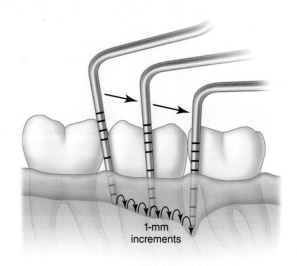

Fig. 20.18 The periodontal probe is "walked" around the tooth in 1-mm steps, establishing contact with the most apical attachment.

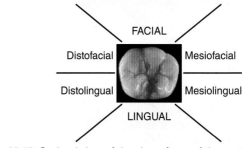

Fig. 20.19 Occlusal view of the six surfaces of the tooth measured for periodontal probing depths.

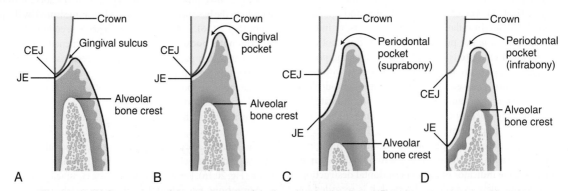

Fig. 20.17 (A) Comparison of the relationship of the junctional epithelium *(JE)* to the cementoenamel junction *(CEJ)* and alveolar bone in health. (B) Gingival pocket or pseudopocket. (C) Suprabony periodontal pocket (periodontitis); JE above alveolar bone. (D) Intrabony periodontal pocket (periodontitis); JE below alveolar bone crest.

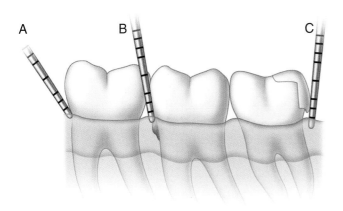

Fig. 20.20 Periodontal probing limitations. (A) Wrong angulation of probe. (B) Probe blocked by calculus. (C) Probe blocked by overhanging restoration. (From Newman MG, Takei HH, Klokkevold PR, Carranza F, eds. *Carranza's Clinical Periodontology*. 11th ed. Saunders; 2012.)

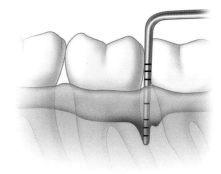

Fig. 20.22 The probe failed to be tilted far enough to keep its end in contact with the tooth surface. The probe is resting on the pocket wall, resulting in an inaccurate probing depth measurement. (Adapted from Newman MG, Takei HH, Klokkevold PR, Carranza F, eds. *Carranza's Clinical Periodontology*. 11th ed. Saunders; 2012.)

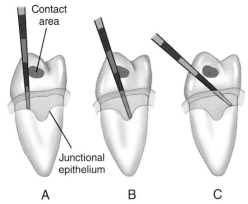

Fig. 20.21 (A) Incorrect technique for probing the interproximal area. (B) Correct technique. (C) Incorrect technique. (Adapted from Perry D, Beemsterboer P, Carranza FA. *Techniques and Theory of Periodontal Instrumentation*. Saunders; 1990.)

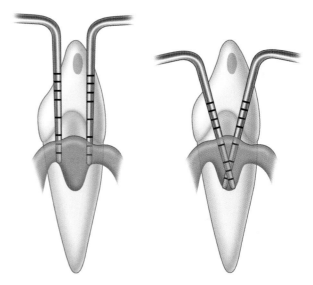

Fig. 20.23 Proximal view of periodontal probing. Vertical insertion of the probe *(left)* may not detect interdental craters; oblique positioning of the probe *(right)* reaches the depth of the crater.

down when exposed to the oral environment, and cementoblasts grow only on root surfaces adjacent to the PDL. Areas of recession may be sensitive because the exposed cementum may be lost, uncovering the underlying dentin. Exposed dentinal tubules are mechanically stimulated (e.g., by tooth brushing), chemically stimulated (e.g., by acidic foods or bacterial plaque biofilm), or thermally stimulated (e.g., by cold air or food at extreme temperatures), producing dentinal hypersensitivity (see Chapter 42).

Noting areas of dentinal hypersensitivity on the patient record provides information for planning dental hygiene therapy; for example, patients may require more time, a local anesthetic agent, or nitrous oxide–oxygen analgesia to provide comfortable and effective instrumentation (see Chapters 23, 43, and 44). During the assessment interview, collecting information about the patient's dentinal sensitivity will assist the hygienist in determining an effective care plan. Providing the patient with desensitizing self-care products and in-office chemotherapeutic agents may provide relief from thermal sensitivity. Patients appreciate the dental hygienist's caring attitude, information, and efforts to reduce their discomfort.

Clinical attachment loss. CAL, the position of the attached periodontal tissues at the base of the pocket, is determined by comparing the distance from the CEJ with the base of the sulcus or pocket (Fig.

20.24). Location of the gingival margin is important in determining the CAL, which includes periodontal pocket depth and recession measurements, if present. When the gingival margin is located at the CEJ, the CAL and the pocket depth are equal. When the gingival margin is apical to the CEJ, the CAL is greater than the pocket depth and equal to the measured amount of recession added to the pocket depth. If a patient has generalized 3 mm of recession and 3-mm pocket readings, then the recession and the pocket readings are added together to obtain the actual CAL of 6 mm (see Fig. 20.24). If these readings are not added together, then the patient may be classified as having slight periodontal disease when 6-mm CAL would actually indicate severe disease. With digital software, this calculation is automatically computed when the gingival margin measurements are entered.

In cases of gingival inflammation or hypertrophy, when the gingival margin is coronal to the CEJ, CAL is less than the pocket depth. To obtain an accurate CAL, enlarged gingival margins above the CEJ must be measured and subtracted from the periodontal pocket measurement (see Fig. 20.24). For example, if a patient has generalized

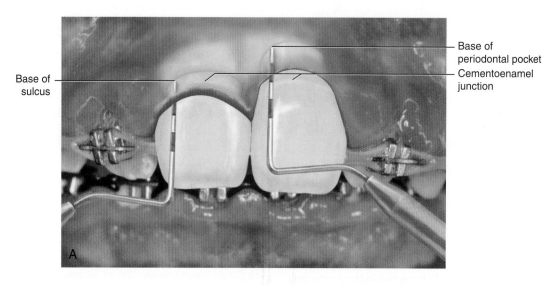

Clinical Attachment Levels

Inflamed gingival margin

Gingival margin
3 mm above CEJ

Pocket reading
6 mm

GM subtracted from pocket reading
(6 − 3 = 3 mm clinical attachment level)

B

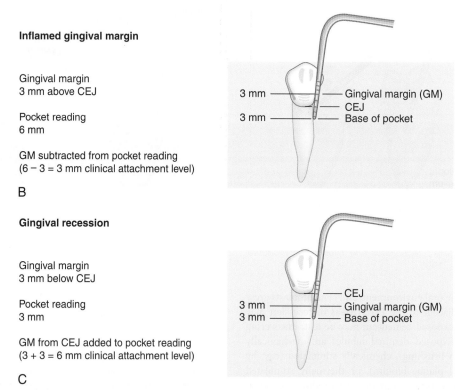

Gingival recession

Gingival margin
3 mm below CEJ

Pocket reading
3 mm

GM from CEJ added to pocket reading
(3 + 3 = 6 mm clinical attachment level)

C

Fig. 20.24 Measuring clinical attachment levels. (A) On the maxillary right central incisor, the inflamed gingival margin hides the cementoenamel junction (CEJ), resulting in a 4-mm pseudopocket (gingival pocket). No clinical attachment loss and no bone loss are exhibited. The base of the sulcus is in a normal relationship to the CEJ and alveolar bone. On the maxillary left central incisor, the gingival margin has receded 2 to 3 mm, exposing the CEJ, and bone loss is evident. Clinical attachment loss of 6 mm and a 5-mm periodontal pocket are demonstrated. (B) Gingival margin is 3 mm above the CEJ (inflamed gingival margin). (C) Gingival margin is 3 mm below the CEJ (gingival recession). (A, Adapted from Newman MG, Takei HH, Klokkevold PR, Carranza F, eds. *Carranza's Clinical Periodontology*. 11th ed. Saunders; 2012.)

6-mm probe readings but 4 mm of the enlarged gingiva is coronal to the CEJ, then the actual CAL is 2 mm. If this 2 mm is not subtracted from the probe reading, then a realistic assessment cannot be obtained. In this situation, a patient with only 2 mm of attachment loss may be misclassified as having more bone loss than has actually occurred. This measurement is achieved with periodontal probe measuring from the CEJ to the gingival crest. Using radiographic images and careful instrumentation will help determine the subgingival location of the CEJ.

Attachment loss (disease activity), not periodontal pocket readings, indicates the progression of periodontal disease and is considered its defining feature. Consequently, regular documentation of comprehensive periodontal assessment in the patient record is important to track periodontal disease activity.

Class	Description
Class I	Involvement is beginning.
	Concavity of furcation can be detected with an explorer or probe, but it cannot be entered.
	Cannot be radiographically detected.
Class II	Clinician can enter the furcation from one aspect with a probe or explorer but cannot penetrate through to the opposite side.
Class III	A through-and-through furcation is involved, but the furcation is still covered by soft tissue.
	A definite radiolucency in the furcation area is visible on a radiographic image.
Class IV	A through-and-through furcation is involved, but the furcation is not covered by soft tissue.
	Furcation is clinically opened and exposed.

Note: Some classifications combine Classes III and IV into a single Class III.

TABLE 20.8 Classification of Mobility

Class	Description
Class I	Tooth can be moved ≤1 mm in any direction.
Class II	Tooth can be moved >1 mm in any direction but is not depressible in the socket.
Class III	Tooth can be moved in a buccolingual direction and is depressible in the socket.

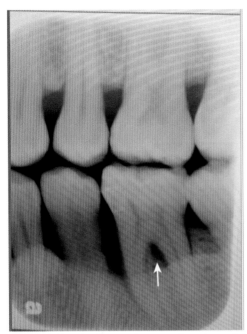

Fig. 20.25 Vertical bitewing image shows a triangular radiolucency in the bifurcation area of the mandibular first molar, indicating furcation involvement *(arrows)*.

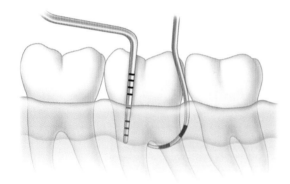

Fig. 20.26 Close-up picture of a Michigan O Probe with Williams markings *(left)* and a Nabers probe *(right)*.

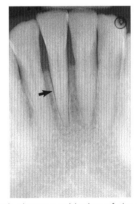

Fig. 20.27 Radiograph shows a widening of the periodontal ligament associated with occlusal trauma *(arrow)*.

Furcation involvement. **Furcation involvement**[14] (or loss of the interradicular bone and PDL attachment of multirooted teeth) is identified, classified, and monitored (Figs. 20.25 and 20.26 and Table 20.7). The patient is informed about areas of furcation involvement and taught home-care techniques to manage these areas (see Chapter 25). The Nabers furcation probe often is used to detect and measure furcation involvement (Fig. 20.26). Radiographic images confirm but do not always accurately reveal this condition until they are severely involved (see Fig. 20.25). Attention to root morphologic structure and instrumentation are important considerations for providing effective periodontal therapy in furcation areas. More information is provided in Chapters 28, 29, and 30.

Tooth mobility. Tooth **mobility** is the degree to which a tooth is able to move in a horizontal or apical direction. Although caused by the loss of PDL and bone support in periodontitis, tooth mobility varies according to diet and stress. Children, young adults, and some women exhibit more tooth movement than individuals in other groups. Although tooth mobility is not a cause of periodontal disease, it may contribute to it. Therefore mobility is evaluated and documented as an important

aspect of periodontal assessment. To test for mobility, the practitioner places an instrument handle on the lingual surface of the tooth and gently applies pressure from the fulcrum finger on the facial surface with another instrument, and then vice versa, to rock the tooth in a horizontal motion (e.g., the handles of a periodontal probe and a mouth mirror). The feeling of movement is most acute at the contact points between two teeth. Mobility classification should be recorded on the dental chart to allow comparative readings at successive appointments (Table 20.8).

Fremitus. **Fremitus** is the vibration or movement of the teeth when in contacting positions from the patient's own occlusal forces. To assess fremitus, the clinician places his or her index finger along the facial aspects of the cervical one-third of each maxillary tooth, and the patient is asked to tap the teeth together. Teeth that are displaced are then identified. At times, a widened PDL space also will be visible radiographically due to excessive occlusal forces (see Fig. 20.27).

Mucogingival conditions and inadequate attached gingiva.
Mucogingival conditions, as discussed earlier in this chapter, are assessed through clinical examination for recession, frenum pulling on the gingiva, and the width of the attached gingiva (Fig. 20.28). A periodontal probe is used as needed to measure the attached gingiva where a potential problem is observed (Fig. 20.29).

Areas with a limited zone of attached gingiva, termed **inadequately attached gingiva** (IAG), are noted, shown to the patient, and explained during the periodontal assessment (see Fig. 20.28). To measure the amount of attached gingiva, a periodontal probe is used to measure the total width of the gingiva from the free gingival margin to the MGJ. Next, the periodontal probing depth is obtained and subtracted from the total width of the gingiva (see Fig. 20.29). The width of attached gingiva is not measured on the palatal side of maxillary teeth because of the inability to differentiate between where attached gingiva ends and palatal tissues begin. IAG exists when less than 1 mm of keratinized attached gingiva is present. Areas with IAG are often sensitive to the patient, are difficult to maintain, and can develop into a mucogingival problem because the thin zone of attachment usually reflects a reduced blood supply and a potential for quick loss of supporting bone and connective tissue. Recession and high frenum or muscle attachments may add to the reduction of alveolar mucosa. These chronic conditions must be recorded and monitored. Although good oral hygiene can maintain periodontal health with almost no alveolar gingiva, high

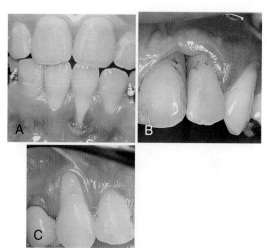

Fig. 20.28 Mucogingival defects. (A) Irregular gingival contours and recession are evident with severe gingival inflammation. (B) Gingival recession, proximal crater formation, and chronic inflammation with fibrotic tissue are exhibited. The bottom of the pocket is beyond the mucogingival junction. (C) Recession on the maxillary canine with a shallow sulcus is present and attached gingiva is absent. (Courtesy Dr. Kenneth Marinak, Adjunct Clinical Instructor, Gene W. Hirschfeld School of Dental Hygiene, Old Dominion University, Norfolk, Virginia.)

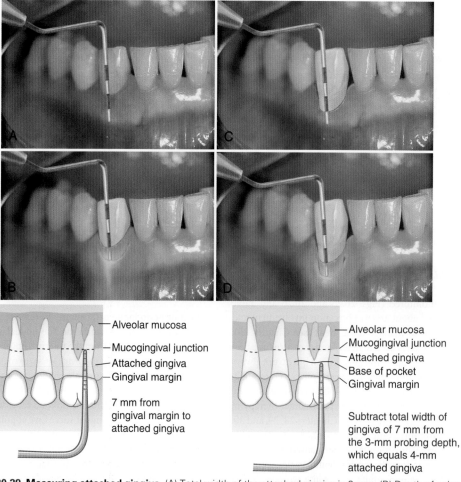

Fig. 20.29 Measuring attached gingiva. (A) Total width of the attached gingiva is 6 mm. (B) Depth of sulcus is 3 mm, with no clinical attachment loss. Therefore 3 mm of attached gingiva is still evident. (C) Total width of attached gingiva is 3 mm. (D) Depth of pocket is 3 mm and 6 mm of clinical attachment loss is evident. Therefore no attached gingiva is demonstrated. (E) Diagram illustrates how attached gingiva is determined.

PROCEDURE 20.1 Periodontal Charting and Assessment

Equipment

Personal protective equipment
Periodontal probe
Nabers probe
Mouth mirror
Dental light
Compressed air

Steps

Use direct and indirect lighting, mouth mirror, and compressed air to determine findings.

Use proper patient and operator body mechanics, appropriate PPE, and infection control protocols. Ask the patient about their health history and any existing conditions.

Gingival recession: Use the periodontal probe to determine the location of the gingival margin in relationship to the cementoenamel junction (CEJ). Recession of ≥1 mm is recorded in the dental chart (see Fig. 20.24).

Measure the periodontal probing depths with the periodontal probe.

a. Insert the tip into the sulcus until gently resting on the junctional epithelium (JE); maintain the tip against the tooth structure.

b. Slightly angle the probe on the proximal surfaces to reach directly apical to the contact point (see Figs. 20.22 and 20.23).

c. "Walk" the tip along the JE in 1-mm increments (see Fig. 20.18).

d. Recognize when deposits, dental restorations, or anatomy obstruct probe measurement readings; manipulate the probe around these obstructions (see Fig. 20.20).

e. Record the locations of bleeding points and suppuration.

f. Record the deepest readings for each of six tooth surfaces: distofacial (DF), facial (F), mesial-facial (MF), distolingual (DL), lingual (L), and mesial-lingual (ML).

g. Where recession is present, record all measurements to reflect the accurate clinical attachment level (CAL).

Furcation involvement: Using a Nabers probe, determine the location and classification of involvement that is present and record (see Table 20.7).

Mobility: Use the handles of two instruments to rock the tooth; classify the amount of movement obtained (see Table 20.8).

Evaluate drifting, extrusion, and misalignment.

Evaluate areas of food impaction.

Evaluate open contacts with dental floss.

Assess fremitus, occlusal disharmonies, and wear facets (see Table 20.4).

Gingival Examination

Record gingival disease entity, severity, and location (see Table 20.2).

Use the correct dental terminology when describing gingival severity and location (see Table 20.6).

Amount of attached gingiva: Subtract the depth of the pocket from the distance from the gingival margin to the mucogingival line (see Fig. 20.28); the difference is the amount of attached gingiva.

<2 mm should be noted as inadequately attached gingiva (IAG).

<1 mm should be noted as no attached gingiva (NAG) in the apical area of the facial aspect of the tooth.

Correlate the radiographic and clinical readings (see Box 20.5).

Periodontal Examination in Periodontal Chart

Record the periodontal status using the appropriate 2017 AAP-EFP periodontal classification.

Record the severity of periodontitis (slight, moderate, or severe).

Record the location of periodontitis (generalized or localized).

Record the service in the dental record under "Services Rendered" (e.g., 8/15/18: Periodontal and risk assessment completed. Explained assessment findings to the patient. Recommended a referral to a periodontist. Provided treatment alternatives, risks, and an opportunity to ask questions.)

AAP, American Academy of Periodontology, *EFP,* European Federation of Periodontology.

---

frenum attachments or the use of the tooth as a crown and bridge abutment may indicate surgical intervention to widen the zone of attached gingiva (Procedure 20.1).

RADIOGRAPHIC ASSESSMENT

Clinical Use of Radiographic Images

Periodontal assessment for a new patient includes an individualized radiographic examination, preferably a full-mouth series, or in specific cases depending on the patient's comprehensive dental needs posterior bitewings with a panoramic examination or posterior bitewings and selected periapical images. A full-mouth intraoral radiographic examination is preferred when clinical evidence of generalized periodontal disease exists.[14] At a recall or periodontal maintenance appointment, the dental hygienist uses clinical judgment to determine the type of radiographic images indicated for the evaluation of periodontal disease. Imaging may consist of, but is not limited to, selected bitewing and/or periapical images of the areas where periodontal disease (other than nonspecific gingivitis) can be clinically demonstrated.

Good-quality radiographic images are indispensable in assessing the amount of alveolar bone present, as well as the pattern, location, and extent of alveolar bone loss. Radiographic images are also helpful in identifying local bacterial biofilm retentive factors involved in periodontal disease, such as calculus and bone loss (Fig. 20.30), furcation involvement, overhanging restorative margins, and dental caries

(Fig. 20.31). Posttreatment radiographic images also can permit the evaluation of the removal of subgingival calculus and overhanging restorations. Not all periodontal defects are visualized on radiographs because the image that is produced is a two-dimensional (2-D) representation of a three-dimensional (3-D) object. Radiographs provide images of alveolar bone changes from past disease and a history of bone destruction, but they do not visualize current disease activity. In addition, soft-tissue changes are not reflected on radiographic images. Because of these limitations, radiographs are always used in conjunction with a thorough clinical assessment. Box 20.5 provides a list of periodontal conditions observed on radiographic images.

Before any radiographic examination, a clinical examination and risk assessment of the patient are conducted. Care is taken to consider the medical, dental, and pharmacologic histories; clinical assessment data; safety concerns; and radiographic history when exposing a patient to radiation.

Selection criteria for patient radiographic exposures should be guided by the use of ALARA (as low as reasonably achievable) principle and are available from various sources. The ADA has collaborated with the U.S. Food and Drug Administration (FDA) to develop the most widely used guidelines.[14] Dental office radiographic exposure policies that fail to recognize the individual's risk for oral diseases, but rather require annual or biannual radiographic images for every patient, are not following the current standard of care practices that optimize patient care and limit radiation exposure.[15]

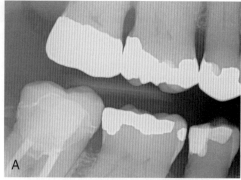

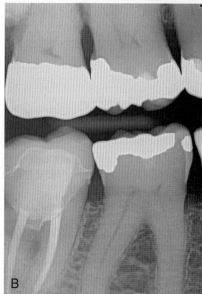

Fig. 20.30 Vertical and horizontal bitewing radiographic images show generalized interproximal bone loss in mandibular left posterior sextants. (A) Horizontal bitewing radiographic image shows calculus tooth #18D. (B) Film placement of a vertical bitewing radiographic image is incorrect, preventing posttreatment evaluation of calculus removal and furcation assessment.

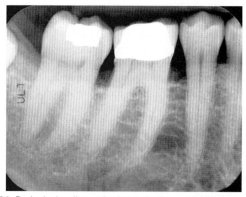

Fig. 20.31 Periapical radiograph shows horizontal bone loss with early furcation involvement on tooth 30.

Selecting Types and Techniques

Periapical and/or vertical bitewing radiographic images provide increased visualization of the periodontium when compared with horizontal bitewing radiographs. Vertical bitewing radiographs are recommended instead of horizontal bitewing images because moderate-to-severe bone loss cannot be adequately imaged on a

| BOX 20.5 | Periodontal Conditions Observed on Radiographic Images |

- Tooth anatomy and crown-to-root ratio
- Confirmation of clinical findings and topography of root surfaces
- Status of the lamina dura
- Remaining bone height
- Changes of periodontal ligament space
- Local irritants such as calculus and overhanging restorations
- Pattern or extent of disease
- Possible furcation involvement
- Disease progression or remission by serial radiographic studies

horizontal bitewing radiograph. When a sensor is positioned vertically instead of horizontally, the area of bone on the radiograph increases by more than 1 cm (Fig. 20.32).

Standard panoramic projections are not recommended for evaluating periodontal disease. Magnification encountered with this type of imaging minimizes its usefulness in accurately detecting bone changes. The paralleling technique is recommended for periodontal disease assessment rather than the bisecting angle technique. The paralleling technique produces more anatomically correct images with more accurate crestal bone height. The bisecting angle technique can create a foreshortened appearance, resulting in an image that may show more or less bone than is actually present.

Three-Dimensional Imaging

New technologies are constantly being explored to facilitate and advance periodontal assessment. One of these recent developments is 3-D imaging or **cone-beam computed tomography** (CBCT). CBCT is similar to a conventional computed tomography (CT) scan, but it is more compact and faster while also greatly reducing the radiation dose.[9] Cone beam technology produces less radiation exposure than conventional CT but significantly more than traditional dental x-ray imaging. Although 2-D radiographs and periodontal probing are currently the evidence-based gold standard for comprehensive periodontal assessment, 3-D imaging is gaining widespread use for implant placement. CBCT has been shown to be useful in periodontal-orthodontic treatment, identifying advanced furcation lesions, root fractures, and root resorption. As new software is developed, this procedure has the potential to improve treatment planning and the standards of care.

Radiographic Interpretation

Radiographically determining changes in the alveolar bone associated with periodontal disease is based on the appearance of the crestal lamina dura and the alveolar bone. In a healthy periodontal environment, the crestal lamina dura radiographically appears as a continuous, radiopaque line running parallel to an imaginary line drawn between the CEJs of the adjacent teeth. In a healthy periodontium, the difference in the distance between the normal alveolar bone crest and the CEJ can range from 0.4 to 2.9 mm. In general, however, a distance greater than 2 mm from the CEJ to the crestal bone is considered evidence of disease. An early radiographic change associated with periodontal disease is a fuzziness or break in the continuity of the lamina dura at the mesial or distal aspect of the interdental area. This change results from a loss of crestal density. As inflammation spreads, a wedge-shaped widening of the PDL occurs, exhibiting a radiolucent area between the tooth and the crestal bone, known as triangulation. The V of the wedge of the triangle points apically. As inflammation spreads deeper into the connective tissue, bone degenerates with a subsequent reduction in bone height.

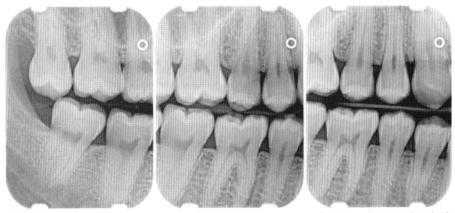

Fig. 20.32 Vertical bitewing images can be used to cover a larger area of the alveolar bone than horizontal bitewing images. (Courtesy Idaho State University, Dental Hygiene, Pocatello, Idaho.)

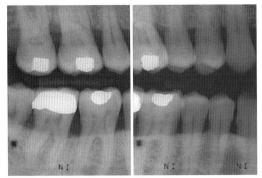

Fig. 20.33 Generalized horizontal bone loss in posterior teeth. Furcation involvement in mandibular molars.

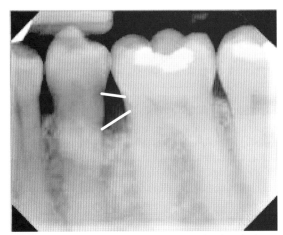

Fig. 20.34 Vertical bone loss, with lines showing level of cemento-enamel junction and bone loss.

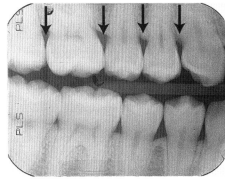

Fig. 20.35 Normal bone is parallel with the bone level and the cemento-enamel junctions *(arrows)* on teeth 2, 3, 4, and 5 and is often confused with bone loss.

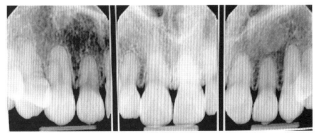

Fig. 20.36 Blunted roots in maxillary anterior teeth.

The pattern of bone loss is described as either horizontal or vertical. The CEJ of adjacent teeth can be used to determine the type of bone loss.
- When bone loss is >2 mm and is parallel to the CEJ of the adjacent teeth, horizontal bone loss is present (Fig. 20.33).
- When bone loss is >2 mm and is diagonally oriented to the CEJ of adjacent teeth, vertical bone loss is present (Fig. 20.34).

If the teeth have erupted at varying levels or are tilted, the lamina dura crest will be oriented slanted to match the variation in crown level. Normal slanting may be confused with bone loss (Fig. 20.35). Bone loss resulting from the inflammation of periodontitis typically does not uniformly occur throughout the mouth, the quadrant, or even on the same

tooth; loss in one area may be more severe than in another. Severity is assessed as a percentage loss of the normal amount of bone. To obtain a percentage loss, the radiographic image and probe are used to measure the total root length—from the CEJ to the root apex. Next, the distance from the CEJ to alveolar crest is determined. The percentage of bone loss is a ratio of these two measurements; that is, the distance from the CEJ to alveolar crest is divided by the total root length. For example, a 6-mm distance from the CEJ to the crest of the bone with a 17-mm root length would equal a 25% bone loss (6 mm divided by 17 mm) (see Table 20.3). Distribution of bone loss should be described as localized or generalized, including the type, vertical or horizontal, as well as a statement of its severity—mild, moderate, or severe (e.g., periodontitis, with generalized mild horizontal bone loss and localized moderate vertical bone loss).

Clinical significance: A patient with short, blunted roots and 6-mm periodontal pockets would not have the same ratio of root-to-bone support as a patient with long roots and a 6-mm pocket (Fig. 20.36). The alveolar support for teeth with short roots would increase the risk of tooth loss from periodontitis; the root length would be less, increasing the risk of tooth loss from periodontitis.

Furcation Involvement

Radiographic images are used to detect changes to interradicular bone in the furcations of multirooted teeth (see Figs. 20.31 and 20.33). When bone in a furcation is destroyed, it appears as a radiolucency in the furcal area. Lack of radiolucency in the furcation does not mean that the disease has not spread to the area. However, the presence of radiolucency in the furcal area does indicate bone loss. The absence of radiographically visible bone loss does not rule out the possibility of furcation involvement. More often, interradicular bone loss is clinically greater than what is radiographically visible. Clinical examinations must always be included to ensure a true representation of furcation involvement. Exposing radiographic images at differing angles also may assist in detecting furcation involvement.

Limitations of Radiographic Images

Radiographs characteristically reveal less bone loss than what has actually occurred; early bone changes are not radiographically visible. Typically, 30% of the bone mineral must be destroyed before it can be seen on a radiographic image. Radiographs confirm clinical findings. For example, if the dental hygienist obtains probing depth readings of 2 to 3 mm but observes bone loss on the radiograph, then probing the depth and recession measurements should be rechecked. In this case, radiographic images provide a check of clinical findings for periodontal probing.

Radiographic images are a record of the patient's periodontal status, showing the history of disease progression, and they provide a basis for comparison with new findings, allowing the dental hygienist to monitor bone levels over time. As part of periodontal risk assessment, the absence of bone loss is associated with a lower risk of future periodontal destruction. However, the presence of bone loss on a radiographic image does not indicate that the patient will experience continued destruction; rather, it indicates an increased risk of future bone loss.

Standardized radiographic images of similar projections are most helpful in making comparisons and for providing objective documentation of clinical findings. For example, periapical projections of posterior teeth should not be compared with subsequent bitewing radiographs because an accurate comparison of bone level cannot be made with two different projection angles. Periodontal probing depths and other clinical findings are subjective assessments, but radiographs present objective data that two or more clinicians can observe at the same time.

Limitations of radiographic imaging in periodontal assessment are as follows:

- Projection factors such as cone-to-film or receptor distance, angulation, technique, and film or receptor positioning can distort or obscure radiographic images. For example, healthy alveolar bone is apically located evenly between 1 and 2 mm to the CEJ, and the alveolar crest should parallel an imaginary line drawn from the CEJ of one tooth to the CEJ of the adjacent tooth. In a radiographic image, this bone position may be distorted by x-ray angulation, erroneously suggesting vertical bone loss.
- Exposure errors such as cone cuts and imbalance of kilovolt peak (kVp) and milliamperage (mA) disguise anatomy and pathosis. Proper exposure uses the widest range of contrast (grays) to ensure that minute changes in bone density and mineralized calculus are shown on the x-ray image.
- Facial and lingual supporting bone are obscured by the radiodense tooth structure. Therefore facial and lingual bone loss cannot be detected on radiographic images.
- Early interdental bone loss is not detectable on radiographs because horizontal alveolar bone loss may not be seen until a significant

percentage of the original bone height and density is lost. By the time bone loss is radiographically observed, it is so far advanced that it is easily clinically detected by probing.

- Bony interdental craters, resulting from vertical bone loss, are not well imaged because facial and lingual ridges of the teeth may be superimposed and because the dense facial and lingual walls of bone obscure the crater. Interdental craters are therefore detected only with the periodontal probe.
- Radiographic images do not show soft tissues or connective tissue attachment and consequently cannot show soft-tissue changes. Pockets cannot be measured from radiographs except by using radiopaque markers, such as a periodontal probe or silver point placed at the depth of the sulcus before exposure.
- Although radiographic images that visualize such conditions as a moth-eaten alveolar crest, discontinuous lamina dura, increased trabeculation, and thickened PDL space suggest periodontal abnormalities, they are not indicators of active periodontitis.
- Although all teeth are radiographically examined for the presence of calculus, radiographic images are not the best indicators of calculus because only highly mineralized deposits may be seen as radiopacities. The best means of detecting calculus is by utilizing an explorer.

ASSESSMENT OF PERIODONTAL DISEASE ACTIVITY

Periodontal disease progression is the pathologic process during which connective tissue attachment at the most apical portion of a periodontal pocket is destroyed. Related to attachment loss is the apical migration of the JE and resorption of alveolar bone. Progression of most forms of periodontitis appears to be associated with qualitative changes in the subgingival flora. Currently, no diagnostic tests reliably identify progressing periodontitis lesions other than longitudinal assessments of radiographic images and probing attachment levels. Disease activity can be measured by host-modulation tests, such as those that test for collagenase enzymes associated with the breakdown of connective tissue. In some circumstances, supplemental testing of the GCF and subgingival microflora are performed, although the usefulness of this information in clinical practice is limited.

Measurement of Attachment Loss

An increase in the distance measured from the CEJ to the base of the sulcus or pocket is currently the best measure for disease progression. Measurement error relates to the fact that the probe's penetration can vary with the design and material used, the insertion force, and the degree of tissue inflammation. In addition, positioning the periodontal probe in exactly the same position from one appointment to another and between clinicians is difficult. The use of standardized equipment and techniques minimizes these limitations.

Clinical Signs of Inflammation

Redness, swelling, BOP, and suppuration have relatively good diagnostic value. Whereas BOP may have some clinical value as an indicator of increased risk of progression when found in conjunction with periodontal pockets, the continuous absence of BOP is a reliable indicator that periodontal health will be maintained.

Supplemental Diagnostic Tests
Salivary Diagnostics

Recent advances in genomic technologies allow for possible saliva-based diagnostics.[16] Although bacterial and genetic tests that use salivary diagnostics are available, more research is needed to determine their practical value in clinical practice. Some salivary diagnostics for periodontal disease are commercially available to identify bacteria associated with periodontal disease. Fragments of bacterial DNA are used in hybridization reactions to probe for complementary DNA in subgingival biofilm samples. In-office tests, although available, do not determine antibiotic sensitivity and only identify organisms for which the tests are sensitive.

GCF flow increases with inflammation. The Periotron, a device that measures GCF, has been used in research but has minimal clinical value other than detecting the presence of fluid in the pocket. GCF contains disease markers, such as inflammatory cytokines (e.g., PGE_2), enzymes (e.g., aspartate aminotransferase, alkaline phosphatase), and tissue breakdown products (e.g., proteinases), that are associated with periodontal disease progression. Tests to identify and quantify these markers in the GCF may prove useful in the future diagnosis of periodontitis because of their association with active disease. Research is ongoing for valid, cost-effective diagnostic testing devices.

Microbiologic Cultural Analysis

Subgingival plaque is sampled and cultured in the laboratory to determine the presence of specific microorganisms—marker bacteria—associated with the progression of periodontitis (e.g., *A. actinomycetemcomitans* and *P. gingivalis*). The advantage of microbiologic testing is its ability to determine antibiotic susceptibility and resistance; however, this method is time consuming and costly and relies on living anaerobic bacterial samples that must be specially handled to survive transport. Consequently, this test is not readily used in private practice settings.

Dental Implants

Implants are monitored for peri-implant health, peri-implant mucositis, peri-implantitis, or peri-implant soft and hard tissue deficiencies. Previous periodontal disease, poor plaque control, smoking, genetic factors, diabetes, residual cement, and excessive occlusal stress are factors increasing the risk of perimucositis and peri-implantitis.

Factors to consider when assessing implant periodontal status include the following[17]:

- BOP
- Suppuration
- Probing depth
- Radiographic bone loss
- Implant mobility

Periodontal probes are used for periodontal assessment of implants (Fig. 20.37). Although some clinicians prefer flexible plastic, gold, or titanium probes to avoid scratching the implant surface, the use of a gentle technique and light pressure is more important than the material used to construct the probe. Signs of bleeding and redness indicate perimucositis, but the presence of exudate should alert the hygienist to the need for further evaluation. A baseline periapical radiograph parallel to the implant is used to determine bone level at initial placement. Subsequent similar radiographic images provide a comparison of bone levels for evaluation of peri-implantitis. Movement of a dental implant may indicate loose or broken components or failed osseointegration. True implant mobility is caused by advanced bone loss.

The dental hygienist must be aware of a patient's placement and location of implants because of the necessity to use instrumentation specifically designed for implants. (See Chapter 31 for more information on implants and peri-implant care.)

RISK FACTORS

Risk factors are attributes or exposures of an individual that significantly increase the risk for the onset and/or progression of a specific

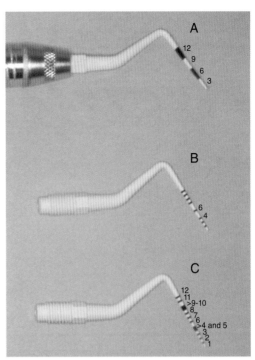

Fig. 20.37 Plastic periodontal probe with three different types of interchangeable tips. (A) Markings at every 3 mm. (B) Markings at 1 to 10 mm, with 4 and 6 absent. (C) Markings at 1 to 12 mm, with 4- to 5-mm band and 9- to 10-mm band.

disease and may affect treatment outcomes. Assessment and analysis of risk factors provide information about a patient's susceptibility to periodontal disease beyond traditional clinical assessment parameters. Many host, environmental, and systemic risk factors modify the body's response to bacterial pathogens in oral biofilm, resulting in a significant variability in individual susceptibility to periodontal disease, its progression, and an individual patient's response to treatment.[2] The number and type of patient risk factors modify the onset, degree, and severity of periodontal disease (Box 20.6). Risk factor assessment is important because conditions associated with increased risks may affect treatment, patient education, and patient management. A clinician bases risk factor assessment on information obtained through patient interviews, through the evaluation of the patient's comprehensive medical dental, and pharmacologic history, and with the clinical and radiographic examinations of the periodontium. Social determinants of health can be considered risk factors since they encompass where patients are born, live, and work and their educational and income level. Comprehensive periodontal assessment, including risk assessment and social determinants of health, is a component of the dental hygiene process of care and provides the basis for formulating a dental hygiene diagnosis, planning, and implementation, as well as the framework for the development of treatment plans that target the risk factors, creating opportunities for enhanced treatment outcomes. Informing and educating patients about their periodontal disease and specific risk factors provides them autonomy with the ability to make informed oral healthcare decisions (Boxes 20.7 to 20.9).

Modifiable Risks

Dental biofilm–induced gingivitis and periodontitis is primarily caused by the host's response to dental plaque bacteria; however, there are risk factors that modify the effect of the dysbiotic plaque biofilm and its effect on the periodontium. The two primary risk factors affecting the progression of periodontitis and the outcomes of treatment are smoking and undiagnosed or poorly controlled diabetes or hyperglycemia. These factors, plus the patient's phenotype, the periodontal destruction in relation to the patient's age, and the amount of biofilm, are included in the grading of periodontitis (see Table 20.4).

Bacterial Plaque Biofilm, Clinical Attachment Loss, and Age

A complex dysbiotic dental plaque biofilm containing anaerobic, Gram-negative bacteria must be present for inflammatory periodontal disease to occur (see Chapter 18). These periodontopathic bacteria, also known as *putative bacteria,* can cause direct tissue damage, resulting from the production of bacterial enzymes and toxins, and can play a major role in the immune system's response and ultimate destruction of periodontal tissues. Nonetheless, the dental hygienist considers bacterial plaque biofilm and calculus, which are always laden with bacteria, in the cause and treatment of periodontal disease. The clinician correlates the signs of periodontal disease, such as inflammatory changes in the gingiva, BOP, CAL, and periodontal pockets, with the presence of deposits.

Previous periodontitis and CAL are risk factors for progressing periodontitis without supportive periodontal (maintenance) therapy. The amount of CAL, radiographic bone loss, and tooth loss due to periodontitis in an individual patient are factors in the staging of periodontitis (see Table 20.3). Severity is determined as follows:

- Incipient (Stage I). CAL 1 to 2 mm, bone loss coronal $\frac{1}{3}$ (<15%), and no teeth lost due to periodontitis
- Moderate (Stage II). CAL 3 to 4 mm, bone loss coronal $\frac{1}{3}$ (15% to 33%), and ≤4 teeth lost due to periodontitis
- Severe (Stages III and IV). CAL ≥5 mm, bone loss extending to middle $\frac{1}{3}$ or apical $\frac{1}{3}$ of the root, and ≥5 teeth lost due to periodontitis

The relationship between the amount and virility of dental biofilm and periodontal destruction affects the risk of disease progression and grading of periodontitis (see Table 20.4). If a patient has heavy plaque and very little CAL, the risk is low (grade A); a patient with biofilm apparently equal to the amount of destruction has a moderate risk (grade B); and a patient with destruction greater than the amount of bacterial biofilm has a high risk (grade C). The amount of dental biofilm present is directly related to poor oral hygiene. This relationship is discussed with patients to emphasize the importance of improved daily oral hygiene techniques. Age, a nonmodifiable risk factor, is also a risk because periodontal attachment loss is cumulative over time. It can be used as one factor to identify whether periodontal disease is rapidly progressive, thus indicating a patient at high risk. If a patient has significant attachment loss at a young age, the progression has been rapid (grade C), whereas incipient attachment loss in an older adult would indicate slow progression of periodontitis.

Tobacco Use

Tobacco use in all forms is one of the most significant risk factors for periodontal disease. Tobacco users have more rapid progression and greater CAL and bone loss, dental calculus formation, and tooth loss than nontobacco users. Heavy smokers (more than 10 cigarettes per day) have greater odds for more severe attachment loss. Surgical and nonsurgical interventions are less effective in those who smoke, and disease recurrence is more common than in nonsmokers. The negative effects of tobacco use on the periodontium are linked with an altered host response, pathogenic bacterial composition, and direct local (heat and/or chemical) damage to periodontal tissues (see Chapter 37).

The effect of tobacco use is an important consideration in periodontal assessment. Clinically, tobacco users exhibit gingiva that is thickened and fibrotic with minimal redness, often without exhibiting obvious signs of inflammation. Reduction in gingival blood flow resulting from constriction of gingival blood vessels results in greater attachment loss and diminished signs of gingival inflammation. In individuals who use smokeless tobacco (chewing tobacco or snuff), gingival recession and oral mucosa tissue changes are common in areas of tobacco placement.

The length of time of tobacco use and the number of smoking exposures are important assessment factors. A direct relationship exists between an increased amount of smoking and an increased loss of attachment (called a *dose-response effect*) and vice versa. Smoking cessation and appropriate periodontal therapy seem to elicit a positive response on the periodontium, but previous damage is not reversible. Research also links secondhand smoke exposure to increased periodontal bone loss. Dental hygienists incorporate smoking cessation strategies into care plans as appropriate (see Chapter 37).

Hyperglycemia (Diabetes)

Diabetes is a chronic, life-long condition that involves increased blood glucose levels and insulin resistance. Irregularly controlled, poorly controlled, or uncontrolled diabetes is a strong risk factor for periodontal disease; however, controlled diabetes does not have the same association with periodontal disease. In type 1 and type 2 diabetes, gingivitis and periodontitis prevalence increases because control of the condition requires challenging dietary and lifestyle changes, regular monitoring, and sometimes medications. Information regarding the control of diabetes is considered during periodontal assessment because high blood glucose levels can increase susceptibility to infections, including periodontitis or periodontal abscesses. Those who maintain desired blood glucose levels have less periodontal attachment and bone loss and respond better to therapy as compared with those with poor control. Evidence also suggests a bidirectional relationship of diabetes and periodontal disease; periodontitis may adversely affect the control of diabetes, and the control of diabetes affects periodontal disease.[18] Research has shown that the risk for periodontitis proportionally increases as the glycemic control decreases. Assessing and monitoring a patient's glycemic control, in addition to improving health literacy, are current best practices for controlling blood sugar and improving oral indices (see Chapter 49 for more information).

Sex Steroid Hormones

Sex steroid hormones (e.g., estrogen, progesterone) have also been reported to cause gingival enlargement in some patients who use them. Gingival enlargement associated with these types of drugs or hormones is also related to an overproduction of collagen by gingival fibroblasts, is co-dependent on oral biofilm, and can generally be minimized with good biofilm control.

Leukemia

In acute leukemia, clinical findings include cervical lymphadenopathy, petechiae, gingival enlargement, and ulcers on the oral mucosa.[2] Severe and persistent inflammation exhibits a red or deep purple color, shiny surface, and spongy texture. In both acute and chronic leukemia, significant bleeding attributable to clotting deficiencies is a characteristic sign. Gingival enlargement may also be present. Local irritants can exacerbate oral manifestations, but they are not prerequisite.

Malnutrition

The role of nutrition in the initiation and progression of periodontal diseases is not clearly known; however, nutrition is related to tissue health and healing. The one nutritional deficiency that is well documented is an ascorbic acid (vitamin C) deficiency, known as scurvy, primarily found in populations without an adequate food supply or those on restricted diets. Oral manifestations of gingival inflammation

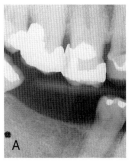
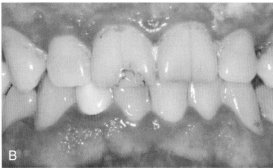
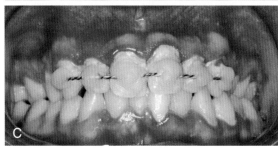

Fig. 20.38 (A) Overhanging restoration on the distal aspect of tooth No. 3, contributing to oral bone loss. (B) Tooth No. 26 crown margin and inflammation. (C) Orthodontic appliances and inadequate oral hygiene, resulting in inflammation.

are present, including severe redness, swelling, and enlarged gingiva that readily bleeds.

Oral Factors Enhancing Plaque Accumulation

The dental hygienist identifies local factors that may increase the accumulation of dental plaque biofilm.

Prominent Subgingival Restoration Margins

Because of the retentive nature of dental plaque biofilm, iatrogenic factors can contribute to the initiation and progression of periodontal disease. Overhanging restorations (Fig. 20.38A), subgingival margin placement of crowns and restorations (Fig. 20.38B), orthodontic appliances (Fig. 20.38C), and fixed or removable partial dentures are examples of iatrogenic factors that may contribute to disease progression because they increase biofilm retention. Local contributing factors serve as biofilm traps, making the removal of oral biofilm difficult and thus increasing the patient's susceptibility to periodontal disease. The dental hygienist works with the dentist and patient to modify these factors.

Hyposalivation

Risk assessment considers patient medications (see Chapter 15). Although some medications, such as tetracycline and nonsteroidal antiinflammatory drugs, have a beneficial effect on the periodontium, others have a negative effect. Xerostomia is associated with more than 500 medications, including diuretics, antihistamines, antipsychotics, antihypertensives, and analgesics. Decreased salivary flow facilitates the accumulation of bacterial plaque biofilm, especially at the cervical one-third of the tooth, and diminishes the immune system's ability to resolve gingival inflammation.

Drug-Influenced Gingival Enlargement

Several categories of drugs, such as calcium channel blockers (e.g., nifedipine), immunosuppressive drugs (e.g., cyclosporine), and anti-seizure drugs (e.g., phenytoin), can cause drug-influenced gingival enlargement.

Other Potential Risk Factors Being Studied
Osteoporosis

The evidence regarding the relationship between osteoporosis and periodontitis is conflicting.[2] Evidence indicates a moderate yet statistically significant greater loss of periodontal attachment in postmenopausal women with osteoporosis or osteopenia than women without the condition. During periodontal assessment, the dental hygienist pays particular attention to bone density, as well as to the bone height in women with a history of osteoporosis, and inquires about regular monitoring of bone density with their physician. For women with osteoporosis who smoke, the risk for tooth loss is extremely high. Research is ongoing to improve an understanding of the effects of osteoporosis on periodontal diseases. (For more information on osteoporosis, see Chapter 47.)

Obesity

The relationship between obesity and periodontitis is compounded by the presence of hyperglycemia in diabetes. Nonetheless, evidence indicates an association exists between obesity and periodontitis.[19] The overall effect appears to be moderate. More studies are needed to clarify the effects of obesity on periodontitis.

Stress

Epidemiologic evidence suggests that negative life experiences and psychologic factors likely contribute to enhanced susceptibility to periodontitis. Uncontrolled or severe psychologic stress is associated with depression of the immune system; studies suggest a link between stress and poor coping skills and periodontal attachment loss. Financial stress in adults with poor coping skills is a risk indicator for more severe periodontal disease. Research is ongoing to determine the link between psychologic stress and periodontal disease.

Gender and Race

Background characteristics that may increase the risk for periodontal disease are race and male gender.[2] Studies report significantly more bone loss, attachment loss, and tooth loss in men than in women, even when considering oral hygiene, age, and socioeconomic status. Other studies suggest that oral hygiene differences between men and women account for the differences in periodontal disease risk.

The greater disease prevalence and increase in susceptibility to aggressive and chronic periodontitis is likely linked to socioeconomic class, which may be more of a factor than race itself. More research is needed to determine the degree to which the susceptibility of periodontal disease is a function of race and gender.

Genetic Marker

An advance in risk factor assessment was the discovery of a genetic marker highly associated with severe periodontal disease.[20] This discovery resulted in the development of a genetic susceptibility test for periodontal disease. The Periodontal Susceptibility Test (PST) analyzes DNA to identify specific variations in interleukin (IL)–1α and IL-1β. A positive result is associated with increased susceptibility to chronic periodontal disease. Studies indicate that approximately 30% of the Caucasian population tests positive for this type of IL-1 gene. A key regulator in the inflammatory process, IL-1 in high concentrations, causes tissue destruction. An overproduction of IL-1 helps explain the more generalized and severe periodontal disease observed in many patients who have a genotype-positive status. The PST can identify patients who are potentially at high risk and therefore have the need for more aggressive treatment and perhaps improved adherence with self-care recommendations. The PST is not a diagnostic test but a prognostic test (i.e., some patients test positive for the genotype but never develop severe periodontal disease; some patients who test negative develop severe periodontal disease). Although genetic testing provides important information concerning the risk of periodontal disease in some populations, the best way to use this test clinically has not been determined. The multifactorial nature of periodontal disease must be considered and explained to the patient when risk is assessed (Box 20.10)

CLINICAL APPLICATION OF RISK ASSESSMENT

A periodontal disease risk assessment form can assist in identifying risk factors, in determining which risks are modifiable versus non-modifiable, and in planning evidence-based treatment interventions to optimize care (Fig. 20.39). Information to complete the risk assessment form is obtained through the comprehensive health and dental history, patient interview, and oral assessment.

A computerized risk assessment tool, available from PreViser Corporation, uses a numeric score from 1 to 5 to predict risk based on nine personal risk factors analyzed via a mathematic algorithm. Evidence suggests the system provides a valid and reliable predictor of periodontitis. This scientific approach to risk assessment may prove beneficial for developing a plan of care based on risk, as well as assessing changes to the risk level over time.

Risk factors increase patient susceptibility for periodontal breakdown; however, even one risk factor may substantially increase the patient's degree of risk. The most significant risk factors are tobacco use, diabetes, poor oral hygiene and self-care behaviors, and genetics or other systemic diseases affecting the immune response.

When periodontal and risk assessment identifies multiple risk factors, suggestions for eliminating or modifying risk factors are addressed, for example, through consultation with a patient's physician to determine whether medications not associated with gingival enlargement can be substituted for those that are. Patients who smoke are counseled to quit or to enroll in tobacco cessation programs based on their state of readiness to change. Patients who are experiencing high levels of psychosocial stress could be provided with stress management strategies and counseled to relieve stress via healthy lifestyle behaviors—for example, exercise, a well-balanced diet, and adequate rest and sleep. Patients with osteoporosis could consult their physicians about the use of weight-bearing exercises, calcium, bisphosphonate medications, and estrogen-replacement therapy (ERT). Patients who test positive with genetic testing may be scheduled for more requested recare visits. When risk factors are identified in the absence of periodontal disease, the patient is educated about his or her increased susceptibility and is encouraged to maintain an effective self-care program, seek frequent maintenance care, cease tobacco use, and reduce other risk factors as appropriate.

Patients with periodontitis and risk factors are aggressively treated, such as scheduled for 2- to 3-month periodontal maintenance care

BOX 20.10 Critical Thinking Scenario A

Synopsis of Patient History

Age: 64

Sex: Male

Height: 5 feet, 8 inches

Weight: 220 lbs

Vital signs

Blood pressure: 150/90 mm Hg

Pulse rate: 80 bpm

Respiration rate: 16 rpm

1. Under care of a physician? Yes ☑ No ☐
   Condition(s): Hypertension; myocardial infarction
2. Hospitalized within last 5 years? Yes ☑ No ☐
   Reason(s): Myocardial infarction; colon cancer surgery
3. Has or had the following: Heart disease, respiratory disease, cancer
   Yes ☑ No ☐
4. Current medications? Plavix, Cardizem, albuterol
5. Smokes or uses tobacco? Yes ☑ No ☐

Health History

A man reports a heart attack 3 years ago and surgery for a malignant tumor in the colon 2 years ago. He was diagnosed with hypertension 10 years ago and reports his physician has requested that he quit smoking, but he reports that he "just can't stop."

Dental History

His last visit was 2 years ago, when he still had dental insurance. The patient reports being told that he had periodontitis and needed a "deep scaling."

Social History

The patient reports being highly stressed by mounting medical bills, which are creating financial difficulties for his family. He is a retired schoolteacher who reports increasing his 30-year smoking habit from approximately one-half pack of cigarettes a day to a full pack.

Chief Complaint

"My wife says I have bad breath and that my teeth seem longer than they used to be."

Supplemental Examination Findings

The patient had a full-mouth series of radiographic images exposed 2 years ago. A recent clinical examination reveals generalized firm, pale, nodular gingiva with moderate enlargement. Heavy subgingival calculus is found throughout the mouth with generalized moderate BOP. Pocket depths have increased from 2 years ago, when the deepest reading was 5 mm.

Periodontal assessment reveals generalized 6-mm pocket depths in all posterior areas; 7-mm pocket depths in the maxillary lingual area; 4-mm pocket depths in all other areas; 3-mm recession on teeth 6, 12, and 13; and 6-mm recession on tooth 28.

Use the case information to answer the following questions:

1. List at least five periodontal risk factors for this patient. Which risk factors are modifiable and which are nonmodifiable?
2. What should you teach this patient about the effects of smoking on his periodontal health?
3. Based on the periodontal assessment findings, what would be the CAL on teeth 24 and 26?
4. What is the patient's periodontal disease status, using the 2017 AAP-EFP classification?
5. What is the most likely explanation for the increased pocket depths found in the maxillary lingual area?
6. What would be the best type of radiographic images to expose for this patient?
7. Teach the patient about the role of the host response in tissue destruction observed in periodontal disease. Role play this dialog with one of your peers.
8. The total width of the attached gingiva on tooth 6 is 12 mm. Is there mucogingival involvement on this tooth? What is the amount of attached gingiva?
9. Teach the patient about the link between periodontitis and coronary heart disease. Role play this dialog with one of your peers.
10. What instrument is best for determining if tooth 30 has furcation involvement? Describe a type IV furcation.

AAP, American Academy of Periodontology; *BOP,* Bleeding on probing; *CAL,* clinical attachment loss; *EFP,* European Federation of Periodontology.

---

visits; referred for earlier periodontal surgery; encouraged to follow a rigorous self-care program, including antimicrobial mouth rinse therapy, oral irrigation, systemic antibiotic medications, local controlled drug delivery, or subantimicrobial doses of doxycycline to control collagenase activity. Eliminating as many risk factors as possible is vital to long-term periodontal health. (For more information on the oral-systemic health connection, see Chapter 21.)

PERIODONTAL SCREENING AND RECORDING

Periodontal screening and recording (PSR) is a method to screen patients for the presence of periodontal disease. This screening tool requires a specially designed probe with a 0.5-mm ball tip color coded from 3.5 to 5.5 mm. The patient's mouth is divided into sextants, and each tooth is probed by walking the probe around the entire sulcus. At a minimum, five areas of the tooth are examined: mesiofacial, midfacial, distofacial, and the corresponding palatal and lingual areas. Only the highest score is recorded for each sextant according to the codes found in Fig. 20.40. Many times the PSR is utilized during clinical trials or during a program evaluation. All patients should receive a comprehensive periodontal assessment annually and patients found to be at high risk should always receive comprehensive periodontal

examinations. All patients should receive a comprehensive periodontal examination annually.

DOCUMENTATION AND RECORD KEEPING

Patient information collected throughout care is recorded at each appointment. Documentation allows the hygienist to monitor the patient's personal oral hygiene efforts, healing, and ongoing oral health and overall health status. Data collected on periodontal and oral hygiene status facilitate the assessment of the patient's skin and mucous membrane integrity of the head and neck, a biologically sound and functional dentition, responsibility for oral health, and conceptualization and problem solving.

Legal and insurance regulations require thorough documentation of the patient's periodontal and general health status at each visit. Documentation protocols are based on current information related to oral biofilm accumulation and the patient's response and compliance (e.g., inflammation, attachment levels [probing depth and gingival recession], furcation involvement, tooth mobility, width of alveolar gingiva, mucogingival problems, bone loss determined from radiographic images). Thorough records demonstrate the dental hygienist's awareness of the patient's periodontal and general health status.

Periodontal Disease Risk Assessment Form

Patient name: _____ Chart #: _____ Date: _____

Assessment date: (Please circle) is this? Base line or Recall

Disease Indicators	(Please circle)		
Existing or previous periodontitis	NO	YES	% sites:
Gingival bleeding	NO	YES	% sites:
Increasing pocket depths	NO	YES	% sites:
Recession	NO	YES	% sites:
Gingival enlargement	NO	YES	% sites:
Interdental papillary changes (blunting, cratered)	NO	YES	% sites:
Suppuration or purulent exudate	NO	YES	% sites:
Furcation involvement	NO	YES	% sites:
Tooth mobility	NO	YES	% sites:
Radiographic evidence of bone loss	NO	YES	% sites:
	YES circled = increased risk		
Nonmodifiable Risk Factors	(Please circle)		
Past history of periodontal disease	NO	YES	
Race	African American may = increased risk		
Gender	MALE	FEMALE	Male = increased risk
Age	Aging may = increased risk		
Family history of periodontal disease	NO	YES	
Genetic disorders or compromised immune system	NO	YES	
DNA testing for periodontal susceptibility	NEGATIVE	POSITIVE	
	YES circled = increased risk		
Modifiable Risk Factors	(Please circle)		
Adequacy of self-care	GOOD	FAIR	POOR
Xerostomia	NO	YES	
Smoking	NO	YES	Amount per day:
Stress	LOW	MODERATE	HIGH
Medications that affect gingival tissues/cause xerostomia	NO	YES	
Poorly controlled diabetes	NO	YES	
Osteoporosis/osteopenia	NO	YES	
HIV and AIDS	NO	YES	
	YES circled = increased risk		
Local Contributing Factors	(Please circle)		
Overhanging restorations	NO	YES	% sites:
Poorly contoured crown margins	NO	YES	% sites:
Ill-fitting fixed/removable appliances	NO	YES	% sites:
Oral jewelry	NO	YES	% sites:
Malpositioned teeth/contacts	NO	YES	% sites:
Calculus	NO	YES	% sites:
Toothbrush abrasion	NO	YES	% sites:
Inadequate attached gingiva	NO	YES	% sites:
Occlusal trauma/fremitis	NO	YES	% sites:
Mouth breathing	NO	YES	
	YES circled = increased risk		

Fig. 20.39 Patient risk assessment for periodontal disease. (From Thomson EM. *Case Studies in Dental Hygiene*. 3rd ed. Pearson-Prentice Hall; 2013. Used with permission.)

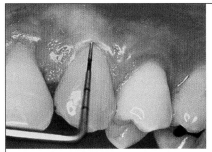
CODE 0

CODE 0

Colored area of probe remains completely visible in the deepest probing depth in the sextant.
- No calculus, bleeding, or defective margins detected
- Gingival tissues are healthy

Treatment recommendations:
Appropriate preventive care

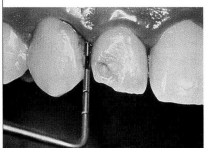
CODE 1

CODE 1

Colored area of probe remains completely visible in the deepest probing depth in the sextant.
- No calculus or defective margins detected
- There is bleeding on probing

Treatment recommendations:
Oral self-care instructions
Appropriate therapy, including:
- Subgingival plaque removal

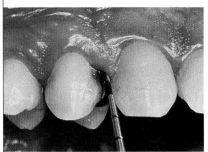
CODE 2

CODE 2

Colored area of probe remains completely visible in the deepest probing depth in the sextant.
- Supra- or subgingival calculus detected, and/or
- Defective margins detected

Treatment recommendations:
Self-care instructions
Appropriate therapy, including:
- Subgingival plaque removal
- Removal of calculus
- Correction of overhanging and defective margins of restorations

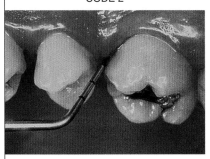
CODE 3

CODE 3

Colored area of probe remains partly visible in the deepest probing depth in the sextant.

Treatment recommendations:
Comprehensive periodontal assessment and charting of the affected sextant are necessary to determine an appropriate treatment plan.
Examination and documentation should include:
- Identification of probing depths
- Mobility
- Gingival recession
- Mucogingival problems
- Furcation invasions
- Radiographs
Note: If two or more sextants score CODE 3, a comprehensive periodontal assessment and evaluation are indicated.

CODE 4

Colored area of probe completely disappears (probing depth greater than 5.5 mm).

Treatment recommendations:
Comprehensive full-mouth periodontal assessment and evaluation are necessary to determine an appropriate treatment plan.

CODE*

The symbol * should be added to sextant score whenever findings indicate clinical abnormalities such as:
- Furcation invasion
- Mobility
- Mucogingival problems
- Recession extending to the colored area of the probe (3.5 mm or greater)

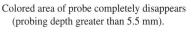
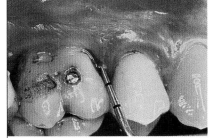
CODE 4

Note: Comprehensive full-mouth examination and charting are necessary to determine an appropriate treatment plan.

Fig. 20.40 Periodontal screening and recording (PSR). (From the American Dental Association, Chicago, Illinois.)

BOX 20.11   Critical Thinking Scenario B

Synopsis of Patient History

Age: 36

Sex: Female

Height: 5 feet, 7 inches

Weight: 135 lbs

Vital signs

   Blood pressure: 120/80 mm Hg

   Pulse rate: 75 bpm

   Respiration rate: 16 rpm

1. Under care of a physician: Yes ☐ No ☑
      Hospitalized within last 5 years: Yes ☑ No ☐
      Reason(s): Childbirth
2. Has or had the following: Heart disease, respiratory disease, cancer Yes ☐ No ☑
3. Current medications: Birth control pills
4. Smokes or uses tobacco: Yes ☐ No ☑

Health History:

Patient has maternal family history of type 2 diabetes mellitus. Patient states she has been diagnosed as "prediabetic," drinks socially one to two times a week, and has no reported allergies. She sees a physician only for annual examinations.

Dental History:

Patient's last visit was 1 year ago when a complete examination was performed and 18 radiographic images were taken. Patient had two carious lesions restored without complications. The dental hygiene assessment determined moderate generalized gingivitis. Dental hygiene therapy and oral hygiene were completed with the recommendation to return in 4 months.

   Patient reports moderate dental anxiety. Patient has a history of cariogenic diet and eats irregularly, snacking as she can at work. Patient's self-reported oral hygiene is fair, brushes one time a day when she can but never flosses.

Social History:

Patient is married, works full-time as waitress, and has three children. Patient reports she has little time for herself.

Chief Complaint:

Patient reports tender gums and bleeding when she brushes; consequently, she has stopped brushing this week.

   Today's periodontal assessment reveals generalized 4-mm pocket depths proximal surface with corresponding bleeding on probing. CAL of 5 mm is due to 1-mm recession on the lingual maxillary anteriors, buccal surfaces of the mandibular cuspids and left bicuspids, and 6-mm pocket depths in the distal areas of the mandibular third molars. Generalized marginal and papillary inflammation with increased erythema and moderate enlargement are evident.

   Use the case information to answer the following questions:

1. List at least three periodontal risk factors for this patient. Which risk factors are modifiable and which are nonmodifiable?
2. What is the patient's periodontal disease status, using the 2017 AAP-EFP classification system?
3. What is the most likely explanation for the pocket depths found on the distal areas of the mandibular third molars?
4. What would be the best type of radiographic images to expose for this patient?

Teach the patient about the role of the host response in the patient's periodontal disease. Role play this dialog with one of your peers.

Teach the patient about the links among periodontal disease, oral hygiene, diet, and stress. Role play this dialog with one of your peers.

AAP, American Academy of Periodontology, *CAL,* clinical attachment loss; *EFP,* European Federation of Periodontology.

The record must provide a baseline documentation of data collected about the patient. Assessment of baseline conditions is repeated at subsequent visits. Changes in conditions are documented, and data are compared with baseline information. Diligent record keeping is key to tracking frequency of care, disease episodes, patient response, and outcomes of care. Trend analysis is based on comparing ongoing findings with baseline data. Longitudinal evaluation is critical for providing optimal care, minimizing legal risks, and meeting third-party requirements for periodontal data on patient needs and treatment outcomes. Moreover, objective notations of patient perceptions, needs, and desires alert other personnel of special considerations and facilitate oral health education and continuity of high-quality care focused on the patient. (Refer to Box 20.11 regarding legal and ethical considerations.)

Documentation

Periodontal status is monitored from appointment to appointment. Documentation of periodontal assessment findings at every visit is essential for accurate diagnosis, periodontal disease management, and risk management. Findings of inflammation, recession, pocket probe readings, aberrant tissue forms, bleeding, suppuration, minimum attached gingiva, tooth mobility, and furcation involvement are recorded. Six-point probing measurements are recorded for each tooth. The practitioner determines improvement or disease progression by comparing data from visit to visit. Comparison of notations facilitates diagnosis, care planning, and long-term monitoring.

The documentation forms should list factors that may negatively affect the outcomes of care. For example, the dental hygienist notes when gingival inflammation, disease progression, and healing may be affected by modifiable and nonmodifiable risk factors. Patient noncompliance, tardiness, cancellations, and missed appointments are recorded to demonstrate that the patient may be responsible for a less-than-satisfactory result (i.e., contributory negligence).

Record-Keeping Formats

Recorded findings provide a graphic display of the patient's periodontal health status and a means to compare previous examinations with the current assessment. Findings of bleeding, recession, furcations, purulence, and mobility are important to include in the electronic periodontal record. An electronic periodontal chart is presented in Fig. 20.41A. Fig. 20.41B displays periodontal measurements from different appointments, which provide a comparison of assessment data for an evaluation of changes in the periodontium. In this view, the clinician is able to select and compare pocket depths, CAL, BOP, and mobility. This type of visual representation allows the clinician to monitor progress of periodontal health over time. Improvement or deterioration of periodontal conditions can be readily determined and shared with the patient. Numerous dental software companies provide electronic data systems with comprehensive formats including health histories, dental and periodontal charting, digital imaging, and monitoring for patient record keeping, practice management, and communication (Fig. 20.42).

DECISION-MAKING MATRIX

Fig. 20.43 illustrates a decision-making matrix used in providing dental hygiene care. Decisions are the result of objective clinical and radiographic information collected and recorded during the assessment

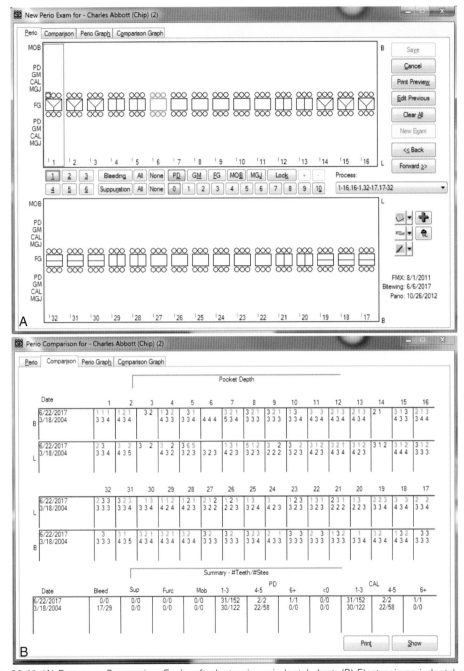

Fig. 20.41 (A) Patterson Companies, Eaglesoft electronic periodontal chart. (B) Electronic periodontal chart showing a comparison of data. Note: the *green numbers* indicate improvement in pocket depths and the *red numbers* highlight deeper measurements.

phase of care, the current research evidence base, and collaboration with the dentist and the patient. Objective assessment data can be further evaluated in follow-up assessments.

The health, dental, pharmacologic, and personal history information influences the choice of treatment modalities. For example, the host defense mechanisms and presence of systemic disease may compromise care results, as can nutritional status, substance use, medications, oral habits, occlusal trauma, oral appliances, and emotional factors. Orthodontic treatment often entails trauma to gingival tissue and compromises oral hygiene. Patient motivation and degree of assumption of responsibility also affect self-care and therapeutic outcomes. Each situation must be assessed to identify the patient's perception of his or her needs, the level of dexterity in oral plaque biofilm control, and the degree of anatomic access to ensure professional and patient self-care efficacy.

The types of periodontal assessment and therapy provided by a dental hygienist are explained in detail in Chapter 33. Data collected during periodontal assessment determine the level of care to be recommended to the patient.

PERIODONTAL INDICES

Quantifying periodontal health can be accomplished in many ways. If the dental hygienist is to survey the prevalence of periodontal disease in a particular population (epidemiologic research), then using the indices used by other researchers is important to ensure that outcomes can be compared. However, to assess a single individual's periodontal status for developing a care plan, a simple, cost-effective, and easily understood method is warranted. Indices can motivate patients to

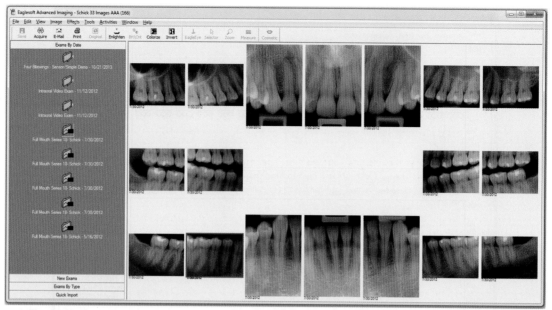

Fig. 20.42 Full-mouth series of radiographic images displayed on a computer monitor using digital technology. (Courtesy Sirona Dental, Inc., Long Island City, New York.)

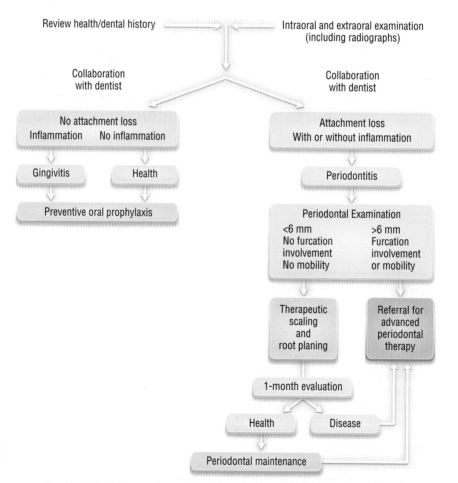

Fig. 20.43 Decision tree for periodontal assessment and treatment of the adult.

improve their self-care behaviors and can provide an easily understood numeric score for comparison between visits. The amount of bacterial plaque biofilm, bleeding, and pocket scores evaluated over time can help patients identify changes in their periodontal health.

Periodontal Indices Used in Larger Populations

Dental hygienists use **periodontal indices** in public health settings and for research epidemiologic studies to quantify the prevalence and incidence of disease in specific populations.

- **Prevalence** means the number of cases existing at a specific point in time per a specified number of persons. For example, the statement, "52% of 1328 college baseball athletes reported using dental floss daily" is a statement of the prevalence of floss use.
- **Incidence** means the number of new cases or diseases per a specified number of persons occurring in a specified time, typically in 1 year. For example, the statement, "50,000 new cases of periodontitis were diagnosed in the United States from 2009 to 2010" is a statement of incidence.
- **Severity** refers to how much destruction is present at one time. For instance, 5 mm CAL is a standard often used to indicate the need for periodontal treatment.

Research uses periodontal and oral hygiene indices as outcome measures when testing the efficacy of approaches to care, for example, in studies testing an antimicrobial toothpaste or a mouth rinse to determine its effectiveness in decreasing gingivitis. Table 20.9 lists some periodontal indices used in research. Usually, the subset of teeth described by Ramfjord is used in evaluating groups of people. Based on large-scale studies, Ramfjord determined that the measurements of teeth 3, 9, 12, 20, 25, and 28 represent the entire dentition. Many indices use these six teeth, the Ramfjord teeth. These indices are called *simplified*. In some studies, missing teeth are not counted; in others, the researcher substitutes the missing teeth with the next most distal tooth. Other indices require substitution by going mesially or to the contralateral tooth. Examiners often use more than one index. Examiners are calibrated, providing reliability, before using any oral index in research. With regard to probing depths, examiners are calibrated to a standard of one measurement being within ±1 mm of the others'

probing depth. Some plaque indices require disclosing solutions rinsed away after application, whereas others require no rinsing or no use of a disclosant. Whether in research, community health practices, or private practices, examiners standardize data-gathering procedures to reach valid results.

Procedures vary with different indices. The Community Periodontal Index of Treatment Needs (CPITN) is of special interest because it provides information on periodontal status and treatment needs. A special periodontal probe with color-coded gradations, designed for this index, has a 0.5-mm ball tip to prevent severing the JE and to allow some tactile sensation as the clinician probes the tooth surface in the pocket. Shallow pockets, less than 3.5 mm, require no special treatment, whereas those represented by reporting a sulcus less than a color-coded gradation from 3.5 to 5.5 mm indicate no special treatment. Deeper pockets measuring within the color gradation require therapeutic scaling. The deepest pockets, where the color-coded gradation cannot be seen (more than 5.5 mm), require complex treatment, described as scaling and root debridement under local anesthesia, with or without surgical exposure for access.

The CPITN assesses sextants or the full mouth, but in epidemiologic studies, only 10 teeth are examined, and only the worst score per sextant is recorded. This approach may underestimate the number of deep pockets in older adult populations who generally have many areas of attachment loss and may overestimate shallow pockets in younger age groups who have many healthy sulcus depths (see Table 20.9 for additional periodontal indices).

Critical Thinking for Comprehensive Periodontal Assessment

Dental hygienists play a key role in periodontal assessment, dental hygiene diagnosis of periodontal disease, related patient education, individualized care planning for the prevention and control of periodontal diseases, implementation of nonsurgical periodontal therapy, and posttreatment evaluation and maintenance. Critical thinking is required for the integration of all periodontal assessment findings as it is critical to these phases of the dental hygiene care process. Boxes 20.10 and 20.11 Critical Thinking Scenarios provide critical thinking exercises to apply the information learned.

TABLE 20.9 Periodontal Indices

Index and Purpose	Procedure for Use	Rating Score and Interpretation
Community Periodontal Index of Treatment Needs (CPITN) (Ainamo, 1982)* To assess priorities for periodontal treatment of an individual or a group	For adults (20 years and older), divide the dentition into sextants. Evaluate all teeth except the third molars. For children and adolescents (7 to 20 years of age), divide the dentition into sextants but evaluate only the first molars in the posterior sextant, the right central incisor in the maxilla sextant, and the left central incisor in mandibular anterior sextant. Use the WHO periodontal probe (CPITN-E probe) marked at 3.5-, 8.5-, and 11.5-mm intervals, color-coding from 3.5 to 5.5 mm, and a ball 0.5 mm in diameter at the working tip. Criteria used: Code 0 = Healthy periodontal tissues Code 1 = Bleeding after gentle probing Code 2 = Supragingival or subgingival calculus or defective margin of filling or crown; gingival inflammation; no probe readings >3 mm Code 3 = 4- or 5-mm probe readings Code 4 = ≥6-mm periodontal pocket Mark one score to represent each sextant. Record only the highest code that corresponds with the most severe condition. Patients are classified (0, I, II, III) into treatment needs, according to the highest coded score recorded during the examination.	Calculations of the number and percentage of individuals with the following can be made: No sextant scoring each code One or two sextants scoring code 1, 2, 3, or 4 Three or four sextants scoring code 1, 2, 3, or 4 Five or six sextants scoring code 1, 2, 3, or 4 Patient classification: I = No need for treatment (code 0) II = Self-care instruction plus scaling (code 1) III = Self-care instruction plus scaling and root debridement, including elimination of plaque retentive margins of fillings and crowns (code 3) IV = II + III + complex periodontal therapy that may include surgical intervention and/or deep scaling and root debridement with local anesthesia (code 4)

Continued

TABLE 20.9   Periodontal Indices—cont'd

Index and Purpose	Procedure for Use	Rating Score and Interpretation
Gingival Index (GI) (Loe and Silness, 1963)* To assess gingival inflammation based on color, consistency, and BOP; based on the assumption that a slight color change is indicative of gingival inflammation	A score of 0–3 is assigned to mesial, distal, buccal, and lingual surfaces of teeth 3, 9, 12, 20, 25, and 28. A blunt instrument, such as a periodontal probe, is used to assess bleeding potential based on the following criteria: 0 = Normal gingiva 1 = Mild inflammation: slight change in color, slight edema; no BOP 2 = Moderate inflammation: redness, edema, and glazing; BOP 3 = Severe inflammation: marked redness and edema; ulceration; tendency to spontaneously bleed Totaling scores around each tooth yields GI score for area; divide by 4, score for tooth is determined. Totaling all scores and dividing by number of teeth examined provides a GI score per person, which can be used on selected or all erupted teeth.	Scoring criteria used: 0.0 = No gingivitis (excellent) 0.1–1.0 = Mild gingivitis (good) 1.1–2.0 = Moderate gingivitis (fair) 2.1–3.0 = Severe gingivitis (poor)
Periodontal Disease Index (PDI) (Ramfjord, 1967)* To measure the extent of periodontal disease (i.e., assesses gingivitis, gingival sulcus depth, calculus, plaque, occlusal and incisal attrition mobility, and lack of contact)	Six teeth are examined: 3, 9, 12, 20, 25, and 28. Criteria used: 0 = Absence of inflammation 1 = Mild-to-moderate inflammatory gingival changes not extending all around the tooth 2 = Mild-to-moderately severe gingivitis, extending all around the tooth 3 = Severe gingivitis characterized by significant redness, a tendency to bleed, and ulceration 4 = Gingival crevice in any of the four measured areas (mesial, distal, buccal, lingual), extending apically to the CEJ but not more than 3 mm 5 = Gingival crevice in any of the four measured areas, apically extending to the CEJ (3 to 6 mm) 6 = Gingival crevice in any of the four measured areas, apically extending more than 6 mm from the CEJ PDI score is obtained by totaling the scores of the teeth and dividing by the number of teeth examined.	Group score of 3.5 = severe gingivitis for epidemiologic purposes. Care must be taken when interpreting the PDI on an individual basis.
Sulcus Bleeding Index (SBI) (Muhlemann and Son, 1971)* To assess clinical signs of inflammation; based on the assumption that BOP is the first clinical sign of inflammation	Four gingival units are scored on each tooth: the marginal gingiva, labial and lingual (M units), and the papillary gingiva, mesial, and distal (P units). Probe each of the four areas. Hold the probe parallel with the long axis of the tooth for the M units and direct the probe toward the col area for the P units. Wait 30 seconds after probing and score using the following criteria: 0 = Healthy appearance of the P and M units, no bleeding on sulcus probing 1 = Apparently healthy P and M units, showing no change in color and no swelling but bleeding from sulcus on probing 2 = BOP and change of color caused by inflammation; no swelling or macroscopic edema 3 = BOP and change in color and slight edematous swelling 4 = BOP and change in color and obvious swelling, or BOP and obvious swelling 5 = BOP and spontaneous bleeding and change in color, significant swelling with or without ulceration Scores for the four units are totaled and divided by 4.	Scores may range from 0 to 5: 0 = Healthy gingiva 5 = Severe gingival inflammation
Eastman Interdental Bleeding Index (Caton and Polson, 1985)* To assess interdental gingival bleeding and to monitor interproximal gingival health	All interdental gingival areas are examined. 0 = Absence of bleeding when a triangular toothpick is horizontally depressed 2 mm interproximally 4 times and checked 15 seconds later 1 = Bleeding after the above procedure	Yields a score that reflects the percentage of bleeding sites. The higher the percentage of bleeding sites, the more generalized the interdental bleeding.

*Original articles establishing reliability and validity.
BOP, Bleeding on probing; *CEJ,* cementoenamel junction; *WHO,* World Health Organization.

KEY CONCEPTS

- Risk factor assessment is important for appropriate targeted care planning that focuses on prevention and treatment, specific risk factors, and reparative therapies.
- The origin of periodontal disease is strongly linked to periodontal pathogens (e.g., *Aggregatibacter actinomycetemcomitans*, *Tannerella forsythia*, and *Porphyromonas gingivalis*). Clinical observations of inflammation and probing depths, the determination of clinical attachment levels, and radiographic images provide primary information for determining periodontal health, diagnosing periodontal conditions, and planning dental hygiene therapy. Dental biofilm–induced gingivitis is a reversible inflammatory periodontal disease without attachment loss and is characterized by any or all of the following tissue changes: redness, edema, enlargement, spongy consistency, and BOP.
- Gingival bleeding is the key clinical characteristic of dental biofilm–induced gingivitis.
- Periodontitis is an inflammation of the periodontium characterized by clinical attachment loss, resulting from the destruction of the periodontal ligament and alveolar bone. It can exhibit periods of exacerbation (i.e., disease activity) and quiescence (i.e., inactivity). Other forms of periodontitis include necrotizing periodontitis and periodontitis as a manifestation of systemic disease.
- Peri-implant diseases include peri-implant mucositis and peri-implantitis.
- The host's immunoinflammatory and immunologic responses to bacteria in oral biofilm is responsible for tissue destruction in periodontal disease.

- Gingival bleeding occurring at sequential continued care visits is associated with an increased risk for periodontal destruction.
- Periodontitis cannot be determined by the appearance of the gingiva, which can appear pale and firm with slight bleeding on probing or fiery red, and boggy, with heavy bleeding. Periodontal pockets can vary from site to site, from tooth to tooth, and even from site to site on the same tooth.
- Radiographic images reveal the amount of alveolar bone present, the pattern, and the extent of bone loss.
- Radiographic images must be used in conjunction with a thorough clinical assessment.
- Vertical bitewing radiographic images are recommended instead of horizontal bitewing exposures for evaluation of periodontitis.
- Continued attachment loss over time, not current clinical attachment loss, indicates a progression of periodontal disease.
- Documentation of periodontal assessment findings at every visit is essential for accurate diagnosis, periodontal disease management, and risk management.
- Individual immune response and susceptibility to periodontal disease varies widely.
- Periodontal risk factors modulate periodontal disease susceptibility and influence the onset, progression, and severity of the disease.
- The most significant periodontal risk factors are smoking, poor oral hygiene, genetics, stress, diabetes, and obesity.

ACKNOWLEDGMENT

The contributors wish to acknowledge Robin Gatlin, RDH, MS, assistant professor, and Kandice Lewis, RDH, MSC, graduate student, with the University of New Mexico, Division of Dental Hygiene, for their thorough reviews.

REFERENCES

1. American Dental Hygienists' Association. Standards for clinical dental hygiene practices: revised 2016. Available at: https://www.adha.org/education-resources/professional-resources/clinical-practice-resources/ Accessed June 20, 2022.
2. Genco R, Bornakke WS. Risk factors for periodontal disease. *Periodontol 2000*. 2013;62:59–94.
3. Caton JG, Armitage G, Berglundh T, et al. A new classification scheme for periodontal and peri-implant diseases and conditions – Introduction and key changes from the 1999 classification. First published: 20 June 2018. Available at: https://onlinelibrary.wiley.com/toc/1600051x/2018/45/S20. Accessed June 20, 2022.
4. Chapple ILC, Mealey BL, Dyke TE, et al. Periodontal health and gingival diseases and conditions on an intact and a reduced periodontium: consensus report of workgroup 1 of the 2017 World Workshop on the Classification of Periodontal and Peri-Implant Diseases and Conditions. *J Clin Periodontol*. 2018;45(suppl 20):S68–S77.
5. Murakami S, Mealey BL, Mariotti A, et al. Dental plaque-induced gingival conditions. *J Clin Periodontol*. 2018;45(suppl 20):S17–S27.
6. Holstrup P, Plemens J, Meyle J. Non-plaque-induced gingival diseases. *J Clin Periodontol*. 2018;45(suppl 20):S28–S43.
7. Papapanou PN, Sanz M, Buduneli N, et al. Periodontitis: consensus report of workgroup 2 of the 2017 World Workshop on the classification of periodontal and peri-implant diseases and conditions. *J Clin Periodontol*. 2018;45(suppl 20):S162–S170.
8. Tonetti MS, Greenwell H, Kornman KS. Staging and grading of periodontitis: framework and proposal of a new classification and case definition. *J Clin Periodontol*. 2018;45(suppl 20):S149–S161.
9. Jepsen S, Berglundh T, Genco R, et al. Primary prevention of peri-implantitis: managing peri-implant mucositis. *J Clin Periodontol*. 2015;42(suppl 16):S152–S157.
10. Berglundh T, Armitage G, Araujo MC, et al. Peri-implant diseases and conditions: consensus report of workgroup 4 of the 2017 World Workshop on the classification of periodontal and peri-implant diseases and conditions. *J Clin Periodontol*. 2018;45(suppl 20):S286–S291.
11. Page RC, Schroeder HE. Current status of the host response in chronic marginal periodontitis. *J Periodontol*. 1981;52:477–491.
12. Hajishengallis G, Korostoff JF. Revisiting the Page and Schroeder model: the good, the bad and the unknowns in the periodontal host response 40 years later. *Periodontol 2000*. 2017;75:116–151.
13. Silva N, Albuslemme L, Bravo D, et al. Host response mechanisms in periodontal diseases. *J Appl Oral Sci*. 2015;23(3):329–355.
14. Karthikeyan BV, Sujatha V, Prabhuji ML. Furcation measurements: realities and limitations. *J Int Acad Periodontol*. 2015;17(4):103–115.
15. American Dental Association, Council on Dental Benefit Programs, Council on Scientific Affairs, U.S. Department of Health and Human Services, Public Health Service, Food and Drug Administration. The selection of Patients for Dental Radiographs. Revised 2012. Available at: https://www.fda.gov/radiation-emitting-products/medical-x-ray-imaging/selection-patients-dental-radiographic-examinations. Accessed June 20, 2022.
16. Lima CL, Acevedo A, Grisi DC, et al. Host-derived salivary biomarkers in diagnosing periodontal disease: systematic review and meta-analysis. *J Clin Periodontol*. 2016;43(6):492–502. 11p. ISSN:0303-6979.
17. Ramanauskaite A, Juodzbalys G. Diagnostic principles of peri-implantitis: a systematic review and guidelines for peri-implantitis diagnosis proposal. *J Oral Maxillofac Res*. 2016;7(3):e8.
18. Glurich I, Nycz G, Acharya A. Status update on translation of integrated primary dental-medical care delivery for management of diabetic patients. *Clin Med Res*. 2017;15(1–2):21–32.
19. Martinez-Herrara M, Silvestre-Rangil J, Silvestre FJ. Association between obesity and periodontal disease. A systematic review of epidemiological studies and controlled clinical trials. *Med Oral Patol Oral Cir Bucal*. 2017;22(6):e708–e715.
20. Nibali L, Di Iorio A, Tu Y-K, et al. Host genetics role in the pathogenesis of periodontal disease and caries. *J Clin Periodontol*. 2017;44(suppl 18):S52–S78.

21

Oral-Systemic Health Connection

Antonio Moretti and Kathryn Bell

PROFESSIONAL OPPORTUNITIES

The oral-systemic health connection has been under investigation for several decades. Our level of knowledge about the interaction between oral and systemic health continues to grow and develop, and it is a safe assumption that new information will continue to emerge to further influence our understanding of these relationships as well as inform the way clinicians practice. It is very important to have a thorough understanding of the oral-systemic connection to educate patients as well as to provide them with evidence-based diagnosis and treatment that will maximize their chances for maintaining both oral and systemic health. It is also critically important for the dental hygienist to remain up to date on current research to maintain an evidence-based practice.

COMPETENCIES

1. Explain why the oral-systemic health connection is important in providing evidence-based care, and discuss how cardiovascular disease, diabetes, and pregnancy can affect oral health.
2. Incorporate periodontal-systemic evidence into treatment and practice, and educate patients about areas of association between periodontal disease and systemic disease as well as how these associations influence the patient's risk of developing periodontal disease and/or systemic disease. Also, determine the need for referrals to primary care providers for dental patients with systemic disease.

INTRODUCTION

Among dental care providers and many patients, it is well known that there are associations between oral diseases and systemic diseases. Dental professionals and the public started to increase their awareness of this problem close to 30 years ago, with several landmark scientific publications, the consequent attention given by the news media, and the ever-growing interest by researchers, dental care providers, and the general population. In particular, periodontal diseases and a group of systemic diseases, such as diabetes, cardiovascular conditions, pregnancy outcomes, and many others, have become the focus of attention. The body of scientific evidence indicates that the association has grown significantly in the last decades. The relationship between periodontal diseases and systemic diseases is complex and is likely to involve various mechanisms ranging from shared genetic susceptibility to direct infectious exposures. Despite all developments, there remains significant difficulty in demonstrating cause-and-effect (causal) relationships among various conditions. We lack large-scale intervention and long-term studies to allow us to reach definitive conclusions, leading to the full practice of periodontal medicine. Nevertheless, we understand enough to educate and guide patients on preventive measures to help improve their intraoral and, potentially, their general health. This chapter aims to update the dental hygienist and other members of the dental profession on this important topic of their daily clinical practices.

To begin interpreting the vast information available in the published literature, one should keep in mind three main topics listed in the Bradford Hill criteria or in the criteria for a causal association between two diseases, both sources that are widely used in public health research: (1) epidemiologic association, (2) **biological plausibility** (the idea that the mechanism of association seems reasonable in light of normal biologic processes), and (3) impact of intervention of one disease on the second disease.[1,2] The same authors have also suggested the critical importance of three main mechanisms that participate in the non oral manifestations of oral diseases, published in 1984:[3] the role of (1) bacteria alone, (2) bacterial products, and (3) inflammatory reaction. It is known that periodontal bacteria travel through the bloodstream to other parts of the body (Fig. 21.1). They also produce multiple detrimental inflammatory mediators such as cytotoxins, proteases, and many others that migrate through the whole body. Furthermore, the inflammatory mediators and byproducts that originate locally will also enter the bloodstream and can affect the overall systemic inflammation. It is also important to emphasize that these oral-systemic associations could be attributable to common risk factors, serving as confounders, and not causally related.

KNOWLEDGE FOR THE ORAL DENTAL CARE PROVIDER AND INTERPROFESSIONAL CARE

It is critical that as healthcare providers, we are able to understand the systemic diseases associated with periodontitis. Dental hygienists and dentists do not receive the same training that physicians, physician assistants, and nurse practitioners do, and they should not act as such. However, interprofessional collaborative efforts with other healthcare providers are fundamental for improving the overall health of patients.

Cardiovascular Diseases

Atherosclerotic cardiovascular disease (ACVD), in which the inside of the arteries narrows with a buildup of deposits called *plaque* or *atheroma*, is responsible for approximately one in five deaths in the United States and is the leading cause of death for both men and women (Fig. 21.2).[4] ACVDs include angina, myocardial infarction (MI), stroke, transient ischemic attack, and peripheral arterial disease (see Chapter 48). It is recommended that oral healthcare practitioners advise patients about the risk of periodontitis for developing an ACVD. Presence of intraoral inflammation may lead to these systemic events. Patients with periodontitis and other risk factors for ACVD, such as hypertension and obesity, need to see a physician at least annually. Dental care providers, together with other healthcare providers, should advise patients on lifestyle modifications, such as diet and exercise.[5]

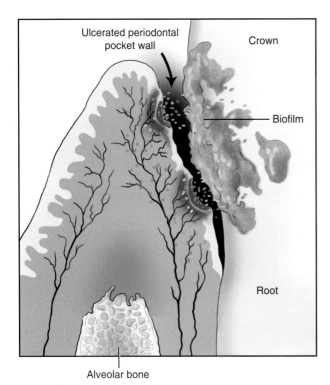

Ulcerated periodontal
pocket wall

Crown

Biofilm

Root

Alveolar bone

Fig. 21.1 Illustration depicting the interface between the gingiva and tooth in a case of periodontal disease. The epithelium of the pocket wall is ulcerated. These ulcerations allow subgingival bacteria in the adjacent periodontal pocket access to the bloodstream for systemic circulation.

Summarized recommendations for oral health professionals in dental practice for people with cardiovascular disease (CVD) include:[6]

- Patients with periodontitis should be advised that there is a higher risk for CVD, such as myocardial infarction or stroke; they should actively manage all their cardiovascular risk factors (smoking, exercise, excess weight, blood pressure, lipid and glucose management, and sufficient periodontal therapy and periodontal maintenance).
- Patients with periodontitis and a diagnosis of CVD should be informed that they may be at higher risk for subsequent CVD complications and, therefore should adhere regularly to the recommended dental therapeutic, maintenance, and preventive regimens.
- Dental providers should collect a careful history to assess for CVD risk factors, such as diabetes, obesity, smoking, hypertension, hyperlipidemia, and hypercalcemia. Dental providers suggest that the patient consult their physician if any of these risk factors are not controlled.
- Oral health education should be provided to all patients with periodontitis, along with a tailored oral hygiene regimen.
- Patients should receive a thorough oral examination, which includes a comprehensive periodontal evaluation, including full–mouth probing and bleeding scores.
- If no periodontitis is diagnosed initially, patients with CVD should be placed on a preventive care regime and monitored regularly (at least once a year) for changes in periodontal status.
- If periodontitis is diagnosed, they should be managed as soon as their cardiovascular status permits.

Diabetes

Diabetes affects more than 37.3 million adults in the United States. It is also estimated that 96 million U.S. adults have prediabetes.[7] **Type**

1 diabetes is the less common form of the disease, in which patients cannot produce enough insulin (approximately 5% of cases). **Type 2 diabetes**, in which patients' bodies cannot use the insulin they produce (90% to 95% of cases), is significantly more prominent. Risk factors for diabetes include being overweight and obesity, which are usually measured using **body mass index (BMI)**, a calculation used to estimate body fat. Additional risk factors include physical inactivity, family history, race (diabetes is more common among Blacks, Hispanic Americans, Native Americans, and Asian populations), age, abnormal cholesterol levels, and history of gestational diabetes.

Diabetes and periodontitis have a bidirectional relationship (see Chapter 49). Chronic presence of systemic inflammation originating from periodontitis may contribute to the initial steps for the development of type 2 diabetes. Inflammation can lead to decreased pancreatic function and can stimulate insulin resistance, leading to hyperglycemia, which is a characteristic of diabetes. The high levels of sugar (hyperglycemia) in the circulating blood lead to high **glycated hemoglobin A1c (HbA1c)** laboratory values. HbA1c values indicate how much sugar is attached to the patient's hemoglobin and are reflective of blood glucose control over the previous few months. Importantly, dental care providers should know the HbA1c levels of their diabetic patients. A normal HbA1c in a nondiabetic patient is below 5.7%. For patients diagnosed with diabetes, an HbA1c of 7% or less is ideal.[8]

Hyperglycemia can negatively affect periodontal diseases. In general, poorly controlled levels of blood glucose can place a patient at high risk for developing infections. The presence of advanced glycation end products (AGEs) leads some body cells to produce inflammatory mediators that can result in hard and soft tissue destruction.

Chapple and Genco[9] have developed the following guidelines for dental care providers who manage patients with diabetes:

- Patients with diabetes should be informed that they are at increased risk for periodontitis. In addition, if they suffer from periodontitis, their glycemic control may become more difficult. They are at higher risk for other complications, such as cardiovascular and kidney diseases.
- Patients with any type of diabetes (type 1 or 2 or gestational diabetes) should receive a comprehensive periodontal examination and have a continual followup plan.
- Children and adolescents diagnosed with diabetes should have at least one annual oral screening for early signs of periodontal involvement, starting at the age of 6 years.
- Diabetic patients with periodontitis should be properly managed by the dental team. In addition, patients with diabetes and no periodontitis should be monitored periodically for possible intraoral changes.
- Diabetic patients with acute oral infections should be treated without delay.
- Diabetic patients with partial or total edentulism should be recommended for tooth replacement treatment to help ensure proper mastication and nutrition.
- Oral health education should be given to all diabetic patients.
- Diabetic patients should be examined for other oral complications, such as dry mouth, burning mouth syndrome, and fungal infections.
- Patients who are at risk of developing type 2 diabetes and have signs of periodontitis should be informed about their risk for diabetes and should have their HbA1c values tested.

Adverse Pregnancy Outcomes

Some of the adverse outcomes for pregnancy are **low birth weight** (<2.5 kg or 5.5 lb), **preterm birth** (<37 weeks), growth restriction, preeclampsia, miscarriage, and/or stillbirth (see Chapter 46). In 2020,

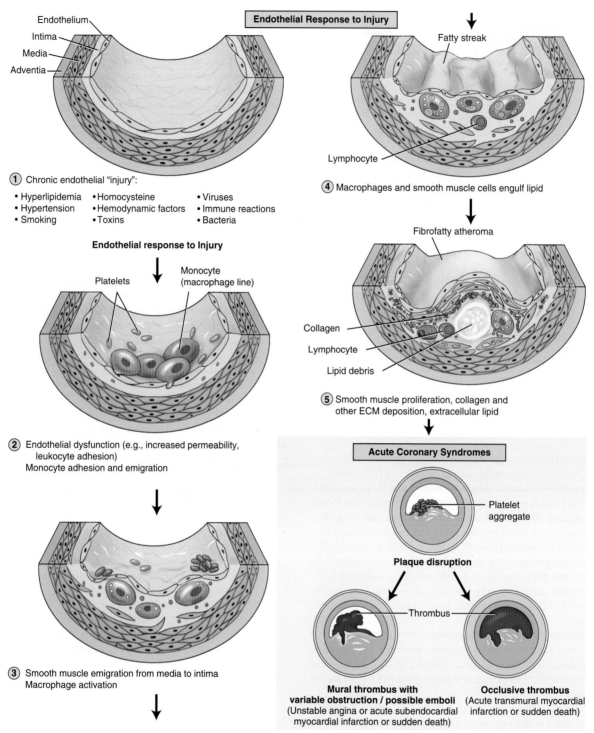

Fig. 21.2 Illustration depicting the development and eventual disruption of an atherosclerotic plaque (atheroma) that can lead to heart attacks (myocardial infarctions) and nonhemorrhagic strokes.

approximately 1 in 10 newborns in the United States were delivered prematurely,[10] and approximately 8% of infants were delivered at a low birth weight.[11] **Preeclampsia** (PE) is a pregnancy complication in which the mother experiences high blood pressure in addition to signs of damage to other organs—often to the kidneys or liver. PE is very dangerous for both the mother and the fetus, with potentially fatal outcomes if left untreated.[12] Adverse pregnancy outcomes (APOs) are generally associated with inflammation and intrauterine infections.[13]

In addition, periodontitis affecting the mother is one possible source of microorganisms and inflammatory mediators that can potentially influence, directly or indirectly, the fetus and the mother.

Dental professionals understand that it is safe to provide diagnostic, preventive, and therapeutic procedures during pregnancy (see Chapter 46). However, obstetric guidelines suggest that elective procedures should be avoided in the first trimester and that the second trimester is the best time to provide dental care. It is important for dental hygienists to understand that it is safe to provide oral healthcare services at any time during pregnancy. Once the patient discloses being pregnant, identify the stage of pregnancy and perform a comprehensive oral and periodontal examination (see Chapter 20). Patients will be clinically classified as having (1) a healthy periodontium, (2) gingivitis, or (3) periodontitis, according to the most recent classification of periodontal and peri-implant diseases and conditions.[14] Recommendations for dental and medical health professionals will be based on the initial diagnosis and on the patient's clinical classification.[13]

Healthy Periodontium

Inform the patient about the potential increase in gingival vascularity, enlargement, and bleeding during pregnancy. Assess the patient's general health for a history of hypertension, diabetes, and cardiovascular diseases, and refer the patient to a physician if necessary (see Chapters 13 and 14). Emphasize oral hygiene instructions, especially at interproximal sites, and consider recommending an antimicrobial dentifrice or mouthrinse. The patient should be assessed again, close to the end of the pregnancy.

Gingivitis

Health promotion (prevention) should be discussed when first meeting the patient. The care provider should treat gingivitis with a dual goal—to reduce both the intraoral bacterial load and the clinical signs of gingival inflammation. A recommendation for an effective antimicrobial dentifrice and mouthrinse is needed, as well as effective mechanical oral hygiene practices. Continue monitoring the patient during the pregnancy and intervene as needed.

Periodontitis

Start with similar health promotion steps as discussed for the patient with a healthy periodontium or with gingivitis. Nonsurgical periodontal therapy should be provided and, if possible, more invasive surgical procedures should be delayed until after the baby is born. If the patient develops areas of significant gingival overgrowth, such as pregnancy gingivitis, then they should be treated accordingly.

Diseases Undergoing Investigation

Linden and collaborators[15] reviewed the scientific evidence of periodontal-systemic associations. They focused on the following diseases and conditions that have had a significant impact on public health: respiratory diseases; chronic kidney disease; rheumatoid arthritis; cognitive impairment (e.g., Alzheimer disease); obesity; metabolic syndrome; and cancer. After reviewing over 100 papers, they noted a lack of consistency and great heterogeneity in the definition of periodontitis used in these studies. When analyzing a more robust data set, with an acceptable definition of periodontitis, very few cross-sectional studies and another group of prospective studies reported significant positive associations between periodontitis and these systemic diseases under investigation. In general, these associations were weak. However, weak associations of two diseases or conditions do not necessarily reject a causal relationship.

Research regarding periodontal disease and systemic health continues. Dental care providers have a legal and ethical responsibility to remain current, using the best evidence to support patient care (Box 21.1).

INCORPORATING PERIODONTAL-SYSTEMIC EVIDENCE INTO TREATMENT AND PRACTICE

To date, the scientific evidence for an association between periodontitis and systemic diseases is robust for type 2 diabetes mellitus and for cardiovascular diseases. In diabetes, a modest but positive trend

---

BOX 21.1   Legal, Ethical, and Safety Issues

- A critical part of evidence-based practice is staying abreast of new developments in research. The research surrounding oral-systemic associations is continually growing and evolving, and it is the responsibility of the practitioner to remain current. Attending evidence-based continuing education courses is a good way for a hygienist to keep their knowledge level current. Additionally, reading peer-reviewed professional journals is a helpful way to maintain current and evidence-based practice. An up-to-date understanding of oral-systemic associations is an expectation of standard of care.
- Another issue involves making referrals and seeking consultations when needed. If a patient has signs and symptoms of a disease for which they have not been previously diagnosed, then it is the responsibility of the clinician to make an appropriate referral to a primary care provider. In addition, if the clinician has concerns or questions about the safest way to plan and proceed with dental treatment, then it is their responsibility to attain an appropriate consultation. (Box 21.2, Critical Thinking Scenario involves a patient with potential referral needs.)

BOX 21.2   Critical Thinking Scenario

You have a 6-year-old male patient today. He weighs 59 pounds and is 42 inches tall, which is categorized as obesity. The child's mother has diabetes. The child's last doctor's appointment was for school vaccinations just after he turned 5 years old.

Answer the following questions regarding this scenario and read the answers after considering them yourself:

1. In addition to relating this child's current dental condition to his mother, what else do you need to discuss?
2. What additional clinical services would you consider providing for this patient?
3. Do you believe a referral is needed at this point and if so, what type?
Answers:
1. Risk of diabetes, the association between diabetes and periodontitis, and the importance of nutrition and physical exercise for general health.
2. Association among obesity, type 2 diabetes, and periodontitis may be related to the effects of these diseases on the immune system and inflammation related to excessive nutrients; importance of changes in nutrition and exercise, such as limiting sweetened beverages, snacks, and fast food; limiting screen time; engaging in physical activity for at least 60 minutes per day; and encouraging family meals.
3. Referral to a primary care provider is recommended for an overall well check and weight management. The results of chairside HbA1c levels should be shared, if significant.

---

supports the fact that periodontal treatment has a positive effect on improved metabolic regulation.[16] It is also known that periodontal treatment (e.g., reduced presence of biofilm and inflammation) has a positive effect on lowering systemic inflammation and improving the condition of the vascular system.

As healthcare providers, we aim to promote overall health for all of our patients. Therefore we must incorporate these concepts as a part of the education and motivation of patients to ensure that they pursue a general healthier status (Box 21.3). A reduction of intraoral biofilm and gingival inflammation remains a relatively simple and cost effective procedure for the dental team. This important intervention, coupled with attention to risk factors for periodontal diseases, can have a very positive long-term effect on the patient's overall health.

BOX 21.3   Client Education Tips

Health literacy is an important aspect of patient education. Many individuals have low literacy and numeracy skills, and it is the responsibility of the clinician to help ensure that the patient understands the information they are given. Although there is a large field of study surrounding health literacy, two easy communication tools to implement into your practice are **plain language** and **teachback**. Plain language simply means using language that is clear and easily understood. This communication approach can be difficult in the healthcare realm, particularly in explaining something as complex as oral-systemic associations. However, keeping the explanations simple will help the patient better understand the information. In the teachback communication approach, the clinician asks the patient to explain the information that they were given. When the patient explains to the provider the information they were just given, the clinician can determine if there is misunderstanding or if the information needs to be explained in a different way.

NATURE OF ASSOCIATIONS BETWEEN PERIODONTAL DISEASE AND SYSTEMIC DISEASES

Atherosclerotic Cardiovascular Disease and Periodontitis

Epidemiologic studies have shown that patients with periodontitis are at an increased risk for developing aortic atheroma (atherosclerotic plaque), coronary artery disease, and atherosclerosis (see Fig. 21.2). These conditions can result in cardiovascular events such as stroke and MI. Periodontal disease can influence the risk indicators for ACVDs, which include serum levels of **C-reactive protein** (CRP), a systemic inflammatory marker, and arterial stiffness, which are risk factors for MI and stroke.[17,18] The primary theory of biologic plausibility surrounding this interaction is that the bacteria from periodontal pockets enter the bloodstream (see Fig. 21.2), which leads to the production of inflammatory mediators that induce systemic inflammation. These mediators are taken up into the **endothelium** (i.e., inner wall of the blood vessels) and contribute to atherosclerotic plaque.[4] The ability of the smooth muscle to respond to nitrous oxide, produced by the endothelial cells, is inhibited, resulting in **arterial stiffness** and formation of the atherothrombotic lesion.[17]

A simple flow chart of the mechanisms of biologically plausible events associating periodontitis and atherothrombogenesis, described by Tonetti and Van Dyke, can be helpful to enhance understanding (Fig. 21.3).[5]

Studies on the ability of periodontal therapy to prevent cardiovascular events have been inconclusive. However, periodontal treatment studies have demonstrated decreased serum levels of CRP and improved endothelial function.[6]

Currently, the evidence supports an association between periodontitis and ACVDs and supports the fact that periodontal therapy can reduce markers of systemic inflammation. However, current evidence is not strong enough to inform patients that periodontal therapy could prevent a cardiovascular event. Patients with periodontitis should pursue periodontal therapy to help reduce oral biofilm and oral inflammation, which should also help achieve a reduction in systemic inflammation. In addition, dental hygienists should encourage healthy habits and discuss techniques for the management of other risk factors for ACVDs (e.g., smoking, poor diet, high blood pressure, high cholesterol level, diabetes, obesity, physical inactivity).

Diabetes and Periodontitis

Research supports a bidirectional relationship between periodontitis and diabetes.[9] This means that patients with diabetes who develop

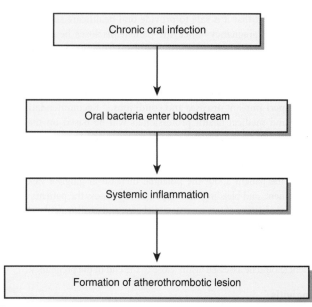

Fig. 21.3 Flowchart outlining the biological plausibility of an association between periodontitis and atherothrombogenesis.

periodontitis will likely have a harder time controlling gingival inflammation and maintaining oral health. Moreover, the more extensive the periodontal inflammation is, the more difficult controlling blood glucose levels will be. Patients who have diabetes are at increased risk of developing periodontitis compared with healthy patients.[9] Thus patients with diabetes, prediabetes, or risk of diabetes need to be educated about this relationship. Patient education should address the benefits of oral self-care, including the daily removal of bacterial biofilm and the use of an antimicrobial mouthrinse or dentifrice for control, and the benefits of healthy dietary and exercise habits, as well as the possible referral for assessment of metabolic health. The main theory of biologic plausibility with this association is systemic inflammation. Systemic inflammation can lead to insulin resistance, which results in an initial increase in insulin production by beta cells. After some time, the beta cells can no longer produce insulin at this increased level and become dysfunctional, leading to lower levels of available insulin and consequently to hyperglycemia. Periodontal bacteria are distributed systemically through the bloodstream, increasing systemic inflammation, and further reducing the body's ability to use available insulin and impeding glucose control.

Periodontal therapy research has demonstrated improvement in blood glucose management. A review conducted by Simpson et al. revealed that currently there is moderately certain evidence that periodontal treatment using subgingival instrumentation improves glycemic control in people with both periodontitis and diabetes by a clinically significant amount when compared to no treatment or usual care.[16] This effect is similar to that of adding an additional medication to manage blood glucose. The consistency within this field of research provides a good foundation for the dental hygienist to be comfortable advising patients with diabetes of the following:

- Patients with diabetes are at increased risk of developing periodontal disease.
- Patients with diabetes have periodontal disease, their blood glucose levels may be more difficult to control.
- Periodontal treatment and maintenance should help improve blood glucose control; however, 3-month intervals for supportive care are recommended.

Adverse Pregnancy Outcomes and Periodontitis

The most commonly studied adverse pregnancy outcomes (APOs) related to periodontitis include preterm birth, a low-birth-weight infant, and preeclampsia. Results of epidemiologic studies support an association between periodontal disease and these APOs, independent of known confounders.[13,19,20] However, the overall level of evidence linking APOs and periodontal disease is generally considered to be modest. Although rates of APOs are higher among patients with periodontitis, periodontal treatment research has been inconsistent in reducing rates of APOs. Because this reversibility has not been established, further research is needed to clarify an understanding of this association.

The following primary theories of biologic plausibility of the association between periodontitis and APOs have been identified:
1. **Direct pathway**, in which oral bacteria reach the fetal-placental unit via the bloodstream or via an ascending infection from the vagina. This infection leads to an immune or inflammatory response, resulting in APOs.
2. **Indirect pathway**, in which inflammatory mediators from the periodontal tissues or liver travel via the bloodstream to the fetal-placental unit. Examples of these mediators include prostaglandin E_2 (PGE_2) and tumor necrosis factor-α (TNF-α). In addition, inflammatory mediators from periodontal tissues may reach the liver, where production of systemic inflammatory mediators (e.g., CRP) increases, affecting the fetal-placental unit.[13,21]

Increases in inflammatory or immune responses can plausibly cause APOs because labor and delivery are initiated by inflammatory signaling. At the end of a pregnancy, the concentration of inflammatory mediators (e.g., PGE_2, TNF-α, interleukin-1β [IL-1β]) in the amniotic fluid increases until it reaches a threshold point. Once this point is reached, rupture of membranes and cervical dilation is induced, leading to the delivery of the newborn. If increased levels of inflammatory mediators are present in the blood at the fetal-placental unit or in the amniotic fluid from an infection, this threshold point may be reached early, leading to preterm birth or a low-birth-weight infant.[21]

The dental hygienist should feel comfortable advising a pregnant patient of the following:
1. Pregnant patients with periodontitis are at increased risk for APOs.
2. Nonsurgical periodontal therapy is safe for pregnant patients.
3. Periodontal treatment should be completed for patients who are pregnant and have periodontitis, with the goal of reducing oral biofilm and signs of inflammation.

Respiratory Diseases and Oral Health

Oral health has been linked to respiratory diseases, particularly pneumonia, and especially in patients confined to hospital or continuous care settings (see Chapter 55). There are several classifications of pneumonia. **Community-acquired pneumonia** (CAP) is when a person who is not in a hospital or care setting is infected and develops pneumonia. **Nosocomial hospital-acquired pneumonia** (HAP) is acquired during a hospital stay, exhibiting symptoms within 48 hours after admission. **Ventilator-associated pneumonia** (VAP) occurs when a patient on a ventilator develops pneumonia 48 hours or longer after intubation; VAP is a subtype of HAP. **Aspiration pneumonia** (AP) occurs when saliva is inhaled into the lungs and an infection results; AP is more common among patients who have difficulty swallowing. Strong and consistent evidence supports an association between increased loads of oral biofilm and pneumonia, specifically with VAP and HAP.[15] The biologic plausibility of this association is relatively simple. A patient on a ventilator has a plastic tube that is passed through the oral cavity and into the lungs, providing a direct route for bacteria to travel into the lungs, resulting in infection. Studies evaluating the efficacy of oral hygiene in preventing HAP have had positive results, and patients who have regular and thorough oral cleaning procedures experience reduced rates of HAP.[15] A review by Lavigne and Forrest, in a position paper from the Canadian Dental Hygienists Association, concluded that the Bradford Hill criteria analysis failed to support a causal relationship between periodontal microbes/oral healthcare and respiratory diseases such as pneumonia.[22] Heterogeneity among studies and lack of consistency in research findings make it difficult to draw firm conclusions regarding the relationship between periodontitis and pneumonia. However, meticulous oral hygiene should be a part of routine care for hospitalized patients, those with difficulty swallowing, or those who are on a ventilator to reduce the risk of pneumonia.

Some limited, weak evidence links periodontitis to chronic obstructive pulmonary disease (COPD); however, additional research into this area is needed. The existing studies do not demonstrate strength of evidence to support a claim of association.[15]

CLINICAL CASE EXAMPLES

To better illustrate the practical application on the importance of the topics discussed in this chapter, three different clinical case examples are presented to the reader (Box 21.4). These cases represent a sample of what a dental care provider may encounter when practicing dental hygiene or dentistry.

BOX 21.4 Clinical Case Examples

Consider the following cases representing a sample of what a dental care provider may encounter when practicing dental hygiene or dentistry.

Case One:

Patient information: A 47-year-old man who works as a clerk in a department store

Health history: Physical status classification is assessed at ASA II (American Society of Anesthesiologists–Class II) and he was diagnosed with type 2 diabetes 5 years before this dental visit. His body mass index (BMI) was 30 kg/m². His last HbA1c level was 9.7%. The only medication that the patient reported taking was metformin to control his diabetes. However, for the last few months before this dental visit, he admitted

not being able to comply with his medication or have a proper diet. Moreover, for the last several months, he reported being very stressed as a result of a contentious divorce from his wife. He had not been eating or sleeping well and also admits to being noncompliant with his oral hygiene routine.

Chief complaint: He came to the clinic as an urgent care patient because of severe generalized pain and discomfort, affecting his gingiva.

Primary intraoral and radiographic findings: Intraorally, extensive redness and swelling of the gingiva are noted, which could not be touched because of severe pain and bleeding. In addition, a fetid odor is originating from his mouth. Radiographically, a generalized presence of interdental calculus is noted as well as two nonsalvageable teeth (18 and 30).

Continued

BOX 21.4   Clinical Case Examples—cont'd

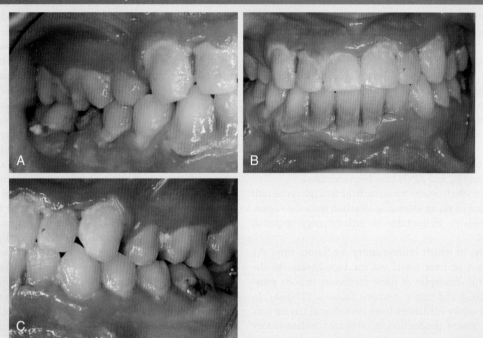

Case One: Pretreatment clinical photographs.

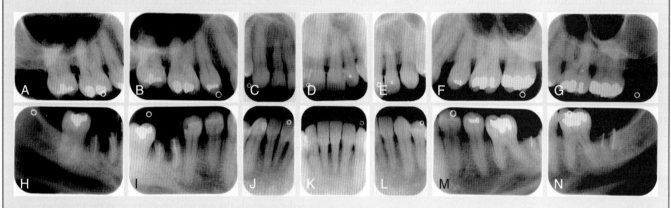

Case One: Radiographic series.

Periodontal diagnosis: The patient is diagnosed with generalized necrotizing periodontal disease.

Treatment provided: Despite the known poor control of his HbA1c level, immediate intervention is needed. Amoxicillin and metronidazole, combined with a chlorhexidine rinse, was initially prescribed to reduce the bacterial load of his oral cavity. He was also advised to improve his overall compliance in relation to his diabetes control. A few days after the initiation of his systemic antibiotics and antimicrobial mouthrinse, he received a full-mouth disinfection (scaling and root planing) and the extraction of teeth 18 and 30. He continued with his medications for a total of 2 weeks.

Treatment outcome and long-term goals: Four months after the initial intervention, the patient has had remarkable improvement in his periodontal health. His probing depths ranged between 1 and 4 mm, with minimal bleeding on probing. He was then placed on a periodontal maintenance protocol every 3 months. At this visit, he reported that his HbA1c returned to acceptable levels (7%) and that his overall lifestyle has improved significantly.

BOX 21.4 Clinical Case Examples—cont'd

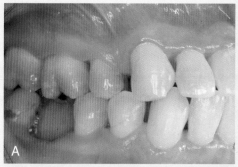
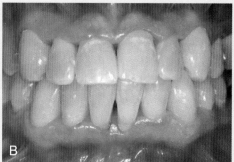
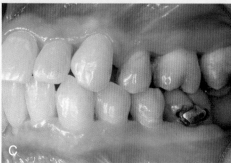

Case One: Posttreatment clinical photographs.

Case Two

Patient information: A 26-year-old woman who works at a hair salon as a stylist

Health history: Physical status classification is assessed at ASA I. She reports having no medical problems and no known drug allergies. She is taking no medications.

Chief complaint: The patient is planning to become pregnant, but she has not had a dental examination or dental prophylaxis for a few years. Her chief complaint is bleeding gums when flossing and sometimes when brushing. She also reports that she wants to have good oral health before becoming pregnant. She said that her physician told her that good oral health may help

prevent pregnancy complications. She reports that she is very interested in having a very healthy pregnancy.

Primary intraoral and radiographic findings: Her initial periodontal examination revealed that she had probing depths ranging from 1 to 5 mm. Multiple posterior sites had 5-mm probing depths. She also had moderate attachment loss associated with some of the moderate pocketing sites. A moderate amount of subgingival calculus was detected in several of the posterior and the mandibular anterior segments of her mouth. Radiographically, very mild horizontal alveolar bone loss, mostly in the posterior sextants, is noted.

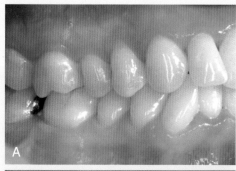
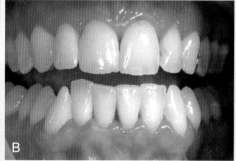
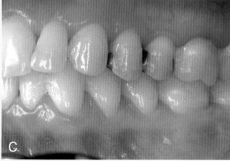

Case Two: Pretreatment clinical photographs.

Continued

BOX 21.4   Clinical Case Examples—cont'd

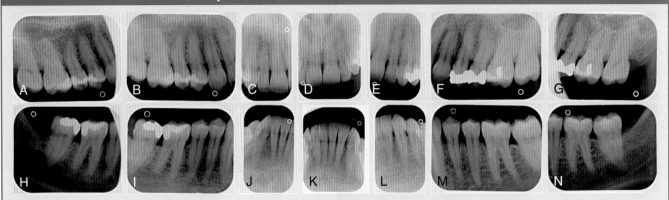

Case Two: Radiographic series.

Periodontal diagnosis: The patient is diagnosed as having localized moderate chronic periodontitis.

Treatment provided: She received localized scaling and root planing, combined with oral hygiene instructions.

Treatment outcome and long-term goals: The reevaluation of her initial periodontal therapy revealed a significantly healthier periodontal condition, with reduced probing depths and almost no bleeding on probing. She was advised to return for periodontal maintenance every 3 to 4 months, especially during her pregnancy.

Case Three

Patient information: A 56-year-old man who is a car mechanic

Health history: His health history reveals a 25-year history of cigarette smoking (between one-half pack to one full pack per day) and a recent (<4 months) history of myocardial infarction (MI). The patient quit smoking since his MI event and he realizes that he needs to treat his severe periodontitis. He is also trying to change his lifestyle to include a healthier diet and better exercise habits.

Chief complaint: His severe periodontitis probably contributed to his recent MI. The patient is also aware that his cigarette smoking habit may have been the primary contributor to both his MI and his severe chronic periodontitis. Tooth 8 was naturally exfoliated recently, attributable to severe mobility and a lack of alveolar bone support.

Primary intraoral and radiographic findings: The patient exhibits generalized probing depths between 3 and 10 mm, accompanied by severe attachment loss. In addition, significant amounts of supragingival and subgingival calculus are noted; most of his teeth had a mobility grade 2 or even a grade 3. Radiographically, the dental care provider observed generalized severe horizontal and vertical alveolar bone loss.

Periodontal diagnosis: The patient is diagnosed as having generalized severe chronic periodontitis.

Treatment provided: As a result of the recent loss of tooth 8, he wanted to replace this tooth temporarily to help with his appearance and speech. An interim removable partial denture was fabricated to temporarily replace tooth 8. More importantly, since the MI event was very recent, a consultation with the medical provider was imperative. Once the medical provider authorized dental hygiene and dental treatment, this patient's treatment included nonsurgical and surgical periodontal therapy.

Treatment outcome and long-term goals: The patient responded well to both nonsurgical and surgical periodontal therapy. However, a few of his posterior teeth were lost during the surgical therapy. Because of the nature of his severe periodontitis, his history of an MI, and his oral hygiene habits, he was initially placed on a strict 2- to 3-month periodontal maintenance protocol.

BOX 21.4 Clinical Case Examples—cont'd

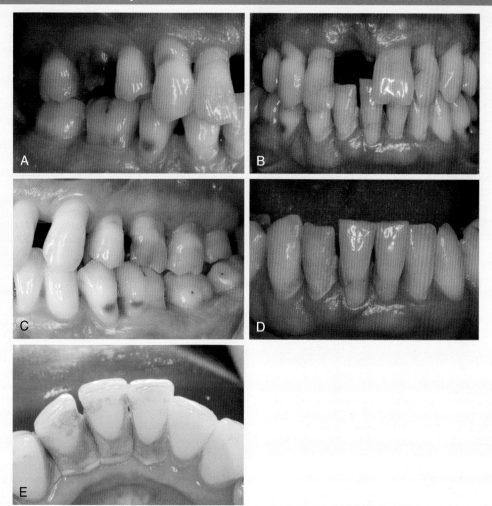

Case Three: Pretreatment clinical photographs.

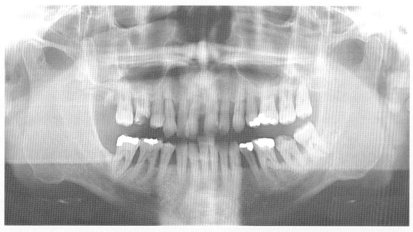

Case Three: Panoramic radiographic image.

KEY CONCEPTS

- ACVD, diabetes, APOs, and pneumonia have been established as areas of association with periodontal disease or oral health.
- Limited or weak evidence suggests associations between periodontitis and rheumatoid arthritis and osteoporosis, chronic kidney disease, obesity, cancer, metabolic disease, obstructive sleep apnea, and cognitive impairment; more robust research is needed.
- A thorough understanding of these areas of association is necessary for patient education.
- Educating patients about their periodontal health and how it relates to systemic health is a critical aspect of patient care.
- Communicating with other healthcare providers to make referrals or request consultations is a necessary aspect of patient care.
- Maintaining an evidence-based practice is expected of dental hygienists, and it is the responsibility of the dental hygienist to remain up to date on oral-systemic knowledge and research.

REFERENCES

1. Bradford Hill A. The environment and disease: association or causation? *Proc R Soc Med*. 58(5):295–300.
2. van Dyke TE, van Winkelhoff AJ. Infection and inflammatory mechanisms. *J Clin Periodontol*. 2013;40(suppl 14):S1–S7.
3. Thoden van Velzen S, Abraham-Inpiin L, Moorer W. Plaque and systemic disease: a reappraisal of the focal infection concept. *J Clin Periodontol*. 1984;11(4):209–220.
4. Centers for Disease Control and Prevention. *Heart disease facts*. Published July 15, 2022. https://www.cdc.gov/heartdisease/facts.htm. Accessed July 27, 2022.
5. Tonetti MS, Van Dyke TE. Periodontitis and atherosclerotic cardiovascular disease: consensus report of the joint EFP/AAP workshop on periodontitis and systemic diseases. *J Clin Periodontol*. 2013;40(suppl 14). https://doi.org/10.1111/jcpe.12089.
6. Sanz M, Marco del Castillo A, Jepsen S, et al. Periodontitis and cardiovascular diseases: consensus report. *J Clin Periodontol*. 2020;47(3):268–288. https://doi.org/10.1111/jcpe.13189.
7. Centers for Disease Control and Prevention. *Diabetes basics*. Published June 21, 2022. https://www.cdc.gov/diabetes/basics/index.html. Accessed July 26, 2022.
8. Mayo Clinic Staff. *A1C Test*. https://www.mayoclinic.org/. Published July 27, 2022. https://www.mayoclinic.org/tests-procedures/a1c-test/about/pac-20384643. Accessed July 26, 2022.
9. Chapple ILC, Genco R. Diabetes and periodontal diseases: consensus report of the joint EFP/AAP workshop on periodontitis and systemic diseases. *J Clin Periodontol*. 2013;40(suppl 14). https://doi.org/10.1111/jcpe.12077.
10. Centers for Disease Control and Prevention. *Preterm birth*. https://www.cdc.gov/. Published July 27, 2022. https://www.cdc.gov/reproductivehealth/maternalinfanthealth/pretermbirth.htm. Accessed July 26, 2022.
11. Centers for Disease Control and Prevention. *FastStats: Birthweight and gestation*. Published July 27, 2022. https://www.cdc.gov/nchs/fastats/birthweight.htm. Accessed July 26, 2022.
12. Mayo Clinic Staff. *Preeclampsia overview*. Published July 27, 2022. https://www.mayoclinic.org/diseases-conditions/preeclampsia/symptoms-causes/syc-20355745. Accessed July 26, 2022.
13. Sanz M, Kornman K. Periodontitis and adverse pregnancy outcomes: consensus report of the joint EFP/AAP workshop on periodontitis and systemic diseases. *J Clin Periodontol*. 2013;40(suppl 14). https://doi.org/10.1111/jcpe.12083.
14. Caton JG, Armitage G, Berglundh T, et al. A new classification scheme for periodontal and peri-implant diseases and conditions – Introduction and key changes from the 1999 classification. *J Clin Periodontol*. 2018;89(S1):S1–S8. https://doi.org/10.1002/JPER.18-0157.
15. Linden G, Lyons A, Scannapieco F. Periodontal systemic associations: review of the evidence. *J Clin Periodontol*. 2013;84(4 suppl):S8S19.
16. Simpson TC, Clarkson JE, Worthington HV, et al. Treatment of periodontitis for glycaemic control in people with diabetes mellitus. *Cochrane Database Syst Rev*. 2022;2022(4). https://doi.org/10.1002/14651858.CD004714.pub4.
17. Schmitt A, Carra MC, Boutouyrie P, Bouchard P. Periodontitis and arterial stiffness: a systematic review and meta-analysis. *J Clin Periodontol*. 2015;42(11):977–987. https://doi.org/10.1111/jcpe.12467.
18. D'Aiuto F, Orlandi M, Gunsolley JC. Evidence that periodontal treatment improves biomarkers and CVD outcomes. *J Clin Periodontol*. 2013;40(suppl 14). https://doi.org/10.1111/jcpe.12061.
19. Papapanou PN. Systemic effects of periodontitis: lessons learned from research on atherosclerotic vascular disease and adverse pregnancy outcomes. *Int Dent J*. 2015;65(6):283–291. https://doi.org/10.1111/idj.12185.
20. Corbella S, Taschieri S, del Fabbro M, Francetti L, Weinstein R, Ferrazzi E. Adverse pregnancy outcomes and periodontitis: a systematic review and meta-analysis exploring potential association. *Quintessence Int*. 2016;47(3):193.
21. Madianos PN, Bobetsis YA, Offenbacher S. Adverse pregnancy outcomes (APOs) and periodontal disease: pathogenic mechanisms. *J Periodontol*. 2013;84(4):S170–S180. https://doi.org/10.1902/jop.2013.1340015.
22. Lavigne SE, Forrest JL. An umbrella review of systematic reviews of the evidence of a causal relationship between periodontal microbes and respiratory diseases: position paper from the Canadian Dental Hygienists Association. *Can J Dent Hyg*. 2020;54(3):144–155.

22

Dental Hygiene Diagnosis

Cynthia C. Gadbury-Amyot and Tanya Villalpando Mitchell

PROFESSIONAL OPPORTUNITIES

Becoming competent in the development of a dental hygiene diagnosis is critical to the practice of dental hygiene. The dental hygiene diagnosis is complementary to the dental diagnosis and provides a framework for collaboration between the dental hygienist and dentist for delivering comprehensive person-centered care. In addition, a dental hygiene diagnosis provides a method for collaborating with other healthcare providers, promoting interdisciplinary patient care.

COMPETENCIES

1. Compare and contrast a dental hygiene and a dental diagnosis using nursing and medicine as a parallel.
2. Discuss the dental hygiene diagnostic process in action and apply the Human Needs and Oral Health-Related Quality of Life models for decision making in the development of a dental hygiene diagnosis.
3. Implement the dental hygiene diagnostic process by identifying interventions that support various dental hygiene diagnoses, write dental hygiene diagnoses, and educate and motivate clients to work toward positive behavior changes.
4. Gather complete data during patient assessment to support recognizable patterns in formulating diagnoses, demonstrating validation and support for the process in providing individualized dental hygiene care.
5. Discuss the outcomes and benefits of dental hygiene diagnoses.

DIAGNOSIS DEFINED

A search in PubMed and Google Scholar for *define diagnosis* leads to thousands of citations. A review of the results quickly shows that diagnosis is associated with medical conditions and diseases. Although the diagnostic process is generic, when applied to the practice of a particular discipline, it becomes a discipline-specific diagnosis. For example, in medicine, a medical diagnosis has traditionally evolved around a disease or medical condition, whereas a nursing diagnosis includes the aspects of a person's response to illness and the effects of the illness on the patient and family.[1] Similar to medicine, a dental or oral diagnosis is problem oriented,[2] whereas a dental hygiene diagnosis first seeks to prevent oral disease and then proceeds to minimize the risk of oral disease and promote wellness. Dentistry continues to operate predominately within a traditional biomedical, paternalistic, disease-oriented environment. Within this environment of practice, there is the assumption that what is considered "normal" for the patient is based on the opinion and judgment of the dentist, with little to no input from the patient. The approach of both nursing and dental hygiene to the diagnostic process uses a holistic, person-centered method that extends beyond considering the disease or medical condition and solicits patient input and collaboration. Particularly relevant to both nursing and dental hygiene diagnoses is the inclusion of **social determinants of health**. Social determinants of health are defined as both "economic and social conditions that influence the health of people and communities."[3] Furthermore, of the factors that influence health, social determinants of health are estimated to account for between 30% and 55% of health of outcomes (see Chapter 2).

Dental Hygiene Diagnosis

To assist communities of interest in defining and outlining the parameters of a **dental hygiene diagnosis**, the American Dental Hygienists' Association (ADHA) released Standards for Clinical Dental Hygiene Practice in 2016.[4] The following is ADHA's definition of dental hygiene diagnosis:

The identification of an individual's health behaviors, attitudes, and oral healthcare needs for which a dental hygienist is educationally qualified and licensed to provide. The dental hygiene diagnosis requires evidence-based critical analysis and interpretation of assessments in order to reach conclusions about the patient's dental hygiene treatment needs. The dental hygiene diagnosis provides the basis for the dental hygiene care plan. (ADHA Standards for Clinical Dental Hygiene Practice—Standard 2: Dental Hygiene Diagnosis)

The Standards are clear that a dental hygiene diagnosis be considered complementary to the dental diagnosis and, likewise, should promote collaboration both within dentistry and with other healthcare professionals to ultimately provide the most comprehensive care for the patient. This chapter discusses the *Human Needs Assessment Form and Dental Hygiene Diagnosis* (Figs. 22.2 and 22.3), and the *Oral Health-Related Quality of Life Assessment, Dental Hygiene Diagnosis, and Care Plan* (Figs. 22.4 and 22.6), and refers to the words "dental hygiene diagnosis." Using Case Study 22.1 in this chapter, a dental hygiene diagnosis has been formed. To explore the extent to which dental hygiene diagnosis is permitted by state, refer to ADHA's *Dental Hygiene Practice Overview: Permitted Functions and Supervision Levels by State*.[5] For example, in the state of Colorado, a dental hygiene diagnosis is a permitted function of the dental hygienist under the category of Direct Access Supervision Levels. The Colorado Dental Hygiene Practice Act states the dental hygienist is able to provide services as they determine appropriate without specific authorization.

Patient
Patient is a 27-year-old Hispanic male.

Chief Complaint
"I have not been to the dentist for over 6 years and have recently been diagnosed with diabetes."

Background and/or Patient History
Background: BP 130/90 mm Hg; HR 82 bpm; RR 20

Medical History
Last physician's visit 3 months ago. Diagnosed with type 2 diabetes with an HbA1C of 7.5%. Diagnosed with high blood pressure 2 years ago.

Medications
- Metformin: 2000 mg/day for type 2 diabetes
Side effect: xerostomia
- Zaroxolyn: 2.5 mg/day for high blood pressure
Side effect: xerostomia

Intraoral and Extraoral Examinations
- Lightly coated tongue
- Large tonsils
- Moderate saliva flow
- Class I molar relationship – 2-mm overbite

Dental History
- Missing teeth #18, #19, #30, #31
- Brushes once a day and uses floss a couple times a week

Periodontal Evaluation
- Stage III, Grade B
- Probing depths 3 to 4 mm in the anterior and 4 to 6 mm in the posterior. Localized 7 mm on tooth #1F and tooth #14DF
- Class II furcation involvement on tooth #2F
- Plaque score is 18%
- BOP score is 68%

Social History
Patient is concerned about his diabetes and noted that his father also is diabetic. Patient perceives his oral health as bad and said he bleeds when brushing. He said he has lost teeth due to caries. He noted that in his culture, seeking oral healthcare is not the norm. Patient does not have dental nor medical insurance but is willing to pay for treatment.

Current Findings
Active caries DO tooth #5; generalized moderate subgingival calculus

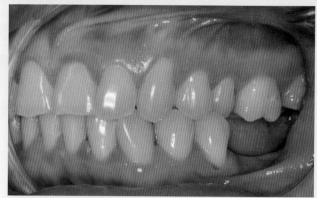

Case Study 22.1 Figure 2 (Left side buccal view)

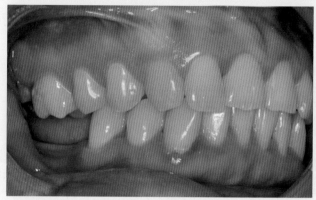

Case Study 22.1 Figure 3 (Right side buccal view)

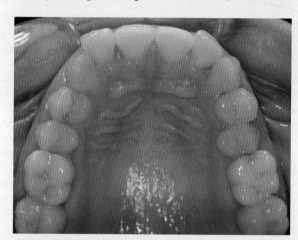

Case Study 22.1 Figure 4 (Upper occlusal)

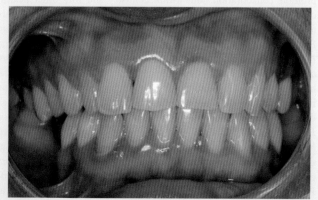

Case Study 22.1 Figure 1 (Frontal teeth in occlusion)

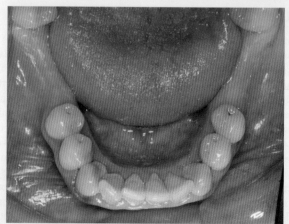

Case Study 22.1 Figure 5 (Lower occlusal)

CASE STUDY 22.1   Synopsis of Patient History—cont'd

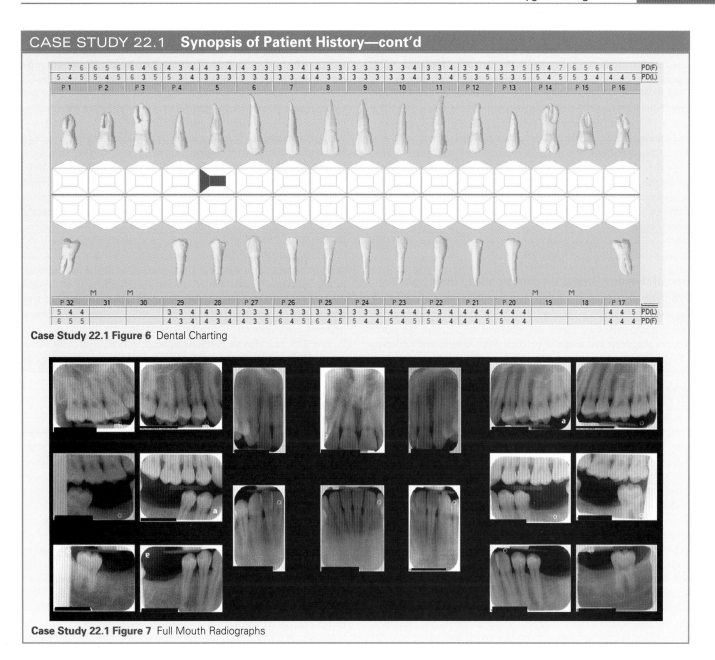

Case Study 22.1 Figure 6 Dental Charting

Case Study 22.1 Figure 7 Full Mouth Radiographs

An illustration of the kind of collaboration called for in the *ADHA Standards for Clinical Dental Hygiene Practice* and the relevance of a dental hygiene diagnosis is made clear by the following example. The first Surgeon General's Report on Oral Health, published in 2000, called attention to how income effects oral health, with those of lower income levels suffering the greatest need.[6] In 2014, Michigan state agencies made a decision to change the water supply of Flint, Michigan, as a money-saving strategy. This decision resulted in contaminated water, including high levels of lead in the drinking water. Subsequent adverse health effects for the residents of the city followed, in particular for those in neighborhoods identified as disadvantaged.[7] This example illustrates how a social determinant of health and low income resulted in a situation that warrants the dental hygienist's consideration when developing a dental hygiene diagnosis. Research has found that excessive lead exposure at young ages can result in cognitive deficits.[8] A

dental hygiene diagnosis, as defined in the *ADHA Standards for Clinical Dental Hygiene Practice*, would consider the need for modifications to oral hygiene instructions aimed at the actual cognitive abilities of the patient rather than age-appropriate instruction. Collaboration with medical professionals to determine the degree of cognitive deficits and working with parents to develop oral hygiene strategies that are realistic would be critical to ensure and maintain oral health. This example illustrates how the *ADHA Standards for Clinical Dental Hygiene Practice* can assist dental hygienists in understanding and using dental hygiene diagnoses. A dental hygiene diagnosis for the situation above would include a holistic, person-centered approach to care. **Person-centered care** is defined as a way of thinking and doing things that sees the people using health and social services as equal partners in planning, developing, and monitoring care to make sure it meets their needs. This means putting people and their families at the center of the decisions and seeing them as experts, working alongside professionals to reach the best outcome.[9] Person-centered care and patient-centered care are often used interchangeably. In the Institute of Medicine (IOM) report, *Crossing the Quality Chasm: A New Health System for the 21st Century*, patient-centered care is one of six pillars defining high-quality care.[10] The IOM report defines patient-centered as "providing care that is respectful of and responsive to individual patient preferences, needs, and values and ensuring that patient values guide all clinical decisions." The *ADHA Standards for Clinical Dental Hygiene Practice* can serve to assist dental hygiene educators working with dental hygiene students on the process and procedure of the development of a dental hygiene diagnosis and care plan. For the licensed practitioner, the *ADHA Standards for Clinical Dental Hygiene Practice* can serve as a guide in the correct application of a dental hygiene diagnosis in support of best practices. Box 22.1 provides an overview of legal, ethical, and safety issues related to the dental hygiene diagnosis.

Dental Hygiene Diagnosis and Expanded Scope of Practice

Legislatively, the *ADHA Standards for Clinical Dental Hygiene Practice* provides understanding, clarity, and guidance on the issue of a dental hygiene diagnosis and scope of practice. Both Oregon and Colorado (2004 and 2009, respectively) authorized the dental hygiene diagnosis as part of the dental hygienists' scope of practice within their practice acts as outlined in ADHA's *Dental Hygiene Practice Overview: Permitted Functions and Supervision Levels by State*.[5] At the time of this writing, 42 US states permit citizens **direct access** to dental hygienists.[11] Direct access involves the ability of the dental hygienist to initiate treatment based on the assessment of a patient's needs without the specific authorization of a dentist. It is worth noting that since the release of the 2000 Surgeon General's Report, the number of states that permit direct access to dental hygienists has grown from 8 to 42. In December of 2021, a followup report, *Oral Health in America: Advances and Challenges*, was released.[12] Many of the key takeaways of the report support greater access to dental hygiene services and legislation that promotes rather than inhibits these efforts. Exploration of the ADHA scope of practice website illustrates efforts by states to advance both settings and dental hygiene services in order to increase access to care (https://www.adha.org/scope-of-practice).[13] The remaining eight states that do not allow direct access are ultimately prohibiting increased access to oral healthcare for their citizens. As direct access has expanded, so have dental hygiene scopes of practice across the country. As the scope of practice expands, it will be critical that the dental hygiene

diagnosis becomes part of the services provided. A review of nursing literature illustrates that with role (i.e., scope of practice) expansion, subsequent revisions in the practice acts have been made to recognize nursing diagnoses.[14] Acknowledgement that the diagnostic process is discipline specific when applied to the practice of that discipline, one would expect to see a similar expansion of practice acts to include dental hygiene diagnosis into the process of care of dental patients. However, the expansion of practice acts to include dental hygiene diagnosis has been slow. One factor contributing to this situation is past actions taken by the Commission on Dental Accreditation (CODA). In 2007, the American Dental Association House of Delegates brought forward a resolution that resulted in the removal of dental hygiene diagnosis from the CODA accreditation standards, a term that had been in the standards since 1998. As a result, CODA removed both dental hygiene treatment plan and dental hygiene diagnosis from the standards for dental hygiene educational programs effective January 1, 2010. At the time of this writing in 2022, CODA standards for dental hygiene education programs include a very limited definition of dental hygiene diagnosis in its *Definition of Terms*: "Dental Hygiene Diagnosis: Identification of an existing potential oral health problem that a dental hygienist is qualified and licensed to treat."[15]

Box 22.2 provides an overview of legal, ethical, and safety issues related to dental hygiene practice acts in the United States, scope of practice, and direct access to dental hygiene services.

DENTAL HYGIENE DIAGNOSTIC PROCESS IN ACTION

In the ADHA *Standards for Clinical Dental Hygiene Practice*, Standard 2 (Dental Hygiene Diagnosis) outlines five aspects of the dental hygiene diagnosis:
  I. Analyze and interpret all assessment data.
 II. Formulate the dental hygiene diagnosis or diagnoses.
III. Communicate the dental hygiene diagnosis with patients or clients.
IV. Determine patient needs that can be improved through the delivery of dental hygiene care.
 V. Identify referrals needed within dentistry and other healthcare disciplines based on dental hygiene diagnoses.

The health professions rely on a *process of care* as a method for providing practitioners with a systematic approach to follow in their care of patients. A methodologic approach to patient care for dental hygiene can be seen in Fig. 22.1—Dental Hygiene Process of Care. Chapters 13 through 21 cover various aspects of dental hygiene assessments, including assessment of the patient health history, dental history, extraoral and intraoral exam, and the periodontal assessment, to name a few. The first step in diagnosis involves a comprehensive assessment and analysis of all the data collected. In alignment with a holistic, person-centered approach to care, dental hygiene assessment should include the collection of not only biologic and physiologic variables (e.g.,

---

BOX 22.1   Legal, Ethical, and Safety Issues Related to Dental Hygiene Diagnosis

The *ADHA Standards for Clinical Dental Hygiene Practice* state that it is only after the dental hygiene diagnosis that the dental hygienists can formulate a care plan that focuses on dental hygiene education, self-care practices, prevention strategies, and treatment and evaluation protocols that focus on patient or community oral health needs. The dental hygiene diagnosis promotes collaboration both within dentistry and with other healthcare professionals to ultimately provide the most comprehensive care for the patient and community. The *ADHA Code of Ethics* further reinforces the importance of interdisciplinary and interprofessional practice.[21] Under "Basic Beliefs" in the *ADHA Code of Ethics*, it states that dental hygiene care is an essential component of overall healthcare and we function interdependently with other healthcare providers. Access the *ADHA Code of Ethics* on the ADHA website to find additional references within the code that further reinforces this commitment to interdisciplinary and interprofessional practice.

BOX 22.2   Legal, Ethical, and Safety Issues Related to the Scope of Practice

Visit the ADHA website to find the information provided on the dental hygiene scope of practice and direct access. Identify the information for the state(s) in which you are licensed or plan to be licensed to practice. Next, find your *state practice act* and compare it to the practice act of another state. Research how dental hygiene scope of practice and direct access are addressed in the practice acts. Discuss whether the state(s) you researched are conducive to or prohibitive to increasing access to oral healthcare through dental hygienists.

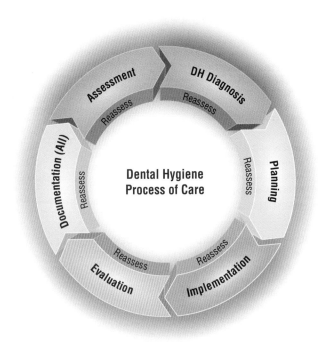

Fig. 22.1 Dental hygiene diagnosis is an integral part of the process of care that provides the basis for the dental hygiene care plan.

medical and dental histories) but also psychologic variables (e.g., effect of oral condition on symptoms, function, and health perceptions) and social variables (e.g., environmental, socioeconomic, and sociocultural influences). Combined, these data are collectively referred to as biopsychosocial data.

When a diagnosis is developed based on biopsychosocial data, it becomes clear that a dental hygiene diagnosis is discipline specific and is a good match to the current healthcare environment referred to as person-centered care. Research has shown that a shared decision-making process between providers and patients results in superior outcomes. Beginning with assessment and ending with evaluation and documentation (see Fig. 22.1), the dental hygienist can follow a process that ultimately results in person-centered, evidence-based, and quality care for the patient. As a component of this process of care, the diagnostic process involves a problem-solving approach to clinical decision making, which helps guide the intellectual activity of the dental hygienist. Two theoretical models developed specifically for the practice of dental hygiene, the Human Needs (HN) Conceptual Model and the Oral Health-Related Quality of Life (OHRQL) Model, are explored below, using Case Study 22.1.

Applying the Human Needs and the Oral Health-Related Quality of Life Models to Diagnostic Decision Making

In Case Study 22.1, a 27-year-old Hispanic male presents for care. The assessment findings include the following: vital signs—blood pressure (130/90 mm Hg), heart rate (82 bpm), and respiration rate (20 rpm). His medical history includes a diagnosis of type 2 diabetes and hypertension. His last physician's visit was 3 months ago. Refer to Case Study 22.1 to see how these theoretical models, Human Needs and Oral Health-Related Quality of Life, can assist the dental hygienist with determining a dental hygiene diagnosis and, ultimately, the development of a comprehensive dental hygiene care plan.

Human Needs Model

With the HN model, the dental hygiene diagnostic process uses eight human needs related to dental hygiene care as its foundation (see

Chapter 2). These eight human needs are assessed using the Human Needs Assessment Form and Dental Hygiene Diagnosis (Fig. 22.2). Note that Fig. 22.2 is a blank form that does not include any patient information. Feel free to use this for practicing both assessment and dental hygiene diagnosis. A review of Case Study 22.1 finds five of the eight human needs as unmet: protection from health risks, skin and mucous membrane integrity of the head and neck, biologically sound and functional dentition, conceptualization and problem solving, and responsibility for oral health (see Fig. 22.3 HN Conceptual Model Assessment Form – Case 22.1). With both the causes and the signs and symptoms identified, the dental hygienist is then able to proceed with a diagnosis. Based on the dental hygiene diagnosis, a care plan is developed and presented to the patient. The care plan should include the patient's goals, dental hygiene interventions, and evaluation. Refer to Chapter 2 to see how the authors have used two fictional cases to apply both the Human Needs Conceptual Model and the Oral Health-Related Quality of Life Models to arrive at dental hygiene diagnoses.

See Box 22.3, where the reader is referred to a patient case study in Chapter 21, Oral-Systemic Health Connection, Box 21.4 – Case Two and directed to the blank Human Needs Assessment Form (Fig. 22.2, Blank HN Assessment Form) to develop a dental hygiene diagnosis.

Oral Health-Related Quality of Life Model

The World Health Organization describes health as a "state of complete physical, mental, and social well-being and not merely the absence of disease and infirmity."[16] **Oral health-related quality of life** is defined in the 2000 Surgeon General's Report as a "multidimensional construct that reflects (among other things) people's comfort when eating, sleeping, and engaging in social interaction; their self-esteem; and their satisfaction with respect to their oral health."[6] While there was mention of oral health-related quality of life in the 2000 Surgeon General's Report, the *2021 Oral Health in America: Advances and Challenges* report shows 21 years later a much greater emphasis being put on the assessment of biopsychosocial measures and how that data is being used in the delivery of person-centered care.[11]

The Oral Health-Related Quality of Life (OHRQL) Model for dental hygiene was introduced in 1998, prior to the 2000 Surgeon General's Report.[17] With the Oral Health-Related Quality of Life (OHRQL) Model, the dental hygiene diagnostic process revolves around the assessment of traditional biologic variables such as medical history and dental history (Fig. 22.4—Blank OHRQL Assessment Form), the oral health-related quality of life assessment, dental hygiene diagnosis, and care plan, and psychosocial variables collected using the OHRQL questionnaire (Fig. 22.5—Blank OHRQL Questionnaire). Note that Figs. 22.4 and 22.5 are blank forms that do not include any patient information. Feel free to use these for practicing assessment, dental hygiene diagnosis, and care plan development. Traditional biologic variables are combined with the psychosocial variables to develop a dental hygiene diagnosis and care plan based on biopsychosocial data. Refer to Figs. 22.6 (OHRQL Assessment Form—Case 22.1) and 22.7 (OHRQL Questionnaire—Case 22.1) to see completed forms that show how this information is collated and developed into a dental hygiene diagnosis and care plan for Case Study 22.1. See Box 22.4, where the reader is referred to a patient case study in another chapter of this book (for example, Chapter 21 Oral-Systemic Health Connection – Case Two) and directed to the blank OHRQL Assessment Form (Fig. 22.4) to develop a dental hygiene diagnosis.

Dental hygiene diagnoses focus on professional care and allow dental hygienists to assess and manage patient conditions within their scope of practice. After diagnosis, goals are developed in collaboration with the patient. It is well documented in the literature that shared decision making results in superior health outcomes.

Human Needs Conceptual Model

ASSESSMENT(circle signs and symptoms present)

1) PROTECTION FROM HEALTH RISKS
- vital signs outside of normal limits
- need for prophylactic antibiotics
- potential for injury
- risk factors
- other _____

5) SKIN AND MUCOUS MEMBRANE INTEGRITY OF THE HEAD AND NECK
- extra-/intraoral lesion
- swelling
- gingival inflammation
- BOP
- interdental CAL (>/= 1m)
- probing depths (>/= 4mm)
- radiographic bone loss
- tooth loss due to periodontitis
- xerostomia
- other_____

2) FREEDOM FROM FEAR AND STRESS
- reports or displays:
  - anxiety about proximity of clinician, confidentiality, or previous dental experience
  - oral habits
  - substance abuse
- concern about:
  - infection control, fluoride therapy, fluoridation, mercury toxicity, other_____

6) BIOLOGICALLY SOUND AND FUNCTIONAL DENTITION
- reports difficulty in chewing
- presents with:
  - defective restorations
  - teeth with signs of disease
  - missing teeth
  - ill-fitting dentures, appliances
  - abrasion, erosion, abfraction
  - active caries
  - other_____

3) FREEDON FROM PAIN
- extra-/intraoral pain or sensitivity
- other_____

7) CONCEPTUALIZATION AND PROBLEM SOLVING
- has questions about DH care and/or oral disease
- other_____

4) WHOLESOME FACIAL IMAGE
- expresses dissatisfaction with appearance
  - teeth - gingiva - facial profile - breath
  - other_____

8) RESPONSIBILITY FOR ORAL HEALTH
- plaque and calculus present
- inadequate parental supervision of oral healthcare
- no dental exam within the last 2 years
- other_____

DENTAL HYGIENE DIAGNOSIS (List the unmet human need, then be specific about the etiology and signs and symptoms evidencing the unmet need)

(Unmet Human Need)	(Etiology – due to…..)	(Signs and Symptoms – as evidenced by…..)	Patient Goal (expected outcome)
Protection from health risks			
Freedom from fear and stress			
Freedom from pain			
Wholesome facial image			
Skin and mucous membrane integrity of the head and neck			
Biologically sound and functional dentition			
Conceptualization and problem solving			
Responsibility for oral health			

DENTAL HYGIENE INTERVENTIONS (target etiologies)

APPOINTMENT SCHEDULE:

CONTINUED CARE RECOMMENDATION:

EVALUATION: (goal met, partially met, or unmet) and supporting evaluative statement

Fig. 22.2 Human Needs Assessment Form and Dental Hygiene Diagnosis (blank—no patient information). (Adapted from Darby ML, Walsh MM. Application of the Human Needs Conceptual Model to dental hygiene practice. *J Dent Hyg* 2000;74(3):230–237.)

Human Needs Conceptual Model

ASSESSMENT (circle signs and symptoms present)

1) PROTECTION FROM HEALTH RISKS

- vital signs outside of normal limits
- need for prophylactic antibiotics
- potential for injury
- (risk factors)
- other _____

5) SKIN AND MUCOUS MEMBRANE INTEGRITY OF THE HEAD AND NECK

- extra-/intraoral lesion
- swelling
- (gingival inflammation)
- (BOP)
- (interdental CAL (>/= 1m))
- (probing depths (>/= 4mm))
- (radiographic bone loss)
- tooth loss due to periodontitis
- (xerostomia)
- other _____

2) FREEDOM FROM FEAR AND STRESS

- reports or displays:
  - anxiety about proximity of clinician, confidentiality, or previous dental experience
  - oral habits
  - substance abuse
- concern about:
  - infection control, fluoride therapy, fluoridation, mercury toxicity, other _____

6) BIOLOGICALLY SOUND AND FUNCTIONAL DENTITION

- reports difficulty in chewing
- presents with:
  - defective restorations
  - teeth with signs of disease
  - (missing teeth)
  - ill-fitting dentures, appliances
  - abrasion, erosion, abfraction
  - (active caries)
  - other _____

3) FREEDON FROM PAIN

- extra-/intraoral pain or sensitivity
- other _____

7) CONCEPTUALIZATION AND PROBLEM SOLVING

- (has questions about DH care and/or oral disease)
- other _____

4) WHOLESOME FACIAL IMAGE

- expresses dissatisfaction with appearance
  - teeth - gingiva - facial profile - breath
  - other _____

8) RESPONSIBILITY FOR ORAL HEALTH

- (plaque and calculus present)
- inadequate parental supervision of oral healthcare
- (no dental exam within the last 2 years)
- other _____

DENTAL HYGIENE DIAGNOSIS

Unmet human need for protection from health risk due to potential risk for medical emergency as evidenced by type II diabetes (metformin 2000 mg/day) with HbA1c 7.5 diagnosed 4 months earlier and hypertension (zaroxolyn 2.5 mg/day) diagnosed 2 years ago, BP 130/90 @ initial visit.

Client Goals	Interventions (target etiologies)	Evaluation
Patient will	Educate on importance of taking medications as prescribed by physician, eating nutritious meal within 2 hours of appointment, and reporting changes in health to reduce risk of a glycemic event. Schedule appointments in the AM.	
• confirm taking daily medications as prescribed by physician, following prescribed diet and any changes in health at the start of each appointment.		

DENTAL HYGIENE DIAGNOSIS

Unmet human need for skin and mucous membrane integrity of the head and neck due to generalized supra- and subgingival plaque biofilm, extrinsic stain, moderate calculus gen. interproximal and lingual sextant 5, immune response to type II diabetes and high blood pressure as evidenced by stage III, grade C periodontitis, radiographic bone coronal to middle 1/3 molar roots (unable to measure interdental CAL with calculus), probing depths 4 to 6 mm posteriors, 7 mm #1 F and #14 DF, gen. horizontal bone loss, % bone loss/age moderate, HbA1c 7.5%, recession 1mm #20, F2 #2F; bleeding index (BI) 68%; gingival inflammation.

Fig. 22.3 Human Needs Assessment Form and Dental Hygiene Diagnosis—with patient information. (Adapted from Darby ML, Walsh MM. Application of the Human Needs Conceptual Model to dental hygiene practice. *J Dent Hyg.* 2000;74(3):230–237.)

Client Goals	Interventions (target etiologies)	Evaluation
The patient will; • reduce probing depths of 5 mm and greater by 1 mm or more by phase 1 re-evaluation and maintain to phase IV maintenance appointment; • reduce BI to less than 10% by phase 1 reevaluation and maintain to Phase IV maintenance appointment; • eliminate gingival inflammation by phase 1 reevaluation. • stabilize clinical attachments to phase IV maintenance appointment.	Phase I nonsurgical periodontal therapy • Periodontal debridement full mouth with powered and hand instrumentation • Local anesthesia • Review/reinforce oral self care • Phase I outcome @ 4-6 weeks • Coronal polish, medium grit paste or air-powder to remove extrinsic stain. • Referral phase II consultation with periodontist following phase I.	

Dental Hygiene Diagnosis

Unmet need for biologically sound and functional dentition due to inadequate oral self-care, generalized plaque biofilm, PI 90%, saliva-reducing medications and frequent snacking, moderate salivary flow by observation, irregular dental care, and impaired ability to utilize molars for proper chewing of food and functionality as evidenced by high risk for caries, active caries, xerostomia causing medication (zaroxolyn), bilaterally missing 1st and 2nd mandibular molars from previous caries.

Client Goals	Interventions	Evaluation
The patient will; • reduce high caries risk to low caries risk by phase IV maintenance continued care visit. • increase protective factors by 4/11. • schedule appointment with dentist of record for restorative needs by 3/14.	Educate on caries risk factors (plaque, diet, saliva) protective factors and the importance of periodic dental examinations. Reinforce brushing 2 x a day and flossing 1 x a day. Discuss the benefits of xylitol-containing gum and self-applied topical fluoride, place on 1.1% NaF toothpaste for pm brushing. Apply professional NaF varnish. Schedule with collaborating dentist to have caries treated.	

Dental Hygiene Diagnosis

Unmet need for conceptualization and problem solving due to lack of knowledge of etiology of periodontal diseases, disease indicators, risk factors, oral-systemic health relationship as evidenced by patient reports never being educated on the importance of oral health, reports his oral health as bad but highly motivated to improve his oral health, patient is unable to explain periodontal disease, role of bacterial plaque biofilm, risk factors that contribute to disease progression, bidirectional relationship of diabetes and periodontitis, and self-care actions to slow disease progression.

Client Goals	Interventions	Evaluation
The patient will; • paraphrase the relationship of bacterial plaque biofilm to the periodontal process, risk factors that impact rate of disease progression and the bidirectional relationship of diabetes and periodontitis by 4/4. • affirm the importance of daily plaque removal and management of blood glucose to minimize risk of progression of periodontitis by 4/4.	Educate on etiology of periodontal diseases, plaque biofilm, impact of diabetes on disease progression and bidirectional relationship of diabetes and periodontitis. Discuss the importance of daily removal of plaque and diabetes management.	

Dental Hygiene Diagnosis

Unmet need for responsibility for oral health due to inadequate oral self-care(technique, infrequency), lack of regular preventive oral health throughout life as evidenced by brushing 2 x day with a medium-bristle brush, flossing 2 to 3 x per week, PI score of 85%. Last dental appointment was 4 years ago, states seeking professional oral healthcare not a cultural norm; however, motivated to improve oral health, seeking dental care on his own.

Fig. 22.3, cont'd

Client Goals	Interventions	Evaluation
The patient will; • demonstrate efficient brushing with a soft bristle brush or power brush and flossing techniques by phase I reevaluation. • reduce PI score to less than 10% by phase I reevaluation. • report brushing 2 x day with soft-bristle brush and flossing 1 x day at phase I reevaluation and maintain to Phase IV maintenance. • schedule phase IV maintenance visit for continuedcare at phase I outcome.	Instruct on brushing with soft bristle brush, flossing technique and frequency. Introduce and instruct on power brush technique. Discuss the importance of regular maintenance appointments to monitor periodontal disease progression.	

APPOINTMENT SCHEDULE:

PROGNOSIS: Short-term prognosis is good as patient seems motivated to improve oral health. Discussed with patient the importance of phase I treatment and adherence to oral self-care recommendations to reduce pocket depths, stabilize bone loss, and decrease hard and soft deposits. Long-term prognosis is fair due to diabetes HbA1c 7.5, age, and localized sites of moderate bone loss and critical pocket depths; however, patient is working with physician to decrease HbA1c and has committed to phase II evaluation with periodontist at the completion of phase I.

SIGNATURES: Patient	Clinician	Date

CONTINUED CARE RECOMMENDATION:

Fig. 22.3, cont'd

BOX 22.3 Critical Thinking Scenario A

Human Needs Assessment and Dental Hygiene Diagnosis
Select a patient case study from one of the chapters in this book. For example, Chapter 21, Oral-Systemic Health Connection, Box 21.4—Case Two. Next, use the Human Needs Assessment Form (Fig. 22.2, Blank HN Assessment Form) to develop a dental hygiene diagnosis. What patient (client) goals could be established? What dental hygiene interventions will you use to help the patient achieve their goals? (If you need assistance filling out the Human Needs Assessment Form on the patient, refer to Fig. 22.3 to see how the form was completed using the information from Case Study 22.1.)

Patient goals—the desired outcome of care—clarify what the patient needs to do to promote, maintain, and achieve oral health and wellness. Planning care is contingent on the dental hygiene diagnosis (see Chapter 23 for treatment and care planning). Interventions are implemented, evaluated, and documented, along with any other relevant information.

USING STANDARDS TO FORMULATE AND VALIDATE DIAGNOSES

Writing Dental Hygiene Diagnoses

After analyzing the patient's data, the dental hygienist reaches one of two conclusions, with each one requiring different actions. First, if the conclusion is that the patient requires treatment, the dental hygienist will collaborate with the patient to formulate, validate, and prioritize a dental hygiene diagnosis before treatment. (Refer to Case Study 22.1 for examples of how the dental hygienist might use the HN and the OHRQL models to take the data collected to formulate and prioritize a dental hygiene diagnosis.) Second, if the conclusion is that the patient does not have an actual problem that requires treatment but has risk factors and risk indicators suggesting that they are at risk for a problem, then a dental hygiene diagnosis

would be targeted toward actions that do not involve treatment but are aimed specifically at alleviating risk. At-risk problems are conditions that should be diagnosed to ensure that actions can be taken to prevent the potential problem from developing. An example of this could be a patient of record who presents for a routine appointment between his freshman and sophomore years of college. As you gather biopsychosocial data, you become concerned about the potential for risky drinking behaviors based on your conversation. You have been trained in the evidence-based practice (EBP), Screening, Brief Intervention, and Referral to Treatment for Substance Use (SBIRT), for substance use, and you decide to administer the AUDIT (Alcohol Use Disorders Identification Test (AUDIT) questionnaire.[18] The results of the AUDIT place the patient in the risky zone. The action suggested for patients identified in this zone is a brief intervention to reduce use. A person-centered discussion using **motivational interviewing** (MI) concepts to raise awareness and enhance motivation to change behavior is employed. If the patient is at risk for potential health problems, there may not be signs and symptoms because the problem has not yet occurred; however, it is still preventable if risk factors are modified.

Patient Education and Motivation

Motivational interviewing is defined as "a collaborative, person-centered form of guiding to elicit and strengthen motivation for change."[19] The premise is to bring the patient into the conversation about a change in behavior; in this case, a change in drinking behavior, in which the patient's reasons for changing are elicited, as opposed to authoritarian and prescriptive advice from the dental hygienist. Metaanalyses can be found in the literature that show motivational interviewing is effective when it comes to changes in behavior. The National Institute on Drug Abuse (NIDA) offers a 1.5-hour online course titled "Blending Initiative Motivational Interviewing and Patient Simulation" (https://nida.nih.gov/nidamed-medical-health-professionals/ctn-dissemination-initiative/blending-initiative-motivational-interviewing-cmece-patient-simulation). Please see Chapter 5—Sustainable Health Behavior Change for more on motivational interviewing.

Validation of Dental Hygiene Diagnoses

To arrive at a valid dental hygiene diagnosis, the dental hygienist can compare observed data (objective and subjective) with an accepted standard. For example, a blood pressure of 130/90 mm Hg may be within the expected range for an individual with hypertension under the control of a physician, but this level is abnormal for a person not under a physician's care. Accepted standards for blood pressure can be found by referring to the American Heart Association (AHA) guidelines (https://www.acc.org/latest-in-cardiology/articles/2017/11/08/11/47/mon-5pm-bp-guideline-aha-2017).

Using the AHA guidelines, the dental hygienist can confirm that the patient in Case Study 22.1 has a blood pressure that would be considered stage 1 for systolic and stage 2 for diastolic (blood pressure:130/90

mm Hg). (Refer to Chapter 13, Personal, Dental, and Health Histories, to find additional resources that can be used to validate a diagnosis of vital signs being within normal limits for Case Study 22.1). Again, find case from another chapter (for example, Chapter 21: Oral-Systemic Health Connection) and use the AHA guidelines to confirm the stage of blood pressure of the patient(s).

In Box 22.5, the accepted standards of practice for periodontal care are the American Academy of Periodontology (AAP) and the European Federation of Periodontology (EFP) 2017 Classification of Periodontal and Peri-Implant Diseases and Conditions. This provides another example of how the dental hygienist can validate the dental hygiene diagnosis. The *ADHA Standards for Clinical Dental Hygiene Practice* offer another resource for validating dental hygiene diagnoses.

ORAL HEALTH-RELATED QUALITY OF LIFE ASSESSMENT, DH DIAGNOSIS AND CARE PLAN

Student Name:	Patient Name:	Chart Number:
I) General Assessment—		Next Appointment:

A Medical Assessment: (refer to patient's medical history.)

B Health Perceptions: (refer to Section I on OHRQL patient questionnaire.)

C Oral Health History: (provide a brief explanation for each)

1 Caries:
- Date of last caries activity
- Fluoride history
- Frequency of caries
- Recurrent, coronal, root, proximal, incipient
- Date and location of last dental exam
- Caries risk assessment -
- History of head and neck radiation therapy-
- Other
- Systemic disease affecting caries-
- Manual dexterity-
- Frequency of restorative care-

Caries / Periodontal:

2 Periodontal:
- Date and location of last prophy—
- Previous periodontal therapy
- Previous case type & disease classification -
- Systemic disease affecting periodontal diseases
- Frequency of preventive and periodontal care (previous recommended maintenance)
- Past response to therapy –
- Other:

Nicotine use–

Alcohol and drug use-

3 Radiographic: (Date of Exposures) If New Patient to SOD—indicate radiographs taken prior to being seen at SOD
- FMX
- BWs
- Pano
- PAs
- Radiographs needed:

II) Patient's Current Oral Status: Patient response. (Circle answer and give brief explanation.)
A. Symptom Status: (refer to Section II on OHRQL pt. questionnaire)
- Dry when eating
- Need liquid to aid in swallowing
- Dry at night
- Tooth pain
- Duration
- Soft tissue pain
- Sensitive to hot/cold/pressure
- Frequency of pain

B. Functional Status: (refer to Section III on OHRQL questionnaire)
- Mobile teeth
- Loose denture
- TMD
- Duration
- Pain
- Go out less
- Others misunderstand words
- Communicate less
- Self-consciousness
- Appearance
- Depression

C. Occlusal: (Based on assessment data)
I   II   III   Overbite: Overjet:
Crowding   • bruxism (clenching, grinding)

D. Individual Characteristics: (refer to Section 4 on OHRQL patient questionnaire)
- Sociocultural:
- Socioeconomic:
- Environmental:

E. Quality of Life: (Based on patient's perceived QOL, indicated impact on DH treatment decisions.)

Fig. 22.4 The Oral Health-Related Quality of Life Model. The oral health-related quality of life assessment, dental hygiene diagnosis, and care plan (blank—no patient information). (Adapted from Williams KB, Gadbury-Amyot CC, Bray KK, et al. Oral health-related quality of life: a model for dental hygiene education, practice and research. *J Dent Hyg.* 1998;72(2):19–26.)

	Put Etiology/CF/RF separate for each item listed in previous column	Everything in this column should show up in the next.	Nothing in this column not already in previous.	
III. Oral Assessment and DH Diagnosis		**IV. DH Care Plan**	**V. Implementation & Evaluation**	ADA code & Fee
Problem/Pathology/Risk Assessment	Etiology	Treatment Selections & HC	Sequence of DH Procedures	
1. Intra/Extra Oral Exam	1 = Primary etiology 2 = Contributing factors/Risk factor)			
2. Dental Evaluation				
3. Periodontal Evaluation • AAP Disease Classification highlight as appropriate Reduced Stable Periodontium Gingivitis-Plaque Induced, Gingivitis Non-Plaque Induced Stage: I, II, III, IV Grade: A, B, C *Annuals of Periodontology*, 2017 • ADA Case Type & Status- **Periodontal Pathologies** • attachment loss: • recession: • pocket formation • bone loss & descriptions: • mobility: • furcation involvement: • gingival description: • BI: • PI: • mucogingival defects: • level of risk for periodontal disease/s)			Referrals/Consults:	
Dental Hygiene Diagnosis				
Dental Hygiene Prognosis				
Outcome Evaluation				
Patient Centered Outcome		Clinical Outcomes:		
Signatures:	Student:	Faculty:	Patient:	Date:

Fig. 22.4, cont'd

The ADHA Standards serve as a resource for dental hygiene practitioners seeking to provide evidence-based practice (EBP) and person-centered care. EBP is best defined by Sackett and colleagues as the conscientious use of current best evidence in making decisions about patient care.[20] EBP includes the integration of scientific evidence, clinical expertise, clinical circumstances, and patient values. The ADHA Standards are put through a rigorous validation process to ensure that they are based on emerging scientific evidence, federal and state regulations, policy development, and changing disease patterns. The ADHA is dedicated to revising these standards as an ongoing commitment to dental hygiene practitioners and the public that they serve; therefore, the dental hygienist can be comfortable using the ADHA Standards from year to year.

For an in-depth review of periodontal staging and grading, complete the course *Aligning the Dental Hygiene Diagnosis with the 2018 AAP Classification of Periodontal and Peri-Implant Diseases* on Dentalcare.com under the Course Listings Topic of Electives, http://www.dentalcare.com.

Recognizing Patterns

Dental hygiene diagnoses should always be based on a cluster of significant information rather than on a single sign or symptom. The danger of arriving at a dental hygiene diagnosis from a single factor is evident from the following example:

The dental hygienist diagnoses an Eastern Indian woman as having an unmet human need for a wholesome facial image. The diagnosis looks to be related to a lack of dental care as evidenced by malpositioned teeth and a prognathic profile, but the observed data may have been misinterpreted. The dental hygienist mistakenly identified the cause as a lack of dental care when it is rooted in the patient's culture, which accepts malocclusion as within the range of normal. The woman has had regular dental care throughout her life but no orthodontic care because of her cultural orientation. Indeed, her human need for a wholesome facial image was met because it was not in deficit from the patient's perspective. Likewise, using the OHRQL questionnaire, the dental hygienist would have discovered that the patient was satisfied with her malocclusion and that it had no negative impact on her oral health-related quality of life since the malocclusion is an accepted norm within her culture. Gathering all data that support a recognizable pattern prevents the dental hygienist from formulating an incorrect diagnosis. (Refer to Box 22.6 to learn how the law can influence the dental hygienist in instances such as malpractice.)

OUTCOMES OF DENTAL HYGIENE DIAGNOSES

Dental hygiene diagnoses facilitate the development of professional autonomy and accountability by focusing on phenomena within the scope of dental hygiene practice and by providing a language for communication. The dental hygiene diagnosis clarifies the role of the dental hygienist and allows for a defined scope and domain of the dental hygiene practice. As the healthcare delivery system continues to change, such as an expanded scope of practice and direct access for dental hygienists, the dental hygiene diagnosis must serve as an integral component of dental hygiene care. With the recognition by dental hygienists that the dental hygiene diagnosis is an essential component of the process of care, patient needs are more accurately communicated, which serves to support the provision of treatment

ORAL HEALTH-RELATED QUALITY OF LIFE QUESTIONNAIRE–STUDENT WORKSHEET

I. HEALTH PERCEPTIONS *General Health* Compared to others your age, how would you rate your general health? • What do you perceive is your biggest problem? *Oral Health* Compared to others your age, how would you rate the condition of your mouth, teeth, or dentures? • What do you think contributes most to your oral condition?	I. PATIENT RESPONSE (give brief explanation of pt. response) *General Health* *Oral Health*
II. **SYMPTOM STATUS** *Dry Mouth* Is your mouth dry, or your amount of saliva too little? *Pain* Do you have any pain or discomfort with your teeth, dentures, or mouth?	II. **PATIENT RESPONSE (circle answer or give brief explanation of patient response)** *Dry Mouth* • Need liquid to aid in swallowing • Dry when eating • Moisture seems too little in mouth • Dry at night *Pain* • Tooth pain • Soft tissue pain • Frequency of pain • Duration • Sensitive to: hot / cold / pressure
III. **FUNCTIONAL STATUS** *Physical Function* Do your teeth, dentures, or mouth interfere with your ability to eat or chew? Do problems with your mouth, teeth, or dentures interfere with your ability to speak? *Social Function* Do problems with your mouth, teeth, or dentures interfere with your interactions with others? *Psychological Function* Do problems with your mouth teeth, or dentures affect the way you feel about yourself?	III. **PATIENT RESPONSE (circle answer or give brief explanation of patient response)** *Physical Function* • Mobile Teeth • Pain • Loose Dentures • TMS • Duration • Others misunderstand words • Repetition *Social Function* • Go out less • Communicate less • Interfere with leisure activities • Interfere with enjoyment of others' company *Psychological Function* • Self-consciousness • Appearance • Relaxation/tension • Depression
IV. **INDIVIDUAL CHARACTERISTICS** *Family/Cultural* Generally speaking, how much do your friends or family members influence the decisions you make about your mouth, teeth, or dentures? <u>Sociocultural influences</u>: <u>Family culture</u>: does the patient's family influence their ability to seek dental care? Influence the patient's values regarding dental care? <u>Community culture</u>: does the patient's living community influence their ability to receive care? Influence the patient's values regarding dental care? Who makes the decisions regarding the patient's ability to seek care and receive treatment? What are the patient's perceptions regarding healthcare? Does the patient value prevention and health promotion? <u>Environmental influences</u> Does the patient have easy access to both medical and dental care? Can the patient transport themselves to receive care or do they rely on others for assistance? Does the patient live independently or do they depend on others for daily functioning? Is their family or living environment conducive to health and healthy habits? (Diet, oral hygiene aids, etc.) Are their overall living conditions conducive to health promotion? (Communication and activities with others, living environment, etc.) Does the patient have fluoride in their drinking water? <u>Economic influences</u> Patient's socioeconomic status (How can this be assessed? What cues are you given?) How do finances influence the patient's ability to receive dental care? Does the patient have insurance coverage for dental care? How does insurance coverage (or lack thereof) influence the patient's decision making regarding dental care? What are the patient's perceptions of healthcare and health promotion as they relate back to finances? Does the patient value health and how does this relate to their financial outlook and status?	IV. PATIENT RESPONSE (give brief explanation of pt. response) *Family/Cultural*

Fig. 22.5 Oral Health-Related Quality of Life Questionnaire (blank—no patient information).

ORAL HEALTH-RELATED QUALITY OF LIFE ASSESSMENT, DH DIAGNOSIS AND CARE PLAN

Student Name:	Patient Name:	Chart Number:

I) General Assessment—Patient is a 27-year-old Hispanic male; chief complaint–none. Patient is new to the SOD.

Next Appointment:

A Medical Assessment: (Refer to patient's medical history.)
Patient was diagnosed 4 months ago with type II diabetes. Patient was diagnosed with high blood pressure 2 years ago. Patient medications include metformin 2000mg/day and zaroxolyn 2.5mg/day. Vitals were WNL –BP: 130/90/ Pulse: 82 Respiration Rate: 20. Patient's last physician's visit was 3 months ago.

B Health Perceptions: (Refer to Section I, on OHRQL patient questionnaire.)
Patient perceives his general health as fair due to high blood pressure and type II diabetes; takes medication to control diabetes and blood pressure. Patient states last dental visit was about 3-4 years ago.

C Oral Health History:

1 Caries:
- **Date of last caries activity** – patient recalls previous caries about 3-4 years ago
- **Fluoride history** – Uses fluoridated toothpaste and fluoridated mouthrinse.
- **Frequency of caries** – patient has active decay and has lost his mandibular 1st and 2nd molars due to caries.
- **Recurrent, coronal, root, proximal, incipient**
- **Date and location of last dental exam** 4 years ago in private practice

- **Caries risk assessment** – High due to infrequent dental care, inadequate home care, existing carious lesions, and frequent snacking.
- **History of head and neck radiation therapy** – None

- **Other** – N/A
- **Systemic disease affecting caries** - None
- **Manual dexterity** – Normal
- **Frequency of restorative care** – Patient mentioned having his mandibular 1st and 2nd molars extracted due to caries.

Caries / Periodontal:
Caries: Moderate caries on #5DO
Periodontal: Stage III, Grade C

2 Periodontal:
- **Date and location of last prophy** – Location unknown. Patient stated it to be about 4 years ago.
- **Previous periodontal therapy** – Unknown
- **Previous case type & disease classification** – Unknown
- **Systemic disease affecting periodontal diseases** – diabetes and HBP

- **Frequency of preventive and periodontal care (previous recommended maintenance)** – Unknown
- **Past response to therapy** – Unknown

- **Other:**

Nicotine use – None

Alcohol and drug use – None

3 Radiographic: (Date of Exposures) **If New Patient to SOD—indicate radiographs taken prior to being seen at SOD**
- **FMX** – today's visit
- **BWs**
- **Pano**

- **PAs**
- **Radiographs needed:** None

II) Patient's Current Oral Status: Patient response. **(Circle answer and give brief explanation.)**

A. Symptom Status: (refer to Section II on OHRQL pt. questionnaire)
- **Dry when eating** – N/A
- **Need liquid to aid in swallowing** – N/A
- **Dry at night** – N/A
- **Tooth pain** – N/A
- **Duration**
- **Soft tissue pain** – N/A
- **Sensitive to hot/cold/pressure** – N/A
- **Frequency of pain**

B. Functional Status: (refer to Section III on OHRQL questionnaire)
- **Mobile teeth** – N/A
- **Loose denture** – N/A
- **TMD** – N/A
- **Duration** – N/A
- **Pain** – N/A
- **Go out less** – N/A
- **Others misunderstand words** – N/A
- **Communicate less** – N/A
- **Self-consciousness** – N/A
- **Appearance** – N/A
- **Depression** – N/A

C. Occlusal: (Based on assessment data)
Bilateral Class I Molar Relation   II   III   **Overbite:** 25% 2mm   **Overjet:** None
Crowding   • **bruxism (clenching, grinding)** - None

D. Individual Characteristics: (refer to Section 4 on OHRQL patient questionnaire)
- **Sociocultural:** Patient is seeking dental care on his own Patient community culture influence their ability to seek dental care because in his Hispanic culture, seeking oral health care is not something of the norm. Oral healthcare is something that is not taught and this could be one of the reasons why the patient has infrequent dental care. Patient values health careand understands he must keep up with medical care due to HBP and diabetes.
- **Socioeconomic:** Patient is willing to pay for dental care and is capable of paying. Patient would like an estimate of how much each appointment would be prior to coming in. Patient does not have dental insurance.
- **Environmental:** Patient does have easy access to medical and dental healthcare as his work schedule is very flexible, but patient does not have neither medical or dental insurance, which makes it hard for him to seek care. Patient can transport himself to and from appointments just fine. Patient is living independently –does not depend on others.

E. Quality of Life: (Based on patient's perceived QOL, indicated impact on DH treatment decisions.)
Patient values his health He was never educated on the importance of oral health so it has never been valued in his life. Patient is determined to improve his oral health. His work schedule it very flexible, allowing him to come to multiple appointments.

Fig. 22.6 The Oral Health-Related Quality of Life Model. The oral health-related quality of life assessment, dental hygiene diagnosis, and care plan—with patient information. (Adapted from Williams KB, Gadbury-Amyot CC, Bray KK, et al. Oral Health-Related Quality of Life: a model for dental hygiene education, practice and research. *J Dent Hyg.* 1998;72(2):19–26.)

	Put Etiology/CF/RF separate for each item listed in previous column	**Everything in this column should show up in the next.**	**Nothing in this column not already in previous.**	
III. Oral Assessment and DH Diagnosis		**IV. DH Care Plan**	**V. Implementation & Evaluation**	**ADA code & Fee**
Problem/Pathology/Risk Assessment	Etiology	Treatment Selections & HC	Sequence of DH Procedures	
1. Intra-/extraoral Exam • Light swelling of submandibular lymph nodes – bilateral • Lightly coated tongue • Small fissures on tongue • Bilateral Class I Molar Relationship • Moderate Salivary Flow • 25% (2mm) Overbite	1= Primary etiology 2= Contributing factors/Risk factor) 1. Lightly coated tongue – patient does not use any type of oral appliance to clean tongue 2. Patient has large tonsils, which can contribute to halitosis.	1. How motivated are you to improve your overall home care now vs. a year ago? (Looking Back) MI: What do you think is causing your tongue to have a white/coated appearance? Preventive Counseling: Educate patient on brushing soft tissue, tongue, to remove all coated bacteria. Inform patient about tongue scraper, Educate patient on xylitol-containing gum can counteract bacteria by preventing the buildup of plaque and that chewing gum can also stimulate the production of more saliva.	Appointment 1: Assessment • Start Check/Vitals • Medical History/Medications • Social History • Social History (Tobacco and Alcohol Assessment) • Preprocedural rinse/chlorhexidine • EO/IO • Intraoral photographs • Full-mouth series • Comprehensive Periodontal Eval. – gingiva, probing, CAL, Bleeding Index (BI), dental charting, calculus charting (radiographic findings will be assessed post appt. #1 in consultation with dentist/periodontist prior to formulating dental hygiene care plan). • Caries Risk Assessment • DDS Exam/consult to address active caries • Discuss initial findings and confirm appt. to present dh care plan. • Preventive Counseling	D0210 D0180 D0603
• Dental Evaluation • #1 – 4, #6 – 16, #17 – 32 sound teeth • Missing #18, #19, #30, #31 • Moderate caries #5 DO • Mild stain • Moderate calculus buildup • High caries risk due to infrequent dental care, inadequate home care, existing carious lesions, and frequent snacking	1. Biofilm (18%) – estimated 18% biofilm was recorded while periodontal probing but proper PI will be recorded when patient is disclosed. 2. Patient has mild stain and moderate calculus buildup due to infrequent dental care and inadequate home care. Last visit was approximately 3-4 years ago. 3. Patient has a moderate salivary flow but poor home care. Moderate salivary flow is a contributor to the patient not having as many carious lesions	MI: 1. Tell me how important it is to you to keep your teeth for a lifetime. (Evocative Question) 2. What do you think has contributed to your current and past caries? Preventive Counseling: Discuss with patient the importance of improving home care to brushing 2x daily and flossing 1x daily. Educate patient on the importance of using a soft-bristle toothbrush instead of a medium. Discuss the benefits of an electric toothbrush rather than a manual. Treatment: Referral to DDS for #5 caries; Disclose patient, record accurate PI and show patient problem areas Have patient demo Oral B power toothbrush with Test Drive Demo c-shaped flossing method Polish full mouth with medium grit paste or air powder polishing to remove moderate stain Apply topical fluoride varnish	Appointment 2: DH Diagnosis and Care • Start Check/Vitals • Review Med HX/Meds, confirm meds taken and meal eaten. • Care Plan Presentation: Inform patient of findings and dental hygiene diagnoses, discuss etiology of dental diagnoses, care plan goals, interventions, prognosis and appointment schedule. • Obtain informed consent. • Preprocedural Rinse/Chlorhexidine • Determine Plaque Index (PI) • Preventive Counseling – Brushing with soft bristle brush 2x day and with floss 1x day • Educate on brushing soft tissue and tongue.	D1330

2.   Periodontal Evaluation
• AAP Disease Classification highlight as appropriate
  Stage: I, II, III, IV
  Grade: A, B, C
  Annuals of Periodontology, 2017
Periodontal Pathologies
• attachment loss: Localized in molar areas, may have more attachment loss but could not accurately record due to calculus buildup
• recession: 1mm on #20
• pocket formation: Generalized 3-4 mm on the anterior teeth and 5-4 mm on the posterior teeth and localized 7 mm pocket depths straight facial of #1, and #14DF
• bone loss & descriptions: Generalized horizontal bone loss
• mobility: None
• furcation involvement: F2 on facial of #2
• gingival description: generalized red pink edematous/ fibrotic gingiva with bulbous interdental papilla
• BI: 68%
• PI: 18%
• mucogingival defects: None
• level of risk for periodontal disease(s): high due to inadequate home care, infrequent dental visits, periodontal pocket formation, and bone loss
	1. Biofilm (18%) – estimated 18% biofilm was recorded while periodontal probing but proper PI will be recorded when patient is disclosed.
	
	Immune Response: recent diabetes diagnosis and HBP
	
	2. Patient has moderate calculus buildup on the lingual surfaces of the mandibular incisors and premolars. Generalized subgingival moderate calculus buildup on the interproximal surfaces of mand./max molars.
	
	Patient brushes 2x day and flosses 2-3x per week. His BI is 68% due to the lack of flossing and the calculus buildup is also contributed inadequate home care.
		MI:
		1.Tell me what you know about Periodontal Disease. (Open - Ended)
		2. May I discuss with you the importance of stopping disease progression? (Teach)
		
		Preventative Counseling:
		Discuss the etiologies of periodontal disease and risk factors contributing to disease. Discuss how the patient can help prevent disease progression and what he can do to maintain it. Educate the patient on the importance of adequate home care and the importance of maintaining regular dental visits.
		
		Discuss treatment of dentition:
		
		Discuss STG & LTG
		SRP 4-8 teeth on all quads (ultrasonic and hand instruments)
		
		4-6 week reevaluation to see improvements in bleeding/plaque index, reduction pocket depths, change in gingival description. Patient will either be on a recare, retreat, or refer based on outcome 4-6 weeks post SRP. Upon completion of treatment, perio consult to evaluate bone loss around tooth #3.
		
		Recommended maintenance – 3 months to stabilize oral health
			Appointment 3: Phase 1 nonsurgical therapy
			• Start Check/Vitals
			• Review Med HX/Meds, confirm meds taken and meal eaten
			• Educate etiology of periodontal disease/plaque/diabetes.
			• Preprocedural Rinse/Chlorhexidine
			• Assess/monitor tissue response to TB/F self-care
			• Preventive Counseling – review & reinforce brushing and flossing, as needed.
			• LA for Quadrant I &4
			• Periodontal debridement Q1 & Q4: Ultrasonic and Hand instrumentation
			• Postop Instructions
			Appointment 4: Phase 1 nonsurgical
			• Start Check/Vitals
			• Review Med HX/Meds, confirm meds taken and meal eaten.
			• Preprocedural Rinse/Chrlorhexidine
			• Assess/monitor tissue response to TB/F self-care and periodontal debridement Q1 & Q4
			• Preventive Counseling – Introduce to power brush
			• LA for Quadrant 2 & 3
			• Periodontal debridement Q2 & Q3 - Ultrasonic and Hand instrumentation
			• Postop Instructions
			Appointment 5: Phase I response to non-surgical therapy/Reeval 4-6 weeks
			• Start Check/Vitals
			• Review Med HX/Meds, confirm meds taken and meal eaten
			• Preprocedural Rinse/Chlorhexidine
			• Periodontal re-evaluation
			• Take PI and BI
			• Measure goals planned to be evaluated
			• Preventive Counseling – review and reinforce TB/F as needed
			• Rretreat/debride residual hard or soft deposits
			• Polish & Floss
			• Apply 5% NaF Varnish
			• Determine recare interval for phase IV maintenance (D4910) and schedule
			• Schedule appointment with periodontists for phase II evaluation
				D1330
				D9210
				D4341
				
				D0171
				
				D1330
				
				D1110
				
				D1206

Dental Hygiene Diagnosis
• Patient presents as a stage III, grade C due to generalized 3-4 mm pocketing on the anterior teeth and 5-4 mm on the posterior teeth with localized 7 mm PD on the straight facial of #1 and #14DF, generalized horizontal bone loss, inadequate home care, infrequent dental visits, and moderate calculus buildup. Patient is high caries risk due to infrequent dental care, inadequate home care, existing carious lesions, and frequent snacking. Modifiable risk factors include inadequate home care, pocket formation and infrequent dental visits. Nonmodifiable risk factors include bone loss.

Dental Hygiene Prognosis
Short-term prognosis is good as the patient seems more motivated to improve oral health. Discussed with the patient the need to keep following appointments for SRP treatment and oral self care recommendations to reduce pocket depths, stabilize bone loss and decrease plaque and calculus deposits. Long-term prognosis is fair due to diabetes HbA1c 7.5%, age and localized sites of moderate bone loss and critical pocket depths; however, patient is working with physician to decrease HbA1c and has committed to phase II consultation at the completion of phase I.

Outcome Evaluation:
Patient Centered Outcome
STG: Improve home care: Report daily brushing 2x day for 2 min. with a soft-bristle toothbrush or powered brush and daily c-shape flossingby re-evaluation/phase I outcome. Reduce PI to less than 10% by phase I re-evaluation.
LTG: Maintain frequent recare appointments and schedule 3-month recare/phase IV maintenance visit for continued care at Phase 1 reevaluation.

Clinical Outcomes:
Reduce 5 mm and greater pockets by at least 1 mm, reduce BI to less than 10% and eliminate gingival inflammation by Phase 1 reevaluation and maintain to recare/phase IV maintenance.

Signatures: Student:	Faculty:	Patient:	Date:

Fig. 22.6, cont'd

BOX 22.4 Critical Thinking Scenario B

Developing a Dental Hygiene Care Plan Using the OHRQL Model

Select a patient case study from one of the chapters in this book, for example, Chapter 21, Oral-Systemic Health Connection—Case Two. Next, use the Oral Health-Related Quality of Life questionnaire (see Fig. 22.5) to first collect psychosocial information (environmental, sociocultural, socioeconomic) and combine this with traditional biomedical assessment data as shown in Fig. 22.4 (dental charting, periodontal charting) to develop a dental hygiene diagnosis and care plan. (If you need assistance filling out the Oral Health-Related Quality of Life Form on the patient, refer to Fig. 22.6 to see how the form was completed using the information from Case Study 22.1) How is this different from the treatment plans that you see in dentistry? What did you learn about the patient from using the Oral Health-Related Quality of Life questionnaire? How can that information be incorporated into the development of a dental hygiene treatment and care plan?

BOX 22.5 Critical Thinking Scenario C

Following a comprehensive assessment, the periodontal status of your 27-year-old patient is stage III, grade B with probing depths 3 to 4 mm in the anterior and 4 to 6 mm in the posterior. There is a localized 7 mm on tooth #1F and tooth #14DF. A review of the radiographs confirms bone loss along with areas of subgingival calculus. To develop a dental hygiene diagnosis that will guide the appropriate dental hygiene care, refer to the American Academy of Periodontology (AAP) website to access the AAP and European Federation of Periodontology (EFP) 2017 Classification of Periodontal and Peri-Implant Diseases and Conditions. Use the Chairside Guide to Periodontitis Staging and Grading to assist in assessment (https://www.perio.org/wp-content/uploads/2019/08/Staging-and-Grading-Periodontitis.pdf).

BOX 22.6 Legal, Ethical, and Safety Issues

Related to Medical Malpractice and the Dental Hygienists

As a licensed healthcare provider, the dental hygienist can be held liable for untreated periodontal disease. The National Practitioner Data Bank (NPDB) was established by Congress in 1986 as a web-based repository of reports on malpractice payments and adverse actions related to healthcare practitioners, providers, and suppliers. Access this database to find instances in which medical malpractice payments have been reported. It is critical that a dental hygienist carry liability insurance and not simply rely on the employer's liability insurance. One of the most cost-effective professional liability insurance plans can be accessed through the ADHA-approved insurance package. Access the ADHA website to explore its professional liability insurance option.

and appropriate referrals to other healthcare providers. The dental hygiene diagnosis is critical for the dental hygienist's communication with healthcare professionals involved in the patient's care, both inside and outside dentistry. This kind of complementary and collaborative approach to patient care needs to become the standard for educational and practice settings. Dental hygiene diagnosis facilitates the delivery of high-quality dental hygiene care and provides a criterion for establishing professional fees. Because dental hygiene diagnoses are based on a diagnostic classification system, communication among oral health professionals is facilitated. Diagnosis facilitates the measurement of clinical outcomes, which has implications for professional accountability, patient education, research, regulatory mechanisms, direct access to care, and direct reimbursement. The use of dental hygiene diagnoses appears promising for the development of a computerized system of dental hygiene diagnosis and care planning, with expansion to a system of cost accounting for dental hygiene practices.

KEY CONCEPTS

- The dental hygiene diagnosis provides the foundation for the dental hygiene care plan.
- A dental diagnosis is problem and disease oriented, whereas a dental hygiene diagnosis takes into consideration both biologic and psychosocial variables that affect patient health and wellness.
- A dental hygiene diagnosis should be considered complementary to the dental diagnosis, thereby promoting collaboration between dental hygiene and dentistry.
- A dental hygiene diagnosis provides the foundation for interdisciplinary patient care, encouraging collaboration among all healthcare professionals in the provision of comprehensive and person-centered care.
- A process of care provides a systematic approach for practitioners to follow in the provision of care to patients. The dental hygiene process of care includes assessment, dental hygiene diagnosis, planning, implementation and evaluation, and documentation.
- The development of a dental hygiene care plan can be guided through the use of theoretical models such as the HN Conceptual Model and the OHRQL Model.

ACKNOWLEDGMENTS

The authors acknowledge Michele Darby and Margaret Walsh for their past contributions to this chapter. The authors wish to acknowledge Cinthia Martinez and Tawnya Guthrie, student dental hygienists at the University of Missouri-Kansas City School of Dentistry, for their assistance with this chapter.

ORAL HEALTH-RELATED QUALITY OF LIFE QUESTIONNAIRE STUDENT WORKSHEET

I. HEALTH PERCEPTIONS *General Health* Compared to others your age, how would you rate your general health? • What do you perceive is your biggest problem? *Oral Health* Compared to others your age, how would you rate the condition of your mouth, teeth, or dentures? • What do you think contributes most to your oral condition?	I. PATIENT RESPONSE (give brief explanation of pt. response) *General Health* Patient perceives his general health as good. Takes a daily multivitamin and actively works out. *Oral Health* Patient perceives his oral health as bad. He mentioned brushing 2x/day and flossing 2 times a week. He also said he bleeds when brushing and had to lose his 1st and 2nd mandibular molars due to caries.
II. SYMPTOM STATUS *Dry Mouth* Is your mouth dry, or your amount of saliva too little? *Pain* Do you have any pain or discomfort with your teeth, dentures, or mouth?	II. PATIENT RESPONSE (circle answer or give brief explanation of patient response) *Dry Mouth* • Need liquid to aid in swallowing - no • Dry when eating - no • Moisture seems too little in mouth - no • Dry at night - no *Pain* • Tooth pain - no • Soft tissue pain - no • Frequency of pain - N/A • Duration only when brushing - N/A • Sensitive to: hot / cold / pressure-none
III. FUNCTIONAL STATUS *Physical Function* Do your teeth, dentures, or mouth interfere with your ability to eat or chew? Do problems with your mouth, teeth, or dentures interfere with your ability to speak? *Social Function* Do problems with your mouth, teeth, or dentures interfere with your interactions with others? *Psychological Function* Do problems with your mouth teeth, or dentures affect the way you feel about yourself?	III. PATIENT RESPONSE (circle answer or give brief explanation of patient response) *Physical Function - no* • Mobile Teeth • Pain • Loose Dentures • TMS • Duration • Others misunderstand words • Repetition *Social Function - no* • Go out less • Communicate less • Interfere with leisure activities • Interfere with enjoyment of others = company *Psychological Function - no* • Self-consciousness • Appearance • Relaxation/tension • Depression
IV. INDIVIDUAL CHARACTERISTICS *Family/Cultural* Generally speaking, how much do your friends or family members influence the decisions you make about your mouth, teeth, or dentures? **Sociocultural influences**: <u>Family culture</u>: does the patient's family influence their ability to seek dental care? Influence the patient's values regarding dental care? <u>Community culture</u>: does the patient's living community influence their ability to receive care? Influence the patient's values regarding dental care? Who makes the decisions regarding the patient's ability to seek care and receive treatment? What are the patient's perceptions regarding healthcare? Does the patient value prevention and health promotion? **Environmental influences** Does the patient have easy access to both medical and dental care? Can the patient transport themselves to receive care or do they rely on others for assistance? Does the patient live independently or do they depend on others for daily functioning? Is their family or living environment conducive to health and healthy habits (diet, oral hygiene aids, etc.)? Are their overall living conditions conducive to health promotion (communication and activities with others, living environment, etc.)? Does the patient have fluoride in their drinking water? **Economic influences** Patient's socioeconomic status (How can this be assessed? What cues are you given?) How do finances influence the patient's ability to receive dental care? Does the patient have insurance coverage for dental care? How does insurance coverage (or lack thereof) influence the patient's decision making regarding dental care? What are the patient's perceptions of healthcare and health promotion as they relate back to finances? Does the patient value health and how does this relate to their financial outlook and status?	IV. PATIENT RESPONSE (give brief explanation of pt. response) *Family/Cultural* Patient is seeking dental care on his own. Patient community culture influence their ability to seek dental care because in his Hispanic culture, seeking oral healthcare is not the norm. Oral healthcare is something that is not taught and this could be one of the reasons why the patient has infrequent dental care. Patients values healthcare. He likes to live a healthy lifestyle by consistently working out, eating a nutritious meal daily, and consuming dietary supplements. Patient is willing to pay for dental care and is capable of paying. Patient would like an estimate of how much each appointment would be prior to coming in. Patient does not have dental insurance. Patient does have easy access to medical and dental healthcare as his work schedule is very flexible, but patient does not have medical or dental insurance, which makes it hard for him to seek care. Patient can transport himself to and from appointments just fine. Patient is living independently – does not depend on others.

Fig. 22.7 Oral Health-Related Quality of Life Questionnaire—with patient information.

REFERENCES

1. Herdman TH. What is the difference between a medical diagnosis and a nursing diagnosis. North American Nursing Diagnosis Association International, Inc. Available at: http://nanda.host4kb.com/article/AA-00266/0/What-is-the-difference-between-a-medical-diagnosis-and-a-nursing-diagnosis-.html. Accessed January 8, 2023.

2. Newsome P, Smales R, Yip K. Oral diagnosis and treatment planning: part 1. Introduction. *Br Dent J.* 2012;213(1):15–19.

3. World Health Organization. Social Determinants of Health. Available at: https://www.who.int/health-topics/social-determinants-of-health#tab=tab_1. Accessed January 8, 2023.

4. *Standards for Clinical Dental Hygiene Practice.* Chicago IL: American Dental Hygienists' Association; 2016. Available at: https://www.google.com/search?q=ADHA+Standards+of+clinical+practice&rlz=1C1GCEA_enUS792US792&sxsrf=ALiCzsaYMaPd6lAUDbWtQqQ0Rrf6LswOOw%3A1667496065237&ei=gfhjY8LjDaizqtsPuMa66A0&ved=0ahUKEwiCqIf1wpL7AhWomWoFHTijDt0Q4dUDCBA&uact=5&oq=ADHA+Standards+of+clinical+practice&gs_lp=Egxnd3Mtd2l6LXNlcnC4AQP4AQEyBRAAGIAEMgUQABiGA8ICBBAAGEeQBghI9xxQ-AhY-AhwAHgCyAEAkAEAmAFKoAGJAaoBATIiAwQgTRgB4gMEEEEYAOIDBCBGGGGACIBgE&sclient=gws-wiz-serp. Accessed January 8, 2023.

5. *Dental Hygiene Practice Act Overview: Permitted Functions and Supervision Levels by State.* Chicago, IL: American Dental Hygienists' Association; 2021. Available at: https://www.adha.org/resources-docs/7511_Permitted_Services_Supervision_Levels_by_State.pdf. Accessed January 8, 2023.

6. US Department of Health and Human Services. *Oral Health in America: A Report of the Surgeon General.* National Institute of Dental and Craniofacial Research, National Institute of Health; 2000. Available at: https://www.nidcr.nih.gov/research/data-statistics/surgeon-general. Accessed January 8, 2023.

7. Hanna-Attisha M, LaChance J, Sadler RC, et al. Elevated blood lead levels in children associated with the Flint drinking water crisis: a spatial analysis of risk and public health response. *Am J Public Health.* 2016;106(2):283–290. https://doi.org/10.2105/AJPH.2015.303003.

8. Levin ED. Crumbling infrastructure and learning impairment: a call for responsibility. *Environ Health Perspect.* 2016;124(5):A79.

9. Walji MF, Karimbux NY, Spielman AI. Person-centered care: opportunities and challenges for academic dental institutions and programs. *J Dent Educ.* 2017;81(11):1265–1272.

10. Institute of Medicine (US). *Committee on Quality of Health Care in America. Crossing the Quality Chasm: A New Health System for the 21st Century.* National Academies Press (US); 2001. Available at: https://nap.nationalacademies.org/catalog/10027/crossing-the-quality-chasm-a-new-health-system-for-the. Accessed January 8, 2023.

11. *Direct Access.* Chicago, IL: American Dental Hygienists' Association; 2022. Available at: https://www.adha.org/sites/default/files/ADHA%20Direct%20Access%20Chart_8-22.pdf#overlay-context=node/578/convert. Accessed January 8, 2023.

12. US Department of Health and Human Services. *Oral Health in America: Advances and Challenges.* National Institute of Dental and Craniofacial Research, National Institute of Health; 2021. Available at: https://www.nidcr.nih.gov/sites/default/files/2021-12/Oral-Health-in-America-Advances-and-Challenges.pdf. Accessed January 8, 2023.

13. Scope of Practice. *American Dental Hygienists' Association*; 2022. Available at: https://www.adha.org/scope-of-practice. Accessed January 8, 2023.

14. Jarrin OF. Core elements of U.S. nurse practice acts and incorporation of nursing diagnosis language. *Int J Nurs Terminol Classif.* 2010;21(4):166–176.

15. Accreditation Standards for Dental Hygiene Education Programs. *Commission on Dental Accreditation*; 2022. Available at: https://coda.ada.org/-/media/project/ada-organization/ada/coda/files/dental_hygiene_standards.pdf?rev=aa609ad18b504e9f9cc63f0b3715a5fd&hash=67CB76127017AD98CF8D62088168EA58. Accessed January 8, 2023.

16. The World Health Organization Quality of Life assessment (WHOQOL): position paper from the World Health Organization. *Soc Sci Med.* 1995;41(10):1403–1409.

17. Williams KB, Gadbury-Amyot CC, Bray KK, et al. Oral health-related quality of life: a model for dental hygiene. *J Dent Hyg.* 1998;72(2):19–26.

18. Johnson JA, Lee A, Vinson D, Seale JP. Use of AUDIT-based measures to identify unhealthy alcohol use and alcohol dependence in primary care: a validation study. *Alcohol Clin Exp Res.* 2013;37(suppl 1):E253–E259.

19. Miller WR, Rollnick S. Ten things that motivational interviewing is not. *Behav Cogn Psychother.* 2009;37:129–140.

20. Sackett DL, Straus SE, Richardson WS, Rosenberg W, Haynes RB. *Evidence-Based Medicine: How to Practice and Teach EBM.* 2nd ed. Churchill Livingston; 2000.

21. *ADHA Code of Ethics.* Chicago, IL: American Dental Hygienists' Association; 2019. Available at: https://www.adha.org/resources-docs/ADHA_Code_of_Ethics.pdf. Accessed January 8, 2023.

23

Dental Hygiene Care Plan, Evaluation, and Documentation

Karen M. Palleschi

PROFESSIONAL DEVELOPMENT OPPORTUNITIES

Patients come to the clinical practice setting with individual needs and challenges that may impact their oral health and quality of life. These patients are trusting that the care provided recognizes and supports those needs, promotes well-being, and is respectful of the patient's desires for health and wellness. The patient's individual needs and challenges, if not addressed, may continue to contribute to further oral health risks or problems. As primary oral healthcare providers, dental hygienists will collaborate with the dentist and interdisciplinary healthcare and community service providers to comprehensively address patients' needs. Dental hygienists provide a valuable service to their patients, using current knowledge and skills to formulate an individualized dental hygiene care plan focused on disease prevention and health promotion and to communicate the plan to the patient, as well as monitor, measure, and professionally document patient care outcomes.

COMPETENCIES

1. Define the planning step of the process of care and differentiate between the dental treatment plan and the dental hygiene care plan. Also discuss the concept of interprofessional collaboration.
2. Discuss the sequence of events in dental hygiene care plan development and, given a case scenario, formulate and evaluate a dental hygiene care plan including:
   - Link the care plan to one or more dental hygiene diagnoses.
   - Write care plan goals.
   - Select professional and self-care intervention strategies.
   - Develop an appointment schedule.
   - Determine attainment of care plan outcomes and write a supportive evaluation statement.
3. Discuss the care plan presentation, maximizing patient involvement, and the patient's potential informed consent and informed refusal as related to dental hygiene care planning.
4. Define the goal of evaluation in the process of care and explain the importance of measuring care plan outcomes including:
   - Discuss how evaluation is integrated into the dental hygiene process of care.
   - Discuss evaluation strategies for monitoring and measuring achievement of care plan outcomes.
5. Discuss documentation in the dental record and its significance to the process of care.

INTRODUCTION

Care planning, evaluation, and documentation are necessary foundational skills of a dental hygienist in contemporary clinical practice. These skills are integral to the dental hygiene process of care and standards of professional practice as defined by the American Dental Hygienists' Association's (ADHA's) Standards for Clinical Dental Hygiene Practice[1] (Fig. 23.1). The Canadian Dental Hygienists Association describes the Dental Hygiene Process of Care (DHPC) as the structural framework that provides the basis for all dental hygiene practices, including patient-specific treatment planning. Similarly, its components include documentation of assessment, dental hygiene diagnosis, a dental hygiene care plan, the recording of interventions, and the required process for evaluation. To this point, the Darby and Walsh textbook has provided the reader with information and strategies for assessing the patient and developing a dental hygiene diagnosis using the Human Needs (HN) and Oral Health-Related Quality of Life (OHRQL) Models. This chapter will cover the steps necessary for care planning, evaluation, and documentation. The reader will see how care planning is dependent on the preceding steps, assessment, and dental hygiene diagnosis and that evaluation and documentation are integrated components of all steps in the dental hygiene process of care. Possessing these skills empowers the dental hygienist in addressing a patient's needs, realizing positive patient care outcomes, and strengthening the patient-clinician relationship. Integrating care planning, evaluation, and documentation into dental hygiene practice, in accordance with the Standards for Clinical Dental Hygiene Practice, can ensure a person-centered approach to care.

PLANNING

The ADHA Standard 3, **planning**, is the process in which diagnosed patient needs are prioritized, patient goals and evaluative measures are established, intervention strategies are determined, and an appointment schedule is proposed. The purpose of planning is to develop a strategy of care that results in the resolution of an oral health problem amenable to dental hygiene care, the prevention of a problem, or the promotion of oral health and well-being. Therefore the term *dental hygiene care plan*, rather than dental hygiene treatment plan, is used intentionally to denote the broad range of preventive, educational, therapeutic, and support services within the scope of dental hygiene practice. In keeping with standards of practice and evidence-based interventions, the dental hygienist engages the patient and/or caregiver of the patient in formulating a person-centered care plan with clearly defined tangible and measurable outcomes. Box 23.1 lists critical foundational skills needed to formulate an effective dental hygiene care plan.

Dental Treatment Plan

The general dentist or dental specialist develops a comprehensive dental treatment plan for the patient. This plan includes the dental diagnosis; all essential phases of therapy to be carried out by the dentist, dental hygienist, and patient to eliminate and manage disease or to promote health; and the prognosis. Components of a comprehensive dental treatment plan, including services that may be performed by the dental hygienist, are shown in Table 23.1. Dental hygiene services

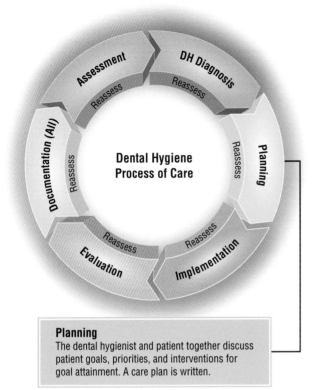

Planning
The dental hygienist and patient together discuss patient goals, priorities, and interventions for goal attainment. A care plan is written.

Fig. 23.1 Planning step of the Dental Hygiene Process of Care.

BOX 23.1 Critical Foundational Skills Needed to Formulate an Effective Dental Hygiene Care Plan

- Use parameters or standards of dental hygiene care.
- Collect, analyze, and interpret comprehensive patient findings.
- Collaborate with the dentist and other **interdisciplinary care providers** (when warranted).
- Integrate evidence-based knowledge and theory, professional judgment, and the patient's values.
- Develop dental hygiene diagnoses.
- Formulate measurable goals and select dental hygiene interventions that support the defined dental hygiene diagnoses.
- Synthesize the aforementioned information into a written plan.
- Communicate oral health needs to patients.
- Position the dental hygiene care plan within the context of the total dental treatment plan.

---

include preventive, therapeutic, supportive, and referral interventions. The dental hygiene care plan supports the overall dental plan. Ongoing collaboration among the dental hygienist, dentist, and other members of the interdisciplinary healthcare team (when warranted) and the patient is critical to attaining a successful outcome.

Collaborative practice between dental hygienists and dentists or teledentistry provides opportunities for similar coordination of patient care. However, dental hygienists providing direct patient care without dentist supervision do not necessarily have access to a dental treatment plan or collaboration with a dentist during care planning. They may formulate the dental hygiene care plan based on the assessment findings and the dental hygiene diagnosis, implement the plan and deliver dental hygiene services, and refer the patient for needed dental care or primary healthcare services. If dental or medical healthcare needs were

urgent, the dental hygienist would refer the patient for assessment and treatment prior to or in conjunction with dental hygiene services.

Interprofessional Collaboration

Interprofessional collaboration (IPC) is the coordinated care of a patient by an **interdisciplinary patient care team**, which is integrated providers from across healthcare disciplines working together to address whole-body patient needs for improved patient outcomes. The literature[2,3] recognizes the role of dental hygienists in IPC, for example, consultation with the primary or specialty provider to coordinate and support the planning of dental hygiene care with the patient's comprehensive health needs, referral for medical evaluation of a suspected undiagnosed condition, and coordination of the planning and delivery of dental hygiene services in an integrated medical-dental setting. See Box 23.2 for an interprofessional education opportunity.

Dental Hygiene Care Plan

The **dental hygiene care plan** is the written blueprint that directs the dental hygienist and patient as they work together to meet the patient's desired oral health outcomes.[4] With new and evolving workforce models expanding scope of dental hygiene practice settings, the contents of the dental hygiene care plan may support a traditional clinician-dentist practice relationship, a collaborative agreement relationship, or direct patient care provision by dental hygienists. In any situation, the care plan supports an integrated approach to the delivery of person-centered, goal-oriented care. The plan is personalized to support the individual's unique oral health needs, general health status, values, expectations, and abilities. The plan identifies all supportive dental hygiene intervention strategies, facilitates the monitoring of patient progress, ensures continuity of care, serves as a vehicle for communication between the IPC team, and increases the likelihood of high-quality care (Box 23.3). See Box 23.4 for a critical thinking scenario for IPC.

The dental hygiene care plan is written immediately following ADHA Standard 2 diagnosis and in conjunction with the overall dental treatment plan or interdisciplinary healthcare plan. The dental hygiene care plan specifies the following:
- Dental hygiene diagnoses
- Goals
- Dental hygiene interventions
- Appointment schedule

During the planning of care, dental hygiene diagnoses are prioritized, and each component of the care plan is developed sequentially and linked to the dental hygiene diagnoses (Fig. 23.2). Establishing this link between the dental hygiene diagnosis, patient goals, and dental hygiene interventions is critical to the outcome of the care plan. When the dental hygienist is confident that the goals and interventions address all of the patient's needs, an appointment schedule is established to support a realistic implementation of the planned interventions.

Each dental hygiene care facility may have its own care plan format. Although formats may differ, the critical point is that the planning process ensures high-quality dental hygiene care. The plan may use standardized abbreviations and key phrases as specified in the policy manual of the healthcare institution with which the dental hygienist is affiliated (Box 23.5).

Sequence of Dental Hygiene Care Plan Development
Linking Care Plan to the Dental Hygiene Diagnosis

A dental hygiene diagnosis is the foundation for care plan development. Chapter 22, Dental Hygiene Diagnosis, looks at two models for diagnosing and care planning patient needs, the HN Conceptual Model and OHRQL Model. Each model suggests that the etiology of oral disease is multidimensional and seeks to identify the underlying

TABLE 23.1   Components of the Overall Dental Treatment Plan

Components	Included in the Dental Hygiene Care Plan
Preliminary Phase	
Emergency care (e.g., relief of pain, treatment of acute periodontal or periapical pathology)	
Removal of nonfunctional and diseased teeth and provisional replacement to restore function as needed (may be postponed to later phases of care)	
Referral for suspected undiagnosed medical condition or risk	X
Nonsurgical Phase: Phase I Therapy	
Patient education and self-care instruction for control of plaque biofilm	X
Dietary guidance (e.g., caries risk management and prevention, tissue healing)	X
Smoking cessation counseling	X
Fluoride and remineralization therapy	X
Placement of pit and fissure sealants	X
Therapeutic periodontal debridement	X
Hard tissue desensitization	X
Correction of restorative and prosthetic irritation factors, excavation of caries and restorations (temporary or final as determined by the prognosis of the tooth and location of the caries)	
Antimicrobial (antiinfective) therapy (local or systemic)	X
Occlusal adjustment, minor orthodontic movement	
Coronal polishing	X
Provisional splinting and prosthesis	
Phase I: Evaluation of Response to Nonsurgical Therapy	
Inquiry of changes in patient's medical health and oral health status (e.g., reassess gingiva, pocket depth, plaque, and calculus), caries risk factors; new concerns or problems	X
Oral hygiene assessment, review and reinforce oral self-care	X
Determine additional nonsurgical and adjunctive therapy (e.g., debride plaque and calculus, hard tissue desensitization as needed)	X
Assess outcome of nonsurgical periodontal therapy, evaluate prognosis, recommend continued care interval	X
Surgical Phase: Phase II Therapy	
Periodontal therapy, including pocket reduction, implant site preparation, and implant placement	
Endodontic therapy	
Restorative Phase: Phase III Therapy	
Final restorative care	
Fixed and removable prosthodontic appliances	
Evaluation of response to restorative procedures (e.g., periodontal status, host response)	
Maintenance Phase: Phase IV Therapy	
Inquiry of changes in patient's medical health and oral health status; comprehensive periodontal examination and charting; new or recurrent disease; patient adherence to oral self-care, caries risk, other pathologic conditions)	X
Supportive, preventive, and therapeutic periodontal maintenance therapy (plaque biofilm and calculus removal)	X
Oral hygiene assessment and self-care education (e.g., review, modify as needed, reinforce)	X
Evaluation and recommendation continued-care interval	X

Adapted from Do, JH, Takei HH, Carranza FA. The Treatment Plan. In: Newman MG, Takei HH, Klokkevold PR, Carranza FA, eds. *Carranza's Clinical Periodontology.* 13th ed. Elsevier; 2019:426–427.

factors that may be contributing to a patient's need or problem.[4,5] Linking the dental hygiene care plan to these factors rather than oral symptoms alone, ensures that care will be comprehensive, humanistic, and focused on individual patient needs. A care plan may include a single or multiple dental hygiene diagnoses.

A dental hygiene diagnosis includes a statement of the problem (health behavior, attitude, or oral healthcare need) that may be addressed within the scope of dental hygiene practice, evidence or risk indicators, and etiology of the problem (see Chapter 22). By focusing on the evidence, risk factors, and contributors to the problem, the clinician is able to develop goals and intervention strategies that best meet the patient's needs.

A philosophic difference in sequencing of *setting goals* and *selecting interventions strategies* exists between the dental hygiene HN Conceptual Model and OHRQL Model. The HN Conceptual Model proposes setting goals, followed by selection of evidence-based intervention strategies. Whereas the OHRQL Model proposes the development of treatment strategies that lead to a discussion with the patient and consideration for defining goals. Either way, the plan is individualized to the patient rather than generic routine care provided to all.

BOX 23.2 Interprofessional Education Opportunity

Invite students from medical, allied health, and behavioral science curriculums to participate in a round-table discussion of a patient case and the role of each discipline in the management of the patient for best health and wellness outcomes. Provide each participant with a case profile and guidelines to prepare for the discussion. Allow participants to individually share their role in patient care. Have the group establish goals or expected outcomes, and propose an interdisciplinary plan.

BOX 23.3 Rationale for Developing a Formal Dental Hygiene Care Plan

- Individualize care.
- Focus care on priorities.
- Facilitate communication and collaboration among the members of the interdisciplinary patient care team.
- Establish patient-centered goals that support attainment of a desired clinical outcome.
- Provide foundation on which an evaluation of patient care outcomes is based.
- Develop roadmap for implementing planned interventions that will achieve the desired outcomes.
- Promote professional practice.

BOX 23.4 Critical Thinking Scenario A

Interprofessional Collaboration

Case Scenario: A 50-year-old female, widowed 2 years ago. Patient's height is 5'6" and weight is 172 pounds. Patient owns and manages a vintage clothing and accessories boutique in the community. Patient reports smoking approximately 3 to 4 cigarettes a day, frequently skips lunch, orders take-out at local restaurants for dinner, and drinks 3 to 4 cups of coffee with milk a day, as well as reports weight gain over the past year. Has recently been diagnosed with prediabetes with an HbA1c of 6.0, hypertension, and elevated cholesterol. Her physician prescribed oral medication to manage the cholesterol (atorvastatin) and hypertension (Avapro), weight loss, and exercise. Patient states concern about her recent health diagnoses and verbalizes the need to get her health back on track. Reports no professional dental care in 4 years. Reason for today's visit is for "teeth cleaning." No chief concern reported, however, and communicated, "I am self-conscious of the appearance of my teeth when I smile and have had a long-time desire to have my teeth straightened." Reports brushing 1× day, occasional flossing and over-the-counter mouthwash for freshening breath. An oral health assessment indicates moderate risk for caries, periodontal risk factors, and diagnosis of Stage I/Grade B periodontitis.

Use critical thinking to propose an *interdisciplinary patient care team* to support this patient's needs for health and wellness, and discuss the role of each care provider.

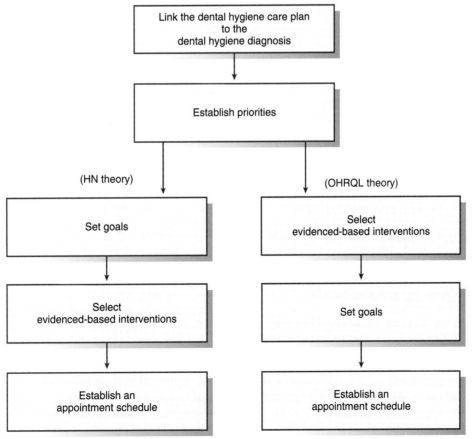

Fig. 23.2 Sequence for developing a care plan. *HN*, Human Needs; *OHRQL*, Oral Health-Related Quality of Life.

BOX 23.5   Characteristics of a Well-Written Dental Hygiene Care Plan

- Reflects goals of care to: (1) develop and maintain the individual's behaviors essential to oral health and the mastery of self-care and the environment; (2) prevent oral disease using primary, secondary, and tertiary preventive interventions; and (3) promote wellness.
- Is consistent with patient needs and readiness to change.
- Identifies a relationship among the dental hygiene diagnoses, patient goals, and interventions.
- Is compatible with the dental treatment plan prepared by the dentist.
- Identifies the dental hygienist's responsibilities, if any, for fulfilling components of the dental treatment plan or interdisciplinary healthcare plan.
- Reflects current standards of evidence-based care.
- Meets the patient's psychosociocultural and physical needs.
- Reflects the dental hygienist's role as clinician, educator, administrator or manager, researcher, and advocate.
- Establishes priorities of care.

Identified evidence-based patient problems may have numerous contributors. Intervention strategies must be selected carefully to ensure that the care plan addresses the fundamental causative factor. For example, a patient may present with dental caries as a result of one or more of the following causes or risk factors:

- Frequency of a cariogenic or acidogenic diet
- Unusual tooth morphologic structure
- Salivary-reducing factors
- Low plaque score
- Inefficient oral self-care techniques or habits
- Sociocultural, environmental, or economic factors (e.g., access to care, availability of fluoride, cost)

In keeping with dental hygiene practice law, the dental hygiene care plan will define patient goals and intervention strategies to resolve or minimize the identified risk for future caries and include a referral to the dentist for treatment of existing caries. Therefore intervention strategies for the prevention of future caries require the establishment of person-centered dental hygiene interventions. Fig. 23.3 provides examples of a dental hygiene diagnosis, goals, and treatment strategies that focus on the unique needs of a patient with dental caries.

Establishing Priorities

In collaboration with the dentist, the dental hygienist considers the dental and dental hygiene diagnoses and determines their urgency.[4] Priorities are based on the degree to which the dental hygiene diagnosis does the following:

- Threatens the patient's well-being; it is important to distinguish patient needs that pose the greatest threat to patient safety, health, and comfort from those that are not life-threatening and/or related to a current oral disease.
- Can be addressed simultaneously with other diagnoses.
- Is a patient priority (chief complaint).

Once these criteria are applied to the dental hygiene diagnoses, the dental hygienist ranks the diagnoses in priority to be addressed. Other than meeting the patient's need for safety (prevention of health risks), which, in some instances, requires preliminary emergency care, dental hygienists most likely would identify the patient's ability to assume responsibility for oral health as a primary priority. Factors influencing how priorities are established include the following:

- Patient values, beliefs, and attitudes
- Healthcare provider philosophy
- Collaborating dentist's goals

- Patient health status
- Whether the patient is experiencing infection, discomfort, anxiety, or pain

Setting Goals

A **care plan goal** is the outcome desired to be achieved through specific dental hygiene intervention strategies to satisfy an identified need or problem.[4] The goals are linked to the dental hygiene diagnosis, thus establishing the parameters for measuring the success of the care plan in meeting the needs of the patient. Although many approaches may be taken, both the HN Conceptual Model and the OHRQL Model provide different views on how a dental hygienist could develop a patient's care plan. Inherent in both models, the care plan establishes a relationship between the pretreatment evidence of a need and posttreatment outcome following implementation of the intervention strategies. This relationship enables the clinician and patient to measure the extent to which a goal has been achieved in terms of changes in the patient's initial behaviors (beliefs, skills, values) and attainment of clinical health outcomes. A dental hygiene diagnosis will have one or more defined goals.

A care plan goal may address cognitive, psychomotor, affective, or oral health status needs (Table 23.2). An oral health status goal defines the desired clinical outcome of care. Patient-centered goals address behaviors or barriers contributing to an unmet need or problem. For example, goals that measure cognitive and psychomotor development are critical to ensuring that the patient is knowledgeable and physically prepared to assume responsibility for self-care; however, these goals alone may not result in the patient making the desired changes in behavior necessary to achieve a resolution in an oral health problem. An affective goal seeks to have the patient internalize the desire to make the necessary modifications in behavior and is critical to the patient achieving a desired clinical or oral health status outcome. Therefore a variety of goal categories are needed to achieve a positive oral health outcome and/or restore an unmet human need. Refer to Chapter 5 to find strategies that can result in sustainable health behavior changes. Fig. 23.4 illustrates the linking of care plan goals to the dental hygiene diagnoses.

Writing goals. Adopting a format for writing care plan goals simplifies the task. Each goal should have a subject, a verb, a criterion for measurement, and a time dimension for evaluation (Box 23.6). Assigning a timeframe to each goal gives the patient and clinician a point of reference for when a goal is measured. Selecting a realistic timeframe for each goal will allow the patient ample time to do the following:

- Internalize information.
- Practice new skills.
- Experience physical and attitudinal changes related to oral health and wellness.
- Assess the importance of these changes to their lifestyle.
- Adopt the new behavior.

Goals evaluated too early restrict the clinician's and the patient's ability to determine the impact of the care provided. Box 23.7 defines guidelines for writing goals for successful patient care outcomes. (See Box 23.8 to analyze the link between dental hygiene diagnoses and the dental hygiene care plan.)

Selecting Dental Hygiene Interventions

Dental hygiene interventions are the evidence-based strategies, preventive services, treatments, products, and referrals that when applied, reduce, eliminate, or prevent a diagnosed need or problem.[1] Interventions, like goals, are linked to the dental hygiene diagnosis or problem. However, interventions address the causative factors, that is, the

Human needs conceptual model: Caries risk for 56-year-old female		

Dental hygiene diagnosis
Unmet Human Need for Biologically Sound and Functional Dentition due to frequency of cariogenic/acidogenic diet, postmenopausal xerostomia, inadequate salivary flow by observation, reports brushing 2 x day with fluoride toothpaste and daily interdental cleaning as evidenced by caries risk assessment indicating high risk associated with disease indicator of recurrent caries, multiple risk factors, few protective factors.

Goal
Patient will exhibit low caries risk at next continued care visit. (oral health status goal)
Patient will report limiting the frequency of high cariogenic/acidogenic food/drinks and increasing protective factors by 6/5. (affective goal)
Patient will report satisfaction with recommended self care strategies for management of dry mouth by 6/5. (affective goal) Patient will complete phase III restorative care with dentist by 6/5. (affective goal).

Interventions
Oral self care:
• Discuss caries process and link to frequency of cariogenic/acidogenic food sources and the role of saliva.
• Recommend OTC saliva stimulating agent as needed
• Recommend dietary guidance to assist in selection of dental healthy choices.
• Recommend a Rx strength sodium fluoride brush-on fluoride toothpaste for pm brushing. Prophylaxis Sodium Fluoride Varnish Refer to dentist for treatment of recurrent caries.

Prognosis: DH prognosis is fair due to patient compliance with recommendations for diet, self-applied fluoride, and salivary substitute. Patient agreed to dietary guidance and verbalized interest in making better food choices. Patient will agreed to scheduling phase III restorative care.

OHRQL model: Caries risk for a 10-year-old male		
Oral assessment and dental hygiene diagnosis		Dental hygiene care plan
Problem/Pathology/Risk Assessment	Etiology	Treatment selection and home care
Intra/Extra oral exam • No significant findings		
Dental evaluation • Caries Risk -High Risk for Pit and Fissure Caries • Dental Exam – Occlusal Caries #19 and #30	Primary: Biofilm – generalized heavy plaque Risk factors: Low Plaque Free Index Score, deep occlusal pits and fissure in molars, brushing frequency (1 x day) and technique, frequency of cariogenic and acidogenic diet, parent responsible for meal preparation and snacks, child prefers sweetened drinks and snacks.	Motivational interviewing: (child) What do you think causes a cavity to occur? (parent) What do you think has caused your son to have cavities? Oral hygiene: Discuss answers to above. Follow up with etiology of plaque. Review proper brushing technique and frequency. Discuss the caries process and diet, Discuss recommendation for dietary guidance to assist parent and child with selection of dental healthy food choices and frequency of consumption. Discuss use of a supplemental fluoride due to high risk for caries. Discuss recommendation for Occlusal Pit and Fissure Sealants #3 and #14. Discuss long term and short term goals Child prophylaxis Topical Fluoride Varnish
Periodontal evaluation • Indicators of health		

Dental hygiene diagnosis
Patient has a healthy periodontium. He is at high risk for dental caries. Mother is responsible for meal planning and preparation. Modifiable risk include diet, daily removal of plaque, deep pits and fissures in molars. Nonmodifiable risks include active caries.

Dental hygiene prognosis
DH prognosis is fair due to patient effectiveness and compliance with oral self care and diet. Parent verbalized interest in making better food choices for family and limiting sugary foods between meals. Parent agreed to scheduling appointment for Pit and Fissure Sealants #3 and #14 as well as phase III restorative care.

Outcome evaluation
Patient-centered outcome: Short term goal: Patient will increase frequency of brushing with a fluoride toothpaste to 2 x day by 6/5. Patient will complete pit and fissure sealant #3 and #14 by 6/5. Long term goal: Patient will increase Plaque Free Index Score to 85% by 6 month continued care visit. Parent will report reduction in the frequency of cariogenic/aciodogenic foods by next continued care visit.
Clinical outcome: Patient will reduce caries risk by next continued care visit.

Fig. 23.3 Example of a dental hygiene diagnosis, goals, and proposed treatment for a patient at risk for dental caries using the dental hygiene Human Needs Conceptual Model and Oral Health-Related Quality of Life Model.

TABLE 23.2 Categories for Care Plan Goals

Care Plan Goal	Category	Definition
Patient-centered	Cognitive goal	Targets an increase in patient knowledge and understanding
	Psychomotor goal	Focuses on patient skill development and skill mastery
	Affective goal	Pinpoints desired changes in patient values, beliefs, and attitudes
Clinical	Oral health status goal	Addresses the signs and symptoms of oral disease (e.g., risk for caries, gingivitis, dentinal hypersensitivity) and reflects a desired oral health or clinical outcome

specific barriers to the patient achieving oral health and wellness. These barriers are defined by the dental hygiene diagnosis and guide in the selection of patient-centered intervention strategies (Box 23.9).

A diagnosed condition or problem may have one or more causative factors requiring one or more intervention strategies. Selecting the proper evidence-based interventions enables the clinician and patient to move toward achieving the proposed care plan goals and resolution of a diagnosed need. Therefore professional dental hygiene care requires the careful tailoring of interventions to meet unique patient needs.

Appointment Schedule

Once the interventions are selected, they are put into action at planned appointments. The **appointment schedule** becomes a guide for implementing the proposed interventions and specifies the following:
- Number of visits
- Time needed for each visit
- Interventions to be implemented at each visit

Number of visits and sequencing of interventions at appointments vary among clinicians and patients. When selected interventions are few and address simple patient needs, the care plan can be implemented in one preventive or wellness visit. When diagnoses, patient goals, and interventions are complex, multiple therapeutic appointments are necessary (Box 23.10).

Scheduling time for educational interventions and the sequencing of self-care strategies must be given consideration during appointment planning. Too often, patient education is squeezed into the end of an appointment as time permits. Effectively addressing the patient's cognitive, psychomotor, and affective needs influences oral health outcomes and the patient's long-term adherence to self-care. Sequencing small increments of instruction into each visit may shape successfully the patient's self-care responsibilities. Box 23.11 suggests strategies for planning patient self-care. (See Box 23.12 for generalized moderate gingivitis using Current Dental Terminology [CDT] code D4346[6,7] and moderate risk for caries.)

Care Plan Presentation

Before presenting the care plan to a patient, the dental hygienist assesses the plan's comprehensiveness and readiness for presentation to the patient (Box 23.13). When the dental hygienist is satisfied, the plan is discussed with the patient. Presentation of the dental hygiene care plan will include the following:
- Nature of the condition
- Proposed care plan

- Risks involved (if any)
- Potential for failure
- Prognosis if the problem goes untreated
- Alternative treatment options

Presentation of the dental hygiene care plan is accomplished best by establishing a collaborative, cotherapeutic relationship with the patient. This philosophy engages the patient in a discussion of the proposed care plan and encourages shared decision making. Patients are more likely to express a commitment to the care plan and willingness to change when they are involved in the process (Box 23.14).

When a care plan includes multiple dental hygiene diagnoses, consider discussing all elements of one dental hygiene diagnosis before introducing a subsequent condition. Engaging the patient in a focused discussion of one condition at a time may be easier for the patient to understand the relationship between the condition and proposed care plan. Continue the discussion by pointing out an etiology or contributor that is common to two or more patient needs and may be addressed by the same proposed treatment or change in behavior. (See Box 23.15 for Patient Education Example: Discussion of Dental Hygiene Diagnoses at Care Plan Presentation for Informed Consent and Fig. 23.5A and B, Case Scenario.)

Most consumers expect to participate in decision making regarding their healthcare needs and know they have the right to accept or refuse services. Therefore the care plan is presented to the patient before preventive and therapeutic dental hygiene services are implemented to ensure that the patient:
- Understands and supports the planned services;
- Recognizes the importance of self-responsibility to the plan; and
- Has realistic expectations of the care plan.

Once the patient agrees, the care plan becomes a legal contract between the dental hygienist and the patient.

Informed Consent

Informed consent is a process of providing a patient with the information needed to make a decision about treatment. The patient's acceptance of care must follow a comprehensive discussion with the healthcare provider regarding the proposed care plan and risks of not receiving care. Informed consent should not be viewed as a one-time activity but as an ongoing process during which the patient is informed continuously and reminded of the terms of care. Box 23.16 lists criteria for informed consent of planned care.

Consent for treatment may be given verbally or in written form. Having an automated informed consent document linked to the dental hygiene care plan ensures that this step will not be overlooked. The patient's written consent is secured by having the patient sign an electronic signature pad that transfers the signature to the informed consent document or by scanning a signed consent document into the patient record. This remains a permanent entry into the patient's dental record. (Refer to Chapter 7, Legal and Ethical Decision Making, for supporting content.)

Informed Refusal

At times, the dental hygienist values specific goals and interventions more highly than the patient does. When this occurs, the dental hygienist explains the professional judgment and decision relative to the goal or intervention, with a clear message that the patient's readiness to change and the wants and needs are equally important to the overall plan. Given all information necessary for a patient to make an informed decision, the possibility exists that a patient may decline all or part of the proposed care plan.

Although troubling, patient refusal must be analyzed to determine how or why the patient arrived at that decision. The clinician should

Human needs conceptual model			
Defined by	Sample human needs diagnoses	Goal statement	Goal category
Specific signs and symptoms (evidence) supporting the existence of an unmet human need; establishes criteria for evaluation of care plan's success in meeting the unmet need of the patient; type of goal is dependent upon the unmet need.	Unmet need for conceptualization and problem-solving due to a knowledge deficit of periodontal disease and its etiology as evidenced by patient misconceptions about periodontal disease process and risk factors.	***Patient-centered goal:*** Patient will describe the periodontal disease process and identify risk factors by 7/10.	Cognitive goal
	Unmet need for responsibility for oral health due to impaired physical ability as evidenced by inability to perform daily oral self care associated with arthritis in hands.	***Patient-centered goal:*** Patient will perform oral self care using a toothbrush and interdental cleaning device with a customized handle grip by end of treatment.	Psychomotor goal
	Unmet need for wholesome facial image due to tooth malalignment and anterior crowding as evidenced by patient reports dissatisfaction with appearance of teeth.	***Patient-centered goal:*** Patient will complete consultation appointment with orthodontic specialist by 3/27.	Affective goal
	Unmet need for skin and mucous membrane integrity of the head and neck due to generalized plaque biofilm as evidenced by generalized moderate gingival inflammation, normal bone patterns and no clinical attachment loss.	***Clinical outcome goal:*** Patient will eliminate gingival inflammation by 6/15.	Oral health status goal
Oral Health-Related Quality of Life model				
Defined by	Sample problem/Pathology/Risk assessment of diagnosis	Sample etiology of diagnosis	Goal statement	Goal category
Patient-centered goal: Etiology and risk factors specific to the identified oral health problem/pathology/ risk assessment.	**Periodontal evaluation** • Generalized slight gingivitis **Periodontal pathologies** • Healthy clinical attachment • Full dentition except for 3rd molars • Normal bone patterns • Gingival description: Slight papillary inflammation • Interdental bleeding on probing	Primary: Biofilm – generalized interdental plaque Risk factors: • Inadequate home care, reports no interdental cleaning • PI of 50%	***Patient-centered goal:*** Patient will describeperiodontal disease, risk factors and the importance of daily removal of bacterial plaque biofilm by end of treatment.	Cognitive goal
			Patient-centered goal: Patient will demonstrate proper flossing technique by end of treatment appointment.	Psychomotor goal
			Patient-centered goal: Patient will reduce PI to less than 10% by next continued care visit.	Affective goal
Clinical outcome goal: Specific signs and symptoms (evidence) of the identified oral health problem/pathology/risk.			***Clinical outcome goal:*** Patient will eliminate gingival inflammation by next continued care visit.	Oral health status goal

Fig. 23.4 Linking care plan goals to the dental hygiene diagnosis using the dental hygiene Human Needs Conceptual Model and Oral Health-Related Quality of Life Model.

engage the patient in conversation, listen, and evaluate the patient's reasons for declining the services. At this time, the clinician may choose to reopen the discussion. If after this discussion the patient makes an **informed refusal**, the clinician should have the patient sign an electronic declaration of informed refusal that remains part of the patient's dental record. A copy of the refusal form can be given or sent electronically to the patient. Box 23.17 suggests patient reasons for refusing care, clinician actions, and documentation strategies of informed refusal.

In some situations, the patient may request care that, in the opinion of the dentist or dental hygienist, is unwarranted, inappropriate,

or dangerous. If the dental hygienist is faced with this dilemma, he or she should refuse to provide the care and encourage the patient to seek a second professional opinion. As a rule, a patient never should be allowed to dictate treatment. (Refer to Chapter 7, Legal and Ethical Decision Making, for supporting content and sample documentation.)

See Procedure 23.1 for steps for dental hygiene planning and Procedure 23.2, Guidelines for Care Plan Presentation. See a Competency Evaluation Form for steps in dental hygiene care planning (https:// evolve.elsevier.com/Pieren/hygiene/).

BOX 23.6 Components of a Care Plan Goal

Subject
- Identifies the patient or patient's caregiver as the person responsible for achieving the goal.

Verb
- Identifies the patient's action desired to achieve the goal.

Criterion of Measurement
- Establishes the observable behavior or tangible desired outcome of the patient.

Time Dimension
- Denotes when the patient is to achieve a goal.
- Target time may be a specific date or statement (e.g., by next appointment, by end of treatment, by next continued care visit).

BOX 23.7 Guidelines for Writing Care Plan Goals

Prepare a goal or set of goals for each dental hygiene diagnosis (Human Needs Conceptual Model).

Support each clinical goal with one or more patient-centered goals.

Ensure that goals, if met, will resolve the problem reflected in the dental hygiene diagnosis.

Collaborate with dentist and interdisciplinary care providers, when warranted, to ensure that the dental hygiene plan is mutually supportive of the dental or interdisciplinary care plans.

Involve patient in goal setting.

Confirm that patient values and is ready to achieve the delineated goals.

Write observable and measurable goals that define patient's target times for demonstrating goal achievement.

Use action verbs such as the following to denote patient behavior expected in the goal:

affirm	decrease	eliminate	increase	replace
attend	define	exhibit	perform	report
choose	demonstrate	explain	plan	stop
communicate	describe	finish	purchase	use
complete	detect	guide	remove	verbalize

BOX 23.8 Critical Thinking Scenario B

Link Between the Dental Hygiene Diagnoses and Dental Hygiene Care Plan

Go to Fig. 23.5 for an example of dental hygiene diagnoses, care plan, and evaluation as applied to the Human Needs Conceptual Model and Oral Health-Related Quality of Life Model using Case Scenario 22.1, Chapter 22, Dental Hygiene Diagnosis, and do the following:

1. Compare and contrast the planning process and discuss how care plan goals and interventions are linked to the dental hygiene diagnoses.
2. Distinguish cognitive, psychomotor, affective, and oral health status goals, and discuss the role of each goal statement in addressing the patient's oral health needs and wellness.

BOX 23.9 Possible Person-Centered Barriers to Personal Health and Wellness

- Lack of knowledge about the disease process or its infectious, chronic nature
- Lack of knowledge about importance of the prevention of oral disease
- Lack of knowledge of the oral-systemic link
- Lack of protective factors
- Skill deficit in oral self-care
- Low value on oral health
- Low self-esteem
- Inadequate financial resources
- Culture as a barrier to professional care
- Presence of other unidentified risk factors

BOX 23.10 Strategies for Formulating an Appointment Schedule

- Time needed for each intervention (e.g., self-care education, prophylaxis versus Phase I therapy or Phase IV therapy)
- Time needed to ensure patient comfort (e.g., pain management, fear, and anxiety concerns)
- Time needed to evaluate care plan goals scheduled to be measured during an appointment
- Logic for grouping interrelated procedures
- Status and severity of patient needs
- Patient's systemic health risks and tolerance for long sessions
- Patient's scheduling requirements (e.g., time of day, transportation limitations)

BOX 23.11 Strategies for Care Planning Self-Care Interventions

- Include self-care education in each visit.
- Link self-care education with related dental hygiene interventions.
- Consider variables such as patient dexterity, skill, knowledge, disabilities, and personal preferences.
- Involve patient during self-care instruction (e.g., ask patient to demonstrate self-care technique intraorally, clarify patient knowledge with open-ended questions, verbalize opinions).
- Encourage patient success (e.g., plan small steps, review, monitor, remediate, reinforce).
- Include parent or caregiver when instructing a young child or patient with special needs.
- Validate patient's ability to obtain recommended oral health aids (e.g., cost, availability).
- Motivate patient to accept responsibility for self-care maintenance.

EVALUATION

Goal of Evaluation

The goal of ADHA Standard 5, **evaluation**, is to measure the extent to which the patient has achieved the goals defined in the dental hygiene care plan, that is, fulfillment of the patient's diagnosed needs[1] (Fig. 23.6). Evaluation is a continuous process of reviewing and interpreting the outcomes of implemented care. The dental hygienist uses these findings to make evidence-based decisions:

- During the implementation of planned interventions for ongoing monitoring of patient progress;

Generalized Moderate Gingivitis Using CDT Code D4346[6,7] and Moderate Risk for Caries

Patient Profile

Eileen is a 27-year-old female, single with no children, and is new to the practice. The patient is scheduled for an initial examination and arrives early to complete a comprehensive health history. No significant findings are revealed except for a chief concern of discolored teeth and bleeding gums. After review of the health history, a comprehensive oral evaluation (D0150) is completed. Findings are as follows:

Vital statistics	Height: 5'4"; weight: 120 pounds; blood pressure: 118/76 mm Hg
Medical history	Good health, no medications. Does not smoke or use tobacco products.
Dental history	Full dentition, third molars were extracted at age 19. No history of restorations. Last preventive appointment was approximately 2 years ago. Eileen states, "I brush 1× a day with nonfluoride toothpaste and medium bristle brush. I don't floss because flossing makes my gums bleed."
Individual characteristics	Patient is a registered nurse at the health center of a local private prep school, full-time employment. Teaches Pilates and yoga classes at a local gym, two evenings a week and Saturday mornings.
Dietary history	Diet rich in fruits and vegetables, chicken, fish, and nuts. Frequently sips on sweet herbal iced tea or hot tea with honey throughout the day. A typical lunch is yogurt, handful of almonds, apple, and iced tea. Enjoys the occasional dish of chocolate ice cream.
Chief concern	"I am self-conscious of the appearance of my front teeth; they look discolored and I have recently noticed my gums sometimes bleed when I brush."
EOE and IOE	No significant findings.
Dental evaluation	No caries; caries risk assessment indicates moderate risk for caries.
Gingival evaluation	Generalized moderate red, enlarged, and edematous gingival margins and bulbous papilla. Modified GI of 3.
Periodontal evaluation	Generalized 3 to 4 mm probe readings; normal radiographic bone patterns; healthy clinical attachment levels; bleeding index (BI) 73%.
Hard- and soft-deposit evaluation	Plaque index (PI) 64%, supragingival calculus lingual sextant; and extrinsic brown stain.

CDT Code, Code on Dental Procedures and Nomenclature.

Dental Hygiene Diagnoses: Suggested Problem Statements

Human Needs (HN) Conceptual Model
Unmet need for conceptualization and problem solving due to _____ as evidenced by _____.
Unmet need for wholesome facial image due to _____ as evidenced by _____.
Unmet need for skin and mucous membrane integrity of the head and neck due to _____ as evidenced by _____.
Unmet need for responsibility for oral health due to _____ as evidenced by _____.

Problem; Pathologic Condition; Risk Assessment

Oral Health-Related Quality of Life (OHRQL) Model
• Intraoral and extraoral examinations: no findings
• Dental examination: moderate risk for dental caries
• Periodontal evaluation: generalized moderate gingivitis; modified GI of 3; periodontal pathologic conditions and risk factors; generalized moderate gingival inflammation, probing depth of 3 to 4 mm, normal bone patterns and healthy clinical attachment levels; BI of 73%, PI of 64%.

Dental Hygiene Diagnoses

1. Select either the HN Conceptual Model or the OHRQL Model and complete the dental hygiene diagnostic statements. (Refer to Chapter 22, Dental Hygiene Diagnosis, for guidance.)
   a. HN Conceptual Model: Complete "due to" and "as evidenced by" statements.
   b. OHRQL Model: Complete etiology for each "problem, pathologic condition, and risk assessment" statement.
   c. OHRQL Model: Complete the dental hygiene diagnosis. (Summarize overall oral health status, and discuss the impact of modifiable and nonmodifiable risk factors on the dental hygiene diagnosis.)
2. Formulate a dental hygiene care plan to address the dental hygiene diagnoses.
3. Discuss the patient's likely prognosis following care plan implementation and propose continued care interval for future preventive appointments.

• At the completion of planned dental hygiene care to determine the patient's prognosis for continued health and recommend a supportive continued cycle of care; and
• At the subsequent cycle of the process of care to measure the patient's continued success at maintaining the previously achieved outcomes and to formulate a supportive care plan.

Evaluation is linked inherently to each step of the process of care and is a critical component of the successful outcome of dental hygiene care. See Procedure 23.3 and the corresponding Competency Form for steps for integrating evaluation into patient-centered care.

Ongoing Monitoring

Ongoing monitoring is the process of continual review and reinforcement of patient progress toward achieving the goals. As the appointment schedule progresses, the clinician continually measures the impact of the intervention strategies on moving the patient toward meeting his or her desired outcomes. Both the dental hygienist and the patient have an active role in this process. For example, a dental hygienist may have performed an intervention competently but if the intervention or therapy was unsuccessful at helping the patient progress toward meeting a desired clinical goal or outcome, a new strategy

BOX 23.13 Dental Hygienist Self-Assessment of Care Plan Readiness for Presentation

- Does the care plan address the patient's diagnosed needs relative to the underlying factors that are amenable to or affect the outcomes of dental hygiene care?
- Does the care plan consider the patient's chief complaint and individual characteristics, such as sociocultural, environmental, and economic influences?
- Has the clinician anticipated patient's possible response to the care plan (e.g., interest, commitment, worry, fear, discontent, lack of enthusiasm) and is prepared for those discussions?
- Has the clinician problem solved best approach to care plan presentation to elicit patient cooperation?
- Is the clinician prepared with strategies to maximize patient involvement?
- Has the clinician anticipated the possibility of patient's refusal to proposed care and is prepared to respond to the patient's concerns?

BOX 23.14 Common Phrases to Maximize Patient Involvement

- "Here is a hand mirror. Let's examine your mouth together."
- "Let's take a look at the images of your mouth on the monitor and review the findings."
- "What is your primary reason for seeking dental hygiene care?"
- "Is this set of treatment priorities acceptable to you?"
- "Is this care plan acceptable to you?"
- "What would you like to achieve as a result of dental hygiene care?"
- "How will you feel if this goal is attained?"
- "Are you satisfied with the plan of care we just discussed?"
- "How important is your oral health?"
- "Where would you like me (dental hygienist) to start?"
- "When and where is it easiest for you to clean your mouth (or your dependent's mouth)?"
- "Can you think of a better way that we can accomplish this goal?"
- "What are you willing to do to keep your mouth healthy?"

BOX 23.15 Patient Education Example: Discussion of Dental Hygiene Diagnoses at Care Plan Presentation for Informed Consent*

"The purpose of today's visit is to share the results of your periodontal examination and discuss dental hygiene treatment options. I see from your dental record that you are scheduled with the dentist to have your tooth with an active cavity restored; that's great. The dental hygiene treatment plan that I am proposing will be complementary to the dental plan to minimize your risk for future cavities and address the health of your gums and supporting structures of your teeth. I would like to begin by talking with you about your gums and the bone surrounding your teeth. Does this sound like a good place to start?" *(Patient replies, "Yes.").*

"You have a diagnosis of stage III/grade C periodontitis. Tell me what you know about periodontal disease." (The dialog continues by affirming patient accuracy and adding patient-centered details describing etiology of periodontal disease.) "Let's take a look at the images of your mouth on the monitor and together review the signs and symptoms that you are exhibiting that lead to this diagnosis." (Clinician's action is to point out gingival changes and radiographic changes in bone health; discuss the significance of other clinical evidence such as bleeding, pockets and attachment loss.) *(Patient replies, "I brush my teeth every day. How did this happen? Am I going to lose my teeth?")*

"The primary cause is the body's inflammatory reaction to bacterial plaque. There is a correlation between the presence of plaque, systemic diseases such as diabetes and hypertension, your immune response, and periodontal disease." *(Clinician educates the patient on the bidirectional relationship of diabetes and periodontitis.) (Patient replies, "I didn't realize that my diabetes could affect the health of my mouth and that the same plaque could affect my ability to control my diabetes and heart health.") (Clinician continues to educate the patient on the findings that are modifiable versus those that are nonmodifiable.)* "Your treatment will be a team approach—the dentist, periodontist, myself *(dental hygienist)*, and you. Your role is very important to the healing and prevention of disease progression. Are you willing to participate in the treatment of your condition?" *(Patient replies, "Yes. I want to do what I can to improve my health.")*

"Great, let's talk about treatment strategies. We are suggesting starting with a review of your brushing and flossing for effectiveness in disrupting plaque biofilm. Efficient removal of plaque each day will help with both conditions. You are already brushing two times a day which is adequate. We would like to change your medium bristle brush to a soft bristle brush. We have included introducing an electric toothbrush. We would like you to increase your flossing to one time a day and can talk about your best time during the day to floss. Can you tell me about your diet?" *(Patient replies, "I am working with my physician to improve my diet and reduce my HbA1c. My physician suggested a plan and I am trying to make more low glycemic food choices.") (Clinician replies, "Sounds like you are taking positive steps for your health.")*

(Clinician continues with recommendations for Phase I nonsurgical therapy, followed by continued treatment with the periodontist.)

"The changes that we are proposing to meet your periodontal health needs will also support lowering your risk for future cavities. Again, plaque is a primary contributor, along with other risk factors such as dry mouth. You are taking a medication whose potential side effect is dry mouth. How frequently do you experience dry mouth in a day? Does this affect you when you eat or swallow? *(Clinician will educate patient on the role of saliva in the caries process, discuss treatment recommendations to address the xerostomia, and daily self-applied topical fluoride.)* "What would you like to achieve after completing the dental hygiene treatment? *(Patient responds, "I would like to save my teeth and improve my oral health.")* "That is a great long-term goal. Together, let's define some measurable goals to help you achieve the outcome that you desire." *(Patient replies, "Okay." Discussion continues with establishing goals and reviewing the detailed appointment schedule, including the monitoring of patient's oral self-care and tissue health.)*

"Are you satisfied with the plan of care we just discussed?" *(Patient replies, "Yes.")* "Do you have any additional questions?" *(Patient replies, "Is the treatment expensive? I don't have dental insurance.)* "We have scheduled time for you to meet with the office manager, who will discuss payment options with you."

*See Fig. 23.5, Case Scenario.

Human Needs Conceptual Model

Assessment See Chapter 22 – Figure 22.1 for completed Human Needs Assessment form

Dental hygiene diagnosis
Unmet human need for protection from health risk due to potential risk for medical emergency as evidenced by Type II diabetes (metformin 2000 mg/day) with HbA1c 7.5 diagnosed 4 months earlier and hypertension (Zaroxolyn 2.5 mg/day), diagnosed 2 years ago, BP 130/90 @ initial visit.

Client goals	Interventions (target etiologies)	Evaluation
Patient will; • Confirm taking daily medications as prescribed by physician, following prescribed diet and any changes in health at the start of each appointment.	Educate on importance of taking medications as prescribed by physician, eating nutritious meal within 2 hours of appointment and reporting changes in health to reduce risk of a glycemic event. Schedule appointments in the am.	**Goal met** at each appointment. Documented in progress notes; 3/27, 4/4, 4/11, 5/18. Patient confirmed medications taken as prescribed by physician and ate nutritious meal within 2 hours of appointment.

Dental hygiene diagnosis
Unmet human need for skin and mucous membrane integrity of the head and neck due to generalized supra– and subgingival plaque biofilm, extrinsic stain, moderate calculus gen. interproximal and lingual sextant 5, immune response to Type II diabetes and high blood pressure as evidenced by Stage III, Grade C periodontitis, radiographic bone coronal to middle 1/3 molar roots (unable to measure interdental CAL with calculus), probing depths 4 to 6 mm posteriors, 7 mm #1 F and #14 DF, gen. horizontal bone loss, % bone loss/age moderate, HbA1c 7.5%, recession 1mm #20, F2 #2F; bleeding index (BI) 68%; gingival inflammation.

Client goals	Interventions (target etiologies)	Evaluation
The patient will; • Reduce probing depths of 5mm and greater by 1 mm or more by Phase 1 reevaluation and maintain to Phase IV maintenance appointment; • Reduce BI to less than 10% by Phase 1 reevaluation and maintain to Phase IV maintenance appointment; • Eliminate gingival inflammation by Phase 1 reevaluation. • Stabilize clinical attachments to Phase IV maintenance appointment.	Phase I nonsurgical periodontal therapy • Periodontal debridement full mouth with powered and hand instrumentation • Local anesthesia • Review/reinforce oral self care • Phase I outcome @ 4–6 weeks • Coronal polish, medium grit paste or air-powder to remove extrinsic stain. • Referral Phase II consultation with periodontist following phase I.	**5/18 Goal met.** Probing depths of 5mm and greater reduced by 1 mm, 7mm probing depths #1 and #14 reduced by 2 mm. **5/18 Goal not met.** BI reduced to 13%, bleeding sites primarily interdental maxillary molars. **5/18 Goal partially met.** Generalized healthy gingiva, localized gingival inflammation maxillary molars.

Dental hygiene diagnosis
Unmet need for biologically sound and functional dentition due to inadequate oral self care, generalized plaque biofilm, PI 90%, saliva reducing medication and frequent snacking, moderate salivary flow by observation, irregular dental care, and impaired ability to utilize molars for proper chewing of food and functionality as evidenced by high risk for caries, active caries, xerostomia, missing 1st and 2nd mandibular molars from previous caries.

Client goals	Interventions	Evaluation
The patient will; • reduce high caries risk to low caries risk by Phase IV maintenance continued care visit. • increase protective factors by 4/11. • schedule appointment with dentist of record for restorative needs by 3/14.	Educate on caries risk factors (plaque, diet, saliva) protective factors and the importance of periodic dental examinations. Reinforce brushing 2 x a day and flossing 1 x a day. Discuss the benefits of xylitol containing gum and self-applied topical fluoride, place on 1.1% NaF toothpaste for pm brushing. Apply professional NaF varnish. Schedule with collaborating dentist to have caries treated.	**3/14 Goal met.** Patient scheduled appointment with dentist to have carious lesion treated. **4/11 Goal met.** Patient has increase protective factors. Patient reported pm brushing with 1.1% NaF toothpaste, satisfaction chewing xylitol gum to stimulate saliva, and makes mouth feel cleaner.

Dental hygiene diagnosis
Unmet need for conceptualization and problem solving due to lack of knowledge of etiology of periodontal diseases, disease indicators, risk factors, oral-systemic health relationship as evidenced by patient reports never educated on importance of oral health, reports oral health as bad but highly motivated to improve, unable to explain periodontal disease, role of plaque biofilm, risk factors that contribute to disease progression, bi-directional relationship of diabetes and periodontitis, and self care actions to slow disease progression.

Client goals	Interventions	Evaluation
The patient will: • Paraphrase the relationship of bacterial plaque biofilm to the periodontal process, risk factors that impact rate of disease progression and the bidirectional relationship of diabetes and periodontitis by 4/4. • Affirm the importance of daily plaque removal and management of blood glucose to minimize risk of progression of periodontitis by 4/4.	Educate on etiology of periodontal diseases, plaque biofilm, impact of diabetes on disease progression and bidirectional relationship of diabetes and periodontitis. Discuss the importance of daily plaque removal and diabetes management.	**4/4 Goal met.** Patient explained in own words the etiology of periodontal disease, risk of disease progression (diabetes) and impact of periodontal inflammation on systemic health. Patient stated slowly changing diet, more low glycemic food choices as recommended by physician. Patient stated recognizes importance of daily plaque removal for oral health and diabetes management.

Fig. 23.5 (A and B) Example of dental hygiene diagnoses, care plan, and evaluation, applied to the Human Needs Conceptual Model and Oral Health-Related Quality of Life Model, using Case Scenario 22.1, Chapter 22, Dental Hygiene Diagnosis.

Dental hygiene diagnosis

Unmet need for responsibility for oral health due to inadequate oral self care (technique, infrequency), lack of regular preventive oral health throughout life as evidenced by brushing 2 x day with a medium bristle brush, flossing 2 to 3 x per week, PI score of 85%. Last dental appointment was 4 years ago, states seeking professional oral health care not a cultural norm however motivated to improve oral health, seeking dental care on his own.

Client goals	Interventions	Evaluation
The patient will; • Demonstrate efficient brushing with a soft bristle brush or power brush and flossing techniques by Phase I reevaluation. • Reduce PI score to less than 10% by Phase I reevaluation. • Report brushing 2 x day with soft bristle brush and flossing 1 x day at Phase I reevaluation and maintain to Phase IV maintenance. • Schedule Phase IV maintenance visit for continued care at Phase I outcome.	Instruct on brushing with soft bristle brush, flossing technique and frequency. Introduce and instruct on power brush technique. Discuss the importance of regular maintenance appointments to monitor periodontal disease progression.	**5/18 Goals met.** Patient purchased a power brush and demonstrated proper adaptation of power brush and dental floss. Reduced PI to 9.8%. Localized plaque molars and sextant 5. Reports adherence to brushing 2x day with power brush and flossing 1 x day. Scheduled Phase IV maintenance continued care visit for 8/29/23

Appointment schedule:

Procedure Codes[6,7]	
D0210 D0180 D0603	***Appointment 1: Assessment – 1.5 hours*** Personal, medical, dental, pharmacologic history; measure vital signs. Confirm meds taken as prescribed and eaten meal. Preprocedural rinse - Chlorhexidine. Perform EOE, IOE. Take intraoral photographs. Full mouth series radiographs. Comprehensive periodontal eval. – gingiva, probing, BI, dental charting, calculus charting (radiographic perio findings will be assessed post appt. in consultation with dentist Caries risk assessment. Dentist examination/consult to address active caries. Discuss initial findings and confirm appointment for presentation of dental hygiene care plan.
D1330	***Appointment 2: Dental hygiene diagnosis and care plan - 1.5 hours*** Review medical history/meds, take BP, confirm meds taken and meal eaten. Preprocedural rinse - Chlorhexidine. Present care plan: Inform patient of findings, discuss dental hygiene diagnoses linking evidence and etiology, care plan goals, interventions, prognosis and appointment schedule. Obtain informed consent. Determine Plaque Index (PI). Oral self care instruction: Brushing with a soft bristle brush 2 x day and flossing 1x day. Educate on caries risk and protective factors. Dispense 1.1% sodium fluoride toothpaste and sample gum with xylitol.
D1330 D9210 D4341	***Appointment 3: Phase I nonsurgical periodontal therapy – 1.5 hours*** Review medical history/meds, take BP, confirm meds taken and meal eaten. Educate on etiology of periodontal diseases, plaque biofilm, bidirectional relationship of diabetes and periodontitis. Reinforce daily plaque removal and diabetes management. Evaluate *goal for unmet need for conceptualization and problem solving* Preprocedural rinse - Chlorhexidine. Assess/monitor tissue response to TB/F self care. Oral self care instruction: Apply disclosing agent, review/reinforce brushing and flossing as needed. Local anesthesia – Q1 and Q4. Periodontal debridement Q1 and Q4: Ultrasonic and hand instrumentation. Postoperative instructions.
D1330 D9210 D4341	***Appointment 4: Phase I nonsurgical periodontal therapy – 1.5 hours*** Review medical history/meds, take BP, confirm meds taken and meal eaten. Preprocedural rinse - Chlorhexidine Assess/monitor tissue response to TB/F self care and periodontal debridement Q1 and Q4. Evaluate *goal for increasing protective factors for caries risk.* Oral self care instruction: Apply disclosing agent, review/reinforce as needed. Introduce power brush. Local anesthesia – Q2 and Q3. Periodontal debridement Q2 and Q3: Ultrasonic and hand instrumentation. Postoperative instructions.
D0171 D1330 D1110 D1206	***Appointment 5: Phase I response to nonsurgical therapy @ 4 to 6 weeks – 1 hour*** Review medical history/meds, take BP, confirm meds taken and meal eaten. Preprocedural rinse – Chlorhexidine. Periodontal reevaluation to measure gingival health, pocket depths, hard and soft deposits, all quadrants. Post treatment Plaque Index and Bleeding Index. Measure goals planned to be evaluated at Phase I reevaluation. Oral self care instructions: Review and reinforce as needed Retreat/debride residual hard or soft deposits. Coronal polish. Apply 5% NaF varnish Determine continued care interval and schedule: Phase IV Maintenance (D4910). Scheduled Phase II evaluation with periodontist.

Prognosis: Short-term prognosis is good as patient seems motivated to improve oral health. Discussed with patient the importance of phase I treatment and adherence to oral self-care recommendations to reduce pocket depths, stabilize bone loss and decrease hard and soft deposits. Long-term prognosis is fair due to diabetes, HbA1c 7.5, age and localized sites of moderate bone loss and critical pocket depths, however, patient is working with physician to decrease HbA1c and has committed to Phase II evaluation with periodontist at the completion of Phase I.

Signatures:	Patient	Clinician	Date

Continued care recommendation: 3 months for Phase IV maintenance to monitor and maintain oral health.

Fig. 23.5, cont'd

Oral Health-Related Quality of Life Model				
See Chapter 22 – Figure 22.1 for completed Oral Health Related Quality of Life Assessment.				
III. Oral assessment and DH diagnosis		IV. DH care plan	V. Implementation and evaluation	ADAcode[6,7] and Fee
Problem/Pathology/ Risk assessment	Etiology	Treatment selections and HC	Sequence of DH procedures	
1. Intra-/extraoral exam • Light swelling of submandibular lymph nodes – bilateral • Lightly coated tongue • Small fissures on tongue • Bilateral class I molar relationship • Moderate salivary flow • 25% (2mm) overbite	1 = Primary etiology 2 = Contributing factors/Risk factor) 1. Lightly coated tongue – patient does not use any type of oral appliance to clean tongue 2. Patient has large tonsils, which can contribute to halitosis.	1. How motivated are you to improve your overall home care now vs a year ago? (Looking back) MI: What do you think is causing your tongue to have a white/coated appearance? Preventive counseling: Educate patient on brushing soft tissue, tongue, to remove all coated bacteria. Inform patient about tongue scraper, Educate patient on Xylitol containing gum can counteract bacteria by preventing the buildup of plaque and chewing gum can also stimulate the production of more saliva.	Appointment 1: Assessment – 1.5 hours • Start check/Vitals • Medical history/Medications • Social history (Tobacco and alcohol assessment) • Preprocedural rinse/ Chlorhexidine • EO/IO • Intraoral photographs • Full-mouth series • Comprehensive periodontal Eval. – gingiva, probing, CAL, Bleeding Index (BI), dental charting, calculus charting (radiographic findings will be assessed post appt. #1 in consultation with dentist/ periodontist prior to formulating dental hygiene care plan). • Caries risk assessment • Dentist exam/consult to address active caries • Discuss initial findings and confirm appt. to present dental hygiene care plan. Appointment 2: DH diagnosis and care plan – 1.5 hours • Start check/Vitals	D0210 D0180 D0603
• Dental Evaluation • #1 – 4, #6 – 16, #17 – 32 sound teeth • Missing #18, #19, #30, #31 • Moderate caries #5 DO • Mild stain • Moderate calculus buildup • High caries risk due to infrequent dental care, inadequate home care, existing carious lesions, and frequent snacking	1. Biofilm (18%) – estimated 18% biofilm was recorded while periodontal probing, but proper PI will be recorded when patient is disclosed. 2. Patient has mild stain and moderate calculus buildup due to infrequent dental care and inadequate home care. Last visit was approximately 3-4 years ago. 3. Patient has a moderate salivary flow but poor home care. Moderate salivary flow is a contributor to the patient not having as many carious lesions	MI: 1. Tell me how important it is to you to keep your teeth for a lifetime? (Evocative question) 2. What do you think has contributed to your current and past caries? Preventive counseling: Discuss with patient the importance of improving home care to brushing 2x daily and flossing 1x daily. Educate patient on the importance of using a soft bristle toothbrush instead of a medium. Discuss the benefits of an electric toothbrush rather than a manual. Treatment: Referral to DDS for #5 caries; Disclose patient, record accurate PI and show patient problem areas Have patient demo oral B power toothbrush with test drive Demo c-shaped flossing method polish full mouth with medium grit paste or air powder polishing to remove moderate stain Apply topical fluoride varnish	• Review Med HX/Meds, confirm meds taken and meal eaten. • Care plan presentation; Inform patient of findings and dental hygiene diagnoses, discuss etiology of dental diagnoses, care plan goals, interventions, prognosis and appointment schedule. • Obtain informed consent. • Preprocedural rinse/ Chlorhexidine • Determine Plaque Index (PI) • Preventive counseling – Brushing with soft bristle brush 2x day and with floss 1x day. • Educate on brushing soft tissue and tongue. Dispense sample gum with xylitol. Appointment 3: Phase I non-surgical therapy – 1.5 hours • Start check/Vitals • Review Med HX/Meds, confirm meds taken and meal eaten. • Educate etiology of periodontal diseases/plaque/ diabetes. • Preprocedural rinse – chlorhexidine	D1330 D1330 D9210 D4341

Fig. 23.5, cont'd

2. Periodontal evaluation • AAP disease classification highlight as appropriate Stage: I, II, III, IV Grade: A, B, C *Annuals of periodontology,* 2017 **Periodontal pathologies** • Attachment loss: Localized in molar areas, may have more attachment loss but could not accurately record due to calculus build up • Recession: 1 mm on #20 • Pocket formation: Generalized 3–4 mm on the anterior teeth and 5–4 mm on the posterior teeth and localized 7 mm pocket depths straight facial of #1, and #14DF • Bone loss and descriptions: Generalized horizontal bone loss • Mobility: None • Furcation involvement: F2 on facial of #2 • Gingival description: Generalized red pink edematous/fibrotic gingiva with bulbous interdental papilla • BI: 68% • PI: 18% • Mucogingival defects: None • Level of risk for periodontal disease/s): High due to inadequate home care, infrequent dental visits, periodontal pocket formation, and bone loss.	1. Biofilm (18%) – estimated 18% biofilm was recorded while periodontal probing but proper PI will be recorded when patient is disclosed. Immune Response: Recent diabetes diagnosis and HBP 2. Patient has moderate calculus buildup on the lingual surfaces of the mandibular incisors and premolars. Generalized subgingival moderate calculus buildup on the interproximal surfaces of mand./ max molars. Patient brushes 2x day and flosses 2–3x per week. His BI is 68% due to the lack of flossing and the calculus buildup is also contributed to inadequate home care.	MI: 1.Tell me what you know about Periodontal Disease? (Open-Ended) 2. May I discuss with you the importance of stopping disease progression? (Teach) Preventative counseling: Discuss the etiologies of Periodontal disease and risk factors contributing to disease. Discuss how the patient can help prevent disease progression and what he can do to maintain It. Educate the patient on the importance of adequate home care and the importance of maintaining regular dental visits. Discuss treatment of dentition: Discuss STG and LTG SRP 4–8 teeth on all quads (ultrasonic and hand instruments) 4–6 week reevaluation to see improvements in bleeding/plaque index, reduction pocket depths, change in gingival description. Patient will either be on a recare, retreat, or refer based on outcome 4–6 weeks post SRP. Upon completion of treatment, perio consult to evaluate bone loss around tooth #3. Recommended maintenance – 3 months to stabilized oral health	• Assess/monitor tissue response to TB/F self care. • Preventive counseling – review and reinforce brushing and flossing as needed. • LA for Quadrants I and 4 • Periodontal debridement Q1 and Q4: Ultrasonic and hand instrumentation • Post op instructions Appointment 4: Phase I non-surgical therapy – 1.5 hours • Start check/Vitals • Review Med HX/Meds, confirm meds taken and meal eaten. • Preprocedural rinse – Chlorhexidine • Assess/monitor tissue response to TB/F self care and periodontal debridement Q1 and Q4. • Preventive counseling - introduce to power brush. • LA for Quadrants 2 and 3 • Periodontal debridement Q2 and Q3 - Ultrasonic and hand instrumentation • Post op Appointment 5: Phase I response to nonsurgical therapy/Re-eval 4–6 weeks – 1 hour • Start check/Vitals • Review Med HX/Meds, confirm meds taken and meal eaten. • Pre-procedural rinse – Chlorhexidine • Periodontal reevaluation • Take PI and BI • Measure goals planned to be evaluated. • Preventive counseling – review and reinforce TB/F as needed. • Retreat/Debride residual hard or soft deposits. • Polish & Floss • Apply 5% NaF Varnish • Determine recare interval for Phase IV maintenance (D4910) and schedule. • Scheduled appointment with periodontist for Phase II evaluation.	D1330 D9210 D4341 D0171 D1330 D1110 D1206

Dental hygiene diagnosis

• Patient presents as Stage III Grade C due to generalized 3–4mm pocketing on the anterior teeth and 5–4mm on the posterior teeth with localized 7 mm PD on the straight facial of #1 and #14DF, generalized horizontal bone loss, inadequate home care, infrequent dental visits and moderate calculus buildup. Patient is high caries risk due to infrequent dental care, inadequate home care, existing carious lesions, and frequent snacking. Modifiable risk factors include inadequate home care, pocket formation and infrequent dental visits. Nonmodifiable risk factors include bone loss.

Dental hygiene prognosis

Short-term prognosis is good as the patient seems more motivated to improve oral health. Discussed with the patient the need to keep following appointments for SRP treatment and oral self care recommendations to reduce pocket depths, stabilize bone loss and decrease plaque and calculus deposits. Long-term prognosis is fair due to diabetes, HbA1c 7.5%, age, and localized sites of moderate bone loss and critical pocket depths; however, patient is working with physician to decrease HbA1c and has committed to Phase II evaluation at the completion of Phase I.

Fig. 23.5, cont'd

Outcome evaluation:	Clinical outcomes:
Patient-centered outcome STG: Improve home care: Report daily brushing 2x day for 2 min. With a soft bristle toothbrush or powered brush and daily c-shape flossing by Phase 1 reevaluation. Reduce PI to less than 10% by Phase I re-evaluation. LTG: Maintain frequent recare appointments and schedule 3month recare/Phase IV maintenance visit for continued care at Phase 1 reevaluation.	Reduce 5 mm and greater pockets by at least 1 mm, reduce BI to less than 10% and eliminate gingival inflammation by Phase 1 reevaluation and maintain to recare/Phase IV maintenance.

Signatures:	Student:	Faculty:	Patient:	Date:

Goal evaluation:
Goals measured at appointment 6 – Phase I reevaluation
Patient-centered outcome: Goals Met, Patient purchased a power brush and reports daily brushing 2x day for 2 minutes with power brush and daily c-shape flossing, reduced PI to 9.8%, localized plaque at gingival margin of molars and sextant 5, and scheduled 3 month continued care visit for Phase IV maintenance. Clinical outcome: Goals partially Met: Probing depths of 5mm and greater reduced by 1 mm, 7 mm probe reading on #1 and #14 reduced by 2 mm. BI reduced to 13%, bleeding sites primarily interdental of maxillary molars, localized sites of gingival inflammation continue at maxillary molars.

Fig. 23.5, cont'd

BOX 23.16 Criteria for Informed Consent of Planned Care

The patient must:
- Be knowledgeable about what the healthcare provider plans to do.
- Have enough information to make a rational choice.
- Give oral or written permission for the plan to be carried out.
- Give consent:
  - For a specific treatment
  - For a procedure that must be legal
  - Under truthful conditions (e.g., consent cannot be obtained through fraud, deceit, misrepresentation, or trickery)
- Be legally competent to give consent for care (In the case of a minor, consent must be given by the parent or legal healthcare decision maker.)

BOX 23.17 Patient Reasons for Refusal of Care, Dental Hygiene Actions, and Documentation of Informed Refusal

Patient Reasons
Cost of service
Fear of pain
Lack of understanding
Low value placed on dental care
Lack of dental insurance coverage

Clinician Actions
Acknowledge patient's concerns.
Clarify proposed plan of care.
Discuss consequences of not receiving recommended care.
Recommend alternative treatment options when appropriate.

Documentation
Include brief explanation of recommended care.
Identify specific treatment procedure being declined.
List risks and consequences to patient's health without treatment.
Indicate date of informed refusal.
Include signatures of patient, dentist, and witness.

PROCEDURE 23.1 Dental Hygiene Care Planning

Steps
- Link care plan to dental hygiene diagnoses.
- Establish priorities of need.
- Set clinical and patient-centered goals.
- Select dental hygiene interventions.
  Note: Philosophic difference exists between the Human Needs (HN) Conceptual Model and Oral Health-Related Quality of Life (OHRQL) Model in the sequencing of setting goals and selecting intervention strategies. The OHRQL Model proposes intervention strategies and then collaborates with the patient to set goals.
- Establish an appointment schedule.
- Present the dental hygiene care plan to the patient.
- Ask the patient to sign an informed consent statement for the care plan (signature pad or hard copy that is scanned).
- Document the completion of this service to the patient's dental record by entering a customized electronic note of presentation and patient acceptance of the care plan; date and sign the entry. For example, "*Clinical and radiographic findings, dental hygiene diagnosis, and care plan were presented and discussed with patient. Patient asked clarifying questions before giving written consent to care plan.*" A supplemental clinical note may be entered to describe additional relevant events such as patient-initiated questions or comments.

---

must be considered. Therefore evaluation of a patient's progress must be ongoing so the clinician can do the following:
- Modify the care plan because the patient is having difficulty in achieving the goal;
- Modify the care plan because the patient is not ready to achieve the goal;
- Continue the care plan because the patient needs more time to achieve the goal; and/or
- Terminate the care plan because the patient has achieved the goal.

Evaluation of Care Plan Goals

Evaluation methods must reflect the intent of the goal statement (e.g., cognitive, psychomotor, affective, oral health status). Each goal is

---

PROCEDURE 23.2   Guidelines for the Presentation of Care Plan

Steps

Define and Discuss the Dental Hygiene Diagnosis

- Engage the patient in a discussion concerning the nature of the problem or condition to determine level of awareness and understanding. Acknowledge what the patient knows and supplement to clarify further.
- Share evidence of observed signs and symptoms of the problem or condition.
- Share suspected causes or contributors such as those observed by the clinician or reported by the patient.
- Consider that most of the discussion time is spent on this step. If the patient is not engaged in this discussion or does not see the link or understand the condition, the remaining steps will most likely be fruitless.

Present and Explain the Proposed Treatment

- Draw a link between the selected interventions and the causes or contributors (modifiable and nonmodifiable) defined by the dental hygiene diagnosis.
- Explain how the intervention strategies support the patient's achievement of the care plan goals and resolution of the problem or condition. Indicate risks and/or potential for failure, if any.
- Differentiate between the patient's responsibilities and the clinician's role.
- Engage the patient in a discussion to confirm acceptance of the proposed interventions. Offer alternative interventions of equal merit, if available. If not, discuss the limitations of alternative treatment approaches.

Discuss the Prognosis of No Treatment

- Consider the dental hygienist's legal and ethical responsibility to ensure that the patient understands how the condition may progress if left untreated or patient is not adherent with responsibility to self-care.

Discuss Care Plan Goals

- Engage the patient in a realistic discussion of what the patient would like to achieve as well as the patient's ability and willingness to make behavior changes (e.g., reverse, stabilize, or prevent a condition; perform a skill).
- Draw a link between the goal statement and dental hygiene diagnosis.
- Confirm that the patient supports the goals.

Discuss the Appointment Schedule

- Consider that the discussion of the appointment schedule comes later in the presentation so that the patient can appreciate the need for multiple appointments.

Discuss Fee Schedule

- Consider that if the fee schedule is presented too early in the discussion, the patient may not be able to focus on the cost per value of the plan, therefore increasing the likelihood that the patient may reject the care plan.

Secure Patient Consent

- Following presentation of the care plan and discussion with the patient, request that the patient provide a written consent to treatment.

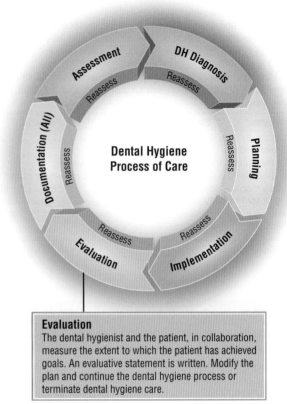

Fig. 23.6 Evaluation step of the dental hygiene process.

concrete evidence that supports the decision. This evaluation statement is recorded in the patient's permanent record and signed and dated by the dental hygienist. The outcome and supporting findings are shared and discussed with the patient. Sample goal statements, evaluation strategies, and evaluative statements for each goal category are displayed in Table 23.3.

Failure to evaluate the outcome of patient care leaves the clinician and patient unaware of the impact that the care plan may or may not have had. Unknown to the clinician and the patient, unresolved patient needs might continue to contribute to a decline in health and wellness. By monitoring and measuring the extent to which patient goals have been achieved, the dental hygienist is able to make evidence-based decisions for continued care.

Modifying or Terminating the Care Plan

When evaluation reveals that the patient has made little progress toward goal attainment (i.e., *goal partially met* or *goal not met*), the dental hygienist reassesses the patient's readiness to change, attitudes, beliefs, and practices and formulates an evaluative statement that defines why the care plan is not successful in achieving the defined goals. The dental hygienist discusses new findings in consultation with the dentist and/or collaborates interprofessionally with members of the interdisciplinary care team, a process that may lead to new diagnoses, revised goals, and alternative interventions. (See Box 23.18 for legal and ethical factors that affect quality dental hygiene care. Box 23.19 suggests potential barriers to the patient achieving care plan goals.)

When evaluation determines successful attainment of patient goals and no new problems are identified, the care plan is terminated. The patient maintains responsibility for continued oral health to the next cycle of care. Written and verbal posttreatment instructions may be

evaluated to determine the degree to which it has been achieved (Fig. 23.7). Based on the new findings, the dental hygienist determines one of the following outcomes:

- Goal met
- Goal partially met
- Goal not met

A written evaluative statement is included, stating the dental hygienist's decision on the degree to which the goal was achieved and

PROCEDURE 23.3 Integrating Evaluation and Documentation Into Patient-Centered Care

Steps

Assess and Diagnose

- Collect and analyze the baseline assessment findings that establish a patient need, providing the foundation for formulating an evaluation strategy.

Plan

- Define care plan goals; that is, define evaluative measures and methodology that address the *clinical evidence* of an unmet need, condition, or problem and *contributing patient behaviors* as defined by the dental hygiene diagnosis.

Implement

- Monitor patient progress toward achieving care plan goals; modify care plan as needed to guide patient toward success.

Evaluate and Document

- Measure and document attainment of care plan goals to determine the prognosis of care, to establish continued-care interval, and to make referrals for additional services as needed.

Continued Care: Assess

- Measure and document patient's outcome at continued care; that is, the patient's long-term success at achieving or maintaining the resolution of an unmet need, condition, or problem addressed by the previous care plan. Measure the previous care plan goals using the new assessment findings to determine goals continue to be met, partially met, or not met. When goals are partially met or not met and a recurrence of an unmet need, condition, or problem is evident, further investigate to determine the underlying contributor. Continue with the process of care.

Continued Care: Diagnose

- Define the dental hygiene diagnosis, based on reassessment findings (e.g., evidence, contributors).

Continued Care: Plan

- Restate or redefine the evaluative measures and methodology to support the continued care dental hygiene diagnosis.
- Select intervention strategies to support patient's continued care needs, with consideration to the identified contributor to the recurrence of an unmet need, condition, or problem.

Continued Care: Implement

- Monitor patient progress toward achieving care plan goals and modify care plan as needed, to guide patient toward success.

Continued Care: Evaluating and Documenting

- Measure and document attainment of care plan goals to determine the prognosis of care, to establish continued-care interval, and to make referrals for additional services as needed.

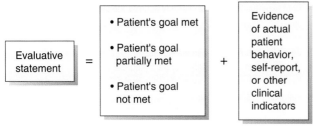

Fig. 23.7 Components of an evaluative statement.

given to the patient as a reminder of self-care responsibilities and signs and symptoms of any possible future problems.

Dental Hygiene Prognosis and Continued Care

A **dental hygiene prognosis** is an evidence-based predictability of the patient's continued health and wellness. The dental hygiene prognosis is contingent on the following:

- Overall appraisal of the evaluative statements
- Patient's continued adherence to recommended self-care and control of plaque biofilm
- Level of optimal oral health achieved
- Systemic health and environmental factors

A favorable prognosis occurs when goals have been met and risk for a new disease or recurrence of the previous condition or problem is low. A prognosis is guarded when risk for a new disease or recurrence of the previous condition is moderate to high. Care plan goals may have been achieved successfully during active therapy; however, a guarded prognosis is determined because of continued risk factors such as smoking or a systemic disease.

At the termination of the dental hygiene care plan, the prognosis directs the determination of a continued cycle of care that will support the patient's efforts to maintain the oral health status achieved during active therapy. Continued-care appointments are scheduled at 2- to 12-month intervals, based on patient need. Periodically, the dental hygienist reviews the continued-care plan and adjusts it as needed.

Outcome at Continued-Care Visit

A **continued-care visit** is a subsequent cycle of the process of care to monitor and support the continued health of a patient. The phrase *continued-care* visit, rather than recare or recall visit, is used to emphasize the supportive role of the dental hygienist in the patient-clinician relationship.

Each continued-care visit begins with assessment and evaluation of the patient to measure continued attainment of the previous care plan goals. Evaluation is integrated into assessment at the continued-care visit to identify and document the following:

- Evidence that the care plan from the previous cycle of care has successfully addressed the patient's needs and attained long-term clinical outcomes
- Evidence of the patient's long-term commitment to continued health and wellness
- Recurrence and etiology of a previous need or condition
- Occurrence and etiology of a new condition or problem that may be present

Evaluative measures are applied to these findings and become the foundation for formulating new dental hygiene diagnoses and a supportive dental hygiene care plan (Table 23.4). Determining long-term outcomes at the continued-care visit is critical to ensuring that the patient's adherence to responsibility for oral health will be reenforced and the recurrence of a previous care plan need will be recognized and addressed. (See Box 23.20 for outcome at continued-care visit.)

DOCUMENTATION

The ADHA Standard 6, **documentation**, is the complete and accurate recording of all collected data, care plan, patient consent for treatment, treatment outcomes, prognosis, continued-care recommendations, and other interactions and information relevant to patient care. Entries

TABLE 23.3 Sample of Goal Statements, Evaluation Strategies, and Evaluative Statements

Goal Category	Goal Statement	Evaluation Strategy	Evaluative Statement
Cognitive	Patient will verbalize the periodontal disease process and identify oral biofilm as the prime causative agent by 9/21.	Ask the patient open-ended questions to measure acquisition of new knowledge.	9/21: Goal met. Patient can describe the role of oral biofilm and the periodontal disease process.
Psychomotor	Patient will demonstrate use of interdental cleaning aid for removal of interproximal soft deposits by 7/12.	Ask the patient to demonstrate a newly learned interdental cleaning technique.	7/12: Goal not met. Patient is having difficulty positioning the interdental aid in most areas of the mouth.
Affective	Patient will report having blood pressure evaluated by physician before rescheduled visit on 10/5.	Ask the patient to report on visit with physician to have blood pressure evaluated and physician recommendations.	10/5: Goal met. Patient reported completing visit with physician and has begun a weight management program as recommended.
Oral health status	Patient will eliminate gingival inflammation and bleeding on probing by end of treatment on 9/10.	Reassess the gingiva and show the patient clinical improvements in oral health.	9/10: Goal met. Gingival findings support health.

BOX 23.18 Critical Thinking Scenario D

Factors That May Detract From the Quality of Dental Hygiene Care

Characteristics of the patient, dental hygienist, and clinical environment interact to enhance or hinder patient goals. The astute dental hygienist identifies positive and negative factors that may affect goal attainment. To facilitate the desired oral health outcome, positive factors are reinforced and negative factors managed. Positive factors include the following:

- Patient who values oral health, is motivated, and has a sense of inquiry
- Dental hygienist who maintains an evidence-based practice
- Work environment that values high-quality healthcare and offers incentives for care that meet or exceed recognized standards of practice
  1. Propose patient, clinician, and environmental variable that may detract from the quality of care.
  2. Discuss possible dental hygiene actions.

BOX 23.19 Potential Barriers to Patient Achieving Care Plan Goals

- Improperly developed goals; goals that, if achieved, do not guarantee problem resolution
- Unrealistic goals for the patient to achieve; immeasurable goals
- Care plan that does not specifically address the patient's goals and unique socioethnocultural characteristics; plan that contains only general information
- Care plan that has not been individualized
- Failure to monitor and address patient progress
- Evaluation method does not support the goal
- Inadequate documentation

TABLE 23.4 Sample of Evaluative Statements for Continued Health at Continued-Care Visit and Action Plan

Stage I/Grade B Periodontitis: Phase I Nonsurgical Therapy and Outcome At Maintenance Phase: Phase IV Therapy

Goal at Phase I	Evaluation at Phase I Evaluation Step	Evaluation at Phase IV Continued-Care Visit	Action Plan
Clinical Goal: The patient will decrease probing depths to 3 mm or less by Phase I evaluation on **4/21:** Patient will stabilize localized CAL of 2 mm to continued care maintenance on **7/24:** **Patient-Centered Goal:** Patient will report daily brushing and flossing by Phase I evaluation on **4/21:** Patient will report no longer smoking by Phase I evaluation on 4/21.	**4/21:** Clinical goal met for decrease in pocket depth, all probing depths are 3 mm or less. **4/21:** Patient-centered goal is met for daily brushing and flossing. **4/21:** Patient-centered goal is partially met for smoking cessation. Prognosis is guarded for continued stable periodontal health and stable CAL. Patient reports a reduction in daily smoking to 3 cigarettes per day, motivation to quit, and has enrolled in a tobacco cessation program for support.	**7/24:** Assessment findings show evidence that all previous care plan goals have been met. CAL are stable at 2 mm and probing depths are 3 mm or less. Patient reports continued adherence to recommended oral self-care and reports no cigarette smoking for 2 months.	Share findings with patient. Praise and reinforce patient's self-care.

Continued

TABLE 23.4   Sample of Evaluative Statements for Continued Health at Continued-Care Visit and Action Plan—cont'd

Preventive Prophylaxis (Modification for Single Appointment)

Goal at Initial Prophylaxis	Evaluation at Initial Prophylaxis	Evaluation at Continued-Care Prophylaxis	Action Plan
Clinical Goal: Patient will decrease moderate risk for caries to low risk by next continued care prophylaxis. **Patient-Centered Goal:** Patient will demonstrate efficient brushing and flossing techniques at end of appointment on 1/22. Patient will increase plaque-free score to 95% at next continued care prophylaxis. Patient will report increasing protective factors by brushing daily with 1.1% self-applied topical fluoride toothpaste and OTC salivary substitute at next continued care prophylaxis.	**1/22**: Patient-centered goal is met for brushing and flossing techniques. Prognosis good for clinical and supporting patient-centered goals being met. Patient demonstrated excellent brushing and flossing skills and appears to be motivated to address oral health needs.	**7/23**: Assessment findings evidence that the previous care plan clinical goal has not been met. Patient continues to demonstrate moderate risk for caries. Supporting patient-centered goals have not all been met. Plaque-free score is 75%; patient reports being inconsistent with interdental cleaning and self-applied topical fluoride toothpaste over the last 2 months. Goal met for OTC salivary substitute, patient reports using daily. Prognosis is guarded for dental health.	Share findings with patient; identify barrier to patient's adherence to recommended self-care. Include the new findings in the dental hygiene diagnosis and formulate care plan to address the new findings.

OTC, Over-the-counter.

BOX 23.20   Critical Thinking Scenario E

Outcome at Continued-Care Visit

A 24-year-old male arrives for a 6-month prophylaxis visit. Outcome at this continued-care appointment reveals that the previous care plan's clinical goal, *patient will eliminate bleeding and inflammation by the next continued care visit,* was not met. The patient is aware that he has gingivitis and understands the periodontal disease process and risk factors. The patient reports brushing 2× a day and flossing each evening as recommended at the previous preventive appointment. Progress notes of the last preventive appointment indicate that the dental hygienist educated the patient about gingivitis and periodontal disease, including etiology and risk factors, demonstrated proper brushing and flossing techniques on a model, instructed the patient on frequency of brushing and flossing, and dispensed a soft bristle brush, sample floss, and written instructions on brushing and flossing.

1. Identify and discuss possible underlying contributors or barriers to the patient not meeting the desired clinical and patient-centered goals.
2. Propose supporting strategies.

---

should represent a chronologic account of all services in accordance with the dental hygiene process of care and proof of a link between each step. Documentation that demonstrates a relationship among assessment, dental hygiene diagnosis, care plan, implemented intervention strategies, and evaluative statements of outcome is legal and ethical evidence that the services rendered supported the patient's individual needs. Table 23.5 suggests guidelines for documenting evidence of a patient-centered process of care in the patient's record.

The goals of documentation are to maintain continuity of care, provide a means of communication among the patient's interdisciplinary care providers, and minimize practitioner risk of malpractice claims.[1] An electronic health record (EHR) has the potential to support these goals. As services are completed, the clinician makes entries into the patient's EHR, thus making needed patient care information available to the IPC team for coordination and communication of services. All entries must be accurate and factual and provide enough detail to describe how the patient progressed through each phase of care. Entries should be objective, concise, legible, and written by the provider who performed the service, signed, and dated. Use of abbreviations and acronyms should be limited to ensure an understanding among subsequent providers.

TABLE 23.5   Guidelines for Documentation in the Patient's Record and Evidence of a Patient-Centered Process of Care

Standards for Clinical Dental Hygiene Practice	Evidence of Services Rendered
Assessment	Demographic patient data; personal, medical, dental, pharmacologic health history; Oral Health-Related Quality of Life questionnaire findings (See Chapter 22, Fig. 22.5); vital signs; current oral self-care practices; oral habits; previous disease classification, if known
	Head and neck examination findings; dental and periodontal examination findings; caries risk assessment and indices; oral self-care skills; intraoral photographs
	Dental radiographs exposed including type, number, date reviewed
	Statement of patient's adherence to previous care plan goals and continued oral health at continued care visit
	Patient's chief concern or reason for visit in patient's own words; patient readiness to change
	Consultation with interdisciplinary patient care team

TABLE 23.5   Guidelines for Documentation in the Patient's Record and Evidence of a Patient-Centered Process of Care—cont'd

Standards for Clinical Dental Hygiene Practice	Evidence of Services Rendered
Diagnosis	**Human Needs Conceptual Model** Statement of unmet need supported by etiology, that is, critical contributing factors followed by signs and symptoms evidencing the deficit **Oral Health-Related Quality of Life Model** Statement reflecting identified problem, pathologic condition, risk assessment and etiology; summarizing overall oral health status, and discussing impact of modifiable and nonmodifiable risk factors
Planning	Written care plan or statement of goals, evidence-based interventions, and appointment schedule supporting the diagnosis Statement of patient involvement in development of care plan Statement of presentation of care plan to patient, patient-clinician discussion of proposed care plan, diagnoses communicated to patient, valid informed consent and/or informed refusal with signatures of patient or legal guardian of patient
Implementation	Detailed implementation of all care provided in chronologic order of appointments (e.g., cognitive, psychomotor, and affective skill development; patient education and oral self-care instructions, objective statement of patient oral self-care skills; patient-clinician interactions; oral and written recommendations, including patient adherence to recommendations; products, oral self-care aids, and literature dispensed for home use, periodontal debridement; anesthesia); referrals (when warranted) to interdisciplinary patient care team for supportive services and followup of referrals Statement of patient's adherence to the appointment schedule (e.g., late arrival, canceled, failed appointments) and when appointment was rescheduled Information and interactions between the patient and practice (e.g., confirmation of appointments or other correspondence by telephone, mail, or electronic communications; emergencies, prescriptions, compliance with scheduled appointments) Periodic reassessment or evaluation during implementation to monitor progress toward achieving proposed outcomes
Evaluation	Evaluative statement of treatment outcome and summary of evaluation methodology Clinician action based on outcome of care Prognosis; statement indicating outcome and prognosis were discussed with patient Recommendation of continued-care interval and referrals; indicating that this was discussed with patient Patient satisfaction survey
Documentation	Conclude each entry with date the service was provided (e.g., month/day/year) and signature of clinician who provided the service and completed the documentation (they should be the same person) Proper correction of an error in previously stored electronic information, mark entry as a *mistaken entry*, add correct information, date and initial entry

BOX 23.21   Legal, Ethical, and Safety Issues

Critical Thinking Activity: Periodic Monitoring of Documentation in Patient Record

Periodic monitoring of patient records can ensure that you are adhering to legal and ethical standards of care or be a reminder that critical patient care evidence of a patient-centered process of care may not be clearly documented. Select a sampling of patient records and complete a quality assurance audit for evidence of the process of care. Refer to Table 23.5 or develop a monitoring tool to guide you in chart review.

BOX 23.22   Legal, Ethical, and Safety Issues

Planning, Evaluation, and Documentation
- Beneficence requires that the dental hygiene care plan uses evidence-based strategies to address actual and patient-centered needs that promote oral health and wellness; requires monitoring and measuring of patient care to ensure positive health outcomes; and requires recommendations for a continued-care schedule that supports patient needs.
- Nonmaleficence is doing no harm; maintaining a safe and supportive patient care environment is expected.
- The planning process must support the patient's autonomy by including the patient in the planning and decision-making process and communicating the recommended care plan to the patient for informed consent.
- Apply risk management strategies to patient record keeping and sharing of patient care information with interdisciplinary patient care providers; comply with state regulations and statutes for record keeping and storage.
- Respect and protect the confidentiality of patient information.

Documented evidence of a patient-centered approach to care is the best defense against a patient's accusation of negligence. Box 23.21 provides a critical thinking activity for periodic monitoring of documentation in the dental record, and Box 23.22 suggests legal, ethical, and safety issues related to planning, evaluation, and documentation.

Documentation may be accomplished by electronically entering a **dental procedure code** or a **customized electronic note** that corresponds to the service and supplementing the entry with a narrative describing relevant events of patient care. Dental procedure codes denote standardized assessment and treatment codes used by the dental profession to indicate services as defined by the American Dental Association (ADA) CDT[6,7] (Table 23.6). A customized electronic note

is designed specifically by the healthcare facility to document a frequently used entry into a patient's EHR (see Fig. 23.8 for an example of entering a dental procedure code). See Procedure 23.4 and corresponding Competency Evaluation Form (https://evolve.elsevier.com/Pieren/hygiene/) for steps for evaluation of care.

TABLE 23.6 Frequently Documented Dental Procedure Codes for Services Provided by the Dental Hygienist

CDT Dental Procedure Codes[6,7]	Description
D1330	Oral hygiene instruction
D1110	Prophylaxis—adult
D1120	Prophylaxis—child
D4346	Scaling in the presence of generalized moderate or severe gingival inflammation—full mouth (absence of periodontitis)
D4341	Scaling and root planing—four or more teeth per quadrant
D4910	Periodontal maintenance
D1206	Topical application of fluoride varnish
D1208	Topical application of fluoride—excluding varnish

CDT, Current Dental Terminology.

Date	Provider	CDT code[6,7] and notes
3/14/2023	RDH2	D0180 - comprehensive periodontal evaluation – new or established patient D0210 - intraoral – complete series of radiographic images D0603 - caries risk assessment and documentation, with a finding of high risk New patient, 27-year-old Hispanic male. No chief concern. Initial personal, medical, dental, pharmacologic health history completed and reviewed with patient. Measured vitals. Last physician visit 3 months ago. Diagnosed 4 months ago with type II diabetes, reported last HbA1c 7.5%. Diagnosed with high blood pressure 2 years ago. Medications: metformin 2000mg/day and Zaroxolyn 2.5mg/day. Patient reported last dental visit and prophylaxis was 4 years ago. Patient confirmed medications taken as prescribed by physician and has eaten within 2 hours of appointment – 2 eggs, wheat toast, and cranberry juice. Preprocedural rinse/chlorhexidine and explained purpose is to reduce MOs. FMS with 4 BW. Preliminary review of dental radiographs indicated generalized horizontal bone loss. Radiographs will be comprehensively assessed in consultation with dentist/periodontist prior to formulating dental hygiene care plan. Performed EOE, IOE. Intra oral photographs taken. Completed comprehensive periodontal evaluation that included examination and charting of; gingival findings, recession, pocket depths, (could not accurately record CAL due to calculus), furcation, dental findings and calculus). Bleeding index 68%. Caries risk assessment. *(Clinician may include summary statement supporting critical findings documented in the patient's dental record* Dentist examination /consult completed; Caries #5DO, bilaterally missing 1st and 2nd mandibular molars, patient stated molars removed due to decay. Dentist discussed future consultation for replacing missing molars. Presented brief overview of initial findings and that radiographs to be reviewed by dentist/periodontist to measure health of the periodontium. Advised patient the dental hygiene care plan and findings will be discussed in detail at next appointment. Discussed medical history of diabetes and hypertension and the importance of taking medications as prescribed by physician and eating a nutritious meal in preparation for each dental visit to reduce risk of a glycemic event. Discussed scheduling morning appointments. Patient agreed best to schedule appointments in am. Next appointment 3/27/2023 for presentation of care plan for informed consent.
3/14/2023	OFF1	Patient scheduled with dentist for treatment caries #5DO on 3/30/2023.
3/27/2023	RDH2	D1330 – oral hygiene instruction Reappointment: Reviewed personal, medical, dental, pharmacologic health history. Patient reported no changes. BP 126/88. Patient confirmed medications taken as prescribed by physician and had eaten a nutritious breakfast within 2 hours of appointment. Preprocedural rinse/Chlorhexidine. Care plan presented for informed consent. Explained to patient the dental hygiene care plan is complementary to the overall dental treatment plan to minimize risk for cavities and address the health of the periodontium. Told patient of high risk for dental decay and Stage III/Grade C periodontitis. Inquired patient's knowledge of periodontal disease. Presented and discussed dental hygiene diagnoses including evidence and etiologies, intervention strategies to address caries risk and periodontal disease and set measurable goals. Discussed the importance of patient's responsibility for oral health and asked patient of willingness to participate in the treatment of condition. Patient replied, "yes, I want to do what I can to improve my health." Praised patient for frequency of brushing (2x day). Discussed recommended self care strategies; soft rather than medium bristle brush, increase flossing to 1x day. Continued with discussion caries risk diagnosis, etiology and risk factor of dry mouth. Explained to patient self care strategies proposed to meet periodontal health needs will support lowering risk for future cavities. Recommended xylitol gum and self applied fluoride. Reviewed detailed appointment schedule for Phase I nonsurgical periodontal therapy including reason for multiple treatment appointments, length of appointments, pain management, monitoring of patient's oral self care and tissue health, 4 to 6 week reevaluation and evaluation with periodontist for phase II care. Patient verbalized wanting to proceed with care. Completed written consent for phase I nonsurgical therapy. *(Clinician will supplement documentation, with details of the discussion including but not limited to knowledge and skill building to ensure understanding, educational strategies and methodology used, patient's comments and questions, clinician responses;* **see Box 23.15, Discussion of Dental Hygiene Diagnoses at Care Plan Presentation for Informed Consent.**) Continued with appointment. Completed plaque index – 90%. Shared finding with patient. Completed oral hygiene instructions for brushing and flossing. Instructed on brushing technique with a soft toothbrush and flossing in a C-shape. Patient practiced intraoral. Dispensed 1.1% sodium fluoride toothpaste and sample gum with xylitol. Next appointment 3/30/2023 restorative and 4/4/2023 Phase I treatment.
3/30/2023	DDS1	D2392 – resin-based composite – two surfaces, posterior D9215 – local anesthesia in conjunction with operative or surgical procedures Reviewed personal, medical, dental, pharmacologic health history. Patient reported no change. BP 126/90. #5 DO, resin-based composite. (type, *agent, concentration, # of cartridges, location of anesthesia).*

Fig. 23.8 Example of documentation of services rendered with evidence of the process of care and informed consent to treatment applied to Fig. 23.5 for the dental hygiene Human Needs Conceptual Model.

4/4/2023	RDH2	D1330 – oral hygiene instruction D9210 – local anesthesia not in conjunction with operative or surgical procedures D4341 – periodontal scaling and root planing – four or more teeth per quadrant, Q1 & Q4 Reappointment: Reviewed personal, medical, dental, pharmacologic health history. Patient reported no changes. BP 128/88. Patient confirmed medications taken as prescribed by physician and had eaten a nutritious breakfast within 2 hours of appointment. Preprocedural rinse/Chlorhexidine. Visually inspected gingiva, no significant change in inflammation resulting from patient's brushing and flossing. Patient verbalized difficulty with flossing due to calculus. Agreed with patient's assessment, stated access will get easier as calculus is removed. Reviewed discussion of etiology of periodontal diseases and plaque biofilm from previous appointment and educated on bidirectional relationship of diabetes and periodontitis. ***Goals met for unmet need for conceptualization and problem-solving. Outcome documented to care plan (evaluation).*** Applied disclosing agent, less plaque evident, reviewed brushing and flossing techniques - adequate. Local anesthesia Q 1 & Q4 (*type, agent, concentration, # of cartridges*). Ultrasonic and hand periodontal debridement Q1 & Q4. Postoperative instructions given to patient. Next appointment 4/11/2023, continue Phase I treatment.
4/11/2023	RDH2	D1330 – oral hygiene instruction D9210 – local anesthesia not in conjunction with operative or surgical procedures D4341 – periodontal scaling and root planing – four or more teeth per quadrant, Q2 & Q3 Reappointment: Reviewed personal, medical, dental, pharmacologic health history. Patient reported no changes. BP 128/86. Patient confirmed medications taken as prescribed by physician and had eaten a nutritious breakfast within 2 hours of appointment. ***Goal met for unmet need for biologically sound and functional dentition. Outcome documented to care plan (evaluation).*** Preprocedural rinse/Chlorhexidine. Patient reported daily brushing and flossing. Assessed tissue response Q1 & Q4 to debridement and patient's daily brushing/flossing. Gingiva are less edematous. Applied disclosing agent, decrease in plaque, localized plaque retentive sites maxillary molars. Shared progress with patient. Patient verbalized disappointment that plaque is present. Stated "working hard to remove plaque." Provided positive feedback to patient for commitment to oral self care and progress. Educated on use of power brush. Reviewed and reinforced flossing technique- adequate. Local anesthesia Q2 & Q3 (*type, agent, concentration, # of cartridges*). Ultrasonic and hand periodontal debridement Q2 & Q3. Postoperative instructions given to patient. Next appointment 5/23/2023 phase 1 reevaluation.
5/23/2023	RDH2	D0171 – reevaluation – post operative office visit D1330 – oral hygiene instruction D1110 – prophylaxis - adult D1206 – topical application of fluoride varnish Phase I response to nonsurgical periodontal therapy/Reevaluation: Reviewed personal, medical, dental, pharmacologic health history. Patient reported no changes. BP 126/88. Patient confirmed medications taken as prescribed by physician and has eaten a nutritious breakfast within 2 hours of appointment. Preprocedural rinse/Chlorhexidine. Completed and documented gingival reassessment, reprobing, CAL, PI, and BI. Measured goals planned to be evaluated at phase I reevaluation. ***Goals for unmet need for skin and mucous membrane integrity of the head and neck (goal met for reducing probing depths of 5mm and greater by 1mm, goal not met for reducing BI to less than 10%, goal partially met for elimination of gingival inflammation). Goals met for unmet need for responsibility for oral health. Outcomes documented to care plan (evaluation).*** Shared all findings and goal outcomes with patient. Reviewed and reinforced power brush and flossing techniques in maxillary molar regions. Debrided residual soft deposits maxillary molars, coronal polish with medium grit paste, applied 5% NaF varnish. Scheduled 3-month continued care visit for Phase IV maintenance 8/29/2023. Scheduled phase II evaluation with periodontist, 6/6/2023.

See Fig. 23.5 for documentation of goal outcomes and evaluative statements to dental hygiene care plan for Human Needs Conceptual Model.

Fig. 23.8, cont'd

PROCEDURE 23.4   Evaluation of Care

Steps

- Identify evaluative criteria and expected outcomes of care.
- Collect evidence to determine extent to which goals are being met.
- Interpret and summarize the findings.
- Write an evaluative statement.
- Propose continued-care options.
- Document the completion of this service to the patient's dental record by entering a customized electronic note of services rendered for outcome of care and recommendation for continued care; date and sign the entry.
- For the Human Needs Conceptual Model, may add a customized note; for example, "Reevaluation of phase I therapy. Goals partially met for unmet need for skin and mucous membrane integrity of the head and neck. Goals met for unmet need for responsibility for oral health."
- Add a supplemental clinical note that supports the aforementioned custom note; for example, "Clinical goals for reducing probing depths of 5 mm and greater by 1 mm are met; eliminating gingival inflammation is partially met; reducing BI to less than 10% is not met. Localized sites of inflammation and bleeding maxillary molars. Supporting patient-centered goals for brushing and flossing technique and frequency, reduction in PI to less than 10% are met. Reinforced importance of oral self-care. Scheduled patient with periodontist for Phase II evaluation. Continued-care interval 3 months."

KEY CONCEPTS

- Planning, evaluation, and documentation are critical dental hygiene foundational skills and integral to ADHA's Standards for Clinical Dental Hygiene Practice.

- The dental hygiene care plan is an evidence-based, patient-centered written proposal formulated to address patient needs and move a patient toward achieving desired oral health outcomes and wellness.

- The dental hygiene diagnosis provides the foundation for care plan development (e.g., establishing care plan goals or expected patient care outcomes, selecting interventions strategies).

- A well-formulated and executed care plan increases the likelihood of a positive patient care outcome.

- Evaluation is the measurement of the extent a patient has achieved the goals as defined in the dental hygiene care plan and of the ongoing processes that occur during implementation of care, at the completion of the care plan, and at the subsequent continued-care visits.

- The goals of documentation are to maintain continuity of care, provide a means of communication among the patient's healthcare team, and minimize risk of litigation by providing evidence of a patient-centered process of care.

REFERENCES

1. American Dental Hygienists' Association (ADHA). Standards for clinical dental hygiene practice, Revised 2016. *Access.* 2016;(suppl):1–15.
2. Bowen, Denise M. Interprofessional collaborative care by dental hygienists to foster medical-dental integration. *J Dent Hyg.* 2016;90(4):217–220.
3. Furgeson D, Inglehart MR, Habil P. Interprofessional education in dental hygiene programs and CODA standards: dental hygiene program directors' perspectives. *J Dent Hyg.* 2017;91(2):6–14.
4. Darby M, Walsh M. *Application of The Human Needs Conceptual Model to Dental Hygiene Practice.* Presented at the 14th International Symposium on Dental Hygiene, Florence, Italy. 1998.
5. Williams KB, Gadbury-Amyot CC, Bray KK, et al. Oral health-related quality of life: a model for dental hygiene. *J Dent Hyg.* 1998;72(2):19–26.
6. American Dental Association. *CDT 2022 Current Dental Terminology.* American Dental Association; 2022.
7. American Dental Association. *CDT 2022 Training Guide for the Dental Team.* American Dental Association; 2022.

24

Toothbrushing

Harold Henson

PROFESSIONAL OPPORTUNITIES

Daily removal of biofilm from the mouth is essential to the maintenance of oral health. A wide variety of manual and power toothbrushes is available, and patients may need guidance in selection of a toothbrush and brushing method most suited to their unique oral needs. Dental hygienists with current product knowledge and evidence-based decision making skills can assist patients in shared decision making, method instruction, reinforcement, and evaluation of effectiveness.

COMPETENCIES

1. Describe characteristics of acceptable manual toothbrush designs.
2. Describe characteristics and modes of action of power toothbrush designs.
3. Discuss toothbrushing instruction, including differentiation among toothbrushing methods including indications, limitations, and impact on oral tissues.
4. Discuss soft and hard tissue lesions, including factors associated with tissue lesions and the significance of a clean tongue and toothbrush.
5. Discuss the dental hygiene process of care and toothbrushing, including the sharing of evidence-based decision making with patients regarding selection and use of a toothbrush based on specific patient needs.

   Self-care or **homecare** refers to behaviors that individuals perform to achieve, maintain, or promote health or oral health. **Oral biofilm** or **plaque control** is the daily removal of bacteria, biofilm, and debris from the teeth, tongue, and adjacent oral tissues as part of an overall preventive program to prevent or control oral diseases. Although 100% removal is not possible, the normal host can tolerate some oral biofilm.

   Mechanical removal of oral biofilm via toothbrushing is the most common means for plaque control. Mechanical cleansing devices such as toothbrushes are indispensable because to date, no chemotherapeutic agents totally prevent the formation of oral biofilm in the mouth. Fair to poor oral hygiene increases the risk of periodontitis by two to five times.[1]

   The use of a dentifrice with toothbrushing does not provide an additional effect for plaque removal, but it does provide twice-daily fluoride application, clean mouth feel, and stain prevention.[2]

MANUAL TOOTHBRUSHES

The most commonly used device for removing oral biofilm, the **manual toothbrush,** is to remove plaque from the facial, lingual, and occlusal tooth surfaces (Box 24.1). Although many features of toothbrushes and toothbrushing methods have been studied, evidence has not demonstrated that any individual manual toothbrush design is consistently superior in removing plaque or preventing and controlling periodontal diseases.[3,4] The individual's motivation and skill are key factors in the effectiveness of toothbrushing.

Parts of the Toothbrush

Manual toothbrushes have several parts, as follows (Fig. 24.1):
- Head—Contains the filaments (bristles) and is approximately 1 to 1.25 inches (25.4 to 31.8 mm) long and 0.33 to 0.37 inches (7.9 to 9.5 mm) wide. Head size is selected based on the size of the patient's mouth rather than age. The head should be large enough to remove plaque efficiently and small enough to reach all areas of the mouth. Contemporary toothbrush head designs are less commonly rectangular and more tapered and oval shaped than earlier designs.
- Handle—Used for grasping the toothbrush by the hand during use; may be aligned in a straight plane, with the toothbrush head angled like a dental mirror, curved, or offset. Consumers may select their preferred handle shape for comfortable use.
- Shank—Connects the head of the toothbrush to the handle.

Toothbrush Filament Design

The toothbrush head contains tufts typically composed of nylon filaments. Tufts are individual bundles of filaments secured in a hole in the toothbrush head. Number and length of filaments in a tuft, number of tufts, and arrangement of tufts vary with toothbrush designs. Less commonly, in-mold tufting has filaments inserted individually into the head. The brushing plane (surface of the toothbrush head used for cleaning the teeth and tissues) may be flat, with all filaments the same length, bilevel, multilevel, rippled, or crisscrossed, with tufts angled in different directions (Fig. 24.2).

Filament design affects toothbrushing efficacy, particularly in difficult to access approximal areas. Angled rather than vertical bristle tuft arrangements have been shown to contribute significantly to more effective plaque removal because they reach farther interproximally.[5]

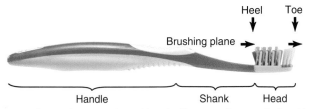

Heel Toe

Brushing plane

Handle   Shank   Head

Fig. 24.1 Parts of a manual toothbrush. (Courtesy Procter & Gamble, Professional and Scientific Relations, Cincinnati, Ohio.)

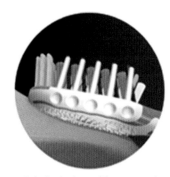

Fig. 24.2 Crisscross bristle design with tongue cleaner on back of the brush head of the Oral-B CrossAction Pro-Health toothbrush. (Courtesy Procter & Gamble, Professional and Scientific Relations, Cincinnati, Ohio.)

Toothbrushing alone does not clean the entire interproximal tooth surface, so interdental cleaning augments toothbrushing for thorough biofilm removal.

It is unclear whether end rounding of bristles has a significant benefit for patients' safety. Toothbrushes containing 40% to 100% end-rounded bristles provide a significant reduction in gingival abrasion compared to toothbrushes with non-end-rounded filaments.[6] Some toothbrushes that claim to have end rounding do not have uniformly rounded bristles. Among manufacturers, significant differences in bristle diameter and bristle shape exist.[7] Dental professionals often recommend toothbrushes with soft nylon filaments, believing that they are less traumatic to the oral tissues and remove as much or more plaque than hard toothbrushes; however, the influence of bristle stiffness on plaque removal and trauma remains unclear.[3] Nylon toothbrush filaments have a range of diameters from 0.15 to 0.4 mm. Stiffness is related primarily to the filament's diameter and length; shorter and wider diameters result in a harder toothbrush. Traditionally, most filaments have been 10 to 12 mm long. A new development in toothbrushes is tapered filaments, claiming better plaque removal and reduced gingival trauma. A systematic review concluded that there is no firm evidence to recommend a tapered filament toothbrush over an end-rounded toothbrush.[8] Many manufacturers vary the type, length, and diameter of the filaments within a single toothbrush head. A multilevel bristle tuft configuration can improve efficacy.[5]

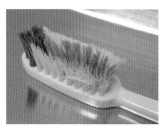

Fig. 24.3 Worn-out toothbrush.

Toothbrush Bristle Wear

Worn toothbrushes have bristles that are splaying, bending, curling, spreading, or matting (Fig. 24.3). Although it makes sense that a worn toothbrush would reduce toothbrush efficacy, evidence supporting this claim is inconclusive.[4] Filament wear varies considerably with different individuals over time; therefore rather than using the usual 2 to 3 months as an indicator for toothbrush replacement, patients must learn to identify visible signs of worn filaments.

POWER TOOTHBRUSHES

Rechargeable **power toothbrushes,** defined by their modes of action, typically are activated by electricity or a battery (Table 24.1). When used properly, power and manual toothbrushes are effective in removing plaque and preventing and controlling gingival disease. A Cochrane systematic review and meta-analysis compared power toothbrushes using several different modes of action with a traditional manual toothbrush (rectangular head with a flat brushing plane). Powered toothbrushes are more effective in plaque reduction (21%) and gingivitis reduction (11%). The weight of the evidence supports the rotation oscillation brushes, which show significant plaque and gingivitis reductions in short-term and long-term studies.[4,9] The Oral-B oscillating rotating power toothbrush has the ADA Seal of Acceptance, having met criteria for rigorous, reproducible data documenting safety and effectiveness. Battery-powered toothbrushes and less expensive rechargeable models increase accessibility of power toothbrushing.

Newer power toothbrushes are available featuring smart technology and associated apps with a variety of features such as smartphone connectivity, visual tracking and feedback, motion sensors, brush replacement reminders, pressure sensors, and coaching programs. These programs use performance feedback and motivation to improve oral hygiene.

Power toothbrushes are safe and effective; therefore a power toothbrush is suitable for almost anyone (Box 24.2). The latest evidence-based research demonstrates that patients' oral hygiene regimen can be individualized by selecting the appropriate power brush program mode.[10,11] Power toothbrushes have a high level of patient acceptance, and clients can be assured of their effectiveness and safety.[3,9,11–13]

TOOTHBRUSHING INSTRUCTION

Toothbrushes require client-specific instructions on thoroughness, duration, frequency, method, and force to achieve an effective technique and adherence. Additionally, when giving instruction, the dental hygienist considers client characteristics such as risk and susceptibility to disease, dexterity, personal values, and preferences. Communication should be appropriate to the patient's or caregiver's age, language, educational level, culture, learning style, and readiness to adopt new behaviors. See the client or patient education tips in Box 24.3, as well as the Critical Thinking Exercise box. Motivational interviewing techniques may improve patient acceptance and behavior change (see Chapter 5).

TABLE 24.1 Power Toothbrushes: General Modes of Action

Action	Description	Examples	Diagram
Oscillating-rotations with microvibrations	Brush head has been developed with a linear magnetic drive, resulting in oscillation-rotations with microvibrations	Oral-B iO**	
Oscillating-rotating	Entire brush head rotates in one direction and then the other; some models also pulsate in and out The Oral-B oscillating rotating power toothbrush has the ADA Seal of Acceptance, having met criteria for rigorous, reproducible data documenting safety and effectiveness.	Oral-B Genius, Pro, and Vitality Conair Opticlean	
Circular	Entire brush head rotates in one direction	Zila Rotadent Procare*	
Sonic	Bristles vibrate side to side or up and down with high amplitude and high frequency; sound waves cause fluid motion	Philips Sonicare[†] Waterpik Sensonic Colgate 360° Advanced Powered Quip Burst	
Ultrasonic	Bristles vibrate at ultrasonic frequencies (>20 kHz)	Emmi-dent Smilex	
Side-to-side	Brush head that moves laterally	Early power models and sonic	

*Rota-dent toothbrush head action. (From Barnes CM. Powered toothbrushes: a focus on the evidence. *Oral Hyg.* 2000;7:3.)
[†]Sonicare toothbrush head action. (From Barnes CM. Powered toothbrushes: a focus on the evidence. *Oral Hyg.* 2000;7:3.)
**Oral-B iO toothbrush head. (Courtesy of Procter and Gamble.)

BOX 24.2 Power Toothbrushes: Indications for Use

Any individual, but particularly those with the following:
- Fixed orthodontic appliances
- Decalcification
- Uncontrolled oral biofilm and periodontal diseases
- Extensive prosthodontics or dental implants
- Dexterity and motivational challenges
- Gingival recession or noncarious cervical hard-tissue lesions
- Caregiver responsibilities

BOX 24.3 Client or Patient Education Tips

- Communicate in a manner appropriate to the patient's or caregiver's age, language, culture, readiness, and learning style.
- Discuss toothbrush selection and toothbrushing methods in relation to the patient's specific needs and oral assessment findings.
- Incorporate interdental cleansing and, if needed, use of an antimicrobial toothpaste or mouthrinse along with toothbrushing.
- Explain the benefits of tongue brushing.
- Correlate toothbrushing effectiveness with presence of oral biofilm, calcified deposits, and gingival disease.
- Discuss gingival recession and noncarious cervical lesions and explain possible causes with patients who exhibit these conditions.
- Use shared decision making when educating patients, sometimes referred to as client cotherapy decisions, about toothbrushing; incorporate patient abilities, values, and preferences.

CRITICAL THINKING EXERCISE

Case Study: Mrs. Truman, a 65-year-old retired schoolteacher from a low-income, rural school district where she has resided for her entire life, is being treated by the dental hygienist. Assessment findings reveal that the patient has generalized heavy oral biofilm, gingival inflammation, and bleeding on probing. Early in the appointment, Mrs. Truman says, "Lately, my arthritis has been particularly bothersome in my hands, and I find it difficult to brush my teeth." Proceed with your counseling of Mrs. Truman regarding her home care. Consider her age, language, educational level, culture, and readiness to adopt new behaviors. What type of toothbrush and toothbrushing method should be recommended for Mrs. Truman and why?

Role-Play Exercise: Working in pairs, one student assumes the role of the dental hygienist and the other student acts as the patient. The dental hygienist interviews the patient about current homecare devices, behaviors, and techniques, and provides patient-specific education and feedback using a sound client-educational approach, possibly motivational interviewing techniques, and the principles of evidence-based decision making. Student pairs can use their dental models for demonstration purposes or, if in the clinical setting, demonstrate techniques intraorally. Students can then reverse roles for both to experience these roles.

BOX 24.4   Legal, Ethical, and Safety Issues

- It is the dental hygienist's ethical responsibility to use the highest level of professional knowledge, judgment, and ability to increase public awareness and understanding of high-quality oral health practices, an ethical principle known as beneficence.
- Beneficent dental hygiene care requires allocation of time for self-care instruction, repetition, reinforcement, and continual assessment of each patient's oral health practices.
- The ethical principle of autonomy requires dental hygienists to listen to and allow for the patient's participation in decision making and to respect the patient's right to make a decision.
- The legal standard of care requires that dental hygienists educate patients about oral self-care considering the patient's age, language, culture, and learning style.
- Care plans should include evaluation of the presence and distribution of oral biofilm and its retentive factors, and patient self-care.
- On completion of care, the dental hygienist documents in the patient's legal record that the patient has been counseled on why and how to perform an effective daily personal oral hygiene program and their level of progress. Confirmation of the patient's understanding also is documented.

Regardless of the toothbrushing method, dental hygienists advise the patient to clean the mouth and tongue thoroughly using a systematic approach. Patients also need to understand the link among oral biofilm, oral and systemic diseases, and the importance of controlling plaque and inflammation. Findings from gingival, periodontal, and dental assessments are reviewed with the patient and correlated with the presence of oral biofilm. Suggestions for improved technique in these areas help patients enhance effectiveness of biofilm removal. Quantitative plaque, gingivitis, and bleeding indices are used to improve patient understanding, monitor self-care, motivate positive behaviors, and measure outcomes of care.

Toothbrushing Duration and Frequency

Dental hygienists teach patients to brush thoroughly for an adequate length of time to remove biofilm efficiently and effectively. There are many possibilities for sequencing, but the individual should be encouraged to select a logical sequence and to use it consistently to avoid omission of any area. This concept is particularly important to instill early in children. Some dental professionals suggest starting toothbrushing on the lingual surfaces of teeth first because of the difficulty in cleaning these areas. Evidence to support superiority of this recommendation is very limited.[14]

Research findings suggest the importance of brushing time. The recommended duration often is a minimum of 2 minutes, and some models of power toothbrushes have 2-minute timers to encourage adherence. The average brushing time is 1 minute or less, but evidence indicates that as brushing times increase, efficacy also increases.[5] Different teaching strategies can be used to encourage longer toothbrushing, such as counting strokes before proceeding to the next area of the mouth or using a timer or a small hourglass.

There is no standard recommendation for how many times per day persons should brush. How often and how much plaque biofilm removal prevents development of dental disease is unknown; however, most people do not remove 100% of the plaque biofilm. Infrequent toothbrushing is associated with severe forms of periodontal disease.[15] From a practical viewpoint, patients are told to brush their teeth at least twice daily to remove plaque and to apply fluoride dentifrice to prevent caries. Following this advice also promotes a feeling of oral freshness.[5] Twice-daily brushing commonly is recommended

to control plaque biofilm that contributes to oral diseases and oral malodor (halitosis), the condition of having unpleasant breath. Brushing before bedtime and after a period of sleep is encouraged (i.e., in the morning and at night). However, decisions about when and how often to brush must be made through a shared decision-making process based on clinical findings and patient preferences. Patients appreciate this ethical approach to cotherapy, including individualized suggestions and autonomy in decision making rather than a standard presentation that may be perceived as a lecture or even an admonishment (Box 24.4).

Toothbrushing Force (Pressure)

Most literature on force applied during toothbrushing has been related to damaging soft tissue (gingival abrasion and recession) and hard tissue (dental abrasion); fewer researchers have examined the effect of force on plaque reduction. Earlier concerns about power toothbrushes applying excessive force and leading to tissue damage are unsubstantiated. Brushing with power toothbrushes applies less force than brushing with manual toothbrushes. Some power toothbrush designs are equipped with indicators or automatic shutoffs when excessive force is applied to the tooth surface, and some manual toothbrush designs incorporate a flexible shaft to contribute to improved safety. This technologic improvement is important because patients are unable to perceive accurately the pressure used. Some clinicians suggest that patients use a fingertip grasp instead of a palm grasp to reduce force during brushing. Evaluating if a patient is exerting excessive toothbrushing force is challenging because of the multifactorial etiology of soft and hard tissue lesions.[3] The dental hygienist makes patient recommendations based on specific patient assessment findings.

Toothbrushing Methods

Table 24.2 summarizes key toothbrushing techniques and indications for use. In general, the Bass and Stillman methods of toothbrushing concentrate on the cervical portion of the teeth and the adjacent gingival tissues. Modification to both methods to add a roll stroke (i.e., modified Bass and modified Stillman) by rolling the toothbrush bristles occlusally to clean the entire facial and lingual surfaces after cleaning the cervical area. The Bass method emphasizes sulcular cleaning, so it is the most commonly recommended toothbrushing method (Fig. 24.4).

More than 90% of people use their own "personal toothbrushing method," typically a scrub technique. Although this method removes oral biofilm from smooth tooth surfaces, it is less effective in other areas and may cause more injury to the soft and hard tissues. Research has not convincingly shown one method to be consistently superior.[3] Specific claims about particular methods producing better outcomes surrounding gingival stimulation, preventing recession, or sulcular cleansing have not been substantiated in the literature.

Selection of the toothbrushing method should depend on patient needs, dexterity, and preferences. Dental hygienists have to assess the

TABLE 24.2   Toothbrushing Methods and Indications for Use

Method	Technique	Indications	
Bass (sulcular)	Filaments are directed apically at a 45° angle to the long axis of the tooth; gentle force is applied to insert bristles into sulcus; use gentle but firm vibratory strokes without removing filament ends from sulcus.	Sulcular cleansing Periodontal health Periodontal disease Periodontal maintenance	
Stillman	Filaments are directed apically and angled similar to Bass method; filaments are placed partly on cervical portion of teeth and partly on adjacent gingiva; short back-and-forth vibratory strokes are employed, and the brush head is moved occlusally with light pressure.	Progressive gingival recession; gingival stimulation	
Charter	Filaments are directed toward the crown of the tooth; filaments are placed at the gingival margin and angled 45° to the long axis of the tooth; short back-and-forth vibratory strokes are used for activation (distinguished from the Bass and Stillman methods in that the bristles are directed away from the gingiva toward the occlusal or incisal edge).	Orthodontics Temporary cleaning of surgical sites Fixed prosthetic appliances	
Roll stroke	Filaments are directed apically and rolled occlusally in a vertical motion.	Used in conjunction with Bass, Stillman, and Charter methods	
Modified Bass, Stillman, and Charter methods	For these methods, add a roll stroke; roll tufts occlusally in a vertical motion after cervical area is cleaned by prescribed method.	Cleaning of entire facial and lingual surfaces	

TABLE 24.2   Toothbrushing Methods and Indications for Use—cont'd

Method	Technique	Indications	
Fones	Filaments are activated in a circular motion.	Young children with primary teeth; otherwise not recommended	
Horizontal Scrub technique	Bristles move back and forth in short horizontal strokes	Occlusal surfaces only; otherwise not recommended due to gingival abrasion	 Occlusal

patient's oral hygiene, level of health or disease, and current toothbrushing practices to make meaningful recommendations. No toothbrushing method can adequately clean interproximal surfaces, and the patient should be made aware that some means of interdental cleansing, and use of an antimicrobial mouthrinse as needed significantly improves oral biofilm and disease control.

For most manual toothbrushing techniques, a fingertip or palm grasp placed on the toothbrush facilitates use as follows:
- The brush head is moved from one group of teeth (two to three teeth) to the next by overlapping with the previously completed group.
- On facial and lingual surfaces of posterior teeth, the toothbrush head is positioned parallel to the arch.
- On anterior teeth, the toothbrush head is placed parallel to the arch when the labial surfaces are brushed; on lingual surfaces, the brush will likely have to be placed parallel with the long axis of the teeth (or vertically).
- On occlusal surfaces, the toothbrush head is pressed firmly into the surfaces so that the filament ends can reach into the pits and fissures as much as possible, and a back-and-forth brushing stroke is used. The brush is advanced section by section until all occlusal surfaces have been cleaned.

Toothbrushing techniques that require brush filament placement on an angle in relation to the teeth are more difficult for patients to achieve consistently. Effective toothbrushing is not easy for most patients, and this additional challenge can limit toothbrushing effectiveness and motivation. When modifying a patient's toothbrushing technique, clinicians must demonstrate the new technique on a mouth model and then in the patient's mouth. This initial demonstration does not replace the need to monitor the patient's actual performance of the new technique to provide feedback and ensure that

the skill is acquired, problems are identified, and errors are corrected over time.

Patients also require instruction with power toothbrushes. Although these instructions vary with manufacturer and design, in general, power toothbrushing is relatively straightforward because the mechanism of action removes the need for the patient to manipulate the toothbrush. Most designs recommend that the patient hold the brush head with a fingertip grasp in place for a few seconds on each tooth or small group of teeth before guiding the brush head slowly to the next tooth or group of teeth and allowing the brush to do the work. The filaments flare slightly while the brush is activated for cleansing the sulcus (Fig. 24.4). The patient must apply sufficient but not excessive pressure, focus on the gingival margin, and keep the toothbrush engaged for a sufficiently long time before moving to the next area.

An individual's dexterity and vision may deteriorate with time, necessitating ongoing assessment and modifications to suggested methods and toothbrush selection. Over time at maintenance appointments, the reinforcement of instruction, observation of patient's technique, and ongoing encouragement are effective means of achieving oral biofilm removal and adherence to professional recommendations.

SOFT AND HARD TISSUE LESIONS

As part of making toothbrushing recommendations, the dental hygienist assesses soft and hard tissues for damage from toothbrushing. Although patients may be removing oral biofilm adequately, they also may be causing trauma from the toothbrushing technique or toothbrush selection. Negative changes in tissues can be detected anywhere in the mouth, although they often are seen on the facial tooth surfaces at the gingival margin.

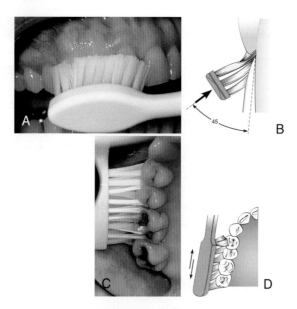

Fig. 24.4 The Bass toothbrushing method. (A) Proper intrasulcular position of brush in the mouth aims the filaments toward and into the gingival sulcus. (B) Diagram shows the ideal placement, with slight subgingival penetration of the filament tips. (C) Place toothbrush so that filaments are angled approximately 45° from the long axis of the tooth. (D) Start at the most distal tooth in the arch and use a vibrating, back-and-forth motion to brush. ([B and D] From Newman MG, Takei HH, Klokkevold PR, Carranza FA. *Carranza's Clinical Periodontology.* 12th ed. Saunders; 2015.)

Soft Tissue Lesions

Vigorous toothbrushing in combination with a hard or stiff toothbrush traditionally has been associated with gingival abrasions and recession. The cause of gingival trauma is multifactorial. The most common toothbrushing factors associated with gingival recession are toothbrushing frequency, use of a horizontal or scrub brushing method, bristle hardness, toothbrushing duration, and frequency of changing a toothbrush.[16] If observed, toothbrush trauma in the form of gingival abrasions can appear as redness, scuffing, or punctate lesions. Over time, if multifactorial influences continue, these early abrasions can lead to more permanent soft tissue lesions, including gingival recession, clefts, or festooning (Fig. 24.5). See the Critical Thinking Exercise box for an exercise related to education for a patient with gingival recession and observed toothbrushing techniques that might relate to this condition.

Although visible gingival abrasions are not a common clinical finding, gingival recession affects 80% to 100% of middle-aged and elderly Americans to some degree. Prevalence and severity of recession increases with age but is not a consequence of aging. Younger individuals also can have aggressive levels of recession. Recession is a concern for several reasons, including its association with increased risk of dentinal hypersensitivity, loss of tooth support, root caries, and aesthetic dissatisfaction.

The cause of gingival recession is multifactorial. Factors include the following:

- Toothbrushing factors (e.g., frequency, direction, force, bristle hardness, duration)
- Anatomic factors (e.g., tooth malposition)
- Pathologic factors (e.g., clinical attachment loss from periodontal disease)

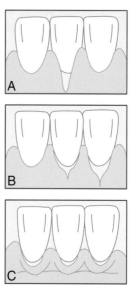

Fig. 24.5 (A) Gingival recession. (B) Gingival clefting. (C) Gingival festooning.

Hard Tissue Lesions

Hard tissue lesions have been attributed to toothbrushing. Tooth **abrasion** is the wearing away of the tooth surface typically located around the cementoenamel junction (CEJ) (see Fig. 24.6). Clinically, tooth abrasions appear as cervical notches surrounding the CEJ, increasing dentinal hypersensitivity and unpleasant aesthetics, and possibly requiring restorations. Cervical defect shapes associated with toothbrushing include V-wedged (most common), U-rounded, and combinations; these defects change shape over time.

Tooth abrasions are distinct from dental **abfractions**, similarly shaped noncarious cervical lesions caused by excessive occlusal loading as teeth flex under pressure, resulting in subsequent loss of hard tooth structure at the CEJ. Difficulty in determining actual causes of tooth abrasions and abfractions has led to use of the term **noncarious**

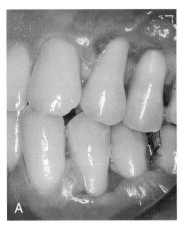
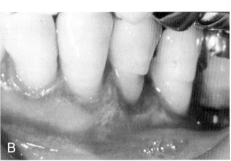

Fig. 24.6 (A) Trauma from vigorous toothbrushing with an abrasive dentifrice. Note trauma to gingival and root surface abrasion and gingival recession. (B) Tooth abrasion attributed to long-term aggressive toothbrushing. (From Newman MG, Takei HH, Klokkevold PR, Carranza FA, eds. *Carranza's Clinical Periodontology.* 12th ed. Saunders; 2015.)

cervical lesion (NCCL), reflecting the multifactorial etiology of the condition. The primary toothbrushing factors associated with NCCL are toothbrushing method and frequency.[13] Despite studies showing an association between hard tissue wear and greater brushing frequency and the use of scrubbing techniques, toothbrushing has only minor influence on cervical wear. In fact, toothpaste is essential to create significant abrasion. Brushing force, bristle stiffness, and duration are other possible contributing factors.

Some patients have NCCLs from demineralization as a result of chemical erosion. There may be a synergistic effect between toothbrushing and previously eroded hard tissue, resulting in more clinically significant lesions than are seen in the absence of dental erosion.

Tongue Cleansing

The dorsum of the tongue is a bacterial habitat. Tongue cleaning reduces the number of organisms, thereby controlling oral malodor, decreasing the opportunity for microorganisms to translocate, improving the patient's taste perception, and contributing to overall oral cleanliness.

Although tongue scrapers and cleansers are available on the market, a typical manual toothbrush or a power toothbrush with a special head can achieve tongue cleansing. Some individuals prefer a tongue cleaning device to reduce the risk of stimulating the gag reflex (see Fig. 24.2).

When using a toothbrush for tongue cleansing, the patient does the following:
- Extends the tongue and, with the toothbrush head placed on the tongue and the bristles angled slightly posteriorly, draws the bristles forward with light pressure
- Repeats brushing motion until the tongue is free of coating

Dental hygienists should advise patients not to scrub the tongue with the toothbrush or a tongue cleaner because tissue trauma could result. Use of an antibacterial mouthrinse after mechanical tongue cleaning further improves tongue hygiene.

Toothbrush Contamination

Toothbrushes can be a mode of indirect transmission for pathogenic organisms. The toothbrush can act as a fomite, an inanimate object that houses and transmits potentially infectious agents. A systematic review of studies related to toothbrush contamination found that toothbrushes of healthy and orally diseased adults become contaminated with potentially pathogenic bacteria from dental plaque, design, environment, or a combination of factors.[17] The important point to consider in relation to patient care is how to reduce toothbrush contamination.

Solid toothbrush designs are less conducive to sustaining colonization of microorganisms than hollow designs. Toothbrush caps and holders or plastic coverings further encourage microbial growth, so air drying is preferred.

Some interventions, such as 0.12% chlorhexidine gluconate, essential oil mouthrinses, 2% sodium hypochlorite, 50% white vinegar, ultraviolet sanitizers, and dishwashers, reduce toothbrush contamination. No studies have confirmed that toothbrush contamination results in disease transmission. Studies are needed to examine specifically contamination in relation to disease transmission in vulnerable populations (e.g., critically ill adults, immunocompromised individuals). It is important that the toothbrush be rinsed and air dried after each use.

THE DENTAL HYGIENE PROCESS OF CARE AND TOOTHBRUSHING

Because oral hygiene instruction is part of the implementation phase of care, the dental hygienist completes the patient's assessment, including current self-care behaviors, type of toothbrush used, frequency and duration of toothbrushing, toothbrush replacement practices, level of satisfaction with tools and technique, and personal values and preferences. As part of oral hygiene instruction, the patient should be asked to demonstrate the toothbrushing method used so that the dental hygienist can observe the patient's technique, skill, and dexterity.

The dental hygienist links information about the patient's self-care with clinical and radiographic observations and identifies the patient's unmet human need deficits related to oral health (dental hygiene diagnoses), along with the corresponding causes, signs, and symptoms. Through this process, the dental hygienist and patient, in shared decision making, formulate a plan of care that includes self-care recommendations (Table 24.3; see Chapter 23). Oral biofilm may be present because the patient has not been able to brush for several hours; conversely, absence of biofilm may be the result of thorough brushing immediately before the appointment rather than an indication of adequate daily plaque removal. Assessment of the soft and hard tissues for signs of oral disease provides the most valid information about the adequacy of self-care.

At times, patients avoid toothbrushing because of discomfort, but avoidance results in oral biofilm maturation. Examples of these patients include those with necrotizing ulcerative gingivitis, acute soft tissue injuries, healing surgical sites, or new dental appliances. In these

TABLE 24.3 Shared Decision-Making Model

Knowledge transfer	Direction: Two-way
	Dental hygienist to patient: Technical knowledge
	Patient to dental hygienist: Patient preferences, beliefs, values, and current practices
Deliberation and decision making	Direction: Bilateral
	Between dental hygienist and patient
	Possibly may include other healthcare providers, caregivers, and family members

situations, special toothbrushing instructions and mouth rinsing with alcohol-free 0.12% chlorhexidine gluconate are indicated.

Patients need positive reinforcement of their attempts to incorporate positive oral health behaviors throughout the process of care. Regardless of the patient's situation, instruction, practice, and reinforcement are indicated at all appointments subsequent to the planning phase. Dental hygienists spend the least amount of educational time with patients for whom they hold the lowest expectations—that is, patients with the highest plaque levels. Dental hygienists should be aware of their personal biases and be accepting of all patients' personal abilities and values.[3]

KEY CONCEPTS

- The manual toothbrush is the most commonly used device for removing oral biofilm from the facial, lingual, and occlusal surfaces.
- A toothbrush that has a small enough head to adapt to all areas of the mouth with a comfortable handle designed to secure a good grasp is desirable.
- Damage to soft and hard oral tissues has a multifactorial etiology; although toothbrush selection and toothbrushing variables contribute to negative effects, dentifrice use and other factors are likely to be more influential.
- Manual toothbrushes and power toothbrushes have greater benefit when dental professionals provide advice and instruction for using these devices.
- Toothbrush replacement should be based on individual wear rather than on time of use.
- Power toothbrushes are more effective than manual toothbrushes; oscillating-rotating power toothbrush designs have been shown to be more effective than traditional manual toothbrushes in reducing plaque and gingivitis.
- Comprehensive toothbrush instruction includes toothbrush selection and replacement, toothbrushing method, evaluation of toothbrushing effectiveness, and tongue brushing.
- Evaluation of toothbrushing effectiveness includes observation of the patient's toothbrushing, disclosing agent use to visualize and quantify plaque, and gingival evaluation for signs of inflammation; corrective measures are undertaken as needed.
- Interdental cleaning, tongue brushing, and, if needed, use of an antimicrobial agent should be planned along with toothbrushing instructions.
- Dental hygienists must be aware of emerging research on toothbrushing and be able to interpret study results critically.

ACKNOWLEDGMENT

The author acknowledges Joanna Asadoorian, Teresa B. Duncan, and Denise M. Bowen for their past contributions to this chapter.

REFERENCES

1. Lertpimonchai A, Rattanasiri S, Vallibhakara SA, et al. The association between oral hygiene and periodontitis: a systematic review and meta-analysis. *Intl Dent J.* 2017. https://doi.org/10.1111/idj.12317.
2. Valkenberg C, Slot DE, Bakker EWP, et al. Does dentifrice use help to remove plaque? A systematic review. *J Clin Periodontol.* 2016;43:1050–1058.
3. Asadoorian J. CDHA position paper on toothbrushing. *Can J Dent Hygiene.* 2006;40:232.
4. Van der Weijden F, Slot D. Efficacy of homecare regimens for mechanical plaque removal in managing gingivitis a meta review. *J Clin Periodontol.* 2015;42(suppl 16):S77–S91.
5. Slot DE, Wiggelinkhuizen L, Rosema NAM, et al. The efficacy of manual toothbrushes following a brushing exercise: a systematic review. *Int J Dent Hygiene.* 2012;10:187.
6. Hennequin-Hoenderdos NL, Slot DE, Van der Sluijs E, et al. The effects of different levels of brush end rounding on gingival abrasion: a double-blind randomized clinical trial. *Int J Dent Hygiene.* 2017;15(4):335–344.
7. Voelker MA, Bayne SC, Ying L, et al. Catalogue of toothbrush head designs. *J Dent Hygiene.* 2013;87(3):118–133.
8. Hoogteijling FCR, Hennequin-Hoenderdos NL, Van der Weijden GA, et al. The effect of tapered toothbrush filaments compared to end-rounded filaments on dental plaque, gingivitis and gingival abrasion: a systematic review and meta-analysis. *Int J Dent Hygiene.* 2018;16(1):3–12.
9. Yaacob M, Worthington HV, Deacon SA, et al. Manual versus powered toothbrushing for oral health. *Cochrane Database Syst Rev.* 2014;6:CD002281.
10. Deacon SA, Glenny AM, Deery C, et al. Different powered toothbrushes for plaque control and gingival health. *Cochrane Database Syst Rev.* 2010;(2):CD004971.
11. Van der Sluijs E, Slot DE, Hennequin-Hoenderdos NL, et al. A specific brushing sequence and plaque removal efficacy: a randomized split mouth design. *Int J Dent Hygiene.* 2016;19:1–7.
12. Zimmermann H, Zimmermann N, Hagenfeld D, et al. Is frequency of toothbrushing a risk factor for periodontitis? A systematic review and meta-analysis. *Community Dent Oral Epidemiol.* 2015;43(2):116–127.
13. Heasmann PA, Holiday R, Bryant A, et al. Evidence for the occurrence of gingival recession and non-carious cervical lesions as a consequence of traumatic toothbrushing. *J Clin Periodontol.* 2015;42(suppl 16):237–255.
14. Frazelle MR, Munroe CL. Toothbrush contamination: a review of the literature. *Nurs Res Prac.* 2012;2012:420630. https://doi.org/10.1155/2012/420630.
15. Adam R, Ram Goyal C, Qaqish J, Grender J. Evaluation of an oscillating-rotating toothbrush with micro-vibrations versus a sonic toothbrush for the reduction of plaque and gingivitis: results from a randomized controlled trial. *Int Dent J.* 2020;70(suppl 1):S16–S21. https://doi.org/10.1111/idj.12569. PMID: 32243576.
16. Thomassen TM, Van der Weijden FG, Slot DE. The efficacy of powered toothbrushes: a systematic review and network meta-analysis. *Int J Dent Hyg.* 2022;20(1):3–17. https://doi.org/10.1111/idh.12563.
17. Wingrove S. Why personalized oral hygiene technology matters. *Compend Contin Educ Dent.* 2022;43(3):f1–4.

25

Interdental and Supplemental Oral Self-Care Devices

Beth Jordan

PROFESSIONAL DEVELOPMENT OPPORTUNITIES

Many people do not floss or use any mechanism for daily removal of bacterial biofilm between their teeth, and they think flossing is the only option. Dental hygienists have the opportunity to help their patients select a preferred and effective method to accomplish this goal. Interdental bacterial biofilm prevention and control is essential to good oral health, especially gingival health.

COMPETENCIES

1. Relate the removal and control of interdental bacterial biofilm to current evidence regarding the prevention of oral disease.
2. Select effective self-care devices including interdental and supplemental self-care devices for each patient based on efficacy, individual client needs, and preferences. Also, discuss oral piercings and their impact on dental procedures, as well as the risks involved.
3. Educate patients as cotherapists in the safe and effective use of self-care devices designed for interdental and subgingival biofilm removal, considering oral conditions, patient preferences, risk factors present, and current evidence.

▶ EVOLVE VIDEO RESOURCE

The following video procedure and technique demonstrations are available for viewing on Evolve (http://evolve.elsevier.com/Pieren/hygiene/):
- Loop Flossing Method
- Spool Flossing Method for Adults
- Using a Floss Holder
- Using a Floss Threader
- Using an Interdental Brush
- Using a Rubber Tip Stimulator
- Using a Tongue Cleaner
- Using a Toothpick in a Toothpick Holder
- Using a Wooden Wedge

Mechanical biofilm control is foundational to preservation of oral health. Toothbrushing methods, power or manual, are best suited for the buccal/facial, lingual, and occlusal surfaces; however, toothbrushes are unable to reach the interdental area to remove food debris and biofilm. The interdental proximal embrasure space of adjacent teeth and the tongue can harbor a host of microbes that can contribute to poor oral health. This is true because of the small spaces between the teeth in normal anatomy, the anatomy of the tooth on the proximal surface, the col area, and the fact that this area is protected by the gingival papilla. The interdental area favors growth and accumulation of mature bacterial biofilm that favors periodontal inflammation. It is especially susceptible; thus the interdental papilla often is first to show signs of host response to inadequate cleaning. The gingival tissues respond within

2 to 4 days to a beginning accumulation of microbial plaque with a classic acute exudative vasculitis.

Removal of plaque biofilm from the spaces where toothbrushing does not reach is important for the following reasons:
1. To prevent periodontal disease—gingivitis commonly begin in the interdental col area, a depressed concave area of nonkeratinized gingival tissue under the contact area of two teeth. The col area connects the lingual and buccal papillae and because of its saddle-like shape it harbors plaque biofilm (Fig. 25.1). The epithelial tissue covering the col area is thin and less resistant to infection. When inflammation is present in this area, the papilla may become red, swollen, or enlarged. Probing depths can become deeper because of the larger interdental papilla and eventually because of connective tissue attachment loss (see Chapter 20).
2. To prevent halitosis—this problem may be caused by interdental and subgingival plaque biofilm as well as microbes on the dorsum of the tongue.

There are numerous devices that are created to help patients' self-care needs. The plethora of products also makes it difficult for patients to decide which device is the appropriate for them. Making individualized recommendations to patients about appropriate selection and use of self-care devices can be challenging. Evidence-based decision making also is challenging because many recommendations that may yield a favorable outcome for the patient are not supported by scientific evidence, simply because of a lack of high-quality evidence at this time.[1] Dental hygienists have an ethical and legal responsibility to use the best evidence in clinical practice and to educate each patient about elements of an individualized oral self-care plan (Box 25.1).

Patients will, therefore, depend on the dental hygienist to help them navigate the "oral care aisle." In many cases, more than one device can provide the desired outcome for a patient. Patient preference and likelihood to use the device then becomes a focal point of discussion. Therefore dental hygienists must remain current and familiar with the different devices, how to use the device, the evidence specific to each device, and the expected results from using the device. This knowledge fosters a conversation between the dental hygienist and patient that leads to a recommendation that produces the favorable outcomes valued by the patient.

SELECTING SELF-CARE DEVICES

Interdental

Historically, self-care recommendations have emphasized flossing to clean the interdental area. Dental floss is designed to clean the interdental surfaces of the teeth. A recent Cochrane review found that flossing plus toothbrushing showed a statistically significant benefit compared to toothbrushing alone for reduction in gingivitis; however, the quality of evidence was rated as low. This finding does not preclude the use of dental floss or tape, especially in a healthy mouth where the interdental

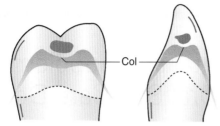

Fig. 25.1 Location of the col, the nonkeratinized epithelial depression connecting the buccal and lingual papillae of teeth, apical to the contact area *(in gray)*. (From Perry DA, Beemsterboer PL. *Periodontology for the Dental Hygienist.* 4th ed. Saunders; 2014.)

BOX 25.1   Legal, Ethical, and Safety Issues

- The legal standard of care requires that dental hygienists educate patients about oral self-care.
- The legal records of the patient should reveal that the patient has been counseled on why and how to perform an effective daily personal self-care program. Specific recommendations of products are noted in the legal records.
- The patient's progress and adherence with recommendations are recorded in the dental record. Alternative methods are recommended and demonstrated if prior instructions are not producing the expected outcomes, or if the patient is not able or willing to use a recommended device.
- Malpractice cases for failure to recognize and treat periodontal disease can be related to failure to inform patients of oral and periodontal conditions, teach adequate plaque biofilm techniques to patients, and provide adequate care and followup. Improper use of devices can cause damage to the hard and soft tissue in the oral cavity. Properly educating and demonstrating the recommended devices to the patient are required and noted in the legal records.
- Autonomy is an ethical principle that applies to self-care instruction; patients always should be given choices regarding self-care devices and provided with evidence-based information to make an informed decision.

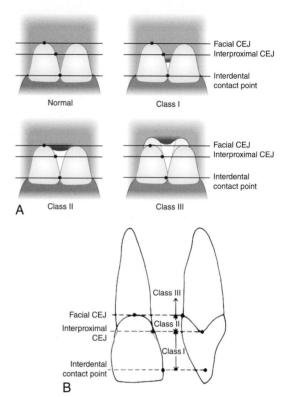

Fig. 25.2 (A) Classification system for papillary height/embrasures. (Redrawn from Robo I, Bitraj E, Mavriqi L. (2017). Gingivo-periodontal Pocket Caused by the Fault Contact Point. *J Dent Sci Ther*, 1(3):12–16. https://doi.org/10.24218/jdst.2017.14). (B) Interproximal view depicting Classification of papillary height/embrasures. (From Nordland, W.P., & Tarnow, D.P. (1998). A classification system for loss of papillary height. *Journal of Periodontology*, 69 10, 1124-6.)

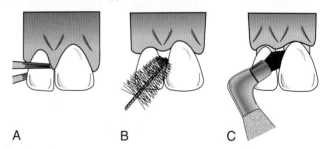

Fig. 25.3 Methods of Cleaning based on embrasure type. (A) Dental floss. (B) Interdental brush. (C) End-tuft brush.

---

gingiva fills the embrasure spaces with shallow sulcus depths, provided the patient has the dexterity and the inclination to use them. However, floss should not be the first or only tool the hygienist uses to prevent and reverse inflammation, as there are other tools and strategies to be employed which bear a stronger body of evidence.

A wide variety of interdental and supplemental plaque control aids is available. Several clinical trials and metaanalyses have shown that alternatives to manual floss such as interdental brushes, floss holders, and power flossers are as effective as or more effective than dental floss at reducing plaque biofilm, bleeding, gingivitis, and/or pocket depths.[2–4] Evidence also indicates that a dental water jet can be as effective or more effective when compared with manual floss for the reduction of interdental plaque biofilm, bleeding, and gingivitis.[5,6] No evidence exists to support interdental biofilm removal in the reduction of dental caries in adults and limited evidence supports potential effectiveness in primary teeth.[7–9]

Expert opinion is that for patients with periodontal disease, the typical recommendation for 2 minutes of brushing is insufficient, especially when adding the interdental cleaning devices to the regimen. In patients with gingivitis, once-daily interdental cleaning is recommended, as well as the use of antimicrobial plaque control agents, which can offer additional advantages (Chapter 27).[10] Dental implants require additional diligence in the matter of plaque control and prevention. Current clinical practice guidelines indicate weak evidence with respect to optimal manual or powered self-care methods around implants; however, supplemental use of antimicrobial agents in dentifrices and mouthrinses is supported.[11]

The tools and parameters used to assess the clinical effectiveness and outcomes of plaque biofilm removal are disclosing solution to better visualize dental deposits and the presence of plaque biofilm, and periodontal assessment for gingival bleeding, probing depths, and attachment levels, as well as other periodontal indices.

When the interdental gingiva is reduced or missing and the embrasures are open (type II and type III) (see Fig. 25.2 for Classification of Embrasures), other methods of interdental cleaning are needed (see Fig. 25.3 for Methods of Cleaning based on Embrasure Type). The dental hygienist evaluates the information gained during the assessment phase of care to select the most appropriate interdental and supplemental aids for the patient. To accomplish this, it is important to keep in mind the following clinical conditions and risk factors:

- Contour and consistency of the gingival tissues
- Probing depths
- Gingival attachment levels
- Size of the interproximal embrasures

- Tooth position and alignment
- Condition and types of restorative work present
- Susceptibility of the patient to disease (risk assessment)
- Level of dexterity and ability to use a device
- Patient motivation
- Cost, safety, and effectiveness of the recommended device
- Patient preference

Once an assessment is made, the dental hygienist reviews the care plan and goals with the patient as a cotherapist to determine which self-care device is most effective. Client education is a key responsibility of the dental hygienist (Box 25.2).

The simplest, least time-consuming procedures that have the potential to effectively control bacterial plaque biofilm and maintain oral health are recommended. If the current self-care regimen is effective in maintaining optimal oral health, the dental hygienist reinforces current practices, documents the products used and frequency of use in the permanent record, and does not introduce anything new to the daily routine. Also, if one device works, the dental hygienist would choose it over two devices that would accomplish the same goal. Studies demonstrate that patient acceptance and effectiveness of self-care recommendations improve when the number of devices is limited.

If a self-care regimen is not effective, the dental hygienist asks the patient why they think the recommendations are not working for them. If the problem is difficulty using the device, the dental hygienist can observe its use and modify, it or select another device that may be easier for that patient to use. If remembering to build the new self-care device into the daily schedule is the problem, the hygienist can recommend strategies for developing a new habit such as linking it with something the patient already does every day. If the patient simply does not want to use the device, other options for interdental cleansing are explored.

The dental hygienist reviews assessment data, including risk factors, and presents new recommendations to the patient. This section contains a summary of a variety of manual or nonpowered interdental and supplemental self-care devices. These devices can help reach areas that the toothbrush is not designed to access, or meet special patient needs based on assessment. They include the following:

- Dental floss and tape
- Floss holders and threaders
- Toothpicks and wooden wedges
- Rubber tip stimulators
- Interdental brushes and tips
- End-tuft, single-tuft brushes
- Tongue cleaners

Benefits of Flossing

The benefit of daily interdental cleaning such as flossing is the reduction or prevention of inflammation caused by the immune response to the toxins produced by interdental plaque biofilm. Comprehensive systematic reviews indicate there is some evidence to support that flossing in addition to toothbrushing reduces gingivitis in comparison with toothbrushing alone; however, the evidence is limited.[8,10] This finding is difficult to understand based on the strong empirical evidence documenting the relationship between plaque biofilm and gingivitis. Perhaps the additional effect of flossing beyond toothbrushing is related to subgingival plaque in the col area, which is not visible for scoring by dental indices used to measure plaque biofilm.[3] Flossing is a difficult skill for most patients to master, and many patients simply do not want to floss. In addition, flossing is recommended for patients with healthy gingiva and normal gingival contour as other devices are more effective in the presence of larger embrasure spaces and periodontal disease. As a result, benefits of floss over toothbrushing alone are not always supported by the evidence.[4] There also is no evidence that flossing reduces the incidence of interproximal caries.[8,9] Fluoride therapy has more impact on interproximal caries, and studies combining the two interventions show no additional benefit from flossing.[8] For more details on caries risk and prevention, see Chapter 19.

Dental Floss and Tape

If dental floss is recommended, the choice of which floss is influenced by the following:

- The tightness of the contact area
- The contour of the gingival tissue
- The roughness of the interproximal surface (e.g., margins of restorations)
- The user's manual dexterity and preference

Today **dental floss** is made of synthetic material monofilaments (e.g., ePTFE or Pebax) (Fig. 25.4) or multifilaments (e.g., nylon) (Fig. 25.5). The benefit of a coated monofilament type of floss is that it slides easily between the teeth and does not fray. The multifilament type allows for separation of the fibers and may fray. This type of floss is available in

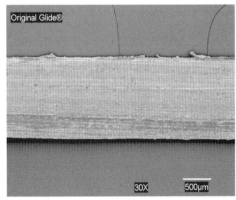

Fig. 25.4 Monofilament floss. (Courtesy of P&G.)

varying widths and may be braided or tufted, waxed or unwaxed. Studies have shown no difference in the effectiveness of unwaxed versus waxed dental floss. Recommendations are based on an individual's ease of use or preference. Waxed floss or monofilament floss may be easier to use for those who have tight contacts. Some flosses are impregnated with flavoring, fluoride, or antimicrobial or whitening agents, though the focus of the floss should remain on its ability to clean.

Dental tape or ribbon is wider and flatter than conventional dental floss. The flat-sided surface of dental tape is preferred by some, particularly when the surface area to be flossed is large (Fig. 25.6).

Tufted dental floss, or variable-diameter dental floss, has been found to be equally as effective as waxed or unwaxed dental floss for removing plaque biofilm. Tufted dental floss is designed to have three continuous segments: a length of waxed or unwaxed dental floss; a shorter segment of cylindric, nylon meshwork; and a relatively rigid nylon needle capable of being threaded beneath the contact or under fixed bridges, or orthodontic wires (Fig. 25.7). The dental floss segment is used in areas of normal gingival contour, and the other segments are used as indicated for site-specific areas (i.e., for crown and bridge abutments and pontics).

Braided or woven floss has more surface area than traditional dental floss for collecting plaque and removing it from teeth. It is intended for cleaning larger embrasures or fixed prosthetics and is sold on a spool or as a precut piece with a stiff nylon end for threading. The intention of woven floss is that when you pull the floss tight, its width decreases to fit through tight contact; then, as you move it between your teeth, if you loosen your grip, it expands and the woven nature of the material traps more plaque. Some floss has a mesh or gauze appearance.

Flossing Methods

The two primary methods of dental flossing are the spool method and the loop method (Procedures 25.1 and 25.2). The spool method starts with all of the floss spooled on one finger of one hand. Then, as each new section is used, the used section is taken up and spooled on the other hand. The loop method ties the two ends of the floss together in a circle to move to a new section. Both methods are designed to avoid using the same section of floss to clean each successive interdental area. Procedure 25.1 reviews the spool method of flossing, a method used by many teens and adults. The spool method of flossing requires manual dexterity. Children may prefer to use the loop method of flossing as described in Procedure 25.2.

It is important to demonstrate wrapping the floss around each tooth to create a "C" shape around the tooth in front of (mesial to) the interdental area being worked and behind (distal to) the interdental area. This allows the floss to cover the most surface area possible.

Proper flossing technique is not easy to master, and detailed instructions must be given and demonstrated. If the patient does not have the ability to master the technique or does not like or want to floss, other devices should be recommended.

Floss Holders and Threaders

Patients who have difficulty mastering string floss techniques for interdental cleaning may find it easier to use a floss holder (Figs. 25.8 and 25.9). **Floss holders** are plastic handles that aid in holding the floss strand. The method of use for floss holders is outlined in Procedure 25.3. If the floss holder is prestrung with floss, it is likely that it is not long enough to form the recommended "C" shape. However, studies have found that use of floss with proper use of a floss holder reduced gingivitis as effectively as use of string floss. In addition, those who used the floss holder preferred using it to traditional flossing techniques for ease of technique.

Another device designed to assist with cleaning under fixed prosthetics or orthodontic bridges and around abutments is the floss threader (Figs. 25.10 and 25.11). A floss threader can either consist of a stiff end of the floss that can be threaded or a separate device to use similar to a sewing needle and thread. A **floss threader** assists in introducing floss between an abutment tooth

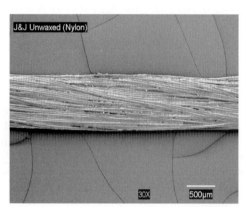

Fig. 25.5 Multifilament floss. (Courtesy of P&G.)

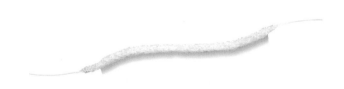

Fig. 25.7 Tufted Floss.

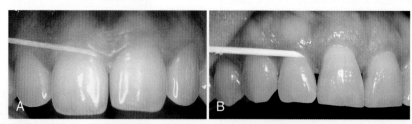

Fig. 25.6 (A) Dental floss. (B) Dental tape. ([A] From Perry DA, Beemsterboer PL. *Periodontology for the Dental Hygienist.* 4th ed. Saunders; 2014. [B] From Newman MG, Takei HH, Klokkevold PR, Carranza FA. *Carranza's Clinical Periodontology.* 11th ed. Saunders; 2012.)

PROCEDURE 25.1 Spool Flossing Method: Adults

Steps

1. Break off a piece of floss 12 to 18 inches long from the spool.
2. Wrap floss around middle fingers; wrap floss around right middle finger two to three times; wrap remaining floss around left middle finger (or vice versa) (part A).
3. For maxillary insertion, grasp floss firmly with thumb and index finger of each hand, using an inch of floss between fingertips (part B). For mandibular insertion, direct the floss down with the index fingers (part C).
4. Use a gentle seesaw motion to pass through the contact area.
5. Wrap tightly in a C shape around the tooth (see Fig. 25.6).
6. Move floss up and down on mesial of tooth three to four strokes, then move above papilla (just below contact); wrap in a C shape on distal surface of adjacent tooth, moving floss up and down three to four strokes.
7. Use a seesaw motion to remove floss through contact.
8. Advance floss to a new area by unwrapping it from the left-hand middle finger and wrapping it onto the right-hand middle finger (or vice versa; see step 2).
9. Repeat steps 3-8 until both interproximal sides of all teeth have been completed.

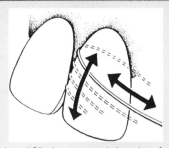

Wrap the floss in a "C" shape around dental surface while pulling side to side and moving up and down. (From Hoag PM, Pawlak EA. *Essentials of Periodontics*. 4th ed. Mosby; 1990.) (See Fig. u25.2.)

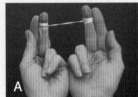 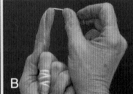 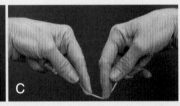

Spooling floss methods (see Fig. u25.1).

PROCEDURE 25.2 Loop Flossing Method: Children

Steps

1. Break off a piece of floss 8 to 10 inches long from the spool.
2. Tie the two ends together in a knot.
3. Follow steps 3-8 until both interproximal sides of all teeth are complete (see Procedure 25.1).
4. Repeat until all teeth have been completed.

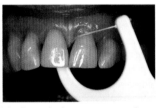

Fig. 25.9 Disposable floss devices are convenient for some patients and may enhance plaque biofilm control.

PROCEDURE 25.3 Use of a Floss Holder

Steps

1. Tightly string floss on holder following the manufacturer's recommendations, or use a prestrung device (see Fig. 25.8).
2. Follow steps 3-8 until both interproximal sides of all teeth are complete (see Procedure 25.1).
3. To move to a new area of floss (Follow steps 3-8 until both interproximal sides of all teeth are complete), the holder must be unwrapped, the floss advanced, and the holder rewrapped.
4. Continue until all teeth are completed.

Fig. 25.8 Variety of floss-holding devices.

used for support of a fixed bridge and a pontic, the artificial tooth that replaces a missing natural tooth. Procedure 25.4 reviews the use of a floss threader.

Dental Water Jets

In studies of patients with fixed orthodontics, implants, crowns and bridges, and gingivitis, and those in a periodontal maintenance

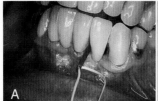
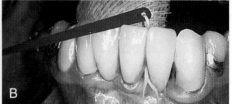

Fig. 25.10 (A) Facial insertion of the threader tip. (B) Threader pulled lingually through the interproximal space.

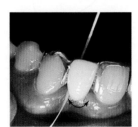

Fig. 25.11 Pulling floss underneath pontic.

PROCEDURE 25.4   Use of a Floss Threader

Steps
1. Break off a piece of floss 4 to 6 inches long from the spool.
2. Thread floss through eye of floss threader, overlapping floss 1 to 2 inches.
3. Grasp threader with thumb and index finger of one hand.
4. Insert tip of threader from the facial surface through an open interproximal area or area between a pontic and an abutment tooth (Fig. 25.10A).
5. Pull floss threader toward the lingual side until threader has passed completely through the interproximal space or under a pontic (only floss is now in the space) (Fig. 25.10B).
6. Slide the floss threader off the floss and remove from mouth.
7. Move floss back and forth several times under the pontic. See steps 8 and 9 of the spool flossing - Procedure 25.1 (Fig. 25.11).
8. Remove floss by letting go with the hand that is on the lingual side and pulling floss toward the buccal side.

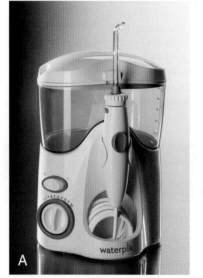
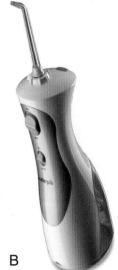

Fig. 25.12 Dental irrigator or water jet, commonly called water flosser. (A) Countertop dental water jet. (B) Cordless dental water jet. (Courtesy Water Pik, Inc, Fort Collins, Colorado.)

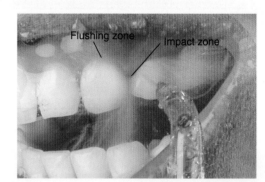

Fig. 25.13 Proper placement of a standard jet tip. (From Daniel SJ, Harfst SA, Wilder RS. *Mosby's Dental Hygiene.* 2nd ed. Mosby; 2008.)

---

program, irrigating the gingival area with a **dental water jet**, or water flosser, that produces pulsating streams of fluid has been reported to reduce plaque biofilm, bleeding, gingivitis, pocket depth, pathogenic microorganisms, and calculus (Fig. 25.12).[5,6,12] On the other hand, dental water jets that produce a steady stream of fluid, as seen with such devices that are attached to a shower or faucet, have not been tested clinically for efficacy in reducing clinical parameters of periodontal disease.

Mechanism of Action

A dental water jet that produces a pulsating stream of fluid (Fig. 25.13) works by impacting the gingival margin with the pulsed irrigant (impact zone) and the subsequent flushing of the gingival crevice or pocket (flushing zone). This **hydrokinetic activity** produces a compression and decompression action that allows the irrigant to reach subgingivally. The majority of studies demonstrating safety and efficacy have been conducted with devices that deliver 1200 pulsations per minute and pressure settings between medium and high (50 to 90 pounds per square inch). Irrigation pressure can be controlled on most devices. Procedure 25.5 outlines basic use of a pulsating dental water jet.

Depth of Delivery of a Solution

The dental water jet has the ability to reach deeper into the periodontal pocket than a toothbrush, interdental aid, or rinsing. This penetration allows for better subgingival cleaning and deeper delivery of antimicrobial agents. Current evidence suggests there is no clinical advantage to the use of an antimicrobial agent; however, there is no disadvantage. The depth to which the solution can reach depends on the tip used. A standard jet tip has been shown to reach 71% in sulcus depths of 0 to 3 mm. Specialty tips designed to be placed slightly below the gingival margin deliver a solution up to 90% in periodontal pockets ≤6 mm (Fig. 25.14).[13]

Interdental Brushes and Tips

Evidence suggests that interdental cleaning with interdental brushes is the most effective method for interdental plaque removal and reduction of inflammation.[2] These brushes should be used from the buccal as well as the lingual aspects.

Interdental brushes are available in various sizes and shapes. The most common brushes are cylindrical or conical/tapered (like an evergreen tree) and designed to be inserted into a plastic, reusable handle that is angled to facilitate interproximal adaptation (Fig. 25.15). Some power toothbrushes come with attachments designed to clean the interproximal area (Fig. 25.16). These attachments are most similar to an end-tufted brush or a large interdental brush. Studies have shown that interdental brushes are equal to or more effective than floss for plaque biofilm removal and for reducing gingival inflammation in type II embrasures, type III embrasures, and exposed furcations.[2] The brush design selected is related to the size of the gingival embrasure or furcation areas. The interdental brush must be slightly larger than the embrasure space so that it can clean the designated area effectively. Interdental brush use is reviewed in Procedure 25.6.

A conical interdental brush may be less effective than a cylindrical brush with respect to lingual approximal plaque control.[14] Rubber-bristled interdental cleaners are shown to be as effective as traditional bristles but are found by some to be more comfortable; therefore they enhanced adherence with daily use recommendations.[15]

Other **interdental tips** are also available in various sizes (Fig. 25.17) and materials, including plastic or foam for plaque biofilm removal in areas similar to interdental brushes. Some interdental tips are designed to fit into smaller areas than a class II embrasure. Tips may be made of foam or other absorbent material that can facilitate delivery of liquid chemotherapeutic agents, such as antimicrobials or desensitizing agents, to the proximal surface. Research in this area is limited. Interdental brushes and tips are available in disposable units designed for travel or use when away from home.

Implant-supported prosthetics or overdenture wearers can benefit from the site-specific use of irrigation and interdental brushes as seen in Figs. 25.18 and 25.19 (Chapter 31).

End-tufted or **single-tufted toothbrushes** are indicated for type II and III embrasures, furcations, large embrasures, and other difficult-to-reach and site-specific areas, such as distal of molars or mandibular anterior lingual. These can also be used around fixed dental appliances because they are designed with a smaller brush head that has a small group of tufts (end-tufted) or a single tuft (single-tufted) (Fig. 25.20). The bristles are directed into the area to be cleaned and activated with a rotating motion, similar to the vibratory motion of Bass toothbrushing. Evidence supports

PROCEDURE 25.5   Use of a Dental Water Jet: Jet Tip

Steps

1. Fill the reservoir with lukewarm water or an antimicrobial agent.
2. Select the appropriate tip and insert into the handle, pressing firmly until it is fully engaged.
3. Adjust the pressure gauge to the lowest setting when using for the first time. Increase as needed or dictated by patient comfort.
4. Place the tip in the mouth, then turn the unit on. Lean over the sink and close the lips enough to prevent splashing while still allowing the water to flow from mouth into the sink.
5. Aim the standard tip at a 90° angle to the long axis of the tooth (see Fig. 25.13); follow manufacturer's instructions for other tip designs (e.g., subgingival or sulcular tips, see Fig. 25.14). Starting in the posterior, follow the gingival margin, pausing between the teeth for a few seconds before continuing to the next tooth. Be sure to irrigate from the buccal and lingual aspects of all teeth.

Read manufacturer's instructions for each model of dental water jet before demonstration.

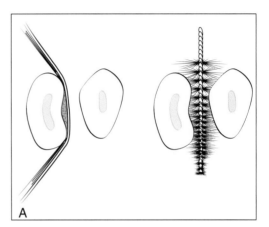

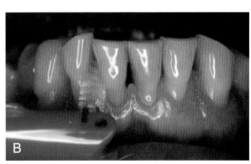

Fig. 25.15 (A) Cleaning of concave or irregular proximal tooth surfaces. Dental floss may be less effective than an interdental brush on long root surfaces with concavities. (B) Proper placement of interdental brush. ([A] From Newman MG, Takei HH, Klokkevold PR, Carranza FA. *Carranza's Clinical Periodontology*. 11th ed. Saunders; 2012. [B] From Perry DA, Beemsterboer PL. *Periodontology for the Dental Hygienist*. 4th ed. Saunders; 2014.)

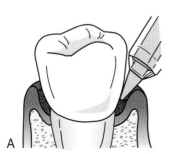
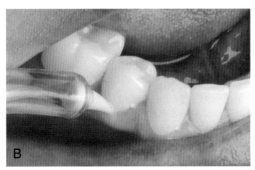

Fig. 25.14 (A) Irrigation with a specialized subgingival tip. (B) Proper placement of a specialized subgingival tip. ([B] From Daniel SJ, Harfst SA, Wilder RS. *Mosby's Dental Hygiene*. 2nd ed. Mosby; 2008.)

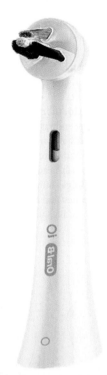

Fig. 25.16 Interproximal power brush head. (Courtesy of P&G.)

PROCEDURE 25.6   Use of an Interdental Brush

Steps

1. Insert bristles into embrasure at a 90° angle to tooth surface (long axis of the tooth) (see Fig. 25.15A).
2. Move brush using in-and-out motion from facial and/or lingual surfaces of appropriate areas (see Fig. 25.15B).
3. Rinse bristles under running water as necessary to remove debris.
4. On completion of use, rinse entire handle and bristles with warm water.

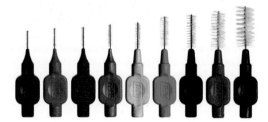

Fig. 25.17 TePe interproximal brushes in a variety of sizes.

interdental brushes for effective biofilm removal and reduction in gingivitis; however, data are lacking specific to end-tufted brushes.

Toothpicks, Toothpick Holders, and Triangular Toothpicks

Some individuals prefer to use toothpicks for control of interdental plaque biofilm, particularly on concave proximal surfaces and exposed furcation areas. **Toothpicks** can be either wooden or plastic. Studies have shown that a household toothpick has no oral health benefit beyond removal of food impacted between the teeth.[3] Safe use of the toothpicks, however, requires sufficient available interdental space because otherwise, they may cause trauma to or blunting of the papilla.

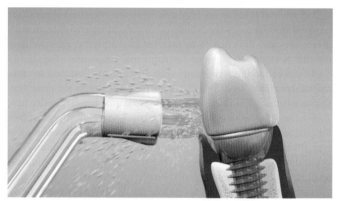

Fig. 25.18 Interproximal tip and irrigator on implant-supported prosthetics. (From Straumann: Home Care – Recommendations for The Straumann® Pro Arch Patient)

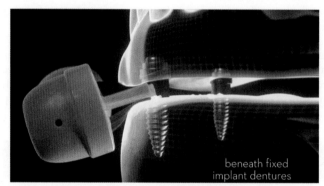

beneath fixed implant dentures

Fig. 25.19 Electric rechargeable interdental brush for implant crown, bridge or fixed implant denture. (Courtesy of P&G.)

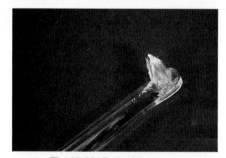

Fig. 25.20 End-tufted brush.

Toothpicks are often too long and wide to reach interproximally from the buccal to lingual surface and have the potential to damage tissue. Patients who use toothpicks for food impaction must be taught proper toothpick use to prevent damage to the gingiva, especially the epithelial attachment (Procedure 25.7). An interdental device should not be directed toward the epithelial attachment or bacteria will be introduced into the nonkeratinized tissue rather than removed. For safe and effective plaque biofilm removal, a toothpick holder or triangular toothpick (wooden wedge) is recommended; however, the same precaution applies. **Toothpick holders** (see Fig. 25.21) are designed to allow use from the facial or lingual aspect and adapt better interproximally and posteriorly when compared with toothpicks alone.

Triangular toothpicks, also called **wooden wedges**, are designed to remove interproximal plaque biofilm from type II and III embrasures. They are recommended for use only from the facial aspect, where the proximal surfaces are exposed by gingival recession, to avoid traumatizing gingival tissue. The use of wooden wedges is reviewed in

PROCEDURE 25.7   Use of a Toothpick in a Toothpick Holder

Steps

1. Insert a round tapered toothpick into the end of an angled plastic holder. Twist toothpick securely into holder and break off longer end of toothpick.
2. Place the toothpick tip at the gingival margin, with the tip pointing at a 45° angle to the long axis of the tooth. Trace the gingival margin around the tooth (Fig. 25.21A).
3. Some patients may be dexterous enough to point the tip at less than a 45° angle into the sulcus or pocket and trace around the tooth surfaces and root concavities. The tip should maintain contact with the tooth at all times. Insertion should stop once the toothpick meets a slight resistance in the space without the teeth being forced apart interproximally or the tissue being impinged. Keeping the tip at the tooth, use a gentle up-and-down motion to clean concave proximal surfaces (Fig. 25.21B).
4. For exposed furcation areas, trace the furcation and use an in-and-out motion to clean the furcation. The tip should maintain contact with the tooth at all times.
5. If debris accumulates on toothpick, rinse under running water.

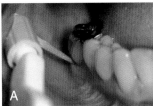 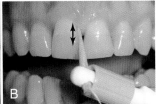

Fig. 25.21 (A) Toothpick tip placed at gingival margin. (B) Gentle up-and-down motion, keeping tip on tooth. (From Newman MG, Takei HH, Klokkevold PR, et al. *Carranza's Clinical Periodontology.* 11th ed. Saunders; 2012.)

PROCEDURE 25.8   Use of a Triangular Toothpick

Steps

1. Place wedge against the proximal surface of a tooth with the base of the wedge triangle toward gingival border and the tip pointing occlusally or incisally at approximately a 45° angle.
2. Use an in-and-out motion interproximally from the facial area only. Apply a burnishing stroke with moderate pressure first to the proximal surface of one tooth and then to the other, about four strokes each. Stop once wedge meets a slight resistance in the space.
3. Trace margin of tissue to remove marginal debris, again with tip pointing occlusally (away from tissue).

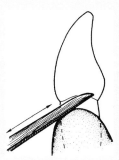

Proper placement of the balsa wood triangular toothpick (wooden wedge) against the proximal surface of a tooth. (From Hoag PM, Pawlak EA. *Essentials of Periodontics.* 4th ed. Mosby; 1990.) (See Fig. 25.21.)

PROCEDURE 25.9   Use of a Rubber Tip Stimulator

Steps

1. Place side of rubber tip interdentally and pointing slightly coronally (45° angle).
2. Move in and out with a slow stroke, rubbing the tip against the teeth and under the contact area.
3. Remove from the interproximal space and trace the gingival margin, with the tip positioned just below the margin, following the contour of the gingiva.

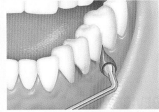

Proper placement of a rubber tip stimulator. (Courtesy Sunstar Americas, Inc, Chicago, IL.)

Procedure 25.8. The key difference between the use of toothpicks and wooden wedges relates to the triangular design of the wedge.

An advantage of using this method of interdental cleaning is that there is no need for a mirror and use requires only one hand. Interdental space must be available for safe use. Triangular toothpicks are inserted interdentally, with the base of the triangle resting on the gingival side, the tip pointing occlusally or incisally, and the sides of the triangle against the adjacent tooth surfaces (see Procedure 25.8). Placing the triangle base against the tissue prevents damage, such as gingival cuts and clefts, to the interdental papilla and gingival margins. The triangular wedge fits the interdental area more snugly and covers a larger surface area, thereby allowing for the removal of plaque biofilm. Systematic reviews have shown that triangular toothpicks are particularly effective in reducing interproximal inflammation and probing depth in patients with periodontitis, but it is unclear whether wooden sticks have a concomitant effect on biofilm removal.

Rubber Tip Stimulators

Interdental stimulators are devices designed primarily for gingival stimulation, not plaque control. The **rubber tip stimulator**, attached to the end of a metal or plastic handle (Procedure 25.9), is used primarily to stimulate the gingiva and to remove plaque biofilm by rubbing it against the exposed tooth surfaces. Research on rubber tip stimulators is limited and inconclusive regarding the efficacy of plaque biofilm removal and reduction of infection.

Massaging the gingiva with a rubber tip or other device can lead to improved circulation, increased keratinization, and epithelial thickening. Whether these gingival changes provide any clinical benefits has not been studied. Improved gingival health resulting from oral hygiene practices has been shown to be related directly to plaque biofilm removal and reduction of risk factors.

Tongue Cleaners

As we seek to aid patients in the prevention and treatment of active oral disease, one area that is often omitted from oral hygiene

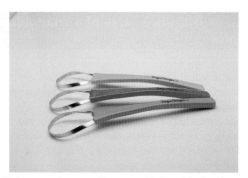

Fig. 25.22 Tongue cleaners. (Courtesy BioCurv Medical Instruments.)

regimens and instruction is tongue cleaning. Tongue cleaning is often overlooked and patients are not aware that the papillae of the tongue harbor bacteria. The dorsal surface of the tongue hosts an abundance of organisms. During the putrefaction of food debris on the tongue, hydrogen sulfide and methyl mercaptan gases are produced. Bad breath, also known as halitosis or malodor, is a common patient complaint. Bacteria on the tongue are one of the primary causes of bad breath. **Tongue cleaners** or scrapers are designed and intended for removal of debris and bacteria from the tongue's dorsal surface (Fig. 25.22).

Brushing the tongue with a toothbrush also can remove bacteria and debris. Some patients may find it difficult to reach the tongue's posterior third with a toothbrush, and the bristles may be too soft to remove moderate to heavy debris adequately. Some may find that a tongue cleaner is easier to use because it does not stimulate the gag reflex as readily as a toothbrush. However, there is insufficient evidence to recommend frequency, duration, or delivery method of tongue cleaning. Further research is needed.[16]

Tongue cleaners come in many shapes, styles, and colors, from a simple plastic strip to a variety of handled devices. Procedure 25.10 outlines use of a tongue cleaner.

Tongue Cleaner Attachments

Powered tongue cleaners have been developed to remove plaque and debris from the dorsum of the tongue and to help control or eliminate malodor. Automation provides a means for additional action that may help patients who have difficulty with dexterity. A tongue-cleaning attachment is available for dental water jets and provides a water flushing action or the delivery of an antimicrobial. Tongue cleaning attachments are also available for some power toothbrushes. No data demonstrate that these devices are better than a manual tongue cleaner.

ADDITIONAL DEVICES

Tooth Towelettes or Finger-Mounted Wipes

Tooth towelettes and finger-mounted wipes are being marketed as a method of plaque biofilm removal when toothbrushing is not possible. The **tooth towelettes** are gauze squares usually treated with some form of mouthwash to freshen breath. The gauze square is held between the thumb and index finger and wiped on the tooth surface, moving from the cervical margin to the incisal or occlusal edge. Facial and lingual surfaces are cleaned at the same time. The finger-mounted wipe is placed over the index finger for the same type of use. These devices are not meant to replace a daily toothbrushing.

PROCEDURE 25.10   Use of a Tongue Cleaner

Steps
1. Hold the handle of the tongue cleaner, or if it is a strip tongue cleaner, wrap in a U shape by holding both ends of the cleaner.
2. Start at the posterior part of the tongue and drag the tongue cleaner to the tip of the tongue. If a gag reflex is triggered, drag from the lateral border of the tongue to the opposite lateral border.
3. Rinse the tongue scraper with water.
4. Repeat step 3 until tongue cleaner is clean on removal, being sure to cover all aspects of the tongue with overlapping strokes.

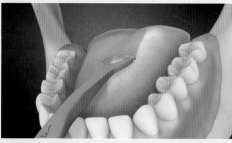

Tongue cleaner. (Courtesy BioCurv Medical Instruments.) (See Fig. 25.22.)

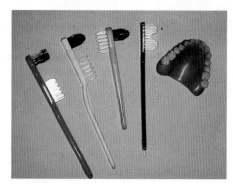

Fig. 25.23 Examples of denture brushes.

Clasp and Denture Brush

Specialty brushes such as the **clasp brush** and **denture brush** have been designed with firm nylon filaments to clean dentures and the clasps of partial dentures (Fig. 25.23). This is because these prostheses are removable and can be cleaned outside of the mouth, where the firmer filaments cannot cause gingival tissue destruction (Chapter 41).

ORAL PIERCINGS

Oral piercing is defined as the cosmetic piercing for the insertion of objects such as rings, studs, or pins. Oral piercings may also include the perioral area such as cheeks, nose, and eyebrows. A needle is inserted through the skin to create an opening through which a piece of jewelry may be worn. An additional oral modification in this category includes tongue splitting, where the tongue is divided into two lateral halves, creating a forked appearance. Among the adolescent populations studied, oral and/or perioral piercings were observed

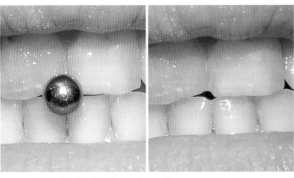

Fig. 25.24 Fracture of maxillary central incisor.

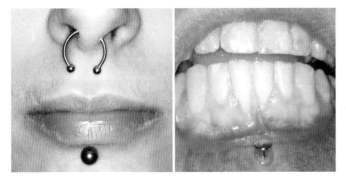

Fig. 25.25 Gingival recession due to Labret piercing.

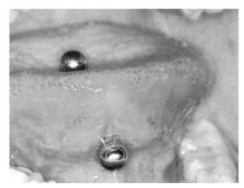

Fig. 25.26 Midline tongue piercing. (From Frese PA. Oral Piercings: Implications for Dental Professionals. Dental Continuing Education Course, updated 2018. Available at: https://www.dentalcare.com/en-us/professional-education/ce-courses/ce423. Accessed November 6, 2018.)

BOX 25.3 **Critical Thinking Scenario**

Scenario: A middle-aged male patient presents with normal gingival contour and localized periodontal probing depths of 4 to 5 mm in the molar areas. His toothbrushing appears to be effective with healthy gingival tissues buccally and lingually, but bleeding on probing occurs in various areas of the mouth where interdental papillae are inflamed. Localized inflammation also is apparent in the mandibular anterior area and around the existing crown and bridge tooth #2–4.

1. What interdental and supplemental devices could be used for effective biofilm removal based on the conditions in various areas of the mouth?
2. Role play discussing these recommendations with a patient and demonstrating the proper technique for use.

---

in a relatively small percentage of young adults. The prevalence was approximately four times higher among females when compared with males.[17] Piercings are made of different materials, usually metal or synthetic materials.

Risks of oral and perioral piercings are due to lack of training of piercing professionals and lack of enforcement of sterilization procedures where infection and life-threatening complications could arise. In the long term, tongue piercings lead to tooth fractures[17,18] (Fig. 25.24). A common risk to individuals with tongue or lip piercings is gingival recession, especially in the mandibular anterior area, with associated alveolar bone loss (Fig. 25.25).[19]

Complications of oral piercings also can occur immediately following the procedure. Short-term risks may include infection, swelling, and bleeding at the site. Piercing is common in the midline of the tongue (Fig. 25.26), the lips (including the labiomental groove and the philtrum), and the cheeks.

Postpiercing instructions include use of an alcohol-free antimicrobial rinse four to five times per day to keep the oral cavity as clean as possible and minimize infection of the pierced site. Cool liquids or ice chips are recommended to minimize swelling. It is recommended to eat small portions of food, slowly. It is important to instruct these patients to gently brush their piercing daily as soon as it is comfortable to do so. Use of nonsteroidal antiinflammatory drugs (NSAIDs) is recommended to control swelling and pain. The patient should be instructed to avoid clicking the jewelry against the teeth and avoid chewing gum and other foreign objects (e.g., fingernails, pens). In addition, patients need to be aware that when they remove the jewelry, food debris and bacteria can accumulate in the hole, posing risk for infection.

Dental hygienists need to be aware of the procedures and risks involved with oral piercings and the social and psychologic reasons that lead people to engage in this practice despite the health risks and oral complications associated with such practices. Hygienists are ideally suited to offer information regarding safe piercings and to provide advice regarding oral hygiene, aftercare, and possible complications.

THE DENTAL HYGIENIST ENGAGING THE PATIENT AS COTHERAPIST

Patients are more likely to adhere to self-care recommendations if they are involved as clients or cotherapists in the selection of devices and agree to mutually determined goals for oral hygiene practices. Dental hygienists have the responsibility for helping their patients select appropriate and effective interdental and supplemental self-care devices. Teaching a patient how to use the device(s) and observing intraoral use is an important element of patient education. Different approaches can be used for patient motivation (Chapter 5), and motivation is requisite for adherence to decisions made. Box 25.3 presents a Critical Thinking Scenario to apply these principles, and Box 25.4 includes an exercise to practice use of interdental and supplemental oral hygiene aids.

ACKNOWLEDGMENT

The author acknowledges Denise M. Bowen, Brenda Parton Maddox, and Deborah M. Lyle for their past contributions to this chapter.

BOX 25.4   Practice Use of Various Interdental and Supplemental

1. Collect various interdental and supplemental self-care devices, review all of the procedure tables in Chapter 25, and practice use of each device on a typodont and, where feasible, in your own mouth.
2. Identify devices that would benefit patients with:
   • Tight interproximal contacts
   • A 3-unit bridge
   • Orthodontics
   • Type II gingival embrasures
   • Type III gingival embrasures
   • A preference for wooden toothpicks
   • A coated tongue
3. Role play providing instructions on the use of the following:
   • Floss, floss threader and holder, dental water jet, interdental tips, brush and stimulator, wood or plastic sticks, toothpick and holder, and tongue cleaner.
   • Various devices designed specifically for periodontal maintenance patients.
   • Various devices used for patients with orthodontics. Demonstrate proper use of the devices on a typodont with fixed orthodontic brackets and wires.
   • Use the PICO process (Chapter 3) and PubMed to gather high-quality evidence on at least one interdental device for biofilm prevention and control, focusing on expected outcomes such as gingival health, improvement in periodontal diseases, and reduced incidence of dental caries.

KEY CONCEPTS

1. Dental hygienists have the opportunity to help their patients select a preferred and effective method to accomplish this goal.
2. Interdental bacterial biofilm prevention and control is essential to good oral health, especially gingival health because the interdental proximal embrasure space of adjacent teeth and the tongue can harbor a host of microbes that can contribute to poor oral health.
3. Dental hygienists must remain current and familiar with the different devices, how to use each device, the evidence specific to each device, and the expected results from using each device.
4. A wide variety of interdental and supplemental plaque control aids is available. Several clinical trials and metaanalyses have shown that alternatives to manual flossing such as interdental brushes, dental water jets, floss holders, and power flossers are as effective as or more effective than dental floss at reducing plaque biofilm, bleeding, gingivitis, and/or pocket depths.
5. When the interdental gingiva is reduced or missing and the embrasures are open (type II and type III), methods of interdental cleaning other than dental floss are needed. The dental hygienist evaluates the information gained during the assessment phase of care to select the most appropriate interdental and supplemental aids for the patient.
6. Bad breath, also known as halitosis or malodor, is a common patient complaint. Bacteria on the tongue are one of the primary causes of bad breath.
7. Dental hygienists need to be aware of the procedures and risks involved with oral piercings, and the social and psychologic reasons that lead people to engage in this practice despite the health risks and oral complications associated with such practices.
8. Patients are more likely to adhere to self-care recommendations if they are involved as clients or cotherapists in the selection of devices and agree to mutually determined goals for oral hygiene practices.

REFERENCES

1. Bidra AS, Daubert DM, Garcia LT, et al. Clinical practice guidelines for recall and maintenance of patients with tooth-borne and implant-borne dental restorations. *J Dent Hyg.* 2016;90(1):60–69.
2. Slot DE, Dorfer CE, Van derWeijden GA. The efficacy of interdental brushes on plaque and parameters of periodontal inflammation: a systematic review. *Int J Dent Hyg.* 2008;6:253.
3. Hoenderdos NL, Slot DE, Paraskevas S, et al. The efficacy of woodsticks on plaque and gingival inflammation: a systematic review. *Int J Dent Hyg.* 2008;6:280.
4. Van derWeijden GA, Slot DE. Oral hygiene in the prevention of periodontal diseases: the evidence. *Periodontol 2000.* 2011;55:105.
5. Husseini A, Slot DE, Van derWeijden GA. The efficacy of oral irrigation in addition to a toothbrush on plaque and the clinical parameters of periodontal inflammation: a systematic review. *Int J Dent Hyg.* 2008;6:304.
6. Rosema NA, Hennequin-Hoenderdos NL, Berchier CE, et al. The effect of different interdental cleaning devices on gingival bleeding. *J Int Acad Periodontol.* 2011;13:2.
7. Poklepovic T, Worthington HV, Johnson TM, et al. Interdental brushing for the prevention and control of periodontal diseases and dental caries in adults. *Cochrane Database Syst Rev.* 2013;12:CD009857.
8. de Oliveira KMH, Nemezio MA, Romualdo PC, et al. Dental flossing and proximal caries in the primary dentition: a systematic review. *Oral Health Prev Dent.* 2017;15(5):427–434.
9. Chapple IL, Van der Weijden F, Doerfer C, et al. Primary prevention of periodontitis: managing gingivitis. *J Clin Periodontol.* 2015;42(suppl 16):S71–S76.
10. Sambunjak D, Nickerson JW, Poklepovic T, et al. Flossing for the management of periodontal diseases and dental caries in adults. *Cochrane Database Syst Rev.* 2011;12:CD008829.
11. Bidra AS, Daubert DM, Garcia LT, et al. Clinical practice guidelines for recall and maintenance of patients with tooth-borne and implant-borne dental restorations. *J Dent Hyg.* 2016;90(1):60–69.
12. Shewale A, Gattani D, Taneja Bhasin M, et al. Adjunctive role of supra- and subgingival irrigation in periodontal therapy. *Int J Pharm Sci Res.* 2016;7(3):152–159.
13. Eakle WS, Ford C, Boyd RL. Depth of penetration in periodontal pockets with oral irrigation. *J Clin Periodontol.* 1986;13:39.
14. Larson HC, Slot DE, Van Zoelen C, et al. The effectiveness of conically shaped compared with cylindrically shaped interdental brushes—a randomized clinical trial. *Int J Dent Hyg.* 2017;15(3):211–218.
15. Hennequin-Hoenderdos NL, van der Sluijs E, van der Wiejden GA, et al. Efficacy of a rubber bristles interdental cleaner compared to an interdental brush on dental plaque, gingival bleeding and gingival abrasion: a randomized clinical trial. *Int J Dent Hyg.* 2018;16(3):380–388.
16. Kuo YW, Yen M, Fetzer S, et al. Toothbrushing versus toothbrushing plus tongue cleaning in reducing halitosis and tongue coating: a systematic review and meta-analysis. *Nurs Res.* 2013;62(6):422–429.
17. Hennequin-Hoenderdos NL, Slot DE, Van der Weijden GA. The incidence of complications associated with lip and/or tongue piercings: a systematic review. *Int J Dent Hyg.* 2016;14(1):62–73. Epub Feb 17, 2015.
18. Frese P. Oral Piercings: Implications for Dental Professionals. Course number 423. www.Dentalcare.com. Last revision 2018. Accessed August 30, 2017.
19. Frese PA. Oral Piercings: Implications for Dental Professionals. Dental Continuing Education Course, updated 2018. Available at: https://www.dentalcare.com/en-us/professional-education/ce-courses/ce423. Accessed November 6, 2018.

26

Dentifrices

Nadia Dubreuil, Elizabeth Michaud-Jobin, and France Lavoie

PROFESSIONAL OPPORTUNITIES

Dental hygiene clients are continually challenged to maintain optimal oral hygiene and prevent oral diseases. Antimicrobial agents used in patients' homecare routines and dental hygiene professional practice can assist mechanical interventions to aid in reducing oral biofilm, periodontal inflammation, and clinical attachment loss. Oral health has a direct impact on overall health and can have serious repercussions for systemic health. The dental hygienist, as a front-line practitioner and change agent, must also address other patient needs, such as treatment of dental hypersensitivity and remineralization therapy. Dental hygienists with current knowledge of antimicrobial, desensitization, and remineralization interventions can effectively make evidence-based recommendations, provide appropriate services, and offer referrals to other oral healthcare providers when necessary.

COMPETENCIES

1. Explain the purpose of a dentifrice and the types of effects that it can produce.
2. Discuss the process of selecting the right dentifrice, including the role of dentifrices in the demineralization and remineralization process.
3. Describe the role of medicinal and nonmedicinal components in dentifrices.
4. Explain the concept of bioavailability.
5. Debate the possible adverse oral health effects of dentifrices.
6. Explain the impact of the pH level of dentifrices.
7. Analyze new trends in dentifrices (vegan, organic, etc.) and their potential effects on oral and global health.
8. Recommend appropriate dentifrices and their uses to meet unique patient needs and address risk factors.
9. Delineate the legal and ethical responsibilities of dental hygienists with regard to dentifrices.

PURPOSE OF A DENTIFRICE

Patients rely on dental hygienists for recommendations on dentifrices that will meet their oral health needs. A **dentifrice**, commonly referred to as toothpaste by clients, is a substance used with a toothbrush or other oral hygiene device to clean the teeth, tongue, and gingiva and to deliver cosmetic and therapeutic agents to the teeth and oral environment. A dentifrice can yield the following types of effects:
- Cosmetic effect: prevents or removes stains, inhibits supragingival calculus formation, whitens teeth, freshens breath, and controls oral malodor.
- Hygienic effect: aids in the removal of food particles and oral biofilm.

- Therapeutic effect: prevents or reverses dental caries; reduces dentinal hypersensitivity, gingivitis, or oral biofilm;[1] and prevents or reduces dental erosion. In addition to the beneficial effects on oral health, the therapeutic, antigingivitis, and antibacterial effects also contribute to maintaining optimal overall health. Combined therapeutic effects are provided by medicinal or active ingredients. Box 26.1 discusses the American Dental Association (ADA)[2,3] Seal of Acceptance and the Canadian Dental Association (CDA)[4] Seal of Recognition.

CHOOSING A DENTIFRICE

The range of dentifrices available over the counter and on the Internet is rapidly increasing and can be confusing for patients and professionals. Over-the-counter (OTC) products have been approved by government authorities (Health Canada, US Food and Drug Administration [FDA]). To be recognized as therapeutic, dentifrices must meet or exceed criteria for safety, quality, and efficacy. Recognized products receive either a Drug Identification Number (DIN) or a Natural Product Number (NPN) in Canada/Natural Drug Code (NDC) in the United States. For example, dentifrices that contain 5000 ppm fluoride are considered a drug, so they receive a DIN. Dentifrices containing 1000 to 1500 ppm of fluoride are considered a natural health product, so they receive an NPN or NDC. In Canada, homeopathic products that have met the scientific requirements established by government authorities receive a Drug Identification Number-Homeopathic Medicine (DIN-HM) on the label.[5,6]

It can be challenging for clients to determine the appropriate dentifrice to meet their needs. Some advertisers use targeted marketing on websites and social media to try to influence consumers to use products that have not been approved by government authorities or even products that are no longer available in the client's country. Some of these dentifrices may pose significant health risks, such as adverse reactions, allergies, and toxicity, depending on their composition. In addition, manufacturers advertise the multiple properties of their products without indicating the minimum concentration of active/medicinal ingredients. Some manufacturers even offer the same product formulation with different packaging and different identified properties (depending on the packaging). In some countries, the lack of indication and research concerning certain properties, e.g., pH and abrasivity level, does not allow clients to identify the product that suits them best.

The choice of a dentifrice should be made according to the therapeutic and personal needs of the patient, including their different health situations and considering scientific evidence (Fig. 26.1, Tables 26.1A–B, 26.2, and 26.3). For example, there are formulations without sodium lauryl sulfate (SLS), which is often listed as a cause of recurrent aphthous ulcers; with sweeteners that do not affect blood glucose (diabetes); with salivary enzymes, lubricants, or salivary stimulants (hyposalivation or xerostomia); and without sodium bicarbonate or sodium chloride (hypertension).

Professionals should ensure that they are up to date on dentifrice options, formulations, and product availability to better advise patients. Dental hygienists should regularly review the patient's personal care regimen and ensure that advice is based on evidence-based research to achieve optimal oral health (Box 26.2).

TRENDS: NATURAL, VEGAN, ORGANIC, BIODEGRADABLE DENTIFRICES

The trend to use natural, vegan, organic, or biodegradable dentifrices aims to limit exposure to chemicals that are known to be toxic to humans and to reduce the ecological footprint.

This trend has resulted in a number of **natural dentifrices**, which are divided into two categories: approved and unapproved. To be approved by governmental authorities, in general:

- **Organic or bio dentifrices** must not contain animal ingredients (e.g., gelatin of porcine origin), potentially toxic molecules, or those that pose a risk to general health (e.g., titanium dioxide).
- **Vegan or vegetarian dentifrices** must be of plant origin. Thus they do not contain products of any animal origin, e.g., calcium from bones or cartilage or even propolis made by bees. Some medicinal plants could be promising vegan ingredients helping with gingivitis, such as *Aloe vera*, *Magnolia officinalis*, and *Curcuma longa*. More studies need to be done in order to establish efficacy for these ingredients.[7,8]
- **Biodegradable dentifrices** must not include polluting ingredients. For example, dentifrices that use microbeads as abrasives are being withdrawn from the international market because of contamination of water and aquatic fauna. Dentifrice containers also follow this trend. Colgate-Palmolive has introduced the first recyclable dentifrice tube. Dentifrice tablets and powders, which come in glass or cardboard containers, are now available to reduce the environmental footprint.

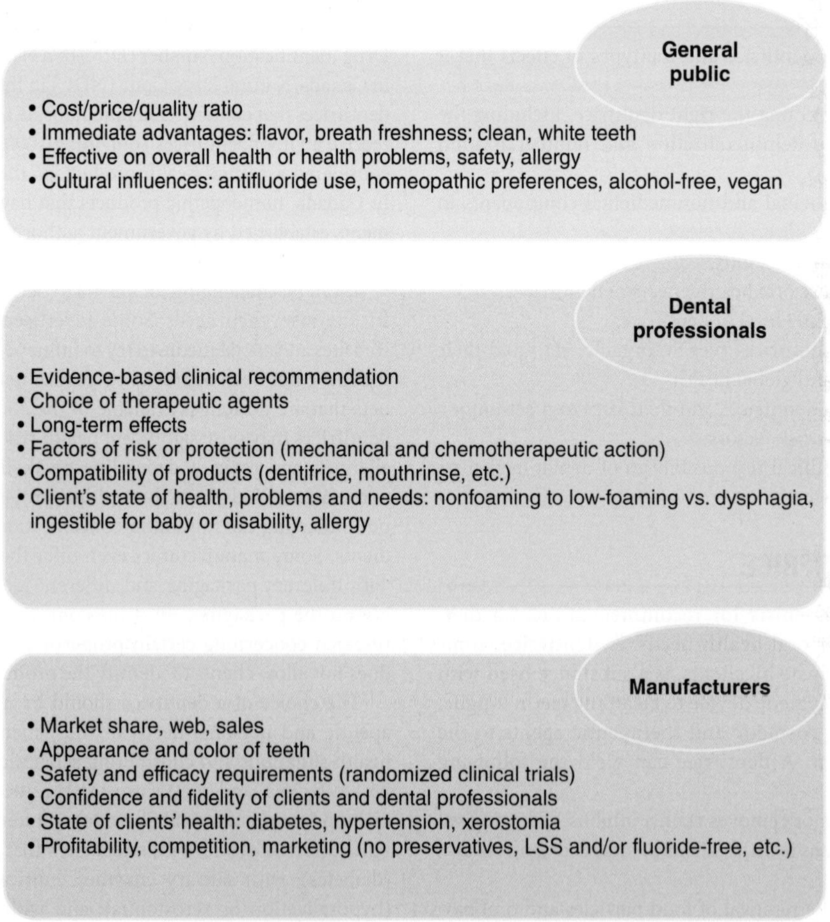

BOX 26.1 ADA Seal of Acceptance or CDA Seal of Recognition

Dentifrices that carry the American Dental Association (ADA) Seal of Acceptance or the Canadian Dental Association (CDA) Seal of Recognition have undergone rigorous testing and research indicating that they are safe and therapeutically effective. These therapeutic effects include antiplaque, antigingivitis, anticaries, antidentinal hypersensitivity, anticalculus, prevent or reduce dental erosion from dietary acids, bad breath control, or a combination of these properties, and have been approved by the US Food and Drug Administration, Health Canada, or other regulatory organizations. The ADA Seal also has been awarded to dentifrices that safely and effectively remove extrinsic tooth stain.

Although it is important to regularly consult these organizations' websites, the absence of a seal does not mean that the dentifrice is not safe and effective; instead, it implies the dentifrice company did not obtain did not or possibly apply for approval. The dental hygienist should compare the dentifrice without a seal to similar products and/or search for evidence regarding these products before recommending them to patients.

General public

- Cost/price/quality ratio
- Immediate advantages: flavor, breath freshness; clean, white teeth
- Effective on overall health or health problems, safety, allergy
- Cultural influences: antifluoride use, homeopathic preferences, alcohol-free, vegan

Dental professionals

- Evidence-based clinical recommendation
- Choice of therapeutic agents
- Long-term effects
- Factors of risk or protection (mechanical and chemotherapeutic action)
- Compatibility of products (dentifrice, mouthrinse, etc.)
- Client's state of health, problems and needs: nonfoaming to low-foaming vs. dysphagia, ingestible for baby or disability, allergy

Manufacturers

- Market share, web, sales
- Appearance and color of teeth
- Safety and efficacy requirements (randomized clinical trials)
- Confidence and fidelity of clients and dental professionals
- State of clients' health: diabetes, hypertension, xerostomia
- Profitability, competition, marketing (no preservatives, LSS and/or fluoride-free, etc.)

Fig. 26.1 Comparison of factors related to the choice of a dentifrice. (Courtesy of France Lavoie.)

TABLE 26.1A Components of Dentifrices: Nonmedicinal Ingredients

Components	Examples
Cleansing and polishing agents	**Phosphate**: calcium pyrophosphate (CalPyro), dicalcium phosphate dihydrate (DCPD), anhydrous dicalcium phosphate, insoluble calcium metaphosphate (IMP) **Carbonates**: calcium carbonate (chalk), sodium bicarbonate **Silica**: silicates, dehydrated silica gels, synthetic amorphous silicates in gel form, perlite **Aluminum compounds**: alumina, hydrated aluminum oxides, aluminum trihydrates, amorphous aluminum silicate **Others**: complex salt of synthetic, methacrylate, clay (China clay, pumice, kaolin, bentonite, volcanic ash), magnesium carbonate, insoluble materials (herbs), microbeads (polyethylene), cuttlebone powder
Humectants	Glycerin, sorbitol, mannitol, propylene glycol, vegetable oils, synthetic cellulose, polyoxyethylene glycol esters (PEG 8), polypropylene glycol ester (PPG), pentatol, xylitol
Water	Distilled water, deionized or oxygenated water, spring water
Binders, gelling agents, or thickeners	**Mineral colloids** Veegum (magnesium aluminum silicate) Sodium aluminum silicate, viscarin **Varieties of clay**: bentonite (derived from volcanic ash), China clay, laponite (inorganic silica clay), kaolin **Natural gums**: arabic or arabic gum, karaya, tragacanth, guar gum, xanthan gum **Seaweed colloids**: alginates (and derivatives), Irish moss extract, sodium or gum carrageenan, agar-agar **Synthetic cellulose**: carboxymethyl cellulose, hydroxyethyl cellulose, hydroxypropyl cellulose, methyl cellulose **Others**: polyethylene glycol (PEG), glycerol carbomer, chitosan, Carbopol
Detergents, surfactants, or foaming agents	Sodium lauryl sulfate (SLS), sodium *N*-lauryl sarcosinate, *N*-lauryl sarcosinate, dioctyl sodium sulfosuccinate, sodium stearyl fumarate, sodium stearyl lactate, sodium lauryl sulfoacetate, sodium cocomonoglyceride sulfonate, cocamidopropyl betaine or betaine de cocamidopropyl, steareth-30, sodium monoglyceride sulfate, ethionates of fatty acid
Flavoring agents or aromatizers	Essential oils (menthol, eucalyptus, peppermint, spearmint), clove oil, aniseed, vanilla, wintergreen, caraway, pimento, citrus, nutmeg, thyme, fennel, cinnamon, linalool, limonene, tea tree oil, bubble gum, mint, fruit flavors (strawberry, grape, etc.)
Preservatives	Alcohols, benzoic acid or benzoates (propyl, sodium, methylparahydroxybenzoates), formaldehydes, phenolic (methyl, ethyl, propyl), parabens (methyl, ethylparaben, etc.), polyaminopropyl biguanide, methylisothiazolinone
Sweeteners	Noncariogenic artificial sweetener, sorbitol, glycerin, sodium saccharin, sodium cyclamate, xylitol, stevia, aspartame, acesulfame, erythritol
Coloring or dye agents	Vegetable coloring, titanium dioxide, chlorophyll, FD&C colors (yellow #5, #6 and #10, green #3, blue #1 and #2, red #3 and #40, acid red #14), covarine blue, cochineal red A

TABLE 26.1B Component of Dentifrices: Active/Medicinal Ingredients

Therapeutic Effect	Therapeutic or Active/Medicinal Agents [Recognized quantity %]
Anticaries	**Fluoride** *Sodium fluoride (NaF)** [0.24%] *Sodium monofluorophosphate (MFP)* [0.76%] *Stannous fluoride (SnF$_2$)* [0.4%] Amine fluoride (AmF) [0.125%] CPP-ACP (Recaldent) with fluoride Fluorocalcium phosphosilicate or F-CSP (BioMin-F) [5% + F 0.1%] **Nonfluoride anticaries components** **Calcium and phosphate derivatives or components**: CPP-ACP (Recaldent) *Calcium phosphosilicate or CSP (NovaMin)* [5%] Hydroxyapatite (HAP) [10%] Calcium derivatives (lactate, carbonate, sulfate) Calcium and phosphates (tricalcium phosphate [TCP], dicalcium phosphate) Phosphate derivatives (trimetaphosphates, glycerophosphates) **Various antimicrobials**: Antibacterial enzymes Metals (zinc, tin) Xylitol [10%]

Continued

TABLE 26.1B   Component of Dentifrices: Active/Medicinal Ingredients—cont'd

Therapeutic Effect	Therapeutic or Active/Medicinal Agents [Recognized quantity %]
Desensitizing	**Chemical action** **Potassium salts [2% minimum to be effective]**: *Potassium nitrate [5%]* *Potassium chloride [3.75%]* *Potassium citrate [5.75%]* **Mechanical action** Strontium acetate hemihydrate [8%] *Stannous fluoride (SnF₂) [0.4%]* *Sodium fluoride (NaF) 5,000 ppm [1.1%]* *Sodium citrate* *CPP-ACP (Recaldent)* Hydroxyapatite (HAP) [10%] ***Bioactive glasses***: *Calcium phosphosilicate or CSP (NovaMin) [5%]* Fluorocalcium phosphosilicate or F-CSP (BioMin-F) [5% + F 0.1%] **Component of**: *Arginine [8%], calcium carbonate [35%] and MFP 1,450 ppm [1.1%]*
Antigingivitis and oral biofilm reduction	Triclosan [0.3%] with [2%] copolymer PVM/MA (Not available in United states and Canada) *Stannous fluoride (SnF₂) [0.4%]* *Chlorhexidine [0.12%]* *Zinc citrate* Zinc chloride *Cetylpyridinium chloride (CPC) [0.05%]* Bioflavonoids EDTA [2.6%] **Essential oils (combined or not)**: Eucalyptol, menthol, methyl salicylate, thymol, tea tree oil, eugenol **Enzymes and proteins (combined or not)**: Lactoperoxidase, glucose oxydase, amyloglucosidase, lysozyme, lactoferrin, potassium thiocyanate
Anticalculus	Copolymer of methyl vinyl ether and maleic anhydride EDTA [2.6%] ***Pyrophosphates or polyphosphates [1%] ADA to [5%] CDA***: *Tetrasodium pyrophosphate* *Disodium pyrophosphate [2%]* *Sodium tripolyphosphate* *Tetrapotassium pyrophosphate* ***Metaphosphate***: *Sodium hexametaphosphate (SHMP) [13%]* *Sodium trimetaphosphate* **Zinc and derivatives**: *Zinc citrate, zinc chloride, zinc sulfate*
Antistain	*Abrasives in dentifrices* *Papain combined with abrasives* *Sodium citrate* *Sodium bicarbonate* **Peroxides**: *Hydrogen peroxide [1%], calcium peroxide* **Phosphates and derivatives**: *Sodium tripolyphosphate* and *pyrophosphate, sodium hexametaphosphate* or *trimetaphosphate*
Erosive protection	All fluorides 1,000 to 1,500 ppm (NaF, MFP, AmF, SnF₂ [0.4%]) NaF [1.1%] combined with calcium and derivatives SnF₂ combined with ACP Bioactive glasses [5%] combined with fluoride [0.1%]

TABLE 26.1B   Component of Dentifrices: Active/Medicinal Ingredients—cont'd

Therapeutic Effect	Therapeutic or Active/Medicinal Agents [Recognized quantity %]
Antihalitosis or malodor (reduction of oral bacteria and the volatile sulfur compounds [VSCs])	Enzymes Chlorine dioxide Sodium bicarbonate Hydrogen peroxide **Zinc and derived:** Zinc citrate [2%] Zinc chloride [0.5%] **Antibacterial agents:** Triclosan [0.3%] with copolymer (not available in the United States and Canada) Stannous fluoride [0.4%]

*Italics denotes acceptance by the ADA or CDA.
ADA, American Dental Association; *CDA*, Canadian Dental Association; *CPP-ACP*, casein phosphopeptide-amorphous calcium phosphate; *PVM/MA*, polyvinylmethoxyethylene and maleic acid.

TABLE 26.2   Allergens Recognized in Dentifrices

Flavoring agents and essential oils*
Mint varieties (peppermint, spearmint, menthol, and carvone or L-carvone), cinnamal or cinnamic aldehyde, cinnamon oil, cinnamyl alcohol, benzyl alcohol, anise or star anise oil, anethole (derived from star anise, anise, and fennel), linalool, tea tree oil (*Melaleuca alternifolia*), strawberries, limonene, cloves, ylang, compositae mix, colophony, unspecified flavors
Other symptoms: recurrent oral ulceration, lichenoid reaction, and oral granulomatosis of the lips

Detergents/surfactant
Cocamidopropyl betaine

Preservatives*
Parabens and derivatives (e.g., methyl and ethyl parabens) currently under high bio surveillance, citric acid and derivatives (zinc or potassium citrate), benzoic acid or benzoates (e.g., propyl and methylparahydroxybenzoate), methylisothiazolinone, benzyl alcohol, formaldehyde, propylene glycol, PEG (8, 12, and 1450)
Other symptoms: irritations

Vitamin E (tocopherol)

Remineralizing agents
Fluoride: Acnelike eruptions, ulcerous stomatitis reaction, discoloration of teeth. If swallowed, it can provoke skin rash, gastrointestinal (GI) upset, headaches, and fluorosis. Excessive dose or maximum tolerated dose (MTD) 0.1 to 0.3 mg/kg can cause nausea, headache, and vomiting.
Lethal dose (LD) > 5 mg/kg
CPP-ACP: Allergy cause by derivative bovine protein

Other allergens
Eggs, milk
Grape extract
Aloe vera
Triclosan, which is withdrawn in Canada and the United States but still available in Europe
Propolis (composed of beeswax): allergy or other symptoms such as dyspnea or labial edema
Xylitol (sweetener): allergy (if derivative of bark of birch) or transitory GI effects
Derivatives of aspirin: acetylsalicylic acid (ASA) as methyl hydroxybenzoate, wintergreen, methyl or sodium salicylate, methyl 2-hydroxybenzoate
Coloring agents: tartrazine (FD&C yellow #5, E102, CI 19140), sunset yellow (FD&C yellow #6, E110, CI 15985), quinoline yellow (FD&C yellow #10, E104, CI 47005), carmoisine (azorubine, acid red #14, E122, CI 14720), cochineal red A (E124, CI 16255), erythrosine (FD&C red #3, E127, CI 45430)
Metals: aluminum, titanium dioxide, tin, silica

*Italic typeface denotes the adverse reactions observed.

TABLE 26.3   Adverse Reactions Associated With Various Ingredients*

Anticalculus: Pyrophosphate derivatives, zinc citrate, sodium hexametaphosphate
Erythema, scaling and fissuring of the perioral area, gingivitis, cheilitis and circumoral dermatitis, dentinal hypersensitivity, soft tissue irritation, ulceration
Detergent: Sodium lauryl sulfate (SLS)
Mucosal desquamation, aphthous ulcerations
Antimicrobial: Stannous fluoride, chlorhexidine, cetylpyridinium chloride
Reversible stains, soft tissue irritation, cheilitis, circumoral dermatitis
Coloring agents: Titanium dioxide (E171 or CI 19140)
If swallowed, it may cause yellow nail syndrome, lymphedema, respiratory symptoms, gastrointestinal inflammation, cancer, neurologic, cardiovascular effects are also possible.
Tartrazine (FD&C yellow #5, E102, CI 19140), sunset yellow (FD&C yellow #6, E110, CI 15985), allura red (FD&C red #40, E129, CI 16035)
May have adverse effects on activity and attention in children
Metals: Zinc, titanium, aluminum, tin, steatite with titane (clay impurities found in natural dentifrices), tripoli, and other heavy metals can be found in the water used to make dentifrice.

*Italic typeface denotes the adverse reactions observed.

BOX 26.2   Data Collection and Documentation

Before recommending a dentifrice, a dental hygienist should check the patient's medical history to eliminate the risk of allergies or adverse reactions and validate the patient's habits (religious beliefs, culture, etc.). Recommendations should be documented in the patient's record and should include product choices (different brands), their concentration, their desired therapeutic effect, and the frequency of use. The patient's signature confirms understanding and acceptance of the recommendations.

An example of an organic, biodegradable, and vegan dentifrice that can be swallowed is Oralpeace.

However, the regulations concerning organic certification are not standardized throughout the world. To obtain organic certification for a product in Quebec, a company must demonstrate that production meets standards according to four principles:

• Health—must support and improve the health of soils, plants, animals, humans, and the planet

- Ecology—must be based on the respect and maintenance of living ecological cycles and systems
- Equity—must be based on relationships that ensure equity in relation to a common environment
- Precaution—must be practiced in a prudent and responsible manner in order to protect the health and well-being of present and future generations.[9]

The lists of tolerated products can also vary depending on the country. For example, tartrazine is prohibited in France, but it is accepted and monitored in Canada and the United States.

RECOMMENDATION ON THE USE OF DENTIFRICES

The use of a dentifrice as well as the quantity to use varies according to age and carious risk, e.g., vulnerable patients (see Table 26.4, Figs. 26.2 and 26.3).[3,4,10] It is recommended to brush teeth twice a day for 2 to 3 minutes. After brushing, the recommendation is to not rinse; instead, simply spit out the excess dentifrice, keeping a thin film on the teeth to allow the active ingredients to continue to have their effect. Similarly, clients should ideally wait 30 minutes or more after brushing before rinsing (even with mouthwash), drinking, or eating to maximize the therapeutic effect.

A child's first preventive visit should take place around 1 year of age or as soon as the first teeth erupt. The dental hygienist will inform the parents of the risks and recommend a dentifrice adapted to the needs of the child. In general, it is recommended that brushing be supervised in children up to 7 years of age or until the child has developed the manual skill to brush. Dentifrices should be stored in a safe place, out of reach of children, to limit the risk of ingestion. For safety reasons, some ingredients are recommended only for those 12 years and older, for example, potassium nitrate[11] and pyrophosphates[12] (see Anticalculus Agents). Some manufacturers suggest stannous fluoride for patients as young as 2, while others recommend waiting until children reach the age of 12 and older.

POTENTIAL DENTIFRICE TUBE CROSS-CONTAMINATION

The opening of the dentifrice tube can be a source of cross-contamination. Bacteria that is responsible for oral and systemic disease can be transmitted when family members' toothbrushes come into contact with the opening of the same tube of dentifrice. The FDA, in the United States, and Health Canada each require that microhostility testing be conducted and that ingredients be added to minimize the risk of cross-contamination. However, each family member should have their own tube of dentifrice

TABLE 26.4   Quantity of Dentifrice per Brushing and per Age According to ADA and CDA Recommendations

	0 to 3 Years	3 to 6 Years	6 to 12 Years	12 Years and Older
Quantity	Grain of rice size	Pea size	Pea size or ½ cm	Pea size, ½ to 1 cm
Weight of dentifrice	0.1 g	0.25 g	0.25 g and over	0.25 g and over
Mg of fluoride	0.1 mg	0.25 mg	0.25 mg and over	0.25 mg and over

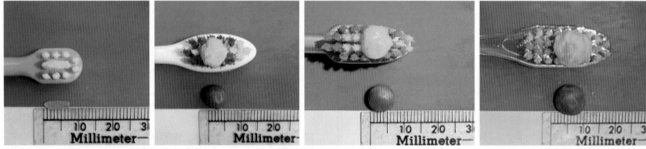

Fig. 26.2 Quantity of dentifrice per brushing and per age according to ADA and CDA recommendations. (Courtesy of Nadia Dubreuil.)

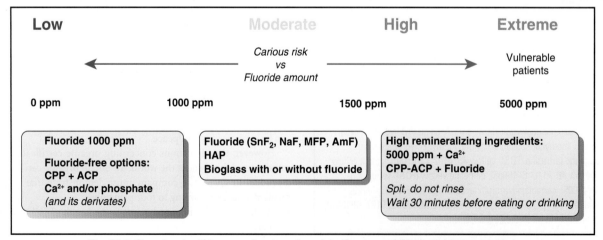

Fig. 26.3 Choosing dentifrice according to carious risk. (Courtesy of Elizabeth Michaud-Jobin.)

to prevent cross-contamination, control infection among people living in the same household or in a daycare center, and meet each family member's unique oral care needs. In the field of public dental health in Canada, it is recommended to dispense individual portions of the appropriate dose of dentifrice onto waxed paper or cardboard so that each child can take their dentifrice without the risk of contaminating the tube or the other children's toothbrushes. These measures are established to prevent the transmission of bacteria responsible for decay, periodontal diseases, and infectious diseases, such as hepatitis B, gastroenteritis, the flu, or even common colds.

FORMS OF DENTIFRICES

Dentifrices come in different forms (Fig. 26.4). A fluoridated liquid gel dentifrice is effective in caries prevention because it reaches the interproximal surfaces and deep grooves of the teeth.[1]

COMPONENTS OF DENTIFRICES

The three main ingredients are humectants, abrasives, and water. Then, in smaller quantities, there are detergents, preservatives, flavors or sweetening agents, binding agents, and medicinal or therapeutic agents. Ingredients may be of natural or synthetic origin (see Table 26.1A–B); however, certain ingredients may result in adverse or allergic reactions

(see Tables 26.2, 26.3, and 26.5 for adverse health effects of dentifrices). Patients with allergies to certain ingredients must be informed of their presence so they can avoid exposure. The list of specific ingredients should be available on the packaging of oral care products and on the manufacturers' website to help patients or dental health professionals identify allergy-inducing ingredients and help avoid the risk of adverse reactions.

Dentifrices consist of complex formulas of medicinal ingredients (known as therapeutic or active ingredients) and nonmedicinal ingredients (inactive ingredients) that must be compatible with each other in order to be effective. A **medicinal ingredient** is intended to produce a therapeutic effect on the hard and/or soft tissues and must improve oral health status in a safe and effective way (e.g., fluoride for caries control) (see Table 26.1B). A **nonmedicinal ingredient** is added to provide a particular flavor or color, prevent bacterial growth, or provide better consistency for the dentifrice (see Table 26.1A).

Nonmedicinal Ingredients
Abrasives
Abrasive agents are used to clean and polish teeth to a smooth, lustrous surface. Patients who brush their teeth without a dentifrice must brush longer because there is no abrasive agent on the toothbrush to help remove soft deposits and stains adequately.[1] Dentifrice powders, tablets, gels, foaming gel, and pastes all contain abrasive agents (Box

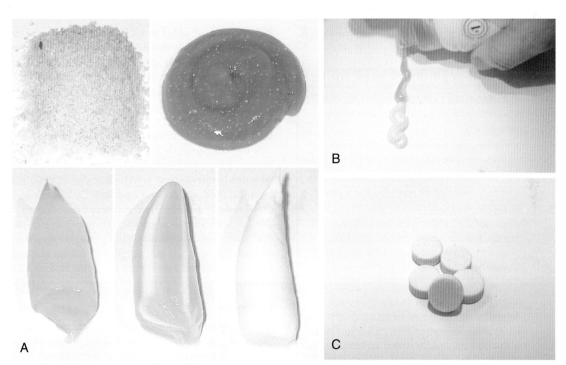

Fig. 26.4 Forms of dentifrices. (A) Powder, liquid gel, gel, gel/paste, and paste. (B) Foaming gel. (C) Tablets. (Courtesy of Nadia Dubreuil, GREDH [Group of Research and Education on Dental Hygiene], Québec, Canada.)

TABLE 26.5 Low Allergenic Flavor Ingredients

Oils	anise, orange, fennel, orange peel
Fruit extracts	orange, banana, pineapple, strawberries, grape orange-mango, mango, apricot, berries

Data from Lavoie F, Feeney N, McCallum L, et al. Evaluation of dentifrices and of variables associated with the choice of a product. *CDHA*. 2007;41:42.

BOX 26.3 The Five Most Common Abrasives

- Phosphates help the dentifrice whiten teeth and make them feel clean.
- Carbonates help to clean and deodorize the mouth and make it smell fresh.
- Silicas mechanically clean teeth and some can thicken the dentifrice. Silicas are chemically compatible with NaF and MFP. Silicas are nonreactive and therefore are used frequently as abrasives in dentifrices.
- Alumina and aluminum compounds are insoluble, with a very high abrasive potential because the particle is irregular and harder than the tooth.
- Other abrasive substances include clay and synthetics, such as vinyl or resins.

26.3). These abrasive agents are either natural or synthetic, and they establish the abrasive capacity of the dentifrice (Table 26.6; Fig. 26.5). If the abrasive capacity of the dentifrice is too low, the abrasive agent is less effective in removing the soft deposits and stains. If it is too high, it may increase the likelihood of scratching tooth structure and/or restored tooth surfaces, initiate or increase hypersensitivity, or cause gingival irritation or abrasion. The risk is especially increased with excessive tooth brushing strength, horizontal brushing technique, and/or the utilization of medium or hard bristles.

The Mohs Hardness Scale, with values ranging from 1 (softest) to 10 (hardest), is useful for understanding abrasiveness of cleaning and polishing agents. Although dentifrice is not measured by the Mohs Hardness Scale, it can be useful to assess the potential abrasiveness—and accompanying risk—of components for unapproved or unregulated dentifrices. Fig. 26.6 shows the Mohs Hardness Scale and compares the hardness of minerals to different dental materials, abrasives, and tooth structures. The threshold of 2.0 to 2.5 is equal to the hardness of dentin, which is often exposed because of gingival recession and noncarious cervical lesions (NCCL). Figs. 26.7 to 26.10 show the NCCL and attrition. The hardness of dentin and cementum is lower than that of enamel due to its lower hydroxyapatite composition.[13] The Mohs scale is useful for understanding the abrasive potential of cleaning and polishing agents. For example, a dentifrice containing alumina (with a hardness of 9.25) is efficient for stain removal but has a higher risk of damaging tooth surfaces because its hardness level is higher than that of the tooth's enamel (4 to 5) and cementum (2.0 to 2.5). Thus alumina

has a very high abrasive potential, especially on teeth with NCCL, where the dentin is exposed.

Dentifrices with a level of abrasiveness of 2% or less are recommended to avoid tooth structure loss on exposed roots; however, even hard agents can be made safe by varying their particle size and shape in the manufacturing process.[14] Children can use a more abrasive dentifrice when their teeth complete their physiologic maturation (hardness level of 4 to 5).

Humectants

A **humectant** is a substance used to retain moisture, prevent air drying, and ensure a chemically and physically stable product. Glycerin, sorbitol, and polyethylene glycols are the three main humectants used in dentifrices. Low concentrations of synthetic cellulose are used as a humectant. In high concentrations, it is used as a binder to stabilize the gel or liquid gel dentifrice formula, and it also acts as a preservative.

Water

The list of dentifrice ingredients seldom specifies the type of water used (deionized, oxygenated, or distilled water). Dentifrices sold as pharmaceuticals contain water that meets the quality norms of the USP standards. Dentifrice tablets do not contain water; instead, they become active after dissolving in the saliva after chewing.

Preservatives

Preservatives are added to inhibit mold and bacterial growth and prolong shelf life. The more water the dentifrice formulation contains, the higher the quantity of preservatives should be. Note that many people are allergic to preservatives. Methylparaben is currently being studied for its obesogenic potential.[15,16]

Binders

Binders are used as thickeners and prevent liquid and solid ingredients in pastes and gels from separating. Gel formulas contain more binders than pastes. "Natural" dentifrice manufacturers tend to replace oil-based binders such as polyethylene glycol (PEG) with plant-based products, such as algae and agar-agar. Chitosan (e.g., Elmex Protection Erosion), a binder used in Europe and derived from shellfish, also has antibacterial properties. When associated with stannous ion (Sn²⁺), chitosan also provides better protection against erosion.[17] However, allergic reactions may occur if the patient is allergic to shellfish. Carboxymethyl cellulose is currently being studied for its obesogenic potential.[15,16]

Detergents

Foaming agents or detergents, called surfactants, are popular in dentifrices to lower surface tension to loosen debris and break up stains. However, SLS can contribute to recurrent aphthous ulcers or irritation

TABLE 26.6	Variables Influencing Dentifrice Abrasiveness
Particle size (grit)	The larger the particles, the more they wear on dental surfaces.
Particle shape	The more irregular the shape, the more dental surfaces are worn and abraded. A round particle is less detrimental to the tooth (see Fig. 26.5; see Table 26.7).
Particle hardness	The harder the particles, the more the dental surfaces are abraded (see Fig. 26.8).
pH level	The more acidic and abrasive, the more the dentifrice increases tooth surface mineral loss, particularly if dentin or cementum is exposed (see Fig. 26.7; see Table 26.7).
Quantity of glycerin and water in dentifrice	The higher the level of glycerin in a dentifrice, the higher its level of abrasiveness as the dissolution of insoluble materials is reduced. The greater the amount of water in a dentifrice, the more soluble particles can dissolve, making them less abrasive to dental surfaces.

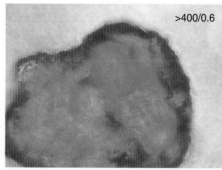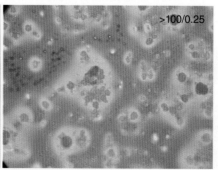

Fig. 26.5 Magnified picture to show irregular size and shape of particles. (Courtesy of GREDH [Group of Research and Education on Dental Hygiene], Québec, Canada.)

of oral mucosa. If such intolerance occurs, it is preferable to use a dentifrice containing cocamidopropyl betaine (e.g., Sensodyne ProNamel or Burt's Bees, Enamel Care). SLS also neutralizes the effects of chlorhexidine gluconate (CHG); therefore, patients using a dentifrice containing SLS should wait at least 30 minutes before using a CHG-containing oral rinse.[2]

Flavoring and Sweetening Agents

Ingredients are added to provide a refreshing flavor and aftertaste and to mask the taste of unpleasant chemical compounds. Xylitol is a sweetener and, in doses greater than 10%, is an effective antimicrobial agent to combat tooth decay and may have antiinflammatory potential (see Box 26.4).[18] Erythritol or stevia alternatives, noncariogenic sweeteners, are also used in the form of dentifrice tablets (DentTabs). However, some natural-origin nutritive sweeteners (polyols) such as sorbitol, xylitol, erythritol, and other nonnutritive artificial substitutes such as sucralose, are currently being investigated for their obesogenic (contributing to obesity) as well as thyroid and pancreatic disruption potential.[15,16] Certain flavors, such as cinnamon, can cause a burning sensation, tissue sloughing, contact stomatitis, intolerances, or allergic reactions.

Hardness	Minerals	Mohs scale	Dental structures	Abrasives	Dental materials
Softer	Talc	1		Potassium and sodium 0.04 to 0.05	
	Gypsum	2	Cementum, dentin : 2 to 2.5	Sodium dihydrate: 2.5 Dicalcium phosphate dihydrate (brushite): 2.5 Sodium bicarbonate: 2.5 to 3 Aluminum trihydroxide: 2.5 to 4 Hydrated silica dioxide: 2.5 to 5	Gold: 2 to 4 Acrylic for prosthesis: 2 to 3
	Calcite	3		Calcium carbonate: 3 Anhydrous dicalcium phosphate: 3.5	Gold alloy type IV: 3 to 4 Composite: 3 to 7
	Fluorite	4	Enamel: 4 to 5	Bioactives glasses 4.5 to 6	Amalgam: 4 to 5
	Apatite	5		Calcium pyrophosphate: 5 Tetracyclic pyrophosphate: 5 Perlite: 5.5 to 7	Composite resin: 5 to 7 Ionomer glass: 5 to 6
	Orthoclase	6		Pumice: 6 to 7 Silica, silica dioxide: 6 to 7	Ceramic: 6 to 7 Porcelain: 6 to 7 Ceramic CAD/CA: 6 to 7
	Quartz	7		Sand (quartz and silica): 7 Aluminum oxide: 7 to 9 Cuttlebone: 7	
	Topaz	8			
	Corundum	9		Alumina: 9.25	
Harder	Diamond	10			

Fig. 26.6 Comparison of hardness scales, abrasives, tooth surfaces, and dental materials. (Courtesy of Nadia Dubreuil. Adaptation of Mohs Scale [1812].)

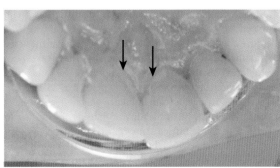

Fig. 26.7 Erosion. (Courtesy of Nadia Dubreuil.)

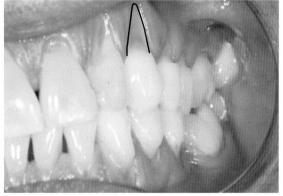

Fig. 26.8 Abrasion. (Courtesy of Nadia Dubreuil.)

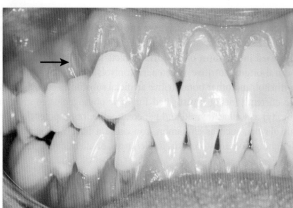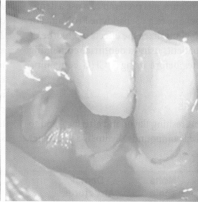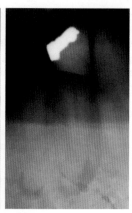

Fig. 26.9 Abfraction and dental fracture caused by abfraction. (Courtesy of Nadia Dubreuil.)

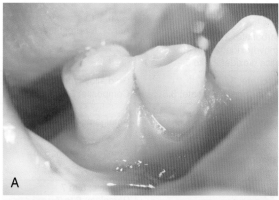

A

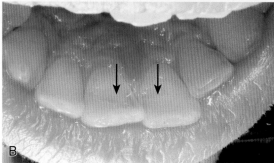

B

Fig. 26.10 Attrition. (A) Occlusal. (B) Lingual. (Courtesy of Nadia Dubreuil.)

Coloring Agents

Dyes make the product more attractive and may be used to obtain an aesthetic effect by optical manipulation. For example, covarine blue is a pigment that is deposited on the teeth to reduce their yellowish appearance. However, some coloring agents can have adverse health effects. Tartrazine (yellow #5), found in some dentifrices, may produce an allergic reaction, especially in patients hypersensitive to aspirin. Care must be taken with the nomenclature used to identify this coloring agent because tartrazine is also identified as E102 in Europe and yellow #5 or CI 19140 in North America.

Copolymers

Polyvinylmethoxyethylene and maleic acid (PVM/MA) copolymer is added into formulations of some dentifrices to increase substantivity, i.e., its duration in the mouth, and prolong the therapeutic effect. For example, Gantrez, the copolymer used with triclosan, is known to extend the antibacterial effect for 12 hours. Chitin is also a naturally

---

BOX 26.4   Xylitol

- Sugar alcohol and sugar substitute that is extracted mainly from birch bark, beechwood, corn cobs, and cane pulp.
- Anticaries, antiinflammatory, and antiplaque properties

---

occurring copolymer that is biodegradable, nontoxic, and comes from the shells of crab, lobster, and other shellfish. Dental hygienists should check for seafood allergies in the medical history to avoid allergic reactions before recommending products with this ingredient.

Therapeutic Effects, Therapeutic Agents, and Medicinal Ingredients

Ingredients added for specific preventive, treatment, or beneficial purposes are referred to as therapeutic agents or medicinal ingredients. For a dentifrice to be considered therapeutic, the manufacturer must follow strict pharmaceutical standards with regard to the quantity and bioavailability of therapeutic agents used, their safety, and their efficacy. The main therapeutic and medicinal agents in dentifrices are found in Table 26.1B. These agents are divided according to the therapeutic effects they provide or the needs of the population they address: anticaries, desensitizing, antigingivitis/antiplaque/oral biofilm reduction, anticalculus, antistain, and antihalitosis agents. In addition, each category is subdivided according to the specific medicinal agent used.

Anticaries and Remineralizing Agents

Fluoride and fluoride compounds. Fluoride is the ingredient that has the strongest evidence supporting its effectiveness in remineralization and caries prevention. Research also suggests that bacteria are less able to adhere to fluorapatite than nonfluoride-treated enamel.[8] Common fluorides found in daily-use dentifrice formulas include stannous fluoride (SnF_2), sodium fluoride (NaF), sodium monofluorophosphate (MFP), and amine fluoride (AmF). Some dentifrices combine multiple fluorides. For example, in some countries, dentifrices can combine SnF_2 with NaF.

A dentifrice with 0.24% NaF has an efficacy equivalent to a dentifrice containing 0.76% MFP (see Table 26.1B). These two concentrations are different because the agents do not have the same molecular weight. Most products contain about 1000 ppm (Box 26.5).[10]

Combinations of agents can influence their effectiveness. Some ingredients increase the bioavailability of fluoride (F) in their formulation. For example, a dentifrice containing cocamidopropyl betaine as a detergent has better bioavailability of F (discussed later) compared with a product containing SLS.[19] The abrasive particle calcium carbonate, combined with sodium MFP, is effective as an anticaries agent. The combination of 1.5% arginine (insoluble calcium compound) and fluoride increases anticaries efficacy.[20] In North America, some dentifrices combine lower concentration of fluoride with bioglass (F-BG) (see the following sections on New Ingredients or New Dentifrices).

Some dentifrice components, such as calcium, SnF_2, MFP, SLS, sodium dodecyl sulfate (SDS), and cocamidopropyl betaine (CAPB), reduce the substantivity and overall effectiveness of CHG; therefore, a patient brushing with a dentifrice should wait for at least 30 minutes before using a CHG-containing product.[2,19] NaF would be compatible with chlorhexidine.[19]

Bioavailability of fluorides. The **bioavailability** of fluoride is defined as the total amount of soluble fluoride, i.e., free ions available for remineralization. This amount of bioavailable fluoride may be less than the total amount of fluoride added to the dentifrice due to the inactivation of some of the fluoride ions by various ingredients in the formulation. For example, it is necessary to add between 0.188% and 0.254% (by weight) to obtain 650 ppm of NaF bioavailability of a dentifrice of about 1000 ppm of fluoride.[11] The bioavailability of fluorides in dentifrices is affected by the following factors:
- Type of fluoride: some types have less bioavailability, such as SnF_2, than others, such as NaF or AmF. Colgate Cavity Protection contains 1100 ppm in the United States and 1450 in Canada.
- Type of abrasive used in the formulation: calcium-based abrasives are only compatible with MFP, while silica is compatible with NaF, SnF_2, and amine fluoride.
- pH level: a pH lower than 6 in dentifrice or in saliva supports the incorporation of fluoride ions.
- Other ingredients: SLS and calcium pyrophosphate may interfere with fluoride effectiveness or bioavailability.

Some manufacturers use cocamidopropyl betaine as a detergent instead of SLS to increase the bioavailability of fluoride ions. Colgate-Palmolive (Prevident Sensitive) and GlaxoSmithKline (Sensodyne ProNamel) use this detergent. Using cocamidopropyl betaine as a detergent improves the availability of fluoride ions and offers better caries protection or remineralization.[19,21]

Nonfluoride anticaries components. In order to offer alternatives to fluorinated products, dentifrices containing calcium and phosphate technologies enhance the bioavailability of calcium and phosphate ions for incorporation into the tooth surface (see Table 26.1B). These minerals aid in the enhancement of remineralization and reduce dentinal sensitivity:
- Calcium sodium phosphosilicate (CSP) or NovaMin, (e.g., Oravive) is a bioglass that releases ions of calcium, phosphate, and sodium when exposed to saliva (pH of approximately 7 or neutral). The sodium is intended to buffer acid in the oral cavity and, over time, the calcium and phosphate ions are available to assist with surface remineralization. These various calcium phosphate compounds are also used for desensitization.
- Hydroxyapatite (HAP) (e.g., X-Pur Remin, SirinMed Hyper Sensitive, Risewell Kids) is deposited on the tooth and in the biofilm. It remineralizes and rebuilds the tooth by releasing calcium ions and phosphates that diffuse into the carious lesion and the rest of the

tooth structure. HAP would be comparable to fluorides for remineralization of weakened enamel.[22] However, remineralization by HAP is most effective on demineralized tooth structures (e.g., caries or after consuming acidic foods or beverages). HAP reduces the potential demineralization of biofilm due to the buffering of pH and therefore protects the tooth from further acid attack. HAP helps to clean the tooth (acts as an abrasive) and reduces the adhesion of plaque after the reconstruction of dental structures. Health Canada certifies that HAP can be safely swallowed by children aged 2 and over.[21]
- A combination of calcium and phosphate is used in dentifrice without fluoride or in combination with fluoride. For example, calcium glycerophosphate (e.g., Nature's Gate, fluoride-free) and dicalcium phosphate (e.g., Wondermint) are used in dentifrice without fluoride. Tricalcium phosphate (TCP) or tricalcium diphosphate is combined with fluoride to enhance remineralization (e.g., Prevident Booster Plus or 3M Clinpro). The casein phosphopeptide (milk protein), combined with amorphous calcium phosphate (CPP-ACP) (e.g., Recaldent in MI Paste), is intended to remineralize teeth and add luster. However, this protein has less efficacy in acidic conditions than in optimal conditions (neutral pH: 7). Patients who are allergic to dairy products must not use CPP-ACP due to the presence of casein.
- Some products combine nonfluorinated components with fluoride in order to improve the remineralization process—for example, CSP with MFP (e.g., Sensodyne Repair & Protect), HAP with MFP (e.g., Signal White Now Sensitive), and CPP-ACP with NaF (e.g., GC MI Paste Plus).

Protection against dental erosion. Enamel that is not enriched with fluoride starts its demineralization at a pH of 5.5. The exposure of enamel to fluorides contributes to the formation of fluorapatite crystals, which are more resistant to acid attacks since the demineralization process for fluorapatite starts at a pH of 4.5. Thus all fluorides contribute to the protection of enamel against dental erosion. However, dentifrices containing SnF_2, combined or not, would provide an additional benefit due to the deposit of tin ions on the surface of the enamel, which would provide additional protection against tooth erosion.[23]

Antimicrobial components targeting caries pathogens. Bacterial flora initiate caries, so some dentifrices contain antimicrobial agents such as polyols (xylitol, sorbitol, and erythritol), complex enzymes and proteins, and minerals to act as anticaries or antibacterial agents (see Table 26.1B). Xylitol, in a therapeutic dose of 1.55 g (minimum of 5 g used daily in the oral cavity) or 10% in dentifrice, decreases *Streptococcus mutans* levels and plaque biofilm and its adhesion to the tooth (Box 26.4). Since *S. mutans* cannot metabolize xylitol, this results in a reduction and inhibition of the growth of *S. mutans* due to the degradation of the cell membrane and consequently a decrease in acidity that demineralizes the tooth structure.[18]

Noncariogenic sweeteners reduce plaque by inhibiting biofilm growth and decrease plaque adhesion by reducing sticky polysaccharides produced by *S. mutans*. They increase oral pH by salivary stimulation and provide antiinflammatory potential by inhibiting proteins related to inflammation.[18] Arginine decreases the risk of caries when it is degraded by certain streptococci (*Streptococcus sanguinis* and *Streptococcus gordonii*) of the biofilm, modifies the composition of the oral microbiota, and decreases the metabolic activity of sucrose by neutralizing its acidifying effect.[20]

Desensitizing Agents

To prevent or reduce hypersensitivity, products with neutral pH and known to be abrasively safe are recommended (see Chapter 42; see Table 26.1B). Patients with dentinal hypersensitivity should choose a low-abrasive and pH-neutral dentifrice, brush no more than twice a day, and avoid any consumption of acidic products immediately before brushing. Otherwise, toothbrushing should be delayed for at least 60 minutes, after consuming any acidic foods or beverages.[24,25]

The availability of chemotherapeutic agents may vary from country to country, e.g., products in North America containing strontium chloride and strontium acetate have been replaced by SnF_2. The mode of action of desensitizing medicinal ingredients are:

- Mechanically blocking dentinal tubules: NovaMin, a calcium sodium phosphosilicate (in Oravive, SootheRx, and DenShield); SnF_2, (Colgate Renewal, Sensodyne Rapid Relief, Crest GUM Detoxify); strontium acetate hemihydrate (Sensodyne Rapid Relief, available in Brazil and China); strontium chloride (Sensodyne Original, available in the United Arab Emirates); a compound with a concentration of 8% arginine, calcium carbonate and MFP (Colgate Pro-Relief) or a high level of fluoride (5000 ppm and above, such as Fluodontyl 13,500 ppm) that promotes remineralization. Mechanical filling of dentinal tubules offers a more durable protection against hypersensitivity than chemical agents due to their retention.
- Chemically preventing depolarization of nerve fibers in the tooth (nerve impulse transmission): potassium nitrate or potassium citrate does this, but unfortunately, its effect is temporary after the client stops using the dentifrice.
- Mechanical and chemical action: a 5000 ppm fluoride product is effective in reducing dentinal hypersensitivity (Colgate PreviDent 5000 ppm Sensitive 1.1% NaF and 5% potassium nitrate).

The various therapeutic agents have demonstrated specific efficacy in relation to the various stimuli (air, cold, and touch). For example, NovaMin technology is said to help with all three stimuli. SnF_2 and HAP are effective in treating tactile and air sensitivities. Arginine, on the other hand, would be effective in treating air sensitivity only.[26]

Antigingivitis and Oral Biofilm Reduction Agents

Daily and effective control of biofilm is very important since it proliferates rapidly, so dentifrices can have antibacterial ingredients (see Table 26.1B) such as triclosan with copolymer, CHG, stannous fluoride (SnF_2), zinc citrate, and others. These antibacterial ingredients help to reduce the risk of cavities and periodontal disease. The antimicrobial effect has an impact on oral and overall health by providing a reduction in chronic inflammation and eliminating certain harmful gram-negative bacteria from the oral microbiota such as *Porphyromonas gingivalis* (Pg). The is necessary to prevent the development of periodontitis and may also help prevent other systemic diseases (see Chapter 21).

Triclosan (not available in the United States and Canada). Triclosan, a bisphenol, is a broad-spectrum antimicrobial agent (most gram-positive and gram-negative bacteria, mycobacterium, strictly anaerobic bacteria, and also against the spore of the fungi of *Candida sp.*) with antiplaque and antigingivitis properties. The mechanism of its antiseptic action consists in acting on the microbial cytoplasmic membrane by inducing leakage of cellular constituent and thereby causing lysis of the microorganism. Scientific evidence has shown that triclosan slows the progression of periodontal disease.

While available in some countries, triclosan (0.3%) with PVM/MA (Gantrez) copolymer (2%) and NaF is no longer available in North America due to potential adverse effects (endocrine-related disturbance, gastrointestinal issues, risk factor for breast cancer, and obesogenic).[8,15,27] In some countries, triclosan is considered a restricted active ingredient due to the detection of traces in water systems.[6] Health Canada notes that triclosan discharged into sewers may endanger the aquatic ecosystem. A dentifrice containing active oxygen and lactoferrin has shown promise in having comparable antiplaque and antigingivitis efficacy to dentifrices containing triclosan.[28]

Chlorhexidine gluconate (CHG or CHX). CHG is an ingredient that effectively controls dental plaque formation and gingivitis.[2] CHG binds to proteins with limited capacity for absorption by the body and is therefore substantive for 12 hours. Its antibacterial action is due to the disruption that it causes to bacteria by increasing the permeability of their cell membranes, thus provoking the lysis of the cells. It is particularly effective against gram-positive and gram-negative bacteria and yeasts.[29] CHG is available in different concentrations. GUM Gingidex dentifrice contains 0.06% CHG and GUM Paroex dentifrice contains 0.12% CHG to control gingivitis and plaque. Both contain 0.05% cetylpyridinium chloride. Curaprox PerioPlus contains a combination of bioflavonoids (citrus extracts) and CHG 0.09%.

Stannous fluoride (SnF_2). This fluoride is recognized as the new gold standard because of its bactericidal and bacteriostatic properties.[8] Stannous fluoride is known for its antiplaque, anticaries, and desensitizing effect as well as for preventing or reducing tooth enamel erosion. SnF_2, when formulated with other ingredients with high bioavailability, has also demonstrated reductions in plaque adhesion and gingivitis. It slows the metabolic production of toxins by binding to gram-negative anaerobes toxins and thus prevents activation of destructive host response, which can reduce gingivitis and bleeding. When it binds to the HAP film, SnF_2 forms a protective shield against dental erosion.

SnF_2 is thought to reduce calculus via its antibacterial and antiplaque action; however, the majority of dentifrices tested in the studies that demonstrated this therapeutic effect also contained anticalculus agents such as metaphosphates (SHMP) and zinc derivatives.[30] Several manufacturers offer a product containing SnF_2. The GC Company has developed a new dentifrice combining SnF_2 and CPP-ACP (e.g., MI Paste ONE Perio). Crest Gum Detoxify has received the ADA Seal of Acceptance for safety and efficacy for all of the above properties except for anticalculus.

Studies have found that SnF_2 is comparable to triclosan.[27,31] However, tin byproducts have the potential to stain the acquired pellicle and cause staining in long-term users of SnF_2 dentifrice.[8] Formulations containing combinations of SnF_2 and SHMP or pyrophosphates would have reduced tooth stain.[30]

Enzymes and proteins. Some dentifrices contain enzymes and/or antibacterial proteins (e.g., Zendium) (see Table 26.1B). They are added to reduce the risk of caries or to compensate for insufficient or absent components in cases of hyposalivation or xerostomia. Recently, Secretory Calcium-binding Phosphoprotein Proline-Glutamine Rich 1 (SCPPPQ1), an antibacterial protein against Pg, was the subject of a study suggesting its inclusion in the composition of dentifrices to seal the epithelial attachment as a natural barrier against the entry of pathogenic bacteria that can access the whole body.[32]

Ethylenediaminetetraacetic acid (EDTA). A specialized formulation of 2.6% EDTA (LIVFRESH Dental Gel [Livionex]) has been shown to have good substantivity and a great ability to diffuse through the biofilm and bind to hydroxyapatite. This binding increases the negative charge of dental molecules, which naturally repel plaque bacteria and neutralize positively charged calcium ions. This EDTA formulation is reported to help reduce periodontal pocket depth, inflammation, and gum bleeding when compared with SnF_2 in patients with stage 1 and 2 periodontitis (in the absence of prior periodontal treatment).[33]

Anticalculus Agents

Polyphosphates, metaphosphates, zinc derivatives, and EDTA. Zinc chloride and zinc citrate are accepted by the ADA as supragingival calculus-inhibiting agents (see Table 26.1B).[2] Polyphosphate (pyrophosphate, sodium tripolyphosphates, sodium triphosphate), metaphosphates (sodium hexametaphosphate or sodium trimetaphosphate), and zinc salts bind to calcium ions to inhibit the mineralization of biofilm before its transformation into supragingival calculus. Livionex has also demonstrated the property to neutralize excess calcium ions in saliva to prevent these ions from precipitating and forming dental calculus.[34] Pyrophosphates, metaphosphates, and zinc derivatives can be added to the antiplaque ingredients (SnF_2). Thus their combination provides an anticalculus effect in addition to the antibacterial effect of SnF_2.

However, pyrophosphates also have undesirable effects. They can cause gingival irritation and, due to their high affinity to bind to HAP in tooth enamel, inhibit the formation of calcium phosphate thus delaying the remineralization process of the tooth. As a result, the period of demineralization may be prolonged, making the tooth more vulnerable to NCCL, caries, and dental hypersensitivity. These adverse effects should be taken into account when recommending a dentifrice and it is the reason that a dentifrice containing pyrophosphate should only be used by people aged 12 years and older.

Antistain or Whitening Effect: Methods of Action

The cosmetic effect of teeth whitening can be achieved by one or a combination of the following actions (Fig. 26.11). The **mechanical action** of abrasive agents prevents or removes extrinsic stains (see Table 26.1A). However, dental hygienists must be cautious when recommending dentifrices containing some abrasives, such as alumina. This abrasive is harder than enamel and cementum and may increase abrasion on root exposures beyond that of a regular dentifrice, especially with rigorous toothbrushing or excessive pressure. An in vitro study has demonstrated that the combination of acidic pH (up to 7), abrasive dentifrice, and toothbrushing significantly increases loss of dental structure.[35] Another in vitro study showed that one whitening dentifrice with hydrogen peroxide and another one with charcoal both caused a decrease in the gloss of polymer composites and also negatively affected their hardness and roughness.[36]

Chemical action helps to break down the organic molecules that make up the stains. It is produced by peroxides or enzymes (papain, bromelain) that oxidize or degrade the pigments bound to the tooth surface.[8] However, the time of exposure to the dentifrice containing peroxide, its instability, and its dilution in saliva and water limits its

effectiveness. Dentifrices with peroxides can also cause hypersensitivity and are not recommended for children under 12.[8] Some agents (e.g., polyphosphate and sodium citrate) prevent or inhibit the redeposit (antiredeposition agents) of organic chromophores on the teeth or inhibit calculus formation.[37] It is assumed that they bind to the enamel surface, preventing redeposition of chromogens after a whitening treatment.[8]

Physical action includes the incorporation of calcium and phosphate (HAP, ACP) on the surface or in the microporosities of the tooth, improving the luster of the tooth and providing a better reflection of light. The addition of dye (covarine blue) induces an optical manipulation, causing a change in color perception from yellow to blue. The following agents contribute to the whitening effect.

Hydrogen and calcium peroxide. Hydrogen or calcium peroxide can remove extrinsic stains, chemically whiten teeth, assist in the control of halitosis, and have antigingivitis properties. As mentioned earlier, any daily whitening dentifrice should have a neutral pH because daily use of acidic dentifrices can damage the teeth and dental restorations, and irritate the gums. Currently, whitening dentifrices containing peroxide have a neutral or basic pH. However, whitening gels intended for use as a single or second step are medium acidic or acidic. They should be used with caution, as demineralized enamel is at greater risk of dental erosion.

Sodium bicarbonate. Sodium bicarbonate, or baking soda, is moderately abrasive when used dry. When dissolved in water or glycerin, it becomes a mild abrasive. Baking soda has also been proven effective to neutralize acids produced by acidogenic bacteria that cause demineralization, control extrinsic staining, reduce halitosis, and have a mild antibacterial effect. In addition, its buffering effect neutralizes other acids of extrinsic origin.[38] It can be combined with hydrogen peroxide for teeth whitening and fluoride for an anticaries effect (Arm and Hammer Extreme Whitening).

Polyphosphates. Anticalculus agents also have the ability to interact with the stained film by removing the stain material and preventing the absorption of new chromogens by depositing a protective layer on the tooth.[8,30]

Charcoal dentifrices. Of various origins, activated charcoal powders and dentifrices have gained a lot of popularity over the years. To date, no scientific evidence currently supports any claims of whitening or antibacterial properties for these dentifrices. Due to its high porosity and the wide surface area of its nanocrystalline form of carbon, the use of powder or charcoal dentifrice without Seal approval could induce a decrease in the bioavailability of fluoride. Charcoal products could lead to several adverse effects including increased tooth roughness, enamel and gum abrasion, hypersensitivity, heightened risk of cavities, tattooing of the marginal gingiva, or interaction with medications (see Fig. 26.12).[39]

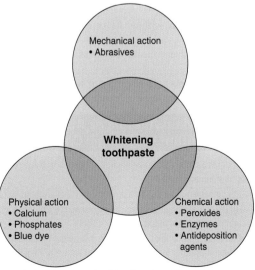

Fig. 26.11 Mode of action of whitening dentifrices. (Courtesy of Nadia Dubreuil.)

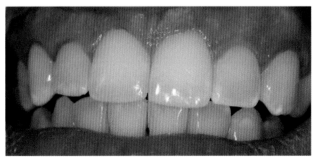

Fig. 26.12 Gum tattooing following the use of activated charcoal powder. The patient used the activated charcoal powder 3 times a week for 6 months. The photo was taken 3 months after the last use of it. (Courtesy of Stéphanie Beaulieu, RHD.)

Antihalitosis Agents

Halitosis is caused by multiple extra- and intraoral factors. Extraoral factors can include odorous foods (garlic, onion), bad habits (smoking), and hyposalivation or xerostomia. Tongue coating, periodontal disease, and poor oral hygiene are the leading intraoral causes of halitosis. An infection in the ear-nose-throat system (sinusitis, tonsillitis) is the second leading intraoral factor, followed by gastrointestinal reflux (gastroesophageal reflux) and endocrine system disorders (diabetes, kidney disease).

In the case of systemic diseases and ear-nose-throat problems, the dental hygienist's intervention is limited, and the patient should be referred to a specialist. When the cause is topical, the dental hygienist may recommend appropriate products to meet the patient's needs more efficiently.

Some medicinal agents act directly on bacteria and anaerobic microorganisms that produce volatile sulfur compounds (VSCs) (see Table 26.1B). Zinc and its derivatives are the most efficient agents to reduce VSCs. They interact with VSCs by degrading them into odorless VSC-free byproducts.[8] Antibacterial agents (triclosan, SnF_2) or oxygenating agents (chlorine dioxide or peroxides) could eliminate the bacteria that can produce VSCs; however, the lack of scientific evidence regarding their efficacy calls into question these alternative therapies.[40]

New Ingredients or New Dentifrices

It is important to be vigilant with the arrival of new products. The dental hygienist and patients are often confronted with aggressive marketing of products sold on the Internet or in pharmacies. These dentifrices are sometimes very expensive ($20 and over).

New dentifrices with new ingredients have appeared on the Internet, containing, for example:

- Fluorided bioactive glasses (F-BG), like BioMin-F (5%) with 530 ppm of fluoride, is a fluorocalcium phosphosilicate (F-CPS) that could increase the duration of fluoride bioavailability (12 hours) while reducing dentinal hypersensitivity.[41,42] However, independent double-blind clinical studies are needed to validate these claims. An in vitro study compared the effectiveness of NovaMin, BioMin, and Remin Pro remineralizing cream for remineralization of an artificial carious-like lesion. The efficacy of the products was similar except for Remin Pro, which demonstrated superior efficacy.[43]

  In Canada, another bioactive glass (Sensi-IP) has been developed and provides desensitizing properties by tubular occlusion. According to an in vitro study, this new ingredient would provide superior occlusion of dentinal tubules compared to NovaMin and Arginine.[44] To date, no double-blind study is available.

- Erythritol is a polyol, compatible with xylitol, that is newly added to dentifrices. In tablet form, erythritol is reported to be more effective than xylitol and sorbitol in reducing the level of *S. mutans*. However, no double-blind studies of erythritol dentifrice are currently available.[45]

- Aragonite, which is derived from ground and processed cuttlebone, is an abrasive softer than enamel and dentin that can prevent and reduce calculus buildup without damaging dental structures. Aragonite nanocrystals, characterized by a relatively high surface area, have sharp angle forms that give an abrasive particle design that are ideal to achieve fragmentation and cutting calculus deposits. This promising new ingredient has shown that a dentifrice containing aragonite (Dr. D-Tart) can also help improve gum health and control stains.[46]

- Biomimetic hydroxyapatite nanocrystal (Biorepair, containing microRepair [15% to 20% HAP]) is composed of zinc-substituted carbonate-hydroxyapatite with superior remineralizing and desensitizing properties compared to dentifrices containing 1400 ppm fluoride. Some of these dentifrices are approved by the Association of Italian Dental Hygienists (AIDI Pro).[22]

- Cannabidiol (CBD), a chemical compound found in cannabis, is believed to improve oral health by inhibiting biofilm formation due to potential antimicrobial properties against gram-negative and gram-positive bacteria. The possible antiinflammatory properties would be induced by its action on the immune response, the complex mechanism of which is not yet fully understood.[47] As of the time of writing this chapter, the FDA does not approve dentifrices containing CBD.[5] In Canada, the sale of dentifrices containing CBD is authorized in certain provinces, but interprovincial export is prohibited.[6] In the United States, these CBD-containing dentifrices and mouthwashes may be available for purchase in states where cannabis is legalized.

DENTIFRICES: ADVERSE HEALTH EFFECTS

A dentifrice has a therapeutic function when it prevents or controls oral disease or condition.[1] It can also be a risk factor if it causes hypersensitivity or erosion or abrasion of dentin (Figs. 26.7 and 26.8). Therefore a dentifrice should be selected based on each patient's specific needs. For example, in addition to the assessment of saliva quantity, a patient with root exposures should be counseled regarding abrasivity, the role of pH, and the source of the product. Thus the choice of dentifrice is an important consideration for the healthcare professional as this product has a direct impact on the patient's dental health, overall health, and quality of life. Assessment of the patient's medical, dental, and pharmacological history is essential to ensure that the patient has no medical conditions, allergies, or medications that would contraindicate a particular dentifrice recommendation.

Medicinal and nonmedicinal ingredients in dentifrice may cause various or combined adverse reactions and affect the overall health of patients with allergies or intolerances. These reactions may occur during or after the use of a traditional or herbal dentifrice. The reaction may occur either after direct contact with the allergen or after exposure to an excessively high dose. Of the ingredients identified in Tables 26.2 and 26.3, flavoring agents are the leading cause of contact allergic reactions, followed by cocamidopropyl betaine and propylene glycol.[2,48] Dentifrices containing unidentified aromatic ingredients should be avoided in patients with allergies or adverse reactions. Box 26.6 provides a complete list of the major allergic or adverse reactions.[49] In addition, Table 26.5 suggests flavoring agents with low allergenicity. Naturally, a dentifrice without flavor has a lower risk of allergic reaction.

Some additional adverse health effects associated with dentifrices are as follows:

- Children and patients with cognitive or swallowing disorders may unfortunately swallow a dentifrice with unsafe ingredients.

BOX 26.6 Main Allergic or Adverse Reactions (Irritant or Allergic Contact)

- Cheilitis: inflamed lips, eczema-like itch, pain, dermatitis, edema, fissured, dryness, swollen and blistering
- Stomatitis: inflamed mouth, acute or chronic, affecting gums (gingivitis), tongue (glossitis), burning mouth sensation or oral pain, redness, swelling, and peeling of the gums, tongue, lips, and cheeks
- Perioral eczema and contact leukoderma: whitening of the skin around mouth
- Contact urticaria: immediate swelling of the lips or eczematous cheilitis
- Dyspnea

- Some ingredients can contribute to hard tissue (abrasion, staining) and sometimes soft tissue damage, especially in patients with gastroesophageal reflux disease (GERD).
- The use of adult dentifrices containing pyrophosphate derivatives in children under 12 increases the risk of caries.[12]
- Low-pH dentifrices that are very abrasive, combined with improper brushing technique, can cause adverse reactions such as dental erosion and abrasion.[35]
- Patients with gingival sensitivity (lichen planus, mucositis) could be sensitive to the acidity of fluoride.[2]
- A bitter taste or taste alteration, burning sensation, gingival abrasion, dry mouth, and enamel erosion are also adverse effects reported by users of cosmetic or whitening dentifrices.[2]
- Gum tattooing can occur in charcoal powder users.[39]

Insoluble, Soluble Materials, and Nanoparticles

Dentifrices contain both insoluble and water-soluble ingredients.[1] Ingredients in dentifrices that cannot dissolve in water are **insoluble materials**. Ingredients that dissolve in water are **soluble materials**, such as sodium bicarbonate. **Nanoparticles** are insoluble and vary in size from 1 to 100 nanometers, which allows them to infiltrate cells or bacteria. Insoluble abrasives, such as silica or alumina, remain intact in water. Some plant extracts such as goldenseal, lithothamnion (seaweed), horsetail, and sage are often found in natural dentifrices and are also insoluble in water. The large amount of insoluble materials contained in dentifrices such as Jasön and Nutrismile C maintains a high rate of abrasiveness. On the other hand, dentifrices with low levels of insoluble matter are often less abrasive, making them mild to dental surfaces (e.g., Aquafresh Whitening).[1,14]

The nanoparticles currently used in dentifrices are HAP, zinc (Zn), silver (Ag)—which is not approved by the FDA in the United States and is restricted by Health Canada—zinc oxide (ZnO), chitosan, casein phosphopeptide-amorphous calcium phosphate (CPP-ACP), bioactive glasses, and charcoal. Some have an antibacterial effect (e.g., zinc), which may contribute to the reduction of caries, gingivitis, and periodontitis. Others increase protection against dental hypersensitivity (e.g., HAP and CCP-ACP). However, some of these particles are known to accumulate in the human body or to disrupt living cells.[50] Some nanomaterials are a risk factor when they cross the brain barrier (e.g., aluminum) or into healthy cells (e.g., titanium dioxide in the placenta).[51] Thus they can be deposited in the brain and contribute to dementia. In several countries, various regulations require manufacturers to mention the presence of nanomaterials on their labels by writing [nano].[6,52] Currently, more research is needed to establish the direct link between the absorption by the oral mucosa of nanomaterials contained in dentifrices and overall health problems.

Advantages and Disadvantages of Higher Abrasive Levels (More Than 2%)

A dentifrice with a high abrasive level can increase abrasion in a patient with exposed root surfaces and can cause dentinal hypersensitivity. However, in a patient without root exposures but with heavy quantities of oral biofilm, a more abrasive dentifrice removes biofilm and acquired pellicle faster than a less abrasive agent. Fortunately, the acquired pellicle reforms quickly and can protect enamel against erosion. The presence and quality of the acquired film is a protective factor.[53] By contrast, using a highly abrasive dentifrice on enamel that has been weakened by mild demineralization can cause the surface enamel to collapse, causing early cavitation.

A highly abrasive dentifrice can also damage the surface of aesthetic restorations and/or titanium implants. Since damaged or rough restorative materials retain bacteria more easily, a dentifrice with low abrasiveness is recommended for persons with aesthetic restorations and/or titanium implants.

Many common brands have slightly higher abrasive levels without being excessive (less than 4%) for patients needing more abrasiveness to effectively remove biofilm (e.g., Crest Gum Detoxify Deep Clean, Colgate Sensitive Pro-Relief Complete Protection). Some dentifrices with natural ingredients, such as Nature's Gate Anise Cream, have an abrasiveness of 6.18%.[14] See Box 26.7 and Table 26.7 for an overview of abrasiveness and the potential loss of dental structures.

Comparison of Methods Used to Evaluate Dentifrice Abrasiveness

The main protocols for testing abrasivity are the **"Relative Dentin Abrasivity"** (RDA) scale and the **"Relative Enamel Abrasivity"** (REA) scale (which is less widely used). Since 2017, the RDA test has been unanimously recognized as an international standard (ISO 11609) and established as the gold standard.[54] In addition to measuring mineral loss after irradiation of a healthy human tooth sample, the test uses profilometry to measure the depth of ridges left after brushing. This standardized scale, whose values vary from 1 to 250, has been simplified into three levels (see Table 26.8).[54]

The RDA test is required of manufacturers prior to marketing a new dentifrice to control quality standards. The RDA is not a safety standard. The ADA does not recommend comparing RDA values between products to compare dentifrices to each other since the RDA values

BOX 26.7 Results from the GREDH's Abrasiveness Scale and Potential Loss of Dental Structures

- Approximately 80% of dentifrices fall below 2% on the Abrasiveness Scale, meaning they do not risk damaging dentin or exposing cementum and of these, about 40% are considered "not very abrasive."
- About 20% of dentifrices are very abrasive.
- Dentifrices such as Tom's of Maine, Clean & Fresh (4.32%), and powder dentifrice Poudre à dent Herbale (9.15%) are more abrasive than enamel (Mohs Hardness Score of 4 to 5) and can damage tooth structures.

TABLE 26.7 Abrasiveness Scale of GREDH and Potential for Loss of Dental Structures

Low abrasive: 0.00% to 0.87%
Moderately abrasive: 0.88% to 1.36%
Abrasive: 1.37% to 1.99%
Very abrasive: 2% and more *2% to 3.99%: risk for dentin and cementum* *4.0% and more: risk for enamel, dentin, and cementum*

TABLE 26.8 Relative Dentin Abrasivity (RDA) Scale

RDA Score	Level of Efficiency on Healthy Dental Structures*
0 to 100	Less efficient to remove tooth stains
100 to 250	Efficient to remove stains
Over 250	Not recommended, damaging for teeth Seal not granted by ADA or CDA

*Clinical dental conditions may influence the level of abrasiveness and should be taken into consideration in professional advice.

are manufacturing standards, not product safety standards,[3] and they do not take into account potential clinical changes in enamel that may affect tooth structure loss.

Dentifrices that have obtained the ADA or CDA Seal of Acceptance have achieved an RDA value of 250 or less. Dentifrices that have obtained an RDA value of 250 or more cannot be marketed because they are too abrasive and are considered dangerous. On the Internet, many dentifrices are marketed without having obtained the ADA or CDA Seal of Acceptance, which means the organizations do not certify that the product meets the Seal safety and efficacy criteria.

When recommending a dentifrice to a patient, in addition to the abrasivity index, dental hygienists must evaluate other important variables in the loss of tooth structure, which is multifactorial. For example, contributing factors include the presence of demineralization, the absence or composition of saliva, an acidic diet, an acidic oral environment due to health problems (eating disorders, gastroesophageal reflux), bruxism, the brushing method and the characteristics of the brush used (hardness of the bristles, electric toothbrush without a pressure indicator), the presence of an acquired film, and root exposures related to the lower hardness of the exposed cementum and dentin compared to the enamel.

The Group of Research and Education in Dental Hygiene (GREDH)[14] uses the single protocol and scale abrasivity, which allows comparison of dentifrices and prophylactic pastes from different manufacturers, taking into account the levels of safety for cement, dentin, and enamel (Table 26.9).

Nonprescription Drug, Natural Health Products, and Cosmetic Products

In Canada and the United States, dentifrices are regulated under the Food and Drugs Act, which is divided into three regulations (Cosmetic Products, Natural Health Products or National Drug Code, Food and Drugs). Dentifrices must meet the standards of the Cosmetic Products or Natural Health Products Regulations. The cosmetic regulations are less stringent than the other two regulations (see Table 26.10).[5,6] Most products will have an NPN number in Canada or an NDC number in the United States, and manufacturers can put a claim on their product, e.g., prevents cavities, reduces dental hypersensitivity, whitening, etc. Some of these dentifrices are available only by prescription in some countries.

To obtain a DIN, the product must meet the requirements of the Food and Drug Regulations and provide a high level of scientific evidence, such as clinical trials, conducted prior to marketing a drug. In the United States, a prescription product must also meet the criteria of the FDA in order to receive an NDC.[55]

Dentifrice pH

The potential of the hydrogen molecule (pH) of a substance is measured on a scale from 1 to 14. Level 1 is very acidic, 7 is neutral, and 14 is very basic (alkaline). The pH of a dentifrice can be beneficial or detrimental to dental structures while interfering in the demineralization–remineralization process (see Box 26.8). The majority of dentifrices have a neutral pH, but a few products have a pH between 3 and 10.[14]

Low or Acidic pH

Advantages for tooth enamel. Acidity of a dentifrice promotes the formation of fluorapatite by facilitating the incorporation of fluoride ions into the enamel crystals. Fluorapatite crystals are characteristically larger, more stable, and less acid soluble. Therefore, a low pH is a desirable characteristic in fluoride dentifrices.[35]

Disadvantages in the case of root exposure or titanium implants. Low pH contributes to the erosion of tooth structure. Because demineralization of dentin and cementum occurs at an average pH of 6.5, dental hygienists must identify root exposures to avoid tooth

TABLE 26.9 Comparison of Dental Products in Terms of Abrasiveness and pH

Products	Abrasiveness (%)	pH
Pursonic, activated coconut, charcoal powder, peppermint and lemon, essential oil powder	11.84	9.06
Herbal tooth powder (polishes and removes calculus from teeth)	9.45	7.14
Denticare Medicom, Pro-Polish, prophy paste, bubble gum, fine	7.03	8.67
Nature's Gate, anise cream, dentifrice	6.18	8.53
Crest Gum Detoxify, Gentle Whitening, dentifrice	2.71	6.28
Crest Pro-Health, Whitening, clean mint, dentifrice	2.69	5.49
Arm and Hammer, Cow Brand, baking soda*	0.98	N/A
Gel-Kam, mint flavor	0.24	3.2
Arm and Hammer, Cow Brand, baking soda with water 1:1	0.06	8.4
Water	0.00	6.9
Hydrogen peroxide USP 3%/10 vol.	0.00	4.9
Baking soda with peroxide 1:1	0.00	8.3

*Dry, without water or any other liquid; assessed using GREDH Scale.[17]
Courtesy of GREDH (Group of Research and Education on Dental Hygiene), Québec, Canada.

TABLE 26.10 Cosmetic, Natural Products, and Food and Drug Regulations

Regulations Standards	Cosmetic Products	Natural Products	Food and Drug
Regulatory reference number	None	NPN or NDC	DIN or NDC
Safety tested (toxicity)	No	Yes	Yes
Therapeutic efficacy tested (action on health)	No	Variable	Yes
Quality tested (controlled manufacturing)	Variable	Yes	Yes
Scientific evidence (level of proof)	None or low	Moderate	High (mandatory clinical trials)
Controlled by the FDA or Health Canada	No or little	Yes	Yes
Product under prescription	No	Variable	Yes
Examples	Charcoal powder	Dentifrices containing medicinal ingredients (see Table 26.1B)	None in Canada and the United States

mineral loss and dentinal hypersensitivity. Low pH can also tarnish titanium implants and affect composite restorations as well as fissure dental sealants.[2]

Neutral and Basic pH

Advantages for teeth and mucous membrane. Because of the similarities to healthy saliva, a neutral or basic pH is less irritating and not cytotoxic to soft tissues and does not demineralize teeth. Saliva and its components serve as a reservoir, ensure the bioavailability of fluoride, provide buffering and immune defense, etc.

Disadvantages for teeth and gums. Dentifrice pH levels are relevant in comparison between products and should be included in the labeling to allow the patient to make an informed choice. Neutral or basic pH levels promote the mineralization of biofilm (calculus formation), which in turn supports the retention of biofilm and extrinsic stains. Most dentifrices have a neutral or basic pH.[14] The pH of acidic or highly acidic dentifrices (approximately 10% of the market) is below the critical threshold of demineralization of enamel. However, a dentifrice with a pH under 6.5 demineralizes and weakens exposed root surfaces. Of available dentifrices, approximately 20% of them are below this critical threshold of demineralization of dentin or cementum.[14]

The combination of toothbrushing, xerostomia, acidity, and high abrasiveness of the dentifrice can further increase the loss of dental substance.[35] According to the ADA, dentifrices bearing the Seal of Acceptance contain a safe level of abrasives, but the organization makes no mention of pH levels.[3] For example, Crest Pro-Health, which carries the ADA Seal of Acceptance, has a pH of 5.5.[3,14] This pH may risk root surface demineralization in patients with gingival recession and hyposalivation. Although important for fluoride uptake, more research is needed on dentifrice pH and its role in remineralization and demineralization of teeth.

Loss of dental substance of chemical origin (erosion) can be increased further by mechanical actions such as toothbrush abrasion (see Box 26.9). Patients experiencing dietary acid or gastroesophageal reflux should wait 60 minutes before toothbrushing to minimize loss of tooth structure.[24] If waiting is not an option, the patient should first rinse with water, at least 0.05% neutral sodium fluoride-containing mouthwash, water and baking soda solution, or magnesium hydroxide solution (Maalox). Other products containing a high content of calcium, such as milk and cheese, can also be used as a buffer to create remineralization effects before toothbrushing. Patients who have cancer or chronic vomiting from bulimia or pregnancy may need the same approach. Patients who are polymedicated or taking medication causing hyposalivation or chronic xerostomia (antidepressant, antihistamine, antihypertensive, antiparkinson, etc.) should use neutral oral care products (dry mouth moisturizers or substitutes—salivary or other products) to help alleviate dry mouth.[2] These products, which are often acidic, should contain minerals and fluoride to help to strengthen tooth enamel. See the Critical Thinking Scenarios in Boxes 26.10 and 26.11.

RECOMMENDING DENTIFRICES TO PATIENTS

When comparing over-the-counter and dentifrices available for purchase on the Internet, it is important for dental professionals to consider the following when recommending products with confidence:

- Considerations for recommending a dentifrice to a client or patient can be found in Box 26.12. It is also important to consider the patient's motivation to brush twice a day with the recommended dentifrices.
- Available dentifrices can have similar abrasiveness to the least abrasive polishing paste analyzed by GREDH[14] (e.g., Nature's Gate Anise Cream at 6.18 abrasiveness compared to the prophy paste of Denticare Medicom [Pro-Polish, bubble gum, fine] at 7.03) (see Table 26.9).
- Products such as water, hydrogen peroxide, and sodium bicarbonate combined with water have no abrasiveness and contain no insoluble materials; however, they differ in pH. Water is neutral, peroxide is acidic with a pH of 4.9, and sodium bicarbonate combined with water is basic.
- Sodium bicarbonate and its relatively high solubility contribute to a low level of abrasiveness.[1] However, it can abrade dentin if used dry because its particles are irregular.
- Some dentifrices contain micronized abrasive particles or nanoparticles to reduce abrasiveness. Theoretically, the smaller the particle size or the finer the grit, the less abrasive the material is, even if it

---

BOX 26.8 Demineralization Thresholds for Dental Structures

- Average pH of 6.5 on cementum and dentin
- pH of 5.5 on enamel (hydroxyapatite)
- pH of 4.5 on fluorapatite enamel

BOX 26.9 Loss of Dental Structures and Noncarious Cervical Lesions (NCCL)

- **Erosion:** Dissolution of organic and inorganic tooth structure as a result of chemical agents (see Fig. 26.7).
- **Abrasion:** Pathologic tooth wear caused by a foreign substance that is harder than the tooth structure (see Fig. 26.8).
- **Abfraction:** Cervical tooth structure loss of noncariogenic origin caused when the tooth is subject to a high occlusal load—that is, the occlusal stress is high enough to cause cervical cracking and mineral loss of tooth structure (see Fig. 26.9).
- **Attrition:** Loss of tooth structure on surfaces resulting from tooth-to-tooth contact (proximal or biting surfaces) from normal (chewing) or pathologic (bruxing or clenching) friction from adjacent or opposite teeth (see Fig. 26.10).

BOX 26.10 Critical Thinking Scenario A

A recall patient indicates they are now being treated for hypertension. The patient notes on the dental history that they brush once or twice a week with baking soda or add baking soda to the dentifrice. What recommendations would you make to this patient as a result of the use of baking soda?

Dental Hygiene Recommendations:
It is important to find out why the patient uses baking soda, for example, halitosis, stains, natural products, etc. When dental hygienists understand the reasons for a patient's habits, they can better analyze patient needs and make better dental and overall health recommendations. According to the American Heart Association, 1 teaspoon of sodium bicarbonate contains nearly 1 gram of sodium. Sodium intake can be an especially important consideration for patients with hypertension. Thus there can be a relationship between the sodium in the patient's dentifrice and overall health. Some people are more sensitive to sodium's effects on blood pressure than others. Consider recommending another dentifrice without baking soda and according to the patient's needs that would be as effective but present less potential health risk for the patient.

BOX 26.11 Critical Thinking Scenario B

A 36-year-old female is pregnant with her third child. In the second trimester, she vomited once every morning upon waking. She has four amalgams and a fully restored implant. Her gums bleed easily (4 sites with 3 PSR [Periodontal Screening and Recording]), and there is calculus on the lingual of sextant 5 and to the buccal of the upper molars. Her last full exam was 2 years ago. She eats three meals a day (no snacks) and drinks little milk. She eats firm cheese and yogurt, which provides her with calcium.

Daily Oral Care: She brushes her teeth twice a day and immediately after vomiting because she does not like the taste that remains in the mouth. She uses a floss holder three times a week. Her dentifrice is a multicare type and she uses about the size of a pea on her electric toothbrush because she does not like the taste. After validating the product, it cannot meet the patient's needs because it does not contain the medicinal ingredients necessary for the observed problems: 0.25% NaF and pyrophosphates (no concentration indicated). The pH is at 6.8 and the dentifrice is moderately abrasive. Moreover, since the patient is pregnant, her oral hygiene is particularly important for the baby. Studies suggest an association between gingivitis and premature delivery and the risk of giving birth to a baby with a low birth weight (see Chapter 21).

Dental Hygiene Treatment Plan:
It is essential to inform the patient of the impact of oral health on her systemic health as well as the potential impact of periodontal diseases on her pregnancy:
- Complete dental prophylaxis.
- Provide treatment over 2 appointments into 1 to 2 weeks in relation to the patient's discomfort in the dental chair. Reassess oral condition in 4 to 6 weeks to check for hygiene improvements and reinforce motivation.

Dental Hygiene Education and Recommendations:
- Explain that adverse pregnancy outcomes, such as low birth weight, are generally associated with inflammation, and that periodontitis affecting the mother is one possible source of microorganisms and inflammation that can potentially influence, directly or indirectly, the fetus and the mother.
- Suggest a multicare dentifrice with a pH higher than 5.5, containing stannous fluoride (remineralization, protection, and prevention of erosion) and zinc (anticalculus) that meet her specific needs. Do not rinse and wait 30 minutes before eating or drinking to allow time for the medicinal agents to act.
- Brush twice a day with the recommended dentifrice with an amount equivalent to the width of the toothbrush (½ to 1 cm).
- Recommend use of the floss holder every day (e.g., early afternoon, during the child's nap) and educate the patient on why it is important to continue despite bleeding.
- Gently clean the tongue, cheeks, and gums.
- Before bedtime, use an undiluted, alcohol-free mouthwash with essential oils for 30 seconds to address gingivitis quickly and to avoid potential complications of premature delivery.

Other Recommendations:
- Do not brush teeth immediately after vomiting. However, it is possible to rinse 30 seconds with bicarbonate and water to change the pH and address the bad taste in the mouth.
- Snack on fresh fruit, vegetables, hard cheese, or nuts to stimulate saliva and gums as needed.

BOX 26.12 Patient Education Tip

In general, the first motivation when buying dentifrices for most patients is to find a product that will make the teeth as white as possible while providing fresh breath. The dental hygienist, while meeting the patient's needs, must ensure that the selected product responds well to the data collected during the clinical examination and is validated by the patient's updated medical history. Each patient has the right to be well informed about the different products that are on the market and to have a recommendation for a product that is in accordance with the patient's culture and daily oral hygiene practices.

BOX 26.13 Critical Thinking Scenario C

A dental hygienist is seeing a regular patient who has no changes or reported health problems in the medical history. The dental history reveals the presence of generalized recessions. The patient has purchased a charcoal whitening dentifrice seen on social media and reports their teeth are more sensitive since using it. They brought the tube and asks if this dentifrice is good for them.

Dental Hygiene Recommendations:
It is important for the dental hygienist to review the tube to verify the presence of medicinal and nonmedicinal ingredients, NPN or NDC and, if there is an ADA or CDA Seal, which certifies that the product meets the organization's safety and efficacy criteria. In addition, the dental hygienist must question and verify the scientific evidence regarding charcoal and other nonmedicinal ingredients to identify potentially harmful effects on the teeth. At the time of writing of this chapter, charcoal dentifrices that do not have an NPN or NDC have not been tested by organizations that test their safety and efficacy. In addition, if dental hypersensitivity develops as a result of using the new product, this charcoal dentifrice is more a risk factor for the patient's oral health, especially considering the presence of generalized recessions in the mouth.

addition, its high composition of proteins, salivary ions, and minerals provides additional protection against erosion. Therefore quality and quantity of saliva play a key role in the process of demineralization and remineralization and should be considered when recommending a dentifrice.[35] In fact, they should be the main variables considered when recommending a dentifrice.
- NCCL can occur by erosion (see Fig. 26.7), abrasion (see Fig. 26.8), or abfraction (see Fig. 26.9). Attrition (see Fig. 26.10) is found on the dental surfaces in contact. Abrasion and erosion have multifactorial causes: the client's choice of dentifrice, frequency of brushing, hardness of the toothbrush filaments, pressure exerted during brushing, direction of the brush strokes, choice of a manual or electric toothbrush, surface substrate brushed (dentin, cementum, or enamel), and reduced or absent salivary flow or the absence of its constituents. In the presence of root exposures, eroded enamel, or enamel weakened by dental caries, remineralizing dentifrices containing a combination of fluoride and minerals such as calcium and a phosphate derivative or HAP (see Fig. 26.3).[22,56]
- When a patient suffers from hyposalivation or xerostomia, a dentifrice containing a copolymer would improve the substantiality of the medicinal ingredients.
- As a precautionary measure, pregnant women should avoid using products containing titanium dioxide, as this nanoparticle crosses the placental barrier and may be harmful to the fetus.
- New trends (charcoal, herbs or medicinal plants, essential oils, probiotics, etc.) require further research to determine their effectiveness or potential risk to dental and overall health.[7,8] For example, Essential Oxygen BR is an organic dentifrice that contains essential oils and plants. See the Critical Thinking Scenario in Box 26.13.

scores very high on the Mohs hardness scale. However, the high amount of abrasives can increase the level of abrasiveness.
- Saliva plays several roles: buffering capacity to neutralize mouth acids, lubrication, predigestion (contains ptyalin), immunity, and potential diagnostic and prognostic tests for oral cancer.[55] In

- Currently, the efficacy of essential oils is controversial due to the purity of the oil, the source of the plant, the part used (root, leaf, etc.), the method of extraction, and preservation of the oils; the scientific value of some studies is limited.[7] On Gard dentifrice by dōTerra is an example of a product that contains essential oils.

KEY CONCEPTS

- It would be medically, legally, and ethically irresponsible for dental hygienists to give information and recommend products without having previously validated the medical records of their patients. Health conditions of patients (hypertension, allergies, or intolerance, hyposalivation or xerostomia, multimedicated, cognitive and physical problems), age (quantity of dentifrices), and their needs (values as vegan, eating, and oral habits) must be considered when recommending a dentifrice.
- The majority of manufacturers produce dentifrices that are effective against calculus, gingivitis, oral biofilm, dentinal hypersensitivity, or a combination of the above, although there are many differences between countries. In addition, many unapproved dentifrices are rapidly emerging on the Internet. It is important to check if the ADA or CDA Seal is on the tube to indicate that the product has been tested by organizations that certify that products meet their safety and efficacy criteria.
- When developing a care plan, the clinician must evaluate whether the product is safe for the health of the patient. It also needs to meet patient needs, taking into consideration root exposure, erosion, abrasion, dental caries, hyposalivation or xerostomia, stains, calculus, and brushing habits (e.g., pressure applied, soft- or stiff-bristled toothbrush, brushing method, etc.).
- Dentifrice variables, including level of abrasion, pH level, insoluble materials, etc., must be considered when recommending dentifrices to patients. While various references are available, select a resource that considers all of these variables so it is useful for a comprehensive comparison of dentifrices.
- Flavoring agents, dyes, and detergents in dentifrices may cause side effects (burning sensation, oral tissue desquamation, aphthous ulcers, intolerance, allergies, altered dental microbiota, etc.). They can have adverse effects on overall health too, provoking allergies, increasing the risk of obesity, altering intestinal microbiota which can be altered by the oral microbiota, etc.

ACKNOWLEDGEMENT

The authors acknowledge Louise Bourassa for her past contributions to this chapter.

REFERENCES

1. Lavoie F, Feeney N, McCallum L, et al. Evaluation of toothpastes and of variables associated with the choice of a product. Comité Dentifrice. Collège François-Xavier-Garneau. *CDHA.* 2007; 41:42.
2. American Dental Association. *ADA/PDR Guide to Dental Therapeutics.* 5th ed. Chicago: ADA; 2009.
3. American Dental Association website. Available at: http://www.ada.org. Accessed July 2022.
4. Canadian Dental Association website. Available at: http://www.cda-adc.ca. Accessed July 2022.
5. U.S. Food and Drug Administration (FDA). U.S. FDA website. Available at: https://www.fda.gov. Accessed July 2022.
6. Health Canada/Santé Canada website. Available at: https://www.canada.ca/en/health-canada. Accessed July 2022.
7. Safiaghdam H, Oveissi V, Bahramsoltani R, et al. Medicinal plants for gingivitis: a review of clinical trials. *Iran J Basic Med Sci.* 2018;21(10):978–991. Available at: https://doi.org/10.22038/IJBMS.2018.31997.7690.
8. Prete BRJ, Barsoum F, Ouanounou A. *Toothpastes in Dentistry: A Review.* Oral Health Group; 2022. Available at: https://www.oralhealthgroup.com/features/toothpastes-in-dentistry-a-review/. Accessed July 2022.
9. Quebec Bio website. Available at: https://quebecbio.com/bio/garanties#fondements. Accessed July 2022.
10. Walsh T, Worthington HV, Glenny AM, et al. Fluoride toothpastes of different concentrations for preventing dental caries. *Cochrane Database Syst Rev.* 2019;3(3):CD007868. Available at: https://doi.org/10.1002/14651858.CD007868.pub3. Accessed July 22, 2022.
11. Natural Health Products Ingredients Database (NHPID) website. Health Canada/Santé Canada. Available at: http://webprod.hc-sc.gc.ca/nhpid-bdipsn/atReq.do?atid=oral.health.sante.bucco.dentaire. Accessed July 2022.
12. Levine RS. Pyrophosphates in toothpaste: a retrospective and reappraisal. *Br Dent J.* 2020;229(10):687–689. Available at: https://doi.org/10.1038/s41415-020-2346-4. Accessed July 2022.
13. Abou Neel EA, Aljabo A, Strange A, et al. Demineralization-remineralization dynamics in teeth and bone. *Int J Nanomed.* 2016;11:4743–4763. Available at: https://doi.org/10.2147/IJN.S107624. Accessed July 2022.
14. Lavoie F, Dubreuil N, Bourassa L, et al. Interactive website descriptive guide of toothpastes, mouthwashes and other products for dental hygiene or oral health. *Group of Research and Education on Dental Hygiene.* Available at: www.grehd.org. Accessed July 2022.
15. Heindel JJ, Howard S, Agay-Shay K, et al. Obesity II: Establishing causal links between chemical exposures and obesity. *Biochem Pharmacol.* 2022;199:115015. Available at: https://doi.org/10.1016/j.bcp.2022.115015. Accessed July 2022.
16. Kassotis CD, Vom Saal FS, Babin PJ, et al. Obesity III: Obesogen assays: Limitations, strengths, and new directions. *Biochem Pharmacol.* 2022;199:115014. Available at: https://doi.org/10.1016/j.bcp.2022.115014. Accessed July 2022.
17. Cicciù M, Fiorillo L, Cervino G. Chitosan use in dentistry: a systematic review of recent clinical studies. *Mar Drugs.* 2019;17(7):417. Available at: https://doi.org/10.3390/md17070417. Accessed July 2022.
18. Gasmi Benahmed A, Gasmi A, Arshad M, et al. Health benefits of xylitol. *Appl Microbiol Biotechnol.* 2020;104:7225–7237. Available at: https://doi.org/10.1007/s00253-020-10708-7. Accessed July 2022.
19. Poppolo Deus F, Ouanounou A. Chlorhexidine in dentistry: Pharmacology, uses, and adverse effects. *Int Dent J.* 2022;72(3):269–277. https://doi.org/10.1016/j.identj.2022.01.005. Accessed July 2022.
20. Zheng X, He J, Wang L, et al. Ecological effect of Arginine on oral microbiota. *Sci Rep.* 2017;7:7206. https://doi.org/10.1038/s41598-017-07042-w. Accessed July 2022.
21. Almohefer SA, Levon JA, Gregory RL, et al. Caries lesion remineralization with fluoride toothpastes and chlorhexidine – effects of application timing and toothpaste surfactant. *J Appl Oral Sci: Revista FOB.* 2018;26:e20170499. https://doi.org/10.1590/1678-7757-2017-0499. Accessed September 2022.
22. Limeback H, Enax J, Meyer F. Biomimetic hydroxyapatite and caries prevention: a systematic review and meta-analysis. *Can J Dent Hyg.* 2021;55(3):148–159. Available at: https://www.ncbi.nlm.nih.gov/pmc/articles/PMC8641555/. Accessed July 2022.
23. Fiorillo L, Cervino G, Herford AS, et al. Stannous fluoride effects on enamel: a systematic review. *Biomimetics (Basel, Switzerland).* 2020;5(3):41. https://doi.org/10.3390/biomimetics5030041. Accessed July 2022.
24. Mouth Healthy website by American Dental Association. Available at: https://www.mouthhealthy.org/en/brushing-mistakes-slideshow. Accessed July 2022.
25. Dubreuil N, Lavoie F, Bourassa L, et al. Les boissons énergisantes. Quels sont les risques sur la santé buccodentaire associés à la consommation des boissons énergisantes chez les 18 ans et plus?. *L'Explorateur. OHDQ. Printemps 2019.* 2019;numéro 1. Available at: https://ohdq.com/public/publications/lexplorateur/sante-buccodentaire-et-les-jeunes-adultes-de-18-a-35-ans/. Accessed July 2022.
26. Martins CC, Firmino RT, Riva JJ, et al. Desensitizing toothpastes for dentin hypersensitivity: a network meta-analysis. *J Dent Res.* 2020;99(5):514–522. https://doi.org/10.1177/0022034520903036.

27. Valkenburg C, Else Slot D, Van der Weijden GA. What is the effect of active ingredients in dentifrice on inhibiting the regrowth of overnight plaque? A systematic review. *Int J Dent Hygiene*. 2020;18:128–141. https://doi.org/10.1111/idh.12423.

28. Cunha EJ, Auersvald CM, Deliberador TM, et al. Effects of active oxygen toothpaste in supragingival biofilm reduction: a randomized controlled clinical trial. *Int J Dent*. 2019;2019:3938214. https://doi.org/10.1155/2019/3938214.

29. Poppolo Deus F, Ouanounou A. Chlorhexidine in dentistry: Pharmacology, uses, and adverse effects. *Int Dent J*. 2022;72(3):269–277. https://doi.org/10.1016/j.identj.2022.01.005.

30. Johannsen A, Emilson CG, Johannsen G, et al. Effects of stabilized stannous fluoride dentifrice on dental calculus, dental plaque, gingivitis, halitosis and stain: a systematic review. *Heliyon*. 2019;5(12):e02850. https://doi.org/10.1016/j.heliyon.2019.e02850.

31. Valkenburg C, Van der Weijden FA, Slot DE. Plaque control and reduction of gingivitis: the evidence for dentifrices. *Periodontol 2000*. 2019;79(1):221–232. https://doi.org/10.1111/prd.12257.

32. Mary C, Fouillen A, Moffatt P, et al. Effect of human secretory calcium-binding phosphoprotein proline-glutamine rich 1 protein on *Porphyromonas gingivalis* and identification of its active portions. *Sci Rep*. 2021;11:23724. https://doi.org/10.1038/s41598-021-02661-w.

33. Kaur M, Geurs NC, Cobb CM, et al. Evaluating efficacy of a novel dentifrice in reducing probing depths in Stage I and II periodontitis maintenance patients: a randomized, double-blind, positive controlled clinical trial. *J Periodontol*. 2021;92(9):1286–1294. https://doi.org/10.1002/JPER.20-0721.

34. Jacobsen P, Novy B. Friction vs chemistry for plaque biofilm management. *Dent Today*. 2021. Available at: https://www.dentistrytoday.com/friction-vs-chemistry-for-plaque-biofilm-management/. Accessed September 2022.

35. João-Souza SH, Lussi A, Baumann T, et al. Chemical and physical factors of desensitizing and/or anti-erosive toothpastes associated with lower erosive tooth wear. *Sci Rep*. 2017;7(1):17909. https://doi.org/10.1038/s41598-017-18154-8.

36. Binhasan M, Solimanie AH, Almuammar KS, et al. The effect of dentifrice on micro-hardness, surface gloss, and micro-roughness of nano filled conventional and bulk-fill polymer composite—a micro indentation and profilometric study. *Materials*. 2022;15(12):4347. https://doi.org/10.3390/ma15124347.

37. Epple M, Meyer F, Enax J. A critical review of modern concepts for teeth whitening. *Dent J*. 2019;7(3):79. https://doi.org/10.3390/dj7030079.

38. Valkenburg C, Kashmour Y, Dao A, et al. The efficacy of baking soda dentifrice in controlling plaque and gingivitis: a systematic review. *Int J Dent Hygiene*. 2019;17:99–116. https://doi.org/10.1111/idh.12390.

39. Brooks JK, Bashirelahi N, Reynolds MA. Charcoal and charcoal-based dentifrices: a literature review. *J Am Dent Assoc (1939)*. 2017;148(9):661–670. https://doi.org/10.1016/j.adaj.2017.05.001.

40. Wylleman A, Vuylsteke F, Dekeyser C, et al. Alternative therapies in controlling oral malodour: a systematic review. *J Breath Res*. 2021;15(2). Available at: https://doi.org/10.1088/1752-7163/abcd2b. Accessed July 2022.

41. Naumova EA, Staiger M, Kouji O, et al. Randomized investigation of the bioavailability of fluoride in saliva after administration of sodium fluoride, amine fluoride and fluoride containing bioactive glass dentifrices. *BMC Oral Health*. 2019;19(1):119. https://doi.org/10.1186/s12903-019-0805-6.

42. Patel VR, Shettar L, Thakur S, Gillam D, et al. A randomised clinical trial on the efficacy of 5% fluorocalcium phosphosilicate-containing novel bioactive glass toothpaste. *J Oral Rehabil*. 2019;46(12):1121–1126. https://doi.org/10.1111/joor.12847.

43. Mohapatra S, Kumar RP, Arumugham IM, et al. Assessment of microhardness of enamel carious like lesions after treatment with Nova Min, Bio Min and Remin Pro containing toothpastes: an in vitro study. *Indian J Public Health Res Dev*. 2019;10:375. Available at: https://www.researchgate.net/publication/338136980_Assessment_of_Microhardness_of_Enamel_Carious_Like_Lesions_After_Treatment_with_Nova_Min_Bio_Min_and_Remin_Pro_Containing_Toothpastes_An_in_Vitro_Study. Accessed July 2022.

44. MacDonald K, Boudreau E, Thomas GV, et al. In vitro evaluation of Sensi-IP*: a soluble and mineralizing sensitivity solution. *Heliyon*. 2021;8(1):e08672. https://doi.org/10.1016/j.heliyon.2021.e08672.

45. Štšepetova J, Truu J, Runnel R, et al. Impact of polyols on oral microbiome of Estonian schoolchildren. *BMC Oral Health*. 2019;19(1):60. https://doi.org/10.1186/s12903-019-0747-z.

46. Al-Hashedi AA, Dubreuil N, Schwinghamer T, et al. Aragonite toothpaste for management of dental calculus: a double-blinded randomized controlled clinical trial. *Clin Exp Dent Res*. 2022. https://doi.org/10.1002/cre2.559.

47. Schofs L, Sparo MD, Sánchez Bruni SF. The antimicrobial effect behind Cannabis sativa. *Pharmacol Res Perspect*. 2021;9(2):e00761. https://doi.org/10.1002/prp2.761.

48. Contact dermatitis institute website. Available at: https://www.contactdermatitisinstitute.com. Accessed July 2022.

49. Dyall-Smith D. Contact reactions to toothpaste and other oral hygiene products. Dermnet New Zealand. Available at: https://dermnetnz.org/topics/contact-reactions-to-toothpaste-and-other-oral-hygiene-products. Accessed July 2022.

50. Carrouel F, Viennot S, Ottolenghi L, et al. Nanoparticles as anti-microbial, anti-inflammatory, and remineralizing agents in oral care cosmetics: a review of the current situation. *Nanomaterials (Basel, Switzerland)*. 2020;10(1):140. https://doi.org/10.3390/nano10010140.

51. Guillard A, Gaultier E, Cartier C, et al. Basal Ti level in the human placenta and meconium and evidence of a materno-foetal transfer of food-grade TiO2 nanoparticles in an ex vivo placental perfusion model. *Part Fibre Toxicol*. 2020;17(1):51. https://doi.org/10.1186/s12989-020-00381-z.

52. *French gouvernement/Gouvernement Français, Comité de la Prévention et de la Précaution (CPP), Nanotechnologie- Nanopaticules: Quels dangers, quels risques?*. 2020. Available at: https://www.ecologie.gouv.fr/sites/default/files/CPP%20-%20Nanotechnologie%20Nanoparticules.pdf. Accessed July 2022.

53. Sälzer S, Graetz C, Dörfer CE, et al. Contemporary practices for mechanical oral hygiene to prevent periodontal disease. *Periodontol 2000*. 2020;84(1):35–44. https://doi.org/10.1111/prd.12332.

54. Organisation internationale de normalisation (ISO). *Médecine bucco-dentaire - Dentifrice - Exigences, méthodes d'essai et marquage*. 3rd ed. Switzerland: ISO 11609; 2017. Available at: https://www.iso.org/fr/standard/70956.html. Accessed July 2022.

55. Zanotti L, Paderno A, Piazza C, et al. Epidermal growth factor receptor detection in serum and saliva as a diagnostic and prognostic tool in oral cancer. *Laryngoscope*. 2017;127(11):E408–E414. https://doi.org/10.1002/lary.26797.

56. Suryani H, Gehlot PM, Manjunath MK. Evaluation of the remineralisation potential of bioactive glass, nanohydroxyapatite and casein phosphopeptide-amorphous calcium phosphate fluoride-based toothpastes on enamel erosion lesion-An Ex Vivo study. *Indian J Dent Res*. 2020;31(5):670–677. https://doi.org/10.4103/ijdr.IJDR_735_17.

27

Antimicrobial Agents for Control of Periodontal Disease

Joanna Asadoorian

PROFESSIONAL OPPORTUNITIES

Dental hygiene patients demonstrate ongoing challenges maintaining optimal oral hygiene and preventing periodontal diseases. Antimicrobial agents used in patients' homecare routines and in dental hygiene professional practice can be adjunctive to mechanical interventions to aid in reducing oral biofilm, dysbiosis, periodontal inflammation, and clinical attachment loss—meaning the agent has a therapeutic effect. Dental hygienists with current knowledge surrounding antimicrobial interventions can effectively make evidence-based recommendations for oral self-care, provide appropriate clinical services, and offer suitable referrals to other oral healthcare providers when necessary.

COMPETENCIES

1. Outline the mechanisms for ensuring efficacy, quality, and safety of periodontal antimicrobial products.
2. Explain the rationale for adjunctive antimicrobial biofilm control.
3. Compare and contrast delivery methods of antimicrobial agents for both home and professional use.
4. Discuss the evidence regarding effectiveness of various active ingredients included in antimicrobial products for the treatment of periodontal diseases.
5. Apply evidence-based indications for use of antimicrobial agents as interventions for the prevention and treatment of periodontal diseases.

▶ EVOLVE VIDEO RESOURCE

View two videos on adjunctive periodontal interventions on Evolve (http://evolve.elsevier.com/Pieren/hygiene/):
- Placing Controlled-Release Drug: Doxycycline Gel
- Placing Controlled-Release Drug: Minocycline Hydrochloride Microspheres

ORAL DISEASE AND BACTERIAL PLAQUE BIOFILM

Periodontal diseases are prevalent inflammatory conditions affecting the periodontal tissues surrounding the teeth leading to destruction of supporting structures, eventual tooth loss, diminished functional dentition, and reduced personal satisfaction. The initiation and progression of many periodontal diseases are related to the interaction between a susceptible host, a pathogenic agent, and environmental factors. Therefore, the prevention and control of periodontal diseases depends, in part, on controlling bacterial dental plaque—or biofilm, which is the main pathogenic etiologic agent of these diseases. Disruption of the dental biofilm, and the prevention of subsequent **dysbiosis**, has predominantly occurred mechanically, through oral self-care methods such as toothbrushing and supported by professional debridement, including scaling and root planing.

Dental hygienists play a key role in care by advising their patients about performing adequate homecare and providing the necessary preventive and therapeutic professional care. However, despite these efforts, many patients require additional, adjunctive antimicrobial therapies. Oral **antimicrobial agents** refer to the incorporation of an active ingredient within a delivery system for preventing, treating, or controlling periodontal diseases. These agents are increasingly being used as adjuncts to customary mechanical methods for biofilm control and treating periodontal diseases.

The total elimination of bacterial plaque is an unrealistic and unwarranted goal. A reasonable approach to prevent and treat periodontal diseases, including both gingival and periodontal involvement, is through methods that reduce oral biofilm to a level below the individual's threshold for disease, thereby preventing dysbiosis and the potential for a subsequent host inflammatory response. Antimicrobial agents contribute to this aim in several ways, including reducing the number of pathogenic organisms and altering their pathogenic potential. Most of the research has been conducted on pathogenic bacterial species, given their role in gingival and periodontal diseases.

Dental hygienists are responsible for recommending and implementing antimicrobial therapies in a shared decision-making relationship with clients and referring patients to other oral healthcare providers when appropriate for possible additional antimicrobial interventions. The indications for antimicrobial use will often emerge during the assessment phase of the dental hygiene process of care. The dental hygienist can then plan for specific antimicrobial interventions while developing the dental hygiene care plan with the client and incorporate these during the implementation phase. During the evaluation phase, it may be determined that antimicrobials should be started, continued, or discontinued.

PRODUCT SAFETY AND EFFICACY

The most important consideration when making recommendations to patients is that interventions are safe and effective. This determination incorporates thinking about the "net benefit" of an intervention, meaning evaluating the weight of the benefit of an antimicrobial agent against its cost and risk of potential adverse effects. Two major organizations in the United States and Canada, the US Food and Drug Administration (FDA) and Health Canada, respectively, contribute to ensuring the safety, quality, and efficacy of oral antimicrobials.

In the United States, the FDA ensures the safety and efficacy of prescription drugs and over-the-counter (OTC) products that make therapeutic claims through federally mandated review and approval processes. A prescription drug must gain premarket approval by the FDA through the New Drug Application (NDA) process, whereas a nonprescription drug product must conform to an already approved monograph specific to its drug category. The FDA develops and reviews active ingredients within therapeutic drug classes and develops an OTC drug monograph for each. This process differs from cosmetic products, which do not require FDA approval prior to being marketed. Some products, including oral health products, are marketed as having both cosmetic and therapeutic benefits. Drug products can be searched through the FDA website for inquiries about the product, including their market status and product labeling.

In Canada, products offered for sale to treat or prevent diseases are regulated by Health Canada within the Health Products and Food Branch (HPFB) under the *Food and Drugs Act*. The HPFB ensures the safety, efficacy, and quality of therapeutic and diagnostic products including prescription and nonprescription drugs, devices, and disinfectants. For prescription oral health products, the manufacturer must provide scientific evidence verifying the product complies with Health Canada's Therapeutic Products Directorate, which is the Canadian federal authority regulating pharmaceutical drugs and medical devices for human use. Drug products can be searched on the *Drug Product Database* to learn more about the status of a particular oral health product (i.e., premarket, marketed, postmarket/canceled) and view its full drug monograph. Nonprescription products, which include many natural health products, are found in the Natural and Non-prescription Health Products Directorate.

In addition to federal approval of prescription and nonprescription drugs and other therapeutic products, the American Dental Association (ADA) Council on Scientific Affairs and the Canadian Dental Association (CDA) provide additional guidance for product selection to oral healthcare providers and the public. The ADA Council on Scientific Affairs evaluates new, nonprescription products for safety and efficacy.[1] Products approved by the FDA may apply to receive the **ADA Seal of Acceptance** (Fig. 27.1A), which is granted to products demonstrating safety and efficacy in accordance with published criteria. Applications for the Seal must include supporting research data demonstrating product safety and efficacy according to specific product category requirements developed by the ADA Council on Scientific Affairs. Specific guidelines for evaluating the effectiveness of a number of oral health products including antimicrobials for the reduction of plaque and gingivitis have been developed and are updated regularly. Oral healthcare products can be searched via the ADA Seal database.

The CDA provides the **CDA Seal Program** (see Fig. 27.1B), which aims to assist consumers by validating manufacturer oral health benefit claims of products to help in making informed choices about products.[2] Manufacturers seeking the CDA Seal must submit an application with evidence supporting the oral health claim for the product. The benefit claim must be measurable, clinically significant, and a result of the preventive, therapeutic, or cosmetic effects of using the product. The CDA conducts an independent expert review to determine the validity of the product benefit claim to award the Seal.

RATIONALE FOR ANTIMICROBIAL AGENTS

It is well established that periodontal health requires a combination of ongoing, supportive, oral hygiene care, including periodontal debridement, and the patient's diligent, daily oral hygiene efforts. Despite the technologic advances and widespread use of mechanical plaque removal tools and aids, individuals continue to have difficulties maintaining adequate oral hygiene to prevent associated biofilm-related diseases, particularly in areas of the mouth that are difficult to access. There is accumulating evidence that some oral antimicrobial agents have a definitive adjunctive benefit for reducing plaque biofilm, dysbiosis, and periodontal inflammation beyond what is accomplished mechanically. It is essential for the dental hygienist to continuously access and critically appraise the literature addressing oral antimicrobial products because new formulations and products are frequently being developed. This information is important for client education and motivation regarding the selection of therapeutic antimicrobial products (Box 27.1).

Delivery Systems and Active Ingredients

Dental hygienists can view oral antimicrobial agents as having two dimensions: (1) the delivery system and (2) the active ingredient (Fig. 27.2). In addition, the delivery system can be subcategorized as being delivered in either a local or a systemic mode. **Local delivery** methods are those where the antimicrobial agent is applied directly to the oral cavity or to a specific location within it. **Systemic delivery** methods are those that are ingested by the patient and delivered via the bloodstream. Further, products falling within these subcategories may be professionally delivered by the dental hygienist, dentist or periodontist, or they may comprise part of the patient's self-care regimen. Modes of delivery can be an intervention applied as a **monotherapy**, meaning

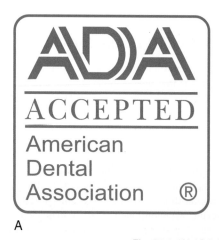

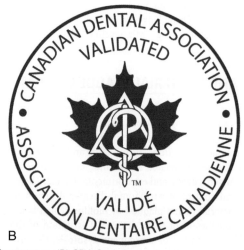

Fig. 27.1 (A) ADA Seal of Acceptance. (B) CDA Seal.

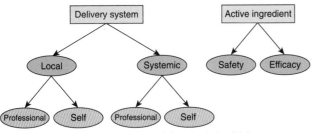

Fig. 27.2 Dimensions of Oral Antimicrobials.

it is used on its own, or, alternatively, antimicrobial therapies can be used in conjunction with others. Antimicrobials, both professionally and self-applied, are typically used adjunctively to mechanical biofilm and calculus control methods rather than as monotherapies. An example of an exception to this is when an antimicrobial rinse is used post-periodontal surgery to control oral biofilm without disturbing the surgical site.

The second dimension of oral antimicrobials is the **active ingredient**. The active ingredient refers to the specific agent, chemical, or drug component within a particular delivery system that is primarily responsible for the therapeutic effect. Active ingredients, alone or in combination, may be applied in numerous ways and found in various delivery systems. See Box 27.2 for an example. The dental hygienist should not assume the proven effectiveness of a specific active ingredient within a particular delivery system ensures this same active ingredient is similarly effective within other delivery systems or within the

TABLE 27.1 Active Ingredient Mechanisms of Action

Category	Description
Antiseptic agents	Usually broad spectrum; kill or prevent propagation of biofilm microorganisms
Antibiotics	Broad or narrow spectrum; inhibit or kill specific or groups of bacteria or modulate host inflammatory response
Modifying agents	Agents that alter the structure and/or metabolic activity of bacteria
Antiadhesives	Products that interfere with the ability of bacteria to attach to the acquired pellicle

same system in different concentrations. Research is required to substantiate other applications of active ingredients.

Active ingredients for periodontal disease prevention and treatment are therapeutically effective in that they disable potentially harmful microorganisms or alter the microflora in several ways (Table 27.1). Some active ingredients exhibit **bactericidal** activity, which means that they kill bacteria directly, or they can exert **bacteriostatic** action, which means that the metabolism or reproduction of the microbe is negatively affected. The term **substantivity** refers to an antimicrobial agent's ability to durably bind with oral tissues and then be released over time aiding in a product's effectiveness. However, some products are effective despite having limited substantivity.

LOCAL DELIVERY METHODS

Self-Applied Modes of Delivery

Self-applied oral antimicrobial agents designed for home use typically have lower concentrations of the active ingredient and are used more frequently as compared with professional delivery systems. The concentration and frequency for product use refers to the dosage and regimen. One of the most common self-applied oral health delivery modes is dentifrice (see Chapter 26). Commonly known as *toothpaste*, **dentifrice** is available mostly as paste or gel and acts as a vehicle for the local delivery of active ingredients. Dentifrice can have both therapeutic and cosmetic effects. In addition to the mechanical plaque removal benefits of toothbrushing, the most important therapeutic effect of toothpaste is the anticariogenic effect of fluoride. Other active ingredients in dentifrices maybe included for the reduction of biofilm and gingival inflammation, hypersensitivity, malodor, discoloration, calculus deposits, and demineralization, but some of these products may require additional research to substantiate their therapeutic claims.

Mouth rinses, commonly known as *oral rinses* or *mouthwashes*, are available for both cosmetic and therapeutic use and are available in prescription and OTC formulations. Therapeutic use of a mouth rinse is primarily dependent on the active ingredients rather than the mechanical action. Potential therapeutic uses include biofilm reduction, the control and reduction of gingival inflammation, caries prevention, and the treatment of oral malodor or halitosis. **Halitosis** is an unpleasant odor emanating from the mouth and can be simply a result of diet, lack of oral hygiene, or inactivity associated with sleeping ("morning breath"), or it can be a more serious and challenging manifestation resulting from advanced periodontal disease, an underlying medical condition or may be idiopathic. Cosmetic use of mouthwash is limited to temporary breath freshening and tooth whitening, and therefore, serious nonresolving cases of halitosis may require a referral to a periodontist or other medical provider.

Therapeutic benefits of mouth rinses vary depending on the active ingredient and the overall effectiveness of the formulation. Increasingly, therapeutic mouth rinses are being recommended as part of patients' oral homecare plan adjunctive to daily mechanical cleansing methods to reduce dental biofilm and gingival inflammation.[3] The active ingredients in mouth rinses may be referred to as *oral antiseptics*. **Antiseptics** are substances that inhibit the growth and development of microorganisms on living tissue and demonstrate very little oral or systemic toxicity or microbial resistance. They typically have a broad antimicrobial spectrum, meaning they are active against a wide range of microorganisms.

It is generally believed that mouth rinses are well accepted by patients because of their ease of use. It is estimated that approximately half of the population in the United States and Canada uses some type of mouth rinse, but many individuals do not use rinses consistently according to manufacturer directions, a point that should be stressed by the dental hygienist in giving oral self-care education. For optimum effectiveness, the correct dosage and regimen must be followed, along with keeping the rinse in the oral cavity for a sufficient time to ensure antimicrobial action occurs. For many products, 1 oz./20 mL, twice daily for 30 seconds, is the recommended protocol, but dental hygienists should refer their patients to the specific manufacturer instructions for every product.

Oral rinsing can reach more inaccessible areas of the oral cavity often missed by mechanical methods. In addition, certain areas of the oral cavity, such as the cheeks and tongue, can be inhabited by microorganisms but often are not mechanically cleansed and can serve as a microbial reservoir for the developing oral biofilm. Because the gel matrix of the biofilm offers protection for inhabiting microorganisms, it is advisable that mechanical cleansing occurs prior to rinsing to enhance the penetration of the rinse. Box 27.3 describes the ideal properties of a mouth rinse. Oral rinses, like dentifrices, have a limited effect on subgingival pathogenic microorganisms because of the inability to penetrate below the gingival margin, which limits the effect on deeper periodontal microbiota and more advanced disease.

Antimicrobial mouth rinses are relatively straightforward to incorporate into patients' homecare routines because of their acceptability and ease of use. However, of the many mouth-rinse products available on the market, few have shown evidence of a clinically important therapeutic benefit.[3] Current research supporting therapeutically effective commercially available mouth-rinse products primarily surrounds three active ingredients: chlorhexidine gluconate, essential oils, and cetylpyridinium chloride.[3]

Chlorhexidine gluconate (CHG) has long been viewed as the gold standard of therapeutic mouth rinses but is available only by prescription (i.e., Peridex 0.12%; PerioGard 0.12%). Additionally, it has reported negative side effects, most notably tooth staining, which requires professional removal, and possible taste alterations and increased calculus accumulation. Together, these factors have limited

its use to a short-term, postsurgical or periodontal therapeutic rinse.[3] The presence of plaque increases CHG side effects and reinforces the need for biofilm removal prior to the start of a CHG mouth rinsing protocol.

CHG strongly binds with the bacterial cell membrane and causes the cell to leak and disrupt its intracellular components. In addition, CHG can interfere with bacterial colonization and cell attachment. These actions undermine biofilm development within the oral cavity. CHG has considerable substantivity in binding to oral tissues, and it remains active for 8 to 12 hours. For prescription CHG mouth rinses, the following should be observed:

- Typically administered in 15-mL dosages for 30 seconds twice daily.
- Allow at least 30 minutes between rinsing with CHG and toothbrushing with toothpaste (either before or after) to avoid an interaction with the toothpaste detergent sodium lauryl sulfate, which causes the deactivation of CHG.
- After CHG use, wait to rinse with water for 30 minutes to avoid removing flavor-masking agents, which decrease the medicinal taste of the drug.

For nonprescription, antimicrobial mouth rinses, the ADA has specific, rigorous criteria that must be met to obtain the ADA Seal of Acceptance, including:

- Studies demonstrating safety and effectiveness
- FDA-approved ingredients
- Assured purity and uniformity
- Packaging and advertising claims supported by science[4]

The guidelines, which are reviewed every 5 years, require studies be at least 3 months in length using placebo controls and demonstrate statistically significant reductions in both plaque and gingivitis outcome measures.[5] Dental hygienists can have confidence in their care planning and making recommendations to their patients when a product has demonstrated its effectiveness in studies meeting these criteria. An OTC mouth rinse formulation that has a fixed combination of four essential oils—eucalyptol 0.092%, menthol 0.042%, thymol 0.064%, and methyl salicylate 0.06% (i.e., Listerine)—has received the ADA Seal for reducing plaque and gingival inflammation outcome measures. Note that in Canada, only three essential oils are listed as active ingredients; methyl salicylate is included as a nonmedicinal ingredient. Considerable research has shown this commercial OTC mouth rinse with this specific combination of essential oils performs well in reducing plaque and demonstrates comparable gingivitis reductions to CHG.[3]

Essential oils (EOs) are components of plants containing phenolic compounds that destroy microorganisms by compromising the cell membrane and inhibiting enzyme activity. Although this specific EO antiseptic formulation has relatively low substantivity compared to CHG, it has multidimensional therapeutic effects:

- Prevents bacteria from aggregating
- Slows bacterial multiplication
- Reduces the bacterial load overall within the oral cavity
- Prevents the plaque mass from maturing
- Reduces the pathogenicity of the plaque mass
- Exerts an antiinflammatory benefit

In long-term (≥6 months) clinical trials, commercially available EO antiseptic mouth rinse has shown whole-mouth mean plaque reductions ranging from 26% to 42% and gingivitis reductions from 16% to over 60% compared to baseline, which is comparable to outcomes measured with CHG.[3] In addition to the demonstrated effectiveness, EO rinse has the advantage of being suitable as a long-term adjunct to mechanical home oral care routines given that it demonstrates:

- No associated stain
- Safety when used as directed
- No changes produced in bacterial composition

BOX 27.3   Ideal Properties of Oral Rinses

- Safe to use over long periods of time
- Palatable to user
- Inexpensive
- Highly soluble and stable in storage
- Effective
- Broad spectrum of effectiveness
- Adequate bioavailability to bacteria
- Minimal side effects
- Adequate retention

- No evidence of opportunistic oral pathogens
- No evidence of antimicrobial resistance

Importantly, the research has shown commercial EO mouth rinse provides an additive benefit to those who are performing toothbrushing and flossing, so it has been recommended for preventative use for virtually all dental hygiene patients, rather than just those presenting with heavy biofilm and/or inflammation.[3] The procedure for rinsing with OTC EO mouth rinse is similar to that for CHG: patients should rinse with 1 oz/20 mL for 30 seconds after brushing and cleansing interproximally, twice daily; no waiting is required between brushing and rinsing, as there are no interactions between toothpaste and this rinse.

Cetylpyridium chloride (CPC)-based mouth rinses contain quaternary ammonium chemical compounds, which are a group of chemicals with antimicrobial properties. Several quaternary ammonium compound–based rinses have been available commercially for many years, with the most well researched being CPC.[3] These mouth rinses can destroy microorganisms by interacting with the bacterial cell membrane, causing it to become permeable and lose its contents. They are bactericidal to Gram-positive and, to a lesser extent, Gram-negative bacteria. CPC oral rinses bind well with oral tissues, but they have lower substantivity compared to CHG. Many CPC formulations are limited to cosmetic use in that clinically significant plaque and gingivitis reductions have not been demonstrated in long-term clinical trials.

Some CPC rinse formulations (i.e., Crest Pro-Health Rinse 0.07% or Colgate Total Rinse 0.075%) have been studied in long-term trials and in systematic reviews and metaanalyses and have demonstrated a benefit as an adjunct to mechanical homecare for plaque and gingivitis reduction.[3] However, CPC rinses reportedly have increased tooth staining. In addition, like CHG rinses, CPC formulations may be inactivated by toothpaste products such as sodium lauryl sulfate. CPC rinses may have breath-freshening qualities and may reduce halitosis.

Other, less well-known active ingredients and novel combinations of well-established agents are the focus of laboratory and clinical research and should be individually evaluated. Many of these products are not yet commercially available to American and Canadian markets. Continually monitoring systematic reviews and clinical practice guidelines surrounding oral rinse formulations is recommended for the dental hygiene clinician.

In addition to the active ingredients found in oral rinses, products may include:

- Water
- Alcohol
- Cleansing agents
- Flavoring ingredients
- Coloring agents

Alcohol (10% to 30% by volume) is included in many formulations to emulsify the antimicrobial ingredients within the rinse. Although the alcohol may have some antiseptic properties, this effect is not considered clinically important.

In general, oral rinses are well tolerated by most individuals, with staining being the most frequently occurring side effect with some formulations. (See Box 27.1 for client education and motivation tips.) Despite some products having a "sharp" taste, diluting the product is not recommended. Tolerance maybe improved with milder, alcohol-free rinses, but research is more limited showing similar clinical effects on plaque and inflammation, and such products must be appraised separately. Despite contradictory reports, research demonstrates there is no increase in oral dryness perception (xerostomia) or a decrease in salivary output with alcohol-containing or alcohol-free EO rinses.[3] In addition, epidemiologic research has not shown an association between regular use of oral rinses, with or without alcohol, and oropharyngeal cancer. Dental hygienists should keep in mind that there is a dose-effect relationship between tobacco smoking and alcohol consumption, especially when combined, and oropharyngeal cancer. It is important to consider the expected benefits of recommending a mouth rinse in relation to potential risks, particularly for patients who engage in high-risk oral health behaviors such as tobacco use and high levels of alcohol consumption.

In addition, alcohol-containing mouth rinses may be contraindicated for some individuals with other conditions, and precautions should be observed:

- Recovering alcoholics should use alcohol-free oral rinses.
- Individuals taking certain antibiotics where gastrointestinal upset may occur should avoid alcohol-containing rinses.
- Individuals not able to expectorate should avoid mouth rinses; ingestion can result in intoxication (where alcohol is present), illness, or fatality; children under 6 years of age should not typically use a therapeutic oral rinse.
- Patients being treated with head and neck radiation and who have mucositis should use bland oral rinses such as sterile water, saline rinse, or a commercial rinse manufactured specifically for these patients due to painful oral ulcerations and sensitivities.
- Individuals on sodium-restricted diets should be aware that some brands of mouthwash may be significant sources of sodium, which can be absorbed; these patients should consult their physicians about the potential impact of such mouthwashes.

New mouth-rinse formulations, some of which are available commercially, have been recommended based on being "natural products" and have been the focus of research to determine their therapeutic value.[3,6] Natural, or more precisely biological and herbal products, typically have a biological origin or are derived from plants, fungi, and algae and may have antimicrobial properties. Many novel natural products have undergone study ranging from short-term, in vitro studies to longer-term clinical trials and in some cases have shown reductions in plaque and gingival inflammation compared to baseline measures and to placebos and other positive controls (Box 27.4).[6–8] Although very few of these formulations consistently perform as well as positive control rinses (i.e., CHG, EO), there is great interest in natural-compound–containing oral rinse formulations. These have the potential to provide low-cost alternatives to more established, commercial products, particularly in less developed countries where access to some plant-based products may be greater.

BOX 27.4 Other Mouth Rinse Ingredients Undergoing Study

- Chitosan
- (Green) Tea
- *Salvadora persica* (miswak)
- Taurolidine
- Pomegranate
- Aloe vera
- Propolis (bee product)
- Turmeric
- Neem tree products
- Cinnamon
- Algae
- Witch hazel
- Povidone iodine
- Other polyherbals

In addition to biological and herbal containing oral rinse products, there has been some interest in vehicles (i.e., supplements) incorporating probiotics. **Probiotics** are live microorganisms that have health benefits for the host when administered alone or in combination. They can have an effect by being antimicrobial to pathogens, regulating the host response, or exerting a competitive exclusion mechanism, meaning that positive microorganisms are favored within the environment and produce a negative effect on pathogens. Although probiotics have been identified as having potential against oral pathogens, research is required to substantiate an effect on periodontal diseases, to determine the strains that are most beneficial, and how to best administer them.

The term **oral irrigation** refers to both powered and manual mechanisms for delivering water or an active ingredient within a solution via an irrigation tip into or around the gingival sulcus or periodontal pocket. This has applications in both the home and professional settings. Home or self-irrigation has been shown to be tolerated without damage to oral tissues. Also referred to as water flossing, it typically makes use of standard jet tips delivering a powered, pulsating stream of fluid (often water) with controlled variable pressure. While home irrigation has been shown to be effective as an adjunct to toothbrushing for improving gingival outcome measures, the research is limited and inconsistent, and therefore remains inconclusive.[9] Much of the research conducted has involved water irrigation suggesting a mechanical effect, but home irrigation devices may have an increased benefit when an antimicrobial agent is incorporated.[10] In addition to disrupting pathogenic microorganisms, irrigation with antimicrobials can positively control host inflammatory mediators. The penetration of the irrigant is dependent on the tip design, the pocket depth, and the patient's ability to access the affected sites. Home irrigation is typically referred to as supragingival irrigation.

Because most home oral healthcare practices, such as toothbrushing and oral rinsing, are minimally effective for the eradication of microbiota within the gingival crevice, subgingival oral irrigation as a delivery vehicle has been recommended to counteract these microorganisms. Needle-like tips called *cannulas* are available and specially designed to be placed below the gingival margin (Fig. 27.3). Although the use of such a tip allows for greater penetration into pockets, it is generally reserved for professional use because these tips require a high level of dexterity to avoid injury and access the specific disease sites.

Professionally Applied Modes of Delivery

Although professional debridement, including scaling and root planing, is recognized as the dental hygienists' standard of care for the prevention and treatment of periodontal diseases, there are some limitations surrounding its effectiveness. Adjunctive, professionally applied antimicrobial agents are aimed at reducing pathogenic bacteria in diseased sites that have resisted healing and for less accessible subgingival areas such as deep pockets, furcations, root concavities, and within the periodontal tissues. Such adjunctive periodontal interventions can be applied locally or systemically.

Locally applied antimicrobial treatments have the benefit of not requiring patient compliance, and the active agent is delivered directly to the affected site in high concentrations while being less invasive to the rest of the body. Professionally applied subgingival irrigation with various antimicrobials, such as povidone-iodine or CHG, has been investigated with mixed results, and positive outcomes have been shown to be only minimally beneficial and are often transient.[11]

Where professional subgingival irrigation is indicated, scaling and root planing should occur first to remove deposits that may interfere with penetration of the irrigant, and only low-level force should be used to prevent excessive penetration into surrounding epithelial tissues. Use of antimicrobials with ultrasonic instrumentation as a form of subgingival irrigation has not demonstrated convincingly beneficial outcomes. Professionally applied irrigants delivered with a cannula can reach the base of periodontal pockets, but active ingredients may not be retained in adequate concentrations for sufficient periods of time, or they may become deactivated by blood products. Because lateral dispersion of the antimicrobial via the cannula is limited, it should be applied circumferentially where indicated. The dental hygienist, together with the patient, will need to carefully weigh the costs of delivering professionally applied subgingival irrigation in relation to the expected clinical benefits.

See Box 27.5 for a critical thinking scenario about professional subgingival antimicrobial irrigation as an adjunctive dental hygiene intervention.

More severe periodontal disease complicates treatment and makes self-care behaviors (e.g., toothbrushing, flossing, mouth rinsing, home irrigation) as well as professional interventions (e.g., mechanical debridement) less effective as pockets deepen and clinical attachment loss increases. Controlled-release drug-delivery methods have been developed to address the limitations of conventional mechanical therapies. **Controlled-release drug delivery** refers to the use of professionally placed intracrevicular devices that provide local drug delivery for sustained periods of time.

Typically, intracrevicular devices consist of an antimicrobial active ingredient placed within a reservoir that controls the rate of drug release and provides sustained administration of the agent directly into the diseased periodontal pocket. In contrast with systemic administration

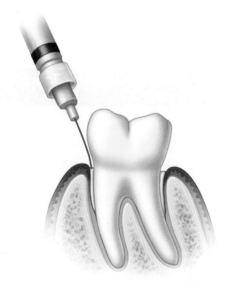

Fig. 27.3 Cannula for Professional Irrigation. (From Newman MG, Takei HH, Klokkevold PR, et al. eds. *Carranza's Clinical Periodontology*. 11th ed. Saunders; 2012.)

BOX 27.5 Critical Thinking Scenario A

Role-play the following scenario with another student: You and your classmate will play the roles of dental hygiene colleagues in general practice together; your classmate recommends using chlorhexidine gluconate (0.12%) as a subgingival irrigant with all patients who have pockets of 4 mm or greater as a routine intervention. What discussion would you and your colleague have about this intervention? Include in your discussion the evidence, or lack of, supporting this intervention.

BOX 27.6 Critical Thinking Scenario B

Visit the website of the American Dental Association (https://ebd.ada.org/en/evidence/guidelines) and view the ADA evidence-based clinical practice guideline. Specifically, look at the accompanying "chairside guide" and explain how this resource can contribute in a practical way to evidence-based decision making and dental hygiene care planning.

(see Systemic Delivery Methods), controlled-release drug delivery results in approximately 1000 times the concentration of the active ingredient within the gingival crevicular fluid (GCF) at the diseased site, but only about one hundredth of the systemic dose reaches the rest of the body. The **minimum inhibitory concentration** (MIC) is a research measurement tool used for these products to describe the lowest concentration of a particular antimicrobial able to inhibit microbial growth during incubation.

Several recently conducted comprehensive reviews and the ADA evidence-based Clinical Practice Guideline, with an accompanying chairside guide (http://ebd.ada.org/en/evidence/guidelines), analyze, summarize, and provide recommendations on several controlled-release drug delivery adjunctive nonsurgical treatments in addition to nonsurgical lasers and systemic antibiotics.[12,13] The ADA guidelines weigh the expected benefit of these products against the risk of adverse events and are especially helpful to clinicians in making suitable product recommendations.[12] The guidelines provide a "level of certainty" for the recommendations based on the amount of quality research included in the review to make the recommendations.[12] Careful determination of interventions should be based on the most current, quality research, the patient's health, the number and severity of sites requiring treatment, the ease of product use, and the degree of required patient adherence to recommendations.

Mechanical debridement alone, including scaling and root planing, within moderately deep pockets (4–6 mm) typically produces a mean pocket-depth reduction of approximately 1 mm and a gain in CAL of 0.5 mm. Sites with pockets over 5 mm in depth, especially those that present with bleeding, should be considered for these adjunctive antimicrobial therapies which include fibers, matrix delivery systems (i.e., films, chips), muco-adhesive gels, microparticulate systems (i.e., microspheres), nanoparticles, and others. Overall, locally delivered controlled-release antimicrobials provide an additional, moderate pocket depth reduction, and clinical attachment level gains from about one-third to one-half millimeter depending on the initial level of disease.

When periodontal disease becomes more advanced, periodontal treatment planning often involves the dental hygienist, dentist, periodontal specialist (periodontist), and the patient. The dental hygienist must be cognizant of the current literature surrounding these antimicrobial products and help in weighing the clinical relevance of the research findings with their patients. The most frequently used and studied locally delivered products are discussed in the following paragraphs, but research is ongoing on novel locally delivered periodontal products.

See Box 27.6 for a critical thinking scenario for using the ADA clinical practice guidelines and the "chairside guide" for developing dental hygiene care plans that potentially incorporate antimicrobial therapies.

Minocycline microspheres (Arestin®) include minocycline hydrochloride (1 mg), which is available in North America as a dry powder (Fig. 27.4). The product is delivered via a syringe-like handle with a preloaded narrow tip inserted subgingivally to the base of the periodontal pocket and immediately adheres within the site. The procedure can be viewed at Procedure 27.1, *The Evolve Video Resources,* and the corresponding *Competency Form* is located on the Evolve website. The

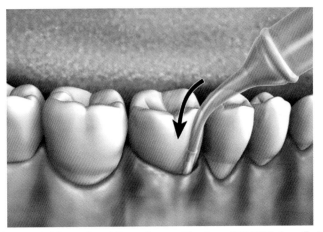

Fig. 27.4 Minocycline Microspheres. (Courtesy TOLMAR Inc, Fort Collins, Col. Atridox is a registered trademark of TOLMAR Inc.)

PROCEDURE 27.1 Placement of Controlled Release Drug: Minocycline Microspheres

Evolve Video Resource and Corresponding Competency Form

---

product is retained within the pocket without periodontal dressing. It well exceeds MIC levels within hours, and it remains active against predominant periodontal pathogens for approximately 14 days while it is slowly resorbed.

According to the ADA guidelines, there is a low level of certainty surrounding the available research conducted on minocycline microspheres because few clinical trials have been conducted, and they show only a small beneficial effect and some associated minor adverse events.[12] Although there is uncertainty surrounding the net benefit, the placement of minocycline microspheres is supported providing it is well considered with the patient regarding its harms versus benefits. Minocycline is from the tetracycline antibiotic family and is contraindicated for individuals with known sensitivity to this category of drug.

Chlorhexidine, a commonly used antiseptic for oral and other applications, is found in several controlled-release vehicles, including chips, gels, and irrigants (0.2% to 2%). The **chlorhexidine chip** (PerioChip®) is a biodegradable 4- to 5-mm hydrolyzed gelatin chip that incorporates 2.5 mg of chlorhexidine D-gluconate for insertion into pockets (Fig. 27.5). The biodegradable chip maintains an average concentration of 125 µg/mL of chlorhexidine within the GCF over a 7- to 10-day period, thereby exceeding the MIC and inhibiting almost all subgingival bacteria. The suppression of subgingival bacterial flora is evident for several weeks after the drug's release.

According to the ADA guidelines,[12] there is a moderate level of certainty surrounding an overall moderate benefit resulting from the chip, but there are potential adverse effects reported that diminish its net benefit. These largely surround oral pain or sensitivity and headache after placement of the chip but typically resolve after a few days. The ADA guidelines recommend the chlorhexidine chip as an adjunctive periodontal antimicrobial, providing it is considered for patients after other, potentially more effective, alternatives have been considered.[12]

The chlorhexidine chip is placed after scaling and root planing, and it is self-retentive after it is exposed to moisture (i.e., GCF). See Procedure 27.2 and the corresponding Competency Form. One chip per pocket site is used and should not be disturbed by homecare regimens for 1 week. The directions included with the product insert should be

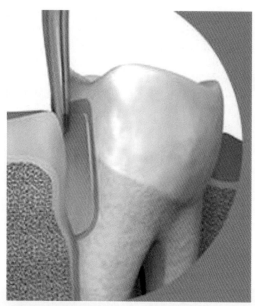

Fig. 27.5 Chlorhexidine Chip.

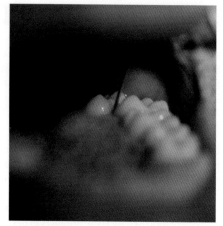

Fig. 27.6 Doxycycline Hyclate Gel.

PROCEDURE 27.3 **Placement of Controlled Release Drug: Doxycycline Gel**

Evolve Video Resource and Corresponding Competency Form

PROCEDURE 27.2 **Placement of Controlled Release Drug: CHX Chip**

Equipment
Personal protective equipment
Mouth mirror
Periodontal probe
Cotton pliers, cotton rolls, dry angles
Scaler(s)
Chlorhexidine chips

Steps
1. Determine need for controlled-release chlorhexidine chip therapy; explain risks and benefits and alternatives to treatment. Obtain informed consent.
2. Review medical and oral history; evaluate contraindications and precautions for treatment.
3. Remove required number of chips from package; note that product is stored at controlled room temperature of 59 to 77°F (15 to 25°C).
4. Isolate and dry area to prevent wetting chip during placement; grasp square end of chip with cotton pliers, and insert subgingivally.
5. Use cotton pliers or an instrument of choice to insert chip into deepest part of pocket.
6. Instruct the client not to floss area for 10 days; inform the client that some moderate sensitivity may be experienced for about 1 week in the area of placement. The client should clean other areas of mouth as usual and call the dental clinic if any pain, swelling, or problem occurs.
7. Schedule reevaluation and/or reapplication, or reevaluation of probe depths and clinical attachment levels may coincide with periodontal maintenance visit.
8. Document the intervention in detail in patient's record under services provided, dating the entry; include tooth numbers and sites and postoperative instructions given.

precisely followed. Because the chip self-resorbs, the need for professional removal is eliminated. The placement of a CHX chip is contraindicated for patients with the rare allergy to chlorhexidine.

Doxycycline hyclate gel (ATRIDOX®) consists of 10% doxycycline hyclate within a gel polymer that flows to the pocket base via cannula

and solidifies into a waxy substance on contact with the moisture of GCF (Fig. 27.6). The product provides controlled release of the antibiotic doxycycline for 7 days. The drug reaches GCF concentrations of more than 1500 mg/mL within hours, and these levels remain well above the MIC for most periodontal pathogens for 7 days. This product will biodegrade negating professional removal.

According to the ADA practice guidelines,[12] a low level of certainty surrounds doxycycline hyclate gel because of the very few controlled trials conducted. Although some research shows a substantial effect (0.64 mm clinical attachment gain) with combined use of the gel and scaling and root planing, other studies showed moderate, minimal, or no effect. There are few potential and reportedly mild adverse effects. Although the net benefit is uncertain, indicating additional research would be helpful for decision making, expert opinion supports its consideration for use.[12]

Doxycycline hyclate gel is available via a two-syringe system; the product is combined manually and then delivered into the pocket via a cannula. The procedure can be viewed at Procedure 27.3, The *Evolve Video Resources* and the corresponding *Competency Form* are located on Evolve. Periodontal dressing can be used to ensure retention particularly for shallower pockets. Doxycycline is a member of the tetracycline family, and therefore any known sensitivity to any drug in the tetracycline family is a contraindication to the administration of doxycycline gel.

CLIENT EDUCATION AND MOTIVATION REGARDING CONTROLLED RELEASE ANTIMICROBIAL INTERVENTIONS

- The dental hygienist must discuss with the client both the potential benefits and possible adverse effects of antimicrobial agents: the expected "net benefit."
- It is important to explain to the client that the measurement and evaluation of clinical parameters—such as plaque, bleeding, gingival, and probing depth scores—will be required as a follow-up (evaluation) after the introduction of an antimicrobial intervention. If clinical outcomes are improved, antimicrobial therapy may no longer be indicated.

LASERS AS ADJUNCTS IN ANTIMICROBIAL PERIODONTAL THERAPY

In addition to controlled released drugs, antimicrobial periodontal treatments also include the nonsurgical use of lasers. *Laser* is an acronym for "light amplification by stimulated emission of radiation," and interest in dental **laser therapy** applications is growing. Dental lasers are classified according to various factors and uses, including:

- Wavelength
- Delivery system
- Emission modes
- Tissue absorption
- Clinical applications

There are various potential applications for lasers in gingival and periodontal therapies, but the research must be reviewed to determine if there is strong evidence to support their broadening use. Lasers marketed and used in dentistry must be federally approved. Currently, scientific research lacks support for the use of lasers as an alternate or adjunctive method for debridement, root planing, or curettage, as it does not provide a consistent additional benefit beyond what is achieved through meticulous scaling and root planing. Specific laser therapies are recommended as an adjunctive antimicrobial treatment augmenting periodontal debridement. Currently approved lasers can reduce subgingival bacterial loads, and some have been shown to contribute to new epithelial attachment.

The ADA evidence-based practice guidelines include recommendations surrounding various laser therapies used for adjunctive periodontal therapy.[12] The photodynamic therapy diode laser (PTD diode laser) can be considered as it has been shown to exert a moderate effect in some studies although other research demonstrated little or no effect. While there is little concern about adverse events, there is much uncertainty remaining about expected benefits, and so PTD diode laser treatment should only be considered for patients after contemplating other, more predictable adjunctive antimicrobial therapies.

For other adjunctive periodontal laser therapies, there is a low level of certainty for their use. Non-PDT diode laser therapy, erbium laser therapy, and the Nd:YAG laser therapy are not recommended in the ADA guidelines because no persuasive evidence of a benefit has been shown.[12] However, dental hygienists will need to keep up to date with the research on laser therapies for the treatment of periodontal diseases as advances in periodontal laser applications are likely.

See Box 27.7 for a critical thinking scenario to demonstrate evidence-based decision making surrounding various locally delivered self and professionally applied antimicrobial therapies.

SYSTEMIC DELIVERY METHODS

Systemically delivered antimicrobials are ingested and then delivered via the bloodstream. Some of these methods are self-delivered, such as fluoridated water for caries prevention (see Chapter 45), whereas many methods require professional administration, such as prescription oral antibiotics. Systemic applications have the advantage of being able to reach more widely distributed pathogens. **Antibiotics** are a type of systemically delivered antimicrobial drug used primarily against bacterial infections. Although some may have antiprotozoal effect, they are ineffective against viruses. They may kill or in some way inhibit the growth of bacteria. Prescription antibiotics delivered systemically for the treatment of periodontitis travel from the bloodstream to the periodontal tissues, eventually reaching the GCF, where they gain access to the subgingival microflora, albeit in low concentrations. Systemic antibiotics for the treatment of periodontal diseases typically should be administered starting the day debridement is completed and continue for a short period of time (i.e., 7 to 21 days).

Several antibiotics have been used systemically either singularly or in combination for the treatment of periodontitis, including:

- Amoxicillin
- Penicillin
- Doxycycline
- Tetracycline
- Azithromycin
- Metronidazole
- Clindamycin

Several comprehensive reviews have been conducted evaluating the benefits of systemic antibiotics on various forms of periodontitis and have showed varying results.[12-15] A Cochrane systematic review and meta-analysis concluded that there was very low certainty evidence to support adjunctive systemic antibiotics to augment nonsurgical periodontal therapy, but other systematic reviews have concluded more beneficial effects.[12-15] While no one antibiotic has been found to be consistently superior to others, metronidazole in combination with amoxicillin showed the best effects. According to the ADA evidence-based clinical practice guidelines, for clients with moderate to severe periodontitis, systemic antimicrobials may provide a small net benefit.[12] However, the guidelines give the intervention a weak recommendation and advise clinicians to consider other treatments first, especially in cases of less severe periodontitis.[12] Systemic antibiotics may be indicated when the periodontal condition is particularly aggressive and/or resistant to healing.

Although systemic administration provides a means of delivering antibiotics to deep periodontal pockets, it is also associated with various contraindications, precautions, and side effects (Box 27.8; see also Box 27.7). Antibiotics are collectively known to cause allergic reactions in some patients. Successful systemic administration requires ongoing patient adherence to the antibiotic protocol; this is a concern because many patients fail to carefully follow prescriptions. Furthermore, the routine use of antibiotics to treat periodontal diseases is not recommended because of concerns about the development of antibiotic-resistant microorganisms. Therefore, as with all interventions to treat periodontal diseases, prescribing systemic antibiotics must be carefully considered based on the evidence, specific clinical situation, and patient considerations.

BOX 27.7 Critical Thinking Scenario C

Develop a case that would support the recommendation of each of the following oral antimicrobial interventions using the most current evidence and patient-specific assessment findings:
- Twice-daily use of over-the-counter therapeutic home oral rinse (Listerine)
- Placement of minocycline microspheres (Arestin)
- Professional use of PTD diode laser

BOX 27.8 Conditions Associated with Systemic Antibiotic Therapy

- Gastrointestinal upset
- Sensitivity to sunlight
- Intrinsic staining in developing teeth
- Potential toxicity to pregnant mother and fetus
- Increase in vaginal candidiasis
- Impaired absorption of some nutrients
- Depressed prothrombin activity
- Potential to render oral contraceptives less effective

As an alternative to systemic antibiotics for the treatment of periodontal diseases, another systemic approach is host modulation of the immune-inflammatory response using a subantimicrobial systemic dose of antibiotics. The term **subantimicrobial systemic dose** refers to the administration of a reduced dose of a drug for purposes other than the elimination of a pathogenic microorganism: in this case, host modulatory therapy. A subantimicrobial dose of doxycycline hyclate (Periostat®) may be administered in low doses (e.g., 20 mg twice daily) over long periods of time (e.g., 6 to 9 months) to inhibit key destructive enzymes involved in the immune-inflammatory response and destruction of periodontal tissues associated with periodontal diseases.

The ADA guidelines state with a moderate level of certainty that a subantimicrobial systemic dose of doxycycline produces a small benefit: a 0.35-mm gain of clinical attachment.[12] A recent systematic review confirms periodontal benefits but with very low to low levels of certainty.[16] Although there is some risk of adverse effects, such as gastrointestinal upset and allergic reactions, the recommendation is in favor of its use. The adjunctive use of subantimicrobial dose antibiotics can be considered particularly for patients with moderate to more severe levels of periodontal disease.

In subantimicrobial low doses, antibiotics are not antibacterial, and no detrimental shifts in the normal periodontal flora or antibiotic resistance have been observed. Despite the reduced dosages, subantimicrobial-dose doxycycline is contraindicated for individuals who are sensitive to the tetracycline antibiotic family. In addition, other side effects and potential adverse reactions are possible and should be reviewed before use.

LEGAL, ETHICAL, AND SAFETY ISSUES

Dental hygienists must adhere to the regulations of their practice jurisdiction when advising patients and implementing specific antimicrobials. In many jurisdictions, certain antimicrobials require a prescription by a dentist and may or may not be administered by a dental hygienist. Regardless of the regulations allowing or restricting dental hygienists' ability to prescribe and implement some antimicrobials, dental hygienists must be prepared to discuss these interventions with their patients based on the most current evidence. It is the responsibility of the oral healthcare team to provide evidence-based information to patients. See Boxes 27.9 and 27.10 for an overview of legal, ethical, and safety issues and for an ethical thinking scenario.

BOX 27.9   Legal, Ethical, and Safety Issues: Overview

- Dental hygienists have a legal and ethical obligation to have a sound understanding of the current literature surrounding personally and professionally applied antimicrobial interventions. Making use of systematic reviews and practice guidelines is helpful for this professional responsibility.
- Patient assessment should include the evaluation of the presence and distribution of bacterial plaque and plaque retentive factors. Care plans should include educational, preventive, and therapeutic interventions to enhance patient oral hygiene and periodontal condition, including the consideration of adjunctive, antimicrobial agents.
- Carefully review the patient's health and dental history to be sure that patients selected for oral antimicrobial therapy have no allergies or drug interactions with the agent being recommended. Instruct patients to keep antimicrobial agents out of the reach of children.
- Dental hygienists are gaining increasing scopes of practice; these may include the administration of antibiotics and the use of periodontal lasers and other adjunctive antimicrobial therapies. Such expansions to dental hygiene practice may require additional education and clinical training.
- Dental hygienists have a legal and ethical responsibility to ensure patients are informed about the benefits and risks of an antimicrobial therapy. They should understand the expected net benefit. Where evidence is lacking, patients should also be aware there is less certainty about beneficial outcomes and risks. The use of evidence-based care incorporating communication techniques for motivating patients about new, beneficial behaviors is required.
- Throughout the dental hygiene process of care, legal records should clearly demonstrate that patients have been educated about their current oral health status and counseled regarding recommendations designed to improve oral health and prevent further deterioration. Records should also include the patient's response to the dental hygiene care plan (i.e., consent), a description of the implementation of interventions, and notes regarding the ongoing evaluation of the patient's progress and treatment outcomes.

BOX 27.10   Legal, Ethical, and Safety Issues: Scenario

You are a recent dental hygiene graduate and a new member of a busy and progressive dental practice. You discover that the dentist is recommending that all new adult patients receive the professional use of a diode laser at their first dental hygiene appointment to assist in what they describe as a "more complete periodontal debridement." Having recently graduated, you understand that this type of laser therapy has not demonstrated consistent and reliable effectiveness and has only a weak level of evidence. So far, only the more experienced dental hygienist in the practice has been using the diode laser during dental hygiene therapy, but you expect that it will not be long before you are scheduled to deliver this service. You are worried because you have never used the equipment. How should you proceed?

KEY CONCEPTS

- Bacterial oral biofilm and periodontal pathogens are the primary initiating etiologic agents in inflammatory periodontal diseases, but it is the host immune-inflammatory response that modulates the progression of disease.
- Although the daily mechanical removal or disruption of dental biofilm and periodic professional removal of plaque-retentive deposits remain the backbone of gingival and periodontal disease prevention and control, oral antimicrobials provide adjunctive benefits that should be considered in dental hygiene care planning.
- Evaluating oral antimicrobial products requires supportive evidence from repeated long-term (≥3 months) clinical trials conducted in homogeneous population groups with comparable interventions and include appropriate controls and outcome measures. Ideally, secondary analysis, including

systematic reviews and metaanalyses and robust clinical practice guidelines, should be available to support these interventions.
- An essential oil antiseptic mouth rinse approaches the efficacy of the gold standard (chlorhexidine gluconate) as an adjunct to mechanical methods for daily plaque control and is considered comparable for gingival improvements without undesired side effects; mouth rinse, with or without alcohol, has not been shown to be linked to oropharyngeal cancer; alcohol-containing mouth rinses are not associated with real or perceived reductions in salivary flow or detrimental changes to pH.
- While there may be a mechanical effect, the research surrounding supragingival irrigation as a homecare adjunct to conventional oral hygiene is limited

REFERENCES

1. American Dental Association; 2017. Available at: http://www.ada.org.
2. Canadian Dental Association. 2017. Available at: https://www.cda-adc.ca.
3. Asadoorian J. Therapeutic oral rinsing with commercially available products. *Can J Dent Hyg.* 2016;50(3):126–139.
4. American Dental Association. *ADA-seal of Acceptance*; 2017. Available at: www.ada.org/science-research/ada-seal-of-acceptance.
5. ADA Council on Scientific Affairs. *Chemotherapeutic Products for Control of Gingivitis; Acceptance Program Requirements: Chemotherapeutic Products for Control of Gingivitis*; June 2016.
6. Chen YW, McGrath RW, Hagg C, et al. Natural compound containing mouth rinses in the management of dental plaque and gingivitis: a systematic review. *Clin Oral Investig.* 2014;18(1):1–16.
7. Asadoorian J. Therapeutic oral rinsing with non-commercially available products: position paper and statement from the Canadian Dental Hygienists' Association, part 2. *Can J Dent Hyg.* 2017;51(1):30–41.
8. Janakiram C, Venkitachalam R, Fontelo P, Iafolla TJ, Dye BA. Effectiveness of herbal oral care products in reducing dental plaque & gingivitis – a systematic review and meta-analysis. 11 *BMC Complement Med Ther.* 2020;20(1):43.
9. Worthington HV, MacDonald L, Poklepovic Pericic T, Sambunjak D, Johnson TM, Imai P, Clarkson JE. Home use of interdental cleaning devices, in addition to toothbrushing, for preventing and controlling periodontal diseases and dental caries. *Cochrane Database Syst Rev.* 2019;4: CD012018. DOI: 10.1002/14651858.CD012018.pub2. Accessed 07 November 2023.
10. Husseini A, Slot DE, Van der Weijden GA. The efficacy of oral irrigation in addition to a toothbrush on plaque and the clinical parameters of periodontal inflammation: a systematic review. *Int J Dent Hyg.* 2008;6(4):304–314.
11. Nagarakanti S, Gunupati S, Chava VK, et al. Effectiveness of subgingival irrigation as an adjunct to scaling and root planing in the treatment of chronic periodontitis: a systematic review. *J Clin Diagn Res.* 2015;9(7):ZE6–ZE9.
12. Smiley CJ, Tracy SL, Abt E, et al. Evidence-based clinical practice guideline on the non-surgical treatment of chronic periodontitis by means of scaling and root planing with or without adjuncts. *J Am Dent Assoc.* 2015;146(7):525–535.
13. John MT, Michalowicz BS, Kotsakis GA, et al. Network meta-analysis of studies included in the clinical practice guideline on the nonsurgical treatment of chronic periodontitis. *J Clin Periodontol.* 2017;44:603–611.
14. Khattri S, Kumbargere Nagraj S, Arora A, Eachempati P, Kusum CK, Bhat KG, Johnson TM, Lodi G. Adjunctive systemic antimicrobials for the non-surgical treatment of periodontitis. *Cochrane Database Syst Rev.* 2020;11: CD012568. DOI: 10.1002/14651858.CD012568.pub2. Accessed 07 November 2023.
15. Teughels W, Feres M, Oud V, Martin C, Matesanz P, Herrera D. Adjunctive effect of systemic antimicrobials in periodontitis therapy: a systematic review and meta-analysis. *J Clin Periodontol.* 2020;47(S22):257–281.
16. Donos N, Calciolari E, Brusselaers N, Goldoni M, Bostanci N, Belibasakis GN. The adjunctive use of host modulators in non-surgical periodontal therapy. A systematic review of randomized, placebo-controlled clinical studies. *J Clin Periodontol.* 2020;47(S22):199–238.

28

Hand-Activated Instrumentation

Joyce Y. Sumi and Michaela T. Nguyen

PROFESSIONAL DEVELOPMENT OPPORTUNITIES

A competent clinician must be proficient in the basics of mechanical debridement by hand instrumentation to provide optimum patient care. Understanding the variations in the common functional parts of all periodontal therapy instruments can aid the clinician in determining the purpose, effectiveness, efficiency, and comfort of use.

COMPETENCIES

1. Discuss the functional components of hand-activated instruments used in nonsurgical periodontal care.
2. Differentiate periodontal treatment and assessment hand-activated instruments.
3. Select design considerations for assessment and treatment instruments based on the periodontal health status and needs of a patient.
4. Relate the basic stroke principles of hand-activated instrumentation to the requirements for effective instrumentation.
5. Discuss treatment instrument selection and criteria considerations in determining the appropriate instrument design and blade size and customize details regarding their sequencing and use for periodontitis-affected teeth.
6. Elucidate the benefits and ethical principles associated with maintaining sharp hand-activated instruments.
7. Describe the application of basic elements of instrumentation skills to optimize effective treatment and minimize risk for injury.
8. Summarize the key elements of comprehensive posttreatment patient education.

EVOLVE VIDEO RESOURCES

Please visit http://evolve.elsevier.com/Pieren/hygiene/ for videos demonstrating the use of various hand-activated instruments, additional practice, and study support tools.

INTRODUCTION

Patients need routine professional therapeutic and preventive procedures to assess and control etiologic agents that cause oral diseases. Hand-activated instruments are used in caring for the full spectrum of patients with healthy and diseased periodontium. The procedure is a widely accepted protocol for the management of periodontal disease.[1] Hand instrumentation continues to be the gold standard for nonsurgical periodontal treatment.[2] The treatment of periodontal inflammation has become essential for both oral and overall systemic health.[3] The increased awareness of the potential transmission of infection from aerosol-generating procedures[4] highlights the need for all clinicians to be proficient in hand-activated instrumentation as well as power scaling.

Dedicated time and training are necessary to develop the knowledge and an experienced skilled approach to successful subgingival instrumentation that avoids harm to the root surfaces[5]. Becoming a competent clinician involves the capability to manage supragingival and subgingival periodontal instrumentation skills for the proper hand-activated instrumentation outcomes for patients and clinicians (Box 28.1).

BASIC DENTAL HYGIENE INSTRUMENT DESIGN: PARTS AND CHARACTERISTICS

A good hand-activated instrument supports three functional parts (Fig. 28.1).

Functional Parts of a Hand Instrument
Handle
- Typically, the longest part of an instrument where clinicians hold or place their grasp.

Shank
- Has two sections, the functional shank and terminal shank, that connect the working end to the handle (Fig. 28.2).

Working End
- The part from the terminal shank to the end of the instrument that comes in contact with the tooth or tissue.

Handle Characteristics

The handle is the information source to transmit vibrations to the clinician's hand. When an instrument is selected, handle specifications primarily benefit clinician comfort and ergonomics. The manufacturer options in the design of the instrument handle can reduce the potential adverse effects of repetitive strain injuries (RSIs) on clinicians by decreasing the demand for excessive pinch forces.[6]

Handles come in wide varieties including removable and nonremovable working ends. An example of this could be a mouth mirror (interchangeable) and a sickle scaler (nonreplaceable).

Material

Hand-activated instruments are made of various metals, resins, or silicones.
- Clinicians have reported handles with resin and silicone materials are more comfortable.[7]

Diameter Size

Size grips have a wide range from small to large (Fig. 28.3).
- Larger-diameter handles can reduce or prevent upper-extremity pain better than the smaller, slender handles.[8]
- Use of too slender handles increases pinch forces and can lead to cramping of the hands.[9]

BOX 28.1 Proper Hand-Activated Instrumentation Outcomes for Patient and Clinician

- Periodontal health for patient will be established and/or maintained when the clinician can effectively apply the fundamental initial and maintenance instrumentation used in periodontal therapy
- The patient will have a comfortable experience when the clinician possesses basic knowledge of instrument designs to meet treatment objectives and is able to minimize trauma to tissues
- There will be an increase in patient health literacy on hand instrumentation procedures when the clinician uses proper hand-activated instrument techniques and educates patient for their comfort, health, and safety
- The patient will have clinically and esthetically pleasing results when the clinician is able to appropriately select instruments for the removal and/or disruption of calculus, biofilm, and stain

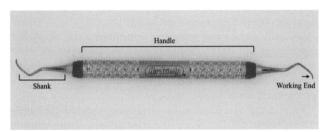

Fig. 28.1 Functional parts of a hand-activated instrument.

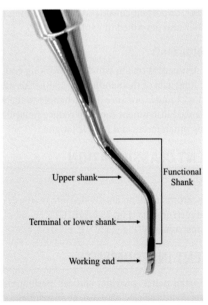

Fig. 28.2 Characteristics of a shank.

- Research has suggested that a 10-mm diameter is optimal.[10,11]
- Larger diameter grips can present challenges to patients that have difficult-access areas and limited mouth-opening ability.

Texture (Knurling) and Shape
Knurling refers to the cut pattern or the relief that assists with the instrument's grasp and control.

Common shapes are round or hexagonal.

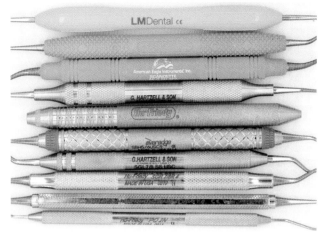

Fig. 28.3 Instrument handle variations in size, shape, pattern, and texture.

- Circumference shape affects the practitioner's comfort level when a suitable surface pattern and material are used.
- Padding and texture of silicone on the handle help decrease muscle stress.[11]

Weight
The two basic types of handles that can affect the weight are either solid or hollow construction.
- Hollow-handled instruments are lighter and less strenuous to use than solid handles.[12]
- Greater tactile sensitivity than solid-handled instruments.

Shank Characteristics
Description
Functional shank (Fig. 28.2)
- The overall shank that starts from the bend nearest the handle to the tip of the working end.
Terminal shank (Fig. 28.2)
- The portion of the functional shank that is from the last bend or curve closest to the working end.

The position of the terminal shank to the working end is important in determining the correct positioning of the angulation of the curet, sometimes referred to as curette, blade. The terminal shank of most instruments is parallel to the long axis of the tooth during usage.

Important differences in shank design help determine the use of each particular instrument.

Length
Shank lengths can range from short to long (Fig. 28.4).

A short lower shank (A and B) is best suited for the following:
- Anterior teeth with shallow probing depths
- Supragingival procedures
- The need to fulcrum close to the area instrumented

A long or extended lower shank (C) is preferred for the following:
- Use on teeth with deep periodontal probing depths or recession
- The need to fulcrum a great distance from the area instrumented

Angle
The shank of an instrument usually has angle configurations that are straight, curved, or bent angles.

Most periodontal instruments have curved or bent shanks in at least one and usually two places (Fig. 28.5). In general, the degree and

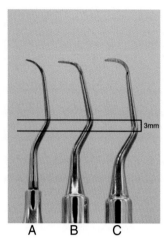

Fig. 28.4 Comparison of Gracey instrument shank lengths. (A) Gracey 1/2. (B) Gracey 5/6. (C) Gracey After-Five series 5/6.

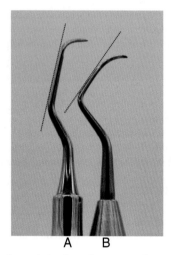

Fig. 28.5 Comparison of shank angles or curvatures. (A) Gracey curet 5/6. (B) Universal curet.

TABLE 28.1	Shank Flexibility
Shank Flexibility	**Usage/Purpose**
Flexible	Detect and remove light subgingival calculus deposits or oral biofilm
Moderately Flexible	Ideal for removal of light to moderate calculus Providing adequate resistance against this type of hard deposit
Rigid	Remove tenacious moderate to heavy calculus Providing firm resistance against this type of hard deposits
Extra Rigid	Remove tenacious and heavy calculus Providing strong and unyielding resistance against this type of hard deposits

Working End

Description

Each working end is designed for a specific task and determines the general purpose of the instrument (Fig. 28.6).

Identically named and numbered instruments can vary among manufacturers with slight differences regarding shape, length, cutting edges, width, strength, bend or curvature, and metallurgy or material of working ends. These details are important considerations when selecting instruments for purchase.

Design names and numbers are identifying marks on the handles. The design name usually indicates the manufacturer, person, or institutional origin of the instrument. The numbers usually indicate the type of working end(s) of the instrument. On double-ended instruments, two numbers follow the name, each designating a working end (e.g., Columbia 13/14). Important considerations in working ends are illustrated in Fig. 28.7 and described in Table 28.2.

Balanced Instruments

A balanced instrument is one in which the working ends are in alignment with the long axis of the handle (Fig 28.8). This allows the most effective transfer of finger pressure on the handle to the working ends. Utilizing a balanced instrument can help reduce musculoskeletal injuries by reducing pinch forces and muscle fatigue.[13]

INSTRUMENT CLASSIFICATION

Description

Dental hygiene care instruments are divided into two basic classifications:
- Assessment instruments (Fig. 28.9A, B, C)
- Treatment instruments (Fig. 28.9D, E, F, G)

ASSESSMENT INSTRUMENTS

Assessment instruments provide clinical periodontal and tooth evaluation information. Basic assessment instrument categories are explorers and periodontal probes. Categories of mouth mirrors include diagnostic instruments such as explorers and probes; however, their use also coincides with treatment instruments.

Mouth Mirror

Design and use. The traditional **mouth mirror** has a handle and mirror, each with a threaded design or cone-socket attachment (Table 28.3). Mirror heads have a variety of sizes from 5/8- to 2-inch diameters. The most commonly used mouth mirror in dental hygiene procedures is the manufacturer sizing of No. 4 and No. 5, which is approximately 7/8 to 1 inch in mirror diameter (Fig. 28.10).

angle of curvature can determine the area(s) in which the instrument is effective.
- Smaller angles and fewer shank bends are more suitable for use on anterior teeth.
- More acute angles and a greater number of shank bends are more suitable for use on posterior teeth.

The implementation of intraoral and extraoral fulcrums can expand the versatility to use straighter shanked instruments in the posterior areas and curved-shanked instruments in the anterior areas.

Flexibility (Strength)

Strength and flexibility are determined by the type of metal and the thickness of the tapered diameter from the handle to the working end. The flexibility of the shank of an assessment instrument, such as a wire-like explorer, is important in transmitting vibrations from the working end to the clinician for increased detection accuracy. In addition, shank flexibility is an important characteristic that determines the strength of the treatment instrument as it transfers the clinician's pressure on the handle and shank to the working end against the tooth surface for calculus removal. The flexibility of the shank is particularly important in dental hygiene procedures (Table 28.1).

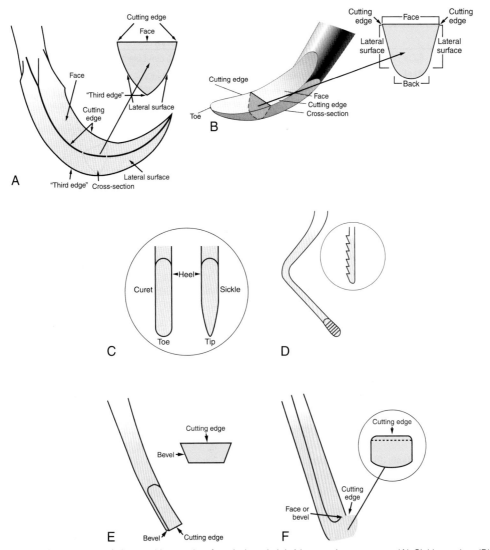

Fig. 28.6 Comparison of the working ends of periodontal debridement instruments. (A) Sickle scaler. (B) Curet. (C) Comparison of curet and sickle working ends. (D) File. (E) Chisel. (F) Hoe. (A, C through F Adapted from Daniel SJ, Harfst SA, Wilder RS. *Mosby's dental hygiene.* 2nd ed. St Louis: Mosby; 2008.)

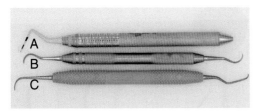

Fig. 28.7 (A) Single-ended instrument with a plastic periodontal probe. (B) Double-ended paired universal curet. (C) Double-ended unpaired instrument with a sickle on one end and curet on the opposite end.

Some considerations for mirror size selection are the following:
- Size of the patient's mouth
- A confined space within to place the mirror and another instrument
- The comfort of the clinician in holding and using a certain size mirror head

The head of the mouth mirror is categorized by the surface shape of the reflective face. The three basic types are the front, concave, or flat style (Table 28.3)

The face of the mirror is most effective when it is free from scratches, debris, and fogging. Surface condensation or fogging is due to the difference in temperature between the mouth and the mirror. Mouth breathing by the patient amplifies the problem. Care must be taken when inserting and using the mirror, as haphazard maneuvers can compromise comfort to the patient. (See Box 28.2 for suggested techniques for mouth mirror management.)

The modified pen grasp typically is preferred to hold the mouth mirror to provide stability during the retraction of the buccal mucosa, the lip, or the tongue (Fig. 28.11). Other grasp options can be used for the various mouth mirror functions (Table 28.4).

Explorer

Design and use. The **explorer** consists of a fine, wire-like tip with a sharp point that comes in a variety of lengths, diameters, and bends. A critical element of an explorer is the tactile sensitivity or the ability to sense the vibrations from the instrument. Explorer designs usually have narrow shank diameters to allow an increased tactile sensitivity to identify physical properties in the mouth. The differences in the curvature of the shank, length, and diameter make different explorers useful

TABLE 28.2 Common Design Specifications of Instrument Working Ends

WORKING END SPECIFICATIONS		
Design of the Blade (Fig. 28.6)	**Face**	Innermost surface of a curet blade
	Back	Opposite surface to the face
	Lateral Surfaces	Surfaces on either side of the face
	Cutting Edges	Sharp edges formed where the face and lateral surfaces meet

	Tip or Toe	• Area where the face, back, and lateral surfaces terminally converge
		  • A pointed end is a tip
		  • Rounded end is a toe

Materials of the Blade	**Stainless Steel**	• Maintain adequate sharpness for periodontal debridement • Do not rust or discolor when sterilized with saturated steam or with formalin-alcohol vapor

	Carbon Steel	• Compared to Stainless Steel:
		  • Feel sharper clinically and hold their sharpened edges longer after prolonged use
		  • More brittle and breaks more easily
		• Follow manufacturer instructions
		  • Dry heat sterilization is typically recommended to prevent corrosion or rusting.

	Stainless Steel Alloy	• Harder than traditional stainless steel • New metallurgy technologies are providing improved options for blade sharpness retention • Reduces the need for sharpening
	Stainless Steel Impregnated With Nitrate	• Do not need sharpening • Discard when coating is lost and become dull (approx. 3 to 4 months)
	Diamond Coated	• Designed for performing final root debridement, polishing root surfaces, and instrumenting furcation areas and other narrow inaccessible areas and when using an endoscope. • Not designed for removal of heavy calculus.
	Implants (Plastic, Graphite, Gold, Solid and Coated Titanium)	Tables 28.6 and 28.8 (Implant Application)
Styles of the Blade Ends	**Single-Ended** (Fig. 28.7A)	Instruments with only one working end
	Double-Ended, Paired (Fig. 28.7B)	Working ends with exact mirror images on the opposite ends
	Double-Ended, Unpaired B (Fig. 28.7C)	Dissimilar working ends that allow two different, distinct functions with two different instruments on the same handle

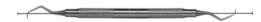

Fig. 28.8 Balanced instrument. Working end is in alignment with the long axis of the handle.

for specific purposes dependent on tissue, calculus, probing depth, tooth alignment, and other details specific to individual patients. Fig. 28.12 shows comparisons of explorer designs for various tasks. Procedure 28.1 outlines the criteria for design, selection, and procedure for use of the explorer.

Use and selection. Heavier, wider, or medium diameter explorers are sturdy. They generally do not deform, bend, or deflect during manipulation under and around caries and metallic margins (Box 28.3).

Fine, elongated diameter explorers allow an increased tactile sensitivity to enhance detection particularly when direct visibility is limited. Those with slightly bent and long designs assist in accessing the increased depths caused by apical migration. Short, curved, or acutely bent explorers help reduce difficulties to adapt to specific surfaces of the tooth. These designs are useful in shallow sulcus areas, around cementoenamel junctions (CEJs), and under contact areas (Box 28.4).

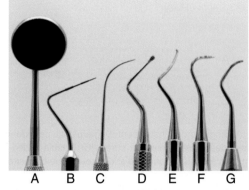

Fig. 28.9 Assessment instruments: (A) Mouth mirror, (B) periodontal probe, (C) explorer. Treatment instruments: (D) File, (E) Hoe, (F) Sickle, (G) Curet.

Tactile exploration is necessary before, during, and after periodontal instrumentation to enhance the quality of care by the clinician. Developing adept tactile skills for detection is as important as skills to remove deposits. Flat, burnished calculus is difficult to visualize

TABLE 28.3 Basic Types of Dental Mouth Mirror Surfaces

Type	Description	Advantage	Disadvantage
Front Surface	Mirror reflection is on the front of a flat glass	Clear image, no distortion	Reflection surface is scratched easily
Concave Surface	Mirror reflection is on the front of a curved glass	Magnified image	Distortion, decreased range compared to front surface
Flat (Plane) Surface (Fig. 28.10A)	Mirror reflection is on the back of a flat glass	Reflection surface resists scratching	Doubled or shadowed image
Rhodium Surface (Fig. 28.10B)	Highly reflective material	Sharp images	Images have less accuracy and brilliance than crystal/HD technology
Crystal/HD Surface (Fig. 28.10C)	Layers of metal oxides for reflective material	±40% brighter clarity and more accurate color than rhodium; less eyestrain	More expensive than traditional surface mirrors

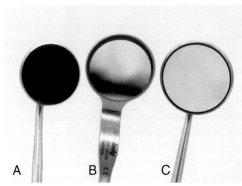

Fig. 28.10 Mouth mirrors in different sizes (A) No. 3. (B) No. 4 HD (C) No. 5.

on radiographs, particularly when deposits are located on facial or lingual surfaces of teeth or obscured by restorations. Light calculus, shallow probing depths, and friable tissue require only a gentle exertion of pressure. Increased pressure is required when trying to distinguish burnished calculus or irregular changes in the root caused by over-instrumentation. After thorough periodontal debridement, pressure from the explorer should be decreased to get an overview of the end product.

Periodontal Probe

See the discussion of periodontal probes in Chapter 20.

Design and use. The **periodontal probe** is a slender, tapered, blunt instrument with millimeter markings to measure and evaluate oral health (Table 28.5). This versatile instrument is useful in determining a wide variety of conditions (Box 28.5).

Personal clinician preference determines the selection of interval of millimeter markings and manufacturer design differences (see Chapter 20) such as color-coded markings of the periodontal probe. See Table 28.5 and Procedure 28.1 for variations of the periodontal probe and criteria for selection, design, and procedures.

A full-mouth probing is essential for accurate and comprehensive dental hygiene diagnosis, care planning, treatment, and referrals (Box 28.2).

Furcation Probe

Design and use. (See discussions of furcation involvement in Chapter 20 and furcation anatomy in Chapter 30.)

The **furcation probe** is a specialized probe instrument designed to adapt to the architecture of multirooted teeth. The typical furcation probe includes a curved shank with a blunted working end to clinically measure the vertical and horizontal depths of a furcation. The most widely used furcation detection instrument is the Nabers probe: the 1N and 2N (Fig. 28.13 and Box 28.7). The 1N is a specialized probe used for the detection and classification of mesial and distal furcations of maxillary molars, whereas the 2N Nabers probe is used for assessing these as well as buccal and lingual furcations.

See Box 28.8 for a critical thinking exercise to review the selection of assessment instruments. In addition, all patients can benefit from individualized education to improve awareness of the signs of oral health and disease in their own mouths (Box 28.9).

TREATMENT INSTRUMENTS

Hand-activated instruments used for calculus removal are **treatment instruments** in periodontal debridement. Differentiating treatment instrument design and function is an important element for providing high-quality care as required by ethical standards (See Box 28.6). The basic modified pen grasp and fulcrum placement techniques generally are used with all treatment instruments (Procedures 28.2 and 28.3).

Curets are typically included as the treatment instrument of choice in nonsurgical periodontal therapy. They typically have one face, two lateral surfaces (one or two cutting edges), and a rounded back and face that join to form a rounded toe (Fig. 28.6). The two main categories of curets are as follows:

- Universal curets
- Area-specific curets

Universal Curet

Design and use. The **universal curet** is a double-ended instrument designed with paired mirror-image working ends (Table 28.6). It is used for supragingival and subgingival periodontal debridement in all areas of the mouth. Universal curet designs have varied shank rigidity, blade curvature, and length (Table 28.6). The universal curet is identified with the following characteristics:

- Two lateral cutting edges on both sides of the flat face (inner surface) form a rounded tip (or toe) at the terminal end of the blade
- The face of the blade is positioned at ≤90° angle to the lower shank
- The blade is formed with the lateral surfaces converging to a rounded back that reduces the chances of trauma to subgingival sulcular tissues and tooth structure
- Both cutting edges are parallel and curved upward toward the toe of the blade (Fig. 28.14A) contrasting with area-specific curets to be discussed next (Fig. 28.14B)

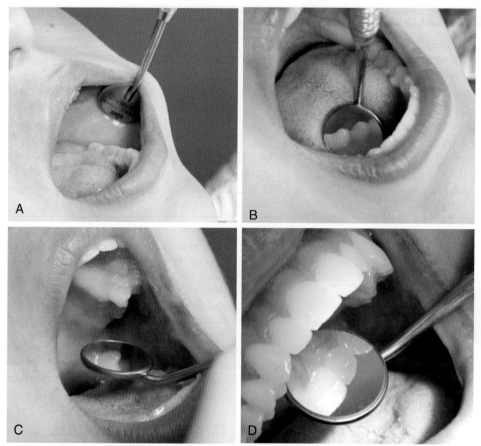

Fig. 28.11 Functions of a mouth mirror. (A) Retraction of buccal mucosa. (B) Indirect vision. (C) Indirect illumination. (D) Transillumination.

TABLE 28.4	**Use of the Dental Mouth Mirror**			
	RATIONALE OF USE AND TECHNIQUES			
Insertion	For patient comfort, enter from the front of the mouth with reflection surface up; avoid contacting teeth, use of excessive pressure of the mirror head against corner of the mouth, gingival tissues, or bony areas			
Surface Condensation	To prevent fogging, warm or wipe mirror surface against buccal mucosa, dip in warm water, mouthwash, or commercial antifog solution with gauze			
Function	**Description**	**Technique**		**Considerations**
Retraction (Fig. 28.11A)	To allow visualization or clearance of the soft tissues, and/or illuminate the working area during instrumentation by moving the lip, tongue, or buccal mucosa	Use modified pen grasp for stability in areas of resistance to the mirror head (Fig. 28.39) After insertion, roll handle to position and establish rest		Face of mouth mirror provide indirect vision head placed on tissues and pulled away from the working site or positioned toward working area to Care given toward corners of the mouth and hitting hard structures
Indirect Vision (Fig. 28.11B)	To view any areas or surfaces of the mouth that cannot be seen directly	Pen grasp option can be used to allow fluid movement of the mirror head around the mouth when there is no resistance and beneficial when examining or comparing large oral areas (Fig. 28.39) Mouth mirror directed toward working site and angled for clinician viewing		Useful on distal surfaces of last molars and mandibular lingual surfaces Face of mirror directed toward working site and angled for clinician viewing Most difficult function to master
Indirect Illumination (Fig. 28.11C)	To use reflective light in a working area to direct additional brightness into an area	Pen grasp optional Light reflected off mirror and directed at the working site		Useful on palatal surfaces of teeth Cannot be used for indirect vision at the same time
Transillumination (Fig. 28.11D)	To reflect light by a shadowing technique that passes the light through teeth or tissues to visualize the various densities	Pen grasp optional Face of mirror placed parallel to teeth, capturing the light to cause a "glow" to the teeth		Useful on anterior teeth for visualizing the contrast of caries and calculus Cannot be used on dense structures

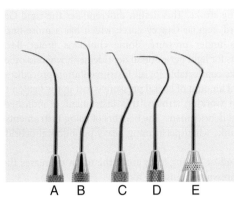

Fig. 28.12 Five typical explorers. (A) No. 3. (B) EXD 11/12. (C) No. 17. (D) No. 23 Shepherd's hook explorer. (E) No. 3H pigtail.

- The curvature of the blades defines the areas in which the instrument is most useful (Table 28.6).
- The handle is not parallel with the lower shank which necessitates closing the angulation for proper use, or slightly tilting the instrument toward the tooth to maintain an angle of ≤90 degrees (Fig. 28.15)

Universal working end/blade selection for anterior teeth (Procedure 28.2). Universal working end/blade selections for the anterior areas have the following considerations:

- Not critical (both working ends may be used)
- Exchanging working ends differ by the degree or angulation of the open blade
  - More open angulation increases traction and reduces burnishing of calculus

PROCEDURE 28.1 Use of Assessment Instruments

	Periodontal Probe	Periodontal Explorer
Equipment	Periodontal probe, mouth mirror	Periodontal explorer (3-A or ODU 11/12), mouth mirror
Grasp	Type: Pen or Modified Pen (Fig. 28.39A, B) Pressure: Light grasp; increase when discerning tooth structure, restorative materials, calculus	Type: Pen or Modified Pen (Fig. 28.39A, B) Pressure: Light to moderate grasp; increase when discerning tooth structure, restorative materials, calculus
Fulcrum and Pressure	Pressure: Relatively light and adjustable Placement: Intraoral, adjacent to tooth being instrumented, cross-arch, opposite arch, extraoral (Figs. 28.40A–E and 28.41A, B)	Pressure: Relatively light/moderate Placement: Intraoral, adjacent to tooth being instrumented, cross-arch, opposite arch, extraoral (Figs. 28.40A–E and 28.41A, B)
Working End Selection	*Periodontal probe:* Typically one working end; however, can be on one end of unpaired instrument	*3-A explorer:* Typically one working end (Fig. 28.12A) *11/12 explorer* (extended for deep periodontal pockets): Paired with two working ends. (Fig. 28.12B) On posteriors, the first bend angles distally • On anteriors, first bend angles toward midsection of tooth
Insertion, Adaptation, Angulation	*Periodontal probe:* (Table 28.5) Insertion: Working end parallel to long axis of tooth until the junctional epithelium is contacted Adaptation: Keep lower 1–3 mm of probe against tooth Angulation: Angle tip area directly under contact (col) at the interproximal area, with shank touching the contact *Furcation probe:* Insertion: Select side of working end that fits parallel and 0° to the long axis of the tooth, not perpendicular Guided by radiographs, previously recorded probing depths, and root anatomy knowledge, negotiate furcation probe into the area of the suspected furcation Adaptation: Gently rotate the probe tip toward the entrance of the furcation and note extent of penetration and classification *Implant probe* (Table 28.5): Insertion: Gently insert into the peri-implant sulcus until slight resistance is met. Maintain light pressure to avoid penetration of the implant mucosal attachment Adaptation: Adapt implant probe to implant surface	Insertion: Insert with lower end of explorer curved toward tooth until the junctional epithelium is contacted Adaptation: Lower 1–3 mm of explorer tip touching root surface
Activation, Stroke Direction, and Efficiency	Activation: Walk probe with gentle pressure along base of sulcus or pocket where the junctional epithelium feels soft and resilient; maintain one side of probe in contact with tooth surface Direction: Small, vertical increments Efficiency: Insert toward distal aspect of tooth; walk distally in small 1-mm increments until distal col area (under contact) of tooth is reached with upper portion of probe straightened and touching contact area Lift probe and reinsert at distal line angle; repeat technique by walking forward to mesial col area Continue throughout mouth buccally and lingually to six deepest readings of distal, buccal or lingual, and mesial surfaces from both buccal and lingual approach	Activation: Begin activation with insertion stroke (vertical) with both a push and pull stroke Light pressure: Friable tissue, light calculus, final assessment Increased pressure: Root irregularities, moderate to heavy calculus, burnished calculus Direction: Multidirectional strokes to assess calculus, burnished deposits, root caries, or restorative margins; upward and downward direction for detecting burnished or sheetlike calculus Efficiency: Long and sweeping strokes; evaluate root smoothness Short strokes: Encountering pieces of calculus or surface irregularities

• Less open angulation decreases inadvertent soft-tissue trauma against wall of pocket

Universal working end/blade selection for posterior teeth (Procedure 28.2). Universal working end/blade selections for the posterior areas have the following considerations:
• Critical (Working ends are not the same for the facial and lingual surfaces in the posterior areas)
• Working end best used for facial surfaces is used for mesial and distal interproximal surfaces of the facial aspect
• Working end best used for lingual surfaces is used for mesial and distal interproximal surfaces of the lingual aspect

Area-Specific Curets

Design and use. **Area-specific curets** are designed with shanks in a variety of strengths and lengths as well as blades of various sizes (Tables 28.7 and 28.8). These variations are to accommodate primarily the subgingival instrumentation needs of periodontally involved dentitions and are named after designers such as Gracey or Langer.

Area-specific curet designs may have specific modifications, with some examples listed below:
• Standard Gracey
• Extended shank Gracey
• Mini-bladed Gracey
• Micro mini-bladed Gracey
• Langer
• Double-Gracey

Area-specific blade design. The area-specific curet has two-bladed sides that come together to form a rounded toe, however, has only one designated cutting edge determined by the longer curved side is the cutting edge (Fig. 28.16).

Area-specific shank design. The shank rigidity of curet instruments is an important characteristic to consider when evaluating the needs of the procedure. Certain manufacturers make the Gracey curet with a rigid and even an extra-rigid shank that sustains the power used

in a working stroke. This design differentiates the rigid Gracey from the standard, regular Gracey curet, which has a more flexible shank that bends under pressure. Some clinicians prefer flexible-shank instruments for light periodontal debridement, whereas others find the rigid shanks comfortable for all instrumentation procedures. Because a significant amount of lateral pressure is lost in the flexion that occurs under firm working strokes, this instrument is indicated for light periodontal debridement. The benefits of using instruments with less-flexible shanks when performing heavy periodontal debridement are as follows:
• Less bend or flexing away from the tooth decreases the required lateral pressure against the tooth.
• Less dissipation of pressure when using elongated, specialized Gracey curets with extended fulcrums distant from the working area.
• More sustained pressure when instrumenting deep periodontal defects.
• Avoidance of injury due to reduced clinician effort with stroke direction needed with heavier deposits (see the discussion of hand, wrist, and finger injuries in Chapter 12).
• Reduces the chance of incomplete or burnished tenacious calculus removal due to more flexing.
• Enhances control without diminishing tactile sensitivity.

Gracey Curet

Design and use. The **Gracey curet** (Table 28.8) is a widely used area-specific curet designed for use in designated areas of the mouth.

Gracey curets consist of nine mirror-image pairs of instruments: the Gracey 1/2, 3/4, 5/6, 7/8, 9/10, 11/12, 13/14, 15/16, and 17/18 (Fig. 28.17). The designation of area-specific curets means that each of the instruments in the collection is designed to scale specific areas of the mouth (e.g., anterior vs. posterior) and specific tooth surfaces (e.g., mesial vs. distal). Gracey curets are particularly effective for instrumentation of teeth with slight to severe periodontitis in individuals who require therapeutic periodontal debridement. Although they are designed for use in designated areas of the mouth (area-specific), it is possible to use Gracey curets in a variety of places.

The basic reason Gracey instruments are ideal for instrumenting periodontitis-affected teeth lies with the relationship of the face of the blade to the lower or terminal shank. Whereas the universal curet's face is at 90°, the Gracey curet face is "offset" at an angle of 60 to 70° to the lower shank (Fig 28.14B). With this angle, the lower shank is parallel to the tooth surface and indicates proper angulation of the cutting edge to the tooth surface.

The Gracey curet blade arcs so that one cutting edge is elongated. This longer curved side of the Gracey curet, as shown in Fig. 28.16A and B, is the correct cutting edge. When the lower shank is perpendicular to the floor with the face of the blade up, this cutting edge is slightly lower than the shorter edge. Together with the basic arc of the blade, this elongation makes Gracey instruments particularly efficient in adapting to root morphology.

Variations of design in area-specific curets affects the selection and criteria for the use of each of the Gracey area-specific curets Table 28.7. Procedure 28.2 outlines the steps for their use.

Extended-Shank Curets

Design and use. The **extended-shank curets** are a modified set of Gracey curets that are exactly like the traditional Gracey curets, except that the lower shank of each instrument is 3 mm longer (Fig. 28.18). The extended length positions the bend in the shank to avoid interference of contact with the tooth and allows access to the base of the pocket. Extended Gracey curets are particularly useful in areas with

TABLE 28.5 Periodontal Probe Design, Use, and Considerations

COMMON DESIGN SPECIFICATIONS OF ALL PERIODONTAL PROBES

Marquis Color-Coded Probe 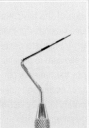	**Shank design:** Thin, round, and tapered **Tip design:** Thin tip • Measurement: Color-coded at 3, 6, 9, and 12 mm • Color coding every 3 mm is easy to read • Markings must be estimated between color bands • Thin tip may penetrate junctional epithelium if too much pressure is applied
UNC-12 and UNC-15 Probe (University of North Carolina) 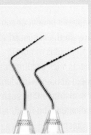	**Shank design:** Thin, round, and tapered **Tip design:** Thin tip • Measurement: UNC-12 and UNC-15 are marked in increments of • 1 mm ending at 12 or 15 mm • UNC-12 color coded at 5 and 10 mm • UNC-15 color coded at 5, 10 and 15 mm • UNC-12 is used for maintenance and UNC-15 for patients with significant attachment loss • Probe with the most markings to manage
Novatech Probe 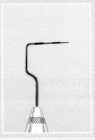	**Shank design:** Upward and right-angled bend **Tip design:** • Measurement: Available in a variety of designs • Paired with different probe ends • Easier access in posterior distal areas (primarily terminal distals), limited to distal surfaces
PSR Screening Probe (World Health Organization Probe) 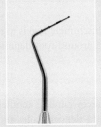	**Shank design:** Thin, round, and tapered **Tip design:** Thin tip with ball tip • Measurement: 0.5, 3.5, 5.5, 8.5, and 11.5 mm • Ball tip (0.5 mm) for patient comfort • Color coded from 3.5 to 5.5 mm • Easy-to-read markings • Markings at 0.5 mm
Nabers Furcation Probe 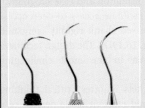	**Shank design:** Round, tapered, and curved **Tip design:** Blunted tip • Measurement: Available with or without measurement markings • Ideal for detection of mesial and distal furcations in maxillary molars. • May feel bulky compared to using a periodontal explorer for furcation detection
Implant Application 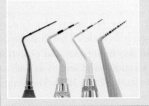	**Shank design:** Thin, round, and tapered **Tip design:** Thin tip or ball tip • Measurement: Color coded and variable measurements depending on manufacturer • Ball tip for patient comfort and less chance of penetration • Color coded: easy-to-read markings • Markings wear away on plastic probes, replaceable probe tip

BOX 28.4 Usage of Fine, Elongated Diameter Explorers

- Detection of supragingival calculus
- Detection of subgingival calculus
- To explore root structures
- To discern external root resorption
- To help distinguish morphologic crown and root anomalies
- To identify cementum irregularities

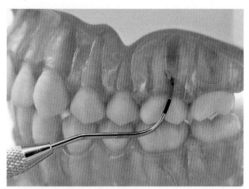

Fig. 28.13 (A) The No. 2 Nabers probe for detection of furcation areas, with color-coded markings at 3, 6, 9, and 12 mm. Probe positioned to assess furcation classification.

BOX 28.5 Usage of the Periodontal Probe

- Measuring probing depths
- Calculate clinical attachment level
- Measure relative attachment level
- Evaluate bleeding tendencies
- Locate calculus
- Demarcate the mucogingival junction
- Determine the amount of keratinized gingiva
- Measure the width of attached gingiva
- Measure gingival recession
- Assess furcation invasion or involvement
- To size atypical or pathologic lesions (Chapter 16)
- Measure distances between teeth

BOX 28.6 Legal, Ethical, and Safety Issues

- It is important for a clinician to have sound knowledge of the basic elements of hand-activated instruments to develop a sound rationale for their use and selection when participating in purchasing. Appropriate dental instruments are essential to provide proper treatment and care to patients.
- The clinician has instruments to assess the severity of the patient's periodontal condition and is educated to make decisions to recommend referrals to other professionals. Not evaluating the periodontal status by lack of full-mouth probing, or the need for referral, can put the patient at risk.
- The clinician should develop familiarity with hand-activated instruments and their function to create safety and efficacy in delivering treatment. Accurate knowledge of designs and functions ensures appropriate use and optimal outcomes for the patient.
- A dull treatment instrument does not provide a therapeutic benefit or contribute to the welfare of the patient when it can increase the likelihood of discomfort, tissue injury, and burnished or inadequate calculus removal.
- The clinician retrieves broken instrument tips, documents such occurrences in the patient record, and communicates with the patient about the incident and any necessary follow-up or referrals. When broken instrument tips cannot be found, a chest radiograph for the patient is indicated. The fractured tip must be treated as an ingested/aspirated foreign object.
- Communicate with patients what they should expect after a periodontal debridement session with hand-activated treatment instruments to assist them in the posttreatment recovery phase.

BOX 28.7 Usage of the Nabers Probe

- Allows subgingival insertion to find the dividing point in multirooted teeth
- Inspects bone support in furcation areas of bifurcated and trifurcated teeth
- Evaluates the extent and depth of the attachment loss in furcations
- Color-coded marking allows furcation classifications more accurately
- Aids in clinical diagnosis of through-and-through furcation areas

such as a mini-curet with a vertical stroke. This instrument also is useful in rounded convexities or concavities found around root depressions and line angles (Box 28.10).

Micro Mini-Bladed Gracey Curets

Design and use. The Micro Mini-bladed Gracey curet is another variation of the mini-bladed curet series with ultra-slender blades and shank rigidity. The blades are usually 20% thinner than mini-bladed Gracey curets to further reduce tissue distention and ease subgingival insertion. Elongated terminal shanks facilitate access to deep access periodontal pockets and slightly increased shank rigidity compared with the mini-bladed Gracey curet (Fig. 26.19D). The design facilitates precise periodontal debridement even in the most challenging periodontal pockets.

Challenging deep periodontal pockets requires critical thinking skills in choosing the most effective and efficient blade designs of a Gracey curet (Table 28.7).

Langer Curets

Design and use. The Langer curets have the bends of a Gracey shank with the blades of a universal curet to scale all tooth surfaces. They typically come in sets of four for use in anterior and posterior areas. Modified versions of the shank rigidity and length as well as standard and mini-bladed types are available (Table 28.8). The design

significant probing depth or recession. Some manufacturers offer a blade thinned by 10% to allow for ease during gingival insertion and to reduce tissue distention. The longer shank often requires an extended fulcrum such as an opposite arch, cross-arch, or extraoral fulcrum. Reinforcement with the nondominant hand often may be helpful for additional control.

Mini-Bladed Curets

Design and use. Another variation of the basic curet is the Gracey **mini-bladed curet**, which has a terminal shank that is 3 mm longer and a working blade that is half the length and slightly thinner than the traditional Gracey curet (Fig. 28.19A and C).

The mini-bladed Gracey curet is particularly useful in areas of narrow, deep pocketing. These situations can present limitations to vertically insert or instrument a long, regular blade straight down into the base of pockets or on interradicular root furcation surfaces. The options in these situations are to use a horizontal stroke with the toe directed to the junctional epithelium or to use a shortened instrument

PROCEDURE 28.2 Use of Curets

	Universal Curet	Area-Specific Curet
Grasp	Type: Modified Pen (Fig. 28.39B)	Type: Modified Pen (Fig. 28.39B)
	Pressure: Secure; responsive to changes by allowing handle (hence blade) to fluidly roll during calculus removal and around root topography such as line angles, convexities, and concavities	Pressure: Secure; responsive to changes by allowing handle (hence blade) to fluidly roll during calculus removal and around root topography such as line angles, convexities, and concavities
Fulcrum and Pressure	Pressure: Stable, moderate with working stroke; increases with tenacity of calculus	Pressure: Stable, moderate with working stroke; increases with tenacity of calculus
	Placement: Intraoral, adjacent to tooth being scaled	Placement: Intraoral, adjacent to tooth being scaled
	Cross-arch, opposite arch, extraoral (Figs. 28.40A–E and 28.41A, B)	Cross-arch, opposite arch, extraoral (Figs. 28.40A–E and 28.41A, B)
Working End Selection	See Table 28.6 to determine anterior vs. posterior usage	See Tables 28.7 and 28.8 for design and selection criteria of area-specific curets
	Posterior: Position universal blade against buccal or lingual surface of tooth and choose end that offers a more closed adaptation	*Gracey:* Position longer, lower cutting edge of offset blade against tooth; for vertical stroke, face of blade toward root surface, lower shank is parallel to the long axis of the tooth or root surface being scaled
	Anterior: Either working end	
Insertion, Adaptation, Angulation	Insertion: Blade in relatively closed position to base of pocket (0° to 10°)	Insertion: Blade in relatively closed position to base of pocket (0° to 10°)
	Adaptation: Adjust first 2 to 3 mm of blade against tooth surface using tactile sensations	Adaptation: Adjust first 2 to 3 mm of blade against tooth surface using tactile sensations
	Angulation: Open blade to between 60° and 80°	Angulation: Open blade to between 60° and 80°
Activation, Stroke Direction and Efficiency	Activation: Resecure grasp and fulcrum to achieve an effective working stroke; modify pressure against tooth by type, amount, and position of calculus and/or tooth irregularity; use the proper fingers to maximize lateral pressure and fluid strokes	Activation: Re-secure grasp and fulcrum to achieve an effective working stroke; modify pressure against tooth by type, amount, and position of calculus and/or tooth irregularity; use the proper fingers to maximize lateral pressure and fluid strokes
	Direction: Vertical, horizontal, and oblique pull stroke; vary stroke directions to complete calculus removal/root planing	Direction: Vertical, horizontal, oblique pull stroke; vary stroke directions to complete calculus removal/root planing
Implant Considerations	Other professional methods for biofilm removal: Subgingival glycine air polishing (see Chapter 32)	Other professional methods for biofilm removal: Subgingival glycine air polishing (see Chapter 32)
	Implant universal curet: Thin, mini-bladed or longer blade if access is needed around restorations (Table 28.6)	Implant area-specific set: Thin, mini- or micro-bladed with longer angled shanks if access is needed around restorations (Table 28.8)
	Healthy: Gentle sweeping, nonaggressive strokes	Healthy: Gentle sweeping, nonaggressive strokes
	Mucositis: Short horizontal strokes, overlapping and/or vertical if accessible and adaptable	Mucositis: Short horizontal strokes, overlapping and/or vertical if accessible and adaptable
	Peri-implantitis and Failing: Thin blade used in slight side-to-side movements to debride around implant threads; refer	Peri-implantitis and Failing: Thin, small blade used in slight side-to-side movements to debride around implant threads; refer

PROCEDURE 28.3 Use of Sickle Scalers

	Straight-Shanked Sickle (Anterior)	Contra-Angled Sickle (Posterior)
Grasp	Type: Modified Pen (Fig. 28.39B)	Type: Modified Pen (Fig. 28.39B)
	Pressure: Moderate grasp	Pressure: Moderate grasp
Fulcrum and Pressure	Pressure: Stable and moderate	Pressure: Stable and moderate
	Placement: Intraoral, adjacent to tooth being scaled	Placement: Intraoral, adjacent to tooth being scaled
	Opposite arch (Figs. 28.40A–E and 28.41A, B)	Cross-arch, opposite arch (Figs. 28.40A–E and 28.41A, B)
Selection of Working Ends based on Design	Based on amount of calculus, tissue tone, probing depth, and correct adaptation	Based on amount of calculus, tissue tone, probing depth and correct adaptation; location can influence blade size; i.e., SCNEVI-4 over S204-SD for periodontally involved patients with heavy calculus (Table 28.10)
	Anterior interproximal surfaces (Table 28.9)	
	Anterior and premolar interproximal areas (Table 28.10)	Use opposite end for alternate sides of tooth
	Sickles with thinner tip designs can be used for calculus located just below tight, anterior contact areas	
Insertion, Adaptation, Angulation	Engage lower edge of interproximal supragingival calculus; however, may extend 1 to 2 mm subgingivally when soft tissue permits	Engage lower edge of interproximal supragingival calculus; however, may extend 1 to 2 mm subgingivally when soft tissue permits
	Adaptation: Lower third cutting edge and tip of sickle closely adapted to tooth surface	Adaptation: Lower third cutting edge and tip of sickle closely adapted to tooth surface
	Angulation: Adjust blade to 80° to 90° against tooth surface.	Engage lower edge of supragingival calculus
		Engage ledge of subgingival calculus by keeping side of tip well adapted to root surface
		Angulation: Adjust blade to 80° to 90° against tooth surface
Activation, Stroke Direction and Efficiency	Activation direction *Supragingival:* Vertical to oblique pull stroke with moderate pressure across tooth surface	Activation direction *Supragingival:* Vertical to oblique pull stroke with moderate pressure across tooth surface
	Activation direction *Subgingival:* Vertical pull stroke using moderate pressure across subgingival area	Activation direction *Subgingival:* Vertical pull stroke using moderate pressure across subgingival area
	Efficiency: Repeat until all gross calculus is removed	Efficiency: Repeat until all gross calculus is removed

TABLE 28.6 Universal Instrument Design, Use, and Considerations

COMMON DESIGN SPECIFICATIONS OF ALL UNIVERSAL CURETS

Instruments (Posterior and Anterior Application)

Barnhart 5/6
Columbia 13/14
Younger Good 7/8

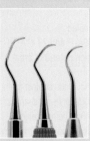

Design:
- Short lower shank
- Rigid or regular flexibility in shank

Use:
- Periodontal debridement of supragingival and subgingival biofilm and calculus

Consideration:
- Use on all anterior tooth surfaces
- Useful in posterior areas with healthy to shallow probing depths

---

Columbia 2R/2L
Columbia 4R/4L
Suter Barnhart 1/2

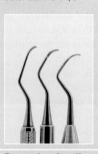

Design:
- Long lower shank
- Rigid or regular flexibility in shank

Use:
- Periodontal debridement of supragingival and subgingival biofilm and calculus

Consideration:
- The more bent the shank, the easier it is to reach interproximally
- The straighter the shank, the easier it is to reach buccally and lingually
- Useful on anterior teeth with moderate pockets and/or recession
- Useful on all posterior tooth surfaces with moderate to deep probing depth

---

Posterior Application

McCalls 17/18
Goldman-Fox 4

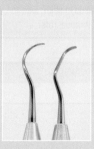

Design:
- Longer lower shank
- Shank: Thick, rigid
- Blade: Thick, heavy

Use:
- Instrumentation of supragingival and subgingival biofilm and calculus

Consideration:
- A less bent, curved shank makes it easier to reach buccally and lingually
- More bent the shank, the better access interproximally
- Useful on all posterior tooth surfaces with moderate to deep probing depth, retractable tissue, and heavy calculus deposits

---

10/11 Loma Linda
R 144 Queen of Hearts

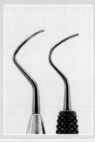

Design:
- Longer lower shank
- Regular flexibility in shank
- Long blade

Use:
- Periodontal debridement of supragingival and subgingival biofilm and calculus

Consideration:
- Use on posterior areas with moderate to deep probing depth.
- Blade design is advantageous for line angles

Universal Implant Instruments

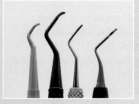

Design:
- Various types of materials and universal curet designs

Use:
- Maintenance instrumentation of supragingival and subgingival biofilm and calculus on all postsurgical dental implants

Consideration:
- No sharpening of working end

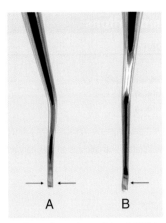

Fig. 28.14 (A) Face of a universal curet is at 90° to its shank. Double cutting edges indicated for the universal curet *(arrows)*. (B) Face of a Gracey curet is offset at a 70° angle to its shank. Comparison shows a single, lower working cutting edge on the downward slope of the Gracey blade *(arrow)*.

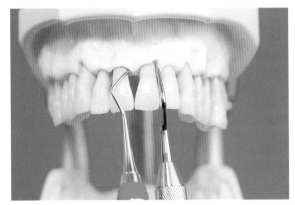

Fig. 28.15 Universal Barnhart 5/6 and Gracey 5/6. The angulation of the two instruments are shown as a result of the differences in the relationships of the face of the blade and the lower shanks.

allows the clinician to adapt and scale both mesial and distal surfaces with the same instrument end.

Additional Modified Gracey Curets

The all-purpose **Double-Gracey curets** are treatment instruments that have the bends of a Gracey shank; however, each working end has two complementary offset blades. These double-bladed Graceys come in sets of four, each able to scale mesial and distal surfaces with one working end (Fig. 28.20). The Double-Gracey curets come in standard and mini-bladed versions.

The **Gracey Curvettes** are area-specific instruments designed with longer shanks and shorter curved blades than the standard Graceys. They enhance adaptation to root surfaces in deep periodontal pockets and furcations. Various manufacturers call the Gracey Curvettes with straighter shanks designed for deep anterior pockets a Sub-0 (Fig. 28.21).

The **Maintenance Gracey curets** are modified area-specific curets for routine maintenance appointments (Fig. 28.22). These designs are useful for patients with tight, healthy tissues, residual pocket depths, and/or recession. Features include a thinner or smaller blade, a slightly closed-angle, and longer lower shanks that allow better access and easier insertion.

Sickle Scaler

Design and use. The **sickle scaler** has a pointed back, two lateral surfaces, two cutting edges, and a face that joins to form a pointed tip (Tables 28.9 and 28.10; see Fig. 28.6A).

The working end is usually 90° to the shank with flat cutting on both sides of the face. The major distinguishing factor from a curet is that the sickle scaler tip always ends in a sharp point. The two forms that the face of the sickle blade can come in are straight and curved.

The sickle shank design can be straight, contra-angled, or curved (Fig. 28.23). Identifying the sharp point of the blade in the curved blade in a contra-angled sickle scaler is important to set it apart from a curet.

The combinations of these design modification features have allowed the sickles to be an important supplement to ultrasonic

TABLE 28.7	Area-Specific Design Variations		
COMMON DESIGN SPECIFICATIONS OF ALL AREA-SPECIFIC CURETS			
Variations	**Options**	**Comparisons**	**Application**
Shank strength	Standard	Slight flexion with increased, firm pressure	Healthy or maintenance patients Light, nontenacious calculus removal
	Rigid and extra rigid	Larger, stronger, less-flexible shank	Moderate to heavy tenacious calculus removal
Shank length (Fig. 28.18)	Standard	Area specificity allows for periodontal debridement of with minimum attachment loss	Healthy or maintenance patients
	Extended	Terminal shank elongated by 3 mm	Deep periodontal pockets
Blade size (Fig. 28.19)	Standard	Upward, curved blade relative to the lower shank Gracey curets have an offset curved blade that produces an elongated cutting edge	Healthy to periodontally involved patients

	Mini	Slightly thinner blade, and length is reduced by approximately
		    50% of the standard blade
			Primarily useful in deep, narrow periodontal pockets
			    and furcations
			Precise debridement of root and tooth surfaces in
			    challenging periodontal pockets

	Micro	Blade length and thickness are reduced by approximately 20%
		    of a mini-bladed curet
			Helpful in tight, narrow periodontal pockets,
			    furcations, and line angles

	Modified Gracey	Reduced blade modifications in length and/or thickness made
		    for easier insertion
			Used for easier access into tight, healthy tissues such
			    as for routine periodontal maintenance case types

TABLE 28.8   Area-Specific Gracey Curet Design, Use and Considerations

INSTRUMENTS (ANTERIOR APPLICATION)

(A) Gracey 1/2
(B) Gracey 3/4
(C) Gracey 5/6

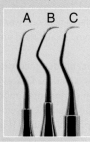

Design:
- Gracey 1/2: Straight shank is similar to but shorter than a Gracey 5/6
- Gracey 3/4: Bent shank is similar to but shorter than a Gracey 7/8
- Gracey 5/6: Straight shank is similar but longer than a Gracey 1/2

Use:
- Periodontal debridement of supragingival and subgingival biofilm and calculus on maxillary and mandibular anterior incisors and canines

Consideration:
- Shorter shank length limits instruments to shallower depths
- If adaptable, Gracey 5/6 and all straight shanks may be used on premolars and molars (opposite arch fulcrums)

Instruments (Posterior Application)

(A) Gracey 11/12
(B) Gracey 15/16

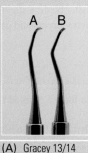

Design:
- Gracey 11/12: Shank is slightly angulated at two points for adaptation to mesial surfaces
- Gracey 15/16: Gracey 11/12 blade on the same shank angulation as the Gracey 13/14

Use:
- Periodontal debridement of supragingival and subgingival biofilm and calculus on maxillary and mandibular molar and premolar mesial surfaces

Consideration:
- Gracey 11/12 and 15/16 are both positioned to reach mesial posterior surfaces, however, the Gracey 15/16 allows increased access to mesial surfaces of molars

(A) Gracey 13/14
(B) Gracey 17/18

Design:
- Gracey 13/14: Shank is angulated for adaptation to distal surfaces
- Gracey 17/18: Slightly longer terminal shank with highly accentuated angles for access to distal posterior surfaces

Use:
- Periodontal debridement of supragingival and subgingival biofilm and calculus on maxillary and mandibular molar and premolar distal surfaces

Considerations:
- The Gracey 13/14 can be used in nontraditional areas such as lingual surfaces when using alternative fulcrums and patient-clinician positions
- Gracey 13/14 and 17/18 are both positioned to reach distal posterior surfaces, however, the Gracey 17/18 allows increased access to distal surfaces of molars with greater periodontal pocket depths

Area-Specific Curets

Langer curets

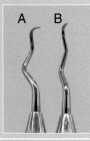

Design:
- Area-specific curet shank design with a universal blade
- Standard (A) and mini-bladed versions (B)
- Standard (A) and extended shanks (B)

Use:
- Periodontal debridement of supragingival and subgingival biofilm and calculus on anterior and posterior teeth

Considerations:
- Design allows instrumentation of both mesial and distal surfaces without changing instruments
- Mini-bladed version is ideal for use in furcations because both cutting edges can be used

Instruments (Implant Application)

Area-Specific Implant

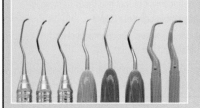

Design:
- Various types of materials

Use:
- Maintenance instrumentation of supragingival and subgingival biofilm and calculus on all postsurgical dental implants

Consideration:
- No sharpening of working end

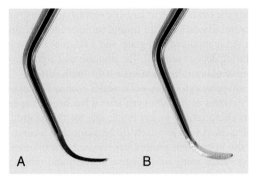

Fig. 28.16 (A) The thin, shorter curved side of the Gracey curet blade is not the working cutting edge. (B) The longer curved side of the Gracey curet blade is the working cutting edge.

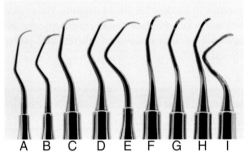

Fig. 28.17 Complete set of Gracey curet designs. Gracey curet (A) 1/2. (B) 3/4. (C) 5/6. (D) 7/8. (E) 9/10. (F) 11/12. (G) 13/14. (H) 15/16. (I) 17/18.

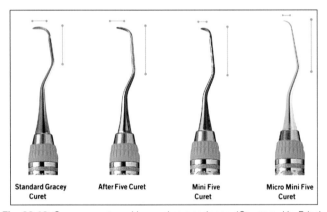

Standard Gracey Curet   After Five Curet   Mini Five Curet   Micro Mini Five Curet

Fig. 28.18 Gracey curet working end comparisons. (Courtesy Hu-Friedy Manufacturing, Chicago, Illinois.)

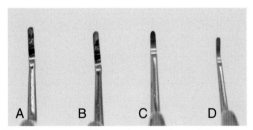

Fig. 28.19 A close-up working end comparison of Gracey curets. (A) Standard. (B) Extended. (C) Mini bladed. (D) Micro mini bladed.

instruments and curets for heavy calculus deposits and accessibility. The curved-bladed sickles are popular because many are thinner with slight shank bends that allow anterior and posterior versatility. The straight-shanked sickle scalers are traditionally anterior instruments.

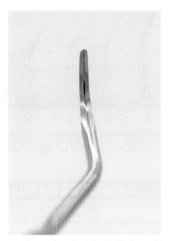

Fig. 28.20 Close-up view of a double-bladed working end (American Eagle Double-Gracey Scandette).

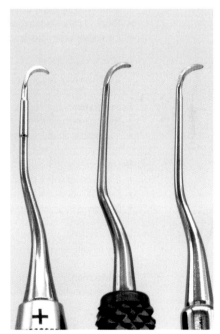

Fig. 28.21 Curevette-style curets: Hu-Friedy Sub-Zero curet *(left)*, Paradise Dental Technologies (PDT) Amazing Gracey™ 00 *(center)*, American Eagle Gracey Access 00-0 curette *(right)*.

They are often single-ended because the same end may be used mesially and distally. The bent or curved shanked sickle scalers may be used for anterior as well as posterior areas of the mouth and are usually double-ended. For anterior teeth, one end is best designed for mesial tooth surfaces and the other end for distal tooth surfaces, however, for posterior teeth, one end can be utilized for both mesial and distal tooth surfaces (Procedures 28.3 and 28.4 and see Tables 28.9 and 28.10).

The advantage of the sickle scaler is its ability to reach between very tight contacts. The disadvantage is that the design does not adapt well to rounded tooth surfaces. Some part of the instrument is not always in contact with the tooth. The V-shaped back can impose on the sulcular

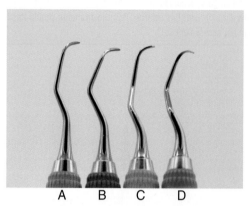

Fig. 28.22 Set of modified maintenance Gracey curets: Hu-Friedy Pattison Gracey Lites (A)1/2. (B) 7/8. (C) 11/12. (D) 13/14 curet.

wall viewing the sickle scaler as largely a supragingival instrument. The need to control adaptation of the tip and cutting edge of this instrument requires a stable modified pen grasp and a fulcrum relatively close to the area during deposit removal. The clinician uses a pull stroke action in a vertical or oblique direction against the tooth surface.

The V shape design of the sickle scaler enables the instrument to be sturdy in terms of strength even after it has been sharpened many times. This characteristic makes it valuable for the removal of heavy calculus (Fig. 28.6) with less likely tip breakage than a curet. The sturdiness of the instrument prompt experienced practitioners who are adept at optionally using sickles supragingivally and subgingivally for moderate to heavy calculus during initial scaling. It is useful subgingivally only in situations where the gingival tissue is not tight around the tooth or when moderate to heavy subgingival calculus is present. The shank strength and 90-degree blade angulation facilitate fracturing and cleaving off deposits. An over-closed angle can shave off subgingival calculus resulting in residual burnished deposits. The curved shanked sickle scalers with a curved blade design are effective for moderate to heavy subgingival calculus removal in anterior and posterior areas (Tables 28.9 and 28.10).

TABLE 28.9 Anterior Sickle Scaler Design and Selection

COMMON DESIGN SPECIFICATIONS OF ALL ANTERIOR SICKLE SCALERS

Instruments (Anterior Application)

U-15
SH 6/7
SHG 6/7

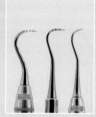

Design:
- Paired, curved sickle design
- Blade: Long, relatively thin with a large, rounded back
- Shank: Short lower shank with slight angulation for accessibility
- Considered as an anterior sickle as blade, shank, and handle within the same plane

Use:
- Use for anterior and premolar supragingival and subgingival calculus removal

Consideration:
- Not recommended for root planing
- If adaptable, all straight shanks may be used on premolars and molars (opposite arch fulcrums)

SH 5/33

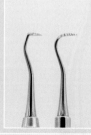

Design:
- Double-ended with a straight sickle on one end and a curved sickle on the other end
- Blade: Relatively thin
- Considered as an anterior sickle as blade, shank, and handle within the same plane

Use:
- Use for anterior and premolar supragingival and subgingival calculus removal

Consideration:
- Not recommended for root planing

SCNevi 1

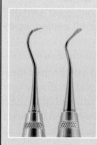

Design:
- An elongated disc end paired with an anterior curved sickle
Shank: rigid

Use:
- Use for anterior lingual supragingival and subgingival calculus and stain removal and a thin curved blade for interproximal instrumentation of biofilm and calculus removal

Consideration:
- Not recommended for root planning
- Recommend on enamel surfaces (gouging may occur on root surfaces with increase pressure)

TABLE 28.10 Posterior Sickle Scaler Design and Selection

INSTRUMENTS (ANTERIOR AND POSTERIOR APPLICATION)

S204SD 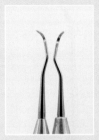	**Design:** • Paired, contra-angle, curved sickle design • Shank: Bent in two places • Blade: Small, about half the width and length of the anterior SH 6/7 sickle scaler • Shank: Bent lower shank **Use:** • Use for supragingival and subgingival calculus removal (where tissue permits) **Considerations:** • Bend in lower shank allows ideal interproximal access in anterior and posterior areas • Short narrow blade allows access subgingivally
SCNEVI 2 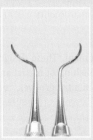	**Design:** • Paired, contra-angle, curved sickle design • Shank: Acutely bent • Blade: Long and thin **Use:** • Use for supragingival and subgingival calculus removal (where tissue permits) **Consideration:** • Bend in lower shank allows ideal interproximal access in anterior and particularly in posterior areas with tight tissue • Bend can be awkward, best used in posterior teeth • Thin blade removes light calculus
Montana Jack Nevi 4 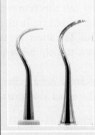	**Design:** • Paired, curved shank, curved bladed sickle design • Blade: Long and thin • Shank: Curved lower shank **Use:** • Use for supragingival and subgingival calculus removal (where tissue permits) **Consideration:** • Curved shank allows ideal interproximal access in anterior and particularly in posterior areas

Instrument (Implant Application)

Sickle Implant Instruments 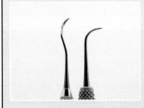	**Design:** • Various types of materials **Use:** • Maintenance instrumentation of supragingival and subgingival biofilm and calculus on all postsurgical dental implants **Consideration:** • No sharpening of working end

Hoe and Chisel Scalers

Design and use. The basic design of the **hoe and chisel scaler** is one with a straight-edged blade at the end. Their purpose is to dislodge large ledges of calculus and remove stains from supragingival surfaces. Smaller designs have allowed for use in deep, narrow subgingival areas or concave root surfaces if tissue distends and permits.

Hoes have a straight or angled shank with a beveled toe that is generally used with a vertical, pull stroke mostly for facial and lingual surfaces of anterior and posterior teeth of the mouth. The working end has one straight cutting edge that intersects the face and beveled toe at 45° to the blade (Fig. 28.24).

Chisels typically have a straight or curved shank that is generally used with a push stroke for between the teeth and facial and lingual surfaces of anterior teeth of the mouth. The working end has a rounded back that flattens out to meet the face of the blade forming the beveled cutting edge at 45° (Fig. 28.25). A pull and push stroke may be used for stain removal on enamel tooth surfaces for anterior lingual surfaces.

File Scaler

Design and use. The **file scaler** consists of a series of miniature hoe blades on a pad attached to the shank. Each blade has an angle of 90 to 105° from the shank (Fig. 28.26A). Each blade possesses sharp corners

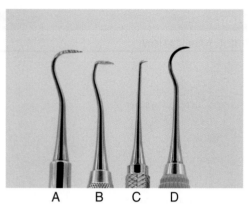

Fig. 28.23 Comparison of various sickle scalers. (A) Curved anterior sickle. (B) Jacquette (double-ended) sickle. (C) Morse anterior sickle. (D) Posterior sickle.

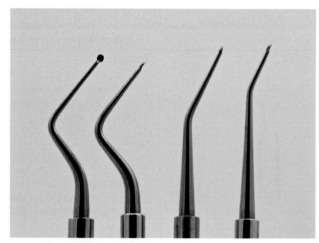

Fig. 28.25 Working end design of chisel instruments.

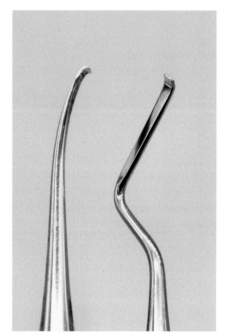

Fig. 28.24 Working end design of hoe instruments.

that require correct adaptation (two-point contact with the working end and shank to the tooth surface) during stroke activation to prevent a hazard to the tooth structure. The file scaler is used supragingivally or subgingivally for crushing or breaking up moderate to heavy subgingival calculus. Roughening up tenacious, burnished calculus helps to prepare the surface, making it easier for the curet to latch onto and break the piece away from the tooth. Although files traditionally have rows of parallel blades on a flat working head, a file also can be diamond coated with the surface like an emery board as a finishing instrument.

The traditional file scaler is a pull stroke instrument that uses a fulcrum close to the immediate working area with the entire series of blades positioned against the tooth surface. Instruments with diamond-coated working end use push and pull strokes with light pressure in a multidirectional manner. Such instruments remove flat, smooth calculus with a sanding motion and significantly reduce root over instrumentation by a curet.

Buccal and lingual designs have universal configurations with paired ends. Mesial and distal diamond-coated working ends can

have concave and/or convex ends on one instrument. These designs are adaptations for the final debridement and polishing of mesial and distal root surfaces, line angles, deep developmental grooves, and furcations.

Furcation Instruments

See the discussion of furcation involvement in Chapter 20, and see Chapter 30 for a review of furcation anatomy.

Design and Use. **Furcation instruments** are specially designed to access small, narrow areas and concave root surfaces. Generally, the purpose of these instruments is not for heavy calculus removal (Fig. 28.26) but for light deposits and finishing of interradicular surfaces (Fig. 28.26). Effective debridement of furcation areas during periodontal maintenance has been shown to help prevent increased bone loss around roots.[5]

Other treatment instruments do not have the classic design characteristics yet have blended adaptations of the discussed categories. Examples are listed below.

- Diamond Tec File Scalers, Hu-Friedy Manufacturing
- Diamond-Tip Curettes, Brasseler USA
- Furcation Files, LM-Instruments
- Quetin (pronounced *kee-tin*) furcation curets (Hu-Friedy)
- O'Hehir Debridement (Hu-Friedy) and New Millennium Curettes (PDT)

Implant Scalers (See Chapter 31)

Dental implants are constructed of biocompatible components that should be maintained by treatment instruments that are made with materials designed to remove deposits without damaging the implant surfaces.[4] (See related sections of Tables 28.5, 28.6, and 28.8.)

Some implant instrument designs are somewhat bulky to access the limited space around the abutment and prosthetic parts. Miniature-bladed design options allow better navigation around the peri-implant tissues and effective adaptation to the implant components (Fig. 28.27).

TACTILE SENSITIVITY

Tactile sensitivity is the ability to sense the vibrations from the instrument to the clinician's fingers on the handle. It is essential to develop the ability to distinguish the degrees of root smoothness and roughness to be an effective clinician. Experience in detecting light calculus, calculus almost completely removed, and burnished calculus is a prerequisite

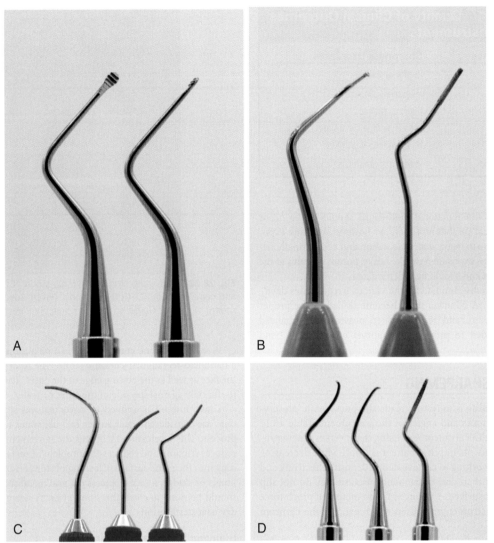

Fig. 28.26 Furcation instruments. (A) Hu-Friedy Hirschfeld files. (B) LM diamond files. (C) Hu-Friedy Diamond Tec file scalers. (D) Hu-Friedy Quetin furcation curets.

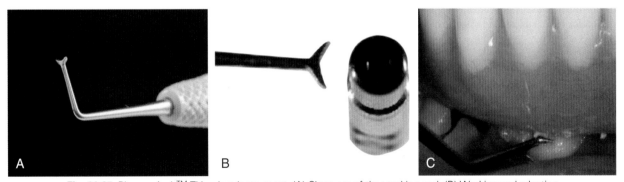

Fig. 28.27 Pineyro Arch™ Ti implant instrument. (A) Close -up of the working end. (B) Working end adapting perfectly to the circular shaped Novaloc Abutment. (C) Working end accessing between prosthesis and gingiva. (Burkhart Dental Supply: Quality Dental Products, Equipment & Service.)

for developing tactile sensitivity. The skill requires attention to stroke direction, tip adaptation, pressure, type of calculus, and type of root surface during an examination.

Tactile sensitivity is important in distinguishing the sulcular soft-tissue wall, the junctional epithelium, and possible osseous exposures. If the explorer contacts soft tissue, it bounces and snags along the wall until the instrument is adapted properly. The nonkeratinized junctional epithelium at the base of the pocket feels different at different states of periodontal health.

- The junctional epithelium in healthy sulci is firm and elastic.
- The junctional epithelium in the inflamed state is soft and easily penetrable with a sharp-pointed instrument.

TABLE 28.11	Quality of Clinical Outcomes With Sharp Instruments	
Sharpness Increases	**Sharpness Decreases**
Calculus removal	Burnished calculus
Tactile sensitivity	Instrument slippage
Patient comfort	Clinician fatigue
Patient safety	Possibility of tissue trauma
Instrument control	Effective lateral pressure
Appointment efficiency	Working time/strokes

- Penetration past the junctional epithelium should never occur during nonsurgical periodontal therapy; however, osseous exposure can occur due to heavy instrumentation and exceptionally friable soft tissue. The exposure feels like heavy, porous calculus at the base of the pocket and should be differentiated.

The tactile skill to discriminate for the various irregularities develops with experience. A clinician must become skilled in the proper modulation of pressure and techniques to possess the enhanced detection skills needed to provide the optimal outcomes in hand instrumentation.

INSTRUMENT SHARPENING

Instrument sharpening is to restore blade sharpness while preserving the original contours and angles of the instrument. Table 28.11 delineates the basic clinical outcome of using sharp versus dull instruments. Sharp instruments improve patient comfort while decreasing clinician fatigue by working to remove dental deposits effectively and are easier to control than dull instruments because they do not slip as readily over tooth surfaces.[1] The need for an increased pinch force occurs when dull instruments are used which exposes the clinician to injury.[14]

The dental hygienist should sharpen the instrument at the first sign of instrument dullness to maintain effectiveness and patient care quality. The manufacturer's guidelines should be referenced for indications on to discard or sharpen their instruments. Traditional sharpening methods are further discussed under each instrument subheading. See Box 28.6 for legal, ethical, and safety issues associated with dull instruments.

Sharpening Stones

Sharpening stones for hand scaling instruments should be part of the nonsurgical periodontal therapy and maintenance armamentarium set-up for chairside sharpening during the procedure. Natural and synthetic sharpening stones for sharpening dental instruments are composed of abrasive crystals that are harder than the metal of the instrument (Fig. 28.28). Diamond-coated sharpening cards are an additional choice for sharpening tools.

Natural and Synthetic (Composition and Ceramic Stones)

The **Arkansas stone**, typically a natural stone with a fine texture, is manufactured in a variety of shapes for sharpening instruments. Conical and cylindrical Arkansas stones are useful for sharpening the face of curets, however, a practice that tends to weaken the blade.

The **India stone**, available as a natural or synthetic stone, comes in a medium texture that removes metal easily, and therefore, the clinician follows its use with an Arkansas stone to provide a polished edge.

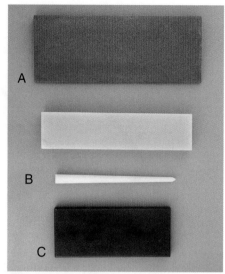

Fig. 28.28 Sharpening stones. (A) India stone. (B) Arkansas stone (flat and cone shaped). (C) Ceramic stone. (From Boyd LRB. *Dental Instruments: A Pocket Guide.* 4th ed. St Louis: Saunders; 2012.)

A synthetic stone **composition** can be a mounted rotary stone or a handheld rectangular **ceramic stone**. The rotary stone is adapted to the face as well as the cutting edge of the curet. The rectangular stone is useful only against the side of the curet or scaler.

Clear, fine oil is applied to cover natural stones while synthetic ones are considered water stones and use water to aid the sharpening process. This lubrication facilitates the movement across these stones, reduces friction, and reduces the problem of metallic particles embedding into the stone surface. Cleaning of stones rids the surface of metal filings or sludge, a mix of excess oil, and metal shavings. This removal should be done to clean the stone prior to steam, chemical vapor, or dry heat sterilization.

Diamond Sharpening Cards

Diamond sharpening cards are credit-card–sized metal plates with a micronized diamond surface. The flat cards are single or double-sided with continuous grit surfaces that range from extra fine to coarse for instrument sharpening (Fig. 28.29).

Sharpening Stone Selection

- Fine-textured Arkansas or medium-textured India stones are preferable for the novice or for sharpening during the patient treatment when little sharpening is required to reestablish a cutting edge.
- Coarsely surfaced stones are preferred when instruments require significant recontouring. Coarsely textured stones require less pressure, fewer strokes, and greater accuracy and remove metal at a faster rate than finely surfaced stones.
- The rotary-mounted stone is useful only when major recontouring of the instrument is required. This mechanical method is considerably more abrasive than coarse handheld stones due to the grinding action of a motor-driven handpiece that activates the mandrel-mounted stone. Disadvantages include the lack of good control, high friction, and rapid wearing of the instrument.
- Diamond sharpening cards are usually slightly more costly than traditional oil and water stones. Their metal construction retains its flatness and the hard diamond grit quickly sharpens the instrument's cutting edges. Attention to adjustments in pressure and strokes prevents unwanted loss of blade.

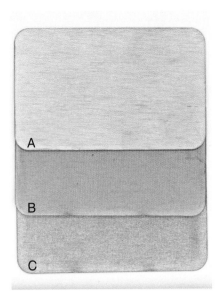

Fig. 28.29 Sharpening diamond cards grit type. (A) Extra fine. (B) Fine. (C) Medium. (Hu-Friedy Manufacturer.)

Sharpening Techniques
Manual Sharpening Technique

Techniques for using handheld sharpening stones consist of using the clinician's dominant hand to initiate movement with either of the following (Fig. 28.30):

- Moving the instrument over the stone (recommended for sharpening flat surfaces such as the sickle scaler)
- Moving the stone over the instrument (recommended for sharpening curets)

Fig. 28.35A compares methods of sharpening the universal curet.

The hand holding the instrument assumes a palm-thumb grasp supported against a firm surface such as a cabinet top, or the clinician's own elbow pulled close to the body to support the wrist and hand holding the instrument. The fingers holding the stone should not wrap around the stone on the long side exposed to the cutting surface but should be positioned behind the cutting surface or at the short end of the stone (Fig. 28.31). Care is observed in stroke length, stone grasp, and instrument grasp when moving the stone against the sharpening instrument to guard against accidental clinician injury. Short, even, continuous strokes keep the instrument on the stone.

Proper angulation of the stone to the surface of the instrument is assumed before initiating the sharpening stroke. Continuous sharpening motions at this constant angle are made across the length of the cutting edge. Stone designs are available to facilitate proper sharpening and are shaped to assist with correct angulation and channels to maintain the original characteristic. The amount of recontouring necessary to produce a sharp blade determines the amount of pressure applied. Greater pressure exerted against the blade with the stone removes more metal. Prudent advice for instrument conservation is to limit sharpening procedures to what is necessary. The last sharpening stroke(s) should be away from the face of the instrument in a downward motion to remove small metal particles called *flash* that adhere to the instrument edges. The practitioner should wipe the blade with a 2-inch × 2-inch gauze square to aid in removing metal shavings and lubricating fluid floating on the instrument surface.

Mechanical Sharpening Technique

A number of manufacturers offer *honing devices* or mechanical tools for sharpening instruments. These types of sharpening equipment

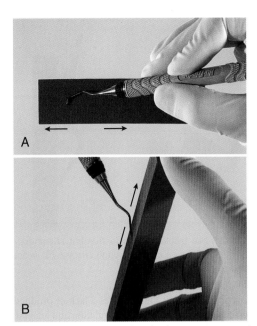

Fig. 28.30 (A) Sharpening by moving the instrument over the sharpening stone. (B) Sharpening by moving the sharpening stone over the instrument.

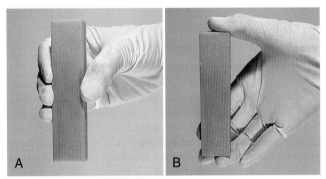

Fig. 28.31 (A) Incorrect finger position on stone; fingertips are exposed to possible injury if stone slips. (B) Correct finger position on stone.

commonly have a stone that automatically activates to move gently across the working end to create a sharp blade. There are also battery-operated sharpening devices that have built-in channel guides for maintaining angulation of the instrument blade against the stone.

Testing for Instrument Sharpness

Testing for sharpness is done by utilizing visual inspection, tactile test, and auditory cues.

- A **visual test** requires a strong light to discern any reflection from a rounded or beveled cutting edge that is seen from the blade of a dull instrument. A sharp instrument will not reflect light if a razor-thin edge at the junction between the face of the blade and the lateral side of the instrument exists (Fig. 28.32A).
- The **tactile test** is when the clinician can detect the catch of a sharpened instrument blade on a hard plastic testing stick when placed at the proper working angulation. When using this method, clinicians must test the instrument fully across the length of the blade and resharpen any area that allows the instrument to slip over the stick (Fig. 28.32B).
- A practiced clinician can use the **auditory test** to recognize a dull instrument by the blade's lack of a distinct pinging sound when tested at the proper blade angulation and adaptation. The

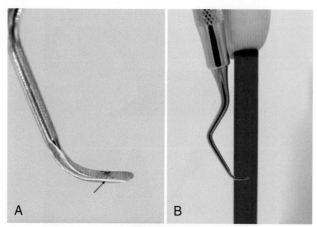

Fig. 28.32 Visual and tactile test for instrument sharpness (A) A dull instrument reflects light on a cutting edge *(arrow)*. (B) A sharp instrument catches on the testing stick.

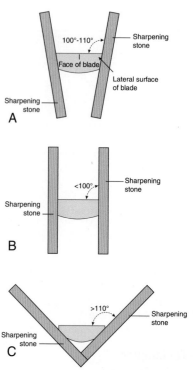

Fig. 28.33 (A) Correct instrument sharpening. (B and C) Common sharpening errors.

experienced practitioner differentiates a lack of productive sound from testing at an improper blade angulation and adaptation.

- The dental hygienist should examine the shape of the blade when sharpening. Instruments sharpened down to moderate or fine dimensions may be used for the healthier individual with little calculus formation. An instrument should be discarded or retipped when it is no longer functional or is a danger to the patient from possible breakage.

Instrument Sharpening Guide

Explorer sharpening techniques.

Explorers that become dull through general use lose tactile sensitivity recognized by the inability to distinguish fine changes in root textures. To sharpen, the explorer is held with a modified pen grasp with the terminal end dragged and rotated 2 to 3 mm while keeping in contact with the stone. The dental explorer should be sufficiently sharpened with two to three rotations. It is important to replace shortened explorers because the length is essential in periodontal procedures.

Universal curet sharpening techniques.

Sharpening of the universal curet includes the cutting edges of each two-sided blade and the rounded toe. The toe is not used as frequently in instrumentation so does not have to be sharpened each time the lateral surfaces require it. The rounded toe of the universal curet should be preserved as long as possible as it is occasionally used to scale the floor of furcation areas or under tooth contacts.

Sharpening the lateral sides. The universal curet is sharpened as follows:

- Positioning the face of the blade of the universal instrument parallel to the floor allows the lower shank to be perpendicular since its blades are set at 90°. The angle of the face to the surface of the stone should be positioned at 100° and 110°. The stone slowly passes across the entire cutting edge at consistent angulation to maintain an evenly sharpened blade. The stone is not lifted from the blade using upward and downward strokes with even pressure. These principles help prevent changing the normal shape of a curet blade. Fig. 28.33 illustrates the cross-sectional views of curet blades resulting from common sharpening errors.

The most common error is to increase the pressure as the stroke nears the toe. The rounded toe of the curet transforms to a point as the lateral sides converge rather than remaining parallel (Fig. 28.34A and B).

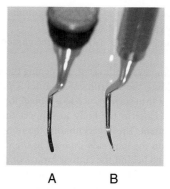

Fig. 28.34 (A) Parallel lateral cutting edge of a Gracey curet 7/8. (B) Converging lateral cutting edge resulting from too heavy pressure of the sharpening stone near the toe of the blade of a Gracey curet 7/8.

The method of moving the stone over the instrument is slightly easier than moving the instrument because the angulation of the lateral surface to the stone is easier to visualize and maintain (Fig. 28.30). The last stroke(s) finishes in a downward motion of the stone tilting slightly toward the back of the instrument, reducing the possibility of a wire edge on the face of the blade. Remove any light film of lubricant and/or sharpening by-products, sludge, that accumulate on the surface of the face.

Sharpening the face. The face of the curet blade may be sharpened with a cone-shaped sharpening stone, the rounded side of a sharpening stone, or a mounted rotary stone. Maintaining even pressure across the face with these methods can be difficult which produces unreliable results. The blade strength of an instrument that uses a pulling action is provided in its dimension from face to back. Removal of too much metal from the face can significantly weaken it.

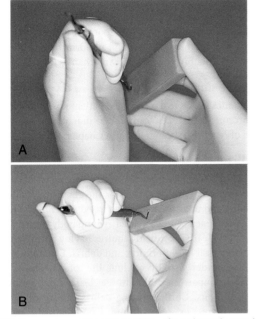

Fig. 28.35 Comparison of handle position of a universal curet (A) and a Gracey curet (B) when the face of the blade is held parallel to the floor for sharpening (from the point of view of the clinician looking down.)

Area-Specific Curet Sharpening Technique

Grasp positions, angulation of 100 to 110°, and the sharpening movement across the blade are the same for the Gracey and universal curets. Positioning the face of the blade of the Gracey instrument parallel to the floor will not allow its handle to be perpendicular since its blades are offset at 60 to 70° to the lower shank. Fig. 28.35 shows a comparison of stone and handle when the face of a Gracey and a universal curet are parallel to the floor. The Gracey curet requires sharpening the blade from the lower, longer cutting edge, and occasionally around the toe. The blades of the instrument should be wiped clean after the sharpening process and before instrumentation. These principles of sharpening also apply to the variations of the Gracey curets.

Sickle Sharpening Technique

Sharpening the sickle scaler requires the stone to remain stationary and the instrument to move over the stone. The stone is secured with the nondominant hand, the instrument is held with a modified pen grasp, and the lateral surface is positioned at an angle of 100 to 110° to the stone. The entire lateral surface on a flat-surfaced sickle scaler lies against the stone. For curved sickle scalers, small portions of the lateral surfaces are sharpened at a time, beginning from the portion nearest the shank. The working hand is stabilized with a fulcrum on the stone, and short, firm strokes are applied for sharpening. Because the sickle scaler has two cutting edges, the instrument is turned over and the procedure is repeated for the other lateral surface of the blade. Occasionally the face of the sickle scaler is sharpened. For this surface, the stone must be either positioned near the edge of the table or held up so that the entire face may be sharpened against the stone surface. Tests for sharpness include the visual or tactile methods described earlier.

File Sharpening Techniques

The file is a difficult instrument to sharpen because of the miniature size of each blade. A tanged file sharpener positioned against each small, flat-bladed surface (Fig. 28.36) accomplishes the sharpening of each blade. For the sharpening procedure, stabilize the instrument and

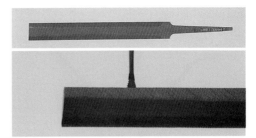

Fig. 28.36 A tanged file for sharpening the file.

the working hand near the instrument to perform light, short, push-pull strokes across each blade.

INSTRUMENT TIP BREAKAGE

Prevention

As sharpening narrows the working end, it is best to discard worn scalers that have become too thin. Other instruments that are subject to easier breakage and are no longer safe to use are ones with developed points of weakness due to uneven sharpening, corrosion, or metal fatigue.

Complications

Instrument tip breakage can cause patient trauma and distress and stress to the clinician. Managing the incident is important to ensure that the patient has not swallowed or aspirated the tip. If so, the clinician is potentially liable and must provide access to medical intervention for the patient. Serious medical problems can result if a foreign object becomes lodged internally.

Managing Instrument Tip Breakage

It is the professional responsibility of the practitioner to address the ethical and safety issues of the patient when managing instrument tip breakage. The clinician must locate and retrieve an instrument tip when it breaks off subgingivally. Instrumentation must stop as soon as the instrument tip has broken and the patient is informed of the situation. To retrieve the small metal fragment, the clinician stops. All low-speed or high-speed aspiration (suction) is discontinued and the patient uses a cup to expectorate in the event the tip is floating in saliva. Techniques for locating the broken piece include the following:

- Reinstrumentation with another instrument from subgingival areas to tease out and catch the broken tip with gauze
- Use of magnetic-tip Periotrievers, shaped like thick explorers or probes, to draw and grab a tip fragment (Fig. 28.37).
- Open-flap periodontal surgery if attempts are unsuccessful for an identified metal tip.

Radiographic examination is helpful during these exploration techniques to locate the metal tip. If the broken tip cannot be clinically located, or if it is not visible on a radiograph of the area, the tip may be outside of the sulcus. The clinician completes a careful visual inspection of the oral cavity looking for the tip and uses gauze squares to wipe out the vestibular areas and areas under the patient's tongue. The clinician informs and presents the recovered tip to the patient to confirm the metal fragment retrieval. The patient is apprised if the tip cannot be located. A chest radiograph is indicated in this situation to rule out the possible aspiration of the fragment. Clinicians should routinely document any instrument tip breakage by noting the specific tooth or site of breakage, incident disclosure to the patient with signature verification, patient response, follow-ups or referrals, and procedure results. See Box 28.4 on the legal, ethical, and safety issues regarding instrument tip breakage. For a scenario to apply best practices for tip breakage should it occur, see Box 28.11.

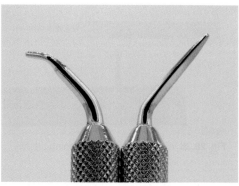

Fig. 28.37 Magnetic broken tip retrievers (Schwartz Periotrievers). Contra-angle tip is for use in furcations; the long tip is for use in pockets.

BOX 28.9 Patient Education and Motivation

Teach patients to visualize health and disease by using a mouth mirror, periodontal probe, or explorer in the patient's own mouth while the patient observes by looking into a hand mirror. "Notice how your gumline is lower in this area. I am using this probe instrument to measure how much your gums have receded." Also explain that bone loss below the gumline can create a deeper pocket that can be difficult to keep clean. Show the patient an area in the mouth where attachment loss has caused a periodontal pocket. Then, show the patient the corresponding bone loss on the radiograph.

HAND-ACTIVATED INSTRUMENTATION FUNDAMENTAL COMPONENTS

A clinician must know the fundamental components to achieve protective and productive hand-activated instrumentation. An improper grasp, joint hypermobility, or an unstable fulcrum can result in excessive pinch forces that will increase the risk for injury.[14] Correct application of these foundational principles facilitates desired outcomes and minimizes occupational injury:

- Clinician/patient positioning
- Body mechanics
- Field of vision
- Grasp
- Fulcrum
- Lateral pressure
- Reinforcement scaling
- Joint hypermobility
- Stroke principles

Attention to fundamental components decreases the development of repetitive strain injuries (see Chapter 12). Self-evaluation throughout the instrumentation process requires that the practitioner monitor the stress effects on the working hand, wrist, elbow, shoulder, neck, back, or spine (Procedure 28.4 and Chapter 12).

Clinician/Patient Positioning

Clinician/patient positioning is the proper location and alignment of the practitioner relative to the patient during treatment. Correct clinician and patient positioning facilitates proper instrumentation technique and achieve a state of musculoskeletal balance that protects the body from strain and cumulative injury (see the section on positioning factors in Chapter 12).

Clock positions commonly describe the clinician's position relative to the patient with the head of the patient at 12 o'clock. Clinicians should place themselves in the proper clock position around the patient that enables them to view and perform treatment inside the mouth while maintaining correct body mechanics (Fig. 28.38).

Body Mechanics

Body mechanics relates to clinician and patient positioning, fulcrums, and reinforcements that seek to minimize practitioner injury (see the discussion of repetitive strain injuries in Chapter 12).

Field of Vision

A clear **field of vision**, keeping the treatment area visible and accessible, is an important basic concept for the clinician. The benefits of good visibility and accessibility are increased safety of the procedure, increased effectiveness, and decreased eye and body strain.

Achieving a clear vision field requires having a visible treatment area clear from oral tissues, fluids, and debris. Examples of oral tissues that can hinder visibility include the tongue, cheek, and lips. Fluids that can impair the ability to see clearly can be water, saliva, blood, or solutions. Compromising debris can be calculus, food, granulation tissues, or even biofilm. The treatment area should remain accessible and unencumbered during the procedure. Having a clear field of vision enhances therapy comfort by decreasing possible tissue trauma and improving the patient and clinician's experience (Procedure 28.4).

Loupes and lights have become common with clinicians for enhanced views of the treatment areas. With the use of loupe magnification, the field of view is the visualized area. Higher magnifications decrease the field of view. Magnification and coaxial illumination (headlights) that focus on the targeted treatment sites may help decrease eye strain and improper body mechanics. Other forms of lights such as fiberoptic handpieces in ultrasonics and even mouth mirrors have augmented improved fields of view.

Grasp

The **grasp** is the precise manner of finger placements to hold an instrument. The basic grasps used in hand-activated instrumentation (Fig. 28.39) are listed below:

- Pen grasp
- Modified pen grasp
- Extended modified pen grasp
- Palm-thumb grasp

Pen grasp

The **pen grasp** (Fig. 28.39A) is used when the exacting or directive type of pressure in periodontal debridement is not required. The thumb and index finger pads are well situated on the instrument handle, but the middle finger slips down, and the instrument rests on the side of the finger near the first knuckle. The pen grasp may be used when light, easy probing, or exploring into non–periodontally involved areas is performed. Added pressure also is possible with this grasp on the mouth mirror for retraction of the buccal mucosa, tongue, or other soft tissues.

Modified pen grasp

The **modified pen grasp** (Fig. 28.39B) is the standard grasp used for dental hygiene instrumentation. When correctly applied, it is a sensitive, stable, and strong grasp because of the tripod effect produced by the position of the thumb, index finger, and middle finger. The thumb pad is placed on the instrument handle. The index finger pad is placed on the instrument at a point slightly higher on the handle than the

PROCEDURE 28.4 Hand-Activated Periodontal Debridement Instrument Fundamental Sequence Guide

Sequence Steps	Process	Reference
1. Initial Grasp	Modified pen grasp	Fig. 28.39B
2. Operator Position "Clock" Positioning	Healthy patient:	Fig. 28.38A–D
	• Right-handed: 8 to 1 o'clock	
	• Left-handed: 4 to 11 o'clock	
	Moderate/Severe periodontal probing depths (mandibular posterior or surfaces facing away of anterior teeth):	
	• Right-handed: 8 to 5 o'clock	
	• Left-handed: 4 to 7 o'clock	
	• Usually requires extraoral fulcrums	
	• Very challenging deep pockets may necessitate standing	
3. Patient Position	Mouth of patient positioned at the height of clinician's waist	Fig. 28.38A–D
	Mandibular: Occlusal plane parallel to floor	
	Maxillary: Occlusal plane perpendicular to floor	
4. Field of Vision	Visibility: Clear working area of oral tissues using retraction, mouth prop; remove fluids or debris using evacuation, air/water syringe, gauze	Fig. 28.11
	Focal lighting: Overhead light, coaxial illumination, fiberoptic handpieces, indirect illumination	
	Enhance visibility: Magnification, loupes	
5. Initial Fulcrum	Locate general fulcrum site:	(Figs. 28.40A–E and 28.41A, B)
	Intraoral (digital): Finger-on-finger, same arch, cross-arch, opposite arch	
	Extraoral (palm): palm-up, palm-down, knuckle-rest, chin	
6. Adaptation*	Insertion (0–10°), reinsertion (angle between insertion and working stroke)	(Figs. 28.45 and Fig. 28.47C)
	Adaptation: Orient lower 1/3 of blade to base of pocket	
7. Angulation*	Tilt blade (60–80°), where a bite of the working end against the tooth surface can be felt, root planing (45–60°)	(Figs. 28.45 and 28.46)
8. Adjusted Fulcrum*	Confirm if a need to reestablish or fine-tune fulcrum placement to cross-arch, extraoral, etc.	(Figs. 28.40, A–E and 28.41A, B)
9. Adjusted Grasp*	Readjust the grasp for adequate lateral pressure before increasing the working stroke pressure	(Figs. 28.42 A, B)
10. Adjusted Operator/ Patient Positions*	Adjust operator (generally 8 to 4 o'clock) and/or patient positioning that allows hand, arm, and shoulder to move as a unit	(Figs. 38.38A-E)
11. Reinforcement Scaling	Dominant: controls adaptation, angulation, working stroke	(Figs. 28-43A-C)
	Nondominant: stability, enhanced pressure, guides instrument	
12. Activation*	Lateral Pressure: Light, moderate, heavy (firm) pressure	(Figs. 28.41 and Fig. 28.48A, B)
	Position for use of thumb, middle finger, and occasionally index finger	
	Initiate exploratory and working stroke as final step of sequence: vertical, horizontal, oblique, basketweave, channel, push, pull	

* Adapted with reference to Analytical Approaches to Root Debridement.

thumb to maximize control of the instrument. The side of the middle finger near the nail bed is placed opposing the thumb and further down the instrument on the shank toward the working end. The middle finger should have a slight downward bend to allow its movement during instrumentation. The instrument handle is positioned between the first and second knuckle of the index finger and not in the web of the hand. These proper finger placements are critical for stroke activation, increase stroke pressure, angulation, and adaptation.

The modified pen grasp is used with the dental explorer. When exploring shallow, light, or obvious calculus, the dental hygienist uses a grasp with light to moderate strength. The grasp should become firmer when more pressure must be exerted against the tooth, or when the clinician must distinguish between tooth structure and burnished calculus.

Once instrumentation is initiated, the modified pen grasp must be reestablished continually on the instrument handle to accommodate the minute rolling of the instrument into and around depressions of tooth structures. Tendency to primarily use the index finger to roll the

instrument will destabilize the modified pen grasp. Efforts to primarily use the thumb and middle finger in the rolling motion will help maintain a constant hold on the instrument to allow proper repositioning of the index finger. Otherwise, the instrument can roll and slip out of the grasp, or the thumb and fingers can end up in an undesirable position on the instrument handle, which may not allow for optimal pressure to be placed against the instrument for adequate assessment or instrumentation.

The thumb, index, and middle fingers also are flexed to allow the instrument to be manipulated in various directions around the tooth surface and to allow equal pressure to be applied against the root structure during the course of the stroke.

The combined use of both fingers, wrist, or arm movements minimizes physical stress to one separate part of the body when instrumenting deep pockets. It is also beneficial to implement a neutral wrist position when possible. The selected instrument, the fulcrum, the area that is being scaled, and the periodontal probing depth determine the degree of movement required for successful instrumentation.

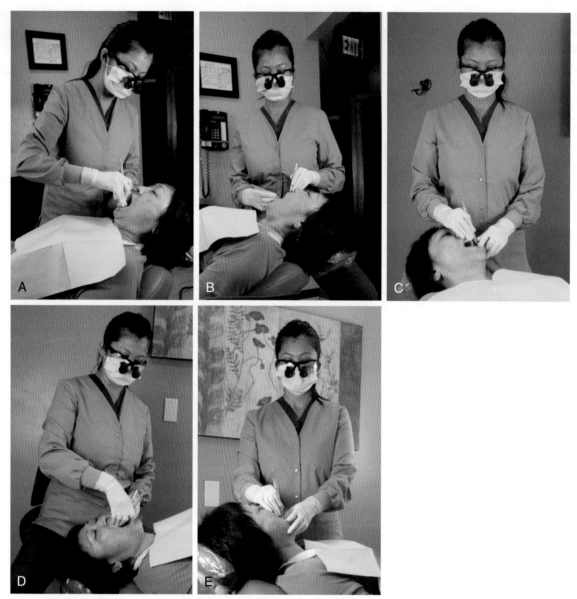

Fig. 28.38 Clinicians can be in a sitting or standing position to perform treatment on patients. Standing position is a useful position when visibility becomes difficult; access to deep pockets is needed, and approach all positions from 8 o'clock to 5 o'clock. (A) Standing at 8 o'clock. (B) Sitting at 9 o'clock, parallel to the patient's head. (C) Standing at 1 o'clock to reach down to the mandible from the maxillary arch with an intraoral, opposite-arch fulcrum. (D) Sitting at 2 o'clock with an intraoral fulcrum on the maxillary arch. (E) Standing at 3 to 5 o'clock to reach down to the mandible from the maxillary arch with an extraoral fulcrum.

BOX 28.10 Critical Thinking Scenario B

1. A dental hygienist, Amelie, is providing periodontal debridement for a patient with periodontal pockets, and moderate to severe inflammation. What hand instrument shank design variations will give the most effective and efficient results? Which instruments would be beneficial in removing the heavy calculus present?

2. In the tray setup, Amelie had regular Gracey curets that she is having difficulty inserting vertically into the deep, narrow pockets of her periodontally involved patient. The root surfaces also have multiple depressions and concavities that are challenging to access. What Gracey blade design variations could she choose that would reduce tissue distention, ease subgingival insertion, and allow adaptation with a vertical stroke?

Extended modified pen grasp

The **extended modified pen grasp** is a subcategory of the modified pen grasp describing the increased length of the grasp on the handle from the working end. The grasp is essentially the same yet the middle finger is positioned on the handle, not the shank. Extraoral, opposite, and cross-arch fulcrums have increased the awareness of the value of an extended modified pen grasp. Extending the grasp further away from the working end allows improved angulation, adaptation, and leverage in the approach for instrumenting deeper periodontal pockets.

Palm-thumb grasp

The **palm-thumb grasp** (Fig. 28.39C) is achieved with all four fingers wrapped tightly around the handle and the thumb placed on the shank in a direction pointing toward the instrument tip. This grasp is

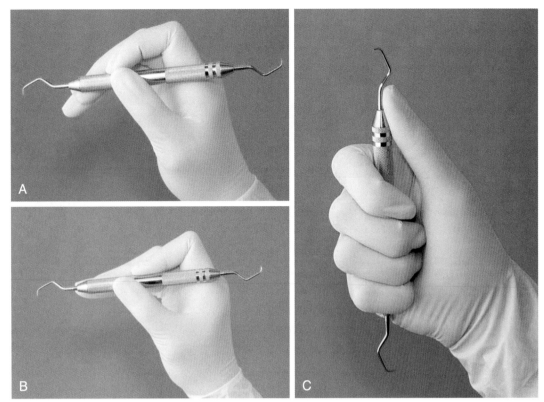

Fig. 28.39 (A) Pen grasp. (B) Modified pen grasp. (C) Palm-thumb grasp.

awkward and uncontrolled because the thumb provides the only source of pressure. The opposing fingers clumsily wrap around the handle and do not provide a means of turning the instrument or modifying the thumb effect. The palm-thumb grasp provides little tactile sensitivity during periodontal debridement procedures; therefore, it is not recommended for supragingival or subgingival periodontal instrumentation. Because the palm-thumb grasp is a very stable grasp that does not allow the instrument to move on its own, it is ideal for use during instrument sharpening. This grasp is also occasionally used to steady high-volume evacuation tips with the nondominant hand during procedures.

Fulcrum

The **fulcrum** is the point at which the working hand is supported and pivots for stability. It is the primary source of strength or leverage on which the finger or hand rests and pushes to hold the instrument with control during stroke activation. All fulcrums should be on a firm tooth or osseous structure for stability and application of force transfer to working strokes.

The most important rule governing fulcrum placement when exploring is that the fulcrum be flexible enough to allow the explorer to move along the surfaces of teeth above and below the gingival margin or contact of the tooth to the apex of the pocket, with correct insertion and adaptation. Not all exploring fulcrums can be used as a scaling fulcrum because a scaling fulcrum needs more stability. The exploratory fulcrum could be located close to the area being explored, cross-arch, or extraorally. As the fulcrum moves farther from the area explored, the clinician's grasp on the instrument handle also moves farther away from the working end. This distance does not diminish one's ability to explore the area, nor does it lessen instrument control. Rather, it enhances access to interproximal regions and deep periodontal pockets.

Applying lateral pressure against the tooth surface with the tip and the anterior third of a sharp blade or pointed instrument necessitates a stable fulcrum. When there is no fulcrum, the instrument uncontrollably slips off the tooth surface when even a slight amount of lateral pressure is exerted. Traditionally, fulcrums have been finger rests that rely on digital focal points for stability and leverage. With the choice of alternate application of extraoral fulcrums, the rest is usually a hand or palm rest against a firm facial surface.

There are two main fulcrum categories used in hand-activated instrumentation:
- Intraoral
- Extraoral

Intraoral fulcrum

The **intraoral fulcrum** is primarily established inside the mouth against a tooth surface and used for instrumenting in shallow pockets. The ring finger pad usually is positioned on the occlusal, incisal, lingual, or facial surface of a tooth close to the one being instrumented. The middle finger should remain in contact with the ring finger even when it is bent during finger flexing or when making digital movements. Stroke control and strength diminish if the middle finger splits away from the ring finger. The stability of a built-up fulcrum is established with the added support of the middle finger (Fig. 28.40A).

Intraoral rests are most stable and powerful when the fulcrum and middle fingers stay close together. Simultaneous finger and wrist motion is used to activate the stroke. The middle-finger fulcrum shortens the arc of movement on activation and results in a shallow stroke that cannot be extended very deep subgingivally. This pivotal stroke closes the blade angulation and promotes finger flexing by the thumb and index finger when attempting to activate a vertical stroke. The diminished ability to maintain proper angulation, control, and power can result in burnishing calculus and clinician fatigue. There is one exception to the middle-finger fulcrum being not as effective as a ring-finger fulcrum. When using a posterior Gracey curet for the distolingual surfaces of the lower left, the ring finger is placed on the buccal of the posterior teeth and the middle finger is placed as an occlusal pivoting point, the fulcrum and

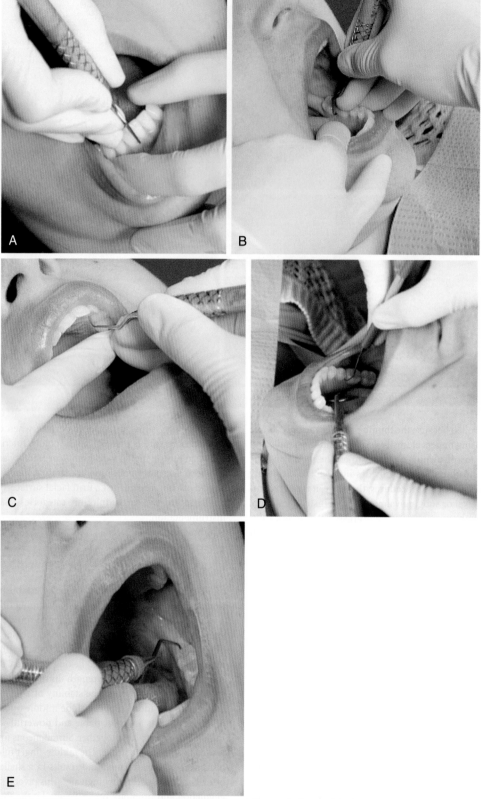

Fig. 28.40 (A) Same-arch fulcrum positioned near area being scaled at 1 o'clock. (B) On the distal/lingual of lower left, ring finger is placed as an occlusal pivoting point. Clinician position is 9 o'clock. (C) Clinician's own finger (finger on finger) used as an intraoral fulcrum. (D) Extraoral, palm-down, opposite-arch fulcrum. Clinician position is at 1 o'clock. (E) Same-arch, opposite-arch, or cross-arch fulcrum. Clinician position is at 9 o'clock.

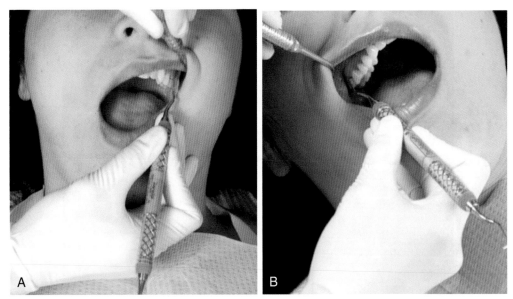

Fig. 28.41 (A) Extraoral, palm-up, cupping-the-chin hand rest. Clinician position is at 9 o'clock. (B) Extraoral, palm-up, opposite-arch fulcrum. Clinician position is at 9 o'clock.

middle fingers remain together, and a hand/wrist motion can be used to create a stable and powerful stroke (Fig. 28.40B).

Depending on the area to be scaled, the angle of access, and the probing depth, intraoral fulcrum placement is as follows:

- The clinician's own finger (finger-on-finger) (e.g., fulcrum on index or thumb), located within the oral cavity (Fig. 28.40C)
- A tooth surface on the opposite arch near the area being scaled (opposite arch fulcrum) (Fig. 28.40D)
- A tooth surface on the same arch but across from the area being scaled (i.e., on the opposite quadrant or cross-arch), creating a cross-arch fulcrum (Fig. 28.40E)
- The index finger of the nondominant hand placed in the vestibule to aid in accessing the distals and buccals, same arch fulcrum (Fig. 28.40F)

Extraoral fulcrum

An **extraoral fulcrum** is one with placement outside of the mouth and is used predominantly when instrumenting teeth with deep periodontal pockets. The extraoral fulcrum uses the broad side of the palm or back of the hand against the chin or outer cheek rather than a small finger point source used in an intraoral fulcrum (Fig. 28.41). The palm or backside of the hand rests with moderate pressure against the bony structures of the patient's face and/or mandible. This extraoral fulcrum may be a palm-up, palm-down, or chin-cup position. This fulcrum provides an excellent means of control and stability. It allows advantageous access into periodontally involved areas that may be cumbersome or physiologically strenuous for the dental hygienist to instrument using intraoral fulcrums. The extraoral fulcrum enables a direct "line of draw" in which the instrument may be pulled straight down, as opposed to rocking with the wrist in areas such as the maxillary posterior regions.

A fulcrum placed away from the immediate working area does not necessarily diminish the stability of the fulcrum. The leverage and lateral pressure may be increased and extended through the length of a long working stroke. Reinforcement from the nonworking index finger or the thumb to the shank or handle close to the instrument's working end easily addresses the control loss from the extended grasp. Finally, the extraoral fulcrum allows the clinician to focus the pulling stroke action to the lower arm, upper arm, and

shoulder. This helps keep a consistent blade adaptation to the tooth surface from the base of the pocket up to the contact. Using instrumentation techniques such as these may protect the clinician from future injury and stress to the nerves, tendons, and ligaments of the wrist and elbow. (See the section on reinforcement scaling later in this chapter.)

Lateral Pressure

Lateral pressure is the pressure of the anterior third of the working end of the instrument against the tooth. This pressure may range from very light to firm, depending on the nature of the tooth surface roughness. Various levels of pressure are necessary during exploratory, scaling, and root planing strokes. Basic principles for applying lateral pressure include the use of the thumb and middle finger during instrumentation (Fig. 28.42). The proper positioning of the clinician and patient with the practiced coordination of the grasp, fulcrum, and basic control of the instrument is important for lateral pressure. The beginning student may have trouble physically applying effective lateral pressure due to the complex coordination of elements.

The degree of lateral pressure affects tactile sensitivity. Exploratory strokes for detection with assessment instruments will benefit with light to moderate pressure. Treatment instruments vary depending on the procedure. Biofilm debridement may require only light pressure, whereas root planing may warrant light to moderate pressure. The removal of calculus deposits can demand light, moderate, and heavy lateral pressure.

Reinforcement Scaling

Reinforcement scaling commonly means that the nondominant hand provides additional support for the instrument instead of holding the mouth mirror. It is used to gain additional instrument stability and control when instrumenting with the intraoral and extraoral fulcrums. The nondominant hand supports the instrument of the working hand, providing additional lateral pressure during instrumentation procedures. The added support from reinforcement may come from the nondominant hand's index finger, thumb, or thenar region (radial palm or fleshy mass on lateral side of palm). The placement of the index finger and thumb may be on or around the instrument between the dominant hand and the working end. The

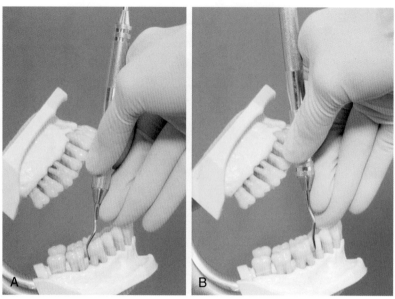

Fig. 28.42 (A) Lateral pressure for No. 30 distal: The thumb is placed against the distal for increased pressure. (B) Lateral pressure for No. 30 mesial: The middle finger is placed against the mesial for increased pressure.

dominant hand must continue to play the major role in exerting control over the instrument. This entails the adapting and angulating of the blade against the tooth surface and the direction in which the instrument is pulled over the tooth.

The names of the reinforcements indicate where the reinforcements originate. Examples of reinforcement scaling in selected mouth areas are shown in Fig. 28.43.

Only treatment instruments, such as curets, typically benefit from the use of reinforcements. Supportive control and lateral pressure are not normally necessary with assessment instruments.

Key benefits of reinforcements are the following:
- Increases stabilization and control accuracy with cross-arch, opposite-arch, and extraoral fulcrums
- Guides and supports the instrument in a longer pull stroke when used with extended extraoral fulcrums
- Provides additional lateral pressure to instrumentation techniques
- Reduces Repetitive Stress Injuries (RSI's) by redistributing the forces that stress components of the musculoskeletal system

JOINT HYPERMOBILITY

Joint hypermobility is an increased range of motions in the joints. Clinicians should be aware of the characteristics to recognize how this condition, commonly referred to as "double jointed," can adversely impact the effectiveness of hand instrumentation (Fig. 28.44A).

Joint hypermobility compromises grasp, fulcrum, and the lateral pressure of a clinician. Adjustments to restore proper angulation, adaptation, and power of the stroke should be made to decrease the risk of burnishing calculus. A hypermobile grasp usually exhibits a collapse or hyperextension of the joint closest to the tip of the index finger and the thumb (Fig. 28.44B). The fulcrums of hypermobile joints can collapse with intraoral same-arch finger rests, affecting stability and leverage. The lateral pressure decreases when fatigue or collapse occurs on either the grasp or the fulcrum. Attaining the proper varied lateral pressure necessary for instrumentation may require increased use of extraoral hand-rest fulcrums and assistance from the nondominant hand. (See Reinforcement Scaling.)

Skillful use of ultrasonic instrumentation for the initial removal of heavy or tenacious calculus may be advantageous to clinicians with joint hypermobility. Conscientious efforts should be made to use the ultrasonic scaler with a traditional tip or use a file to fracture and remove as much calculus as possible before finishing with hand-activated instruments in order to avoid overstressing hypermobile joints with excessive pressure.

STROKE PRINCIPLES

Description

A **stroke** is the movement of the instrument over the tooth surface. Stroke principles include the basic principles of angulation, adaptation, and activation.

Instrument Insertion

Insertion is the act of placing an assessment or treatment instrument into subgingival areas. The purpose of insertion may be to measure a sulcus or pocket, classify furcation involvement, explore the subgingival areas, or scale and/or root plane subgingival areas. This procedure must be done with precision to be nontraumatic and accurate. All sharp-pointed instruments warrant extreme care when inserting the point directly toward the junctional epithelium. Excessive pressure can cause a perforation through the attachment apparatus yet can also be caused by an improper grasp, fulcrum, or lack of contact point with the instrument.

Straight instruments, such as the periodontal probe, should keep the working end and side of the tip in constant contact with the root when inserting. A delicate touch using light pressure is required when probing or initially exploring subgingivally. The junctional epithelium offers a moderate amount of resistance, feels slightly elastic to the touch, and gives with a slight amount of pressure when exploring with an instrument. Pressure on the instrument may be increased after the pocket topography is understood, to interpret cementum irregularities, calculus, and restorative margins. When inserting a curved explorer, the tip points apically and the side of the tip should be in contact with the tooth surface explored. Care must be taken to avoid directing the

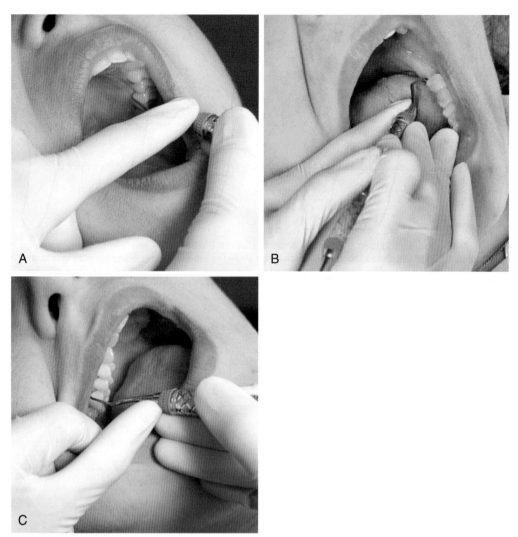

Fig. 28.43 (A) Index finger reinforcement. Left maxillary mesial surface from the lingual approach. Clinician is at 9 o'clock. Position of the working hand is extraoral fulcrum, palm down. The position of the reinforcement hand shows the index finger on the instrument applying pressure in the same direction of lateral pressure in which the dominant hand is working. (B) Index finger reinforcement. Mandibular left posterior distal line angle from lingual approach. Clinician is at 8 o'clock to 9 o'clock position. The working hand is positioned cross arch of the area being scaled. The index finger of the reinforcement hand is positioned on the instrument. (C) Thumb reinforcement to stabilize instrument—right maxillary posterior mesial surface from facial approach. Clinician is at 9 o'clock position.

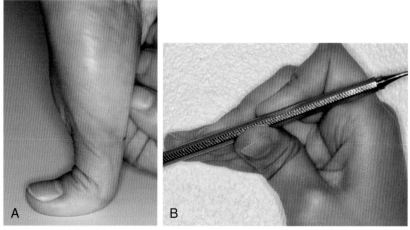

Fig. 28.44 (A) Collapsed thumb bent at 90° demonstrating hypermobility. (B) Modified pen grasp on an instrument with collapsed thumb. (From Sumi JY, Pattison AM, Nguyen M. Impact of joint hypermobility. Dimensions of dental hygiene. *Journal of Professional Excellence* 2017;15(5):23–24, 26, 28.)

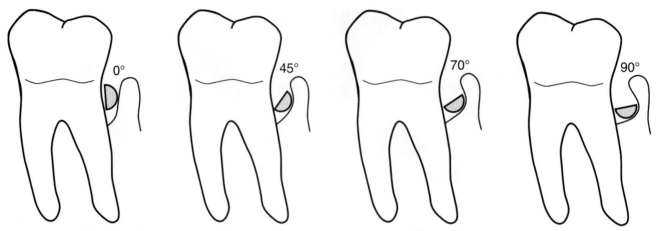

Fig. 28.45 Subgingival Angulations. Insertion angle of close to 0° is ideal for insertion of working end into the pocket; a 45° cutting edge to tooth angulation is too closed to remove calculus, and burnishing is likely to occur; a 70° cutting edge to tooth angulation is ideal for debridement; a 90° cutting edge to tooth angulation is too open, with potential for damaging adjacent tissues. (Adapted from Daniel SJ, Harfst SA, Wilder RS. *Mosby's Dental Hygiene.* 2nd ed. St Louis: Mosby; 2008.)

point right at the root surface. This can result in tissue distention with the rounded bend, inaccurate deposit assessment, and possible root surface scratching. The only time this is done intentionally is when root caries or furcation involvement is suspected and a technique to detect burnished subgingival calculus. Careful insertion of a bladed treatment instrument into subgingival areas involves closing the angle of the cutting edge of the blade relative to the tooth surface. This avoids tissue trauma with the opposite side of the blade to reach the base of the pocket on the down stroke of insertion. The closed blade angulation for the insertion of a curet is from 0° to 10°. The angulation of insertion for a sickle scaler is usually much less than the "working" angulation (see Angulation) but slightly more than 10°.

Instrument reinsertion is the act of returning the instrument down into the subgingival areas after an assessment or working stroke. The reinsertion stroke angulation is slightly less open compared with that of a working stroke. The instrument's working end should remain in contact with the tooth until instrumentation is complete.

A common error with the reinsertion stroke is lifting the instrument from the tooth surface during the act of reinsertion. The pressure of the working stroke should be released to ensure reinsertion to the base of the pocket. Reinsertion follows the same initial insertion guidelines to avoid tissue trauma and to allow repositioning of the blade accurately for continuous, overlapping strokes.

Angulation

Angulation is the relationship between the working end of an instrument and the tooth surface.

The angulation of a bladed instrument refers to the incline of the cutting edge to the tooth surface during a working stroke (Fig. 28.45). Specifically, this is the measurement from the face of the blade to the tooth surface scaled. A "working" angulation is defined as the angle of the cutting edge of the blade against the tooth that produces a grip to the tooth surface. An angle that is closed closer to 45° tends to slide over the tooth surface while an angle opened closer to 90° increases the bite to the tooth (Fig. 28.46).

It is often necessary to modulate blade angulation. An example of such a situation is heavy calculus located only at the base of a 6-mm pocket with smooth cementum directly above. Angulation of the blade of a curet is more closed and the pressure applied is heavier at the base of the pocket to remove the calculus. The angulation is more open and the

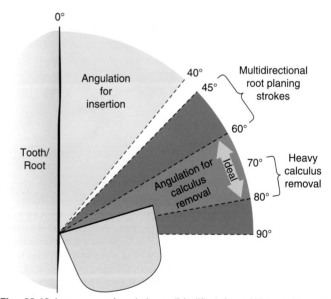

Fig. 28.46 Instrument Angulations. (Modified from Wolters Kluwer Health/Lippincott Williams & Wilkins 2008)

pressure applied is lighter toward the gingival margin for root planing. Several more strokes at less than 80° follow for periodontal debridement and root planing from the junctional epithelium to the CEJ. The likely result of improper instrument angulation is residual calculus.

Designs of various treatment instruments can affect the angulation. The cutting edge of the sickle scaler should be greater than 45 and less than 80° to the tooth surface.

Adaptation

Adaptation is the placement of the working end of an instrument onto the tooth surface. Proper adaptation allows the optimal performance of an instrument without causing harm. It can vary due to the various designs of instruments.

Assessment Instruments

Assessment instrument adaptation refers to the alignment or placement of the side of the first few millimeters of the periodontal probe

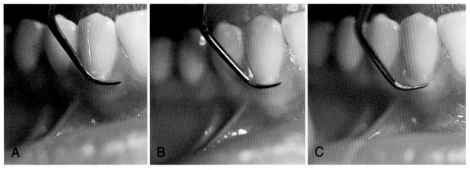

Fig. 28.47 Comparison of various adaptations of bladed instrument. (A) Upper third of blade. (B) Middle third of blade. (C) Lower third of blade.

or straight explorer against the tooth. The lack of alignment with the tooth surface can intrude into the soft tissue to cause patient discomfort. Proper adaptation of assessment instruments provides accurate measurements or correct information about the tooth surface. Erroneous probing depths and misinterpretations of the presence of calculus deposits or cementum irregularities can arise from poor adaptation.

The periodontal probe and the explorer are thin, pointed instruments by design to facilitate tactile sensitivity and access deep, subgingival pockets. The tip and fine, delicate working ends of explorers should be in close contact with the tooth structure when reaching under tight tooth contacts to detect acquired deposits and assess the presence of root irregularities. Close alignment avoids excessive distention and pressure against subgingival tissues and the inadvertent use of the appropriate side of the instrument tip instead of the point.

Treatment Instruments

Treatment instrument adaptation is the close relationship of the working blade to the tooth surface used for periodontal debridement. The most effective adaptation position causing the least amount of hard- or soft-tissue damage occurs when the lower third of the working blade remains in contact with the tooth surface during periodontal debridement procedures. The surface may become gouged or over-instrumented if only the toe or tip is in contact with the tooth or if too much pressure is activated directly on the tooth. Tissue trauma to the sulcular epithelium can occur only if the middle or upper third of the blade is in contact with the tooth surface leaving the lower third and the toe off the tooth (Fig. 28.47A and B)(Fig. 28.47C).

A double-ended bent shank sickle scaler has one side that can best correctly adapt the blade to the tooth surface and maintain a shank position parallel to the plane of the tooth surface scaled. The angulation of the cutting edge to the tooth surface should be greater than 45 and less than 80° to the tooth surface (Fig. 28.46).

The principle of adapting the lower third of the blade of a curet becomes more critical when instrumenting periodontitis-affected teeth. Most instrumentation difficulties lie in the continuous process to conform instruments to the varying convexities and concavities found with root morphology. Furcation involvement, close root proximity from multiple-rooted teeth or adjacent teeth, and tooth alignments contribute to the complications in instrumentation. Adaptation of the lower third of the blade can be aided in these situations with a smaller working end such as a micro mini-bladed curet or choosing an alternative method such as a diamond-coated file.

Activation

Activation is the movement of the working end against the tooth surface to perform the instrument's task. This operational motion simultaneously uses a combination of the forearm, wrist, hand, and/or fingers for instrument usage. The coordinated use of the wrist, hand, and fingers may be sufficient for assessment instruments while the inclusion of the forearm to aid with calculus removal may be necessary.

Stroke Types

Exploratory Stroke

The **exploratory stroke** is used for detection and is usually performed with an explorer or periodontal probe. The curet also may perform an exploratory function to assess the tooth surface during actual periodontal debridement. An exploratory stroke may use light to firm lateral pressure, as follows:

- Light lateral pressure is useful for detecting light spicules of subgingival calculus, as firm lateral pressure is insensitive for fine-deposit exploration.
- Moderate to firm lateral pressure is recommended for the detection of flat, burnished, or smooth calculus or distinguishing restorative margins from tooth anatomy.
- Light, medium, or firm lateral pressure will probably detect the calculus if it occurs in the form of ledges.

Scaling Stroke

The **scaling stroke** is a working stroke movement used for removing calculus from supragingival and subgingival areas. The curet is the instrument of choice for definitive periodontal debridement. Lateral pressure used with scaling stroke ranges from light to firm, however, firm pressure is far greater during scaling than during exploring. Instrument action may change quickly from a scaling stroke to an exploratory stroke to break off calculus but not to over instrument. It also allows for assessing areas previously treated without having to stop and pick up an explorer and reserve the use of an explorer after completion of deposit removal in major areas (Box 28.12).

Lighter lateral pressure during scaling strokes is indicated for light and easy-to-remove calculus and detection. Calculus deposits that are dense and tenacious make instrumentation more difficult than with light calculus deposits.

The practitioner increases the lateral pressure of the scaling stroke as the tenacity and density of the calculus increase. Too little lateral pressure on instrumentation may cause burnishing of tenacious calculus on cementum. Evaluating the changes on the root surface during instrumentation with the curet using exploratory strokes or by using a dental explorer will indiscriminately avoid applying too much lateral pressure causing unnecessary gouging and over-instrumentation of root surfaces.

Root Planing Stroke

The **root planing stroke** is used for removing embedded calculus from cemental surfaces and smoothing root surfaces. The porous nature of

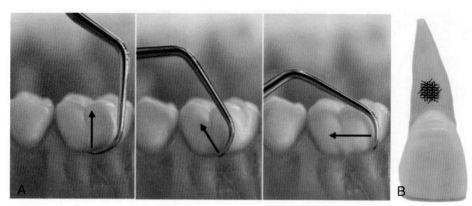

Fig. 28.48 (A) Three basic stroke directions: vertical *(left)*, oblique *(middle)*, and horizontal *(right)*. (B) This diagram illustrates cross-hatching strokes with vertical, horizontal, and oblique stroke directions.

residual calculus and the rough areas of the root act as retention areas for the periodontopathic microorganisms.[15] Patient's ability to achieve and maintain soft-tissue health maintain is improved because oral biofilm control is easier when the roots are smooth.

Successful root planing requires efficacious control; smoothing subgingival surfaces evenly along the entire root surfaces, knowledge of root morphology; and tactile sense of the area the curet has covered on the root surface. The root planing stroke is a longer stroke than the scaling stroke and may begin with firm lateral pressure if there is significant root roughness to smooth. The change to lighter lateral pressure should occur rather quickly as the curet moves to even out the cementum surface.

The cementum thickness varies, but it is thinnest at the cervical third of the tooth (0.02 to 0.05 mm). The tooth structure has such a thin covering of cementum that it leads to dentin exposure and dentinal hypersensitivity (Chapter 39). The dental hygienist must explore the area carefully and use lateral pressure discriminately during scaling and root planing with the purpose of removing only subgingival calculus and altered cementum, smoothing the root surface and removing as little healthy cementum as possible to achieve optimal results while avoiding hypersensitivity during the process. (See the discussion of clinical and therapeutic endpoints in Chapter 33.)

Stroke Movements
Stroke Direction and Pressure
Subgingival assessments are aided by the direction and pressure of the strokes. For accurate identification and removal of deposits, a combination of three basic stroke directions is used with assessment and treatment instruments, as follows (Fig. 28.48A):
- **Vertical** stroke direction is parallel to the long axis of the tooth.
- **Horizontal** stroke direction is perpendicular to the long axis of the tooth.
- **Oblique** stroke direction is diagonal across the long axis of the tooth.

Combinations of stroke directions are termed **cross-hatching** or a "basket weave" of strokes (Fig. 28.48B). Varying stroke direction allows a greater possibility for detection and removal of burnished or smooth calculus because the instrument may catch one side of the calculus when all other sides may be smooth.

Stroke pressure is defined by the direction of the working pressure in relation to drawing toward or away from the clinician. These strokes are as follows:
- Pull
- Push

The pull and push stroke direction may be vertical, horizontal, or oblique. The typical working stroke of the curet, sickle, file, and hoe is performed with a pull stroke. The push or insertion stroke with working pressure is not useful with treatment instruments. This stroke causes unnecessary patient discomfort and has the potential to violate the integrity of the patient's intact junctional epithelium by forcing dental calculus and oral biofilm through the membrane, potentially causing a periodontal abscess. A push stroke with most treatment instruments can promote burnishing calculus because of the blade adaptation and angulation. Some treatment instruments are designed for the push stroke.

An efficient stroke direction is best to keep moving forward in the direction of the toe of the instrument. Channel scaling is the continuous, systematic overlapping of working strokes. This progressive movement of the instrument is the most effective technique for complete calculus removal.

Stroke Length
Stroke length consideration is determined by tissue tone, tooth morphology, and periodontal probing depth measurements. Loose and inflamed tissue accommodates the movement of long, sweeping, overlapping strokes. Healthy tissue or fibrotic in tone and positioned tightly against the tooth are short, overlapping, well-adapted strokes.

Shallow pockets with little recession generally restrict the stroke length. Deep periodontal pockets have an increased root surface area from the clinical attachment allowing greater flexibility in the extent of the stroke. Periodontal conditions with significantly more exposed root surface area with gingival recession give more opportunity to vary the length of the stroke.

Calculus removal demands short, overlapping pull strokes and a firmly planted fulcrum for effective clinician-controlled movement of the instrument. Shorter strokes allow increased pressure and are more reliable at managing the curvatures of root surfaces because they do not pass over deposits in root depressions as easily as longer strokes.

Root planing begins following the removal of most of the calculus. The overlapping stroke becomes longer with decreased pressure to maximize root coverage. Long stroke lengths can maintain a controlled and effective movement in relatively flat areas.

TREATMENT INSTRUMENT SELECTION

A knowledgeable clinician develops the important skill to choose appropriate treatment instruments by assessing various considerations and criteria of the case to make informed choices (Box 28.12).

Considerations and Criteria
Treatment Objective
The **treatment objective** begins to narrow the instrument selection. Primary decision making for the desired outcome includes identifying

During instrumentation, a dental hygienist notices that the instrument's tip broke off subgingivally. What are the proper ethical and legal procedures the hygienist should follow? How should this situation be explained to the patient?

Review components of stroke principles and features of shank designs and types of instruments available for moderate to heavy calculus. What are these components, and how does this help ensure complete calculus removal? Which instruments facilitate removal of heavier calculus?

if a natural tooth, a restored tooth, or a dental implant is to be treated.[12] Time constraints and appointment therapy endpoints of removing gross deposits or root planing assist in this decision making.

Type of Calculus

Assess the **type of calculus** with the quantity and quality of the deposits. Quantity includes descriptions such as light, moderate, heavy, grainy, rough, spicules, sheets, ledges, and rings. Quality includes descriptions such as porous, dense, tenacious, and burnished (Procedure 28.5).

In the presence of heavy, tenacious subgingival calculus, one type of treatment instrument option is the rigid curet. Within this category of treatment instrument, there is a range in variation among manufacturers of the same instrument (e.g., differences in blade size, length, shape, and metallurgy) (Box 28.10).

Tissue Assessment

Instrument selection relies heavily on **tissue assessment** of the periodontal health. This entails considerations such as the clinical attachment loss, probing depths, the amount of attached gingiva, and the presence of mucogingival involvement. Equally as important is the evaluation of the gingival tissues for consistency, size, and the texture that allows retractability allowing instrument insertions.

Tooth Surface

Tooth surfaces can determine instrument selections as many are designed for use in specific areas. This category includes location within the oral cavity (anterior, posterior, maxillary, or mandibular), the specific site on the tooth (mesial, distal, buccal, facial, lingual, palatal, and all line angle areas), tooth morphology (furcations, depressions, and prominent cementoenamel junctions), and location of deposits to be removed (supra- or subgingival accumulations).

Technique Preferences

Technique preferences refer to the comfort and personal preferences of a clinician. Instrument familiarity and clinician traits are also factors that influence instrument selection. For example, a clinician may select area-specific curets, which require different instruments for different tooth areas, for instrumentation in advanced periodontal disease cases. For a prophy, a clinician may choose universal curets to instrument all surfaces for more efficiency in terms of time management. Other factors that may define instrument selection may be if the clinician has finger hypermobility or hyperflexibility conditions, or if the clinician prefers instruments made with materials that reduce or eliminate the need for sharpening.

Task Challenges

Task challenges that influence instrument selection include not only the periodontal disease severity but other situations such as tooth alignments, root proximity, the patient's limited ability to open the mouth, or an overactive lip and tongue.

Curet Selection

Choosing the best-suited curet instruments for successful subgingival instrumentation is critically important. The various metal properties and the strength and lengths of shanks and blades are significant considerations in the decision making. Instrument selection relies on experience using different periodontal debridement instruments, the quantity and quality of calculus, the severity of periodontal involvement, gingival retractability, root morphology complexities, and overall accessibility. Variations require customization of basic instrumentation techniques to treat a particular individual successfully. Customizing instrumentation in periodontitis-affected areas allows the clinician to reach almost any area of the mouth, reach both sulcus areas and deep periodontal pockets, and manage difficult root anatomy with the control and strength needed for effective care.

Instrument Blade Selection

The most important factor in subgingival instrumentation is choosing the blade size to successfully scale the total root surface in the limited pocket space. The same factors that dictate general instrument selection influence choosing the width and thickness of the blade (Procedure 28.5).

The correct working end of the selected instrument is determined by the tooth surface to be scaled. Some instruments have a universal working end (i.e., used on all tooth surfaces) such as the periodontal probe and the No. 3-A EXD explorer. Other instruments have working ends that work well on particular areas (i.e., mesial and distal surfaces, mainly anterior teeth) such as the straight-shanked sickle scaler. The majority of treatment instruments are site-specific with a definite side of the blade used against a particular tooth surface (Box 28.11).

Customizing Instrumentation for Periodontitis-Affected Teeth

Customizing instrumentation successfully depends on finding the correct fulcrum. The dental hygienist should use an analytic approach to accomplish this (Procedure 28.4).

If the tooth surface shape changes to the degree that one fulcrum position no longer works, an alteration of the fulcrum accommodates the change. With experience, adjustments are made within seconds.

It is important to allow for variations in probing depths or alterations in root anatomy, which affect the amount and direction of lateral pressure that can be applied to the root surface. For instance, as probing depth increases on the distal aspect of a mandibular molar from 3 mm to 10 mm, the dental hygienist may find a change in the root surface plane from a vertical to a slightly more oblique or horizontal inclination. Such slight changes in the tooth surface plane alter stroke effectiveness. By readjusting the fulcrum as the instrument maneuvers into deeper probing depths, the practitioner is able to produce effective lateral pressure.

The more periodontally involved the tooth is, the more the dental hygienist needs to fulcrum away from the working site.

POSTTREATMENT INSTRUCTIONS

Posttreatment instructions are general instructions given to the patient on the management of any discomfort and healing after treatment. It is an important responsibility to provide information that will help with the safety and comfort of the patient, especially after initial therapy. Good communication of posttreatment instructions must be tailored toward the empathetic support, cultural sensitivity, and health literacy levels required for the patient.[16] Elements should include

PROCEDURE 28.5 Treatment Instrument Selection Guide

Periodontal Condition	Healthy Preventive	Gingivitis Therapeutic	Early/Moderate Periodontitis Therapeutic	Advanced Periodontitis Therapeutic
Supragingival and Subgingival Soft Deposits				
Acquired Pellicle Biofilm Material Alba Food debris	Type 0/1 inflammation* Powered instruments[†] Universal curets: • thin blade, flexible shank	Type 2/3 inflammation* Powered instruments[†] Universal curets: • thin-medium blade, flexible shank	Type 0/1 inflammation* Powered instruments[†] Universal curets: • thin-medium blade, flexible shank Type 2/3 inflammation* Powered instruments[†] Universal curets: • medium-thick blade, flexible shank	Type 0/1 inflammation* Powered instruments[†] Universal curets, area-specific curets: • standard, mini, and/or micro thin-medium blade, standard shank Type 2/3 inflammation* Powered instruments[†] Universal curets, area-specific curets; • standard, mini, and/or micro medium-thick blade, standard–rigid shank, standard–extended length shank
Supragingival Calculus				
Light-Moderate-Heavy Including D4355	Powered instruments[†] Sickles, hoes, chisels Universal curets: • Blade: thin-medium • Shank: flexible-rigid		Powered instruments[†] Sickles, hoes, chisels Universal curets: • Blade: medium-thick • Shank: rigid Area specific curets: • Blade: standard medium-thick • Shank: rigid–extra rigid, standard length	
Subgingival Calculus				
Light (roughness and localized spicules)	Type 0/1 inflammation* Powered instruments[†] Sickles Universal curets: • Blade: thin-medium • Shank: flexible-rigid Area-specific curets: • Blade: standard, thin-medium standard Shank: flexible-rigid, standard length	Type 1/2 inflammation* Powered instruments[†] Sickles Universal curets: • Blade: thin-medium • Shank: flexible-rigid Area-specific curets: • Blade: standard, thin-medium standard • Shank: flexible-rigid, standard length	Type 1/2 inflammation* Powered instruments[†] Sickles Universal curets: • Blade: thin-medium • Shank: rigid Area specific curets: • Blade: standard, mini, and/or micro thin-medium • Shank: rigid–extra rigid shank, standard-extended length • Furcation instruments Type 2/3 inflammation* Powered instruments[†] Sickles Universal curets: • Blade: medium-thick • Shank: rigid Area specific curets: • Blade: standard, mini, and/or micro medium-thick • Shank: rigid–extra rigid, standard–extended length shank • Furcation instruments	

PROCEDURE 28.5 Treatment Instrument Selection Guide—cont'd

Periodontal Condition	Healthy Preventive	Gingivitis Therapeutic	Early/Moderate Periodontitis Therapeutic	Advanced Periodontitis Therapeutic
Moderate (Light spicules and localized ledges)	N/A	Type 1/2 inflammation* Powered instruments† Sickles Universal curets: • Blade: medium • Shank: rigid Area-specific curets: • Blade: standard, medium • Shank: flexible-rigid, standard length shank	Type 2/3 inflammation* Powered instruments† Sickles Universal curets: • Blade: medium-thick • Shank: rigid Area specific curets: • Blade: standard, mini, and/or micro medium-thick • Shank: rigid–extra rigid, standard–extended length shank • Furcation instruments	
Heavy (Moderate ledges and/or rings including burnished)	N/A	Type 1/2 inflammation* Powered instruments† Sickles Universal curets: • Blade: medium • Shank: rigid Area specific curets: • Blade: standard, mini, medium • Shank: flexible-rigid, standard length shank	Type 2/3 inflammation* Powered instruments† Sickles Files Universal curets: • Blade: medium-thick • Shank: rigid Area specific curets: • Blade: standard, mini medium-thick • Shank: rigid–extra rigid, standard-extended length • Furcation instruments	Type 2/3 inflammation* Powered instruments† Sickles Files Universal curets: • Blade: medium-thick • Shank: rigid Area specific curets: • Blade: standard, mini and/or micro medium-thick • Shank: rigid–extra rigid, standard-extended length • Furcation instruments

* Löe and Silness gingival inflammation index
† Powered instruments can include ultrasonics, supra/subgingival air polishers, lasers
Type 0: No inflammation
Type 1: Mild inflammation—slight change in color, slight edema but no bleeding on probing
Type 2: Moderate inflammation—redness, edema, and bleeding on probing
Type 3: Severe inflammation—marked redness and edema, ulceration with tendency to spontaneous bleeding

explanations of the recovery phase, usual expectations, and anticipating the patient's needs.

Details of posttreatment instructions are particularly imperative for initial therapy (Table 28.12).

DENTAL PERIOSCOPY

Although costly, **dental perioscopy**, fiberoptic imaging of the periodontal pocket, allows subgingival visualization for diagnosis as well as treatment.[17] Using dental perioscopy, the clinician magnifies, visualizes, and accesses deep subgingival calculus, root fractures, and the periodontal pocket's internal wall. Magnification is from 20× to as high as 40×, depending on the distance between the object and the lens.

The system is composed of a disposable sterile sheath that houses a fiberoptic endoscope, provides continuous irrigation, and has a metal soft-tissue shield that keeps the soft tissue away from the tube. The system includes a flat-panel HD color display monitor and a small-footprint transport system (Fig. 28.49), and video-out source connections allow users to employ a digital system to record and later view endoscopic images if desired.

Under endoscopic magnification, black calculus ledges are actually white, porous, and crystalline in appearance, and subgingival calculus sheets may occur in colors from golden brown to black. Dental perioscopy has shown a direct relationship with tissue inflammation and the presence of subgingival calculus deposits. Direct visualization has shown the degree of inflammation of tissues is greater in areas of calculus deposits covered with biofilm than in areas of biofilm alone.[17]

This system of visualization during root surface instrumentation improves clinical assessment of results over traditional tactile assessment methods.[17] Clinicians experienced with the system indicate an extraordinary ability to visualize and instrument deep, narrow pockets, depressions, line angles, and furcations. Although this method demands that the clinician learn new techniques, patients have no increase in discomfort for the calculus detection procedure of the endoscope when compared to probing.[18] The process also is educational, because patients see the intricacies of their disease and treatment on the monitor and judge the effectiveness of oral self-care procedures. To view the endoscope in place subgingivally, visit decisionsindentistry.com/applications-limitations-periodontal-endoscopy

Periodontal instrumentation with visualization is significantly more accurate and specific than instrumentation without visualization. In addition to traditional treatment instruments, nontraditional periodontal instruments such as diamond-coated instruments (Fig. 28.26) are being used with success when the clinician is able to view areas of burnished calculus. Even with visualization, successful instrumentation is still dependent on the clinician's ability to use a variety of fulcrums, stroke directions, and periodontal instruments.

TABLE 28.12 Posttreatment Instructions for Initial Therapy

Day of Treatment Procedure

Rinsing	Gentle swishing; rigorous rinsing can increase clot removal and bleeding
Oral Hygiene	Normal oral hygiene routine except for treated site (gentle rinsing only)
Diet/Eating	Eating should be avoided while numb; selection of comfortable softer foods if necessary
Smoking/Vaping	If possible, smoking/vaping should be avoided for 7–10 days as it may delay healing

Possible Expectations; Contact Clinician if Increasing Symptoms Occur

• Bleeding	Slight bleeding is observed by pink saliva which slowly decreases; moistened caffeinated teabag pressure for 10 minutes if bleeding persists
• Discomfort	Slight tenderness, throbbing, or aching gradually decreases; recommend warm salt-water rinses; ibuprofen or Advil
• Recession	Gingival shape changes can occur with decreased inflammation and tightening of tissues
• Sensitivity	Root surfaces along the gingival marginal area may have thermal sensitivity; recommend desensitizing products
• Tooth mobility	Slight increase in mobility can occur if severe periodontal conditions exist; may decrease with improved gingival health
• Abscess formation	Localized increase in tenderness and swelling may develop; advise to contact clinician

Day After Treatment Procedure

Oral hygiene	Normal oral hygiene routine can gently be resumed and increased to usual pressure as tolerated

Supplemental Instructions

Follow-up appointment	Periodontal health is to be reassessed in 4–6 weeks after periodontal debridement treatment is completed
Contact clinician	Prolonged pain, visible swelling, bleeding, fever, adverse or allergic reactions, excessive patient discomfort or concerns

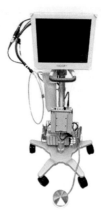

Fig. 28.49 The Zest Solutions, Danville Materials, LLC Perioscopy System (PS).

KEY CONCEPTS

- The basic functional components of hand-activated instruments are the handle, the shank, and the working end.
- Dental hygiene hand instruments are divided into two classifications. The assessment instruments include the mouth mirror, periodontal probe, and explorer. The basic treatment instruments include universal curets, area-specific curets, sickles, hoes, files, and chisels.
- Primary design considerations important for treatment instrument selection are the blade (design, shape, and size) and the shank (length, curvature, and flexibility). These can significantly affect use and effectiveness of hand-activated instruments.
- The stroke principles of hand instrumentation are angulation, adaptation, and activation.
- Treatment objectives, periodontal conditions, type and location of accumulations, and technique preferences of the clinician are some of the factors that determine the appropriate instrument selection design and blade size.
- A dull instrument can be considered an unethical practice as it can compromise the benefits to the patient by increasing the likelihood of discomfort, tissue injury, and the result of burnished calculus.
- Application of basic instrumentation skills of proper clinician/patient positioning, body mechanics, the field of vision, hand grasp, and proper lateral pressure help reduce injury risk optimizes benefits for the clinician and the patient.
- The importance of the patient education of posttreatment instructions by the clinician is to ensure the safety and comfort of their patient.

ACKNOWLEDGMENTS

The authors acknowledge Anna M. Pattison for providing advice on current assessment and treatment instruments.

Instruments provided by Hu-Friedy Manufacturing, Paradise Dental Technologies, L-M Instruments, Brasseler USA, and American Eagle Instruments.

REFERENCES

1. Krishna R, De Stefano JA. Ultrasonic vs. hand instrumentation in periodontal therapy: clinical outcomes. *Periodontol 2000.* 2016;71(1):113–127.
2. Lin Z, Strauss FJ, Lang NP, et al. Efficacy of laser monotherapy or non-surgical mechanical instrumentation in the management of untreated periodontitis patients. A systematic review and meta-analysis. *Clin Oral Invest.* 2021;25:375–391.
3. Cobb CM, Sottosanti JS. A re-evaluation of scaling and root planing. *J Periodontol.* 2021;92(10):1370–1378. Epub 2021 Mar 16.
4. Pierre-Bez AC, Agostini-Walesch GM, Bradford Smith P, et al. Ultrasonic scaling in COVID-era dentistry: a quantitative assessment of aerosol spread during simulated and clinical ultrasonic scaling procedures. *Int J Dent Hyg.* 2021;19(4):474–480.
5. Graetz C, Schützhold S, Plaumann A, et al. Prognostic factors for the loss of molars—an 18-years retrospective cohort study. *J Clin Periodontol.* 2015;42(10):943–950.
6. Sanders MJ, Turcotte CA. Ergonomic strategies for dental professionals. *Work.* 1997;8(1):55–72. WOR-1997-9107.
7. Hayes MJ. The effect of stainless steel and silicone instruments on hand comfort and strength: a pilot study. *J Dent Hyg.* 2017;91:40–44.
8. Rempel D, Lee DL, Dawson K, Loomer P. The effects of periodontal curette handle weight and diameter on arm pain: a four-month randomized controlled trial. *J Am Dent Assoc.* 2012;143(10):1105–1113. jada.archive. 2012.0041.

9. Suedbeck JR, Tolle SL, McCombs G, et al. Effects of instrument handle design on dental hygienists' forearm muscle activity during scaling. *J Dent Hyg*. 2017;91:47–54.

10. Dong H, Barr A, Loomer P, Rempel D. The effects of finger rest positions on hand muscle load and pinch force in simulated dental hygiene work. *J Dent Educ*. 2005;69(4):453–460.

11. Simmer-Beck M, Branson BG. An evidence-based review of ergonomic features of dental hygiene instruments. *Work*. 2010;35(4):477–485.

12. Bidra AS, et al. Clinical practice guidelines for recall and maintenance of patients with tooth-borne and implant-borne dental restorations. *J Dent Hyg*. 2016;90:60–69.

13. Hayes M, Cockrell D, Smith DR. A systematic review of musculoskeletal disorders among dental professionals. *Int J Dent Hyg*. 2009;7(3):159–165.

14. Gehrig JS, Sroda R, Saccuzzo D. *Fundamentals of Periodontal Instrumentation & Advanced Root Instrumentation*. 8th ed. Wolters Kluwer; 2019.

15. Eick S, ed. *Oral Biofilms*. Karger Medical and Scientific Publishers; 2020.

16. Walker KK, Jackson RD, Maxwell L. The importance of developing communication skills: perceptions of dental hygiene students. *J Dent Hyg*. 2016;90:306–312.

17. Kuagn Y, et al. Effects of periodontal endoscopy on the treatment of periodontitis: a systematic review and meta-analysis. *J Am Dent Assoc*. 2017;10:750–759.

18. Poppe K, Blue C. Subjective pain perception during calculus detection with use of a periodontal endoscope. *J Dent Hyg*. 2014;88(2):114–123.

29

Ultrasonic Instrumentation

Marie D. George and Dani Botbyl

PROFESSIONAL OPPORTUNITIES

Learn how to implement effective ultrasonic therapy and inform patients and colleagues about why ultrasonic instrumentation is being used.

COMPETENCIES

1. Value the role of ultrasonic instrumentation in accomplishing the objectives of periodontal debridement in terms of the advantages and indications.
2. Relate the mechanisms of action of ultrasonic instruments to effective debridement of the tooth/root surface.
3. Compare and contrast magnetostrictive and piezoelectric ultrasonic scaling instruments.
4. Discuss the acoustic power produced by an ultrasonic scaler.
5. Apply information about the relationship of key operational and technique variables to the mechanisms of ultrasonic debridement.
   - Produce a level of acoustic power suitable for the treatment objective through proper adjustment of the operational variables.
   - Consider the influence of tip design on clinical performance to guide tip selection based on the treatment objective and the anatomy of the treatment site.
6. Execute proper ultrasonic instrumentation technique with any tip design in any area of the dentition.
7. Discuss assessment and management of using ultrasonic instrumentation for patient care.

INTRODUCTION

Ultrasonic instrumentation in dentistry originated in an era when the primary objective for preventing and treating periodontal disease was the successful removal of calculus from teeth. Ultrasonic instrumentation was implemented as an adjunct to manual (hand) instrumentation and was the key armamentarium for the removal of heavy supragingival calculus. The removal of subgingival calculus and subsequent intentional removal of cementum and dentin to achieve a "glass like root surface" was completed manually, with sharp bladed instruments.

Today, contemporary periodontal therapy recognizes gingivitis and periodontitis as chronic inflammatory disease processes that are initiated and perpetuated by periodontal pathogens encased within subgingival biofilm and, accordingly, aims to resolve the inflammation and promote stabilization of the periodontal tissues through routine periodontal debridement (PD) procedures implemented both professionally and at home by the patient. The objectives of professional PD are noted in Box 29.1.

PD can be accomplished by manual and/or ultrasonic instrumentation. Ultrasonic instrumentation, by tip design and mechanisms of action, provides several advantages over manual instrumentation in meeting the objectives of PD. These advantages include:

- Greater predictability and efficiency of biofilm disruption. To optimize mechanical disruption of biofilm, particularly at the microscopic level, maximum contact between the treatment surface and working end of the instrument tip is required, regardless of the type of instrument used. The cylindrical shape of the blunt ultrasonic tip better conforms to the curvatures of the tooth surface than does the straight bladed edge of a manual instrument. Consequently, the greater degree of contact achieved by the ultrasonic tip, the vibratory motion of the tip, and the biophysical forces produced by ultrasonic instruments are more conducive to thorough and efficient disruption of plaque biofilm than the mechanisms of manual instrumentation, which are intended to cut calcified deposits from the tooth surface.
- Conservation of tooth structure. PD requires a light touch or gentle form of instrumentation to achieve plaque biofilm removal without over instrumentation of the root surface. Using a bladed instrument at an appropriate force to effectively disrupt biofilm without inherent cementum removal is difficult to ascertain and maintain, requires constant effort by the clinician, and is influenced by the integrity of the cutting edge. In contrast, the mechanisms of ultrasonic debridement, combined with the ability of the clinician to modify variables (such as power level, lateral pressure, and tip design) minimize root surface alteration without compromising the effectiveness and efficiency of biofilm disruption.
- Greater procedural efficiency. The time it takes to finish a debridement procedure using manual instruments increases with severity of disease, whereas a PD procedure that uses a protocol including the appropriate combination of ultrasonic instruments (no hand instruments) is completed significantly quicker regardless of disease severity.[1]

Given the pathogenesis of periodontal disease and the advantages of ultrasonic technology, the use of ultrasonic instrumentation for PD has evolved to become a standard of care.[2]

Clinicians should use critical thinking to choose the best instrumentation approach to PD, given the armamentarium available at the time therapy is provided. Box 29.2 provides a Critical Thinking Scenario for your consideration. After contemplating the Scenario, reflect on the Legal, Ethical, Safety Responsibility presented in Box 29.3.

ULTRASONIC INSTRUMENTATION MECHANISMS OF ACTION

The term **ultrasonic** applies to sound (**acoustic**) energy having a frequency above the highest that is audible to the human ear, which is 20 kilohertz (kHz) (Fig. 29.1). Ultrasound is used in many different fields in a variety of ways. For example, sonography used in obstetrics applies ultrasound waves to penetrate a gel medium and measure the reflection signature of the fetus, whereas the ultrasonic cleaning of jewelry or dental instruments uses ultrasound waves to supply focused energy to disrupt the tarnish or debris.

In ultrasonic scaling instruments, electrical current is converted into high-frequency vibrations that cause **oscillation** (forward and backward movement) of the tip. This high-frequency movement of the tip produces both mechanical and biophysical forces capable of disrupting and removing deposits from the tooth surface. These forces (Table 29.1) are the *mechanisms of action* of ultrasonic instruments.

Mechanical

The primary mechanism of ultrasonic deposit removal is mechanical. The high-frequency oscillating action of the blunt tip contacting the deposit (biofilm or calculus) mechanically disrupts or fractures the deposit.

Irrigation

An irrigant (typically water) is used with ultrasonic instruments to counteract any frictional heat generated by the oscillating tip against the tooth surface. The irrigant creates a continuous flow, or lavage, which has been demonstrated to remove loosely attached biofilm and endotoxin from the root surface, in addition to flushing debris from the treatment site.

Cavitation and Acoustic Microstreaming

Cavitation and acoustic microstreaming are biophysical phenomena generated by the vibrating tip transmitting ultrasonic energy into the irrigating water. These hydrodynamic forces are produced simultaneously and act synergistically to disrupt plaque biofilm.[3,4]

Cavitation is characterized by the formation and explosive collapse of microscopic bubbles in a flowing liquid, resulting from forces acting on the liquid (Fig. 29.2). The violent collapse of the microbubbles forms high-velocity liquid jets that aid in debriding biofilm from the tooth surface.[3]

Acoustic microstreaming occurs near any object in oscillatory motion in liquid, including ultrasonic scaler tips and cavitation bubbles, and is characterized by a vigorous swirling motion of fluid (Fig. 29.3).[4]

ULTRASONIC SCALING TECHNOLOGIES

In dentistry, ultrasonic scaling units are either **magnetostrictive** or **piezoelectric** in nature. It is essential for clinicians to be cognizant of each technology, as both will likely be used during one's career.

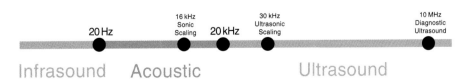

Fig. 29.1 Range of sound frequencies. Frequencies >20 kHz are ultrasonic. (Reprinted from George MD, Botbyl D, Donley TD, Preshaw PM. *Ultrasonic Periodontal Debridement: Theory and Technique, 2nd Edition.* Wiley; 2023. Reproduced with permission of John Wiley & Sons, Inc.)

Magnetostrictive Devices

The distinguishing components of a magnetostrictive ultrasonic scaler (Table 29.2) are the insert and handpiece. The **insert** is composed of a stack of thin nickel strips soldered together at the ends and attached by a connecting body to a tip (Fig. 29.4). The handpiece (Fig. 29.5) surrounds the nickel stack of the insert with copper wire, which generates an alternating magnetic field upon application of electrical current. In response to the electromagnetic energy, the nickel stack elongates and contracts along its length, producing longitudinal vibrations that travel through the connecting body to the tip, resulting in high-frequency oscillation of the tip (Figs. 29.6 and 29.7). Popular brands of magnetostrictive scalers are shown in Figs. 29.8 and 29.9.

Piezoelectric Devices

A piezoelectric ultrasonic scaler is differentiated (Table 29.2) by a tip which screws onto the handpiece using a torque wrench (Fig. 29.10). The handpiece contains a crystalline (ceramic or quartz) disc which expands, then contracts in response to an alternating application of current, producing vibrations that result in high-frequency oscillation of the tip (Fig. 29.11). Popular brands of piezoelectric scalers are shown in Figs. 29.12 and 29.13.

OPERATIONAL VARIABLES OF ULTRASONIC SCALING UNITS

Whether ultrasonic vibrations are produced by magnetostriction or by piezoelectricity, powered scaling units share common operational variables that influence the mechanisms, and thereby, success of ultrasonic debridement (Table 29.3). With an understanding of the effect of each variable on both deposit removal and the root surface, the clinician can appropriately adjust the variables to meet the treatment objective.

Operating Frequency

Specific to ultrasonic scalers, the **operating frequency** of the unit is the number of complete back-and-forth cycles (strokes) the oscillating tip completes per second, measured in kilohertz. Common operating frequencies are 30 kHz (30,000 strokes/sec; magnetostrictive and piezoelectric) or 25 kHz (25,000 strokes/sec; magnetostrictive only). Adjustment of the operating frequency by the clinician is neither necessary nor possible.

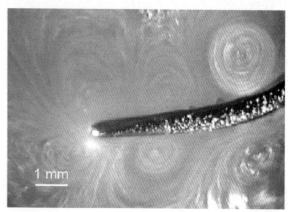

Fig. 29.3 Video-captured digitized image of a magnetostrictive insert (P-12) showing acoustic microstreaming as demonstrated by the movement of zinc stearate particles floating on the water surface into which the scaler tip is oscillating at 10.5 μm displacement amplitude. (Khambay BS, Walmsley AD. Acoustic microstreaming: detection and measurement around ultrasonic scalers. *J Periodontol*. 1999;70(6):626–631. Reproduced with permission of American Academy of Periodontology.)

TABLE 29.1	Ultrasonic Debridement Mechanisms of Action
Mechanical	Vibratory action of the oscillating blunt tip against the deposit disrupts or ablates the deposit from the tooth surface
Irrigation	Lavage action of water flowing over tip flushes biofilm from the tooth surface and debris from the treatment site
Cavitation	Removal/disruption of biofilm by shock waves resulting from the implosion of bubbles
Acoustic microstreaming	Removal/disruption of biofilm by turbulent currents of water surrounding the tip

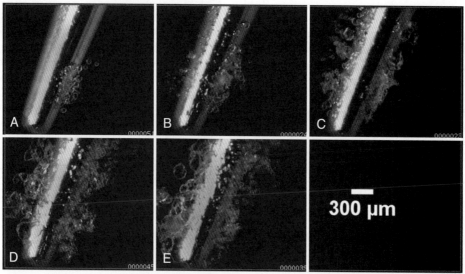

Fig. 29.2 High-speed images of microbubbles around piezoelectric scaler tip 10P at various power settings: (A) power 5, (B) power 7, (C) power 10, (D) power 15, (E) power 20 (maximum power setting). (Vyas N, Dehghani H, Sammons RL, et al. Imaging and analysis of individual cavitation microbubbles around dental ultrasonic scalers. *Ultrasonics*. 2017;81:66–72.)

TABLE 29.2   Components of Ultrasonic Scaling Devices

Component	Description MAGNETOSTRICTIVE	Description PIEZOELECTRIC
Insert or tip	**INSERT** – An insert is composed of a stack, connecting body and tip. The stack is a collection of thin nickel strips soldered together at the ends and attached by a connecting body to a metal tip. The stack of the insert is the element that is connected to the handpiece.	**TIP** – A stack and connecting body do *not* exist. The metal tip has threads at its base and is screwed into the handpiece by a torque-controlled wrench.
Handpiece	Holds the insert to surround the nickel stack in a spiral of copper wire which generates a magnetic field upon application of electrical current, resulting in magnetostriction of the stack	Embeds ceramic or crystal discs that encircle a metal bar. The terminal end of the bar is threaded to allow attachment of the tip.
Base unit	Houses controls that regulate power level and water flow; provides connection between foot switch and handpiece	Houses controls that regulate power level and water flow; provides connection between foot switch and handpiece
Foot switch	When engaged, sends electrical current through base unit to the handpiece, activating movement of the tip	When engaged, sends electrical current through base unit to the handpiece, activating movement of the tip

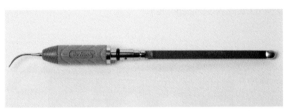

Fig. 29.4 A magnetostrictive insert. (Reprinted from George MD, Botbyl D, Donley TD, Preshaw PM. *Ultrasonic Periodontal Debridement: Theory and Technique*, 2nd Edition. Wiley; 2023. Reproduced with permission of John Wiley & Sons, Inc.)

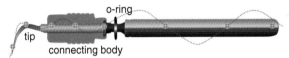

Fig. 29.7 Longitudinal vibrations travel from the nickel stack through a connecting body to the tip of the insert. The crosshairs denote points of no vibration or movement, referred to as nodal points or antinodes. (Reprinted from George MD, Botbyl D, Donley TD, Preshaw PM. *Ultrasonic Periodontal Debridement: Theory and Technique,* 2nd Edition. Wiley; 2023. Reproduced with permission of John Wiley & Sons, Inc.)

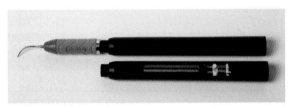

Fig. 29.5 The handpiece of a magnetostrictive unit contains a spiral of copper wire (visible in the lower, cutout handpiece), which surrounds the stack once the insert is seated in the handpiece. (Reprinted from George MD, Botbyl D, Donley TD, Preshaw PM. *Ultrasonic Periodontal Debridement: Theory and Technique,* 2nd Edition. Wiley; 2023. Reproduced with permission of John Wiley & Sons, Inc.)

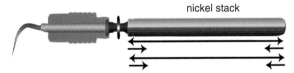

Fig. 29.6 Diagram of a magnetostrictive insert. Application of an electromagnetic field to the stack of nickel strips results in magnetostriction—elongation then contraction—of the nickel stack along its length, producing longitudinal vibrations. (Reprinted from George MD, Botbyl D, Donley TD, Preshaw PM. *Ultrasonic Periodontal Debridement: Theory and Technique,* 2nd Edition. Wiley; 2023. Reproduced with permission of John Wiley & Sons, Inc.)

Power Input

The amount of electrical power input to the unit is adjustable by manipulating the power setting of the unit. The power setting influences the range of movement, or stroke length, produced by the oscillating tip. Stroke length is measured as the **displacement amplitude**, meaning

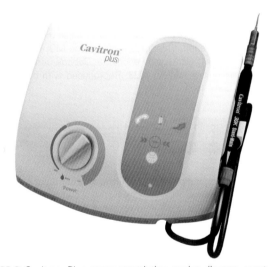

Fig. 29.8 Cavitron Plus magnetostrictive scaler. (Image courtesy of Dentsply Sirona.)

how far the tip is displaced from a position of zero movement and is measured in microns (μm) (Fig. 29.14A), with the greatest displacement amplitude occurring in the active area of the tip[4] (Fig. 29.14B).

There is a positive correlation between power setting and displacement amplitude, meaning that an increase in power will increase the displacement amplitude and vice versa.[5] The power level controls on current ultrasonic scaling devices may be in the form of a knob, push button, or touch screen and use linear or numeric scales, ranging from low to high, to provide an estimate of the displacement amplitude produced (Fig. 29.15).

The extent to which increasing or decreasing power affects the displacement amplitude of the tip varies according to the design of the tip. At any given power setting, different tip designs, and even

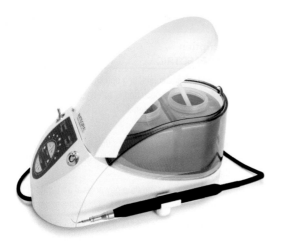

Fig. 29.9 Integra magnetostrictive scaler. (Image courtesy of Parkell, Inc.)

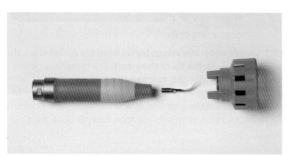

Fig. 29.10 Handpiece of a piezoelectric unit to which the tip is attached using the torque wrench. (Reprinted from George MD, Botbyl D, Donley TD, Preshaw PM. *Ultrasonic Periodontal Debridement: Theory and Technique,* 2nd Edition. Wiley; 2023. Reproduced with permission of John Wiley & Sons, Inc.)

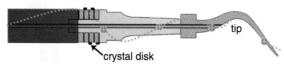

Fig. 29.11 Diagram of a piezoelectric ultrasonic handpiece. Application of an alternating electrical current to the crystalline disc causes it to expand, then contract, producing longitudinal vibrations that travel to the attached tip. Crosshairs denote nodal points (antinodes) or points of no movement or vibration. (Reprinted from George MD, Botbyl D, Donley TD, Preshaw PM. *Ultrasonic Periodontal Debridement: Theory and Technique,* 2nd Edition. Wiley; 2023. Reproduced with permission of John Wiley & Sons, Inc.)

different tips of the same design, will oscillate with different displacement amplitudes.[6]

Water Flow Rate

An adequate supply of water to the tip is needed to minimize the production of frictional heat, generate a lavage, and maximize the occurrence of cavitation and acoustic microstreaming. To achieve this, a flow rate of 20 to 30 mL/min is sufficient. However, the water control on current ultrasonic scaling devices does not measure the flow produced in mL/min but instead, quantifies the flow rate as low to high, using a control knob located on the front of the unit or a rotatable ring located at the base of the handpiece. To produce an adequate flow rate, clinicians should adjust the water control until droplets are intermittently released from the tip at a medium power setting (Fig. 29.16).

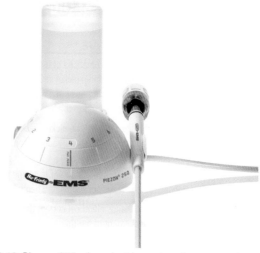

Fig. 29.12 Piezon 250 piezoelectric scaler. (Image courtesy of Hu-Friedy Mfg Co., LLC, Chicago, IL.)

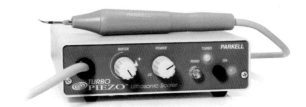

Fig. 29.13 TurboPIEZO piezoelectric scaler. (Image courtesy of Parkell, Inc.)

TABLE 29.3	**Ultrasonic Scaler Operational Variables**
Variable	**Description**
Operating Frequency	The number of back-and-forth strokes the tip oscillates per second, measured in kilohertz. Typically fixed at resonant frequency of 30 or 25 kHz
Power Input	Adjusts the displacement amplitude (stroke length) of the oscillating tip, thereby influencing the amount of force and cavitation/microstreaming generated by the tip
Water Flow Rate	Adjusts the amount of water (or other irrigant) flowing through the handpiece and over the oscillating tip
Tip Diameter	Width of the active area (terminal 2 to 4 mm) of the scaling tip; indicates the mass of the tip
Tip Shape	Shape of the active area in cross section; typically described as rectangular or circular (cylindrical)

Tip Design

As the diameter and shape of the tip used have a direct impact on both the mechanical and biophysical (cavitation/microstreaming) mechanisms of action, these elements of tip design are considered operational variables and therefore are introduced here.

Diameter refers to the width or thickness at the **active area** (terminal 2 to 4 mm) of the tip. Three categories of tip diameter are described in Table 29.4.

Shape refers to the shape of the active area in cross section, being either rectangular or circular (Fig. 29.17). Tip shape is independent

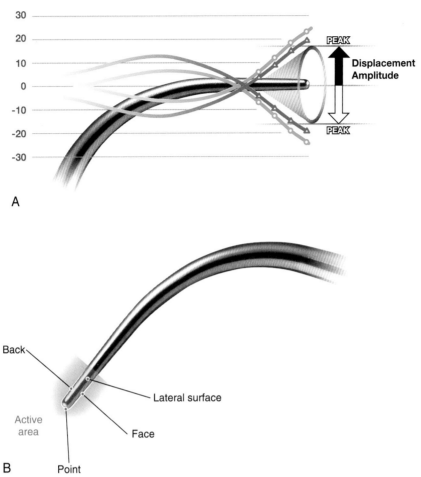

Fig. 29.14 (A) Plotting the maximum vibration along the length of the scaler tip (values shown are the mean of 10 readings ± 1 standard deviation) demonstrates how far the tip is displaced from a position of zero movement. Displacement amplitude is measured as half the peak-to-peak displacement of the tip and is greatest at the free, unconstrained end of the oscillating tip. (Lea SC, Felver B, Landini G. Ultrasonic scaler oscillations and tooth-surface defects. *J Dent Res.* 2009;88(3):229–234. Modified with permission of Sage Publications.) (B) The active area of the tip (highlighted in *gold*) extends approximately 4 mm in length from the terminal end of the tip. (Reprinted from George MD, Botbyl D, Donley TD, Preshaw PM. *Ultrasonic Periodontal Debridement: Theory and Technique,* 2nd Edition. Wiley; 2023. Reproduced with permission of John Wiley & Sons, Inc.)

of the diameter of the tip; slim-diameter tips with a rectangular cross section exist, as do standard-diameter tips with a circular cross section.

ACOUSTIC POWER

As previously explained, the power setting of an ultrasonic unit controls the amount of electrical power being supplied to the magnetostrictive or piezoelectric transducer. In contrast, the term **acoustic power** refers to the overall amount of energy—mechanical and biophysical combined—emitted at the tip. As the operational variables influence the level of acoustic power, a solid understanding of their synergistic actions is necessary in order to operate the ultrasonic scaler at a level of acoustic power suitable for the indicated treatment objective.

Mechanical Mechanism of Action

The efficiency of the vibrating tip in mechanically disrupting the biofilm or ablating the calculus deposits correlates to the amount of lateral force exerted by the tip. The force exerted is influenced by several factors: (1) the power setting, which determines displacement amplitude/stroke length; (2) diameter (mass) of the active tip; and (3) shape of the active tip (Table 29.5). Clinically, one must consider the correlation of

these variables in regard to both the mechanical removal of biofilm and calculus and the effect on the root surface. Increasing degrees of force result in an increase in the depth and volume of root surface defects[5] or lack of ideal preservation of root structure. Additionally, excessive force has the potential to create discomfort and sensitivity for the patient.

To better comprehend the correlation of these variables, consider a rectangular-shaped tip. The surfaces of a rectangular tip meet to form an edge; because of its reduced surface area, this edge exerts a greater output of energy (greater force) compared to a circular tip. At any given power setting, the force is greater with the use of a standard-diameter (vs. slim-diameter) tip and if that standard tip is rectangular, the net force is increased even more.

Biophysical Mechanisms of Action (Cavitation and Microstreaming)

The efficacy and extent of biofilm disruption is relative to the amount of cavitation and acoustic microstreaming occurring in the water surrounding the oscillating tip. In general, greater displacement amplitude (power level) and wider diameter tips produce higher levels of cavitation/microstreaming. However, to be useful in the debridement of

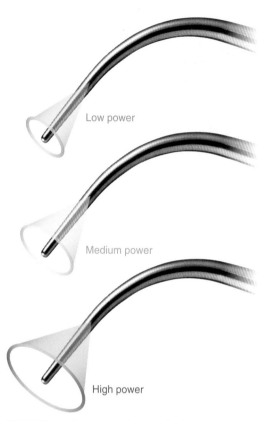

Low power

Medium power

High power

Fig. 29.15 Effect of power setting on displacement amplitude (stroke length) of tip. (Reprinted from George MD, Botbyl D, Donley TD, Preshaw PM. *Ultrasonic Periodontal Debridement: Theory and Technique,* 2nd Edition. Wiley; 2023. Reproduced with permission of John Wiley & Sons, Inc.)

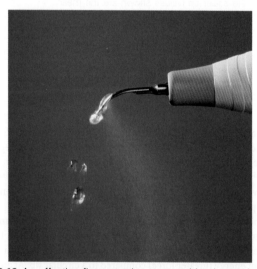

Fig. 29.16 An effective flow rate demonstrated by the production of intermittent droplets at the activated tip at a medium power setting. (Reprinted from George MD, Botbyl D, Donley TD, Preshaw PM. *Ultrasonic Periodontal Debridement: Theory and Technique,* 2nd Edition. Wiley; 2023. Reproduced with permission of John Wiley & Sons, Inc.)

biofilm from a root surface, these hydrodynamic events need to occur at lower power settings and with slimmer diameter tips (reduced force to preserve the root surface). It has been demonstrated that the lateral pressure applied to maintain contact between the tip and tooth increases the amount of cavitational activity occurring at lower power settings, especially with slimmer diameter tips.[3]

TABLE 29.4 **Categories of Ultrasonic Tips by Diameter**	
Diameter	**Traits**
Standard ("Scaling")	• Greater mass • Wide in diameter • Either circular or rectangular in shape • Straight geometry
Slim ("Thin" or "Perio-")	• Less mass • Reduced in diameter; ~30%–40% narrower than standard-diameter tips • Either circular or rectangular in shape • Straight or curved geometry
Ultraslim ("Extra-thin")	• Least mass • Narrowest in diameter; ~40% thinner than slim-diameter tips • Circular in shape • Straight geometry

Producing an Appropriate Level of Acoustic Power

In order to accomplish efficient deposit removal without overinstrumentation of the root surface, it is essential for the clinician to operate the ultrasonic scaler at the minimum effective acoustic power level. The minimum level of acoustic power needed will vary according to the type of deposit to be removed because the scaling of calculus requires different working parameters than does debridement of biofilm. Therefore instrumentation is implemented in two stages through modification of the operational variables (Table 29.6).

The intention of the scaling stage is to remove or reduce substantial and/or tenacious calculus deposits to a lesser degree. To accomplish this efficiently, a standard-diameter tip oscillating at medium to medium-high displacement amplitude/stroke length (power level) is generally indicated.

Debridement instrumentation then follows in a conservative manner to definitively remove light calculus and plaque biofilm. This requires working parameters that minimize root surface damage while at the same time produce optimal levels of cavitation and microstreaming. Accordingly, a slim or ultraslim diameter tip oscillating at medium displacement amplitude/stroke length (power level) should be used.

ULTRASONIC TIP SELECTION

As with hand instrumentation, a variety of tip designs is required to properly implement ultrasonic root surface debridement. Unlike hand instruments, the classification of ultrasonic instruments is not standardized among manufacturers, making tip comparison and selection by name difficult. Selection of a proper tip is streamlined by examining key design features common to all ultrasonic tips (Table 29.7).

Tip dimension and tip shape were previously defined in the discussion of operational variables. The geometry of the tip is descriptive of the number of planes that the shank of the tip crosses, being either one or two. A tip that extends in only one plane is geometrically straight, whereas a tip with a curved (semispiral) design extends into a second plane (Fig. 29.18). Curved tips are area specific (Table 29.8) and labeled as either left or right (Fig. 29.19) according to the direction of the curve. Use of an area-specific curved tip is indicated for the debridement of curved or concave surfaces; the arc of the tip improves access to and contact with such anatomy. For this reason, curved tips are often used on posterior roots and furcation surfaces; noting the design also prevents the point from coming in

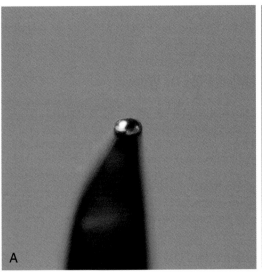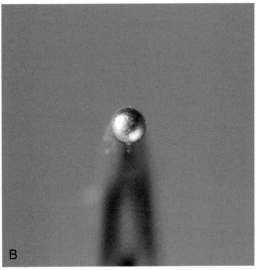

Fig. 29.17 The shape of an ultrasonic tip in cross section may be (A) rectangular or (B) circular. (Reprinted from George MD, Botbyl D, Donley TD, Preshaw PM. *Ultrasonic Periodontal Debridement: Theory and Technique,* 2nd Edition. Wiley; 2023. Reproduced with permission of John Wiley & Sons, Inc.)

TABLE 29.5 Influence of Operational Variables on Net Force Exerted by Oscillating Tip

Increases Net Force	Decreases Net Force
Higher displacement amplitude/ power setting	Lower displacement amplitude/power setting
Wider tip diameter	Narrower tip diameter
Rectangular tip shape	Circular tip shape

TABLE 29.6 Variable Modification per Stage of Instrumentation

Operational Variable	Scaling Stage	Debridement Stage
Displacement amplitude	Medium to medium-high	Medium
Tip diameter	Standard	Slim or ultraslim
Tip shape	Circular or rectangular	Circular

TABLE 29.7 Key Design Features of Ultrasonic Tips

Tip Feature	Description	Impact
Diameter	Width of the active area of the tip (standard, slim, ultraslim)	• Degree of force • Amount of cavitation • Degree of contact
Shape	Shape of the active area in cross section (circular or rectangular)	
Geometry	Number of planes crossed by the shank (one or two)	• Access to treatment site • Degree of contact
Profile	Number of bends in active area (single, double, triple)	

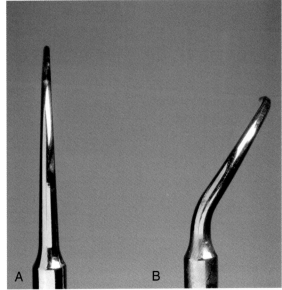

Fig. 29.18 The geometry of an ultrasonic tip may be (A) straight or (B) curved. (Reprinted from George MD, Botbyl D, Donley TD, Preshaw PM. *Ultrasonic Periodontal Debridement: Theory and Technique,* 2nd Edition. Wiley; 2023. Reproduced with permission of John Wiley & Sons, Inc.)

TABLE 29.8 Left and Right Curved Tip Use Guide

Arch	Surface	SEXTANT		
		Right	Anterior	Left
Maxillary	Buccal/facial	LEFT Curved	RIGHT Curved	RIGHT Curved
	Palatal	RIGHT Curved	LEFT Curved	LEFT Curved
Mandibular	Lingual	LEFT Curved	RIGHT Curved	RIGHT Curved
	Buccal/facial	RIGHT Curved	LEFT Curved	LEFT Curved

*using traditional operator positions

direct contact with the splayed roots. The unique ability of the point of curved tips to avoid contact with cementum and dentin prevents damage of the root surface and discomfort of the patient.

The profile of the tip relates only to straight tips and indicates the number of bends placed in the shank to facilitate adaptation of the active area to the tooth surface. While a single-bend design is most conventional, double- or triple-bend tips are also available to facilitate adaptation around line angles and into interproximal spaces (Fig. 29.20).

Given that the primary mechanism of ultrasonic debridement is mechanical, the clinician must consider, in addition to the influence of tip design on the force produced, how the design of the tip impacts access to the treatment site and the degree of contact made with the treatment surface.

The degree of contact required will vary as the disruption of calculus and biofilm require different levels of contact to engage the deposit. A greater degree of contact (key for accessing biofilm) is achieved when the design of the tip *conforms* to the contours of the treatment site. Therefore tip selection is made according to (1) the type of deposit to be removed (stage of debridement) and

(2) the anatomy of the treatment site (Table 29.9).[7] After reviewing the criteria for tip selection, consider the critical thinking situation provided in Box 29.4 and the key concept regarding universal tip designs in Box 29.5.

Monitoring Tip Wear

With use, the ultrasonic tip will wear, becoming reduced in length. As this reduction in length occurs in the active area, a reduction in the displacement amplitude results and decreases clinical performance of the tip. Therefore tip wear should be monitored at regular intervals, using wear guides specific to the brand of tip. Manufacturers suggest replacement when 50% (2 mm) of the original tip length is lost as this loss of 50% in active tip yields a 50% reduction in tip performance. One millimeter of tip length loss equates to a 25% reduction in active tip and performance, making replacement after 1 mm of length loss reasonable for slim-diameter tips.

Specialty Tips

A few tips with unique features have been developed for specific applications. Carbon fiber or plastic tips are safe for use on the smooth titanium portion of implants and therefore can also be used safely around restoration margins. Plastic ultrasonic tips are not recommended for use on implant threads (nonsmooth or coated titanium). Tips coated

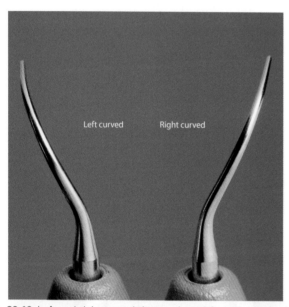

Fig. 29.19 Left and right curved tips as viewed from the back of the tips, with the points of the tips directed away. (Reprinted from George MD, Botbyl D, Donley TD, Preshaw PM. *Ultrasonic Periodontal Debridement: Theory and Technique,* 2nd Edition. Wiley; 2023. Reproduced with permission of John Wiley & Sons, Inc.)

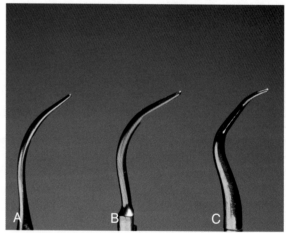

Fig. 29.20 Comparison of the various bends placed in the shank of a straight ultrasonic tip. (A) Single bend; (B) double bend; (C) triple bend. (Reprinted from George MD, Botbyl D, Donley TD, Preshaw PM. *Ultrasonic Periodontal Debridement: Theory and Technique,* 2nd Edition. Wiley; 2023. Reproduced with permission of John Wiley & Sons, Inc.)

			TIP FEATURE			
Stage of Debridement	**Type of Deposit**	**Contour of Tooth Surface**	**Diameter**	**Shape**	**Geometry**	**Profile**
Scaling	Moderate-heavy calculus	Flat or curvaceous All coronal surfaces All root surfaces	Standard	Circular or rectangular	Straight	1–3 bends
Debridement	Biofilm/light calculus	Flat or minimally curvaceous All coronal surfaces Anterior root surfaces	Slim or ultraslim	Circular Rectangular (coronal surfaces only)	Straight or curved	1 or 2 bends Triple bend (on coronal surfaces only)
		Highly curvaceous posterior root surfaces	Slim	Circular	Curved	Not applicable to curved tips

TABLE 29.9   Tip Selection Guide

with fine or medium grit diamonds are indicated for use only during open flap (surgical) debridement to enhance calculus removal; their use during nonsurgical debridement is contraindicated because of the significant risk of root surface removal by the diamond coating.

ULTRASONIC INSTRUMENTATION TECHNIQUE PRINCIPLES

Implementation of ultrasonic instrumentation follows technique principles that differ considerably from manual scaling and more closely resemble exploring and probing techniques (Table 29.10). It is important to note that these principles apply regardless of the design of the tip.

Grasp

As during exploring, digital activation and a light pen grasp is used to control the tip. Correct placement of the grasp is determined by first balancing the handpiece between the thumb and forefinger; once

---

BOX 29.4 Critical Thinking Scenario B

A relatively new tip is designed to be slim in diameter, rectangular in shape, and with a triple-bend profile. Based on what you have learned about the influence of each of these design features—diameter, shape, and profile—on acoustic power, discuss during which stage and on what surfaces use of this tip is indicated.

BOX 29.5 "Universal" Tip Designs

It has been a common practice for certain ultrasonic tips to be labeled as "universal," implying that the tip can be used anywhere in the dentition, and for either scaling or debridement. Universal tips are geometrically straight, with one bend (aka #10) but may be cylindrical or rectangular in cross section, and standard or slim in diameter. Given that diameter and shape of the tip significantly influence the level of acoustic power emitted and the degree of contact made, a truly universal tip design cannot and does not exist.

---

balance is established, the thumb, index, and middle fingers are placed into a pen or modified pen grasp (Fig. 29.21).

Finger Rest

When using ultrasonic instruments, finger rests are needed for stabilization, not leverage. An ideal finger rest for any given treatment area will enable the clinician to maintain the appropriate tip adaptation as the active tip is advanced across all surfaces of the treatment site. A variety of finger rests can be used but in general, a finger rest that is more distant rather than closer to the treatment site works best. Split and cross-arch fulcrums, opposite-arch, and extraoral fulcrums are also very useful (Fig. 29.22). Of note, a balanced ultrasonic grasp should first be established, with that grasp leading to a finger rest position. The finger rest position should not be chosen before grasp is determined.

Adaptation

The oscillation pattern of the active tip ranges from near-linear to elliptical depending on tip design. Slimmer tips typically oscillate in a broader (elliptical) manner, whereas wider and rectangular-shaped tips

---

TABLE 29.10 Ultrasonic Periodontal Debridement Technique Principles

Principle	Description
Grasp	Balanced pen or modified pen
Finger rest	Established at a distance from treatment site for stabilization
Adaptation	Adapt appropriate surface of the active tip • Vertical orientation • Horizontal orientation
Angulation	0° to 15° to tooth surface
Lateral pressure	Light pressure applied to maintain contact with tooth
Insertion	At gingival margin (or outer edge of deposit if supragingival)
Stroke	Constant and varied in direction; implement channeling

---

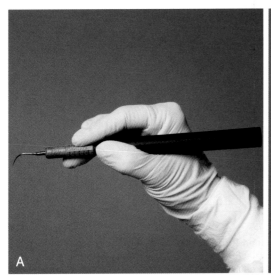
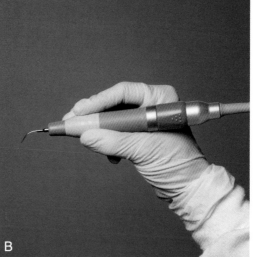

Fig. 29.21 At the point of balance, the thumb, index, and middle fingers form a standard pen grasp of (A) magnetostrictive or (B) piezoelectric handpiece. (Reprinted from George MD, Botbyl D, Donley TD, Preshaw PM. *Ultrasonic Periodontal Debridement: Theory and Technique,* 2nd Edition. Wiley; 2023. Reproduced with permission of John Wiley & Sons, Inc.)

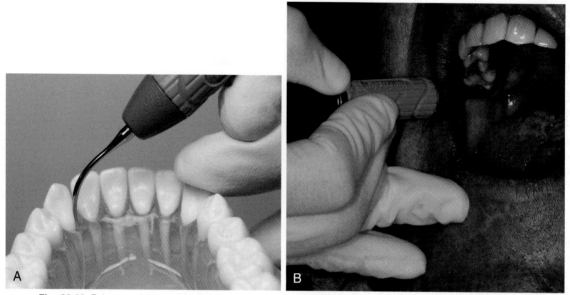

Fig. 29.22 Fulcrums that provide stabilization at a distance from the treatment site include (A) the cross-arch fulcrum and (B) the extraoral fulcrum. (Reprinted from George MD, Botbyl D, Donley TD, Preshaw PM. *Ultrasonic Periodontal Debridement: Theory and Technique,* 2nd Edition. Wiley; 2023. Reproduced with permission of John Wiley & Sons, Inc.)

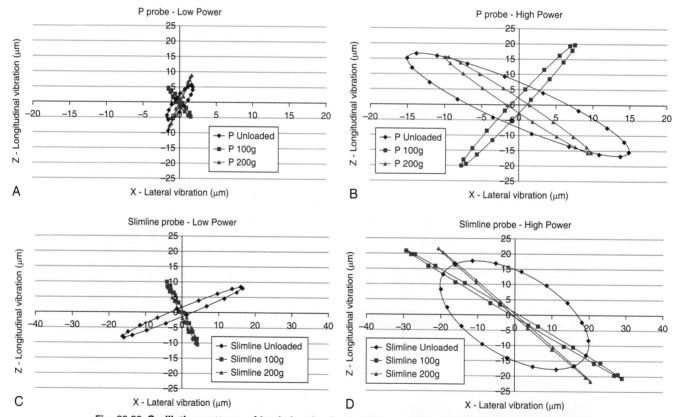

Fig. 29.23 Oscillation patterns of loaded and unloaded P (broad/flat) and Slimline (slim/cylindrical) tips at high and low generator powers. Note the variation in the transverse movement of the elliptical pattern, from near-linear to broad. (Lea et al., 2009a. Reproduced with permission of John Wiley & Sons, Inc.)

move in a narrower (near-linear) pattern (Fig. 29.23).[6,8] When the tip is stroking in an elliptical pattern, any surface of the tip (back, face, or lateral surfaces) can be adapted to the tooth surface. This is significant; it gives the clinician the ability to adapt the surface which best conforms to the anatomy of the treatment site, achieving a greater degree of contact and increasing the efficiency and thoroughness of the debridement procedure (Fig. 29.24).

At some treatment sites, it will not be possible to adapt the surface that best conforms to the anatomy. In this situation, the tip surface most readily available to the treatment surface is used (Fig. 29.25). The point of the tip should only be used against heavy supragingival deposits, as explained in Box 29.6.

Several orientations are used during ultrasonic instrumentation to adapt the tip to the surface.

Vertical Adaptation

The primary adaptation technique used during ultrasonic debridement positions the active tip in vertical orientation. As with periodontal

> ### BOX 29.6 Safety Issue Related to the Point of the Tip
>
> Because of its reduced surface area, the point of the tip exerts a concentrated output of force. It can be used to break heavy or tenacious calculus deposits from coronal surfaces, but the point should never be directed toward the root surface, as significant root surface damage can occur.

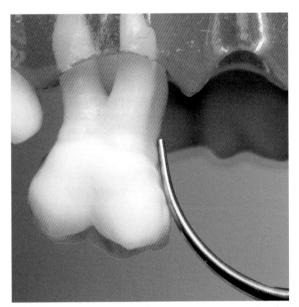

Fig. 29.24 The degree of conformity to the mesial concavity of a maxillary molar achieved by adapting the back of a curved tip. (Reprinted from George MD, Botbyl D, Donley TD, Preshaw PM. *Ultrasonic Periodontal Debridement: Theory and Technique,* 2nd Edition. Wiley; 2023. Reproduced with permission of John Wiley & Sons, Inc.)

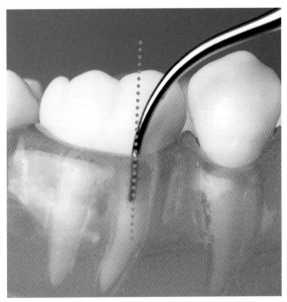

Fig. 29.26 Vertical adaptation. (Reprinted from George MD, Botbyl D, Donley TD, Preshaw PM. *Ultrasonic Periodontal Debridement: Theory and Technique,* 2nd Edition. Wiley; 2023. Reproduced with permission of John Wiley & Sons, Inc.)

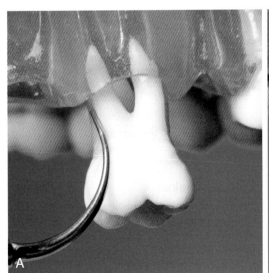
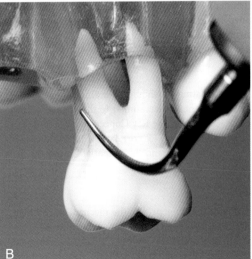

Fig. 29.25 In a distal concavity, (A) adaptation of the convex back of the tip is ideal but impossible to achieve; as an alternative, (B) the lateral surface of the tip is adapted. (Reprinted from George MD, Botbyl D, Donley TD, Preshaw PM. *Ultrasonic Periodontal Debridement: Theory and Technique,* 2nd Edition. Wiley; 2023. Reproduced with permission of John Wiley & Sons, Inc.)

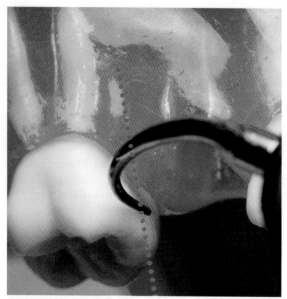

Fig. 29.27 Horizontal adaptation. (Reprinted from George MD, Botbyl D, Donley TD, Preshaw PM. *Ultrasonic Periodontal Debridement: Theory and Technique,* 2nd Edition. Wiley; 2023. Reproduced with permission of John Wiley & Sons, Inc.)

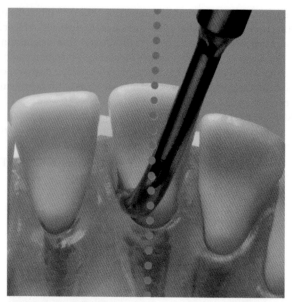

Fig. 29.28 Oblique adaptation. (Reprinted from George MD, Botbyl D, Donley TD, Preshaw PM. *Ultrasonic Periodontal Debridement: Theory and Technique,* 2nd Edition. Wiley; 2023. Reproduced with permission of John Wiley & Sons, Inc.)

probing, the point of the ultrasonic instrument is directed toward the base of the pocket (Fig. 29.26). Vertical orientation is indicated for the instrumentation of all subgingival and supragingival surfaces (excluding interproximal spaces), using any surface of the tip.

Vertical adaptation promotes the active tip reaching the full depth of the treatment site and allows the clinician to readily advance the tip throughout the treatment area with minimal repositioning.

Horizontal Adaptation

Horizontal adaptation is used to adapt the back and the face of the active tip area to surfaces within the interproximal space (Fig. 29.27).

Oblique Adaptation

Oblique adaptation is the orientation required to remove deposits with a bladed instrument. Although the lateral surface of the active tip can be positioned in this manner, doing so hinders rather than optimizes the instrumentation process and therefore is not recommended (Fig. 29.28).

Angulation

The active area of the oscillating tip should be maintained at a 0° to 15° angulation to the treatment surface, similar to the angulation of a periodontal probe (Fig. 29.29). Per the Key Concept presented in Box 29.7, opening this angulation beyond 15° correlates with an increase in undesirable root surface alterations and the potential for patient discomfort and sensitivity.

Lateral Pressure

As adequate oscillation of the tip generates the mechanisms of ultrasonic debridement, the degree of lateral pressure applied to the ultrasonic tip is significantly less than that applied to a bladed instrument. The degree of lateral force that optimizes efficient deposit removal while minimizing root surface alterations will vary between 0.5 and 2 N depending on the type of deposit engaged (Table 29.11). Because it is not possible for clinicians to measure the amount of force being applied to the tip, the minimal degree of force (0.5 N) is similar to if

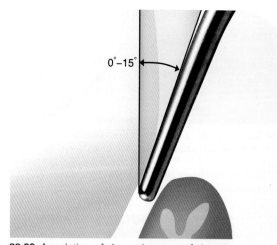

Fig. 29.29 Angulation of the active area of the ultrasonic tip to the tooth surface is 0° to 15°. (Reprinted from George MD, Botbyl D, Donley TD, Preshaw PM. *Ultrasonic Periodontal Debridement: Theory and Technique,* 2nd Edition. Wiley; 2023. Reproduced with permission of John Wiley & Sons, Inc.)

not slightly less than the force applied with an exploratory stroke, with the maximum degree of force (1 to 2 N) being slightly greater than that used with an exploratory stroke.

Working Stroke

Once the adaptation/orientation position of the tip is established, the clinician proceeds with deliberate and methodical working strokes intended to contact as much of the involved tooth/root surface as possible. The working stroke used during ultrasonic instrumentation is comparable to an erasing motion, with the strokes generated being bidirectional, equally distributed, short, overlapping, and constant (Box 29.7).

The direction of the working strokes will vary according to tooth surface and orientation of the active tip (Table 29.12).

TABLE 29.11 **Lateral Pressure Guide**

Stage of Debridement	Type of Deposit	Lateral Pressure	Explanation
Scaling	Moderate calculus	Exploratory (0.5 N)	To keep root surface alterations to a minimum while using a standard-diameter tip at higher power setting
Debridement	Minimal calculus, plaque biofilm	Slightly greater than exploratory (1–2 N)	To optimize the occurrence of cavitation at the active area of a slim-diameter tip

BOX 29.7 **Key Concept: Characteristics of the Ultrasonic Working Stroke**

Bidirectional: Oscillation of the tip disrupts/removes deposit regardless of stroke direction. Accordingly, ultrasonic working strokes are bidirectional, such as forward and backward or upward and downward.

Equally distributed: The distance the tip moves in each direction of the bidirectional stroke should be equal; the forward (or upward) motion should not be longer than the backward (or downward) motion.

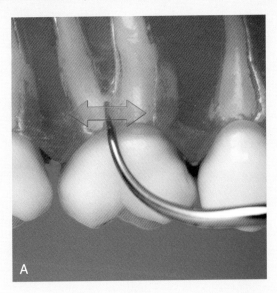

Short: To facilitate thorough debridement of as much surface area as possible, the bidirectional working stroke should not exceed 2 to 3 mm in total length (0.5 to 1.5 mm in each direction), with even shorter strokes necessary in narrow areas or pockets.

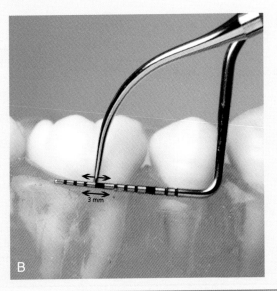

Overlapping: Also, to facilitate thoroughness, the working strokes must overlap as the tip is navigated, both in and out of the pocket and across the surface being treated.

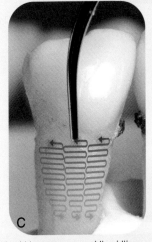

Constant: Stroking should be constant, avoiding idling on any one spot to prevent frictional heating that may be uncomfortable for the patient and damaging to the tooth. A controlled stroke implemented at a slower speed is preferred to faster strokes that are more difficult to control.

All images in this box reprinted from George MD, Botbyl D, Donley TD, Preshaw PM. *Ultrasonic Periodontal Debridement: Theory and Technique*, 2nd Edition. Wiley; 2023. Reproduced with permission of John Wiley & sons, Inc.

TABLE 29.12   **Ultrasonic Working Strokes Guide**

	Tooth Surface	Adaptation Method	Stroke Direction
A	Buccal/facial and lingual/palatal crown and root surfaces	Vertical	Horizontal
B	Interproximal root surface	Vertical	Oblique
C	Interproximal surfaces of crown	Horizontal	Vertical
D	Tenacious or heavy supragingival calculus	Point	Tapping

All images in this table reprinted from George MD, Botbyl D, Donley TD, Preshaw PM. *Ultrasonic Periodontal Debridement: Theory and Technique*, 2nd Edition. Wiley; 2023. Reproduced with permission of John Wiley & Sons, Inc.

Insertion and Advancement

Because the oscillating tip disrupts the deposit as it is engaged, stroking begins at the gingival margin and continues as the tip is advanced subgingivally, while a technique described as **channeling** is implemented (Fig. 29.30). Channeling refers to the methodical movement of the ultrasonic tip within a defined space or "channel;" the depth of the channel is the base of the pocket and the width of the channel should not exceed 2 to 3 mm. The tip is advanced to the base of the pocket using the stroke pattern indicated (see Table 29.12); upon reaching the base of the pocket, the tip is retreated back toward the gingival margin by stroking along the same path taken

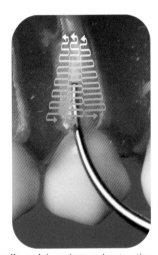

Fig. 29.30 Channeling. Advancing and retracting the tip across the treatment surface by way of channels promotes contact of the active area of the tip with all segments of the involved surface. (Reprinted from George MD, Botbyl D, Donley TD, Preshaw PM. *Ultrasonic Periodontal Debridement: Theory and Technique,* 2nd Edition. Wiley; 2023. Reproduced with permission of John Wiley & Sons, Inc.)

for advancement. As the tip returns to the gingival margin, it is then advanced proximally to begin debridement of the next channel. This approach provides a methodical means for the active area of the tip to engage with as much tooth surface as possible, promoting thorough debridement of the involved site.

ULTRASONIC INSTRUMENTATION IMPLEMENTATION

By implementing the following three strategies, instrumentation can be completed in the most thorough and efficient manner.

Work by Sextant

Although treatment is often planned by quadrant, executing instrumentation by sextant is more efficient as it reduces the frequency of changing tips per stage (scaling/debridement) and per location (anterior/posterior) and requires fewer changes in operator position.

Advance Toward Operator

Instrumentation should begin on the tooth in the treatment area most distant from the operator and advance toward the operator. In posterior sextants, then, instrumentation begins on the most posterior tooth; in anterior sextants, it begins with the tooth farthest from the operator, which will differ for left- and right-handed clinicians (Fig. 29.31).

Advance by Transitioning

Instead of readapting the ultrasonic tip to specific points of adaptation on each tooth (distal line angle of posterior tooth/midline of anterior tooth), as is done with a bladed instrument, the ultrasonic tip is advanced through the treatment area in an efficient sequence using appropriate surfaces of the active tip. The instrumentation sequence is initiated at the distal line angle of a posterior tooth or the midline of an anterior tooth (Fig. 29.32).

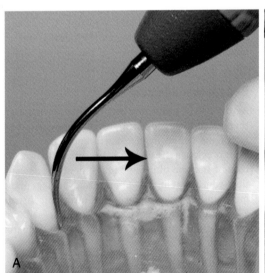
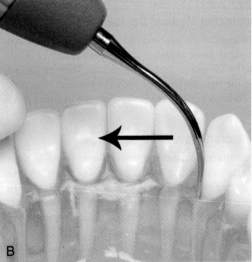

Fig. 29.31 Instrumentation advances toward the operator in anterior sextants from the tooth farthest from the operator, which will differ for (A) right-handed versus (B) left-handed operators. (Reprinted from George MD, Botbyl D, Donley TD, Preshaw PM. *Ultrasonic Periodontal Debridement: Theory and Technique,* 2nd Edition. Wiley; 2023. Reproduced with permission of John Wiley & Sons, Inc.)

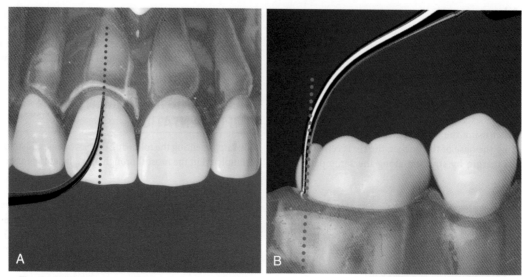

Fig. 29.32 To initiate a sequence of instrumentation, the tip is adapted at (A) the midline of an anterior tooth and (B) the distal line angle of a posterior tooth. (Reprinted from George MD, Botbyl D, Donley TD, Preshaw PM. *Ultrasonic Periodontal Debridement: Theory and Technique,* 2nd Edition. Wiley; 2023. Reproduced with permission of John Wiley & Sons, Inc.)

From these initial points of adaptation, five fundamental transitions in adaptation are made to move the tip from one tooth surface to the next: transition to proximal root surface; transition to interproximal surface; transition to buccal/lingual surface; transition to next tooth; and transition from interproximal surface (Table 29.13).

Using these transitions in a logical sequence optimizes the debridement procedure by ensuring that all surfaces are engaged and with a tip surface that maximizes contact, facilitating predictable and efficient removal of deposits.

PATIENT ASSESSMENT AND MANAGEMENT

Presence of Implanted Medical Devices

Modern implanted medical devices, including pacemakers, implanted defibrillators, and vagus nerve stimulators, have been tested for functional interference by ultrasonic dental instruments. There is general agreement among the manufacturers of such devices that ultrasonic instruments pose no known risk to the proper function of any of these implanted devices.[7]

Presence of Restorations at Diseased Sites

All periodontal instruments have the capacity to modify the surfaces of restorative materials, depending on the hardness of the restorative material and the degree of force exerted during instrumentation. In addition to avoiding direct application of the oscillating tip to a restoration, proper application of ultrasonic instrumentation as presented in this chapter, including use of appropriate power level, lateral pressure,

and technique, minimizes alteration of both tooth/root surfaces and restoration surfaces.

Aerosol Management

Preprocedural rinses, personal protective equipment, and high-volume evacuation (HVE) contribute to minimizing cross contamination by the splatter, droplets, and aerosol generated during ultrasonic instrumentation. Ultimately the goal of HVE is to collect aerosols at the source before they enter the ambient air (the space outside the oral cavity) and reach the clinician. The degree of aerosol reduction is dependent on the HVE device, the positioning of the HVE device, and the main vacuum unit and system's ability to pull large volumes of air. In 2021, Agostini-Walesch et al. reported a 99% reduction in particles using an HVE device with a single large-bore opening, with the placement of the opening very close to the ultrasonic tip (Fig. 29.33).[9]

Patient Management

As the use of ultrasonic instrumentation increases in periodontal therapy and expands into preventive procedures (routine prophylaxis), the dental hygienist will encounter patients who have not been previously treated with an ultrasonic instrument or who may request that the ultrasonic instrument not be used. In either situation, educating the patient on the advantages of ultrasonic debridement, and/or what to expect with ultrasonic instrumentation can go a long way in curbing any anxiety or unease the patient may have. Information to include in the dialog with the patient is provided in Box 29.8.

TABLE 29.13 Transitions Guide*

Step	Transition	Figure	Description
1	TO proximal root surface	A	From the point of initiation (distal line angle), the lateral surface of the tip is advanced to the distal root surface; an oblique stroke pattern and channeling technique is used to debride the distal root surface.
2	TO interproximal surface	B	As the most posterior tooth does not contact another tooth at the distal aspect, the distal interproximal surface is next debrided, maintaining vertical adaptation of the tip and horizontal or oblique strokes.
3	TO buccal/lingual surface	C	From the distal surface, the lateral surface of the tip is advanced across the distal line angle and buccal surface using a horizontal stroke pattern and channeling technique.
4	TO proximal root surface	D	As the mesial line angle is crossed, the back of the tip adapts to the mesial root surface; an oblique stroke pattern and channeling technique are used to debride the mesial root surface.

Continued

TABLE 29.13   **Transitions Guide–cont'd**

Step	Transition	Figure	Description
5	TO interproximal surface		Once subgingival debridement is completed, the back of the tip maintains contact with the mesial surface as the tip is transitioned from vertical to horizontal adaptation; vertical strokes are used to debride the mesial surface of the crown.
6	TO next tooth		Instrumentation then advances to the next tooth by horizontal adaptation of the face of the tip to the distal surface of the crown; vertical strokes are used to debride the distal surface of the crown.
7	FROM interproximal surface		Maintaining contact with the distal surface, the tip is transitioned to vertical adaptation of the lateral surface to begin debridement of the distal root surface using oblique strokes and channeling technique. From this step, instrumentation continues, following steps 1–7, until the designated treatment area is completed.

*Exemplifying instrumentation sequence in the maxillary right posterior sextant.

All images in this table reprinted from George MD, Botbyl D, Donley TD, Preshaw PM. *Ultrasonic Periodontal Debridement: Theory and Technique*, 2nd Edition. Wiley; 2023. Reproduced with permission of John Wiley & Sons, Inc.

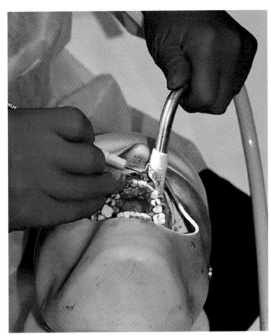

Fig 29.33 Using HVE on a dental simulation unit demonstrated a 99% reduction in particles. Note the size of the HVE opening and the close proximity of the opening and the ultrasonic tip. (Agostini-Walesch, 2022. Reproduced with permission from the American Dental Hygienists Association.)

BOX 29.8   Client or Patient Education Tips

From a patient's perspective, ultrasonic instrumentation may be accepted as a logical technologic advancement from a manual to an automated therapeutic approach or, for a patient who is already wary of dental treatment, disdained as potentially painful because of the automation and noise. In either case, an explanation of how the instrument works and what the patient may experience will favor patient acceptance of the therapy.

"The tip of this instrument vibrates to break up the plaque, much like the power toothbrush that you use but at a higher frequency. The tip also produces a spray of water to flush out the pocket, so I will be using the suction as I work. Because the high-frequency vibration of the tip is doing all of the work, I do not need to apply any pressure to your teeth. Although it will be slightly noisy, you should not feel any discomfort."

KEY CONCEPTS

- Ultrasonic debridement is accomplished by both mechanical and biophysical disruption of the plaque biofilm.
- Operating variables, including power level, tip design, and lateral pressure, should be modified according to the stage of debridement (scaling of calculus or root surface debridement) to optimize deposit removal and minimize alteration to the root surface.
- The instrumentation technique used with an ultrasonic instrument significantly differs from that used with manual instruments.
- A variety of tip designs is necessary to properly implement ultrasonic debridement therapy.

REFERENCES

1. Johnston W, Paterson M, Piela K, et al. The systemic inflammatory response following hand instrumentation versus ultrasonic instrumentation—a randomized controlled trial. *J Clin Periodontol*. 2020;47(9):1087–1097.
2. Suvan J, Leira Y, Moreno Sancho FM, Graziani F, Derks J, Tomasi C. Subgingival instrumentation for treatment of periodontitis. A systematic review. *J Clin Periodontol*. 2020;47:155–175.
3. Vyas N, Wang QX, Manmi KA, Sammon RL, Kuehne SA, Walmsley AD. How does ultrasonic cavitation remove dental bacterial biofilm? *Ultrason Sonochem*. 2020;67:105–112.
4. Vyas N, Dehghani H, Sammons RL, et al. Imaging and analysis of individual cavitation microbubbles around dental ultrasonic scalers. *Ultrasonics*. 2017;81:66–72.
5. Lea SC, Felver B, Landini G. Three-dimensional analyses of ultrasonic scaler oscillations. *J Clin Periodontol*. 2009;36(1):44–50.
6. Lea SC, Felver B, Landini G. Ultrasonic scaler oscillations and tooth-surface defects. *J Dent Res*. 2009;88(3):229–234.
7. George MD, Botbyl D, Donley TG, Preshaw PM. *Ultrasonic Periodontal Debridement: Theory and Technique*. 2nd ed. John Wiley & Sons, Inc; 2023.
8. Pecheva E, Sammon RL, Walmsley AD. The performance characteristics of a piezoelectric ultrasonic dental scaler. *Med Eng Phys*. 2016;38(2):100–203.
9. Agostini-Walesch GM, Pierre-Bez AC, Marcelli-Munk G, et al. Aerosols in ultrasonic instrumentation: comparison of particle spread utilizing saliva ejectors versus high-volume evacuation. *J Dent Hyg*. 2021;95(3):18–24.

30

Root Morphology and Instrumentation Implications

Rachelle Williams

PROFESSIONAL OPPORTUNITIES

A dental hygienist's comprehension of root morphology is essential for the treatment and maintenance of periodontitis and acquired abnormalities/conditions. According to the National Health and Nutrition Examination Survey, an estimated 48% of adults aged 30 years and older have periodontitis, which increases to 65% in older adults aged 65 and older.[1] The high prevalence of periodontitis translates to a high percentage of exposed root surfaces. The application of instrumentation related to exposed root surfaces is essential to successful outcomes of nonsurgical periodontal therapy and periodontal maintenance treatments.

COMPETENCIES

1. Discuss general morphologic characteristics.
2. Consider the significance of cementoenamel junction location in periodontal assessment.
3. Discuss root surface texture, root shapes, and teeth with one, two, or three roots.
4. Associate furcation size and location with successful periodontitis treatment outcomes.
5. Describe root concavities and tooth alignment and how both relate to accessing root surfaces.
6. Consider and document variations in root form during periodontal assessment procedures and integrate into individualized patient treatment planning.

INTRODUCTION

Various assessment instruments (e.g., the periodontal probe, Nabers probe, dental explorer) are used for assessing root surface characteristics. Ultrasonic inserts and hand-activated instruments designed to reach anatomic root structures (e.g., precision thin and microprecision thin inserts; curved slimline inserts: extended-shank and mini- or microbladed area-specific curettes) allow for proper adaption during instrumentation (see Chapters 28 and 29). Current periapical and vertical bitewing radiographs provide information on the number of roots, shape, and variation; furcation location; bone height and contour; calculus, caries, and defective restorations; and other contributing factors that may influence root instrumentation (see Chapter 20). An anatomically correct model of the dentition with transparent gingiva is helpful for visualizing anatomy of individual roots and positioning within the alveolar processes.

ROOT TERMINOLOGY

The **anatomic root** of a tooth is the part of the dentin covered by cementum and embedded in the alveolar bone; it begins at the cementoenamel junction. The end of the root is called the **root apex**, and the area surrounding the apex is the **periapex**. At the apex is an opening, the **periapical foramen**, where the blood vessels and nerves enter the **pulp (root) canal**.[2]

Teeth have one, two, or three roots. Teeth with two or three roots have an unbranched portion called the **root trunk**. The area where the root trunk branches into two roots is the **furcation** or **furca**. The opening into the furcation is the **furcation entrance** (Fig. 30.1).

The most coronal portion of the furcation is the **furcation roof**, which is often more coronal than the furcation entrance. The area between the roots of a two- or three-rooted tooth is the **interfurcal** or **interradicular area**.

When the junctional epithelium has migrated apically and there is clinical attachment loss, portions of the anatomic root are included in the definition of a **clinical crown**, the unattached portion of a tooth. The concept of cervical, middle, and apical thirds is used when discussing root anatomy (Fig. 30.2).

CEMENTOENAMEL JUNCTION

The **cementoenamel junction** (CEJ) or cervical line is a structure that the dental hygienist must be able to identify subgingivally with an instrument. In a healthy mouth, the CEJ is located within 1 mm of the free gingival margin and is covered slightly by free gingiva. The CEJ is the fixed landmark in the identification of the amount of attached gingiva. Subgingival identification of the CEJ is a competency that requires knowledge of root anatomy, development of tactile skill, and experience. Tactile, nonvisual indicators of the CEJ may include the following:

- Rougher root texture, because cementum is not as smooth as enamel.
- Location between the convex cervical third of a crown and the flatter root surface.
- Facial and lingual contours of the CEJ on anterior and premolar teeth are convex; on molars, the CEJ is less convex.
- An apical dip of the CEJ, called the cervical enamel projection (CEP), may be present toward the furcation on molars.
- Proximal curvature of the CEJ is more pronounced on both maxillary and mandibular anterior teeth compared to posterior teeth (Table 30.1).
- Proximal curvature of the CEJ is more pronounced on the maxillary posterior teeth compared to mandibular posterior teeth (Table 30.1).
- The CEJs on anterior teeth have a curvature which is V-shaped toward the incisal surface and more prominent on the mesial surface of incisors, especially the maxillary central incisor. These areas are particularly difficult to instrument because of limited proximal access, which may contribute to incomplete deposit removal. Deposit removal at the curvature of the CEJ on the proximal surface of anterior teeth can be achieved by turning the toe end of a curette, or ultrasonic insert

TABLE 30.1	Cementoenamel Junction
Anterior proximal curvature of the CEJ is more pronounced on both maxillary and mandibular anterior teeth compared to posterior teeth. Posterior proximal curvature of the CEJ is more pronounced on the maxillary teeth compared to mandibular teeth.	Maxillary Teeth Cementoenamel junctions (CEJs; maxillary). (Courtesy of the Department of Dental Hygiene, Idaho State University.) Mandibular Teeth Cementoenamel junction (mandibular). (Courtesy of the Department of Dental Hygiene, Idaho State University.)

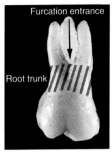

Fig. 30.1 Root terminology: root trunk entrance. (Courtesy of former Department of Dental Hygiene, Marquette University.)

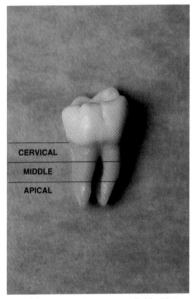

Fig. 30.2 Portions of the anatomic root are divided into cervical, middle, and apical thirds. (Courtesy of the Department of Dental Hygiene, Idaho State University.)

into the most incisal portion, which may be very narrow. The end of a scaler may be needed to access this area. See Box 30.1 for a Critical Thinking Activity regarding clinical assessment of the CEJ.

ROOT SURFACE TEXTURE

Surface textures of crowns and roots differ, owing to different degrees of enamel and cementum mineralization and how they are altered by oral biofilm. Enamel (anatomic crown) is comparable to glazed pottery: smooth, hard, and glassy when unaltered. Cementum (anatomic root), in contrast to enamel, has a moderately hard pourous texture. Cementum can be altered by loss of periodontal attachment, biofilm by products, and unintentional injury by patient or clinician through:
- Use of ultrasonic instruments and curettes during debridement
- Use of scaling instruments with pointed tips on root surfaces (pointed tips should *not* be used on root surfaces)
- Removal of varying amounts of cementum and exposure of dentin during root planing, resulting in dentinal hypersensitivity (see Chapter 42).

ROOT SHAPES

Roots of permanent teeth vary from one individual to another. For instrument placement on root surfaces, the following are considered:
- Individual root morphology
- Position of the teeth in the alveolar bone
- Interference from crown contours
- Patient's periodontal status
- Instrument design

BOX 30.1 Critical Thinking Scenario A

Materials: Anatomically correct typodont with clear gingiva; 11/12 explorer (explorer of choice); see Table 30.1 and its figures for reference.
1. Implement correct exploration techniques to locate the interproximal CEJ on one maxillary incisor, premolar, and molar. Use tactile sensitivity and Table 30.1 maxillary teeth figure for guidance.
2. Implement correct exploration techniques to locate the interproximal CEJ on one mandibular incisor, premolar, and molar. Use tactile sensitivity and Table 30.1 mandibular teeth figure for guidance.

Critical thinking: What differences did you discover in the location of CEJs on the anterior teeth versus the posterior teeth? What challenges did you experience when attempting to locate the CEJ? What modifications will you make to locate the CEJ on the teeth of a patient?

Limited knowledge of root morphology can result in detrimental effects on the periodontium. See Box 30.2 for an overview of ethical and safety issues.

TEETH WITH ONE ROOT

All anterior teeth, maxillary second premolars, and mandibular first and second premolars have one root. Comprehension of the

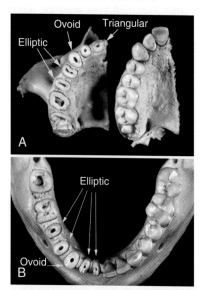

Fig. 30.3 Root shapes in cervical cross-section. (A) Maxillary teeth: triangular, elliptic, and ovoid. (B) Mandibular teeth: elliptic and ovoid. (Courtesy of former Department of Dental Hygiene, Marquette University.)

characteristics associated with one-rooted teeth provides clinicians with the knowledge necessary for instrumentation adaption.

Characteristics of teeth with one root include the following:

a. Cone shape, with facial, lingual, and proximal surfaces converging (tapering) apically, with different degrees of convergence widest in the cervical third and tapering to a small apex.[3]
   - Distal inclination from a facial (lingual) view
b. Cervical cross-sections (i.e., crown cut off the root horizontally at CEJ) are triangular, ovoid, or elliptic (Fig. 30.3).[3]
   - **Triangular:** Appears to be three-sided with broad (equal) facial, mesial, and distal surfaces and a narrow lingual surface. Proximal surfaces converge markedly to the lingual surface (e.g., maxillary central incisors). Proximal surfaces of roots that are narrower on the lingual than the facial surface (both triangular and ovoid root shapes in cervical section) are instrumented more readily from the lingual surface because of greater access.
   - **Ovoid:** Oval, egg-shaped, with facial surface broader than lingual surface; proximal surfaces are equal and broader than either facial or lingual surface (e.g., canines).
   - **Elliptic:** Proximal surfaces are relatively equal; facial and lingual surfaces are approximately the same size but smaller than the proximal surfaces. Root dimensions are broad from the facial and lingual view and narrower from the mesial and distal view. Roots of mandibular incisors and maxillary premolars are elliptic in cervical cross-section.
c. In midroot sections, root shapes are generally the same as in cervical sections, although smaller.

Roots that are triangular or ovoid in cross-section have smaller lingual than facial surfaces because of proximal surface convergence (taper) toward the lingual surface. Cervical cross-section shapes may be altered by the presence of root concavities. The cervical half of a conical root has more than 50% of the root surface area because of the convergence of surfaces apically.[3] See Box 30.3.

TEETH WITH TWO OR THREE ROOTS

For periodontal assessment and instrumentation, each root of a multi-rooted tooth is treated individually—that is, a two-rooted tooth is like having two single-rooted teeth. Therefore, exploration and instrumentation of each root will require mesial and distal adaption. Extended shank or minicurettes are ideal for instrumentation into the limited spaces between root branches (the first two figures in Table 30.2).

In addition, the complexity of unbranched root trunks and furcations must be considered. Posterior teeth are more difficult to reach, and the clinician's competence influences the therapeutic outcome. Characteristics of the teeth with more than one root are given as follows.

a. Maxillary first premolars:
   - Generally have two roots (facial and lingual)
   - Furcations on the mesial and distal sides (see the third and fourth figures in Table 30.2)
b. Maxillary molars:
   - Have three roots—mesiobuccal, distobuccal, and palatal (lingual)
   - Furcations on the buccal side between the mesiobuccal and distobuccal roots, on the mesial side between the mesiobuccal and palatal roots, and on the distal side between the distobuccal and palatal roots (see the fifth through seventh figures in Table 30.2)
   - Radiographic assessment of the roots can be compromised owing to the complex root anatomy of the mesiobuccal, distobuccal, and palatal roots (radiographs show the image only from a facial or lingual view)
c. Mandibular molars:
   - Have two roots—mesial and distal
   - Furcations on the buccal and lingual surfaces between the mesial and distal roots (see the eighth and ninth figures in Table 30.2)
   - Roots on second molars are more likely to have longer root trunks, be closer together, and have more distal orientation
d. Maxillary and mandibular molar roots in cervical cross-section are larger and have more variation in appearance (Fig. 30.3).
   - Both may show slight depressions where furcations or proximal root concavities begin.

TABLE 30.2   Multirooted Anatomy and Instrumentation

Multirooted Instrumentation

Each root of a multirooted tooth is instrumented individually: each root has a mesial and distal surface, and therefore instrumentation on each root is mesial adaption and distal adaption.

Tooth No. 3 ML

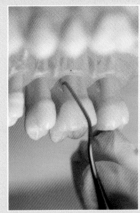

Multirooted instrumentation (maxillary first molar) (Courtesy of the Department of Dental Hygiene, Idaho State University.)

Tooth No. 30 L

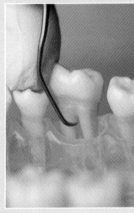

Multirooted instrumentation (mandibular first molar) (Courtesy of the Department of Dental Hygiene, Idaho State University.)

Maxillary Premolar Root and Furcation Anatomy

Maxillary premolars have two roots with mesial and distal furcations.

Tooth No. 5 M

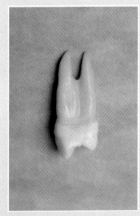

Root and furcation anatomy (maxillary first premolar mesial surface) (Courtesy of the Department of Dental Hygiene, Idaho State University.)

Tooth No. 5 D

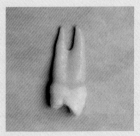

Root and furcation anatomy (maxillary first premolar distal surface) (Courtesy of the Department of Dental Hygiene, Idaho State University.)

TABLE 30.2   Multirooted Anatomy and Instrumentation—cont'd

Maxillary Molar Root and Furcation Anatomy

Maxillary molars have three roots: mesiobuccal, distobuccal, and palatal (lingual). Furcations are located on the buccal, mesial, and distal root surfaces.

Tooth No. 3 B

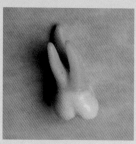

Root and furcation anatomy (maxillary first molar buccal surface) (Courtesy of the Department of Dental Hygiene, Idaho State University.)

Tooth No. 3 M

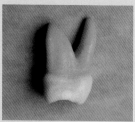

Root and furcation anatomy (maxillary first molar mesial surface) (Courtesy of the Department of Dental Hygiene, Idaho State University.)

Tooth No. 3 D

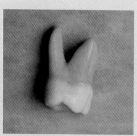

Root and furcation anatomy (maxillary first molar distal surface) (Courtesy of the Department of Dental Hygiene, Idaho State University.)

Mandibular Molar Root and Furcation Anatomy

Mandibular molars have two roots with buccal and lingual furcations.

Tooth No. 30 B

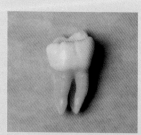

Root and furcation anatomy (mandibular first molar buccal surface) (Courtesy of the Department of Dental Hygiene, Idaho State University.)

Tooth No. 30 L

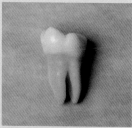

Root and furcation anatomy (mandibular first molar lingual surface) (Courtesy of the Department of Dental Hygiene, Idaho State University.)

B, Buccal; *D,* distal; *L,* lingual; *M,* mesial.

- The root trunk of a maxillary molar has more equal sides and appears somewhat rhomboidal in shape, with the more prominent "corner" being the mesiobuccal.
- The root trunk of a mandibular molar is more rectangular in shape, with the mesial distal width being greater than the facial lingual width.
- Generally, roots are elliptic when a cervical cross-section is shown after the furcation.[3]

See Box 30.4.

FURCATIONS

Furcations generally begin as a shallow depression on the root trunk that gradually opens into a space between the roots; this opening may be too narrow for instruments. Initially, changes in root trunk anatomy or beginning furcations can be felt by the working end of a dental explorer and then, as the periodontal status changes and as the space widens, furcations are readily appreciated by a Nabers probe. Furcations are difficult to access with traditional scaling and root planing instruments because their working ends are too large. Rather, precision thin and furcation inserts for ultrasonic instruments, microbladed and minibladed curettes with smaller and narrower working ends, curettes with extended shanks, and furcation curettes are used to debride furcation areas (Table 30.3; see Chapters 28, 29, and 33).[4] Instrumentation techniques for class II, III, and IV furcation involvements include instrumenting the furcation area as if there were two or three distinct roots. For limited access, use furcation or ultrasonic instruments. A very narrow furcation entrance can be enlarged surgically with burs by a periodontist.

Furcation characteristics are as follows:
- The more cervical the furcation, the more stable the tooth because of root divergence (separation).
- Furcations are generally more cervical on first molars; first molar root trunks are shorter than second or third molar root trunks.
- Furcations close to the CEJ are more likely to become involved with periodontal disease, although access for instrumentation is easier (shallower) and therefore such disease has a more favorable posttherapy prognosis.
- Furcations close to the apex are less likely to result in furcation involvement; however, instrument access is more difficult (deeper) and posttherapy prognosis is less favorable.
- Furcation involvement occurs when there is a loss of attachment apical to the furcation and is classified according to extent (see Chapter 20 for classification of furcations).

It is important to know the expected furcation location in horizontal and vertical directions. Horizontally, most furcations are located midway on the root trunk. The mesial furcation of a maxillary first molar generally is located more toward the lingual surface in a horizontal direction and, therefore instrumentation of the mesial furcation of this tooth is easier from the lingual approach (see the first figure in Table 30.3). Vertically, furcations on a maxillary premolar are in the apical third to half (see the third and fourth figures in Table 30.2). Furcations on a maxillary molar are near the junction of the cervical and middle thirds of the root (see the fifth through seventh figures in Table 30.2). Furcations on the mandibular second and third molars are slightly more apical than on the first molars (Table 30.4).

ROOT CONCAVITIES

Root concavities are shallow vertical depressions on root surfaces. They protect the tooth from forces that could rotate it in its alveolus and provide more root surface area and direction for periodontal fiber attachment. Root concavities complicate root instrumentation access and make it more difficult to place the cutting edge of the instrument on the root surface. Root concavities most frequently occur on proximal root surfaces (proximal root concavities) (Table 30.5).[2]

Maxillary first premolars have a mesial concavity extending from the CEJ to the furcation. The pronounced mesial concavity is often missed by clinicians during instrumentation and requires adaption of a periodontal instrument (Table 30.6, first figure). Maxillary first molars have a concavity on the lingual surface of the palatal root (lingual concavity) (see Table 30.6, second figure). Molars may have root concavities on the surface of their root toward the furcation (furcal concavities).[2] If there are (anatomic) concavities cervical to or with class I furcation involvement, scale the area with very small strokes and turn the toe into the concave area that marks the initial stages of division. Horizontal strokes may also be implemented (best access is from the lingual concavities).

Horizontal instrumentation adapts to the lingual maxillary concavity and mandibular buccal/lingual concavities for thorough deposit removal (see Table 30.6, second and third figures). Adaption of periodontal instruments into concavities is essential for thorough calculus and biofilm removal.[2]

See Box 30.5.

TOOTH ALIGNMENT

Assessment of the alignment of the teeth within an arch is essential to adapting instruments subgingivally. Tooth size, prominence of its crown, contact areas, and the convergence of root surfaces determine the amount of space and interproximal bone. In a healthy mouth, the mandibular anterior teeth have the narrowest amount of space and bone. In a diseased mouth, if loss of bone is accompanied by gingival recession, there is more access for instrumentation. When teeth have

TABLE 30.3 Furcation Instrumentation

Extended shank and minibladed Gracey curettes adapting into furcations

Tooth No. 3 ML

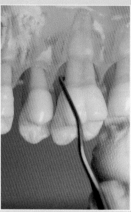

Furcation instrumentation (maxillary first molar mesial furcation) (Courtesy of the Department of Dental Hygiene, Idaho State University.)

Tooth No. 3 DL

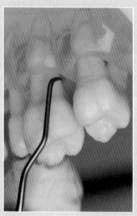

Furcation instrumentation (maxillary first molar distal furcation) (Courtesy of the Department of Dental Hygiene, Idaho State University.)

Tooth No. 30 L

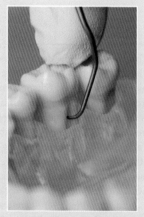

Furcation instrumentation (mandibular first molar lingual furcation) (Courtesy of the Department of Dental Hygiene, Idaho State University.)

D, Distal; L, lingual; M, mesial.

insufficient space, crowding occurs, making instrument positioning difficult. Teeth with close or altered root proximity may have minimal or no proximal space and long proximal root contact, which may significantly influence oral hygiene, periodontal health, and subgingival instrumentation.[4]

The position of teeth within the alveoli is also a factor in root instrumentation. **Axial positioning** is the relationship of an imaginary vertical line representing the long axis of a tooth in relationship to a horizontal plane.[4] The functions of this positioning are to bring the maxillary and mandibular teeth into an interarch relationship that

TABLE 30.4 Permanent Posterior Tooth Furcations

Furcations

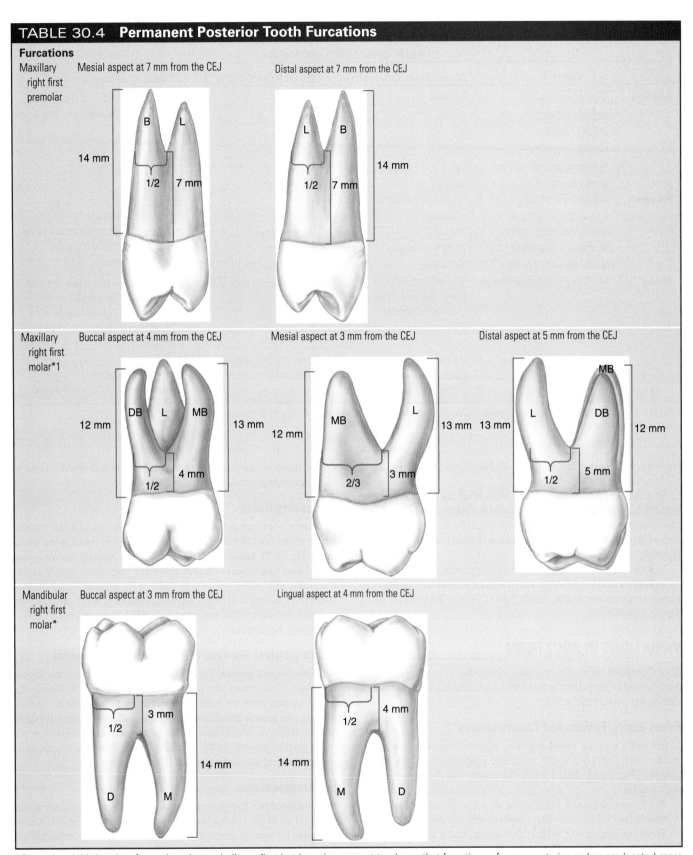

Maxillary right first premolar

Mesial aspect at 7 mm from the CEJ

B L
14 mm
1/2 7 mm

Distal aspect at 7 mm from the CEJ

L B
14 mm
1/2 7 mm

Maxillary right first molar*1

Buccal aspect at 4 mm from the CEJ

DB L MB
12 mm 13 mm
4 mm
1/2

Mesial aspect at 3 mm from the CEJ

MB L
12 mm 13 mm
3 mm
2/3

Distal aspect at 5 mm from the CEJ

MB
L DB
13 mm 13 mm 12 mm
1/2 5 mm

Mandibular right first molar*

Buccal aspect at 3 mm from the CEJ

3 mm
1/2
14 mm
D M

Lingual aspect at 4 mm from the CEJ

4 mm
1/2
14 mm
M D

*Second and third molars for each arch are similar to first but have longer root trunks so that furcations of more posterior molars are located more apically and with roots closer together, creating tighter furcation entrances.
CEJ, Cementoenamel junction; *D*, distal; *DB*, distobuccal; *L*, lingual; *M*, mesial; *MB*, mesiobuccal.
Adapted from Nelson S. *Wheeler's Dental Anatomy, Physiology, and Occlusion.* 10th ed. Philadelphia: Elsevier; 2015.

TABLE 30.5   Root Concavities

		ROOT CONCAVITY LOCATIONS		
	Tooth	**Mesial Root Concavity**	**Distal Root Concavity**	**Clinical Application**
Anteriors	Maxillary centrals	Not likely	No	Maxillary anteriors have greater lingual access for instrumentation
	Maxillary incisors	Variable	Variable	
	Maxillary canine	Yes	Yes (deeper)	
	Mandibular centrals	Yes	Yes (deeper)	
	Mandibular incisors	Yes	Yes (deeper)	
	Mandibular canine	Yes	Yes (deeper)	
Premolars	Maxillary first premolar	Yes (deeper, extends from crown to furcation)	Yes	Mesial of maxillary first premolar—common area for burnished calculus
	Maxillary second premolar	Yes	Yes (deeper)	Important to adapt the toe of the cutting edge into the concavity to avoid burnishing calculus
	Mandibular first premolar	Yes 50% of the time	Yes (deeper)	
	Mandibular second premolar	No (unlikely)	Yes (deeper)	
Molars	Maxillary first and second molars	Mesiobuccal root—yes Buccal root trunk—concavity leading to furcation Lingual root—lingual concavity	Distobuccal root—variable	Distal of maxillary first molar—common area for burnished calculus Instrumentation—greater access of proximal surfaces from the lingual surfaces
	Mandibular first and second molars	Mesial root—yes (slight) Buccal and lingual root trunk—concavity leading to furcation	Distal root—variable	Crowns of all mandibular posterior teeth are inclined lingually and make instrument placement more difficult

Adapted from Scheid RG, Weiss, G. *Woelfel's Dental Anatomy*. 9th ed. Lippincott Williams & Wilkins; 2016.

facilitates incision and mastication and distributes forces throughout the bones of the skull.

In a faciolingual dimension, the roots of all the teeth except the mandibular posteriors have a more lingual inclination than the crowns. Mandibular posterior crowns are more lingually inclined than roots that are more facial in orientation, making biofilm removal in this area especially difficult for patients.

In a mesiodistal dimension, the roots of the canines, premolars, and molars have a distal inclination, which is more pronounced posteriorly. Incisor roots do not incline distally.[4] See Client or Patient Education Tips in Box 30.6.

VARIATIONS IN ROOT FORM

Root alterations, anomalies, or abnormalities should be recognized and documented in the patient record for instrumentation adaptations and subsequent patient education.

Fused Roots, Fusion, and Concrescence

Molar roots may be **fused** together, especially second and third molar roots, and are a result of limited space during tooth development (Fig. 30.4). Fused roots frequently can be observed on radiographs.[2]

- Teeth may be joined together in an anomaly called fusion, in which two tooth buds fuse together during development and form one large tooth with a large crown and a single root that has two pulp canals. This fusion must be confirmed by radiographs.
- Concrescence occurs when two adjacent teeth become joined by cementum after they have been formed.

- For fused or concrescence roots, use the toe end of the curette to instrument the area of junction of the roots.

Accessory Roots

Accessory roots are extra roots. Sometimes the mandibular permanent canines are bifurcated into facial and lingual roots in the apical third (Fig. 30.5). Maxillary first premolars can have three roots—two buccal and one lingual. Buccal roots are very thin, which makes treatment difficult if periodontal disease is present. Third molars sometimes have extra roots. Accessory roots may be assessed via radiographs and are instrumented only if the attachment level is apical to their occurrence.[2]

Palatogingival Grooves (Palatoradicular Grooves)

A **palatogingival groove** (Fig. 30.6) extends apically from the lingual concavity of the crown of a permanent maxillary incisor, usually the lateral incisor, onto the root, often resulting in an isolated, narrow pocket. This groove provides challenges in instrumentation, is highly biofilm retentive, and is susceptible to periodontal disease. For the palatogingival groove, use the toe end of a micro-, mini-, or extended-shank curette to access the groove.[5]

Hypercementosis

Hypercementosis, the excessive formation of cementum in the apical third to half of the tooth after the tooth has erupted (Fig. 30.7), may be caused by trauma, chronic inflammation of the pulp, or metabolic disturbances. It is assessed radiographically. If areas of hypercementosis are exposed with apical migration of the junctional epithelium, decisions about the extent of root instrumentation will be more difficult.[4]

TABLE 30.6 Concavity Instrumentation

Tooth No. 5 ML: An extended shank curette with a miniblade was adapted using a vertical stroke to the mesial concavity of the maxillary first premolar. A horizontal stroke in this area would also be effective.

Tooth No. 3 L and Tooth No. 30 L: An extended shank curette with a miniblade was adapted using a horizontal stroke on the lingual surface concavities of the maxillary and mandibular first molars. Vertical strokes in these areas would also be effective.

Tooth No. 5 ML

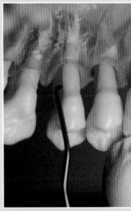

Concavity instrumentation (maxillary first premolar mesial concavity) (Courtesy of the Department of Dental Hygiene, Idaho State University.)

Tooth No. 3 L

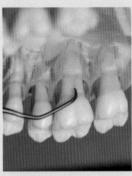

Concavity instrumentation (maxillary first molar lingual concavity) (Courtesy of the Department of Dental Hygiene, Idaho State University.)

Tooth No. 30 L

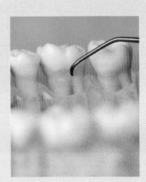

Concavity instrumentation (mandibular first molar lingual concavity) (Courtesy of the Department of Dental Hygiene, Idaho State University.)

L, Lingual; *M*, mesial.

Cervical Enamel Projections

Cervical enamel projections (CEPs) are apical extensions of the CEJ toward the furcation of a molar (Fig. 30.8).[2]

CEPs are classified by degree of extension, as follows:

- Grade I CEPs extend slightly toward the furcation and occur frequently.
- Grade II CEPs approach the area of root separation.
- Grade III CEPs extend into the furcation.
- Grade IV CEPs are the same as grade III CEPs, plus the furcation is visible because of recession.

Periodontal attachment loss is more likely in CEP areas because periodontal fibers do not form the same type of attachments to enamel as to cementum. Most isolated furcation involvements in otherwise healthy dentitions are found to be related to CEPs. A CEP can be removed surgically to expose dentin and facilitate reattachment of periodontal fibers.

Enamel Pearls

Enamel pearls, most frequently seen on maxillary molars, are droplets of enamel in the furcation area (Fig. 30.9). They are thought to be due to a genetic error in the developing root sheath as it reaches the

BOX 30.5 Root Anatomy Exercise

Materials: Two plastic typodont maxillary and mandibular molars or two autoclaved extracted permanent maxillary and mandibular first molars; flat black hobby paint, nail polish, or liquid calculus; glitter or fine sand; black crayon; posterior area-specific curettes; tray cover; gauze square.

Preparation: For each molar, apply flat black hobby paint, nail polish, or liquid calculus to the root cervical third of the distal half of the tooth; while it is wet, sprinkle glitter or fine sand on the painted area (simulates deposit, altered cementum); color the mesial half of the root with crayon (simulates subgingival biofilm/slime layer).

Classroom Setting:
1. Identify natural or plastic first molar and hold it in the correct orientation (may also reinsert the plastic molars into the typodont).
2. Select the appropriate curette for the area and remove deposit from root trunk and roots of the molars.
3. Observe how each root is approached as if it were a single tooth and how each of the surfaces must be approached.
4. Count number of strokes needed to remove the deposit.

Clinical Setting:
1. Complete the classroom setting steps using maxillary and mandibular right first molars for ultrasonic instrumentation and maxillary and mandibular left first molars for hand instrumentation with posterior area-specific curette.
2. Reflect on the challenges of root morphology adaption with the ultrasonic tip compared to the curette.

BOX 30.6 Client or Patient Education Tips

- Root morphology variations must be discussed with the patient.
- Educate patients about root morphology and related periodontal structures as a rationale for recommended self-care behaviors, products, and devices.
- Individualize oral self-care methods and appropriate adjunctive aids to patient's anatomy.

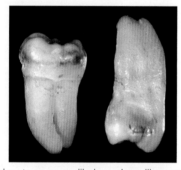

Fig. 30.4 Fused roots on a mandibular and maxillary molar. (Courtesy of former Department of Dental Hygiene, Marquette University.)

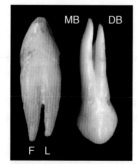

Fig. 30.5 Accessory roots on a mandibular canine and maxillary first premolar. *DB,* Distobuccal; *F,* facial; *L,* lingual; *MB,* mesiobuccal. (Courtesy of former Department of Dental Hygiene, Marquette University.)

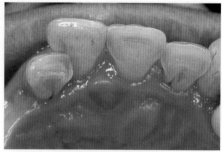

Fig. 30.6 Palatogingival groove on a maxillary lateral incisor. (Courtesy of Gay Derderian, BA, DDS, MSD, Marquette University School of Dentistry.)

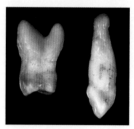

Fig. 30.7 Hypercementosis. (Courtesy of former Department of Dental Hygiene, Marquette University.)

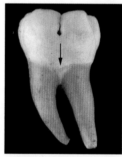

Fig. 30.8 Cervical enamel projection on a mandibular first molar. (Courtesy of former Department of Dental Hygiene, Marquette University.)

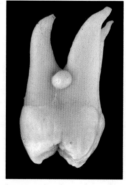

Fig. 30.9 Enamel pearls near the furcation of a maxillary molar. (Courtesy of former Department of Dental Hygiene, Marquette University.)

furcation area. Because periodontal fibers will not attach to enamel, enamel pearls may encourage periodontal disease. Exploration of an enamel pearl sometimes can be puzzling if it is not visible on radiographs because it may feel like subgingival calculus.

Dilaceration

Dilaceration is a sharp bend in the root surface caused by the displacement of the root during tooth development (Fig. 30.10).

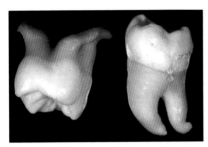

Fig. 30.10 Dilaceration. (Courtesy of former Department of Dental Hygiene, Marquette University.)

BOX 30.7   Charting Examples

- *Charting Example 1:* No. 30 facial, Class II furcation with 6-mm pocket depth present; used slim ultrasonic insert and 11–14 Gracey curette for full furcation instrumentation; spoke with patient at length regarding homecare requirements, prognosis, and need for follow up treatment; no anesthesia; patient tolerated well; reinforced OHI; referred to dentist of record.
- *Charting Example 2:* No. 3, Class II furcation with 6-mm pocket depth present, used ultrasonic instrumentation and curettes for full furcation instrumentation; access easiest from lingual aspect; reinforced OHI; advised of need for periodontal referral/evaluation; referred to dentist of record.

BOX 30.8   Critical Thinking Scenario B

Apply knowledge of root anatomy and instrumentation to answer the following questions (see Tables 30.1 through 30.6):
1. The patient exhibits generalized light subgingival deposits as you are exploring the maxillary premolars with an explorer.
   a. Where would a concavity be on the root surface?
   b. What if these teeth were the mandibular premolars instead?
2. During the assessment of the maxillary first and second molars, you have identified 5-mm interproximal pockets and a 2-mm recession.
   a. Are you likely to encounter furcation involvement? Discuss your response.
   b. If so, what would you use to detect a furcation, explore the furcation, and instrument (root plane and debride) within the furcation?
   c. Where would a concavity be on the root surface? Are there instrumentation modifications or techniques to assist in reaching the concavities?
3. While you are completing an oral assessment, you identify 4-mm CAL buccal and lingual on the mandibular molars.
   a. Are you likely to encounter furcation involvement?
   b. How does the axial positioning of the mandibular molars affect instrumentation of the lingual surfaces?

Documentation of Variations in Root Form

Root variations must be recorded in the patient's chart, discussed with the patient, and accounted for in the plan of care as they influence treatment, referral, and self-care recommendations. Dental hygienists document oral healthcare to minimize the risk of malpractice claims and provide a means of communication between providers. Documentation is considered a legal record of treatment and includes all aspects of care provided. Box 30.7 provides examples of clinical charting notes

---

PROCEDURE 30.1   Root Morphology and Implications for Root Instrumentation

Assumption
The clinician has mastered instrumentation procedures from Chapter 20, Periodontal Assessment and Charting; Chapter 28, Hand-Activated Instrumentation; and Chapter 29, Ultrasonic Instrumentation.

Steps
Select ultrasonic insert and area-specific curettes for use on cementum and root surfaces.
1. Make a mental image of the unseen portion of the tooth to be instrumented and the width and height of the adjacent alveolar bone.
2. Review periodontal parameters recorded on the periodontal assessment form.
3. Observe clinical and radiographic alignment of the tooth and adjacent teeth.
   General Characteristics of Roots and Their Implications for Instrumentation
1. Adapt instrument so that it follows the long axis of the root and the taper or convergence of root surfaces apically. For curettes, use the terminal shank of the instrument as a guide to maintain parallelism. For periodontal probe and universal ultrasonic inserts, use working end to maintain parallelism.
2. Adapt instrument to the taper or convergence of the proximal surfaces toward the lingual surface. If the convergence of the proximal surfaces is pronounced, as in maxillary anterior teeth and maxillary molars, approach more of the proximal surfaces from the lingual surface.
3. Adapt instrument so that it also accounts for the position of the tooth in the alveolar bone and the patient's position in the chair.
4. Use multidirectional strokes, alternating horizontal, vertical, and oblique stroke directions.
5. Adapt instrument to the lingual inclination of mandibular posterior teeth by slightly angling instrument shank toward the lingual surface.
6. Use alternative instrument placement or an alternative instrument for very narrow spaces (e.g., posterior curette on an anterior tooth or, rarely, a scaler).

Root Morphology Instrumentation
See Tables 30.4 and 30.5 for location of furcations and concavities requiring instrument adaption.

Specific Characteristics of Roots and Their Implications for Instrumentation
See Tables 30.1 through 30.6.
   Adapt toe end of instrument's cutting edge to proximal root concavities with small overlapping strokes that are channeled gradually into the concave area from facial and lingual approaches. If tooth has more than one root, adapt instrument similarly to the slight concave area approaching the furcation.
   Adapt instrument into furcations.
   Refer to the dentist of record when Class II or higher furcation involvement is found.

Variations
Use the toe end of the curette to instrument palatogingival grooves and junction of concrescence roots.

KEY CONCEPTS

- Root assessment, instrumentation, and management require thorough knowledge of root morphology.
- Periodontal assessment includes the identification of root anatomy and root surface characteristics before the development of the plan for care.
- Incisors, canines, and all of the premolars except the maxillary first premolars have one root.
- Approximately 60% of maxillary first premolars have two roots (one facial and one lingual), with furcations on the mesial and distal surfaces.
- Mandibular molars have two roots, one mesial and one distal, with furcations on the facial and lingual surfaces.
- Maxillary molars have three roots (mesiobuccal, distobuccal, and lingual), with mesial, facial, and distal furcations.
- Teeth with more than one root have a root trunk before root division.
- The division area is called the *furca;* a furcation entrance may be very narrow.
- The cementoenamel junction on posterior teeth has much less pronounced curvatures on all surfaces.
- Cementum is not as hard as enamel; only instruments with a rounded toe should be used on it.
- The number and shape of the roots determine the selection and adaptation of assessment, scaling, and root planing instruments.
- Root surfaces converge (taper) apically; there is more root surface area in the cervical third than in the apical or middle thirds.
- More of the proximal surface of a single-rooted tooth with broader facial than lingual surfaces can be reached from the lingual approach because of the proximal convergence toward the lingual side.
- The horizontal and vertical location of the furcation determines selection and placement of instruments.
- Root surfaces may have shallow, longitudinal vertical depressions (concavities), which add curvature and dimension to instrumentation.
- Axial positioning of each individual tooth in its alveolus is considered when instruments are adapted on root surface.

that should be included in addition to all other required charting entries (e.g., date, medical and dental history updates, vital signs). See Box 30.8. See Procedure 30.1 to apply your knowledge of root morphology and instrumentation.

ACKNOWLEDGMENT

The author acknowledges Lynn Bergstrom Bryan, Merry Greig, and Marilyn Beck for their previous contributions to this chapter; the Department of Dental Hygiene at Idaho State University for technical assistance in the preparation of the photographs; Eric Gordon, previously at Idaho State University, for the professional photography; and the Department of Dental Informatics at the Marquette University School of Dentistry for technical assistance in the preparation of the photographs from past editions used for this edition.

REFERENCES

1. Eke P, Thornton-Evans G, Wei L, Borgnakke W, Dye B, Genco R. Periodontitis in US adults: National Health and Nutrition Examination Survey 2009–2014. *J Am Dent Assoc.* 2018;149(7):576–586.
2. Scheid RG, Weiss G. *Woelfel's Dental Anatomy.* 9th ed. Lippincott Williams & Wilkins; 2016.
3. Nelson SJ. *Wheeler's Dental Anatomy, Physiology and Occlusion.* 10th ed. Saunders/Elsevier; 2015.
4. Blue CM. *Darby's Comprehensive Review of Dental Hygiene.* 9th ed. Elsevier; 2020.
5. Nield-Gehrig JS. *Fundamentals of Periodontal Instrumentation and Advanced Root Instrumentation.* 9th ed. Lippincott Williams & Wilkins; 2000.

31

Dental Implants and Peri-implant Care

Diane M. Daubert and Russell I. Johnson

PROFESSIONAL DEVELOPMENT OPPORTUNITIES

The number of patients with dental implants has increased dramatically in the past 10 years and will only continue to increase in the future. It is critical for the dental hygienist to have a thorough understanding of biology, planning, assessment, and maintenance procedures for dental implants in order to successfully treat patients.

COMPETENCIES

1. Describe the background of dental implants and discuss the indications, contraindications, and patient selection of dental implants.
2. Explain the basic steps in implant treatment planning, placement, and maintenance.
3. Understand the role of the dental hygienist in relation to implant maintenance.
4. Define peri-implant health, peri-implant mucositis, and peri-implantitis and explain how to make the diagnoses.
5. Detail the need for compliance with proper at-home implant care.
6. Discuss professional maintenance of dental implants.

BACKGROUND

Traditionally, tooth loss had required replacement with either a removable denture or a fixed bridge. This required preparation of adjacent teeth and restoration of teeth that may have not otherwise required restoration. Dental implants have provided an alternative that, many times, may be more conservative to existing tooth structure, decrease the need for endodontic therapy, and provide easier access for hygiene.

The use of dental implants to replace missing teeth has become a mainstay in today's dental practice. Popularized by P. I. Branemark between the 1960s and 1980s for use in completely edentulous patients and then for single tooth replacement, the addition of dental implants to the treatment planning process has provided an alternative to conventional fixed and removable prosthodontics, and implants are now, in many cases, considered the standard of care. The dental implant provides many advantages in the present dental setting, but meticulous understanding of the planning, components, maintenance, and complications is vital to successful long-term outcomes.

Dental implants provide a method for stabilizing a prosthesis to the supporting hard and soft tissue. Despite variations, this stabilization is generally achieved by three main components: the dental implant, abutment, and prosthesis (Fig. 31.1). The dental implant is placed beneath the mucosa, within bone, and relies on a predictable, stable, and long-term connection to this supporting bone. This connection is defined as **osseointegration**, which is the apparent direct attachment or connection of osseous tissue to an implant without intervening fibrous connective tissue. This interface must remain stable with functional loading throughout the life of the implant.

The **abutment** is a supplemental component of a dental implant that is used to support and/or retain a fixed or removable prosthesis. This abutment comes in many shapes and sizes, depending on the type of restoration. With fixed restorations, an abutment may be integrated into the prosthesis as one piece, may be used as an angle-correcting component, or could simulate a tooth preparation to allow cementation of a crown. Removable prostheses often use prefabricated abutments to create a connection between the implant and the prosthesis, such as a Locator abutment. Abutments are also the transmucosal component responsible for the healthy transition and soft tissue interface between the implant platform and the oral environment; thus proper design and maintenance is essential.

The **prosthesis** can be completely supported by the implant, as in the case of a single or multiunit fixed prosthesis. Or, it may be retained by the implant and supported by the soft tissue, as in the case of a removable prosthesis, such as an implant-retained overdenture.

INDICATIONS, CONTRAINDICATIONS, AND PATIENT SELECTION

Regardless of the cause of the tooth loss, the replacement of a tooth with a dental implant can certainly be considered. However, functional or aesthetic concerns should be analyzed critically as opposed to indiscriminate tooth replacement. Thorough treatment planning should be accomplished, starting with an evaluation of the patient's health and medical condition. Medical consults and health should be achieved prior to surgical intervention whenever feasible. Although many relative and absolute contraindications to implant placement have been recommended, lack of high-level evidence exists, and most are instead based on clinical observations and biologic plausibility. Generally accepted contraindications to dental implant placement include psychosis, active periodontal disease, smoking more than 10 cigarettes per day, and uncontrolled systemic disease such as diabetes or rheumatoid arthritis as well as a history of head and neck radiation or use of bisphosphonates.[1] Of course, a well-educated patient who understands and is willing to participate in the treatment and maintenance process must also be taken into consideration.

STAGES OF TREATMENT

For the most successful dental implant outcomes, a restoratively driven interdisciplinary approach to treatment planning is necessary. In general, the treatment team consists of the patient, the surgeon, and the restorative team. The restorative team, which includes the dental hygienist, is responsible not only for the prosthesis fabrication but also for long-term implant maintenance and evaluation. Following proper planning, the treatment sequence can be summarized as follows: (1) the extraction of the tooth and a healing period of 3 to 6 months; (2) the surgical placement of the implant, followed by another healing period of 3 to 6 months; and (3) the restorative process. There may be significant variations to this summary on the basis of such factors as the individual's specific condition, the implant location, the bone quality and quantity, and the practitioner's expertise. After the completion of the implant restorative procedures, it is critical to initiate well-planned dental hygiene and maintenance protocols.

Presurgical Workup

After a thorough evaluation of the patient's overall health, all of the active dental disease should be addressed or treatment planned in an appropriate sequence with the planned dental implants. The presurgical workup usually includes diagnostic study models, radiographic imaging, and a wax-up or virtual modeling of the anticipated tooth position. In addition to bitewing and periapical films, a panoramic radiograph or a cone-beam computed tomography scan is often required for better visualization of the anatomic landmarks and assessment of the available bone for implant placement, especially associated with critical anatomic landmarks (maxillary sinus, nasal cavity, inferior alveolar nerve, mental foramen, mandibular lingual undercut, roots of adjacent teeth, etc.).[2] If the patient is a candidate for orthodontic therapy, this should be discussed and addressed prior to implant placement

given the ability to reposition teeth but the inability to alter an implant position once osseointegrated.[3]

Virtual Treatment Planning

Much of this diagnostic workup and treatment planning can now be done virtually. The objective of this workup is to determine the implant position in relation to the planned prosthesis, the anatomic landmarks, the available bone volume, and the need for any site development prior to implant placement. Three-dimensional or virtual implant treatment planning allows the surgeon to better visualize a patient's bony anatomy in three dimensions for dental implant placement by using cone-beam computed tomography scanning (Fig. 31.2A). Pertinent vital structures, including nerves, sinuses, soft tissue thicknesses, and the available bone volume, can be visualized while virtually placing a dental implant using computer planning software (Fig. 31.2B).

Surgical Procedure

A surgical guide that transfers the planned information should be used during implant surgery to help with precise placement of the implant based on the planned restorative outcome (Fig. 31.3). An incision is made in the gingiva and/or mucosa to provide access to the underlying alveolar bone, and implant sites are prepared using a series of drills that mimic the implant length and width. These site preparations are referred to as the implant osteotomy (Fig. 31.4). The implants are then placed and stabilized within the osteotomy sites at a preplanned location and angulation that is suitable for the final prosthesis. The initial stability, also referred to as insertion torque, of the implant at the time of placement is often used to determine the ability to place a temporary restoration at the time of surgery, the need for complete covering of the implant to allow for healing without exposure of the implant to the oral cavity or even the length of time that is provided for healing. The implant is typically allowed to heal for 3 to 6 months, undergoing the physiologic processes needed for osseointegration with the surrounding bone.

Stage Two Surgery and Mucosal Interface

Traditionally, implants were left buried under the mucosa during the initial healing period of 3 to 6 months. This requires a second surgical procedure to "uncover" the implant and place a transmucosal abutment that allows access through the soft tissue to the implant platform. However, many implants are now placed with a transmucosal abutment, or even a temporary restoration in certain circumstances, at the time of surgery, depending on the need for grafting at the time of placement or adequate initial stability. Wound care and oral hygiene are critical during this healing period. The healing abutment protrudes through the mucosa and allows for the healing and formation of a mucosal

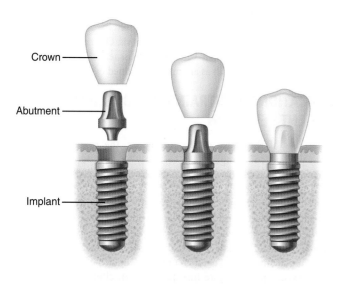

Crown

Abutment

Implant

Fig. 31.1 Components of a dental implant.

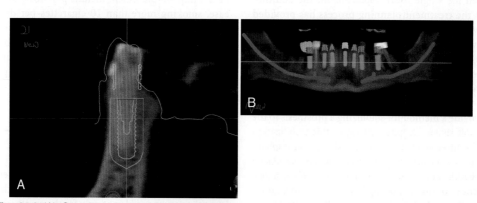

Fig. 31.2 (A) Cone-beam computed tomography for implant planning. (B) Virtual planning for implant placement.

collar around the abutment, which creates access for the connection of prosthetic components to the implant (Fig. 31.5).

Restoration/Prosthesis

Fabrication of a prosthesis is often falsely considered the final step in implant therapy, when maintenance is a key and ongoing factor for implant success and survival. Prosthesis design is, however, a critical step to create both a functional and aesthetic result for the patient while also creating a cleansable and maintainable interface for the patient and maintenance team. Fabrication often requires several appointments to achieve a desirable fit. Design factors of importance besides shade and contour include texture, material, emergence profile, interproximal space, and tissue contact to allow appropriate daily oral biofilm removal. Oral hygiene instruction should be provided before, throughout, and after the prosthetic appliance placement to achieve optimal outcomes. This discussion of maintenance beforehand aids in setting expectations, educates the patient that implants are not problem-free

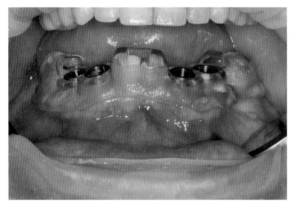

Fig. 31.3 Surgical guide for implant placement.

and will require maintenance, and ensures the patient is a suitable recipient for a dental implant.

MATERIALS AND DESIGN

Understanding implant maintenance requires an understanding of implant as well as prosthetic materials and designs. It is futile to discuss all materials and designs in use today as this is presently an ever-changing area of dentistry. However, key materials and designs are discussed and considered in this chapter.

Dental Implant Materials

Dental implants have traditionally been made of either commercially pure titanium or a titanium alloy of titanium, aluminum, and vanadium. Other alloys, carbons, and ceramic implants have been manufactured and are even available to the dental market today, but they make up a minor share of implants currently in use. Historically, non–root-form implants had been used with limited success (subperiosteal, blade, staple, etc.), but root-form implants have been the standard for implant therapy since the 1980s. The macrogeometry of root-form implants may be parallel walled, tapered, threaded, or smooth surface. The "top" of the implant, referred to as the implant platform, may have either an internal or external connection and may be at the bone level or at the tissue level (Fig. 31.6). "External hex" implants were the standard connection before internal connections became available. Favor has tended toward internal connection implants for several reasons, including decreased incidence of screw loosening and distribution of lateral masticatory forces into the walls of the implant rather than on the narrow abutment screw.

The implant-abutment interface is an area with variation that can mislead a clinician without thorough knowledge of current designs. The implant platform is generally in direct contact with the base of the abutment. Microscopically, even with the most intimate fit, a gap

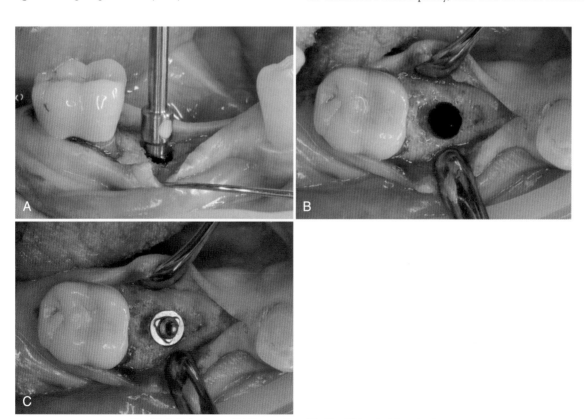

Fig. 31.4 Osteotomy. (A) Preparation, (B) site, (C) implant in osteotomy.

is present. This is referred to as a "microgap," which is large enough to allow for bacterial colonization. It has been shown that the location of this microgap is associated with peri-implant bone loss. When the microgap is moved toward the center of the implant, in the case

of "platform-switching," the bone loss appears to be slightly less. Thus two designs to be aware of are a platform-matched and a platform-switched implant-abutment interface. To the untrained eye, this can appear either that the abutment is the wrong size for the implant or that it may not be completely seated (Fig. 31.7).

Implant Restorative Connections and Materials

The restoration of a single implant is commonplace in dental practices. A single crown may be fabricated for cementation to an abutment, which mimics a tooth preparation or standardized form thereof as previously discussed, or the crown could be fabricated in combination with the abutment, which eliminates the need for cement as the crown would be screwed to the implant. This is termed a "screw-retained crown," as compared to a "cement-retained crown." The benefit of a screw-retained crown is retrievability of the restoration and lack of cement, which in excess, can be a significant risk factor for peri-implant bone loss (Fig. 31.8). A screw-retained crown is not always possible, however, when implant angulation is not ideal. In the case of poor implant angulation, a custom abutment may be fabricated to correct angulation and allow a cement-retained crown to be delivered without a screw access hole. Cement is worth discussion at this point as it has a role in peri-implant disease but can be challenging to distinguish clinically and in radiographs, depending on the type of cement used. Many studies have been published reviewing cement and its use in implant dentistry.[4] Recommendations are often made for a zinc-containing cement (Temp-bond, ZOE, or zinc phosphate) because of its radiopacity, improved visibility on radiographs, dissolution over time, and ease of removal. Many resin cements are in use and some are not visible on radiographs, leading to a need for meticulous attention during cementation and during maintenance visits by the hygienist.

Abutment materials are generally gold-alloy, titanium, or zirconia, a white ceramic material. Titanium will appear slightly less radiopaque than the other two materials. Dark abutment materials (titanium or

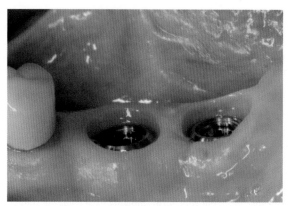

Fig. 31.5 Implant/mucosal interface.

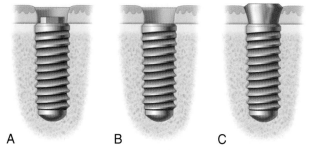

Fig. 31.6 (A) Bone-level external hex connection, (B) internal hex connection, and (C) tissue-level implant.

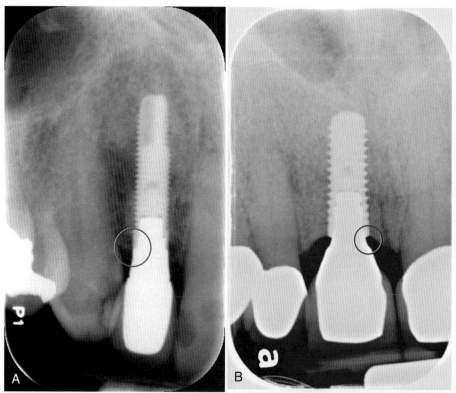

Fig. 31.7 Radiographic appearance of (A) non–platform-switched and (B) platform-switched implants.

alloys) may lead to a dark soft tissue appearance if there is bone loss, recession, or thin tissue overlying the abutment (Fig. 31.9).

Crown materials are similar to those routinely used in traditional tooth-borne crown and bridge restoration.

Edentulous Restoration

Patients with extensive tooth loss or edentulism can experience great improvements in lifestyle with the addition of dental implants. Restoration with implants can typically be broken into a removable tissue-supported prosthesis that is retained by implants (i.e., Locator abutments), a removable implant-supported prosthesis also retained by the implants (i.e., Dolder bar) (Fig. 31.10), or a fixed implant prosthesis that is screwed to the implants and only removed by the dental provider.

Removable prostheses are often fabricated similarly to traditional dentures, using acrylic, polymer, or composite prosthetic materials, with the possible addition of an internal metal framework to decrease

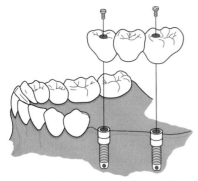

Fig. 31.8 Screw-retained restorations. (From Worthington P, Lang BR, Rubenstein JE. *Osseointegration in Dentistry: An Overview.* Quintessence; 2003.)

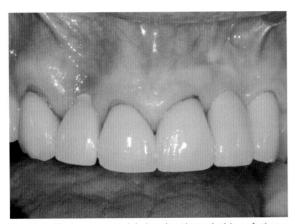

Fig. 31.9 Abutment material showing through thin soft tissue.

the risk of fracture. Fixed prostheses are commonly fabricated with acrylic, metal-ceramic, or zirconia materials.

Removable prostheses are generally acceptable for patients who have increased hygiene demands and need improved access to their implants and soft tissues or who have limited dexterity, so a fixed prosthesis would prove challenging. This would allow removal and ease of access to peri-implant tissues. Removable prostheses may also prove beneficial when additional lip support is needed for aesthetic purposes. The main advantage to a removable prosthesis is the ability to replicate prosthetic hard and soft tissues without concern for a "ridge-lap" or uncleansable prosthesis as the prosthesis can be removed and cleaned at any time. Disadvantages include wear and need for replacement of retentive elements and need for daily removal for tissue health.

Alternatively, design considerations for fixed prostheses in edentulous patients require more attention to hygiene and maintenance as they cannot be removed by a patient. Oftentimes, a full-arch prosthesis is designed with aesthetics as a primary consideration, which may lead to a lack of hygiene space between the soft tissue and the prosthesis. Worse yet, the prosthesis may be designed with a ridge lap that will not allow floss or oral care devices to contact the depth of a concave intaglio (tissue-contacting) surface. Designs should be established to have a convex intaglio surface, access at implant locations for probing and evaluation, and access for hygiene. If a patient is unable to access any area of the prosthesis at a recall examination, oral hygiene instruction and/or modification of the prosthesis by the restorative dentist should be completed.

See Box 31.1 for a Critical Thinking Scenario related to patient selection criteria for dental implants.

IMPLANT MAINTENANCE AND THE ROLE OF THE DENTAL HYGIENIST

Complex dental restoration creates complex maintenance needs. Dental hygienists must be experts at dental implant hygiene maintenance so that they can educate clients throughout and after dental implant therapy. The dental hygienist is a critical member of the implant team from the implant planning phase, when the patient should be informed of risk factors and establish good oral hygiene practices, throughout the surgical and restorative phase, when oral hygiene procedures will change periodically because of healing, and continuing through the maintenance phase of treatment to ensure the best chance of success

---

BOX 31.1   Critical Thinking Scenario A

With colleagues, discuss the characteristics of current edentulous and partially edentulous patients. Which ones would be good candidates for dental implants and why? Which patients are poor candidates and why?

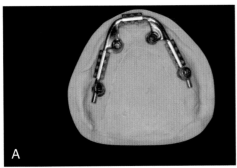
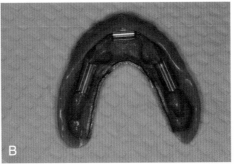

Fig. 31.10 (A) Dolder bar attachment for implant-supported denture. (B) Implant denture.

TABLE 31.1   Dental Hygiene Implant Maintenance Guidelines

Presurgery
1. Risk assessments
   a. Smoking >20 cigarettes/day
   b. HbA1c levels >8%
   c. Current use of IV antiresorptive agents
   d. History of irradiation to the head and neck
   e. Periodontal disease active or poorly controlled
2. Oral hygiene instruction
3. Smoking cessation

Postsurgery
1. Wound care instruction
2. Chlorhexidine rinse as prescribed by surgeon
3. Meticulous oral hygiene in all areas of mouth but avoid area of surgery
4. Use of ultrasoft toothbrush after 1 week in area of surgery
5. No probing until after healing and insertion of prosthesis

Post–Implant Restoration—Healthy Implant
1. Biologic maintenance
   a. Extra- and intraoral exam
   b. Probe implant using gentle force, plaque index, gingival index, bleeding on probing
   c. Radiographs taken post insertion of restoration and annually or as needed
   d. Biofilm and hard deposit removal with implant-appropriate instruments such as glycine powder air-polishing
2. Mechanical maintenance
   a. Detailed examination of implant and prosthesis including removable components
   b. Decision to remove fixed prosthesis is made by restorative dentist based on patient's ability to perform oral hygiene
3. Home care instruction for both fixed and removable restorations
   a. Patient-specific recommendations for oral hygiene aids or topical agents
   b. Removable appliances should be cleaned daily using a commercial denture cleaner

Peri-implantitis Mucositis Treatment (4-mm Probing and Bleeding on Probing)
1. Risk assessment
2. Probe implant using gentle force, plaque index, gingival index, bleeding on probing
3. Consider taking a radiograph if one has not been taken in past year
4. Thorough biofilm removal and oral hygiene instruction
5. Shorten maintenance interval to 3 or 4 months

Peri-implantitis Treatment (5 mm With Bleeding on Probing and ≥2 mm Radiographic Bone Loss)
1. Refer to surgeon for evaluation and possible surgical treatment of peri-implantitis

joint panel from the American College of Prosthodontists, the American Dental Association, the Academy of General Dentistry, and the American Dental Hygienists' Association.[5] These guidelines were established after a review of the literature and assessment of the level of evidence available for clinical recommendations. These guidelines are divided into professional maintenance covering both biologic and mechanical maintenance and at-home maintenance. The guidelines support the hygienist's important role in maintaining dental implants.

IMPLANT ASSESSMENT OVERVIEW

The dental hygienist evaluates, identifies, and documents the following during the maintenance visit, with emphasis on signs and symptoms of oral problems, risk factors, and issues associated with the dental implant:
- Changes in the health history
- Oral mucosa conditions
- Discomfort, pain, or complaints related to the implant
- Color, texture, and overall condition of the mucosal peri-implant tissues, as measured by the following:
  - Attached peri-implant tissue
  - Periodontal probing depths
  - Bleeding on probing
  - Presence of exudate in sulci around abutments
  - Amount of oral biofilm and calculus formation
  - Oral hygiene knowledge and behaviors
  - Mobility and occlusal interference
  - Change in radiographic marginal bone height surrounding the fixture compared to time of restoration insertion
  - Presence of mechanical problems with prosthetic components

Following the assessment of the implant, the dental hygienist will determine if the implant is healthy or whether peri-implant disease is present, which is followed by the dental hygiene treatment plan and designation of the appropriate maintenance interval. Details of each part of the assessment follow.

Peri-implant Tissue Assessment

Assessment of the dental implant and surrounding supporting structure is critical in order to determine the state of health or disease and establish the appropriate dental hygiene treatment plan. This assessment will start with a visual inspection of the soft tissue to look for signs of inflammation. The mucosa around an implant varies distinctly compared to the mucosa/gingiva around natural teeth. Natural teeth have a **biologic width**, a physical attachment that includes epithelial and connective tissue attachment directly to the tooth surface via Sharpey fibers. The supracrestal and periodontal ligament fibers help to create a barrier to resist periodontal breakdown. Implants, however, lack the same attachment and resistance to breakdown, having only circular fibers present, creating a tissue collar. Another significant variation is the decreased blood supply around implants as there is no periodontal ligament or blood supply coming from the periodontal space (Fig. 31.11).

A soft tissue collar that consists of keratinized or nonkeratinized mucosa will surround dental implants. The distinction is important since the color will vary depending on whether this tissue is keratinized, with the nonkeratinized tissue appearing redder, even in a state of health. Fig. 31.12 shows an implant with the appearance of healthy soft tissue that is keratinized and an implant lacking keratinized mucosa, respectively. Signs of inflammation therefore will not be dependent on color alone but also on swelling, contour of the tissue margin, and bleeding on probing.

Probing Implants

The periodontal probe is an important tool in the evaluation of dental implants. It is widely used as a diagnostic tool for assessment of dental

for the dental implant. During each maintenance visit, the hygienist will be called on to perform assessment, education, and biofilm removal procedures. Just like teeth, implants can develop problems in the supporting soft tissue or bone that surrounds them and in addition, they may have mechanical problems involving the components of the implant and restoration. An overview of the hygienist's role at each stage during implant treatment is found in Table 31.1.

In order to provide practitioners with a framework for the maintenance of dental implants, a set of clinical practice guidelines for patients with implant-borne dental restorations were developed by a

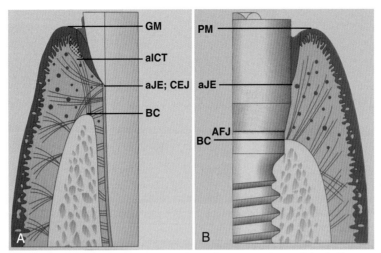

Fig. 31.11 Biology of implants and teeth. (A) The sulcular tissue around a tooth is similar to an implant, and so is the junctional epithelial zone. The connective tissue zone, which attaches to the cementum on a natural tooth, is completely different around the implant. (B) The peri-implant tissues exhibit histologic sulcular and junctional epithelial zones that are similar to those of a natural tooth. The primary difference is the lack of connective tissue attachment and the presence of primarily two fiber groups (rather than the 11 seen with a natural tooth). (From Misch CE. *Dental Implant Prosthetics.* Mosby; 2005.)

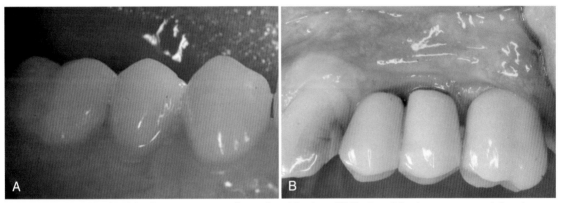

Fig. 31.12 (A) Keratinized mucosa surrounding a dental implant. (B) Nonkeratinized mucosa around dental implants.

implants reported throughout the literature. The American Academy of Periodontology recommends both probing and radiographic assessment in order to diagnose peri-implant disease and states that the initial probing should be done once the final restoration has been placed using a traditional probe with light (25 N) force. Likewise, the 2017 World Workshop on Periodontal Diseases and Conditions consensus group states that probing is essential for diagnosis and that probing using a light force will not damage the peri-implant tissues (Fig. 31.13).[6]

It is essential to have a baseline probing depth because unlike healthy teeth, the implant probing depth may be greater than 3 mm initially due to the depth of implant placement or prosthesis design. In fact, it is not possible to define a range of probing depths compatible with health since peri-implant health can exist around implants with reduced bone support.[6] However, a baseline reading is imperative in order to assess the change. It is clear that an increase in probing depth over time is associated with attachment loss. In addition to assessing changes in probing depth, the periodontal probe is used to assess the presence of bleeding on probing and suppuration. Probing depth, bleeding on probing, and suppuration are important elements in the diagnosis of peri-implant disease.

Historically, there has been some controversy regarding the use of a probe on implants. This stems from the concerns that periodontal

probing can break down the fragile epithelial attachment around the dental implants or scratch the titanium surface. The available research does not suggest any harm to the implant surfaces or to the prognosis of the implant with careful and proper periodontal probing. While the use of a plastic probe has been suggested, there is no evidence that it is necessary. It is imperative, however, that there be consistency in the type of probe and angulation used within the dental office in order to have validity in the interpretation of changes in recorded probing depths. It is also important to have the radiographs available when probing, as implant diameter is variable and the size of the prosthesis does not indicate the width of the implant (Fig. 31.14).

Radiographic Assessment of Implants

Periodic radiographs are necessary for the assessment of dental implant bone levels. It has been recommended that radiographs be taken at the time of the implant fixture placement, at the time of the prerestorative check, after the final prosthesis is inserted, annually for the first several years, and periodically after that time. It is important to note that some initial bone remodeling will occur in the first year, and it is considered within normal limits to see remodeling of up to 1 mm (Fig. 31.15). In addition, the limitations of conventional radiographs must be considered as radiographs have limited use in assessing changes on the buccal

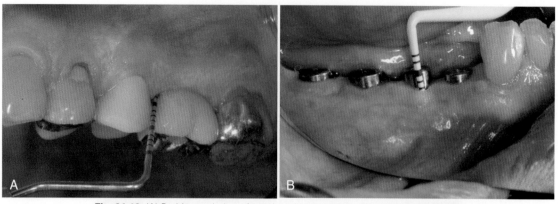

Fig. 31.13 (A) Probing technique for a dental implant and (B) use of plastic probe.

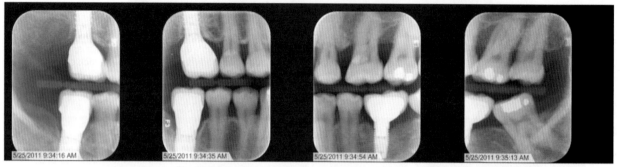

Fig. 31.14 Importance of radiographs for probing implants.

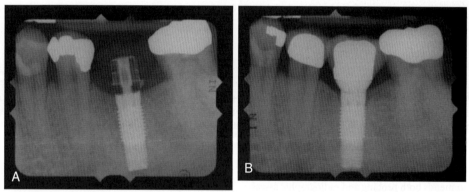

Fig. 31.15 Initial remodeling following implant placement: (A) at placement and (B) at 1 year.

and lingual surfaces and will give the appearance of less severe bone loss, underscoring the need for probing in addition to radiographic assessment.

Assessment of Prosthetic Components

A detailed examination of the prosthesis and prosthetic components and patient education about any foreseeable problems is part of the maintenance visit. All dental implants have some prosthetic component that will need evaluation at the maintenance visits, ranging from a single tooth prosthesis to complex implant-borne restorations in which fixed or removable appliances must be checked for stability. The dental hygienist is in the position to evaluate and refer the patient to the restorative dentist when mechanical complications arise with the prosthesis, just as the patient would be referred to the surgeon if there are biologic complications. **Mechanical complications** include loose or fractured screws connecting to the implant or abutment; worn or missing O-rings, clips, or Locator caps; fractured porcelain; and fractured implants.

Implants may also have iatrogenic complications such as excess cement and inadequately seated restorations (Figs. 31.16 and 31.17). In addition, radiographic and soft tissue evaluation is required to recognize periapical implant complications that may appear clinically as a sinus tract and arise from a surgical complication such as implant placement that damages an adjacent root, or a lesion that arises from a residual cyst subsequent to prior endodontic problems (Fig. 31.18). Although radiographs are useful in diagnosing these complications, problems occurring on the buccal and lingual surfaces may be undetected without the addition of the clinical examination of the implant and prosthetic components.

In patients with implant-supported prostheses, the decision to remove the prosthesis during the maintenance visit is based on individual assessment. If the patient is able to clean adequately, demonstrates good oral hygiene, and the implants are stable, the prosthesis may not be removed at all. Fig. 31.19 shows an implant-supported fixed denture that is designed to allow the patient to floss around the implants. The restorative dentist will determine if the prosthesis needs to be

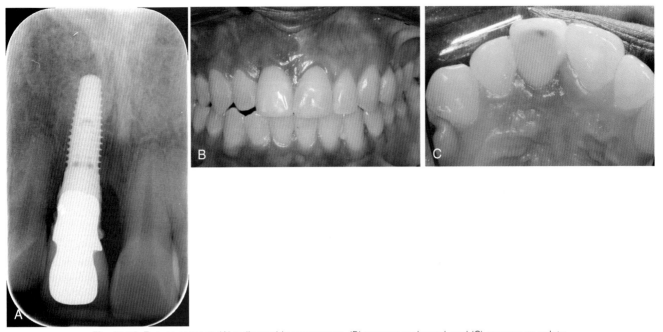

Fig. 31.16 Excess cement: (A) radiographic appearance, (B) mucosa on buccal, and (C) mucosa on palate.

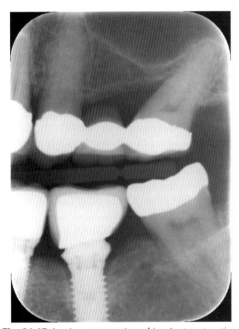

Fig. 31.17 Inadequate seating of implant restoration.

Mobility and Occlusal Interference

Mobility should be assessed at each implant maintenance visit. This is accomplished with the standard method using the blunt ends of an instrument such as a probe or mirror handle on either side of the implant or implant crown and gently attempting to move it back and forth. Unlike teeth that are held in by periodontal ligaments, allowing for some physiologic movement, implants are in direct contact with bone and if osseointegration has been successful, there will be no movement. If the implant is mobile, it is no longer integrated and has failed. It may be, however, that a mobile crown is related to a loose or fractured abutment screw and the implant body is fully integrated with the bone. Additional assessment, including a current radiograph, will be needed to make this determination. A radiolucency surrounding the entire implant indicates loss of integration.

Occlusion should also be assessed for interference. Excessive occlusal forces are associated with implant prosthesis fractures and implant failures. Many times, complications involving porcelain fractures can be prevented by using an occlusal guard to protect the restorations. If the patient is using an occlusal appliance or night guard, advise them to bring it in for the maintenance visits so that it can be evaluated for fit and signs of wear, and the patient can be advised of the appropriate home care for the appliance.

PERI-IMPLANT DISEASE

Dental implants are widely used to replace missing teeth, but they are not exempt from biologic complications. Peri-implant inflammation can occur around the implant abutment if biofilm accumulates. The pathogenesis of peri-implant inflammation, like periodontitis, is believed to be of bacterial etiology. There are two separate disease entities that can occur in the supporting structure of a dental implant, peri-implant mucositis and peri-implantitis. **Peri-implant mucositis** has been defined as a reversible inflammatory reaction that resides in the mucosa and does not include loss of supporting bone. In peri-implant mucositis, bleeding on probing must be present (Fig. 31.21). **Peri-implantitis**, an inflammatory reaction that is associated with loss of bone around an implant that is in function, is thought to be more difficult to reverse (Fig. 31.22).

removed and will reattach the prosthesis after the cleaning. In some cases, the prostheses may need to be reassessed to facilitate at-home maintenance. Fig. 31.20 shows significant inflammation surrounding a fixed implant bridge with limited access for the patient to successfully clean the implants, and the resulting improvement after modification of the prosthesis. If the implant-borne restoration needs to be removed to access the implants during the cleaning, replacing them with new screws should be considered rather than reusing the old ones. In many cases, the patient may not be aware that there is a loose abutment screw, O-ring, or clip that needs replacement, but they may be aware that the crown or overdenture feels loose. In other cases, the loose feeling may be due to a fractured implant screw or even a fractured implant fixture. In these cases, it is imperative to have the restorative dentist involved in the implant assessment.

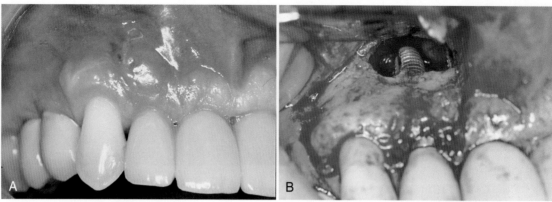

Fig. 31.18 Periapical peri-implantitis: (A) clinical appearance and (B) defect seen at surgery.

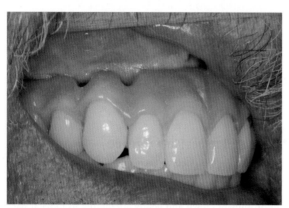

Fig. 31.19 Implant-supported denture designed for adequate access for self-care.

Historically, the criteria used for the diagnosis of peri-implantitis have varied widely, which could potentially hinder diagnosis and early referral for treatment. Some definitions used a specific probing depth, such as greater than 4 mm, and coupled that with different amounts of radiographic bone loss. The 2017 World Workshop on Periodontal Diseases and Conditions provides standards for diagnosis of peri-implant diseases, stating that the diagnosis includes the presence of bleeding and/or suppuration on gentle probing, increased probing depth compared to previous examinations, and the presence of bone loss beyond initial crestal bone remodeling.

In the absence of previous examination data, probing depths of ≥6 mm and bone level ≥3 mm apical of the most coronal portion of the intraosseous part of the implant are used to make the diagnosis.[6] These definitions imply that the initial dental implant healing was uneventful and that osseointegration was achieved as anticipated. It is important to note that bony destruction can progress without any notable impact on implant mobility since osseointegration is generally maintained apically to the peri-implantitis defect. Mobility of the implant indicates the complete loss of osseointegration and total implant failure.

The diagnosis for both peri-implant mucositis and peri-implantitis is made by gentle probing to detect probing depth, presence of bleeding on probing and/or suppuration, and radiographic assessment to determine the presence or absence of bone loss.

See Box 31.2 for a Critical Thinking Scenario related to clinical assessment of dental implants.

The prevalence of both peri-implant mucositis and peri-implantitis is substantial. A recent systematic review reports the prevalence of peri-implantitis to be 18.5%.[7] Risk factors have been identified that include poor oral hygiene, a history of periodontal disease, smoking,

diabetes, radiographic calculus or excess cement, poor bone quality, and occlusal overloading.[8,9] In addition, disruption of the titanium dioxide surface layer of the implant may lead to corrosion and increase the risk of peri-implant disease. With the high prevalence of disease, it is important that the patient be educated regarding the risk factors and need for frequent monitoring and biofilm removal.

It is difficult to define the continuum between inflammatory changes of peri-implant mucositis and peri-implantitis. Therefore, peri-implantitis management may be equally challenging (Box 31.3). Peri-implant mucositis may respond well to nonsurgical treatment modalities such as mechanical debridement, whereas there is a limited response to non-surgical mechanical debridement alone in peri-implantitis cases.

AT-HOME IMPLANT CARE

During the initial planning stages and throughout treatment, the need for compliance with oral self-care recommendations should be emphasized. Unfortunately, many patients view the dental implant as a new tooth that will tolerate mistreatment better than a natural tooth. This myth must be dispelled and the patient must realize that the soft tissue around the dental implant needs as much or more daily oral care to control plaque biofilm as the gingival tissue around a natural tooth. Some dental implant candidates have lost their natural teeth as a result of significant oral risk factors for periodontal disease. These individuals may also be at risk for peri-implant inflammation or failure of the dental implant, and they need education about the modification and control of those risk factors.

Ongoing oral self-care education should be customized on the basis of patient preferences and with regard to implant location; the prosthetic design and the ease of biofilm removal between the appliance and gingival tissue; patient motivation, compliance, and manual dexterity; and peri-implant tissue health. The dental hygienist should regularly observe the patient's oral self-care technique and monitor the oral tissues to ensure that the patient is not causing trauma with an oral hygiene aid.

Brushing

Patients should be advised to clean their existing natural teeth and implants two times daily with a soft toothbrush directed at a 45° angle toward the soft tissues. A soft toothbrush is especially important because titanium is a softer material than natural tooth, and the abutment surface can be damaged with hard-bristled toothbrushes, thereby facilitating oral biofilm accumulation. In cases where keratinized mucosa is minimal or lacking, the patient should also be advised to be gentle to prevent trauma to the delicate mucosa that surrounds the abutment. Power brushes may be prescribed for

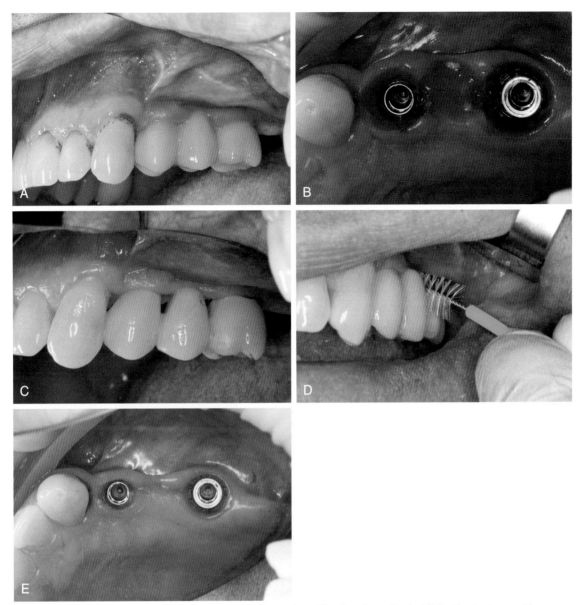

Fig. 31.20 Inflammation due to inadequate access and modification of prosthesis. (A) Peri-implant mucositis, (B) inflammation in implant/mucosal interface, (C) improved access, (D) Proxi-Brush, and (E) resolution of inflammation after modification.

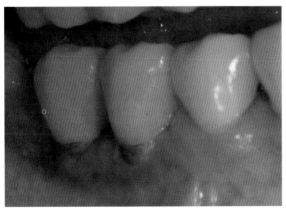

Fig. 31.21 Peri-implantitis mucositis.

patients, with the same recommendations regarding minimal use of force to prevent trauma.

With the fully edentulous patient, additional devices such as the end-tuft toothbrush and sulcus brush may help the patient to focus on one implant at a time (Fig. 31.23).

Removable Prostheses

Patients with implant-supported removable dental prostheses should be advised to clean their removable prosthesis at least twice daily using a soft brush with a professionally recommended denture-cleaning agent. They should be advised to remove the prosthesis while sleeping and store it in the prescribed cleaning solution.

Floss

Additional oral hygiene devices may be recommended, depending on the specific needs of the patient and design of the prosthesis. A general

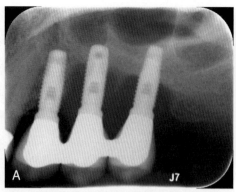
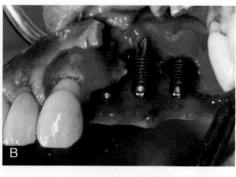

Fig. 31.22 Peri-implantitis: (A) radiographic appearance and (B) extent of bone loss seen at surgery.

BOX 31.2 **Critical Thinking Scenario B**

You have been performing maintenance on a patient's implants for 5 years and they have been stable. The patient comes in for a 3-month visit and you have increased probing depth with bleeding and suppuration. Discuss what additional diagnostic data you would gather and what treatment is indicated.

BOX 31.3 **Legal, Ethical, and Safety Issues**

Dental hygienists must assess for peri-implant mucositis and possible peri-implantitis at each professional dental implant care session. In addition, the hygienist must review the patient's at-home maintenance and assess whether there are problems associated with the implant that are related to oral hygiene or whether there are mechanical or iatrogenic problems associated with the prosthetic components.

Patients should be referred to a general dentist, a periodontist, or an oral and maxillofacial surgeon for implant treatment planning when peri-implantitis is diagnosed or when prosthetic or surgical treatment is needed.

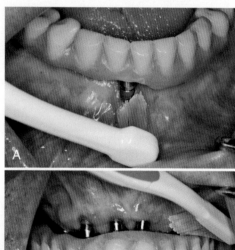
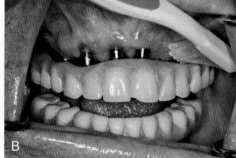

Fig. 31.23 End-tuft toothbrush application for dental implant (A) and sulcus toothbrush (B).

---

recommendation is to keep things as simple as possible so that the patient will be able to comply with the recommendations. A patient who is advised to use multiple aids in addition to brushing may be overwhelmed.

If abutments are spaced close to each other, dental floss or tape should be used to clean their proximal surfaces at least once daily (Fig. 31.24). The floss is placed around the implant, crisscrossed, and pulled in a shoe-shining motion to clean the abutment. Floss or tape can be used in conjunction with a floss threader to allow easy access through the embrasure or limited areas. Other types of interdental cleaning devices may be advised, such as water flossers (Fig. 31.25) and air flossers if the patient has less dexterity and is not interested in or is unable to perform regular flossing (see Chapter 25).

See Box 31.4 for a Critical Thinking Scenario related to dental implant maintenance.

Plastic Nylon-Coated Interdental Brush and Foam Pads

The interproximal areas of dental implants can be reached with a cone-shaped or cylindrical interdental brush, foam tip, or Proxi-Tip (Fig. 31.26). To avoid alteration of the abutment surface, nylon-coated wires are required rather than metal-wired brushes. Interdental brushes should be discarded when the nylon coating has worn down to the metal wire. The interdental brush can be used from the facial or lingual

areas and interproximally. Interdental brushes are recommended for use at least one time daily.

Dentifrice

Abrasive dentifrice can alter the abutment surface; therefore patients should be advised to brush twice daily using low-abrasive toothpaste. Toothpastes that carry the American Dental Association Seal of Acceptance or the Canadian Dental Association Seal of Recognition meet this criterion for low abrasiveness. See Chapter 26.

Antimicrobial Agents

Systematic reviews have supported the short-term use of 0.12% chlorhexidine rinse either postsurgically or as an adjunct to the maintenance procedure when inflammation and biofilm are present. It should be noted, however, that recent evidence shows that when chlorhexidine is used to decontaminate a diseased implant, it is adsorbed on the titanium surface and may prevent reattachment of bone cells. If the practitioner chooses to prescribe chlorhexidine for the implant patient, it should be used as a short-term adjunct to mechanical oral hygiene procedures. To target the delivery of the

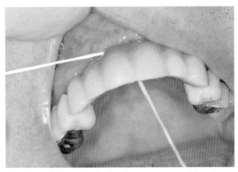

Fig. 31.24 Use of floss under implant-supported fixed prosthesis.

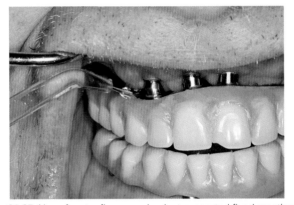

Fig. 31.25 Use of water flosser on implant-supported fixed prosthesis.

BOX 31.4   Critical Thinking Scenario C

You have a patient with an implant-supported superstructure retained by four maxillary implants. The patient presents with inflammation and bleeding on all four implants and visible plaque and says that she is trying to clean them but can't get floss under the denture. Discuss what you would use to assess and clean the implants, and what advice you would give the patient.

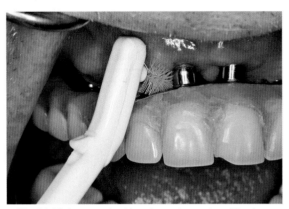

Fig. 31.26 Interproximal brush used on a dental implant.

chlorhexidine to a specific site, a cotton swab, a soft toothbrush, an interdental brush, or a subgingival irrigator may be used for the delivery to the site. Rinsing with 0.12% chlorhexidine gluconate reduces both gram-positive and gram-negative oral bacteria for up to 5 hours after use with the 30-seconds-twice-a-day protocol, thereby resulting in less peri-implant gingivitis and bleeding; however, the use of chlorhexidine gluconate as a rinse for more than a month may cause staining of the natural teeth or the prosthetic appliance.

PROFESSIONAL MAINTENANCE

Thorough biofilm removal is extremely important for long-term success. Patients who are not enrolled in maintenance programs have been found to have a higher incidence of peri-implantitis.[10] In addition, a retrospective review of 1020 implants found that regular maintenance reduced failure by 90% and irregular maintenance reduced failure by 60% over no maintenance.[11] The dental hygienist should advise the patient to obtain a dental professional examination visit at least every 6 months as a lifelong regimen. Patients at a higher risk based on age, ability to perform oral self-care, or biologic or mechanical complications of remaining natural teeth should be advised to obtain professional examinations more frequently depending on the clinical situation.

Dental Hygiene Strategies for Dental Implants

Titanium implants are highly biocompatible because of the titanium dioxide layer that forms on the surface of the implant when it is first exposed to oxygen. When the titanium dioxide layer initially forms, it is only 1 to 2 nm thick, but it continues to grow slowly, reaching a thickness of 25 nm in 4 years. It is the presence of this thin

passive oxide film that provides chemical stability and protects the bulk metal from further oxidation or corrosion. When attempting to remove biofilm, calculus, or cement, scratching or gouging the titanium surface should be avoided because this not only will create an area that becomes more retentive to biofilm accumulation and its bacterial byproducts, but it also will disrupt the titanium dioxide surface layer, providing the potential for titanium corrosion and loss of biocompatibility.

Dental hygiene strategies for cleaning implants must be devised with the material in mind rather than through the prism of natural teeth. Calculus formation does not occur as frequently on implants and abutments as it does on natural teeth. Biofilm formation does occur frequently and it is the biofilm that inducesing the inflammatory process. This means the hygienist must leave behind the paradigm of instrumenting every bit of implant surface and assess whether the implant needs instrumentation at all or whether a minimally invasive biofilm removal technique will be indicated.

Air Polishing

Air polishing with erythritol or glycine powder has been shown to be a safe and effective method of biofilm removal from the implant surfaces that will not damage the implant. In addition, air polishing with both of these powders can be used to reach subgingivally and will reach areas that are difficult to access with instruments, such as under the implant support superstructure beneath a fully edentulous fixed prosthesis (Fig. 31.27). A subgingival tip for erythritol or glycine powder can be used to access deeper pockets in a nonsurgical manner. When neither calculus nor cement is present on the implant, air polishing will be all that is needed for effective biofilm removal. For more information on air polishing, refer to Chapter 32.

Implant Instrumentation

Removal of biofilm is an integral part of treatment, yet the hygienist must keep in mind that traditional periodontal instruments may disrupt the titanium dioxide and abrade the implant surface, leading to a surface that accelerates the accumulation of biofilm. When

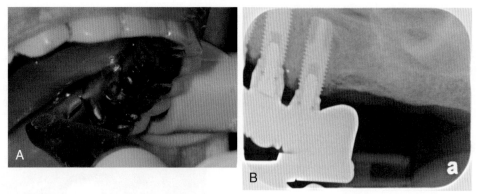

Fig. 31.27 Air polisher used to access under fixed-detachable implant-supported prosthesis: (A) clinical and (B) radiographic appearance of prosthesis.

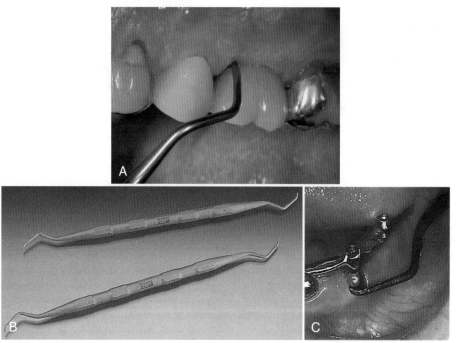

Fig. 31.28 Implant hand instruments: (A) titanium curet, (B and C) graphite-filled curet. (Courtesy Steri-Oss, Yorba Linda, CA. C–F, Courtesy Hu-Friedy, Chicago, IL.)

instrumentation is required to remove calculus or cement, there are several types of instruments available for implant maintenance. Instrument rigidity and design, prosthetic appliance design, location of deposit, and calculus tenacity should be carefully assessed before making an instrument selection. Ultimately, the deposit must be removed in order to maintain implant health using the least disruptive method.

Various instruments have been developed specifically for use when scaling dental implants (Fig. 31.28). There are a large variety of commercially available instruments that use various materials as alternatives to metal curets, including plastic, graphite, Teflon-coated, gold-coated, titanium-coated, and solid titanium alloy. Much research has focused on the effect of these instruments on the smooth surface of the abutment or implant neck and the rough surface of the implant body. Systematic review of surface alterations following the

use of different mechanical instruments allows for assessment of a large number of studies, resulting in a strong body of evidence supporting the use of nonmetal instruments as the instruments of choice for smooth and rough surfaces.[12] Plastic instruments, however, have been shown to leave behind a deposition of debris that may interfere in restoration of osteoblast attachment to the surface. Titanium curets have been shown to produce only minimal smooth surface alteration over prolonged treatments and avoid the debris accumulation associated with plastic curets. In some cases, a titanium curet may be necessary because of the location and tenacity of the deposit. Because the titanium abutment surface can be easily abraded, the following are strongly contraindicated for use on dental implants: stainless steel curets and scalers, metal tip inserts of sonic and ultrasonic scaling instruments, and rubber cup polishing with flour of pumice or abrasive paste.

Sonic and Ultrasonic Instrument Tips

Specialized tips have been developed for sonic, ultrasonic, and piezoelectric-powered instrumentation of dental implants to minimize damage to the titanium surface (Fig. 31.29). It has been shown that the plastic tips can cause mild to moderate surface alterations compared to severe alterations caused by the metallic tips. An additional consideration regarding the use of sonic and ultrasonic implant tips is that the use of the tips may affect the cell viability of osteoblasts, causing the viability to be lower when compared to manual instrumentation of implants. (Box 31.5). More research is needed in this area, and it is important for the dental hygienist to stay tuned to the current evidence-based research.

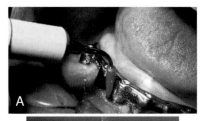
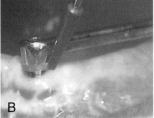

Fig. 31.29 Ultrasonic scaler tip for implants. (A, Courtesy Dentsply, York, PA. B, Courtesy Tony Riso Company, North Miami Beach, FL.)

Nonsurgical Treatment of Peri-implant Disease

The progression from peri-implant mucositis to peri-implantitis is difficult to determine (Fig. 31.30). Therefore, it is important to treat the signs of inflammation as soon as they are present. Peri-implant mucositis is reversible and can be successfully treated nonsurgically with control of the etiologic factors and thorough biofilm removal. Patients should be monitored regularly and all treatments should disrupt the submucosal biofilm. Once a lesion has progressed to peri-implantitis, nonsurgical treatment alone has limited efficacy. If nonsurgical treatment does not resolve or arrest bone loss, surgical therapy may be considered. Before surgical therapy, however, local and systematic factors such as poor oral hygiene, smoking, and periodontitis should be under control.

Surgical Treatment of Peri-implant Disease

Surgical therapy is superior to nonsurgical therapy in resolving peri-implantitis and therefore may ultimately be required. Surgical therapy includes granulation tissue removal and thorough cleaning of the contaminated surface and may include bone grafting to obtain defect fill. Patients should be advised that there is little evidence suggesting what treatment is best for peri-implantitis and, in some studies, the recurrence rate was up to 100%. Since it is a chronic disease, retreatment may be necessary.

BOX 31.5 **Legal, Ethical, and Safety Issues**

Never provide periodontal debridement around implants with the use of metal scalers or sonic and ultrasonic scalers (unless the ultrasonic or sonic tip is specially designed for implants).

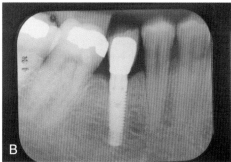
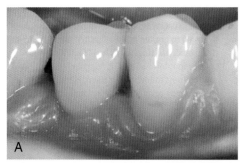
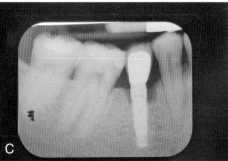

Fig. 31.30 Progression from mucositis to peri-implantitis: (A) clinical appearance of mucosa, (B) implant at 1 year postprosthesis insertion, and (C) 5.5 years postprosthesis with radiographic bone loss and peri-implantitis.

KEY CONCEPTS

- Dental implants provide an alternative to missing dentition. Dental hygienists must be able to recognize good candidates who will benefit from this investment and discuss the risks and benefits of dental implant placement with potential candidates.
- Osseointegration is a unique biologic phenomenon in which living bone cells fuse to the metal titanium.
- The dental hygienist should be able to distinguish differences between bone-level and tissue-level implants and between cement and screw-retained restorations.
- Dental implants require regular maintenance in order to decrease the risk of peri-implantitis and implant loss. The dental hygienist emphasizes and describes the importance of daily oral self-care and professional dental hygiene care to dental implant patients.
- The dental hygienist recommends strategies for cleaning dental implants with appropriate oral hygiene aids.
- Neither stainless steel instruments nor metal ultrasonic or sonic instruments are recommended for dental implants. Stainless steel instruments and abrasive home care tools may cause scratches and irregularities on the implant, thereby leading to faster oral biofilm accumulation and inflammation. Plastic, titanium, or graphite instruments may be used for scaling dental implants. The dental hygienist must know which instruments are safe for titanium metal. Some mechanized instrument manufacturers market plastic tips that can be used with dental implants.
- Periodontal probing is necessary in order to diagnose implant health, mucositis, or peri-implantitis. A baseline probing depth is required after the prosthetic insertion in order to detect later changes. Gentle force is indicated when probing.
- The dental hygienist must know the definitions of peri-implant health, peri-implant mucositis, and peri-implantitis and understand that probing depth alone cannot be used to make any of those diagnoses.
- Risk factors for peri-implant disease and implant loss should be assessed at each visit. The patient should be advised of the risks and recommendations should be made regarding those risks that can be modified, such as smoking, glycemic control, and poor oral hygiene.
- When peri-implantitis or mechanical implant complications are noted, they must be called to the attention of both the patient and the dentist and the appropriate referrals made.

ACKNOWLEDGMENT

The author acknowledges Mehran Hossaini-Zadeh and Vivian L. Young-McDonald for their past contributions to this chapter.

REFERENCES

1. Diz P, Scully C, Sanz M. Dental implants in the medically compromised patient. *J Dent.* 2013;41(3):195–206.
2. Greenstein G, Cavallaro J, Tarnow D. Practical application of anatomy for the dental implant surgeon. *J Periodontol.* 2008;79(10):1833–1846.
3. Smalley WM. Implants for tooth movement: determining implant location and orientation. *J Esthet Dent.* 1995;7(2):62–72.
4. Staubli N, Walter C, Schmidt JC, et al. Excess cement and the risk of peri-implant disease—a systematic review. *Clin Oral Implants Res.* 2017;28(10):1278–1290.
5. Bidra AS, Daubert DM, Garcia LT, et al. Clinical practice guidelines for recall and maintenance of patients with tooth-borne and implant-borne dental restorations. *J Dent Hyg.* 2016;147(1):67–74.
6. Berglundh T, Armitage G, Araujo MG, et al. Peri-implant diseases and conditions: consensus report of workgroup 4 of the 2017 World Workshop on the Classification of periodontal and peri-implant diseases and conditions. *J Periodontol.* 2018;89(suppl 1):S313–S318.
7. Rakic M, Galindo-Moreno P, Monje A, et al. How frequent does peri-implantitis occur? A systematic review and meta-analysis. *Clin Oral Invest.* 2018;22:1805–1816.
8. Daubert DM, Weinstein BF, Bordin S, et al. Prevalence and predictive factors for peri-implant disease and implant failure: a cross-sectional analysis. *J Periodontol.* 2015;86(3):337–347.
9. Derks J, Tomasi C. Peri-implant health and disease. A systematic review of current epidemiology. *J Clin Periodontol.* 2015;42(suppl 16):S158–S171.
10. Costa FO, Takenaka-Martinez S, Cota LO, et al. Peri-implant disease in subjects with and without preventive maintenance: a 5-year follow-up. *J Clin Periodontol.* 2012;39(2):173–181.
11. Tran DT, Gay IC, Diaz-Rodriguez J, et al. Survival of dental implants placed in grafted and nongrafted bone: a retrospective study in a university setting. *Int J Oral Maxillofac Implants.* 2016;31(2):310–317.
12. Louropoulou A, Slot DE, Van der Weijden FA. Titanium surface alterations following the use of different mechanical instruments: a systematic review. *Clin Oral Implants Res.* 2012;23(6):643–658.

32

Tooth Polishing and Whitening

Jennifer A. Pieren, Bryn Taylor, and Lauren DeSantis

PROFESSIONAL OPPORTUNITIES

Stain removal and tooth whitening address the concerns of many dental hygiene patients because they want cleaner, brighter smiles. Subgingival biofilm removal with air polishing also contributes to periodontal health in patients with periodontitis or during periodontal maintenance therapy. Dental hygienists with current knowledge and skills to facilitate these patient goals safely and effectively can provide valuable services for these patients.

COMPETENCIES

1. Discuss rubber-cup tooth polishing technique and armamentarium selection for various patient conditions, and perform the procedure on a patient.
2. Discuss air polishing technique and armamentarium options for various patient conditions, and perform the procedure on a patient.
3. Describe client or patient education and motivation in relation to extrinsic stain removal procedures.
4. Discuss teeth whitening, including at-home products and in-office techniques. Consider the hygienist's role in in-office whitening procedures.
5. Value the legal and ethical principles that apply to tooth polishing and whitening services.

INTRODUCTION

Patients dissatisfied with the appearance of their teeth often seek solutions by making an appointment for a professional oral prophylaxis and/or tooth whitening. When these patients come to their dental hygiene appointment, the first step is to identify the source of their concerns. If stain is the problem, the dental hygienist determines its cause because polishing cannot change some stains, whereas it may improve others to varying degrees. Identifying the type of stain might also lead to the discovery of patient factors that contribute to tooth stain, for example, smoking or drinking tea (see Chapter 18). If tooth polishing and/or whitening can address the stain, the dental hygienist selects the least damaging method to address the concern and discusses the options with the patient. At times, more than one method may be indicated. If tooth polishing or whitening addresses the stain, the dental hygienist can mention potential restorative options and make an appropriate referral as needed.

At times, dental hygienists perform tooth polishing for therapeutic rather than cosmetic reasons. It therapeutically removes bacterial plaque biofilms not removed by instrumentation or

the patient. Air polishing with glycine powder is beneficial to remove subgingival microbiota and biofilm in periodontal pockets. Whether addressing cosmetic concerns or therapeutic needs of patients, these services are important components of comprehensive dental hygiene care.

Refer to Chapter 18 for a review of extrinsic and intrinsic tooth stains and their causes and Chapter 26 for a review of abrasive agents used in dentifrices and prophylaxis polishing pastes. The focus of this chapter is stain removal and management.

EXTRINSIC STAIN MANAGEMENT

Recognition of extrinsic stain and appropriate treatment can address the patient's esthetic goals. Rubber-cup polishing and air polishing are the two primary procedures for the management of extrinsic stains or discolorations on the outside of the tooth from external sources. Rubber-cup tooth polishing for extrinsic stain removal has no therapeutic value in terms of periodontal health. Although it is a cosmetic concern, tooth stain is not a pathologic condition.

RUBBER-CUP TOOTH POLISHING

Rubber-cup polishing is the removal of extrinsic tooth stains after scaling, when indicated, using a low-speed dental handpiece, a prophylaxis angle with a rubber cup and bristle brush, and a prophylaxis paste or another cleaning or polishing agent. Rubber-cup polishing also is known as **coronal polishing** because the technique focuses on the crowns of the teeth. Patients generally accept this traditional method for the removal of extrinsic tooth stain and it is easy to learn and perform. Polishing is a fundamental procedure in the delivery of oral prophylaxis. Although the process of polishing seems simple, it involves several issues for consideration.[1] The polishing of teeth and dental restorations is important for patient satisfaction and may contribute to success in the prevention and treatment of oral disease.

Years ago, all patients had their teeth polished after scaling and debridement or as a sole procedure for teeth cleaning. This practice has changed over the years because of possible adverse effects on the tooth surfaces, restorations, and soft tissues. In some patients, tooth polishing is contraindicated. **Selective polishing**, or selective stain removal, focuses on the tooth surfaces with visible stains after scaling and debridement is completed, especially when polishing may cause damage or when polishing is contraindicated. The dental hygienist applies the tooth polishing procedure selectively by polishing only those tooth surfaces with stain, avoiding newly erupted teeth, cementum, dentin, demineralized areas, and restored tooth surfaces that have the potential for being damaged by the process.

Choosing a Prophylaxis Paste

One of the key factors to safe and effective tooth polishing is choosing the appropriate prophylaxis paste. Most pastes have splatter-free formulations. Some products come with a finger ring to hold the cup of prophylaxis paste, or rings can be purchased separately. The particle size (also known as *grit*) of prophylactic pastes affects the cleaning rate and scratch pattern produced on a tooth surface. Fine grit yields the least amount of surface abrasion, even if the abrasive material is high on the Mohs Hardness Scale, whereas coarse grit, the most abrasive, can scratch and roughen surfaces, potentially making them more likely to accumulate oral biofilm and stain. Abrasives are classified as coarse, moderate, fine, or superfine, based on the size of the particles measured in microns (Fig. 32.1). There is no industry standard for defining superfine, fine, medium, or coarse grit; however, ratings are based on the particles being passed through a standardized sieve that allows a specific size of particles to pass. The meaning of these labels can vary from manufacturer to manufacturer.

Larger abrasive particles are more coarse: ≥100 micrometers (μm), coarse; 20 to <100 μm, medium; and <20 μm, fine (Table 32.1)[2]; 1 micron equals 1000 μm. Clearly, there is a significant difference between the degree of abrasiveness for coarse and fine pastes on tooth surfaces and restorations, and a great deal of variation exists in medium grit pastes. Prophylaxis pastes with a smaller particle size, such as those found in fine or superfine paste, will increase tooth surface cleanliness, luster, and smoothness. Prophylaxis pastes containing fluoride,

remineralizing agents, whitening ingredients, or desensitizing agents are available; however, there is a need for more evidence to support the efficacy of these products. The US Food and Drug Administration (FDA) classifies polishing pastes without drug components as devices for cleaning and polishing teeth. When a manufacturer adds drugs, the FDA has determined that the prophylaxis paste functions as an abrasive agent intended to clean and polish the teeth, whereas the drug component plays a secondary role, augmenting the safety and/or effectiveness of the prophylaxis paste, rather than its therapeutic component.[3]

Dental hygiene practice articles assert that many dental hygienists inappropriately use the same polishing paste for every patient, regardless of the grit size and the patient's needs. The worst-case scenario in dental hygiene practice is to use a coarse polishing paste on every patient to remove the entire range of stain—from light to heavy—to save time. This theory is contrary to the professionally recommended, evidence-based method of using the finest polishing paste grit that will achieve the desired result, and, in the few instances where stain requires a coarse grit for stain removal, following the coarse grit paste with a progression to medium grit and then to fine grit. Unfortunately, some product lines include only medium and coarse grit pastes, so look for available products with fine grit paste. Two-step, single-dose products are available with the disposable paste cup containing coarse and finer grit pastes. Coarse grit polishing pastes can cause dentinal hypersensitivity, tooth roughness, and damage to restorations, so their use is unethical unless necessary for removing heavy tenacious stain and followed with less abrasive polishing agents.[4]

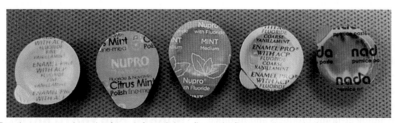

Fig. 32.1 Prophy pastes—in order from left to right—fine grit, fine-medium grit, medium grit, coarse grit, and pumice paste. (Courtesy Lauren DeSantis.)

TABLE 32.1	Abrasives Used for Rubber-Cup Tooth Polishing in Dental Hygiene Practice	
Abrasive Agent	**Mohs Hardness Value***	**Application**
Aluminum silicates	2	Is used as a polishing agent, has no excessive abrasion, and is compatible with dental fluoride compounds
Calcium carbonate (chalk or whitening)	3	Is used as a polishing agent, has no excessive abrasion, and is compatible with dental fluoride compounds
Superfine pumice (flour of pumice)	6 to 7	Is used as a cleaning agent in prophylaxis paste for oral biofilm and stain removal, and for polishing tooth enamel, gold foil, dental amalgam, and acrylic resin
Tin oxide (putty powder, stannic oxide)	6 to 7	Is used for polishing teeth and metallic restorations; is mixed with water or glycerin to form a mildly abrasive paste
Silica or sand (silex [silicon dioxide])	6 to 7	Used for heavy stain removal; it effectively cleans tooth surfaces with low abrasion and high cleaning capability
Zirconium silicate (zircon)	6.5 to 7.5	Used in dental prophylaxis pastes and to coat abrasive discs and strips
Corundum (aluminum oxide [alumina])	7 to 9	Is used for polishing composites, highly filled hybrid composites, acrylic resin, and porcelain restorations and custom trays; is bonded to discs or paper strips and impregnated into rubber wheels and points
Diamond	10	Is used in polishing paste and on ceramic, porcelain, and resin-based composite materials and metal-backed abrasive strips and furcation files

*Mohs Hardness Value is the standard for the hardness of abrasives and substrates; the higher the value, the harder or more abrasive the material. For comparison, cementum is 2 to 3, dentin is 3 to 4, and enamel or apatite is 5 to 6.

The following five variables influence efficiency, effectiveness, and tooth structure loss during extrinsic tooth stain removal with a rubber cup:

1. **Abrasiveness of the prophylaxis paste (or other abrasive agent) used during the procedure:** The harder the abrasive, the greater the rate of abrasion. Always use the least abrasive agent to accomplish stain removal.
2. **Quantity of abrasive agent:** The greater the amount of abrasive particles applied, the greater the rate of abrasion. Water or humectants suspend abrasive agent particles in the paste to decrease both the quantity of abrasive particles and the frictional heat generated by the procedure. Never use a dry abrasive agent on tooth enamel.
3. **Contact time of the rubber cup or bristle brush on the tooth surface:** The longer the contact time, the greater the rate of abrasion and frictional heat. Always use short, intermittent contact between the rubber cup and the tooth or restorative materials.
4. **Speed or revolutions per minute (rpm) of the rubber cup or bristle brush:** The greater the speed of the rotating rubber cup, the greater the rate of abrasion and frictional heat generated. Always use low speeds no greater than 3000 rpm.
5. **Applied pressure or force of the rubber cup or bristle brush on the tooth surface:** The greater the force applied to the rubber cup against the tooth, the greater the rate of abrasion and frictional heat generated. Always use a light intermittent touch when polishing tooth surfaces and restorations.

To preserve tooth structure and prevent damage to teeth and restorative materials, start with the least abrasive agent and amount of agent, with the least amount of contact time, at the lowest speed, and with the least amount of pressure to remove the extrinsic stain and to avoid tooth surface damage. A clinician can increase any of these variables if necessary to achieve the desired clinical outcome.

Effects on Oral and Dental Tissues

Rubber-cup polishing removes the microscopic outer layer of tooth enamel. Because the highest fluoride concentration is in the outermost layer, performing routine rubber-cup polishing could remove the fluoride-rich outer enamel layer. However, minerals in saliva continuously remineralize enamel. Using a fluoride-containing toothpaste, gel, or mouthrinse, as indicated, on a daily basis also is important for remineralization, especially for patients with moderate or high caries risk. The amount of enamel lost during rubber-cup polishing is minimal, even when repeated over time; however, root surfaces may be at risk of tooth wear over time because cementum and dentin are softer than enamel. Stain on root surfaces is often removed with ultrasonic or sonic scaling devices set on low power. Moreover, tooth sensitivity to rubber-cup polishing may occur in cervical areas because of the thinness of enamel in these areas and exposed dentin or cementum. Demineralized tooth areas, or white spots, lose significantly more surface structure during polishing than intact enamel. All of these conditions require fluoride therapy, depending on caries risk assessment (see Chapter 19).

Irritation of soft tissues can result from rubber-cup polishing if the tissues are inflamed; particles of the abrasive agent can embed in the gingiva and delay healing. Trauma to gingiva also can occur with improper technique, especially if the rubber cup is used at a high speed or with excessive pressure and/or is kept in one place too long. Pressure should be enough to flatten one edge of the cup so that it slips into the sulcus but not enough so that the entire lip of the cup is flat. Pulpal discomfort also may occur if pressure, speed, and abrasiveness of the polishing paste are sufficient to generate heat, especially in newly erupted teeth with wide pulpal chambers.

Effects on Restorations and Titanium Implants

Rubber-cup polishing may damage restorations by making surfaces rough. Dental hygienists need to refer to the dental charting to determine the location of all aesthetic restorations, as some of them can be difficult to detect clinically. Gold, amalgam, conventional composites, and microfilled composites exhibit surface roughness after polishing with a prophylaxis paste. Therefore prophylaxis pastes designed for cosmetic restorations and less abrasive polishing techniques, such as slow speed and light, intermittent pressure, are recommended. Polishing a dental implant with an abrasive agent is not recommended because it could cause damage, and stain does not readily form on these implants. Plaque biofilm removal from titanium implants requires the use of oral hygiene aids or subgingival air polishing. Despite clinical improvements, research indicates that peri-implant mucositis may not be resolved completely by professionally administered plaque removal. The addition of antimicrobials and daily self-care practices may improve outcomes, although specific recommendations require additional study.[5]

To prevent damage to teeth, restorations, and soft tissues, adhere to the following principles:

1. Use proper technique to reduce unnecessary abrasion. Control the time, speed, and pressure during tooth polishing procedures.
2. Select the least abrasive polishing agent that will remove the stain and remaining plaque biofilm after self-care demonstration, scaling, and debridement.
3. Avoid polishing when contraindicated (Box 32.1).

Prophylaxis Angle and Dental Handpiece Technique

A bristle brush or rubber polishing cup is inserted into a disposable or reusable, sterilizable (e.g., stainless steel) prophylaxis angle attached to a low-speed, ergonomically designed handpiece and is used for coronal polishing (Fig. 32.2). Many practices use disposable angles to save time required for sterilization of stainless steel angles, although these devices often are sterilized together. Some disposable prophylaxis angles come prepackaged with prophylaxis paste; however, this packaging may not favor selection of the paste grit for each patient.

The head of the prophylaxis angle has one of the following:

- Rubber cup (screw-type, latch-type, or snap-on, or on a disposable prophylaxis angle) used on all tooth surfaces
- Flat or pointed bristle brush (screw-type, latch-type, or snap-on, or on a disposable prophylaxis angle) used for stain removal on occlusal surfaces and in fossa

---

BOX 32.1   Contraindications and Precautions to Rubber-Cup Polishing

Contraindications

Absence of extrinsic stain
Newly erupted teeth, especially primary teeth
Enamel hypocalcification or hypoplasia
Enamel demineralization and active unrestored caries lesions
Areas of recession where cementum or dentin is exposed
Areas of dentinal hypersensitivity
Acute gingival or periodontal inflammation
Allergy to ingredients in paste

Precautions Needed

Use a special polishing agent on restored tooth surfaces, such as composite, bonding, glass ionomer, porcelain, gold, or titanium.
Consider particle impaction risk immediately after deep scaling, periodontal debridement, or root planing when gingival tissues may be irritated.

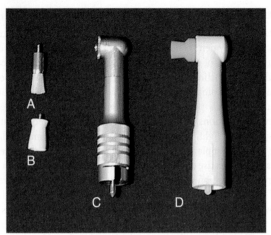

Fig. 32.2 (A) Bristle brush. (B) Rubber polishing cup. (C) Sterilizable prophy angle. (D) Disposable prophy angle. (From Bird DL, Robinson DS. *Modern Dental Assisting.* 12th ed. Elsevier; 2016.)

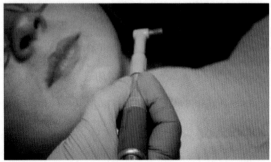

Fig. 32.3 Pen grasp used for dental handpiece. (Dental hygiene procedures videos, St Louis, 2015, Saunders.)

Rubber cups can use prophylaxis paste, or paste-free abrasive-impregnated rubber prophylaxis polishing cups are available for use without paste. A soft cup is recommended, so flaring of the edge of the cup provides easy reach into the sulcus or interproximal areas. These angles might maintain a smooth surface finish when applied to composite resin and enamel; however, research is limited. Latex-free disposable cups and brushes also are available for tooth polishing when patients report a latex allergy.

Handpieces with a prophy angle and prophy cup or brush are used with a pen grasp (Fig. 32.3), using overlapping strokes to cover the areas of stain on the tooth surfaces (Fig. 32.4). Manufacturer's directions provide guidance for cleaning, lubricating, and sterilizing handpieces and stainless steel prophylaxis angles. Disposable prophylaxis angles allow for disposal after each use. Procedure 32.1 outlines the materials and procedures for rubber-cup polishing. The Evolve Video Resources and the corresponding Competency Form are located on Evolve (http:/evolve.elsevier.com/Pieren/hygiene/).

Critical Thinking Scenario

Box 32.2 provides a Critical Thinking Scenario to practice an appropriate approach to rubber-cup polishing for extrinsic stain removal.

Legal, Ethical, and Safety Issues

Use critical thinking to choose the best approach and agents for tooth polishing. Box 32.3 provides an overview of the legal, ethical, and safety issues, and Box 32.4 provides an ethical thinking scenario.

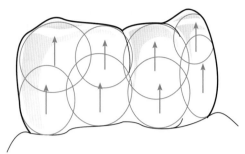

Fig. 32.4 Use of overlapping strokes to ensure complete coverage of the tooth. (From Bird DL, Robinson DS. *Modern Dental Assisting.* 12th ed. Elsevier; 2016.)

BOX 32.2 **Critical Thinking Scenario A**

Rubber-Cup Polishing

Oral assessment reveals the presence of generalized tobacco stain and localized plaque biofilm and calculus in the mandibular anterior and maxillary teeth. Your patient reports smoking a pack of cigarettes a day. When you complete the examination and self-care instructions, you begin the implementation phase of your dental hygiene care.

1. What approach would you take for instrumentation?
2. What grit(s) of polishing paste would you use?
3. When would selective polishing be appropriate for this patient?

Hand-Activated and Sonic or Ultrasonic Scaling

Hand-activated instruments, such as curets and sickle scalers, are designed primarily for calculus removal, but they also can be used for extrinsic stain removal (see Chapter 28). When stain adheres to calculus, removal is efficient along with the calculus. Because scaling instruments have small tips, they can remove stain in areas inaccessible to a rubber cup. However, they can remove cementum on root surfaces, so overinstrumentation should be avoided. When moderate-to-heavy stain is present on root surfaces, the dental hygienist selects the stain removal approach with the least alteration of exposed cementum or dentin. As much stain as possible should be removed during scaling and debridement. The less root structure removed, the less chance of root surface sensitivity after the procedure.

Ultrasonic scaling and sonic scaling (see Chapter 29) to remove extrinsic stain have the same advantages and disadvantages as when they are used for calculus removal. Efficiency and efficacy are the primary benefits for selecting these instruments for stain removal. In addition, a slender tip is able to remove stain on occlusal surfaces in areas of anatomic concavities and rotated or overlapped teeth. Studies on the effects of hand-activated instruments versus sonic and ultrasonic instruments indicate that hand instruments remove root irregularities that can harbor plaque and calculus. Sonic and ultrasonic instruments remove less of the tooth structure but leave a rough surface. However, both techniques are equally effective in removing stain, plaque, and calculus deposits. Using low power with precision thin tips designed for periodontal debridement is the safest choice when instrumentation is required for stain or calculus removal on exposed root surfaces.

AIR POLISHING

Air polishing is a method of stain and biofilm removal that uses a specially designed device with a handpiece that delivers a spray of warm water and prophy powder under pressure (Figs. 32.5 and 32.6). Air polishing has several advantages over traditional rubber-cup polishing

PROCEDURE 32.1 Rubber-Cup Polishing

Equipment

Safety glasses for patient

Personal protective equipment (PPE)

Polishing paste, esthetic restoration polishing paste, and low-abrasive tooth-paste

Prophylaxis angle and toothbrush

Low-speed handpiece

Rubber cups and pointed bristle brushes

Mouth mirror and air-water syringe

Saliva ejector or high-volume evacuation (HVE) tip

Dental floss or tape

Floss threader (if needed)

Gauze squares

Disclosing solution (optional)

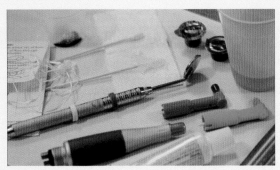

Rubber-cup polishing tray setup. (Dental hygiene procedures videos, St Louis, 2015, Saunders.)

Steps

Preparation and Positioning

1. Evaluate patient's health and pharmacologic history to determine need for precautions or treatment alterations.
2. Identify tooth surfaces indicated and contraindicated for polishing. Always polish esthetic restorations first and then polish teeth.
3. Educate patient about tooth stains, polishing procedure, and stain prevention (as needed).
4. Select polishing abrasive, based on type of stain and oral restorations, and assemble basic setup.
5. Wear appropriate PPE and provide protective eyewear for patient.
6. Have patient tilt the head up and turn slightly away when polishing maxillary and mandibular right buccal surfaces of posterior teeth (left buccal surfaces if practitioner is left-handed), and maxillary and mandibular left lingual surfaces of posterior teeth (right lingual surfaces if practitioner is left-handed).

Grasp

7. Use modified pen grasp (see Fig. 32.3).
8. Rest handpiece in V of hand.
9. Have all fingers in contact as a unit.

Fulcrum

10. Establish fulcrum close to working area.
11. Place fulcrum on ring finger.
12. Use moderate fulcrum pressure.

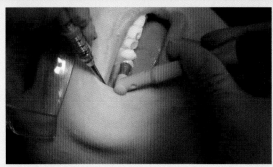

Rubber polishing cup adaptation technique. (Dental hygiene procedures videos, St Louis, 2015, Saunders.)

Adaptation

13. Angle rubber cup to flare at gingival margin and interproximally.
14. Adapt rubber cup to reach distal, facial, and lingual or mesial surfaces.
15. Adapt cup to each tooth by rotating handpiece or pivoting on fulcrum as necessary.
16. Adapt brush to occlusal surface.

Stroke

17. Fill cup with paste and apply evenly to surfaces to be polished.
18. Place cup on tooth; activate handpiece by gently stepping on rheostat. Stroke from the gingival third to the incisal third with just enough pressure to make the cup flare while using wrist-forearm motion to polish the teeth.
19. Use low speed and intermittent dabbing overlapping strokes with light-to-moderate pressure in a cervical-to-occlusal or incisal direction (see Fig. 32.4).
20. Remove rubber cup from tooth at completion of stroke; readapt cup for next stroke.
21. Hold mirror in nondominant hand to retract buccal mucosa. Instruct patient to close mouth halfway and tilt head slightly toward the ceiling. Polish buccal surfaces of maxillary right posterior quadrant.
22. Polish teeth systematically as indicated. Begin with restorations needing polishing. Then polish facial surfaces of maxillary teeth, lingual surfaces of maxillary teeth, buccal surfaces of mandibular teeth, and lingual surfaces of mandibular teeth needing coronal polishing.
23. Rinse patient's teeth as indicated, based on presence of prophylaxis paste.
24. Floss patient's teeth with abrasive agent still on teeth, then rinse.

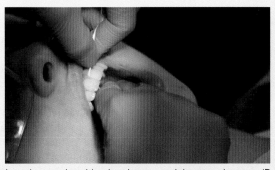

Flossing the teeth with abrasives remaining to cleanse. (Dental hygiene procedures videos, St Louis, 2015, Saunders.)

Continued

PROCEDURE 32.1   Rubber-Cup Polishing—cont'd

25. Apply fluoride therapy, if indicated (see Chapter 19).

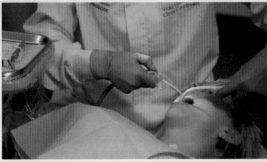

Rinsing the teeth to remove abrasive particles. (Dental hygiene procedures videos, St Louis, 2015, Saunders.)

26. Document completion of service in record under "Services Rendered," and date the entry (e.g., "Removed tobacco stain with rubber-cup polishing on No. 6-11 L, 22-27 F and L; patient removed oral biofilm from remaining teeth with a soft toothbrush and fluoride gel toothpaste. Flossed all teeth. Applied fluoride varnish. Advised patient to avoid hot foods or beverages for 4 to 6 hours.").

BOX 32.3   Legal, Ethical, and Safety Issues Related to Tooth Polishing

1. Nonmaleficence requires that all recommended guidelines on the safe use of rubber-cup air polishing and tooth bleaching must be followed to minimize patient risk for possible damage to teeth, restorations, and soft tissues.
2. Patients have the right to autonomy, so they must be informed of and consent to procedures that may harm tooth structure, oral soft tissues, and restorations before performing these procedures.
3. Employ risk management strategies for treating medically compromised or immunocompromised patients must be followed for air polishing.
4. State statutes specifying the laws governing polishing teeth by allied dental personnel must be followed. Delegation of extrinsic stain removal procedures to dental assistants in states where assistants are not legally allowed to perform them is illegal. An ethical issue arises when delegation to dental assistants is legal but a lack of background knowledge or skill exists.
5. Adhere to state statutes regarding the dental hygienist's role in in-home or in-office bleaching procedures.
6. Provide information about tooth staining prevention for beneficent care and patient autonomy.
7. Document procedures and patient recommendations or goals as legally required.

BOX 32.4   Critical Thinking Scenario B

Ethics

Your schedule is overly full and you are behind schedule. Your midafternoon patient has heavy stain generalized with moderate supragingival and subgingival calculus on the lingual surfaces of all mandibular teeth and the buccal surfaces of maxillary molars. You use ultrasonic instrumentation for deposit and stain removal, but some tenacious stain remains. As you are preparing for tooth polishing, the receptionist notifies you that your next patient has arrived. There is coarse prophylaxis paste in your drawer that would facilitate its removal, but you do not have time to follow up with medium and fine grit pastes. The dental assistant offers to polish for you. Although this procedure is legal in your state, you know she has not had formal training in this procedure. You want to do your best to avoid excessive wait time for the next patient and provide the highest quality service for this patient. What is your most ethical pathway? Why is that the best decision, given the circumstances?

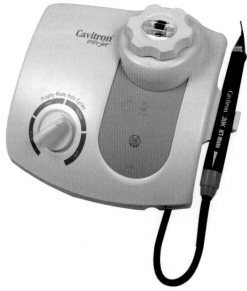

Fig. 32.5 Prophy-Jet and ultrasonic scaler. (Courtesy DENTSPLY Preventive Care Division, York, PA.)

Therapeutic Effect

Subgingival polishing with glycine powder has multiple benefits. Research on subgingival air polishing with glycine powder has suggested that it is as effective as or more effective than traditional hand

methods. It requires less time than traditional polishing when used supragingivally, removes stain three times as fast as hand scaling, and creates less operator fatigue. Air polishing also is preferred for cleaning and removing extrinsic stain from pits and fissures before placing dental sealants.

Air polishing can be performed supragingivally to remove stain and biofilm but also subgingivally to remove biofilm with a low abrasive prophy powder such as glycine.[6] See Procedure 32.2 for details of air polishing using the following three types of techniques:
- **Supragingival:** with a standard air-polishing handpiece to remove stain and biofilm
- **Shallow subgingival (up to 4 mm):** with a standard handpiece using glycine or erythritol powders and angled toward the sulcus for biofilm removal
- **Subgingival (probing depths of up to 9 mm):** with a subgingival nozzle using glycine or erythritol powder

Although polishing typically occurs after hard deposit removal, subgingival air polishing is recommended prior to hard deposit removal.[7]

PROCEDURE 32.2 Air-Polishing Techniques

Equipment

Appropriate air-polishing powder and low-abrasive prophy powder
Appropriate air-polisher device and nozzle and toothbrush
Dental floss or tape
Mouth mirror, air-water syringe
Disclosing solution
Lubricant for patient's lips
Saliva ejector and high-volume evacuation (HVE) tip
Safety glasses for patient
Personal protective equipment (PPE)

Steps

Preparation and Positioning

1. Evaluate patient's health and pharmacologic history to determine need for antibiotic premedication and contraindications to air polishing.
2. Identify tooth surfaces and restorations indicated and contraindicated for polishing and agents to be used.
3. Educate patient about air-polishing procedure.
4. Assemble high-speed evacuation and saliva ejector.
5. Verify that slurry exits from device tip when held outside the mouth; adjust saliva ejector as necessary.
6. Use appropriate PPE, and provide protective eyewear for patient.
7. Clinician, patient, and equipment must be in appropriate position for each area.

Grasp

8. Use modified pen grasp.
9. Rest handpiece in V of hand.
10. Have all fingers in contact as a unit.
11. Tuck excess cord around pinkie finger, if desired.

Fulcrum

12. Use external soft tissue fulcrums.

Select and Implement the Appropriate Adaptation and Step From the Following Three Techniques and Devices:

Adaptation and Stroke for Supragingival Polishing With DENTSPLY Cavitron Prophy-Jet

13. Activate foot pedal per manufacturer's instructions for appropriate combined air-water-powder spray.
14. At about 3 to 4 mm from tooth surface and at correct angulation, use constant circular sweeping motions, from proximal to proximal; pivot nozzle to surface being polished; polish several teeth for 1 to 2 seconds each and rinse. Surfaces without stain are cleaned with a toothbrush and low-abrasive toothpaste.

Adaptation and Stroke for Shallow Subgingival Polishing With Hu-Friedy/EMS Air-Flow Standard Handpiece (1 to 4 mm)

13. Activate foot pedal per manufacturer's instructions for appropriate combined air-water-powder spray.
14. At 3 mm from tooth surface and at 45° angulation to the gingival margin, use a constant half-circle "smiley face" motion, from proximal to proximal, moving incisally for 3 to 5 seconds per tooth.

Adaptation and Stroke for Subgingival Polishing With Hu-Friedy/EMS Air-Flow With Subgingival Nozzle (up to 9 mm)

13. Insert tip of nozzle into the depth of pocket; pull nozzle 1 mm from base.
14. Activate foot pedal per manufacturer's instructions for appropriate combined air-water-powder spray; move nozzle in continuous vertical motion for 5 seconds until nozzle is removed from pocket. Remove calculus with power and hand scaling.
    - **Note:** Check your applicable regulations. At the time of publication, the US Food and Drug Administration has approved the subgingival nozzle for up to 5 mm in the United States, and Health Canada has approved it for up to 9 mm in Canada.

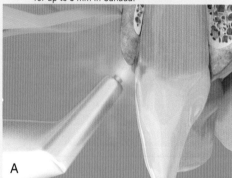

A

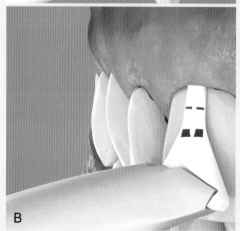

B

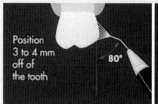
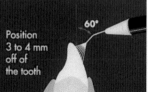
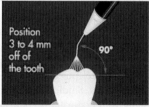

Recommended angulations of Prophy-Jet nozzle to tooth surface. (Adapted from DENTSPLY Preventive Care Division, York, PA.)

Continued

PROCEDURE 32.2   Air-Polishing Techniques—cont'd

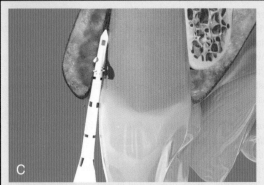

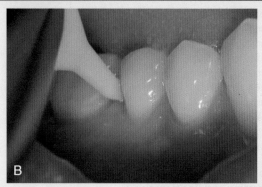

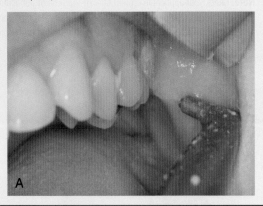

Subgingival air flow therapy with standard nozzle (A) and subgingival nozzle illustrations (B-C). (Courtesy Electro Medical Systems Corporation Dallas, TX.)

Subgingival air flow therapy with standard nozzle (A) and subgingival nozzle (B) intraoral photographs. (Courtesy I-Chung [Johnny] Wang)

Other

15. Rinse with water; floss all teeth (or have patient do so and evaluate their flossing technique).
16. Evaluate effectiveness with disclosing solution, compressed air, and good lighting.
17. Provide professionally applied topical fluoride treatment as indicated.
18. Dispose of single-use items according to federal, state, and local regulations.
19. Properly disinfect and sterilize all other equipment.
20. Document completion of service in patient's record under "Services Rendered" and date the entry (e.g., "Removed tobacco stain with supragingival air polishing using glycine powder on No. 6-11L, 22-27L; removed patient oral biofilm from remaining teeth with a soft toothbrush and fluoride toothpaste. Flossed all teeth. Applied fluoride varnish. Advised patient to avoid hot foods or beverages for 4 to 6 hours.").

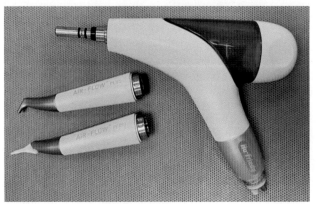

Fig. 32.6 Air polishing handpiece and nozzles. (Courtesy Lauren DeSantis.)

and ultrasonic instrumentation at removing biofilm up to 4 mm with a standard handpiece and up to 9 mm with a subgingival nozzle. It is also less damaging to the root surfaces than those therapies.[8,9] Subgingival air polishing with glycine can disrupt biofilms and improve outcomes when used in peri-implant mucositis and peri-implantitis treatment (see Chapter 31 for further discussion on implants).[10] Subgingival air polishing with erythritol powder also shows promising antibacterial and therapeutic effects. Studies have suggested that the effectiveness of air polishing with erythritol is comparable with that of mechanical debridement, is less damaging, and can be used as an adjunct during active periodontal therapy and as an alternative to conventional mechanical debridement during supportive periodontal

therapy.[7,11,12] It is reported that subgingival polishing with erythritol and glycine powder was tolerated by the patients better than hand or ultrasonic instrumentation.[7,12]

Choosing an Air-Polishing Device and Powder

Hygienists should identify the correct air-polishing device for the selected air-polishing powder; not all air-polishing devices can accommodate all powder options. Check with the manufacturer to determine the appropriate powders for the device selected for treatment. In addition, a special nozzle and handpiece are necessary for subgingival air polishing.[8]

For safe and effective air polishing, the dental hygienist must choose the appropriate prophy powder (Fig. 32.7). Powders indicated for supragingival use have particle shapes or hardness that make them effective at stain removal, but their abrasiveness contraindicates their use subgingivally. Subgingival powders are the least abrasive powders and are minimally abrasive to the root surface and dental materials. These powders are also appropriate for supragingival stain and biofilm removal. One disadvantage of using a minimally abrasive powder for supragingival stain removal is that it can take longer to achieve optimal stain removal on extensive stain as compared with the more abrasive powders. Any powder should be used for the minimum amount of time needed to achieve the desired result and prevent damage.[6,8] A summary of the available evidence on the powders follows.

Sodium bicarbonate:
- Is indicated for supragingival use.
- Is safe for use on orthodontic brackets.
- Causes significant surface defects in restorations.

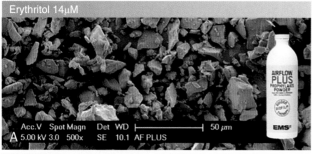

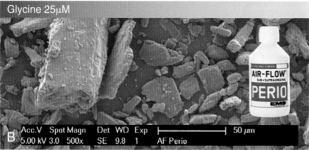

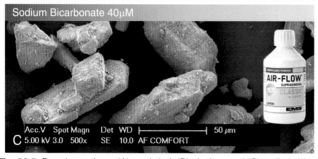

Fig. 32.7 Powder options: (A) erythritol, (B) glycine, and (C) sodium bicarbonate. (Courtesy Electro Medical Systems Corporation Dallas, TX.)

Calcium carbonate:
- Is indicated for supragingival use.
- Causes defects in intact enamel.
- Causes significant surface defects in restorations.
Aluminum trihydroxide:
- Is indicated for supragingival use.
- Is capable of causing defects in intact enamel.
- Causes significant surface defects in restorations.
Calcium sodium phosphosilicate:
- Is indicated for supragingival use.
- Is capable of causing defects in intact enamel.
- Causes significant surface defects in restorations.
- May help with dentinal sensitivity.
Glycine:
- Is indicated for supragingival and subgingival use.
- Is safe for use on the gingiva and mucosa.
- Is safe for use on implants.
- Is safe for orthodontic brackets.
- Is perceived to be more comfortable than other powders.[6,9]
Erythritol:
- Is indicated for supragingival and subgingival use.
- Is safe for use on implants.
- Is safe for orthodontic brackets.
- Is the least abrasive powder.
- Is perceived to be more comfortable than other powders.[8,13]

Effects on Oral and Dental Tissues

Currently, air polishing may be less damaging and a more efficient means of removing stain on enamel when compared with rubber-cup

polishing. Gingival bleeding and abrasion are the most common soft tissue effects of air polishing. These outcomes are temporary and healing occurs quickly. However, the tip of the air polisher should be pointed away from the gingiva to avoid tissue trauma when using sodium bicarbonate, calcium carbonate, aluminum trihydroxide, or calcium sodium phosphosilicate powders. Even with subgingival powders, 5 seconds of treatment per subgingival site and continuous movement are recommended to minimize damage to hard- and soft-dental tissues when using a subgingival nozzle (see Procedure 32.2).[8-10]

Patients report a salty taste when sodium bicarbonate prophy powder is used, but it is not objectionable if the water-to-powder ratio is adjusted properly. Laying a moist gauze square on the tongue may prevent tongue irritation and an excessively salty taste. Rinsing with water or mouthwash also helps reduce the salty taste. Another option is using a flavored powder or another type of powder.[6]

Effects on Restorations and Titanium Implants

The effects of air polishing on restorative materials have been researched extensively and continue to evolve. Air polishing with sodium bicarbonate, calcium carbonate, aluminum trihydroxide, or calcium sodium phosphosilicate powders resulted in significant surface defects in restorations comprised of various materials. Accordingly, extended use of air polishing on all restorative dental materials should be avoided. Except as noted above, avoid any air polishing on or near the following:
- Amalgam alloy and other metal restorations to prevent a matte finish, surface roughness, morphologic changes, and structural alterations
- Composite restorations to prevent surface roughness or pitting
- Porcelain, gold alloy, and glass ionomer restorations to prevent surface roughness, staining, pitting, and loss of marginal integrity[6,9]
- Dental implants, except with glycine or erythritol powder, which can be used safely on implant surfaces.

Research suggests that subgingival air polishing with glycine can disrupt biofilms and improve outcomes in peri-implant mucositis and peri-implantitis sites (see Chapter 31 for further discussion on implants).[10] Although recent research suggests that air polishing supragingivally with sodium bicarbonate powder does not seem to negatively affect the biocompatibility of titanium dental implant surfaces, these findings conflict with previous studies. Additional research is needed to confirm these recent findings and the clinical ramifications.[8,10,14]

Safety Issues

Literature identifies air-polishing safety concerns for the patient, hygienist, and others in the treatment area. Patient concerns include the following:
- Systemic problems from absorption of sodium bicarbonate prophy powder (other powders are an option for sodium-sensitive patients)
- Respiratory difficulties and potential for infection from inhaling contaminated aerosols, especially in patients with respiratory diseases
- Stinging of the lips from the concentrated spray
- Eye problems from spray entering the eyes, especially if contact lenses are worn (safety goggles are recommended)

These problems can be managed by coating a patient's lips with a protective lubricant, using appropriate technique including safety suction devices, removing contact lenses, wearing safety glasses, and placing a protective drape over the patient's nose and eyes.

It is important for the body to maintain a specific pH balance. Some individuals cannot adjust if this balance is disturbed. Due to the potential absorption of sodium bicarbonate by the oral mucosa, air-polisher manufacturers caution against using the sodium bicarbonate prophy powder during air polishing with such patients. Limited information is available on the systemic effects of prophy powder absorption from air-polishing powders.[6,8]

Because of the significant rise in aerosols generated with air polishing, additional health hazards can exist for patients and healthcare professionals present during or after a procedure. To decrease potential risks, hygienists should adhere to standard precautions, including the following:

- Wear appropriate PPE, including a well-fitting face mask with recommended bacterial filtration efficiency (BFE) scores of 74% to 98% (see Chapter 10).
- Use high-volume evacuation, which reduces aerosols more effectively than a saliva ejector.
- Disinfect contaminated surfaces as far away as 6 feet from the immediate treatment area to help prevent cross-contamination between patients. Contaminated surfaces, if not covered with disposable plastic drapes, should be cleaned and disinfected with an approved high-level surface disinfectant. To ensure safety of hygienists and patients, follow the Centers for Disease Control and Prevention (CDC) guidelines for infection control (see Chapter 10) for polishing procedures.
- Air polishing is included in the dental hygiene care plan only after a careful review of the patient's health and dental history and a thorough examination of the oral hard and soft tissues. A synopsis of the medical contraindications to air polishing can be found in Box 32.5.[6,8]

Air-Polishing Technique

Materials and sequence of steps for air polishing are outlined in Procedure 32.2, based on the manufacturer's guidelines for the device (e.g., Cavitron Prophy-Jet, DENTSPLY Preventive Care Division, York, PA; and Air-Flow, Hu-Friedy Mfg. Co., LLC, Chicago, IL/Electro Medical Systems Corporation, Dallas, TX). Manufacturers' directions should be followed for maintenance and care of equipment.

Client Education and Motivation

Before extrinsic stain removal procedures, the dental hygienist encourages patients to remove all visible plaque biofilm with assistance and a demonstration to improve awareness of the areas needing concentration during daily self-care practices. All patients with tooth stains can benefit from individualized education linking tooth stains with lifestyle, diet, and oral hygiene practices (Box 32.6) (Chapters 18 and 25).

Tooth stains often adhere to plaque biofilm and calculus deposits, so education regarding their prevention and control often is indicated when extrinsic stain is present on the teeth. There is strong evidence indicating that powered toothbrushes reduce plaque and gingivitis more than manual toothbrushing. Some evidence supports flossing in combination with toothbrushing for reducing gingivitis; however, interdental brushes are most effective for interproximal plaque biofilm removal when embrasure spaces allow for their use. Food choices; medications; chromogenic bacteria; and tobacco, marijuana, or betel nut or leaf use cause extrinsic stains on teeth, so discussing these choices and habits is important. A suggestion for more frequent visits for professional prophylaxis or periodontal maintenance might also be indicated. The use of goal setting, self-monitoring, and planning are effective interventions for improving oral hygiene and related behaviors.

INTRINSIC STAIN MANAGEMENT

Although intrinsic stains and discolorations incorporated within the tooth structure cannot be removed by scaling or polishing, they may

---

BOX 32.5   Medical Contraindications and Precautions to Air Polishing

- Low-sodium diet or history of hypertension (for sodium-containing prophy powder only)*
- Respiratory illness that limits swallowing or breathing
- Communicable disease that can be transmitted via contaminated aerosols
- Renal insufficiency or end-stage renal disease
- Immunocompromising conditions
- Addison disease
- Cushing disease
- Metabolic alkalosis†
- Medications such as mineralocorticoid steroids, antidiuretics, or potassium supplements†
- High-risk patients needing antibiotic premedication may have to be premedicated for air polishing.
- Patients wearing contact lenses should remove them first and wear safety glasses.

*Air polishing can be performed with sodium-free prophy powder.
†Precautions are needed, but these are not strict contraindications.

BOX 32.6   Patient Education Example: Stain Prevention

"I understand your concern about the color of your teeth. Of course, we will remove the stains from your teeth today by removing the soft plaque deposits and calcified deposits from your teeth, and we will use a paste to clean and polish your tooth surfaces afterward. I would like to make some suggestions to help you prevent these brown stains on your teeth in the future. Would you be interested in hearing about these options?" *(Client replies, "Yes.")*

"Stain often attaches to soft and hard deposits on the teeth, so some changes in your daily oral hygiene might help prevent staining. Research shows that power toothbrushes are more effective than manual toothbrushes. Have you tried one? *(A "no" response would indicate a recommendation.)* We also suggest you use something each day to clean between your teeth, primarily for prevention and control of gum disease. Would you like to review flossing or possibly consider a different device? *(Dialog continues after these questions are answered, based on client responses.)*

"Brown stains on the teeth are usually caused by foods or substances that would also stain your clothing, such as tobacco, marijuana, red wine, tea, coffee, soda, and some drugs like the active ingredient in your toothpaste. We can evaluate your toothpaste choice and make a recommendation. *(Client replies, "That would be great.")* Are there any other habits or substances that you suspect might be causing the stain on your teeth? *(Client reports, "I frequently drink tea.")* Well, you might consider less frequent tea exposures throughout the day or coming in for professional care more frequently for stain removal."

"When considering options for preventing stain, which daily self-care practices and/or other changes would seem realistic for you to try? *(Patient sets goals.)*

"Those goals are great. Try to keep track of your adherence to these changes and goals, and we will evaluate their impact on your tooth color next time you come for an appointment."

---

be managed by tooth whitening with a chemical oxidizing agent to lighten tooth discolorations or by restorative procedures. Recognition of intrinsic staining and appropriate treatment can address the patient's aesthetic goals. Intrinsic tooth stain severity and the patient's level of concern about tooth color and appearance usually determine which stain management method is recommended. These methods are discussed later in this chapter.

TOOTH WHITENING

Tooth whitening, also known as bleaching, is a viable alternative for stain management for intrinsic stains. Tooth whitening is a cosmetic procedure that uses a chemical oxidizing agent to lighten the tooth discoloration. Carbamide peroxide (most are 10% to 38% concentration but some can range up to 44%) and hydrogen peroxide (5% to 40% concentration) are two of the most common oxidizing agents used for tooth whitening.[2] Many techniques, ranging from over-the-counter (OTC) products to professionally dispensed whitening to in-office laser systems, are available and vary significantly in cost to the patient. In general, whitening products can be categorized as OTC home-use products, professionally dispensed home-use products, and professionally applied in-office products.

All whitening procedures must be approached with caution.[15–17] The dental hygienist must understand the processes involved in tooth whitening and educate the patient on the expectations and considerations of whitening prior to treatment. The dental hygienist's role is summarized in Box 32.7.

Over-the-Counter Home-Use Whitening Products

- A variety of OTC products are marketed and available directly to patients to whiten their teeth at home. Common products include toothpastes (see Chapter 26), mouthrinses (see Chapter 27), tray delivery options (see Fig. 32.8), whitening strips, and an increasing number of products available from nondental suppliers such as social media retailers, salons, and spas. Generally, OTC options have lower concentrations of whitening agents than products available to dental professionals. Some OTC whitening products have advantages over professionally supervised and dispensed products, and they can be less expensive and comparable in whitening efficacy to professionally dispensed products. Some OTC products are a cause for concern in terms of efficacy and safety due to the potential for overuse and abuse by uninformed patients.
- Some commercial whitening kits contain an oxidizing agent and materials to form a "boil and fit" mouth tray. The oxidizing gel may seep out of improperly fitted trays and harm soft tissues. Similarly, improperly placed whitening strips can cause gingival irritation.
- An acidic prerinse found in some kits can damage enamel.
- Patients may not know how to deal with side effects they may encounter (e.g., tooth sensitivity, gingival irritation). Patients with extreme tooth sensitivity are poor candidates for tooth whitening.
- Without a comprehensive oral examination to determine the etiology of the stain and the safest and most appropriate method to use in its treatment, patients may neglect to seek appropriate care for an undiagnosed oral problem. For example, a dark area on a tooth may be due to a carious lesion or a tooth in need of a root canal, and whitening would not remedy either situation. Encourage patients to seek professional advice to whiten teeth.[2,15,16]
- Some individuals seek advice regarding tooth whitening options from their primary care providers. Dental hygienists can enhance knowledge of other healthcare professionals about safe and effective OTC products and professionally administered tooth-whitening options. See Box 32.8 for an interprofessional education scenario.

Professionally Dispensed Home-Use Whitening Products

Professionally dispensed home-use whitening products include professional-strength whitening strips and tray delivery options, which

---

BOX 32.7 Dental Hygienist's Role in Tooth Whitening

- Assess the patient's oral self-care and provide patient education regarding bleaching.
- Recommend homecare to reduce dentinal hypersensitivity as needed (prophylactically and/or after treatment).
- Determine the cause of the stain and any allergies to ingredients in the bleaching agents.
- Assist the patient with setting realistic expectations (e.g., pretreatment and posttreatment comparisons using a shade guide, intraoral photographs, computer imaging, intraoral video camera).
- Assess for conditions that contraindicate bleaching (e.g., presence of gingival recession, extreme tooth sensitivity, tooth cracks [depending on their direction and depth]). Fiberoptics or an intraoral camera can verify and measure enamel cracks.
- Assess for any signs of caries or defective restorations that must be addressed before bleaching.
- Evaluate translucency of teeth for alternative whitening procedures; highly translucent teeth may appear more gray than white after bleaching.
- Use radiographs, percussion, thermal testing, and electrical pulp testing to help determine vitality, size of pulp, and the most appropriate method to meet patient needs.
- Remove soft and hard deposits before tooth-bleaching procedure.
- Take impressions, fabricate custom bleaching trays for home use, and provide instructions.
- If dental practice act permits, provide in-office bleaching.

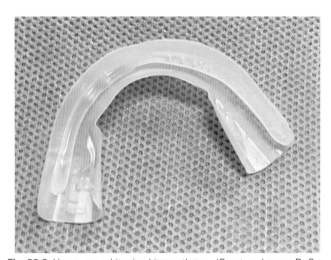

Fig. 32.8 Home-use whitening kit mouth tray. (Courtesy Lauren DeSantis.)

---

are similar to their OTC counterparts but with stronger concentrations of the whitening agent. Professional-strength whitening strips are available for patients to use at home. Alternatively, professional-strength tray delivery options commonly involve the in-office fabrication of a custom mouth tray (see Chapter 38), dispensing of the appropriate whitening agent, and patient education on home use with a prescribed frequency and time period. The dentist monitors the patient until the desired outcome is achieved. Home whitening with a custom-fitted tray and whitening agent is the superior tooth whitening method because of product innovations that control dentinal hypersensitivity and loss of enamel. It is lower in cost to the patient than in-office bleaching and it has the most scientific evidence supporting its effectiveness. It does require patient

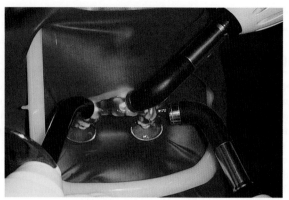

Fig. 32.9 In-office bleaching procedure with a rubber dam, bleaching gel, and a resin-curing light as the heat source. (From Hatrick CD, Eakle WS. *Dental Materials: Clinical Applications for Dental Assistants and Dental Hygienists.* 3rd ed. Elsevier; 2016.)

adherence to the protocol for a good outcome. In most cases, a thickened oxidizing agent, usually 10% to 38% carbamide peroxide, is loaded into a flexible polyvinyl, custom-made tray that the patient wears 2 to 10 hours a day or overnight for a 6- to 28-day period.[2,16]

Home whitening is effective in producing a lightened tooth surface, but patients should be informed that the degree of change, especially with tetracycline-stained teeth, may be unpredictable. Therefore, patient expectations must be clarified before any treatment. Patients need to know the following:

- Stains in the yellow-to-brown range respond better than stains in the blue-to-gray range.
- Teeth with horizontal bands or striations of various colors, as seen with tetracycline-stained teeth, may bleach at different rates, making enamel defects more noticeable.
- Although the teeth may look lighter, they may not necessarily be whiter, owing to their normal intrinsic tooth color.
- Tooth-colored restorations subjected to bleaching will not change color and may no longer match the color of the teeth after the bleaching procedure.
- Whitening is temporary and additional treatments may be necessary in 1 to 3 years, which carry a cost and time commitment for the patient. Longevity of whitening varies from patient to patient.
- The tooth surface becomes more porous with whitening and thus daily OTC fluoride toothpaste and mouthrinse or gel are recommended while using bleaching agents.[15]

PROFESSIONALLY APPLIED TOOTH WHITENING PROCEDURES

Professionally applied tooth whitening is any whitening procedure performed in the office by a dental professional. A variety of techniques exist for professionally applied tooth whitening and may differ based on a number of factors: etiology of the stain, tooth vitality, and the number of teeth needing the procedure (e.g., single tooth, multiple teeth, one arch, both arches). Office time involved, patient preference and compliance, cost, provider preference, and oral assessment findings are additional factors to consider when selecting the most appropriate procedure.

The techniques for professionally applied tooth whitening of vital teeth can be used individually or in combination with home whitening procedures to enhance the desired effect. For a nonvital tooth or teeth, the procedure is usually intracoronal and may be combined with one of the procedures indicated for vital teeth.[2]

In-Office Whitening Techniques

The exact technique for in-office whitening depends on the specific system used (Fig. 32.9 provides one example). Manufacturers of in-office

bleaching systems have specific instructions for using their products, which should always be followed. In general, the bleaching procedure for vital teeth involves the following:

- Protection of the patient's lips, eyes, clothing, and gingiva (with placement of a rubber dam) and/or protection of the gingival tissues (with a protective gel) is necessary.
- Teeth may or may not be etched before placing the bleaching agent. Although some manufacturers may recommend etching to enhance the whitening effect, etching has been reported to contribute to additional complications, including sensitivity and surface wear.[2]
- A gel, varnish, or liquid bleaching agent is applied to the enamel surface. If the liquid form is used, gauze squares saturated with the bleaching agent are placed on the facial surfaces. The bleaching agent is allowed to remain on the teeth for about 30 to 60 minutes. A heat source, visible light-curing lamp (resin curing light), plasma arc, light-emitting diode (LED), xenon-halide light, or laser may be applied to catalyze the oxidizing agent and accelerate the chemical reaction.[2,15,16] The value of the heat or light source has not been established in the literature.
- Local anesthesia must never be used during bleaching. Patient discomfort is monitored at all times to avoid tissue burns or excess heat buildup in the pulp. Analgesics may be recommended for the first 24 hours postoperatively if tooth sensitivity is experienced.
- At the end of the procedure, any excess bleaching agent should be removed with water before removing the rubber dam. Topical fluoride may be professionally applied or recommended for daily home use.

The in-office bleaching procedure lasts from 30 to 60 minutes and may involve 1 to 3 appointments at 2- to 4-week intervals until teeth sufficiently lighten or no further color change is noted. This time interval between appointments allows for pulpal irritation to subside. Patients should be informed that white spots on the tooth may become whiter and result in a blotchy appearance. If tooth-colored restorations are necessary, it is advisable to wait 2 to 3 weeks to determine the correct color shade. In addition, this waiting period can prevent failed restorations that are due to inadequate bond strength since resin bonds can be weakened significantly by tooth-whitening procedures.[2]

Intracoronal Bleaching

Intracoronal bleaching, a method of in-office bleaching, is used only for bleaching endodontically treated teeth. With both of the following techniques, the bleaching agent is placed within the tooth. To enhance the final effect, both nonvital bleaching methods may be combined with the professionally applied or in-home whitening methods for vital teeth:

- **Thermocatalytic:** In the thermocatalytic bleach method, the bleaching agent is usually 30% to 35% hydrogen peroxide, sodium perborate, or sodium hypochlorite. The agent is placed within the coronal portion of the pulp chamber with a cotton pellet after the cervical portion has been sealed with zinc phosphate or zinc oxide–eugenol cement to prevent penetration of the bleaching agent into the dentinal tubules and the possibility of cervical resorption. Heat (e.g., heat lamp, heated instrument, electric heating device, ultraviolet light) is applied to hasten the reaction.

- **Walking:** In the walking bleach method, a paste of sodium perborate and hydrogen peroxide is placed in the coronal portion of the pulp chamber, the tooth is sealed, and the patient is seen again in a week. At that time, the paste may be reapplied if further alteration in color is necessary. Often only a small amount of color change can be achieved, but it may be sufficient to satisfy the patient. This procedure is technique sensitive; failure to follow exact protocols may result in severe pain during or after the procedure. If the cervical area is not sealed well, cervical resorption may occur.[2]

Microabrasion

Microabrasion is a procedure that removes superficial dark stains or mineralized white spots of enamel. It is more effective on mild stains than in moderate or severe cases. This procedure involves removal of a thin layer of enamel and uses a paste of abrasives and hydrochloric acid on a specially designed prophy angle attachment. Some commercially prepackaged kits are available. Although considered effective, this procedure is technique sensitive, may require multiple applications of the abrasive paste and hydrochloric acid, and removes some tooth structure. Burns, sensitivity, pulpal damage, and noticeable removal of the outermost fluoride-rich layer of tooth enamel can occur. It is sometimes difficult for the dentist to determine the exact amount of enamel to remove, and a restorative procedure may be needed if the stain is deep. Long-term studies are not available. Home-use bleaching products may be recommended after microabrasion to enhance whitening.

SIDE EFFECTS OF TOOTH WHITENING

Short-term side effects are usually minimal and disappear at the end of treatment. The most common side effects are mild thermal tooth sensitivity and gingival irritation. Reversible pulpitis can occur due to the easy passage of the hydrogen peroxide through the enamel and dentin to the pulp, resulting in temporary tooth sensitivity.[15,16] Using a prescription, self-applied fluoride gel or mouthrinse and a shortened bleaching exposure time may decrease sensitivity. Patients with recession should not have bleaching because of the possibility of exposed dentin, which provides the hydrogen peroxide a direct route to the pulp. Approximately 10% of the population exhibits a gap between the cementum and the enamel, leaving exposed dentinal tubules that can lead to extreme sensitivity. Gingival irritation may occur if the bleaching tray is overfilled or improperly fitted or if the whitening strips are improperly placed. Using a syringe dosage system, a highly viscous gel, a properly fitted tray, or properly placed whitening strips can prevent excess material from coming into contact with the gingiva.

Occasionally, sore throats, tooth pain, tingling of tissues, and headaches are reported as side effects of tooth whitening. Slight morphologic changes in the enamel have also been noted with vital bleaching gels. Research, however, showed that 10% carbamide peroxide did not significantly alter enamel microhardness.[15,16] Although localized microstructural and chemical changes were seen, they were not clinically significant. However, long-term overuse of whitening products can decrease enamel hardness.

Although wide variations in data exist concerning composite restorations, some composites may be more susceptible to alterations, and some high-concentration bleaching agents are more likely to cause these alterations. These changes, however, are unlikely to be clinically significant. No effects on porcelain or ceramic materials have been reported. Whitening of teeth containing amalgam restorations is not contraindicated but should be approached with caution because some changes in amalgam have been noted.

Another possible side effect involves the temporomandibular joint (TMJ). When fabricating the bleaching tray, a thin material should be used to avoid interference with the patient's occlusion. No long-term systemic effects have been identified.[15,16] Box 32.9 provides a complete list of contraindications.

In addition to the general side effects, professionally applied tooth whitening procedures carry additional potential side effects due to the concentration of the whitening agent and the application of a catalyst. Gingival burns and tooth sensitivity can occur. While reversible pulpitis can occur during whitening, the pain resolves as the whitening is discontinued and the inflammation subsides. The use of the light as a catalyst may cause significant photosensitivity and hyperpigmentation in persons taking acne medication, antidepressants, anticancer drugs, antipsychotics, diuretics, hypoglycemics, and nonsteroidal antiinflammatory drugs (NSAIDs). Skin should be shielded for these patients.

RESTORATIVE MANAGEMENT OF STAINED TEETH

Deep stains, mottled or pitted teeth, and grayish-blue stains may need restorative procedures by the dentist, such as composite bonding, veneers, or full crowns to provide the patient with a more aesthetic appearance than can be achieved by whitening or microabrasion. All whitening of teeth should be done before restorative procedures to ensure that crowns, bondings, and veneers will match the new enamel shade. Although these procedures can achieve the patient's goals, restorative procedures are typically not recommended just to make teeth whiter. They involve the removal of tooth structure and should be considered on a case-by-case basis only after normal conservative methods have been deemed ineffective or inappropriate (see Chapter 39).

LEGAL AND ETHICAL ASPECTS OF TOOTH WHITENING AND INTRINSIC STAIN MANAGEMENT

The dental or dental hygiene practice act, rules, and regulations in each jurisdiction determine the extent of the dental hygienist's legal involvement in whitening or restorative services and should be consulted before any clinical whitening service is provided. If the whitening system is defined as a topical medication under the dental practice act, then dental hygienists may, in some states, provide in-office whitening.

BOX 32.9 Contraindications to Tooth Whitening[2,16,18]

- Pregnant or nursing*
- Allergy to any of the ingredients
- Medications that cause photosensitivity or hyperpigmentation (important if a light will be used as a catalyst)
- Large, defective restorations (should be replaced before bleaching)
- Gingival, periodontal, or mucosal conditions that could be irritated by using a bleaching tray or rubber dam
- Inability to provide informed consent or follow instructions
- Recession†
- Cervical erosion†
- Enamel cracks†
- Tooth sensitivity†
- Dental caries†

*No research is available on these population groups because they generally are not used as research participants.
†Tooth sensitivity may increase.

BOX 32.10 Critical Thinking Scenario C

Tooth Whitening

Mr. Jones, age 58, comes to the office as a new patient. His medical and dental history indicates that he has not received dental care in several years but he lists his chief complaint as "I want whiter teeth." An examination reveals that Mr. Jones has multiple carious lesions, generalized heavy subgingival calculus, and generalized inflammation that will require multiple appointments to resolve. He has generalized heavy biofilm and extrinsic stain. He reports that he quit smoking last year after a cancer scare and continues daily coffee consumption. He is attending a class reunion in 2 months and wants to have a nice, white smile. He reports running daily and prides himself on being a fit individual. He is well groomed and works in sales.

Hygienist: Mr. Jones, you have several restorative needs and periodontal problems that need to be addressed before your teeth can be whitened.

Patient: OK. The cleaning today will take care of that, right? How long will it take to whiten my teeth? I was hoping to have that done today.

Hygienist: Mr. Jones, you are not a candidate to whiten your teeth at this point, but we will do everything we can, with your consent, when the dentist discusses your restorative treatment plan to facilitate your goal before your reunion. We want you to look your best.

Patient: Can I just use the whitening strips I can get at the drugstore?

Questions

What could you do to enhance this patient's understanding of his treatment needs (e.g., provide individualized education; start a discussion about your findings; show examples in his own mouth; discuss how your goals both align health and esthetics and propose a plan to meet them; explain how stabilizing oral health will help meet esthetic goals; explain why oral health needs are stabilized before initiation of whitening)?

How can you motivate Mr. Jones in the short and long term? Role play a dialog to focus on the items he values—health and appearance—and apply to his current dental needs; explain how oral systemic health is related.

Some state dental practice acts specifically state that only licensed dentists may use a laser in connection with a whitening process.

Tooth whitening and stain management options, including risks and benefits of each method that is appropriate, should be discussed with the patient. Patients must be informed and able to make autonomous decisions about their healthcare under professional ethics standards. Box 32.10 provides a Critical Thinking Scenario regarding dilemmas that can be faced when patients with a high-level oral health need tooth whitening.

KEY CONCEPTS

- Select rubber-cup polishing, air polishing, and bleaching based on patient needs and goals.
- Although not a pathologic concern, tooth stain is a cosmetic concern.
- Selective polishing is the practice of limiting polishing procedures to only those tooth surfaces with stain, avoiding newly erupted teeth, cementum, dentin, demineralized areas, and restored tooth surfaces that could be damaged by the process.
- Subgingival air polishing with glycine powder offers a therapeutic benefit to the treatment of patients with periodontal diseases and implants.
- Knowledge of the indications, contraindications, and various in-home and in-office techniques for esthetic management of extrinsic and intrinsic stains is essential for patient education.
- For tooth stain removal and management, the dental hygienist must use the least abrasive and most effective technique and product to achieve the desired clinical outcome.

ACKNOWLEDGMENT

The authors acknowledge Marylou E. Gutmann, Michele Darby, Margaret Walsh, and Denise M. Bowen for their past contributions to this chapter.

EVOLVE RESOURCES

Please visit http://evolve.elsevier.com/Pieren/hygiene/ for additional practice and study support tools.

REFERENCES

1. Sawai MA, Bhardwaj A, Jafri A, et al. Tooth polishing: the current status. *J Indian Soc Periodontol*. 2015;19(4):375–380.
2. Eakle WS, Bastin KG. *Dental Materials: Clinical Applications for Dental Assistants and Dental Hygienists*. 4th ed. Elsevier; 2021.
3. Combined products. Jurisdictional Update: dental prophylaxis pastes with drug components. Federal drug Administration.gov. Available at: https://www.fda.gov/combination-products/jurisdictional-updates/jurisdictional-update-dental-prophylaxis-pastes-drug-components; 2018. Accessed February 28, 2023.
4. Barnes CM. Follow the evidence: evidence-based polishing protocols. *Dimens Dent Hyg*. 2015;13(11). 36, 38.
5. Schwarz F, Becker K, Sager M. Efficacy of professionally administered plaque removal with or without adjunctive measures for the treatment of peri-implant mucositis. A systematic review and meta-analysis. *J Clin Periodontol*. 2015;42(suppl 16):S202–S213.
6. Graumann SJ, Sensat ML, Stoltenberg JL. Air polishing: a review of current literature. *J Dent Hyg*. 2013;87(4):173–180.
7. Shrivastava D, Natoli V, Srivastava KC, et al. Novel approach to dental biofilm management through Guided Biofilm Therapy (GBT): a review. *Microorganisms [Internet] 2021*. 1966;9(9). https://doi.org/10.3390/microorganisms9091966.
8. Rothen M. The tipping point for air polishing. *Dimens Dent Hyg*. 2016;14(10):30. 32, 35.
9. Cobb CM, Daubert DM, Davis K, et al. Consensus conference findings on supragingival and subgingival air polishing. *Compend Contin Educ Dent*. 2017;38(2):e1.
10. Schwarz F, Becker K, Bastendorf KD, et al. Recommendations on the clinical application of air polishing for the management of peri-implant mucositis and peri-implantitis. *Quintessence Int*. 2016;47(4):293–296.
11. Sultan DA, Hill RG, Gillam DG. Air-polishing in subgingival root debridement: a critical literature review. *J Dent Oral Biol*. 2017;2(10):1–7.
12. Abdulbaqi HR, Shaikh MS, Abdulkareem AA, Zafar MS, Gul SS, Sha AM. Efficacy of erythritol powder air-polishing in active and supportive periodontal therapy: a systematic review and meta-analysis. *Int J Dent Hygiene*. 2022;20:62–74. Available from: https://onlinelibrary.wiley.com/doi/abs/10.1111/idh.12539.
13. Bühler J, Amato M, Weiger R, et al. A systematic review on the patient perception of periodontal treatment using air polishing devices. *Int J Dent Hyg*. 2016;14(1):4–14.
14. Louropoulou A, Slot DE, Van der Weijden F. Influence of mechanical instruments on the biocompatibility of titanium dental implants surfaces: a systematic review. *Clin Oral Implants Res*. 2015;26(7):841–850.
15. Kwon SR, Wertz PW. Review of the mechanism of tooth whitening. *J Esthet Restor Dent*. 2015;27(5):240–257.
16. American Dental Association (ADA). *Whitening*. Available from: www.ada.org/resources/research/science-and-research-institute/oral-health-topics/whitening; Accessed February 28, 2023.
17. Irusa K, Abd Alrahaem I, Ngoc CN, Donovan T. Tooth whitening procedures: a narrative review. *Dentistry Review*. 2022:100055. Available at: https://www.sciencedirect.com/science/article/pii/S2772559622000207.
18. American Academy of Pediatric Dentistry. *Policy on the Use of Dental Bleaching for Child and Adolescent Patients. The Reference Manual of Pediatric Dentistry*. American Academy of Pediatric Dentistry; 2022:127–130.

33

Decision Making Related to Nonsurgical Periodontal Therapy

Kathleen O. Hodges

PROFESSIONAL OPPORTUNITIES

The provision of nonsurgical periodontal therapy (NSPT) is part of every dental hygiene practitioner's responsibility to patients. Efficacious delivery of NSPT is the cornerstone of quality periodontal therapy for patients with gingivitis or periodontitis. The dental hygienist has the opportunity to provide advice about person-centered self-care in combination with professional periodontal debridement and adjunct therapies to aid in restoring health to the periodontium.

COMPETENCIES

1. Compare and contrast concepts of dental hygiene care for patients with various classifications of periodontal health and disease, including scaling, oral prophylaxis, root planing, periodontal debridement, host modulation therapy, and therapeutic endpoints.
2. Describe the assessment, diagnosis, and care planning involved with NSPT.
3. Detail the current classifications of periodontal diseases and discuss how each classification might progress and respond to NSPT given risk factors, systemic health, self-care, and adherence to periodontal maintenance recommendations.
4. Discuss oral hygiene instructions for self-care.
5. Describe the process of appointment planning for NSPT and plan implementation of nonsurgical periodontal therapy, including mechanical nonsurgical pocket therapy, chemotherapy for periodontal diseases, and/or full mouth disinfection.
6. List the reasons a patient may need a referral to a periodontist and discuss surgical intervention. Also, discuss the rationale and procedure for reevaluation following NSPT and its relationship to the decision regarding followup care including possible referrals.
7. Explain how dental insurance benefit plans relate to case presentations and implementation of nonsurgical periodontal therapy.
8. Consider factors that influence decisions regarding periodontal maintenance therapy and suggest appropriate intervals based on individual patient needs.

BASIC CONCEPTS IN NONSURGICAL PERIODONTAL THERAPY

Nonsurgical periodontal therapy (NSPT) encompasses the control of oral biofilm through self-care and professional periodontal debridement (scaling and root planing), supplemented by adjunctive therapy with antimicrobials or host modulation agents as needed, for the treatment of periodontal diseases involving natural teeth and implant replacements. The aim is to attain periodontal health in the least invasive and most cost-effective manner, and NSPT is often the means used to accomplish this objective. Health is assessed by evaluating clinical parameters including bleeding on probing for no/minimal presence, erythema and edema, or suppuration (see Chapter 20).

The goals of periodontal therapy follow:
- To preserve, maintain, and improve the natural dentition, implants, periodontium, and peri-implant tissues.
- To achieve health, comfort, aesthetics, and function.

Oral biofilm disruption or removal alone will not resolve inflammation in all cases. Supragingival biofilm control alone will not control microorganisms in periodontal and peri-implant disease, especially in the presence of periodontal pockets. Therefore self-care for supragingival and subgingival biofilm disruption and control must occur simultaneously with professional therapy to enhance the outcomes of NSPT. For more involved cases in which NSPT does not resolve the disease process and achieve health, periodontal surgery is recommended. For this reason, NSPT also is called *phase I of periodontal therapy* or *initial therapy* (see Chapter 23).

The purposes of NSPT are as follows:
- Eliminating or suppressing infectious microorganisms
- Eliminating or controlling infection to prevent reinfection
- Establishing an environment that helps resolve inflammation
- Modifying host and environmental risk factors for periodontal diseases
- Employing antimicrobial agents when indicated (see Chapter 27)

Scaling—the instrumentation of the crown and root to remove oral biofilm, calculus, and stains—is the procedure indicated for the treatment of patients with healthy gingiva or gingivitis.

Oral prophylaxis combines both supragingival and subgingival scaling with stain and biofilm removal. This procedure is preventive in nature, not therapeutic, as is NSPT. The dental hygienist performs oral prophylaxis for patients diagnosed with periodontal health- or biofilm-induced gingivitis. See Box 33.1 for a reminder about ethics, legality, and safety in regard to providing oral prophylaxis.

Scaling and root planing (SRP) is a definitive procedure to remove cementum or surface dentin characterized by roughness related to subgingival deposits or impregnated with calculus, thus contaminated with toxins or microorganisms. The objective of therapeutic SRP is to remove as little root structure as possible to return adjacent tissues to health.

Periodontal debridement is the removal of all subgingival oral biofilm and its byproducts, biofilm retentive factors, and calculus-embedded cementum during instrumentation while preserving as much tooth surface as possible. Biofilm retentive factors include calculus and overhangs that are clinically detectable, whereas calculus-embedded cementum can only be evaluated through clinical detection as well. Other terms for periodontal debridement include root debridement and subgingival debridement. This intervention focuses on the removal of all biofilm retentive factors while preserving tooth structure and using judgment with regard to root roughness; therefore the evaluation of healing 4 to 6 weeks after debridement is critical. Because oral biofilm is a primary causative factor for inflammatory forms of periodontal diseases, gingivitis, periodontitis, implant perimucositis, or peri-implantitis, subgingival plaque biofilm removal is essential. The removal of calculus is important because calculus is a risk factor for periodontal diseases, particularly in relation to its oral biofilm retentive nature.

Periodontal debridement strives to achieve tissue healing with minimal iatrogenic damage (e.g., damage from professional treatment) to the soft tissue and the cementum. In addition to periodontal debridement, antimicrobial agents (via local delivery such as in dentifrices and mouthrinses, controlled-release drug delivery, or systemic delivery) are adjuncts used to suppress infectious microorganisms and inflammation (see Chapter 27).

Host modulation therapy targets the host's role in host-bacteria interactions primarily involving the destruction of connective tissue in the gingiva, the periodontal ligament, and the alveolar bone in a periodontal pocket during the development and progression of periodontal disease.

The **therapeutic endpoint** is the restoration of gingival health, a reduction in pocket depth, and a gain in or maintenance of a stable clinical attachment level. These parameters occur only after a 4- to 6-week healing interval after successful periodontal therapy. This appointment, called **periodontal reevaluation**, is scheduled to reassess the clinical parameters of health after NSPT. Without a reevaluation visit, assessment and documentation of the therapeutic endpoint of active therapy cannot take place. An alternative approach is to evaluate the therapeutic endpoint 4 to 6 weeks post therapy in a segment of the mouth (e.g., a quadrant or half of the mouth) during appointments for treatment of new segments.

Assessment, Diagnosis, and Care Planning

For a discussion of periodontal assessment, see Chapter 20. A comprehensive evaluation and risk assessment should occur after initial therapy and *at least* annually. Decisions about frequency are based on the assessment of disease extent, the stability or progression of the condition, the patient's oral self-care practices, risk factors (e.g., systemic health), and the host response to therapy.

The **periodontal diagnosis** is determined after analyzing information collected during the assessment phase of therapy. To classify periodontal disease on the natural dentition, the practitioner first differentiates between gingival disease and more advanced forms, such as periodontitis, which are largely determined based on clinical features, severity (the amount of clinical attachment/bone loss/tooth loss), complexity (probing depth and type of bone loss), and extent (localized, generalized, molar/incisor pattern), among other factors (see Chapter 20).[1,2] Patients may simultaneously have areas of health, gingivitis (on an intact or reduced periodontium), and periodontitis with initial, moderate, severe, or advanced destruction (staging I to IV) that is slowly, moderately, or rapidly progressing (grading A, B, C).[1,2] See Table 33.1 for a review of staging and Table 33.2 for a review of grading of periodontitis.[3] The periodontal diagnosis might also include differentiation of health or disease around implants (peri-implant mucositis or peri-implantitis).[4] In addition, other conditions may exist, such as acute gingival infection, a periodontal abscess, or systemic diseases that often require specific knowledge for appropriate care by the clinician. The periodontal diagnosis is dynamic and can change over time based on clinical assessment, treatment, risk/modifying factors, and outcomes.

Periodontal diagnosis is a part of the dental hygiene diagnosis (see Chapter 22). NSPT relates to a variety of unmet human needs, but the

TABLE 33.1   Periodontitis Staging[3]

Periodontitis Stage**	Severity Interdental CAL at Site of Greatest Loss	Severity Radiographic Bone Loss	Severity Tooth Loss	Complexity Local
Stage I	1 to 2 mm	Coronal third (less than 15%)	None due to periodontitis	*Maximum probing depth 4 mm or less *Mostly horizontal bone loss
Stage II	3 to 4 mm	Coronal third (15% to 33%)	None due to periodontitis	*Maximum probing depth 5 mm or less *Mostly horizontal bone loss
Stage III	5 mm or greater	Extending to midthird of root and beyond (greater than 33%)	Four or fewer due to periodontitis	In addition to stage 2 complexity: *Probing depth 6 mm or greater *Vertical bone loss 3 mm or greater *Class II or III furcation involvement *Moderate ridge defect
Stage IV	5 mm or greater	Extending to midthird of root and beyond (greater than 33%)	Five or more due to periodontitis	In addition to stage 3 complexity: Complex rehabilitation needed due to: *Masticatory dysfunction *Secondary occlusal trauma (Mobility degree 2 or greater) *Severe ridge defect *Bite collapse, drifting, flaring *Fewer than 20 teeth (10 opposing pairs)

**Extent and Distribution—Add to stage as descriptor: describe extent as localized (fewer than 30% of teeth involved), generalized, or molar/incisor pattern.

TABLE 33.2   Periodontitis Grading[3]

Periodontitis Grade	Primary Criteria	Primary Criteria	Grade Modifiers	Risk of Systemic Impact***	Biomarkers***
	Direct evidence of progression-Longitudinal data (radiographic bone loss or CAL)	Indirect evidence of progression-% bone loss/age *Case phenotype	Risk factors *Smoking *Diabetes	*Inflammatory burden *High sensitivity CRP (hsCRP)	*Indicators of CAL/bone Loss *Saliva, gingival crevicular fluid, serum
Grade A: slow rate of progression	Evidence of no loss over 5 years	*Less than 0.25 *Heavy biofilm with low levels of destruction	*Nonsmoker *Normoglycemic/no diagnosis of diabetes	Less than 1 mg/L	?
Grade B: moderate rate of progression	Less than 2 mm over 5 years	*0.25 to 1.0 *Destruction commensurate with biofilm	*Smoker/fewer than 10 cigarettes/day *HbA1c less than 7% in patients with diabetes	1 to 3 mg/L	?
Grade C: rapid rate of progression	Greater than 2 mm over 5 years	*Greater than 1.0 *Destruction exceeds expectations given biofilm**	*Smoker/10 cigarettes or more/day *HbA1c 7% or greater in patients diagnosed with diabetes	Greater than 3 mg/L	?

**Clinical patterns suggestive of periods of rapid progression and/or early onset disease (e.g., molar/incisor pattern: lack of expected response to standard bacterial control therapies).
***Needs to be substantiated with specific evidence; might be integrated in the future as evidence becomes available.

clinical parameters of periodontal disease focus on the human need for skin and mucous membrane integrity of the head and neck. Bleeding on probing, gingival inflammation, pocket depth, and attachment/bone loss are all deficits related to this need, and each requires interventions such as self-care education and NSPT. In addition to the Human Needs Model, the Oral Health-Related Quality of Life Model provides another framework for developing a dental hygiene diagnosis, with consideration of biopsychosocial variables unique to each patient (Chapter 22). NSPT has been shown to significantly improve oral health-related quality of life. Long-term followup studies showed reductions in pain, psychological discomfort, and physical disability.[5]

The sequencing of therapeutic procedures follows a traditional model of dental care planning, including plans for periodontal therapy, that involves four phases (see Chapter 23, Table 23.1). NSPT is part of *phase I therapy* (also referred to as *initial therapy, initial preparation,* or *antiinfective therapy*). Much of phase I therapy is the responsibility of the dental hygienist who is working in concert with the general dentist or periodontist. It includes the NSPT and the reevaluation of NSPT 4 to 6 weeks after completion. *Active therapy* involves nonsurgical care, surgical care, or both, depending on the needs of the patient. Active therapy includes phase I care; in addition, it can extend to phase II care, periodontal surgery. Phase III involves restorative care. Phase IV, which encompasses periodontal maintenance (PM), is not part of active therapy.

After a series of appointments for NSPT (and surgery, if indicated) with successful outcomes, the dental hygiene process of care continues with reassessment, dental hygiene diagnosis, planning, implementation, evaluation, and documentation of care that moves from active therapy to maintenance therapy. **Periodontal maintenance (PM)**, which is also known as *supportive periodontal therapy, supportive periodontal care,* or *continued care,* is an extension of the periodontal therapy performed at selected intervals to assist the patient with the maintenance of oral health. It continues at patient-dependent intervals for the life of the dentition or its implant replacements. PM may

be discontinued and active therapy reinstituted if recurrent disease is detected.

Periodontal disease states that are refractory are indications for bacterial culturing and subsequent systemic antibiotic therapy, in addition to mechanical periodontal debridement. The term *refractory,* although not a disease form or classification, refers to periodontal disease states that continue to progress despite patient adherence to recommended oral self-care and professional care that yields successful clinical outcomes for most cases. Biomarkers might be useful for early detection and grading of periodontitis for patients who are more susceptible to periodontitis, less responsive to self-care and mechanical therapy, and likely to have periodontitis impact systemic diseases.[3]

- When planning care, after the patient accepts decisions regarding interventions, appointments are scheduled for appropriate periodontal care (see Chapter 23). The number, sequence, and length of the appointments are determined to meet the patient's individual needs. For periodontitis, the staging should be the basis for decision making for the patient's care plan interventions, while the grading of the case should be the basis for the individual plan of care.[6] Although Table 33.3 is not all inclusive, it outlines common periodontal disease features and treatment options for the natural dentition in addition to highlighting where surgical intervention may be required.

Periodontal Disease States

Periodontal disease classifications include health, gingival diseases and conditions including plaque-induced gingivitis, periodontitis, and other conditions affecting the periodontium, as well as dental implant diseases and conditions. In initial to moderate stages of periodontitis (stages I and II) without complexity factors such as furcation involvement or significant modifying factors such as poorly controlled diabetes or smoking, periodontal disease responds in a relatively predictable manner to NSPT directed at reducing disease-causing bacteria, given coinciding self-care. It is noted, however, that

TABLE 33.3	Clinical Features and Interventions for Common Periodontal Diseases*	
Case	**Clinical Features**	**Interventions**
Plaque-induced gingivitis	Oral biofilm present at gingival margin • Disease begins at margin • Bleeding on probing ≥ 10 • Probing pocket depth ≤ 3 mm* • No clinical attachment loss* • No radiographic bone loss* • Change in gingiva (erythema and edema present) • Changes reversible with oral biofilm control	Oral self-care education • Daily self-care for removal of biofilm • Periodontal debridement or scaling • Correction of biofilm retentive factors • Home irrigation and/or twice-daily mouthrinsing with effective antimicrobial agent, as needed
Periodontitis (excluding necrotizing or as a manifestation of systemic diseases)	Most prevalent in adults; also occurs in children and adolescents • Amount of destruction is consistent with presence of local factors or may be inconsistent and manifest as rapid attachment and bone loss • Subgingival calculus and bacterial subgingival oral biofilm present • Variable microbial pattern • Different rates of progression; may be periods of rapid progression • Further classified on the basis of stage (severity, complexity, extent) and grade (progression, modifiers, systemic impact, biomarkers) • Can be associated with *local* predisposing factors • May be modified by risk factors (smoking, diabetes, inflammatory burden)	Elimination, alternation, or control of risk factors • Self-care education • Periodontal debridement (SRP) • Chemotherapeutics, as needed; control of risk factors • Locally delivered antimicrobials, as needed • Host modulation therapy as needed • Reevaluation for surgery needs • Cotherapy with medical colleagues

*Will change with reduced periodontium nonperiodontitis or stable/reduced periodontium periodontitis patients
See Chapter 20.

there is a spectrum of disease progression rates ranging from rapid bursts of destruction around specific teeth in short periods of time to many bursts of destruction at a high rate.[3] For the treatment of initial to moderate disease states without confounding factors, the focus of NSPT is oral self-care education and the mechanical disruption of oral biofilm and biofilm retentive factors to reduce microbial load and the host's inflammatory response. (Note: chronic inflammatory response of the host is indirectly responsible for the destruction of collagen and bone.) For the treatment of peri-implant mucositis and peri-implantitis without confounding factors, the focus of care is oral self-care, biofilm removal and control, and antiinfective therapies. Oral self-care is ultimately the patient's responsibility, whereas comprehensive NSPT care plans, including effective periodontal instrumentation, antimicrobial interventions, and followup evaluation, are the clinician's responsibility.

The treatment of biofilm-induced gingivitis includes oral self-care education and supragingival and subgingival debridement (scaling), along with antimicrobial and antiplaque agents. The correction of plaque biofilm and calculus retentive factors is also essential; these include overhanging margins, open margins, overcontoured crowns, narrow embrasure spaces, open contacts, ill-fitting fixed or removable partial dentures, dental caries, and tooth malposition. At times, the surgical correction of gingival deformities that hinder the patient's oral self-care addresses challenges with the control of the oral biofilm.

Therapy for periodontitis with the initial to moderate loss of periodontal support includes active therapy (i.e., NSPT) and PM. Systemic diseases, modifiers, and risk factors are considered in the care plan because they affect the therapeutic outcome of NSPT (see Chapters 20

and 21). Diseases and conditions, modifiers, or risk factors that affect the host response affect the initiation and progression of periodontal diseases (e.g., diabetes mellitus, Down syndrome, obesity, osteoporosis, human immunodeficiency virus infection, arthritis, smoking, emotional stress and depression, and medications). When systemic diseases and conditions are present, consultation with the patient's physicians may be appropriate to determine the status. Oral self-care and periodontal debridement are the main therapeutic foci, and they are crucial to a successful long-term clinical outcome. Antimicrobial, chemotherapeutic, or host modulation agents or devices might be useful adjuncts when treating periodontitis with coexisting gingivitis. Implant therapy is initiated during the initial phase of care and may be considered in phase II or III therapy.

Periodontal surgery is also a problem-focused therapy aimed at enhancing root debridement and tissue regeneration, and reducing gingival recession for individuals with effective self-care practices. Surgery may be indicated for severe or advanced periodontal sites; however, most cases of initial and moderate involvement can be treated nonsurgically, provided access to subgingival deposits and biofilm retentive factors is achievable. If the results of initial therapy resolve the periodontal infection and conditions, then PM is scheduled. If the results of initial therapy do not resolve the periodontal condition or if conditions exist that indicate periodontal surgery (e.g., furcation involvement and mobility, deep pockets), a referral to a periodontist is indicated (see Referral to a Periodontist).

When severe or advanced periodontitis is present, additional considerations for initial therapy may be necessary; these include subgingival microbial analysis, antibiotic sensitivity testing, and the extraction of hopeless teeth. In some cases, optimal results may not be attainable because of the patient's health, age, systemic condition, and extent of disease; initial therapy may, in fact, be the endpoint of periodontal care.

Some cases of periodontitis progress at more rapid rates than others. The grades of periodontitis classify the rate of progression based on direct evidence of progressions as follows.

Grade A: slow, no evidence of attachment loss for 5 years

Grade B: moderate, <2 mm of loss over 5 years

Grade C: rapid, ≥2 mm of loss over 5 years,[3] previously called aggressive periodontitis (see Table 33.2 for a detailed overview of periodontitis grading).

Rapidly progressing periodontitis (staged appropriately and graded as C) often manifests with an early onset, rapid disease progression, thin biofilm, and localized incisor or molar destruction, while these patients can be medically (clinically) healthy.[3] Traditional NSPT is the basic therapeutic modality for rapidly progressing periodontitis; however, initial periodontal therapy alone often is not effective for controlling the host response to specific pathogens. Other care planning considerations include the following:

- A general medical evaluation to determine if systemic disease is present
- A consultation with a physician/specialist to coordinate medical and periodontal care
- The modification of risk factors
- Adjunctive antimicrobial chemotherapeutic therapy, including systemic antibiotics
- Adjunctive host modulation
- Microbiologic identification
- Antibiotic sensitivity testing
- A determination of genetic susceptibility (see Genetic Markers in Chapter 20)

Tooth extraction and occlusal therapy may also be part of the comprehensive care plan. The PM interval should be short (i.e., 1 to 3 months) to slow rapid disease progression. Monitoring of disease progression may require time to determine the rate of attachment loss, control of risk factors, and comparisons of former periodontal examination data is critical. Referral to a periodontist is often indicated.

Cases of biofilm-induced peri-implant mucositis and peri-implantitis are treated with oral biofilm removal and control to eliminate bleeding on probing and restore health. Antiinfective therapy is recommended for reducing inflammation and suppressing disease progression. Smoking, diabetes mellitus, and radiation therapy could modify results of therapy for perimucositis and chronic periodontitis, poor biofilm control, and irregular maintenance (i.e., supportive implant therapy) are risk factors for areas of peri-implantitis. Perimucositis generally resolves in 3 or more weeks. Progression of peri-implantitis is faster than that of periodontitis and should be considered in establishing maintenance intervals. Peri-implantitis is a consideration for referral to a periodontist and/or oral surgeon and surgery may be indicated (see Chapter 31).[4]

Appointment Planning (see Chapter 23)

One major consideration that affects the appointment plan during NSPT is the use of pain control or anxiety management strategies. Need must be established based on assessment data and patient-related factors (Table 33.4). Pain control modalities might require more appointment time, and this time consideration affects care planning. The length of the appointment could vary from 40 to 90 minutes, depending on patient needs. In general, NSPT takes more time than oral prophylaxis or PM. The most important factor for determining the success of periodontal therapy is the thoroughness of the root surface debridement and the patient's oral hygiene care, so appointments should allow

TABLE 33.4 Determining the Need for Local Anesthetic Agents During Nonsurgical Periodontal Therapy*	
Factor	**Comment**
Periodontal Assessment Factors	
Pocket depth of >4 mm	Use to improve accessibility and visibility Increases patient comfort and operator confidence
Tissue tone or consistency	Enhances access where tight, nonelastic tissue exists adjacent to deep pockets or challenging root anatomy Increases the turgor of the gingiva when injected into an edematous interdental papilla
Pocket shape/topography	Will enhance access where cratering exists near the epithelial attachment or for narrow infrabony pockets
Furcation involvement	Use to improve accessibility and visibility Pain control increases patient comfort and operator confidence
Root anatomy	Consider anatomic variations (see Chapter 30): • Complex root anatomy due to deep periodontal pockets • Increased root sensitivity • Gingival recession • Abrasion
Inflammation	Inflamed tissue that may or may not be painful and bleed Incidental soft tissue curettage will occur inadvertently
Hemorrhage	Use vasoconstrictor for hemostasis, such as with bleeding on probing or spontaneous hemorrhage
Patient-Related Factors	
Pain threshold	If threshold is low, use for pain control and anxiety reduction
Sensitivity	Determine the type of sensitivity (i.e., pulpal or soft tissue)

*Always assess the patient's health, dental, and pharmacologic histories before the selection and use of pain control agents. Noninjectable anesthetics are also available.

Adapted from Hodges K (Ed.). *Concepts in Nonsurgical Periodontal Therapy.* Delmar Cengage Learning; 1998. Carlene Paarmann, Chapter 9—Use of Pain Control Modalities, Table 9.6, p. 237.

ample time and sequencing for thorough periodontal debridement while providing for patient comfort and self-care education.

Case Presentation and Informed Consent (See Chapters 7 and 23)

The primary objectives of a case presentation are the following:

- To encourage collaborative treatment between the patient and the clinician
- To satisfy legal responsibilities

Through case presentation and the gaining of informed consent, the clinician is able to communicate the following to the patient:

- The patient's periodontal risk and assessment findings that indicate disease, similar to risk factor discussions for other chronic disease states

- How NSPT differs from oral prophylaxis and the need for reevaluation and PM for long-term success
- The extensive nature of periodontal debridement and a rationale for the number of appointments and the time involved are critical to the achievement of an optimal outcome
- The need for pain control or conscious sedation/analgesia and an explanation of why this is necessary

Box 33.2 outlines a case scenario for critical thinking about informed consent for NSPT.

IMPLEMENTATION OF NONSURGICAL PERIODONTAL THERAPY

Implementation includes the delivery of preventive and therapeutic procedures identified in the individualized care plan to meet the patient's needs. Preventive and therapeutic entities of NSPT such as self-care education, manual and mechanized instrumentation, chemotherapeutic interventions, pain control strategies (if indicated), and stain-removal procedures are performed as needed.

Oral Hygiene Instructions for Self-Care

Regular oral self-care and motivation of each patient as a cotherapist in NSPT is an important factor in treatment outcomes. Oral self-care is a critical aspect of dental hygiene care, and therefore oral hygiene instruction is extensively covered in this textbook by the references to the chapters with more detailed information. Examples of oral hygiene instructions include toothbrushing technique, selection and use of an interdental aid or special oral hygiene aids, and the need for a therapeutic dentifrice or mouthrinse with a specific antimicrobial agent (see Chapter 24 on toothbrushing, Chapter 25 about interdental and supplemental oral self-care devices, Chapter 26 on dentifrices, and Chapter 27 covering antimicrobial agents for control of periodontal diseases).

Other preventive services include nutritional counseling or tobacco cessation counseling as a part of treatment and control of periodontal diseases (see Chapters 36 and 37). In some cases, dental case management requires motivational interviewing or other behavioral change therapies (see Chapter 5) to identify and modify behaviors interfering with positive health outcomes or patient education to improve health literacy (i.e., individualized, customized communication to assist patients in making appropriate health decisions to improve oral health literacy; acknowledging economic circumstances and different cultural beliefs, values, attitudes, traditions and language preferences; and adopting information and services to these differences). See Box 33.3 for important concepts about patient self-care.

A summary of a Clinical Practice Guideline (CPG) for treatment of stage I to III periodontitis based on a systematic review of evidence is presented in Table 33.5 for consideration.[6] This guideline does not include treatment of gingivitis, stage IV periodontitis, necrotizing periodontitis, periodontitis as manifestations of systemic diseases, and mucogingival conditions.[6] This CPG suggests three steps for periodontal care, the first step being guided behavior change for successful removal of supragingival biofilm and risk factor control (i.e., oral hygiene instructions for self-care). The second step is controlling, reducing, or eliminating the subgingival biofilm and calculus via subgingival instrumentation and adjuncts, if appropriate. The third step is retreatment of nonresponsive areas through NSPT or surgery, or both. These steps correlate to interventions delivered during the implementation phase of dental hygiene care.

Supportive interventions for achieving the ultimate goals of NSPT include overhang removal (margination), desensitization, nutritional counseling, tobacco cessation counseling, dental caries risk assessment and management, and occlusal therapy. Therapeutic procedures in NSPT may include the following:

- **Mechanical nonsurgical pocket therapy:** SRP; periodontal debridement with the use of hand-activated and power-driven instruments (see Table 33.5; Chapter 28—Hand-Activated Instrumentation; and Chapter 29—Ultrasonic Instrumentation).
- **Chemotherapy for periodontal disease:** the use of systemic, topical, and locally delivered antimicrobials (also known as *antiinfective, chemotherapeutic therapy*) or host modulation agents (e.g., subantimicrobial doses of doxycycline) to selectively target the host-pathogen interaction (see Table 33.5 and Chapter 27).

Full-mouth treatment modalities include full-mouth scaling or periodontal debridement and **full-mouth disinfection (FMD)**.[7] FMD involves the SRP of all pockets within a 24-hour time period. FMD may include the application of 0.12% chlorhexidine gluconate to all periodontal pockets, followed by twice-daily 30-second mouthrinsing with 0.12% chlorhexidine gluconate for 2 months. The rationale underlying FMD is that the traditional method of four consecutive appointments for SRP without proper disinfection may allow for the reinfection of previously disinfected pockets by pathogenic bacteria from an untreated region of the mouth. FMD, however, has the potential for an acute systemic inflammatory response.[6] Considerations for FMD depend on patients' needs and preferences, the practitioner's skills and experience, practice-setting logistics, and cost effectiveness. Full-mouth scaling is similar to FMD; however, chlorhexidine is not used.

Interventions for subgingival biofilm and calculus control (reduction or elimination) are identified as the second step in the CPG. The recommendations are based on evidence regarding SRP alone and SRP plus adjuncts (see Table 33.5).[6]

TABLE 33.5 Summary of Treatment of Stage I to III Periodontitis: Clinical Practice Guidelines[6]

Step and Intervention	Recommendation	Comments
1—Guided behavior change through motivating the patient to successfully remove supragingival biofilm and risk factor control		• Insufficient alone to treat periodontitis • Is foundation for optimal response and long-term stability • May include supragingival biofilm control, interventions to improve oral hygiene, adjunctive therapies for gingival inflammation, professional mechanical biofilm removal and risk factor control
• Supragingival biofilm control by patient	A to use	• Use same guidelines as for gingival inflammation during all steps of periodontal therapy and periodontal maintenance • Recommend manual or power brushes • Recommend interdental brushes for gingival inflammation • Recommend other interdental aids when interdental brushes inappropriate
• Strategies for motivation for self-care	A to use	
• Psychological methods for motivation for self-care	O have not shown a significant impact	• Motivational interviewing and cognitive behavioral therapy have not shown a significant impact. • Unclear • Additional research needed
• Supragingival biofilm control by a professional	A to use	Use for plaque-induced gingival inflammation and periodontitis
• Risk control	A to use	• Diabetes control interventions (A to use) • Smoking cessation is recommended (A to use) • May consider stress reduction, dietary counseling, weight loss, or increased physical activity (O—unclear, additional research needed)
2—Controlling (reducing/eliminating) subgingival biofilm and calculus (subgingival instrumentation) only in teeth with loss of periodontal support and/or pocket formation.		• Cause-related therapy • May include adjunctive: physical or chemical agents, host-modulating agents, subgingival local delivery antimicrobials, or systemic antibiotics
• Subgingival instrumentation	A to use	• Performed with hand or power instruments in combination or alone (A to use) • Quadrant over multiple visits versus full mouth procedure within 24 hours (B to use)—evidence of systemic implications (i.e., acute systemic inflammatory response with full mouth protocols). Note: full mouth disinfection not analyzed.
• Chemical agents (antiseptics)*	O may be considered	• Chlorhexidine for limited time periods often studied • Unclear if antiseptics should be a general recommendation for initial therapy • May need to optimize mechanical biofilm control before considering • Considerations may be made with FMD and/or systemic antimicrobials. • Consider adverse effects and cost
• Local-delivery sustained-release chlorhexidine*	O may be considered	
• Local-delivery sustained-release antibiotics*	O may be considered	
Systemic antibiotics • Routine use • Generalized periodontitis in stage III young adults	• A not to use • O may be considered	Metronidazole and amoxicillin had most pronounced effects on clinical outcomes; however, with highest frequency of side effects.
• Lasers*	B not to use	Evidence grouped into two categories: wavelength ranges of 2780 to 2940 nm or 810 to 980 nm
• Antimicrobial photodynamic therapy (aPDT)*	B not to use	Evidence grouped into two categories: wavelength ranges of 660 to 670 nm or 800 to 900 nm
• Probiotics*	B not to use	
• Systemic subantimicrobial dose doxycycline (SDD)*	B not to use	Up to 40 mg per day
• Local statins*	A not to use	For example, atorvastatin, simvastatin, rosuvastatin gels
• Systemic/local bisphosphonates*	A not to use	
• Nonsteroidal antiinflammatory drugs*	A not to use	Well-known risk of long-term side effects
• Omega-3 polyunsaturated fatty acids (PUFA)*	A not to use	
• Local metformin drugs*	A not to use	

*As adjuncts to subgingival instrumentation
Strength of Recommendation: grading scheme
A = strong recommendation **to use** or **not to use**
B = recommendation **to use** or not to use
O = **open recommendation, may be considered**

From Sanz M, Herrera D, Kebschull M, et al. Treatment of stage I-III periodontitis—the EFP S3 level clinical practice guideline. *J Clin Periodontol.* 2020;47(Suppl 22):S4–S60.

Mechanical Nonsurgical Pocket Therapy

The basis of successful NSPT is not the treatment modality but rather the detailed thoroughness of the periodontal debridement and the patient's standard of self-care. These principles remain the foundation for NSPT; evidence that supports adjunctive therapies alone is not as strong as evidence that supports meticulous mechanical therapy and self-care. Advanced hand-activated instrumentation is an extension of basic instrumentation. Instrumentation in pockets of 6 mm or greater that are adjacent to furcation involvement and those with tooth mobility is significantly impaired when providing NSPT; therefore subsequent periodontal surgery should be considered. Options for treating areas affected by destructive periodontal disease include the standard armamentarium such as hand-activated or ultrasonic instruments. The clinician will select instruments on the basis of the following:

- Type of deposit or oral biofilm retentive factor
- Probing depth
- Inflammation
- Tissue tone (resilience, consistency, and texture)
- Access
- Root morphology (see Chapter 30)
- Pocket topography (shape)

Clinicians are challenged to stay abreast of the most recent developments in hand-activated and power-driven designs and to evaluate their effectiveness for periodontal debridement through clinical use and evidence-based decision making.

CLINICAL OUTCOMES OF PERIODONTAL DEBRIDEMENT

Despite documented incomplete calculus and endotoxin removal, nonsurgical instrumentation has been shown to arrest periodontitis (i.e., the host can now manage the microbial challenge). After periodontal debridement and SRP, the loss of clinical attachment at sites with initially shallow pockets and a gain in the attachment level at sites with deeper pockets are common. The loss of attachment after NSPT at shallow sites relates to overinstrumentation and overzealous self-care. In addition, thinner gingival margins experience more loss, and instrumentation at deeper sites adjacent to shallow sites can damage the shallow sites. Clinical attachment loss in shallow sites (1 to 3 mm) is minimal.

Evidence has shown that mean clinical attachment loss was 0.1 mm per year for adults; however, for those with periodontitis, the loss was 0.6 mm per year.[8] Generally, for periodontitis, an average improvement in clinical attachment of approximately 0.5 mm is expected with SRP. When SRP is combined with various adjunctive therapies (single or combination), clinical attachment level improvements for periodontitis are between 0.2 and 0.6 mm.[9] Tooth loss was found to be 0.20 per year for adults; however, tooth loss with moderate periodontitis was 0.17, and with severe periodontitis was 0.38 per year, representing a twofold increase over moderate cases.[8]

Pocket depth reduction is a desired result to enhance patient self-care, and it is greater initially after surgery than after SRP; however, over time, the differences become insignificant in initial to moderate periodontitis cases (i.e., stages I and II). These findings highlight the need for clinicians and patients to understand the expected outcomes of mechanical therapy during NSPT, the need for continued care at appropriate PM intervals, and the potential need for additional treatment.

Clinicians use bleeding on probing as an indicator of disease activity because it is an early and accurate sign of gingival inflammation. There is a correlation between bleeding on probing and risk for future clinical attachment loss; bleeding sites have higher odds for attachment loss and greater prevalence for progressive severe attachment loss.[1] The absence of bleeding is a reliable criterion for *periodontal disease stability* (i.e., control of local and systemic factors, minimal bleeding on probing, optimal improvements in periodontal pocket depth and attachment levels, control of modifying factors, and a lack of progressive destruction).[10] *Periodontal disease remission/control* is achieved when there is a reduction of inflammation and improvement in periodontal pocket depth and attachment levels, and not optimal control of local or systemic contributing factors.[10]

Mechanical NSPT predictably reduces the level of inflammation and hence the high levels of proinflammatory mediators (e.g., matrix metalloproteinases, cytokines, and prostaglandins) that cause the breakdown of bone and collagen. After periodontal debridement and SRP, several additional outcomes are considered:

- Effective oral self-care practices slow or inhibit microbial repopulation of subgingival periodontal pockets. The presence of supragingival oral biofilm facilitates the repopulation of pockets, with high percentages of spirochetes and motile rods within 4 to 8 weeks.
- Shifts toward subgingival health are transient; therefore PM at timely intervals is needed to sustain positive effects.

Evidence at 6 to 8 months post instrumentation revealed a mean periodontal pocket reduction of 1.7 mm and for sites greater than 6 mm, the mean reduction was 2.6 mm. The proportion of closed pockets was 74% and the bleeding on probing reduction was 63%.[6]

As previously discussed, furcation involvement associated with periodontitis presents a particularly challenging environment for accomplishing the objectives of mechanical therapy that eventually affect the longevity of these teeth. Problems with mechanical therapy adjacent to furcation involvement typically include the following:

- Identification during the periodontal assessment
- Furcal anatomy (Fig. 33.1) (see Table 30.4)
- Lack of access
- Persistence of pathogenic microflora

These same factors affect the patient's ability to perform oral self-care. Retreatment of furcation involvement with mechanical therapy, as identified in Fig. 33.1 and use of adjunctive therapies might be needed, as well as site-specific continued self-care education to enhance patient outcomes.

Factors affecting the assessment and instrumentation of furcation involvement include the location in relation to the cementoenamel junction, width of the separation of roots, vertical and horizontal dimensions, enamel projections, and the relationship of the gingiva and bone. In the initial stage of periodontitis, furcation invasion may be present on a multirooted tooth with a 4-mm periodontal probe

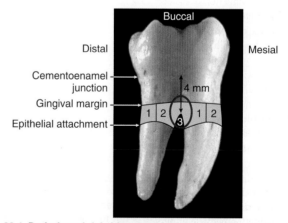

Fig. 33.1 Periodontal debridement of a furcation. The distal surface of each root is instrumented *(area 1)*. The buccal, lingual, and mesial surfaces are then treated *(area 2)*. Finally, the concavity is debrided *(area 3)*.

reading, normal gingival contour, and attachment loss of only 2 to 4 mm. On mandibular molars, the furcation entrance is located only 3 mm from the cementoenamel junction. The width of the separation of roots is important because the diameter of a curette is larger (i.e., .75 to 1.1 mm) than some furcation entrance diameters (i.e., buccal of maxillary first molars is 0.5 mm; buccal and lingual of mandibular first molars is 0.75 mm to 1 mm; second molars have closer root proximity than first molars). Narrow and thin probes, curettes and ultrasonic tips, as well as specialized instruments, are indicated to aid in effective instrumentation (see Chapters 28 and 29). Referral to a periodontist for appropriate surgery (open flap debridement, regeneration, tunneling, bicuspidization, or root resection/hemisection) might be indicated when bleeding on probing, inflammation, and deep pocket depth persist adjacent to the defect or when enamel projections or pearls exist.

Aggressive instrumentation to remove endotoxin on any root surface is unwarranted because endotoxin is loosely bound to the root surface. In addition, treated root surfaces become recontaminated over short time periods. Another outcome of mechanical instrumentation to consider is the role that root surface roughness plays in microbial recolonization and in the achievement of the desired clinical endpoint. Both surface-free energy and roughness play major roles in the initial adhesion and retention of microbes. These findings particularly apply to supragingival root surfaces; however, they are also important to subgingival root surfaces. Clinicians need to achieve the smoothest root surface in the presence of probable deposits on the root surface without resorting to overinstrumentation.

Clinical and Therapeutic Endpoints

There are two endpoints of care for NSPT. The **clinical endpoint** measures the tooth surface's preparation for the healing of adjacent tissues. This endpoint is determined immediately after closed NSPT (instrumentation) by exploring the subgingival environment. The *therapeutic endpoint* is determined at the reevaluation visit and includes the measurement of critical criteria such as probing depth, clinical attachment level, and gingival inflammation accompanied by bleeding on probing. Goals for the therapeutic endpoint are pocket closure defined by probing pocket depth of 4 mm or less and absence of bleeding on probing.

The topography of the tooth surface is the best criterion for decision making about the clinical endpoint because the removal of subgingival oral biofilm and its byproducts cannot be measured clinically. The clinical endpoint for the majority of patients is a tooth surface that is devoid of detectable biofilm retentive factors. When deciding if instrumentation is complete, the clinician considers the following:

- The self-evaluation of instrumentation technique
- Progress toward the removal of the irregularity
- Probable root anatomy in the areas (see Chapter 30)
- The radiographic appearance of the tooth surfaces
- The extent of gingival inflammation
- The severity of the periodontitis
- The generalized characteristics of the calculus and other oral biofilm retentive factors

When root roughness and irregularity are not changing despite appropriate detailed instrumentation and the unchanging nature of the tooth surface is not reasonably explained (e.g., tenacious calculus), the clinician stops instrumentation and waits for reassessment by an explorer and endoscope at the 4- to 6-week reevaluation appointment. Endoscopic therapy, if available, enhances the ability to reassess difficult and refractory areas (see Chapter 28). If the area warrants further instrumentation because of persistent bleeding on probing, indicating inflammation, then instrumentation continues. This decision-making process and evaluation build the clinician's experience base and

expertise with regard to the provision of NSPT. During active therapy or reevaluation, it is important to document in the patient's record any questionable areas to ensure completion at the next visit.

It is important to note that periodontal debridement includes the removal of all oral biofilm retentive factors, including the removal of detectable calculus, until the outcome attained is periodontal health. The removal of 100% of calculus and diseased cementum is not possible or even desirable because of the resulting tooth structure loss and probable dentinal hypersensitivity. Although meticulous periodontal debridement may remove some cementum, aggressive root planing to remove cementum intentionally is not recommended.

Calculus removal is critical to the success of periodontal therapy because calculus retains oral biofilm. There is not one simple standard for assessing these endpoints because the patient's systemic health, risk/modifying factors, immune response, and self-care practices influence healing. Sound professional judgment determines these endpoints of NSPT. Intentionally leaving detectable calculus constitutes unethical or substandard care.

Evaluation

Evaluation occurs continually during active therapy; however, final evaluation of the outcomes of NSPT occurs during the reevaluation visit, where the initial assessment data is compared with data at the completion of care. The clinician is determining the effectiveness of therapy and patient self-care. Presumably, reexamination of areas has occurred during initial/active therapy because the multiple visits allow the clinician to examine periodontal debridement in a previously treated sextant, quadrant, or half-mouth. The clinician has had the opportunity to reexamine gingival healing via color and shape changes as well as bleeding on probing, deposit removal, oral self-care practices, and the results of diagnostic testing or medical screening. Care plan revisions during initial/active therapy reflect any new information gained through continual evaluation.

The purposes of a reevaluation are as follows:

- To evaluate the patient's response to therapy and to recommend additional therapy, as needed
- To make a final periodontal diagnosis and prognosis by modifying the presumptive diagnosis, if indicated. If a 5-year period of treatment is reached or can be reevaluated based on previous data, the grading can be reconsidered.

The reevaluation visit includes the following:

- Reassessing the periodontal data and risk/modifying factors to evaluate host response and self-care practices
- Reeducating and motivating patients
- Removing residual deposits or biofilm retentive factors
- Debriding unresponsive areas as indicated by bleeding on probing or gingival inflammation
- Performing any supportive intervention, such as desensitization or antimicrobial therapy
- Reassessing the maintenance interval and adjusting it, if indicated See Box 33.4 for a reevaluation sequence that can be used in practice.

Conditions diagnosed initially as plaque-induced gingival disease should demonstrate a reduction in bleeding on probing, reduced gingival inflammation, stable clinical attachment levels, and a reduction in clinically detectable oral biofilm to a level that is compatible with gingival health. Factors reassessed if the resolution of these conditions does not occur include the following:

- Self-care practices
- Periodontal disease risk/modifying factors
- Systemic disease status
- Residual calculus and oral biofilm
- Oral biofilm retentive factors

BOX 33.4   Reevaluation Appointment Guide

Assessment
- Probe depth measurements (expected healing is 1 to 2 mm)
- Bleeding on probing (should be <10%)
- Gingival description (should be healthy)
- Soft tissue assessment information (should be healthy)

Periodontal Diagnosis
- Reevaluation of the presumptive diagnosis

Care Planning: Decision Making for the Appointment
- Localized periodontal debridement
- Need for generalized periodontal debridement; appointment for additional care visit
- Incorporate adjunctive care; local controlled delivery of antibiotic, antimicrobial rinse, desensitization therapy, and so on
- Referral to periodontist or another specialist
- Set periodontal maintenance or continued care interval
- Reinforce self-care (teach; focus on skill or management deficiencies)

Implementation
- Delivery of care as planned
- Quality of care

BOX 33.5   Factors to Consider for Reevaluation

- Bleeding on probing
- Gingival inflammation
- Depth, number, and location of periodontal pockets
- Clinical attachment loss
- Furcation involvement and mobility
- Tooth loss
- Expected patient response to oral self-care recommendations
- Presumptive or preliminary diagnosis and dental hygiene diagnosis
- Other complicating factors, such as restorative needs or occlusion
- Systemic disease and risk/modifying factors present
- Cotherapy goals for NSPT and degree of adherence to recommendations
- Likelihood of disease progression

- Adherence to the continued care interval
- Disabilities that may limit self-care

The expected outcomes for conditions initially diagnosed with periodontitis include reductions of the following:

- The periodontal probing depth
- Inflammation (or its resolution)
- Bleeding on probing (or its resolution)

Treated patients are periodically staged to monitor progress. Complexity factors that contributed to initial staging should be resolved; therefore clinical attachment level and radiographic bone loss will determine the stage. The stage will not retrogress to a lower stage, however, because the original complexity factors need to be reconsidered in PM.[1] If no response is apparent, further evaluation of the affected sites or the patient's case is imperative.

Nonresponse with some periodontitis cases requires retreatment, with another PM visit scheduled at the appropriate interval or the return to active therapy. For patients with rapid progression of periodontitis, the stability and control of the disease are the objectives of reevaluation. If control is not possible, then slowing the progression of disease is the next alternative.

Most patients who have completed initial or active NSPT should be reevaluated to assess whether the objectives of NSPT were met. The inclusion of reevaluation in a care plan is dependent on multiple factors assessed during initial therapy (Box 33.5). It is critical to evaluate systemic conditions, risk/modifying factors, forms of the disease, pockets ≥6 mm, advanced bone loss or attachment loss, furcation involvements, or tooth mobility. Adherence to self-care recommendations requires discussion of the need for the reevaluation visit as an essential part of the NSPT care plan at the time of case presentation and informed consent. The reevaluation visit can be considered as part of the initial periodontal debridement (i.e., SRP) fee or as a separate fee. The appointment may also entail other procedures, such as pit and fissure sealants, stain removal, coronal polishing, tooth whitening, desensitization, and fluoride therapy, to maximize the patient's time and the hygienist's productivity.

In practice, the time for a reevaluation appointment varies but often requires at least 30 minutes; it may be longer if other services are included in the care plan. An additional appointment for nonresponse or retreatment is indicated because 30 minutes will not be adequate. Nonresponse identifies a new problem, for retreatment and reeducation, or for referral for a medical evaluation, if indicated. Explanations for the nonresponse focus on the potential reasons for the lack of healing, including incomplete periodontal debridement, systemic disease, inadequate self-care, smoking, diabetes, or the use of inappropriate self-care aids. More than one course of action (a multifaceted approach) addresses nonresponse because several factors might be involved. The clinician could retreat the area, reevaluate the self-care aids recommended or used, or use a chemotherapeutic antimicrobial agent (e.g., home oral irrigation, local delivery of antibiotics or antimicrobials) in the area, or refer for periodontal surgery. These additional therapies precipitate the need for more discussion and patient decision making (i.e., informed consent).

At the conclusion of the reevaluation visit, the first PM visit is established as follows:

- 8 to 10 weeks after the reevaluation visit, with the achievement of the objectives of care; this interval is 3 to 4 months after the last appointment for periodontal debridement.
- 4 weeks after the last appointment for periodontal debridement, if the objectives of care are not reached (or if risk/modifying factors for continuing periodontal destruction exist). In this case, with a diagnosis of initial to moderate periodontitis (stage I or II), the patient is returned to the initial phase of care rather than maintenance. Severe and advanced cases (stage III or IV) may require referral to a periodontist.

Reevaluation is the only mechanism for determining if inflammation has been eliminated and whether probing depth is reduced and level of attachment maintained. It is also important because the appropriate person-centered PM interval can be established.

Referral to a Periodontist

The decision to care for the patient in the general dental practice or to refer to a periodontal practice is made on the basis of the following:

- The type, severity, complexity, and grading of the patient's disease
- The dental hygienist's acquired experiences
- The time allotted to maintain periodontally involved cases

For example, if the periodontal diagnosis is advanced periodontitis (stage IV) or a rapidly progressing form of the disease, referral to a periodontist is indicated. Most likely, severe periodontitis (stage III) cases will be referred to a periodontist due to deep pocket depth, vertical bone loss, or class II or III furcation involvement, particularly if resolution of inflammation does not occur. A patient with moderate periodontitis (stage II) may be referred to the periodontist if complicating risk factors exist and if the severity, complexity, or extent of disease is progressing. Some practitioners use the "5-mm standard" as a factor when referring; this means that a loss of attachment of 5 mm or greater represents a loss of bone support of about one-half of the root length of the average tooth (i.e., approximately between 33% and 66%). It is then the responsibility of the dental hygienist to strive to maintain the patient's periodontal health and to inform the patient when that goal was not achieved. This standard should be considered when inflammation persists. Conversely, deep pockets without inflammation can remain stable over long periods of time with PM.

Some patients decline referral because of geographic constraints, cost, or the fact that they do not want to go to a new office setting. Others may fear or object to surgery. Documentation of the referral to the periodontist and the patient's response in the dental record is imperative.

Most periodontists are willing to alternate visits for PM with the general practitioner. Patients with severe or advanced disease or rapidly progressing disease will probably be maintained at the periodontist's office and be referred to the general dentist once every 3, 6, 9, or 12 months for restorative examination, depending on the patient's caries risk. Box 33.6 provides a case scenario for a patient referral from a general dental practice to a periodontist.

Surgical Intervention

Forms of severe to advanced periodontitis need to be reevaluated often to determine whether the goals of periodontal therapy are being achieved and maintained. Therapeutic goals for these patients include the following:

- Resolution/reduction of gingival inflammation
- Decrease in periodontal probing depths
- Maintenance of or a gain in attachment level
- Radiologic resolution of osseous defects
- Occlusal stability
- No additional tooth loss
- Oral biofilm reduction to a level that is acceptable to the host response

Surgery should be considered when nonsurgical therapy is unsuccessful in reaching treatment goals—for example, in the following circumstances:

- When a need for enhanced access for the removal of causative factors exists
- When diseased sites with deep periodontal pockets persist
- When the regeneration or reconstruction of the periodontal tissues (e.g., osseous defects) is indicated

Periodontal debridement and self-care education should be completed to control active disease prior to surgery. The patient should also be following self-care recommendations on a routine basis. It is

important to complete initial therapy prior to the surgical phase of care for three key reasons:

- NSPT assessment gauges the healing expected with surgery.
- NSPT prepares the tissues for surgery by reducing inflammation and improving the tissue tone. In turn, this healing allows surgery to be more effective and predictable in relation to incisions, flap elevation, bleeding, and suturing. In general, initial therapy preceding surgery enhances case prognosis.
- Initial therapy might decrease the number of teeth or sites involved in the surgery.

Additional Nonsurgical Interventions

Systemic antimicrobials or antibiotics are not used routinely for patients with periodontitis. Indications include refractory cases or rapidly progressing periodontitis (grade C). Their administration is not a substitute for meticulous periodontal debridement coupled with effective self-care. Antibiotics are selected based on the patient's medical history, dental status, current medications, and results of microbial analysis, if performed. These treatments are best incorporated as part of NSPT in conjunction with instrumentation of subgingival biofilm, starting on the day of debridement completion and continuing as directed. It is important that directions for use be discussed with patients to provide a clear understanding of purpose, dosage, time of administration, and possible side effects. Systemic antimicrobials are used discriminately because of side effects, microbiologic adverse effects, and bacterial resistance concerns.

See Table 33.5 for additional information about controlled-release and systemic antibiotics in treatment of periodontal diseases staged as I to III.[6] Chlorhexidine, as an antiseptic, may be considered for limited time periods in specific periodontitis cases; however, there is a need for more research to assess the role of chlorhexidine in nonsurgical management of peri-implant mucositis and peri-implantitis to determine effectiveness.[11] While laser therapy interventions have potential to improve outcomes of nonsurgical subgingival instrumentation, depending on the wavelength and settings used, there is insufficient evidence to recommend application as an adjunct to subgingival instrumentation.[6] Box 33.7 provides a reminder about ethics, legality, and safety in regard to interventions for NSPT.

PERIODONTAL MAINTENANCE

PM is planned after the active phase of periodontal care at appropriately timed intervals that are based on patient needs. *Periodontal maintenance* is the preferred term for what is also referred to as *supportive periodontal therapy* or *periodontal recall*. Although the dentist or collaborating supervising healthcare professional might have ultimate responsibility for PM, the dental hygienist also has the responsibility to provide comprehensive and individually timed PM for patients who have participated in NSPT. PM continues for the life of the dentition or its implant replacements and this recommendation must be explained to patients who have NSPT, emphasizing that periodontal diseases are never cured but are stable or controlled. Patients with gingivitis and periodontitis have a chronic disease entity that must be controlled by frequent periodontal care and daily self-care.

BOX 33.6 Critical Thinking Scenario B

Referral
Discuss the factors considered when referring a patient of many years from a general dentist to a periodontist. Role play the dialogues that you would use to explain why a patient should seek the expertise of a periodontist for the treatment of severe to advanced periodontitis associated with 4- to 8-mm pocket depth, clinical attachment levels of 5 mm or more, furcation involvement in multiple areas, and periodontal risk factors of smoking and type 2 diabetes.

BOX 33.7 Legal, Ethical, and Safety Issues

The dental hygienist uses evidence-based decision making to select and recommend appropriate interventions for care. The dental hygienist must remain current by continually evaluating recent evidence through appropriate online searching strategies and continuing education.

Goals of Periodontal Maintenance

- To prevent or minimize the recurrence and progression of periodontal disease among patients who have been treated for gingivitis, periodontitis, or peri-implantitis
- To prevent or reduce the incidence of tooth loss
- To increase the probability of locating and treating other diseases and conditions

Intervals for Periodontal Maintenance

Patients with gingivitis who are in good general health, who do not have a history of attachment loss, and who maintain their oral health status have continued care appointments every 4 to 6 months, usually for supragingival and subgingival scaling for biofilm, calculus, and stain removal. For patients with periodontitis, an interval of 3 months or less is ideal for PM. Part of the rationale for 3-month intervals is that after periodontal pathogens are suppressed, they return to pretreatment levels in 9 to 11 weeks; however, this interval varies significantly among patients. The PM interval is customized for the patient based on the patient's self-care adherence, extent of disease, systemic contributions to disease, risk/modifying factors, and consent. Factors that influence patient consent to a specific interval are cost, third-party benefits, motivation, cooperation, and personal values and needs.

It is clear that PM after active therapy is needed and results in positive outcomes.[12–14] There is, however, no evidence to support one specific interval for all patients following periodontal care; evidence supports intervals of 3 to 12 months based on the patient's risk profile and periodontal conditions after active therapy.[6] Evidence often supports the 3- to 4-month interval. For advanced disease, a 1- to 2-month interval might be initially suggested. Therefore intervals should be evaluated frequently for adequacy. Adherence to the suggested interval is key to efficacious PM.

Components of Care

The components of PM should be similar at each PM visit; however, the extent of these services may vary depending on patient adherence, the length of time in PM, and the extent of gingivitis or periodontitis. Table 33.6 presents a summary of the assessments used for a PM visit to address associated risk factors.

Appointment Time

The time required for effective PM varies with regard to the following:
- Number of teeth and implant replacements
- Self-care efficacy
- Motivation
- Cooperation
- Systemic health
- Previous frequency of PM
- Instrumentation needs
- Adjunctive therapy needs
- History of periodontal disease
- Practitioner skill

Refer to Table 33.7 for evidence-based CPG for some interventions in PM.[6] In practice, 60 minutes is probably adequate for a PM visit; however, 45 minutes may suffice in some cases, and others may require 90 minutes. It is challenging in the practice sector to establish a reasonable fee, to work with insurance carriers, and to explain needs to the patient. Insurance carriers and/or plans might not provide partial or full coverage for the needed annual PM appointments. In this case, the patient's out-of-pocket expenses and the consequences of inadequate PM are discussed.

NONSURGICAL PERIODONTAL THERAPY AND DENTAL BENEFIT PLANS

Dental benefit plans (dental insurance) influence the patient's reimbursement for NSPT. The dental hygienist needs to know or have available the current ADA procedure codes and descriptors of these codes.[15] See Table 33.8[15] for how to relate the dental hygiene process of care to procedures. The dental hygienist needs to know the following:
- Professional philosophy regarding third-party payment as well as that of the practice setting and employer, if applicable
- Common dental terms associated with procedure codes and filing insurance claims for NSPT
- Procedure codes for nonsurgical periodontal, diagnostic, preventive, implant, and adjunctive services (see Table 33.8[15])
- How to decide which procedure(s) are needed for each patient (Fig. 33.2)
- Third-party insurance carriers in the geographic location of the clinical practice setting
- Enhanced coverage-of-benefits letters used (if not, letters can be developed)
- The individual responsible for filing insurance claims, explaining insurance-related issues to the patient, and communicating with insurance companies
- Use of medical procedure codes, if appropriate
- How to maximize insurance benefits
- Recommendations for optimal dental hygiene care are not dependent on insurance reimbursement
- Special dental case management considerations related to teledentistry or additional person-centered self-care education sessions needed to comprehensively address individual patient needs

The dental hygienist is a source of information about procedures related to and insurance coverage for periodontal services. The dental hygienist may explain the relationship between the fees for service and third-party insurance benefits and the patient's responsibility for the NSPT fee charged. Treatment plans are developed according to professional standards and patient needs, not according to the provisions of the patient's insurance policy. This philosophy ensures that patients receive appropriate care.

A specific periodontal diagnosis is used for insurance reporting whenever appropriate; an extensive range of therapies exists for periodontal therapy, and no single treatment is effective for everyone. In fact, one section of the mouth may require one type of therapy while another area requires a different therapy. Therefore the description of disease in one quadrant of the mouth as reported on the insurance claim may differ from that reported for another area.

Medical procedure codes might be used when applicable. These procedure codes are from the American Medical Association's Current Procedure Terminology Code Set and the Healthcare Common Procedure Code Set. All medical diagnosis codes are from the International Classifications of Diseases, Clinical Modification (ICD-10-CM) Code Set. The use of medical codes for reimbursement of services by oral healthcare providers should expand in the future.

It is useful to develop a fee-for-service schedule for dental hygienists that includes the following:
- Classifications of periodontal diseases
- The ADA dental procedure codes (updated annually)
- Medical procedure codes, if appropriate
- Descriptions of the services
- The fees or ranges of fees charged

This schedule provides standardized fees for service among dental hygienists working together in the same practice or environment and enhances communication with the office manager(s) or administration personnel. Although there are ADA codes for various supportive

TABLE 33.6   Periodontal Maintenance Assessment Criteria, Procedures, and Associated Risk Factors

Criteria	Procedure	Risk Factors to Evaluate
Health and pharmacologic history	Review and update the following: • Need for prophylactic antibiotics • Assessing if medications have been taken as prescribed • New diseases or medications • Need for medical consultation • Smoking and diabetes status	Age of patient Smoking status Diabetes status Systemic diseases and conditions such as cardiovascular disease, osteoporosis, pregnancy, or immunosuppression Stress
Dental history	Review and determine chief complaint	Lack of adherence with the continued care interval
Extraoral and intraoral soft tissue assessment	Examine for significant pathology	Dependent on type of pathology
Restorative assessment	Evaluate prostheses (including implants), caries activity and risk, and restorations	Overhangs or ill-fitting restorations Failing implant
Periodontal assessment	Examine gingiva for color, contour, consistency, texture, position, and mucogingival involvement	Inflammation Progressive recession Minimal or no keratinized gingiva
	Probing depth	1- to 2-mm increase Moderate to deep probing depths
	Attachment loss	Extent and severity of disease; type of disease present; changes in attachment level (loss of less than 2 mm over 5 years or 2 mm or greater over 5 years) (grade B or C, respectively)
	Radiographs	Changes in bone levels (0.25 to 1.0% loss/age or 1.0% or greater bone loss/age) (grade B or C, respectively) Vertical bone loss Presence of dental caries
	Bleeding with probing	Presence indicates inflammation and risk
	Furcation involvement	Presence indicates risk; the more advanced the furcation involvement, the more risk
	Mobility	Presence indicates risk; the more advanced the mobility, the more risk
	Tooth loss	Presence indicates risk
	Suppuration	Presence indicates risk
Deposit accumulation (consider case phenotype for grading)	Evaluate location and extent of supragingival oral biofilm	Presence of supragingival oral biofilm is strongly correlated with gingivitis
	Supragingival and subgingival deposits	Pathogenicity of microorganisms present in the subgingival environment (i.e., microbiologic monitoring) Lack of adherence with oral self-care Calculus (i.e., biofilm retentive factor)
Radiographic assessment	Evaluate the following: • Risk of advancing disease • Clinical findings, especially progressive attachment loss • Patient radiographic history	Advancing radiographic bone loss

Adapted from Hodges K (Ed.). *Concepts in Nonsurgical Periodontal Therapy.* Delmar Cengage Learning; 1998. John S. Mattson, Chapter 16—Periodontal Maintenance, Table 16.1, p. 443.

services (e.g., local anesthetic, root desensitization), not all dental plans provide reimbursements for these services. In fact, there are variations in insurance coverage by different carriers as well as among different plans from the same carrier with regard to services covered, frequency of payment for services, and maximum fee reimbursed. For example, some insurance plans reimburse for PM every 3 months, whereas others do not. Practice management computer software programs help staff members and dental hygienists to assess reimbursement rates; however, the ultimate responsibility for the fee rests with the patient.

Compliance or Adherence

The less threatening a health problem appears to be to the individual, the less likely the compliance. Time-consuming therapies or recommendations and the absence of symptoms affect compliance. A main patient-reported reason for noncompliance with PM was inadequate information and motivation; rate of compliance was variable (between 3.3% and 86.8%) and smoking was associated with a lower level of compliance.[12] Other reasons for nonadherence include self-destructive behavior, fear, economics, health beliefs, stress, and perceived professional indifference.

TABLE 33.7 **Summary of Treatment of Stage I to III Periodontitis: Clinical Practice Guidelines for Supportive Periodontal Care[6] (Periodontal Maintenance).**

Intervention	Recommendation	Comments
Supragingival biofilm control by patient	A to use	• An appropriate design of manual or powered toothbrush and interdental cleaning devices should be based on patient's needs and preferences **(A to use)** • Powered toothbrushes may be considered **(0)** • Interdental brushes should be used as adjuncts to toothbrushing if anatomically possible **(A to use)** • Flossing is not recommended as the first choice for interdental cleaning (B not to use) • Other interdental aids can supplement toothbrushing **(B to use)**
Strategies for motivation for self-care	A to use	Use same information for the first step (initial therapy)
Physical exercise, dietary counseling, and lifestyle modifications aimed at weight loss	O statement unclear	• Unclear • Additional research needed
Risk factor control	A to use	• Tobacco smoking cessation **(A to use)** • Promotion of diabetes control **(B to use)**
Adjunctive antiseptics/chemotherapeutic agents for gingival inflammation	O may be considered	• Considered as part of a personalized treatment approach • Mainly dentifrices and mouthrinses or both • Consider cost, taste, etc. • Consider unwanted effects (staining, burning, etc.) • Consider potential negative effects (nitric oxide pathway, blood pressure) • Frequency and duration of use must be determined
Professional mechanical plaque removal	B to use	
Replace professional plaque removal with alternative methods	B not to use	Example—Er:YAG laser treatment
Use of adjunctive methods for professional mechanical plaque removal	B not to use	Examples—Subantimicrobial dose doxycycline, photodynamic therapy

Strength of recommendation: grading scheme
A = strong recommendation **to use** or **not to use**
B = recommendation **to use** or not to use
O = **open recommendation, may be considered**
From Sanz, M, Herrera D, Kebschull, M et al. Treatment of stage I-III periodontitis—the EFP S3 level clinical practice guideline. *J Clin Periodontol.* 2020;47(Suppl 22):S4–S60.

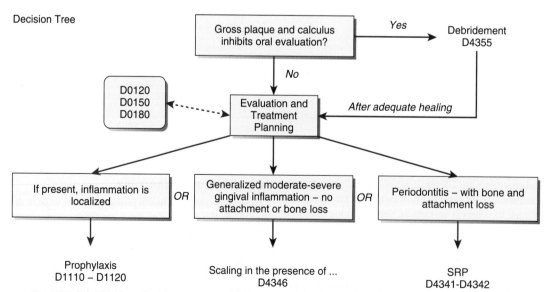

Fig. 33.2 Decision tree for procedure codes for scaling, and scaling and root planing. (American Dental Association. Guide to reporting D4346, 2. November, 2021. ©2021 American Dental Association. All rights reserved. Reprinted with permission)

TABLE 33.8   The Relationship Between the Dental Hygiene Process of Care and Procedures

General Information

The American Dental Association (ADA) has developed the publication *Current Dental Terminology (CDT®)* to enhance standardized language and effective communication about procedures in dentistry.

- The CDT® content is commonly referred to as "procedure codes" by oral health professionals.
- CDT® is published annually in print, e-copy and app formats.
- Federal HIPPA law requires that CDT® codes be used in electronic healthcare transactions.
- Oral health professionals can submit suggestions for new codes and updates to current codes annually to the ADA. ADA's Council on Dental Benefit Programs, dental specialty organizations, third-party payers, and others in the dental community can also make requests for changes through ADA.
- This CDT® publication contains three components for each procedure or service: a code, nomenclature and descriptors. Each code has corresponding nomenclature and a descriptor.
- The *codes* are five-digits starting with a D and four numbers (XXXXX) that relate to specific nomenclature and descriptors of procedures.
- *Nomenclature* is the term used to describe the procedure such as scaling and root planing.
- *Descriptors* are definitions of the nomenclature or procedure including indications for use such as time and age as well as payment limitations.
- The ADA, ADHA and others provide continuing education, in various formats, about the CDT® publication and its' application for oral health care professionals.
- The codes, nomenclature and descriptors are used throughout the United States by insurance companies (third party payers), Medicaid and Medicare for reimbursement for care.
- Coverage for procedures is dependent on a patients' insurance company and specific plan.
- Software such as Dentrix® and Eaglesoft® have licenses to incorporate the CDT® information into proprietary software for use by providers.
- ADA nor the CDT® codes set fees for service; fees for service are set by the provider.

Process of Care	Comments about Procedures
Assessment There are codes for diagnostic clinical oral evaluation services that pertain to NSPT. The nomenclature "evaluation" is used to indicate assessment procedures.	• There is a periodic oral assessment (evaluation) to determine a patients current dental and medical health since a previous evaluation that includes periodontal screening. • There is a comprehensive assessment (evaluation) for new and returning patients that includes periodontal assessment. • Detailed oral assessment (evaluation) is another procedure that focuses on a problem such as a periodontal-prosthetic condition or a condition requiring consultation from multiple disciplines. • A comprehensive periodontal assessment (evaluation) is a separate code and procedure for patients with symptoms of periodontal diseases and associated risk factors (i.e. smoking or diabetes). This code includes evaluation of periodontal conditions as well as probing and charting. • Consultation with a medical health care professional has a code and descriptor.
Diagnosis There are no codes for diagnosis.	• Best practices suggest a periodontal disease(s) diagnosis, via staging and grading, be assigned to each patient and to each insurance claim related to NSPT.
Care Planning There are no codes for care planning.	• Multiple codes are applied to care or procedures outlined in a care plan. For example, codes for assessment, radiographs, scaling and root planing, implant maintenance and HbA1c testing might all be used at one appointment. There is no specific code for care planning.
Implementation There are codes for preventive and nonsurgical periodontal therapy services that pertain to NSPT.	• Codes and descriptors exist for prophylaxis for an adult or a child. • Preventive codes and descriptors exist for nutritional or tobacco counseling. • There is a code and descriptor for oral hygiene instructions (self-care) including education about tooth brushing, interdental cleansing, and special aids. • Periodontal scaling and root planing procedures have codes based on number of teeth involved and quadrant location for the care. SRP is therapeutic and not prophylactic and might be definitive and/or part of presurgical procedures. • A code and descriptor have been identified for full mouth scaling with generalized moderate or severe gingival inflammation. • Another code and descriptor are available for full-mouth debridement to facilitate comprehensive periodontal evaluation and diagnosis. • Localized delivery of antimicrobial agents with a controlled-release device has a related code and descriptor, per tooth. • Other treatment a patient might consent to includes HbA1c testing, microbial specimen processing, saliva sample collection and testing, and genetic testing. Each of these procedures has a related code(s) and descriptor. • Periodontal maintenance has a separate code and descriptor from other procedures in NSPT. • Care for implants includes codes for maintenance procedures when prostheses are removed and reinserted post cleansing. • Scaling and debridement of single implants with inflammation or mucositis without flap entry is denoted by another code and descriptor. • There is a code and descriptor for local anesthesia not with operative or surgical procedures. • Application of desensitizing medicaments has a code and descriptor. • Application of desensitizing resin for cervical and/or root surface per tooth has a code and descriptor. • Dental case management using motivational interviewing has a corresponding code and descriptor. • Dental case management employing patient education to improve oral health literacy has a code and descriptor. • There are codes for tele-dentistry that is synchronous or asynchronous.
Evaluation There are no codes for evaluation.	• While there is not a specific code(s) for evaluation for NSPT, some miscellaneous codes might apply to treatment rendered at a reevaluation or evaluation appointment. Also, evaluation occurs throughout treatment; therefore, a code might apply to an indicated procedure such as desensitization, delivery of antimicrobial agents, and/or salivary sampling.
Documentation There are no codes for documentation.	• It is incumbent on the provider to ensure the procedure codes used for treatment correspond with the services rendered and documented in the patient's record of services.

The success of long-term PM is impressive; after 10 years, bleeding on probing and periodontal pocket depth were found to be maintained and the mean number of teeth lost was only 2.6.[13] Also, noncompliant patients had a 26% increased risk for tooth loss when compared with compliant patients.[14]

To improve patient adherence to professional recommendations, the following are suggested:

- Enhance client education about cotherapy and *therapeutic* need.
- Discuss the patient's risk/modifying factors and level of control.
- Keep recommendations simple yet thorough, and have the patient implement them in small steps.
- Target recommendations for oral self-care devices and strategies for the patient's conditions.
- Minimize the number of aids needed.
- Incorporate motivational interviewing and other evidence-based strategies for motivation.
- Incorporate adjunctive therapy only after meticulous conventional therapy (instrumentation) so as not to burden the patient with additional time commitments or costs.
- Pay attention to patient questions and needs.
- Remind patients of their appointments.
- Inform patients, in written form, about the disease and appropriate self-care practices.
- Provide positive reinforcement.
- Target potential noncompliers early.
- Ensure dentist, periodontist, and physician/specialist involvement as necessary.

Contemporary electronic communication mechanisms can easily send email reminders, text message reminders, and educational information to patients in an attempt to enhance adherence.

Fig. 33.3 offers a brief summary of decisions about treatment for periodontitis.[3,6,16] In conclusion, all stages of periodontitis require initial therapy of debridement/scaling and root planing of the teeth and periodontal sulcus in conjunction with self-care or oral hygiene instructions.[17] Generally, scaling and root planing is performed at the same time as education to teach patients how to remove the consistently renewed plaque biofilm, and education is evaluated, reviewed, and reinforced at every appointment.[17] The NSPT is the responsibility, clinically and ethically, of the dental hygienist and dentist or periodontist. Also, the patient's adherence to self-care recommendations is needed for clinical success.

There is general agreement that plaque biofilm is the initial cause of periodontal diseases and there is a renewed interest in calculus having a direct role in periodontal inflammation and destruction.[17] It is also clinically and ethically important during NSPT that reevaluation occur, and it might be that periodontal conditions have improved; however, inflammation has not been eliminated.[17] The cause of the inflammation and compromised healing might be inadequate removal of deposits. In this case, scaling and root planing can be repeated with or without incorporation of an endoscope or videoscope or through surgical access.[17]

A patient will be placed in PM only when inflammation is eliminated. If inflammation or active disease persists, advanced therapy might be indicated. Referral to a periodontist or other appropriate specialist is a consideration.

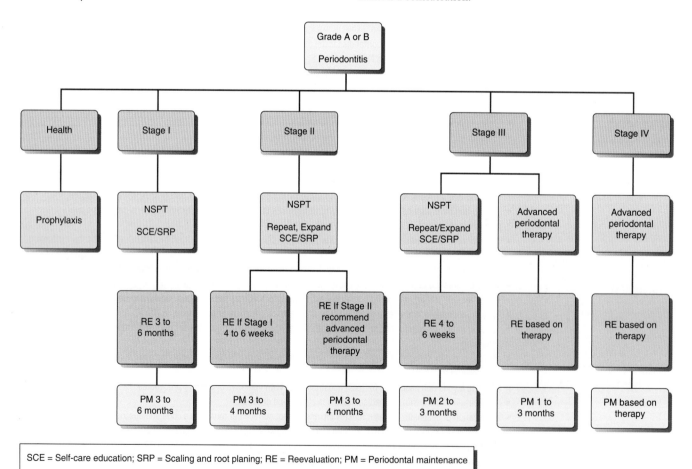

SCE = Self-care education; SRP = Scaling and root planing; RE = Reevaluation; PM = Periodontal maintenance

Fig. 33.3 Decision tree for treatment of Grade A and B periodontitis. Grade C periodontitis is considered for advanced periodontal therapy (i.e., specialty-level care and management regardless of who provides the care).

KEY CONCEPTS

- Outcomes for periodontal health include the absence of or minimal bleeding on probing and inflammation, as well as the maintenance of periodontal attachment over time.
- Gingivitis is the presence of inflammation on an intact or stable/reduced periodontium; it is treated with oral prophylaxis or scaling in the presence of generalized moderate or severe gingival inflammation (i.e., scaling and stain management).
- Periodontitis, characterized by loss of clinical attachment and supporting bone, indicates nonsurgical periodontal therapy (NSPT), surgery, or both.
- NSPT includes oral biofilm removal and control, supragingival and subgingival scaling and root planing (i.e., debridement), and the use of chemotherapeutic agents. The host's response to care must be assessed and risk factors modified.
- Periodontal debridement is the removal of subgingival oral biofilm and its byproducts, clinically detectable biofilm retentive factors, and detectable calculus-embedded cementum sufficient to allow for the healing of adjacent periodontal tissues.
- The therapeutic endpoint is the restoration of gingival health, a reduction in pocket depth, and a gain in or stabilization of the clinical attachment level.
- Periodontal infection detrimentally influences overall health.
- Periodontal assessment is the foundation for the provision of successful periodontal care, which includes NSPT, periodontal maintenance (PM), and referral to the periodontist.

- NSPT is phase I periodontal therapy; it is the responsibility of the dental hygienist who is working in concert with the general dentist or the periodontist.
- Disease states of gingivitis and periodontitis usually progress slowly and can respond to NSPT in a predictable manner; however, periodontitis that progresses at a rapid rate does not always respond in a predictable manner.
- Periodontal diagnosis is determined by analyzing information during the assessment phase of therapy; this includes the patient's health, dental history, and pharmacologic history as well as disease classification based on staging and grading.
- Evaluation occurs throughout NSPT, and the reevaluation of the full mouth occurs 4 to 6 weeks after the initial therapy of certain intraoral areas or of the case to determine stability or control and assignment to PM.
- PM follows the active phase of therapy, is appropriately timed based on patient needs, and continues for the life of the dentition or the implant replacements.
- PM prevents or minimizes the recurrence and progression of periodontal diseases, prevents or reduces tooth loss, and increases the chances of locating and treating other diseases and conditions.
- Patients with gingivitis and adequate oral self-care can maintain their oral health when PM is performed every 6 months or less, depending on severity and extent of disease progression.
- Patients with periodontitis require a 3- to 4-month interval or less for PM, depending on severity and extent.

REFERENCES

1. Trombelli L, Farina R, Silva CO, et al. Plaque-induced gingivitis: case definition and diagnostic considerations. *J Periodontol.* 2018;89(suppl 1):S46–S73.
2. Papapanou PN, Sanz M, Buduneli N, et al. Periodontitis: consensus report of workgroup 2 of the 2017 world workshop on the classification of periodontal and peri-implant diseases and conditions. *J Periodontol.* 2018;89(suppl 1):S173–S182.
3. Tonetti MS, Greenwell H, Kornman KS. Staging and grading of periodontitis: framework and proposal of a new classification and case definition. *J Periodontol.* 2018;89(suppl 1):S159–S172.
4. Berglundh T, Armitage G, Araujo MG, et al. Peri-implant disease and conditions: consensus report of workgroup 4 of the 2017 world workshop on the classification of periodontal and peri-implant diseases and conditions. *J Periodontol.* 2018;89(suppl 1):S313–S318.
5. Khan S, Khalid T, Bettiol S, et al. Non-surgical periodontal therapy effectively improves patient reported outcomes: a systematic review. *Int J Dent Hygiene.* 2021;19:18–28.
6. Sanz M, Herrera D, Kebschull M, et al. Treatment of stage I-III periodontitis—the EFP S3 level clinical practice guideline. *J Clin Periodontol.* 2020;47(suppl 22):S4–S60.
7. Eberhard J, Jepsen S, Jervoe-Storm PM, et al. Full-mouth treatment modalities (within 24 hours) for chronic periodontitis in adults. *Cochrane Database Syst Rev.* 2015;4:CD004622.
8. Needleman I, Garcia R, Gkranias K, et al. Mean attachment level, bone level and tooth loss: a systematic review. *J Periodontol.* 2018;89(suppl 1):S120–S139.

9. Smiley CJ, Tracy SL, Abt E, et al. Systematic review and meta-analysis on the nonsurgical treatment of chronic periodontitis by means of scaling and root planing with or without adjuncts. *JADA.* 2015;146:508.
10. Lang NP, Bartold PM. Periodontal health. *J Periodontol.* 2018;89(suppl 1). S9–S16.
11. Liu S, Li M, Yu J. Does chlorhexidine improve outcomes in non-surgical management of peri-implant mucositis or peri-implantitis? A systematic review and meta-analysis. *Med Oral Patol Oral Cir Bucal.* 2020;25(5):e608–e615.
12. Amerio E, Mainas G, Patrova D, et al. Compliance with supportive periodontal/peri-implant therapy: a systematic review. *J Clin Periodontol.* 2020;47:81–100.
13. DeWet LM, Slot DE, Van der Weijden GA. Supportive periodontal treatment: pocket depth changes and tooth loss. *Int J Dent Hyg.* 2018;16:210–218.
14. De Oliveira Campos IS, de Freitas MR, Costa FO, et al. The effects of patient compliance in supportive periodontal therapy on tooth loss: a systematic review and meta-analysis. *J Int Acad Periodontol.* 2021;23: 17–30.
15. American Dental Association. *CDT 2024 Current Dental Terminology.* Chicago. *ADA.* 2023.
16. Harrel SK, Cobb CM, Sottosanti JS, et al. Clinical decisions based on the 2018 classification of periodontal diseases. *Compendium.* 2022;43:52–56.
17. Harrel SK, Cobb CM, Sheldon LN, et al. Calculus as a risk factor for periodontal disease: narrative review on treatment indications when the response to scaling and root planing is inadequate. *Dent J.* 2022;10:195.

34

Acute Gingival and Periodontal Conditions

Antonio Moretti and Rebecca Wilder

PROFESSIONAL OPPORTUNITIES

A dental hygienist must be able to recognize and care for patients with acute gingival and periodontal conditions. Patients must be educated regarding the need for immediate treatment of these common conditions and the expected outcomes of care.

COMPETENCIES

1. Compare and contrast periodontal and periapical abscesses, including their etiology, signs, symptoms, and treatment.
2. Explain the etiology, signs, symptoms, and treatment of herpetic infections.
3. Discuss the etiology, signs, symptoms, and treatment of pericoronitis.
4. Explain the etiology, signs, symptoms, and treatment of necrotizing periodontal diseases.

INTRODUCTION

The dental hygienist is frequently in a position to identify urgent gingival and periodontal conditions in need of treatment. A major part of care provided in these situations is recognizing the disease process. Postponement of appropriate care can result in prolonged pain, further periodontal tissue destruction, and potential tooth loss, as well as a serious burden on the body caused by the infection and inflammation. Acute periodontal diseases typically have a rapid onset (24 to 48 hours), mostly involving pain and/or discomfort that make the patient seek professional care. These conditions may be correlated to preexisting gingivitis or periodontitis. In addition, they can be either localized or generalized. The dental hygienist should also consider a possible involvement of an underlying systemic condition as a potential contributing factor to the problem.

ABSCESSES

An abscess is a localized accumulation of purulence (pus) within an organ, tissue, or other pocket in the body. Oral abscesses are distinguished by location, originating either in the periodontium (gingival or periodontal abscess) or from within the tooth (periapical abscess; Fig. 34.1). It is sometimes challenging to clearly distinguish between the different abscesses because the associated facial pain and tenderness to the tooth can be similar; however, each has unique characteristics for further differentiation. These abscesses can also occur around dental implants. See Chapter 31, which is dedicated to dental implants and peri-implant care.

Periodontal Abscess

A periodontal abscess is a localized accumulation of purulence within the periodontal tissues.[1] Periodontal abscesses are distinguished by

location (i.e., either gingival or periodontal pockets) and by the course of the disease (i.e., acute or chronic).

- A **gingival abscess** is a periodontal abscess that is confined to the marginal gingiva and that often occurs in previously healthy gingival areas.
- A **periodontal abscess** is a deeper infection (it affects the root structure more so than a gingival abscess) associated with periodontal pockets, furcations, and alveolar bone loss (Fig. 34.2).
- An **acute periodontal abscess** is a lesion with expressed periodontal breakdown occurring over a limited period of time and with easily detectable clinical symptoms.[1] It is characterized by pain, swelling, and other symptoms that lead the patient to seek urgent care (Fig. 34.3).
- A **chronic periodontal abscess** is a long-standing infection that often is associated with a sinus tract. This opening permits drainage of the infection and a decrease in acute symptoms such as pain and swelling, thus making the abscess chronic in nature. The sinus tract, which is an abnormal channel that connects the abscess to another space or to the surface, is also called a **fistula** (Fig. 34.4).[1,2]
  See Box 34.1.

Periodontal abscesses are also classified by number as either a single abscess or multiple periodontal abscesses.

- A single abscess is usually caused by local factors that lead to acute or chronic symptoms.
- Multiple abscesses have been related to factors such as medically compromised systemic health, poorly controlled diabetes type 2, and systemic antibiotic therapy for situations that are not related to oral health.[1]

The importance of recognizing and treating patients with periodontal abscesses cannot be overemphasized. A retrospective study of tooth loss caused by a periodontal abscess demonstrated that 55% of teeth with a periodontal abscess were maintained for an average of 12.5 years (range, 5 to 29 years).[1] The importance of recognizing the disease process and encouraging patients to follow through with treatment is significant to a major goal of dental hygiene practice: preserving oral health.

Microbiology of the Periodontal Abscess

Bacteria play a crucial role in the formation and progression of periodontal diseases. Accordingly, while periodontal abscesses are complex mixed infections that can vary from person to person and from one site of infection in the mouth to another within the same person,[3-5] all periodontal abscesses share a characteristically complex pathogenic microbiota similar to that associated with periodontitis. In these pathogenic microbiota, the majority of the bacteria changes from approximately 75% gram-positive facultative rods and cocci associated with gingival health to one harboring approximately 74% gram-negative rods.[5]

Those microbial species most associated with abscesses are listed in Box 34.2.

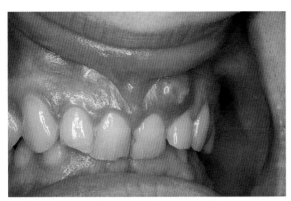

Fig. 34.1 An example of an oral abscess: a collection of purulence within the oral tissues. (Regezi J, Sciubba J, Jordan R. *Oral Pathology: Clinical Pathologic Correlations*. 6th ed. Saunders; 2012.)

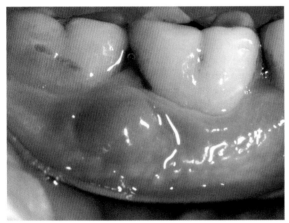

Fig. 34.2 Periodontal abscess associated between the apices of the mandibular first and second molars. (Fehrenbach M. *Illustrated Anatomy of the Head and Neck*. 5th ed. Saunders; 2017.)

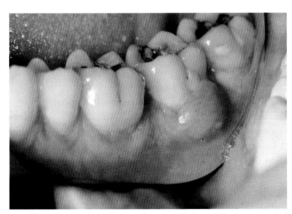

Fig. 34.3 Mandibular right first molar presenting with acute periodontal abscess. (Gutmann J, Lovdahl P. *Problem Solving in Endodontics: Prevention, Identification, and Management*. 5th ed. Mosby; 2011.)

Characteristics and Treatment of Periodontal Abscesses
Acute Periodontal Abscess

The acute periodontal abscess is a localized accumulation of purulence in the gingival wall of a periodontal pocket. It usually occurs on the lateral aspect of the tooth, and it clinically appears edematous, red, and shiny. It may have a domelike appearance or come to a distinct point. Fig. 34.3 depicts an example of an acute periodontal abscess with these characteristics. Acute abscesses are frequently associated with preexisting periodontal disease. The anatomic features of periodontal

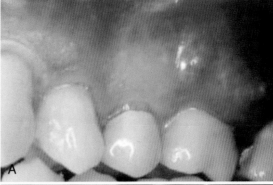
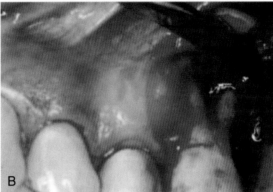

Fig. 34.4 Chronic periodontal abscess. (A) Inflammatory exudate drained continuously through the opening of the pocket. (B) On surgical opening of the defect, an extensive furcation involvement was seen. (Courtesy of Dr. Philip R. Melnick. In Perry D, Beemsterboer P, Essex G, eds. *Periodontology for the Dental Hygienist*. 4th ed. Elsevier; 2014.)

BOX 34.1 Critical Thinking Scenario A

A 30-year-old patient who has not been treated for several years arrives for a dental hygiene appointment. The patient wants to have their "teeth cleaned today" but tells you about some pain and sensitivity in the lower right quadrant and a tooth that feels "high" in that same area. The pain is intermittent but "very bothersome." After taking the patient's medical and pharmacologic histories, you determine that the patient is in good general health, with no systemic illnesses and is taking no medications. Your intraoral findings indicate that the patient has redness and swelling on the buccal surface of tooth No. 30. The gingival architecture appears normal and there is no sinus tract, but pus can be elicited from the site by gentle finger pressure.
A. What condition is most likely causing the patient's symptoms?
B. What is the most likely treatment for the condition?
C. What dental hygiene diagnosis should be addressed first for this patient?

BOX 34.2 Microbial Species Most Associated With Periodontal Abscess

- *Porphyromonas gingivalis*
- *Prevotella intermedia*
- *Tannerella forsythia* (formerly *Bacteroides forsythus*)
- *Fusobacterium nucleatum*
- *Aggregatibacter (Actinobacillus) actinomycetemcomitans*
- *Capnocytophaga ochracea*
- *Eikenella corrodens*
- *Campylobacter recta*
- *Selenomonas* species
- *Treponema denticola*

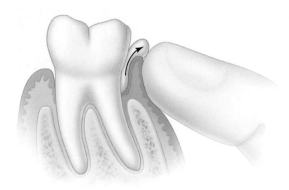

Fig. 34.5 Gentle digital pressure may be sufficient to express purulent discharge.

pockets—a pocket depth of at least 5 mm, furcation involvement, and complex pocket anatomy—may predispose the patient to occlusion of the pocket orifice. This occlusion permits an exacerbation of infection in the pocket wall as well as pus formation. Purulent exudate can often be expressed from the pocket with gentle finger pressure (Fig. 34.5).[1,4] If the pocket continues to drain through the open orifice, it can stabilize and become a chronic infection that drains exudate to relieve pressure in the surrounding tissues.

Abscess formation can also occur when a foreign body becomes lodged in the pocket.[1] An exacerbated inflammatory reaction then occurs. Conversion to the chronic state rarely occurs when foreign objects, such as peanut skins or popcorn hulls, are embedded in the pocket, thus provoking the acute response.

Incomplete scaling that leaves residual calculus at the base of treated pockets has been suggested as a cause of periodontal abscesses.[1] It is postulated that the pocket orifice tightens from improved gingival health, thereby leaving the calculus and associated biofilm to infect the deeper pocket tissues. This perspective is a commonly held belief, but few data support it. Some clinicians also believe that the indiscriminate use of an antibacterial mouthwash such as chlorhexidine without an initial mechanical debridement of the periodontal pockets also has the potential to cause multiple periodontal abscesses. The elimination of bacteria at the gingival margin area can "seal" the pocket and favor growth of the pathogenic anaerobic or facultative anaerobic bacteria. In an analysis of 29 individuals who sought treatment at a postgraduate periodontics clinic and who had been diagnosed with periodontal abscess, 18 (62%) had untreated periodontal disease, 7 (24%) were on periodontal maintenance, and only 4 (14%) reported a history of recent scaling and root planing. Of these 29 individuals, 27 were diagnosed with moderate to severe periodontitis (stages II and III); the other two had initial periodontitis (stage I). The mean probing depths of these abscesses were quite deep (7.3 mm, with a range of 3 to 13 mm), and the abscesses were mostly associated with molar teeth.[4] Given the number of abscesses treated, one would expect to see a much larger proportion of patients returning shortly after scaling and root planing appointments if incomplete treatment was a major cause of acute exacerbation.

In another study, four types of periodontal treatments were compared and abscess rates were noted. Quadrants treated with supragingival scaling alone developed abscesses to a far greater extent than those treated with subgingival scaling and root planing or those treated with periodontal surgery.[1] These data suggest that abscess formation is more associated with deep pockets and untreated disease than with recent scaling and root planing treatment. It is also known that residual calculus and plaque biofilm are often left in pockets after even the most thorough scaling and root planing, especially in deep pockets.[1] This information highlights the following three points:

1. It is extremely difficult to remove all calculus from root surfaces associated with deep probing depths.
2. The clinician should debride and scale as completely as possible, with the intention of removing all subgingival deposits.
3. Supragingival scaling alone is totally inadequate for periodontal treatment and may predispose periodontal patients to multiple acute abscess formation.

Signs and symptoms. Acute periodontal abscess may be associated with any tooth in the mouth. Abscesses appear as shiny, red, raised, and rounded masses on the gingiva or mucosa. Abscesses can point and drain through the tissue or simply drain through the pocket opening. Purulent exudate is usually apparent around the abscess opening or it can be expressed by finger pressure. Box 34.3 lists the signs of acute periodontal abscesses.

The patient also may report that the tooth "feels high," because it may become slightly extruded as a result of swelling.[1] Radiographs may be helpful for locating a preexisting area of bone loss and can suggest the origin of the abscess. However, the infection moves through the soft tissue in the direction of least resistance, so the external features may appear at some distance from the affected tooth.[1]

Treatment. Treatment consists mainly of drainage and the appropriate use of antimicrobial agents. The acute phase of the disease must be managed to alleviate pain and prevent the spread of infection. The abscess must be drained, either through the pocket opening or through an incision. Drainage through the pocket opening is less invasive; this is commonly performed by the dental hygienist. The tooth or teeth in the affected area are anesthetized and scaled. Postoperative instructions call for rest, fluid intake, and warm saltwater rinses to help reduce swelling. The patient is scheduled to return in 24 to 48 hours or longer for reevaluation of the area and to plan for required followup treatment (e.g., periodontal surgery to eliminate the problem area).[1]

The dentist often delegates the initial treatment of the acute abscess that does not require surgical intervention to the dental hygienist. However, sometimes treatment requires an incision and reflection of the tissue (i.e., surgical flap procedure) to provide access to perform a more thorough debridement. If the patient is febrile or if lymphadenopathy is present, the dentist prescribes antibiotic therapy. Fig. 34.6 shows an example of debridement therapy for acute periodontal abscess.

Repair potential for acute periodontal abscesses is usually excellent. After treatment, the gingival appearance returns to normal within 6 to 8 weeks. Bone defect repair requires approximately 9 months. Bone is lost rapidly during the acute phase; however, with immediate problem recognition and proper treatment, the lost tissue can largely be regained.[1] The positive nature of clinical results from healing further emphasizes the importance of the recognition and treatment of acute abscesses by the dental hygienist.

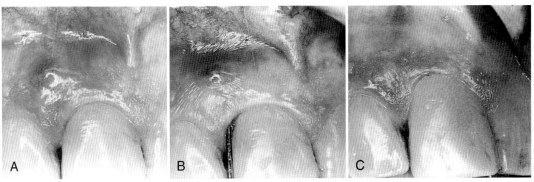

Fig. 34.6 Treatment of acute periodontal abscess. Acute abscesses can often be successfully treated without surgical intervention. (A) Abscess associated with tooth #9 showing swelling and a nondraining fistula. Clinically, the tissue appears very red. (B) Probe in place to show 9-mm pocket depth before scaling, root planing, and curettage. (C) Healing after 1 month shows normal tissue architecture and little recession. A 7-mm periodontal pocket is still present, but surgical reduction would result in nonaesthetic recession. This situation can continue indefinitely with good homecare and frequent periodontal maintenance. (Courtesy of Philip R. Melnick.)

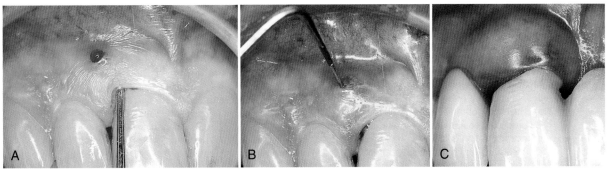

Fig. 34.7 Chronic periodontal abscess. (A) Draining through a sinus tract. (B) Probe inserted to show communication to periodontal pocket. (C) Draining through the periodontal pocket. (Courtesy of Philip R. Melnick.)

Chronic Periodontal Abscess

A chronic periodontal abscess resembles an acute periodontal abscess in that there is an overgrowth of pathogenic organisms in a periodontal pocket that drains inflammatory exudate.[1,2] Chronic abscesses have an opening within the oral cavity, either through the periodontal pocket or through a sinus tract that permits constant drainage. The chronic periodontal abscess is usually painless or it may cause dull, intermittent pain; however, the patient may recount previous episodes of painful acute infection.[1,2] Fig. 34.7 provides examples of draining chronic periodontal abscesses.

Signs and symptoms. The signs and symptoms of chronic periodontal abscesses are similar to those of acute periodontal abscesses; however, the pain level can be the distinguishing feature (Box 34.4). The dental hygienist must assess exudate associated with the periodontium as being indicative of a possible chronic abscess to ensure that appropriate dental referral and treatment are provided.

Treatment. Treatment of a chronic periodontal abscess is similar to treatment of an acute periodontal abscess. Scaling (usually requiring local anesthesia in the abscessed area) must be performed. The patient returns within 24 to 48 hours or longer for further diagnosis. The dentist must determine the need for additional periodontal treatment to reduce the pocket depth and to address other periodontal defects. Additional treatment usually includes pocket reduction periodontal surgery, but it may also include tooth extraction and more frequent periodontal maintenance visits. Some chronic periodontal abscesses are better treated initially by gaining surgical access.[1,6] Fig. 34.8 shows the surgical treatment sequence for a chronic periodontal abscess.

BOX 34.4 Signs and Symptoms of Chronic Periodontal Abscess

- Inflammatory exudate seeping into the oral cavity without inducement or when digital pressure is applied to the pocket or sinus tract
- Reddened and swollen gingival tissue in the area
- Varying degrees of pain (a chronic draining abscess is rarely painful)

The dental hygienist plays a very significant role in educating the patient about the condition's chronic nature. The patient is informed of the likelihood of increased bone loss and future acute episodes if no further treatment is performed in addition to the need for frequent maintenance care that includes scaling, root planing, and daily plaque biofilm control. Often, the discussion of the risk of rapid bone loss during acute episodes of abscess helps the patient value the need to seek further care to better preserve the teeth.[4]

Gingival Abscess

Gingival abscess usually occurs in previously disease-free areas, and it is often related to the forceful inclusion of some foreign body into the area. Gingival abscesses are most frequently found on the marginal gingiva and are not associated with deeper tissue pathology.[1,4]

Signs and symptoms. Gingival abscess can be observed on the marginal gingiva; Box 34.5 includes a list of signs and symptoms of this condition. An exudate-filled lesion that is not associated with the

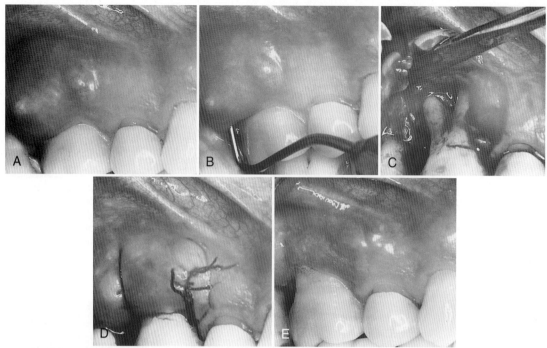

Fig. 34.8 Surgical treatment of a chronic periodontal abscess associated with a furcation. (A) Abscess associated with tooth #3 exhibits swelling and a fistula that is not draining. The tissue is very reddened, and the patient has intermittent, severe pain. (B) Periodontal probe inserted to show the depth of the pocket and determine its association with the buccal furcation. (C) Flap reflected to permit access for debridement. Note the extent of the bone loss and the depth of the furcation involvement. (D) After debridement, the flap is sutured in place. (E) Healing after 1 month shows tissue returned to normal color and consistency and no evidence of the fistula. Note the recession that occurred after surgical treatment. This patient must keep the teeth clean and return for frequent periodontal maintenance visits to preserve the tooth. (Courtesy of Philip R. Melnick.)

BOX 34.5 Signs and Symptoms of Gingival Abscess

- Reddened tissue (marginal gingiva)
- Swelling (pus-filled lesion)
- Pain

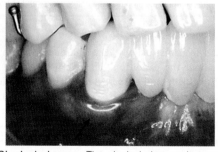

Fig. 34.9 Gingival abscess. The gingival abscess is associated with the marginal gingiva and is often the result of presence of a foreign body. Note the swelling and color change of the marginal gingiva. (Courtesy of Philip R. Melnick.)

sulcular epithelium is often clearly seen. Fig. 34.9 shows a gingival abscess in the otherwise healthy periodontium of a teenager.

Treatment. The gingival abscess must be drained and the foreign object removed by the dentist or periodontist. The acute lesion is incised and irrigated with saline solution. Sutures are not usually required. Warm saltwater rinses are recommended for postoperative therapy at home. The patient must return for postoperative observation in about 24 hours or longer, at which time the swelling should be greatly reduced and the acute tenderness subsided.

PERIAPICAL ABSCESSES

Periapical abscesses or lesions of endodontic origin are among the most common dental emergencies.[2] Periapical abscesses are also referred to as dentoalveolar, apical, periapical, apical periodontitis, or endodontic abscesses.[1,2] The periapical abscess begins as a local inflammation in the pulp and the periodontal ligament, and grows into a larger histopathologic lesion characterized by destruction of the periapical tissues.[2] The periapical abscess represents an infection burden in the teeth of 17% to 65% of cases following unsuccessful endodontic treatment.[2–5] The condition is often asymptomatic, and its treatment might not always be adequate in eliminating the infection.

In 2012, a systematic review of cross-sectional studies showed a very high prevalence of periapical radiolucency (1 per patient) and also a very high prevalence of endodontic treatments (2 per patient). Thus a significant portion of the population may have retained teeth through root canal treatment but with remaining periapical lesions, presenting a potential dental source of infection.[2] Dental hygienists need to recognize this possibility and monitor these potential dental concerns in their patients.

Microbiology of the Periapical Abscess

The dental pulp and the periodontium are connected via three main avenues of communication: exposed dentinal tubules, small portals of exit from the root surface, and the apical foramen. Inflammatory

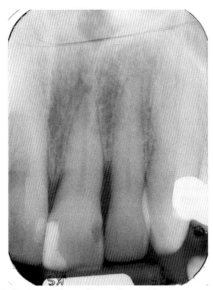

Fig. 34.10 Periapical lesions. The radiographic appearance of a periapical abscess associated with tooth #9 shows the classic appearance of radiolucency at the root apex. Note that the periodontal ligament does not appear to be intact around the tooth apex. (Courtesy of Edward J. Taggert.)

BOX 34.6   Signs and Symptoms of a Periapical Lesion

- Sharp pain that is likely to be intermittent
- Sinus tract/fistula often present
- Swelling of tissues in a localized area
- Redness of tissues in a localized area
- History of restoration, trauma, or other source of tooth infection
- Rounded radiolucency at tooth apex that appears later in the disease process

---

TABLE 34.1   Treatment Strategies for Abscesses

Cause	Condition of the Pulp	Treatment
Endodontic	Nonvital	Endodontic
Periodontal	Vital	Periodontal
Endodontic	Nonvital	Endodontic; first observe and then later institute periodontal therapy, if necessary

---

BOX 34.7   Critical Thinking Scenario B

A 45-year-old patient arrives at the dental office without an appointment and complains of severe pain. You seat the patient and determine that they are in good general health, have no systemic illnesses, and are taking no medications. Intraoral examination reveals a large, pointed fistula on the buccal surface of tooth #3, about one-third of the way toward the tooth apex. The patient has been treated for periodontal disease in the past, including in some areas that required periodontal surgery, and they have many teeth that have been restored with amalgam and composite restorations. There is a large mesial-occlusal-distal amalgam with a lingual extension on tooth #3. The radiograph you just took shows no obvious apical pathology.

A. What condition is most likely causing the patient's symptoms?
B. What should the dental hygiene component of overall dental treatment that day include?
C. What dental hygiene diagnosis should be addressed first for this patient?

---

processes in the periodontium associated with necrotic dental pulps have a clear infectious cause. The inflammatory processes are directed toward infectious components released from bacterial growth and bacterial disintegration in the root canal system.[5] When the pulp becomes infected, it elicits an inflammatory response in the periodontal ligament at the apical foramen and/or adjacent to openings of the small portals of exit.[1,2,4] Inflammatory byproducts of pulpal origin may permeate through the apex or through smaller canals in the apical third of the root canal system and exposed dentinal tubules and trigger an inflammatory vascular response in the periodontium.[5]

Characteristics and Treatment of Periapical Abscesses

It is sometimes difficult to distinguish a periapical abscess from an acute periodontal abscess because the associated facial pain and tenderness to the tooth are similar. Periapical abscess commonly results from pulpal tissue infection as a result of caries, traumatic tooth fracture, or dental procedure trauma. When assessing an abscess to determine its origin, it is helpful to know that 85% of tooth pain is pulpal and that 15% is periodontal. In addition, many teeth with periapical abscesses are nonvital, which is a distinguishing sign.[2]

Signs and Symptoms

Periapical abscess is mainly a radiographic finding.[2] It is most identifiable on radiographs as a rounded radiolucency at the apex of the tooth. Fig. 34.10 shows the typical appearance. However, early on in abscess formation, the radiographic changes are often not easily detectable. If the periapical abscess drains through a sinus tract in the cortical bone or through the periodontal ligament, it is likely to be much less identifiable on radiographs. Periapical abscesses that drain through the periodontal ligament can resemble acute periodontal abscesses because their symptoms are very similar: both exhibit reddened soft tissue, swelling, and a sinus tract opening. It is often difficult to determine if the fistula opens into the periodontal pocket or goes to the apex of the tooth (Box 34.6).[2]

Treatment

Periapical abscess treatment requires either endodontic treatment to remove the infected tooth pulp and replace it with inert material such

as gutta percha or tooth extraction. Untreated endodontic abscesses can lead to severe cases of brain abscess or fasciitis of the neck or chest wall that can be life-threatening.[2] The dental hygienist has a responsibility to inform patients with untreated periapical abscesses of the risk associated with delaying treatment. Patients without acute symptoms caused by abscess draining are likely to need a clear understanding of the disease process so that they pursue care and avoid further tissue destruction and ill effects from the infection. Table 34.1 summarizes abscess treatment strategies.

See Box 34.7.

Combination Abscess

The periodontium is continuous. Pathology at the tooth's apex (i.e., infection of the pulp) can extend to the marginal tissues, and infection originating in the periodontal tissue can progress to the pulp through openings at the apex or through lateral canals. A true combination of periodontal and periapical abscess is present when both of these infectious processes are present. Fig. 34.11 illustrates a combinational abscess.

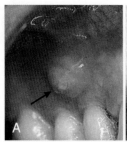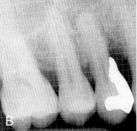

Fig. 34.11 Combined periapical and periodontal abscess. The combined abscess is associated with tooth #5. It could have occurred from the spread of pathologic microorganisms from the deep pockets to the tooth pulp, the caries process, or trauma from the placement of the very deep restoration. (A) The sinus tract (fistula) emerges into the oral cavity. (B) Radiolucency at the apex and significant bone loss appear on the radiograph. (Courtesy of Philip R. Melnick.)

HERPETIC INFECTIONS

More than 80 herpesviruses have been identified, 8 of which are known human pathogens.[7,8] Herpes simplex viruses (HSVs) belong to the ubiquitous Herpesviridae family of viruses, which contains HSV-1, HSV-2, varicella-zoster virus, cytomegalovirus, and Epstein-Barr virus, as well as human herpesviruses and Kaposi sarcoma–associated herpesvirus (type 8).[7,8] Herpesvirus infection occurs worldwide, has no seasonal variation, and affects only humans naturally.

The prevalence of HSV-1 infection increases gradually from childhood, reaching 60% to 95% prevalence among adults. Primary HSV-1 infection in oral and perioral sites usually manifests as gingivostomatitis, whereas virus reactivation in the trigeminal sensory ganglion gives rise to mild cutaneous and mucocutaneous disease; this is often called *recurrent herpes labialis*.[7,8]

Primary Herpetic Gingivostomatitis

Irrespective of the viral type, HSV primarily affects the skin and mucous membranes.[7] **Primary herpetic gingivostomatitis (PHGS)** is the most common orofacial manifestation of HSV-1 infection, and it is characterized by oral and perioral vesiculoulcerative lesions.[7] Although herpetic gingivostomatitis is a self-limiting disease, affected individuals may experience severe pain and be unable to eat or drink. The virus is spread by physical contact, but there is no documentation that it can be spread through the airborne droplet route, contaminated water, or contact with inanimate objects. Most people encounter the virus and never show signs or symptoms of primary infection.[7] Up to 90% of the population have antibodies to HSV-1.[7]

PHGS typically develops after the first-time exposure of seronegative individuals or among those who have not produced an adequate antibody response during a previous infection with either of the two HSVs.[7,8] The majority of infections are subclinical. Although PHGS typically affects children between the ages of 1 and 5 years, occasional cases of primary infection affecting adults also occur.[7] Infants are passively protected through maternal immunity for the first 6 months of life. The clinical manifestations of the infection, whether from HSV-1 or HSV-2, may lead to primary oral infection; nearly all are caused by HSV-1.[6,7] The majority of HSV-1-induced primary orofacial infections are subclinical and therefore unrecognized.[6] Symptomatic PHGS is typically preceded or accompanied by a sensation of burning or paresthesia at the inoculation site, cervical and submandibular lymphadenopathy, fever, malaise, myalgia, appetite loss, dysphagia, and headache. The most characteristic signs at presentation are acute generalized marginal gingivitis, with the inflamed gingiva appearing erythematous and edematous. Most patients with primary herpetic infections never

experience the secondary or recurrent forms. In healthy individuals, primary infection has an excellent prognosis, with recovery expected within 10 to 14 days.[6] Nevertheless, the painful herpetic ulcers in the mouth associated with primary infection often cause a reduction in food and fluid intake, thereby increasing the chances for the health risks that accompany this disease. Nutritional deficits can be critical in children and infants. Serious dehydration is not uncommon, and this can lead to infant hospitalization.

Signs and Symptoms

Acute herpetic gingivostomatitis is recognized by a set of characteristic systemic and intraoral signs and symptoms (Box 34.8). The vesicular eruptions may occur on the skin, the vermilion border, or the oral mucous membranes. Intraorally, they may appear on any mucosal or gingival surface, the hard palate, and the alveolar mucosa or any other oral soft tissue area.[7] The discrete grayish vesicles rupture and coalesce within 24 hours to form ulcers. The ulcers have a red, elevated, halolike margin with a depressed yellow or gray central area. They are teeming with shedding virus. Fig. 34.12 exemplifies the intraoral appearance of primary herpetic infection in a teenager. The disease is commonly associated with systemic symptoms including fever, malaise, headache, and cervical lymphadenopathy.[7,8]

The recognition of PHGS is based on knowledge of the appearance of the ulcers and the assessment of systemic manifestations. Diagnostic tests, such as culturing for herpesvirus by the patient's physician, can be conducted for confirmation of the presence of the virus, but these are not done routinely. Because PHGS is a highly infectious disease, the dental hygienist, the patient, and the patient's parents (in the case of children) must work together to prevent the transmission of the virus to family members and other members of the oral healthcare team. Fig. 34.13 shows a presentation of a herpetic infection on the facial skin and eyes.

Treatment

The treatment of gingival inflammation and any other elective dental care should be postponed until the PHGS has run its course. The patient is assessed by the dentist to obtain a definitive dental diagnosis. The management of acute herpetic gingivostomatitis is entirely supportive because of the infectious nature of the disease and the fact that it runs its course in 7 to 10 days. The patient should be instructed to rest, take fluids, and make every effort to eat a nutritious diet, including soft, nutrient-dense foods. The patient should also try to perform oral hygiene as much as possible at home, cleaning the teeth at home with an extra-soft toothbrush if it can be tolerated.[1,2,4] Over-the-counter topical anesthetics and systemic nonsteroidal antiinflammatory agents can be used to minimize discomfort. The patient can swab topical anesthetics onto the lesions for controlled local delivery. Topical anesthetics should be used cautiously and as directed with children because of the health risks associated with them.

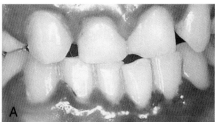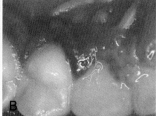

Fig. 34.12 Primary herpetic gingivostomatitis. This oral infection of the mouth is characterized by bright red gingiva, vesicles, and pain. (A) Facial gingiva showing swelling and color change. (B) Lingual view of the premolar and anterior teeth showing coalesced vesicles. (Courtesy of Philip R. Melnick.)

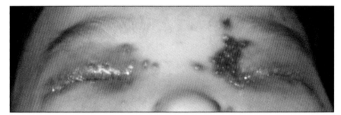

Fig. 34.13 HSV blepharitis presenting as a vesicular lesion with surrounding erythema. HSV conjunctivitis. The follicular reaction is often unilateral, recurrent, and worsens with topical corticosteroids. (Mannis M, Holand E. *Cornea* (2 vols). 4th ed. Elsevier; 2016.)

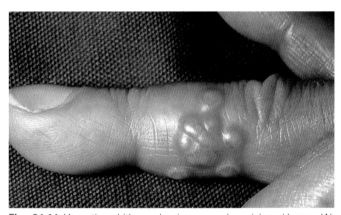

Fig. 34.14 Herpetic whitlow, classic grouped vesicles. (James W, Berger T, Elston D. *Andrews' Diseases of the Skin.* 12th ed. Elsevier; 2016.)

Professional care should not be performed because of the risk of transmission of the virus to other head and neck areas of the patient or to the dental hygienist and other workers. Even if the hygienist was previously exposed to the herpesvirus or has had an episode of initial infection with or without recurrent lesions, they can still be inoculated with the virus by an inadvertent finger puncture with an HSV-contaminated instrument. This infection could result in the development of herpetic whitlow (Fig. 34.14). Herpetic whitlow is a recurrent herpetic finger lesion that can be extremely painful and debilitating. The whitlow can last many weeks longer than the usual 2-week course of herpesvirus infection in the oral tissue.[7]

See Box 34.9.

Recurrent Oral Herpes Simplex Infections

After primary infection, latent HSV reactivates periodically, migrating from the sensory ganglia to cause recurrent oral or genital herpes.[7,8] These recurrences are known as **recurrent herpetic lesions**. Despite the high prevalence of HSV-1 in the population, only 15% to 40% of seropositive patients ever experience symptomatic mucocutaneous

---

BOX 34.9   Critical Thinking Scenario C

A patient arrives for a 4-month continued-care appointment. They are very excited to be leaving tomorrow for a 6-month stay in Europe and eager to have dental hygiene maintenance care completed before leaving. You notice a 6-mm round, crusted lesion on the patient's lower lip, with some vesicles on the edge. The patient says they have never had such a sore before and that it was hurting a few days ago but is fine now. They request that you cover the lesion with petroleum jelly so that it will not crack during treatment.

A. What condition is most likely present on the patient's lip?
B. What is the dental hygiene care protocol for the patient?
C. What dental hygiene diagnosis should be addressed first for this patient?

BOX 34.10   Signs and Symptoms of Recurrent Herpetic Infection

- Prodromal symptoms of burning or tingling at the site
- Ulcer on the lip or the perioral skin
- Pain
- Vesicles early in the course of the infection
- Crusting of the ulcer surface as it heals

---

recurrence.[1,7,8] An individual's genetic susceptibility, immune status, age, anatomic site of infection, initial dose of inoculums, and viral subtype appear to influence the frequency of recurrence. Compared with primary infections, recurrent episodes are milder and shorter in duration, with minimal systemic involvement.[7]

Patients often arrive for dental hygiene appointments when they have recurrent herpetic lesions. These lesions are quite common, as previously mentioned, and they do not interfere with activities of daily living, so patients are frequently unaware of the nature of the event. The typical recurrent lesion is on the lip and is referred to as *herpes simplex labialis*. Common names such as fever blister and cold sore reflect the public's understanding of what precipitates these recurrences. Unfortunately, these are extremely innocuous names for lesions with serious potential effects for the dental hygienist.

Signs and Symptoms

Patients often have prodromal symptoms of burning, tingling, or pain at the site where the lesion recurs (Box 34.10). Within hours of the prodromal symptoms, vesicles appear, which become ulcerated and coalesce into a large ulcer or ulcers. The lesions heal without scarring in about 14 days, and they can recur as often as once per month. Typically, lesions will recur in the same place on the vermilion border and on the skin around the face. Fig. 34.15 shows an example of recurrent herpetic lesions.

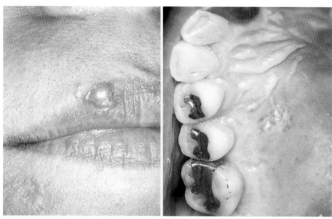

Fig. 34.15 Clusters of recurrent herpes simplex vesicles. *Left*, on the lip; *right*, on the hard palate, both present 2 to 3 days, in different patients. (Goldman L, Schafer A. *Goldman-Cecil Medicine.* 25th ed. Elsevier; 2016.)

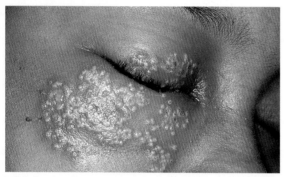

Fig. 34.16 Recurrent herpes simplex erupted around the eye of this 11-year-old male. The cornea was not involved and vesicles crusted over in less than a week. (Cohen B. *Pediatric Dermatology.* 4th ed. Saunders; 2013.)

Treatment

Recurrent lesions shed vast amounts of herpesvirus. For this reason, the dental hygienist must not treat the patient while the lesions are present. Sometimes, this can be very disconcerting because it requires reappointing a patient who may have waited months for an appointment. However, the dental hygienist is placed at great risk of inoculation, just as with primary herpetic infections. Not only are herpetic whitlow lesions a possibility, but the virus is also shed in the saliva, which means that spatter during treatment can be hazardous. Fig. 34.16 shows an example of a recurrent herpetic infection around the eye.

Herpetic lesion treatment is entirely supportive. There are some antiviral agents available by prescription (e.g., acyclovir) that the patient may benefit from using. These agents may reduce the extent and duration of the recurrence. The dental hygienist should inform the patient of this possibility and refer the patient to a physician or dentist for further information.

It is extremely important for the patient to be educated about these lesions and about their responsibility for preventing the spread of infection. Patients who have common recurrences are often aware of the prodromal symptoms and should be informed to call and reschedule dental appointments after the disease runs its course. Box 34.11 presents additional information for treatment of patients with recurrent intraoral herpetic lesions.

Recurrent intraoral herpetic lesions can almost always be easily distinguished from the more commonly occurring **aphthous ulcers**.

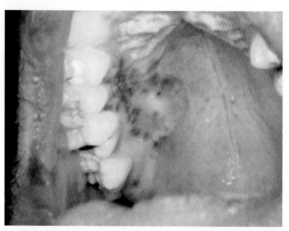

Fig. 34.17 Painful recurrent herpes simplex reactivation, shown on the third day. The lesions resolved without specific antiviral treatment in 7 days. (Silverman S. Mucosal lesions in older adults. *J Am Dent Assoc.* 2007;138:S41.)

Reviewing patient history for recent trauma or illness may be helpful, but either lesion can result. The more distinguishing characteristic is that recurrent herpetic lesions almost always occur on the gingiva or the hard palate, and aphthous ulcers almost always appear on the movable mucosa.

See Box 34.12 for related legal, ethical, and safety issues.

PERICORONITIS

Pericoronitis is soft tissue inflammation associated with a partially erupted tooth. It may be acute, subacute, or chronic in nature.[9] The most commonly affected tooth is the mandibular third molar, but maxillary third molars and other teeth that are the most distal in the arch have been associated with the disease. The tissue flap that either

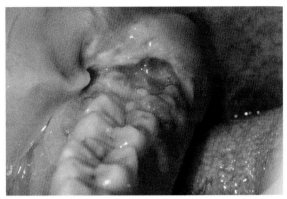

Fig. 34.18 Pericoronitis. Painful erythematous enlargement of the soft tissues overlying the crown of the partially erupted right mandibular third molar. This condition is most commonly found in the third molar region and can be extremely painful. (From Chi A, Neville B, Allen C, Damm D. *Oral and Maxillofacial Pathology.* 4th ed. Saunders; 2016.)

> ## BOX 34.13   Signs and Symptoms of Acute Pericoronitis
>
> - Extreme pain
> - Swelling of the operculum and gingiva associated with the most distal tooth in the arch
> - Redness
> - Purulent exudate
> - Foul taste
> - Swelling of the cheek
> - Cervical lymphadenopathy
> - History of recurrence

completely or partly covers the associated tooth is called an **operculum**. The space between the tissue flap and the tooth is an ideal location for food debris to collect and bacteria to grow. As bacteria increasingly infect the area, the tissue responds by becoming extremely inflamed and painful.[9] There is constant inflammation in the area, so it is always considered subacute or chronically infected, even if the acute symptoms are not present.[9]

Acute pericoronitis involves an extremely high degree of inflammation in the local area. As inflammation increases, the tissue swells, and this can interfere with the complete closing of the jaws. This interference can lead to added trauma, increased inflammation, and severe pain. The tissue becomes quite red, suppuration is evident, and the pain can radiate to the throat and ear.

This disease is a common problem associated with young adults, and it has been considered to be a serious problem for military personnel, most of whom are in the 17- to 26-year-old age group. In fact, 20% of dental emergencies reported by the military during World War II and 16% of those from the Vietnam conflict were acute pericoronitis.[1] Fig. 34.18 shows an example of acute pericoronitis.

Signs and Symptoms

Oral areas that have an operculum are predisposed to pericoronitis and typically exhibit chronic signs of the disease, increased redness, and some exudate (Box 34.13). The tissue may be so swollen that it interferes with mastication, and it is easily traumatized during eating. The infection can extend very deeply into the tissues and cause peritonsillar abscess formation, cellulitis, and Ludwig angina.[9] These signs are rare sequelae, but they emphasize the importance of recognition and lesion treatment.

> ## BOX 34.14   Critical Thinking Scenario D
>
> A patient comes to the dental office without an appointment, complaining of extreme pain in jaw. In fact, the patient can hardly open the mouth. A review of the patient's medical and pharmacologic histories shows that the patient is in good general health and takes no medications. Intraoral findings reveal extremely reddened and swollen gingiva on the mandibular right posterior area. The patient complains of a bad taste in the mouth and says that the condition "comes and goes," but that this is the worst pain they have experienced. The patient has many large amalgam restorations and appears to have a partially submerged molar in the quadrant.
> A. What is the most likely emergency condition?
> B. How should the dental hygiene component of the overall dental treatment begin?
> C. What dental hygiene diagnosis should be addressed first for this patient?

A review of military studies documents the extent of symptoms associated with pericoronitis. In a military study of 359 recruits, pain, swelling, and redness were present in every instance. Purulent exudate was reported in half of the cases, few patients bled on palpation, and no individual in that population had a fever. In addition, two-thirds of 25 cases in the naval population reported previous episodes of pericoronitis, which suggests that pericoronitis is often a recurrent problem.[8]

Treatment

A number of considerations are involved when treating pericoronitis, including the severity of the case, whether it is a recurrence, and possible systemic complications. The dentist may ask the dental hygienist to participate in the care of the patient with pericoronitis, which requires multiple visits.

Initial dental management is aimed at treating symptoms, with the goal of making the patient more comfortable. The infected area is debrided, usually by gentle flushing with warm water or dilute hydrogen peroxide delivered in a disposable irrigating syringe with a blunt needle. Topical anesthetic is applied first. Tissue manipulation may be difficult and uncomfortable for the patient, but the tissue needs to be lifted away from the tooth to permit as much debridement as is tolerable at the first treatment appointment.[1] After this initial debridement, the patient is instructed to rest at home, use warm saltwater rinses, and drink fluids to avoid dehydration. The dentist may prescribe antibiotics if the patient is febrile or if there is cervical lymphadenopathy. The patient is asked to return the next day. At the second visit, the area is irrigated again and instrumented if possible, and more thorough homecare is initiated. A marked improvement is usually observed at the second appointment.

After the acute condition has resolved, the patient is assessed by the dentist to determine further treatment. Dental treatment may include the extraction of the offending third molar or operculum removal to produce a more normal gingival contour if the tooth is to be retained.[9]

The presence of any operculum is assessed and viewed with suspicion. Some amount of inflammation is almost always present, and the potential for acute exacerbations is likely. The dental hygienist informs patients about the potential issues associated with the condition to permit them to understand the situation and take responsibility for their oral health.

See Box 34.14.

NECROTIZING PERIODONTAL DISEASES

Necrotizing ulcerative periodontal diseases are opportunistic gingival infections that are associated with lifestyle risk factors (e.g., stress, tobacco use) as well as with systemic conditions (e.g., blood dyscrasias, acquired immunodeficiency syndrome, Down syndrome).[10] These diseases have been widely reported, and they are not uncommon in nonindustrialized countries.[10] Classical diagnostic features include ulceration and necrosis of the interdental papillae, pain, and spontaneous gingival bleeding. Necrotizing ulcerative periodontal diseases are clinically recognizable diseases that are distinct from chronic periodontitis. The diseases were first described by Vincent during the late 19th century and were so common among troops fighting in trenches in Europe during World War I that the name *trench mouth* was adopted. They were primarily seen in young adults.[10] The condition is not communicable, infectious, or spread through direct contact.

Until 1999, the condition was most commonly called *acute necrotizing ulcerative gingivitis* or just *necrotizing ulcerative gingivitis*. However, the condition is often associated with attachment loss, which makes the term *gingivitis* inaccurate, so it is now referred to as *necrotizing ulcerative periodontitis*. It is not certain whether the conditions involving attachment loss are separate diseases from those confined to the gingiva, so the consensus is to use the more general disease name of *necrotizing periodontal diseases*.

Necrotizing ulcerative periodontal diseases are recognized to be recurrent diseases with complex bacteriology consisting of a large proportion of spirochetes and gram-negative organisms. The consistent presence of specific bacteria, fusobacteria, and spirochetes has suggested that the cause could be explained in microbiologic terms. These organisms invade the tissue, which causes the characteristic appearance of the disease. Other contributory factors implicated include poor oral hygiene, mouth breathing, smoking, stress, sepsis, malnutrition, and systemic diseases, including hormonal imbalance and alterations in lymphocyte and neutrophil function.[10]

Signs and Symptoms

Necrotizing ulcerative periodontal diseases have specific clinical characteristics that distinguish them from other forms of acute oral infections. The clinical appearance of the disease is one of cratered or "punched-out" papillae, very reddened gingivae, and pain. There is often a collection of debris, dead cells, and bacteria on the gingival surface, which appears gray and that is referred to as the pseudomembrane. The gingival lesions may be localized to specific areas or generalized throughout the mouth, and they progressively destroy the gingiva and the underlying periodontal structures. Patients frequently exhibit an extremely offensive and fetid breath odor that can be smelled anywhere in a room that is occupied by the patient. They may also complain of a thick or pasty texture to the saliva. In addition, the acute lesions can be extensive and cover parts of the face, as is seen in developing countries in association with malnutrition. Fig. 34.19 shows the clinical oral features of necrotizing ulcerative periodontitis.

The three most reliable criteria for recognizing the disease are as follows:
1. Pain (this is a hallmark of the condition)
2. Acute necrosis and ulceration of the interproximal papillae
3. Bleeding

Other symptoms have also been recognized as being strongly associated with the disease (Box 34.15).

Stress is often related to both the initial occurrence and recurrence of this disease. The role of the psychologic factors involved with stress is not well understood, but it has been postulated that changes in the immune system that occur at stressful times predispose certain individuals to an exuberant bacterial response that results in necrotizing ulcerative disease.

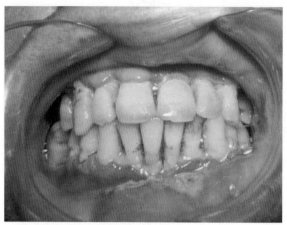

Fig. 34.19 Necrotizing stomatitis. (Courtesy of Joseph L. Konzelman, Jr, DDS, Augusta, GA.)

BOX 34.15   Signs and Symptoms of Necrotizing Ulcerative Periodontitis

- Necrosis of interproximal papillae of the gingiva
- Bleeding
- Pain
- Fetid odor
- Pseudomembrane over the gingiva
- Cervical lymphadenopathy
- Fever

Treatment

The course of a single episode of necrotizing ulcerative periodontitis is usually short but painful. Patients come to the oral care setting most often as a result of the associated pain. Because of the cyclic and recurring nature of the disease, treatment focuses on microbial control through mechanical debridement by both the patient and the clinician. It also requires consultation with the patient's physician because of possible predisposing systemic factors, such as human immunodeficiency virus infection.[7,8] Treatment should progress daily during the acute phase of the disease because the pain often inhibits thorough cleaning by the patient or the dental hygienist at one time. Treatment includes periodontal debridement with ultrasonic scalers, plaque biofilm control, and 0.12% chlorhexidine rinses twice daily. The dentist may prescribe a systemic antibiotic if fever and lymphadenopathy are present. The recommended treatment sequence is described in Table 34.2.

Given the signs and symptoms, most patients with necrotizing periodontal diseases have head and neck pain and inflammation of the skin and mucous membranes, which can affect their conceptualization and problem solving. Patient health, oral health, and well-being are the keys to the successful treatment of these diseases. Patients must be knowledgeable about the roles of stress, bacteria, and nutrition in the disease process and encouraged to take control of their oral health and lifestyle behaviors. Suggestions to identify stress management techniques and to improve nutrition (see Chapter 36) are necessary components of dental hygiene care.

Box 21.4 (Chapter 21) depicts a clinical case of necrotizing periodontitis with initial diagnosis and treatment outcomes.

See Box 34.16.

Table 34.3 provides a summary comparison of acute gingival and periodontal conditions.

TABLE 34.2 Treatment Regimen for Necrotizing Ulcerative Periodontitis

Day 1	First visit: oral therapy	Scale and debride as much as possible. Mechanized (ultrasonic) instruments may be tolerated better than hand-activated scalers. Use topical anesthetic as needed. Provide plaque control instruction. Recommend frequent rinsing at home with a mixture of warm water and 3% hydrogen peroxide to soothe and oxygenate the pseudomembranous plaque.
Day 1	Systemic therapy	Review the patient's health history for underlying conditions, and consult with the patient's physician as needed. Antibiotic use (e.g., penicillin, erythromycin, metronidazole) is indicated if the patient has fever and cervical lymphadenopathy.
Day 2	Second visit	Pain should be reduced considerably. Continue to remove calculus to the limit of the patient's pain tolerance. Oral hygiene instructions should be reinforced. The home rinsing regimen should be continued.
Days 4 to 7	Third visit	Therapeutic scaling and root planing should be completed, taking as many appointments as necessary. Oral hygiene must be reinforced. Hydrogen peroxide rinses can be discontinued. Continue the patient on 0.12% chlorhexidine mouth rinse twice daily for 2 to 3 weeks.
Month 1	Reevaluation for continued care	Reinforce oral hygiene. Scaling and root planing if necessary. Meticulous and regular debridement by the patient and the dental hygienist must occur to control bacterial pathogenicity. Cratering frequently occurs and can result in significant gingival defects that should be evaluated by the dentist for possible surgical correction.
Month 3	Periodontal maintenance therapy	Regular professional mechanical dental hygiene care should be encouraged to minimize the risk of recurrence. Continued care interval should be 2 to 4 months.

BOX 34.16 Critical Thinking Scenario E

A 20-year-old patient comes to the dental office complaining of severe pain in their mouth. You determine that the patient has no systemic illnesses, and you examine their oral tissues. Your findings are extreme redness and swollen gingiva throughout the mouth and small, grayish ulcers on the gingiva and mucosa in several areas.

A. What condition is most likely causing the patient's symptoms?
B. What is the most likely treatment for the condition?
C. What dental hygiene diagnosis should be addressed first for this patient?

TABLE 34.3 Summary Comparison of Acute Gingival and Periodontal Conditions

Cause	Risk Factors	Signs and Symptoms	Prevention and Management
Acute Periodontal Abscess			
Periodontal pathogens	Deep pockets Untreated periodontal disease	Swelling Redness Pain Exudate Sinus tract may occur	Education about the disease Therapeutic scaling and root planing Referral for further treatment
Chronic Periodontal Abscess			
Periodontal pathogens	Deep pockets Untreated periodontal disease	Sinus tract Exudate Pain Swelling Redness Acute episodes	Education about the disease Therapeutic scaling and root planing Referral for further treatment

Continued

TABLE 34.3   Summary Comparison of Acute Gingival and Periodontal Conditions—cont'd

Cause	Risk Factors	Signs and Symptoms	Prevention and Management
Gingival Abscess			
Foreign object	Unknown	Swelling Redness Pain Exudate	Education to prevent recurrences Referral for incision and drainage of abscess Removal of causative agent
Periapical Lesions			
Caries Periodontal disease Tooth fracture Traumatic dental procedures	Dental caries Periodontal disease Traumatic injury	Pain Swelling Sinus tract	Education to reduce likelihood of recurrences Referral for definitive endodontic treatment
Combined Periodontal Abscess			
Caries Periodontal disease Tooth fracture Traumatic dental procedures	Dental caries Periodontal disease	Pain Swelling Bone loss	Education to reduce likelihood of recurrences Referral for definitive endodontic and periodontal treatment
Acute Herpetic Gingivostomatitis			
Herpes simplex virus	Age	Ulcers with halos Pain Systemic symptoms	Reappointment for dental procedures Education to prevent transmission to others Supportive care until the virus has run its course
Recurrent Herpetic Lesions			
Herpes simplex virus	History of recurrences Change in immune status	Ulcer on lip or perioral tissues	Reappointment for dental procedures Supportive treatment Education about antiviral drugs Referral to physician
Acute Pericoronitis			
Bacterial plaque	Partially erupted molars Operculum	Pain Swelling Redness Foul odor	Education to pursue treatment and prevent recurrences Debridement and irrigation of area
Necrotizing Ulcerative Diseases			
Pathogenic bacteria	Systemic disease Stress Smoking	Pain Bleeding Fetid odor Redness Pseudomembrane Cratered papillae	Education to prevent recurrences Debridement over multiple appointments Definitive scaling as soon as possible Consultation with physician

KEY CONCEPTS

- A periodontal abscess is a treatable and often preventable disease process.
- A lesion of endodontic origin is a serious infection that requires consultation and referral for immediate treatment. Left untreated, a lesion of endodontic origin could develop into a brain abscess or fasciitis of the neck or chest wall, which can be life threatening.
- Periodontal abscesses have a pathogenic microflora similar to that associated with periodontal diseases.
- When treating periodontal abscesses, dental hygienists should scale and debride as thoroughly as possible.
- Abscesses can point and drain through the tissue or simply drain through the periodontal pocket opening.
- Infection moves through tissue along the pathway of least resistance; therefore, clinical features of the infection may appear at a distance from the affected tooth.

- Pain may be the key feature for distinguishing between periapical and periodontal abscesses. Periapical pain is sharp, severe, intermittent, and hard to localize; periodontal pain is constant, less severe, and localized.
- Primary and recurrent herpetic infections are serious but self-limiting conditions that require the postponement of elective dental hygiene and dental treatment. Dental hygiene care should not be performed on a patient with a herpetic infection because of the risk of transmission of the virus to the dental hygienist and other workers.
- Pericoronitis at any stage is a serious infection that requires referral and definitive treatment.
- Necrotizing periodontal diseases are complex processes that benefit from the dental hygiene process of care.

ACKNOWLEDGMENT

The authors acknowledge Dorothy A. Perry and Birgitta Söder for their past contributions to this chapter.

REFERENCES

1. Herrera D, Alonso B, De Arrabia L, et al. Acute periodontal lesions. *Periodontol 2000*. 2014;65:149–177.
2. Rotstein I. Interaction between endodontics and periodontics. *Periodontol 2000*. 2017;74:11–39.
3. Socransky SS, Haffajee AD. Periodontal microbial ecology. *Periodontol 2000*. 2005;38:135.
4. Herrera D, Roldçn S, Sanz M. The periodontal abscess, a review. *J Clin Periodontol*. 2000;377:386.
5. Rajasekaran M, Nainar DA, Alamelu S, et al. Microbiological profile in Endodontic-periodontal lesion. *J Oper Dent Endod*. 2016;1(1):25–29.
6. Parameter on acute periodontal diseases. *J Periodontol*. 2000;71:863–866.
7. Fatahzadeh M, Schwartz RA. Human herpes simplex virus infections: epidemiology, pathogenesis, symptomatology, diagnosis, and management. *J Am Acad Dermatol*. 2007;57:737.
8. Slots J. Human viruses in periodontitis. *Periodontol 2000*. 2010;89:110.
9. Yamalik K, Bozkaya S. The predictivity of mandibular third molar position as a risk indicator for pericoronitis. *Clin Oral Investig*. 2008;12:9.
10. Folayan MO. The epidemiology, etiology, and pathophysiology of acute necrotizing ulcerative gingivitis associated with malnutrition. *J Contemp Dent Pract*. 2004;5:28.

35

Pit and Fissure Sealants

Matt Crespin

PROFESSIONAL OPPORTUNITIES

As the settings where dental hygienists provide care expand, ensuring dental hygienists are skilled in the placement of dental sealants is critical. Dental hygienists play a key role in delivering preventive care to children and adolescents at high risk for dental caries.

COMPETENCIES

1. Describe the professional development opportunity provided by pit and fissure sealants and the role pit and fissure sealants play in primary and secondary prevention. In addition, discuss retention of sealants and contraindications to sealant placement.
2. Select an appropriate sealant material based on the clinical setting, the oral environment, and the individual needs of the patient.
3. Compare and contrast autopolymerized versus photopolymerized sealants, as well as filled versus unfilled sealants.
4. Describe legal and safety issues related to dental sealants and describe the procedure for sealant placement.

INTRODUCTION

The dental hygienist plays an important role in the detection, recognition, and management of dental caries. The placement of pit and fissure sealants is an integral part of comprehensive caries management.

A **pit and fissure sealant** is a thin plastic resinous coating that acts as a physical barrier to oral bacteria and carbohydrates (Fig. 35.1). The grooves found on occlusal surfaces of posterior teeth are risk factors for dental caries because they harbor debris and bacterial biofilm. Sealants can be placed on sound occlusal surfaces where there is no clinically detectable lesion as part of a primary prevention strategy, or they can be placed over **noncavitated carious lesions (NCCLs)** (i.e., initial, early, or white spot carious lesions visually confined to the enamel) as part of a secondary prevention program (Box 35.1). The sealant bonds primarily by mechanical retention to the enamel surface and forms a protective layer so that caries-producing bacteria cannot colonize within pits and fissures. By contrast, **cavitated lesions** are tooth surfaces that have invaded the dentin and cannot biologically repair themselves. These lesions penetrate enamel and/or extend into the underlying dentin and should be treated restoratively.

Approximately 90% of dental caries occur in the pits and fissures of permanent teeth with molars being the most susceptible.[1] Children and adolescents who have sealants placed on sound occlusal surfaces or on NCCLs experience an 80% reduction in the risk of developing new carious lesions, compared with those that do not receive sealants.[1] Moreover, after more than 7 years of followup studies, children and adolescents with sealants had a caries incidence of 29%, whereas those without sealants had a caries incidence of 74%.[2] Sealants have also been shown to be more effective in reducing the incidence of occlusal caries

in primary and permanent molars of children and adolescents when compared with fluoride varnish.[3] This benefit has been seen on both sound occlusal surfaces and noncavitated occlusal carious lesions.[3] Although sealants are considered most frequently in children and adolescents, they also can benefit adults without decay or fillings in their molars.

Despite their effectiveness at preventing and controlling the progression of occlusal caries, dental sealants are underused, especially in children at high risk for dental caries[4] (see Chapter 19). Only 40% of children aged 6 to 11 years have dental sealants. Children living in poverty receive sealants at a lower rate than children living in higher-income homes.[4] From 1999 to 2004 to 2011 to 2016, sealant use increased about 75% among children 6 to 11 from low-income families, reaching 39% in 2011 to 2016. Even with these increases, sealant use for these children remained below that of higher-income children (45% sealant use).[4]

School-based sealant programs are effective in decreasing the incidence of dental caries.[1] They typically target children at high risk for dental caries and focus primarily on those in the second and sixth grades because these children are most likely to have newly erupted permanent molars.[5] Dental hygienists working in these programs can deliver sealants to children who otherwise would not have access to preventive dental care (Table 35.1). School-aged children without sealants have almost three times as many cavities in first molars compared to children with sealants.[6] Applying sealants in schools for about 7 million children from low-income families could save up to $300 million in dental treatment costs.[6]

As part of the dental hygiene process of care, the dental hygienist should assess the patient's caries risk (see Chapter 19). The clinical

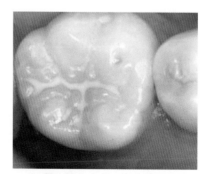

Fig. 35.1 A dental sealant.

BOX 35.1 Indications for Sealant Placement

- Sound occlusal surfaces of primary and permanent molars
- Noncavitated occlusal lesions of primary and permanent molars

TABLE 35.1 Recommendations for School-Based Sealant Programs

Topic	Recommendation
Indications for sealant placement	Seal sound and noncavitated pit and fissure surfaces of posterior teeth, with first and second permanent molars receiving the highest priority. Premolars and primary teeth at higher risk for caries may also be sealed.
Tooth and surface assessment	Differentiate cavitated and noncavitated lesions: • Unaided visual assessment is appropriate and adequate. • Dry teeth with cotton rolls, gauze, or compressed air, when available, before making assessments. • Do not use a sharp explorer under force. • Radiographs are unnecessary. • Other diagnostic technologies are not required.
Sealant placement and evaluation	Clean the tooth surface: • Toothbrush prophylaxis is acceptable. • Air abrasion or enameloplasty are not recommended. Use four-handed technique when feasible. Seal teeth of children, even if followup evaluation cannot be ensured. Evaluate sealant retention within 1 year.

component of caries risk assessment involves both a visual and a tactile examination. The clinician cleans and dries the teeth to evaluate the pits and fissures. Sharp explorers are not recommended for caries detection because they may cause a cavitation in any demineralized surface of the enamel. However, a dull explorer or a ball probe can be dragged along the occlusal surface to evaluate whether the surface is rough or smooth.[7] Sound occlusal surfaces of primary and permanent molars are assigned an International Caries Detection and Assessment System (ICDAS) code of 0 and are recommended for sealant placement (Fig. 35.2).[2] This intervention can prevent decay from occurring, especially if the patient is at high risk for dental caries.[3] NCCLs are demineralized areas confined to the enamel and are characterized by a change in color, glossiness, or surface structure. These lesions are assigned an ICDAS code of 1 or 2 and are also recommended for sealant placement because they are at risk for caries progression (Fig. 35.2).[2] Clinically, noncavitated lesions appear as white demineralized lines or spots or areas of yellow-brown discoloration around the pits and fissures of teeth (Fig. 35.3).

CONTRAINDICATIONS TO SEALANT PLACEMENT

If there is radiographic evidence of proximal dental caries, then sealant placement in occlusal pits and fissures is contraindicated. The patient must be referred to a dental care provider who can restore the tooth.

American Dental Association Caries Classification System.

	Sound	Initial		Moderate		Advanced	
Clinical Presentation	No clinically detectable lesion. Dental hard tissue appears normal in color, translucency, and gloss.	Earliest clinically detectable lesion compatible with mild demineralization. Lesion limited to enamel or to shallow demineralization of cementum/dentin. Mildest forms are detectable only after drying. When established and active, lesions may be white or brown and enamel has lost its normal gloss.		Visible signs of enamel breakdown or signs the dentin is moderately demineralized.		Enamel is fully cavitated and dentin is exposed. Dentin lesion is deeply/severely demineralized.	
Other Labels	No surface change or adequately restored	Visually noncavitated		Established, early cavitated, shallow cavitation, microcavitation		Spread/disseminated, late cavitated, deep cavitation	
Infected Dentin	None	Unlikely		Possible		Present	
Appearance of Occlusal Surfaces (Pit and Fissure)*,†	ICDAS 0 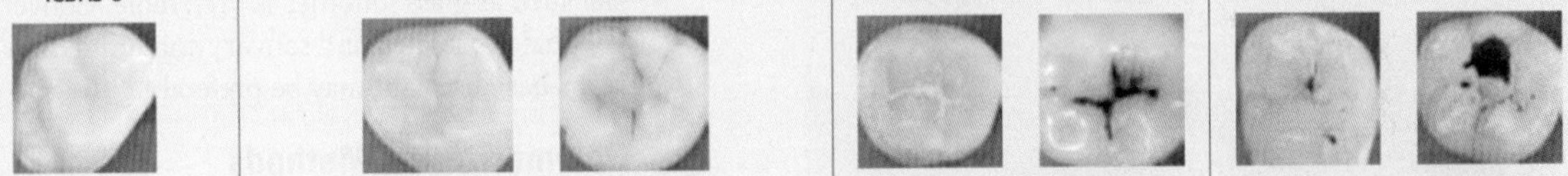	ICDAS 1	ICDAS 2	ICDAS 3	ICDAS 4	ICDAS 5	ICDAS 6
Accessible Smooth Surfaces, Including Cervical and Root‡							
Radiographic Presentation of the Approximal Surface§	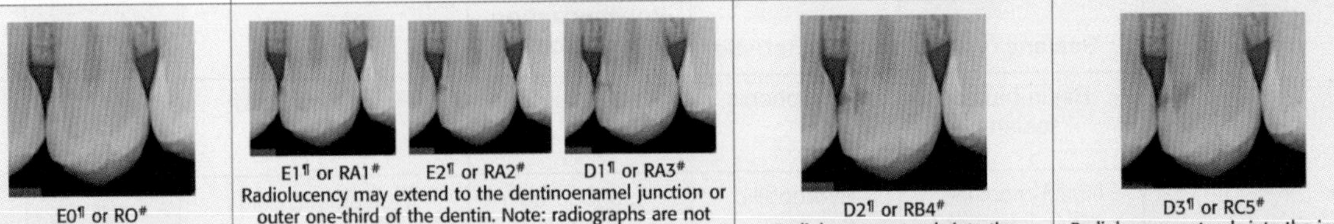 E0¶ or R0# No radiolucency	E1¶ or RA1# E2¶ or RA2# D1¶ or RA3# Radiolucency may extend to the dentinoenamel junction or outer one-third of the dentin. Note: radiographs are not reliable for mild occlusal lesions.		D2¶ or RB4# Radiolucency extends into the middle one-third of the dentin		D3¶ or RC5# Radiolucency extends into the inner one-third of the dentin	

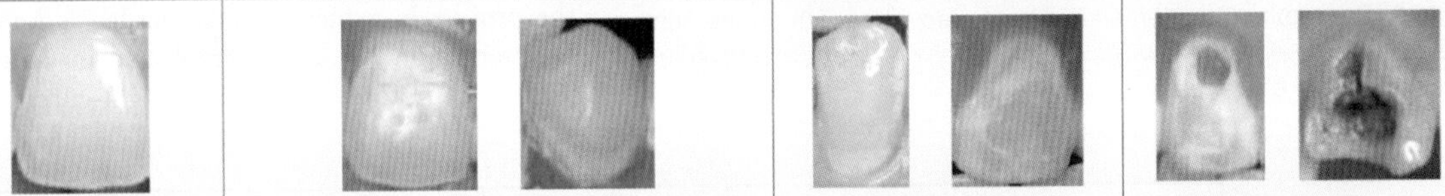

* Photographs of extracted teeth illustrate examples of pit-and-fissure caries.
† The ICDAS notation system links the clinical visual appearance of occlusal caries lesions with the histologically determined degree of dentinal penetration using the evidence collated and published by the ICDAS Foundation over the last decade; ICDAS also has a menu of options, including 3 levels of caries lesion classification, radiographic scoring and an integrated, risk-based caries management system ICCMS. (Pitts NB, Ekstrand KR. International Caries Detection and Assessment System [ICDAS] and its International Caries Classification and Management System [ICCMS]: Methods for staging of the caries process and enabling dentists to manage caries. *Community Dent Oral Epidemiol* 2013;41[1]:e41-e52. Pitts NB, Ismail AI, Martignon S, Ekstrand K, Douglas GAV, Longbottom C. ICCMS Guide for Practitioners and Educators. Available at: https://www.icdas.org/uploads/ICCMS-Guide_Full_Guide_US.pdf. Accessed April 13, 2015.)
‡ "Cervical and root" includes any smooth surface lesion above or below the anatomical crown that is accessible through direct visual/tactile examination.
§ Simulated radiographic images.
¶ E0-E2, D1-D3 notation system.[33]
# R0, RA1-RA3, RB4, and RC5-RC6 ICCMS radiographic scoring system (RC6 = into pulp). (Pitts NB, Ismail AI, Martignon S, Ekstrand K, Douglas GAV, Longbottom C. ICCMS Guide for Practitioners and Educators. Available at: https://www.icdas.org/uploads/ICCMS-Guide_Full_Guide_US.pdf. Accessed April 13, 2015.)

Fig. 35.2 International Caries Detection and Assessment System (ICDAS) chart. (From Young DA, Nový BB, Zeller GG, et al. The American Dental Association Caries Classification System for clinical practice: a report of the American Dental Association Council on Scientific Affairs. *J Am Dent Assoc.* 2015;146(2):79–86.)

SEALANT RETENTION

The ability of pit and fissure sealants to prevent dental caries is highly dependent on their ability to be retained on the tooth surface (**sealant retention**). Adhesive systems placed under resin-based sealants can increase retention but require an additional step prior to sealant placement.[8] First, the tooth surface must be etched; second, a primer is applied to make the tooth more susceptible to the adhesive resin; and finally, the adhesive resin is applied. Self-etching adhesive materials are available, although more evidence is needed to indicate equal retention when compared with the conventional approach.[9] The adhesive resin copolymerizes with the primer and sealant material, thus enhancing sealant retention. These bonding agents increase the time and cost of the procedure. Therefore they would not be recommended for use in a public health setting.

Salivary contamination during placement can also affect sealant retention and is the most common reason for sealant failure. In situations when dry isolation is difficult, such as a partially erupted tooth, a hydrophilic material (e.g., GI sealant) is preferable. If the tooth can be properly isolated with a rubber dam or cotton rolls, then a resin-based sealant is preferable to ensure long-term retention.[3] Other factors affecting sealant retention rates include clinician inexperience and lack of patient cooperation.

TYPES OF SEALANTS

Sealants can be classified by type (glass ionomer versus resin), by polymerization method (autopolymerized versus photopolymerized),

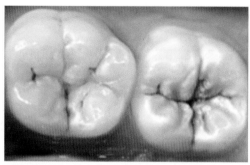

Fig. 35.3 The tooth on the left should be sealed. The tooth on the right should be restored. (Courtesy Steve Eakle, University of California–San Francisco School of Dentistry.)

or by filler (filled versus unfilled). There are four types of sealant material: (1) resin-based sealants, (2) polyacid-modified resin sealants, (3) glass ionomer cements, and (4) resin-modified glass ionomer sealants. These materials release fluoride in varying degrees (Fig. 35.4). Current research indicates that the fluoride released from sealant materials has the properties to be effective in controlling the progression of dental caries, but the added benefit of the fluoride is not proven.[10]

Resin-based sealants (RBSs) are urethane dimethacrylate (UDMA) or bisphenol A-glycidyl methacrylate (bis-GMA) monomers. They harden by either autopolymerization or photopolymerization. They are **hydrophobic** (repel water) and must be applied to a completely dry surface. Consequently, RBS are aerosol generating, and placement using four-handed technique reduces aerosols and increases retention.[3]

Glass ionomer sealants (GISs) are cements that bond directly to enamel and are used for their fluoride-releasing properties. They are **hydrophilic** and can be placed when moisture control is an issue. Glass ionomer sealants are five times more likely to not be retained than RBS and should be monitored by the dental provider for ongoing retention.[3]

Polyacid-modified resin sealants are also known as *compomers*. They combine resin-based material found in traditional resin-based sealants (*comp-*) with the fluoride-releasing and adhesive properties of glass ionomer sealants (*-omer*).[3] They are hydrophobic and must be applied to a completely dry surface.

Resin-modified glass ionomer sealants are essentially glass ionomer sealants with resin components. This type of sealant has similar fluoride-releasing properties as glass ionomer sealants but has a longer working time and is hydrophilic.[3]

Current research indicates that no single sealant material is superior to another in preventing and/or arresting occlusal caries.[3] When choosing a sealant material, clinicians must assess the clinical environment (i.e., private practice versus public health setting), the individual needs of the patient, ability for ongoing evaluation of retention, and the oral environment. In situations where dry isolation is difficult, such as a partially erupted tooth or a noncompliant patient, a hydrophilic material such as glass ionomer is preferable. Conversely, if the tooth can be adequately isolated and salivary contamination is not a concern, then a resin-based sealant may be preferable.[3]

Polymerization Methods

The process by which sealants harden is known as *polymerization*. Polymerization can be accomplished by **autopolymerization** (self-curing) or **photopolymerization** (light-curing).

Sealant Type	Characteristic	Polymerization method	Etchant	Increasing fluoride release
Resin-based sealant	Hydrophobic	Light cured	Phosphoric acid	
Resin-modified glass ionomer sealant	Hydrophilic	Light cured	Polyacrylic acid (dentin conditioner)	
Polyacid-modified resins	Hydrophilic	Light cured	Phosphoric acid	
Glass ionomer cements	Hydrophilic	Self-cured	Polyacrylic acid (dentin conditioner)	

Fig. 35.4 Sealants with increasing fluoride release. (Courtesy Dr. Pia Staana, Foothill College, Los Altos Hills, CA.)

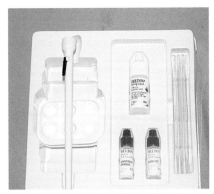

Fig. 35.5 Universal monomer and catalyst with mixing well and mixing stick.

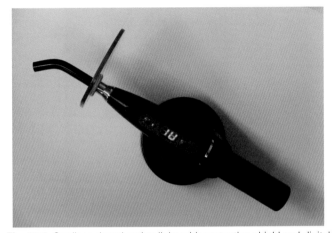

Fig. 35.6 Cordless dental curing light with protective shield and digital timer.

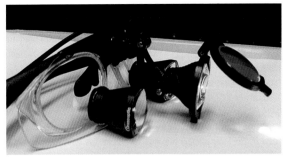

Fig. 35.7 Protective shield attached to clinician's loupe light.

BOX 35.2 Critical Thinking Exercise A

Patient Profile: Evan is a 14-year-old boy with Down syndrome. His mother, a single parent, raises Evan alone.

Chief Complaint: "My mom brought me here to see if I have any new cavities."

Health History: Evan has "glue ear," which causes sounds to be muffled, and he wears eyeglasses. He also has mitral valve prolapse.

Dental History: Evan has composite fillings on teeth 3 and 19 that were placed 6 months ago. Teeth 18 and 31 have erupted, but teeth 2 and 15 are unerupted. He also has macroglossia.

Social History: He is a freshman in high school and a member of the student council.

Oral Self-Care Assessment: Evan brushes his teeth twice a day and uses a fluoride toothpaste. His toothbrushing technique is not monitored by his mother.

1. Would you recommend sealant placement for Evan? If so, what type of sealant material would you use? (Consider resin-based versus glass ionomer, filled versus unfilled, and self-cured versus light cured.) Which teeth would you seal and why?
2. Does Evan need to take antibiotic premedication prior to sealant placement?
3. What explanation can you give for why teeth 2 and 15 are unerupted?
4. What educational tips can you provide to Evan's mother regarding his future dental needs?

Autopolymerized sealants have two components: a universal liquid monomer and a catalyst (Fig. 35.5). When these two components are mixed together, they harden (polymerize). Polymerization starts as soon as mixing begins, and the material hardens within 60 to 90 seconds. Autopolymerized sealants are commonly used in school-based sealant programs because there is no special equipment required.

Photopolymerized sealants harden when exposed to a light-curing unit. Because no mixing time is required, the clinician controls the start of polymerization. Curing time is usually 20 to 30 seconds, depending on the manufacturer. Glass ionomer sealants do not require light curing; however, they will set faster with the use of a curing light.

There are a variety of **light-curing units** (LCUs) available: light-emitting diode (LED), plasma arc curving (PAC), tungsten halogen, and laser. These lights come with special filters that protect the clinician's eyes from potential retinal damage (Fig. 35.6). Otherwise, the clinician can wear a protective shield over their loupe light (Fig. 35.7). It is important to periodically measure the light intensity output of the unit, which can be done with a dental radiometer. If the output intensity of the curing light is less than 280 milliwatts per square centimeter (mW/cm²), the polymerization process of the monomer will be incomplete and early loss of the sealant may occur. Other factors that can decrease the output of the unit are residual sealant material retained on the tip of the curing light and/or a plastic barrier that covers the light tip. An LCU that operates at full capacity will ensure that a secure bond is obtained between the sealant material and the enamel surface being sealed.

Filled sealants contain particles of glass or quartz to increase the sealants' strength and resistance to abrasion and occlusal wear. Sealants with fillers tend to be more viscous, thus affecting their ability to flow easily into the pits and fissures. Filled sealants are harder and more resistant to the patient's occlusion; therefore they may need to be mechanically adjusted.

Unfilled sealants do not contain particles, so they are less resistant to wear over time. They usually adjust on their own, which makes them ideal for use in a public health setting. There is no difference in the retention rates between filled and unfilled sealants. See Boxes 35.2 and 35.3 to help develop critical thinking skills regarding selection of sealant material depending on clinical findings and practice setting.

Sealant Color

Sealants are available as clear, tinted, opaque, or white. Color sealants are easier for the clinician to see during application and to reevaluate during recall appointments. The addition of color to sealants material does not affect their retention. Sealants may be available in a tinted format in the liquid phase that change color when polymerized.

Legal and Safety Issues Related to Dental Sealants

It is legal in all 50 states for dental hygienists to place sealants. Since most dental sealants are placed on children and adolescents, it is the responsibility of the dental hygienist to obtain informed consent from the parent or guardian prior to sealant placement. The American Dental Association (ADA) evaluates the safety and effectiveness of sealant

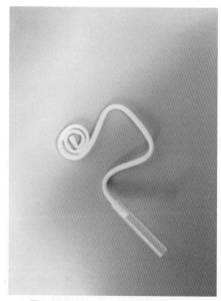

Fig. 35.8 Hygoformic saliva ejector.

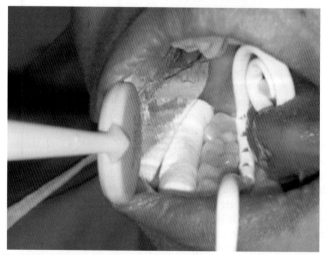

Fig. 35.9 Proper isolation and placement for moisture control, using Dri-Angles, cotton rolls, and a Hygoformic saliva ejector. (Courtesy Dr. Pia Staana, Foothill College, Los Altos Hills, CA.)

materials. The concern that sealants might exhibit adverse effects is primarily associated with the presence of bisphenol A (BPA) in the sealant material. BPA has been associated with estrogen-like effects that may lead to hormonal reactions in the patient. Current evidence suggests that the trace amount of BPA found in the saliva after sealant placement does not place patients at risk. There have been no findings of systemic BPA or increased estrogen production after sealant placement.[11] Breathing air exposes people to about 100 times more BPA than dental sealants.[12] Aside from an allergic reaction to the sealant material, there are no known side effects to placing sealants. Box 35.4 provides the legal and safety issues associated with dental sealants.

Client Education

Prior to sealant placement, it is important for patients to understand that although dental sealants are effective in reducing caries when compared with teeth without sealants, they are not permanent. Their integrity must be reassessed at each recare visit and replaced if missing or defective (Box 35.5). Sealants are not a replacement for caries preventive procedures such as fluoride treatments, effective self-care practices, use of antimicrobials, and/or modification of risk factors.

PROCEDURE FOR SEALANT PLACEMENT

Proper sealant placement is necessary for a patient to maintain a biologically sound and functional dentition. It is important to follow manufacturer's instructions because the technique varies depending on the product. The patient should wear tinted safety glasses to protect the eyes from the curing light, and a four-handed technique with an assistant is helpful in maintaining a dry working field and reducing aerosols. A rubber dam is effective for tooth isolation when working on several teeth in a quadrant; however, bibulous pads (e.g., Dri-Angles) placed over the Stensen duct, cotton rolls placed in the vestibules and at the sides of the tongue, and using a traditional or Hygoformic saliva ejector are also effective for moisture control (Figs. 35.8 and 35.9). There are various suction/isolation devices available on the market that can assist in moisture control. After isolating the tooth, the occlusal surfaces must be cleaned. A toothbrush used alone or a slow-speed handpiece and prophy brush are effective to remove any debris from the occlusal surfaces. Following cleaning, the tooth is then dried. Once isolated, cleaned, and dried, the tooth is then etched. Acid etches come in concentrations ranging from 15% to 50% and are in liquid, gel, or semigel form. Liquid etches flow easily but are hard to control; gel etches are easy to see but are more difficult to rinse; and semigel etches are easy to see, easy to control, and rinse well. The acid etch works to create micropores in the enamel and helps with sealant retention. Liquid etches are applied with a small brush, sponge, or cotton pellet using a small dabbing motion. It is important to keep the tooth surface moist for the entire etching time (15 to 60 seconds). When using a gel or semigel etchant, it is applied with a manufacturer's supplied syringe (Fig. 35.10). It is critical that the etchant does not touch the soft tissues as this can cause an acid burn. After acid etching, the tooth must be rinsed and dried again for 15 to 20 seconds. A properly etched surface will have a chalky appearance. If this does not occur, then the etchant must be reapplied. The sealant material is then applied into the pits and fissures. Care must be taken not to overfill them. It is also important not to overmanipulate the material as doing so can cause bubbles to occur. Once placed, the sealant is either self-cured or light-cured. The final step is to check the occlusion and adjust the sealant as necessary.

Detailed methods for the placement of photopolymerized and auto-polymerized sealants are described in Procedures 35.1 and 35.2.

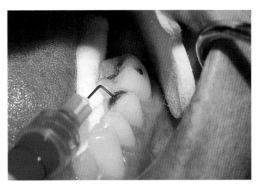

Fig. 35.10 Acid etching solution in gel form.

PROCEDURE 35.1 Applying Light-Cured (Photopolymerized) Sealants

Equipment

Mouth mirror
Explorer
Cotton forceps
Traditional or Hygoformic saliva ejector
Sealant kit
Cotton rolls and rubber dam
Air-water syringe tip
Dri-Angles
High-speed evacuation tube
Low-speed handpiece or air-polishing device
Bristled brush
Floss
Light protective shield
Patient protective eyewear
Personal protective equipment
Light-cure unit
Round finishing burr
Articulating paper

Steps

1. Assemble sealant armamentarium.

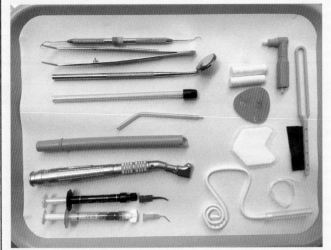

Armamentarium for pit and fissure sealant. (Courtesy Dr. Pia Staana, Foothill College, Los Altos Hills, CA.)

2. Provide patient with filtered protective eyewear. Wear personal protective equipment.
3. Identify tooth or teeth to be sealed.
4. Polish the intended surface with a bristled brush attached to a low-speed handpiece. Rinse with water.

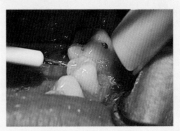

Rinsing tooth surface.

5. Isolate teeth with a rubber dam, or place Dri-Angle over Stensen duct and insert cotton rolls. Place saliva ejector into patient's mouth.
6. Dry the site to be sealed with compressed air that is free of oil and moisture.

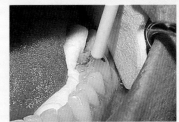

Drying tooth surface before applying acid etching solution.

7. Apply phosphoric acid to the clean, dry tooth surface. Etch the tooth for 10 to 20 seconds. If using a liquid etchant, apply it with a brush. If using a gel etchant, apply it and leave undisturbed.
8. Rinse etched surfaces for 30 to 60 seconds using a water syringe and high-speed evacuation. If gel etchant is used, rinse for an additional 30 seconds.

Continued

PROCEDURE 35.1   Applying Light-Cured (Photopolymerized) Sealants—cont'd

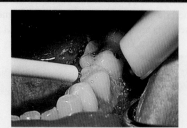

Rinsing etched tooth surface.

9. Using cotton forceps, replace cotton rolls and Dri-Angles as they become wet.

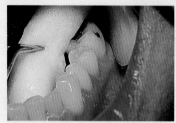

Removing wet cotton rolls.

10. Dry the treatment site with compressed air for 10 seconds. Evaluate etched surface.

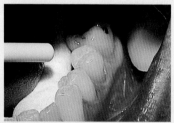

Drying etched surface.

11. Apply hydrophilic primer and dry with compressed air.
12. Apply liquid sealant over the pits and fissures at less than 90 degrees. Allow the sealant to flow into the etched surfaces.

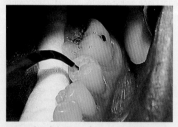

Applying sealant material.

13. Apply light-cure tip to sealant. Place tip of light source 2 mm from sealant.

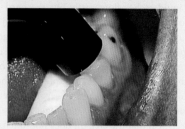

Curing sealant material.

14. Check manufacturer's instructions for time before advancing the light to another area. After the polymerization process, evaluate the sealant with an explorer and check for hard, smooth surface and retention. Set sealant appears as a thin, polymerized film.
15. Check sealant for imperfections (e.g., incomplete coverage, air bubbles). If detected, reetch tooth for 10 seconds; wash and dry teeth, and apply additional sealant material.

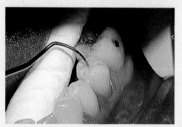

Checking sealant for coverage and/or imperfections.

16. Check occlusion with articulating paper to detect high spot areas. Remove excess filled sealant material with a finishing burr.

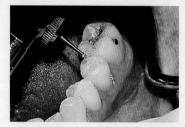

Adjusting sealant with round burr.

17. Remove any residual unsealed liquid sealant with dry gauze. Floss treated teeth.
18. Apply topical fluoride.
19. Record type of sealant and teeth sealed in patient's dental record.
20. Evaluate sealants at each recare appointment.

PROCEDURE 35.2   Applying Self-Cured (Autopolymerized) Sealants

Equipment

Mouth mirror
Explorer
Traditional or Hygoformic saliva ejector
Self-cure sealant kit
Gauze
Cotton rolls and rubber dam
Air-water syringe tip
Dri-Angles
High-speed evacuation tube
Low-speed handpiece or air-polishing device

Bristled brush
Floss
Personal protective equipment
Protective barriers

Steps

1. Follow steps 1 to 10 as described for light-cured sealants in Procedure 35.1.
2. Mix one drop of universal liquid and one drop of catalyst liquid in mixing well. Follow manufacturer's directions, especially when sealing more than two teeth.

PROCEDURE 35.2 Applying Self-Cured (Autopolymerized) Sealants—cont'd

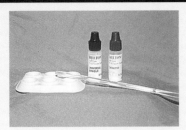

Liquid monomer and catalyst for autopolymerized sealants

3. Mix for 10 to 15 seconds or as specified by manufacturer's instructions.
4. Apply sealant with brush over pits and fissures. Working time is 45 seconds.
5. Allow sealant to set for 60 to 90 seconds or according to manufacturer's instructions.
6. Follow steps 14 to 20 as described for light-cured sealants in Procedure 35.1.

KEY CONCEPTS

- Sealants are safe and effective in reducing the incidence of caries in sound occlusal surfaces and noncavitated carious occlusal lesions of children and adolescents compared with the nonuse of sealants or fluoride varnishes.
- Sealant use should be increased, along with other preventive interventions, especially in individuals at elevated risk for developing dental caries.
- Choice of sealant material should be based on the individual needs of the patient and the oral environment; no sealant material is superior to another in regard to caries prevention.
- It is important to follow manufacturer's instructions when applying sealants.
- Economic data indicate that the benefits of school sealant programs outweigh their costs when the programs target individuals at high risk for developing dental caries.

REFERENCES

1. Community Preventive Services Task Force. *Preventing Dental Caries: School-Based Dental Sealant Delivery Programs.* US Department of Health and Human Services, Community Preventive Services Task Force; 2016. https://www.thecommunityguide.org/sites/default/files/assets/Oral-Health-Caries-School-based-Sealants_0.pdf.
2. Wright JT, Tampi MP, Graham L, et al. Sealants for preventing and arresting pit-and-fissure occlusal caries in primary and permanent molars. A systematic review of randomized controlled trials-a report of the American Dental Association and the American Academy of Pediatric Dentistry. *J Am Dent Assoc.* 2016;147(8):631–645.
3. Wright JT, Crall JJ, Fontana M, et al. Evidenced-based clinical practice guideline for the use of pit and fissure sealants. American Academy of Pediatric Dentistry, American Dental Association. *Pediatr Dent.* 2016;38(5):E120–E136.
4. Centers for Disease Control and Prevention. *Oral Health Surveillance Report: Trends in Dental Caries and Sealants, Tooth Retention, and Edentulism, United States, 1999–2004 to 2011–2016.* Centers for Disease Control and Prevention, US Department of Health and Human Services; 2019.
5. Griffin SO, Naavaal S, Scherrer C, et al. Evaluation of school-based dental sealant programs: an updated community guide systemic review. *Am J Prev Med.* 2017;52(3):407–415.
6. Centers for Disease Control and Prevention. Dental Sealants Prevent Cavities—Vital Signs. 2016. Available at: https://www.cdc.gov/vitalsigns/pdf/2016-10-vitalsigns.pdf. Accessed Nov 7, 2023.
7. Gooch BF, Griffin SO, Gray KS, et al. Preventing caries through school-based sealant programs. Updated recommendations and reviews of evidence. *J Am Dent Assoc.* 2009;140:1356–1365.
8. Young DA, Novy BB, Zeller GG, et al. American Dental Association Council on Scientific Affairs. The American Dental Association Caries Classification System for Clinical Practice: a Report of the American Dental Association Council on Scientific Affairs. *J Am Dent Assoc.* 2015;146(2):79–86.
9. Botton G, Morgental CS, Scherer MM, et al. Are self-etch adhesive systems effective in the retention of occlusal sealants? A systematic review and meta-analysis. *Int J Paediatr Dent.* 2016;26(6):402–411.
10. Bagherian A, Shirazi AS, Sadeghi R. Adhesive systems under fissure sealants: yes or no? A systematic review and meta-analysis. *J Am Dent Assoc.* 2016;147(6):446–456.
11. Cury JA, deOlivia BH, dos Santos AP, et al. Are fluoride releasing dental materials clinically effective in caries control? *Dent Mater.* 2016;32:323–333.
12. American Dental Association. Sealants. Available at: https://www.mouthhealthy.org/all-topics-a-z/sealants. Accessed Nov 11, 2022.

36

Nutritional Counseling

Kylie J. Austin

PROFESSIONAL OPPORTUNITIES

As the correlation between overall health and oral health becomes more evident, dental hygienists have a significant role in educating clients about this relationship. Gathering information about a patient's dietary intake allows the clinician to evaluate the patient's nutritional status using recommended dietary guidelines. Dental hygienists who can use this information to identify key factors in the overall health–oral health relationship can effectively provide nutritional counseling to promote positive behavior changes for their patients.

COMPETENCIES

1. Apply knowledge about a patient's personal, medical, and dental histories to formulate a comprehensive nutritional assessment.
2. Evaluate a patient's nutritional status using nutritional assessment data and the United States Department of Agriculture's (USDA's) MyPlate guidelines.
3. Demonstrate comprehensive and individualized nutritional counseling for individuals at risk of dental caries, periodontal disease, or nutrient deficiencies.
4. Compare and contrast the nutritional needs of various patient populations, including variations in nutritional requirements throughout the life span.

Diet and nutrition are vital oral health components. **Nutritional counseling** is the process by which a clinician works with patients to assess their dietary intake and then identifies areas where change is recommended. It can be used in the oral healthcare setting to help patients achieve and maintain optimal oral health and develop healthful behaviors that promote overall health. When providing nutritional counseling to dental patients, dental hygienists must consider a variety of individual factors, including age, sex, culture, socioeconomic status, lifestyle influences, dental knowledge, existing systemic conditions, medications, allergies, and special dietary considerations.[1]

As healthcare professionals who treat patients on a frequent and ongoing basis, dental hygienists can identify dietary issues and intervene as necessary. Dental hygienists must be knowledgeable about nutrition, oral manifestations of nutritional deficiencies, and effects on oral health. However, for nutritional concerns outside the scope of dental hygiene practice, referral to a registered dietitian or nutrition professional is recommended (Box 36.1). An official diagnosis of nutritional deficiency or metabolic disease should only be made by a physician after extensive data collection.

NUTRITIONAL ASSESSMENT

Nutritional assessment is the systematic collection of information to identify the need for nutritional counseling and make the appropriate recommendations and referrals. The assessment is comprehensive, taking a patient's personal, health, and dental histories into consideration. The patient's personal history can reveal information regarding educational, cultural, financial, and environmental influences on food intake. The health and pharmacologic histories identify health factors and medications that interfere with an individual's ability to eat or the body's ability to absorb nutrients. The dental history provides information about caries susceptibility, fluoride use, and dentition concerns that may affect food intake. These findings, along with a dietary assessment, direct the dental hygienist in the role of nutritional counselor. Every patient can benefit from nutritional counseling, but those most often targeted include patients who are:

- At high risk for dental caries, enamel erosion, or periodontal disease
- Exhibiting oral manifestations of a possible nutritional deficiency
- Undergoing periodontal or oral maxillofacial surgery
- At risk for osteoporosis
- Diagnosed with osteopenia

Health and Pharmacologic History

Questions normally included in a comprehensive health history provide clues to nutritional status, lifestyle behaviors, and overall health (see Chapter 13). The health history should acknowledge conditions and medications that interfere with food digestion, absorption, and metabolism. The dental hygienist should also ask detailed questions about dietary supplements, vitamins, and herbal preparations and discuss any recent illnesses, changes in health behaviors, or diet modifications with their patients.

Height and Weight

Height and weight are important components of the health history as they are used to determine a patient's **body mass index (BMI)**. BMI measurement is calculated by dividing a patient's weight in kilograms by height in meters.[2] It reflects weight in relation to height (Table 36.1).[2] Although a BMI measurement does not reflect how much of the weight is fat, it does give a measurement associated with health risks such as heart disease, hypertension, diabetes, and cancer (Box 36.2). Calculation of BMI is the most practical method to integrate into patient care, making use of the reported height and weight during the health history interview. The US Department of Health and Human Services National Heart, Lung, and Blood Institute has an online BMI calculation tool that can be accessed at https://www.nhlbi.nih.gov/health/educational/lose_wt/BMI/bmicalc.htm.

Waist circumference (see Table 36.1) also can be used to indicate health risk. Waist circumference is a numeric measurement of the waist that provides a prediction of risk above and beyond the BMI. It is used most effectively in patients who are categorized as normal or overweight on the BMI scale. A female with a waist measurement of 35 inches or greater and a male with a waist measurement of 40 inches or greater are associated with upper body obesity. Upper body obesity is correlated strongly with heart disease and type 2 diabetes.

Another useful and simple calculation is ideal body weight. Ideal body weight calculators are available online to assist with calculating the ideal body weight based on a patient's height. Although commonly used, these are not the most accurate method because they do not take age, ethnic origin or body habitus into consideration.

Exercise Patterns

Activity levels ascertained during the health history interview may be used to determine daily caloric needs more accurately. Along with anthropometric measures such as height and weight, activity levels can be entered into one of the online interactive tools such as the USDA's MyPlate[3] Plan to determine an individual's caloric needs and provide patients with recommendations for a healthy lifestyle. Individualized plans can be determined using the MyPlate checklist available at https://www.myplate.gov/widgets-sm/myplate-daily-checklist-input-start.

An approximate daily caloric expenditure can be useful in planning for weight loss or weight gain. However, the primary goal in the dental setting is to identify nutritional concerns that may contribute to

systemic or oral disease risk—not to modify weight. Patients interested in modifying their weight should be referred to a nutrition professional.

Prescription Medications and Dietary Supplements Intake

An assessment of the ingestion of prescription medications, as well as vitamin and mineral supplements, provides insight into oral manifestations such as xerostomia, lichenoid reactions, candidiasis, cheilitis, and glossitis. Dietary supplements and herbal products are used routinely by dental patients. Many of these products have effects on the oral tissues that may interfere with dental care, so it is essential that the dental hygienist update and review these nonprescription medications before treatment. Increased bleeding, elevated blood pressure, and delayed wound healing are potential effects that may occur.

DIETARY ASSESSMENT

Dietary assessment is the identification of current dietary practices and dietary requirements of the patient. Dietary assessment includes frequency of food intake, methods of food preparation, cultural or religious dietary considerations, and exercise or activity levels. Dietary assessment is based on the *Dietary Guidelines for Americans* provided through the USDA's food guidance system titled MyPlate.[3] Types of dietary assessments include the dietary history, a food frequency questionnaire, and a computer dietary analysis.[4]

Dietary History

A **dietary history** may consist of a 24-hour food record; a food frequency questionnaire; or a 3-, 5-, or 7-day dietary history, in which the patient records all foods and drinks consumed within the defined timeframe (Procedure 36.1). The dietary history determines a patient's

---

BOX 36.1 Legal, Ethical, and Safety Issues

Dental hygienists play an integral role as members of an interprofessional healthcare team. They have the unique opportunity to potentially treat patients multiple times per year; therefore they might be among the first healthcare professionals to identify a nutrition-related disease or deficiency.

- Dental hygienists should refrain from practicing nutritional assessment or counseling that is beyond the scope of their practice (e.g., weight management, development of comprehensive dietary plans, metabolic disease control, eating disorders).
- Refer patients with signs of nutrition-related diseases or deficiencies to a physician or licensed nutrition professional.
- Alert patients to potential signs and symptoms of nutritional deficiencies and refer them to a physician for diagnosis.
- In the patient's record, document all information provided to the patient during nutritional counseling for oral disease prevention and health promotion.

BOX 36.2 Body Mass Index (BMI) Categories

- BMI less than 18.5 is an indication of being underweight.
- BMI of 18.5 to 24.9 is considered within the normal range.
- BMI of 25 to 29.9 is in the overweight category.
- BMI of 30 and above is considered obese.

TABLE 36.1 Nutrition-Related Formulas and Calculations

Formula or Calculation	Definition	Use	Disadvantage
Body Mass Index (BMI) Weight in kilograms ÷ height in meters^2 or Weight in pounds × 703 ÷ height in inches^2	Measurement of weight in relation to height	Useful in determining if patient is underweight or overweight	Does not measure lean tissue in relation to fat; for example, bodybuilders may have a higher BMI owing to a larger amount of lean tissue but are not overweight or obese.
Waist Circumference For men, 40 inches; for women, 35 inches	Measurement of waist used to determine central obesity	Useful in determining health risks if a patient is overweight or obese	Incorrect placement of the tape measure could produce inaccurate result.
Ideal Body Weight (Hamwi Equation) For men, 106 pounds for the first 5 feet of height and 6 pounds for each inch above 5 feet; or 6 pounds subtracted for each inch under 5 feet For women, 100 pounds for the first 5 feet and 5 pounds for each inch above 5 feet; or 5 pounds subtracted for each inch under 5 feet	Determines ideal body for height of individual	Useful in determining if patient is underweight or overweight	Does not measure lean tissue in relation to fat. A patient may be considered underweight but may still have excess fat.

PROCEDURE 36.1   Food Record Instructions for Dental Patients

Steps

1. Record everything you eat or drink for the suggested period of time (3, 5, or 7 days) in a notebook, on a single piece of paper, or using an online tracking tool or application.
2. Include one weekend day.
3. Try to record as soon after eating as possible. Indicate whether foods are consumed as meals or consumed between meals. Record time consumed.
4. Indicate any oral hygiene regimens incorporated throughout day (e.g., brush teeth after meals, chew gum with xylitol, rinse with antiseptic mouth rinse).
5. Exclude days that you are sick, dieting, or fasting for medical or religious purposes.
6. Be as specific as possible when recording the amounts consumed. When possible, use measuring terms to indicate sizes of servings, such as cup (C), tablespoon (T), teaspoons (tsp), and ounces (oz). Also, try to include all ingredients when consuming a dish with multiple ingredients.
7. Record all added sauces, gravies, condiments, and extras such as sugar or cream.
8. Indicate food preparation method (e.g., baked, fried, grilled, broiled).
9. All gum, hard candies, cough drops, or mints should be recorded, and indicate if sugar-free.
10. Use brand names whenever possible and include restaurant names if food is consumed outside the home.
11. Record all liquids consumed and indicate if sugar-free.

usual intake over a period of time and is a screening tool to identify those in need of nutritional counseling. The clinician can create a simple form to be distributed to the patient or use one of several sample forms that are available online. There are also websites and smartphone applications that allow patients to track their dietary history online. These resources typically result in greater compliance and more accurate reporting because the patient can immediately and conveniently document food and drinks consumed from any location using a smartphone or other electronic device.

Dietary History Best Practices

A dietary history can be obtained through a face-to-face interview with the patient or a self-administered form. The 24-hour dietary history usually requires 10 to 15 minutes for the dental hygienist to complete as it simply entails asking the patient to recall all food and drinks consumed during the previous 24 hours. This method does not require the patient to possess a long memory. It also minimizes the likelihood that the patient will alter their diet if it is given unannounced. However, the 24-hour dietary recall may not be representative of the person's usual food intake. For most people, workdays, weekends, and holidays influence food intake considerably.

When administering a 3-, 5-, or 7-day dietary recall, the patient and the dental hygienist should determine the length of time the diet will be documented. The shorter the period, the less likely it is that the record will reveal usual eating patterns; however, the longer the period, the more likely that the patient will lose interest and fail to record detailed information for the duration of the timeframe. Regardless of the timeline selected, it is recommended that both weekdays and weekends are included so that variations based on the day of the week are captured in the recall.

An advantage of the face-to-face dietary recall is that it serves as a teaching session. Accuracy as well as content can be discussed during the session, and factors that affect eating habits can be determined. Although not always practical in the dental hygiene care setting, food

models such as measuring cups and spoons can help the patient recall the amount of food consumed and should be used when possible to capture serving sizes more accurately.

DIETARY EVALUATION

On completion of the dietary history, the dental hygienist and the patient should evaluate the diet for intake adequacy. Diets may also be evaluated for cariogenic potential to determine if the patient is considered at high risk for caries.

Evaluation of Diet Adequacy Using MyPlate

Using MyPlate recommendations (http://www.myplate.gov), foods consumed are categorized into each of the five food groups. The average number of servings for a patient's diet, based on the dietary history, should be compared with the recommended servings on MyPlate (Fig. 36.1). Individual caloric needs are determined based on age, sex, and activity level. Once energy needs are established, the dental hygienist can compare an individual's intake to the specified amount recommended by MyPlate[3] to assess the patient's dietary adequacy. This information is useful in identifying individuals in need of general nutritional counseling.

Evaluation of the Cariogenic Potential of the Diet

The cariogenic potential of the diet may be analyzed further by calculating the amount of acid produced in the diet (Fig. 36.2). Each sugar exposure, defined as any sweet or sugar-sweetened solid food or liquid, is circled in red. The total number of liquid and solid sugar exposures ingested over a 3-, 5-, or 7-day period is tallied and multiplied by the appropriate time interval. The number of liquid sugar exposures ingested over the period is multiplied by 20 minutes, and the number of solid sugar exposures ingested over the period is multiplied by 40 minutes. This resulting figure is divided by the number of days assessed to determine the amount of time daily that the teeth are subjected to an acid exposure. The total daily acid production is calculated by adding the daily acid production from liquid and solid sugars. Sugars consumed at the same time are considered one acid exposure (e.g., ice cream and cake eaten for dessert equals one acid exposure). Sweet foods or liquids eaten 20 minutes apart are recorded as 2 acid exposures. Calculating the number of acid exposures further illustrates the cariogenic potential of the patient's diet.

Computer Dietary Analysis

All dietary records have the potential for computer analysis. There are various programs available, and the choice often depends on the information obtained, its purpose, and the type of computer hardware available. Some programs are designed for research and provide everything from bar graphs to merging data for community-based programs. Most computer programs provide information on caloric intake, as well as deficient or excess nutrient amounts. Some programs analyze sugar intake, including percentage of sugars in the diet (e.g., simple versus complex carbohydrates).

NUTRITIONAL COUNSELING

Using the information obtained from the health history and dietary assessment, the dental hygienist and patient formulate a plan for nutritional counseling. Box 36.3 contains suggestions for performing nutritional counseling in the oral care setting.

Patient Education and Motivation

Like other types of patient education performed in the dental setting, dental hygienists should use motivational interviewing techniques

COMPARE YOUR DIET TO
MYPLATE: STEPS TO A HEALTHIER YOU

GRAINS

1 serving =
1 slice bread
1 cup dry cereal
1/2 cup pasta or rice

A
B

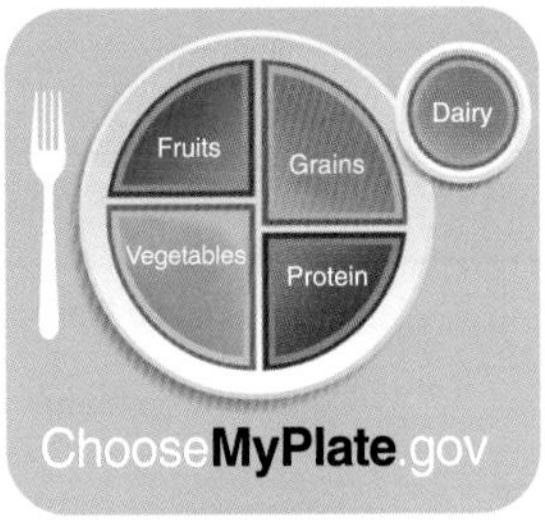

MEAT AND BEANS

1 serving =
1 ounce lean beef, fish, poultry
1/2 cup cooked beans
1/2 ounce nuts or seeds
1 tablespoon peanut butter

A
B

ChooseMyPlate.gov

VEGETABLES

1 serving =
1/2 cup cooked veggies
1 cup raw veggies
3/4 cup juice

A
B

FRUITS

1 serving =
1 medium piece
1 cup raw
1/2 cup juice

A   B

MILK

1 serving =
1 cup milk or yogurt
1 1/2 ounces cheese
1 1/2 cups frozen yogurt,
   cottage cheese

A   B

How much do you need?
Sedentary, female, or older adults: Check off only the "A" boxes for each food group
Teenage boy or active male: Check off all the "A" and "B" boxes for each food group

DETERMINE YOUR CARIES RISK

Using the list of what you eat on a typical weekday:
1. CIRCLE all the sweets, crackers, soda, juice, etc.
2. In the table below, put a CHECKMARK by the appropriate category for each of
   the items you circled that was consumed at the end of a meal or between meals.
3. ADD up the number of checks in each frequency box and multiply by the caries risk.

FOOD	No. times consumed per day (put checkmarks for each food)	Caries risk
Liquid Soft drinks, fruit juice, fruit-flavored drinks, energy drinks, sports drinks, mochas, lattes, sugar, honey, nondairy creamer, ice cream, sherbert, gelatin, flavored yogurt, pudding, custard, popsicles		_____ × 1 =
Solid and sticky Cake, cupcakes, donuts, sweet rolls, pastry, canned fruit in syrup, bananas, cookies, crackers, pretzels, potato chips, dry cereal, fat free and regular cereal/granola bars, chocolate candy, caramel, toffee, jelly beans, chewing gum, jelly, marshmallows, jam, raisins, and fruit leather		_____ × 2 =
Slowly dissolving Hard candies, breath mints, antacid tablets, cough drops, Altoids, Tums		_____ × 3 =
	TOTAL SCORE	_____

PUT YOUR SCORE ON THE CARIES RISK LINE BELOW

LOW RISK   0–1   2–4   5–7   8–9   >9   HIGH RISK

Fig. 36.1 Form to assess adequacy of the diet and calculate the cariogenic potential of the diet from a 24-hour food diary. (Courtesy Dr. L. Boyd. Adapted from C. Palmer, Tufts University School of Dental Medicine, 1998.)

Form of Sugar	When Eaten	1st Day	2nd Day	3rd Day	4th Day	5th Day	Total
Liquid (e.g., soda, sugar in coffee)	With meals						
	Between meals						
Solid (e.g., cookie, candy)	With meals						
	Between meals						

Grand total = ______ (Sugar in liquid form)

Grand total = ______ (Sugar in solid form)

______ (Liquid exposure) × 20 minutes (pH below 5.5) = ______ (Acid production) 5 DAYS = ______ (Daily liquid acid production)

______ (Solid exposure) × 40 minutes (pH below 5.5) = ______ (Acid production) 5 DAYS = ______ (Daily liquid acid production)

Total daily acid production = ______ (Liquid acid production total) + ______ (Solid acid production total) = ______ (Total time tooth is exposed to acid daily (demineralization))

Fig. 36.2 Form to calculate the cariogenic potential of the diet from a 5-day food diary. (Adapted from Nizel AE, Papas AS. *Nutrition in Clinical Dentistry*. 3rd ed. Saunders; 1989.)

BOX 36.3 Client or Patient Education Tips

- Maintain a separate space in the office for discussions of diet. This space ensures that infection control is maintained and provides a more casual and relaxed atmosphere for discussions of nutritional issues.
- Show plastic examples of foods to help patients conceptualize the size of a portion.
- Present a set of measuring spoons and cups to help demonstrate portion sizes.
- Laminate an 11" × 14" picture of MyPlate to use as a teaching tool. With a wipe-away marker, checkmarks can be placed in the appropriate sections to illustrate dietary choices from a dietary recall. The laminated picture also makes it easy to maintain infection control.
- Provide brochures and information about the US Dietary Guidelines, MyPlate, and the dietary recommendations from the American Diabetes Association, American Heart Association, and American Cancer Society.

to yield successful behavior changes in their patients. Tailoring the instruction to meet the patient's desires and goals will result in better compliance by the patient. Chapter 5 contains best practices for motivational interviewing strategies.

The clinician should begin by reviewing results of the nutritional assessment and discussing how those compare with dietary guidelines and recommendations. Areas of nutritional deficiency should be noted and incorporated into the counseling session. From there, the patient and dental hygienist should collectively determine areas where improvements could be made and brainstorm methods to implement those suggestions. Finally, a strategy for evaluating the effectiveness of the counseling should be determined and reflected upon during future dental hygiene visits. Discussion topics for the session could include the following:

- Explain how positive lifestyle changes related to healthy eating habits and exercise can benefit overall health and periodontal health.
- Explain the recommended *Dietary Guidelines for Americans* and the USDA MyPlate as the basis for appropriate food choices.
- Emphasize that decreasing the amount and frequency of simple sugars consumed promotes oral health, weight management, and systemic health.
- Discuss how healthy, nutrient-dense snack foods can be substituted for snacks that promote dental caries.
- Explain how nutrient needs change during the life cycle and at times of stress, such as periodontal and oral surgery.

Identifying Nutritional Deficiencies

Nutritional problems become evident both orally and systemically. A **primary nutritional deficiency** is caused by inadequate dietary intake of a nutrient. Once identified, this type of deficiency can be corrected with dietary assessment, followed by nutritional counseling that promotes proper selection and intake of nutrients. A **secondary nutritional deficiency** is caused by a systemic disorder that interferes with the ingestion, absorption, digestion, transport, and use of nutrients. This type of deficiency is more complex, and referral to a physician and a registered dietitian is necessary for treatment.

Often, a dental hygienist is one of the first to notice manifestations of nutrient deficiencies because they observe signs in the oral cavity. Tables 36.2 through 36.5 list the most common vitamins and nutrients involved in oral health and signs or symptoms of a deficiency. The tables also include dietary sources for recommendation if patients need to increase their intake. After potential dietary deficiencies and excesses are identified, the dental hygienist and patient work collaboratively to develop a dietary program that promotes optimal oral health. When dietary modifications are made, the following should be considered:

- The overall nutritional adequacy should be maintained by conforming to the USDA MyPlate[3] for at least the recommended number of servings from each of the food groups.
- The diet should vary as little as possible from the normal dietary pattern.

TABLE 36.2 Vitamins Associated With Structure and Calcification of Hard Tissues—Sources, Human Deficiency and Excess Syndromes, and Oral Implications

Nutrient	Dietary Source	Deficiency Syndrome	Oral Implications of Deficiency	Excess or Other
Vitamin A (fat soluble)	Only in animal foods (beef liver is an excellent source) Beta carotene: carrots, melon, squash, sweet potatoes, spinach	Growth failure, xerosis, keratomalacia	Enamel hypoplasia, defective dentin formation	Excess may cause headache, vomiting, severe liver damage, and defects in long bone formation.
Vitamin D (fat soluble)	Synthesized in skin exposed to sunlight	Rickets, osteomalacia	Enamel hypoplasia, loss of lamina dura	Excess may cause vomiting and diarrhea and hypercalcemia.
Vitamin E (fat soluble)	Vegetable seed oils, widely distributed in foods	Anemia, neuropathy, myopathy	Loss of resistance to inflammation in periodontium	Excess may inhibit vitamin K functions, causing problems with blood clotting.
Vitamin K (fat soluble)	Synthesized by intestinal bacteria: green leafy vegetables, soybeans, beef liver	Defective blood clotting	May be involved in bone formation	High doses of synthetic form may cause oxidation of membrane lipids and severe jaundice in infants.
Vitamin C (water soluble)	Citrus fruits, papaya, cantaloupe, broccoli, potatoes, strawberries	Scurvy	Inhibition of formation of fibroblasts, osteoblasts, and odontoblasts	Excess can cause gastrointestinal distress and interfere with vitamin B_{12} absorption.

From US Department of Agriculture, US Department of Health and Human Services. *Dietary Guidelines for Americans 2020–2025*. 9th ed. US Government Printing Office; 2020. Available at: https://www.dietaryguidelines.gov/sites/default/files/2021-03/Dietary_Guidelines_for_Americans-2020-2025.pdf. Accessed August 1, 2022.
National Institutes of Health Office of Dietary Supplements. *Dietary Supplement Fact Sheets*. Available at: http://ods.od.nih.gov/factsheets/list-all. Accessed August 1, 2022.

TABLE 36.3 Minerals Associated With Structure and Calcification of Hard Tissues—Sources, Human Deficiency and Excess Syndromes, and Oral Implications

Nutrient	Dietary Source	Deficiency Syndrome	Oral Implications of Deficiency	Excess or Other
Calcium	Milk and milk products, sardines, clams, turnip and mustard greens, broccoli	Rickets, osteomalacia, osteoporosis, stunted growth	Tooth exfoliation due to osteoporosis in alveolar bone	Excess may cause constipation.
Phosphorus	Meat, poultry, fish, eggs, milk products, chocolate	Rickets, osteomalacia	Possible failure of reparative dentin formation	Symptoms associated with excess are rare; problems appear to occur only when calcium-to-phosphorus ratios are altered significantly in infants.
Magnesium	Nuts, legumes, cereal grains, chocolate, blackstrap molasses, spinach	Growth failure, neuromuscular dysfunction, personality changes, muscle spasms	Reduced formation of alveolar bone, hypoplasia of enamel, widening of periodontal ligament space, gingival hyperplasia	Acute toxicity from excessive intravenous administration results in nausea, depression, and paralysis.
Fluoride	Mackerel, salmon, shrimp, meat, potatoes, wheat, sardines	Osteoporosis, osteosclerosis	Dental caries	Excess results in fluorosis.

From US Department of Agriculture, US Department of Health and Human Services. *Dietary Guidelines for Americans 2020–2025*. 9th ed. US Government Printing Office; 2020. Available at: https://www.dietaryguidelines.gov/sites/default/files/2021-03/Dietary_Guidelines_for_Americans-2020-2025.pdf. Accessed August 1, 2022.
National Institutes of Health Office of Dietary Supplements. *Dietary Supplement Fact Sheets*. Available at: http://ods.od.nih.gov/factsheets/list-all. Accessed August 1, 2022.

- The diet should meet the body's requirements for essential nutrients as generously as the diseased condition can tolerate.
- The diet should accommodate the individual's cultural and religious beliefs and practices, likes and dislikes, food habits, and other environmental factors, without interfering with the objectives.

The use of the *Dietary Guidelines for Americans*[1] in conjunction with the USDA MyPlate[3] guides the necessary dietary modifications by promoting balance among all food groups. The dental hygienist should also try to tailor recommendations to the patient's lifestyle. Although most healthy patients have similar nutrient needs, stages within the life cycle may require special consideration, including pregnant women, infants, children, and older adults (Box 36.4). Moreover, the dental hygienist should consider patients' special nutritional needs related to their risk for caries, periodontal disease, and oral surgery.

TABLE 36.4   Vitamins Associated With Soft Tissue, Including Oral, Salivary, and Taste Function—Sources, Human Deficiency and Excess Syndromes, and Oral Implications

Nutrient	Dietary Source	Deficiency Syndrome	Oral Implications of Deficiency	Excess or Other
Vitamin B$_1$, thiamine (water soluble)	Pork, sunflower seeds, legumes	Beriberi, muscle weakness, tachycardia, enlarged heart, edema, anemia, neuropathy, myopathy	Glossitis, gingival tissue discoloration	Excessive doses may cause headache, convulsions, cardiac arrhythmia, and anaphylactic shock.
Vitamin B$_2$, riboflavin (water soluble)	Beef liver, lean steak, mushrooms, ricotta cheese, milk	Photophobia, dermatitis, anemia	Cheilosis, glossitis, edema of pharyngeal and oral mucous membranes, angular stomatitis	No toxicity symptoms are reported.
Vitamin B$_6$, pyridoxine (water soluble)	Sirloin steak, navy beans, potatoes, bananas	Dermatitis, neurologic symptoms of confusion, drowsiness, neuropathy	Glossitis	Excess causes sensory and peripheral neuropathy; minimal dose, at which toxicity occurs, is not defined.
Vitamin B$_{12}$ (water soluble)	Meat, fish, shellfish, poultry, milk	Megaloblastic anemia (pernicious anemia), degeneration of peripheral nerves, skin hypersensitivity	Glossitis, eventual disappearance of the filiform and fungiform papillae; glossopyrosis	No effects from excessive doses have been reported.
Niacin (water-soluble B vitamin)	Tuna, beef liver, chicken breast, mushrooms	Pellagra, diarrhea, dermatitis, dementia	Stomatitis, atrophic changes of filiform and fungiform papillae, tongue smooth and shiny	Large doses used in the treatment of hypercholesterolemia; excess may cause facial flushing and release of histamines, which may be detrimental to asthmatic patients
Folate (water-soluble B vitamin)	Brewer's yeast, spinach, asparagus, turnip greens, lima beans, beef liver	Megaloblastic anemia, increased risk of spina bifida and neural tube defects during pregnancy	Glossitis, chronic periodontitis, *Candida* infection; cleft lip and cleft palate	Large doses may cause kidney damage; may mask symptoms of vitamin B$_{12}$ deficiency and may provoke seizures in patients taking anticonvulsants.
Pantothenic acid (water-soluble B vitamin)	Widespread in foods, egg yolk, liver, kidneys	Deficiency very rare, numbness and tingling of hands and feet	May impair healing of oral tissue	Diarrhea is the only reported effect from excessive doses.
Biotin (water-soluble B vitamin)	Synthesized in intestinal tract	Deficiency very rare, anorexia, nausea, depression, dermatitis	Glossitis, lingual and mucous pallor, patchy atrophy of lingual papilla	No effects from excessive doses have been reported.
Vitamin C (water soluble)	Synthesized in intestinal tract	Scurvy	Weakened collagen formation, leading to gingivitis and poor oral wound healing	Overdose may cause diarrhea and kidney stones.
Vitamin A (fat soluble)	Synthesized in intestinal tract	Xerosis, keratomalacia	Decreased salivary secretion and xerostomia; delayed or impaired wound healing	Excess may cause fetal birth defects, headache, vomiting, severe liver damage, and defect in long bone formation.
Vitamin E (fat soluble)	Synthesized in the intestinal tract	Anemia, neuropathy	Loss of integrity in cell membranes of mucosa	Can act as an anticoagulant and may increase the risk of bleeding problems.

From US Department of Agriculture, US Department of Health and Human Services. *Dietary Guidelines for Americans 2020–2025*. 9th ed. US Government Printing Office; 2020. Available at: https://www.dietaryguidelines.gov/sites/default/files/2021-03/Dietary_Guidelines_for_Americans-2020-2025.pdf. Accessed August 1, 2022.

National Institutes of Health Office of Dietary Supplements. *Dietary Supplement Fact Sheets*. Available at: http://ods.od.nih.gov/factsheets/list-all. Accessed August 1, 2022.

Cultural Sensitivity

Culture should be a part of every assessment and counseling session (see Chapter 6). Different beliefs and lifestyles exist in society and each should be accorded respect. There are many different population subgroups, and these groups often have specific cultural, ethnic, or religious beliefs and practices to consider (Box 36.5). The culturally competent dental hygienist maintains knowledge of different cultures and remains sensitive to their beliefs and practices.

NUTRITIONAL NEEDS OF SPECIAL PATIENT POPULATIONS

Nutritional Needs During Pregnancy

All stages of pregnancy require an increase in nutrient and energy intake, but the most relevant to fetal oral health may be the first and second trimesters, when the development and calcification of teeth occur. Bone growth, which is equally important, occurs primarily

TABLE 36.5   Minerals Associated With Soft Tissue Including Oral, Salivary, and Taste Function—Sources, Human Deficiency and Excess Syndromes, and Oral Implications

Nutrient	Dietary Source	Deficiency Syndrome	Oral Implications of Deficiency	Excess or Other
Sodium	Table salt, meat, seafood, cheese, milk, bread, vegetables	Muscle atrophy, poor growth, weight loss	Thirst, dry, sticky tongue and mouth	High sodium intake may affect calcium excretion.
Potassium	Avocadoes, bananas, dried fruits, wheat bran, eggs, dairy products	Muscular weakness, mental apathy, cardiac arrhythmias, paralysis, adrenal hypertrophy, decreased growth rate	None	Hyperkalemia is toxic, resulting in severe cardiac failure.
Chloride	Table salt, seafood, eggs, meat, milk	Failure to thrive in infants, muscle weakness, hypokalemia, metabolic acidosis	None	No excess effects have been noted.
Iron	Organ meats, clams, oysters, legumes, enriched and/ or whole grain cereals and breads	Fatigue, palpitations on exertion, anemia, decreased resistance to infection	Pallor of lips and oral mucosa, angular cheilitis, atrophy of filiform papillae, glossitis	Excess causes damage to tissues, including liver and other organs.
Zinc	Wheat germ, oysters, beef liver, dark meat or poultry	Poor wound healing, subnormal growth, skin inflammation, anemia, retarded development of reproductive organs	Abnormal taste and smell; increased susceptibility to periodontal disease; flattened filiform papillae; congenital defect cleft lip and palate	Acute toxicity produces metallic taste, nausea, vomiting, epigastric pain, abdominal cramps. Can result in renal damage, pancreatitis, and even death.
Iodine	Iodized salt, saltwater shellfish, spinach, pumpkin, broccoli, chocolate	Hypothyroidism or Graves disease, cretinism, increase in blood lipids	Delayed eruption of primary and secondary teeth, an enlarged tongue, and malocclusion commonly occur in cretinism; craniofacial growth and development is also altered	Can cause enlargement of thyroid gland. Toxicity symptoms are similar to deficiency symptoms.

From US Department of Agriculture, US Department of Health and Human Services. *Dietary Guidelines for Americans 2020–2025*. 9th ed. US Government Printing Office; 2020. Available at: https://www.dietaryguidelines.gov/sites/default/files/2021-03/Dietary_Guidelines_for_Americans-2020-2025.pdf. Accessed August 1, 2022.

National Institutes of Health Office of Dietary Supplements. *Dietary Supplement Fact Sheets*. Available at: http://ods.od.nih.gov/factsheets/list-all. Accessed August 1, 2022.

BOX 36.4   Critical Thinking Scenario A

A 16-year-old female patient arrives for a new patient hygiene appointment. Upon review of the personal and health histories, she quietly whispers that she has been struggling with an eating disorder. Recognizing signs and symptoms of nutritional deficiency as a result of this condition, you recommend that she schedule an appointment with her physician to obtain treatment. She states that she is afraid to tell her parents and therefore does not want to be referred to a physician. What ethical principles should be considered in this situation? How would you proceed?

---

in the second and third trimesters, when most of the calcium that is essential for this process is transferred from mother to fetus. In most cases, the exception being an underweight or teenage pregnancy, the woman's energy requirement increases by approximately 350 to 450 kilocalories a day. Unlike energy needs, however, vitamin and mineral requirements nearly double. Prenatal nutrient supplements recommended by the patient's obstetrician ensure that the developing fetus receives adequate vitamins and minerals to promote healthy bone and tooth development.

During pregnancy, the mother may experience changes in taste and smell, food cravings, and food aversions that do not necessarily reflect real physiologic needs. These pregnancy-related experiences, along with varying levels of nausea, create a potential for nutrient imbalance.

Fortunately, the developing fetus is usually not at risk during these short episodes because a healthy mother provides the essential nutrients from her own nutrient stores. However, a prolonged nutrient deficiency poses a problem.

The dental hygienist treating a pregnant female reinforces the recommendations of the obstetrician. Reinforcement of the importance of eating nutrient-dense foods along with meticulous oral hygiene minimizes the occurrence of pregnancy-associated gingivitis, pregnancy granulomas, and giving birth to premature low-birth-weight infants.

Nutritional Needs During Infancy and Childhood

Nutrient intake and food choices during infancy and childhood influence growth patterns. Undernutrition, overnutrition, and improper nutrient amounts can set the pattern for a lifelong struggle with weight, developmental delays, or social discrimination. Children need calories for growth and development, and they often grow in spurts. Children are born with an innate sense of how much food they require. Parents who advocate finishing an entire meal may be causing their children to override their internal sense of satiety. The simplest advice is the provision of nutrient-dense foods, regular mealtimes, and the achievement of a balanced diet by offering a variety of foods from all food groups.

Unless a child has extenuating medical circumstances, children should not ingest significant amounts of alternative sweeteners. Artificial sweeteners should not be part of the diet of infants or children under 2 years of age. Although alternative sweeteners may appear

BOX 36.5 Examples of Dietary Considerations for Various Populations

African American
- Incidence of lactose intolerance is high.

Asian
- Incidence of lactose intolerance is high.

Buddhism
- Vegetarianism is prevalent with five pungent foods excluded: garlic, leeks, scallions, chives, and onion.

Hinduism
- Primarily vegetarian with certain geographic exceptions.

Islam
- No unclean foods (e.g., carrion, dead animals, swine) are consumed.
- Only halal-processed meat may be consumed.
- No carnivorous animals with fangs, birds of prey, and land animals without ears (e.g., frogs, snakes) are consumed.
- Pork and pork products, such as gelatin, are prohibited.
- Alcoholic beverages and alcohol products are prohibited.

Latino
- Incidence of lactose intolerance is high.

Native American
- Incidence of lactose intolerance is high.
- Incidence of diabetes is high.

Alaskan Natives
- Obesity and diabetes mellitus are common.

Orthodox Judaism
- Prohibits consumption of swine, shellfish, and carrion eaters.
- Kosher foods are consumed.
- Fruits, vegetables, and cereal products can be consumed with no restrictions.

Vegetarianism
- Often motivated by philosophical reasons, religious influences, or a desire for healthier lifestyle.
- Lacto-vegetarians do not eat meat, fish, poultry, or eggs but can consume milk, cheese, and other dairy products.
- Lacto-ovo-vegetarians can also consume eggs.
- Vegans do not consume any food of animal origin.
- Megaloblastic anemia is often a concern in vegans owing to deficiency of vitamin B_{12}, which is only found in animal products.
- On the whole, vegetarians should pay special attention to ensure they get adequate calcium, iron, zinc, and vitamins B_{12} and D.

Adapted from Food and nutrient delivery. Planning the diet with cultural competence. In Mahan LK, Raymond JL, Escott-Stump S, (eds.) *Krause's Food and the Nutrition Care Process.* 13th ed. Saunders; 2012.

desirable to parents because of their anticariogenic properties, good oral hygiene care, fluoridation, and healthy snack choices can reduce the risk of dental caries without exposing children to these sweeteners.

The focus of nutritional counseling for children in the oral care setting is primarily caries control. In addition, the importance of vitamins and minerals responsible for bone growth should be included in discussion with the child and caregiver. As children age, their preference

for beverages often changes from milk and juices to carbonated beverages. Dairy products, some of the best sources of calcium, phosphorus, and magnesium, are essential for adequate bone and tooth formation. Replacing dairy products with carbonated beverages eliminates the primary source of these nutrients and could adversely affect the bone growth and tooth development of children and teenagers.

Nutritional Needs of Older Adult Patients

Significant nutritional issues in older adults include a reduced energy requirement and an increased need for certain vitamins (D, E, B_6, B_{12}, and folate) and minerals (calcium, magnesium, iron, and zinc) (see Chapter 47). Older adult patients may not be as active and therefore may not require the same amount of energy intake as an average patient. The decrease in energy and increase in nutrient needs means that the older adult patient may need guidance in choosing nutrient-dense foods such as whole grains, breads, and pastas. Along with complex carbohydrates, fruits and vegetables are a natural source of the vitamins and minerals that promote tissue growth and regeneration.

The consumption of nutrient-dense foods is essential to the older adult diet. Sources of high-quality protein such as eggs, dairy products, and well-cooked meats, chicken, and fish should be promoted as an important part of the diet. Protein also provides a good source of vitamin B_{12}, which is often deficient in older adults. Pernicious anemia and burning mouth syndrome are commonly noted in older adult patients with a diagnosed deficiency of vitamin B_{12}. Vitamins A, C, and B_6 can be obtained from a diet rich in cooked green vegetables and potatoes. Fresh fruit is also a good source of vitamins and minerals and can be tolerated if the fruit is ripe or peeled. Table 36.6 lists oral signs and symptoms of possible nutrient deficiencies in older adults.

Indirect factors can also play a role in nutrient deficiencies for the older adult population. Since many older adult patients lack dental insurance, they may be unable to afford regular dental care. Periodontal disease, carious teeth, and ill-fitting dentures can be painful and restrict the older individual's ability to chew and swallow food. Hot or cold foods can aggravate oral disease conditions, and xerostomia can make chewing and swallowing food difficult. In addition, crisp or fibrous foods that require significant force when biting or chewing also can cause pain. Therefore older adults may choose soft foods such as cakes, cookies, and breakfast cereals, which can contribute to dental decay.

Finally, guidance should be given to older adults to achieve optimal nutrition. Referral to a registered dietitian may be indicated. Community-based services such as Meals on Wheels, congregate meal sites, and shopping assistance provide an opportunity for socialization and assistance for those who are disabled or who lack transportation. Also, modifications applied to oral hygiene aids for people with manual dexterity problems can be applied to eating utensils to increase the likelihood of adequate nutritional intake.

Nutritional Needs of Patients With a High Risk of Dental Caries

Nutritional counseling for dental caries prevention must emphasize decreasing the frequency with which sugar is consumed and replacing cariogenic foods with nutritionally sound foods. Although sugar consumption is an important factor in caries risk assessment[5] (see Chapter 19), the following factors are also involved in the development of dental caries:

- Acid-producing microorganisms (e.g., *Lactobacillus, Streptococcus mutans*)
- Cariogenic diet
- Susceptible tooth surface
- Salivary factors

TABLE 36.6   Signs of Nutritional Deficiencies in Older Adults

Clinical Signs	Possible Deficiency	Comments
Skin		
Edema	Protein, thiamine	Is common in protein-calorie malnutrition as a result of aging
Poor tissue turgor	Water	Pellagra or hemochromatosis may develop.
Dermatitis	Protein	None
Keratosis	Vitamin A, essential fatty acids	None
Pigmentation	Niacin	Loss of lubrication or dryness of skin can develop.
Petechiae	Vitamin A, vitamin C	None
Xerosis	Essential fatty acids	None
Eyes		
Dull, dry conjunctiva	Vitamin A	Can lead to other eye problems, including blindness
Keratomalacia	Vitamin A	Usually results in blindness
Bitot spot	Vitamin A	Is associated with night blindness
Corneal vascularization	Vitamin A	None
Photophobia	Riboflavin, zinc	Sensitivity to light is extreme; individuals who suffer from migraines may experience this condition. Other eye problems such as night blindness may be present.
Tongue		
Magenta tongue	Riboflavin	None
Fissuring, raw	Niacin	May also be caused by food irritants, antibiotic administration, and/or uremia
Glossitis	Pyridoxine, folacin, iron, vitamin B_{12}	Is seen if anemia is not pronounced
Fiery red tongue	Folacin, vitamin B_{12}	None
Pale tongue	Iron, vitamin B_{12}	Is seen in severe cases
Atrophic papillae	Riboflavin, niacin, iron	Is also seen with ill-fitting dentures or food irritants and is a result of aging
Lips and Oral Structures		
Angular fissures, scars, stomatitis	B-complex, iron, protein, riboflavin	Is also seen with ill-fitting dentures
Cheilosis	B_6, iron, niacin, riboflavin, protein	Could also be a result of fungal infections
Ageusia, dysgeusia	Zinc	Certain conditions and medications can contribute; is also seen with ill-fitting dentures
Swollen, spongy, bleeding gums	Vitamin C	Is also associated with an altered sense of smell if not edentulous

Nutritional counseling for dental caries prevention targets the elimination or reduction of fermentable carbohydrates from the diet. Dissolving foods that sit on the teeth for extended periods of time and solid, sticky foods that do not readily clear from the mouth contribute the greatest risk. Frequent consumption of fermentable carbohydrates and acidic beverages subjects the tooth enamel to repeated acid exposures. The demineralization process weakens the tooth and can lead to the formation of dental caries as well as enamel erosion. (See Chapter 17 for types of caries and Chapter 19 for a review of the caries process.) Snacks that are selected as a healthy alternative still contribute to demineralization and subsequent caries formation. Examples include low-calorie carbonated beverages, juices, and sticky foods such as baked chips, pretzels, granola, and dried fruit. Box 36.6 includes recommendations and strategies for reducing the cariogenic potential of an individual's diet.

Nutritional Needs of Patients Undergoing Surgery

In a healthy adult, creation of new proteins and breakdown of existing proteins closely balance one another. Typically, well-nourished, healthy individuals experience very few complications and require

BOX 36.6   Dietary Recommendations for the Reduction of Dental Caries

- Limit the use of fermentable carbohydrates to mealtime. Consume foods higher in protein and fat to help buffer and neutralize plaque acids.
- Reduce the frequency of cariogenic and acidogenic foods if susceptible to caries.
- Between-meal snacks should consist of protective, noncariogenic foods such as raw vegetables. Raw, unrefined foods in the vegetable and fruit group require chewing. The chewing action increases the salivary flow, thus aiding in the removal and dilution of sugars and their harmful byproducts.
- Use as few concentrated sweets as possible in the preparation of foods.
- Do not eat sweets before bedtime unless the teeth are brushed afterward. Salivary flow decreases at night and foods are not cleared as readily from the mouth as they are during waking hours. Acid left undisturbed remains in the mouth for 1.5 to 2 hours.
- Limit natural sugars; they are as detrimental to the tooth surface as refined sugars.
- Avoid sticky foods; they are retained in the mouth longer than nonsticky foods.
- Encourage consumption of sugar-free gum with xylitol after meals if brushing is not an option.

minimal dietary modifications. However, periodontal, oral, and maxillofacial surgical patients are often unable to consume an adequate amount of recommended nutrients because of a temporary or permanent loss of function. Other patients, such as chronic alcoholics, extremely underweight individuals, or those taking steroids or immunosuppressants, may have depleted their stores of nutrients. These individuals may need to postpone surgical procedures 1 to 2 weeks or until more favorable nutritional levels are achieved. Immunocompromised individuals, as well as those with complex health histories, should be referred to a registered dietitian for more in-depth analysis and guidance before surgery. A team effort between the dental hygienist and a registered dietitian ensures a more positive treatment outcome.

To optimize immune function to promote healing and overall health, patients should be instructed in proper postsurgical nutritional rehabilitation. Presurgical nutritional education provided by the dental hygienist should include the following:

- Discussion of the patient's present food intake pattern and recommended caloric needs based on height, weight, and activity level using MyPlate[3] as a guide
- Review of adequate nutrients to enhance and facilitate the healing process
- Consideration of the extent of surgery, potential discomfort, and patient's ability to eat after the surgery; food preferences and dislikes also should be taken into account

In addition to caloric and protein requirement increases, there also may be an increase in select nutrient needs because of blood loss, increased catabolism, and tissue regeneration that occurs after surgery. The first 1 to 3 days after surgery, high-calorie, high-protein, full-liquid diets consisting of choices such as powdered skim milk that can be used to fortify milk, soups, puddings, milkshakes, broth, and fruit or vegetable juices may be necessary. Patients may then progress to a mechanical soft diet. This is a regular diet that is modified to a consistency that makes foods easier to consume. A mechanical soft diet consists of soft, ripened, chopped, ground, mashed, and pureed foods. This type of diet may be recommended for 3 to 7 days or until the patient is able to consume a regular diet. Small, frequent meals ensure adequate intake. Raw fruits and vegetables and foods with seeds or nuts should be avoided; bland foods should be encouraged to avoid irritating the tissue. Eight glasses of fluid are also recommended. It is always preferable to obtain nutrients through a food source, but in cases in which the patient is unable to ingest the required nutrients adequately, a liquid form of supplemental nutrition such as Ensure or Boost may be acceptable. If supplemental liquid nutrition is indicated, patients should be educated on the high sugar content and the need for meticulous oral hygiene. Liquid and soft diets are not indicated for simple procedures such as tooth extractions. These diets are recommended more commonly for patients who require periodontal surgery, jaw surgery, intermaxillary fixation, or temporomandibular joint surgery.

A practical patient education program is accomplished using the USDA MyPlate[3] and *Dietary Guidelines for Americans.*[1] Quick calculations and charts provided by MyPlate[3] can be used as visual aids for patient education. Individualized meal plans that incorporate caloric, protein, and other suggested nutrient needs postsurgically are an excellent resource in the dental setting. Often, it is easier to obtain

compliance when patients are presented with an actual list of foods or meal plans to follow. The dental hygiene clinician can provide only basic recommendations. Referral to a registered dietitian is indicated to develop a comprehensive meal plan that meets individual needs. The Academy of Nutrition and Dietetics is an exceptional resource for examples of full liquid and mechanical soft diets designed to provide optimal calories and nutrients for surgical patients. It is also a great source for locating a local registered dietitian for referrals (http://www.eatright.org).

Nutritional Needs of Patients with Osteoporosis

A thorough health history, dental hygiene assessment (intraoral examination, periodontal charting, radiographs), and dietary analysis help to identify patients at risk for osteoporosis (see Chapter 47). These individuals must be encouraged to consume at least three cups of calcium food sources daily. The preferred calcium source is dairy products and foods fortified with calcium, such as orange juice. Calcium bioavailability from dairy foods is excellent, especially when consumed with a meal (see Table 36.3). Emphasis also needs to be on vitamin D to promote optimal calcium absorption. Tables 36.2 and 36.3 provide a list of the minerals and vitamins essential for calcified structures. For individuals who have inadequate intake of dairy, a calcium supplement may be indicated. The dose should be taken in halves to ensure proper absorption (e.g., 500 to 600 mg taken twice daily). For an individual at risk of or diagnosed with osteoporosis, referral to a physician or a registered dietitian may be recommended to verify that calcium needs are being met.

Nutritional Concerns of Overweight and Obese Patients

Obesity is a growing concern in children, adolescents, and adults. Currently, more than one-third of US adults and approximately 17% of children and adolescents ages 2 to 19 years are obese.[6] Obesity is defined as having a BMI greater than or equal to 30 (see Table 36.1). Obesity is associated with many chronic diseases, including periodontal disease. It is beyond the role of the dental hygienist to create diet plans for use in weight loss. However, as healthcare providers, it is the dental hygienist's responsibility to educate patients on health promotion, disease prevention techniques, and habits that benefit oral health and overall health. Patients may be educated on positive lifestyle changes as they relate to healthy eating habits and exercise, the link between obesity and diabetes and periodontal health, and the impact of systemic health on oral health. Referral to a physician and/or a registered dietitian is indicated for those patients interested in weight loss.

Bariatric surgery is common in this population. After surgery, it is recommended that these individuals eat small meals throughout the day, and beverages should be consumed separately from meals. Although this method of consuming foods and beverages optimizes the digestion process for the bariatric surgery patient, the frequency and timing of foods and beverages can increase the risk of caries. In addition, nutrient deficiencies may occur as a result of surgical alterations to the gastrointestinal tract; thus healing after periodontal therapy or surgery may be affected. Collaboration with the medical team to ensure the most favorable patient outcome is recommended.

BOX 36.7 Critical Thinking Scenario B

Older Adult Patient

Patient Profile

Name: Mr. Conrad Farmer

Age: 71 years old

Sex: Male

Height: 5'11"

Weight: 160 pounds

Race: African American

Health History

Has high blood pressure, rheumatoid arthritis, and depression.

Pharmacologic History

Is currently taking atenolol and amlodipine (Norvasc) for blood pressure, trazodone for depression, and celecoxib (Celebrex) for rheumatoid arthritis.

Dental History

Presents to the dental clinic with carious lesions on the facial surfaces of teeth 3, 14, 15, and 18 and the mesial surface of tooth 24. He has moderate supragingival calculus and slight to moderate subgingival deposits. He has generalized bleeding with 5-mm pockets noted on the mesial and distal surfaces of all posterior teeth.

Chief Complaint

"My mouth is really dry, and I have a few teeth that ache a little."

Social History

Patient is a retired widower; he lost his wife to cancer a year ago. He and his wife never had children. He does not have any extended family in the local area.

Dietary Assessment

Mr. Farmer frequently keeps cinnamon hard candies in his mouth to stimulate his saliva. He also sips on soda throughout the day to keep his mouth moist.

Since Mr. Farmer's wife died, he has cooked for himself. His cooking skills are minimal. Breakfast usually consists of a whole-grain bagel or muffin. Lunch is usually a sandwich of some sort with a bowl of soup. Dinner is often a frozen dinner. However, he often skips the evening meal because he does not like eating alone at night. He snacks frequently throughout the day on pretzels, trail mix, and cheese-flavored snack crackers. To take the edge off his hunger before he goes to bed, Mr. Farmer often snacks on peanut butter crackers or his personal favorite—a bowl of chunky chocolate banana ice cream. He drinks coffee continuously throughout the day and likes it with three table-spoons of sugar and lots of cream.

Nutritional Risk Factors

- Snack choices have a sticky consistency and contribute to the risk of caries.
- Frequently consumes acidic beverages.
- Lacks variety and balance in his diet.
- Slow-dissolving candies promote caries.
- Cariogenic food choices coupled with decreased salivary function.

Dental Hygiene Diagnosis

- Unmet need for responsibility for oral health due to inadequate homecare and dietary habits as indicated by presence of carious lesions, bleeding points, and bone loss.
- Unmet need for protection from health risks due to a lack of nutrient-dense foods in the diet and skipping meals.
  1. Do you have any recommended interventions for Mr. Farmer's dietary practices?
  2. What snacks would you suggest to replace some of the cariogenic choices? What questions would you ask Mr. Farmer prior to suggesting alternative foods to him?
  3. Access the Internet to find some community nutrition services that you may recommend to Mr. Farmer.

BOX 36.8 Critical Thinking Scenario C

Patient With Rampant Dental Caries

Patient Profile

Name: Kathleen Mulvaney

Age: 8 years old

Sex: Female

Height: 3'10"

Weight: 55 lbs (25 kg)

Race: Caucasian

Health History

Patient has experienced several childhood illnesses, including chickenpox, measles, and mumps, and frequent sore throat and common cold symptoms. Patient was injured on the school playground at age 6 years and underwent treatment for fractures of the right leg and arm.

Pharmacologic History

Because of frequent cold symptoms and sore throats, client regularly ingests over-the-counter cough drops. Her favorite flavors are cherry and honey lemon. These cough drops are not sugar-free.

Dental History

Because of her health history and subsequent treatment for illness and injury, Kathleen's parents have not taken her to the dentist often in an effort to avoid "overtraumatizing" her. Intraoral examination reveals rampant caries of

remaining primary teeth with the largest lesions in the molar area. Radiographic examination shows decay throughout the mouth. Permanent tooth development appears to be normal. Erupted molars have incipient lesions with some surfaces requiring class I restorations at this time.

Chief Complaint

"My friends at school make fun of my teeth because they are black. Sometimes it's hard to chew." Patient does not appear to be experiencing pain at this time.

Dietary History

Food frequency questionnaire indicates that client has a high intake of foods containing added sugars and appearing in the moderate to high cariogenic potential category. Using MyPlate, the client can point out most foods in her diet and indicates that she adds sugar to her breakfast cereals and on top of the fruit she eats with lunch. Patient loves raisins and dried fruit as a snack. She keeps a little bag in her desk at school in case she gets hungry during the day. Patient's favorite snack is a bowl of chocolate ice cream, which she has every night before bed. Patient drinks regular cola with each meal except breakfast. Friends eat candy bars, but Kathleen prefers gummy bears, Dots, Sour Patch Kids, and other sticky fruit candies.

Social History

Patient is the youngest child in a family of six. Parents work outside the home. Family status is middle class with occasional financial challenges because of

BOX 36.8   Critical Thinking Scenario C—cont'd

the large family. Patient stays after school until picked up by older siblings. Because of work and social obligations, parents have left most of the child-care responsibilities to older siblings. Previous injuries and chronic illnesses have promoted a special reward system at home of sweet desserts and ice cream before bed. Limited parental supervision has caused client to adopt the diet and habits of her older siblings who enjoy regular cola with meals instead of milk. Patient appears to understand the importance of a healthy diet and appears receptive to adjusting her habits "as long as my parents say it's okay."

Nutritional Risk Factors

- Preferred snack foods have high concentration of added sugars and limited nutritional value.
- Snack habits (e.g., dried fruits available throughout the day) promote caries.
- Choice of beverage with meals is unsatisfactory for promoting growth and development.
- Limited parental supervision allows for poor food choices.

Dental Hygiene Diagnoses

- Deficit in the need for biologically sound and functional dentition due to poor dietary choices and poor oral hygiene care as evidenced by rampant decay.
- Deficit in the need for responsibility for oral health due to lack of parental supervision and infrequency of dental visits as evidenced by parental self-reports.

1. Given the history and dental hygiene diagnosis, develop a comprehensive overall dental hygiene care plan, including client goals, nutritional counseling plan, interventions, and evaluative measures. What factors would you use as motivators to change behavior? Share your approach to care with your peers.
2. Access the Internet. Find at least three sites that you could recommend for nutritional information appropriate for children, teenagers, adults, and senior citizens.
3. How might your nutritional counseling plan change, depending on the cultural influences of the patient? Consider the cultures represented in your community.

KEY CONCEPTS

- A patient's nutritional status assessment is part of a comprehensive dental hygiene treatment.
- Nutritional counseling helps patients develop healthful eating behaviors.
- Dietary assessment is the identification of the patient's current dietary practices and dietary requirements. Dietary assessment includes a dietary history that may be gathered through a 1-, 3-, 5-, or 7-day recording of food intake. Dietary assessment may provide clues to overall health through analysis of nutrient content.
- Factors that may influence an individual's food selection include age, sex, ethnicity, cultural influences, socioeconomic status, educational level, and lifestyle.
- Cultural sensitivity is an essential part of dietary assessment and nutritional counseling.
- Pregnancy, infancy, childhood, the aging population, and overweight patients have specific nutritional needs, and hygienists should counsel these patients or their caregivers on nutrition as it relates to dental health.
- Dietary assessment and nutritional counseling promote healing postoperatively in patients undergoing periodontal or oral and maxillofacial surgery.
- Minimizing the amount of sugar consumed and replacing cariogenic foods with nutrient-dense foods decrease the risk of dental caries.

ACKNOWLEDGMENTS

The author acknowledges Stacy Long and Lisa F. Harper Mallonee for their past contributions to this chapter.

REFERENCES

1. U.S. Department of Agriculture, U.S. Department of Health and Human Services. *Dietary Guidelines for Americans 2020–2025*. 9th ed. U.S. Government Printing Office; 2020. Available at: https://www.dietaryguidelines.gov/sites/default/files/2021-03/Dietary_Guidelines_for_Americans-2020-2025.pdf. Accessed August 1, 2022.
2. Centers for Disease Control and Prevention. Body Mass Index (BMI). Available at: https://www.cdc.gov/healthyweight/assessing/bmi/index.html. Accessed August 1, 2022.
3. U.S. Department of Agriculture. MyPlate. Available at: https://www.myplate.gov/. Accessed August 1, 2022.
4. Shim J-S, Oh K, Kim HC. Dietary assessment methods in epidemiologic studies. *Epidemiol Health*. 2014;36:e2014009. https://doi.org/10.4178/epih/e2014009.
5. Gustafsson BE, Quensel CE, Lanke LS, et al. The Vipeholm Dental Caries Study: the effects of different levels of carbohydrate intake on caries activity in 436 individuals observed for five years. *Acta Odontol Scand*. 1954;11:232.
6. Centers for Disease Control and Prevention. Overweight and Obesity. Available at: https://www.cdc.gov/obesity/data/adult.html. Accessed August 1, 2022.

37

Tobacco Cessation

Victoria V. Patrounova

PROFESSIONAL OPPORTUNITIES

Dental hygienists are in a great position to screen for effects of tobacco use and have an ethical obligation to address tobacco use with individual patients, community groups, and students at schools as it affects oral and overall health and success of dental treatment. Clients should be educated on a continual basis about health risks, the significance of secondhand smoke, and the connection between tobacco use and oral cancers and diseases. Dental hygienists should motivate patients to quit tobacco and nicotine use and provide cessation options. They can refer patients to effective programs or, with additional training, provide behavioral interventions themselves. Public health dental hygienists can collaborate interprofessionally with other healthcare providers to screen for health effects of tobacco use or educate various populations within their communities.

COMPETENCIES

1. Describe the prevalence of the use of tobacco and nicotine products among different segments of the population.
2. Describe adverse systemic and oral health effects of different nicotine and tobacco products in terms as they would be explained to a patient or community group.
3. Accurately communicate to patients the scientific evidence to allow patients to make informed decisions to quit and refrain from using tobacco.
4. Identify various aspects of nicotine addiction.
5. Apply knowledge of treatment programs for nicotine addiction, the Five A's approach, and motivational interviewing for counseling patients to become tobacco-free. In addition, discuss statewide tobacco use quitlines.
6. Evaluate level of dependence and recommend appropriate pharmacologic strategies, including nicotine replacement therapies, to prevent tobacco use and aid in cessation.
7. Encourage local governmental agencies, dental and dental hygiene organizations, community leaders, and insurers to support health promotion and policy making for smoking prevention and cessation, and discuss the dental hygienist's role in the community related to tobacco.

INTRODUCTION

Tobacco is the leading cause of preventable illness and death in the United States. Each year, more than 480,000 individuals die due to smoking or exposure to environmental (secondhand) smoke.[1] Tobacco use has been causally associated with negative effects on fetal growth and development, declining health status, and illnesses involving every major organ of the body.[2] These illnesses include many types of cancer;

cardiovascular, metabolic, and respiratory diseases; and birth defects, such as orofacial clefts. Exposure to secondhand smoke is also linked to cancers, respiratory and cardiovascular diseases, and adverse effects in infants and children.[2] Illnesses attributable to tobacco use result in annual costs of more than $300 billion in the United States, including over $225 billion in direct medical costs.[3] However, the Centers for Disease Control and Prevention (CDC) reported an all-time low of 12.5% of US adults who smoked cigarettes in 2020. This rate has declined from 15.1% since 2015.[3] This decrease in smoking by US adults demonstrates great progress in tobacco control efforts, including comprehensive smoke-free laws, increases in tobacco product prices, and access to cessation services.

Yet, there are still missed opportunities in the dental setting. Many dental professionals feel unprepared to implement tobacco cessation interventions for a number of reasons, including lack of time, knowledge, and experience with tobacco cessation intervention techniques.[4] The *Healthy People 2030* has established an objective to reduce "illness, disability and death due to tobacco use and secondhand smoke."[5] Efforts of healthcare providers should address the higher prevalence of smoking among American Indians/Alaskan Natives, people with behavioral health conditions, LGBTQ patients, and people with lower incomes and education levels.[5] While current use of nicotine and tobacco products among middle and high school students has declined in 2019–2020, the prevalence (13.4%) is higher than in the adult population.[6] All healthcare providers should assess and advise against the use of **tobacco and nicotine products** such as cigars, hookahs (water pipes), electronic cigarettes, and smokeless tobacco products to increase the likelihood of tobacco cessation. Studies have shown that even brief tobacco cessation interventions by healthcare providers can improve a patient's chance of quitting smoking, but cessation often requires a series of behavioral interventions.[7]

Tobacco cessation occurs when a person stops tobacco use with the goal of achieving permanent abstinence. Although some tobacco users achieve abstinence during an initial quit attempt, the majority typically cycle through multiple periods of abstinence and then **relapse**, i.e., revert back to regular tobacco use. All tobacco contains nicotine, a highly addictive drug that creates physical and psychological dependence. Tobacco dependence makes it difficult for individuals to stop tobacco use even if they have health problems and want to quit. **Tobacco dependence** is a chronic disorder characterized by a vulnerability to relapse that persists for months. The relapsing nature of this disorder requires the need for ongoing care rather than just a one-time intervention.[8] As with other chronic conditions (e.g., periodontal disease and diabetes), dental hygienists who encounter tobacco-dependent patients are encouraged to provide ongoing advice, counseling in a compassionate manner, and referrals as needed. Numerous effective treatments and resources are available to assist dental hygienists in promoting and setting up a plan for tobacco cessation.[8] Such resources include telephone support and quitlines (1-800-QUIT-NOW or 800-784-8669), websites (www.smokefree.gov), mobile-based interventions (LIVESTRONG MyQuit Coach, Quit It Lite, among others), and social media support groups. According to the National Institute on Drug Abuse, "technology-based cessation interventions are particularly relevant to young adults aged 18 to 25."[9]

SYSTEMIC HEALTH EFFECTS

Although nicotine is responsible for addiction, it is other chemicals in tobacco and tobacco smoke—*N*-nitrosamines, aromatic hydrocarbons, polonium 210, carbon monoxide, and many more—that have the most detrimental effects on health. At least 69 chemicals are known to be associated with different types of cancer.[10] During the inhalation process, smokers inhale tar and absorb these chemicals contained in tobacco smoke. These toxins enter the bloodstream and are distributed to tissues throughout the body. This exposure to chemicals threatens the health and shortens life expectancies of smokers and those who inhale environmental smoke.[10] Box 37.1 lists numerous adverse systemic health effects associated with tobacco use.

Smokeless tobacco products, such as snuff, snus, and chewing tobacco, are perceived as safer than cigarettes or other smoked tobacco products because their use is not associated with lung cancer and respiratory diseases. Oral snuff is finely ground tobacco, packaged either loose or in a teabaglike sachet (Fig. 37.1). As with other tobacco products, oral snuff contains cancer-causing chemicals, such as *N*-nitrosamines, aromatic hydrocarbons, metals, and polonium 210. Chewing tobacco is made up of more coarsely shredded tobacco leaves. Snus is a smokeless tobacco product that originated in Sweden. While Swedish snus uses less harmful pasteurized tobacco, American snus is similar to chewing tobacco and contains cured tobacco (Fig. 37.2). According to the CDC, smokeless tobacco products can increase the risk of oral diseases, certain types of cancer, and the risk of death from heart disease and stroke, and cause nicotine poisoning in children.[11]

Tobacco product manufacturers control the amount of free nicotine available for uptake into the body by controlling the pH of their products through the addition of alkaline-buffering agents. Free nicotine is ionized nicotine that passes rapidly through the oral mucosa into the bloodstream and brain. Free nicotine is formed in an alkaline environment; therefore the higher the pH of a smokeless tobacco product, the more free nicotine is available. For example, at a neutral pH of 7.0, there is no free nicotine available; however, at a pH of 8.0, about 60% of the nicotine is ionized and available for use by the body to create dependence. Usually, new users start with products that contain low amounts of free nicotine to avoid the unpleasant side effects of nicotine toxicity (e.g., nausea and vomiting). Eventually, as a result of nicotine dependence, many individuals need to use products with higher amounts of free nicotine. Table 37.1 shows the pH of popular oral snuff brands and the percentage of free nicotine available in each brand. Brands with high levels of available free nicotine are very addictive, making it difficult for individuals to quit.

One of the alternative tobacco products that is popular among high school and college students is the **hookah** or **water pipe**. Hookah came to the United States from the Middle East, where smoking hookah is a popular social activity. When smoking hookah, tobacco (*shisha*) is roasted, and the user inhales both the tobacco and charcoal smoke. The smoke passes through the water chamber into a rubber hose with a mouthpiece (Fig. 37.3). Many erroneously believe that the water filters out all the toxins contained within the shisha tobacco. Unfortunately,

BOX 37.1   Adverse Health Effects of Cigarette Smoking

Oral Diseases and Conditions
- Gingival recession
- Impaired healing after periodontal treatment and surgeries
- Oral mucosal lesions (e.g., oral leukoplakia, nicotine stomatitis)
- Periodontal disease
- Tooth staining

Cardiovascular Disease
- Abdominal aortic aneurysm
- Atherosclerosis
- Coronary heart disease
- Peripheral arterial disease
- Stroke

Respiratory Disease
- Chronic obstructive pulmonary disease (e.g., asthma, chronic bronchitis)
- Emphysema

Increased Cancer Risk
- Bladder
- Blood (acute myeloid leukemia)
- Cervix
- Colon and rectum (colorectal)
- Esophagus
- Kidney and ureter
- Larynx
- Liver
- Oral and oropharynx, including parts of the throat, tongue, soft palate, and tonsils
- Pancreas
- Stomach
- Trachea, bronchus, and lung

Obstetrics and Pediatrics
- Ectopic pregnancy
- Low birth weight
- Orofacial clefts in infants
- Preterm (early) delivery
- Stillbirth (death of the infant before birth)
- Sudden infant death syndrome (SIDS; known as crib death)

Other Chronic Diseases
- Blindness, cataracts, age-related macular degeneration
- Diabetes
- Erectile dysfunction
- Pneumonia
- Rheumatoid arthritis

hookah smokers are exposed to carbon monoxide, heavy metals, tar, and carcinogens.[12] One session of smoking hookah usually lasts an hour, and users inhale more smoke than those who smoke traditional cigarettes because the smoke is humidified and less irritating due to passing through the water chamber. Several types of cancer, including lung and oral cancer, cardiovascular and respiratory diseases, and obstetric and perinatal complications, as well as periodontal disease and complications after oral surgeries, have been linked to hookah smoking.[13] Hookah smoking also presents a unique risk of spreading infectious diseases such as tuberculosis and hepatitis if the mouthpiece

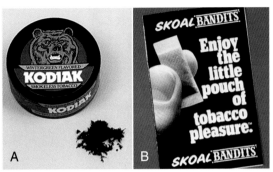

Fig. 37.1 Examples of oral snuff products. (A) Packaged loose. (B) In a teabaglike sachet.

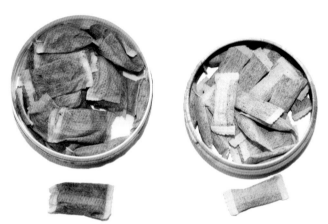

Fig. 37.2 American (L) and Swedish (R) Snus.

TABLE 37.1 **The pH and Percentage of Free Nicotine in Oral Snuff Brands**

Brand	pH	Percentage of Available Free Nicotine
Copenhagen	8.0	57%
Skoal Fine Cut	7.5	29%
Skoal Long Cut (varying brands)	7.2	23%
Skoal Bandits	5.4	<1%

is not changed or disinfected after each use. Annual hookah use has declined in recent years, but a new form of electronic hookah smoking has been introduced recently.[12]

Since 2014, the most commonly used nicotine products among youth have been electronic nicotine delivery systems (ENDS).[14] ENDS (also known as **electronic cigarettes**, e-cigarettes, tanks, electronic hookah, or vapor pens) provide nicotine without combusting tobacco or inhaling tar. The simple act of inhaling or pressing a button activates an e-cigarette; it heats up and converts a liquid mixture (*e-liquid*) into an aerosol (commonly termed *vapor*). Many e-cigarette users refer to themselves as vapers. In fact, when asked about tobacco use, e-cigarette users often deny smoking and refer to their use of e-cigs as vaping. E-cigarettes vary greatly in design and price, but some of them resemble conventional cigarettes, cigars, or pipes (Fig. 37.4). Many rechargeable e-cigarettes can be refilled and modified to deliver customized e-liquid. E-liquids typically contain propylene or polyethylene glycol, glycerin, additives, flavorings, and nicotine. E-cigarettes are not

considered a tobacco product because e-liquid is not directly derived from tobacco leaves. However, in 2016, the US Food and Drug Administration (FDA) finalized a rule extending the agency's authority to regulate e-cigarettes and other products, including cigars, hookahs, pipes, and dissolvable tobacco, that meet the legal definition of a tobacco product. E-cigarettes are perceived as less harmful than traditional cigarettes, but they can affect oral and systemic health. Recent research shows negative effects on respiratory, gastrointestinal, cardiovascular, and immune systems. E-cigarettes can also cause mechanical injuries (from battery explosions) (Fig. 37.5) and poisoning.[15] In 2019–20, significant numbers of EVALI (e-cigarette or vaping use–associated lung injuries) associated with adding cannabis oil to e-liquids were reported.[16]

ORAL HEALTH EFFECTS OF TOBACCO USE

Use of any tobacco or nicotine products has detrimental effects on oral health and can lead to changes in oral tissues.[17] The dental hygienist should be able to identify and discuss with patients the visible effects of their tobacco use. All relevant findings should be documented in the dental record. For example, both cigarette and pipe smokers may have nicotine stomatitis on the palate (Fig. 37.6). Smoking can also lead to tooth staining, melanosis, delayed healing, and increased risk for caries, leukoplakia, and oral cancer. Smokeless tobacco users typically have oral mucosal lesions and gingival recession associated with placement of smokeless tobacco in the vestibule (Fig. 37.7). The oral mucosal lesions are white, hyperkeratinized, and wrinkled; they often disappear if tobacco use is terminated at an early stage. Smokeless tobacco use can also cause halitosis, enamel erosion, and root-surface dental caries due to sugar content in smokeless tobacco[17] (see Box 37.1 for a list of the oral effects of tobacco use).

Tobacco use is the most important risk factor for the development of periodontal disease, increase in severity, and poor outcomes after treatment, as well as failure of osteointegration of dental implants.[18,19] Clinical manifestations of tobacco-induced periodontal disease and their biological bases are presented in Table 37.2. Smoking and sun exposure and alcohol use are risk factors for head, neck, skin, and lip cancers (see Chapter 50); therefore it is important to have a thorough health history and extraoral and intraoral examinations. Dental hygienists are ethically obligated to address patients' tobacco use and inform them about any tobacco-related tissue changes. Changes should be described to patients as they might not be aware of oral effects of tobacco use (Critical Thinking Scenario 1, exercise 1).

SUCCESSFUL TOBACCO CESSATION

Nicotine is what makes tobacco products addictive. It is absorbed in the bloodstream from tobacco or nicotine products, leading to dependence. Addiction to nicotine makes it very difficult to quit, and most users will try multiple times to quit before they succeed. The hallmarks of **nicotine addiction** are as follows:
- Compulsive use
- Use despite its harmful effects
- Pleasant (euphoric) effects
- Difficulty with quitting or controlling use
- Recurrent cravings
- Tolerance
- Physical dependence
- Relapse after abstinence[19]

Helping a tobacco-using client achieve abstinence requires an understanding of the different aspects of nicotine addiction.

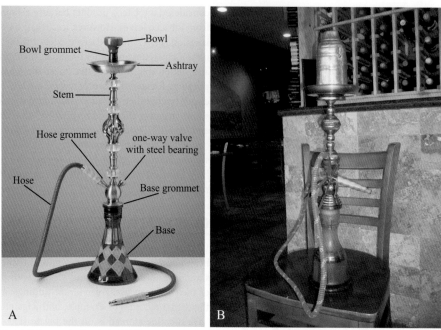

Fig. 37.3 (A) Parts of a hookah. (B) Example of a hookah. ([A] Copyright iStock Getty Images [istock.com]; [B] Courtesy Victoria Patrounova.)

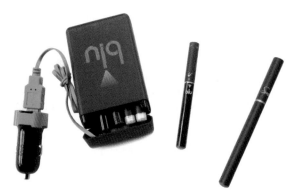

Fig. 37.4 Example of e-cigarettes. (Courtesy Victoria Patrounova.)

Physical Aspects of Nicotine Addiction

The physical aspects of nicotine addiction include reinforcing effects, tolerance, and physical dependence.[19]

Reinforcing Effects

Nicotine causes the brain to release chemicals such as dopamine, norepinephrine, acetylcholine, vasopressin, serotonin, and beta-endorphins. These chemicals produce effects in the brain that cause the user to experience pleasure, both anxiety and tension reduction, a sense of well-being when the user feels down, stimulant effects (perks up the user when tired), short-term memory improvement, and appetite suppression. These neurochemical rewards that nicotine provides a tobacco user are called **reinforcing effects**,[19] which increase tobacco users' desire to continue using tobacco.

Tolerance

With chronic exposure to nicotine, brain cells adapt to compensate for the actions of nicotine. This process is called neuroadaptation. **Tolerance** results from neuroadaptation; over time, a given level of nicotine eventually has less of an effect on the brain and a larger dose is needed to produce the same rewarding effects. As a result, the longer

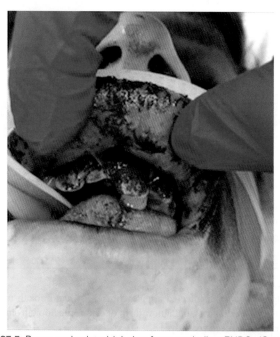

Fig. 37.5 Burns and related injuries from exploding ENDS. (Courtesy of Wang KS et al. from "Adolescent Vaping-Associated Trauma in the Western United States.")

individuals use tobacco, the more nicotine they need to achieve the desired reinforcing effects.[19]

Physical Dependence

Although the brain adapts to function normally in the presence of nicotine, it also becomes **physically dependent** on nicotine for that normal functioning. When nicotine is not available, brain function becomes disturbed, which results in **withdrawal symptoms** (Table 37.3). Symptoms peak within 12 to 24 hours and last 2 to 4 weeks if tobacco use is discontinued. Not all individuals experience withdrawal symptoms, and the degree of discomfort from withdrawal also varies. In general, the nicotine withdrawal symptoms produced by nicotine abstinence require clients to resume their tobacco use to prevent withdrawal symptoms going forward. Although individuals initially use tobacco for the reinforcing effects of pleasure, enhanced cognitive performance, and mood modulation, tobacco use often ends up dominating their lives. Because tobacco use produces tolerance and physical dependence, it results in addiction and the loss of control over use. This loss of control is the result of the individual's intense need to use tobacco to self-medicate to prevent withdrawal symptoms.[19] In general, the highly dependent tobacco user poses the greatest challenge to cessation efforts; this type of client usually requires pharmacotherapy in combination with intense behavioral counseling.

Psychological, Behavioral, Sensory, and Sociocultural Aspects

Psychological, behavioral, sensory, and sociocultural aspects of nicotine addiction also sustain tobacco use.[19]

Psychological Aspects

Psychological aspects of nicotine addiction relate to a tobacco user's need to use tobacco to cope with stress, depression, or boredom. Many tobacco users perceive their tobacco as a friend that is always with them, providing a sense of well-being, comfort, and passive entertainment.

Behavioral Aspects

Behavioral aspects of nicotine addiction relate to responses that tobacco users develop from having experienced various forms of gratification from tobacco use in certain situations.[19] When a

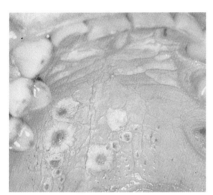

Fig. 37.6 Nicotine stomatitis on the palate of a smoker.

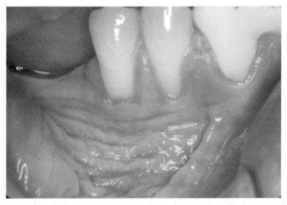

Fig. 37.7 Gingival recession and hyperkeratosis of the vestibular mucosa that developed after the use of chewing tobacco. (Courtesy Dr. Jerry E. Bouquot, DDS.)

CRITICAL THINKING SCENARIO 1

Patient: Mr. A

Profile: A 45-year-old male has a preventative oral care appointment with a dental hygienist. He has been dipping snuff since he was 18. He reports having three to five drinks every week.

Social history: He works for an oil company and frequently travels.

Health history: He has had no systemic conditions and takes no medications.

Supplemental note: On clinical examination, a wrinkled 10 × 20 mm mixed red and white lesion is found on the vestibular right labial mucosa; it extends to the alveolar mucosa and attached gingiva on the mandible. Recession on teeth 28 and 29 is noted. The patient reports that he places oral snuff in that area. He was unaware of the lesion, and the lesion was asymptomatic.

Exercise 1

1. What is the most likely diagnosis and prognosis for Mr. A's lesion?
2. Practice describing tobacco-related lesions (e.g., nicotine stomatitis, melanosis, hyperkeratinization) to a patient who is unaware of the oral effects of tobacco in the mouth.

Exercise 2

1. Is Mr. A at risk of other oral and systemic conditions?
2. How would you incorporate clinical findings into your tobacco cessation counseling advice?
3. Working with a classmate, practice the Five A's approach for Mr. A and provide feedback.

TABLE 37.2 Tobacco-Induced Periodontal Tissue Changes

Changes With Use	Biological Basis for Changes	Tissue Changes With Abstinence
Pale tissue color	Increased vasoconstriction	Increased blood flow
Decreased bleeding	Oxygen depletion	Initially more bleeding and erythema
Thickened fibrotic consistency; minimal erythema relative to extent of disease	Compromised immune response: • Fewer and impaired polymorphonuclear neutrophils • Reduced immunoglobulin G antibodies	Healthier consistency and anatomy
Gingival recession around anterior sextants	Increased collagenase production	
Greater probing depths, bone and attachment loss, and furcation invasion	Reduction of bone mineral; impaired fibroblast function	Stabilization of attachment levels
Refractory status: continued use	Impaired wound healing	

tobacco user encounters these environmental cues or stimuli, they serve as situational reminders of tobacco use (e.g., after a meal, work breaks, when drinking alcohol or coffee) and its associated pleasure or other reinforcing effects. They then generate a strong urge to use tobacco, known as a **learned anticipatory response**. Such learned anticipatory responses can last 6 months or longer after physical dependence has been overcome, and they are often responsible for relapse. For successful cessation, tobacco users have to learn to anticipate situational cues that will trigger the desire to use tobacco and plan alternative rewards and ways to cope with these triggers.

Sensory Aspects

Puffing on a cigarette, vaping, or having a dip of a specific size and texture in the mouth provides oral gratification, which relates to the sensory aspect of nicotine addiction. Because of the sense this oral gratification provides, the use of nontobacco oral substitutes (e.g., chewing gum, sunflower seeds) is important to the quitting process.[19] In addition, because nicotine is an appetite suppressant, individuals often increase their food intake when they reduce their nicotine exposures. Individuals who successfully stop their tobacco use gain 10 pounds on average. Drinking a lot of water, exercising, and eating a balanced diet can help these individuals avoid this weight gain.[19]

Sociocultural Aspects

Sociocultural aspects of nicotine addiction that pose challenges to cessation include peer pressure, the influence of family members, and a social network that supports and accepts tobacco use.

HELPING CLIENTS BECOME TOBACCO-FREE

When a healthcare provider assists clients with their efforts to stop using tobacco, all aspects of nicotine addiction must be confronted and alternative coping strategies identified. Being supportive and assisting the client with problem solving are critical to the promotion of tobacco cessation.

The Five A's Approach

The **Five A's approach** is an evidence-based strategy geared toward helping clients become tobacco-free. This approach, developed by the National Cancer Institute and the Agency for Healthcare Research and Quality, involves *asking* clients about tobacco use, *advising* users to quit, *assessing* their readiness to quit, *assisting* with the quitting process, and *arranging* followup.[19] Table 37.4 provides sample language for the dental hygienist to use while performing components of the Five A's. This approach serves as a model for brief, effective interventions that have been successfully implemented in both medical and dental care environments.[19] A team approach that involves all office staff members facilitates the success of the Five A's strategy.

Ask

It is important to identify all tobacco users and ask each patient about tobacco use systematically at every visit. Cues or prompts, such as chart icons or codes, are recommended to remind the hygienist to ask each patient.

Advise

The dental hygienist advises all tobacco users to quit to protect their health. Such advice should be clear, nonjudgmental, and related to something immediately relevant to the client. Personalizing cessation advice with findings visible to the client provides a teachable moment that can motivate the patient to decide to make a quit attempt.[19] It is

TABLE 37.3 Nicotine Withdrawal Symptoms and Suggested Behavioral Coping Strategies

Symptoms	Mechanisms for Coping
Cravings	Realize cravings last only 20 to 30 minutes; "I can wait them out."
	Consider thinking responses (e.g., "I can do this, and I will.")
	Use distraction techniques (e.g., exercise, read)
	Avoid triggers (e.g., people, places, things associated with former habit)
	Use substitutions (e.g., chew gum, drink water, hand doodling)
Irritability, frustration, anger, depression	Accept referral to a counselor or support group
	Exercise
	Breathe deeply and then slowly exhale
	Reward self for maintaining abstinence (e.g., every day, first week, anniversaries)
Anxiety	Perform aerobic exercise
	Visualize positive action or thing
	Relax and perform breathing exercises
Depression, sad mood	Accept referral to physician, counselor, or support group
	Engage in a hobby; reward self
	Exercise
Insomnia	Avoid caffeine
	Perform aerobic exercise (but not within 2 hours of bedtime)
	Perform breathing and relaxation exercise; meditate
Difficulty concentrating	Perform breathing and relaxation exercise; meditate
	Perform aerobic exercise
Hunger or weight gain	Chew xylitol gum or eat xylitol hard candy
	Eat a well-balanced diet
	Exercise
	Drink water

appropriate to discuss actual and potential adverse health effects associated with tobacco use. After providing the advice component, however, the dental hygienist replaces the discussion of negative health effects with discussions about the benefits of quitting to enhance the patient's motivation to stop tobacco use (Box 37.2).

Assess

For all patients who report tobacco use, the dental hygienist determines which tobacco users are willing and ready to make a quit attempt. To assess readiness to quit, the dental hygienist simply asks clients if they would like to stop their tobacco use during the next month. Whether patients respond yes or no will determine the appropriate strategy for assisting with the quitting process.[19]

As individuals attempt to stop tobacco use, **relapse** often occurs. The dental hygienist encourages patients to view relapse as a learning opportunity because what is learned from each quit attempt can be applied to the next one. Fig. 37.8 provides a summary and suggested dental hygiene interventions.

Assist

The manner in which the dental hygienist assists a patient with quitting tobacco use depends on the client's readiness to quit (see Fig. 37.8). Whether or not patients are ready to quit, it is critical that the dental hygienist engage them by applying **patient-centered communication**.[19,20]

TABLE 37.4   The Five A's Approach to Tobacco Cessation (Revised)

Approach	Suggested Actions and/or Language	Time Required
Ask	*Gather information on the patient's tobacco use.* "I take time to ask all of our patients about tobacco use because it is important." "Tell me about your tobacco habit (types, frequency)."	1 minute
Advise	*Deliver a strong, clear, personalized message to quit at every appointment and show patients the visible effects of tobacco use in their own mouths.* "There have been some tissue changes in your mouth and your periodontal disease is getting worse since your last visit. Smoking is affecting your health. The best thing that I can do for you today to protect your health is to advise you to stop smoking."	30 minutes
Assess (readiness to quit)	*Assess a person's willingness to change behavior.* "Would you like to try to quit smoking in the next month?" "How ready are you to quit (on a scale of 1–10)?"	30 seconds
Assist	*Provide assistance based on the patient's readiness to quit.* *Patients who are in the preparation or action stage will be the most receptive.* *For patients who are not ready to quit:* Provide a brief intervention or a motivational interview.	3 to 5 minutes
Arrange	*For patients who are not ready to quit:* "If it is okay with you, I'd like to check in with you at your next dental appointment to see where you are in your decision making." (Document patient's response in chart.) *For patients who are ready to quit:* Refer client to 1-800-QUIT-NOW and provide information about a community-based tobacco cessation program in the area. (Document in chart to check on the patient's quitting progress.) Help with quit plan, nicotine-replacement therapies (NRTs). Establish a followup system (e.g., a call, letter, postcard, referral).	3 to 5 minutes

Adapted from the US Department of Health and Human Services. *Treating Tobacco Use and Dependence.* US Department of Health and Human Services Publication No. 69-0692, Washington, DC, US Government Printing Office; 2000.

BOX 37.2   Benefits of Stopping Tobacco Use

- I won't have the smell of tobacco on my breath or stains on my teeth.
- I will save money.
- It will reduce my chances of getting mouth cancer.
- My friends and family want me to quit.
- I'll be setting a good example for my children.
- I'll feel more in control of my life.
- I'll feel more liberated and self-assured that I can set goals and accomplish them.
- It will reduce my chances of heart trouble.
- It will reduce my chances of gum disease.
- It will reduce my chances of hypertension and circulatory problems.
- It will increase my chances of being around to support my family and of seeing my children grow up.
- Between 2 weeks and 3 months after quitting smoking, circulation improves, walking becomes easier, and lung function increases up to 30%.
- One year after quitting smoking, the risk of coronary heart disease decreases to one-half that of a smoker.
- Five years after quitting smoking, the risk of stroke is reduced to that of a person who has never smoked.
- Fifteen years after quitting smoking, the risk of coronary heart disease is similar to that of people who have never smoked.

Characteristics of patient-centered communication include the following:

- *Collaborating, not persuading:* The dental hygienist–patient relationship involves a partnership that honors the patient's experience and perspectives. The dental hygienist seeks to create a positive interpersonal atmosphere that is conducive to change while not being coercive.
- *Eliciting information, not imparting information:* The dental hygienist's tone is not one of imparting information but rather, of drawing out motivation for change from the person. Patients do most of the talking and dental hygienists listen carefully.
- *Emphasizing the client's autonomy, not the authority of the expert:* Responsibility for change is left with the client.[19]

Arrange

Arranging a followup contact is comparable to the evaluation phase of the dental hygiene process of care (see Chapter 23). During followup contacts, the dental hygienist checks on where patients are in their thinking process about quitting or how they are coping with the quitting process. For those who have made an unsuccessful quit attempt, modifications (e.g., a new quit date, different pharmacological adjuncts, new coping strategies) may be introduced. New goals may need to be set.[5,19] (Practice the Five A's approach in Critical Thinking Scenario 1, exercise 2.)

Assisting Clients Who Are Not Ready to Quit

For patients who are not ready to stop their tobacco use within the next month, the primary goal is to help them think about the benefits of stopping tobacco use versus the benefits of continuous use. When the benefits of stopping outweigh the benefits of using, the patient will make a decision to quit. For this goal to be accomplished, a brief intervention or a motivational interview is recommended.

Brief Intervention

The goal of a brief (about 3-minute) intervention is to communicate acceptance of the patient's decision not to attempt quitting at this time and to provide information about the benefits of stopping tobacco use.[20]

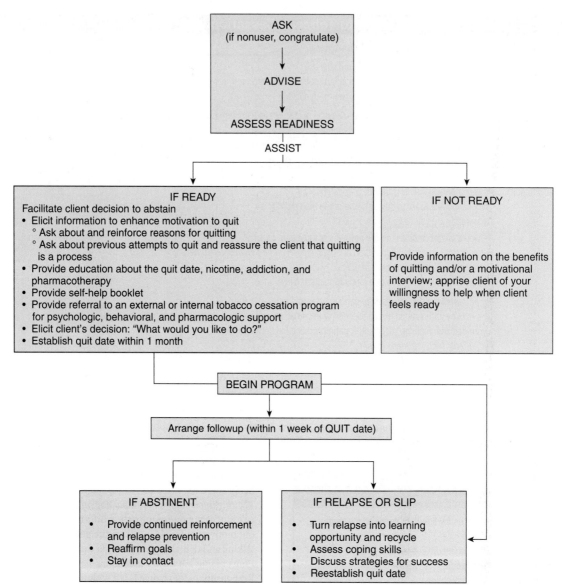

Fig. 37.8 Tobacco intervention flowchart.

When a patient refuses an offer of help, the dental hygienist does the following:

- Responds by stating, "I understand that you are not ready to stop smoking now, but if you don't mind, I would like to give you some information on the benefits of stopping for you to consider" (see Box 37.2). This statement communicates to patients that they have been heard and that the dental hygienist understands that they are not ready to stop now. In addition, the dental hygienist offers information to help move patients in the direction of making a decision to quit someday.
- Reassures the patient by stating, "When you decide to try to stop, if you want, we can help you."
- Asks permission to check in again at the next visit to see where the patient is in the decision-making process by stating, "Would it be all right if I check in with you at your next dental hygiene care appointment regarding your thinking about all this?"
- Makes a note in the chart to check in again at the next dental care visit.[20]

Motivational Interview

A **motivational interview** is a form of patient-centered counseling style for addressing patients' ambivalence about change that

can trap them in their tobacco use. It is a compassionate and collaborative conversation about change where the provider respects the autonomy of the patient and tries to evoke the patient's own motivation. Ambivalence is a normal stage in the quitting process (see Chapter 5). After ambivalence is resolved, little else may be required for the patient to decide to stop tobacco use. Attempts to force the resolution of ambivalence by direct persuasion to stop can lead to strengthening the very behavior that the clinician intended to diminish. For example, nagging may increase smoking if users perceive that their personal freedom is being infringed. Discovering and understanding a person's motivations for tobacco use are important first steps toward promoting change. The four general principles of the motivational interview—expressing empathy, developing discrepancy, rolling with resistance, and supporting self-efficacy—are outlined in Table 37.5.

The goal of motivational interviewing is to ask the patient to voice the arguments for change; this is known as **change talk**. Change talk includes *desire, ability, reasons for concern,* and *need for change,* as well as *commitment/action/taking steps* towards change (DARN-CAT). Tools for eliciting change talk include four strategies referred to by the acronym **OARS**.[19,20]

TABLE 37.5 Principles of the Motivational Interview

Express empathy	• Listen to the patient with a desire to understand, and with no expression of judging, criticizing, or blaming. • Use reflective listening to seek a shared understanding. Summarize by stating, "So, you think smoking helps you maintain your weight?" • Normalize the patient's feelings and concerns by stating, "Many people worry about managing without cigarettes." • Support the patient's autonomy and right to choose or reject change.
Develop discrepancy	• Highlight the discrepancy between the patient's present behavior and expressed priorities, values, and goals by stating, "It sounds like you are very devoted to your family. How do you think your smoking is affecting your children?" • Reinforce and support "change talk" and "commitment" language. • Build and deepen the patient's commitment to change by stating, "There are effective treatments that will ease the pain of quitting, including counseling and many medication options."
Roll with resistance	• Avoid arguing and use reflection when the patient expresses resistance by stating, "It sounds like you are feeling pressured about your smoking." • Express empathy by stating, "You are worried about how you would manage withdrawal symptoms." • Ask permission to provide information.
Support self-efficacy	• Help the patient identify and build on past successes by stating, "You were fairly successful the last time you tried to quit and remained smoke-free for 3 months." • Offer options for achievable small steps toward change: • Call the quitline (1-800-QUIT-NOW) for advice and information. • Read about quitting benefits and strategies. • Suggest changes in smoking patterns (e.g., no smoking in the home). • Ask the patient to share ideas about quitting strategies.

Adapted from Tobacco Use and Dependence Guideline Panel. *Treating Tobacco Use And Dependence: 2008 Update.* US Department of Health and Human Services; May 3, 2008. Clinical Interventions for Tobacco Use and Dependence.

These tools are as follows:

- *Open-ended questions:* During the motivational interview, the dental hygienist allows patients to express themselves by asking open-ended questions. For example, "What do you like about tobacco use?" or "What kind of roadblocks come to mind when you think about stopping smoking?" Patients should be doing most of the talking.
- *Affirming change talk:* This strategy reinforces and focuses on patient comments that support stopping tobacco use. The dental hygienist shows appreciation and understanding. For example, "That's a good point. Do you have any other concerns?"
- *Reflective responding:* Restating or rephrasing what patients say acknowledges to patients that they are heard. For example, "So, one of the most important considerations for you is how your smoking may affect your daughter."
- *Summarizing results of the dialog:* This strategy brings closure to the session. For example, "So, if I understand you so far, you enjoy smoking because it relaxes you, but you have some real concerns that it is beginning to affect your health and that you may be a negative role model for your daughter. It is clear that you have overcome a number of challenges in your life and you will be able to resolve this issue of smoking once you make up your mind. If it is all right with you, I'd like to check in with you at your next appointment to see where you are in your thinking about all of this. Just know that if you decide to try to stop smoking, we can help."

Assisting Patients Who Are Ready to Stop Tobacco Use

For patients who state that they are ready to quit during the next month, the dental hygienist provides referral for more intensive assistance either to internal or external tobacco cessation resources (e.g., telephone quitlines, online support groups, behavioral counseling, smartphone applications, and websites). A list of tobacco cessation programs within the community should be developed for use in the referral of clients. When clients choose to stop using tobacco, all dental team members lend support by providing positive reinforcement.

Statewide Tobacco Use Quitlines

Tobacco-use telephone quitlines are excellent external resources for referral for tobacco cessation assistance; they can be accessed from any state in the United States. They offer easy access at no cost to the client, and they address ethnic and geographic disparities. Many tobacco users prefer quitlines over face-to-face programs because telephone and online counseling is more convenient and provides anonymity. Key factors that increase quitline effectiveness include the use of trained counselors, a proactive format in which staff initiates contact and followup, and the combination of the quitline with client self-help materials and approved pharmacotherapy (Critical Thinking Scenario 2.)

CRITICAL THINKING SCENARIO 2

1. Research the websites of the American Dental Association (ADA), Canadian Dental Association (CDA), American Dental Hygienists' Association (ADHA), Canadian Dental Hygienists Association (CDHA), and World Dental Federation for resources to use during chairside tobacco cessation counseling.
2. Develop a referral guide with local tobacco treatment programs and local quitline telephone numbers.

KEY ELEMENTS OF INTENSIVE TOBACCO CESSATION TREATMENT PROGRAMS

Whether the dental hygienist refers the client to an intensive (i.e., multiple-appointment) tobacco cessation treatment program within the dental setting or within the community, key elements shared by high-quality tobacco cessation programs are listed in Box 37.3 and discussed in detail in the following sections.

Assessment

Initially, the tobacco cessation counselor assesses clients' motivation to quit, reasons for quitting, previous quit attempts, nicotine dependence level, tobacco use patterns in a typical day (i.e., number of dips, chews,

---

BOX 37.3   Key Elements of Intensive Tobacco Cessation Treatment Programs

- Assessing the following:
  - Motivation to quit
  - Reasons for quitting
  - Previous quit attempts
  - Nicotine dependence
  - Patterns of tobacco use
  - History of mood disorders
  - Contraindications for pharmacotherapy
- Setting a quit date
- Establishing a plan for quitting
- Offering coping skills training
- Encouraging the enlistment of support from others
- Recommending pharmacologic agents
- Preventing relapse
- Following up

---

cigarettes used per day, and associated cravings and mood states), mood disorder history, and pharmacotherapy contraindications. The assessment is used to tailor quit plans to individual needs. The following information relates to this assessment process.

Motivation to Quit

Motivation is fundamental to changing behavior. A client's level of motivation to stop tobacco use is often a good predictor of outcome.[19] To enhance clients' motivation and to measure their motivation to quit, the provider reads the following question and asks clients to circle an answer:

On a scale of 0 to 10, how important would you say it is for you to stop your tobacco use?

Not at all important   0   1   2   3   4   5   6   7   8   9   10   Extremely important

---

The circled number then serves to measure clients' initial motivation, and it is used to monitor motivation to stop tobacco use at subsequent appointments. The number also serves as the basis for a discussion to increase clients' motivation to quit. For example, if a client circles the number 5, the provider might say, "Great! But why did you circle a 5 rather than a 3?" This open-ended question requires clients to talk positively about their motivation to quit, which serves to enhance their motivation. In general, asking clients why they circled a *higher* number rather than a *lower* number on the importance of quitting scale triggers clients to respond positively about their motivation to quit.

Reasons for Quitting

To enhance the motivation to quit, the provider also asks clients about their reasons for wanting to stop their tobacco use. The provider may suggest that clients write these reasons down because motivation may be high but wane somewhat with time. Remembering a patient's reasons for quitting enhances motivation and provides an incentive to get through the tough times during the quitting process. Strong motivation is essential for tobacco users who are trying to quit, and success is unlikely without it.[19]

Previous Quit Attempts

The provider assesses clients' previous quit attempts by asking them about problems they encountered. If nicotine replacement or other pharmacological adjuncts were used, it is important to find out what happened. When discussing quit attempts, the provider promotes

clients' positive self-images by telling clients something along the lines of the following, "Quitting tobacco is a process that takes most people several tries before they are able to quit for good. You learn something new about yourself and quitting with each try."

Nicotine Dependence

There are many ways to assess nicotine dependence. Recommended evidence-based questions to ask clients include the following:

- "How many cigarettes do you smoke per day?"
- "Do you use tobacco within 30 minutes of waking?"
- "Do you find it difficult not to smoke in places where it is not permitted?"
- "Do you smoke when you are so ill that you are in bed most of the day?"

Based on "yes" responses to these questions, the level of dependence can be determined (Fig. 37.9).

Nicotine dependence can be assessed based on the number of tobacco products used, smoking patterns, and withdrawal symptoms. To minimize discomfort from nicotine withdrawal, it is important for nicotine-dependent tobacco users to wean themselves off nicotine before the quit date rather than to stop abruptly (i.e., cold turkey). Strategies that combine behavioral treatment and FDA-approved cessation medication achieve the best outcomes for nicotine-dependent clients.[9]

Patterns of Tobacco Use

To assess patterns of use in a typical day, clients recall each cigarette, chew, dip, or e-cigarette that they have during a typical day. Beginning with the first use of the day, the time of day that tobacco is usually used, and the situation in which the use occurs, is recorded. Clients are asked to do the following:

- Rate their desire or craving for each recorded tobacco use on a scale of 1 to 10, with a score of 1 representing "I do not crave it at all" (the lowest craving) and a score of 10 representing "I have to have it" (the strongest craving). Tobacco users with lower craving scores are easier to eliminate, and it is recommended that clients give them up first during the weaning process.
- Describe their mood at each recorded tobacco use by indicating a number between 1 and 10, with the scores representing the following: 1 = relaxed; 2 = bored; 3 = angry; 4 = happy; 5 = stressed; 6 = excited; 7 = tired; 8 = sad; 9 = hungry; and 10 = irritable.

Understanding the level of craving and the client's mood when tobacco is used helps establish a quit plan and identifies coping strategies to prevent relapse after the client quits. After working with the client to monitor tobacco use on a typical day, the provider may suggest that the client monitor tobacco use over a week and fill out a tobacco diary with the following information to track tobacco use for 7 days (Fig. 37.10). The client and provider can discuss the tobacco diary at the followup appointment.

History of Mood Disorders

According to the National Alliance on Mental Health, in 2020, approximately 21% of adults in the United States have mental illness, and these individuals are twice as likely to smoke and to smoke more heavily than people without such a condition.[21,22] Some individuals may use tobacco to self-medicate for depression or anxiety because nicotine is a mood elevator. However, recent research indicates that smoking can worsen the symptoms of mental illness and that quitting tobacco is associated with improvements in mental health and does not interfere with behavioral health treatment.[22] Although smoking can reduce the effectiveness of some psychiatric medications, requiring higher doses to achieve the same results, quitting can decrease signs of depression, anxiety, and stress and improve behavioral health outcomes.[22]

1 Smoker Pre-Treatment Diagnostic Profile

Additional ACCP resources on Disc* or, www.tobaccodependence.chestnet.org*

Loma Linda University School of Dentistry

AMERICAN COLLEGE OF CHEST PHYSICIANS®

Diagnostic Factors	Mild	Moderate	Severe	Very Severe
Daily Cig Use	< 5	6–19	20–40	>40
1st Cig in AM	> 60 mins.	31–60 mins.	6–30 mins.	0–5 mins.
Nicotine Withdrawal Symptoms: (See 0–48 point NWS Scale*)	Intermittent, 11–20	Frequent 21–30	Constant, 31–40	Constant, >40
FTND* (Fagerstrom Test for Nicotine Dependence*)	2–3	4–5	6–7	8–10
Health and Psych History	Healthy	Healthy	≥1 Chronic Medical Disease OR ≥1 Psychiatric Disease	≥1 Chronic Medical Disease AND/OR ≥1 Psychiatric Disease

Note: if answers fall in multiple categories, utilize the most severe category for treatment medications.

Adapted from the American College of Chest Physicians Tobacco-Dependence Treatment Tool Kit, 3rd Ed., © 2010, with permission

ver: 1.0

2 Initial Tobacco Treatment Medications: Determined by Diagnostic Profile (Side 1)

Treatment Goal: Suppress nicotine withdrawal symptoms and keep suppressed.

Options	Mild	Moderate	Severe (1 or More)	Very Severe (Multiple)
Controller*	Nicotine Patch OR	Varenicline, w/no Relievers OR	Nicotine Patch* (Standard, Individualized, or High-Dose*) AND/OR Bupropion-SR	Varenicline AND Bupropion-SR AND/OR
	Bupropion-SR OR	Nicotine patch OR		
	Varenicline	Bupropion-SR	Nicotine patch AND/OR Bupropion-SR	High Dose Nicotine Patch AND/OR
Reliever†	OR	AND/OR	AND/OR	AND
As needed	NG, NL, NNS, NI	NG, NL, NNS, NI	NG, NL, NNS, NI	Multiple Reliever Medications
Step-Down/ Maintenance	• Gradually reduce medications one at a time. • Monitor to maintain No nicotine withdrawl symptoms. • Some patients will need indefinite use of Controller or Reliever Medications to maintain zero nicotine withdrawl symptoms and no tobacco use.			

*Controller Medications: Foundation, slow-acting medication to suppress nicotine withdrawal symptoms
†Reliever Medications: Rapid-acting medications to suppress break-through nicotine withdrawal symptoms; include NG=Nicotine Gum, NL=Nicotin Lozenge, NNS=Nicotine Nasal Spray, and NI=Nicotine (Oral) Inhaler
Rx Dosages: Bupropion-SR 300 mg daily; Varenicline, Starter Pack, 0.5-mg tablets, Continuing pack, 1-mg tablets, w/a maintenance dose of 2 mg daily. Duration: Minimum 6–24 weeks to as long as needed to keep nicotine withdrawal symptoms suppressed.

Adapted from the American College of Chest Physicians Tabacco-Dependence Treatment Tool Kit, 3rd Ed., © 2010, with permission

ver: 1.0

Fig. 37.9 Tobacco Medication Guidelines developed by Loma Linda University and the American College of Chest Physicians to determine dependence status and to select tobacco treatment medications. (Loma Linda University School of Dentistry.)

Day	Time used	Place used	Activity done at time used	Mood (e.g., bored, happy, stressed)	Intensity of cravings (1-10)	Tobacco used
1						
2						
3						
4						
5						
6						
7						

Fig. 37.10 An example of a tobacco diary.

Contraindications to Pharmacotherapy

As a chronic disease, tobacco dependence can be treated with multiple clinical modalities, including medications. Clinical practice guidelines for treating tobacco use and dependence state the following:

Numerous effective medications are available for tobacco dependence, and clinicians should encourage their use by all patients attempting to quit smoking—except when medically contraindicated or with specific populations for which there is insufficient evidence of effectiveness (i.e., pregnant/breastfeeding females, smokeless tobacco users, light smokers, and adolescents).[8]

TABLE 37.6	Over-the-Counter Pharmacotherapies for Tobacco Cessation*			
Pharmacotherapy	**Contraindications**	**Dose**	**Duration**	**Administration**
Nicotine gum	Unstable coronary syndrome (ischemia, serious arrhythmias, angina) Recent myocardial infarction (MI) Pregnancy[†] Lactation[†] Stomach ulcer Temporomandibular joint disease (TMD) Dentures, dental appliances, loose teeth	1 to 20 cigarettes/day: 2-mg gum (≤24 pieces/day) ≥25 cigarettes/day: 4-mg gum (≤24 pieces/day)	Weeks 1 to 6: chew one piece of gum every 1 to 2 hours and at least nine pieces/day during the first 6 weeks Weeks 7 to 9: chew one piece of gum every 2 to 4 hours Weeks 10 to 12: chew one piece of gum every 4 to 8 hours	Instruct patient not to chew nicotine gum as regular gum; begin chewing slowly until tingling or peppery taste in mouth; then move the gum between the inside of the cheek in the vestibule until the tingling subsides.
Nicotine lozenge	Recent MI Unstable coronary syndrome Pregnancy[†] Lactation[†] Stomach ulcer Oral thrush or lesions	Based on time of first cigarette: Within 30 minutes of waking, begin with a 4-mg lozenge. After 30 minutes of waking, begin with a 2-mg lozenge. Consume 5 to 20 lozenges/day.	Up to 12 weeks Weeks 1 to 6: use one lozenge every 1 to 2 hours Weeks 7 to 9: use one lozenge every 2 to 4 hours Weeks 10 to 12: use one lozenge every 4 to 8 hours	To use the lozenge, place it in the mouth and allow it to dissolve slowly. Do not chew or swallow lozenges. Once in a while, use the tongue to move the lozenge from one side of the mouth to the other. It should take 20 to 30 minutes to dissolve. Do not eat while the lozenge is in the mouth.
Nicotine patch[‡]	Recent MI Unstable coronary syndrome Pregnancy[†] Lactation[†] Psoriasis or eczema	≥10 cigarettes/day 21 mg once daily 14 mg once daily 7 mg once daily or 15 mg once daily 10 mg once daily 5 mg once daily ≤10 cigarettes/day 14 mg once daily 7 mg once daily	 6 weeks 2 weeks 2 weeks 6 weeks 2 weeks 2 weeks 6 weeks 2 weeks	Apply to clean, dry, nonhairy area of skin (typically upper arm or shoulder). Apply new patch upon awakening and wear patch for 24 hours unless vivid dreams or insomnia occur (then remove patch before bedtime).

*The information contained in this table is not comprehensive. See package inserts for additional information.
[†]Only on the advice of your healthcare provider.
[‡]Recommendations for NicoDerm CQ.
Adapted from https://www.quit.com/ and Center for Tobacco Independence www.tobaccoindependence.org.

TABLE 37.7	Prescription Pharmacotherapies for Tobacco Cessation			
Pharmacotherapy	**Contraindications**	**Dose**	**Duration**	**Administration**
Nicotine nasal spray	Hypersensitivity Caution with hypertension, cardiovascular or peripheral vascular diseases Hyperthyroidism, insulin-dependent diabetes Rhinitis, nasal polyps, or sinusitis	One 0.5 mg spray in each nostril to provide 1 mg/dose	8 doses/day initially Initiate with 1 to 2 doses/hour; at least 8 doses/day Do not exceed 5 doses in 1 hour or 40 doses in 24 hours	Tilt head back. Do not sniff, swallow, or inhale through the nose as the spray is being administered
Nicotine oral inhaler	Unstable coronary syndrome (ischemia, serious arrhythmias, angina) Caution with hyperthyroidism, pheochromocytoma, insulin-dependent diabetes Asthma, allergy to menthol	10 mg/cartridge (4 mg delivered)	At least 6 cartridges/day for 3 to 6 weeks Do not exceed 16 cartridges/day	Inhale deeply into back of throat or puff in short breaths. As the user inhales or puffs through the mouthpiece, nicotine turns into vapor and is absorbed into the mouth and throat. Use inhaler longer and more often at first to help control cigarette cravings.

The information contained within this table is not comprehensive. Please see package inserts for additional information.

BOX 37.4   Preparing to Quit Cold Turkey

- Have a positive attitude that the quit date will be the last day tobacco will ever be used.
- Tell others and ask for their support.
- Practice going without tobacco at a time when its use would be common or enjoyable and use coping skills.
- Plan rewards.

BOX 37.5   Strategies to Cope With Cravings and Temptation to Use Tobacco

Action Responses
- Avoidance—Get away
- Distraction—Do something
- Alternatives—Exercise
- Relaxation—Deep breathing
- Use of oral substitutes—Nontobacco
- On the quit date—Change routine

Thinking Responses
- Positive thinking—I know it's difficult, but I can do it! I will succeed.
- Delay—I won't have a cigarette now. I'll decide again in an hour.
- Rewards—I am proud of myself, so I will reward myself every day for the first week and on anniversaries.

To identify special circumstances, the provider assesses the presence of any contraindications to FDA-approved medications. Tables 37.6 and 37.7 list contraindications for specific pharmacological agents.

Setting a Quit Date

Counselors or healthcare providers encourage clients to set a quit date within a 2-week period from the time that they decide to quit.[8] Then between the time clients decide to quit and their actual quit date, they can get ready to quit: inform their family and friends, get rid of tobacco products, and stock up on nontobacco oral substitutes. Low-stress times, such as a day when there are no work deadlines, might be a better time to quit. Some individuals will select a date of particular significance to them, such as a birthday or anniversary. On the quit date, total abstinence is essential.

Choosing a Method

After a quit date is set, the provider helps the client establish a method to get ready to quit and to cope with the quitting process. The two basic methods of quitting tobacco use are cold turkey and gradual nicotine reduction. Cold turkey is the approach of quitting tobacco use abruptly on the client's quit date (Box 37.4). Gradual nicotine reduction is the approach that slowly and systematically reduces the amount of nicotine clients use so that they will have fewer symptoms of withdrawal on their quit date. Nicotine reduction can be accomplished by gradually tapering down smoking.

Tapering down use is a method of systematically reducing the number of tobacco uses by cutting out the "easiest to quit" cigarette, increasing intervals between smoking, and scheduling the reduction of tobacco uses by 1 or 2 every few days; tapering may also be accomplished with nontobacco oral substitutes. When clients get to the point at which they are using half of their original amount of tobacco, they can try to quit cold turkey. For clients who choose to taper down their tobacco use, the provider refers to their pattern of use on a typical day as recorded in a diary during the assessment phase of counseling. On the basis of the diary information, the provider suggests that clients start cutting back on those cigarettes or dips with the lowest craving scores (see Table 37.3 for lists of some helpful suggestions for behavioral strategies to cope with nicotine withdrawal and the temptation to use tobacco). Specific coping strategies that clients use and the rewards they plan for themselves on their quit day and for the first week without tobacco use are noted in the client record.

Coping Skills Training

Coping skills training involves helping clients identify action responses (i.e., things they can do) and thinking responses (i.e., things they can say to themselves) to avoid tobacco use when tempted (Box 37.5).

Action Responses

The following strategies are suggested action responses to cope with the temptation to use tobacco.

Avoidance. Clients may help prevent relapse by avoiding situations in which their potential for using tobacco is high, such as socializing with other tobacco users and avoiding food and beverages that trigger smoking and places where they typically smoked before. During these high-risk situations, cravings and temptations may be strong and the motivation to stop using tobacco may waver.

Distraction. Since a craving usually disappears after a few minutes, teaching clients to focus their attention on doing something else can help them cope with cravings. For example, when a craving arises, clients could engage in physical activity or behavior that is incompatible with smoking (e.g., walking, jogging, swimming, or gardening), call a friend, brush their teeth, or engage in their favorite hobby.

Alternatives. Exercise can help with the stress and irritability that commonly occur when quitting tobacco use. Clients are encouraged to do stretching and relaxation exercises at the beginning and end of each day. Goals for exercise should be realistic. Examples vary from simple exercises like taking the stairs rather than the elevator to attending regularly scheduled group classes.

Relaxation. Taking 10 slow, deep breaths when having a craving can help to allow the few minutes for a craving to pass. Breathing slowly and deeply in through the nose and out through the mouth is a technique to suggest to clients. Deep breathing also helps with stress and tension.

Use of oral substitutes. The provider helps clients make a list of nontobacco oral substitutes (e.g., sunflower seeds in the shell, fruits, raw vegetables, flavored toothpicks, or xylitol-based candy) to use when they have a strong craving for tobacco. Clients are counseled to stock them where they normally keep their tobacco. They are also instructed to throw out all tobacco products and to stock up on nontobacco substitutes the night before they quit.

On the quit date. Clients are encouraged to change their daily routine on the quit date to break away from tobacco triggers and decrease the temptation to use tobacco. It is important for clients to make plans to keep busy, such as scheduling an exercise class to boost energy and stamina or a dental hygiene care appointment during which they can receive preventive oral care along with words of encouragement.

Thinking Responses

Thinking responses are the client's thoughts about quitting tobacco use. Some thinking responses that the client can use to cope with the temptation to use tobacco are listed in Box 37.5.

Positive thinking. Providers encourage clients to be as supportive of themselves as they would be of their best friends. When a negative thought or self-doubt comes to mind (e.g., "I can't do this"), providers instruct clients to substitute a positive thought such as, "I know it's difficult, but I *can* do this. I just need to get through today or the next hour." In addition, clients need to be encouraged to think in terms of "getting rid of" an addiction rather than "giving up" tobacco.

Delay. Providers encourage clients to tell themselves, "I won't have a cigarette now. I'll decide again in an hour." In the meantime, if clients

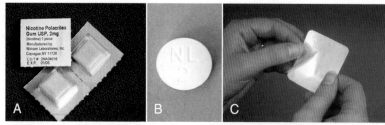

Fig. 37.11 US Food and Drug Administration–approved over-the-counter nicotine replacement therapies for smoking cessation. (A) Nicotine gum. (B) Nicotine lozenge. (C) Transdermal nicotine patch.

find something else to do to get their minds off the craving, by the time an hour passes, the craving is more likely to go away.

Rewards. Clients are encouraged to choose rewards for themselves every day for the first week they are tobacco-free and to reward themselves on anniversaries to avoid the feeling of deprivation while quitting tobacco. For example, they could buy something they really want (e.g., new music, magazine, or book) with the money they save by not buying tobacco. Rewards can also be free, such as visiting a friend or enjoying time at the beach.

Support From Others

Clients are encouraged to tell family, friends, and coworkers that they are trying to quit tobacco use and to request understanding and support.[20] If clients who are trying to quit are feeling irritable, family members and friends will be more understanding if they are informed about the situation. These individuals can help clients by not offering tobacco, by providing support and reinforcement to refrain from tobacco use, and by encouraging them if things are not going well.

Relapse Prevention

Although nicotine withdrawal lasts only 2 to 4 weeks, the temptation to use can last for years.[8] To prevent relapse, it is critical for clients to identify at least three tough situations in which they know they will be tempted most and then plan ahead regarding what they will do instead to remain tobacco free. In addition, because drinking alcohol is highly associated with relapse, providers often encourage clients to review their alcohol use and consider abstaining from alcohol during the quitting process.

Followup Contact

Initial followup occurs on the quit date, during the first week after the quit date, and within the first month of the quit date. Additional followup contacts are scheduled as needed in person, by telephone, or through online forums. During followup, the provider congratulates the client on their success. For clients who have experienced a slip (i.e., the use of tobacco but not a resumption of regular tobacco use), it is important to transform the event into a learning situation. For example, clients may have learned that they really cannot be around friends who smoke or drink and that they need to focus on nontobacco stress reduction techniques. The provider helps clients identify what caused the slip or relapse and think about what they can do to prevent a recurrence. If a full relapse has occurred, a new quit date needs to be set and the client should recommit to not smoking. Ongoing support is critical. For some clients seeking cessation assistance in the dental setting, referral to a more specialized intensive tobacco cessation program may be appropriate.[20]

US FOOD AND DRUG ADMINISTRATION–APPROVED PHARMACOLOGICAL ADJUNCTS

Based on the level of dependence, clients are advised about pharmacological support to facilitate the quitting process (see Fig. 37.9). The

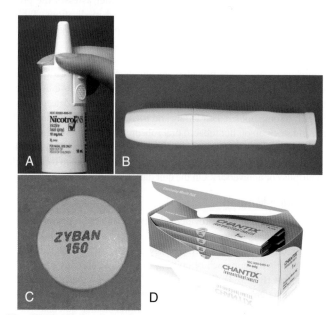

Fig. 37.12 US Food and Drug Administration–approved nicotine and nonnicotine prescription pharmacological therapies for smoking cessation. (A) Nicotine nasal spray. (B) Nicotine oral inhaler. (C) Zyban. (D) Chantix.

dental hygienist may recommend over-the-counter (OTC) nicotine replacement therapies (NRTs) and other prescription FDA-approved adjuncts. The different types of OTC NRTs for smoking cessation are shown in Fig. 37.11, and their use and related contraindications are listed in Table 37.6. Fig. 37.12 shows the FDA-approved nicotine and nonnicotine prescription pharmacological therapies for smoking cessation. Such adjuncts are helpful for diminishing cravings and other withdrawal symptoms, which allows clients to concentrate on action responses and thinking coping strategies to resist the temptation to use. Clients, however, need to be cautioned that no pharmacological adjunct is a magic bullet.

Nicotine Replacement Therapy

The purpose of **nicotine replacement therapy** (NRT) is to provide some blood concentration of nicotine to reduce or eliminate withdrawal symptoms so that clients can focus on the psychosocial and behavioral changes necessary to stop their tobacco use.[20] However, there may be a period of trial and error to determine the optimal dose of NRT to avoid nicotine withdrawal symptoms while, at the same time, preventing **nicotine toxicity** (i.e., nicotine overdose). Nicotine replacement products must be used according to manufacturers' instructions. Individuals must discontinue all tobacco use before starting NRT to prevent nicotine toxicity, during which the client may experience stomach upset, nausea, or vomiting (Box 37.6)

- Provide team members with in-service training about the adverse health effects of tobacco use and the Five A's approach.
- Suggest mechanisms for program incorporation.
- Designate a program coordinator to do the following:
  - Facilitate team involvement.
  - Publicize the program to patients.
  - Order literature.
  - Implement an office-wide system that ensures patient's tobacco use status is queried and documented.
  - Ensure patient followup.
  - Reinforce documentation in the dental record.
  - Create a tobacco-free environment by posting signs and ordering magazines that do not advertise tobacco products.

Current OTC nicotine replacement products are the nicotine transdermal patch system, nicotine polacrilex gum, and the nicotine lozenge (see Fig. 37.11). Prescription products that are available include nicotine nasal spray and the nicotine oral inhaler (see Figs. 37.12A and B). All types of nicotine replacement products enhance abstinence when used properly and in conjunction with cognitive behavioral counseling. In general, nicotine replacement products are contraindicated for individuals with underlying cardiovascular disease, especially those who have experienced recent myocardial infarction, life-threatening arrhythmias, or severe or worsening angina. Nicotine toxicity can also result if clients overuse nicotine replacement products.

Transdermal Nicotine Replacement Therapy (Patch)

Transdermal nicotine patches are marketed for 24-hour use. One advantage of the patch is that it delivers a constant dose of nicotine to the bloodstream at a constant rate. A small percentage of individuals who have used the 24-hour patch have reported sleep interrupted by nightmares, which is an indication of nicotine toxicity. If this side effect occurs, the dose of nicotine should be reduced either by removing the patch during sleeping hours or by using a lower-dose patch. Clients may also experience dermatitis as a side effect of using the patch and it should be avoided in patients with dermatological conditions such as psoriasis, eczema, and atopic dermatitis. Directions for use require the client to place a new patch each day on a nonhairy site of the upper body or upper outer arm. No single site should be used again until more than a week has passed. Patches work on a dosing-down principle, and the aim is to gradually discontinue use over the course of 12 weeks (see Table 37.6). The person is eventually weaned off nicotine completely. Dose modification may be required based on the client's weight. For oral healthcare providers, consultation with the patient's physician is advised, particularly if the patient has systemic disease. In general, compliance is easier to achieve with the patch than with other forms of NRT that require more behavior modification.

Nicotine Polacrilex (Gum)

Nicotine gum is available OTC in 2- or 4-mg doses, and the dose should be based on the client's smoking pattern. The aim is to gradually discontinue use of the gum over a 3-month (12-week) period (see Table 37.6).

Proper gum use requires chewing the gum very slowly because the nicotine is absorbed through the oral mucosa (in an alkaline environment) and not the gut (in an acidic environment). The individual should stop chewing at the first sign of a peppery, minty, or citrus taste or tingle, and then park the gum between the cheek and the gingiva.

Overchewing can result in nicotine toxicity. Success with nicotine gum is greater with a fixed dosage schedule throughout the day to prevent craving rather than using gum when a craving arises. Often, if a person waits until a craving arises, they will relapse to tobacco use because a cigarette or dip provides more rapid absorption of nicotine into the blood compared with gum. To avoid withdrawal and relapse, nicotine gum is sometimes used in the morning in combination with the patch when the patch is first placed. This action enables the user to receive a quick boost of nicotine with the addition of gum to prevent breakthrough cravings.

Nicotine Lozenge

The nicotine lozenge is available OTC in 2- or 4-mg doses. The lozenge provides 25% more nicotine than the equivalent nicotine gum dose because the lozenge dissolves in the mouth completely in 20 to 30 minutes. Clients should stop eating and drinking 15 minutes before using a lozenge or gum and avoid using acidic beverages (e.g., coffee, juice, wine, and sodas) to allow better absorption. Like gum, it is used on a regular schedule (every 1 to 2 hours) throughout the day to prevent cravings. The initial dose is based on the time of the first cigarette after waking. Those who have a history of having their first cigarette within 30 minutes of waking begin with the 4-mg lozenge. The aim is to discontinue use gradually over 12 weeks on a schedule similar to that used for gum (see Table 37.6 for the schedule). To achieve maximum effectiveness and avoid adverse side effects similar to those reported with the improper use of gum, the person using a lozenge should not chew or swallow it.

Nicotine Nasal Spray

Nicotine nasal spray is available by prescription only due to the rapid absorption of its nicotine through the nasal mucosa and its potential for abuse (see Fig. 37.12A). Of all of the nicotine replacement products, nicotine spray provides the fastest nicotine delivery into the bloodstream. Each dose delivers 0.5 mg of nicotine in each nostril. A daily fixed schedule begins with one or two doses per hour, with at least eight doses daily for the first 6 to 8 weeks. The aim is to gradually discontinue use over an additional 4 to 6 weeks (see Table 37.7).

Nicotine Oral Inhaler

The nicotine oral inhaler is available by prescription only (see Fig. 37.12B). It consists of a mouthpiece and a plastic cartridge that deliver 4 mg of nicotine vapor. The nicotine is absorbed across the oropharyngeal mucosa and should not be inhaled into the throat or lungs. The inhaler is most effective if it is puffed frequently over 20 minutes. A person may use up a cartridge all at once or puff on it for a few minutes at a time until the nicotine is finished. At least eight cartridges per day for 3 to 6 weeks are recommended. The schedule can be adjusted based on individual preferences, and the dose can be increased to 16 cartridges a day. The aim is to discontinue use gradually over an additional 6 to 12 weeks (see Table 37.7).

Combination Nicotine Replacement Therapy

The nicotine patch is a long-acting formulation that produces relatively constant levels of nicotine. Short-acting, rapidly absorbed formulations, such as nicotine gum, lozenge, inhaler, and spray, are often used to supplement the patch to prevent or control breakthrough cravings or withdrawal symptoms. These short-acting formulations allow for acute dose titration as needed for severely nicotine-dependent tobacco users (see Fig. 37.9). Some tobacco users with moderate and severe dependence will require additional prescription medications such as bupropion (Zyban) or varenicline (Chantix) to achieve abstinence (see Figs. 37.12C and D). These medications can be prescribed by a dentist or physician and require monitoring of the patient for side effects such as sleep disturbances, psychiatric symptoms, and depression (see Table 37.7). Recommendations for NRTs and nonnicotine pharmacological agents should be made according to the client's level of dependence (Critical Thinking Scenario 3).

CRITICAL THINKING SCENARIO 3

Patient: Mrs. Z

Profile: A 38-year-old female patient reports smoking about one pack of cigarettes per day for 20 years. She reports having a first cigarette within 30 minutes of waking and having a hard time staying away from cigarettes when in smoke-free areas or when sick.

Social history: Mrs. Z is a housewife who hides her smoking from her kids.

Health history: She takes medication for depression.

Oral health behavior: She reports brushing three times a day and using mints and mouthrinse.

Supplemental note: She is interested in replacing restorations that have become "too yellow" and tooth whitening.

1. How would you personalize your advice?
2. If Mrs. Z is not interested in quitting, what parts of the Five A's approach would you use in your tobacco cessation counseling message?
3. What are the ethical and legal implications of providing aesthetic services without providing tobacco cessation counseling?

DENTAL HYGIENIST'S ROLE

Dental hygienists are often the strongest proponents of tobacco intervention activities in their employment settings. Four key steps are necessary to ensure the successful incorporation of tobacco intervention programs into clinical settings: (1) generating team support, (2) designating a coordinator, (3) creating a tobacco-free environment, and (4) addressing reimbursement issues.

BOX 37.7 Legal, Ethical, and Safety Issues

- As oral healthcare providers, dental hygienists are ethically obligated to address patients' tobacco use and its relationship to their oral health and overall well-being.
- Because tobacco use is a life-threatening habit, all tobacco-using patients must be informed of its detrimental effects, and educated and guided toward abstinence.
- The links among tobacco use, oral cancer, and periodontal disease are undisputed. Patients who are diagnosed with oral cancer and periodontal disease could potentially sue providers who have not informed them of the relationship among tobacco use, oral cancer, and periodontal disease.
- With the current emphases on prevention and health promotion, tobacco use interventions are a standard of care and are therefore expected behaviors of oral health professionals.

The dental hygienist's role related to tobacco extends beyond the immediate clinical environment. Given its magnitude as a public health issue, tobacco use commands dental hygienists' actions at both the professional and societal levels. Ethically, dental hygienists are committed to the health and well-being of society (Box 37.7). Involvement with tobacco-related issues helps with the improvement in the overall health of members of society. The effort to reduce tobacco use in the United States must include collaborative efforts with other healthcare professionals (e.g., dentists, nurses, counselors, and public health professionals) at the local, state, and national levels. Dental professionals need to encourage local government agencies, youth organizations, dental and dental hygiene organizations, community leaders, insurers, and families to support tobacco control efforts in their community and advocate for policy changes and community-based initiatives that would reduce tobacco use. This support includes advocating for the following:

- Laws restricting the marketing of tobacco and nicotine products
- Increases in taxes on tobacco/nicotine products
- Reimbursement of tobacco use cessation services through dental insurance plans
- Programs that provide comprehensive tobacco-use cessation counseling
- Tobacco-use cessation training and continuing education courses for all healthcare professionals
- Funding of research on the health effects of novel tobacco products such as e-cigarettes
- School- and community-based tobacco use prevention programs
- Tobacco dependence education in dental and dental hygiene curricula
- Ordinances that encourage tobacco-free environments.

KEY CONCEPTS

- Tobacco contains nicotine, an addicting drug that changes brain chemistry.
- Tobacco use is the number one cause of preventable disability and death.
- There are numerous adverse systemic and oral health effects of tobacco use.
- Nicotine addiction is a physical, psychological, behavioral, and sensory dependence that makes it very difficult for a person to stop tobacco use.
- The Five A's approach, which involves a brief and effective tobacco cessation intervention, is a methodology endorsed by the National Institutes for Health for implementation by oral health and medical care teams in private practice and community settings.
- Characteristics of patient-centered communication are collaboration, elicitation of information, and emphasis on client autonomy.
- Motivational interviewing is a form of patient-centered communication to help clients get unstuck from the ambivalence that traps them in their tobacco use.
- When the benefits of quitting tobacco use outweigh the benefits of continuing tobacco use, a person will make a decision to quit.
- Motivation is fundamental to changing behavior. Asking patients why they circled a higher number rather than a lower number on a 1-to-10 scale rating the importance of their reasons to quit (10 indicates the highest motivation) requires patients to talk positively about their motivation to quit and serves to enhance their motivation.
- Nicotine withdrawal lasts 2 to 4 weeks.
- Pharmacological adjuncts help reduce or eliminate nicotine withdrawal symptoms so the person trying to quit can focus on behavioral and psychological factors that support abstinence from tobacco use.
- High-quality, intensive tobacco cessation treatment programs include several key elements such as assessment, choosing methods of quitting, and coping skills training.
- The dental hygienist's role related to tobacco issues extends beyond providing immediate clinical care.

RECOMMENDED ONLINE RESOURCES

- **Clearing the Air.** https://smokefree.gov/sites/default/files/pdf/clearing-the-air-accessible.pdf
- **American Dental Association.** https://www.ada.org/resources/research/science-and-research-institute/oral-health-topics/tobacco-use-and-cessation
- **Cessation Materials.** https://www.cdc.gov/tobacco/quit_smoking/cessation/index.htm
- **Tobacco Smoking Cessation in Adults, Including Pregnant Persons: Interventions.** https://www.uspreventiveservicestaskforce.org/uspstf/recommendation/tobacco-use-in-adults-and-pregnant-women-counseling-and-interventions
- Tobacco Use Cessation Services and the Role of the Dental Hygienist—A CDHA (Canadian Dental Hygienists Association) position paper. https://www.cdha.ca/pdfs/Profession/Resources/1004_tobacco.pdf
- **FDI Tobacco Cessation Guide for Health Professionals in English, Arabic, Spanish and French.** https://www.fdiworlddental.org/fdi-tobacco-cessation-guide-health-professionals
- **Tobacco Treatment Specialist services—Mayo Clinic.** https://www. youtube.com/watch?v=5EDaA26unVw

ACKNOWLEDGMENT

The author acknowledges Margaret Walsh and Kirsten Jarvi for their contributions to this chapter.

REFERENCES

1. Centers for Disease Control and Prevention. Current Cigarette Smoking Among Adults in the United States. Available at: https://www.cdc.gov/tobacco/data_statistics/fact_sheets/adult_data/cig_smoking/index.htm#references. Accessed July 3, 2022.
2. US Department of Health and Human Services. Smoking Cessation: A Report of the Surgeon General. Available at: https://www.hhs.gov/sites/default/files/2020-cessation-sgr-full-report.pdf. Accessed July 3, 2022.
3. Centers for Disease Control and Prevention. Cigarette Smoking in the United States – Data and Statistics on Smoking – Campaign Resources – Tips From Former Smokers – Smoking & Tobacco Use. Available at: https://www.cdc.gov/tobacco/campaign/tips/resources/data/cigarette-smoking-in-united-states.html. Accessed July 3, 2022.
4. Davis JM, Ramseier CA, Mattheos N, et al. Education of tobacco use prevention and cessation for dental professionals – a paradigm shift. *Int Dent J.* 2010;60(1):60–72.
5. Tobacco Use. Healthy People 2030. Available at: https://health.gov/healthypeople/objectives-and-data/browse-objectives/tobacco-use. Accessed July 27, 2022.
6. Centers for Disease Control and Prevention. Youth and Tobacco Use. Available at: https://www.cdc.gov/tobacco/data_statistics/fact_sheets/youth_data/tobacco_use/index.htm. Accessed July 22, 2022.
7. Stead LF, Buitrago D, Preciado N, et al. Physician advice for smoking cessation. *Cochrane Database Syst Rev.* 2013;(5):CD000165. Accessed December 12, 2017.
8. Fiore MC, Jaén CR, Baker TB, et al. *Treating tobacco use and dependence: 2008 update. Quick Reference Guide for Clinicians.* US Department of Health and Human Services. Public Health Service; 2009.
9. NIDA. What are treatments for tobacco dependence? Available at: https://nida.nih.gov/publications/research-reports/tobacco-nicotine-e-cigarettes/what-are-treatments-tobacco-dependence; 2021. Accessed July 4, 2022.
10. American Cancer Society. Harmful Chemicals in Tobacco Products. Available at: https://www.cancer.org/healthy/cancer-causes/tobacco-and-cancer/carcinogens-found-in-tobacco-products.html Accessed July 4, 2022.
11. Centers for Disease Control and Prevention. *Smokeless Tobacco: Health Effects.* Centers for Disease Control and Prevention. Available at: https://www.cdc.gov/tobacco/data_statistics/fact_sheets/smokeless/health_effects/index.htm. Accessed July 4, 2022.
12. Centers for Disease Control. *Hookahs.* Centers for Disease Control and Prevention. Available at: https://www.cdc.gov/tobacco/data_statistics/fact_sheets/tobacco_industry/hookahs/index.htm#:~:text=Hookah%20Smoke%20and%20Cancer&text=Hookah%20tobacco%20and%20smoke%20contain,%2C%20bladder%2C%20and%20oral%20cancers.&text=Tobacco%20juices%20from%20hookahs%20irritate,risk%20of%20developing%20oral%20cancers. Accessed July 22, 2022.
13. El-Zaatari ZM, Chami HA, Zaatari GS. Health effects associated with waterpipe smoking. *Tob Control.* 2015;24(suppl 1):i31–i43.
14. Centers for Disease Control. Available at: https://www.cdc.gov/tobacco/data_statistics/fact_sheets/youth_data/tobacco_use/index.htm#:~:text=E%2Dcigarettes%20have%20been%20the,in%20the%20past%2030%20days. Accessed July 22, 2022.
15. Hua M, Talbot P. Potential health effects of electronic cigarettes: a systematic review of case reports. *Prev Med Rep.* 2016;4:169–178.
16. Centers for Disease Control and Prevention. Outbreak of Lung Injury Associated With the Use of E-Cigarette, or Vaping, Products. Available at: https://www.cdc.gov/tobacco/basic_information/e-cigarettes/severe-lung-disease.html. Accessed July 22, 2022.
17. American Dental Association. Tobacco Use and Cessation. Available at: https://www.ada.org/resources/research/science-and-research-institute/oral-health-topics/tobacco-use-and-cessation#:~:text=Cigarette%20smoking%20can%20lead%20to,periodontal%20disease%2C%20and%20tooth%20staining. Accessed October 26, 2023.
18. Silva H. Tobacco use and periodontal disease-the role of microvascular dysfunction. *Biology.* 2021;10(5):441. https://doi.org/10.3390/biology10050441. PMID: 34067557. ; PMCID: PMC8156280.
19. Walsh MM, Ellison J. Treatment of tobacco use and dependence: the role of the dental professional. *J Dent Educ.* 2005;69:521.
20. Miller W, Rollnick S. *Motivational Interviewing: Preparing People for Change.* Guilford Press; 2002.
21. National Alliance on Mental Illness. Mental Health by Numbers. Available at: https://www.nami.org/mhstats#:~:text=21%25%20of%20U.S.%20adults%20experienced,represents%201%20in%2020%20adults. Accessed July 25, 2022.
22. Centers for Disease Control and Prevention. *What We Know: Tobacco Use and Quitting Among Individuals with Behavioral Health Conditions.* Centers for Disease Control and Prevention; 2022. Available at: https://www.cdc.gov/tobacco/disparities/what-we-know/behavioral-health-conditions/index.html.

38

Impressions for Study Casts and Custom-Made Oral Appliances

Kimberly Bastin

PROFESSIONAL DEVELOPMENT OPPORTUNITIES

The responsibility to take preliminary dental impressions, related bite registration, and fabricate custom-made oral appliances often falls on the dental hygienist. In some states, the dental hygienist's scope of practice includes taking final impressions and constructing custom-made oral appliances such as mouthguards and whitening or fluoride trays.

COMPETENCIES

1. Define "dental impression," list the main types of dental impressions, and make appropriate clinical judgments regarding the uses of dental impressions in dental hygiene practice, including alginate impressions. Use the criteria for evaluating the acceptability of a dental impression.
2. Discuss dental casts, including gypsum products.
3. Differentiate between the uses and benefits of various custom-made removable oral appliances used by patients for preventive and active dental treatment.
4. Compare and contrast the types of oral surgical splints and stents and their uses.
5. Use patient assessment findings to determine the need for a custom-made oral appliance.
6. Educate patients regarding the maintenance of custom-made oral appliances.

INTRODUCTION

A **dental impression** is a negative reproduction of the teeth and surrounding tissues of the oral cavity used to create an accurate or exact three-dimensional positive reproduction of the teeth and surrounding tissues of the oral cavity. This positive reproduction is a *study model, diagnostic cast,* or *die.* There are three main types of dental impressions used in dentistry: a preliminary impression, a final impression, and a bite registration. **Preliminary impressions** are *accurate* reproductions of the patient's mouth used to construct study models for diagnosing, documenting a patient's dental arches as part of permanent records, and enhancing client education as a visual aid. Preliminary impressions also are useful to construct diagnostic casts for the construction of removable oral appliances. **Final impressions** are more detailed reproductions of the patient's tooth structures and surrounding tissues used to make casts and dies. A dental laboratory technician uses casts and dies in the construction of inlays, onlays, crowns, bridges, partial or full dentures, and restorations placed on titanium implants. A **bite registration** is an impression made of the teeth occluded by biting into wax, polysiloxane, or other material to record the occlusal relationship between arches. The occlusal relationship is essential when establishing articulation of a maxillary and mandibular cast.

Custom-made oral appliances are trays or stents used for the targeted delivery of materials (e.g., tooth-whitening products, home fluoride application, other desensitizing agents); for the fabrication of provisional restorations, orthodontic retainers, and aligners; and for the protection of oral structures from bruxism and contact sports (mouthguards). Oral **surgical stents** are guides that provide communication between the surgeon and the restoring dentist to guide the placement of an implant at the ideal prosthetic position and angulation. This chapter provides an overview of concepts related to making dental impressions, study models, diagnostic casts, bite registrations, and custom-made oral appliances. The reader should consult a text about dental materials for complete information about the properties and manipulation of specific types of dental materials.

DENTAL IMPRESSIONS

Impression Trays

Because dental impressions have many uses in oral healthcare, there are various types of impression trays available to deliver and position impression material into the mouth. Impression tray designs vary for different areas of the mouth and include quadrant trays, which cover half an arch, and full trays, which cover the complete maxillary or mandibular arch (Fig. 38.1). Tray selection depends on the purpose of the impression. Metal, plastic, or disposable Styrofoam trays are available in standard small, medium, and large sizes for children and adults. Some trays have perforations to promote a mechanical lock with the impression material (Box 38.1 and Procedure 38.1). The metal trays are typically cleaned and sterilized for multiple uses, while the plastic and Styrofoam trays are considered disposable and only used for one patient.

Traditional Alginate Impression Material

The impression material that is most widely used in dentistry for preliminary impressions is irreversible hydrocolloid (*hydro,* meaning "water," and *colloid,* meaning "gelatin"). Because hydrocolloid is in a water suspension, the product is considered **hydrophilic,** a term that means "loves water." Hydrocolloids can exist in a sol (solution) or a gel (solid) state. Depending on the type of hydrocolloid used, the physical change from sol to gel is either reversible (changed by thermal factors) or irreversible (changed by chemical factors). Gelation is the transformation from sol to gel.[1,2]

Irreversible hydrocolloids do not change their physical state after gelation. **Alginate** is an irreversible hydrocolloid powder and water impression material that changes from a sol to a gel state by means of a chemical reaction. Cool water is added to the potassium alginate powder and mixed to produce a sol. The impression material reaches the gel state after the chemical setting reaction in the patient's mouth. After the impression reaches the gel state, the clinician removes it from

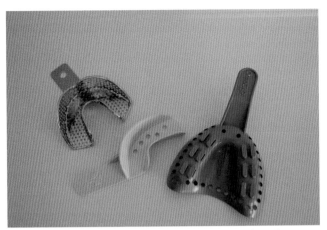

Fig. 38.1 Types of impression trays; full arch and quadrant.

the mouth. Alginate materials are ideal for preliminary impressions in which accurate detail is important. However, these materials are not appropriate for final impressions that require exact fine detail for the precise fabrication and fit of a restoration.[1,2]

Packaging and Storage

Alginate impression material is available either in premeasured packages or in bulk canisters. The premeasured packages are more expensive, but they save time by eliminating the need to measure the powder and provide a consistent mix. Because the powder deteriorates when exposed to elevated temperatures or water, it is important to store the powder in a tightly closed container in a cool, nonrefrigerated place. Use of the individual premeasured packages immediately upon opening avoids water condensation on the powder from humidity in the air. Properly stored alginate impression material has a shelf life of about 1 year.

Although an alginate impression does not change its physical state after gelation, it is subject to distortion caused by even slight changes in its physical surroundings. Thus alginate impressions must be "poured up" within an hour after taking them. The potential for dimensional change is due to the water component of the material. For example, if left exposed to the room environment uncovered, the impression may shrink owing to **syneresis** (the loss of water) from evaporation. **Imbibition** is the uptake of water in the presence of moisture. It is recommended that a disinfected impression be wrapped in a slightly moistened towel and placed in a plastic biohazard bag or unwrapped in a **humidor** (a covered container with a moist environment) to cause the least amount of distortion. Because of the loss of water and resultant dimensional changes

upon pouring with gypsum products, alginate impressions can only be poured once.[1,2]

Water/Powder Ratio

When alginate powder stored in canisters is used, a plastic scoop for dispensing the powder and a calibrated plastic cylinder for measuring the water are supplied by the manufacturer (Fig. 38.2). It is important to use the manufacturer's measuring devices as sizing may be different depending on the product. Caution should be used when dispensing and mixing the product; a mask should be worn to protect the clinician from inhaling potentially hazardous particles contained within the powder. Accurate measurements of both the powder and water are critical for a successful impression. The powder should be fluffed in the canister by turning the container end over end before measuring, and the measuring scoop must be full and level, which can be accomplished by tapping the scoop and leveling with a spatula. The water must be carefully measured in the provided measuring cylinder. Mandibular alginate impressions generally require two scoops of powder and two measure lines of water. A large mandible may require three scoops of powder to three measure lines of water. A maxillary impression generally takes three scoops of powder and three measure lines of water. The water/powder ratios can also be based off of impression tray size. The small and medium trays may accommodate two scoops of powder and two measures of water, while a large tray would accommodate three scoops of powder and three measures of water.[1,2]

Setting Time

The time needed to mix the impression material, load the tray, and seat it in the patient's mouth is called the **working time**. The time required for gelation, after which the impression tray is removed from the mouth, is called the **setting time**. Alginate impression material is available in regular-set powder (a working time of 2 minutes and a setting time of up to 4.5 minutes) and fast-set powder (a working time of 1.25 minutes and a setting time of 1 to 2 minutes). Currently, there are several brands of color-changing alginate available. The color-coded handling sequence guides the clinician in the mixing, loading, and setting of the material. When the alginate powder is mixed with water, it changes color to purple; it changes color to pink when it is time to load the tray and to place it into the mouth; and it changes to white at gelation.

The alginate powder is mixed with room-temperature water (68° to 70°F or 20° to 21°C). Altering the temperature of the water is the best way to control the working and setting time of the material. Cooler water increases the working and setting time; warmer water decreases these times. Powder is incorporated into the water to wet the powder completely and then vigorously spatulated against the sides of the mixing bowl until a smooth, creamy consistency is achieved. The clinician should carefully follow the manufacturer's instructions to allow the chemical reaction to proceed effectively. Loading the tray and insertion should take no more than 1 minute. The objective is for the impression material to reach the final gel state in the patient's mouth. If the gelation of the material begins before the complete seating of the impression, distortion of the final product is likely. Procedure 38.2 describes the details for mixing alginate impression material. Table 38.1 presents factors that affect gelation and therefore the success of the impression.[1]

Silicone Alginate-Alternative Materials

Alginate-alternative materials are becoming increasingly popular in the fabrication of preliminary impressions. These materials have the elasticity of alginate and the dimensional stability of polyvinyl siloxane impression materials, enabling pouring and repouring of models at any time from immediately after disinfection to up to several weeks later. The option to delay or repeat pours enhances the flexibility of

PROCEDURE 38.1 Selecting the Correct Impression Tray Size and Preparing It for Use

Equipment
Personal protective equipment
Antimicrobial mouth rinse
Lip protectant
Maxillary and mandibular impression trays
Mouth mirror
Utility (rope) wax

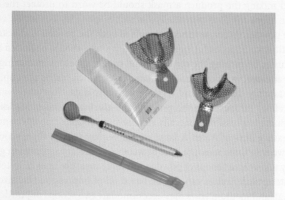

Equipment for selecting and preparing an impression tray.

Steps

Preparation

1. Gather all necessary supplies.
2. Position yourself at the side and in front of patient, and seat the patient in an upright position.
3. Explain the procedure to the patient. Have the patient remove any removable oral appliances.
4. Place protective eyewear on the patient.
5. Don personal protective equipment. Disinfect hands and don gloves.
6. Lubricate the patient's lips with a small amount of protectant. Petroleum jelly is not recommended as it can degrade some gloves.

Mandibular Tray Selection

7. Inspect the patient's mouth to estimate tray size. Note teeth out of alignment, tori/exostosis, and length of dental arch that may require additional tray adaptation for patient comfort.
8. Instruct the patient to tilt chin down. Retract the patient's lip and cheek with index and middle fingers of nondominant hand and at the same time, turn the tray sideways and distend the lip and cheek on the opposite side of the mouth with the side of the tray to gain entry into the patient's mouth. Insert the tray with a rotary motion.

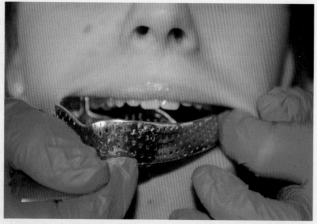

Inserting the impression tray during try-in.

9. Ensure that the tray is centered over the lower teeth by placing the handle at the midline, usually between the central incisors and in line with the center of the chin. If there is a midline shift, the handle may not line up between the central incisors, but the nose and chin can be utilized as a guide for centering the tray.
10. Instruct the patient to raise the tongue. Lower the tray and at the same time retract the cheek to make certain the buccal mucosa is not caught under the rim of the tray.
11. Check to be sure that the tray covers the teeth and soft tissue. Lift the front of the tray to make certain that the area posterior to the retromolar pad is covered and that there is enough room to allow for 2 to 3 mm of impression material in the facial and lingual surfaces of the teeth. If necessary, adapt the tray borders with utility (rope) wax to extend into the depth of the vestibule or extend the posterior length of the tray.
12. Reselect a larger or smaller tray as needed.

Maxillary Tray Selection

13. Repeat steps 7 and 8; include an evaluation of the height of the palatal vault.
14. Center the tray by placing the handle between the central incisors, in line with the center of the nose and chin.
15. Bring the front of the tray about 2 to 3 mm anterior to the incisors.
16. Seat the tray first by lowering the handle toward the mandibular teeth.
17. Make sure that all the posterior teeth and soft tissue, including the maxillary tuberosity, are covered. Check that laterally there is enough room to allow for a 2- to 3-mm space between the inside of the tray and the facial and lingual surfaces of the teeth.
18. Retract the patient's lip and raise the anterior portion of the tray into place. The tray should fit to the depth of the vestibule and not impinge on soft tissue.
19. Reselect larger or smaller tray as needed.

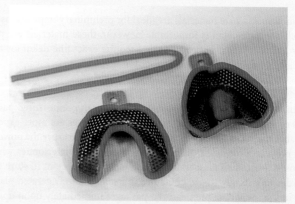

Impression tray extended with utility wax. (From Eakle WS, Bastin KG. *Dental Materials, Clinical Applications for the Dental Assistant and Dental Hygienist.* 4th ed. Elsevier; 2021.)

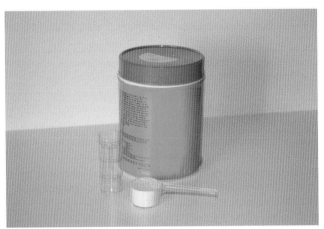

Fig. 38.2 A plastic scoop and water cylinder are supplied by the manufacturer with each canister of alginate powder.

this product when making multiple molds or time constraints prevent immediate pouring of the impression.

The materials are available in smaller automix cartridges for extruder mixing guns with mixing tips and in 380-mL volume cartridges for automatic mixing machines. The extruder tips eliminate the need for mixing and the resultant cleaning. The convenience and flexibility of these products comes with a price; they are roughly 6 to 8 times more expensive than traditional alginate products.

Digital Impressions

New processes are being introduced in dental practices for the purpose of obtaining impressions using digital technologies. These technologies obtain three-dimensional (3-D) imaging of the mouth and other pertinent oral structures needed for impressions. An intraoral scanner uses a beam of infrared light to create accurate 3-D records by use of a stream of video images or a series of static images (Fig. 38.3). The digital impressions are considered a clinically acceptable alternative to traditional impression methods.[2]

PROCEDURE 38.2 Mixing Alginate

Equipment

Personal protective equipment
Alginate powder
Measuring scoop (provided by manufacturer)
Room-temperature water
Vial for measuring water (provided by manufacturer)
Wide-blade mixing spatula
Flexible rubber mixing bowl

Steps

1. Read the manufacturer's directions for the dispensing and manipulation of the alginate.
2. Place one measure of room-temperature water into the flexible mixing bowl for each scoop of alginate. The water-to-powder ratio should always be one to one (1:1). Check temperature of water to ensure that it is at room temperature. Use warmer water to accelerate the setting of the mix and cooler water to slow the setting of the mix. Altering temperature of water may cause variances in the quality and detail of the impression.
3. Shake or fluff the alginate by turning the container end over end two or three times. Ensure the lid is closed tightly and the scoop has been removed prior to fluffing the material.
4. Overfill the correct scoop with powder; tap the scoop with the side of the spatula. Scrape the excess from the scoop with the spatula.
5. Sift the powder into the water, and stir this with the spatula until all the powder is moist. The chemical reaction begins when the alginate touches the water. A clinician should expedite the process of adding alginate to water to ensure proper time is allotted to mix materials and take impression.
6. Cup the flexible rubber bowl in the palm of your nondominant hand with the opening of the bowl facing your wrist. Firmly spread the alginate between the spatula and the side of the rubber bowl. Spatulate the mixture vigorously using a back-and-forth hand motion, spreading the material against the sides of the bowl (similar to the process of spreading icing on a cake). Use both sides of the spatula and rotate the bowl with your fingers during spatulation.
7. Spatulate vigorously for 30 seconds for fast-set products and gather the material together. Use the spatula to collect the mixture and spread it out again. Repeat until a smooth, creamy consistency is achieved within the designated mixing time for either the normal-set or fast-set alginate.

8. Gather the material into one mass, and wipe it on the inside edge of the mixing bowl.

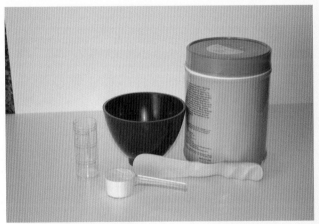

Equipment for mixing alginate impression material.

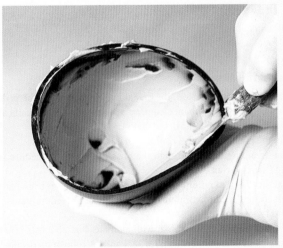

Proper consistency of mixed alginate impression material. (From Eakle WS, Bastin KG. *Dental Materials, Clinical Applications for the Dental Assistant and Dental Hygienist.* 4th ed. Elsevier; 2021.)

TABLE 38.1	Factors That Affect Gelation
Factor	**Comments**
Ratio of water to alginate powder	Manufacturer's directions must be followed carefully. The water/powder ratio must be precise. Too much water in the mix will make a weak impression that will tear easily during removal from the mouth as a result of tension. Too little water creates a grainy impression that will cause an inaccurate reproduction of the oral tissues. If the container holding the alginate is not fluffed before measuring, too much powder will be dispensed, which will result in a grainy impression.
Water temperature	Water temperature affects gelation time. If the water is too warm, the product will gel at a faster rate, resulting in poor detail in the impression. If the water is cool, the product will gel at a slower rate and the final impression will be more accurate in detail. In hot, humid climates, it is recommended to use cooler water and to refrigerate the bowl and spatula.
Spatulation technique	Proper mixing (spatulation) will determine setting time. A mechanical device that automatically mixes the material can be used. Too much spatulation will decrease the strength of the impression material because the gel is broken as it forms. Too little spatulation decreases strength up to 50% and will cause a grainy impression that is inaccurate in details of the mouth.
Tray movement	Movement of the tray during gelation causes distortion of the impression. It is important to hold the impression tray steady in the mouth during gelation.
Removal of impression	Premature removal of impression from the mouth creates an inaccurate impression because the material has not fully gelled. The most frequent result of premature removal is inaccuracy of the incisor teeth. The elasticity of alginate increases with time, and a better impression results from the clinician being patient. Rocking the tray back and forth to release it from the patient's mouth may cause distortion of the impression.
Improper storage of impression	The impression should be poured within 1 hour. Leaving the impression unprotected from the environment can result in imbibition or syneresis. After disinfection, maintain the integrity of the impression (if it cannot be poured with a gypsum product) by immediately wrapping it in a damp towel or storing it in a humidor. A humidor is a closed plastic container with a moist bottom layer of paper towels that creates a humid environment.

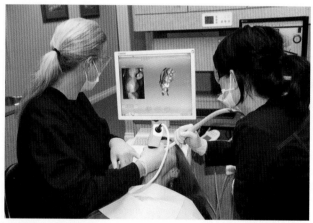

Fig. 38.3 Intraoral digital scanner used by the dental auxiliaries to obtain a digital impression. (From Rosenstiel SF, Land MF. *Contemporary Fixed Prosthodontics*. 5th ed. Elsevier; 2016.)

BOX 38.2   Mouth Areas to Precoat With Alginate

Precoat the following areas with a small amount of alginate to prevent excessive air bubbles on the tooth surfaces and to customize areas not adequately covered by the insertion of the impression tray:
- Occlusal surfaces
- Tooth surfaces adjacent to edentulous areas
- Areas of erosion, abfraction, or abrasion
- Vestibular areas
- High palatal vaults

BOX 38.3   Criteria for a High-Quality Alginate Impression

- No visible voids, tears, or debris
- Clear and distinct detail of desired structures
- All teeth and alveolar process recorded
- Retromolar pad area or maxillary tuberosity present
- Alginate material firmly attached to tray
- Adequate peripheral roll

Impression Taking

Before taking the impression, the dental hygienist explains the procedure to the patient to enhance comfort and cooperation. Specifically, education includes the following:
- That the material will feel cool and that it will gel quickly
- That breathing deeply through the nose during the procedure will help them to relax
- That they need to refrain from talking after the tray has been placed
- That if they need to communicate during the procedure, raising a hand is best

Box 38.2 lists areas to precoat with alginate. Box 38.3 lists criteria for a quality impression. Procedures 38.3 and 38.4 illustrate details for making mandibular and maxillary dental impressions, respectively.

The impression of mandibular teeth should be taken first because gagging is less likely in the mandibular area and enhances trust in the clinician for the maxillary impression (see Box 38.4 for additional suggestions to minimize gagging).

Disinfecting Impressions

Dental impressions must be disinfected before placing them in the office laboratory or sending them to a commercial laboratory as they are contaminated. Rinsing the impressions with water is an essential step in disinfection as it removes saliva, blood, and debris from the surface. Excess water is shaken from the impression and an appropriate disinfectant is used to adequately cover all surfaces of the impression. After the required disinfection time, thoroughly rinse

Equipment

Personal protective equipment

Antimicrobial rinse

Lip protectant

Occupational Safety and Health Administration (OSHA)–approved disinfectant

Alginate powder

Powder measuring scoop (provided by manufacturer)

Water dispenser (provided by manufacturer)

Wide-blade mixing spatula

Flexible rubber mixing bowl

Selected and adapted mandibular impression tray

Utility (rope) wax

Saliva ejector

Steps

Preparation

1. Gather all necessary supplies. Seat the patient upright and explain the procedure. Have patient take out any removable oral appliances.

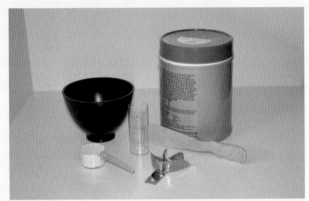

Scoop for alginate powder, water dispenser, mixing bowl, spatula, and stock impression tray.

2. Check the patient's health history to determine any risk factors that may complicate the procedure.
3. Place protective eyewear on the patient.
4. Don personal protective equipment.
5. Lubricate the patient's lips with a small amount of moisturizer.
6. Combine appropriate measures (2 or 3) of room-temperature water with appropriate scoops (2 or 3) of alginate, and mix the alginate.

Loading the Tray

7. Quickly gather half the alginate in the bowl onto the spatula. Wipe the alginate onto one side of the tray from the lingual side, working from the posterior toward the anterior. Fill to an area just below the rim. Quickly press the material down to the base of the tray.
8. Gather the remaining half of the alginate in the bowl onto the spatula and load the other side of the tray in the same way.
9. Moisten your fingers with cold water and smooth over alginate.

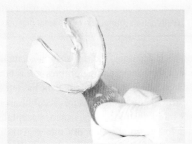

The mandibular impression tray filled with alginate and smoothed. (From Eakle WS, Bastin KG. *Dental Materials: Clinical Applications for the Dental Assistant and Dental Hygienist.* 4th ed. Elsevier; 2021.)

10. Ask the patient to swallow any saliva mouth prior to placing alginate in the mouth. (This swallowing will help to remove excessive saliva that may interfere with the detail of the occlusal anatomy.)
11. Take a small amount of impression mixture from the spatula and quickly apply to the occlusal surfaces of the teeth and undercut areas.

Seating the Tray

12. Place yourself at the 8 o'clock position (4 o'clock position if left-handed), and ask the patient to tilt the chin down, making the occlusal plane parallel to the floor.
13. Turn the impression tray sideways.
14. Retract the patient's lip and cheek with fingers of nondominant hand. Turn the tray sideways when placing it in the mouth, and distend the lip and cheek on the opposite side of the mouth with the side of the tray.
15. Center the tray over the teeth and center the handle in line with the center of the patient's chin.
16. Align the tray 2 to 3 mm anterior to the incisors. Press down the posterior portion of the tray first and then seat the anterior portion of the tray directly down by rocking the tray from posterior to anterior. This seating pattern will move the alginate from the posterior to anterior and keep the material from flowing to the back of the throat. Instruct the patient to raise the tongue toward the roof of the mouth and move it to left and right.

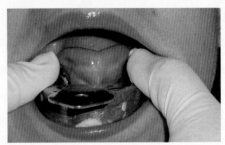

The mandibular impression tray is seated completely in the arch with the tongue lifted out of the way.

17. Instruct the patient to relax the lips and to breathe normally. If the patient struggles to stay open, they can rest their teeth on the clinician's fingers without applying biting pressure.
18. Hold the tray steady in place until the material has gelled. Apply firm bilateral pressure with the middle fingers and use the thumbs to support the jaw.

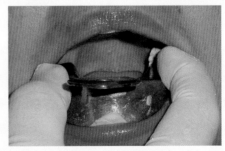

Holding the mandibular impression tray.

Removing the Impression

19. Place the fingers of nondominant hand on top of the tray. The index finger of the nondominant hand rests on the incisal surface of the maxillary anterior teeth.
20. Move the index finger of other hand along the buccal mucosa posteriorly between the impression and the peripheral tissues. The index finger is

Continued

PROCEDURE 38.3   **Making a Mandibular Preliminary Impression—cont'd**

placed under the posterior facial portion of the tray to lift the tray and break the seal between the impression and the teeth. Grasp the handle of the tray with the thumb and index finger of the dominant hand, and use a firm lifting motion. Be cautious not to apply too much force, which could hit the opposing teeth.

21. Remove the tray by turning it slightly sideways to remove it from the patient's mouth.
22. Evaluate the impression for accuracy.

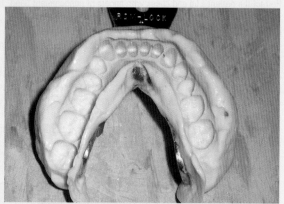

The mandibular impression. (From Eakle WS, Bastin KG. *Dental Materials, Clinical Applications for the Dental Assistant and Dental Hygienist.* 4th ed. Elsevier; 2021.)

Postimpression Care
23. Give the patient water to rinse the mouth.
24. Gently rinse debris from the impression under a stream of cold water. This is the most critical step to prepare for the disinfection process.
25. Spray the impression with an approved disinfectant within 10 to 15 minutes. Follow the manufacturer's recommended procedure.

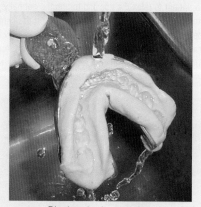

Rinsing the impression.

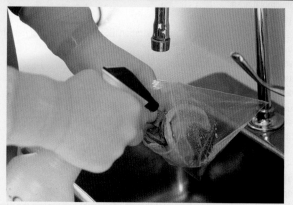

Spraying the rinsed impression with an approved disinfectant. (From Eakle WS, Bastin, KG. *Dental Materials, Clinical Applications for the Dental Assistant and Dental Hygienist.* 4th ed. Elsevier; 2021.)

26. Wrap the impression in a moist paper towel and place it in a precaution bag before pouring it up or placing it in a humidor; label with patient's name. Prepare the laboratory prescription if sending the impressions to the dental laboratory.

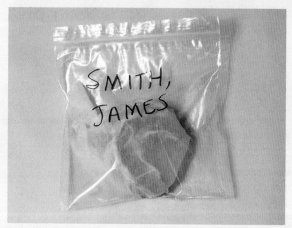

Labeled impression stored in precaution bag. (From Eakle WS, Bastin, KG. *Dental Materials, Clinical Applications for the Dental Assistant and Dental Hygienist.* 4th ed. Elsevier; 2021.)

27. Remove any remaining alginate from patient's mouth with floss, scaler, or explorer.
28. Remove any alginate from patient's face and lips with a warm cloth.
29. Return any removable oral appliances to patient.
30. Document completion of this service in the patient's electronic record under "Services Rendered." For example, "9-1-19 Alginate impression for diagnostic casts."

   Rationale: This documentation ensures the integrity of the patient's record for both the patient's health and the protection of the legal practitioner.

the impression to remove all disinfectant prior to pouring gypsum into the mold.

Bite Registration

When impressions of both dental arches are made, an accurate registration of the patient's normal centric occlusion (interocclusal record) is also needed. **Centric occlusion** is the maximal stable contact of the maxillary and mandibular arches' occluding surfaces when the jaws are closed. This can be recorded with a wax-bite registration or silicone impression materials. Silicone impression materials are superior to bite registration

materials due to their accuracy and dimensional stability. The bite registration is made at the time the initial impression is taken to articulate the models or diagnostic casts after the patient has left the office. Then trimming of the articulated models ensures accurate articulation.

When a wax-bite registration is selected, **baseplate wax** and **wax wafers** are used to record the patient's bite registration (Procedure 38.5 and the corresponding Competency Form). These waxes are pliable at room temperature. Baseplate wax comes in 1- to 2-mm-thick red or pink sheets, and wax bite wafers are horseshoe shaped, come in multiple colors, and some have foil laminated between layers to lessen

PROCEDURE 38.4 Making a Maxillary Preliminary Impression

Equipment
Personal protective equipment

Antimicrobial rinse

Lip protectant

Occupational Safety and Health Administration (OSHA)–approved disinfecting solution

Alginate powder

Powder measuring scoop (provided by manufacturer)

Water dispenser (provided by manufacturer)

Wide-blade mixing spatula*

Flexible rubber mixing bowl*

Selected and adapted maxillary impression tray

Utility (rope) wax

Saliva ejector

Steps
Preparation
1. Gather all necessary supplies. Seat and prepare the patient.
2. Measure 2 to 3 units of room-temperature water and 2 to 3 scoops of alginate, depending on size of impression tray, and mix the alginate.

Loading the Tray
3. Load the maxillary tray in one large increment by gathering all of the alginate on the spatula, and load from the posterior end of tray. Use a wiping motion to bring the material forward with the spatula, being careful to place the bulk of the material in the anterior palatal area of the tray. Fill to an area just below the edge of the tray or wax rim if added.
4. Be careful not to overfill the posterior portion of the tray that rests against the palate.
5. Moisten your fingers with water and smooth surface of the alginate.

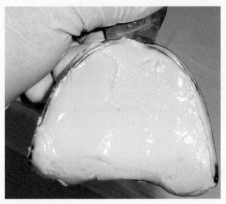

The maxillary impression tray is filled with alginate. The filled tray is smoothed on the surface.

Seating the Tray
6. Position yourself at the 11 o'clock position (1 o'clock position if left-handed), and instruct the patient to tilt head forward and chin down, making occlusal plane parallel to the floor.
7. Retract the lips and cheek with fingers of nondominant hand. With the dominant hand, turn the impression tray sideways and at the same time, distend the lip and cheek on the opposite side of the mouth with the side of the tray.
8. Center the tray over the patient's teeth, and center the handle at the midline, in line with the center of the patient's nose.
9. Seat the back of the tray against the posterior border of the hard palate to form a seal. Place the tray one-quarter inch or 6 mm anterior to incisors, and seat posterior to anterior direction.

10. Gently pull the patient lips out and move them up and over the tray as it is seated. This process aids in the flow of the alginate up into the vestibule.

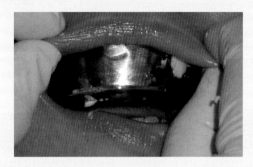

The maxillary alginate impression is placed in the arch. The maxillary lip is lifted and positioned outside the tray.

11. Place your middle fingers over the premolar areas, and hold them down over the impression tray with the index finger and the thumb.
12. Instruct the patient to breathe slowly through the nose and to form an "O" with the lips.
13. Hold the tray in place until the material has completely gelled.

Removing the Impression
14. Place an index finger under the posterior facial portion of the tray to break the seal between the impression and the teeth.
15. Place the index finger of the nondominant hand on the incisal surface of the mandibular anterior teeth.
16. Move the index finger of your other hand along the buccal mucosa posteriorly between the impression and the peripheral tissues. The index finger is placed under the rim of the tray to lift and break the seal between the impression and the teeth. Grasp the handle of the tray with the thumb and index finger of the dominant hand to lower it from the maxillary teeth.
17. Remove the tray by turning it sideways to take it out of the patient's mouth.
18. Evaluate the impression for accuracy.

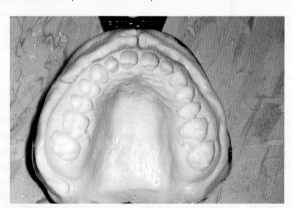

The maxillary impression. (From Eakle WS, Bastin KG. *Dental Materials, Clinical Applications for the Dental Assistant and Dental Hygienist.* 4th ed. Elsevier; 2021.)

Postimpression Care
19. Give the patient water to rinse the mouth.
20. Gently rinse debris from the impression under a stream of cold water. This is the most critical step to prepare for the disinfection process. Spray the impression with an approved disinfectant within 10 to 15 minutes. Follow the manufacturer's recommended procedure.

Continued

PROCEDURE 38.4 Making a Maxillary Preliminary Impression—cont'd

21. Wrap the impression in a moist paper towel and place it in a biohazard bag before pouring it up or in a humidor, and label with patient's name. Prepare the laboratory prescription if sending the impressions to the dental laboratory.
22. Remove any remaining alginate from patient's mouth with floss, scaler, or explorer.
23. Remove any alginate from patient's face and lips with a warm cloth.

24. Return any removable oral appliances to patient.
25. Document completion of this service in the patient's electronic record under "Services Rendered." For example, "9-1-19 Alginate impression for diagnostic casts."

    Rationale: This documentation ensures the integrity of the patient's record for both the patient's health and the protection of the legal practitioner.

---

* If the same bowl and spatula are reused from the mandibular impression, they must be thoroughly cleaned and dried to prevent contamination of the maxillary mix with the set material from the previous impression mix.

BOX 38.4 Guidelines to Minimize Gagging During Impression Taking

- The gag reflex is located on the posterior third of the tongue. It is important to keep material from flowing onto this area.
- Seat the maxillary tray from posterior to anterior to direct the flow of impression material anteriorly away from the soft palate.
- Place a wax dam on the posterior border of the maxillary tray to help contain the material.
- Avoid overfilling the tray with impression material. Fill to the level just below the wax beading of the tray rim.
- Seat the patient upright. During the insertion of the tray, instruct the patient to bend the head forward with the chin tilting down.
- Avoid using too small of a tray because the material will flow out of the confines of a tray that is too small to accommodate the needs of the arch.
- Use a calm, confident, yet gentle approach and work efficiently.
- Instruct patients to breathe slowly and deeply through the nose, to point their toes, and to pinch the skin between the index finger and the thumb.

---

distortion from the patient biting through. The most common technique used for obtaining a bite registration is to have clients close the teeth into wax softened by warm tap water.

Legal, Ethical, and Safety Issues box (Box 38.5) includes an overview of legal, ethical, and safety issues related to dental impressions.

DENTAL CAST

Once the impression has been taken, the next step is the fabrication of a dental cast. A **cast** is a three-dimensional model (positive reproduction) of the teeth and surrounding tissues of the patient's maxillary and mandibular arches created from a dental impression. The accuracy and detail of the model will be dependent on the impression material utilized and technique of the clinician. Gypsum products are used to make dental casts. A **diagnostic cast** or *study model* frequently is constructed of plaster or stone and used for treatment planning, case presentation, tracking of treatment progress, patient education, and construction of custom-made oral appliances (trays, splints, and stents). Stone that is strong enough for fabrication of indirect restorations or prostheses is desirable for constructing **working casts** or *master casts*. A **die** is a replica of a prepared tooth or teeth made from the densest of the gypsum products. Dental laboratories use these exact replicas in the construction of cast restorations (Procedure 38.6).

Gypsum Products

Gypsum is a powdered hemihydrate, which means there is one-half part water to one part of calcium sulfate. When mixed with water, the hemihydrate crystals form clusters that grow during the setting process. The interlinking of the crystals results in a stronger and harder final product. There are three types of gypsum products for pouring

casts: model plaster, dental stone, and high-strength stone. These materials consist of hemihydrate crystals that vary in size, shape, and porosity. Varying the amount of water used to mix the gypsum product determines the physical properties of the product, including strength, hardness, abrasion resistance, dimensional accuracy, reproduction of detail, and solubility. Size, shape, and porosity of the gypsum particles determine the amount of water required to mix the product. An increase in the amount of water needed to mix the product will result in a weaker final product. Working casts and dies require the most resistance to stresses and thus higher properties of strength, abrasions resistance, and accuracy.

Plaster, a beta calcium sulfate hemihydrate (plaster of Paris), has very porous crystals that are large and vary in shape. Because of its porosity, it requires the most water when mixing compared with the other types of gypsum products. It is used for pouring preliminary impressions to construct models when strength is not critical but a detailed reproduction of the mouth is required (e.g., study models).[1,2]

Dental stone, an alpha calcium sulfate hemihydrate, is stronger than plaster. Its crystals are uniform in shape and are smaller and less porous than plaster. Dental stone is used when a stronger working diagnostic cast is needed to make oral appliances, orthodontic retainers and aligners, custom trays, and provisional restorations. High-strength stone has very dense crystals and requires the least amount of water for mixing. High-strength stone has a hardness that makes it ideal to create casts and dies used in the production of crowns, bridges, and indirect restoration. Both plaster and stone are mixed by hand with a spatula or mechanically with a vacuum mixer, which eliminates trapping air into the mix.[1,2] (For a thorough explanation of the technique for pouring an impression and additional use of gypsum products, please refer to a text on dental materials.)

CUSTOM-MADE REMOVABLE ORAL APPLIANCES

A removable oral appliance is a device or tray used for various dental and medical procedures. In dentistry, custom-made oral appliances (*trays, guards, aligners, splints,* and *stents*) most frequently are placed intraorally for targeted delivery of materials, protection of oral structures, movement of misaligned teeth, and determination of implant placement.

Wearing the appliance serves the following purposes:
- The application of fluoride, desensitizing, and tooth-whitening products
- The protection of the teeth, mucosa, and bone to alleviate tooth surface wear and sports-related orofacial injuries
- Orthodontic alignment for tooth movement
- The control of obstructive sleep apnea (OSA)

Home Fluoride Trays

Construction of home fluoride trays facilitates the targeted delivery of topical fluoride for patients with high caries risk and patients

PROCEDURE 38.5   Making a Wax-Bite Registration

Equipment

Personal protective equipment

Bite registration wax (baseplate wax or wax wafer)

Wide-blade laboratory knife

Heat source (warm water, Bunsen burner, or torch)

Flexible mixing bowl will be required to hold water if selected as heat source

Air-water syringe

Occupational Safety and Health Administration (OSHA)–approved disinfectant

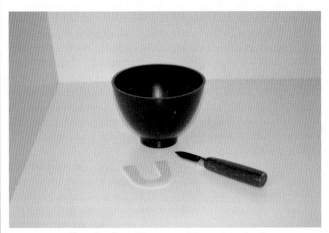

(Supplies for taking a wax-bite registration.)

Steps

Preparation

1. Gather all necessary supplies. Seat the patient upright and explain the procedure.
2. Reassure the patient that the wax will be warm, not hot.
3. Measure the length of the wax needed by placing the wax over the biting surfaces of the teeth. If the wax extends past the last tooth, use the laboratory knife to shorten its length after removing the wax from the patient's mouth.
4. Soften the bite registration wax in hot water or with another heat source (e.g., Bunsen burner or torch).

Seating

5. Place the softened warm wax over the maxillary occlusal surfaces and instruct the patient to bite together on posterior teeth gently and naturally into the wax.
6. Allow the wax bite to cool in the mouth. If necessary, air from the air-water syringe can be used to cool the wax.

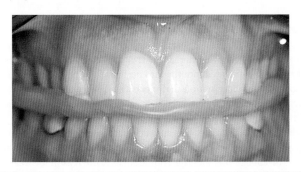

Wax-bite registration in the patient's mouth. (From Eakle WS, Bastin KG. *Dental Materials, Clinical Applications for the Dental Assistant and Dental Hygienist.* 4th ed. Elsevier; 2021.)

Removal

7. Remove the wax carefully when it has cooled by grasping the sides extending past the buccal of the teeth and gently pulling.

Post–Wax-Bite Care

8. Inspect the wax to be sure it represents the patient's bite. Chill in cold water until firm.
9. Write the patient's name on a piece of paper and keep it with the wax-bite registration.
10. Disinfect wax-bite registration with an OSHA-approved disinfectant.
11. Store the wax-bite registration with the impressions or casts until it is needed for the trimming of the casts.
12. Document completion of this service in the patient's electronic dental record under "Services Rendered." For example, "9-1-19 Bite Registration for diagnostic casts."

Rationale: This ensures the integrity of the patient's record for both the patient's health and the protection of the legal practitioner.

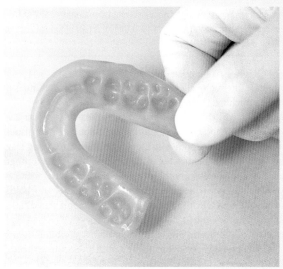

Wax-bite registration. (From Eakle WS, Bastin KG. *Dental Materials, Clinical Applications for the Dental Assistant and Dental Hygienist.* 4th ed. Elsevier; 2021.)

experiencing hypersensitivity. The design of these custom appliances maintains the fluoride solutions or desensitizing agents in close proximity to the dentition to maximize remineralization and desensitization. The tray is fabricated from an impression to fit the patient's dentition to ensure the solution covers all targeted teeth. These trays are very similar to whitening trays in their oral criteria and their construction.

Tooth-Whitening Trays

Patients often seek oral healthcare to improve their appearance. A continued focus on self-image in the media has increased the demand for cosmetic dental procedures. The smile and appearance of the teeth dominates our image-conscious society and is an important factor to meet a person's human need for a wholesome facial image.

BOX 38.5   Legal, Ethical, and Safety Issues

- In most states, dental hygienists can legally make preliminary dental impressions and, in some states, can legally make final impressions. It is the responsibility of the dental hygienist to practice within the scope authorized by state law.

- Impression trays can be a source of cross-contamination. They are semicritical instruments because they become contaminated by saliva. If the tray is disposable, it must be discarded after use or try-in. Reusable trays should be cleaned to remove any gypsum or impression materials and then sterilized for reuse. Surface areas the contaminated try comes in contact with are also considered contaminated. (See Chapter 10 for infection control recommendations.)

- The manufacturers' protocols for product uses and disinfection as well as the written handling instructions called Safety Data Sheets (SDSs) according to OSHA laws should be read and followed. SDS warnings for alginate include eye irritation, congestion, and irritation of throat, nasal passages, and upper respiratory system. Health conditions aggravated by exposure to alginate powder include the lung diseases bronchitis, emphysema, asthma, and silicosis. Long-term exposure to alginate may produce silicosis because of the crystalline silica element of the diatomaceous earth ingredient. Dustless alginate powder is now available. To prevent possible complications associated with the handling of alginate, clinicians must wear eye protection and a mask when dispensing and mixing the material.

- Study models and diagnostic casts are retained as part of the patient's permanent record.

Consequently, the removal of tooth discoloration or whitening is often the reason individuals seek oral healthcare.

Many tooth-whitening procedures require the patient to use a whitening tray. See Chapter 32 for information about dentist-dispensed home-use and in-office tooth whiteners. The tooth-whitening tray is a custom-made device constructed in the same manner as a mouthguard using an acrylic material. Tooth-whitening trays are filled with carbamide or hydrogen peroxide gels for tooth bleaching. The tray holds the whitening solution against the targeted teeth to help prevent dilution of the solution by oral fluids.

However, not all teeth will respond similarly to whitening procedures (see Chapter 32). Yellow teeth whiten the best, brown teeth less well, and gray teeth may not whiten well at all. Tetracycline stain and fluorosis may not respond to whitening; however, treatment with a combination of tooth whitening, microabrasion, and cosmetic restorative dental procedures might be options. In addition, some whitening techniques may result in tooth sensitivity, which typically subsides when the whitening is discontinued. Professionally fabricated whitening trays deliver office-supplied desensitizing products to address tooth sensitivity.

Some tooth-whitening systems on the market do not require a tray for delivery. Tooth-whitening strips are a viable option for patients who cannot tolerate trays or who wish only a small change to the color of their dentition. Procedure 38.6 describes construction of a custom-made tray.

Athletic Mouthguards

An athletic **mouthguard** is a protective appliance that covers the teeth and palate and extends to the depth of the vestibule to stabilize the mandible to absorb energy during contact sports or other recreational activities. Athletic mouthguards most commonly cover only the upper dentition, but some activities may call for protection of the lower arch as well. Mouthguards are an important preventive service provided by dental hygienists to help meet the patient's human need for protection from health risks. Dental hygienists should also discuss prevention of injuries with their patients during client education (Box 38.6).

Wearing a mouthguard serves the following purposes:

- *The protection of teeth and oral tissues*; tooth fracture, lip, tongue, or other soft tissue injury.

- The protection of the maxilla and mandible, the temporomandibular joint (TMJ), and the head and neck against intracranial pressure changes and bone deformation during contact sports.[3-4] Blows transmitted to the TMJ during athletic competition can be absorbed and distributed throughout the mouthguard while preventing contact between the maxillary and mandibular teeth is prevented.

- *A protective device to prevent or diminish the incidence of concussion.* Although the use of an athletic mouthguard is primarily for the protection of the teeth and orofacial structures, ongoing studies indicate that a properly fitted mouthguard with 3 mm or greater thickness may reduce the incidence of mild traumatic brain injury/concussion injury. **Concussion** injury is the alteration of consciousness and/or disturbance in vision and equilibrium caused by a direct blow to the head, rapid acceleration and/or deceleration of the head, or direct blow to the base of the skull from a vertical impact to the mandible.

- *The prevention of tooth avulsion.* More than 5 million teeth are avulsed yearly in the United States; the most frequent injuries occur in 8- to 15-year-olds.

- The provision of an occlusal cushion against trauma.

The ADA and five different health organizations suggest that a properly fitted mouthguard be worn while individuals participate in contact and nonimpact sports. Nonimpact sports (e.g., weightlifting) require mouth protectors due to the clenching of teeth involved in these strenuous sports (Box 38.7 includes a list of sports in which participants should wear mouth protection).[3]

Box 38.8 summarizes the types of athletic mouthguards available. The following are mouthguard guidelines:

- They should be of adequate thickness (3 mm or greater) in all areas to reduce impact forces

- They should have a snug fit that is retentive to prevent dislodging on impact

- They should extend into the vestibules and provide full dentition coverage that equals the athletic demands of the wearer

- They should be constructed with US Food and Drug Administration (FDA)–approved materials

- The recommended life of a mouthguard is limited to one season of play.

The National Collegiate Athletic Association (NCAA) and many K–12 division schools as well as community recreational sports teams mandate the use of mouthguards. The American Dental Association (ADA) Council on Scientific Affairs encourages patient education about the benefit of mouthguard use. A dental office or dental laboratory custom-fabricated mouthguard performs best; however, the use of an over-the-counter option that meets the ANSI/ADA standards may offer the patient a safe method of protection where cost is a barrier to compliance.

The dental hygienist has an important responsibility to educate the patient in the prevention of sports and recreational activity injuries. The educational message should include the reason for wearing a mouthguard, the types available, the fact that the mouthguard must be used during any sports activity, and proper cleaning and maintenance of the device (see Box 38.8).

Custom-Made Mouthguards

Dental professionals believe the most superior type of mouthguard is one custom made to the patient's mouth. The advantages of fit, ease

PROCEDURE 38.6 Constructing a Custom-Made Oral Appliance (a Single-Layer Mouthguard, Fluoride Tray, or Tooth-Whitening Tray)

Equipment

Personal protective equipment

Lip lubricant

Polyurethane mouthguard material, 4 × 4 square

Long-shank acrylic bur in a laboratory engine

Matches

Diagnostic casts

Crown and collar or iris scissors

Hanau torch

Vacuum forming machine

Laboratory knife

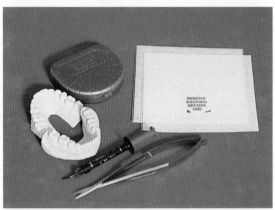

Supplies for constructing a custom-made oral appliance. (From Eakle WS, Bastin, KG. *Dental Materials, Clinical Applications for the Dental Assistant and Dental Hygienist*. 4th ed. Elsevier; 2021.)

Steps

1. Don personal protective equipment.
2. Trim the diagnostic cast according to the appliance being fabricated. For a whitening and fluoride tray, the case should be trimmed where the base extends 3 to 4 mm past the gingival border and the vertical height is minimal. For a mouthguard, the cast should maintain the area of the vestibules and palate. A hole can be cut into the palate to allow air exchange on the vacuum former. Spray the cast with silicone lubricant.

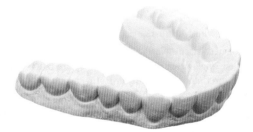

Trimmed cast. (From Eakle WS, Bastin KG. *Dental Materials, Clinical Applications for the Dental Assistant and Dental Hygienist*. 4th ed. Elsevier; 2021.)

3. Place the vacuum-forming machine under a hood fan for control of organic emissions.
4. Prepare the machine. The perforated vacuum plate and the sides of the hinged frame should be lightly sprayed with silicone lubricant.
5. Open the hinged frame and center the polyurethane tray material onto the lower frame.

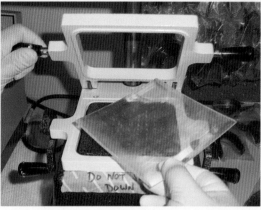

Open the hinge and place the material.

6. Close the frame and secure the frame with the latch knob.
7. Grasp both handles of the locked hinged frame and lift it until it clicks into position, approximately 3 inches above the vacuum plate. Some machines require a turning of the knob on the right to lock the hinged frame in place.
8. Swing the heating unit to the center position and turn on the heating element switch at the base of the unit.
9. Center cast on the vacuum plate. Some units have extra holes at the front and back of the machine; place the cast between these holes.
10. Do not leave the machine unattended. Watch the material as it heats for 1 to 2 minutes until it sags one-half inch below the hinged frame.

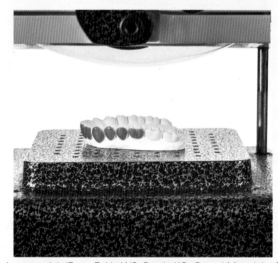

Sagging material. (From Eakle WS, Bastin KG. *Dental Materials, Clinical Applications for the Dental Assistant and Dental Hygienist*. 4th ed. Elsevier; 2021.)

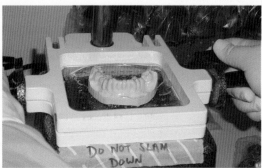

Hinged frame pulled over vacuum plate.

Continued

PROCEDURE 38.6   Constructing a Custom-Made Oral Appliance (a Single-Layer Mouthguard, Fluoride Tray, or Tooth-Whitening Tray)—cont'd

11. Swing the heating unit out of the way and turn the switch off. The heating element can be left in the front position in instances when the clinician is in a hurry to seat the tray material; however, this provides an opportunity for injury.
12. Turn on the vacuum motor.
13. Grasp both handles of the hinged frame and pull it down over the vacuum plate. The material will be draped over the cast.
14. Allow the vacuum to pull the tray material around the cast for approximately 10 seconds.
15. Turn off the vacuum switch.
16. Release the hinged frame knob and open the frame and hold by the edges to remove it from the vacuum plate.
17. Hold the splint and cast under running, cold water for at least 30 seconds or allow the cast and tray material to cool on the vacuum former platform.
18. Cut excess material just below the depth of the periphery to remove it from the cast.
19. Use small, sharp crown and collar scissors or iris scissors to trim approximately 0.5 mm away from the gingival margin. Scallop the tray at the gingival margin on the facials for whitening or fluoride trays. Mouthguard material should go to the height of the mucobuccal fold, no scalloping necessary.

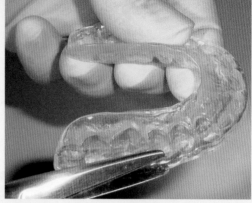
Trimming material away from the gingival margin.

20. Wearing a mask and safety goggles, trim the mouthguard with an acrylic bur in a laboratory engine. The margin of the tray should be rounded and smoothed out.
21. Use a low flame to gently readapt the margins and remove any excess flash from trimming.

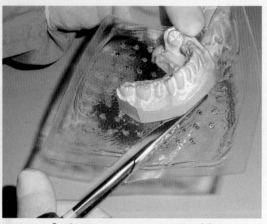
Cutting away gross excess material.

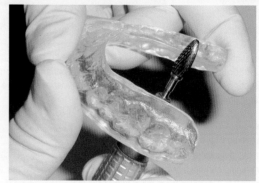
Trimming mouthguard material with an acrylic bur.

---

of speech, comfort, retention, minimal interference with breathing, and protection from concussion by a blow to the jaw make this type of appliance superior to patient-fabricated mouthguards.

Single-Layer Mouthguards

Vacuum-formed thermoplastic polymers are useful to make mouthguards called *single-layer mouthguards*. They are fabricated from one sheet of polyurethane or soft ethylene vinyl acetate (EVA) acrylic, are custom fitted, allow for breathing and speech, and do not deform over time or with use. Heating of the EVA plastic sheet allows pliability for suctioning by a vacuum former machine over a stone model (positive reproduction) of the patient's dentition. These vacuum-formed mouthguards, custom fabricated by dental staff or laboratory technicians, are superior to the store-bought stock or boil-and-bite mouthguards. Although the store-bought and boil-and-bite mouthguards provide protection, they are not adequate for full-contact sports such as football, wrestling, or boxing (see Procedure 38.6).

Multiple-Layer Mouthguards (Pressure Laminated)

Multiple-layer mouthguards made of EVA are recommended for full-contact sports. Two or three fused layers of EVA material are heated and pressure-laminated over a stone model (positive reproduction) of the patient's dentition to achieve the necessary thickness. At a minimum,

---

BOX 38.7 Sports Dentistry Facts

Facts From the American Academy of Pediatric Dentistry (AAPD)

- Dental injuries are the most common type of preventable orofacial injury sustained during participation in contact sports. About 32% of injuries in children occurred during sports activities.
- Sports injuries result in an annual estimated cost of $500 million. Sports injuries also result in 20 million lost days of school. Athletes were 60 times more likely to suffer harm to teeth not wearing a mouth guard.
- 67% of parents admit their child does not wear a mouthguard during organized sports.

Facts From the American Dental Association

- A properly fitted mouthguard may reduce the chances of sustaining a concussion from a blow to the jaw.
- Mouthguards should be worn at all times during practice, games, and competition.
- Non–mouthguard users have twice the risk of orofacial injury. Prevalence of dental trauma among non–mouthguard users is between 48% to 59%, with coronal fracture and tooth avulsion being the most frequent injuries.
- Contact your local dental society and association for information on dentists and mouthguard programs in your area.

BOX 38.9 Results of Bruxism and Clenching

- Abfraction lesions
- Exostosis to support the teeth
- Gingival recession
- Gingival clefting
- Headaches
- Impaired hearing
- Limited range of motion of mandible
- Excessive linea alba and/or tongue crenation
- Temporomandibular joint (TMJ) pain
- Periodontal pockets
- Tenderness of the muscles of mastication
- Tinnitus
- TMJ disorders
- TMJ noise with movement
- Tooth fracture
- Tooth mobility
- Tooth sensitivity
- Tooth wear facets (attrition)

BOX 38.8 Types of Athletic Mouthguards Available

Stock Type
"One size fits all," purchased over the counter, inexpensive, offers the least protection

Boil and Bite
Formed by heating the material, purchased over the counter, inexpensive, offers little protection

Custom Vacuum-Formed Single-Layer Mouthguard
Fabricated in the dental office or dental laboratory using a preliminary cast of the patient's dentition, custom fit, moderately expensive, provides moderate protection; not recommended for contact sports

Pressure-Laminated Multiple-Layer Mouthguard
Fabricated in the dental laboratory using a preliminary cast of the patient's dentition, custom fit, expensive, provides the best protection

---

mouthguards should have a labial thickness of 3 mm, palatal thickness of 2 mm, and occlusal thickness of 3–4 mm. Most over-the-counter athletic mouthguards have an average thickness of 1.65 mm, providing little occlusal protection. In addition, many of the boil-and-bite mouthguards are cut off at the posterior by the patient, preventing proper posterior occlusal coverage.

Parafunctional Occlusal Forces

Parafunctional occlusal forces result when there is tooth-to-tooth contact made when the patient is not in the act of mastication. This is not an activity related to normal function and has a reported prevalence of 8% to 31% in the general population. **Clenching** is the continuous or intermittent forceful closure of the maxillary teeth against the mandibular teeth. **Bruxism** is the forceful grinding of the teeth. Bruxism and clenching are often subconscious habits that usually occur during sleep. Clenching often occurs during nonsleeping hours. Patients frequently

have no conscious knowledge of their parafunctional habits or the detrimental effect on their dentition. Studies indicate that a growing percentage of the adult population experiences nocturnal teeth grinding. Occlusion discrepancy between centric occlusion and centric relation is thought to be one cause of nocturnal bruxism and clenching. Stress is a major contributing factor in both parafunctional habits and may increase the frequency and intensity of either. Central nervous system disorders such as Parkinson disease and Huntington disease can contribute to nocturnal bruxism. Many individuals experience clenching and bruxism, but the degree of either determines the sequelae. Box 38.9 lists the possible sequelae of bruxism and clenching. Severe bruxism may result in loss of vertical dimension of occlusion. This bite collapse can result in painful temporomandibular joint dysfunction (TMD) and changes to facial appearance.

The dental hygienist has responsibility to evaluate the dentition and record evidence of occlusal stresses. Intraoral assessment includes examination of the teeth for the presence of wear on the teeth; craze lines and wear facets are an indication of current or past grinding patterns. Patients may also report tooth sensitivity, waking with their teeth clamped together, and/or fatigue of facial muscles upon waking. These symptoms may be a result of clenching, grinding, or both.

Treatment of Parafunctional Occlusal Forces

Treatment for parafunctional occlusal forces may be both reversible and irreversible. Reversible treatment is conservative, noninvasive, and causes no permanent changes in the structure or position of the jaw or teeth. Most therapies attempt reversible interventions, but treatment needs may progress to irreversible procedures. Irreversible treatment is invasive and causes permanent changes in the structure or position of the jaw or teeth.

Reversible procedures. **Appliance therapy** is the use of removable oral appliances in a variety of situations. Dental appliances such as nightguards or day guards treat bruxism and clenching. Although wearing of an oral appliance will not prevent clenching or bruxing, evidence suggests that wearing a nightguard during sleep will decrease damage to the teeth and relax strained muscles which result from bruxing and clenching habits.

Irreversible procedures. Orthodontics may be recommended to properly align teeth when malocclusion is noted. In cases of severe malocclusion, orthognathic surgery may be necessary. Equilibration therapy (occlusal adjustment) is used to adjust the occlusion of the teeth by recontouring occlusal enamel and existing restorations with dental burs. This adjustment permanently removes the occlusal discrepancy, thereby removing the occlusal stresses from the teeth. In some cases, reduction of the tooth structure is not ideal and the placement of full-coverage restorations may be necessary for permanent change in the vertical relationship between the teeth to eliminate damaging occlusal contact.

Nightguards and Day Guards—Occlusal Guards

A **nightguard** or **day guard** may be made of soft or hard materials that fit over the maxillary or mandibular dentition to protect the teeth by absorbing the forces of parafunctional habits. The appliance is most frequently worn during sleep; however, some patients identify clenching patterns during the day and are advised to wear the appliance during waking hours when they feel themselves clenching. The purpose of these appliances is the following:

- Absorb the forces of clenching or grinding
- Minimize loss of tooth structure (attrition)
- Ease muscle hyperactivity
- Reduce pressure on the TMJ
  There are several nightguard and day guard designs.
- A single-layer athletic mouthguard may be used as an inexpensive nightguard or day guard to temporarily change the neuromuscular behavior and produce muscle relaxation in mild clenching and bruxism. This appliance usually lasts less than 1 year. However, the occlusion cannot be adjusted, and the mouthguard can actually encourage an increase in these parafunctional habits.
- Full occlusal coverage nightguards or day guards are fabricated in hard acrylic to cover the occlusal surfaces. These small, low-profile nightguards or day guards are fabricated and adjusted by a dentist. The appliance fully covers either the maxillary or the mandibular teeth and is adjusted appropriately to the patient's occlusion. The life span for full occlusal coverage nightguards and day guards varies from 3 to 10 years.
- A new type of guard is the dual-laminated nightguard. It combines two layers of material with a soft inside and hard acrylic outside. The soft material is comfortable against the teeth, and the hard outside acts as a protective shell against the patient's parafunctional habits. Patient feedback is very promising for this type of device.

Contributing factors to the development of periodontal diseases include those risk factors that cause direct damage to the periodontium from occlusal forces as well as those that increase plaque biofilm retention. Dental hygienists identify risk factors and include education and options for treatment in the care plan. The fabrication of nightguards and day guards usually requires two appointments. At the first appointment, the clinician makes accurate alginate impressions. The alginate impressions are poured in class I dental stone to create diagnostic casts. A centric relation bite registration is made to enable placement of the casts on an anatomic articulator that simulates tooth occlusion and TMJ positioning. Then the dental laboratory uses the articulated models for fabrication of the appliance by a dental technician.

Sleep Guards for Sleeping Disorders

Sleep disorders comprise a growing group of medical conditions that are more common in the general population than previously known. Snoring and OSA are two sleep disorders that the patient may wish to discuss with the dental hygienist. Mild to moderate forms of snoring

and OSA may successfully be treated intraorally with an oral splint, known as a **snore guard**, to be worn at night. A well-designed hard acrylic resin snore guard fits over the maxillary dentition to reposition the mandible. The appliance works by advancing the mandible anteriorly to prevent the tongue from obstructing the oropharynx and stabilizes the mandible in this forward position during sleep. Considerable evidence exists to suggest that OSA, bruxism, chronic pain, and TMD are linked.

Orthodontic Aligners

Many children and adults seek orthodontic treatment to realign or straighten their teeth for cosmetic and malocclusion purposes. The evaluation of the patient's occlusion is a component of the assessment phase of the dental hygiene process of care. Properly aligned teeth and proper occlusion are beneficial to the patient's overall periodontal health. The malpositioned dentition is destructive to the teeth, periodontium, TMJ, and surrounding muscles. Tooth malposition often compromises the patient's ability to maintain the cleanliness of the oral cavity and the health of the dentition. Correcting these malocclusions is important to prevent and minimize the tissue injury associated with trauma from occlusion. The movement of teeth that have drifted can provide improved adjacent tooth position before tooth replacement with an implant or other appliance.

A new approach to the traditional band, bracket, and archwire type of orthodontic movement uses clear aligners to straighten the teeth. The clear, soft plastic aligners are provided to the patient as a series of custom-made trays that gradually and gently shift the teeth into place using planned movements by the dentist. The brackets or archwires are no longer used, resulting in the elimination of the need to make adjustments. The patient inserts a new set of aligners approximately every 1 to 2 weeks, advancing them to the next stage of treatment, until the treatment is complete. Patients wear aligners for 20 to 22 hours per day and remove them for eating and homecare. The aligners apply the right amount of force at the right time to move the teeth horizontally and vertically and rotate them as needed.

As the treatment with the clear aligners progresses, tooth movement is regularly monitored by the dentist and the next series of aligners is delivered. The treatment typically takes approximately 12 to 18 months for adults and is comparable in time to that of traditional bonded orthodontic appliances for teens. This system is not recommended for severe crowding or spacing or when patient compliance is a concern. It is best suited for adults and responsible teens.

Because the aligners are removed for homecare, the patient is able to brush and floss normally for better periodontal health. The smooth plastic aligner eliminates the gingival irritation often caused by sharp metal or plastic brackets and archwires. Orthodontic aligners may be an acceptable orthodontic treatment for adults who are seeking an invisible method to align their teeth and who feel traditional orthodontic treatment is too embarrassing or disruptive.

ORAL SURGICAL SPLINTS AND STENTS

Periodontal Splints

Periodontal splints are used to stabilize mobile teeth to prolong their presence in the mouth. Periodontal splinting of teeth joins adjacent teeth to convert them into a single unit that can withstand occlusal forces better than an individual tooth.

Surgical Splints

Surgical splints are orthopedic devices used to cover the graft donor site for protection after the harvesting of tissue for periodontal soft-tissue graft surgery.

Oral Surgical Stents

Oral surgical stents provide communication between the surgeon and restoring dentist to facilitate placement of an implant at the ideal position and angulation for the prosthetic.

CUSTOM-MADE ORAL APPLIANCES AND DENTAL HYGIENE TREATMENT PLANNING

Through a thorough clinical assessment, the dental hygienist identifies conditions requiring a custom-made oral appliance and addresses them in the care plan. The clinician is able to recommend the appropriate treatment options or refer the patient for a consultation. See the Critical Thinking Exercises box for critical thinking activities related to custom-made oral appliances.

CRITICAL THINKING EXERCISES RELATED TO CUSTOM-MADE ORAL APPLIANCES

1. Apply knowledge of various types of custom oral appliances to the following conditions to select and provide a rationale for the appliance of choice:
   a. Desire for whiter teeth
   b. Malpositioned teeth not requiring orthodontics
   c. Playing contact sports
   d. Bruxism or clenching
   e. High caries risk
2. Review the factors that affect alginate impression materials. Manipulate alginate material in the lab by purposefully varying the factors in your procedure. What is the outcome?
3. Visit your local pharmacy and athletic store. Review the types of athletic mouth protectors available over the counter. How would you educate your patient about these products in comparison to a custom-made mouthguard?
4. Interview a coach who works with high school athletes about the school's guidelines for wearing a mouthguard for each sport sponsored by the school. How are the athletes educated about the importance of wearing a mouthguard for protection of their teeth and possibly against symptoms of concussion?
5. Joseph is a healthy 27-year-old male who works in an urban setting as an attorney. He reports grinding his teeth while sleeping. Your exam revealed generalized attrition, with craze lines on the teeth. To prevent any further tooth damage, you provided client education regarding tooth attrition, tooth fracture, and tooth loss.
   a. What would you say to this patient about these conditions, his bruxism, and options for treatment?
   b. During your discussion, the client informed you that he is a "gagger." How would you factor this information as well as your clinical findings into your dental hygiene care plan? Write a care plan for Joseph, including dental hygiene diagnosis, client goals, interventions, and methods of evaluation.

BOX 38.10 Removable Oral Appliance Patient Care Instructions

- Remove the appliance and brush with a soft toothbrush and liquid soap or a nonabrasive toothpaste designed to be safe for the material.
- Soaking solutions should only be used with hard acrylic types of appliances.
- Store the appliance when not in use in a well-ventilated plastic container. A sealed container will promote mold growth. Be sure to keep appliance in a safe place away from children or pets.
- Wash the storage container weekly with soap and water.
- Store the appliance in a room-temperature area; heat may distort a soft appliance.
- Do not purposely chew on the appliance; this habit will likely distort the appliance and will adversely affect its fit.
- Evaluate the appliance for signs of wear. Replace it when you see holes or tears, or when the appliance does not fit or is not able to be retained in the mouth.

After identifying the damages resulting from parafunctional occlusal forces, the clinician will be able to recommend a custom-made oral appliance appropriate to mediate the excessive forces to the teeth and the periodontium. Malpositioned teeth increase plaque biofilm retention and can contribute to periodontal and dental deterioration. The correction of this malpositioning with the appropriate appliance will greatly improve the patient's ability to maintain their dentition and periodontal health.

MAINTENANCE OF A REMOVABLE ORAL APPLIANCE

The dental hygienist is most frequently responsible for the education of the patient in proper care of the removable oral appliance. The patient cleans these appliances minimally once daily with a soft or extra-soft bristled toothbrush and water or a cleaner approved for removable appliances. Evidence suggests that toothpaste is too abrasive for use on removable appliances, causing microscopic scratches that provide an environment for increased bacterial growth. Soaking solutions for hard acrylic oral appliances are also available and are recommended for periodic use. Box 38.10 gives instructions for patient care of their oral appliance. It is important to educate patients on proper appliance care and to assess functionality of the appliance at each subsequent assessment appointment. The clinician may instruct patients to bring the appliance with them to continuing appointments for evaluation of the integrity of the appliance.

KEY CONCEPTS

- A dental impression is used to create an accurate three-dimensional positive reproduction of the teeth and surrounding tissues called a *diagnostic cast, study model,* or *study cast.*
- There are three main types of dental impressions used in dentistry: a preliminary impression, a final impression, and a bite registration.
- Loading and inserting the impression tray should take no more than 1 minute. The objective is for the impression material to reach the gel state in the patient's mouth.
- Impression trays are seated in a posterior to anterior direction to avoid triggering the gag reflex, prevent the excess material from going toward the back of the mouth, and move the impression material forward, ensuring complete coverage of the oral structures with alginate.
- Stone casts and plaster models are made of gypsum products; stone casts are stronger than plaster models.
- Safety precautions must be used when handling alginate and gypsum materials.
- Baseplate wax and wax wafers are used for the bite registration procedures (interocclusal record).
- Dental hygienists recommend and construct mouthguards for patients at risk for sports-related dentofacial injury. Properly fitted professionally manufactured mouthguards reduce tooth avulsion, facial bone fractures, temporomandibular joint (TMJ) injuries, and concussions.
- Signs and symptoms of bruxism and clenching may include craze lines, abfraction lesions, exostosis, gingival recession, headaches, TMJ noise with movement, limited range of motion of jaw, excessive linea alba and tongue crenation, tenderness of muscles of mastication, tinnitus, TMJ disorders, tooth fracture, tooth mobility, tooth sensitivity, and attrition.
- Bruxism and clenching is treated with reversible and irreversible therapies. Reversible therapies include biofeedback, drug therapy, oral appliances, physical therapy, and heat and cold therapy. Irreversible therapies include occlusal equilibration, orthodontic therapy, and orthognathic surgery.
- Sleep disorders are treated in the dental practice using a snoreguard. A snoreguard reduces snoring by repositioning the mandible and tongue. Snoreguards may treat some cases of mild to moderate obstructive sleep apnea by repositioning the mandible and tongue.
- Dental hygienists are responsible for educating patients about indications for oral appliances. Maintenance of the appliance is also important to teach patients who wear them.

ACKNOWLEDGMENT

The author acknowledges Carol Dixon Hatrick for past contributions to this chapter.

REFERENCES

1. Eakle WS, Bastin KG. *Dental Materials Clinical Applications for Dental Assistant and Dental Hygienists.* 4th ed. Elsevier; 2021.

2. Sakaguchi R, Ferracane J, Powers J. *Craig's Restorative Dental Materials.* 14th ed. Elsevier; 2019.

3. American Academy of Pediatric Dentistry. *Policy on Prevention of Sports-Related Orofacial Injuries. The Reference Manual of Pediatric Dentistry.* American Academy of Pediatric Dentistry; 2021:110–115.

4. American Dental Association Online. Available at: https://www.ada.org/resources/research/science-and-research-institute/oral-health-topics/athletic-mouth-protectors-mouthguards. Accessed July 2022.

39

Restorative Therapy

Ann Mora and Sheila Kensmoe Norton

PROFESSIONAL OPPORTUNITIES

Restorative dentistry is an interesting and exciting component of clinical practice for dental hygienists where deemed legal within the dental hygiene scope of practice. Dental hygienists can restore teeth using direct restorative methods for placement of amalgam and composite restorations. The goal of this chapter is to provide an overview of the process and procedures for general restorative dentistry. Even without the legal ability to perform restorative procedures, there is value for all dental hygienists in having a working knowledge and understanding of these processes to relay treatment options and restorative care information to their patients.

COMPETENCIES

1. Discuss the variety of educational requirements that can provide pathways for licensure for dental hygienists and other dental personnel to practice restorative dentistry. In addition, describe the collaborative role of the dental hygienist in restorative dentistry.
2. Detail the rationale for restorative therapy.
3. Describe both direct and indirect restorations, and list the principles of cavity classification and preparation.
4. Discuss the rationale, moisture control, accessibility, visibility, disadvantages, and contraindications of dental isolation.
5. Describe how restorative material type, location of restoration, and the presence of a proximal contact impact appropriate decision making with regards to matrix system choice.
6. Describe bonding agents, bases, liners, and cavity sealers.
7. Compare and contrast the differences between amalgam and composite materials and techniques, including preparation design, matrix systems, armamentarium differences, and finishing techniques.
8. Describe intermediary crowns, gingival retractions, temporary or interim restorations, and luting agents.
9. Discuss why the restorative care cycle demands ongoing assessment, evaluation, documentation, and continued care.

RESTORATIVE THERAPY PROVIDERS

Each state's or province's laws, rules, and regulations dictate the legal services that a dental hygienist can provide, the level of supervision required, and the settings in which these services can be delivered. Restorative therapy legally requires diagnosis and treatment planning by a licensed dentist.[1]

A variety of educational requirements provide pathways that can lead to licensure for dental hygienists and other dental personnel to practice restorative dentistry. These extended care provider roles were created as a meaningful solution to the problem of dental access for underserved communities by providing care for diverse populations.

Restorative Function Endorsement (RFE) Dental Hygienists and Expanded Functions Dental Auxiliaries (EFDAs) can provide restorative treatment limited to the placement and finishing of amalgam and composite restorations following cavity preparation and treatment planning by a dentist. Alaska was the first state in the United States to use the **Dental Hygiene Therapist (DHT)** and **Dental Health Aid Therapist (DHAT)**. Minnesota was the first state to create an **Advanced Dental Therapist** with dual licensure for dental hygienists as dental therapists. These oral healthcare providers are considered **midlevel dental providers** or **midlevel oral health practitioners** because they provide more extensive dental hygiene and dental care to include cavity preparations, removal of decay, placement of direct restorations, and simple extractions under the supervision of a consulting dentist. Several states have provisions for dental hygienists to provide restorative care with special permits in addition to their license to practice dental hygiene. The title of these permits varies—for example, extended access dental hygiene restorative endorsement, expanded functions permit, restorative endorsement, and extended care permit.

The number of states passing legislation to allow various dental personnel to perform restorative treatment is changing each year, highlighting the importance of continued advocacy in favor of increasing access to oral healthcare, promoting diversity in the workforce, and expanding opportunities for professional growth. Washington State is unique as it is the only state that requires competence in restorative procedures for *initial* licensure as a dental hygienist. Consultation with your state or provincial licensing agency is recommended.[2]

State by state, dental hygienists, usually with special permits, are permitted to perform a broad range of restorative therapies that include but are not limited to the following:
- Placement and removal of dental dams and alternative isolation
- Placement and removal of matrices and wedges
- Placement of cavity bases, liners, and sealers
- Placement and finishing of direct restorations to include amalgam, composite, and glass ionomer and compomer materials
- Placement and cementation of stainless steel crowns
- Placement and removal of retraction cord
- Fabrication, placement, cementation, and removal of temporary restorations

Dental hygienists in all states and practice settings provide educational information about restorative therapies. Therefore it is important for dental hygienists to understand the rationale and goals of restorative therapy, the types of restorations, maintenance of restorative dental materials, and the procedures involved in the restorative process.

RATIONALE FOR RESTORATIVE THERAPY

When a patient's need for a biologically sound and functional dentition is lacking, the optimal course of action would be to intervene and restore the dentition to a state of health, support the maintenance of health and function, and provide esthetic modification. Restorative therapy includes the restoration of damaged tooth structure, defective restorations, esthetic modifications, and anatomic and physiologic abnormalities. In many cases, restorative therapy prevents tooth loss by halting disease progression. It is used in conjunction with antimicrobial therapy and dietary counseling to eliminate the bacterial infection that causes dental caries. Common caries prevention therapies include application of fluoride, silver diamine fluoride, amorphous calcium phosphate, and sealants. Xylitol products and salivary aids can also be prescribed as an adjunctive home care regimen. Restorations replace and reestablish proper embrasure spaces and contact position. This in turn prevents food impaction, tissue irritation, and destabilization of the teeth. Because of all these benefits, restorative care improves our patients' oral health and quality of life.

Defective Restorations

Defective restorations no longer restore the dentition to an acceptable state of form and function. Although restorations can be either temporary or permanent, no restoration can be considered truly permanent due to the extreme oral cavity conditions. Patient responsibilities of oral hygiene care and dietary factors contribute to the need for repair and replacement of restorations if self-care practices need improvement or when high caries risk is present. Physical properties of restorative materials make them susceptible to alteration and deterioration. Certain materials, however, have withstood the test of time and are recognized more readily for their longevity. Gold restorations are within the dentist's scope of practice and when used properly, they are durable and compatible in the oral environment. Their resistance to corrosion, nonirritating chemistry, similarity to enamel in texture, modulus of elasticity, and wear resistance are qualities that other materials often lack. Amalgam remains the longest-lasting restorative material and it is still commonly used as a restorative material in dentistry because of its cost effectiveness, versatility, workability, and clinical longevity (Fig. 39.1A). However, expansion over time, masticatory forces, and tooth-to-tooth contact eventually can cause wear and breakdown of amalgam restorations (Fig. 39.1B). Due to their ability to match tooth colors, composite restorations are a popular choice for esthetics; however, over time, they have a greater rate of recurrent decay. Placement of composite restorations is significantly more technique sensitive compared with amalgam restorations. Although isolation would be best practice for all restorations, composite restorations are negatively affected by blood, saliva, and moisture. Material costs and extended time due to additional steps required during placement result in higher costs. Some types can shrink during the curing process, therefore requiring meticulous technique in the bonding and placement phases to obtain desired long-lasting results. Recurrent caries of crown and bridge restorations may be related to inadequately sealed margins or the use of antiquated cements that have been found to dissolve in the oral environment, leading to the need for replacement or repair.

Defective restorations, however, may not always be related to the restorative material. Defective restorations also can be caused by iatrogenic means. **Iatrogenic** is defined as caused by the practitioner. Placement techniques of the clinician can result in overhangs, open margins, poor contours, and open proximal contacts. These are the result of improper placement technique, poor judgment, and lack of attention to detail (Figs. 39.2 and 39.3). Iatrogenic restoration defects are avoidable; thus they do not meet the requirements for the standard of care. (See Box 39.1.)

Esthetic Appearance

Restorative therapy is an important factor in meeting a patient's need for a satisfactory esthetic result. Missing, broken, or obviously decayed

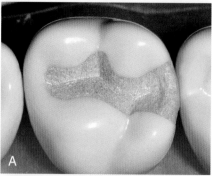
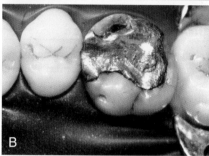

Fig. 39.1 (A) A quality amalgam restoration has proven longevity. (B) This older amalgam restoration exhibits marginal breakdown.

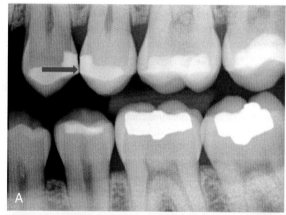
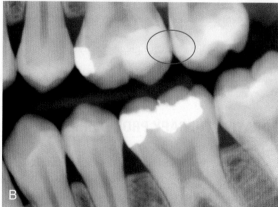

Fig. 39.2 Proper formation of interproximal anatomy is influenced by the clinician's placement technique. (A) Note the *arrow* indicating malformed embrasure spaces, contact, and poor interproximal contours often caused by using an improper matrix system. (B) Note the *circle* indicating the proper replication of embrasure spaces, contact, and interproximal contours.

teeth are often the reasons individuals seek dental treatment. Dental anomalies such as diastemas, mottled enamel, congenital tooth defects, and intrinsic tooth discolorations such as tetracycline staining may require restorative treatment to improve appearance (Fig. 39.4). One main disadvantage of metallic restorations has been esthetics. When appropriate, the dentist and patient may opt for nonmetallic restorations, such as composite, glass ionomer, porcelain, or ceramic due to their appearance of natural dentition.

Occlusion

The occlusal relationship influences the function and health of the dentition. Restorative treatment can improve a patient's occlusion. Occlusal adjustment, the selective reduction of enamel, may be indicated to improve occlusion. The occlusal adjustment procedure is performed by a dentist who has in-depth knowledge of occlusion. Adjustment may be necessary when previous restorations have been completed with poor contour. When teeth become misaligned because of the loss of adjacent or opposing teeth, it may be necessary to replace or recontour them. Either process would establish a stable, functional occlusion by

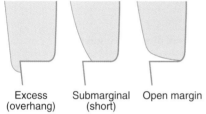

Excess   Submarginal   Open margin
(overhang)   (short)

Fig. 39.3 Note possible defects at the gingival margins of restorations. It may be possible to remove an overhang without replacing the restoration; however, restorations with short and open margins require replacement.

BOX 39.1 Critical Thinking Scenario A

Ethics
After you have completed the amalgam restoration on tooth #30-MO, the marginal ridge chipped when the occlusion was being checked. The fracture has left a slight open contact that can lead to food impaction and tissue irritation as well as loss of confidence by the patient. What procedure is needed to correct this problem? What should you tell the patient? If your schedule does not permit redoing the restoration that day, what should you do?

---

realigning the occlusal forces to be more parallel to the long axis of the teeth (Fig. 39.5). Crown and bridge restorative work may be necessary to restore occlusion in dentitions with extensive damage that cannot be treated with occlusal adjustment.

Mastication

The most basic function of teeth is to chew food, which begins the process of digestion. Patients with compromised dentition may identify difficulty chewing as a chief concern. Quality of life may be affected when missing teeth, defective restorations, or carious lesions compromise an individual's ability to process food, thereby affecting their nutrition.

COLLABORATIVE ROLE OF THE DENTAL HYGIENIST

During the assessment phase of dental hygiene care, tooth damage and its causes may be identified and communicated to the dentist. In addition, based on assessment of the patient's oral hygiene status and oral health behaviors, the dental hygienist plans, implements, and evaluates oral disease prevention and health promotion strategies for the patient (Chapters 22 and 23). These strategies may then be communicated to the dentist to aid in the decision-making process regarding selection of restorative materials and procedures that most benefit the patient's needs and desires.

Delivery of Restorative Therapies by Expanded Functions Dental Hygienist

Originally, the dental hygienist was chiefly responsible for the prevention of oral disease. This origin explains why today the dental hygienist is recognized as an oral disease preventive and health promotion specialist.

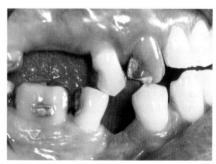

Fig. 39.5 Tooth loss has resulted in pathologic occlusion from tooth movement (tip, drift, and extrusion).

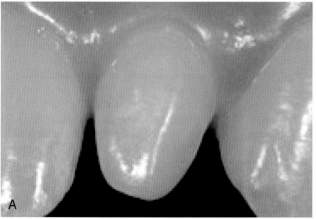
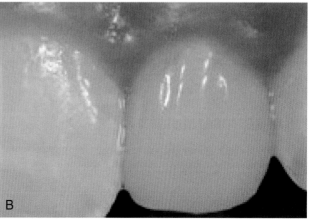

Fig. 39.4 Peg laterals are a common dental anomaly. (A) Pretreatment. (B) Posttreatment of tooth No. 10 with a direct composite and Bioclear matrix system. (Courtesy of Bioclear by David Clark, Tacoma, WA.)

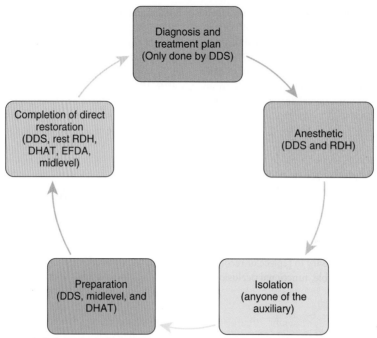

Fig. 39.6 Collaborative roles of dental personnel in placement of direct restorations.

However, in the 1960s and 1970s, the dental hygienist's role began to encompass the delivery of nonsurgical periodontal therapy, pain and anxiety control, and restorative therapies. Washington was the first state to legislate educational requirements to include restorative and local anesthetic delivery in the dental hygienist's education in 1971. The primary focus of the dental profession became improving the oral health of the public through the elimination and treatment of dental caries. Therefore the rationale for the initial delegation of restorative services was to provide a mechanism to respond to an expanding need and demand for dental care, broadening dental hygienists' role and responsibilities. More recently, the scope of dental hygiene practice has been expanded to improve access to oral healthcare for underserved populations.

Participation of the RFE dental hygienist (RFEDH) in the delivery of restorative therapy affords a unique collaborative opportunity for the dentist and RFEDH in oral healthcare delivery. The efficient use of the dentist, dental hygienist, RFEDH, EFDA, and dental assistant allows all members of the team to contribute their expertise, which ensures high-quality, cost-effective restorative treatment. Fig. 39.6 illustrates the collaborative integration of the roles of the dentist and dental auxiliaries throughout the delivery of restorative care.

Educational programs prepare hygienists to practice according to their state, province, or territorial laws, which can vary dramatically throughout a country. Hygienists seeking licensure in other states may be required to take an intensive continuing education course and additional board exam to obtain restorative function endorsement or initial licensure. Dental hygienists have the legal and ethical responsibility to always know and practice within the scope of the law.

TYPES OF RESTORATIONS

Restorations are categorized by the technique required for placement of the restorative material. These placement techniques have been classified as direct and indirect.

Direct Restorations

Direct restorations are placed and formed directly in a cavity preparation. These restorations typically are placed in increments, adapted closely to the cavity walls, and shaped to the desired contours based on patient anatomy and occlusion. Shaping is completed with instruments to carve or manipulate materials when they are still in a soft or unset state, and with rotating instruments such as burs and discs when the restorative materials are in a hard or set state. Materials commonly used in direct restorations include moldable substances such as amalgam, composite (resin), and resin-modified glass ionomer. In addition, preformed stainless steel crowns (SSCs), strip crowns, and zirconia preformed crowns (used in pediatric dentistry) are also considered direct restorations. Restorative procedures that have been delegated legally to dental hygienists fall within the direct restoration category. Table 39.1 outlines the uses, advantages, and disadvantages of direct restorative materials.

Indirect Restorations

Permanent restorations that are fabricated outside the mouth and cemented in are considered **indirect restorations**. Gold and porcelain crowns, inlays, and onlays are examples of indirect restorations. Indirect restorations fall within the scope of practice of dentists rather than dental hygienists. However, dental hygienists often provide education to patients regarding these procedures, especially when recommended in their dental treatment plan. There are currently two techniques used for the fabrication of indirect restorations. One is to fabricate the crown on a reproduction or die of the prepared teeth. This restoration is shaped by preparing the desired form in wax and then casting this form in metal using the lost wax technique. Porcelain fused to metal restoration (PFMs) are formed by building the restoration to shape on a metal understructure on the die with porcelain powder and then solidifying the mass in a special "firing" oven. All-porcelain crowns are "stacked" directly on the die without the aid of a metal substructure. The advantage of an all-porcelain crown is its lifelike nature and appearance, and the disadvantage is its strength. Because indirect restorations are rigid, solid objects, the cavity preparation must be designed specifically to allow for complete seating of the restoration at the time of permanent cementation. The second technique for fabrication of indirect restorations is by computer-aided design and computer-aided manufacture (CAD-CAM), which

TABLE 39.1   Direct Restorations

Material	Primary Area of Use	Main Advantages	Main Disadvantages
Amalgam	Posterior	Ease of placement Low cost Longevity	Color Patient acceptance
Composite	All areas	Esthetics Patient acceptance	Technique sensitive Needs isolation Proper proximal contact
Resin-modified glass ionomer	Primarily Class V	Release of fluoride ions Ease of placement Bonds to enamel and dentin	Easily abraded
Preformed stainless steel crowns	Primary molars/anteriors Permanent molars/premolars	Longevity Low cost alternative	Esthetics Temporary for permanent teeth
Composite strip crowns	Primary anteriors	Esthetics Less costly than zirconium	Sensitive to oral fluids
Preformed zirconium crowns	Primary anteriors	Esthetics	High cost

can be emailed to a lab or prepared chairside using a computer. With a specialized intraoral camera, the dental professional or laboratory technician takes a digital picture of the tooth before and after the preparation (Fig. 39.7). This digital image contains three-dimensional information about the size of the tooth, the defect being restored, the adjacent teeth, and the opposing arch. The dental professional then designs the desired restoration directly on a computer screen using CAD-CAM software. Once the pertinent information has been entered, a tooth-colored block of ceramic material is milled using the computer image, and the indirect restoration is created at chairside.[3] Table 39.2 outlines the uses, advantages, and disadvantages of indirect restorative materials.

Cavity Preparation

Black's Classification System, the ADA's Caries Classification System, and the Complexity Classification System, presented in Chapter 17, are used to describe the type and location of dental caries and dental restorations. These systems expedite communication among those involved in the delivery of dental services. A critical step in restoring the dentition is the preparation of the cavity. A basic understanding of the principles and instrumentation of cavity preparation supports the dental hygienist as a collaborative member of the team.

Principles of Cavity Preparation

Although in most jurisdictions, the dental hygienist with a permit to deliver restorative care is not responsible for cavity preparation without an advanced degree or credential, there is value in understanding the systematic procedure of cavity preparation based on biomechanical principles. GV Black cavity preparations typically follow these steps:
1. *Establish outline form*—provides the framework of the restoration. The preparation must extend to sound tooth structure.
2. *Obtain resistance and retention form*—shaping the internal aspects of the preparation.
3. *Obtain convenience form*—allows access to the carious lesion.
4. *Remove caries*—establishes a disease-free environment.
5. *Finish enamel*—smooths walls and margins, which support the desired marginal seal between the restoration and the tooth.
6. *Cleansing of the cavity preparation*—removal of debris prior to placement of the bonding agent and/or the restorative materials.

Each tooth and cavity presents a unique challenge. The severity of the carious lesion influences the complexity of the cavity preparation process. However, these fundamental steps in cavity preparation result

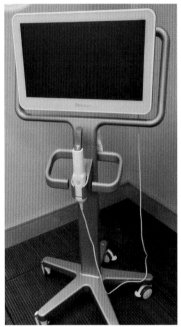

Fig. 39.7 This iTero intraoral scanner unit produces 3D digital dental impression scans quickly and efficiently. (Courtesy of Ann Mora, RDH, BASDH, Olympia, WA.)

in a preparation ready for a restoration. Because of the increased frequency of composite restorations, not all of GV Black's principles of cavity design apply to current conservative dentistry principles. Continual changes are being made to preparations designed for composite restorations. Bonding agents, used with composite restorations have replaced retentive undercuts needed for amalgam restorations, as well as the need for retention pins within the dentin. No sharp angles are required for composite restorations, and altered preparation techniques and requirements can accomplish caries removal interproximal without excessive tooth structure removal. The "Clark Class II" is an example of a cavity preparation using beveled margins, which maximize enamel surfaces available for bonding. This design has also proved to decrease bulk fracture (Fig. 39.8).[4,5] This figure represents the changes that have occurred in tooth preparations from GV Black's in the late 1800s to Clark's 2005.

Material	Primary Area of Use	Main Advantages	Main Disadvantages
Gold alloy	Posterior (inlay, onlays, and crowns)	Durability Contours	Color
Porcelain	All (inlay, onlays, and crowns)	Esthetics Wide range of color	Marginal seal Abrades opposing teeth
Porcelain fused to metal	All crowns	Esthetics Wide range of color	Marginal seal Abrades opposing teeth
CAD-CAM restorations	All (inlay, onlays, and crowns)	Esthetics	Marginal seal Texture Expensive equipment

TABLE 39.2 **Indirect Restorations**

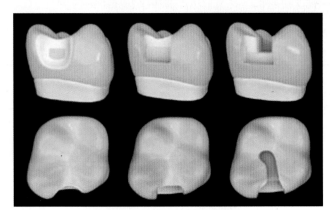

Fig. 39.8 Preparation modifications. Left to right: Clark 2005 composite preparation uses bevels to increase bondable surface area; Simonsen 1990s composite slot preparation with rounded corners; GV Black 1890s amalgam preparation. (Courtesy of Bioclear by David Clark, Tacoma, WA.)

Dental hygienists should have knowledge of the embrasure spaces and identification of cavosurface margins (occlusal, gingival, buccal, lingual) to communicate or record the correct location in need of repair or margination, which is a procedure for removal of excessive restorative material from margins of restorations.[3]

DENTAL ISOLATION

Rationale

The purpose of dental isolation is to improve the quality and comfort of restorative dental treatment. In most states, any dental hygienist or dental assistant can place dental isolation with proper training and practice. Currently, numerous methods of isolation are available. Dental dams are the oldest and most universally accepted method of isolation, but they are used infrequently because they are perceived as being time consuming and having negative patient acceptance. Alternative isolation products are available: for example, Isolite® dental isolation systems by Zyris, Inc; OptraGate and OptraDam by Ivoclar Vivadent; and HandiDam by Aseptico (Fig. 39.9).

The goal of any isolation used in restorative care is as follows:
- Moisture control
- Accessibility and visibility
- Patient and operator protection and infection control

Moisture Control

The moisture control property of the dental dam and its alternatives ensures the essential dryness of the operating field. The bonding of crowns and composite resins to the tooth structure is negatively affected

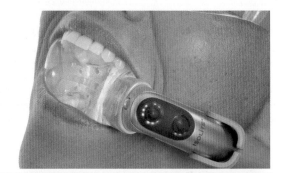

A

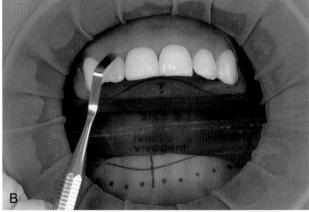

B

Fig. 39.9 (A) The Zyris Isolite® Pro dental isolation system provides hands-free continuous suction, retraction, and airway protection. Paired with their posterior mouthpiece, this system offers multiple levels of brightness and a true amber "cure-safe" light to prevent premature curing of resins. (B) OptraDam Plus is a fast and easy method of isolation with an integrated frame that is punched as a dental dam for quadrant isolation. (A, Courtesy of Zyris, Inc. Santa Barbara, CA. All rights reserved. B, © Ivoclar Vivadent AG, Schaan, Liechtenstein.)

by moisture contamination and cleanliness of the prepared surface. Composite materials are adversely affected when exposed to moisture, saliva, or blood during placement. Zinc-containing amalgam can undergo delayed expansion if placed in a wet or contaminated environment.

Accessibility and Visibility

The dental dam and other isolation devices provide accessibility and visibility by retracting the gingival tissue surrounding the site of restoration and by retracting the cheeks, lips, and tongue from the field of operation. The color of dental dams provides excellent contrast with the tooth structure and reduces glare from the moist surfaces of the oral tissues.

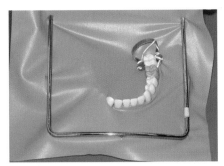

Fig. 39.10 Dental dam isolation: universally accepted as the standard for isolation and cross-contamination.

Patient and Practitioner Protection

To fully protect the patient and dental personnel, a physical barrier must be placed. The dental dam and similar isolation methods protect oral tissues from instruments and medicaments that may cause injury. Providing a physical barrier limits the possibility of patients aspirating or swallowing debris and materials associated with restorative care and treatment (Fig. 39.10). In addition, dental dams are universally accepted as an aid in the infection control process for the protection of dental personnel from contaminated aerosols.

Disadvantages

The disadvantages of the dental dam most often cited are time consumption and patient objection. The efficient practitioner overcomes the perception of the procedure as time consuming. The quality of restorations completed with the dental dam should outweigh perceived inconvenience. Patient objections usually can be minimized with communication and education.

Contraindications

Dental dam application may be contraindicated because of cracks or fissures of the commissures, respiratory congestion, claustrophobia, or acute or severe asthma. Latex allergy in the past was a concern; however, latex-free dental dam material is currently widely available and utilized.

MATRIX SYSTEMS

Function

Matrix placement for any restorative procedure is the key to a quality restoration. Various matrix systems are used in dentistry, depending on the classification of the cavity preparation and material being placed. The location, absence of adjacent teeth, and personal preference can also be determining factors when selecting a matrix system. All matrix systems are designed to reproduce the proximal wall(s) removed during the preparation of the tooth. Cavity classifications generally needing a matrix for restoration are Classes II, III, and IV. Matrix systems include bands and wedges. Some matrix systems can be utilized for both amalgam and composite restorations. All systems recommend the use of wedges for the interproximal spaces. Wedges assist with the separation of teeth and aid in proximal contour and contact and in the prevention of overhangs when placing the restorative material. Any matrix band has the ability to be modified and used in specialty situations.

After the cavity preparation is complete, an ideal matrix system is placed to do the following:
- Confine the restorative material during insertion, thereby allowing adequate condensation or application of the selected material

- Provide a framework for reconstruction and contouring of interproximal tooth anatomy
- Support establishment of proper proximal contacts
- Prevent overhangs

Matrix Systems for Amalgam Restorations

The matrix system most typically used for Class II amalgam restorations is the Tofflemire retainer and bands. This system is composed of a Tofflemire retainer and metal matrix bands of various widths and

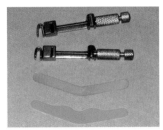

Fig. 39.11 Tofflemire retainer shown with standard matrix band and extension band for deep gingival preparations.

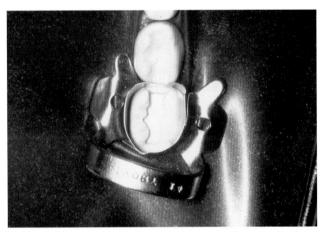

Fig. 39.12 T-band matrix bands can be placed on the same tooth as a dental dam clamp.

shapes, dependent upon the cavity preparation depth and tooth circumference, and wedges (Fig. 39.11). Smaller bands are made for primary teeth. Retainerless systems are available and used when the dental dam clamp interferes with the positioning of the Tofflemire retainer (Fig. 39.12). AutoMatrix, ReelMatrix, Denovo, and T-Bands matrix systems can be viable options (Fig. 39.13). Generally, metal matrix bands are required for amalgam restorations. The Tofflemire matrix system is the most popular and versatile (Procedure 39.1).

Matrix Systems for Composite Restorations

Matrix systems used for composite restorations are dependent on the cavity classification. Class II composite restorations, like Class II amalgam restorations, require the use of a matrix and wedge to restore anatomic proximal contours and contact areas. Composite materials differ from amalgam in their ability to establish a proximal contact. Composite resins cannot be condensed to achieve a proper contact. Therefore in order to achieve ideal contact, interproximal pressure is applied with a specialized pressure ring. This ring creates tooth separation and stretches the periodontal fibers, aiding in restoring the correct proximal contact and contours. Since the 1990s, sectional pressure matrix systems have evolved, and they are used currently to meet this challenge. The ultrathin sectional matrix band is applied only to the interproximal area and is used in combination with a pressure ring. The sectional bands typically are anatomically shaped to achieve the proper proximal contours and can be metal or plastic. They come in various shapes, sizes, and heights and are selected by location and depth of the cavity preparation (Fig. 39.14). The silicone-covered tines and ring apply pressure to the interproximal space to attain tooth separation during placement of the composite resin material. Interproximal

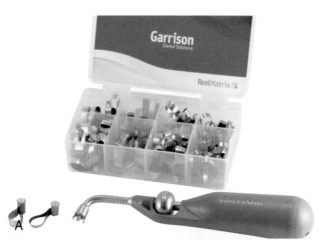
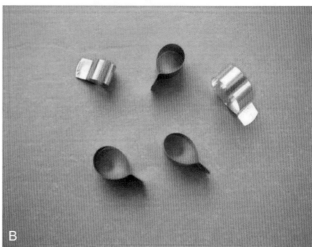

Fig. 39.13 (A) ReelMatrix is the modern version of the Automatrix system. ReelMatrix bands are available in metal as well as plastic. (Courtesy of Garrison Dental Solutions, Spring Lake, MI.) (B) Denovo matrix band available for pedodontic teeth as well as adult.

PROCEDURE 39.1 Placing a Tofflemire Matrix System and Wedge

Equipment
Personal protective equipment
Protective eyewear for patient
Tofflemire retainer
Tofflemire matrix bands
Wooden wedges
Cotton pliers
Burnishing instrument
Metal-cutting scissors

Steps
1. Evaluate the prepared tooth.
2. Select a matrix band that best encloses all lateral aspects of the cavity and extends 1 to 2 mm above the adjacent marginal ridge and 1 mm beyond the gingival margin.
3. Select a Tofflemire retainer.
4. Loop band in fingers so that ends match. The convergent opening (smaller) of the loop should be positioned next to the gingiva (dental dam).
5. Position locking vise approximately one-quarter inch from end of retainer and free locking screw (spindle) from band slot in the locking vise.

6. Position loop in retainer (leading with the occlusal edge of the band); insert matched ends into the slots in the locking vise and the loop into the appropriate guide channel. When positioned, the guide channels of the retainer open toward the gingiva. The loop of band should exit guide channel to allow the loop to be positioned from the preferred side of the tooth (usually the facial side).
7. When inserting band into the retainer, first insert the wider occlusal aspect of the band so that the retainer is seated with the slots of the retainer toward the gingiva.

Placement of band in retainer slot with occlusal aspect of loop being inserted first, followed by tightening of the locking nut.

8. Secure matrix band by advancing the locking screw (smaller nut).
9. Shape matrix loop into a rounded form: (1) insert an instrument handle through the loop, (2) pinch the band between the instrument handle and your thumb, and (3) rotate your wrist as you pinch the band.

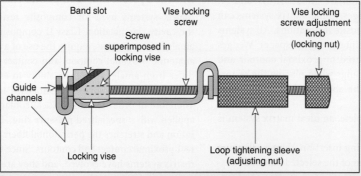

Diagram of the Tofflemire retainer.

PROCEDURE 39.1 Placing a Tofflemire Matrix System and Wedge—cont'd

10. Position loop around tooth with slots of the Tofflemire and narrow aspect of band toward the gingiva; brace lingual aspect of loop with thumb of opposite hand; gently tighten band by rotating the adjusting nut (larger nut).
11. Examine placement of band to ensure that it extends occlusally 1 to 2 mm beyond the adjacent marginal ridge; it also should extend apically approximately 1 mm beyond the gingival margin without impinging on soft tissue.

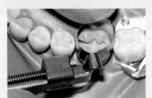

Initial placement of band after it has been rounded over prepared tooth. Finger pressure supports lingual aspect of band.

12. Moisten wedge(s) and place into the lingual embrasure between band and adjacent tooth, slightly beyond the gingival margin. Apply steady pressure on base of the wedge to move it in a facial direction to desired position. Numerous pretrimmed wedges are available for selection.

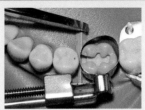

After insertion, the handle of the cotton pliers is used to position the wedge firmly.

13. Burnish internal aspect of band against the adjacent tooth (or teeth) with a burnishing instrument.
14. Conduct a final evaluation of cavity preparation with matrix system in place. Ensure that the matrix is secured below the gingival margin.

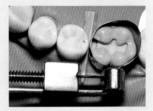

Final preparation and matrix system.

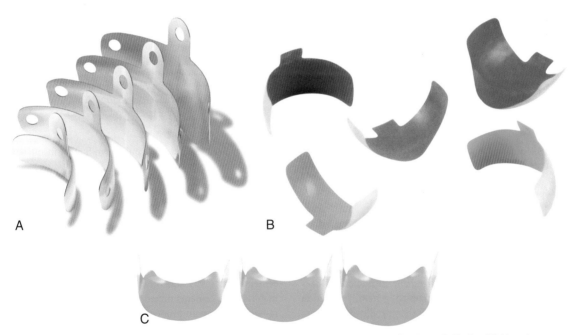

Fig. 39.14 (A) Palodent matrix system bands of varying sizes and widths. (B) Garrison 3D Fusion Slickbands are coated to prevent bonding and to help identify various sizes easily. (C) Composi-Tight 3D clear bands allow curing through the bands. (A, Courtesy of Dentsply/Sirona, York, PA. B and C, Courtesy of Garrison Dental Solutions, Spring Lake, MI.)

contacts established with a sectional matrix system and separation ring result in more predictable proximal contacts and contours. When a Class II MOD restoration is restored, two sectional matrix bands and two separation rings are applied.[5] Pressure rings and bands continue to be tailored by manufacturers for placement on premolar teeth, wide interproximal preparations, and gingival extended preparations. Brands such as Bioclear, Garrison, Palodent, and Triodent systems are some options, and all use sectional matrices and interproximal pressure rings (see Fig. 39.15).[6] These systems allow improved curing ability without the circumferential metal matrix band. Bioclear was the first to design a system that uses contoured Mylar bands suitable for posterior placement.

The Tofflemire system can be used for a Class II composite when ultrathin bands (precontoured or standard) are used with wooden wedges to create interproximal pressure. Contouring of these bands is required to achieve proper gingival contours. A sectional matrix cannot be used without a proximal contact; therefore, circumferential options would be used. Mylar matrix bands are typically used for Class III and IV composite restorations. Currently, shaped Mylar matrix bands are available (Fig. 39.16A). In addition, specialty matrix

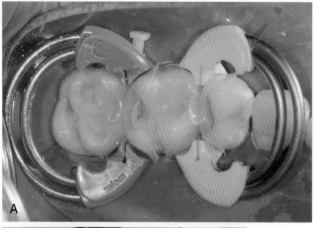

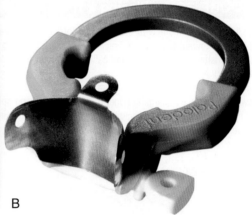

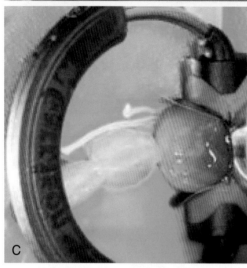

Fig. 39.15 (A) Bioclear Twin Ring system uses twin Nitinol wires to provide strong, even tension for tooth separation. When two rings are required, they can be placed as shown or stacked. (B) Palodent Plus matrix systems have the ring, contoured bands with tabs for placement, and stackable wedges. (C) Composi-Tight 3D system has soft faces to adapt to the interproximal embrasure spaces. (A, Courtesy of Bioclear by David Clark, Tacoma, WA. B, Courtesy of Dentsply/Sirona, York, PA. C, Courtesy of Garrison Dental Solutions, Spring Lake, MI.)

systems are offered for Class V composite restorations (Fig. 39.16B). See Box 39.2 for a Critical Thinking Scenario on matrix system and band selection.

Wedges

Significant changes have been made to the traditional wooden wedge (Fig. 39.17). Various types of wedges include shaped wooden and a variety of plastic that are specifically designed for the diverse sectional pressure matrix systems available. Wedges are triangular to fit into an interproximal space and are available in numerous sizes and adaptations. For ideal adaptation, wedges are generally placed in the largest embrasure, typically the lingual, thereby allowing a more complete wedge placement. A properly shaped and positioned wedge does the following:

- Gently displaces dental dam and gingival papilla in an apical direction
- Supports the matrix band in the proximal space without encroaching on the contact area
- Specialty plastic wedges adapt the band to the interproximal root morphology and the gingival cavity margin
- Wooden wedges provide slight tooth separation that supports the attainment of a positive proximal contact (see Procedure 39.1).

BASES, LINERS, AND SEALERS

Before placing a dental restoration on vital teeth, preservation and protection of the dental pulp is the primary concern. Vital dentin is a dynamic tissue. At a microscopic level, it is easy to understand how a gentle stream of air may cause injury to a delicate pulp that is covered by a paper-thin thickness of dentin. In particular, deep areas of decay must be treated to protect the pulp from further insult; bases and liners provide such protection.

Bases

Base materials are placed in the deepest areas of the cavity preparation to provide protection for the pulp and support beneath restorations. The materials must be strong enough to resist occlusal forces, provide thermal insulation, and, in the case of amalgam restorations, resist firm condensation. This category of material can include glass ionomer cements and less frequently, zinc phosphate cement. Cement-based materials are cements mixed to a thick consistency, placed, and often reprepared to attain proper cavity preparation form. The rationale for use of cement-base materials is preventing sensitivity; however, this is questionable because of their acidic nature. Sealing the dentinal tubules to prevent microleakage is believed to be far more important in controlling postoperative sensitivity than is physical insulation. In comparison, glass ionomer cements release fluoride, require less time to prepare, and bond directly to dentin, achieving a desirable seal. Most glass ionomer cements are available in a self-dispensing form and do not require manual mixing. However, when these cements are prepared manually, mixing and manipulation times are critical.

Liners

Liners are liquidlike materials applied in a thin coating to the internal portion of the cavity preparation. Glass ionomer liners have become the material of choice here as well, with their versatile ability to release fluoride, bond to tooth structure, and promote the health of the pulp. Calcium hydroxide preparations were once most commonly used; however, they have been virtually replaced by glass ionomer materials.

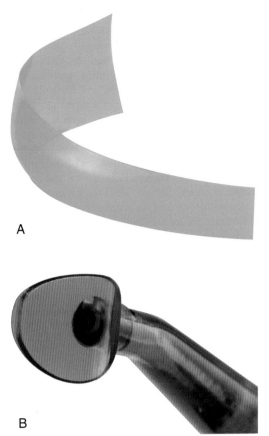

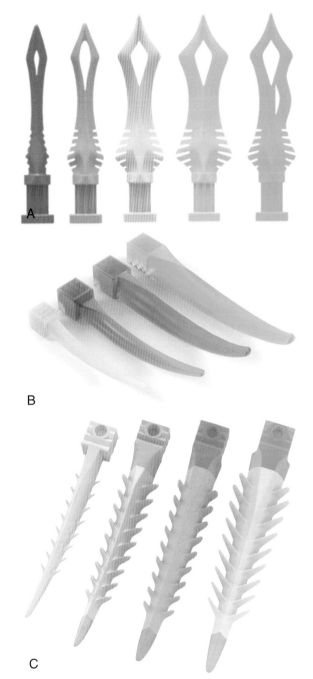

Fig. 39.16 (A) Blue View Vari Strip has a variable height and curved incisal/gingival contour to help create correct interproximal anatomy. (B) Blue View cervical matrix helps to shape a Class V restoration while allowing curing through the matrix. (Courtesy of Garrison Dental Solutions, Spring Lake, MI.)

BOX 39.2   Critical Thinking Scenario B

Matrix System and Band Selection

The dental treatment plan for your 13-year-old patient includes tooth #14 needing an MO composite restoration. How would you go about selecting the matrix system and the matrix band?

Answers

1. Evaluation of the dentition. Do you have a proximal contact for the sectional matrix system? Is #15 present to place the dental dam clamp on and #13 fully erupted to have a contact?
2. How extensive is the caries? How do you determine the size? Deep gingival caries would require the sectional band with the extension, or a very shallow preparation could use a narrow band.
3. Are there issues with bleeding or isolation?

Liners can be used in the cavity preparation for insulation. Glass ionomer bases and liners must be placed prior to dentin sealers to allow them to bond to the dentin (Fig. 39.18).

Cavity Sealers[3]

Cavity sealers are used to seal dentinal tubules and to protect the pulp from chemical irritation. Sealing of dentinal tubules is accomplished by using bonding resins or liners. Following tooth preparation, microscopic amounts of tooth particles, biofilm, and debris are left, which is known as the **smear layer**. Once the smear layer is removed with an acid etch, dentin bonding agents provide a hybridization bond

Fig. 39.17 (A) Bioclear Diamond Wedges have cutouts to allow the wedge to collapse when inserted and spring open once through the embrasure. This creates a complete marginal seal. (B) A+ Wedges with Astringent eliminate the need to apply astringent separately to prevent bleeding: astringent is incorporated into the wedge itself. (C) Composi-Tight 3D Fusion Ultra Adaptive Wedges help to adapt the band to the root concavities. (A, Courtesy of Bioclear by David Clark, Tacoma, WA. B and C, Courtesy of Garrison Dental Solutions, Spring Lake, MI.)

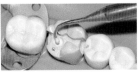

Fig. 39.18 Placement of liner material in the deeper areas of the cavity preparation.

formed between the restorative material and the tooth structure, which is deemed the **hybrid layer**. The hybrid layer has been found to better seal tubules and provide some retentive strength for resin composites when used. Sealers can be used under amalgam restorations as well to prevent absorption of the metallic restorative material by sealing the dentinal tubules.

DIRECT RESTORATIONS

Dental Amalgam Restorations

Amalgam remains an acceptable restorative material for posterior teeth. This reputation is based on decades of clinical evaluation, during which it has proven to be a durable material even when placed in compromised circumstances. Its longevity is related directly to proper cavity preparation, attention to basic principles of manipulation, and condensation in a moisture-free environment. Some countries have discontinued use due to environmental or health concerns (e.g., Denmark and Norway). Scientific studies have not verified these concerns without question, and its use is permitted in the United States and Canada.

Materials

According to the American Dental Association (ADA), dental amalgam has served as a safe, durable, and affordable material in restorative dentistry for more than 150 years.[7] **Dental amalgam** is a compound of an alloy—a mixture of metals, mainly silver, copper, tin, and zinc—with mercury. Mercury makes up approximately 50% of the amalgam mixture and functions to wet the alloy particles, causing the mass to undergo metallurgic changes and hardening. Early amalgams were unpredictable in their clinical longevity and particularly subject to delayed expansion (creep), corrosion, and margin deterioration. Current-generation, low-copper amalgam materials show marked improvement in stability, strength, and margin integrity. Amalgam alloy powders were developed with spherical particle shapes to decrease the mercury needed for wetting, with lathe-cut particles for additional strength, or with a blend of spherical and lathe-cut particles (dispersed or admix) that provides both advantages. Selection of amalgam type and setting time is a matter of personal preference. Necessary armamentarium for amalgam restorations include a triturator to mix the amalgam capsules (Fig. 39.19A), an amalgam well to place the material in, an amalgam carrier to place the material in the cavity preparation (Fig. 39.19B), condensing instruments to pack and adapt the amalgam into the cavity preparation and seal the margins (Fig. 39.19C), and bladed carving (Fig. 39.19D) and burnishing instruments to shape the amalgam into the anatomically correct form that restores tooth function (See Procedure 39.2).

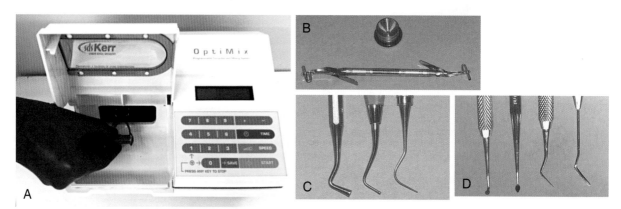

Fig. 39.19 (A) Amalgam capsule is placed in the triturator. Mixing time is set according to manufacturer's instructions. (B) Amalgam well and carrier. (C) Large and small amalgam condensers. (D) Common amalgam carvers. As pictured left to right, cleoid, discoid, 1/2 Hollenback, and Baum interproximal carver.

PROCEDURE 39.2   Placing an Amalgam Restoration

Equipment

Personal protective equipment
Protective eyewear for patient
Isolation materials
Triturator
Amalgam well
Amalgam carrier
Amalgam capsules
Condensing instruments
Tofflemire matrix system
Carving and burnishing instruments
Articulating paper

Steps

1. Pretest access to cavity by holding condenser nibs in confined areas of preparation to verify accurate condenser selection.
2. Adjust triturator settings for speed and time of mix according to manufacturer's recommendations.

3. Secure amalgam capsule in triturator locking device; close protective lid.
4. Mix amalgam, then remove capsule; open it over a catch tray and dispense mix into the amalgam well.
5. Examine mixed amalgam; note time or set a timer for 3 minutes.
6. Load small end of amalgam carrier; dispense a portion into the most confined area of the preparation.

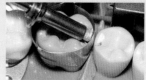

Small increments of amalgam are expressed into the proximal box of the cavity preparation.

7. Using small condensers and a stable hand position, firmly adapt the amalgam into all internal cavity features and over margins.

PROCEDURE 39.2   Placing an Amalgam Restoration—cont'd

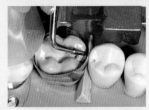

Initial condensation is begun with a small condenser in the proximal box.

8. Continue to add increments; gradually increase condenser size; remove any mercury-rich surface by lateral scooping motions of the condenser nib.
9. Triturate fresh amalgam as needed; continue to add increments and condense to build a moderate excess over cavity margins.

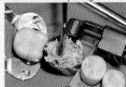

The cavity is overfilled with amalgam, and a large condenser is used to complete condensation.

10. Rub and grossly shape the occlusal surface with a few firm strokes using a large ball or egg-shaped burnisher.

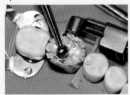

Burnishing of the overfilled amalgam.

11. Carve and suction away excess amalgam.
12. Establish marginal ridge height and outer contours next to matrix band by carving with an explorer or similar fine, sharp instrument. Carve excess amalgam away rapidly and recover occlusal margins.

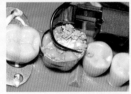

Marginal ridge height and outer contours are established with an explorer.

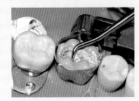

Excess amalgam is removed and occlusal margins are recovered with a carver.

13. Release matrix band from retainer by loosening band tightener and locking nut; remove wedges.

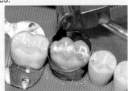

The wedge has been removed, and the retainer loosened from the band.

14. While maintaining gentle pressure on the marginal ridge with a large amalgam condenser, lift matrix band from unrestored proximal area first, then finally from the restored area.

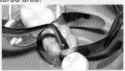

An amalgam condenser is used to stabilize the marginal ridge during the removal of the band.

15. Explore gingival margin for excess (overhang); carve away excess with a fine-bladed instrument (an interproximal carver).

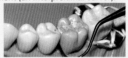

Gingival margin is checked for excess amalgam with an explorer.

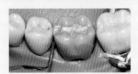

Excess amalgam at the gingival margin is carved away.

16. Carve proximal and outer contours to final form. Recover all margins. At margins, all cutting strokes should be directed parallel to margins to maintain a seal and avoid overcarving. Tooth surface is used as a guide by resting the carving edge on it as shaving strokes are made. Carve occlusal anatomy to general form, keeping pits and grooves shallow.
17. Remove rubber dam; caution patient against biting at this time.
18. Wipe patient's lips; suction mouth to remove saliva; isolate operating site with cotton rolls.
19. Insert articulating paper over area and have patient "gently tap back teeth together."
20. Carve away marking spots on the amalgam until centric occlusion is reestablished as it was before the procedure; remark the occlusion as necessary, carving away high spots each time with a carver or round bur if the amalgam has set up.

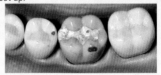

The occlusal markings show that the contact on amalgam, although present, is lighter than that on the natural tooth. As a result, the operator does not need to further reduce the occlusal contact.

21. Insert ribbon and have patient gently grind the back teeth; make sure the patient moves teeth in all functional directions. Remove markings until presurgical contacts are restored.
22. Finalize carving and burnish carved amalgam to create a smooth finish. Rinse and suction away all debris; caution patient to avoid chewing on restored tooth for 24 hours.
23. After putting patient in an upright position, have patient "tap-tap-tap" again, then look at the new restoration for shiny spots. Repeat procedure; have patient grind the teeth for lateral movement. Adjust high spots as necessary.
24. Caution patient that discernible high spots should be adjusted to avoid fracture.

Considerations for Use

While research into the safety of dental amalgam use is ongoing, a statement made by the US Food and Drug Administration (FDA) and supported by the ADA recommends not placing amalgams in children, especially those under 6 years of age, nursing and pregnant women, and people with existing neurological disease or impaired kidney function.[8,9]

The FDA also does not recommend removal of existing amalgam restorations that are clinically sound unless it is deemed medically necessary by a healthcare professional due to the potential temporary increase in mercury vapor exposure released during the removal process, coupled with the potential loss of healthy tooth structure.[9]

Mercury Hygiene and Dental Personnel

Care exercised in preventing bodily harm from mercury ingestion or inhalation is termed mercury hygiene; disregard for mercury's toxic potential may produce injury and disease. However, in decades of use, careful handling and the use of preencapsulated amalgam continues to make its use safe. Individuals primarily at risk from mercury exposure are dental personnel. Common sense and the use of personal protective equipment (PPE) provide a more than adequate margin of safety. Safety begins with well-ventilated work and storage spaces and special filters and detectors to monitor mercury vapors. All handling of amalgam mixes should be done gloved and over a deep tray to contain loose particles and promote easy cleanup of scrap amalgam. Carpeting in the work area is not recommended because vacuuming of scrap amalgam may release mercury vapors. Careful examination and cleaning of trays, amalgam wells, chair seams, and other susceptible areas may reveal small scrap particles that should be recovered safely and stored. In addition, chairside evacuation traps should be cleaned routinely and amalgam scrap properly stored. Disposal of amalgam capsules and other contaminated materials should be done in compliance with state and local environmental and safety policies. In many states, amalgam separators are required to be installed in central vacuum systems.

Mercury Hygiene and the Patient

Significant patient exposure to mercury is negated by the brevity of the dental appointment and by controlled placement of the amalgam. Dental dam isolation provides the best control of the working area. All scrap is removed readily when the dam is in place, and thorough suctioning of particles is recommended. The molecular bonding of mercury with alloy prevents the release of mercury in a significant quantity. Practitioners may routinely restore teeth with amalgam under the assurance that if they exercise reasonable care, no harm will come to the professional staff or their patients. Some individuals have attempted to discredit the benefits of amalgam and the virtues of dentists who recommend it. Claims that dentists are poisoning their patients have not been demonstrated or proven scientifically. Except in the rare case of patient allergy to mercury, dental professionals may continue to provide restorative care using amalgam.[9]

Dental Composite Restorations

Dental composite is a tooth-colored restorative material composed of resin matrix and filler particles. It is a common choice for many dentists and patients and is the most widely used esthetic material.

Material

The matrix of a dental composite resin is a polymer, usually bis-GMA or a similar monomer. Polymerization, the chemical reaction that links the monomers together, is activated by light energy or a chemical reaction (a paste and catalyst mixture). Dual-cure composites combine activation by light curing and chemical reaction to be used where light

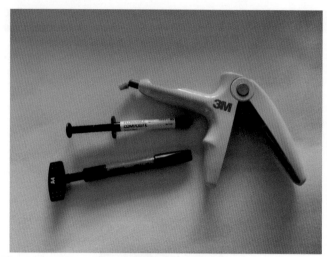

Fig. 39.20 Dispensing methods for composite materials available are dental composite unidose applicator gun with capsules and syringe delivery of standard and flowable composite.

cannot penetrate, such as in an endodontic canal. Light-cure materials are the most widely used. When cured, this matrix material forms a solid mass, but without fillers, it is soft, weak, and prone to wear. It can absorb water, stain, and discolor. To make a stronger material acceptable for posterior composite restorations, manufacturers minimize the matrix content and maximize the filler content. Filler particles, which include silicate glass, quartz, or zirconium silicate, are coated with silane for adhesion and coupling to prevent dislodging of particles. Particle shapes and sizes vary and determine the strength and polishability of the cured composite. Other components of composite include photopolymerizable synthetic organic resin matrix; radiopaque fillers, such as barium, which are added to make the composite restorations visible on radiographs; and colors to allow shade matching. There are several types of composite materials, most of which are classified by the size and/or type of filler particle, such as microfilled, hybrid, and nanofilled composites.[3] Various dispensing systems are available (Fig. 39.20).

Considerations for Use

While composite resin use in dentistry is increasing and research is ongoing, current statistics reveal limited longevity alongside potential health risks. Concerns related to possible exposure to bisphenol-A (BPA), which is associated with several systemic diseases, exist with use of dental composites containing BisGMA. Composite resin materials have been found to accumulate more biofilm on their surfaces compared to other direct restorative materials (e.g., amalgam and glass ionomer). The inevitable enzymatic and hydrolytic degradation of dental composite components coupled with polymerization shrinkage promotes secondary caries formation, leading to a higher frequency of restoration replacement. Ongoing research is also being done on the effects of incomplete monomer conversion due to inadequate polymerization.[10]

Preparation and Bonding

Composite placement procedures and cavity design are unique. Composite preparations allow for **minimally invasive dentistry**, the removal of minimal tooth structure to access and remove decay while maintaining the ability to bond to enamel and support a restoration. This concept, known as micromechanical or enamel bonding, has become the basis for procedures such as the routine placement of direct composite restorations, pit and fissure sealants, and bonded veneers. By maximizing the enamel surfaces available with modified tooth preparation designs and bevels, significant retention can be achieved. The enamel surface is shaped with instruments such as rotary burs or diamonds to establish the desired design. The smear layer and remaining biofilm can be identified with disclosing solutions and removal accomplished with a specialized air polisher with aluminum trihydroxide, in conjunction with the application of an acidic conditioning agent.[4,5] Acid etching roughens the surface, preparing it for bonding. Thorough rinsing and air drying gives the etched enamel a frosty appearance, which indicates it is ready to receive a primer and/or bonding resin prior to a composite restoration.

Compared with enamel bonding, dentin bonding is far less predictable. Most cavities extend into dentin, making the treatment of this tissue surface questionable. Lack of inorganic structure results in a weaker bond to organic collagen fibers. The composition of dentin presents special challenges for those attempting to bond to it. Dentin is more organic than enamel and, when instrumented, leaves a surface covered with microscopically observable debris. This smear layer may interfere with bonding at the dentin-composite interface. In addition, trace amounts of moisture from the dentinal tubules are present on the dentin surface. Because restorative resins are incompatible with moisture (**hydrophobic**), numerous adhesive systems that tolerate minimal amounts of water (**hydrophilic**) have been developed to chemically unite the composite with the moist dentin surface. Hybridization bonding is the bond between the dentin and the composite material. Multiple generations of bonding agents have been introduced to increase dentin and enamel bond strength, decrease time needed, and minimize operator errors in placement. Dental bleaching products have been found to adversely affect the bond strength of composites; therefore it is recommended that the patient stop bleaching 1 to 2 weeks before restorative treatment that involves bonding agents.

Curing Lights

A curing light is required to initiate polymerization of the resin matrix. Types of curing lights include light-emitting diode (LED), quartz tungsten halogen, plasma arc, and argon laser. The light is in the blue wavelength range and is transmitted from its electrical source via a fiberoptic bundle to the tip of a small wand that is positioned on the tooth surface (Fig. 39.21). An intensity of 400 mW/cm^2 or higher is considered adequate. This allows for a curing depth of 2 mm.[3] Some curing light manufacturers tout a higher intensity curing light with a deeper cure depth; however, there is evidence that this may be hazardous to the health of the pulp due to overheating. The wavelengths produced by the curing light have been shown to damage the retina and must be screened to protect the operator and assistant. Protective shields for screening are typically attached to the wand.

Composite Placement Instruments

Composite placement instruments are designed to carry, shape, and mold soft composite materials. They may have flat, nonbladed paddle or smooth, burnisher-type ends to shape, rather than condense or carve the composite (Fig. 39.22). Selection of instruments is based on the location of the cavity preparation and personal preference. Teflon-coated or anodized instruments have been developed specifically to facilitate placement of composite material without adherence to the instrument due to its tacky consistency.

Composite Restoration Placement

Patient demands for natural-looking teeth have resulted in use of composite material for restoring anterior and posterior teeth. The placement of composite restorations is extremely technique sensitive. In addition to the need for careful isolation and moisture control, accurate

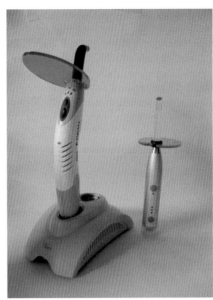

Fig. 39.21 Examples of light sources for polymerization. Orange shield should be used to protect operator and assistant.

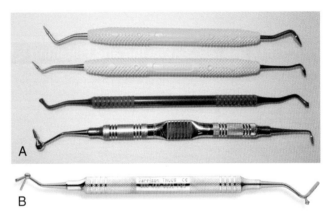

Fig. 39.22 (A) Various composite instruments with paddle and blunt ends for manipulating composite. Composite instruments are typically coated with a nonstick surface. (B) The Garrison multifunctional composite instrument has four instruments in one.

manipulation of the matrix band for Class II, III, and IV restorations is critical for a successful restoration. Reestablishing the correct proximal contact and contours is the biggest challenge facing the clinician in these procedures.[11] To place a composite restoration, the clinician must first select the desired shade of composite and then place isolations such as a dental dam or Isolite for optimal moisture control. After selection and placement of the matrix system, base, and liners as needed, the bonding agent is applied. It is critical to be aware of the bonding product being used and mindful of the techniques required, as all generations are different. Depending on the generation of bonding material, variations of 1-step, 2-step, and 3-step systems are available (Fig. 39.23). Materials requiring etch/no etch, separate or combined primer and bond, and rinse/no-rinse products are available. It is critical to follow the manufacturer's instructions. Polymerization of the bonding resin to form the hybrid layer is the final step prior to placement and curing of the composite. Placement of composite material is generally limited to 2-mm increments. Incremental placement allows for complete curing and the formation of proper occlusal contours prior to curing. Incremental placement, when done correctly, has been found to reduce the incidence of gaps and voids due to polymerization shrinkage. Even though Class II composite restorations are challenging to place and technique sensitive, dentists and patients frequently prefer them because of their esthetic nature. Procedure 39.3 outlines placement and finishing techniques for Class II composite restorations.

The average cavity preparation is typically 5 mm or less in depth. A growing subset of composites, known as bulk fill composites, have

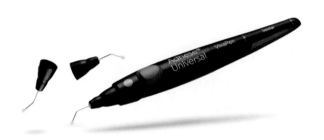

Fig. 39.23 Adhese Universal VivaPen is an example of the newest generation of bonding agents used for direct and indirect bonding procedures. It can be used as a one-step or with etch, depending on the procedure. (© Ivoclar Vivadent AG, Schaan, Liechtenstein.)

been created to allow depth of placement in a single increment up to 5 mm. Bulk fill composite materials can be placed in a variety of ways beyond the standard composite gun and compule extrusion method. Some bulk fill composites such as Sonic Fill use sonic vibration to transform the stiff composite into a less viscous material, much like a vibrating machine aids with pouring gypsum without bubbles or voids (Fig. 39.24). The Bioclear method, founded by David Clark, DDS, uses a composite heater to allow better flow of the material in one seamless increment, decreasing time needed for the layering technique and finishing. Bioclear recommends injection molding, which places all material interproximally in one step (Fig. 39.25).[5]

After the final contours are established with finishing burs, polishing is completed with specialized rubber points, discs, and cups as needed. Composite sealers are available as a final step to fill in any surface irregularities left behind after the polishing process, which minimizes potential for stain and wear (Box 39.3).

Class III cavity preparations are made with emphasis on conservatism in outline form. The plastic nature of the composite material allows it to be placed under virtually no force, and specifically designed instruments are available for placement and finishing. In the maxillary anterior area, access is dependent on the location of the caries but is usually from the lingual direction, and care is taken to preserve the marginal ridge whenever possible. In deep restorations, dentin

PROCEDURE 39.3   Placing and Finishing a Class II Composite

Equipment
Personal protective equipment
Protective eyewear for patient
Isolation materials
Glass ionomer cavity liner or sealer as needed
Conditioning agent (acid gel)
Primer/bonding system of choice
Composite
Matrix system: sectional matrix system or Tofflemire retainer with precontoured band
Dispensing syringe
Curing light and protective shields
Plastic instruments
Finishing and polishing armamentarium (e.g., burs, discs, brushes, pastes, etc.)
Articulating paper
Photo series features Triodent V3 sectional matrix system, standard microfilled composite material. (All photos courtesy of Sheila Norton BS, RDH, and Ann Mora, RDH, BASDH.)

Steps
1. Question patient regarding expectations; explain nature of composites.
2. Select composite shade, place small amount of material on the tooth near the lesion, and cure it; involve patient in shade selection.
3. Place dental dam.
4. After cavity preparation, apply cavity liner, sealer, and/or base as needed.
5. Place matrix and wedge to obtain tight seal at gingival margin. If using a Tofflemire system, refer to Procedure 39.1. To use a sectional ring matrix system, select an appropriate-sized sectional matrix band. Place the band between the preparation and the adjacent tooth. Place wedge from direction of largest embrasure (usually from the lingual).

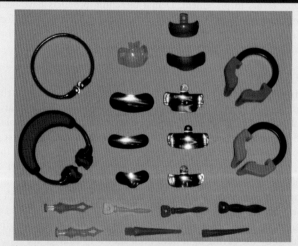

Sectional matrix systems are available from various manufacturers in a variety of sizes and designs to adapt to a variety of tooth preparations. Matrix retainers come in various sizes to adapt to specific locations (e.g., molar, premolar, anterior). Matrix bands are available in a variety of different shapes and materials (e.g., premolars, molars, deep cervical preps, primary molars). Various plastic wedges are designed to adapt to the interproximal contours of the tooth. (Courtesy of Ann Mora, RDH, BASDH, and Sheila Norton, BS, RDH.)

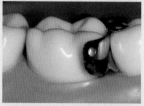

The band should extend 1 mm beyond the gingival cavosurface margin and to the height of marginal ridge. (Courtesy of Ann Mora, RDH, BASDH, and Sheila Norton, BS, RDH.)

PROCEDURE 39.3   Placing and Finishing a Class II Composite—cont'd

6. Use forceps to place the pressure ring. Ring forceps are specific to chosen pressure matrix system. The ring is typically placed over the plastic wedge; placement can vary with the chosen system. The tines of the ring should be positioned below the height of contour to prevent dislodging of the system.

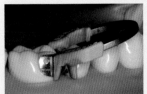

Using ring placement forceps, spread the ring and place tines carefully over the wedge to ensure the band is tight against the tooth to provide a tight seal. (Courtesy of Ann Mora, RDH, BASDH, and Sheila Norton, BS, RDH.)

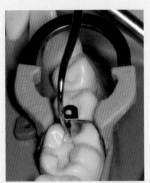

Use an explorer to check the seal of the band at the gingival floor. Also check the height of the band and ensure contact with the adjacent tooth. With the system shown, the bent placement tab approximates the adjacent marginal ridge height. (Courtesy of Ann Mora, RDH, BASDH, and Sheila Norton, BS, RDH.)

7. Examine the cavity preparation carefully and develop a mental picture of the outline form of the preparation as well as the anatomy of the adjacent tooth surface. Remember the location of the cavosurface margins in order to avoid overfilling, as using a tooth-colored material can make it difficult to visually identify flash during finishing.
8. Because prime/bonding systems (collectively called adhesives) differ, it is important to follow the directions from the respective manufacturer. Etch, prime, and bond the tooth preparation before placement of composite restorative materials. The proper use of adhesives is critical to the success of composite restorations due to creation of the hybrid layer. There are different types of adhesives (e.g., total etch, prime and bond, all-in-one).

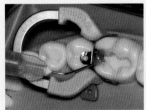

A conditioner/etchant (37% phosphoric acid) is initially placed on enamel, followed by dentin surfaces due to their differences in surface porosity resulting in varying rates of etching placed,

rinsed, and dried in accordance with manufacturer's recommendation. (Courtesy of Ann Mora, RDH, BASDH, and Sheila Norton, BS, RDH.)

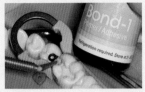

Primer and bonding agent are applied and light cured according to manufacturer's instructions. (Courtesy of Ann Mora, RDH, BASDH, and Sheila Norton, BS, RDH.)

9. Many clinicians promote the application of a flowable resin to line the floor of the proximal box. There is some evidence that it improves the adaptation of this area and minimizes the potential for voids. The flowable composite is applied by ejecting a small amount across the gingival floor of the preparation. A thickness of only 0.5 mm is needed. After light curing flowable per manufacturer's instructions, the next step is to layer the composite material into the preparation.
10. Incrementally fill: Composite is added in incremental layers of no more than 2 mm to allow complete photopolymerization. Incremental placement minimizes material shrinkage which can occur with certain types of composite. Keeping each layer of composite thin means that the cumulative effects of this distortion will be less problematic.

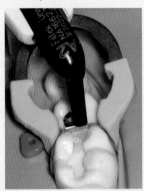

After the proximal box has been filled and cured up to the level of the pulpal floor, the remainder of the prep is filled incrementally and cured. The size of the preparation will determine the number of layers needed. Incremental layers should be no thicker than 2 mm for the light to cure the composite completely. (Courtesy of Ann Mora, RDH, BASDH, and Sheila Norton, BS, RDH.)

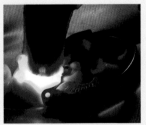

Each layer should be cured per manufacturer's instructions as close to the composite as possible. (Courtesy of Ann Mora, RDH, BASDH, and Sheila Norton, BS, RDH.)

Continued

PROCEDURE 39.3 Placing and Finishing a Class II Composite—cont'd

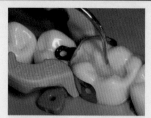

For conservative preparations, a two-layer technique can be used. Start by placing and anatomically shaping composite material from the lingual cavosurface margin sloped toward the buccopulpal line angle of the preparation and cured. (Courtesy of Ann Mora, RDH, BASDH, and Sheila Norton, BS, RDH.)

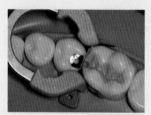

Follow with placement and anatomical shaping of a second composite increment from the buccal cavosurface margin to the central groove. Use of this technique results in a well-shaped composite that will need minimal finishing and polishing. (Pink-colored material used for visual demonstration of layering technique courtesy of Ann Mora, RDH, BASDH, and Sheila Norton, BS, RDH.)

11. Depending on the depth of the preparation multiple layers may be required. The anatomy is shaped by using appropriate composite instruments. Keeping the tip in the central groove and angling the instrument up to the cavosurface margin, pat/tamp the material in place. Excess material is wiped up and over the cavosurface margin.

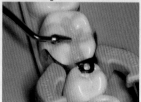

There are a variety of instruments that can be used to help shape the anatomy when approaching the occlusal layer. (Shown using PDT's CSS-6 composite instrument courtesy of Ann Mora, RDH, BASDH, and Sheila Norton, BS, RDH.)

12. Round and contour the height of the marginal ridge. An explorer or paddle-shaped blade can be used to remove excess composite from and around the matrix band. Again, cure the composite.

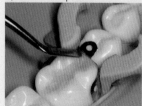

Developing the height and shape of the marginal ridge before curing. (Shown using PDT's CSS-2 composite instrument courtesy of Ann Mora, RDH, BASDH, and Sheila Norton, BS, RDH.)

13. Remove the matrix system. After removal, cure the interproximal area from both the buccal and lingual aspects according to manufacturer's

instructions. This provides a final cure to ensure that those areas previously shielded by the metal matrix band are cured fully.

14. Finishing and polishing posterior composite resins can be accomplished immediately after polymerization of composite restorations using any of the variety of composite supplies available. Check the proximal area for overhangs, proper contour, and contact. Using light shaving strokes, a gold knife or Bard-Parker blade can be used to remove minor overhangs that may remain.

15. A flame-shaped finishing bur or composite disc can be used to correct over-contoured areas and remove flash in other areas. Polish the entire surface of the restoration with composite polishing points followed by a composite polishing paste in a rubber cup.

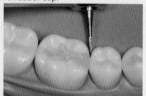

A flame-shaped finishing bur is used here to shape the marginal ridge, embrasures, and proximal contact areas. (Courtesy of Ann Mora, RDH, BASDH, and Sheila Norton, BS, RDH.)

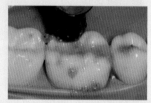

Polishing paste designed specifically for composite resin is shown here as the final step in polishing. (Courtesy of Ann Mora, RDH, BASDH, and Sheila Norton, BS, RDH.)

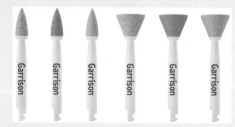

Many excellent polishing points, cups, and discs are available for finishing and polishing composite resin. As with all polishing abrasives, begin with the most abrasive, graduating to the least abrasive, taking care not to generate excessive heat. (Courtesy of Garrison Dental Solutions, Spring Lake, MI.)

16. Check the proximal contact with floss.

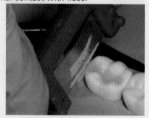

If it is too tight, a finishing strip or tapered bur can be used to correct it. (Photo features ContactEZ interproximal strip courtesy of Ann Mora, RDH, BASDH, and Sheila Norton, BS, RDH.)

PROCEDURE 39.3 Placing and Finishing a Class II Composite—cont'd

17. After assessing the restoration, remove the dental dam.

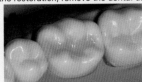

Check the restoration for any excess or deficiencies, proper proximal contour and contact, no voids, and smooth surface finish. Remove the rubber dam and check occlusion. (Courtesy of Ann Mora, RDH, BASDH, and Sheila Norton, BS, RDH.)

18. Evaluate the occlusion with articulating paper and adjust as required. If occlusal adjustment is required, repolish the areas that were adjusted.
19. The clinician should inform the patient of the following:
    • They may experience some minor discomfort of the tissues around the restored tooth because of irritation from the gingival wedge and the finishing of the gingival margin area.
    • Desiccation of the tooth may make the tooth look lighter, resulting in a temporary mismatch of the composite shade selection. After a few hours, the tooth will rehydrate and the composite color will blend with the natural tooth.
20. Document procedure.

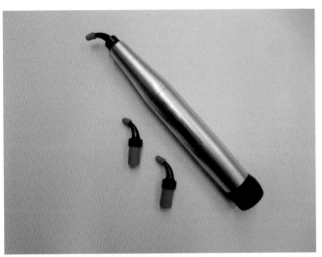

Fig. 39.24 Sonic Fill handpiece and composite capsules use sonic vibration to allow the material to flow for bulk fill technique.

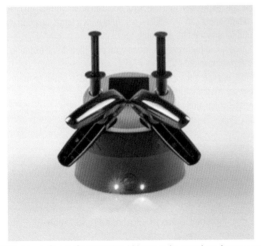

Fig. 39.25 Heat Sync Composite Warmer is used to heat composite to allow better flow of the composite for Clark injection molding technique. (Courtesy of Bioclear by David Clark, Tacoma, WA.)

coverage with glass ionomer helps decrease microleakage and the possibility of sensitivity by bacterial invasion (Procedure 39.4).

A major challenge in restorative dentistry is the treatment of decay at the gingival margin. Abrasion, erosion, dental caries, or a combination of these can create defects that are difficult to restore properly.

BOX 39.3 Critical Thinking Scenario C

Material Selection

You have a new 19-year-old patient in the office for an initial visit. When assessing the radiographs, you notice generalized interproximal caries. You discussed the patient's diet with them, and they relay that they drink two sodas and two energy drinks per day with no desire to change the habit.

Answers

1. What information would you relay to the patient regarding restorative materials? What are the best options, given the patient's diet history?
2. What would you suggest to them if their desire was composite restorations?

These defects often require isolation with special dental dam retainers, matrix bands, instruments, or cord. Class V restorations frequently extend into the gingival sulcus and have weak bond strength. This weak bond strength is due to being primarily located in dentin. Restorative material and cavity preparation techniques should be carefully selected.

Resin-Modified Glass Ionomer

Glass ionomers are available as cavity liners as well as definitive restorations, although one disadvantage is that they undergo dissolution when exposed to saliva and blood. To compensate for the tendency to dissolve and improve their use as a restorative material, glass ionomers have been modified. The improved product is called *resin-modified glass ionomer (RMGI)*. All glass ionomer dental materials release fluoride ions. As a result, recurrent caries are rarely seen at the margin of an RMGI restoration. RMGIs offer enhanced esthetics, less solubility, and greater strength than regular glass ionomers but retain some of their fluoride-releasing characteristics. RMGIs are an important class of materials for restoration of primary teeth, for Class V restorations, and in patients with a high caries risk.

Materials

Resin-modified glass ionomers are composed of fluoroaluminosilicate glass particles and polyalkenoic acid that set through both an acid-base reaction and photopolymerization between the filler and the resin. A great benefit is that this material bonds to prepared dentin and enamel tooth structure.

Considerations for Use

While there are many benefits to using resin-modified glass ionomer, it is important to note that it can degrade over time via chemical erosion through exposure to fluoride due to the glass particle and

PROCEDURE 39.4 Placing and Finishing a Class III Composite Restoration

Equipment
See equipment list for Class II composite restoration (Procedure 39.3).

Steps

1–4. Repeat steps 1 through 4 listed for Class II composite restorations (Procedure 39.3).

5. Position matrix band and wedge of choice between the preparation and the adjacent tooth.

6. Dry tooth and apply etchant to the entire cavity surface according to manufacturer's instructions. Rinse with an air-water spray for at least 15 seconds; dry with forced-air drying.

7. Inspect the peripheral etched pattern.

8. Apply thin coats of chosen primer/bond to etched surfaces according to manufacturer's instructions and lightly dry.

9. Apply a thin coat of bonding resin if applicable to primed surface; spread resin over etched enamel with a small brush or microbrush followed by a gentle stream of air.

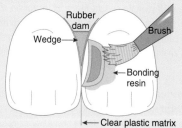

The etched enamel receiving a coat of bonding resin. A matrix separates the cavity from the adjacent tooth and is contoured and stabilized by a wedge placed interproximally.

10. Polymerize bonding resin with curing light per manufacturer's instructions; light wand should be as close as possible without direct contact. Careful inspection of cured bonding resin will reveal a slightly tacky surface. This very thin layer of resin is unable to polymerize completely because of the influence of air. It will polymerize rapidly once covered by composite or a matrix strip and reexposed to the curing light.

11. Remove cap from composite dispensing device; express small amount of selected composite onto a small paper pad; replace cap. Many systems are preencapsulated.

12. With a composite placement instrument or preencapsulated mixture placed in dispensing gun, place increment of composite (no more than 2 mm thick) in preparation; adapt to walls and margins; cure this first increment per manufacturer's instructions.

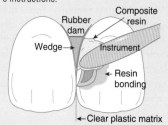

Placement of increments of composite into the preparation. The composite must be adapted into the recesses of the cavity and built against the matrix and cavity walls.

13. Continue to add and cure increments, building form to a slight excess in contour. In small cavities, final form may be achieved by firmly wrapping clear matrix against tooth and curing through it; remove wedge and matrix.

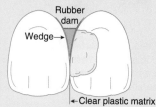

Cavity filled to slight excess, cured, and prepared for finishing.

14. Contour restoration with finishing burs and discs, exercising care to avoid tooth damage.

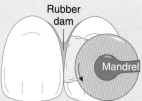

Contouring the composite with a disc to achieve the final form. The wedge and matrix have been removed.

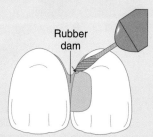

Damage to the tooth structure occurs if due caution is not exercised with the use of a bur in the finishing procedure.

15. Remove the dental dam and check for occlusal prematurities on restoration. Lingual high spots can be reduced carefully with a large, round finishing bur or a football-shaped fine diamond.

16. Polish accessible parts of restoration with polishing discs; examine gingival sulcus and remove debris.

17. If desired, apply resin surface coating with a cotton pellet or foam applicator; cure per manufacturer's instructions.

18. Show patient finished restoration.

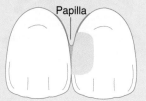

Finished Class III composite restoration.

19. Document procedure.

polysalt composition of the material matrix, creating a rough surface that encourages adherence of biofilm. Increased surface roughness of a restoration can also lead to discoloration.[12] In addition to gradual degradation, the incorporation of resin presents the potential issue of shrinkage during light curing that may contribute to margins that are not completely sealed.[13] There is evidence that a 3-minute delay in light curing after placement may allow the initial chemical reaction time to form sufficient bond strength prior to photopolymerization in lesions that did not undergo a surface pretreatment, resulting in lower rates of marginal microleakage.[14]

Indications for RMGI Restorations

Indications include root caries; Class V abrasion and erosion (gingival margin) lesions in permanent teeth; and Class I, II, III, and IV restorations in primary teeth (Procedure 39.5).[15]

Finishing and Polishing Restorations

Both amalgam and composite restorations can benefit from polishing. **Finishing** refers to producing the final shape and contour of a restoration and **polishing** refers to buffing the restoration in order to reduce scratches, resulting in a smooth surface.[3] The purpose of finishing and polishing restorations is to produce a restoration that can be cleaned easily by the patient, thereby decreasing plaque retention and the possibility of recurrent decay.

Finishing and Polishing Amalgam Restorations

Polished amalgam retains less oral biofilm and resists tarnish and corrosion better than unpolished amalgam. Over time, the amalgam hardens completely and can be polished to a high degree of smoothness; it is

recommended that amalgam restorations be allowed to set completely (at least 24 hours) before finishing or polishing.

During the polishing procedure, care must be taken to minimize heat generated by rotary instruments such as burs, rubber cups, and points as they contact the amalgam. Heat can harm the pulp, leaving the tooth hypersensitive. The metallurgy of the amalgam also can be affected adversely. The use of water while polishing minimizes the heat generated.

During amalgam finishing, marginal irregularities are removed, and areas of roughness are smoothed. During amalgam polishing, the surface is smoothed to a high luster using a sequence of abrasives from coarse to fine grit. Abrasives used during finishing are coarser than abrasives used during polishing.[3] When an amalgam restoration is finished, it is followed by polishing. If finishing is not indicated, polishing can be done alone.

Polishing the amalgam may be accomplished in two ways. The first option is by using a pumice and tin oxide slurry. The slurry mix of pumice and water is prepared in a dappen dish, and using a brush or rubber cup, the amalgam is polished to a smooth, satin appearance. The tooth

---

PROCEDURE 39.5 Placing a Resin-Modified Glass Ionomer (RMGI) for Class V Restoration

Equipment
Personal protective equipment
Protective eyewear for patient
Isolation materials
RMGI
Polyacrylic acid/conditioner
Pumice
Polishing cup
Composite placement instruments
Carving instrument
Bonding resin
Special protective varnish
Curing light and protective shields
Matrix system

Steps
1. Examine lesions; assess need for local anesthetic agent.
2. Select shade of restorative material to be used.
3. Place dental dam.
4. Place gingival retraction cord as needed.
5. According to manufacturer's instructions, apply conditioner to abrasion lesion (approximately 15 seconds); rinse thoroughly for 15 seconds with a strong air-water spray, and dry lightly, ensuring a moist surface.
6. Mix glass ionomer according to manufacturer's directions or triturate preencapsulated RMGI.
7. Rapidly fill cavity to slight excess, using a plastic instrument to place material to desired shape and contours; if desired, position a cervical matrix over cavity to hold cement against tooth; light-cure per directions using protective shield.

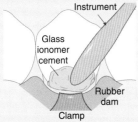
Placement of the resin-modified glass ionomer to overfill the cavity slightly.

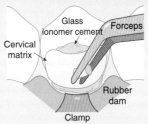
Alternative technique utilizing clear cervical matrix over the cavity and expressing excess resin-modified glass ionomer at the edges of the matrix.

8. Remove matrix, if used.
9. Contour restoration with finishing burs and discs; take care to avoid damage to tooth root.

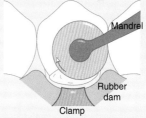
Final contouring of the restoration with a disc.

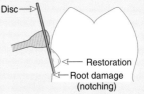
Root damage from improper disc use.

10. Apply thin coat of bonding resin/protective varnish per manufacturer's instructions to protect restoration surface and cure.
11. Remove dental dam and cord; examine gingival sulcus and remove debris.
12. Show final result to patient.
13. Document procedure.

is rinsed and dried, and a mix of tin oxide and water or rubbing alcohol is prepared. The amalgam is polished with the slurry, using a clean brush or rubber cup. The tooth is rinsed and dried, and the restoration should be evaluated for a smooth, shiny finish. The second method is accomplished using rubber cups and points incorporated with abrasive particles. They are available in three color-coded grits based on degree of abrasiveness: brown, green, and yellow-banded green. The cups are designed to be used on the proximal surfaces, while the points are used on the occlusal surfaces. Using a light intermittent touch and low-to-moderate rotary speeds with water to minimize heat generation, they polish restorations quickly and are a less messy alternative to the slurry mixes. Brown abrasive cups and points, the most abrasive of the three, are used first to polish the occlusal, proximal, and then the facial and lingual surfaces, followed by the decreasing abrasiveness of the green and yellow-banded "super greenie" cups and points. The final step is evaluating the restoration for a smooth, shiny finish (Procedure 39.6).

Finishing and Polishing Composite Restorations

The purpose of finishing and polishing composite restorations is to create a smooth, plaque-resistant surface with optimal esthetics and contours. Unlike amalgam restorations, composite restorations can be finished and polished immediately after placement. The finishing procedure involves removal of flash (overextension of composite material), smoothing the margins, occlusal adjustment, and refining of the anatomy. Polishing refers to producing a smooth, shiny finish. Many products are available, including burs, finishing strips, discs, points, cups, pastes, and brushes.[3] The process is the same as other finishing and polishing procedures, which involves progressing from coarse to fine abrasives.

Finishing concave surfaces such as pits and fissures and lingual fossae is best accomplished with an egg- or football-shaped diamond or finishing bur, using smooth, intermittent strokes on the composite material. A convex surface, such as the facial and lingual areas, is done best with a flame-shaped bur to contour the surfaces, smooth margins, and remove flash. Metal or plastic finishing strips, which come in a variety of sizes, grits, and designs, help to finish the interproximal areas (Fig. 39.26). The finishing procedure is evaluated before moving on to polishing. The composite restoration should be smooth, with the flash removed, original occlusal anatomy reproduced, and occlusion registered correctly with articulating paper. When polishing composite restorations, finer abrasives are needed, less material is removed, and it results in a high shine. Polishing points, discs, or cups and brushes impregnated with aluminum oxide or diamond particles are used to smooth and polish composite resins. Aluminum oxide and diamond polishing pastes are also available as optional final steps. Evaluation of the polished composite restoration is important, including checking for a smooth, scratch-free surface with a shiny appearance. Optimal finishing and polishing enhances the esthetics of composite restorations and decreases plaque accumulation, leading to healthier tissues. (See Chapter 32, Table 32.1, Abrasives Used for Rubber Cup Tooth Polishing in Dental Hygiene Practice.)

INTERMEDIARY CROWNS

SSCs, preformed zirconium, resin-veneered SSCs, composite strip, and polycarbonate crowns are primarily used when primary teeth can no longer support direct restorations and/or have pulp involvement.[16] SSCs are also available for permanent molar dentition as an intermediary restoration when financial considerations prevent use of permanent cast restorations. Zirconium, veneered stainless steel, composite strip, and polycarbonate crowns can all provide an esthetic option for primary anterior areas (Figs. 39.27 and 39.28). Preformed or uncrimped SSCs are available for anterior and posterior primary teeth and permanent molars. These materials have varying longevity, which should be

---

PROCEDURE 39.6 Finishing and Polishing Amalgam Restorations

Equipment
Personal protective barriers
Isolation materials
Finishing burs
Carving instruments
Handpiece
Rubber polishing cups and points (or flour of pumice and polishing powders)

Steps
1. Question patient regarding occlusion and tooth sensitivity since restoration was placed.
2. Explain value of polished versus unpolished restoration to the patient.
3. Examine amalgam for burnish marks; adjust occlusion as necessary with a round finishing bur.
4. Refine occlusal margins with a sharp discoid carver, drawn in shaving strokes parallel to margins.

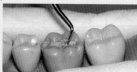

Using a stroke parallel to the margin, a sharp carver refines occlusal margins of the amalgam.

5. Using low to moderate speeds and intermittent brief strokes, polish amalgam with abrasive-impregnated rubber cups and points. Begin with most abrasive

and end with least abrasive. Maintain wet field during polishing procedures to avoid overheating pulp; avoid overpolishing established occlusal contacts.

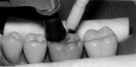

A rubber polishing cup is used to polish the marginal ridge and cusp slopes. An air/water stream is used as a coolant.

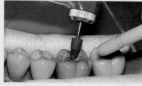

A rubber polishing point is used to polish pits and grooves.

6. Rinse mouth of debris.
7. Show patient polished restorations.

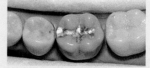

A polished amalgam.

8. Document procedure.

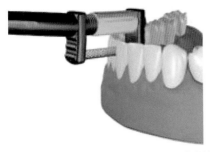

Fig. 39.26 Fit Strip allows for a variety of diamond finishing strips for interproximal finishing of composites. (Courtesy of Garrison Dental Solutions, Spring Lake, MI.)

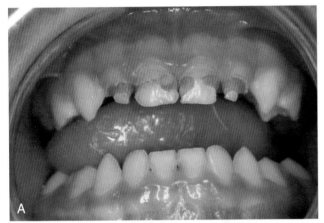

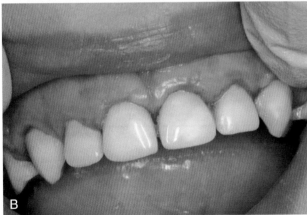

Fig. 39.27 (A) Clinical photograph exhibiting severe anterior decay in primary dentition. (B) Final treatment results utilizing composite strip crowns. (A and B, Courtesy of Ann Mora, RDH, BASDH.)

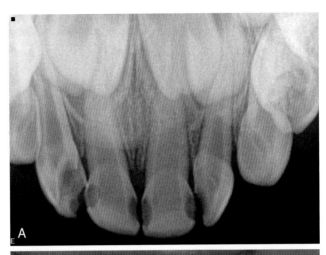

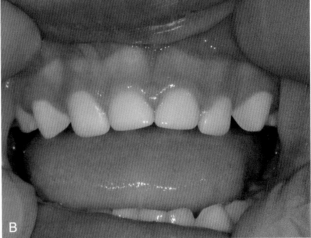

Fig. 39.28 (A) Radiograph of established anterior pediatric caries. (B) Preformed zirconia crowns used to restore severe cases of caries on pediatric anterior teeth. (A and B, Courtesy of Ben Ruder, DDS.)

considered when deciding on treatment. In some jurisdictions, dental hygienists are able to place intermediary crowns, as this procedure falls within their scope of practice. (See Box 39.4).

Materials and Armamentarium

Materials needed include the following:
- SSCs (preformed or standard)
- Trimming scissors
- Crimping and contouring pliers
- Dental handpiece and burs for adjusting and finishing
- Glass ionomer cement
(See Procedure 39.7.)

BOX 39.4 Critical Thinking Scenario D

Pediatric Crown Selection
Your 3-year-old patient presents with early childhood caries on all anterior teeth and will require crowns because of the extent of the caries. You are consulting the parent on the best treatment options. What should be considered?

Answers
1. What are the options? SSC, premade zirconium, or composite strip crowns are available in your office.
2. Is the parent concerned with esthetics?
3. How would SSCs affect the child until the age of 6 or 7?

GINGIVAL RETRACTION

The use of retraction cord is twofold. It is an essential first step for the fabrication of an indirect restoration in the making of an accurate impression, and it is used to isolate and provide retraction for Class V restorations. Gingival tissue management ensures that the margins of the preparation are captured appropriately in the impression. Gingival retraction, through the use of retraction cord around the preparation, is a critical step in achieving the desired impression. Retraction

PROCEDURE 39.7   Placing a Stainless Steel Crown

Equipment
Personal protective equipment
Protective eyewear for patient
Isolation materials
Stainless steel preformed crowns
Crown trimming scissors
Crimping and contouring pliers
Cement
Floss
Articulating paper

Steps
1. Evaluate prepared tooth for size.
2. Correct size is selected by measuring the mesiodistal width between contact points of a matching tooth in mouth.
3. Choose smallest crown that will fit.
4. To seat, place crown lingually and adapt it over the occlusal and buccal aspects of prepared tooth.
5. Use firm pressure to seat crown. You may hear an audible click as it springs over gingival undercut area of preparation.
6. To evaluate fit, observe marginal gingiva. It will blanch somewhat with a well-fitting crown. If excess blanching is observed, crown will have to be trimmed.
7. In a properly seated crown, margin should extend approximately 1 mm subgingivally. To trim crown, scribe a line where marginal gingiva hits crown with an explorer.
8. Trim crown 1 mm below scribed line. Use crown scissors or an abrasive wheel to trim crown.

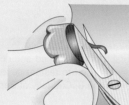

Trim the margin of the crown with crown scissors.

9. Use contouring pliers followed by crimping pliers to adapt edge of crown for a tighter fit.

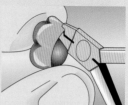

Crimping pliers are used to adapt the margin of the crown.

10. Seat crown once more to evaluate fit.
11. Crown is now ready to be cemented.
12. Fill the entire crown with cement.

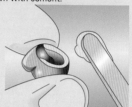

Overfill the crown with cement.

13. Excess cement will flow out from margins as crown is seated.
14. Use an explorer, a scaler, and knotted floss to remove excess cement.

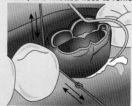

Use knotted floss and a scaler or explorer to remove excess cement after seating the crown.

15. Check occlusion using articulating paper.
16. Document procedure.

---

cord relaxes the gingival tissue, thereby expanding the gingival sulcus to allow impression material into the gingival crevice to capture the gingival margins of the preparation. Retraction cord placement is also recommended when using 3D intraoral imaging scans for impressions. Although dental hygienists and EFDAs in some jurisdictions may place gingival retraction cord and take the final impression, indirect restorations must be placed by a dentist (Procedure 39.8).

TEMPORARY OR INTERIM RESTORATIONS

Rationale for Use

Temporary or interim restorations offer patient comfort and tooth protection while a patient waits for delivery of a permanent restoration by providing the following:
- Coverage of exposed dentin to prevent tooth sensitivity, plaque biofilm accumulation, caries, and pulpal involvement
- Prevention of unwanted tooth movement
- Ability of patients to eat and speak normally
- Maintenance of the health and contours of the adjacent gingival tissue
- Means of addressing cosmetic or functional preferences and concerns of the patient

Temporary Materials and Placement Techniques

Reinforced zinc oxide with eugenol (ZOE) readily restores intermediate-size cavities that require a more durable material; it is prepared with a mixture of zinc oxide powder and eugenol liquid. The insulating properties of the hardened zinc oxide mass and the obtundent sedative effect of the eugenol result in a material that protects the vital pulp against chemical and thermal insults. Reinforced ZOE is relatively easy to prepare and place and is reliable for interim periods of a few months. ZOE is not recommended when a bonded restoration or composite is to be placed. The eugenol oil penetrates the dentinal tubules and affects the bond strength of the permanent restoration. Noneugenol materials are available for these situations.

Capsules are triturated, or a powder and liquid are mixed on a nonabsorbent pad according to the manufacturer's instructions. Firm pressure on the spatula is needed to mix the material thoroughly. Properly mixed, the material is thick and claylike. Once mixed, the material is rolled into a ball, divided into increments, and firmly packed into the preparation until it is full (Procedure 39.9).

Custom-Made Acrylic Resin

The custom-made acrylic resin temporary restoration is recommended for complex restorations such as inlays, onlays, veneers, and crowns.

PROCEDURE 39.8 Placing Gingival Retraction Cord

Equipment

Personal protective equipment
Protective eyewear for patient
Examination kit (mouth mirror, explorer, periodontal probe, cotton pliers)
Dappen dish
Scissors
2 × 2 gauze
Cotton rolls or dry angles
Retraction cord hemostatic agent
Retraction cord of various sizes
Astringent and coagulation liquid

Steps

1. Estimate circumference of preparation; cut a piece of bottom cord to encompass preparation margins.
2. Cut a piece of top cord that is approximately one-half inch longer than bottom cord and thicker in diameter. The top cord is longer and thicker than the bottom cord because it provides primary lateral tissue displacement necessary for satisfactorily allowing injection of impression material.
3. Soak bottom and top cords in hemostatic agent; place cords on a dry 2 × 2 gauze to remove excess solution.
4. Isolate site with cotton rolls and/or dry angles.
5. Using bottom cord, lasso tooth with loop around lingual aspect of the tooth.

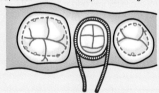

Retraction cord looped around the lingual of the prepared tooth.

6. Start placement of bottom cord in one of the interproximal areas using a periodontal probe; while periodontal probe holds packed cord in place, side of the explorer rotates the cord into sulcus.

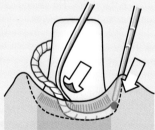

Periodontal probe holds packed cord in place while side of explorer rotates cord into place in the sulcus.

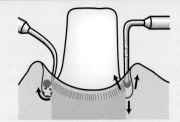

Cord placement is achieved by gently rolling cord down tooth into the gingival sulcus and below gingival margin of the preparation. Avoid forceful apical pressure on cord.

Explorer on left properly permits the cord to roll into place, but the round-ended instrument on the right permits the cord to pop up improperly on the sides.

7. Proceed in a methodic manner around the tooth, ending on the facial surface. Work from one end of cord to the other; avoid skipping around. Excess cord should be cut at this point to avoid overlapping.
8. With bottom cord in place, take top cord and lasso tooth, with loop around the lingual aspect of tooth.
9. Start placement of top cord in one of the interproximal areas; proceed with placement technique described in steps 6 and 7. Depending on the gingival status, the top cord placement may not be below the gingival margin of the preparation. A small end of the top cord will extend out of the sulcus after it has been placed around circumference of tooth.

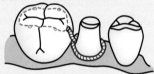

A small end of the top cord extends out of the sulcus.

This technique permits the reproduction of the tooth anatomy. A limitation of this technique is that the tooth restored must be intact enough to allow adequate retention of the temporary restoration. However, the final product is durable, smooth, and comfortable and can last for several weeks to several months.

Preformed Stock Crown (Metal or Polycarbonate)

Preformed stock crowns make useful temporary crowns. These crown forms are trimmed readily, modified for fit, and provide a satisfactory alternative to the custom-made acrylic crown previously discussed. The final product is extremely durable; polycarbonate crowns are tooth colored and available for anterior and premolar teeth, and metal preformed crowns are available for molar and premolars. All temporary crowns need to be cemented with temporary cement. Patients should be advised of the importance of maintaining the temporary while waiting to receive the permanent restoration.

LUTING AGENTS

Indirect restorations are fabricated in the dental laboratory on dies made from impressions or digital scans of prepared teeth. These restorations include crowns and inlays made of rigid materials such as metal, ceramic, or porcelain. When these restorations are seated completely, all margins should be smooth, with no gaps between tooth and restoration. However, a very small space exists between the restorations

PROCEDURE 39.9   Preparing Reinforced Zinc Oxide and Eugenol Temporary Restoration

Equipment

Personal protective equipment
Protective eyewear for patient
Isolation materials
Tofflemire matrix system
Petrolatum
Reinforced zinc oxide and eugenol
Nonabsorbent mixing pad
Plastic instruments
Cotton pellets and rolls, dry aids
Finishing burs
Carving instruments
Articulating paper

Steps

1. Isolate operating site as appropriate.
2. Prepare Tofflemire matrix system. Apply thin coat of petrolatum on the inside of the matrix band; position matrix, secure it, and place interproximal wedges as needed.
3. Use manufacturer's instructions for measuring and mixing. Premeasured capsules are available and are mixed with a triturator.
4. Prepare mix; when material reaches consistency of firm clay, carry an ample amount to cavity with a plastic instrument. Firmly adapt rubbery material to all walls of cavity with a placement instrument.

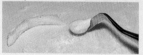

Properly mixed reinforced zinc oxide with eugenol ready for placement.

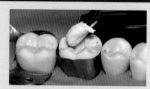

Reinforced zinc oxide with eugenol being placed in cavity preparation.

5. Fill cavity to slight excess; shape occlusal anatomy by using a moist cotton pellet in cotton pliers to create a general anatomic form.
6. When material has hardened, remove wedge(s), retainer, and matrix band; support the restoration with a condenser using apical pressure while removing the band.
7. Check proximal and gingival margins for excess material and remove with sharp, narrow-bladed carving instrument.
8. Remove isolation materials; evaluate premature occlusion on temporary restoration with articulating paper and adjust as necessary with large, round bur and carving instruments.

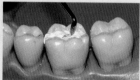

Final adjustment to the occlusal aspect of the temporary restoration with a carver.

9. Examine gingival sulcus for debris and remove as necessary; excess material at gingival margin can be removed using a bladed instrument such as the 1/2 Hollenbeck or IPC carver.

---

and the tooth that is filled with a luting agent (cement) that when set, prevents the indirect restoration from loosening. Dislodging forces of occlusion and mastication are resisted by this firm interface of cement. Without a proper luting agent, restorations leak, loosen, and fail.

Glass Ionomer Cement

The chemical adhesion of this material to the tooth surface and relative ease in handling has led to the popularity of glass ionomer as a luting agent. When compared with zinc phosphate, it is less acidic and more compatible with the dental pulp. It inhibits recurrent caries through the slow release of fluoride. The mixing and working times for the chemical-cured glass ionomer cement are short, so the dental team must be efficient when luting restorations with glass ionomer cement. GI cements are available in a trituratable capsule that is also used for dispensing. Mixing can also be accomplished on a nonabsorbent paper pad in accordance with the manufacturer's instructions. The luting cement is mixed to a much less viscous state than the glass ionomer cement base material or restorative material previously described.

Resin Cements

Chemical-cured resin cements are used when strength of bonding is needed and light activation is not possible (e.g., cementation of cast posts, cores, and Maryland bridges). The bond strength of resin cements is much greater than that of other cements, but handling characteristics are more sensitive and the working time is shorter. The modified resin cements are also useful for cementation of complete metal or metal-ceramic crowns to be placed on tooth preparations with minimal retentive features.

Zinc Phosphate Cement

Zinc phosphate, the oldest of the luting agents, can be used for cementation of most indirect restorations. However, its use has been largely replaced by glass ionomer and resin cements.

Temporary Cements

Temporary restorations can be cemented with a variety of temporary cements. Historically, ZOE was preferred; however, with the need to avoid oils such as eugenol for bonded restorations, noneugenol products are used. These materials vary in hardness and retaining abilities and are selected accordingly. Temporary cements are most commonly contained in small tubes and have a fluid-paste consistency. Equal amounts of base and catalyst are expressed onto a small pad and rapidly mixed. The cement is applied to cover the inside of the restoration (usually a temporary restoration), which is then seated and held in place until the cement has hardened. Excess hardened cement is removed with an instrument such as an explorer or curette. Again, ZOE is not recommended when a bonded restoration or composite is to be placed.

DOCUMENTATION

Restorative treatment must be documented accurately in the patient's record, including all procedures involved in the restorative treatment. Documentation may include but is not limited to the tooth number; surfaces and location of the restoration; anesthetic agents and medications; isolation procedures; base, liner, and bonding agents; and restorative material used (the brand and shade of composite or RMGI), complications, and patient education. When restorative treatment

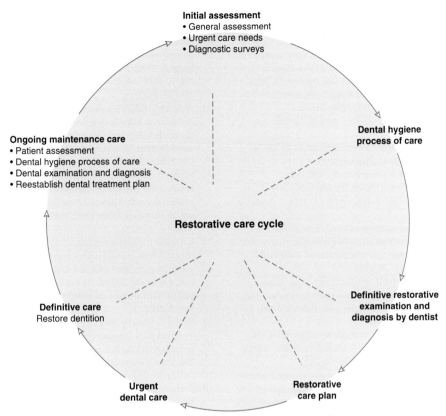

Initial assessment
• General assessment
• Urgent care needs
• Diagnostic surveys

Dental hygiene process of care

Ongoing maintenance care
• Patient assessment
• Dental hygiene process of care
• Dental examination and diagnosis
• Reestablish dental treatment plan

Restorative care cycle

Definitive restorative examination and diagnosis by dentist

Definitive care
Restore dentition

Urgent dental care

Restorative care plan

Fig. 39.29 Comprehensive restorative care cycle.

dictates special precautions for future treatment, specific details should be recorded.

EVALUATION

The restorative care cycle demands ongoing assessment and evaluation (see Fig. 39.29). Appropriateness of treatment must be judged from the perspectives of the professional and the patient. The professional must be responsible for proper manipulation and technical quality of the restoration, and the patient should be prepared to address issues such as comfort, function, and appearance.

MAINTENANCE OR CONTINUED CARE

Assessment is an ongoing component of restorative therapy. During continued-care appointments, the dental hygienist thoroughly reviews the medical and dental histories of the patient, assesses the outcomes of preventive and restorative care, and evaluates the patient's current oral health status. Assessments at the continued-care appointment that include evaluation and maintenance of existing restorations provide optimal restorative care outcomes for the patient.

Please visit the website at http://evolve.elsevier.com/Pieren/hygiene for additional information on restorative techniques included in the chapter.

ACKNOWLEDGMENTS

The authors acknowledge Cheryl A. Cameron and Richard B. McCoy for their past contributions to this chapter. The authors thank Sarah Hill, BS, RDH, EPDH, CDA; Brenda Wertman, RDH, MPH; Linda McKay Clover, RDH, and Lindsey Markegard Johnson, BS, RDH, MBA for chapter review.

KEY CONCEPTS

- Restorative therapies restore the dentition to a state of health, support the maintenance of health, and provide esthetic modifications to the dentition.
- The dental hygienist's role in restorative therapies continues to expand.
- Cavity preparations for amalgams and composites are different. GV Black preparations are ideal for amalgam restorations; however, changes are continuing to be made to provide minimally invasive dentistry and increase longevity for composites.
- Dental isolation is necessary for composite restorations to avoid contamination by saliva or blood.
- The dental dam is an isolation technique used to control moisture, improve accessibility and visibility, and protect the patient and operator with an impervious barrier for aspiration and cross-contamination. Other methods are available.
- Amalgam is a durable and safe restorative material to restore primarily Class I, II, and V preparations.
- Composite is a popular tooth-colored restorative material used for Class I, II, III, IV, and V restorations.
- Glass ionomers and resin-modified glass ionomers release fluoride ions and are indicated for the restoration of root caries, Class V abrasion and erosion lesions, and Class I and II caries on primary teeth.
- Stainless steel, composite strip, and zirconium preformed crowns are durable restorations for the primary dentition with multisurface caries.
- Gingival retraction is essential for making an accurate impression of gingival margins of an indirect restoration. It can also be useful when placing a Class V restoration.
- Temporary restorations ensure patient comfort, provide tooth and gingival protection, and prevent tooth movement during the period between initial and final tooth preparation and restoration placement.
- Luting agents are used to cement indirect restorations and prevent the restoration from leaking and dislodging.

REFERENCES

1. American Dental Hygienists' Association. Dental hygiene practice act overview: Permitted functions and supervision levels by state. Available at: https://www.adha.org/wp-content/uploads/2023/05/ADHA-Practice-Act-Overview-5-2023.pdf. Published May 2023. Accessed October 24, 2023.

2. American Dental Hygienists' Association (ADHA). Restorative Duties Chart. Available at: https://www.adha.org/wp-content/uploads/2022/11/7516_Restorative_Duties_by_State.pdf. Published April 2016. Accessed December 26, 2022.

3. Eakle WS, Bastin KG. *Dental Materials: Clinical Applications for Dental Assistants and Dental Hygienists*. 4th ed. Elsevier; 2020.

4. Clark DJ. The injection-molded class II restoration. *Dent Today*. 2018;37(5):109–112. Available at: https://www.dentistrytoday.com/the-injection-molded-class-ii-restoration/. Published May 1, 2018. Accessed December 26, 2022.

5. Clark DJ. The seven deadly sins of traditional class II restorations. *Dent Today*. 2017;36(1):119–121. Available at: https://www.dentistrytoday.com/the-seven-deadly-sins-of-traditional-class-ii-restorations/. Published January 1, 2017. Accessed December 26, 2022.

6. Clark DJ. An improved quadrant class II composite technique. *Dent Today*. 2017;36(5):99–101. Available at: https://www.dentistrytoday.com/an-improved-quadrant-class-ii-composite-technique/. Published May 1, 2017. Accessed December 26, 2022.

7. American Dental Association. Amalgam. Available at: https://www.ada.org/resources/research/science-and-research-institute/oral-health-topics/amalgam. Published April 21, 2021. Accessed May 30, 2022.

8. American Dental Association. The American Dental Association reaffirms its position on dental amalgam. Available at: https://www.ada.org/en/about/press-releases/2020-archives/the-american-dental-association-reaffirms-its-position-on-dental-amalgam. Published September 24, 2020. Accessed May 27, 2022.

9. U.S. Food and Drug Administration. FDA issues recommendations for certain high-risk groups regarding mercury-containing dental amalgam. Available at: https://www.fda.gov/news-events/press-announcements/fda-issues-recommendations-certain-high-risk-groups-regarding-mercury-containing-dental-amalgam. Published September 24, 2020. Accessed May 27, 2022.

10. Aminoroaya A, Neisiany RE, Khorasani SN, et al. A review of dental composites: challenges, chemistry aspects, filler influences, and future insights. *Compos B Eng*. 2021;216:108852. Available at: https://doi.org/10.1016/j.compositesb.2021.108852. Published July 1, 2021. Accessed May 27, 2022.

11. Shuman I. Achieving successful proximal contacts with direct composite. Available at: https://www.dentalacademyofce.com/dace/coursereview.aspx?url=3227%2FHTML%2F1611cei_Shuman_Composites_web%2Findex.html&scid=16544. Published November 2016. Accessed December 26, 2022.

12. Seung-Hwan O, Seung-Hoon Y. Surface roughness and chemical composition changes of resin-modified glass ionomer immersed in 0.2% sodium fluoride solution. *J Dent Sci*. 2021;16(1):389–396. https://doi.org/10.1016/j.jds.2020.07.002. Published January 2021. Accessed June 5, 2022.

13. Rayapudi JJ, Sathyanarayanan R, Carounanidy U, John BM. Evaluation of noncarious cervical lesions restored with resin-modified glass ionomer and glass carbomer: a single-blind randomized controlled clinical trial. *J Dent Res*. 2021;11(1):8–15. https://jsd.sbvjournals.com/doi/JSD/pdf/10.5005/jp-journals-10083-0940. Published January 2021. Accessed June 5, 2022.

14. Shafiei F, Yousefipour B, Farhadpour H. Marginal microleakage of a resin-modified glass-ionomer restoration: interaction effect of delayed light activation and surface pretreatment. *Dent Res J (Isfahan)*. 2015;12(3):224–230. https://www.ncbi.nlm.nih.gov/pmc/articles/PMC4432604/#__ffn_sectitle. Published May 2015. Accessed June 5, 2022.

15. Graham L. Glass ionomers in modern clinical practice. *Dent Today*. 2017;36(2):130–133. Available at: https://www.dentistrytoday.com/glass-ionomers-in-modern-clincial-practice/. Accessed December 26, 2022.

16. Shuman I. Pediatric crowns: from stainless steel to zirconia. Available at: www.ineedce.com; 2016. https://www.dentalacademyofce.com/dace/coursereview.aspx?url=3222%2FHTML%2F1611cei_Shuman_PediatricCrowns_web%2Findex.html&scid=16525. Published November 2016. Accessed December 26, 2022.

40

Orthodontic Care

Beth Jordan

PROFESSIONAL DEVELOPMENT OPPORTUNITIES

Dental hygienists with an understanding of the underlying indications, process, and goals of orthodontic treatment often help prepare the patient for the orthodontic treatment. This role includes identifying potential candidates and discussing what to expect during the process. Dental hygienists help patients maintain dental and periodontal health during and after orthodontic treatment.

COMPETENCIES

1. Discuss malocclusion, including the effects of malocclusion.
2. Assess and evaluate the need for a referral for orthodontic care.
3. Educate patients and guardians to understand normal developmental changes versus orthodontic needs and describe various orthodontic considerations that affect dental care.
4. Describe the biomechanics of tooth movement.
5. List and describe the three types of orthodontic treatment.
6. Detail the uses of a variety of orthodontic appliances.
7. Identify risks associated with orthodontic treatment and communicate how to mitigate or manage the risks.
8. Discuss the need for dental collaboration when dealing with alternative orthodontic treatment to address restorative, periodontal, and implant needs.
9. Instruct patients on effective self-care regimens to address hard and soft tissue concerns during treatment.

INTRODUCTION

The hygienist identifies facial and dental abnormalities that can be corrected orthodontically and advises patients of treatment benefits and risks. In addition, it is the role of the hygienist to aid the patient with compliance, motivation, and maintaining oral health during the treatment phase (Box 40.1). This chapter provides an overview of the basic concepts involved in orthodontics and recommendations for specific self-care techniques for patients undergoing orthodontic treatment. The specifics of orthodontic treatment planning are beyond the scope of dental hygiene practice and thus this chapter.

Orthodontics is a dental specialty that deals with the recognition, prevention, and treatment of conditions involving irregularities of the teeth, jaws, and face, and their influence on the physical and mental health of the individual. The goals of orthodontics are as follows:
- Establish or maintain a normal functioning occlusion
- Improve or maintain good facial aesthetics
- Promote long-term stability
- Establish the best physiologic position of the condyle in the temporomandibular joint
- Establish periodontal health

The American Association of Orthodontists recommends that an orthodontist examine a child by the age of 7 years.[1] This recommendation is based on three main factors:
- Posterior occlusion is established when the first permanent molars erupt. It is at this time that basic occlusal relationships can be evaluated.
- Incisors have begun to erupt, leading to identification of crowding, deep or open bites, or other jaw discrepancies.
- For some, early detection and interceptive treatment can lead to more effective treatment plans and identify psychosocial impacts of maligned or missing/impacted teeth.

Malocclusion is not a disease state. Rather, it is any deviation from the normal relationship of the maxillary arch or teeth to the mandibular arch or teeth, termed *malocclusion*. For a discussion of types of malocclusion, see Chapter 17. Malocclusion can occur in the sagittal plane, the transverse plane, or the occlusal plane (Fig. 40.1).

There are two origins of malocclusion. The first is founded in genetic discrepancies. These genetic discrepancies can be either skeletal or dental. Some examples of genetic malocclusion are overcrowding, supernumerary teeth, narrow jaw, and premature or late exfoliation. An example of strictly dental malocclusion is individual tooth placement or tipping of teeth within the arch or a posterior crossbite.

Malocclusion can be a combination of skeletal and dental causes. For example, a posterior crossbite is a malocclusion in the transverse plane of space where the buccal cusps of the maxillary teeth are lingual to the buccal cusps of the mandibular teeth, unlike the normal relationship between the maxillary and mandibular teeth (Fig. 40.2). If the palate is too narrow or the mandible is too wide and if the teeth are in an appropriate position, the crossbite has a skeletal cause. If the palate is of adequate width, but the maxillary posterior teeth incline lingually, the crossbite is dental in origin. The malocclusion is of skeletal and dental origin if both the relationship of the jaws and the alignment of the teeth are involved. A less severe difference in width can result in teeth that occlude end to end in the posterior. See Figs. 40.3 and 40.4 for examples of malocclusion and related facial discrepancies.

The second cause of malocclusion is caused by trauma or parafunctional habits. Examples include thumbsucking, clenching, grinding, and other habits outside of the range of normal speech and mastication that affect normal growth and development patterns.

EFFECTS OF MALOCCLUSION

Malocclusion can affect individuals as follows:
- Psychosocial problems caused by poor facial aesthetics or poor word enunciation
- Oral function problems, such as difficulties with chewing, swallowing, and speech

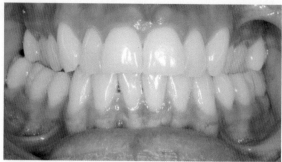

Fig. 40.2 Posterior crossbite, which is a malocclusion in the transverse plane. (From Alfonso M, Dolce C. *New and Evolving Concepts in Orthodontics*. Courtesy of Procter & Gamble Company; 2017. https://www.dentalcare.com/en-us/professional-education/ce-courses/ce524.)

BOX 40.1   Patient or Client Education Tips

- The dental hygienist remains current regarding evidence-based options and directions for use of oral hygiene, antimicrobial, fluoride and nonfluoride caries-preventive agents, and care of fixed and removable appliances (Tables 40.1 and 40.2), so this information can be reinforced with the patient and the hygienist can answer questions the patient or parent may have.
- Stress the importance of regular dental hygiene visits throughout orthodontic therapy.
- The hygienist identifies facial and dental abnormalities that can be corrected orthodontically and advises patients of treatment benefits and risks.
- It is the role of the hygienist to aid the patient with compliance, motivation, and maintaining oral health during the treatment phase.
- Explain changes that are occurring during treatment and the importance of retention after treatment.
- Discuss the need for further periodontal and/or prosthodontic procedures.
- Work carefully with clients (patients and parents or caregivers) to develop a self-care regimen that is acceptable and effective; to limit dietary sugars; to use home fluoride rinses and dentifrices; and to clean removable appliances.
- Reinforce the importance of following procedures and attending orthodontic appointments as recommended by the orthodontist.

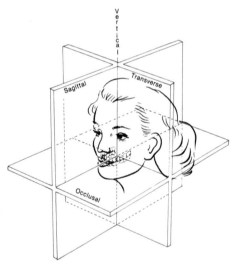

Fig. 40.1 Perspective view of the planes of reference normally employed for orthodontic examination. The alignment of teeth and the asymmetry of the dental arches are best seen in projection against the occlusal plane; profile and facial aesthetics along with anteroposterior and vertical relationships are best studied in projection against the sagittal plane; and transverse dentofacial relationships are best evaluated in projection against the transverse plane. (From Graber LW, Vanarsdal RL Jr, Vig KWL. *Orthodontics: Current Principles and Techniques*. 6th ed. Mosby; 2016.)

- Increased biofilm, debris, and stain retention contributing to periodontal disease (i.e., gingival recession, mucogingival problems, alveolar defects)
- Injury caused by trauma to and breakage of malpositioned teeth
  - Temporomandibular dysfunction, a chronic impairment or discomfort of the function of the temporomandibular joint (TMJ)

ASSESSING AND EVALUATING FOR REFERRAL FOR ORTHODONTIC CARE

When assessing the patient for referral treatment, the dental hygienist must be able to identify features and patterns of normal growth and development versus abnormal as indications for referral. Assessment commonly includes visual and radiographic, intraoral and extraoral inspection, and evaluation of function. However, the orthodontist will do an orthodontically oriented set of analyses consisting of visual inspection, palpation, photographs, casts or digital study models, and a set of radiographs or three-dimensional (3D) imaging. This next section is an overview of the factors for consideration in orthodontic evaluation.

Medical History

The patient's medical history can include information related to a potential need for orthodontic referral. Examples of medications with orthodontic consideration are antiseizure drugs such as phenytoin that sometimes produce gingival hyperplasia that may slow tooth movement, or bisphosphonates that may slow down bone turnover. Many children with asthma are mouth breathers, and a correlation has been observed between mouth breathing in children and higher palatal vaults, greater overjets, and posterior crossbite incidence.[2]

Intraoral and Extraoral Assessment

The dental hygienist classifies occlusion and assesses the dentition for malocclusion or malalignment during the intraoral examination (see Chapter 17). Primary and permanent **tooth eruption patterns**, primate spaces, or the process in tooth development in which the teeth enter the mouth and become visible should be evaluated for appropriate or altered sequencing. Overretention or early loss of primary teeth, trauma, crowding, or malposed teeth can be reasons for an orthodontic referral. Although it may seem basic, simply counting the teeth present intraorally as well as radiographically can help identify orthodontic needs.

Functional status of the TMJ and occlusion are key determinants for orthodontic evaluation; therefore, their assessment, as well as observing speech and articulations patterns, is an important component of the intraoral and extraoral examination (see Chapters 16 and 17). A thorough clinical interview and physical examination is indicated to detect signs and symptoms of temporomandibular disorder (TMD). Restricted range of jaw movement, clicking and pain in the TMJ, and tenderness of muscles of mastication are all signs of TMJ dysfunction that should be evaluated and noted during the oral assessment.

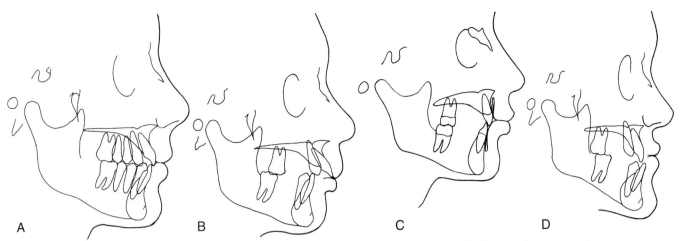

Fig. 40.3 Sagittal evaluation of the dentition focusing on the molar Angle classification and the amount of overjet. (A) Class I occlusion, (B) Class II, Division 1 occlusion, (C) Class II, Division II occlusion, (D) Class III occlusion. (From McDonald RE, Avery DR, Dean JA. *Dentistry for the Child and Adolescent.*; 2004.)

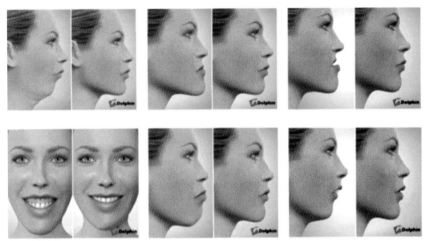

Fig. 40.4 Examples of facial discrepancies.

Photographs

The orthodontist or orthodontic dental assistant will take a standard series of intraoral and extraoral photographs. These photographs include: (1) full face with lips relaxed, (2) full face smiling, (3) a smiling profile, and (4) a nonsmiling profile both left and right. The purpose of extraoral photographs is to evaluate facial symmetry, profile, and quality and esthetics of smile and gingiva. The midline of the maxilla is assessed in relation to the philtrum and the nasal column (Fig. 40.5). The profile photographs assess anteroposterior discrepancies of the maxilla and mandible. In addition, they reveal the posture of the lips and the position of the incisors. An example of profile evaluation is when the lips appear prominent in the profile or when the lips are separated by more than 3 to 4 mm when at rest. The separation of the lips to this extent is called **lip incompetence** (Fig. 40.6). This condition can be caused by incisors that are protrusive. Patients may be able to close their lip; however, this may cause "mentalis strain."

To evaluate vertical facial dimensions, horizontal lines are drawn through the bottom of the chin, the base of the nose, the eyebrows, and the top of the forehead/hair line to produce three zones of equal height (Fig. 40.7). An imaginary line drawn along the inferior border of the mandible should incline downward at only a slight degree. A steep incline

of the mandible correlates with an anterior open bite and a long face. A flat mandibular plane correlates with a deep overbite and a short facial height (note that in Fig. 40.7 the line drawn with arrows at both ends illustrates a slight degree of incline or normal vertical facial dimensions).

Standard intraoral photographs include right and left lateral retracted views, maxillary and mandibular occlusal views, an anterior bite position, and an anterior profile. These capture anterior and posterior occlusal relationship, tooth spacing, and overall tooth placement such as overjet and overbite (Fig. 40.8).

Radiographs

Panoramic radiographs are used to examine the perioral structures for the presence of pathology or for supernumerary, congenitally missing, or impacted teeth (Fig. 40.9). A **lateral cephalometric** radiograph is used to assess the facial and jaw proportions and the skeletal relationship of the jaws to each other and to the base of the cranium, and to determine the need to reposition the anterior teeth. Cephalometric analysis is conducted by identifying anatomic points on the radiograph, measuring their separation, and using those data to compare to known measurements (Fig. 40.10). The use of cephalometrics in orthodontics is valuable because although two cases of malocclusion may appear similar clinically or on a study model, significant differences in the two cases become apparent when the skeletal components of the malocclusion are analyzed. Taken

TABLE 40.1   **Examples of Common Fixed Orthodontic Appliances**

Passive and Active Appliances

Archwire	Held in place by brackets bonded to the tooth. Placed into the bracket that is bonded to the tooth. Held in place by a ligature, typically a elastic band. Applies pressure to the tooth.	Applies pressure.	Orthodontic Archwire. (Photo courtesy of Ortho Technology, Inc) 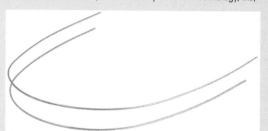
Twin Brackets	Bonded to the tooth. Metal or acrylic. May be placed on buccal or lingual surface.	Holds archwire. Requires elastic ligature.	Twin Brackets. (Photo courtesy of Ortho Technology, Inc.) 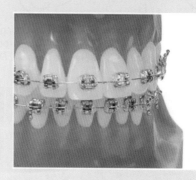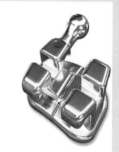
Bands	Bonded to the tooth to securely hold the archwire.	Usually on molars.	Orthodontic Bands. (Courtesy of Dolphin Imaging & Management Solutions [www.dolphinimaging.com].) 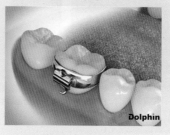
Ligatures	Small ties or rings made of wire or elastic.	They fasten the archwire to the bracket.	Ligatures. (Photo courtesy of Henry Schein Orthodontic) 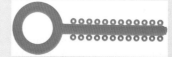
Self-Ligating Brackets	Require no additional ligature, therefore reducing friction.	Holds archwire. No ligature required.	Self-Ligating Brackets. (Graber, L.W. and L., V.K.W. (2023) Orthodontics: current principles and techniques. Philadelphia: Elsevier - Health Sciences Division.) 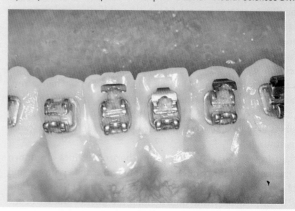

TABLE 40.1	Examples of Common Fixed Orthodontic Appliances—cont'd		
Buccal Tube	Metal tube welded to the cheek side of a molar band.	Tube that holds the end of a lip bumper, headgear, or other appliance.	Buccal Tube. (Courtesy of Dolphin Imaging & Management Solutions [www.dolphinimaging.com].) 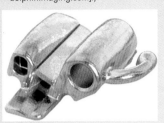
Transpalatal Appliance (TPA) Passive holding device or active with loop		Holds upper molars in place to stabilize their position or rotate molars.	Transpalatal Appliance (TPA). Specialty Appliance. (Courtesy of Dolphin Imaging & Management Solutions [www.dolphinimaging.com].) 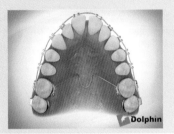
Temporary Anchorage Device	A microimplant inserted through the buccal ridge, where elastic band chains can be attached.	Used to correct mild to moderate anterior open bite and or vertical excess problems. May reduce the need for orthognathic surgery.	Temporary Anchorage Device. (Courtesy of Dolphin Imaging & Management Solutions [www.dolphinimaging.com].) 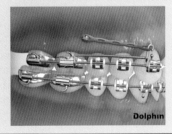

before, during, and after orthodontic therapy, cephalometric radiographs can be used to assess changes in dental and skeletal relationships.

Cone beam computed tomography (CBCT) is a special type of x-ray equipment used when regular dental or facial x-rays are not sufficient. This technology produces 3D images of the teeth, soft tissues, nerve pathways, and bone in a single scan. It provides practitioners with a 3D image of the location and anatomy of teeth and craniofacial anatomy. A full CBCT can be used and has the capability to extract a panoramic or lateral cephalometric radiograph (Fig. 40.11).

Impressions/Study Casts

Impressions of the maxillary and mandibular arches must be taken, along with a wax-bite registration, to assess the occlusion, the symmetry of the form of the dental arches, and the symmetric positioning of the individual teeth within the arches (see Chapter 38). Digital study models are typically used in orthodontics today. Digital models can be used to generate stereolithography (.stl) files that can be used to print a 3D model, if necessary. CBCT images can be used to generate digital models as well.

DEVELOPMENTAL AGES

- **Skeletal age** is the development of the skeletal system.
- **Chronologic age** is the patient's age in years and months.
- **Dental age** refers to the maturation of the teeth, including clinical eruption.

The correlation among these three factors is assessed when orthodontic treatment is planned. The occlusion depends not only on the eruption, shift, and position of the teeth but also on the skeletal growth of the mandible and the maxilla. The dental and skeletal ages can be used to make decisions about the timing of orthodontic treatment or the extraction of primary teeth. The degree of calcification and the stages of tooth development give the clinician information about abnormal sequences so that preventive measures can be taken.

Adolescence is a stage of tremendous growth and development. The timing of orthodontic treatment during adolescence must be planned carefully to take advantage of a rapid increase in the rate of growth (i.e., the growth spurt) that occurs during these years. Most orthodontists prefer to begin orthodontic treatment earlier than the adolescent years.

The skeletal age of a child is important to know because orthodontic treatment often involves manipulation of the growth of the maxilla or mandible. If the orthodontist knows that a child has a significant amount of growth remaining, treatment procedures to modify this remaining growth can be planned. However, if the orthodontist finds that the child has advanced skeletal growth for age, treatment options other than the manipulation of the growth of the jaws must be planned.

ORTHODONTIC CONSIDERATIONS[3,4]

Altered Eruption Sequence

Knowledge of eruption patterns enables the dental hygienist to recognize abnormalities that may predispose a child to orthodontic

TABLE 40.2	Examples of Common Fixed Orthodontic Appliances for Jaw Development or Expansion		
Nance Holding Appliance (NPA) passive holding device	Holds upper molars in place to stabilize their position or rotate molars.	Maintains maxillary space holding 3 and 14. Acrylic button provides additional stability.	Nance Holding Appliance (NPA). (Courtesy of Dolphin Imaging & Management Solutions [www.dolphinimaging.com].) 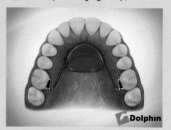
Palate Expander	Can also be removable. Requires activation by turning a key in an expansion screw.	Widens the maxilla slowly by stretching the soft cartilage of the palate over the course of months.	Palatal Expander. (Courtesy of Dolphin Imaging & Management Solutions [www.dolphinimaging.com].) 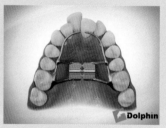
Herbst Appliance	A metal tube that connects the mandible and maxilla to create Class I occlusion.	Help the jaw develop in a forward direction by controlling the mandible's position in relation to the maxilla. Can be removable like headgear (see Removable).	Herbst Appliance. (Courtesy of Dolphin Imaging & Management Solutions [www.dolphinimaging.com].) 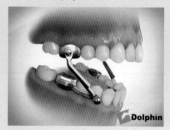
Bluegrass, Crib, or Tongue Guard Appliance	Used to block tongue thrust, train a correct swallow, or arrest thumbsucking habit.		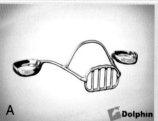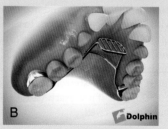(A-B) Bluegrass, Crib, or Tongue Guard Appliance. (Courtesy of Dolphin Imaging & Management Solutions [www.dolphinimaging.com].)

TABLE 40.2 Examples of Common Fixed Orthodontic Appliances for Jaw Development or Expansion—cont'd

Common Removable Appliances

Headgear	Class II correction (excess growth of maxilla/deficient growth of mandible).	Allows extrusion or intrusion of maxillary first molar.	(A–B) Headgear. (Courtesy of Dolphin Imaging & Management Solutions.)
Reverse Headgear or Protraction Facemask	Used for Class III occlusion correction (deficient growth of maxilla/excess growth of maxilla).	Accelerates maxillary growth by using the chin and forehead for support to allow the maxilla to pull ahead of the mandible.	(Courtesy of Dolphin Imaging & Management Solutions [www.dolphinimaging.com].)(A and B) Reverse Headgear or Protraction Facemask. (Courtesy of Dolphin Imaging & Management Solutions [www.dolphinimaging.com].)
Chin Cup	Normal maxilla. Prognathic mandible.	Restricts mandibular growth.	Chin Cup. (Courtesy of Dolphin Imaging & Management Solutions [www.dolphinimaging.com].)

problems. Sequence of eruption is more important than age timing. The size of permanent teeth is accommodated by the spacing of the deciduous dentition, the growth of the alveolus, and the eruption of the maxillary incisors. This understanding of development can also reassure concerned parents of patients.

Overretained Primary Teeth

Overretention of the primary teeth requires orthodontic consideration (Fig. 40.12). A permanent tooth should erupt when three-fourths of its root is completed. If the primary tooth still has significant root structure remaining at this time, it should be extracted if the permanent

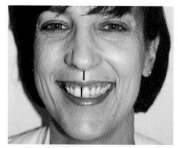

Fig. 40.5 Midline discrepancy described by the relationship of the midline of the maxilla to the philtrum. In this case, the midline of the maxilla deviates to the patient's right.

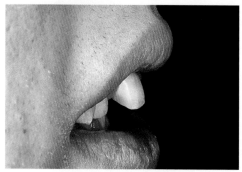

Fig. 40.6 Lip incompetence.

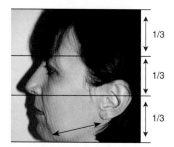

1/3

1/3

1/3

Fig. 40.7 Three zones equal height.

tooth is present. This problem typically occurs when the permanent tooth bud develops in a position that is too far lingual to the primary tooth or when a primary molar root is still intact and prevents exfoliation. Alternatively, this primary tooth may not have a replacement, because the permanent tooth is congenitally missing. A radiograph is required to make this determination.

Congenitally Missing Teeth

Congenitally missing teeth are an additional problem seen during the permanent dentition. The teeth most likely to be congenitally missing are the mandibular second premolars and the maxillary lateral incisors. Whether the condition is unilateral or bilateral, a congenitally missing tooth will cause the dental arch to develop asymmetrically, even if the primary tooth remains. Missing permanent teeth can be managed by the orthodontic closure of the space, the replacement of the tooth (or teeth) with a bridge, or the placement of a dental implant.

Early Loss of Primary Teeth

Premature primary tooth loss resulting from severe caries or trauma will create an alignment problem because existing adjacent or opposing teeth will drift into the space of the missing tooth. The loss of a tooth is considered premature if it occurs 6 months before the permanent

tooth is expected to erupt. If a primary second molar is lost prematurely and the first permanent molar tips mesially, it is possible that the permanent first molar will close all space available for the permanent second premolar. To prevent the loss of space caused by the drifting of adjacent teeth, an appliance to maintain the space of the missing tooth is used (Table 40.3).

Early primary tooth loss, however, will delay eruption of the permanent tooth because a layer of dense bone and tissue forms over the developing tooth. The permanent tooth should be given the chance to erupt on its own, but it may not do so until after the root is completely formed. The surgical excision of the overlying gingiva or forced eruption by placing an attachment on the permanent tooth may be required if the tooth fails to eventually erupt on its own.

Crowding of Mandibular Incisors

A slight space deficiency in the arch for the eruption of permanent mandibular incisors will result in mild crowding and malalignment of these teeth. A phase of slight mandibular incisor crowding is considered normal, however, until a child approaches the age of 10 years. Space then becomes available to eliminate this crowding after the mandibular canines erupt for the following reasons:

- The distance between the canines will increase slightly because the incisors erupt not only incisally but also facially, thereby increasing the length of the arch.
- The mandibular canines move distally into the **primate spaces**, naturally occurring spacing between primary teeth, thus creating more room for the alignment of the incisors. Primate spaces are located between the lateral incisors and canines on the maxilla and between the canines and first molars or canines and first premolars in the mandibular arch.
- Permanent premolars are smaller than primary molars they replace, allowing distal drift of the canines. This is called "leeway space."

If crowding of the permanent mandibular incisors is severe, these processes will not create enough space to relieve the crowding. The most common form of malocclusion, in fact, is an Angle Class I malocclusion with crowding of the incisors. Crowding in primary teeth is almost certainly indicative of crowding in permanent dentition. Growth of the alveolar processes is adequate to provide room for the permanent teeth. The permanent incisor teeth are each 2 to 3 mm larger mesiodistally than the primary incisors that they replace. See Critical Thinking Exercise box.

CRITICAL THINKING EXERCISE

Client: T.J. Langer

Profile: T.J. is a 5-year-old boy who has come with his mother for a dental hygiene appointment.

Chief Complaint: His mother is concerned that there is spacing between T.J.'s upper front teeth and between some of his lower teeth. She asks you if he will need braces to close these spaces.

Social History: T.J. lives with both parents.

Medical History: Asthma controlled by inhalers.

Dental History: On inspection, you notice that the spaces are between the maxillary lateral incisors and the canines and between the mandibular canines and first molars. You also notice that the primary second molars are in an end-to-end relationship.

Supplemental Notes: The family lives in a fluoridated community.

- What would you say to T.J.'s mother about his potential need for orthodontic treatment?

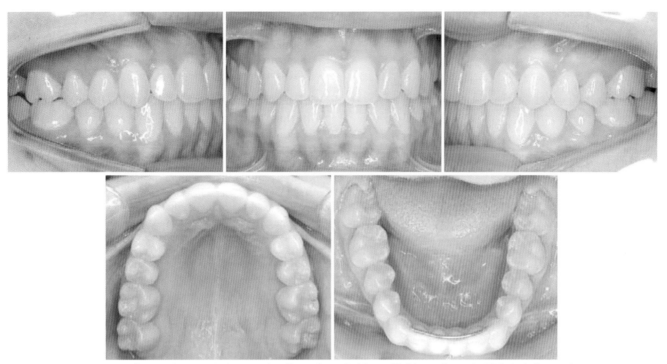

Fig. 40.8 Series of intraoral photographs. (From Saga A, Maruo IT, Maruo H, et al. Clinical challenges in treating a patient with deviated dental midlines and delayed root development of the mandibular left second premolar. *Am J Orthod Dentofacial Orthop.* 2009;135(4):S103.)

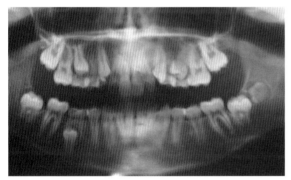

Fig. 40.9 Panoramic radiograph is taken to evaluate the dentition for the presence and location of the permanent teeth, pathology, and temporomandibular joint conditions.

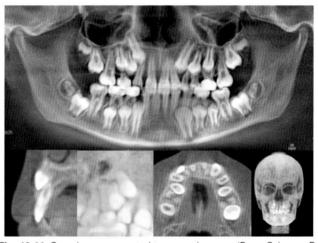

Fig. 40.11 Cone beam computed tomography scan. (From Calogero D, Alfonso M. *Orthodontics: A Review Analysis of Occlusion.* CE course. https://www.dentalcare.com/en-us/professional-education/ce-courses/ce202/panoramic-radiograph.)

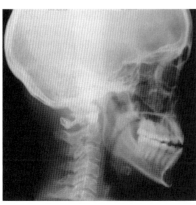

Fig. 40.10 Lateral cephalometric radiograph is taken to evaluate the impact of skeletal and dental-skeletal relationships.

Tooth Crowding

Patients with crowding during the mixed dentition may experience early loss of the primary canines. The severe crowding and malalignment of the anterior teeth cause the roots of the primary canines to be resorbed by the eruption of the permanent lateral incisors. Affected patients may be treated with expansion of the dental arches or by serial extraction therapy.

Methods for expansion of the dental arches include orthodontic and orthopedic approaches.

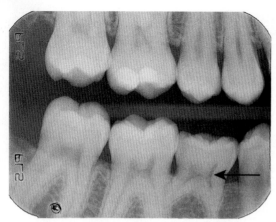

Fig. 40.12 Retained primary second molar.

The goal of **orthodontic expansion** is to widen the maxilla. At early intervention this occurs prior to palatal skeletal fusion. This skeletal expansion allows for improved stability. Once the maxillary suture has fused, **dental expansion** can produce similar broadening by tipping the crowns of the teeth facially with the use of conventional fixed appliances in addition to removable expansion appliances (Table 40.2). If the desired expansion width cannot be achieved via mechanical means, more advanced techniques (e.g., surgery) may be required. Relapse may occur after treatment because forces applied by the cheek musculature can tip the teeth back to their original lingual positions.

Orthopedic expansion is achieved by applying forces so the underlying skeletal structures can be expanded without movement or tipping of teeth within stationary alveolar bone. The goal of orthopedic expansion during the mixed dentition is to reduce the need for the extraction of permanent teeth by establishing adequate arch length and promoting an optimal skeletal relationship between the maxilla and the mandible. Various types of appliances are used for orthopedic expansion (see Table 40.2).

For children with severely crowded teeth, decisions are made during the early period of mixed dentition about whether there will be adequate space within the arches for all the permanent teeth. For patients who have a Class I molar relationship, a normal overbite, and normal skeletal relationships, **serial extraction** is a treatment option in which select teeth are extracted at planned points in time to reduce crowding during the transition from the primary dentition to the permanent dentition. Serial extraction is almost always treatment planned as extraction of a premolar in each quadrant, where the goal is to have the canines erupt in the position of the first premolars that were extracted. A second phase of fixed orthodontic therapy must also follow serial extraction. The second phase of fixed orthodontic therapy, however, can be expected to be less complex than it would have been if the extractions had not been completed.

Midline Diastema

In contrast with the crowding of mandibular incisors, spacing typically occurs in the maxillary incisors, seen as a slight diastema, or naturally occurring space between the permanent central incisors. In this phase, the maxillary incisors fan out, leaving space. If the midline diastema is 2 mm or less in size, it is likely to close as the maxillary lateral incisors and canines erupt.

Most children with a maxillary midline diastema at age 9 will have complete closure of the diastema by the age of 16 without any orthodontic intervention. If, however, the size of the diastema is more than 2 mm, total closure may not occur. A diastema of more than 2 to 3 mm in size may be caused by the following:

- A midline supernumerary tooth
- A midline soft tissue or intrabony lesion
- Missing lateral incisors
- A tooth-size discrepancy (e.g., peg lateral incisors)
- Low labial frenum attachment

Malposed and Lingual Eruption of the Permanent Anterior Teeth

The permanent maxillary and mandibular incisor tooth buds develop lingual to the existing primary teeth. As a result, the permanent mandibular incisors may erupt malposed and lingual to the primary incisors, even in children with normal spacing (Fig. 40.13). The permanent maxillary lateral incisor is also particularly prone to eruption lingual to its ideal position in the arch. The extraction of the primary canines may be needed to allow for labial positioning of the lateral incisors with an orthodontic appliance.

Impacted Canines

While the third molars are the most likely teeth to be impacted within the bone, the maxillary canine is next (Fig. 40.14). Depending on the impaction severity, the canine may erupt normally after primary canine extraction. If this is not expected to be successful, an impacted canine can be surgically exposed, bracketed, and brought into occlusion orthodontically after space in the arch has been created. The age of the patient also must be considered when making the treatment decision. The older the patient, the more likely the tooth will be ankylosed (fused to the bone), thus making orthodontic movement impossible.

Lack of Leeway Space for the Eruption of the Permanent Premolars

Exactly opposite to the situation in the permanent anterior teeth, the permanent premolar teeth are smaller than the primary molars that they replace. This additional space, called the *leeway* or *E space,* is on average 5 mm in size in the mandibular arch and 3 mm in size in the maxillary arch. When the primary second molars are lost, the first permanent molars will rapidly shift mesially into this leeway space, thereby contributing to an ideal Class I occlusion in the permanent dentition. If a problem of crowding of the permanent dentition is apparent in the child at this time (i.e., at approximately 11 years of age), the orthodontist may choose to prevent the mesial drifting of the permanent molars by maintaining the leeway space with the use of a space maintainer.

The following variations in the eruption sequence of the permanent dentition are signs of the need for early orthodontic treatment:

- Mandibular second molars erupt before the mandibular second premolars, thereby reducing the space available for the second premolars.
- Maxillary canines erupt around the same time as the maxillary premolars, thus causing the canines to be displaced labially.
- The eruption of a permanent tooth on one side without eruption of the same tooth on the other side within a 6-month time frame indicates the need to take a radiograph of the unerupted tooth to determine if some physical obstruction is present.

BIOMECHANICS OF TOOTH MOVEMENT

Although there are micromovements considered normal in our dentition, why do our teeth seem to remain stable? Equilibrium theory is an engineering theory applied in orthodontics. An object will move only if forces of unequal magnitude are applied to it. If an object remains in position, the forces acting on it must be equal in magnitude and therefore in equilibrium. The light forces of the tongue, cheeks, and lips that are applied while at rest are the most effective for determining tooth position.

TABLE 40.3 Examples of Orthodontic Appliances: Tooth Separators and Space Maintainers

Elastic Separators	Usually elastic.	Used to create mesial distal spaces to allow placement of bands.	Elastic Separators. (Courtesy of Dolphin Imaging & Management Solutions [www.dolphinimaging.com].)
Band and Loop Space Maintainer	Allows adequate room and shape for permanent tooth eruption.	Prevents space closure.	Band and Loop Space Expander. (Courtesy of Dolphin Imaging & Management Solutions [www.dolphinimaging.com].)
Lip Bumper		Used to gain mandibular anterior space. Moves molars toward the back of the mouth and allows anterior teeth to drift forward without the constant pressure from the lower lip. Can be fixed or removable.	Lip Bumper. (Courtesy of Dolphin Imaging & Management Solutions [www.dolphinimaging.com].)

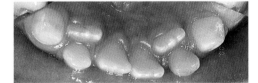

Fig. 40.13 Permanent tooth eruption lingual to primary mandibular anterior teeth.

A tooth will move when light pressure is consistently exerted on the tooth. This pressure results in bone being resorbed on the pressure side of the movement of the tooth and new bone growing in and slowly hardening behind the movement of the tooth (Fig. 40.15). This new bone holds each tooth in its new position. The duration of the force applied is more important for causing tooth movement than the strength of the force applied. To affect the position of the teeth, the force must be applied for at least 6 hours per day.

The periodontal ligament (PDL) consists of collagenous fibers, undifferentiated mesenchymal cells, and the fibroblasts and osteoblasts into which they differentiate; nerve fibers; blood vessels; and tissue fluids. These constituents function together to support the teeth during

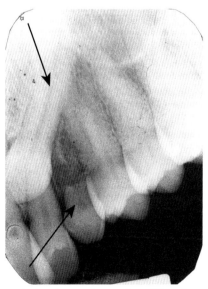

Fig. 40.14 Impacted canines and resorption of the primary canine root.

normal function, in addition to making orthodontic tooth movement possible. The PDL space is filled with the same extracellular fluid that is found in all tissues of the body. This fluid allows the PDL to function as a shock absorber during normal function.

When light, sustained force is applied to a tooth, the tooth moves in the socket within seconds, which expresses fluid from the PDL space. The PDL becomes compressed between the tooth and the alveolar wall, and pain is felt. Within a few minutes after pressure is applied, altered blood flow occurs, in addition to changes in oxygen levels and the release of cellular mediators such as prostaglandins and cytokines within the PDL. After 6 hours of sustained pressure, cellular activity in the PDL, including differentiation into osteoclasts and osteoblasts, occurs. This needed pressure explains why a force must be applied to a tooth for at least 6 hours per day to result in tooth movement.

Osteoclasts must form within the PDL to remove bone from the area adjacent to the compressed part of the PDL ahead of the movement. These osteoclasts attack the lamina dura and remove bone on the pressure side during a process called **frontal resorption**. Osteoblasts are needed to then remodel bone on the pressure side of the tooth as well as to form new bone on the side to which tension is applied. Both osteoclastic and osteoblastic activities are stimulated by prostaglandin E, an inflammatory mediator important to tooth movement.

Light and continuous forces that produce only frontal resorption are ideal. Clinically, however, it is likely even with the lightest force that some areas of PDL necrosis and undermining bone resorption will develop, temporarily weakening the base or foundation needed for tooth support. If undermining bone resorption does occur, tooth movement will occur about 10 days after activation. A period of another 10 to 14 days is then needed to allow for repair and regeneration of the PDL before force should be applied again. Based on this process, orthodontic appointments are typically made no more frequently than every 4 weeks and typically every 6 weeks to allow healing and to prevent damage to the teeth or bone that could occur.

ORTHODONTIC TREATMENT

The types of intervention are categorized into three treatment types. Phase I or early intervention, also called interceptive orthodontics, may be recommended to correct certain dental malocclusions that develop early. Some orthodontic problems such as underbites *and* crossbites, deep overbites, severe crowding, severely protruded front teeth, and narrow jaws are easier to correct at a younger age. Early intervention also can correct harmful habits such as thumbsucking, tongue thrusting, and speech problems, reducing the risk of tooth trauma to protruded front teeth. In addition, early interceptive orthodontics may help avoid the removal of permanent teeth in the final phase of orthodontic treatment and reduce the bullying caused by abnormally "crooked teeth."

Some examples of interceptive orthodontics are expansion of the upper jaw to correct a crossbite, early removal of baby teeth to facilitate the proper eruption of the permanent teeth, maintaining space for permanent teeth after a premature loss of a baby tooth, and reducing protrusion of upper front teeth to decrease the likelihood of fracture from trauma. The purpose is to fix problems that are most easily corrected at an early age and to make the future treatment easier. Early correction often leads to easier and more predictable treatment after all of the permanent teeth have erupted. Phase II, also called the corrective phase of orthodontics, is considered active treatment and is usually full braces in permanent dentition.

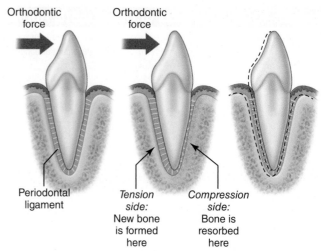

Fig. 40.15 Biomechanics of tooth movement.

To put it simply, phase I takes care of the initial structural (skeletal) corrections such as palatal expansion (see Table 40.2) so that braces can make more refined (dental) corrections and finish the job. Between phases I and II, patients may wear a retainer or space maintainer to maintain their progress (Tables 40.3 and 40.4), and they should continue visiting their orthodontist so they can check on jaw and tooth development.

Orthodontic treatment on average lasts about 24 months, depending on the severity of treatment needed. The final phase of treatment is also referred to as the retentive phase. The retention phase of treatment will last a minimum of 6 months or for years. However, permanent retention can be achieved through use of an archwire bonded directly to the lingual surfaces of anterior teeth.

ORTHODONTIC APPLIANCES

How do we artificially replicate and sustain the gentle forces needed to create the desired movement? Table 40.1 shows a variety of appliances that are used to create and sustain these forces.

Activated Archwire

The metal of the archwire is unique. Unlike traditional metals that become more malleable when warmed, the unique composite of metals in the archwire tries to revert to its original shape. When the archwire is ligated to the tooth, usually with elastomers, this constant light pressure is enough to generate the desired movements.

Plastic Tray Aligners

Very precise cast study models are taken and images are scanned into the computer. This digital model allows the patient's teeth to be replicated and manipulated digitally, and therefore corrected virtually. The clinician has the ability to view the 3D models from malocclusion to correction. The patient's treatment plan can be reviewed, movement by movement and aligner by aligner, and corrections can be made before the treatment plan is validated by the clinician. These aligners are worn about 20 hours per day and are 0.25 to 0.3 mm in thickness. The patient receives a new set of aligners every 1 to 2 weeks over the course of their treatment time. These removable aligners are not capable of treating all types of orthodontic needs and are not ideal for patients who are uncooperative with wearing them as required. However, they are more hygienic and less obvious.

TABLE 40.4 Examples of Orthodontic Appliances: Retainers and Aligners

Lingual Retainers	A stainless steel wire that is bonded to the lingual surfaces of teeth, Most commonly, mandibular anterior canine to canine.	Long-term control of orthodontic alignment, Particularly during the late growth that occurs between the ages of 16 and 20.	Lingual Retainers. (Courtesy of Dolphin Imaging & Management Solutions [www.dolphinimaging.com].)
Hawley Appliance Retainer	Worn on the maxillary arch. Consists of a thin acrylic palatal component that clasps on the molar teeth and a labial metal wire that typically surrounds the six anterior teeth and has adjustment bows at the canine.	Retains movement and prevents relapse of maxillary anterior teeth. The bow can also be adjusted to close spaces between anterior teeth that were banded.	Hawley Appliance Retainer. (Courtesy of Dolphin Imaging & Management Solutions [www.dolphinimaging.com].)
Essix Retainer	Thin plastic retainer that fully covers all maxillary teeth	Retains movement and prevents relapse.	Essix Retainer. (Courtesy of Dolphin Imaging & Management Solutions [www.dolphinimaging.com].)
Plastic Tray Aligners	A sequence of trays that apply pressure similar to the action of, and may be used in lieu of, the archwire and brackets.	Applies pressure.	Plastic Tray Aligners. (Courtesy of Dolphin Imaging & Management Solutions [www.dolphinimaging.com].)

Clear aligners have demonstrated an advantage over traditional braces in cases where there is segmented tooth movement and potentially shorter treatment duration but had disadvantages compared to braces in terms of torque control and other types of fine movements and stability.[5] It is up to an experienced provider to determine which course of treatment is best for the patient. There are many direct-to-consumer clear aligner companies that may or may not involve a dental professional, let alone an orthodontic specialist. While there is no "one size fits all" approach to orthodontics, orthodontic treatment involves the movement of biological material, which could lead to potentially irreversible and expensive damage such as tooth breakage and or tooth gingival tissue loss, incorrect occlusion, TMJ concerns, and other issues if not done correctly. As well, there may be underlying issues involved in correction beyond simple tooth movement. Therefore it is highly recommended that a patient consult with a properly trained professional.

ORTHODONTIC EFFECTS AND TREATMENT RISKS

Effects of Orthodontic Force on the Maxilla

The sites of maxillary growth where growth modification may be effective are the sutures where the maxilla is attached to the cranium and the midpalatine suture area. To counter excessive maxillary growth, forces would be applied to oppose the natural soft tissue forces that place tension on and separate the craniofacial sutures. To treat deficient growth, forces would be applied to enhance the natural forces that stimulate maxillary growth.

Extraoral headgear appliances are used to restrain maxillary growth (see Table 40.2). The appliance must be worn at least 8 hours per day, and wearing it for 12 to 14 hours per day is preferable. Physiologic reasons exist for wearing headgear at night. More growth hormone is secreted in children at night than during the day. The growth of the long bones of the body has been found to be greater at night than during the day. Although it is not known if facial bones grow in the same pattern, it is reasonable to expect that they do. As a result, the use of headgear to modify skeletal growth is more effective at night than during the day.

Effects of Orthodontic Force on the Teeth and the Periodontium

Constant resorption and repair of dentin and cementum occur during orthodontic movement. Cementum and dentin are removed during periods of force application and replaced by cementum during periods of rest. As a result, the tooth root is remodeled during optimal orthodontic tooth movement in the same manner as alveolar bone is remodeled. Remodeling, however, will not occur if more serious damage develops, such as the damage that may occur at the root apex, where portions of cementum or dentin may actually break away from the root. These portions will be resorbed by the body and will not be replaced. The permanent loss of root structure occurs only at the root apex. This apical root resorption appears radiographically as a loss in the length and apical blunting of the root (Fig. 40.16). Some loss of root length will occur in almost every individual who is treated orthodontically, and this is usually of little clinical significance. At times, however, the severe loss of one-third to one-half of the root length occurs from even routine orthodontic tooth movement. Although the cause of this type of resorption is not clear, some individuals are found to be more prone to resorption than others. The use of low-force wires has reduced the occurrence of root resorption when they are placed low on the teeth and move the teeth slowly. The maxillary and mandibular incisors are the most frequently affected teeth.

Orthodontic therapy is not associated with an increase in the loss of alveolar bone. The only situation in which bone loss is exacerbated by orthodontic tooth movement is when teeth are moved in a patient who has active periodontal infection. When periodontal disease has been controlled before and during orthodontic treatment, improved tooth position and placement will actually improve the osseous contours as well. This improvement is demonstrated by the uprighting of mesially drifted second molars to allow for the construction of crown and bridge prostheses. As the tooth is uprighted during orthodontic treatment, the osseous contours on the mesial aspect of the tooth are improved because the crestal bone is uprighted along with the tooth (Fig. 40.17).

Increased tooth mobility is expected during orthodontic treatment. PDL fibers become disorganized and detached from the bone and the root cementum, and the adjacent bone must remodel. Radiographs taken during treatment will reveal widened PDL spaces. However, excessive mobility may be an indication that too much force is being applied, thereby causing too much undermining bone resorption. If a tooth becomes extremely mobile during therapy, all force

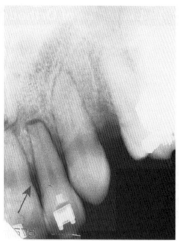

Fig. 40.16 Apical root resorption.

should be discontinued until the mobility is reduced to moderate levels. Usually, this problem can be corrected without causing permanent damage.

Pain is the result of the development of ischemic areas within the PDL. Tenderness with the chewing of firm foods is caused by the mild pulpitis that occurs and by inflammation at the tooth apex. The greater the force applied to the tooth, the greater the amount of pain expected because larger areas within the PDL will undergo sterile necrosis. If light forces are applied, painful symptoms can be relieved by having the patient chew gum during the first 8 hours after the adjustment. Chewing temporarily displaces the teeth enough to allow some blood flow through the compressed areas of the PDL, thereby preventing the buildup of metabolites that stimulate pain receptors.

Gingival Recession

When the arch is expanded by labial movement of the teeth to relieve crowding problems (see Table 40.2), the risk of gingival recession is increased. Labial movement of the teeth may result in the development of a dehiscence in the bone. The labial gingiva becomes thin, and recession begins. Recession can progress rapidly if the labial keratinized gingiva is thin or nonexistent (Fig. 40.18).

Nonkeratinized Tissue

Aphthous ulcers or other soft tissue lesions can result from the friction of the braces rubbing against the soft tissue of the mouth, or a broken wire. In these cases, wax can be dispensed to patients to protect this softer tissue.

Gingival Inflammation and Overgrowth

While rare, a patient may experience an acute mucosal reaction due to hypersensitivity or allergy to metals used in orthodontic treatment. The most common cause is nickel.[6] A common presentation of this reaction is the presence of a lichenoid plaque on the buccal mucosa adjacent to the offending antigen.[7] Even more unusual would be a cutaneous display.

More commonly, the typical chronic inflammatory condition that arises is periodontal inflammation, which causes teeth to move more slowly. Keeping the soft tissues healthy can prevent prolonging treatment time. In addition, successful nonsurgical management of severe postorthodontic gingival enlargement and erythema consists of intensive periodontal therapy, consisting of oral hygiene instruction, scaling, and periodontal debridement, and by targeting the primary etiologic factor—bacterial biofilm—so periodontal health can

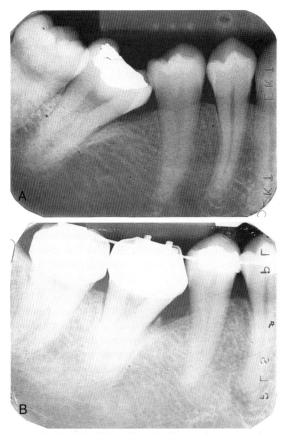

Fig. 40.17 (A) Mesial drifting of tooth No. 31 into extraction space. Note the bony defect on tooth No. 31. (B) Note the improvement in the contour of the alveolar bone near tooth No. 31 mesial as the tooth is uprighted.

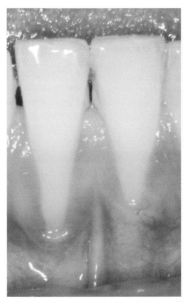

Fig. 40.18 Gingival recession on teeth Nos. 24 and 25. (From Chatzopoulou D, Johal A. Management of gingival recession in the orthodontic patient. *Semin Orthod.* 2015;21(1):15–26. Copyright © 2015 Elsevier, Inc.)

be restored without the need for surgical intervention. Reducing the bacterial load will give the biologic natural healing capacity of the body the opportunity to stabilize the periodontal condition and, thus should be considered as the first line of intervention before a surgical approach

is taken. However, if unresolved, surgical measures such as excision and resection of overgrown tissue to restore a biologically correct and maintainable tissue are indicated (Fig. 40.19).

Decalcified Enamel or "White Spot" Lesions

Occurring under and adjacent to orthodontic bands and brackets, the white spot lesion (WSL) is early caries (Fig. 40.20). These early lesions may be reversible after appliances are removed, especially if the lesion has a smooth surface. If the lesion is visible only when the tooth is dried, it likely involves the enamel only. If the WSL is visible without drying, demineralization has progressed deeper within the enamel, although a relatively intact outer enamel surface remains. A sharp explorer should not be used to probe the intact surface of a WSL, because the intact outer surface may be broken by the explorer, thereby requiring restoration of the lesion. If the lesion continues to progress, the outer surface will break down and form an open carious lesion.

Pulp

Properly applied orthodontic forces will, at most, minimally affect the dental pulp. A mild transient pulpitis may occur and is usually experienced by patients as discomfort during the first few days after appliances are **activated** (i.e., adjusted to apply desired pressures). Occasionally, however, a loss of pulpal vitality may occur during orthodontic treatment, with poor control.

Retention and Relapse

The elastic gingival fibers contribute to the equilibrium of forces applied to the teeth. When stretched into new positions by the orthodontic movement of teeth, these fibers, especially the transseptal fibers, will contribute to the teeth relapsing back into their original positions after treatment completion. A periodontal surgical procedure completed to incise the gingival fibers (i.e., fibrotomy) and/or the placement of a permanent wire retainer bonded to the lingual surfaces of the anterior teeth can prevent the relapse of teeth after orthodontic movement (see Table 40.4).

Retention of the teeth after orthodontic treatment is necessary for the following reasons:
- Gingival and periodontal tissues need time to reorganize after the appliances are removed.
- Soft tissue pressures from the tongue, lips, and cheeks may contribute to relapse if the musculature has not had time to adapt to the new occlusion and if tooth position is unstable.
- Skeletal growth can continue to affect the occlusion as it did before treatment, depending on the age of the patient.

Sufficient time for the reorganization of the gingival and periodontal tissues is necessary because orthodontic tooth movement causes widening of the PDL and disruption of the supporting collagen fibers. This change in the PDL is evidenced clinically by the mobility of the teeth that are present when appliances are removed. The teeth are not only mobile at treatment completion but also susceptible to displacement as a result of forces applied by the surrounding soft tissues and the occlusion. Reorganization of the periodontium takes 3 to 4 months and can occur only when each tooth is able to respond individually to the forces of mastication. Retainers should be worn full time for the first 3 to 4 months after treatment and removed during eating only (see Table 40.4). The natural flexion of the individual teeth during eating will encourage periodontal tissue remodeling and a reduction in tooth mobility. If a fixed retainer is placed, it should not be so rigid that the natural flexion of teeth within the alveolar process cannot occur.

Retention after the correction of severe malalignments should be continued for at least 12 months because of the slow remodeling of the gingival fibers. After 3 to 4 months, however, removable retainers are not required on a full-time basis. Permanent retention may be required for teeth that are not able to tolerate the forces of the lips, cheeks, and tongue. For patients who are still growing, retention should be maintained until growth has stopped. The dental hygienist must encourage the patient to follow strictly the orthodontist's recommendations for the use of retainers. If any indication of relapse is noted, the patient must be referred to the orthodontist.

Orthodontic relapse can occur because adult skeletal growth is a process that continues throughout life. Facial growth in adults follows the same growth pattern that is seen in adolescents. Although the magnitude of change that occurs each year in the adult is small, the cumulative effect over the decades is significant. The growth patterns that contributed to a malocclusion in the first place continue into adulthood and can contribute to the relapse of orthodontic treatment results. Adult patients may express discouragement about the relapse that can result after years of wearing braces as a teenager and may attribute it to inadequate orthodontic treatment.[3]

WORKING COLLABORATIVELY WITH OTHER ORAL HEALTHCARE PROVIDERS

Use of Orthodontics for Periodontal and Restorative Treatment

Working collaboratively with a periodontist or other practitioner, the orthodontist can establish an environment that will ultimately house an aesthetic and functional restoration. Periodontal factors, such as the width and height of bone and the shape of the gingiva, are all considerations in periodontal care that can be treated in a multidisciplinary approach collaborating with an orthodontist. Orthodontics can enhance hard and soft tissue volume and height.

This benefit is useful when collaborating for restorative fixed prosthetics. Orthodontics can provide a means to a more robust foundation for natural or implanted teeth as well as improve the aesthetic outcomes of restorative and cosmetic procedures or osseous defects (Fig. 40.21). For example, uprighting molars can improve defect(s) and allow space for easier maintenance of periodontal health.

Implant Site Development

The quality and quantity of alveolar bone and gingival tissues in potential implant recipient sites is a major determinant of the long-term prognosis of the implant fixture (See Chapter 31—Dental Implants and Peri-implant Care). The primary stability of a dental implant is directly related to the amount of alveolar bone available at the time of implant placement. Implants should be placed in preexisting bone and can be supported by regenerative bone, either allograft or autogenous transplant. However, if the alveolar ridge is insufficient, orthodontic forces may be applied to the site to generate bone and create more ideal bone for the implant recipient site, especially in the anterior region, where aesthetics play a major role in treatment planning.

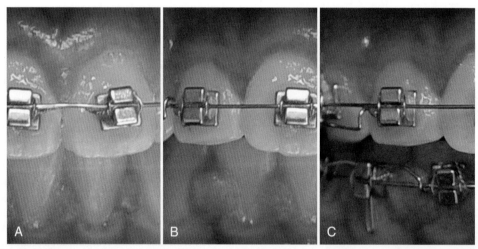

Fig. 40.19 Gingival overgrowth in orthodontics. (A) Mild, (B) moderate, and (C) severe. (From Gong Y, Lu J, Ding X. Clinical, microbiologic, and immunologic factors of orthodontic treatment-induced gingival enlargement. *Am J Orthod Dentofac Orthop.* 2011;140(1):58–64. Copyright © 2011 American Association of Orthodontists.)

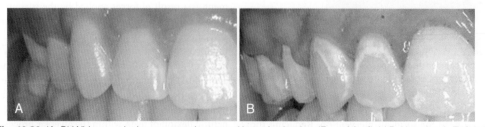

Fig. 40.20 (A–B) White spot lesions on anterior caused by orthodontics. (From Maxfield B, Hamdan A, Tüfekçi E, et al. Development of white spot lesions during orthodontic treatment: perceptions of patients, parents, orthodontists, and general dentists. *Am J Orthod Dentofac Orthop.* 2012;141(3):337–344. Copyright © 2012 American Association of Orthodontists.)

If a hopeless tooth is orthodontically extruded before it is extracted, the extrusion can improve marginal bone levels before implant placement. This also improves the aesthetics of the gingival margin after placement (Fig. 40.22).

Orofacial Myology and Speech Therapy

An orthodontist may also work with an orofacial myologist, who is trained to recognize orofacial myofunctional disorders (OMDs) and can provide individualized therapy for nasal breathing, tongue rest position, and correct swallowing. Because of the nature of OMDs, several orofacial structures and processes can be affected, including proper palatal formation, dental occlusion, facial growth and development, breathing, sleeping, speech, and swallowing patterns (see Table 40.2). Treatment for many OMDs exists in the form of orofacial myofunctional therapy (OMT), which typically consists of retraining exercises for the lips, tongue, or facial muscles, as well as behavior modification or elimination. The goal of OMT is to correct improper orofacial muscle movements and postures and to restore natural functioning. The role of the dental hygienist is to identify these patterns early in development in order to make appropriate referrals. Some dental hygienists also have training and certification in OMT.

A speech pathologist could assess for atypical orofacial functions and initiate speech therapy, if needed. As with any myofunctional program, patient and family willingness and adherence to treatment and self-care recommendations are important to assess before initiation.

Autogenous Transplantation

Dental autotransplantation or autogenous transplantation is defined as the surgical repositioning of one tooth from one position to another,

within the same person. This procedure could involve the transfer of impacted, embedded, or erupted teeth into extraction sites or into surgically prepared sockets.

In specific clinical situations, when extraction is orthodontically indicated or supernumerary teeth are present, donor teeth may be used for transplantations, avoiding prosthetic or implant therapy. Because placement of osseointegrated implants is contraindicated when alveolar bone is growing, transplantation of available teeth remains a suitable choice for replacing missing teeth in the young patient.

Autotransplantation of teeth has been widely used in young patients, most commonly in cases of severe impactions, early loss of permanent teeth, or congenital aplasia.[8] A tooth with incomplete root development and maintained PDL that has the capability of further growth promotes alveolar bone development in the receptor area. The stage of root development and the size of the crown of a donor tooth are considered. In the case of maxillary incisors, the teeth most frequently involved in trauma, a mandibular first or second premolar appropriate in mesiodistal dimension might be used to replace a lost central incisor. Later, an adequate reconstruction of the crown with composite resin or an artificial crown to resemble normal anatomy is needed. Then, resulting space can be closed orthodontically. Most frequently, a wisdom tooth is transferred to the site of a hopeless molar because of its late development compared to the other teeth.

The Role of the Dental Hygienist in Orthodontic Treatment

The satisfaction of successful completion of orthodontic treatment can be diminished by the presence of periodontal or restorative treatment needs that can arise with lack of effective oral hygiene. The Hippocratic Oath and the ethical principle of nonmaleficence require practitioners to address these potential periodontal or restorative issues as priorities over correcting malocclusions. See Box 40.2, which outlines legal, ethical, and safety issues related to the dental hygienist's role in orthodontic therapy.

After initial referral and throughout active treatment, the patient must continue to have comprehensive oral examinations. In fact, some patients may need to appoint with the hygienist more frequently if they have difficulty managing their self-care. Alternatively, some orthodontists employ a dental hygienist to assist with biofilm management and promote self-care. Orthodontic care is truly a partnership with the referring practitioner, the patient, and, for minors, parents/caregivers. It is important for professional dental hygiene care to be coordinated with orthodontic appointments (Box 40.3).

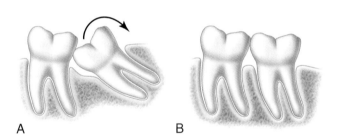

Fig. 40.21 (A–B) Uprighting a molar to improve the contour of the alveolar bone. (From Bathla S. *Textbook of Periodontics*. Jaypee Brothers Medical Publishers; 2017. http://www.jpmedpub.com/bookdetails.aspx?SearchTxt=periodontics&OBookID=2413.)

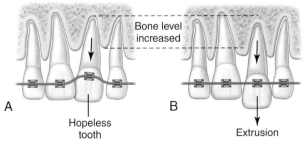
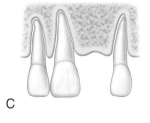
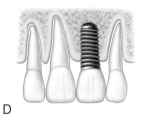

Fig. 40.22 (A) Hopeless tooth identified as needing extraction. (B) Tooth is orthodontically extruded. (C) Tooth is extracted. (D) Implant is placed to replace missing tooth. (From Bathla S. *Textbook of Periodontics*. Jaypee Brothers Medical Publishers; 2017. http://www.jpmedpub.com/bookdetails.aspx?SearchTxt=periodontics&OBookID=2413.)

(see Chapter 24—Toothbrushing, and Chapter 25—Interdental and Supplemental Oral Self-Care Devices).

BOX 40.2 Legal, Ethical, and Safety Issues

- The ethical principle of beneficence requires comprehensive oral health services throughout the process of dental hygiene care.
- The ethical principle of autonomy requires a dental hygienist to carefully consider options for self-care and oral hygiene aids and to involve the client(s) as cotherapist(s) in the selection and management of appropriate regimens and devices.
- The dental hygienist or receptionist maintains communication with the orthodontic office regarding mutual patients, or coordinates that communication with the receptionist. In this communication, the orthodontist is advised of the date of the last appointment with the dental hygienist for oral assessment and preventive care, any changes in the health history, any changes in the patient's oral health, dental care recommended or completed, recommendations provided for self-care including oral hygiene and home-use fluoride, and any problems with the orthodontic appliances noted (e.g., loose brackets or bands, wires impinging on tissues). Any radiographs taken also need to be transmitted electronically to the orthodontist's office.
- The dental hygienist carefully evaluates young patients to identify malocclusions that might benefit from early orthodontic intervention and brings any findings to the attention of the collaborating dentist and parents or caregivers. Failure to note such malocclusions could result in the need for more lengthy orthodontic treatment with less favorable results; therefore it violates the ethical principle of nonmaleficence.
- When seeing a patient for maintenance visits after orthodontic therapy has been completed, the dental hygienist continually evaluates the dentition for retention or relapse. If any areas of relapse in the malocclusion are noted, the patient, dentist, or orthodontists, as appropriate, must be advised and the patient referred back to the orthodontist for evaluation.
- The law requires thorough and accurate documentation of all dental hygiene care provided as well as any client education, observations about adherence to recommendations, and referrals.

BOX 40.3 Planning Dental Hygiene Visits With Orthodontic Appointments

Several hours after an appliance is activated during an orthodontic visit, a patient may feel a mild aching sensation and sensitivity to pressure, so chewing a hard food is painful. This pain will likely last for 2 to 4 days and then disappear until the appliance is again adjusted. Pain after orthodontic adjustments varies among individuals. Pain levels and tolerance vary among patients. When planning dental hygiene appointments with patients who are undergoing orthodontic treatment, it is generally more comfortable for a patient to be seen *before rather than immediately after* orthodontic adjustments. Scaling procedures are particularly uncomfortable for teeth that are already painful as a result of an orthodontic adjustment.

During the dental hygiene visit, in addition to thorough plaque control and self-care instruction, the orthodontic patient should undergo additional assessment to evaluate the environment of the appliances. Examples of these additional assessments include noting soft or hard tissue trauma due to ill-fitting appliances, as well as evaluation of tooth mobility or orthodontic appliance mobility. Appliance bond failure can be detected by gently rocking each tooth with the blunt handle ends of two instruments. Remember, failed cement seals can lead to caries under the band or bracket. The dental hygienist should know the directions for oral hygiene and care and use of removable appliances, so these directions can be reinforced with the patient as well as answering questions the patient or parent may have

ORAL HYGIENE AND ORAL HEALTH EDUCATION CONSIDERATIONS

The most difficult area for an orthodontic patient to keep clean is the area from the bracket to the gingival margin; this is above and beyond the typical interproximal challenges. Although it has been stated that fixed orthodontics do not cause periodontal damage if basic principles are followed and patients are compliant with good oral hygiene, a significant percentage of orthodontic patients experience oral hygiene challenges and demonstrate adverse effects from poor biofilm control during treatment.

Consequences of poor oral hygiene and nonadherence to self-care recommendations during orthodontic treatment affect the quality of the end result. In addition, these behaviors prolong treatment times. This information might serve as a motivation for orthodontic patients.

Self-care is challenging enough in the general population, but it is especially challenging for the adolescent population, which comprises the majority of patients being treated. During orthodontic treatment, there are so many more obstacles requiring attention that slacking on homecare has far worse consequences than in nonorthodontic populations. The introduction of fixed orthodontic appliances induces a rapid increase in the volume and composition of biofilm as well as periodontal indices. The two main therapeutic challenges the orthodontic patient faces are caries and poor gingival health. Inflammation and persistent gingivitis are common and can lead to gingival overgrowth and contribute to periodontal breakdown.

The presence of fixed orthodontic appliances places patients in a moderate- to high-risk category for caries (see Chapter 19). The patient is considered to be at moderate risk for dental caries simply as a result of the presence of fixed orthodontic appliances alone, even if the patient has had neither incipient nor cavitated caries during the past 3 years. The presence of dental caries in the orthodontic patient who also has additional risk factors such as poor oral hygiene, nonfluoridated water, or xerostomia places the patient at high risk for experiencing further dental caries.[9]

After 3 months, with good oral hygiene, caries risk can stabilize due to host microbial reestablishment. However, if left unchanged, poor oral hygiene can increase the risk for both periodontal and carious breakdown.[3,4] If the patient is not able or willing to maintain good oral care, the braces may have to be removed and treatment delayed.

Effective oral hygiene regimens should include at least several of the following interventions:

- Mechanical biofilm management devices: brushing, interdental cleaning aids, oral irrigation, regular preventive dental hygiene care
- Pharmacotherapeutic:
  - Fluoride to prevent caries
  - Antimicrobials to reduce pathogens associated with caries and periodontal disease
- Sealants and placement of fluoride-containing glass ionomer cements under bands
- Nutritional counseling
- Motivational communication

Mechanical Biofilm Control

A variety of toothbrush designs are available. For example, one style includes brushes with middle rows of bristles that are shorter to allow the bracket to fit easily while the outer bristles reach the enamel and gingiva. Manual brushes are helpful tools to remove biofilm. Electric toothbrushes are a good idea for nearly any patient and particularly so for orthodontic patients. The use of an electric toothbrush

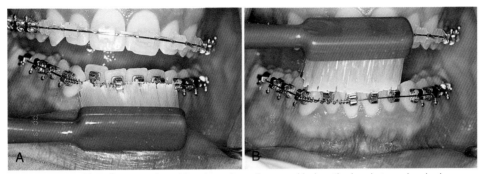

Fig. 40.23 Use of a manual toothbrush to clean above and below the brackets and archwire.

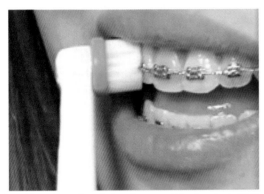

Fig. 40.24 Use of an electric brush around the bracket. (OrthoEssentials, © 2018 Procter & Gamble Company, Cincinnati, Ohio.)

is recommended. An electric toothbrush with the orthodontic head and interdental tip is more effective at controlling plaque biofilm as well as helping patients brush for the recommended 2 minutes. In addition, electric toothbrushes may promote gingival health better than manual toothbrushes in orthodontic patients (Figs. 40.23 and 40.24).[9,10]

Interdental cleaning presents a particular challenge for the patient with fixed appliances. Various oral hygiene aids were detailed in Chapter 25. Superfloss, Gumchucks, and Platypus are all brand-name products that make flossing under the archwire easier. If the patient has large cervical embrasures as a result of a history of periodontal disease, or because of the stage of orthodontic movement, electric or manual interproximal brushes may be more effective for biofilm control. Interdental cleaning devices are an alternative aid for interproximal biofilm removal (Figs. 40.25 and 40.26). Patients often find a dental water jet easier to use than floss or other interdental aids, and a special low-power orthodontic tip is available for the water jet and should be used. The irrigating stream should be directed perpendicularly to the long axis of the tooth rather than into the gingival sulcus. For young patients, teaching the parents to assist with oral hygiene around the child's appliances is recommended.

When orthodontic treatment is planned prior to placement and fabrication of a fixed prosthetic, it is often necessary to place a fixed retainer or space maintainer between abutments to maintain the pontic space. The same aids used for plaque biofilm removal around fixed retainers on the anterior teeth can be used around the wires that retain the pontic space.

Antimicrobial Agents for Biofilm Control

During active therapy and post debonding, regular twice-daily topical application of stannous or sodium fluoride over-the-counter

dentifrice and rinse is recommended for caries prevention. Stabilized stannous fluoride dentifrice delivers additional benefits compared to sodium fluoride because the stannous ion serves as an antimicrobial agent for its antigingivitis effect. Evidence exists to support stannous fluoride dentifrices in reducing inflammation. A systematic review comparing gluconate chelated stannous fluoride to NaF or MFP demonstrated a 51% reduction in gingival bleeding in 3 months when using stannous fluoride,[10] while another meta-nalysis found 83% less enamel surface loss with the use of stannous fluoride versus arginine or NaF,[11] both of which are common needs for orthodontic patients.

Evidence supports the use of mechanical biofilm control combined with antimicrobial dentifrices or mouth rinses to achieve better antiplaque and antigingivitis outcomes than mechanical biofilm control on its own (see Chapter 27). The rinses with strong evidence supporting antiplaque efficacy contain chlorhexidine, essential oils with an antiseptic formulation, and cetylpyridinium chloride (CPC).

Fluoride Recommendations

Clinical practice guidelines by the ADA regarding professionally applied and prescription-strength, home-use topical fluoride agents were based on a systematic review of fluoride used for caries prevention including varnishes, gels, foams, and pastes.[12] For caries risk, 2.26% fluoride varnish or 1.23% APF gel, or a prescription-strength, home-use 0.5% fluoride gel or paste or 0.09% sodium fluoride mouth rinse for patients aged 6 years or older were recommended. Only 2.26% fluoride varnish was recommended for children younger than 6 years of age.[13]

To prevent demineralization of enamel and resultant WSLs during orthodontics, daily use of a 5000-ppm fluoride toothpaste may be recommended.[14] Moderate evidence, based on a single study, also exists to support fluoride varnish applied every 6 weeks during fixed orthodontic treatment for the prevention of early decay or demineralized white lesions.[15] Once the WSLs occur and are detected during or following orthodontic therapy, the monthly use of fluoride varnish and casein phosphopeptide–amorphous calcium phosphate (CPP-ACP) can help to ameliorate WSL.[16] Prevention of WSLs is the best approach. Because regular dental hygiene visits are recommended throughout orthodontic therapy for oral assessment and preventive services, oral hygiene, antimicrobial, and fluoride recommendations can be reinforced and monitored.

The demand for tooth whitening has grown exponentially over the past 20 years, and 90% of requests by patients in the United States are made to orthodontists.[17] The dental hygienist might encounter this request, as most orthodontists refer their patients to the general dental practice for this service. When effectiveness and stability are desired, tooth whitening should be recommended after completion

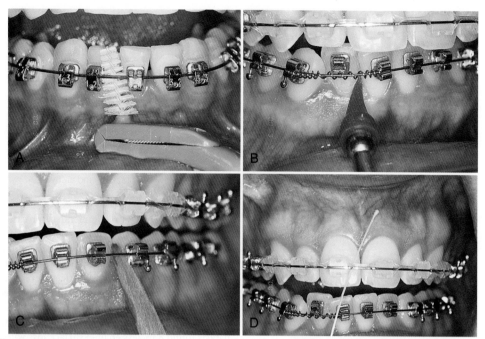

Fig. 40.25 (A) Use of an interdental brush to clean around brackets. (B) Use of a rubber-tip stimulator to disrupt plaque and to massage the papillae. (C) Use of a wooden wedge to remove plaque and stimulate gingiva. (D) Use of a floss threader to place floss under the archwire.

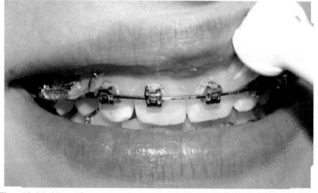

Fig. 40.26 Use of an electric rechargeable toothbrush with an interdental tip. (Hillmann C. Orthodontics 101 for the Dental Professional. CE course No. 413. https://www.dentalcare.com/en-us/professional-education/ce-courses/ce413.)

of orthodontic treatment. If patients request whitening during orthodontic treatment, **it should be discouraged**. Whitening while in orthodontics may results in bracket detachment, loss of enamel color uniformity revealed after fixed orthodontic appliances are removed.

The patient should be informed of possible risks, and frequent professional oral assessment and fluoride varnish treatments should be recommended.

Dietary Counseling

Because plaque biofilm control is more difficult for the patient who wears fixed orthodontic appliances, sugar and sticky carbohydrate intake should be minimized during the period of active treatment. If sweets are eaten, they should be eaten as part of a meal to limit the number of acid attacks throughout the day. The dental hygienist informs the patient that foods that cannot be removed from the fixed orthodontic appliances may lead to dental caries, white spots, and unattractive food debris accumulation. In high-risk patients, a more formalized approach to dietary counseling may be needed (see Chapter 36).

Motivational Communication

It has been stated that the value of treatment is significantly compromised without an efficient patient self-care routine to control plaque levels. Therefore it is imperative that behavior management is seen as a part of both prevention and therapy of periodontal diseases. While there is not a one-size-fits-all approach, it is well documented that traditional paternalistic teaching or lecturing puts the patient in a reactive versus proactive approach.[18] The clinician's role is to guide or coach their patients. This is covered in more detail in Chapter 5—Sustainable Health Behavior Change.

Questions that are open-ended and allow patients to create their own solutions can aid compliance (see Chapter 5). Patients might also be asked to rate their own oral health at each visit to assess their own perceptions in relation to actual oral assessment findings (Fig. 40.27). Oral hygiene and health as well as any instructions for care should be recorded at each visit.

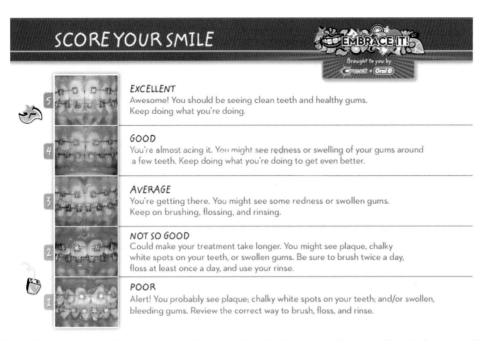

Fig. 40.27 System for patient scoring of their own oral health. (Courtesy of Procter & Gamble Company, Cincinnati, Ohio. From Hillmann C: *Ortho 101 for the Dental Professional*. CE course No. 413, last updated June 10, 2020. www.dentalcare.com/en-us/professional-education/ce-courses/.)

KEY CONCEPTS

- Evaluation of the occlusion includes not only the relationship of the teeth to one another as categorized by Angle I, II, and III classifications but also the skeletal relationship of the maxilla and mandible to each other.
- Children's skeletal development as well as their chronologic age must be determined in order to take advantage of growth modification procedures. Such procedures are most effective when applied during the preadolescent growth spurt. Growth modification can be used to restrain maxillary growth, enhance mandibular growth, and/or expand the palate to correct transverse discrepancies and create more space within the arch.
- The sequence of tooth eruption is more important than the date of eruption. In the primary dentition, spacing is preferred. Primate and developmental spaces provide room for the developing permanent teeth. A lack of space in the primary dentition indicates that the permanent dentition will be crowded.
- Tooth development and eruption of the permanent teeth occurs as a result of cellular activities within the periodontal ligament. Eruption is a process that continues at various rates throughout life. The primary dentition plays a critical role in the optimal eruption of the permanent teeth.
- The position of the teeth within the dental arches is affected by an equilibrium of forces applied by the tongue, cheeks, and lips while at rest, the elastic gingival fibers, and the periodontal ligament. The duration of the force applied is more important in determining tooth position than the strength of the force.
- Light, sustained orthodontic forces result in optimal tooth movement through a process of frontal resorption. Heavy forces result in some necrosis of the periodontal ligament followed by undermining resorption, a process that will delay tooth movement 7 to 14 days.
- Orthodontic treatment planning is a complex process that must take into consideration a patient's chief complaint. It also is based on the clinical judgment and experience of the orthodontist. It may be impossible to achieve all orthodontic goals. The dental hygienist must be aware of this potential limitation when seeing a patient for maintenance after treatment has been completed.

- Properly applied orthodontic forces will affect the dental pulp, cementum, and dentin to a minimal degree. Apical root resorption occurs in almost all orthodontic cases, but it is usually not clinically significant.
- Orthodontic brackets are made of metal, ceramic, or plastic material and are attached directly to the teeth through bonding or attached to stainless steel bands that are cemented around the teeth.
- Comprehensive orthodontic treatment consists of three phases: leveling and alignment, correction of molar relationships and space closure, and finishing and settling of the occlusion.
- Client education, including the patient and the parent or caregiver, is particularly important during orthodontic therapy. The dental hygienist must help the client develop skill in removing plaque biofilm from around the orthodontic appliances as well as in understanding the treatment procedures that are needed to ensure an optimal result.
- The dental hygienist plays a key role in preparing the patient for orthodontic treatment as well as maintaining the client's oral health during and after orthodontic treatment. The dental hygienist may complete data collection procedures, including taking the medical and personal histories, completing periodontal and dental chartings, taking radiographs, and preparing study models.
- For the orthodontic patient with active periodontal disease, the dental hygienist must complete periodontal debridement and provide daily self-care education to eliminate infection and restore health at home.
- For the orthodontic patient with caries risk, the dental hygienist must complete through biofilm removal and discuss at-home biofilm control, as well as offer daily self-care education and product usage recommendations.
- During treatment, the client must be seen regularly by the dental hygienist for clinical maintenance procedures and followup on homecare recommendations.

ACKNOWLEDGMENTS

The author wishes to acknowledge the former chapter authors, Lee-ann Branscome Simmons, BSDH, MS, and Margaret M. Walsh and Denise Bowen, in addition to Dr. Greg Asatrian as SME for content review.

REFERENCES

1. American Association of Orthodontists Consumer website. Available at: https://www3.aaoinfo.org/blog/when-should-your-child-see-an-orthodontist/. Accessed Dec 29, 2022.
2. Tanaka L, Dezan C, Chadi S, et al. The influence of asthma onset and severity on malocclusion prevalence in children and adolescents. [serial online] *Dental Press J Orthod.* 2012;17(1):50–51. Accessed August 15, 2017. Available from: Dentistry & Oral Sciences Source, Ipswich, MA.
3. Graber TM, Vanorsdall RL, Vig KWL, et al. *Orthodontics: Current Principles and Techniques.* 6th ed. Mosby; 2016.
4. Proffit WR, Fields HW, Larson B, Sarver DM. *Contemporary Orthodontics.* 4th ed. Mosby; 2018.
5. Ke Y, Zhu Y, Zhu M. A comparison of treatment effectiveness between clear aligner and fixed appliance therapies. *BMC Oral Health.* 2019;19(1):24.
6. Schultz JC, Connelly E, Glesne L, Warshaw EM. Cutaneous and oral eruption from oral exposure to nickel in dental braces. *Dermatitis.* 2004;15(3):154–157.
7. Zigante M, Rincic Mlinaric M, Kastelan M, Perkovic V, Trinajstic Zrinski M, Spalj S. Symptoms of titanium and nickel allergic sensitization in orthodontic treatment. *Prog Orthod.* 2020;21(1):17.
8. Ali FM, Kahn MI, Kota Z, et al. Autotransplantation of teeth: a review. *Am J Med Dent Sci.* 2013;1(1):25–30.
9. Al Makhmari SA, Kaklamanos EG, Athenasiou AE. Short-term and long-term effectiveness of powered toothbrushes in promoting periodontal health during orthodontic treatment: a systematic review and meta-analysis. *Am J Orthod Dentofacial Orthop.* 2017;152(6):753–766.e7.
10. Biesbrock A, He T, DiGennaro J, Zou Y, Ramsey D, Garcia-Godoy F. The effects of bioavailable gluconate chelated stannous fluoride dentifrice on gingival bleeding: meta-analysis of eighteen randomized controlled trials. *J Clin Periodontol.* 2019.
11. West NX, He T, Zou Y, DiGennaro J, Biesbrock A, Davies M. Bioavailable gluconate chelated stannous fluoride toothpaste meta-analyses: effects on dentine hypersensitivity and enamel erosion. *J Dent.* 2021.
12. Sälzer S, Slot DE, Dörfer CE, et al. Comparison of triclosan and stannous fluoride dentifrices on parameters of gingival inflammation and plaque scores: a systematic review and metaanalysis. *Int J Dent Hyg.* 2015;13:1–17.
13. Weyant RJ, Tracy SL, Anselmo T, et al. Topical fluoride: executive summary of the updated clinical recommendations and supporting systematic review. *J Am Dent Assoc.* 2013;144(11):1279–1291.
14. Sonesson M, Twewtman S, Bondemark L. Effectiveness of high-fluoride toothpaste on enamel demineralization during orthodontic treatment-a multicenter randomized controlled trial. *Eur J Orthod.* 2014;36(6):678–682.
15. Benson PE, Parkin N, Dyer F, et al. Fluorides for the prevention of early tooth decay (demineralized white lesions) during fixed brace treatment. *Cochrane Database Syst Rev.* 2013;12:CD003809. pub3.
16. Lapenaite E, Lopatiene K, Ragauskaite A. Prevention and treatment of white spot lesions during and after fixed orthodontic treatment. *Stomatologija.* 2016;18(1):3–8. Review.
17. Slack ME, Swift Jr EJ, Rossouw PE, et al. Tooth whitening in the orthodontic practice: a survey of orthodontists. *Am J Orthod Dentofacial Orthop.* 2013;143(4 suppl):S64–S71.
18. Suvan JE, Sabalic M, Araújo MR, Ramseier CA. Behavioral strategies for periodontal health. *Periodontol 2000.* 2022;90(1):247–261. Epub 2022 Aug 1.

41

Fixed and Removable Dental Prostheses

Leeann R. Donnelly and Caroline T. Nguyen

PROFESSIONAL OPPORTUNITIES

Tooth loss can occur at any age and for a variety of reasons. Dental hygienists may encounter a patient with a fixed or removable dental prosthesis almost daily, and therefore a good understanding of how and why tooth loss is restored will aid in patient care and education.

COMPETENCIES

1. Describe the demographics, risk factors, and psychologic factors associated with tooth loss.
2. Describe the hard and soft tissue changes associated with tooth extraction.
3. List and describe the types of prosthodontic prostheses and discuss the challenges associated with the replacement of missing teeth.
4. Explain implications for dental hygiene care with removable prostheses, including occlusion and fit, irritations, and lesions that can occur.
5. Explain the importance of regular professional care and personal home care for individuals with fixed or removable prostheses. Also, discuss the nutritional considerations for individuals with fixed and removable dental prostheses.

INTRODUCTION

Normally, individuals are not conscious of the critical daily functions of teeth—eating, speaking, facial expression, and appearance. Once the teeth are lost, the person quickly realizes that eating becomes more difficult, speech is not as distinct, and facial tissues lose support, which ultimately impairs appearance and other people's perceptions of the person.

The term **edentulous**, derived from the Latin word *edentatus*, means being without teeth or lacking teeth. Although the percentage of people with tooth loss increases with age, it is not uncommon to find younger adult patients with prostheses. A **prosthesis** is a fixed or removable appliance that is designed to functionally and cosmetically replace a missing natural tooth or teeth. Although maintaining the oral health of patients with tooth loss entails the same basic preventive and therapeutic care elements as provided for patients with a complete dentition, those with missing teeth have specialized needs. Dental hygienists must be knowledgeable about how to meet the specialized needs of patients with prostheses.

DEMOGRAPHICS OF TOOTH LOSS

Changing patterns in oral disease, professional care, and attitudes toward healthcare have decreased the number of completely edentulous individuals. Nevertheless, surveys indicate that edentulism occurs in nearly 5% of the adult American population, suggesting that the provision of complete dental prostheses is still common in the oral healthcare environment and may remain so, given longer life spans and the growing older adult population.[1] At present, approximately one in five adults aged 65 years or older in the United States and Canada are completely edentulous.[1,2] Although edentulous rates have been dropping, these figures suggest that dental hygienists are likely to encounter edentulous patients within any dental hygiene practice setting.

RISK FACTORS FOR TOOTH LOSS

Major risk factors that contribute to a person's edentulous status include:
- Dental caries
- Periodontal diseases
- Low socioeconomic status
- Inadequate access to professional oral care
- Low frequency of professional oral care
- Poor daily oral hygiene

The primary reason for tooth loss before age 35 is dental caries. After age 35, periodontal diseases increasingly contribute to tooth loss. Oral cancer, the corresponding treatment for oral cancer, and oral injuries also contribute to tooth loss.

OTHER FACTORS ASSOCIATED WITH TOOTH LOSS

Psychologic Factors

Patient attitude and values influence the success of care, and the edentulous or the partially edentulous person is no exception. The patient may not have a wholesome facial image because of tooth loss, fear of aging, decreased sexuality, feelings of insecurity, fear of rejection, loss of self-esteem, and unrealistic expectations for tooth replacement. Loss of self-esteem is especially related to patients in whom tooth loss is attributed to oral cancer and oral cancer treatments. Human responses associated with tooth loss include the five stages of bereavement, behavioral changes, embarrassment, and loss of dignity. These responses must be considered when providing care for edentulous or partially edentulous patients.

Physiologic Factors

Although prostheses can restore many oral functions when a person experiences tooth loss, remodeling of the orofacial tissues is inevitably encountered. Prostheses placement introduces unfamiliar forces that contribute to the following:
- Residual ridge and alveolar bone resorption
- Oral mucous membrane remodeling
- Loss of orofacial muscle tone

Hard and Soft Tissue Changes

After tooth extraction, major bony changes, such as residual alveolar ridge resorption, occur within the first year and continue throughout life. Correlation between the degree of alveolar bone resorption and the duration of being edentulous is well documented. Metabolic bone disease, postmenopausal osteoporosis, and a calcium-poor diet also contribute to severe mandibular atrophy in edentulous individuals.[3]

Generally, older individuals resorb bone at faster rates than younger individuals because of anatomic, metabolic, functional, and prosthetic factors. Problems that arise as a result of residual bone resorption are magnified as the person ages. For example, severe mandibular alveolar ridge resorption may expose the contents of the mandibular canal and cause increased discomfort from the prosthesis. In addition, compression of an exposed mental nerve at or near the crest of the alveolar ridge with only a thin layer of oral mucosa overlying it may cause pain and paresthesia of the lower lip and chin. During assessment, if the dental hygienist identifies changes to the hard and soft tissues that may impact chewing, the fit of the prosthesis, speech difficulties, or the potential for decreased comfort and quality of life, immediate dental referral is indicated.

Resorption of alveolar ridges diminishes stability and retention of the prosthesis as the bony ridges continue to flatten with time. Generally, bony changes observed in the mandibular arch differ significantly from those in the maxilla. The resorption rate is greater in the mandible than in the maxilla. Occasionally, irregular patterns of alveolar ridge resorption create numerous sharp spikes, especially in the mylohyoid ridge. Considerable pain can develop if the mucous membrane covering becomes trapped between the hard prosthesis base and sharp bone surfaces.[4]

Other bony irregularities from either growth abnormalities or alveolar resorption may create undesirable consequences and should be noted. **Exostoses**, benign bony outgrowths, frequently occur on the hard palate and/or lingual aspect of the mandibular alveolar ridge and are known as **palatal tori** and **mandibular tori**, respectively. Their proper surgical removal before prosthesis construction can prevent irritation to the tori's overlying oral mucosa. Similarly, large maxillary tuberosities can lead to uncomfortable bony undercuts and an unsatisfactory fit of the prosthetic appliance.

TYPES OF PROSTHODONTIC PROSTHESES

Individuals can have missing teeth replaced by dental implants (see Chapter 31) or by fixed or removable dental prostheses. Transition from a natural dentition to a completely or partially artificial dentition is a major life event that most individuals find challenging. This situation can affect a patient's stress and anxiety levels due to a esthetic concerns as well as reduced mastication abilities, which limit the ability to enjoy favorite foods, negatively impacting quality of life. If these concerns are not addressed or if patients believe that their needs cannot be met, successful prosthodontic therapy may be jeopardized.

Several types of prostheses ranging from partial to complete can be fabricated to meet patients' needs. The **partial denture** is used to replace some but not all of the natural teeth (Fig. 41.1A). Partial dentures may be fixed or removable. A **fixed partial denture** is either cemented permanently to natural teeth or screwed to dental implants or abutments and is commonly called a bridge (Fig. 41.1B); it cannot be removed by the patient.

Components of fixed partial dentures include the following:
- **Abutment**: Tooth or teeth or implant(s) used to anchor the prosthesis and support the pontic(s)
- **Pontic**: Artificial tooth or teeth that occupy the edentulous space and replace the missing tooth or teeth

Removable partial dentures (Fig. 41.2) can be removed and replaced by the patient. This type of prosthesis may be supported by

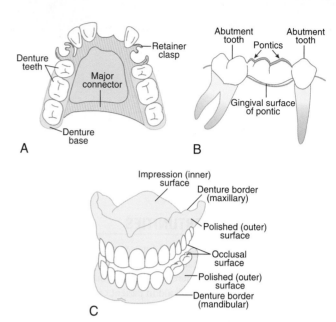

Fig. 41.1 Types of prostheses. (A) Removable partial denture. (B) Fixed partial denture or bridge. (C) Complete denture.

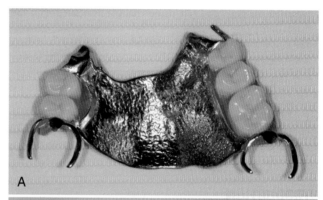
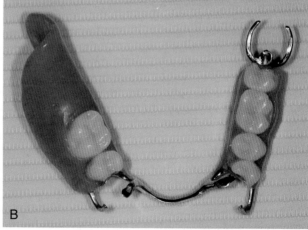

Fig. 41.2 Maxillary (A) and mandibular (B) removable partial denture. (Courtesy Dr. Caroline Nguyen, maxillofacial prosthodontist, National Dental Examining Board of Canada, Ottawa, Canada.)

retainer clasps around the natural teeth (Fig. 41.3). **Removable complete dentures** (Fig. 41.4; see also Fig. 41.1C) replace the entire dentition and associated structures of the maxilla or mandible.

If a removable dental prosthesis is designed for a patient who has undergone oral cancer surgery, it also may need to function as an obturator. An **obturator** (Fig. 41.5A) is a prosthesis that closes an opening or communication between the nasal and oral cavity (Fig. 41.5B), which may have been caused by the removal of a cancerous tumor, created by an accident, or the result of a congenital anomaly

such as a congenital cleft palate. In such cases, the obturator aids in retaining foods and fluids in the mouth and keeping them out of the nasal passage.

Implant-supported overdentures (Figs. 41.4C and D) are removable complete dentures designed to fit over implant fixtures that are inserted partially or entirely into living bone. The prosthesis can be clipped to the implants using attachments or retained by magnets. The increased stability and retention derived from this type of prosthetic appliance has renewed the hopes of the edentulous population for an acceptable alternative to natural teeth (see Chapter 31).

CHALLENGES ASSOCIATED WITH REPLACEMENT OF MISSING TEETH

Although **prosthodontic therapy** can give the edentulous or partially edentulous individual a biologically sound and functional dentition, success depends on the patient's attitude and commitment. At the outset, the patient must understand the limitations of teeth replacements and their effectiveness as substitutes for natural teeth. Patients need to be informed about the physical manifestations of bone resorption related to facial appearance, potential speech difficulties, and the effects of tooth replacement

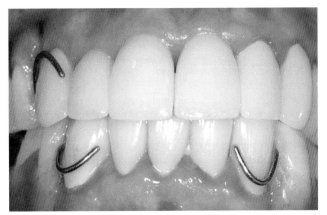

Fig. 41.3 Removable partial denture with clasps in the mouth. Note some plaque biofilm can be seen between the mandibular anterior teeth. (Courtesy Dr. Caroline Nguyen, maxillofacial prosthodontist, National Dental Examining Board of Canada, Ottawa, Canada.)

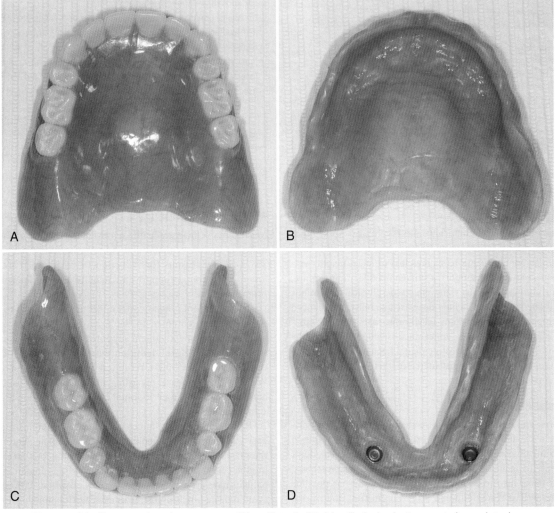

A

B

C

D

Fig. 41.4 Maxillary complete denture cameo (A) and intaglio (B). Mandibular implant supported complete denture cameo (C) and intaglio (D). (Courtesy Dr. Caroline Nguyen, maxillofacial prosthodontist, National Dental Examining Board of Canada, Ottawa, Canada.)

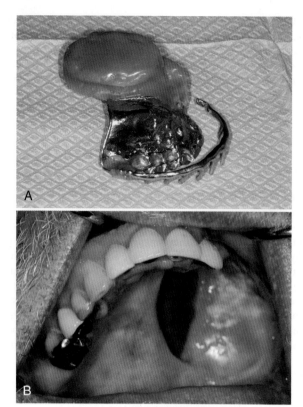

Fig. 41.5 (A) Obturator. (B) Corresponding oral defect. (Courtesy Dr. Caroline Nguyen, Maxillofacial prosthodontist, National Dental Examining Board of Canada, Ottawa, Canada.)

BOX 41.2 Critical Thinking Scenario A

Judith King, 75 years old, lives with her 80-year-old husband in a long-term care facility close to the dental office. She usually schedules continued-care appointments annually, but it has been 2 years since her last visit. On her health history, Mrs. King reports that she missed last year's visit because of a stroke. She is partially paralyzed on the right side, which is her dominant side. Mrs. King also has experienced some facial paralysis as a result of the stroke. Her current medications include an anticoagulant and diuretic. Mrs. King wears a maxillary removable complete denture and a mandibular removable partial denture. She has retained her mandibular anterior teeth from canine to canine. During assessment, the hygienist finds moderate-to-heavy biofilm and food accumulations in the right buccal vestibule. Mrs. King has light-to-moderate calculus accumulations on the remaining natural teeth. Periodontal probing depths are 3 mm or less, with bleeding on probing and no gingival recession. The maxillary denture appears to fit well but the underlying palatal tissue is red. The mandibular denture appears to be loose and has a broken supporting clasp.

Develop a dental hygiene diagnosis, patient goals, and a dental hygiene care plan including interprofessional collaboration strategies for Mrs. King.

on masticatory efficiency. If realistic expectations and goals for care of prostheses are outlined early, the patient can adapt successfully to their artificial dentition. Patient education is essential for this adaptation, and dental hygienists need to ensure that they explain and document discussed options for the replacement of missing teeth and refer the patient to the dentist for evaluation and treatment(s) (Boxes 41.1 and 41.2).

Physical Appearance

Alveolar bone resorption dramatically affects physical appearance and facial image. Modifications in appearance often are visible after extensive alveolar bone resorption, such as loss of facial height (vertical dimension), reduced lip support, a sunken maxillary appearance, and increased chin prominence. The effects of physical alterations attributed to bone resorption include decreased stability, unbalanced occlusion, temporomandibular joint (TMJ) disorders, and dissatisfaction with appearance. Usually, appearance is judged critically by patients themselves; however, the astute dental hygienist who focuses patients on their positive attributes increases their self-esteem and reduces their anxiety and stress.

Speech Disturbances

Speech patterns are affected by loss of teeth, loss of associated periodontal structures, and acquisition of prostheses. Transient speech articulation difficulties and oral resonance problems are expected but soon disappear. To facilitate speaking with a new dental prosthesis, patients need to be instructed to talk to people as often as possible for practice, as well as read aloud and articulate in front of a mirror regularly. If a speech disturbance persists longer than a few weeks, the prosthesis may be ill fitting and reevaluation by a dentist or denturist might be warranted. A speech deficit can also arise in conjunction with

bone resorption because a loosely fitting prosthesis is more difficult to control.

Masticatory Efficiency

Masticatory efficiency with removable partial prostheses is estimated to be 20% of that of individuals who have a natural dentition.[3] Two primary reasons for reduction in masticatory abilities are (1) loss of periodontal support and stability and (2) loss of periodontal proprioception.

The periodontal ligament support area is critical to the stability of a prosthesis confined to one arch only. However, in edentulous people, periodontal ligament support is one-fourth to one-half of the support of the natural dentition. Further, proprioception is a major component of the body's reception and interpretation of sensation. Without this feedback regarding movement and position from the baroreceptors in the periodontal ligaments, chewing ability declines significantly.[4]

Biting and chewing forces also decrease significantly and can be nearly five times less in people who wear complete dentures. Although the mastication muscles are adequate, the mucous membrane covering the edentulous ridge cannot withstand the pressures exerted. The patients have greater success with a new prosthesis if they are taught to avoid repeated incision using anterior teeth, gum chewing, and sticky foods. Patients also need to be instructed to consume food in smaller pieces, lengthen chewing time, and evenly distribute food to both the left and right posterior sides of the mouth while chewing (Box 41.3).[5]

> ## BOX 41.3 Patient or Client Education Tips
>
> **Patients with Removable Dentures**
> - Instruct patient to consume foods in smaller pieces, lengthen chewing time, evenly distribute food to both the left and the right sides of the mouth while chewing, and avoid incision with anterior denture teeth.
> - Instruct the prosthodontic patient to avoid chewing gum or eating sticky foods.

Educating patients to practice these behaviors is critical to masticatory efficiency and prosthesis stability.

FACTORS AFFECTING THE ORAL MUCOSA OF PROSTHESIS-WEARING INDIVIDUALS

Systemic Diseases and Conditions

Poor general health results in prosthesis-related problems, such as friable denture-bearing mucosa. Decreased tolerance to stress, impaired healing, emotional strain, and medications related to poor systemic health adversely affect oral soft tissues. Systemic conditions that may require modifications of dental hygiene care include cardiovascular diseases, hypertension, allergies, psychologic problems, and chronic diseases such as diabetes, anemia, and postmenopausal osteoporosis.

Medications taken for systemic diseases or conditions can affect a patient's oral condition and must be assessed and documented during each appointment (see Chapters 13 and 15). Hormones, digitalis, nitroglycerin, diazepam (Valium), and chlordiazepoxide (Librium) are among the many medications that can affect the oral environment of the edentulous patient. Uncontrollable tongue and facial movements may develop with psychotropic medications. Drugs such as cortisone, thyroid hormone, and estrogen may perpetuate a chronic mucosal tissue soreness. Xerostomia, a common side effect of diuretic, antihypertensive, and antidepressant drugs, interferes with complete denture retention and stability as a result of a loss of mucosal lubrication.[6]

Xerostomia (Dry Mouth)

Xerostomia is the subjective perception of a dry mouth and/or lack of saliva by the patient. It might or might not be correlated with hyposalivation measurements. Extreme difficulties experienced by the edentulous patient with dry mouth warrant an understanding of the critical role of saliva in the oral health maintenance. Normal salivary flow aids in denture retention and function. A thin film of saliva provides adhesive action as well as lubrication and cushioning effects. When the mouth becomes dry, movement of the denture can cause frictional irritation of the denture-bearing mucosa. Other symptoms may arise as a result of oral dryness, including altered taste perceptions, cracked lips, a fissured tongue, swallowing and speech difficulties, and burning mouth syndrome.[6] Although the exact cause of xerostomia may be difficult to identify, the most common factors associated with it are as follows:

- Sjögren syndrome
- Emotional and anxiety states
- Negative fluid balance
- Selected nutritional and hormonal deficiencies
- Acquired immunodeficiency syndrome (AIDS)
- Anemia
- Polyuric states
- Drugs or medications
- Therapeutic radiation

Diminished salivary output is not associated directly with increased age; therefore other factors must be considered if xerostomia is observed in older adult patients.

Xerostomia Management

Professional care for the denture patient with xerostomia can be challenging because most remedies provide only temporary relief (see Chapter 52). The dental hygienist may recommend saliva substitutes and frequent sips of water, especially during meals, to keep the mouth lubricated and to provide temporary symptomatic relief. Also, coating the tissue surface of dentures with silicone fluid or denture adhesive material, sucking on ice chips, and using xylitol or sugarless mints are recommended for the management of soft tissue dryness. Moisturizing products to recommend include oral lubricants, mouth rinses, sprays, and lozenges. If the patient's medications are suspected of being the cause of the xerostomia, contacting the physician to find possible alternative treatment options could be beneficial.[6]

Cholinergic drugs, such as oral pilocarpine, decrease symptoms associated with xerostomia by increasing salivary flow. This prescriptive medication is effective in patients who have undergone head and neck radiation therapy or who have Sjögren syndrome and experience a severe dry mouth. Although oral pilocarpine has not been tested extensively in denture-wearing populations, it may be of value for those individuals with dry mouth.[6] This treatment option may be discussed with the patient's dentist or physician and then presented to the patient.

REMOVABLE DENTAL PROSTHESES OCCLUSION AND FIT

The state of the oral mucosa overlying the edentulous ridges directly affects the comfort of removable partial and complete dentures. A thick mucosal covering is more resilient and provides more padding than thin mucosa. Unfortunately, dental interventions for minimizing discomfort associated with friable mucosa are limited. Soft-lining materials, such as tissue conditioners and resilient liners, comprised of soft, flexible elastomer polymers, may alleviate discomfort for some individuals as they palliatively treat chronic soreness and protect supporting tissues from functional and parafunctional occlusal stresses. Dentures with a flexible elastomer require special care because these soft materials cannot be cleaned effectively, and debris can accumulate and support halitosis, a disagreeable taste, and the growth of *Candida albicans*. Soft liners can also precipitate alveolar ridge resorption, especially on the mandible, which can lead to dentures more rapidly becoming unretentive and unstable and needing to be replaced more often. Most professionals recommend using a soft brush with soap and water or a nonabrasive denture cleanser (see Chapter 52). Oxygenating and hypochlorite-type denture cleansers can damage resilient liners and tissue conditioners, and therefore patients must be cautioned about their use.[7]

ORAL HYGIENE

Many oral mucosal conditions in denture wearers are associated with improper oral hygiene care, extended denture wear, or poor prosthesis fit. The patient's oral mucosa reveals information about daily self-care. Accumulation of biofilm, stain, and calculus on the denture and oral mucosa leads to offensive odors and mucosal irritations, such as the following:

- **Denture stomatitis**: Inflammation of the oral mucosa underlying the denture; characterized by redness, pain, and swelling
- **Papillary hyperplasia**: Abnormal increase in the volume of tissue as a result of irritation

- **Chronic candidiasis**: Long-standing *C. albicans* infection (see Chapter 52 on the prevention and treatment of oral candidiasis)

Presence of any of these conditions mandates that the patient be educated about oral hygiene interventions to maintain the health of mucosal tissues. Specific oral hygiene techniques and products are presented in Chapters 24, 25, 26, 33, and 52.

Continuous Wear of Removable Dental Prostheses

Masticatory stress exerted by removable partial and complete dentures may compromise residual alveolar ridges and oral mucosa. In addition, the risk for an inflammatory condition increases if the tissues are not allowed to rest. Therefore patients are advised to remove their dentures overnight or for 8 hours during each 24-hour period. While out of the mouth, dentures must be cleaned thoroughly and placed in a container, either dry or submerged in a cleansing solution. Storing dentures dry is an effective method to prevent the growth of bacteria and fungi with no clinically significant change to denture fit.

REMOVABLE DENTAL PROSTHESES–INDUCED ORAL LESIONS

Understanding the soft tissue response to removable prostheses enables the dental hygienist to assess the patient's skin and mucous membrane integrity of the head and neck. The soft tissues associated primarily with dentures are the tongue, floor of the mouth, cheeks, lips, and mucosa overlying the edentulous ridge.

Denture-bearing tissues react differently from individual to individual. For example, differences in the mucosa thickness in conjunction with varying degrees of keratinization can be expected in the mouth of the denture-wearing patient. Some edentulous patients develop a denture-induced fibrous hyperplasia as a result of fibrous tissue proliferation after alveolar bone resorption under an ill-fitting prosthesis (Fig. 41.6). Although detection is sometimes difficult because of nearly normal color and texture, this flabby hyperplastic tissue is identified by palpating freely movable tissue over edentulous ridges or on the vestibular mucosa.[7]

If fibrous tissue proliferation is observed, the dental hygienist refers the patient to the dentist for evaluation and treatment. Depending on the severity of hypermobile tissue, treatment may involve a period of tissue rest, prosthesis adjustment, and/or surgical removal to reduce the excess tissue. Keratinization of edentulous alveolar ridges may be completely absent or may progress to a hyperkeratinized state. This **focal (frictional) hyperkeratosis**, classified as a hyperkeratotic white

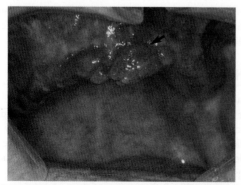

Fig. 41.6 Prosthesis-induced fibrous hyperplasia. Chronic denture-induced trauma or irritation has resulted in an overgrowth *(arrow)* of soft tissue. The chief complaint from the patient was an ill-fitting denture. (Courtesy Dr. Catherine Poh, oral pathologist, faculty of dentistry, University of British Columbia, Vancouver, Canada.)

lesion of the oral mucosa, usually resolves with time on discontinuation of the underlying trauma.[7]

Although it is highly unlikely that chronic irritation resulting from ill-fitting prostheses causes oral carcinoma, trauma induced by removable dentures and other mechanical irritations probably accelerates the disease progression. The dental hygienist must be especially attentive to potential oral cancer signs and symptoms, such as ulceration or erosion, induration, fixation, chronicity, lymphadenopathy, leukoplakia, and erythroplakia that do not get better within 2 weeks after prostheses adjustments (see Chapter 50).

Denture-induced lesions are subdivided into the following three categories according to causative factors and clinical features[7] (Table 41.1):

- Reactive or traumatic (Fig. 41.7)
- Infectious (Figs. 41.8A and 41.9)
- Mixed reactive and infectious (Fig. 41.10)

Reactive or Traumatic Lesions

Reactive or traumatic lesions commonly are secondary to either acute or chronic injury. Lesions in this category are ulcers (see Fig. 41.7), focal (frictional) hyperkeratosis, and denture-induced papillary hyperplasia (see Fig. 41.10). Fig. 41.11 shows an overexuberant repair response that produces hyperplastic tissue. This condition often is painless, but pain may develop if the fibrous lesion is traumatized or ulcerated. Surgical removal of the irritating factor is an effective method of treating reactive lesions.[7] Palliative treatment can include over-the-counter products such as Rincinol and Ameseal.

Infectious Lesions

The most common inflammation of the removable dental prosthesis–bearing mucosa is **denture stomatitis** (see Fig. 41.8). Despite minimal pain associated with this condition, it often is referred to inappropriately as *denture sore mouth*. With a predilection for females the condition has an incidence of 20% to 40% of the edentulous population and occurs in up to 65% of older adults who wear complete maxillary dentures.[7] It is most commonly due to patients wearing their prostheses continually or overnight and not allowing their supporting tissues to rest.

Angular cheilitis is a mixed bacterial and fungal infection typically caused by *Staphylococcus aureus* and *C. albicans* (see Fig. 41.9A,B). The condition results from small amounts of saliva accumulating at the commissural angles, which promotes the colonization of yeast. Clinically, angular cheilitis appears as cracked, eroded, and encrusted commissural folds and may cause moderate pain. Often, it is secondary to overclosure resulting from a reduction in the patient's vertical dimension. Vitamin B (riboflavin) deficiency, resulting from inadequate nutrition, also can cause angular cheilitis.

Denture stomatitis can, in most cases, resolve spontaneously by instructing the patient to remove their removable dental prostheses overnight. For more persistent infections, dental treatment requires correcting the prosthesis to eliminate trauma and prescribing antifungal drugs to eliminate the *Candida* infection. Dental hygiene care to prevent recurrence includes patient instruction in thorough daily mechanical cleansing of the infected prosthesis as well as chemical immersion of the prosthesis in chlorhexidine or a weak sodium hypochlorite solution (Box 41.4). Sodium hypochlorite damages metal and never should be used when metal is part of any oral appliance. It can also damage nylon implant attachments and should not be used with implant-supported overdentures. Moreover, if the sodium hypochlorite is too concentrated or if the denture is soaked for more than 10 minutes, it can bleach the colored portion of the resin base and discolor soft liner materials. Other denture cleansers include nonabrasive denture pastes, commercial denture cleansers, and vinegar. Household cleaners other than a weak sodium hypochlorite solution never should

TABLE 41.1 Dental Hygiene Diagnoses Related to Deficits in the Need for Skin and Mucous Membrane Integrity of the Head and Neck in Dental Prostheses–Wearing Patients

Oral Soft Tissue Lesion	Causes	Evidence (Signs and Symptoms)
Reactive Lesions		
Acute ulcers	Ill-fitting prosthesis Chemical agent irritation: • Denture adhesive • Denture cleanser • Self-medication	Yellow-white exudates Red halo Varying pain and tenderness
Chronic ulcers	Same causes as above	Yellow membrane Elevated margin Little or no pain
Focal (frictional) hyperkeratosis	Chronic rubbing or friction of prosthesis	White patch Asymptomatic
Denture-induced fibrous hyperplasia (epulis fissuratum, denture hyperplasia)	Ill-fitting prosthesis	Folds of fibrous connective tissue Varying color Asymptomatic Typical on vestibular mucosa at denture flange contact
Infectious Lesions		
Denture stomatitis (denture sore mouth)	Chronic *Candida albicans* infection Poor oral hygiene care Continuous wear of prosthesis Ill-fitting prosthesis Systemic factors: • Anemia • Diabetes • Immunosuppression • Menopause • Systemic antibiotic medications Chemical agent irritation: • Denture adhesive • Denture cleanser • Self-medication • Denture base allergy	Generalized redness of mucosa Velvetlike appearance Pain and burning sensations Typical under maxillary denture
Angular cheilitis	Chronic *C. albicans* infection Pooling of saliva in commissural folds Riboflavin deficiency	Fissured at angles of mouth Eroded Encrusted Moderate pain
Mixed Lesions		
Papillary hyperplasia	Chronic *C. albicans* infection Chronic low-grade denture trauma	Multiple round-to-ovoid nodules: • Cobblestone appearance • Generalized red mucosa background • Rarely ulcerated • Typical under maxillary denture

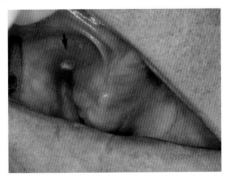

Fig. 41.7 Reactive or traumatic lesion. A traumatic ulcer *(arrow)* resulting from elongated buccal flange of the upper complete denture. (Courtesy Dr. Catherine Poh, oral pathologist, faculty of dentistry, University of British Columbia, Vancouver, Canada.)

be used to clean oral appliances (see the section Removable Dental Prosthesis Cleansers).

Most removable dental prosthesis–related infections, including denture stomatitis, are caused by a **chronic candidiasis** infection and are treated using a topical antifungal agent such as nystatin. Prescribed by the dentist for use at home, nystatin cream is applied to affected tissues and the dentures to eliminate the fungi. A nystatin oral troche may also be prescribed and has the added benefit of treating oropharyngeal tissues. To be effective, topical antifungal agents must be used by the patient for approximately 1 week after the disappearance of clinical symptoms.

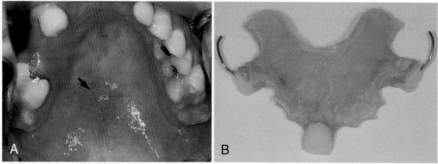

Fig. 41.8 (A) Infectious lesions. *Arrow* points to chronic candidiasis on upper palate (erythematous area). (B) Upper partial denture worn by patient. (Courtesy Dr. Catherine Poh, oral pathologist, faculty of dentistry, University of British Columbia, Vancouver, Canada.)

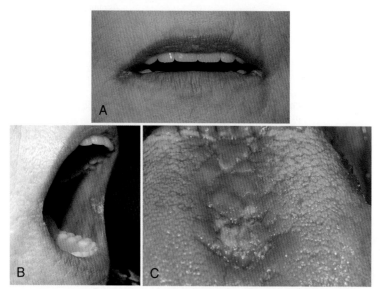

Fig. 41.9 Oral candidiasis. (A and B) Angular cheilitis. Note bilateral irregular white plaques on an erythematous base on mouth commissures. (C) Candidiasis on dorsum surface of tongue (erythematous and depapillated area at the center). (Courtesy Dr. Eli Whitney, certified specialist in oral medicine and oral pathology, faculty of dentistry, University of British Columbia, Vancouver, Canada.)

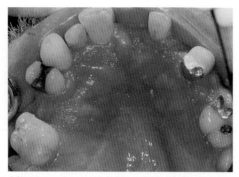

Fig. 41.10 Mixed reactive and infectious lesions. Palatal papillary hyperplasia is associated with candidiasis. Note that the generalized granular erythematous change of the palatal mucosa matches the shape of a repeatedly relined removable partial denture. Also, note denture-induced papillary hyperplasia of the palate. (Courtesy Dr. Catherine Poh, oral pathologist, faculty of dentistry, University of British Columbia, Vancouver, Canada.)

A chronic *Candida* infection is primarily responsible for the development of denture stomatitis, although recent studies implicate bacteria as the causative agent: gram-positive *Streptococcus* species and *Lactobacillus*, *Bacteroides*, and *Actinomyces* species. Other contributing

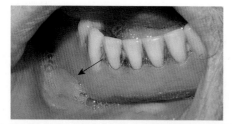

Fig. 41.11 Prosthesis-induced fibrous hyperplasia (epulis fissuratum). Chronic denture-induced trauma has resulted in leaflike masses *(arrow)* of soft tissue that overgrow the denture flange. (Courtesy Dr. Catherine Poh, oral pathologist, faculty of dentistry, University of British Columbia, Vancouver, Canada.)

factors include biofilm accumulation on dentures; chronic, low-grade soft tissue trauma resulting from ill-fitting dentures; an unbalanced occlusal relationship; and continuous wearing of the denture at night. In some circumstances, systemic conditions such as diabetes, anemia, menopause, malnutrition, and nutrient malabsorption in the digestive tract can predispose an individual to a *Candida* infection.

Chronic candidiasis appears more often on the palatal mucosa than on the mandibular alveolar mucosa (see Fig. 41.8). Clinical features demonstrate variations in surface texture ranging from a smooth, velvety appearance to a more nodular or hyperplastic form. With severe infections, surfaces may appear eroded with small confluent vesicles. Characteristically, the bright-red color of the denture-supporting mucosa is confined within a well-defined denture border.

Mixed Reactive and Infectious Lesions

Trauma and infection are causative factors contributing to mixed reactive and infectious lesions, such as papillary hyperplasia (see Fig. 41.10). A cobblestone appearance describes the granular papillary projections that result from a hyperplastic tissue response. This condition can predispose or potentiate the growth of *C. albicans* under the prosthesis and further complicate the problem. Surgical removal, antifungal agents, soft-tissue conditioners and liners, and strict oral hygiene measures are all options to resolve the lesions (Box 41.5).

IMPORTANCE OF REGULAR PROFESSIONAL CARE

Patients who are edentulous and have removable dental prostheses may not recognize the need for regular professional care. A critical role for the dental hygienist is to encourage regular maintenance care and to recognize oral changes that often go unnoticed by the patient. Periodic maintenance care provides an excellent opportunity to identify denture-related tissue lesions and refer patients for dental evaluation and treatment. Although studies have demonstrated no correlation between cancer at specific sites and the wearing of removable dentures, denture irritation may be a cocarcinogenic factor in predisposed individuals.[8]

Some patients erroneously perceive that prostheses last a lifetime without further modifications; however, in reality, adjustments are needed annually, and new dentures are needed every 4 to 8 years. Hence education is a priority for the denture-wearing individual. (Box 41.6).

DENTAL HYGIENE CARE FOR INDIVIDUALS WITH REMOVABLE DENTAL PROSTHESES

From the outset, the patient must be educated regarding expectations, oral hygiene practices, prosthetic use and care, and regular periodic maintenance appointments. Also, the dental hygienist needs to educate the patient about the causes of bone resorption and suggest methods of minimizing the rate of resorption, including removal of dentures at night, regular evaluation to ensure well-fitting dentures, and a calcium-rich diet. Resorption rates vary enormously among individuals, and well-fitting prostheses decrease the rate of resorption. Local factors, including trauma, can affect the resorption rate so that the denture becomes ill fitting.

Successful prosthodontic therapy also greatly depends on patients who possess a sense of responsibility regarding their oral health status. The dental hygienist encourages patients to set personal goals for oral health and suggests behavior patterns and techniques that are compatible with their lifestyle, cultural customs, values, and physical capabilities.

The dental hygienist assesses loss of retention, stability, and support of the prosthesis and calls problems to the dentist's attention (Procedure 41.1 and the corresponding Competency Form). The dental hygienist also documents biologic, psychologic, and social issues, informs the patient and the dentist, and recommends daily self-care to prevent further tissue destruction.

The newly edentulous patient commonly requires a denture adjustment within the first 6 to 12 months. Thereafter, annual continued care

PROCEDURE 41.1 Professional Care for Patients With Removable Dental Prostheses

Equipment
- Protective barriers
- Prophy cup and bristled brush
- Low-speed handpiece
- Antimicrobial mouth rinse
- Tin oxide
- Mouth mirror
- Hand mirror
- Gauze
- Tongue blades
- Small plastic bag
- Stain and calculus remover solution
- Ultrasonic cleaning unit

Steps
Assessment
1. Update patient's health history to identify systemic disorders, current medications, and conditions that may affect care and patient's ability to wear the prosthesis.
2. Review patient's personal history records; note details such as age, occupation, and culture.
3. Review patient's dental history.
4. Ask patient to explain prosthesis-related problems they have experienced; listen attentively to complaints.
5. Perform caomprehensive assessment of head and neck.
6. Assess the TMJ and associated musculature as patient opens and closes mouth and slides jaw from side to side.
7. Assess extraoral soft tissues.
8. Assess intraoral soft tissues for evidence of local denture trauma or systemic diseases, and record lesion color, texture, size, contour, and presence of pain.
9. Visually inspect the prosthesis for cleanliness, and palpate prosthesis-bearing mucosa with prosthesis out of the mouth.
10. Assess the structure and form of the alveolar ridges.

11. Document changes in associated structures, including the tongue, floor of the mouth, and oropharynx.
12. Assess oral hygiene status.
13. Ask patient to displace the prosthesis away from supporting tissues. The posterior border seal of the maxillary denture is checked by attempting to pull the anterior teeth forward.
14. Assess stability of the prosthesis with respect to its position during normal oral functions.
15. Indicate changes in occlusion and articulation.

Dental Hygiene Diagnosis
16. Analyze objective and subjective assessment data.
17. Present significant findings to patient and dentist.

Planning
18. Determine a dental hygiene care plan and goals to be achieved in consultation with patient and dentist.

Implementation
19. Review self-care and dental care; suggest methods for improvement.
20. Counsel patient on adequate nutrition.
21. Fill a small plastic bag with cleaning solution, label with patient's name, submerge the prosthesis in it, and place the bag in an ultrasonic cleaning unit.
22. Lightly polish the prosthesis with an extremely fine polishing agent (tin oxide) *on external surfaces only,* and thoroughly rinse under warm water (when appropriate).

Evaluation
23. Discuss continued-care intervals. Emphasize the importance of regular professional care.
24. Measure the achievement of goals established at the previous dental hygiene care appointment.
25. Formulate an evaluative statement regarding the level of goal attainment.
26. Document services in patient's record under "Services Rendered," and date entry.

is essential to denture longevity and meets the need for denture duplication, rebasing, or replacement. Individuals with poor oral hygiene may require more frequent visits.

Patients need to be advised of the importance of daily care of their dentures and the associated soft tissues. Procedure 41.2 and the corresponding Competency Form provide instructions for daily oral care for individuals with removable prostheses. Procedure 41.3 and the corresponding Competency Form provide an overview of instructions for daily oral care for individuals with fixed prostheses. Verbal and written instructions reinforce the homecare regimen, especially for older adults. A simple reminder to rinse the dentures and mouth after each meal helps reduce accumulation of food debris and biofilm. Written instructions or other formal educational materials that include proper denture hygiene and cleansing of the oral tissues provide specific, tangible recommendations for maintaining oral health. Pertinent information to teach the patient is presented in the section on patient education issues. At continued-care visits, the dental hygienist assesses the patient's ability to perform meticulous oral hygiene care at home (Box 41.7).

REMOVABLE DENTAL PROSTHESIS CLEANSERS

Maintaining denture hygiene is essential to promote aesthetics, control malodor, and prevent and treat oral infections in the patient. Proper hygienic care can be confusing for the patient because of the many

products available for home use, as well as the various in-office procedures used to maintain good hygiene. Commonly available denture cleansers include the following:
- Chemical soak cleansers
- Antimicrobial cleansers
- Ultrasonic cleaning devices

Table 41.2 describes common cleansers that are available. When selecting a cleanser, patient and prosthesis safety are paramount. Abrasive powders and pastes, including toothpastes, are not recommended for cleaning dentures because of the potential for the patient to use these products incorrectly, thus damaging the prosthesis. Denture acrylic can become abraded, and this abrasion may alter the denture fit if a hard-bristle brush or extreme vigor is used when the prosthesis is cleaned.

Prosthesis cleanser efficacy depends partially on the patient's dexterity. Brushing with a nonabrasive denture paste is suitable for the patient who is motivated and has the dexterity to clean all denture surfaces thoroughly; however, this cleansing method is the most difficult, especially for physically challenged or older adult patients. Chemical-soak cleansers can be alternatives to mechanical cleansing. Alkaline peroxide and hypochlorite solutions can be recommended for dentures with and without metal components, respectively. The majority of clinical studies report hypochlorite solutions to be an effective soaking method for dentures constructed with only acrylic materials. Caution, however, must be taken to avoid the use of hypochlorite solutions on

PROCEDURE 41.2 Daily Oral and Denture Hygiene Care for Individuals With Removable Prostheses

Equipment
- Soft denture brush, soft intraoral toothbrush, antimicrobial mouth rinse
- Basin
- Denture cup
- Towel
- Diluted sodium hypochlorite solution (for removable complete dentures) or commercial denture cleanser (for removable partial dentures and implant-supported dentures)
- Warm water
- Wall-mounted mirror
- Soft nylon toothbrush

Steps
1. Explain the importance of daily care for both dentures and soft tissues.
2. Describe the consequences of oral and denture hygiene neglect.
3. Summarize the patient's responsibilities in monitoring oral function and health status.
4. Advise against the use of denture home-repair kits and encourage the patient to return to the dentist for proper care.
5. Discourage use of denture adhesives with a stable and retentive prosthesis. Under dentist's supervision, a small amount of adhesive (3 to 4 pea-sized drops) may be applied to the inner surface that directly contacts the oral mucosa. Denture adhesives are not normally used with partial removable dentures.
6. Remind the patient to brush dentures after each meal and before going to bed or, at the very least, to rinse dentures under running water.
7. Teach self-examination of dentures for proper fit, denture deposits, and abraded inner and outer surfaces.
8. Teach patient that some commercially available denture powders and pastes are too abrasive for dentures and are not recommended for use.
9. Suggest daily use of fresh denture immersion cleansers. Recommend a diluted sodium hypochlorite solution as a cleanser for complete dentures. Soak complete dentures for 5 to 10 minutes and rinse thoroughly. Partial dentures benefit from alkaline peroxide solutions found in many denture cleansing products, usually in the form of a tablet. Soak partial dentures for 15 minutes or overnight, and rinse thoroughly. Change solutions daily.
10. Teach the patient to remove dentures when possible and at night while at rest.
11. Assemble supplies.
12. Fill basin with water and line with a small towel.
13. Gently remove dentures and rinse away saliva and loose debris. In the case of complete dentures, remove any denture adhesive material.
14. Firmly grasp dentures in palm of one hand and hold over water-filled basin.
15. Demonstrate use of a denture brush with a mild soap solution or nonabrasive denture paste to remove accumulations on the inner impression and outer polished surfaces, and adapt brush as necessary.
16. Rinse dentures and brush under running water to completely remove all denture cleanser.
17. Inspect dentures for any remaining biofilm, food debris, or cleanser by visual and tactile examination.
18. Place prostheses in a denture cup.
19. On removal of dentures, rinse mouth with warm water, antimicrobial mouthrinse, or saline solution.
20. Teach the patient to use a soft toothbrush or soft cloth daily to clean edentulous mucosa and tongue by employing long strokes in a posterior-to-anterior direction.
21. Teach patient to use thumb and index finger to massage edentulous tissues daily by applying pressure and then releasing it continually along the ridge. Mechanical and vibratory stimulation with the sides of multitufted soft toothbrush filaments can provide similar results.

PROCEDURE 41.3 Daily Oral Care for Individuals With Fixed Dental Prostheses

Equipment
- Soft toothbrush
- Interdental cleaners such as variable-diameter floss, dental floss, dental yarn, floss threaders
- Antimicrobial mouth rinse
- Wall-mounted mirror

Steps
1. Assemble supplies.
2. Explain the importance of daily self-care for fixed dental prostheses, remaining natural teeth, and periodontal tissues.
3. Describe the consequences of oral and prosthesis hygiene neglect.
4. Summarize the patient's responsibilities in monitoring oral function and health status.
5. Teach the patient to brush the natural teeth and fixed prosthesis after each meal and before going to bed. Patients benefit from flossing remaining natural teeth and fixed prosthesis and using an antimicrobial mouth rinse daily.
6. Demonstrate use of a soft toothbrush to remove biofilm and gross debris from fixed prosthesis and remaining natural teeth (see Chapter 24).
7. Demonstrate use of a suitable interdental aid to cleanse under the pontic and around abutments and natural teeth (see Chapter 25).

BOX 41.7 Critical Thinking Scenario D

Andrea Smith, an 84-year-old widow, visits the dental office twice a year for regular dental and dental hygiene assessments and care. She has a maxillary removable partial denture that replaces her lost molar teeth on both the right and left sides of the arch, as well as replacing her two maxillary central incisors. Mrs. Smith has retained most of her mandibular teeth except her left second premolar and left first molar. These teeth have been replaced with a fixed partial dental prosthesis or bridge. She is in relatively good health and takes no medications. At her current continued-care appointment, she has heavy biofilm deposits around her bridge but light-to-moderate deposits around her remaining natural teeth. She has light calculus deposits localized to the mandibular anterior teeth. On assessment, the hygienist finds periodontal probing depths ranging from 3 to 4 mm, with a 6-mm pocket on the mesial surface of the second molar, which serves as an abutment for her bridge. There is 2 mm of recession generalized. Mrs. Smith states that her removable partial denture fits well and that she rarely removes it. Mrs. Smith is reluctant to remove her prosthesis during your appointment.

Develop a dental hygiene diagnosis, patient goals, and a dental hygiene care plan for Mrs. Smith.

any metal-containing prostheses. Table 41.3 presents the variety of oral appliances and dental prostheses that also can be cleansed by these denture cleaning methods. (Refer to Box 41.3 for Client or Patient Education Tips for the care and cleansing of removable dentures.)

TABLE 41.2 Removable Dental Prostheses Cleansing Products

Product	Mechanism of Action	Advantages	Disadvantages
Chemical Cleansers			
Alkaline hypochlorite	Dissolves mucins and organic substances of prosthesis biofilm matrix.	Bactericidal cleanser. Fungicidal cleanser. Bleaches stains. May inhibit calculus formation.	Corrodes metals. Odor and taste may be unacceptable. May bleach acrylic if used in high concentration or for prolonged periods.
Alkaline peroxide	Mechanical cleansing effect is caused by the release of oxygen (bubbling).	Provides some antibacterial effect. Removes stains.	Harmful to soft liners. Not very effective in removing calculus.
Antimicrobial Cleansers			
Chlorhexidine gluconate solution	Antimicrobial action is caused by chemical agent.	Antibacterial cleanser. Antifungal cleanser.	Provides temporary relief of denture stomatitis symptoms. Stains denture teeth.
Ultrasonic cleaning devices	Ultrasonic sound wave action creates vibrating and bubbling effect.	Removes biofilm. Enhances effectiveness of chemical cleansers.	Commonly an in-office procedure. Efficacy of ultrasonic action is uncertain.
Microwave radiation (in-office use only)	Electromagnetic waves kill microorganisms.	Bactericidal cleanser. Minimal negative effect on resilient liners.	High temperatures can affect dimensional stability of a denture.

TABLE 41.3 Comparison of Various Oral Appliances and Dental Prostheses*

Appliance	Definition	Purpose
Removable complete (full) denture	Prosthetic appliance designed to replace an entire arch of missing teeth and the surrounding alveolar bone; can be inserted and removed by the patient	Replaces teeth (form, function, and appearance) in fully edentulous dental arches.
Removable partial denture	Prosthetic appliance designed to replace several missing teeth and the surrounding alveolar bone; can be inserted and removed by the patient	Replaces teeth (form, function, and appearance) in partially edentulous dental arches.
Implant-supported overdenture	Prosthetic appliance designed to fit over osseointegrated implant fixtures	Replaces teeth (form, function, and appearance) in fully edentulous or partially edentulous dental arches.
Immediate denture	Prosthetic appliance placed immediately after all remaining teeth are extracted from a fully dentate or partially edentulous arch	Replaces teeth (form, function, and appearance) in fully edentulous dental arches.
Fixed partial denture (bridge)	Prosthetic appliance designed to replace one or several missing teeth; permanently cemented or screwed in place and removed only by the dentist	Replaces teeth (form, function, and appearance) in fully or partially edentulous dental arches.
Athletic mouth guard (mouth protector)	Oral appliance designed to protect the teeth and head from trauma during contact sports	Prevents oral and facial injury.
Bleaching trays	Custom-made stent in the shape of the teeth and dental arch for carrying the bleaching or whitening agents	Holds the whitening agent against the tooth surfaces.
Bruxing guard (nightguard and day guard)	Hard acrylic appliance that fits over all or just several of the maxillary or mandibular teeth to create a functional occlusion or to relax the muscles; may be worn at night or during the day	Controls tooth attrition. Eases muscle hyperactivity and pressure on temporomandibular joint.
Fluoride tray (custom)	Custom-made stent in the shape of the teeth and dental arch for carrying the fluoride agent to the tooth structure	Holds the prescription agent against the tooth surface to decrease caries risk.
Oral habit appliance	Oral appliance used to interfere with habits such as thumb sucking, tongue sucking, or tongue thrusting	Prevents the habitual behavior from occurring.
Orthodontic appliance or repositioner	Oral appliance used for tooth movement and the treatment of malocclusion	Provides tooth movement and stabilization.
Stent	Device used after periodontal surgery to support and protect the oral tissues and/or to hold a medicinal or other desired agent in a particular area	Stabilizes general tissue during periodontal surgery. Holds anesthetic or antiseptic agents in the area of the surgical site.
Sleep apnea or snoring appliance	Flexible, custom-made device that positions the jaw forward during sleep	Opens the airway during sleep. Prevents snoring.
Space maintainer	Fixed or removable oral appliance to maintain a space created by premature tooth loss	Maintains an open space in the dental arch caused by premature tooth loss until the permanent tooth can erupt.

*See also Chapter 38.

NUTRITIONAL CONSIDERATIONS FOR INDIVIDUALS WITH FIXED AND REMOVABLE DENTAL PROSTHESES

The edentulous person's ability to adapt to a denture greatly influences eating pleasure, eating proficiency, and overall health. The quality and quantity of nutritional intake are not necessarily modified in the edentulous individual. Nonetheless, if the prosthesis is ill fitting, nutritional status may suffer. Eating can become a chore and less pleasurable.

Nutritional deficiencies are seldom noticed and therefore infrequently corrected. For example, a patient deficient in B-complex vitamins may have symptoms of atrophic glossitis; angular cheilitis; or cracking, fissuring, or ulceration of the lips. These clinical signs may be interpreted as a chronic *C. albicans* infection rather than a nutritional deficiency. Although nutritional deficiencies are difficult to identify, the dental hygienist must be cognizant of changes related to them in some denture wearers and can facilitate success of prosthodontic therapy by assessing the patient's nutritional status. After assessment, the dental hygienist informs the dentist of potential nutritional problems and either refers the patient to a dietitian or provides dietary counseling to ensure that nutritionally rich foods, such as vegetables, meats, beans, fish, and fruits, are not ignored (see Chapter 36).

Nutritional Factors

Key nutritional factors for patients include the following:
- Negative water balance and its effect on oral structures
- Negative calcium balance and its effect on alveolar bone
- Nitrogen-protein imbalance and resulting muscle weakness and oral tissue fragility

Water is essential for all body functions. Therefore evidence of tissue dehydration can be recognized throughout the body, especially in older adults, as wrinkled skin, loss of muscle mass, decreased sweat and sebaceous gland secretions, dry eyes, xerostomia, and a smooth, atrophic tongue. The best dietary recommendation for dehydrated patients is to consume vegetable soup because water and nutrients are retained more effectively in this form.

A negative calcium balance results in osteoporosis, which can precipitate rapid and extensive resorption of the alveolar ridges. A deficit in calcium intake, absorption, or transport may be responsible for the bony changes. Low-fat milk and milk products are good dietary sources of calcium.

Protein depletion not only affects muscle mass but also may increase tissue fragility and lip cracking. A decrease in mastication muscle mass and strength is especially evident in older adults and can be monitored by placing the finger in the vestibule of the mouth and asking patients to clench their teeth. Patients are encouraged to maintain a high-protein diet (e.g., meat, fish, beans, tofu, legumes) to maintain muscle mass.

Undoubtedly, food nutritional quality depends on the preparation method. Variations in food preparation result from the patient's physical capabilities, living conditions, and cultural preferences. Therefore dietary advice should include cooking instructions that maximize the nutritional value of the diet with consideration of individual circumstances and preferences. For example, meat and fish are most nutritious when broiled or boiled rather than fried. In addition to limiting saturated fat intake, boiling foods breaks down complex proteins into more easily digestible components. On the other hand, fried protein-rich foods lose some nutritional value because the protein coagulates and becomes more difficult to digest.

Nutrition and the Edentulous Older Adult

For the edentulous older adult, diet is of great concern (see Chapters 36 and 47). Essential nutrient deficiency magnifies the tissue friability and diminishes repair potential observed in geriatric patients. Older adults may have low incomes, inadequate kitchen facilities, loneliness, poor physical health, and other conditions that predispose them to poor nutritional habits. A lack of knowledge and interest in proper nutrition also contributes to malnutrition. The older adult's dietary intake often is affected by wearing dentures, and deficiencies in protein, calcium, and B-complex vitamins may be present. Normally, these nutrients are essential in the maintenance and repair of oral tissues and bone. Many older adults have a limited ability to digest and absorb food. This problem can be exacerbated by ill fitting prostheses, which may result in chewing difficulties and diminish consumption of fibrous foods. Therefore, digestion, absorption, and the use of nutrients are impaired. Two common dietary tendencies of the older edentulous person are the following:
- Preference for a soft diet high in carbohydrates and refined sugar
- Consumption of fewer protein-rich and high-fiber foods

For these reasons, the dental hygienist routinely assesses nutritional habits and suggests healthy food alternatives to promote weight control and a nutritionally balanced diet (Table 41.4). This assessment and counseling can be accomplished effectively if simple, well-defined, concise guidelines are constructed so that no major changes in food habits and preferences are made. The patient and the dental hygienist can set

TABLE 41.4 Nutritional Guidelines for Maintenance of Oral Health in Edentulous and Partially Edentulous Patients	
Nutritional Goal	**Rationale**
Eat a variety of foods.	Essential for repair and maintenance of structurally and functionally competent body parts; increases likelihood of getting necessary nutrients.
Select foods high in complex carbohydrates: fruits, vegetables, whole-grain bread, and cereals.	Blood glucose levels rise less if complex carbohydrates are consumed rather than simple sugars. Also, fiber in these foods promotes normal bowel function and may reduce serum cholesterol levels.
Protein-rich foods, including lean meat, poultry, fish, dried peas, and beans are required daily.	Maintains strength and integrity of tissues, especially when patient is exposed to physiologic stress.
Obtain calcium from dairy products; some nondairy foods also contain substantial amounts of calcium.	Calcium intake is critical to maintaining bone mass. Alveolar bone is an early site of calcium withdrawal if dietary calcium intake is low.
Consume fruit juices containing vitamin C and citrus fruit daily.	Essential for repair and healing of wounds and for absorption of other vitamins and minerals.
Limit intake of processed foods high in saturated and hydrogenated fats and sodium.	Evidence links high fat intake to heart disease, certain cancers, and obesity. High sodium intake may cause hypertension.
Limit intake of bakery products high in fat and simple sugars.	Bakery products are often high in calories and/or low in nutrients.
Drink eight glasses of water daily.	Essential for all body functions.

See also Chapter 36.
Adapted from Zarb GA, Hobkirk JA, Eckert SE, et al. *Prosthodontic Treatment for Edentulous Patients.* 13th ed. Mosby; 2013.

nutritional goals, taking into account lifestyle, financial resources, and cultural preferences. With the edentulous patient, nutritional deficits should always be considered during determination of factors that contribute to a denture-related problem.

KEY CONCEPTS

- A prosthesis is a fixed or removable appliance that is functionally and cosmetically designed to replace a missing tooth or teeth.
- People who wear dental prostheses receive an oral examination periodically to monitor the health of hard and soft tissues, functional integrity of the prosthesis, and changes that may be warranted. Frequency should be based on the patient's risk factors for disease.
- A removable dental prosthesis should be marked with the wearer's name or identification number, especially if the person lives in an institutional setting.
- Just like natural oral structures, the dental prosthesis and oral cavity of the wearer must be thoroughly cleansed daily.
- Risk factors for edentulism include caries, periodontal disease, low socioeconomic status, inadequate access to professional care, low frequency of care, and poor daily oral hygiene.
- Loss of natural teeth is associated with fear of aging, decreased sexuality, feelings of insecurity, fear of rejection, loss of self-esteem, and unrealistic expectations for tooth replacement.
- Oral changes related to tooth loss include resorption of the residual ridge and alveolar bone, oral mucous membrane remodeling, and loss of orofacial muscle tone.
- Patients who lose teeth face challenges in their physical appearance, speech, and masticatory efficiency.
- Removable dental prosthesis–induced oral lesions include fibrous hyperplasia, focal hyperkeratosis, denture stomatitis, chronic candidiasis, angular cheilitis, and papillary hyperplasia.
- Patient education is a priority for patients wearing prostheses and oral appliances. Patients must know how to clean the mouth and prosthesis or oral appliance to maintain their oral health.

REFERENCES

1. Slade GD, Akinkugbe AA, Sanders AE. Projections of US edentulism prevalence following 5 decades of decline. *J Dent Res.* 2014;93(10):959–965.
2. Health Canada. Report on the Findings of the Oral Health Component of the Canadian Health Measures Survey 2007–2009 (Technical Report) [accessed July 2022]. Available: H34-221-2010-eng.pdf (publications.gc.ca).
3. Carlsson GE, Persson G. Morphological changes of the mandible after extraction and wearing of dentures: a longitudinal, clinical, and x-ray cephalometric study covering five years. *Odontol Revy.* 1967;18:27.
4. Avila-Ortiz G, Elangovan S, Kramer KW, Blanchette D, Dawson DV. Effect of alveolar ridge preservation after tooth extraction: a systematic review and meta-analysis. *J Dent Res.* 2014;93(10):950–958. https://doi.org/10.1177/0022034514541127. Epub 2014 Jun 25. PMID: 24966231; PMCID: PMC4293706.
5. Moynihan P, Varghese R. Impact of wearing dentures on dietary intake, nutritional status, and eating: a systematic review. *JDR Clin Transl Res.* 2022;7(4):334–351. doi: 10.1177/23800844211026608.
6. Nguyen CT, MacEntee MI, Mintzes B, Perry TL. Information for physicians and pharmacists about drugs that might cause dry mouth: a study of monographs and published literature. *Drugs Aging.* 2014;31(1):55–65.
7. Regezi JA, Sciubba JJ, Jordan R. *Oral Pathology: Clinical Pathologic Correlations.* 7th ed. Saunders; 2016.
8. Bugshan A, Farooq I. Oral squamous cell carcinoma: metastasis, potentially associated malignant disorders, etiology and recent advancements in diagnosis. *F1000Research.* 2020;9.

42

Dentinal Hypersensitivity

Mina C. Kim and Juliana J. Kim

PROFESSIONAL OPPORTUNITIES

Correctly diagnosing and treating dentinal hypersensitivity is a valuable service the dental hygienist can provide to the many patients that live with sensitive teeth. There are a variety of professionally and self-administered agents the dental hygienist can apply or recommend to alleviate symptoms. If these options prove to be insufficient, the dental hygienist can refer their patients to a general dentist or periodontist who can recommend more invasive treatment options, such as restorative therapy, root coverage, or laser therapy.

COMPETENCIES

1. Distinguish between dentinal hypersensitivity and other sources of tooth pain.
2. Discuss oral conditions associated with dentinal hypersensitivity, elucidate the teeth and risk factors most likely contributing to dentinal hypersensitivity, and describe the prevalence and distribution of dentinal hypersensitivity.
3. Explain the specific clinical and radiographic criteria that must be present to arrive at a diagnosis of dentinal hypersensitivity.
4. Describe the management of dentinal hypersensitivity, including the indications and effectiveness of various treatment options.

INTRODUCTION

Tooth pain and sensitivity are common patient complaints in the oral care environment. Several conditions may elicit a pain response; the nature and extent of pain vary substantially, individually and among persons. Therefore, an assessment of oral sites using a standardized approach is critical to identifying an appropriate cause and, in response, managing the problem correctly. **Dentinal hypersensitivity** is characterized by short, sharp pain arising from exposed dentin that occurs in response to stimuli, typically thermal (both hot and cold), evaporative, tactile, osmotic, or chemical, and is characterized by symptoms that cannot be ascribed to any other form of dental defect or pathologic condition (Box 42.1).

ETIOLOGY AND NATURE OF DENTINAL HYPERSENSITIVITY

Tooth development results in the following cementum-to-enamel relationships:

- Cementum overlaps the enamel (approximately 60% to 65% of time).
- Cementum and enamel meet without overlap (30% of time).
- Cementum and enamel do not meet (5% to 10% of time) but with no exposed dentin.
- Enamel overlaps the cementum (1.6% of time).

The histologic differences associated with dentinal hypersensitivity are important because dentin is comprised of numerous thin tubules that transverse from the pulp to the outer dentinal surface. Two types of sensory nerve fibers, known as A-fibers and C-fibers, are known to extend 10% to 15% of the distance from the pulpal side of the dentinal tubule to the dentinoenamel junction. A-fibers are myelinated and therefore transmit stimuli faster than unmyelinated C-fibers. Stimulation of these sensory nerve fibers results in tooth pain. **A-delta fibers** are comprised of small myelinated fibers that evoke a sensation of well-localized sharp pain and are thought to be responsible for dentinal hypersensitivity. Similarly, **A-beta fibers** are susceptible to the same types of stimuli but respond more sensitively to electrical stimulation. In contrast, the stimulation of the **unmyelinated C-fibers** results in a dull, poorly localized, aching type of pain that is usually associated with pulpal pain. Thus the activation of specific fibers results in different types of tooth pain.

Hypersensitive dentin has the following characteristics:
- Dentinal tubules open to the oral cavity
- Large and numerous dentinal tubules
- Thin, poorly calcified, or breached smear layer (i.e., deposit of salivary proteins, debris from dentifrices, and/or other calcified matter that occludes dentinal tubules)

In nonsensitive dentin, the smear layer covers the opening of the dentinal tubules or mineral compounds physically occlude the tubules, thereby reducing the ability of stimuli to induce fluid flow (see the following section on Hydrodynamic Theory) and thus stimulating nerve conduction to the pulp. Therefore the loss or removal of a smear layer may result in exposed tubular nerve fibers, leading to a pain response. Nonsensitive dentin also is found to have fewer dentinal tubules present at the surface than sensitive dentin.[1] Scanning electron photomicrographs verify that hypersensitive dentin has eight times as many open dentinal tubules and twice the diameter of open tubules as nonsensitive dentin. These findings serve as the basis for treatment options.

Hydrodynamic Theory

Many theories have been proposed through the years to explain the etiology of dentinal hypersensitivity, including the transducer theory, modulation theory, "gate" control theory, vibration theory, and

BOX 42.1 Common Stimuli in Dentinal Hypersensitivity

- Cold (frozen drinks, ice cream, cold air)
- Heat (coffee, tea)
- Sweets (candy, chocolate)
- Acid (citrus fruits, grapes)

hydrodynamic theory. The most accepted theory today is the hydrodynamic theory. Brannstrom was the first to provide evidence to support this widely accepted hydrodynamic theory that explains the pain of dentinal hypersensitivity.[2] The hydrodynamic theory proposes that stimuli (e.g., thermal, tactile, chemical) are transmitted to the pulp surface via movement of fluid within the dentinal tubules. This fluid movement acts as a transducing medium that conveys peripheral stimuli to free A-delta nerve endings near the odontoblastic layer of the pulp-dentin interface. Subsequently, this reaction is interpreted as tooth pain by the individual with dentinal hypersensitivity (Fig. 42.1).

For dentinal hypersensitivity, an open dentinal tubule channel must traverse from the exposed dentin surface to a vital pulp. The exposed dentin necessary for such hypersensitivity is most commonly the result of gingival recession or enamel loss. When gingival recession occurs, cementum is exposed. This exposed layer of cementum is thin and labile and easily abraded or eroded away, thus offering little protection against sensitivity.

ORAL CONDITIONS ASSOCIATED WITH DENTINAL HYPERSENSITIVITY

Causes of Gingival Recession

The most common cause of dentinal hypersensitivity is gingival recession, where as soon as the thin layer of cementum below the CEJ is exposed, it becomes nonviable and is lost, leaving dentin exposed, which leads to its hypersensitivity. However, the cause of gingival recession is multifactorial, and its appearance is most commonly the result of more than one factor acting together.[3] (Fig. 42.2) Epidemiologic studies have identified the following factors associated with gingival recession:

- *Age.* The frequency of gingival recession increases with age. In fact, all or almost all older adults have some recession.[3] Gingival recession in younger age groups generally is localized. The relationship between age and increasing gingival recession may be due to the cumulative effect and longer presence of etiologic factors. Prevention of subsequent root caries in older patients indicates recommendations for twice-daily brushing with a fluoride dentifrice, application of a fluoride varnish or chlorhexidine-thymol varnish, and if indicated, frequent continuing care.[4] Identifying the cause of localized recession in younger patients and providing oral health education or interventions to ameliorate the effects of these behaviors or conditions is potentially an important aspect of dental hygiene care.
- *Tooth type.* The most common areas for localized gingival recession are on the buccal surfaces of the canines, premolars, and mandibular anterior teeth. In premolars and molars, recession had been associated with the presence of misaligned teeth in this area with thin, fenestrated, or absent labial alveolar bone as a predisposing factor to recession. Recession commonly presents with plaque and calculus deposits or inadequate oral hygiene. Tooth anatomy and tooth position also may affect the thickness of the labial plate. Although not considered a singular cause, orthodontic treatment may move the tooth through the buccal plate, predisposing it to recession.

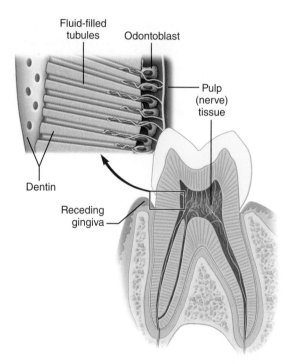

Fig. 42.1 Structure of dentinal tubules.

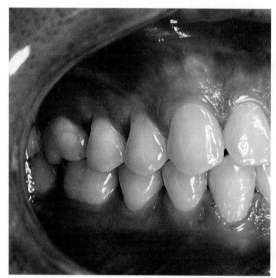

Fig. 42.2 Recession of maxillary premolars. (Courtesy Dr. Mina C. Kim.)

- *Bacterial plaque biofilm.* The most common factor associated with gingival recession is plaque.[3] Poor oral self-care results in plaque-induced gingivitis as inflammation breaks down gingival epithelium and connective tissue. Gingivitis also can progress to attachment loss and result in recession.
- *Trauma from traumatic toothbrushing.*[3] Gingival trauma caused by traumatic toothbrushing and/or injury from abrasive dentifrices, or a combination of both, may be risk factors. The technique, frequency, duration, and force of brushing and toothbrush filaments have been associated with recession, although more evidence is needed to conclusively state a causal relationship. A horizontal toothbrushing stroke or scrubbing and vigorous or forceful toothbrushing may be damaging.[3] There is no evidence to substantiate a difference in the use of manual or powered toothbrushes.[5]

- *Occlusal trauma.* Occlusal discrepancies appear to contribute to gingival recession and gingival clefts.[6] Sources of occlusal trauma include a poorly equilibrated bite and bruxism. Many patients who show evidence of bruxism also show gingival recession. Occlusal forces may exacerbate a preexisting periodontal lesion and possibly lead to further recession.
- *Dental restorations.* Poorly contoured restorations can be plaque traps that cause recession. Sound fillings can also cause recession when margins are placed at the gingiva or subgingivally, which is often necessary to completely remove caries.[7]
- *Smokers.* Cigarette smoking is a known risk factor for periodontitis due to decreased blood flow and greater chance of recession for smokers versus nonsmokers. Vaping is also shown to cause gum disease as nicotine is a vasoconstrictor. However, it is unknown if vaping causes recession.
- *Piercings.* Oral piercings can cause trauma to the teeth and gingival recession by the pulling of the piercing.[8]

Causes of Enamel Loss

Hard tissue loss exposing dentin leads to dentin hypersensitivity. The loss of enamel above the cementoenamel junction (CEJ) is a prerequisite for dentin exposure. Researchers have found that enamel loss may be due to the following causes, either acting individually or together:

- *Attrition.* Sites of tooth structure wear are found commonly on the incisal or occlusal surfaces of teeth caused by masticatory forces. Unless malocclusion is involved, it is highly unlikely that attrition is observed at the buccal sites.
- *Abrasion.* Toothbrush variation (i.e., stiffness and configuration of the bristles), together with force, method, frequency, abrasiveness of toothpaste, and duration of brushing, results in tooth structure loss. When the teeth are brushed, enamel has been found to abrade 25 times more slowly than dentin and 35 times slower than cementum.
- *Erosion.* Tooth structure loss caused by a chemical process is most responsible for enamel loss. Intrinsic erosion is caused by acid regurgitation associated with medical and psychologic disorders (e.g., bulimia, acid reflux disease, morning sickness). Extrinsic erosion also may result from dietary factors that contribute to a highly acidic oral environment (e.g., frequent consumption of acidic, carbonated, or fruit drinks, or frequent sugar consumption).
- *Abfraction.* The ongoing flexion, tension, and compression forces exerted in the cervical area of a tooth from mastication and occlusal trauma can result in cracking and eventual loss of cervical tooth structure. Bruxism is a common cause of abfraction.

Additional Causes of Dentinal Hypersensitivity

- *Periodontal therapy.* Nonsurgical and surgical periodontal therapy reduces inflammation, increases clinical attachment levels, and often results in gingival recession.[9] In addition, periodontal surgery such as open flap debridement may necessitate apical repositioning of the gingival margin to reduce deep periodontal probing depths. These procedures can remove layers of protective cementum and dentin, thus exposing tubular dentin and causing sensitivity.
- *Vital teeth bleaching.* In-office and at-home procedures using peroxides to enhance the esthetic appearance of teeth, known as tooth bleaching or whitening, are popular. Tooth sensitivity is a common associated side effect.[10] The degree of sensitivity can be affected by the frequency of application or concentration of bleaching agents. Clinicians should recommend that patients follow manufacturer's instructions for usage time and frequency, and use concurrent fluoride therapy to strengthen enamel while bleaching teeth at home and prior to in-office bleaching.

PREVALENCE AND DISTRIBUTION OF DENTINAL HYPERSENSITIVITY

Reports of dentinal hypersensitivity occur in patients of all ages. The prevalence is thought to be anywhere from 4.8% to 62.3% and is more common in young adults. As an individual ages, the prevalence of dentinal hypersensitivity decreases because of an increase in secondary and tertiary dentin that forms a barrier to the pulp;[11] reduction in pulpal chamber size, vascularity, and pulpal nerve fibers; and dentinal sclerosis (i.e., reduction of the dentinal tubule lumen as a result of the deposition of intratubular dentin).

Dentinal hypersensitivity is most prevalent on the buccal cervical regions of teeth. Similarly, these same sites have a predilection for gingival recession and are the areas where the enamel is the thinnest. Thus gingival recession and loss of enamel appear to be related to the initiation of dentinal hypersensitivity.

Persons with moderate-to-severe sensitivity exhibit hypersensitivity at the same tooth sites. Individuals who are right-handed tend to clean their left-sided teeth more vigorously than their right-sided teeth, contributing to unilateral hypersensitivity.

DIAGNOSIS

Many oral conditions exhibit symptoms similar to dentinal hypersensitivity. Conditions such as chipped or fractured teeth, dental caries, pulpal pathologic conditions, incorrect placement of dentin adhesives, traumatic occlusion, or leaking, fractured, or failing restorations require completely different treatments from dentinal hypersensitivity. It is vitally important for the treating practitioner to understand that dentinal hypersensitivity is a diagnosis of exclusion. Therefore a thorough clinical and radiographic examination must be conducted to exclude these conditions and to arrive at a differential diagnosis of dentinal hypersensitivity (Box 42.2). For a diagnosis of dentinal hypersensitivity to be made, specific clinical and radiographic criteria must be present.

Clinical Criteria

Clinical findings that might be associated with dental sensitivity include the following:

- Sensitivity or pain when a stimulus is applied (e.g., hot, cold, tactile)
- Exposed dentin at the site of sensitivity
- No clinical signs of dental caries
- No evidence of fracture lines in tooth structure
- Restoration margins flush with tooth structure

Radiographic Criteria

Radiolucency may be present at the cervical third of the tooth where pain is reported, indicating possible abrasion, erosion, abfraction, or radiolucent restorative material. However, one or more of the following findings must be confirmed clinically to exclude dental caries:

- No pulpal inflammation or apical pathologic condition
- Absence of distinct fracture lines
- No radiolucent areas under restorations

In addition, it is important to not confuse cervical burnout as a pathological radiolucency.

Additional Testing

Salivary tests for flow and buffering capacity can be completed to evaluate the patient's ability to flush and neutralize acids and promote remineralization necessary to occlude tubules. Fluoride therapy, dietary counseling, and, if indicated, salivary stimulants or substitutes should be recommended (Fig. 42.3).

BOX 42.2 Characteristics of Hypersensitive Versus Nonsensitive Dentin

Hypersensitive Dentin
- Ends of dentinal tubules are open to the oral cavity.
- Tubules are larger and more numerous than in nonsensitive dentin.
- Smear layer is thin, poorly calcified, or breached.

Nonsensitive Dentin
- Fewer dentinal tubules at tooth surfaces are present than in sensitive dentin.
- Either a smear layer is present or tubules are occluded by mineral compounds.

Teledentistry

In the age of COVID-19, teledentistry has become much more widely used (see Chapter 65). Since dentinal hypersensitivity can cause severe pain, being able to properly diagnose and manage symptoms can be a great service to our patients.

When examining patients, we should use the same parameters as that done in a nonvirtual practice setting, such as recording the chief complaint, history of present illness, and medical history. Pictures and videos can help rule out certain conditions. If dentinal hypersensitivity is suspected, patients can apply desensitizing agents at home until they are able to visit in person. Make sure to always stress that a telehealth visit does not replace an in-person dental visit when patients have pain.

Some additional considerations to remember are the following (see Chapter 65):

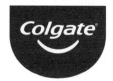

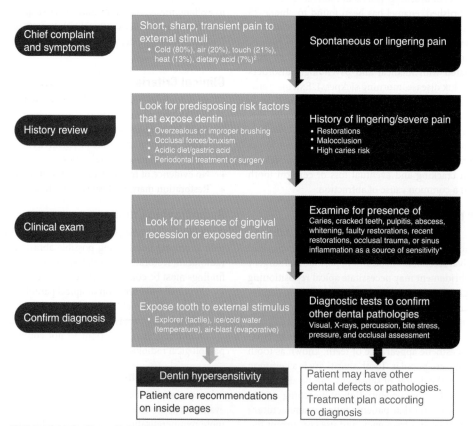

Fig. 42.3 Decision tree. (Courtesy of Colgate.)

- Be knowledgeable about telehealth regulations in your state
- Ensure platforms used to communicate with patients are secure (many EMRs offer this)
- Be cognizant of billing

MANAGEMENT OF DENTINAL HYPERSENSITIVITY

Managing dentinal hypersensitivity requires identification of the condition's cause and risk factors (Box 42.3). Failure to address the reason for an individual patient's pain or discomfort can result in inadequate and/or unnecessary therapy.

After a cause is established, the patient needs to be educated about behaviors that exacerbate symptoms of dentinal hypersensitivity.

BOX 42.3 Factors That Contribute to Dentinal Hypersensitivity

Factors that may expose dentin or opening tubules that are already blocked or sealed include the following:
- Gingival recession
- Loss of enamel
- Toothbrush abrasion
- Erosion
- Abfraction
- Acidic foods
- Periodontal surgery
- Occlusal hyperfunction
- Cusp grinding
- Instrumentation (e.g., root planing, scaling, extrinsic stain removal)
- Cosmetic tooth whitening (see Chapter 32)

BOX 42.4 Patient or Client Education Tips

- Explain multifaceted causes of dentinal hypersensitivity and modifiable risk factors.
- Discuss dietary information and monitor acidic and sugary fruits and beverages that may contribute to hypersensitivity.
- Explain significance of oral biofilm control, effective toothbrushing, interdental cleaning, and using low-abrasive fluoride dentifrices for sensitive teeth.
- Explain use of an ultrasoft toothbrush without the application of a toothpaste.
- Suggest dabbing a desensitizing dentifrice on the most sensitive areas of the tooth at bedtime.

Behavior modification to prevent further recession should be discussed, including improved oral hygiene; dietary choices such as avoiding carbonated beverages, acidic foods, and extremes in hot and cold foods; use of a daily fluoride mouth rinse and a low-abrasive, fluoride dentifrice for sensitive teeth; and cessation or reduced frequency or concentration of home bleaching (Box 42.4).

Treatment options include self-applied (at-home) desensitizing agents and professionally applied (in-office) desensitizing procedures, restorations, and surgeries.[12] Desensitizing agents used in treatment are classified by modes of action (Tables 42.1 and 42.2). The four mechanisms of action include the following:[11]

- Physical occlusion of dentinal tubules through particles to block the neural stimulus of the pulp tissue
- Chemical occlusion of dentinal tubules by the precipitation of minerals at the entrance of the dentinal tubules (examples of agents to use include oxalate compounds, strontium chloride, calcium phosphate–based compounds, fluorides, silver nitrate fluoride, and hydroxyethyl methacrylate [HEMA])
- Nerve desensitization to block pulp tissue nerve transmission, using potassium-based compounds to depolarize neural synapses
- Photobiomodulation using laser therapy to increase the metabolism of odontoblasts stimulating the formation of tertiary dentin

Without effective daily oral biofilm control and control of an acidic oral environment, the desensitizing effects of these agents are limited.

Self-Applied Desensitizing Agents

Self-applied desensitizing agents should be recommended to manage mild-to-moderate dentinal hypersensitivity (Fig. 42.4; see also Table 42.1). These agents are cost effective, safe, noninvasive, convenient, and simple to use at home. Dental hygienists should inform their patients with sensitive teeth that regular and continuous applications are needed to manage sensitivity.

Frequent and regular applications of a desensitizing dentifrice are necessary to avoid recurrence of symptoms. Of the potassium salts, potassium nitrate is the most common desensitizing agent in over-the-counter dentifrices; it works by depolarizing the nerve. Other ingredients that have been shown to be effective desensitizing agents in dentifrices include stannous fluoride, arginine, and strontium acetate.

Stannous fluoride (0.4% or 0.454%), a known antihypersensitivity ingredient, has been formulated into gels and toothpastes for daily use in controlling pain associated with dentinal hypersensitivity. Stannous fluoride produces the rapid onset or formation of a protective smear layer and the precipitation of calcium fluoride crystals, which physically block exposed dentinal tubules and hence act as a desensitizing agent against acidic or other environmental challenges. Clinical studies have shown that subjects who brushed twice daily with a 0.454%

TABLE 42.1 Self-Applied Desensitizing Agents and Their Mode of Action

Active Ingredients	Mechanism of Action	Examples of Products
5% potassium nitrate	Depolarizes nerves, resulting in reduced excitability of the nerves and making the nerves unresponsive to stimulus.	Colgate Sensitive Colgate PreviDent 5000 (prescription needed), Sensodyne Crest Sensi-Relief Tom's of Maine Sensitive Toothpaste (sodium lauryl sulfate-free)
0.4% stannous fluoride	Chemically occludes dentinal tubules.	Colgate Gel-Kam Crest Pro-Health Sensitive & Enamel Shield Crest Sensi-Repair & Prevent Toothpaste
8% arginine, calcium carbonate	Physically blocks the tubules by sealing them.	Colgate Sensitive Pro-Relief
Strontium acetate or strontium chloride	Nerve impulses are desensitized, and dentinal tubules are chemically blocked.	Sensodyne Rapid Relief (GlaxoSmithKline)

TABLE 42.2	Some Professionally Applied Desensitizing Agents		
Active Agent	**Mechanism of Action**	**Examples of Products**	**Comments**
38% silver diamine fluoride	Forms silver ion salts that chemically block the dentinal tubules without staining; sodium fluoride has added benefit of caries prevention.	Advantage Arrest (Elevate Oral Care)	Technique is sensitive and will stain active caries lesions black; evidence supports effectiveness in desensitization, caries prevention, and caries arrest; both products have FDA approval.[10]
Sodium fluoride	Physically blocks or occludes dentinal tubules.	Colgate Duraphat Colgate PreviDent 3M ESPE Vanish Varnish Enamel Pro Varnish (Premier) NUPRO White Varnish (Dentsply Sirona)	Is indicated and effective for caries prevention. Is FDA approved as a treatment for dentinal hypersensitivity; limited evidence is available.
Arginine and calcium carbonate	Physically blocks or occludes dentinal tubules.	Colgate Sensitive Pre-Procedural Desensitizing Paste	Is recommended before scaling and root planing; is used as a polishing paste on hypersensitive sites; additional evidence is needed for determining its effectiveness as a prophylaxis paste.
Strontium acetate and strontium chloride	Chemically blocks dentinal tubules.	Zarosen Desensitizing Cavity Varnish Dentinal Tubuli Seal (Cetylite)	Is recommended before scaling, before and after extrinsic stain removal, after cavity preparation, before crown and bridge cementation, and before pin and after seating; appears effective in the treatment of dentin hypersensitivity, but more evidence is needed.
Hydroxyethyl methacrylate (HEMA) and glutaraldehyde (Gluma)	Bonding resin seals and desensitizes nerves within dentinal tubules.	GLUMA Desensitizer (Kulzer) HemaSeal-G Desensitizing Solution (Germiphene Corporation)	No mixing or curing is involved; has a strong smell and taste; some are used in conjunction with bonding adhesive systems and crown and bridge luting agents; appears effective in the treatment of dentine hypersensitivity, but more evidence is needed.
Calcium compounds, including CPP-ACP	May seal dentinal tubules; however, assumption is based on enamel remineralization through release of soluble calcium and phosphate precipitate.	MI Paste (GC America) NUPRO NUSolutions (Dentsply Sirona)	Is a prophylaxis paste that cleans, occludes tubules, and desensitizes; evidence is limited to support effectiveness in desensitization.
Dimethacrylate and trimethacrylate resins	Mechanically protects exposed dentin areas.	Seal&Protect (Dentsply Sirona)	Is a light-curing resin sealant; appears effective in the treatment of dentine hypersensitivity; more evidence is needed.

CPP-ACP, Casein phosphopeptide–amorphous calcium phosphate; *FDA*, US Food and Drug Administration.

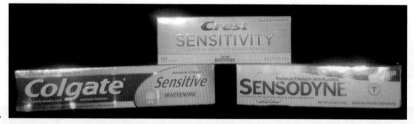
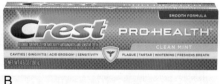

Fig. 42.4 Some commonly used desensitizing dentifrices, with active ingredients supported by the evidence. (A) Examples with potassium nitrate. (B) Example of 0.454% stannous fluoride dentifrice. ([B] Courtesy Proctor & Gamble.)

stannous fluoride dentifrice experience reduced hypersensitivity.[3,11] It is important to note that stannous fluoride formulations can stain teeth.

Dentifrices containing 8.0% arginine and calcium carbonate have also been shown to relieve dentinal hypersensitivity by occluding the dentinal tubules. This occlusion occurs when the arginine component triggers physical adherence of the calcium carbonate to the exposed dentin surface and to the inner surfaces of dentin tubules, thereby inducing deposition of calcium and phosphate-rich materials on the dentin surface and occluding the dentin tubules. Studies demonstrate that toothpastes containing 8.0% arginine and calcium carbonate are effective in the everyday treatment of dentin hypersensitivity when used twice daily during routine brushing.[3,11]

Strontium acetate (10%) in dentifrices has been shown to be more effective than fluoride dentifrices and negative controls in pain reduction from dentinal hypersensitivity. Moderate evidence supports its use. The active ingredient chemically blocks dentinal tubules. Twice-daily use is recommended.

Self-applied desensitizing agents also are marketed as gels and rinses. The active agents for these products are various fluoride compounds, such as sodium fluoride, sodium silicofluoride, and stannous fluoride; however, sodium fluoride dentifrices and gels are not as effective as other desensitizing agents. Some dentifrices have the American Dental Association (ADA) Seal of Acceptance for treatment of dentinal hypersensitivity. With any desensitizing product, long-term relief requires continued use of fluoride-containing substances to permanently seal off the exposed tubules with calcium fluoride particles.

Professionally Applied Desensitizing Agents

Evidence to support professionally applied desensitizing products appears to be effective in the treatment of dentin hypersensitivity; however, additional evidence is needed to support one agent or modality over another.[3] In-office products and procedures include varnishes and precipitants, bonding agents containing HEMA, polymerizing agents, and laser therapy.

Before any desensitizing treatment, hard and soft deposits should be removed from the tooth surfaces. Periodontal debridement in areas of recession with dentinal hypersensitivity may cause considerable discomfort, in which case teeth should be anesthetized before mechanical treatment (Procedure 42.1 and corresponding Competency Form). A complete discussion of potential side effects and likelihood of successful pain relief and evidence supporting the selected procedure or product is legally and ethically required for informed consent (Box 42.5).

Varnishes

- *5% sodium fluoride varnish.* Fluoride varnishes temporarily occlude dentinal tubules because the material is lost over time. This desensitizing agent is effective for caries prevention, but evidence is weak for relief of dentinal hypersensitivity.[3,6]

Other agents in varnishes, such as chlorhexidine, and fluoride glass ionomer varnishes have limited evidence supporting their effectiveness.

Precipitants

- *8% arginine and calcium carbonate.* After scaling, application of an in-office desensitizing paste containing arginine–calcium carbonate to teeth exhibiting sensitivity has been demonstrated to be effective in providing immediate relief; however, evidence for the agent used in a paste is limited. As with polishing teeth, the paste should be applied using a prophylaxis cup on a prophy angle and using low speed and a moderate amount of pressure. The paste is burnished into exposed tubules to occlude them.
- *Casein phosphopeptide (CPP)–amorphous calcium phosphate (ACP).* When applied orally, this nanocomplex has great affinity for bacterial biofilm. It also binds to soft tissues, pellicle, and hydroxyapatite and, subsequently, releases calcium and phosphate ions when challenged by an acid attack. It is thought that this ion release leads to a precipitate that plugs open dentinal tubules; however, limited evidence supports this assumption. CPP-ACP formulations in prophylaxis pastes are approved for desensitization claims by the US Food and Drug Administration (FDA).
- *Calcium sodium phosphosilicate (CSP).* NovaMin is the brand name of the bioactive glass CSP. This inorganic chemical binds to tooth surfaces and delivers calcium, phosphorus, sodium, and silica to replace lost minerals. When the glass particles come in contact with saliva, calcium and phosphate ions are released. A calcium-phosphate layer forms and crystallizes as new hydroxyapatite. Dentinal tubules are occluded in the process, and desensitization is supported by a moderate level of evidence that CSP may be effective. This agent is approved by the FDA for desensitization claims.

Primers Containing Hydroxyethyl Methacrylate

Although few controlled clinical trials have been conducted on the efficacy of HEMA-containing primers, desensitizing agents containing either 5% glutaraldehyde and 35% HEMA in water or 35% HEMA in water alone are popular.

- *5% glutaraldehyde, 35% HEMA in water.* Studies regarding a primer containing 5% glutaraldehyde and 35% HEMA in water (e.g., Gluma, Gluma 2000) have shown mixed results regarding its effectiveness in reducing dentinal hypersensitivity in the long term. More evidence is needed to document effectiveness of this formulation.

Polymerizing Agents

- *Glass ionomer cements (GICs).* GICs are used in cervical abrasions and abfractions for the treatment of dentinal hypersensitivity. GICs are effective in treating hypersensitivity if they cover the affected area.

PROCEDURE 42.1 Administration of Desensitizing Agents

Equipment

- Isolating materials (cotton rolls, gauze, dry angles)
- Cotton applicators
- Dappen dish
- Personal protective equipment
- Desensitizing agent

Steps

1. Assemble armamentarium for desensitization.
2. Explain rationale, procedure, and limitations of desensitizing agent to client.
3. Identify sensitive sites requiring desensitization treatment.
4. Remove oral biofilm and debris from tooth surfaces before desensitizing agent is applied.
5. Isolate area with cotton rolls and dry dentin surface by blotting with gauze.
6. Dispense and apply the desensitizing agent according to manufacturer's instructions.
7. Evaluate treated areas for success; reapply if necessary.
8. Discard materials according to infection control procedures.
9. Record treatment in "Services Rendered" section of dental record, including tooth number, region of treatment, agent used, and patient response.
10. Educate patient about supplementary procedures for controlling sensitivity.

BOX 42.5 Legal, Ethical, and Safety Issues

- Properly assess the client's hypersensitivity to rule out alternative causes of pain.
- Begin with the most noninvasive treatment options and advance to more invasive procedures (e.g., root coverage, laser) only when less invasive options have proven insufficient in alleviating symptoms.
- Document the problem, product recommendation, instructions provided, and client's response to care (e.g., adherence, product success, adverse effects) in the dental record.
- Evaluate clinical outcomes of treatment and document degree of effectiveness.
- Comply with the individual state practice act regarding dental hygienists' scope of practice in terms of product recommendation, use, and clinician application.

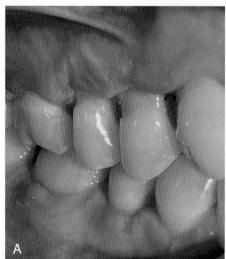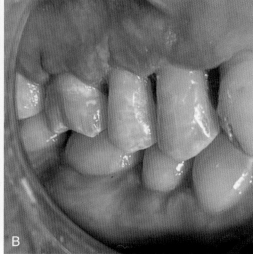

Fig. 42.5 Composite restorations of maxillary premolars (A) before restorations; (B) after restorations. (Courtesy of Dr. Mina C. Kim.)

- *Adhesive resin bonding primers.* Adhesive resin bonding primers decrease dentin permeability by occluding the open dentinal tubules. Resin primers come in either a two- or one-bottle system. The product is gently rubbed on the hypersensitive dentin for approximately 10 seconds, air-dried, and cured, and the procedure possibly is repeated.

Lasers

In studies, lasers are shown to reduce dentinal hypersensitivity compared to placebos in the short term. The mechanism by which laser treatment works is debated, but one theory proposes that lasers can seal dentinal tubules. Laser therapy is relatively quick and safe, and one treatment can reduce or eliminate dentinal hypersensitivity.[13]

Restorations

Desensitizing agents either occlude the open tubule or inactivate the nerve. Restorations may be placed to cover exposed dentin and restore tooth anatomy, especially when a esthetics are important. In extreme circumstances, it may be necessary to remove the pulp and perform root canal therapy or extract the tooth. These last two options are indicated for reasons in addition to dentinal hypersensitivity, such as inability to restore the tooth, severe periodontal destruction, overeruption, or a esthetics (Fig. 42.5).

Periodontal Plastic Surgery

Over the years, numerous techniques have been developed to surgically correct gingival recession. Procedures range from use of juxtaposed gingiva to guided tissue regeneration and tissue-engineered, human fibroblast–derived dermal substitute; however, the most common and predictable procedure for the treatment of Miller class I and II defects is the **subepithelial connective tissue graft**. This procedure, which harvests autologous connective tissue and places it on top of the exposed root, has been reported to increase patient clinical attachment and decrease dentinal sensitivity (Case Study 42.1 and Fig. 42.6). Allografts (donated from a cadaver) and synthetic materials can also be used.

CONCLUSION

Many dental patients suffer from the problem of dentinal hypersensitivity. It is important for a patient to be evaluated for these symptoms

CASE STUDY 42.1   Case Study of Patient Treated With a Connective Tissue Graft to Control Dentinal Hypersensitivity

- CM has come to the practice complaining of severe sensitivity to cold air and fluids around tooth 22 over the past 5 months and, as a result, has avoided toothbrushing or flossing in that area. Periodontal assessment reveals localized erythema, oral biofilm accumulation, and recession of 2 mm. In addition, tooth 22 has a extrinsic staining and cervical abrasion. CM acknowledges a history of aggressive tooth brushing.
- CM's care plan includes oral self-care instructions, with emphasis on the modified Bass brushing technique with a sensitivity toothpaste, scaling and root planing under a local anesthetic, and use of a soft-bristled toothbrush to improve gingival health before periodontal surgery.
- A connective tissue graft procedure is performed to provide a thicker gingival biotype buccal to tooth 22. Before surgery, CM reports a Visual Analog Scale (VAS) value of 10 when tooth 22 is subjected to a cold air blast from an air-water syringe.
- Six weeks after the surgical procedure was performed, CM reports that VAS value improved to 5.

and informed of the treatment options available. A patient's habits also factor into this process since they may be contributing to the problem and if not changed, the condition may persist. Most often, dentinal hypersensitivity occurs as a result of recessed gingiva with exposed dentinal tubules. Once the tubules are exposed, the patient experiences pain due to thermal, tactile, and osmotic stimuli. Desensitizing treatments should be delivered systematically. Preventive and over-the-counter treatments, such as desensitizing toothpastes, are a good place to start and can later be complemented by in-office treatments.

Dentinal hypersensitivity can be difficult to diagnose and treatment should always start with the most conservative option. Currently, there is not a standard way to treat the condition, but studies suggest that dentinal tubule occlusion and nerve desensitization are the most effective methods.[12]

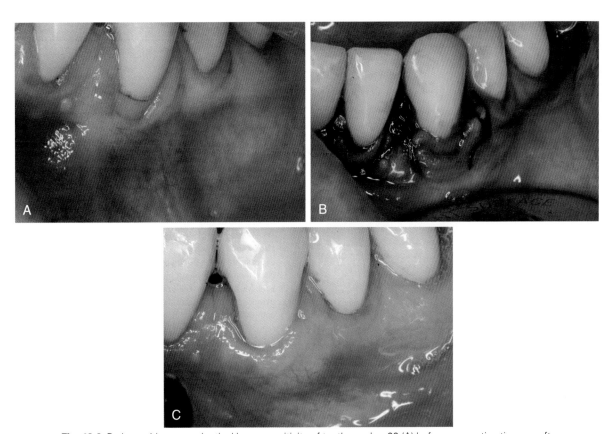

Fig. 42.6 Patient with severe dentinal hypersensitivity of tooth number 22 (A) before connective tissue graft; (B) immediately after connective tissue graft; (C) 8 weeks after connective tissue graft. (Courtesy Dr. James E. Jacobs.)

CRITICAL THINKING EXERCISES

Use Fig. 42.7 and the following information to answer the questions about this case.

Patient Profile: A 32-year-old female single mother of two boys (ages 2 and 4), who is an emergency care nurse.

Chief Complaint: "My teeth are very sensitive when I eat or drink cold foods and beverages."

Health History: No significant findings are revealed.

Pharmacologic History: The patient takes the following medications:
- Ortho Tri-Cyclen (norgestimate and ethinyl estradiol)
- Wellbutrin SR (bupropion hydrochloride 100 mg)
- Imitrex (sumatriptan succinate 50 mg)

Dental History:
- Regular 6-month continued-care appointments
- History of frequent aphthous ulcers
- Brushes twice daily
- Flosses once daily

Clinical Examination Findings:
- Absence of soft tissue pathologic conditions
- Absence of clinical carious lesions
- Light to moderate calculus
- Localized attrition along anterior incisal surfaces

- Localized recession and cervical abrasion evident on teeth 6, 7, 11, 22, 23, 26, and 27
- Crowns on 8 and 9

Radiographic Findings:
- Incipient enamel lesions (distal aspect of tooth 3, mesial aspect of tooth 15, distal aspect of tooth 19)
- Linear radiolucent areas along the cementoenamel junction (CEJ) of premolar teeth 28 and 29; consistent with the clinically observed posterior cervical abrasion

Given the patient profile, chief complaint, and examination findings, answer the following questions:

1. What patient characteristics indicate that she is at risk for dentinal hypersensitivity?
2. What are some common explanations for gingival recession?
3. What dental conditions must be considered to arrive at a differential diagnosis?
4. Based on the differential diagnosis determined by you and the dentist, what are the treatment options?
5. What special self-care instructions will relieve the client's symptoms of sensitive teeth? What specific products may reduce the occurrence of aphthous ulcers?

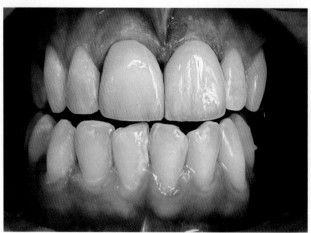

Fig. 42.7 Intraoral photo of a young woman. Note accumulation of oral biofilm, gingival recession, crowns, and attrition. (Courtesy of Dr. Stacy A. Spizuoco.)

KEY CONCEPTS

- Assessment of etiology and risk factors is critical to accurately identify dentinal hypersensitivity.
- Hypersensitive dentin has the following characteristics: dentinal tubules open to the oral cavity; large and numerous dentinal tubules; and thin, poorly calcified, or breached smear layer (i.e., deposit of salivary proteins, debris from dentifrices, and other calcified matter).
- Abfraction is damage resulting from the ongoing flexion, tension, and compression forces exerted in the cervical area of a tooth as a result of mastication and occlusal trauma. These forces result in cracking and eventual loss of cervical tooth structure.
- Dentinal hypersensitivity is characterized by short, sharp pain arising from exposed dentin that occurs in response to stimuli, typically thermal (both hot and cold), evaporative, tactile, osmotic, or chemical, and that cannot be ascribed to any other form of dental defect or pathologic condition.
- The hydrodynamic theory proposes that stimuli (e.g., thermal, tactile, chemical) are transmitted to the pulp surface via movement of the fluid or semi-fluid materials in the dentinal tubules.
- Desensitization and prevention measures are incorporated into the client's care plan and daily self-care regimen.
- Most persons experiencing dentinal hypersensitivity can be treated with self-applied desensitizing dentifrices; however, if the sensitivity persists, bonding agents for desensitization and restorative interventions can reduce sensitivity.
- Dental hygienists have a role in the management of dentinal hypersensitivity, which includes staying informed of best evidence and new products, selecting treatments that meet the patient's needs, and educating patients about effective self-care habits (see Box 42.3).

ACKNOWLEDGMENT

The authors acknowledge Dr. Dimitrios Karastathis for his past contributions to this chapter.

REFERENCES

1. Absi EG, Addy M, Adams D. Dentine hypersensitivity. A study of the patency of dentinal tubules in sensitive and non-sensitive cervical dentine. *J Clin Periodontol*. 1987;14(5):280.
2. Brannstrom M. A hydrodynamic mechanism in the transmission of pain-produced stimuli through dentine. In: Anderson DJ, ed. *Sensory Mechanisms in Dentine*. Pergamon Press; 1963:73–79.
3. Sarpangala M, Suryanarayan MA, Shashikanth H, et al. Etiology and occurrence of gingival recession—an epidemiological study. *J Indian Soc Periodontol*. 2015;19(6):671–675.
4. Heasman PA, Ritchie M, Asuni A, et al. Gingival recession and root caries in the aging population: a critical evaluation of treatments. *J Clin Periodontol*. 2017;44(suppl 18):S178–S193.
5. Sanz M, Baumer A, Buduneli N, et al. Effect of professional mechanical plaque removal on secondary prevention of periodontitis and the complications of gingival and periodontal preventive measures: consensus report of group 4 of the 11th European Workshop on Periodontology on effective prevention of periodontal and implant diseases. *J Clin Periodontol*. 2015;42(suppl 16):S214–S220.
6. Krishna PD, Sridhar SN, Solomon EG. The influence of occlusal trauma on gingival recession and gingival clefts. *J Indian Prosthosdont Soc*. 2013;13(1):7–12.
7. Paniz G, Nart J, Gobbato L, et al. Clinical periodontal response to anterior all-ceramic crowns with either chamfer or feather-edge subgingival tooth preparations: Six-month results and patient perception. *Int J Periodontics Restorative Dent*. 2017;37(1):61–68. https://doi.org/10.11607/prd.2765. PMID: 27977819.
8. Covello F, Salerno C, Giovannini V, Corridore D, Ottolenghi L, Vozza I. Piercing and oral health: a study on the knowledge of risks and complications. *Int J Environ Res Public Health*. 2020;17(2):613. https://doi.org/10.3390/ijerph17020613. PMID: 31963636; PMCID: PMC7013412.
9. Aimetti M. Nonsurgical periodontal treatment. *Int J Esthet Dent*. 2014;9(2):251–267.
10. DeGeus JL, Wambier LM, Kossatz S, et al. At home vs in-office bleaching. *Oper Dent*. 2016;41(4):341–356.
11. Favaro Zeola L, Soares PV, Cunha-Cruz J. Prevalence of dentin hypersensitivity: systematic review and meta-analysis. *J Dent*. 2019;81:1–6. https://doi.org/10.1016/j.jdent.2018.12.015. Epub Jan 11, 2019. PMID: 30639724.
12. Moraschini V, da Costa LS, dos Santos GO. Effectiveness for dentin hypersensitivity treatment of non-carious cervical lesions: a meta-analysis. *Clin Oral Investig*. 2018;22:617–631.
13. Mahdian M, Behboodi S, Ogata Y, Natto ZS. Laser therapy for dentinal hypersensitivity. *Cochrane Database Syst Rev*. 2021;7(7):CD009434. https://doi.org/10.1002/14651858.CD009434.pub2. PMID: 34255856; PMCID: PMC8276937.

43

Local Anesthesia

Gwen Lang and Laurie Bercasio

PROFESSIONAL OPPORTUNITIES

Learning how to confidently administer safe, gentle, and effective local anesthesia is the goal of a professional dental hygienist so that patients are comfortable during dental hygiene therapy. Dental hygienists who use these techniques will quickly establish themselves as caring, trustworthy professionals. Comfort during nonsurgical periodontal therapy is one of the most valuable patient-centered services the dental hygienist can provide.

COMPETENCIES

1. Discuss the physiologic mechanism of nerve conduction and the primary action of local anesthetics as it relates to pain management and patient comfort.
2. Evaluate various topical and local anesthetic agents and their indications/contraindications for safe and effective use.
3. Describe the local anesthetic armamentarium components, including the procedures for appropriate setup and breakdown.
4. Determine anatomical landmarks, nerves, and areas anesthetized after applying safe and effective procedural techniques for each injection.
5. Describe various local and systemic complications that may develop despite preanesthetic patient assessment and adherence to recommended procedures for local anesthesia administration.

▶ EVOLVE VIDEO RESOURCE

Videos on local anesthesia techniques and procedures are available for viewing on Evolve (http://evolve.elsevier.com/Pieren/hygiene/).

INTRODUCTION

The term *anesthesia* is often preceded by either *local* or *regional*. Either phrase is correct; each indicates that a specific area is anesthetized and that the patient is conscious, unlike in general anesthesia, in which the patient is unconscious. Therefore, the use of either term is appropriate, and they can be used interchangeably, although *local anesthesia* appears to be more commonly used.

Administration of intraoral local anesthetic (LA) when needed during dental hygiene care allows the dental hygienist to provide local anesthesia to alleviate pain and the potential stress and anxiety that can be associated with it, to meet the patient's human needs, and improve oral quality of life. **Local anesthesia** is the loss of sensation in a well-circumscribed area of the body resulting from the depression of excitation in nerve endings or the inhibition of the conduction process in peripheral nerves.[1] LA agents used in clinical practice today prevent both the generation and conduction of nerve impulses. Essentiall, the LA agent provides a chemical roadblock between the source of the impulse (e.g., toothache) and the brain. The impulse is unable to reach the brain and is therefore not interpreted as pain or discomfort by the patient. Local anesthesia differs dramatically from general anesthesia in that local anesthesia produces loss of sensation without inducing a loss of consciousness.[1]

Not all dental hygiene patients require local anesthesia. Those receiving preventive oral prophylaxis or even periodontal maintenance care may experience little or no discomfort; however, LA administration usually is required if the dental hygiene care plan includes therapeutic scaling and root planing or if a patient is simply experiencing undue tooth or soft tissue sensitivity. In addition, the dental hygienist may collaborate with the dentist to provide local anesthesia in preparation for restorative or surgical periodontal therapy. Moreover, in some states, a hygienist can collaborate with a dentist in alternative practice settings as a Registered Dental Hygienist, Expanded Function Dental Auxiliary (EFDA), or a Dental Therapist (DT). In all instances, services will depend on effective pain management and LA administration, especially if restorative care, pulpotomies, or simple extractions are within the scope of practice. Clinicians in alternative practice settings primarily work with underserved populations such as low-income patients and those with special needs, which improves access to healthcare, the workforce equity gap, and efforts to meet human needs.[2]

PHYSIOLOGY OF NERVE CONDUCTION

To understand how LA agents work, the dental hygienist needs to be familiar with the physiology of nerve conduction. Two principal ions are needed for nerve conduction: potassium (K^+) and sodium (Na^+). Because these two ions are positively charged, they normally exist in equal concentrations across a membrane; however, in a nerve cell, this equilibrium does not exist (Fig. 43.1, *Phase 1*). Because of a sodium pump located within the cell membrane, the positively charged sodium molecules are forced outside the nerve cell. As the sodium leaves the intracellular fluid, a state of negativity is created inside the nerve cell. At the same time, the extracellular fluid, which has received the sodium, becomes positive. Once the sodium ion is transported out of the cell, it is not able to diffuse back into the intracellular fluids because of the relative impermeability of the nerve membrane to this ion. Although the nerve membrane is freely permeable to the potassium, this ion remains within the nerve cell because the negative charge of the nerve membrane restrains the positively charged ion by electrostatic attraction. The nerve is polarized, or in a resting state or at resting potential, when this balance exists between positive sodium ions on the outside of the nerve membrane and positive potassium ions on the inside of the membrane. Polarization of the membrane continues as long as the nerve remains undisturbed.

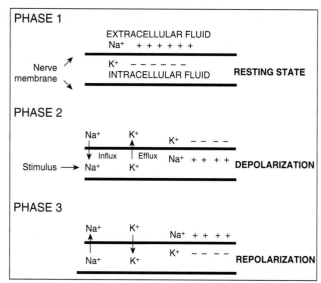

Fig. 43.1 Rapid sequence of changes, depolarization, and repolarization is termed *action potential.*

TABLE 43.1	**Amide Local Anesthetics Proprietary Names and Generic Names**	
Generic Name	**United States**	**Canada**
Articaine	Articadent, Orabloc, Septocaine, Zorcaine	Astracaine, Orabloc, Septanest, Ubestesin, Ultracaine, Zorcaine
Bupivacaine	Marcaine, Vivacaine	Marcaine, Vivacaine
Lidocaine	Xylocaine, Lignospan, Octocaine	Lignospan
Mepivacaine	Carbocaine, Polocaine, Isocaine, Scandonest	Polocaine, Scandonest
Prilocaine	Citanest	Citanest

From Malamed SF. *Handbook of Local Anesthesia.* 7th ed. Elsevier; 2020.

A stimulus, which may be chemical, thermal, mechanical, or electrical in nature (such as pain), produces excitation of the nerve fiber and therefore a change in the ion balance (Fig. 43.1, *Phase 2*). During this phase, referred to as **depolarization**, the nerve membrane becomes more permeable to the sodium ion. Consequently, the positive sodium ions move rapidly across the nerve membrane into the inside of the nerve cell. During this influx of sodium, the potassium ions diffuse from the inside to the outside of the nerve membrane.

Thus, during depolarization, the ion balance of the nerve cell reverses. On the interior of the nerve membrane are the positive sodium ions, whereas on the exterior of the nerve cell are the potassium ions. The inside of the nerve is now electrically positive compared with the outside of the nerve.

Immediately after depolarization, the permeability of the membrane to the sodium ion once again decreases (Fig. 43.1, *Phase 3*). This situation is referred to as repolarization. During this phase, the sodium pump actively transports the sodium ion out of the nerve cell while potassium ions diffuse into the nerve cell. Thus, the nerve's resting potential is reestablished. This rapid sequence of changes, depolarization and repolarization, is termed *action potential.*

Once the resting potential of the nerve membrane is disrupted by a stimulus, such as pain, and depolarization occurs, the impulse must be transmitted along the nerve fiber. This impulse propagation is achieved when the ion changes during depolarization produce a new electrical equilibrium. These ion changes in turn produce local currents that flow from the depolarized segment of the nerve to the adjacent resting area. As a result of this electrical current flow, depolarization begins in this previously resting area and continues propagating itself along the entire length of the nerve fiber. Thus, the depolarization step begins a chain reaction that continues the action potential along the nerve. In this manner, the impulse is propelled along the nerve fiber to the central nervous system (CNS).[3]

Mechanism of Action of LA Agents

Two common theories of how LAs block nerve conduction are the membrane expansion theory and specific receptor theory, with the latter being more widely accepted.[1] According to the specific receptor theory, LAs block the influx of sodium (Na^+) ions along the nerve membrane by binding to the structural proteins or specific receptors, which prevents the nerve from reaching its firing potential. The primary action of LA drugs is in reducing the nerve membrane permeability to the Na^+ ions. The nerve membrane remains impermeable to the Na^+ ions despite the introduction of a stimulus to the nerve. Because the Na^+ ions remain on the outside of the nerve cell and are unable to enter the nerve membrane, an action potential never occurs. The nerve cell remains in a polarized state (resting state) because the ionic movements responsible for the action potential do not develop. Thus, the action of depolarization that is required to initiate or to continue nerve impulse transmission (propagation) is blocked. An impulse that arrives at the blocked nerve segment is unable to be transmitted to the brain and is therefore not interpreted as pain or discomfort by the patient.

LOCAL ANESTHETIC AGENTS

Although many drugs are classified as LAs, only a few are used in dentistry. **Ester LAs** are used as topical anesthetics (primarily benzocaine). Currently, the injectable LA agents employed in North America consist exclusively of amides (Table 43.1).[1]

Metabolism (Biotransformation) and Excretion

The mechanism by which LA agents are metabolized is important because the overall toxicity of an agent depends on the balance between the agent's rate of absorption into the bloodstream at the injection site and the rate of the agent's removal from the blood through the processes of tissue uptake and metabolism.

Most amide LAs undergo biotransformation in the liver by microsomal enzymes.[3] Therefore, the liver function of a patient influences the rate of biotransformation of an amide drug. Those patients with impaired liver function are unable to metabolize amide LAs at a normal rate, thereby leading to excessive levels of the agent in the blood, which increases the potential for toxic overdose.

The metabolic products of amide LAs are almost entirely excreted by the kidneys. In addition, a small amount of a given dose of LA agent is excreted unchanged in the urine. Amides are usually excreted in their original form in small concentrations in the urine. Patients with significant renal impairment or those undergoing renal dialysis may be unable to efficiently remove the unchanged form of the LA compound or its breakdown products from their blood. This renal impairment leads to elevated LA blood levels and an increased potential for toxicity (see the later discussions on selection of LA agents, preanesthetic patient assessment, and systemic complications).[3]

VASOCONSTRICTORS

All LA agents presently used in dentistry produce some degree of **vasodilation** (relaxation of the blood vessel wall resulting in increased blood flow to the injection site). After LA injection into the tissues, the following reactions occur:

- Accelerated LA absorption into the bloodstream, causing the anesthetic to be carried away from the injection site
- Higher amounts of LA in the blood, with greater risk for an overdose reaction
- Decreased duration of action and decreased LA effectiveness because it diffuses away from the administration site more rapidly
- Increased bleeding at the injection site because of the increased blood flow to the area[3]

Since dental hygiene care often involves soft tissue manipulation, hemorrhage is a frequent result, especially when inflammation is present. LA use without vasoconstrictors can be problematic because the vasodilating properties of the anesthetic actually increase bleeding at the site of the injection. To counteract the vasodilating properties of LA agents, the dental hygienist can elect to use an LA with a vasoconstrictor to minimize bleeding during dental hygiene care. Vasoconstrictors are drugs that constrict the blood vessels and thus control blood flow in the area of the injection. Vasoconstrictors are important additions to an LA solution because **vasoconstriction** leads to the following:

- Slowed rate of LA absorption into the bloodstream, thus keeping it at the injection site longer and producing lower levels in the bloodstream
- Lower LA amounts in the blood, thereby decreasing the risk for an overdose reaction (or reducing the potential for systemic toxicity)
- Increased duration of action and increased LA effectiveness as higher concentrations of the agent remain in and around the nerve for a longer period
- Decreased bleeding at the injection site (hemostasis) from the decreased blood flow to the area[3]

Vasoconstrictors are an important addition to an LA solution because they decrease the potential toxicity of the anesthetic solution while increasing the duration and effectiveness of pain control. For example, the addition of 1:100,000 or 1:200,000 epinephrine to 2% lidocaine increases the duration of pulpal and hard tissue anesthesia from approximately 10 minutes to 60 minutes. Dental treatment appointments are frequently 60 minutes in length, and therefore vasoconstrictors may be necessary to provide a pain-free state for patients during completion of dental hygiene care.

For pain control when providing dental hygiene care, nerve blocks, such as the posterior superior alveolar (PSA) or inferior alveolar nerve block (IANB), are frequently the technique of choice. To derive the bleeding control benefits from the vasoconstrictor, however, the drug must be administered, via local infiltration, directly into the area where the bleeding is occurring or is expected to occur. For example, to provide pain control to the maxillary molars and the buccal tissue over these teeth, a PSA nerve block is administered. The anesthetic agent is deposited posterior and superior to the posterior border of the maxilla, some distance from the area being anesthetized. If hemostasis is needed on the buccal tissue over any of the molars, however, the administration of a local infiltration into the area is necessary even though the anesthesia may be profound. Fortunately, only small volumes of solution are required (approximately 1 mL) for hemostatic purposes.[1]

Mechanism of Action

The sympathetic nervous system component of the autonomic nervous system, in addition to other functions, controls the dilation and constriction of various blood vessels throughout the body. Adrenalin, also known as *epinephrine,* is one of the naturally occurring agents responsible for sympathetic nervous system activity.[1] The LA vasoconstrictors used are chemically identical to or very similar to adrenalin produced naturally during sympathetic nervous system stimulation. Therefore, because the actions of the vasoconstrictors so closely mimic the action of the sympathetic autonomic nervous system, they are referred to as *sympathomimetic* or *adrenergic* agents.

Throughout body tissues, adrenergic receptors are found that are stimulated by the chemicals released by the sympathetic nervous system or a sympathomimetic agent (drug). These receptor sites are divided into two major categories: alpha and beta. Activation of the alpha receptors by a sympathomimetic agent (drug) results in smooth muscle contraction and vasoconstriction in blood vessels.

Activation of the beta receptors by a sympathomimetic agent (drug) produces smooth muscle relaxation and cardiac stimulation. Beta receptors have been further characterized as $beta_1$ and $beta_2$. Activation of $beta_1$ receptors increases cardiac rate and force, whereas $beta_2$ receptors are responsible for bronchodilation and vasodilation. Those changes resulting from beta-receptor stimulation are undesirable side effects of sympathomimetic drug incorporation into LA solutions. These beta effects are potentially hazardous.[4]

Concentrations

Vasoconstrictor concentrations are most often expressed as a ratio, such as 1 part per 100,000. For example, the concentrations for epinephrine (adrenaline) are as follows: 1:50,000; 1:100,000; and 1:200,000. The least concentrated solution that produces effective pain control should be used.[1,3] Otherwise, clinical manifestations of excessive vasoconstrictor use may cause tissue necrosis and sloughing (Fig. 43.2).

Epinephrine

Epinephrine is available as a synthetic and is also obtained from the adrenal medulla of animals. Whereas a variety of vasoconstrictors are used presently in oral healthcare, epinephrine is the most potent and widely employed. It is the standard by which all other vasoconstrictors are measured. Of all the concentrations available, epinephrine 1:100,000 is the most commonly used. Epinephrine 1:200,000 or even 1:250,000 is thought to be optimal for prolongation of pain control but has the least effect on hemostasis. The most concentrated, 1:50,000 epinephrine, provides the greatest hemostasis with just a few drops into a bleeding site (i.e., papilla); however, it does not increase pain control quality or duration any more than a 1:100,000 concentration. For most procedures in the typical patient, the epinephrine concentration that is preferred is 1:100,000 as it provides hemostasis and similar pain control to other anesthetics.[1]

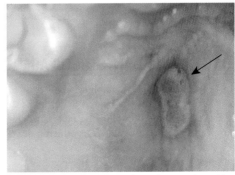

Fig. 43.2 Sterile abscess (*arrow*) on the palate produced by excessive vasoconstrictor use. (From Malamed SF. *Handbook of Local Anesthesia.* 7th ed. Elsevier; 2020.)

TABLE 43.2	Recommended Maximum Doses of Vasoconstrictors			
Concentration (Dilution)	Maximum Recommended Dose per Appointment for Healthy Patients	Number of Cartridges for Healthy Patients (ASA I)	Maximum Recommended Dose per Appointment for Patients with Cardiovascular Disease (AS III or IV)	Number of Cartridges for Patients with Cardiovascular Disease
1:50,000 epinephrine	0.2 mg	5.5	0.04 mg	1.1
1:100,000 epinephrine	0.2 mg	11.1	0.04 mg	2.2
1:200,000 epinephrine	0.2 mg	22.2	0.04 mg	4.4
1:20,000 levonordefrin	1.0 mg	11.1	0.2 mg	2.2

From Malamed SF. *Handbook of Local Anesthesia.* 7th ed. Elsevier; 2020; Logothetis D. *Local Anesthesia for the Dental Hygienist.* 3rd ed. Elsevier; 2022.

There are few contraindications to vasoconstrictor administration in the concentrations in which they are found in dental LAs. Because there is always concern about the systemic effects, however, it is recommended that the less-concentrated solution be used, particularly with patients known to be cardiovascularly compromised.[3] For all patients, however, the benefits and risks of including a vasoconstrictor in the LA solution must be weighed against the benefits and risks of using an anesthetic solution without a vasoconstrictor. (See later sections on preanesthetic patient assessment and systemic complications.)

Side Effects and Overdose

Epinephrine overdose (due to high amounts in the blood) can result from CNS stimulation. Clinical manifestations include increasing fear and anxiety, tension, restlessness, throbbing headache, tremor, weakness, dizziness, pallor, respiratory difficulty, and palpitation. With increasing epinephrine levels in the blood, cardiac dysrhythmias, ventricular fibrillation, dramatic increase in blood pressure, and stroke are rare but possible. Because of epinephrine's rapid inactivation, overdose reactions are usually brief. Nevertheless, in cardiovascularly compromised patients, it is prudent to limit or avoid exposure to vasoconstrictors if possible. Table 43.2 lists the maximum recommended doses (MRDs) of epinephrine.[1]

Levonordefrin

Levonordefrin is approximately one-sixth (15%) as potent a vasoconstrictor as epinephrine and therefore is used in a greater concentration of 1:20,000. It is similar to using epinephrine in 1:50,000 or 1:100,000 concentrations. Patients taking tricyclic antidepressants should not receive levonordefrin (or norepinephrine), which is an absolute contraindication. With large doses, patients may experience serious side effects, including exaggerated responses. In the United States, it is available with mepivacaine in a 1:20,000 dilution.[1] Norepinephrine (Levarterenol), a vasoconstrictor with similar action, is no longer available in the United States and Canada.

SELECTION OF A LOCAL ANESTHETIC AGENT

Table 43.3 lists the LAs and the combinations of vasoconstrictors that are currently available in the United States and Canada. The dental hygienist must weigh the following factors when determining the appropriate anesthetic agent to use during dental hygiene care:

- The duration of action of the LA agent, the length of time that pain control is needed, and half-life
- The need for pain control after treatment
- The patient's health status

- Current medications and/or natural supplements being taken by the patient
- An LA allergy (e.g., vasoconstrictors with sulfites)[5]

Duration of Action, Length of Time Pain Control Is Needed, and Elimination Half-Life

An important consideration when selecting an LA agent for pain control during dental hygiene care is the LA agent's duration of action coupled with the length of time that pulpal and soft tissue pain control is needed. The elimination half-life, or the time it takes for 50% of the LA agent to be metabolized and removed from the body, is also an important consideration due to the potential for toxicity. An LA agent such as articaine has a much shorter half-life (27 minutes) due to metabolism by plasma esterase in the blood. After two half-lives, 75% of the drug will be removed and after three half-lives, more than 87% will be eliminated, and so forth until the drug is no longer present in the body. In comparison, lidocaine has a longer half-life (approximately 90 minutes) before 50% is metabolized by the liver. In some instances, articaine may be the safer drug if the need to reinject later in the appointment is desired, but for nonsurgical periodontal therapy appointments, the average patient can tolerate twice as much 2% lidocaine as articaine before the MRD is reached.[1,3] The dental hygienist will have to carefully weigh the risks versus benefits for each patient. Table 43.3 lists the commonly used LA agents, their approximate duration of action of anesthesia, and their elimination half-lives.

In addition to the presence or absence of a vasoconstrictor, several other factors described in the following sections may affect both the duration and depth of the anesthetic agent's action, either increasing or, more commonly, decreasing the drug's effectiveness.

Variation in Response to the Agent Administered

Although most individuals respond predictably to an anesthetic agent (e.g., the duration of pulpal anesthesia after administration of 2% lidocaine with epinephrine 1:100,000 is approximately 60 minutes), some patients exhibit either a longer or a shorter duration of action than anticipated. This variation in response is normal and is simply a variation in the individual's reaction to the anesthetic agent.

Accuracy of the Administration of the Agent

Accuracy becomes significant when a substantial amount of soft tissue must be penetrated to reach the nerve to be anesthetized. For example, the IANB involves advancing through 20 to 25 mm of soft tissue before reaching the nerve, thereby influencing the accuracy of the injection. When injecting where it is not necessary to penetrate a large amount of tissue to block the nerve, however, such as with a supraperiosteal, accuracy is seldom a problem.

TABLE 43.3 Commonly Used Local Anesthetic Agents, Duration of Pulpal and Soft Tissue Anesthesia, and Half-Life

	Short Duration Approx. 30 Minutes Pulpal	Intermediate Duration Approx. 60 Minutes Pulpal	Long Duration 90+ Minutes Pulpal	Soft Tissue Minutes	Half-life Hours
Lidocaine	z				1.6 hours (96 minutes)
2% + epinephrine 1:50,000		X		180–300	
2% + epinephrine 1:100,000		X		180–300	
Mepivacaine					1.9 hours (114 minutes)
3% plain	X 20 minutes supraperiosteal 40 minutes nerve block			120–180	
2% + levonordefrin 1:20,000		X		180–300	
Prilocaine					1.6 hours (96 minutes)
4% plain	X 10–15 minutes supraperiosteal 40–60 minutes nerve block			90–120 supraperiosteal 12–240 nerve block	
4% + epinephrine 1:200,000		X		180–480	
Articaine					0.5 hours (27 minutes)
4% + epinephrine 1:100,000		X (60–75 minutes)		180–360	
4% + epinephrine 1:200,000		X (45–60 minutes)		120–300	
Bupivacaine					2.7 hours (162 minutes)
0.5% + epinephrine 1:200,000			X	240–540 (up to 720)	

Adapted from Malamed SF. *Handbook of Local Anesthesia.* 7th ed. Elsevier; 2020, and Logothetis D. *Local Anesthesia for the Dental Hygienist.* 3rd ed. Elsevier; 2022.

Condition of the Soft Tissues at the Site of Drug Deposition

Anesthetic duration is increased in areas of decreased vascularity. Conversely, the presence of inflammation or infection increases vascularity and often decreases the anesthetic agent's duration of action as a result of more rapid absorption.

Anatomic Variation

The injection techniques described in this chapter are based on a "normal" anatomy. Of course, anatomic variations from this norm can exist and may decrease the duration of LA action. Anatomic variations in the maxilla that may account for failed effectiveness and shortened duration include the following:

- Extradense alveolar bone
- Palatal roots of maxillary molars that flare more than normal to the midline of the palate, thus affecting the anesthetic's action on these roots
- An unusually low zygomatic arch, common in children, which prevents anesthesia or lessens its duration in the first and second molars

Anatomic variations in the mandible that are cause for concern include the following:

- The height of the mandibular foramen
- A wide, flaring mandible
- A wide ramus in the anterior-posterior direction
- A long ramus in the superior-inferior direction
- Bulky musculature or excess adipose tissue
- Accessory innervation to the mandibular teeth[1]

Suggestions for overcoming these variations in anatomy when administering anesthetic solution are discussed in the section on mandibular injection techniques.

Type of Injection Administered

In oral healthcare, there are three major types of injections used to obtain local anesthesia. A local infiltration (intraseptal) injection deposits solution closest to smaller terminal nerve endings; a field block (supraperiosteal) deposits the solution near large terminal nerve branches; and a nerve block involves the deposition of solution close to a main nerve trunk, often at some distance from the treatment area. When an anesthetic solution is administered, both pulpal and soft tissue anesthesia are sustained for a longer period of time when a nerve block, rather than a supraperiosteal injection, is administered. For example, if 2% lidocaine with 1:100,000 epinephrine is administered, a nerve block can provide approximately 60 minutes of pulpal anesthesia, whereas a supraperiosteal injection may provide only 40 minutes of anesthesia. To achieve the desired duration, however, the recommended minimal volume of anesthetic must be administered.

Need for Pain Control After Treatment

Although the need for pain control after dental hygiene care may be limited, long-duration agents may be administered if posttreatment discomfort is a factor. Anesthetic agents, such as 4% prilocaine with 1:200,000 epinephrine, can provide 3 to 8 hours of soft tissue anesthesia, whereas 0.5% bupivacaine with 1:200,000 epinephrine can alleviate posttreatment discomfort for 4 to 12 hours. These agents can be administered before dental hygiene care is begun or even at the end of the care to allow for maximum posttreatment anesthesia. These drugs should not be given to children or to people who are mentally or physically disabled because these individuals may lack the ability to refrain from chewing or biting their lip, cheeks, or tongue. Use critical thinking to consider the legal, ethical, and safety issues that can accompany use of pain control in a dental hygiene setting (Box 43.1).

PREANESTHETIC PATIENT ASSESSMENT

An evaluation of the patient's health history and current health status is an essential prerequisite to dental hygiene care and meeting the patient's human needs for freedom of health risks, fear, stress, and pain. The dental hygienist must ascertain if any conditions represent contraindications or require alterations to the dental hygiene care plan in order to avoid or minimize risk to the patient. Furthermore, the administration of local anesthesia and vasoconstricting agents provides an additional rationale for a thorough health history and health status review since LAs and vasoconstrictors, like all drugs, exert actions on multiple body systems.

Utilizing the following assessment tools will help to evaluate the patient's ability to receive treatment and local anesthesia: the health history, dental history, dialogue history, physical exam (vital signs), and the American Society of Anesthesiologists (ASA) psychological and physiological risk assessment (see Chapters 13, 14, and 15 for more detailed discussions). Also essential to the preanesthetic assessment is a history of allergic responses and identification of current medications. Collection of these data guides the dental hygienist in determining the appropriateness of administering an LA agent or vasoconstrictor, seeking medical consultation, recommending psychosedation (nitrous oxide-oxygen sedation), and modifying the dental hygiene care plan. A thorough preanesthetic patient assessment helps prevent or minimize complications and medical emergencies.[4]

Contraindications to local anesthesia and vasoconstrictors are divided into two categories: absolute and relative. **Absolute contraindications** require that the drug in question not be administered to the individual under any circumstances.[1] The administration of such a drug is contraindicated in all situations because it substantially increases the possibility of a life-threatening risk for the patient. An example is a documented LA allergic reaction.

A **relative contraindication** means that the drug in question may be administered to the patient after careful weighing of the risks of using the drug against its potential benefits, and if an acceptable alternative drug is not available. The smallest clinically effective dose, however, always should be used.

BOX 43.1   Legal, Ethical, and Safety Issues

Scenario: Yvonne is a 27-year-old patient who works in the tech industry. Her treatment plan for today includes scaling and root debridement of the maxillary anterior teeth with local anesthesia. She insists the dental hygienist use the same long-acting anesthetic (bupivacaine at 1:200,000) that was used for her past oral surgery procedure because she plans to have an upper lip piercing immediately after her hygiene appointment and would like to be numb for this procedure.

What are the legal, ethical, and safety issues that the hygienist needs to consider?

Comments: It is the legal responsibility of the dental hygienist to practice within the scope authorized by state law concerning local anesthetic agent delivery. At first glance, it may seem appropriate to grant the patient's request; however, the type of local anesthesia and concentration that she is requesting would be unsafe and may set her up for postoperative injuries to the oral mucosa due to its long duration period, and there is no indication for posttreatment anesthesia. Providing anesthesia for reasons other than for the prescribed treatment is unethical.

Patient Health Status

Although LAs and vasoconstrictors are considered relatively safe drugs when administered properly, certain health conditions require limiting or eliminating their use. Table 43.4 summarizes those health conditions that affect the selection of an LA or vasoconstrictor and appropriate actions that the dental hygienist may take.[3]

Few health conditions, such as documented allergy or uncontrolled hyperthyroidism, are absolute contraindications to vasoconstrictors in the concentrations found in LA solutions used in oral healthcare; however, the dental hygienist must carefully consider the benefits versus the risks of administering a vasoconstrictor to patients with a history of hypertension, cardiovascular disease, or controlled hyperthyroidism because often the risks outweigh the benefits.

Current Patient Medications (Prescription, Nonprescription, Herbal, and/or Natural Supplements)

A drug interaction occurs when one drug modifies the action of another drug. A drug may potentiate or diminish the action of another drug and may alter the way in which another drug is absorbed, metabolized, or eliminated from the body.[1,4] Although LAs and vasoconstrictors exhibit few interactions with other drugs, the dental hygienist should consult a prescription and/or nonprescription drug reference, of which electronic versions are now widely used, when a patient reports using any medications. This practice enables the clinician to assess both the drug's activity and the drug-to-drug interactions between the LA and vasoconstrictor and the prescribed medication. In doing so, the dental hygienist meets the patient's human need for protection from health risks. If further questions remain regarding the use of an LA or vasoconstrictor while a prescribed medication is being taken, the dentist or the individual's physician should be consulted.

Table 43.5 summarizes those medications that may affect the selection of an LA or vasoconstrictor and appropriate actions the dental hygienist may choose.

While LAs have few interactions with other prescribed drugs, procaine has been cited as interfering with the action of antiinfective sulfonamide drugs. When CNS depressants or cardiovascular system (CVS) depressants are being taken by an individual, it is recommended that doses of LAs be kept to a minimum because they may cause further depression.[1,4]

TABLE 43.4   Health Conditions That Require Special Consideration when Local Anesthetics and/or Vasoconstrictors Are Administered

Health Condition	Type of Contraindication	Reason for Modification	Local Anesthetics and/or Vasoconstrictor Dose/Drug Modification
Cardiovascular disease	Relative	Vasoconstrictors will enhance the cardiovascular effects; ASA III patients are treatable with appropriate drug modifications	Limit vasoconstrictor to cardiac dose; 0.04 mg per appointment for epinephrine; 0.2 mg per appointment for levonordefrin; do not use 1:50,000 epinephrine
Diabetes	Relative	Vasoconstrictors directly oppose effect of insulin, possible changes in blood levels of glucose; amounts used in dentistry are generally safe and do not significantly raise blood sugar levels	Use with caution; limit the dose of vasoconstrictor for patients with uncontrolled "brittle" diabetes
Controlled hyperthyroidism	Relative	Sensitivity to vasoconstrictors, increasing their effect	Surgically corrected or medication-controlled patients respond normally to vasoconstrictors
Sickle cell anemia	Relative	No dental treatment during a crisis; vasoconstrictors will increase stress	Routine dental care appointments should be short. Use of local anesthesia is acceptable. The inclusion of small amounts of epinephrine (1:200,000) should be limited to treatment where profound anesthesia is warranted and to obtain hemostasis.
Significant liver disease	Relative	Amides primarily metabolized in the liver increase possibility of toxic overdose	Reduce dosage of amides metabolized in the liver; articaine is preferred
Renal dysfunction	Relative	Slight risk of toxicity with severe renal dysfunction	Use local anesthetics but judiciously
Malignant hyperthermia	Relative	Life-threatening syndrome caused by general anesthetics	Medical consultation is recommended; use amides but reduce dosage
Methemoglobinemia	Relative	Potential for clinical cyanosis	Use amides but avoid prilocaine or topical benzocaine
Atypical plasma cholinesterase	Relative	Inability of esters to be metabolized in the plasma by cholinesterase enzymes	Should not be given ester-derivative anesthetics
Pregnancy	Relative	Anesthetics are not teratogenic and pose little danger to the fetus	For the most conservative approach, use lidocaine or prilocaine anesthetics only after first trimester

From Logothetis D. *Local Anesthesia for the Dental Hygienist.* 3rd ed. Elsevier; 2022.

TABLE 43.5   Medications That Affect the Selection of Local Anesthetic Agents or Vasoconstrictors

Medication	Type of Contraindications	Drugs to Avoid	Potential Problem(s)	Action or Alternative Drug
CVS depressants, CNS depressants	Relative	Large doses of LAs	Increased depression of CVS or CNS	Minimize dose of LA
Tricyclic antidepressants	Relative	Large doses of vasoconstrictors	Potentiate the action of epinephrine and increase blood pressure	Epinephrine concentrations of 1:200,000 or 1:100,000 used judiciously or mepivacaine 3% or prilocaine 4%
Phenothiazines	Relative	Large doses of vasoconstrictors	Potentiate the action of epinephrine and increase blood pressure	Epinephrine concentrations of 1:200,000 or 1:100,000 used judiciously or mepivacaine 3% or prilocaine 4%
Beta-receptor blockers	Relative	Large doses of vasoconstrictors	Potentiate the action of epinephrine and increase blood pressure	Epinephrine concentrations of 1:200,000 or 1:100,000 used judiciously or mepivacaine 3% or prilocaine 4%
Adrenergic neuron blockers	Relative	Large doses of vasoconstrictors	Potentiate the action of epinephrine and increase blood pressure	Use vasoconstrictor judiciously—as low dose as possible
Sulfonamides	Relative	Esters	Esters inhibit action of sulfonamides	Amides

CNS, Central nervous system; *CVS,* cardiovascular system; *LA,* local anesthetic.
Adapted from Malamed SF. *Handbook of Local Anesthesia.* 7th ed. Elsevier; 2020.

There are many conflicting reports of drug-to-drug interactions between vasoconstrictors and prescribed medications, but it is recommended that the dental hygienist proceed cautiously when administering a vasopressor to a person who is being treated with any of the drugs listed in Table 43.5.

Currently, none of the drugs described in the following paragraphs poses an absolute contraindication to the administration of a vasoconstrictor; however, it is recommended that the dental hygienist exercise caution by administering the smallest dose that is clinically effective (such as that recommended for persons at cardiovascular risk) or eliminating the vasopressor entirely. If the dental hygienist is uncertain about the inclusion of a vasoconstrictor in the LA solution, consultation with the patient's physician is advisable.

Tricyclic Antidepressants

Tricyclic antidepressant medications (e.g., amitriptyline, imipramine) have been cited as possibly potentiating the action of epinephrine and norepinephrine and resulting in an increase in blood pressure.[1,4] Similarly, phenothiazines categorized as antipsychotic drugs (e.g., prochlorperazine) are often prescribed for treatment of anxiety or nausea and, when combined with vasoconstrictors, may also cause an exaggerated increase in blood pressure.

Beta-Receptor Blockers

Beta-receptor blockers such as propranolol and nadolol (note that these generic drugs end in "olol") decrease systolic and diastolic blood pressures.[1] When these drugs are combined with epinephrine from an LA injection, however, significant increases in blood pressure may result.

Adrenergic Neuron Blockers

Adrenergic neuron blockers such as guanethidine and reserpine also are used to lower blood pressure through interference with the normal release of norepinephrine.[1] When these drugs are combined with a vasoconstrictor, the effects of the vasopressor may be exaggerated, resulting in an increase in blood pressure.

Allergies

An allergy is a hypersensitive reaction acquired through exposure to a specific substance (allergen); reexposure to the allergen increases one's potential to react.[1] A documented LA allergy, however, represents an absolute contraindication and must be investigated for authenticity. Table 43.6 summarizes allergies that affect the selection of an LA agent or vasoconstrictor and appropriate alternative drugs the dental hygienist may choose. A true allergic response to a pure amide drug is extremely rare. A true allergy to amides may exist; however, a verifiable occurrence is virtually nonexistent.

Allergic reactions have been documented for various dental cartridge contents. Sodium bisulfite and metabisulfite are antioxidants that are incorporated into LA solutions to act as preservatives for the vasoconstrictor. In addition to their use in LA cartridges, these agents are often sprayed on fruits and vegetables to keep them appearing fresh. They also are included in a variety of canned foods. Allergy to the bisulfites has been reported.[5] Patients with a history of asthma may be particularly susceptible to an allergic response. If a patient reports a history of sulfite sensitivity, the dental hygienist should be alerted to the possibility of a similar response if a sulfite is included in the dental cartridge. Although sodium bisulfite or metabisulfite is found in all dental cartridges containing a vasoconstrictor, these agents are not included in solutions in which there is no vasopressor. Therefore, it is recommended that the dental hygienist administer LAs containing no vasoconstrictor to patients with a history of sulfite sensitivity.[1]

MAXIMUM RECOMMENDED DOSES OF LOCAL ANESTHETICS

All drugs, if administered in excess, can produce an overdose reaction. The exact dose or the blood level at which a toxic reaction occurs is impossible to predict because biologic variability greatly influences how individuals respond to a drug. Recommended maximum doses, however, can be calculated to serve as a guideline for the dental hygienist. A **maximum recommended dose (MRD)** is the maximum drug amount that can be safely administered to a healthy individual. Maximum doses of injectable LAs should be determined after consideration of the following factors:

- *Patient's age.* Individuals on both ends of the age spectrum (i.e., the young child or the older adult) may be unable to tolerate normal doses. Therefore, the dose of LA should be decreased accordingly.
- *Patient's physical status.* The calculated dose must be adjusted for patients with compromised health. For example, a patient with significant liver or renal dysfunction needs to be given a reduced dose of LAs.
- *Patient's weight.* The larger the individual (within limits), the greater the drug distribution. When administering a normal LA dose to a large individual, the blood drug level is lower than that in a small person. Therefore, a larger dose can be safely given. Although this rule is generally true, there may be exceptions, and care must always be exercised.[1]

Table 43.7 lists the MRD by manufacturers and approved by the US FDA. Table 43.7 also includes the milligrams of LA per cartridge for the available LA agents. It is important to note that the maximum doses are expressed in terms of milligrams per pound of body weight. The dental hygienist must be familiar with the relationship among solution percentage, the number of milligrams of solution contained per cartridge, the patient's body weight, and the MRD dose per pound. With this information, the hygienist can calculate the maximum dose and the number of cartridges that can be safely administered.

Box 43.2 provides examples of how to calculate maximum doses and numbers of LA cartridges to be administered to various patients when only one LA is used. Box 43.3 provides similar calculation examples for when multiple drugs are used.[1]

TABLE 43.6   Allergies That Affect the Selection of Local Anesthetic Agents or Vasoconstrictors

Reported Allergy	Type of Contraindication	Drugs to Avoid	Potential Problem(s)	Alternative Drug
Local anesthetic (LA) allergy, documented	Absolute	All LAs in same chemical class (esters vs. amides)	Allergic response, mild (e.g., dermatitis, bronchospasm) to life-threatening reactions	LAs in different chemical class (esters vs. amides)
Sodium bisulfate or metabisulfite	Absolute	LAs containing a vasoconstrictor	Severe bronchospasm, usually in asthmatics	LA without vasoconstrictor

TABLE 43.7 Maximum Recommended Doses (MRDs) of Local Anesthetics Available in North America

MANUFACTURER'S AND U.S. FOOD AND DRUG ADMINISTRATION MAXIMUM RECOMMENDED DOSE

Local Anesthetic	mg/kg	mg/lb	Maximum Recommended Dose (mg)
Articaine			
With vasoconstrictor	7.0	3.2	None listed
Bupivacaine			
With vasoconstrictor	None listed	None listed	90
With vasoconstrictor (Canada)	2.0	0.9	90
Lidocaine			
With vasoconstrictor	7.0	3.2	500
Mepivacaine			
No vasoconstrictor	6.6	3.0	400
With vasoconstrictor	6.6	3.0	400
Prilocaine			
No vasoconstrictor	8.0	3.6	600
With vasoconstrictor	8.0	3.6	600

CALCULATION OF MILLIGRAMS OF LOCAL ANESTHETIC PER DENTAL CARTRIDGE (1.8-mL CARTRIDGE)

Local Anesthetic	Percent Concentration	mg/mL	×1.8 mL = mg/cartridge
Articaine	4	40	72*
Bupivacaine	0.5	5	9
Lidocaine	2	20	36
Mepivacaine	2	20	36
	3	30	54
Prilocaine	4	40	72

*Cartridges of articaine hydrochloride in the United States read, "Minimum content of each cartridge is 1.7 mL."
From Malamed SF. *Handbook of Local Anesthesia.* 7th ed. Elsevier; 2020.

BOX 43.2 Calculation of Maximum Doses and Number of Cartridges (Single Drug)

Patient: 22 Years Old, Healthy, Female, 110 lb (50 kg)
LA: lidocaine HCl + epinephrine 1:100,000
Lidocaine 2% = 36 mg/cartridge
Lidocaine: 7.0 mg/kg = 350 mg (MRD)
No. of cartridges: manufacturer: 350/36 = approx. 9¾

Patient: 40 Years Old, Healthy, Male, 200 lb (90 kg)
LA: articaine HCl + epinephrine 1:200,000
Articaine 4% = 72 mg/cartridge
Articaine: 7.0 mg/kg = 630 mg (MRD)
No. of cartridges: manufacturer: 630/72 = approx. 9.0

Patient: 6 Years Old, Healthy, Male, 40 lb (20 kg)
LA: mepivacaine HCl, no vasoconstrictor
Mepivacaine 3% = 54 mg/cartridge
Mepivacaine: 6.6 mg/kg = 132 mg (MRD)
No. of cartridges: manufacturer: 130/54 = approx. 2.5

From Malamed SF. *Handbook of Local Anesthesia.* 7th ed. Elsevier; 2020.
HCl, Hydrochloride; *MRD*, manufacturer's maximum recommended dose.

BOX 43.3 Calculation of Maximum Doses and Number of Cartridges (Multiple Drugs)

Patient: 100 lb (45 kg) Female, Healthy
LA: mepivacaine 2% + levonordefrin 1:20,000
Mepivacaine 2% = 36 mg/cartridge
Mepivacaine 6.6 mg/kg = 297 mg (MRD)
Patient receives 2 cartridges = 72 mg, but anesthesia is inadequate
Doctor wishes to change to articaine 4% + epinephrine 1:100,000
How much articaine can this patient receive?
Articaine 4% = 72 mg/cartridge
Articaine: 7.0 mg/kg = 315 mg (MRD)
Total dose of BOTH LAs should not exceed the lower of the two calculated doses or 297 mg.
Patient has received 72 mg mepivacaine can still receive 225 mg of articaine
Therefore 225 mg/72 mg per cartridge = approx. 3.0 cartridges of articaine 4% + epinephrine 1:100,000

From Malamed SF. *Handbook of Local Anesthesia.* 7th ed. Elsevier; 2020.
MRD, Manufacturer's maximum recommended dose.

Fortunately, maximum doses are unlikely to be reached for most dental hygiene procedures. If the dental hygiene care plan involves scaling and root planing a quadrant, the administration of one to two cartridges often suffices. There is seldom a need to administer more than four cartridges during any appointment involving dental hygiene care.

In addition to considering the MRD, the dental hygienist must follow other procedural guidelines to increase safety during local anesthesia administration and to prevent an overdose reaction. These guidelines include the following:

- Careful evaluation of the patient's health history
- Use of a vasoconstrictor whenever possible
- Aspiration before LA deposition
- Use of a slow injection technique
- Use of the smallest amount of drug necessary

A more detailed discussion of these guidelines can be found in the section on procedures for a successful injection and complications.

ARMAMENTARIUM

Armamentarium, the equipment essential for the administration of an LA agent, includes the following:

- Syringe
- Needle
- Cartridge of LA agent
- Supplementary armamentarium

Syringe

The syringe is the component of the local anesthesia armamentarium that holds the needle and cartridge of anesthetic (thus allowing the solution to be delivered to the patient). Several types of syringes may be used for local anesthesia administration, as follows:

1. Reusable
   a. Breech-loading metallic cartridge-type
      - Aspirating
      - Nonaspirating
      - Self-aspirating
   b. Computer-controlled anesthetic delivery system
   c. Pressure-type
   d. Jet injector
2. Disposable

The syringes most often employed in oral healthcare are the reusable aspirating syringe and the self-aspirating syringe.[1]

Reusable Breech-Loading Metallic Cartridge-Type Aspirating Syringe

The reusable breech-loading metallic cartridge-type aspirating syringe is the most commonly used syringe for administration of an intraoral LA agent (Fig. 43.3).

The needle is affixed to the threaded portion (or needle adaptor) at one end of the syringe. At the other end, a thumb ring and finger rest provide the dental hygienist with a means to grasp and control the syringe. The body of the syringe holds the cartridge of anesthetic solution. The aspirating syringe is characterized by a barbed piston, also referred to as the *harpoon*. The harpoon engages the rubber or silicone stopper of the cartridge of anesthetic. The harpoon allows the dental hygienist to exert negative pressure on the thumb ring to assess the location of the lumen of the needle, a procedure referred to as *aspiration. Therefore, a nonaspirating syringe (Fig. 43.4) that does not have a harpoon should never be used for dental anesthesia.* If the needle lumen rests within a blood vessel, blood appears in the cartridge after negative pressure is applied to

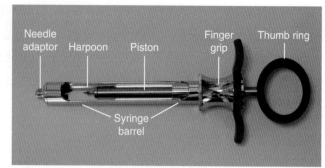

Fig. 43.3 Example of breech-loading metallic cartridge-type syringes. (Courtesy of J. E. Bercasio Photography.)

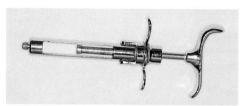

Fig. 43.4 Nonaspirating syringe. Not to be used for dental local anesthesia.

BOX 43.4   Advantages and Disadvantages of the Metallic Breech-Loading Aspirating Syringe

Advantages	Disadvantages
- Visible cartridge - Aspiration with one hand - Autoclavable - Rust resistant - Long lasting with proper maintenance	- Weight (heavier than plastic syringe) - Syringe may be too big for small operators - Possibility of infection with improper care

From Malamed SF. *Handbook of Local Anesthesia.* 7th ed. Elsevier; 2020.

the thumb ring. If this occurs, the dental hygienist needs to withdraw the needle, replace the cartridge of anesthetic solution and the needle, and repeat the procedure. Positive pressure on the thumb ring injects the anesthetic solution into the tissues. Advantages and disadvantages are listed in Box 43.4. A plastic, autoclavable, nonrusting model also is available.[1]

Reusable Breech-Loading Metallic Cartridge-Type, Self-Aspirating Syringe

The importance of aspirating before injecting an anesthetic solution is widely accepted, and the self-aspirating syringe was developed to aid the oral healthcare provider in completing this important step. This type of syringe achieves the negative pressure necessary for aspiration via the elasticity of the rubber diaphragm in the anesthetic cartridge. When the cartridge is placed in the syringe, the diaphragm rests against a metal projection inside the syringe; this projection also directs the needle into the cartridge (Fig. 43.5).

Pressure exerted by the dental hygienist on the thumb disc (Fig. 43.6) or on the plunger by way of the thumb ring moves the cartridge slightly toward the metal projection, thereby stretching the rubber diaphragm. When the pressure is released, the cartridge rebounds slightly, thus producing enough negative pressure within the cartridge to achieve aspiration. Therefore, the dental hygienist does not need to

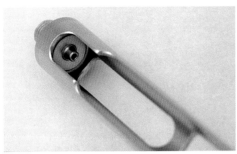

Fig. 43.5 A metal projection within the barrel depresses the diaphragm of the LA cartridge. (From Malamed SF. *Handbook of Local Anesthesia*. 7th ed. Elsevier; 2020.)

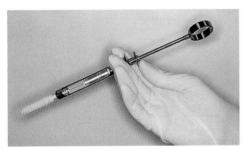

Fig. 43.6 Pressure exerted on the thumb disc (as shown in figure) or the thumb ring increases pressure within the cartridge. Aspiration occurs when the pressure is released.

BOX 43.5   Advantages and Disadvantages of the Computer-Controlled Local Anesthetic Delivery Systems (C-CLAD)

Advantages	Disadvantages
• Precise control of flow rate and pressure produces a more comfortable injection, even in tissues with low elasticity (e.g., palate, attached gingiva, periodontal ligament) • Increased tactile "feel" and ergonomics from the lightweight handpiece • Nonthreatening appearance • Automatic aspiration • Rotational insertion technique minimizes needle deflection	• Requires additional armamentarium • Cost

Adapted from Malamed SF. *Handbook of Local Anesthesia*. 7th ed. Elsevier; 2020.

---

pull back on the thumb ring to aspirate, as is necessary with an aspirating syringe.

Computer-Controlled LA Delivery

Several Computer-Controlled LA Delivery (C-CLAD) systems are used in dentistry today.[1] Box 43.5 lists the advantages and disadvantages of the C-CLAD systems. For example, the Wand STA (formerly known as the Wand) is a C-CLAD system that can be used instead of the traditional breech-loading aspirating syringe (Fig. 43.7). The Wand STA has several unique features. The handpiece is light and ergonomic; it is held in a pen grasp instead of a

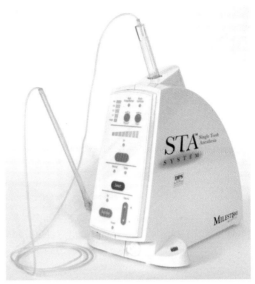

Fig. 43.7 Computer-controlled LA delivery device with lightweight handpiece: the Wand STA, Single Tooth Anesthesia system. (From Logothetis D. *Local Anesthesia for the Dental Hygienist*. 3rd ed. Elsevier; 2022. Courtesy of Milestone Scientific.)

palm grasp, allowing a higher level of comfort and control for the clinician. The handpiece is also good for use with fearful patients because it looks nothing like the traditional syringe and therefore is much less threatening. The LA delivery is controlled by a computer that regulates the agent's flow rate and the pressure of the deposition. The computer-controlled rate allows for creation of an anesthetic pathway immediately in front of the needle as it moves through the soft tissues, resulting in a high level of comfort for the patient. Particularly with administration of palatal injections, the Wand STA can greatly increase patient comfort and acceptance of local anesthesia procedures.

To initiate anesthetic delivery and aspiration, the clinician controls the computer via a foot pedal. Because the clinician is able to control the needle with the fine muscles of the hand rather than the large muscles required to operate a traditional syringe, the clinician can penetrate the soft tissues by gently rotating the needle back and forth between the thumb and fingers (bidirectional rotation) rather than by the typical linear penetration. This technique has two advantages: (1) by allowing the bevel to cut into the tissues by rotating, the technique causes no tearing of the tissue on penetration; and (2) the bidirectional rotation results in less needle deflection as the tissue is penetrated. This decrease in needle deflection can increase the effectiveness of the injection because the needle is more likely to be at the desired deposition site.[1]

An addition to the C-CLAD system is the Dentapen, a handheld, battery-operated device. Among the features and benefits are: three rates of injection (slow [90 sec/mL], medium [60 sec/mL], and fast [30 sec/mL]), ergonomic and lightweight, compatible with needle of choice, two different handles which give the operator flexibility in a traditional syringe or a penlike grasp, cordless and without a foot petal, and two modes of flow (continuous or gradual increase). Overall, the Dentapen is a viable option for more comfortable delivery of local anesthesia.[1,3]

Alternative Syringes

Several other types of syringes that the dental hygienist may encounter include a pressure-type syringe, the jet injector syringe (needleless), and the disposable syringe.

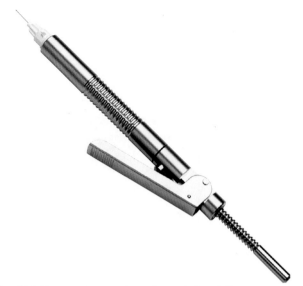

Fig. 43.8 Pressure-type syringe for periodontal ligament injection. (From Logothetis D. *Local Anesthesia for the Dental Hygienist*. 3rd ed. Elsevier; 2022. Courtesy of Septodont, New Castle, Delaware.)

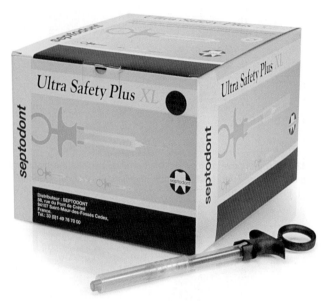

Fig. 43.9 Disposable safety syringe. (Courtesy of Septodont, Lancaster, Pennsylvania.)

Pressure-Type Syringe

The pressure-type syringe is used when providing pulpal anesthesia to one tooth on the mandible (Fig. 43.8). A standard aspirating syringe can be used as well, but the main advantages of the pressure syringe include delivery of measured doses, decreased tissue resistance, and a protected cartridge. A pressure-type syringe is equipped with a trigger mechanism that delivers a measured dose (0.2 mL) of anesthetic solution and allows the administrator to more easily express the solution despite significant tissue resistance. This type of syringe permits easy administration of the solution; however, patient discomfort may ensue during the injection and after the anesthesia has worn off due to the lack of operator control in depositing the solution.[3]

Jet Injector Syringe

The jet injector syringe is needleless and is used to deliver 0.05 to 0.2 mL of topical anesthetic agent to the mucous membranes at a high pressure (2000 psi) via small openings called *jets*. This would be used prior to the administration of nerve blocks or supraperiosteal injections with a conventional syringe and needle. Its disadvantages include the patient's dislike of the jolt of jet injection and possible postinjection discomfort that may follow. Properly applied topical anesthetics accomplish the same objectives as the jet injector.[1]

Disposable Safety Syringe

Traditional disposable plastic syringes are most often used for intramuscular or intravenous drug administration and typically would not be employed by the dental hygienist. Because of the risks of accidental exposure to contaminated needles, disposable safety syringes were developed (Fig. 43.9). A retractable disposable sheath covers the needle until use and then locks over the needle once it is removed from the tissue.

Care and Handling of the Syringe

Recommendations for the care of reusable syringes used for LA administration follow:

- The syringe should be sterilized after each use, following the appropriate infection control protocol. Deposits resembling rust and/or blood may accumulate on the syringe. Such deposits may be removed by ultrasonic cleaning or scrubbing (see Chapter 10).

- The syringe should be dismantled and all threaded joints should be lubricated after several exposures in the autoclave.
- The piston and harpoon may be replaced if the harpoon loses its sharpness and fails to engage the rubber stopper of the cartridge.[1]

Problems with the Syringe

- *Bent harpoon.* The syringe harpoon must be sharp and straight to embed the cartridge's rubber stopper. If the harpoon is bent, it may fail to engage the rubber stopper accurately, making aspiration unreliable.
- *Disengagement of the harpoon from the rubber stopper of the cartridge during aspiration.* Disengagement may ensue if the harpoon is dull or if the dental hygienist applies excessive pressure to the thumb ring during aspiration. With regard to aspiration, only a gentle retraction of the thumb ring is needed; forceful action is not required.
- *Difficulty aspirating because of practitioner's hand size.* When using an aspirating syringe, dental hygienists must be able to stretch the fingers and thumb to retract the syringe thumb ring. If this cannot be done effectively, reliable aspiration does not occur. Therefore, it is important that the syringe fits the practitioner's hand. Most syringes are similar in their dimensions, but variations do exist. When selecting an aspirating syringe, it is beneficial to hold the syringe and test your ability to aspirate efficiently. If this is not possible, a self-aspirating syringe should be selected.

Needle

The **needle** is the component of the armamentarium that delivers the anesthetic agent from the cartridge and into the tissues. Virtually all needles used in oral healthcare today are made of stainless steel, are presterilized by the manufacturer, and are disposable.

Parts of the Needle

Needles used for LA administration have several components (Fig. 43.10). The **bevel** (Fig. 43.11) is the angled surface of the needle point that is directed into the tissues. The shaft is the length of the needle from the point to the hub. The syringe adaptor with hub is a plastic or metal piece that attaches the needle onto the syringe. To attach a plastic-hubbed needle to a syringe, the dental hygienist must concurrently

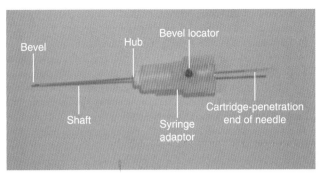

Fig. 43.10 Parts of the dental LA needle. (Courtesy of J.E. Bercasio Photography.)

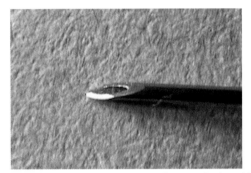

Fig. 43.11 Bevel of the needle. Barbs may form on the bevel if bone is contacted forcefully. (Courtesy of J.E. Bercasio Photography.)

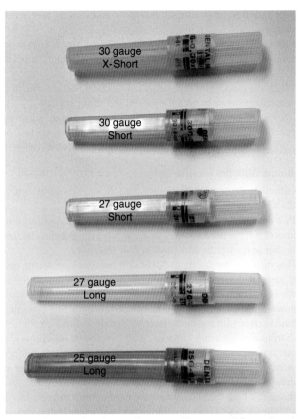

Fig. 43.12 Color coding by needle gauge. (Courtesy of Septodont, Lancaster, Pennsylvania)

push and screw the needle onto the syringe. The cartridge-penetrating end of the needle enters the needle adaptor component of the syringe and engages the rubber diaphragm of the LA cartridge. This sterile needle is packaged in a plastic encasement consisting of two protective shields. A colored shield or needle guard protects the part of the needle that is inserted into the tissues, and a clear or white protective cap covers the syringe and cartridge end of the needle.

Gauge

The gauge is the diameter of the lumen of the needle. The higher the gauge number, the smaller the lumen diameter. Therefore, a 30-gauge needle has a smaller internal diameter than a 27-gauge needle. The most commonly employed needles in oral healthcare are the 25-, 27-, and 30-gauge needles.

A common assumption is that a larger-diameter needle (e.g., 25-gauge) is more uncomfortable to the patient on insertion than a smaller-diameter needle (e.g., 30-gauge); however, this assumption is untrue. Research suggests that people cannot distinguish among a 25-, a 27-, and a 30-gauge needle when injected with each.[1]

Actually, larger-gauge needles (e.g., 25-gauge) have several advantages over smaller-gauge needles. Less deflection occurs when the larger-gauge needle passes through the tissues. Because it is larger and more rigid, it can be guided to the deposition site with minimal deviation, thus ensuring greater accuracy and a higher rate of injection success. This needle rigidity is particularly important with injections requiring significant penetration of the soft tissues, such as the IANB. Although needle breakage is uncommon with disposable needles, it is less likely to occur with a larger-gauge needle. Another advantage of larger-gauge needles is the ability to aspirate and thereby reduce the possibility of intravascular injections.

Opinions vary, but many authorities conclude that aspiration is easier and more reliable through the larger lumen (e.g., 25-gauge) compared to diameters too narrow to adequately aspirate (e.g., 30-gauge).[1]

Blood may be aspirated through a 25-, 27-, or 30-gauge needle, but more pressure is required when a larger gauge number (e.g., 30-gauge) is employed. This difficulty in aspirating may decrease the reliability of the aspiration and increase the likelihood of the harpoon becoming disengaged from the rubber stopper. Therefore, it is recommended that the dental hygienist use a 25-gauge needle for those injections that pose a high risk for aspiration or when a significant depth of soft tissue must be penetrated (e.g., IANB, PSA, or mental or incisive nerve blocks). The 27-gauge needle may be used for all other injections, provided the possibility of aspiration and the depth of tissue penetration are minimal. The 30-gauge needle is not recommended. In the United States, needles are color coded by gauge (Fig. 43.12).

Length

Lengths of needles can vary. The most common needle lengths used in oral healthcare are the short (approximately 1 inch or 20 to 25 mm) and the long (approximately 1⅝ inches or 30 to 35 mm) as measured from the hub to the needle tip.[1,3] Choice of needle length depends on accessibility of the area to be anesthetized. Long needles are preferred for those injections that require penetration of a significant thickness of soft tissue (e.g., IANB). Short needles are indicated for injections in which smaller thicknesses of tissue are to be entered.

Care and Handling of the Needle

Recommendations for the care and handling of disposable needles used for LA administration are as follows:
- Never use a needle for more than one patient.
- Change the needle after the administration of approximately three or four injections on the same patient. Some clinicians recommend changing the needle even more often. The stainless steel becomes dull after several injections, causing each succeeding tissue

penetration to be potentially traumatic and causing postinjection soreness.

- Cover the needle with a protective sheath when it is not being used—both before the injection and immediately upon completion of the injection.
- Watch the position of the uncovered needle tip at all times to prevent needle injury to both the patient and the operator.
- Dispose of needles in an approved sharps container. These rigid, puncture-proof, leak-resistant containers need to be disposed of in accordance with federal, state, and local regulations (see Chapter 10).[1]

Problems With the Needle

The dental hygienist may encounter the following problems with the needle when administering LA agents:

- *Pain on insertion.* Patients may experience tissue discomfort during insertion if the needle is dull; to avoid this pain, the clinician needs to change the needle after three or four insertions.
- *Pain on withdrawal.* Patient discomfort may occur when the needle is being withdrawn from the tissues if any barbs are on the needle tip. Although barbs may be the result of the manufacturing process, most are caused by the needle tip contacting bone or any hard surface with too much force.[1,3] Therefore, checking for needle sharpness or presence of barbs on all subsequent injections is recommended and addresses the human need for patient comfort and satisfaction. To check for needle sharpness, the practitioner may draw the needle tip backward across a sterile piece of gauze. When the needle barb snags the gauze, the needle needs to be replaced. In addition, a needle should never be pushed forcefully against bone.
- *Needle stick exposure of the clinician.* For prevention of an accidental needle stick injury, the needle should be capped with a protective shield before being used and immediately on injection termination. If a needle stick exposure occurs, follow the percutaneous exposure protocol and postexposure evaluation procedure outlined in Chapter 10.
- *Needle breakage.* Refer to the later section on local complications.

Cartridge

The cartridge is the component of the armamentarium that contains the LA drug in addition to other ingredients. The LA cartridge is often referred to as a *carpule* by oral health professionals; however, this term is a registered trademark name for the anesthetic cartridge manufactured by Cook-Waite Laboratories.[1]

Parts of the Cartridge

The cartridges used for LA administration have four components (Fig. 43.13):

- The rubber stopper or plunger is located on one end of the cartridge and is the part in which the harpoon of an aspirating syringe

is embedded. This component is pushed into the glass cylinder by pressure on the syringe thumb ring, thereby ejecting the LA solution through the needle. During manufacturing, the rubber stopper is often treated with silicone to allow it to traverse the glass cylinder without sticking. In an unused LA cartridge, the rubber stopper end is slightly indented from the glass cylinder rim (Fig. 43.14). Cartridges that do not exhibit this characteristic should not be used because it is an indication that the solution has been contaminated. This topic is discussed in detail in the later section on problems.

- On the opposite end of the cartridge is a diaphragm into which the needle penetrates. The diaphragm is made of a semipermeable material, usually rubber, that allows solutions to diffuse into the cartridge (see Fig. 43.13B).
- An aluminum cap fits securely around the cartridge neck, holding the diaphragm in place.
- The glass cylinder makes up the cartridge body on which the cartridge contents, the solution amount, and the manufacturer's name are imprinted. Also, several manufacturers now place a color-coded band around the glass cylinder to aid in drug identification.

Ingredients

Several ingredients collectively form the anesthetic solution. The LA drug or combination of drugs is, of course, the primary reason for the dental cartridge. Although the LA molecule is stable and can withstand being boiled or processed in an autoclave without breaking down, the other ingredients and dental cartridge components are more fragile; therefore, it would not be safe to process in an autoclave.

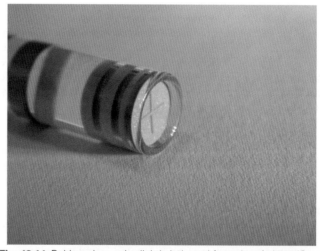

Fig. 43.14 Rubber plunger is slightly indented from rim of glass. (Courtesy of J.E. Bercasio Photography.)

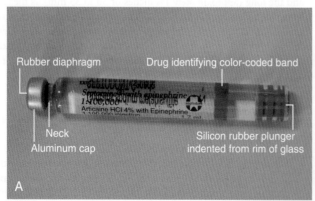

Rubber diaphragm

Drug identifying color-coded band

Neck

Aluminum cap

Silicon rubber plunger indented from rim of glass

A

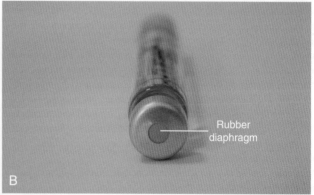

Rubber diaphragm

B

Fig. 43.13 (A) Components of the LA cartridge. (B) Rubber diaphragm. (Courtesy of J.E. Bercasio Photography.)

A vasoconstricting drug in various concentrations is incorporated in some anesthetic cartridges. This component increases the safety and the duration of action of the LA agent. Vasoconstrictor-containing cartridges also have a preservative for the vasoconstrictor. The agent most often employed is sodium bisulfite, which prevents biodegradation of the vasoconstrictor by oxygen.

Sodium chloride is added to the dental cartridge to make the solution isotonic with the body tissues. Finally, distilled water is incorporated into the anesthetic solution to produce a sufficient volume of solution in the cartridge. Cartridges available in the United States contain a total of 1.8 mL of solution; however, it is important to note that manufacturers can only guarantee a minimum amount of 1.7 mL of solution. During hygiene licensure examinations, candidates must be mindful of these differences when performing calculations for recommended doses.[3]

Cartridge Care and Handling

LA cartridges are packaged either in a vacuum-sealed metal canister containing 50 cartridges or in boxes that include 10 sealed units of 10 cartridges each, referred to as a *blister pack*. Regardless of how the cartridges are packaged, it is recommended that the cartridges be stored in their original container at room temperature in a dark place until use. Exposure to prolonged heat or direct sunlight results in accelerated solution deterioration, particularly the vasoconstrictor. In addition, if kept in these original containers, the cartridges remain clean and uncontaminated.

It is not necessary to prepare a cartridge before use. The LA solution is sterilized during the manufacturing process, and bacterial cultures taken from exterior cartridge surfaces immediately after opening a container usually fail to produce bacterial growth.[1] If the oral healthcare provider is concerned about the cartridge exterior, all components may be wiped with a disinfectant approved by the American Dental Association (ADA) and Environmental Protection Agency (EPA). Plastic cartridge dispensers are also available to aid in disinfecting cartridges. They can hold 1 day's supply of cartridges with the diaphragm or aluminum cap placed downward. Gauze moistened with a disinfectant is placed in the center. When assembling the armamentarium for LA administration, the oral healthcare provider may wipe the diaphragm end of the cartridge with the moistened gauze.

Cartridges should never be immersed in liquid disinfectant or sterilant. These solutions may diffuse through the semipermeable material of the diaphragm and contaminate the cartridge contents or may corrode the aluminum cap. In addition, LA cartridges should not be processed in the autoclave. Neither the labile vasoconstrictor nor the seals of the cartridge can withstand the extreme temperatures.

Cartridge warmers that bring the LA solution to body temperature to promote patient comfort during administration are commercially available; however, they are neither necessary nor recommended. LAs stored and injected at room temperature are not uncomfortable for patients. Indeed, an overheated cartridge may cause a burning sensation during the injection and may destroy the heat-sensitive vasoconstrictor, thus producing a shorter anesthesia duration.

Each box or canister is marked with an expiration date by the manufacturer. This expiration date also appears on the individual cartridges. Cartridges should not be used beyond the expiration date because injection with an outdated LA solution may result in patient discomfort and unreliable anesthesia.

A product identification package insert is placed in all LA containers. It includes important information about the LA agent, including dosages, contraindications, warnings, care and handling, and more. It is imperative that the dental hygienist be familiar with this material to ensure patient safety and comfort.

Problems

Problems are seldom encountered with cartridges, but the following may be noted:

- *Bubble in the cartridge.* Small bubbles (1 to 2 mm in diameter) may at times be seen in a cartridge. These bubbles consist of nitrogen gas that was bubbled into the anesthetic solution during the manufacturing process to prevent oxygen, which destroys the vasoconstrictor, from being trapped in the cartridge. The bubbles are harmless and may be ignored. A larger bubble (larger than 2 mm) in the cartridge, however, is an indication that the solution has been frozen. In this case, the stopper may also extend beyond the cartridge end (extruded). Because solution sterility is no longer guaranteed, the cartridge should not be used.
- *Extruded stopper.* As noted previously, an extruded rubber stopper accompanied by a large bubble in the cartridge is an indication that the solution has been frozen. Having a stopper that extends beyond the rim of the glass cylinder with no bubble present is often a sign that the cartridge was stored in a disinfectant and the solution has diffused through the diaphragm into the cartridge. This means that the contents are contaminated and the cartridge should be discarded.
- *Sticky stopper.* Because rubber stoppers are more frequently being treated with silicone during manufacturing, stoppers that stick have become less of a problem. To minimize the sticky stopper problem, cartridges should be stored at room temperature.
- *Corroded cap.* Aluminum cap corrosion may be observed if the cap has been immersed in quaternary compounds such as benzalkonium chloride. If disinfecting the cartridge is necessary, an ADA- and EPA-approved disinfectant is recommended. Cartridges exhibiting corrosion should not be used.
- *Rust on the aluminum cap.* The presence of rust signifies that a cartridge has broken or leaked in the metal container. The metal container rusts and deposits appear on the cartridge cap. A cartridge that has a rust deposit should not be used and each cartridge in the container should be carefully inspected.
- *Broken cartridge.* Cartridge breakage may occur if the cartridge has been fractured during handling. Damaged containers should be returned to the supplier. Before being used, each cartridge is checked for signs of cracked or chipped glass. The area surrounding the stopper and the cylinder-cap interface need to be carefully examined. If a fractured cartridge is subjected to the pressure of an injection, it may shatter. Fortunately, the introduction of the color-coded band around the glass cylinder has minimized such occurrences by reinforcing the glass.
- A broken cartridge may result if excessive force is used when the dental hygienist engages the harpoon of an aspirating syringe. The harpoon is engaged by gently pressing the thumb ring and piston into the rubber stopper. If it is necessary to use more pressure to embed the harpoon, the dental hygienist should use one hand to cover the glass cartridge.
- Pressure on the syringe thumb ring may cause the cartridge to break if the syringe harpoon is bent or the needle is bent and not perforating the cartridge diaphragm. Thorough examination and proper armamentarium preparation before use prevent cartridge breakage from occurring. One should never apply excessive pressure on the dental cartridge if significant resistance is met.

- *Leakage during injection.* An off-center perforation of the needle into the cartridge diaphragm produces an oval-shaped puncture. When positive pressure is applied to the plunger, anesthetic solution may leak through the perforation. It is important to carefully insert the needle into the cartridge diaphragm so that a centric perforation occurs and to prevent leakage during the injection.
- *Burning on injection.* Refer to the later section on local complications.[1]

Supplementary Armamentarium

In addition to the syringe, needle, cartridge, and needle recap safety device, other items are needed to effectively administer LAs. These include topical antiseptic, topical anesthetic, applicator sticks, gauze, and a hemostat or cotton pliers.

Topical Antiseptics

Topical antiseptics may be applied to the mucosal surface at the injection site to reduce the risk of introducing surface microorganisms into the tissue, which could result in inflammation and infection. Betadine (povidone-iodine) and Merthiolate (thimerosal) are agents commonly used for this purpose.[1] A small quantity of the agent is placed at the injection site for 15 to 30 seconds before topical anesthetic placement and the initial needle penetration. Sterile gauze use for wiping the surface is considered an adequate

alternative, with topical antiseptic application as an option for further microbe reduction. Because postinjection infections may occur, the use of a topical antiseptic should be considered, especially when administering LA agents to individuals who may be immunosuppressed.[1]

Topical Anesthetic Agents

Topical anesthetic agents are applied to the mucous membrane before the initial needle penetration to anesthetize the terminal nerve endings and thus promote patient comfort during the injection procedures (Fig. 43.15). For maximum effectiveness, the topical anesthetic agent is placed at the penetration site, on dried tissue, for 1 to 2 minutes.

The concentration of agents used for topical application is high to facilitate diffusion of the drug through the mucous membranes (usually 2 to 3 mm). Therefore, only small amounts applied to a limited area are used to avoid toxicity. Both ester and amide topical anesthetic agents are available. They are prepared in the form of gels, ointments, solutions, or sprays. Topical anesthetic sprays that deliver a continuous stream until deactivated may potentially deliver a very high anesthetic agent dose and are therefore not recommended. Those sprays that deliver a measured dose limit the amount that can be expelled and are much preferred.

Oraqix is an amide topical anesthetic with 2.5% lidocaine and 2.5% prilocaine (see Fig. 43.15C). Oraqix is a periodontal gel that

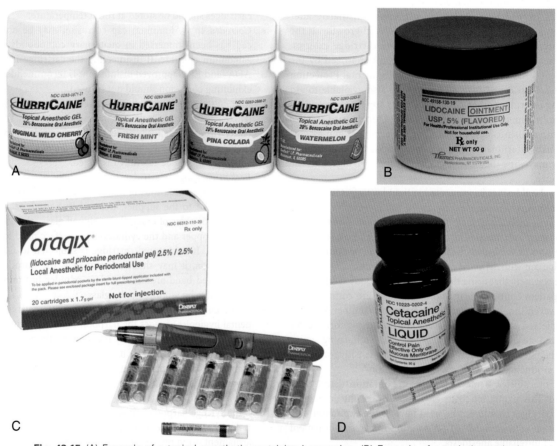

Fig. 43.15 (A) Example of a topical anesthetic containing benzocaine. (B) Example of a topical anesthetic containing lidocaine (DentiPatch). (C) Example of Oraqix, containing lidocaine and prilocaine. (D) Example of Cetacaine liquid. (A, Courtesy Beautlich LP, Pharmaceuticals, Waukegan, Illinois. B, Courtesy Septodont, New Castle, Delaware. C, From Logothetis, D. *Local Anesthesia for the Dental Hygienist.* 3rd ed. Elsevier; 2022. Courtesy of DENTSPLY Pharmaceutical, York, Pennsylvania. D, Courtesy of J.E. Bercasio Photography.)

is FDA approved for intraoral use and is available by prescription. Oraqix comes in a cartridge that is inserted into a specially designed dispenser for administration. The cartridge has a safety collar that prevents loading of the product into a standard dental syringe. This product has unique thermosetting properties. It is fluid at room temperature, which ensures delivery subgingivally but becomes a gel at body temperature, which keeps it at the site. Oraqix contains no epinephrine, has a 30-second onset, and the anesthetic benefits will last on average 20 minutes. A maximum dose of five cartridges per hygiene appointment is advised, and also caution is advised when administering to nursing mothers (Procedure 43.1).[6]

PROCEDURE 43.1 Oraqix Topical Anesthetic Application for Use During Scaling and Root Planing

Equipment
Personal protective equipment
2.5% lidocaine and 2.5% prilocaine cartridge
Oraqix dispenser
Blunt tip applicator
Cotton pliers/hemostat
2 × 2 gauze

Steps
1. Assemble armamentarium.

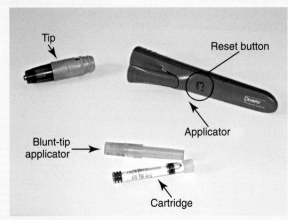

Oraqix armamentarium. From top left: applicator tip, applicator body, blunt tip applicator in blue cap, and cartridge of Oraqix topical gel. (Courtesy of F. O'Brien Photography.)

2. Place blunt tip applicator into the tip of the Oraqix dispenser and turn it to lock in place.

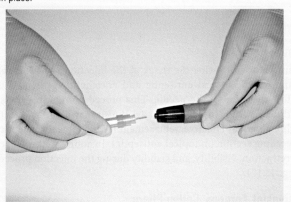

Connect blunt tip applicator with applicator tip. (Courtesy of F. O'Brien Photography.)

3. Press reset button on body of handle.

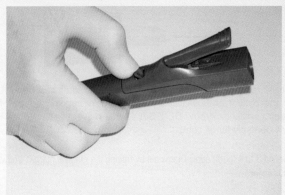

Press reset button on body of handle. (Courtesy of F. O'Brien Photography.)

4. Load the cartridge stopper, end-first, into the body of the handle and join the tip to the applicator body. Twist to lock it in place.

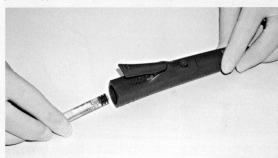

A

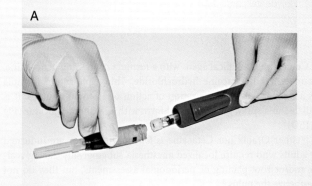

B

(A) Load the cartridge stopper end first into the main applicator body. (B) Join the tip to the applicator. Twist to lock in place. (Courtesy of F. O'Brien Photography.)

Continued

PROCEDURE 43.1   Oraqix Topical Anesthetic Application for Use During Scaling and Root Planing—cont'd

5. Partially remove the blunt tip applicator cap in order to bend the tip into a shape to suit individual patient or clinician needs.

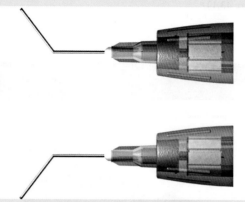

Partially remove the cap on the blunt tip applicator and bend it to suit the patient and clinician's needs. (From Oraqix: Product information available from DENTSPLY Pharmaceuticals, York, PA. www.dentsplydental.com)

6. Select 3 to 4 teeth, apply Oraqix gel by tracing the gingival margin, and wait 30 seconds.

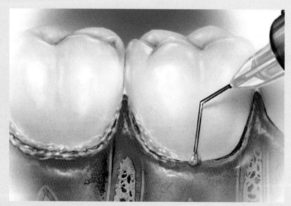

Apply gel by tracing the gingival margin. (From Oraqix: Product information available from DENTSPLY Pharmaceuticals, York, PA. www.dentsplydental.com)

7. Then move the blunt tip applicator directly into the periodontal pocket and fill it with the Oraqix gel.

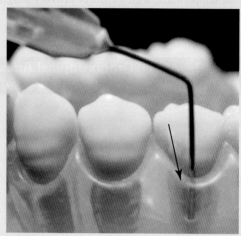

Move the blunt tip applicator directly into the periodontal pocket and fill it with the gel. (From Oraqix: Product information available from DENTSPLY Pharmaceuticals, York, PA. www.dentsplydental.com)

8. For a detailed demonstration, go to Evolve Resource Videos to view a video of the application process.

Cetacaine is a topical agent with a formula containing benzocaine, butamben, and tetracaine hydrochloride. This triple-action formula has a rapid onset with a duration of action of 30 to 60 minutes. It is available in a spray, gel, and liquid form with a syringe applicator (Fig 43.15D).

Neither Oraqix nor Cetacaine *is for injection.* They are indicated for adults who require localized anesthesia subgingivally during scaling and/or root planing or periodontal assessments, but they do not anesthetize the pulps.[3]

Cotton-Tipped Applicator Sticks

Cotton-tipped applicator sticks are needed for topical antiseptic and anesthetic agent application. They also may be used to apply pressure to the tissue before and during palatal injections (Fig. 43.16).

Gauze

Gauze is used to wipe the tissue at the injection site before application of the topical antiseptic and anesthetic agents and again before insertion of the needle. This procedure removes the saliva and debris from the injection site. It also may serve as a suitable, although not as effective, replacement for the topical antiseptic (see preceding section on topical antiseptic). In addition, the gauze aids in retraction, visibility, and stability during the injection procedures (Fig. 43.17).

Hemostat, Forceps, Cotton Pliers

Hemostats, forceps, or cotton pliers are the components used in the unlikely event of a needle breakage during administration which must be retrieved from the soft tissues (Fig. 43.18). These instruments are also used to remove rubber stoppers when they fail to disengage from the harpoon during dismantling of the syringe.

PREPARATION OF ARMAMENTARIUM

Loading and Unloading the Metallic or Plastic Cartridge-Type Syringe

Proper loading of the syringe is essential to prevent complications associated with the syringe, cartridge, and needle and to ensure patient safety and comfort during LA administration (Procedure 43.2 and Evolve Resource Video).

Unsheathing and Resheathing the Needle

A needle should only be uncovered (unsheathed) at the time of LA administration. Therefore, the needle is always covered with its colored protective cap. Concerns regarding the possibility of a needle stick exposure have led to the formulation of guidelines for resheathing needles. Oral healthcare providers are most often injured with needles when the needle is being resheathed after an injection.[1] At this time, the needle is contaminated with blood, saliva, and debris, and the potential for disease transmission exists. A variety of techniques have been suggested, but currently the use of recapping

devices is trending to replace the scoop technique; a one-handed "scoop" technique for sheathing the needle is recommended if no recapping devices are available (see Procedure 43.2). The one-handed resheathing technique or an approved mechanical device should be consistently used by the dental hygienist whether or not the needle has been contaminated.

Devices such as shields and needle sheath props are available to aid in preventing accidental needle stick exposure (see Step 12 in Procedure 43.2). Dental hygienists should be familiar with the devices available and determine which technique or mechanical device is most acceptable to them.

Dismantling the Armamentarium

At the completion of the dental hygiene care appointment, the local anesthesia armamentarium needs to be dismantled. Procedure 43.3 describes the sequence for properly unloading the syringe. In regard to cartridge disposal, cartridges generally fall into three categories which include general waste, pharmaceutical waste, and medical waste. Empty, nonbroken cartridges can be discarded into the regular trash. Cartridges that contain residual pharmaceutical liquid are put in a container labeled "pharmaceutical waste." Cartridges with blood are considered medical waste and should be placed in a sharps container for regulated waste. However, the Occupational Safety and Health Administration (OSHA) states, "The ultimate disposal of pharmaceutical vials must be in accordance with municipal, state and federal regulations (e.g., those of the Environmental Protection Agency, EPA)."[7]

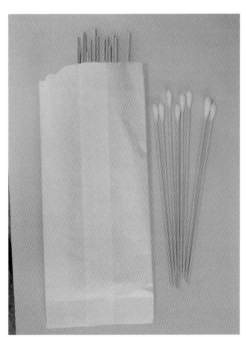

Fig. 43.16 Cotton-tipped applicator sticks. (Courtesy of J.E. Bercasio Photography.)

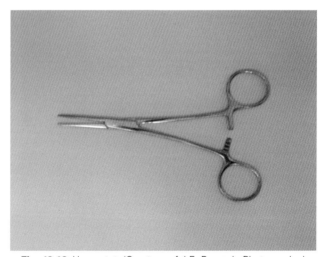

Fig. 43.18 Hemostat. (Courtesy of J.E. Bercasio Photography.)

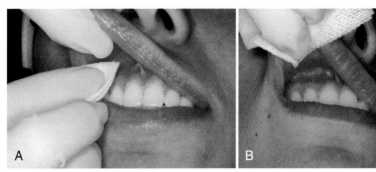

Fig. 43.17 Gauze is used (A) to wipe mucous membrane at site of needle penetration and (B) to aid in tissue retraction if necessary. (From Malamed SF. *Handbook of Local Anesthesia.* 7th ed. Elsevier; 2020.)

Equipment

Personal protective equipment
Syringe
Needle
Gauze
Anesthetic cartridge
Topical antiseptic or sterile gauze (optional)
Topical anesthetic
Cotton-tip applicator
Hemostat or cotton pliers

Steps

1. Assemble armamentarium.

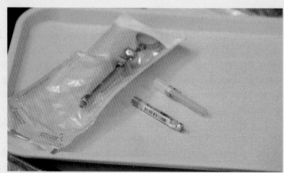

Armamentarium: sterile syringe, cartridge, and needle. (Dental Hygiene Procedures Videos, St Louis, 2015, Saunders.)

2. Remove the sterilized syringe from its container and inspect to ensure the harpoon is sharp and straight.
3. Retract the piston.

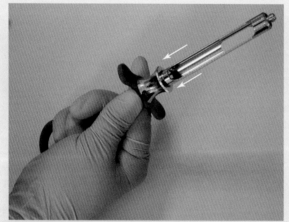

Retract the piston. (Courtesy of J.E. Bercasio Photography.)

4. Insert the cartridge.

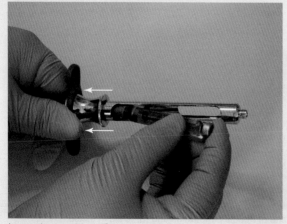

Insert the cartridge. (Courtesy of J.E. Bercasio Photography.)

5. Engage the harpoon. Use the thumb as shown to engage the harpoon in the plunger with gentle finger pressure. Another technique is to grasp the thumb ring in the palm of the hand and simultaneously rotate the harpoon while applying gentle pressure to engage it.

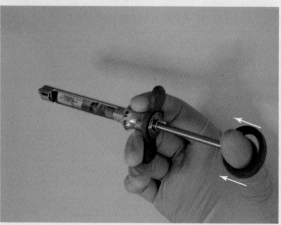

Engage the harpoon in the plunger with gentle finger pressure. (Courtesy of J.E. Bercasio Photography.)

Although no longer recommended, some clinicians may engage the harpoon by using gentle pressure on the plunger and use the other hand to cover the glass as a precautionary measure should the cartridge glass break.

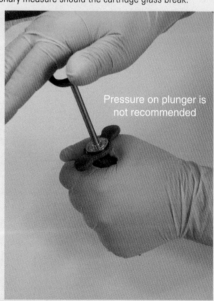

Pressure on plunger is not recommended

Caution: excessive force may cause the cartridge to break. (Courtesy of J.E. Bercasio Photography.)

6. Remove the small clear or white plastic protective shield that covers the cartridge end of the needle.

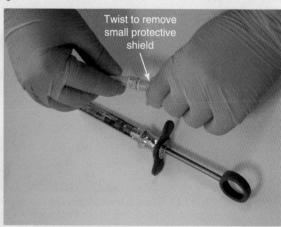

Twist to remove small protective shield

(Courtesy of J.E. Bercasio Photography.)

7. Screw the colored plastic-hubbed needle onto the syringe while simultaneously pushing it into the metal needle adapter of the syringe.

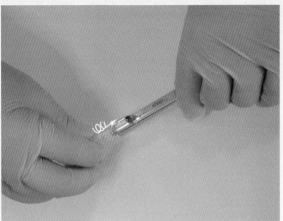

(Courtesy of J.E. Bercasio Photography.)

8. Check for flow of solution.
   a. With transparent protective shields, proper flow is easy to confirm by looking at expelled drops through the clear cap.
   b. With solid color protective shields, direct the needle away from the body, keep the hand at the needle hub, and loosen the colored plastic protective cap from the needle. Use a one-handed technique with the dominant thumb and index finger to pinch the cap to remove.

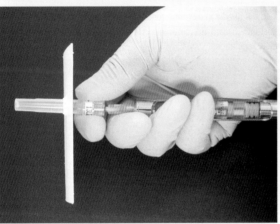

(Courtesy of J.E. Bercasio Photography.)

   Let the cap slide off the needle and onto a piece of sterile gauze if not using a recapping device.

   Expel a few drops of solution to test for proper flow and recap the needle using a safe recapping device.

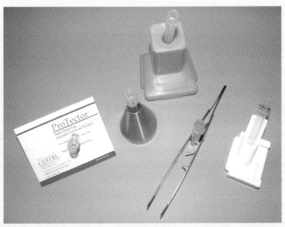

Examples of recapping devices. (From Logothetis D. *Local Anesthesia for the Dental Hygienist.* 3rd ed. Elsevier; 2020.)

9. If using the scoop technique, follow steps A and B:
   a. Hold the syringe with one hand and glide the needle into the colored plastic cap lying on the instrument tray. Never attempt to hold cap with other hand because this may lead to an accidental needle stick exposure.
   b. Tilt the syringe upward to allow the cap to slide down to the hub and cover the needle. If the cap starts to slip off the needle, do not attempt to stop it with the other hand. Instead, let the cap fall on the instrument tray and begin the process again.

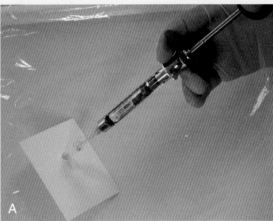

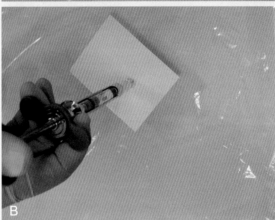

One-handed "scoop" technique for recapping needle. (Courtesy of J.E. Bercasio Photography.)

10. The syringe is now ready for use.

PROCEDURE 43.3   Unloading the Breech-Loading Metallic or Plastic Cartridge-Type Syringe

Equipment

See Procedure 43.2.

Steps

1. Retract the piston and pull the cartridge away from the needle with your thumb and forefinger as you retract the piston until the harpoon disengages from the plunger.

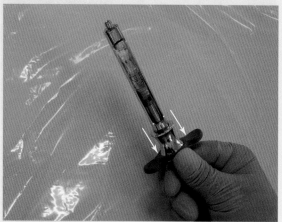

Retract the piston. (Courtesy of J.E. Bercasio Photography.)

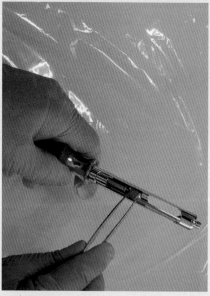

If stopper remains on harpoon, use cotton pliers to safely remove it. (Courtesy of J.E. Bercasio Photography.)

2. Remove the cartridge from the syringe by inverting the syringe, permitting the cartridge to fall free.

3. Carefully unscrew the recapped needle, being careful not to accidently discard the metal needle adaptor.

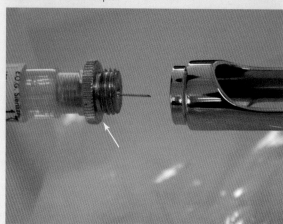

When discarding needle, check to be sure that the metal needle adaptor (arrow) from the syringe is not inadvertently discarded too. (Courtesy of J.E. Bercasio Photography.)

4. Place the needle in a sharps container that is rigid, puncture proof, and leak resistant. Discard the cartridge in a container according to recommended waste regulations.

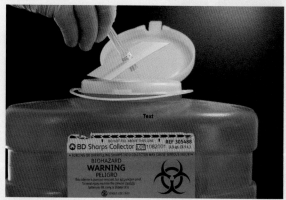

Needles and cartridges with a positive aspiration are considered infectious. (Courtesy of J.E. Bercasio Photography.)

TRIGEMINAL NERVE

Sensory innervation of the face and neck is supplied by the trigeminal nerve (fifth cranial or V), which is the largest of the twelve cranial nerves (Fig. 43.19). The three divisions of the trigeminal nerve include the ophthalmic (V_1), the maxillary (V_2), and the mandibular (V_3) divisions. Because of the vicinity of facial nerves to many vital structures in a compact area, the efficacy and safety of nerve blocks are based on precise and detailed knowledge of the anatomical relationships of the selected nerve, its deep and superficial courses, and the final sensory territories. For each nerve block, the dental hygienist should have thorough knowledge about practical anatomy, indications, technique, and complications.

Ophthalmic Division (V_1)

The ophthalmic nerve, the first and smallest division of the trigeminal nerve, branches off the trigeminal (semilunar or Gasserian) ganglion and forms three branches: the nasociliary nerve, the frontal nerve, and the lacrimal nerve. This division of the trigeminal nerve innervates tissues superior to the oral structures, including the eye, nose, and frontal cutaneous tissues. It has only sensory function. Of the three divisions of the trigeminal nerve, the ophthalmic is the least important to intraoral local anesthesia administration.

Maxillary Division (V_2)

The maxillary division of the trigeminal nerve, which is entirely sensory in function, arises from the trigeminal (semilunar or Gasserian)

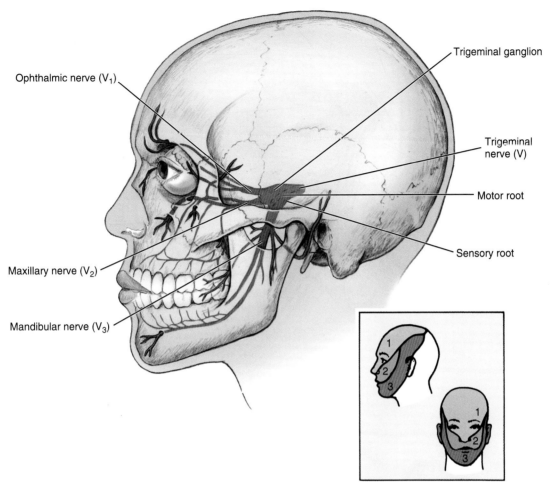

Fig. 43.19 Trigeminal nerve distribution. (From Fehrenbach MJ, Herring SW. *Illustrated Anatomy of the Head and Neck*. 6th ed. Elsevier; 2021.)

ganglion, exits the cranium via the foramen rotundum, and then passes into the pterygopalatine fossa, where it gives off several branches (Fig. 43.20). Only those branches pertinent to intraoral local anesthesia are discussed.

Pterygopalatine Nerves

Two branches pass through the pterygopalatine ganglion and form the greater (anterior) palatine nerve and the nasopalatine (NP) nerve (see Fig. 43.20). The greater palatine (GP) nerve enters the oral cavity on the hard palate via the GP foramen and innervates the palatal soft tissues and bone of the posterior teeth. The NP nerve leaves the pterygopalatine ganglion and passes forward and downward, entering the oral cavity through the incisive foramen. This nerve provides sensory innervation to the lingual bone and soft tissues in the premaxilla (canine to canine).

Posterior Superior Alveolar Nerve

The PSA nerve (Fig. 43.21) descends from the main trunk of the maxillary nerve just before it enters the infraorbital (IO) canal. Most often, there are two PSA branches that pass downward on the posterior surface of the maxilla. An internal branch enters the PSA foramen, located on the superior portion of the maxillary tuberosity. This branch provides sensory innervation to the pulpal and osseous tissues and the periodontal ligaments of the maxillary third, second, and first molars (usually with the exception of the mesiobuccal root of the first molar). An external branch of the PSA nerve remains on the outer surface of

the maxilla and continues downward to innervate the facial gingiva of the maxillary molars and the adjacent vestibular mucosa.

Branches of the Infraorbital Nerve

The maxillary nerve continues anteriorly after having given off the PSA nerve and enters the IO canal. At this point, the maxillary nerve is referred to as the *infraorbital nerve* (see Fig. 43.21). Two branches may descend from the IO nerve: the middle superior alveolar (MSA) and the anterior superior alveolar (ASA) nerves.

The MSA nerve branches off the IO nerve within the IO canal. This nerve provides sensory innervation to the maxillary premolars, the mesiofacial root of the first molar, the periodontal tissues, and the facial soft tissue and bone in the premolar area. The MSA nerve is present in approximately 28% of individuals.[8] In its absence, these areas are innervated by the PSA nerve or, more commonly, the ASA nerve.

The ASA nerve descends from the IO nerve just before the latter's exit from the IO foramen. The ASA nerve provides innervation to the central and lateral incisors, the canine, the periodontal tissues, and facial soft tissue and bone over these teeth. In those individuals without an MSA nerve, the ASA nerve most often provides innervation to the premolars and possibly the mesiofacial root of the first molar.

Mandibular Division (V₃)

The mandibular nerve, the third and largest division of the trigeminal nerve, both has a sensory root and carries the motor root for the trigeminal nerve (Fig. 43.22). The sensory root arises from the trigeminal

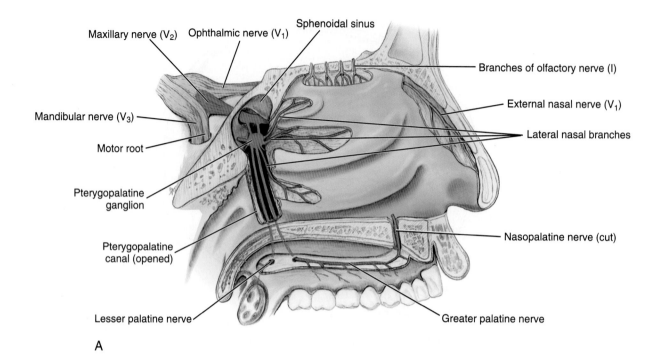

A

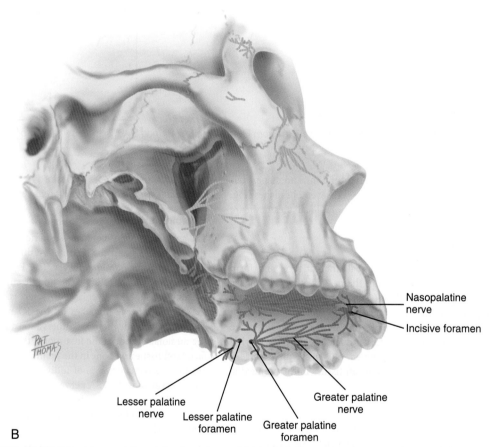

B

Fig. 43.20 (A) Maxillary nerve and its palatine branches, which include the greater, lesser, and nasopalatine nerves, are highlighted from a medial view of the lateral nasal view and opened pterygopalatine canal with the nasal septum removed, thus severing the nasopalatine nerve. (B) From an oblique lateral view of the skull and its hard palate. (From Fehrenbach MJ, Herring SW. *Illustrated Anatomy of the Head and Neck.* 6th ed. Elsevier; 2021.)

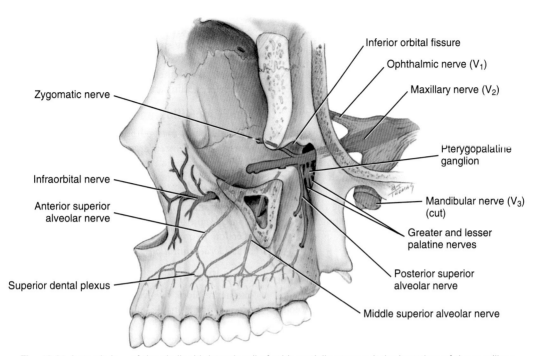

Fig. 43.21 Lateral view of the skull with lateral wall of orbit partially removed; the branches of the maxillary nerve are highlighted. (From Fehrenbach MJ, Herring SW. *Illustrated Anatomy of the Head and Neck*. 6th ed. Elsevier; 2021.)

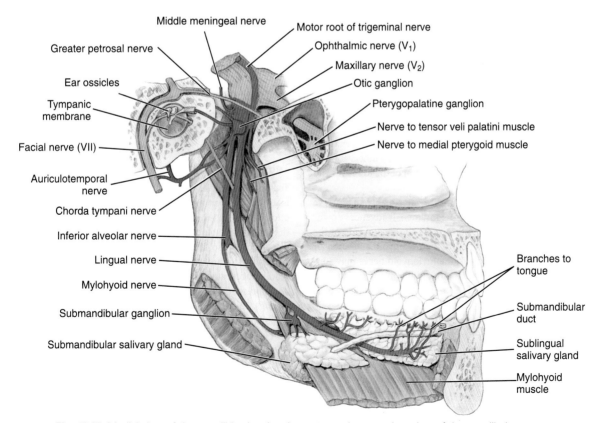

Fig. 43.22 Medial view of the mandible showing the motor and sensory branches of the mandibular nerve. (From Fehrenbach MJ, Herring SW. *Illustrated Anatomy of the Head and Neck*. 6th ed. Saunders; 2021.)

ganglion, after which it is joined by the motor root. Both roots emerge from the cranium via the foramen ovale and at this point, they unite to form the main trunk of the mandibular nerve.

The trunk then divides into an anterior branch and a posterior branch. The nerves arising from these branches that relate to intraoral local anesthesia are described in the following paragraphs.

Branches of the Anterior Division

The anterior division is smaller than its posterior counterpart and contains primarily motor fibers. The motor component innervates the muscles of mastication: the masseter, the temporalis, and the lateral and medial pterygoid. The sensory component of the anterior division is the buccal nerve. At the level of the occlusal plane of the mandibular molars, it crosses the anterior border of the ramus and branches to innervate the buccal gingiva of the mandibular molars (Fig. 43.23).

Branches of the Posterior Division

The posterior division of the mandibular nerve is primarily sensory, but it also has a small motor component. The posterior division branches related to mandibular anesthesia are the lingual and inferior alveolar nerves (see Fig. 43.23).

The lingual nerve emerges between the lower head of the lateral pterygoid and medial pterygoid muscles and lies between the ramus and the medial pterygoid muscle in the pterygomandibular space. It turns anteriorly, where it enters the oral cavity and innervates the anterior two-thirds of the tongue, the mucous membranes of the floor of the mouth, and the lingual gingiva of the mandible.

The inferior alveolar nerve runs posterior and parallel to the lingual nerve within the pterygomandibular space, where it enters the mandibular foramen. Within the mandible, the inferior alveolar nerve travels in the mandibular canal and innervates the pulpal and osseous tissues of the mandibular teeth in the quadrant and facial soft tissues anterior to the first molar. Throughout its course, the inferior alveolar nerve is accompanied by the inferior alveolar artery and vein.

As the inferior alveolar nerve reaches the mental foramen, it divides into two terminal branches. The incisive nerve is a direct extension of the inferior alveolar nerve, continuing anteriorly within the mandibular canal. It innervates the pulpal and osseous tissues of the mandibular premolars, canine, and lateral and central incisors and the facial periodontal tissues of the teeth.[3,8]

The mental nerve branches from the inferior alveolar nerve, exits the mandible via the mental foramen, and provides sensory innervation to the facial soft tissues, mucous membranes, and skin of the lower lip and chin.

The mylohyoid nerve branches from the inferior alveolar nerve before the latter enters into the mandibular foramen. It advances downward and forward in the mylohyoid groove on the medial side of the ramus and provides motor innervation to the mylohyoid and anterior digastric muscles. In some individuals, the mylohyoid nerve may supply accessory sensory innervation to the mandible in the incisor and molar areas, particularly the mesial root of the first mandibular molar.

LOCAL ANESTHESIA TECHNIQUES

When choosing the appropriate injection to be administered, the dental hygienist needs to consider the area to be treated, the procedure to be performed, the extent of anesthesia necessary, and the patient's needs and comfort. The three major types of injections—local infiltration, field block, and nerve block—are differentiated by the deposition site of the anesthetic solution and the area to receive treatment.

Local Infiltration (Intraseptal)

A **local infiltration** injection involves placement of the anesthetic solution close to the smaller terminal endings of the nerve fibers in the immediate area to be treated (Fig. 43.24). An example would be the injection of anesthetic solution into an interproximal papilla before therapeutic scaling and root planing (i.e., papillary).

Field Block (Supraperiosteal Injection)

The **field block** method of obtaining anesthesia involves the deposition of solution near large terminal nerve branches (Fig. 43.25). The resulting anesthesia is more circumscribed, most often involving one tooth and the tissues surrounding the tooth. Treatment is away from the site of the injection. The deposition of anesthetic solution above the apex of a maxillary tooth, such as the maxillary right central incisor, is an example of a field block or is correctly called a **supraperiosteal** injection. In oral healthcare, the field block is often incorrectly referred to as a *local infiltration*.

Nerve Block

The **nerve block** involves the deposition of anesthetic solution close to a main nerve trunk, often at some distance from the treatment area (Fig. 43.26). This injection type most often anesthetizes a larger area than that of a field block. Examples include a PSA nerve block and an IANB.

When dental hygiene care is to be performed in a small, isolated area, infiltration anesthesia may be the best choice, whereas a field block is the injection of choice when one or two teeth are to be treated. When the dental hygiene care plan involves a sextant or quadrant, nerve block anesthesia is recommended.

PROCEDURES FOR A SUCCESSFUL INJECTION

The goal for each LA administration is, of course, to give a safe, comfortable injection for control and elimination of painful sensations during and after dental hygiene care. It is ironic, however, that a procedure meant to control pain for patients is often reported to be the most dreaded. Although the prospect of receiving an intraoral injection provokes fear and apprehension in many individuals, LA agent administration need not be painful. There are technical and communication components to an atraumatic injection, and dental hygienists who embrace the following will establish themselves as revered professionals.

Technical Aspects

Technical strategies include using a topical anesthetic before needle insertion, depositing a few drops of anesthetic solution, waiting 5 seconds before cautiously advancing the needle, and slowly depositing the anesthetic solution; these techniques help minimize or eliminate discomfort. Also, it is essential to maintain complete control over the syringe at all times so that tissue penetration may be accomplished readily, accurately, and without inadvertent nicking of tissues. Fig. 43.27 presents hand positions for injections.

Figs. 43.28 and 43.29 illustrate some hand rests and finger rests that can be used to stabilize syringes.

Fig. 43.30 presents incorrect techniques to be avoided.

Communication Aspects

The ethical principle of beneficence supports the idea that dental hygienists have the obligation to reduce pain to the best of their ability. It is a common experience for patients to have pain or anxiety associated with receiving local anesthesia. If patients perceive their hygienist as sincere and caring, they are more likely to trust the hygienist,

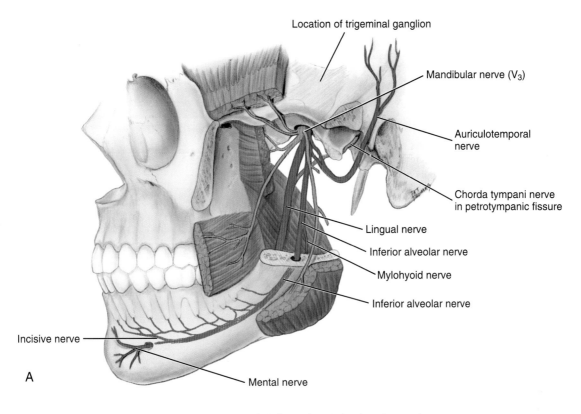

Location of trigeminal ganglion

Mandibular nerve (V₃)

Auriculotemporal
nerve

Chorda tympani nerve
in petrotympanic fissure

Lingual nerve

Inferior alveolar nerve

Mylohyoid nerve

Inferior alveolar nerve

Incisive nerve

Mental nerve

A

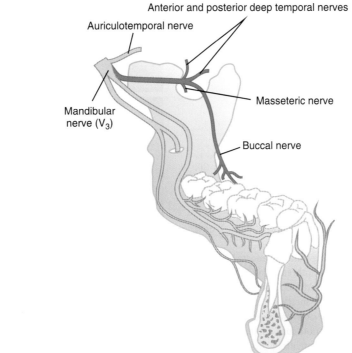

Anterior and posterior deep temporal nerves

Auriculotemporal nerve

Masseteric nerve

Mandibular
nerve (V₃)

Buccal nerve

B

Fig. 43.23 (A) The pathway of the posterior trunk of the mandibular division of the trigeminal nerve. (B) Pathway of both anterior (*red*) and posterior (*yellow*) trunks of mandibular nerve or 3rd division of the trigeminal nerve. (From Fehrenbach MJ, Herring SW. *Illustrated Anatomy of the Head and Neck.* 6th ed. Elsevier; 2021.)

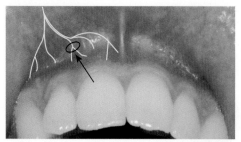

Fig. 43.24 Local infiltration. The area of treatment is flooded with LA. An injection is made into the intraseptal area *(arrow)*. (From Malamed SF. *Handbook of Local Anesthesia*. 7th ed. Elsevier; 2020.)

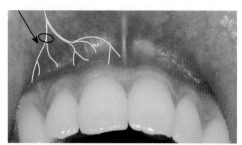

Fig. 43.25 Field block. Local anesthetic is deposited near the larger terminal nerve endings *(arrow)*. (From Malamed SF. *Handbook of Local Anesthesia*. 7th ed. Elsevier; 2020.)

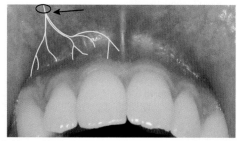

Fig. 43.26 Nerve block. LA is deposited close to the main nerve trunk, located at a distance from the site of injection. (From Malamed SF. *Handbook of Local Anesthesia*. 7th ed. Elsevier; 2020.)

thereby reducing anxiety and lessening the likelihood of pain. This is one of the benefits of good communication.

Communication aspects include keeping patients informed of the procedures in a calm manner and using nonthreatening language to minimize apprehension and promote trust and cooperation. For example, telling patients, "I'm applying the topical anesthetic to the tissue so that the remainder of the procedure is more comfortable," uses words with less-threatening (more positive) connotations to place a positive idea in the patient's mind about the impending procedure. Saying "administer the local anesthetic" in place of "give an injection" or "give a shot," and using the word *discomfort* rather than the word *pain* are recommended. Avoid saying "This will not hurt," because patients often only hear the word *hurt*, ignoring the rest of the statement.[4] Taking the extra time to communicate in a less-threatening manner typically reduces fear and results in a more comfortable procedure for the patient. Box 43.6 provides Patient Education and Communication Tips.

Procedure 43.4 presents steps to ensure comfort, safety, and success common to all injections. Although each injection is unique with regard to anatomic considerations, these steps should be employed

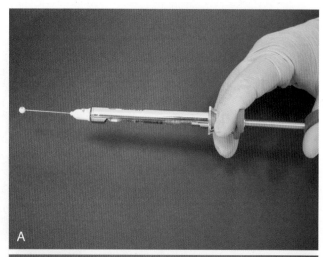

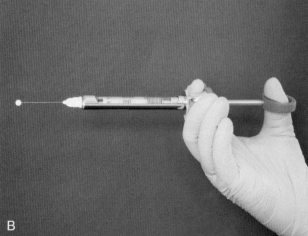

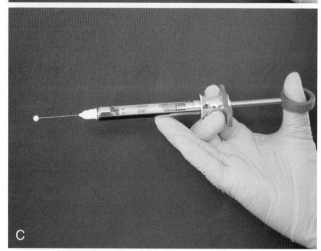

Fig. 43.27 Hand positions for injections. (A) Palm down: poor control over the syringe; not recommended. (B) Palm up: better control over the syringe because it is supported by the wrist; recommended. (C) Palm up and finger support: greatest stabilization; highly recommended. (Courtesy of J.E. Bercasio Photography.)

regardless of the injection being administered. Not every injection is successful and totally free of discomfort because the patients' reactions and hygienists' skills vary; however, if the steps in Procedure 43.4 are followed, the patient and the dental hygienist will enjoy the benefit of the safest and least traumatic injection possible.

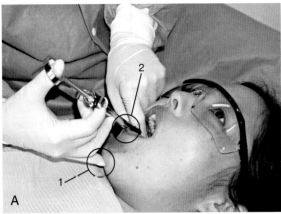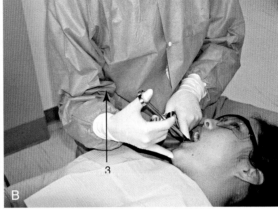

Fig. 43.28 (A) Use of the chin *(1)* as a finger rest, with the syringe barrel stabilized by the patient's lip *(2)* during a right inferior alveolar nerve block. (B) When necessary, stabilization may be increased by drawing the clinician's arm in against the chest *(3)*. (Courtesy of F. O'Brien Photography.)

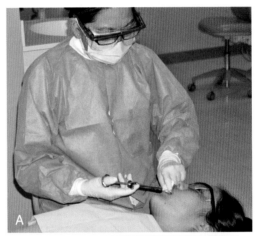

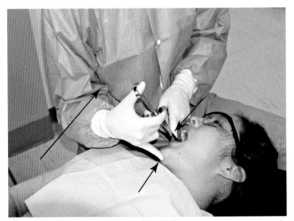

Fig. 43.29 Syringe stabilization of a right posterior superior alveolar nerve block: syringe barrel on the patient's lip, one finger resting on the chin, and one on the syringe barrel *(arrows)*. Upper arm is kept close to the clinician's chest to maximize stability. (Courtesy of F. O'Brien Photography.)

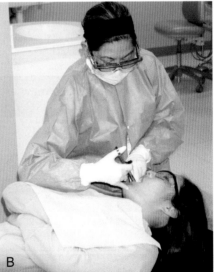

Fig. 43.30 (A) Incorrect position: no hand or finger rest for stabilization of syringe. (B) Incorrect: clinician resting elbow on patient's arm. (Courtesy of F. O'Brien Photography.)

BOX 43.6 Patient Education and Communication Tips

Advantages of Receiving Local Anesthesia

"Jody, I noticed your teeth and gums are sensitive when I probe. I want you to be as comfortable as possible during our appointment today. I recommend that I numb the area with a local anesthetic, which will help you relax and help me to deliver the best care to you. I use a gentle technique. Would you like me to proceed with the local anesthesia?"

(Patient seems hesitant.)

"You seem hesitant. Let me explain how I am going to ensure your maximum comfort during your treatment. I will use a topical gel that numbs the surface of the gum, I will proceed slowly with depositing the solution, and I will coach you through the process. If it becomes too uncomfortable, I will stop when you give me the signal for me to stop."

(Patient nods her head and her facial expression indicates readiness to proceed.)

"Shall I proceed?"

(Patient replies, "Yes, I'm ready.")

PROCEDURE 43.4   Basic Techniques for a Successful Injection

Equipment

See Procedure 43.2.

Steps

1. Assess health history. Take vital signs (including blood pressure, heart rate [pulse], respiratory rate, and temperature, at a minimum).
2. Confirm care plan.
3. Check armamentarium.
4. Load the syringe and determine the syringe window and needle bevel orientation. The large window of the cartridge should face the clinician, and the bevel of the needle should face the bone to decrease risk of injuring the periosteum if the bone is contacted.
5. Expel a few drops to check for free flow of solution.
6. Position the patient in a supine position (head and heart parallel to the floor) with the feet elevated slightly.

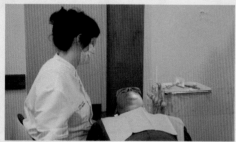

(Dental Hygiene Procedures Videos, St Louis, 2015, Saunders.)

7. Communicate with the patient to place positive ideas in the patient's mind about the injection. Tell the patient about the reasons for topical anesthetic (e.g., "I am applying a topical anesthetic to the tissue so that the remainder of the procedure will be much more comfortable"). Do not use words with a negative connotation, such as *injection, shot, pain,* or *hurt.* Instead, use less-threatening terms such as *administer the local anesthetic.*
8. Visualize or palpate to locate the penetration site.
9. Dry the needle penetration site with sterile gauze.

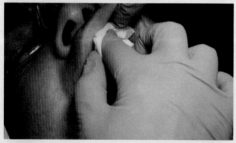

(Dental Hygiene Procedures Videos, St Louis, 2015, Saunders.)

10. Apply topical anesthetic to needle penetration site for 1 to 2 minutes.

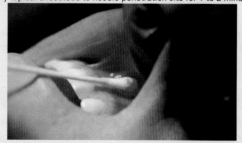

(Dental Hygiene Procedures Videos, St Louis, 2015, Saunders.)

11. In the case of palatal injections, when placing topical anesthetic on the injection site, apply considerable pressure with the cotton swab for a

minimum of 1 minute before the injection. Move the swab immediately adjacent to the penetration site and maintain pressure at this site during the injection. (See Fig. T13.2 in Table 43.13 and Fig. T14.2 in Table 43.14.)

12. After the topical anesthetic swab is removed from the tissue, dry the penetration site.
13. Pick up the prepared LA syringe and establish a firm hand rest. Never place the arm holding the syringe directly on the patient's arm or shoulder.
14. Make the tissue taut at the penetration site by retracting it (except on the palate) using sterile gauze, aiding both visibility and atraumatic needle insertion.

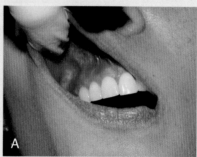

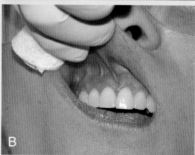

(From Logothetis D. *Local Anesthesia for the Dental Hygienist.* 3rd ed. Elsevier, Inc; 2022.)

15. Keep syringe and needle out of the patient's line of vision.
16. Gently insert the needle into the mucosa until the bevel is completely under the tissue.

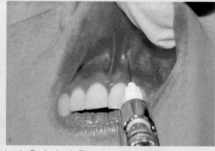

(From Logothetis D. 3rd ed. Elsevier, Inc; 2022.)

17. Observe and communicate with the patient. Watch for any signs of discomfort or distress.
18. Deposit a few "comfort" drops of anesthetic solution, pause for 5 seconds, and then advance the needle a few millimeters. Repeat process as you slowly advance to the deposition site. Communicate with the patient by saying, "To make you more comfortable, I will slowly deposit the anesthetic. To help you relax, please breathe slowly."
19. Aspirate on arrival at the deposition site by pulling the thumb ring back gently. Movement of only 1 or 2 mm is needed. Tip of needle must remain unmoved.
20. For most injections, rotate barrel of the syringe about 45°, and aspirate a second time to ensure that the needle is not located inside a blood vessel.

PROCEDURE 43.4   Basic Techniques for a Successful Injection—cont'd

and abutting against the wall of the vessel, providing a false-negative aspiration. In highly vascular areas, a triple aspiration is recommended.

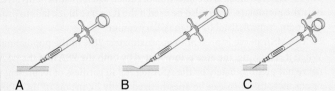

A   **B**   **C**

Intravascular injection of LA. (A) Needle is inserted into lumen of blood vessel. (B) Aspiration test is performed. Negative pressure pulls vessel wall against bevel of needle; therefore, no blood enters syringe (negative aspiration). (C) Drug is injected. Positive pressure on plunger of syringe forces LA solution out through needle. Wall of vessel is forced away from bevel, and anesthetic solution is deposited directly into lumen of blood vessel. (From Malamed SF. *Handbook of Local Anesthesia.* 7th ed. Elsevier, Inc; 2020.)

21. If no blood appears (negative aspiration), slowly deposit the LA solution at a rate of 1 mL/min for approximately 2 minutes for a full cartridge (see part A [*arrow*]).

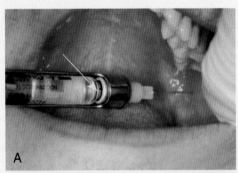

A

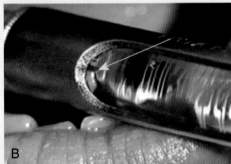

B

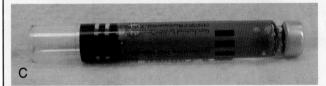

C

(A) Negative aspiration. With the needle in position at the injection site, the administrator pulls the thumb ring of the harpoon aspirator syringe 1 or 2 mm. The needle tip should not move. Check the cartridge at the site where the needle penetrates the diaphragm *(arrow)* for bubble or blood. (B) Positive aspiration. A slight reddish discoloration at the diaphragm end of the cartridge *(arrow)* on the aspiration usually indicates venous penetration. (C) Positive aspiration. Bright red blood rapidly filling the cartridge usually indicates arterial penetration. (From Malamed SF. *Handbook of Local Anesthesia.* 7th ed. Elsevier, Inc; 2020.)

22. If blood appears in the cartridge (positive aspiration), slowly withdraw the needle and communicate with your patient (see parts B and C). Replace the cartridge and the needle and proceed with the injection.

23. Observe and communicate with the patient. Watch for any signs of discomfort or distress. Reassure the patient with statements such as, "I am depositing the solution slowly, so this procedure will be comfortable for you."

24. Slowly withdraw the needle when the indicated amount of anesthetic has been deposited.

25. Resheath the needle using a recapping device (preferred) or the scoop technique (see the last two figures in Procedure 43.2). It is recommended to change to a new needle after 3 to 4 injections.

26. Observe the patient.

27. Rinse the patient's mouth.

28. Massage the tissue over the injection site when indicated.

29. After 2 to 3 minutes, use a probe or rounded back of an instrument to test for anesthesia: first touch an area that is *not* anesthetized, then, second, touch the area that is anesthetized. The patient should have little or no sensation in the anesthetized area.

30. Reassure the patient that numbness, tingling, and a sense of swelling or the tooth feeling different are normal responses.

31. Include both verbal and written postoperative instructions—for example, "Avoid eating and drinking until all the feeling in your mouth returns to normal. If you need to eat or drink, carefully chew on the side that is not numb and only drink room temperature beverages." Advise patient of the expected amount of time their mouth will feel numb.

32. Record the injection(s) in the patient's chart, including:
    a. Area anesthetized and specific injection(s) given
    b. Type of anesthetic used and type of vasoconstrictor and its concentration (ratio)
    c. Gauge and type of needle(s) used
    d. Total amount of solution administered (in milligrams and/or total cartridges)
    e. Time the drug was administered
    f. Patient reaction
    g. Postoperative instructions were given both verbally and in writing

It is important to remember that no drug ever exerts a single action and no clinically useful drug is entirely devoid of toxicity. The potential toxicity of a drug rests in the hands of the user. With practice and proper knowledge, good anesthetic skills can be achieved and help reduce any complications or adverse reactions for the patient.

MAXILLARY ANESTHESIA INJECTION TECHNIQUES

The injection techniques available to anesthetize the maxillary teeth, the facial hard and soft tissues, and the palatal tissues include supraperiosteal injection, ASA nerve block, MSA nerve block, IO nerve block, PSA nerve block, anterior middle superior alveolar (AMSA) nerve block, GP nerve block, and NP nerve block.

Supraperiosteal Injection

A supraperiosteal injection, a field block, more commonly and incorrectly referred to as a *local infiltration,* involves depositing anesthetic solution near the apex of a single tooth, thus providing anesthesia of the tooth and the immediate surrounding area. This injection is most often used to anesthetize maxillary teeth. The rather thin, porous nature of the bone in the maxilla facilitates diffusion of the anesthetic solution from the deposition site to the apex of the tooth to be treated.

By contrast, the mandible consists of much denser bone, which prevents diffusion of the anesthetic agent to the apices of the posterior teeth, therefore precluding the supraperiosteal injection in this area. A supraperiosteal injection may be used to anesthetize the central and lateral teeth in the mandible because the bone in this area is thinner and nutrient canals may be present. Fig. 43.31 shows hand rests that may be used for a maxillary supraperiosteal injection, ASA, and MSA nerve blocks.

Indications for this injection include the need for pulpal anesthesia of maxillary teeth when only a limited number of teeth are to be treated and for soft tissue procedures to be performed on a circumscribed area. Because the anesthetic and vasoconstrictor are deposited so near the area to be treated, this injection provides effective hemostasis, which is often needed during dental hygiene care. Conversely, if there is infection or severe inflammation in the area, administration of the anesthetic solution at a distance from the area of inflammation (i.e., nerve block) provides better and safer pain control because of the presence of more normal tissue conditions at the deposition site. Furthermore, if a large area involving several teeth needs to be treated, the supraperiosteal injection is not suitable because of the need for multiple needle insertions and the necessity of administering large volumes of anesthetic solution.

Table 43.8 and the Evolve Video Resource summarize the criteria pertinent to a supraperiosteal injection and provide tips for success.

Anterior Superior Alveolar Nerve Block

The ASA nerve block is recommended for pain management when treatment is to be done only on the maxillary anterior teeth. Table 43.9

and the Evolve Video Resource describe the criteria specific to the ASA nerve block.

Middle Superior Alveolar Nerve Block

The MSA nerve block is the injection of choice when treatment involves only the premolars. It can also be used if the IO nerve block fails to provide pain control distal to the maxillary canine.

The MSA nerve is present in approximately 28% of the population. When it is missing, the area is innervated by both the PSA and the ASA nerve but predominately by the ASA nerve.[8] Regardless of its presence or absence, this area can be anesthetized easily by means of the MSA technique described in Table 43.10. This table and the Evolve Video Resource provide the guidelines for administering an MSA nerve block and suggestions to ensure success.

Infraorbital Nerve Block

Whereas the ASA and the MSA nerve blocks can be employed by oral healthcare professionals when they are anesthetizing the maxillary anterior and premolar teeth, the IO nerve block is the injection of choice for many when pain control is provided to this area.[1] Human needs should be considered when selecting this injection in regard to treatment planning and the patient's comfort level with the possible effects of local anesthesia on the lower eyelid and nose.[3] The IO nerve block provides both pulpal and facial soft tissue anesthesia of the maxillary central incisor through the premolars in approximately 60% of individuals.[1] One injection of 0.9 to 1.2 mL of solution provides pain control in a relatively large area, effectively minimizing needle penetrations and volume of solution administered. Despite these advantages, this injection is not used as often as indicated because many operators are fearful of injuring the patient's eye. This fear, however, is unfounded, and when the appropriate procedures are followed, this injection is highly effective and safe.

Table 43.11 and the Evolve Video Resource describes the criteria applicable to the IO nerve block and includes directions for locating the IO foramen and directing the needle and anesthetic solution to the nerve.

Posterior Superior Alveolar Nerve Block

The PSA nerve block, employed to anesthetize the maxillary molars, is preferred to supraperiosteal injections because it minimizes both the number of injections required and the volume of anesthetic solution administered. Also, because the anesthetic solution is deposited into an

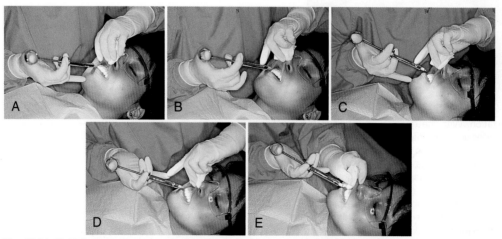

Fig. 43.31 (A–E) Syringe orientation and hand rests and finger rests that may be used for a maxillary supraperiosteal injection and anterior superior alveolar and middle superior alveolar nerve blocks. (Courtesy of F. O'Brien Photography.)

TABLE 43.8 Supraperiosteal Injection

Nerves Anesthetized	Large Terminal Branches of Dental Plexus
Areas anesthetized	Entire region innervated by the large terminal branches of the plexus: Pulp of the tooth Facial or lingual gingiva and periodontium (Fig. T8.1) **Fig. T8.1** Areas anesthetized. (From Fehrenbach MJ, Herring SW. *Illustrated Anatomy of Head and Neck.* 6th ed. Elsevier, 2021.)
Needle gauge and length	25-gauge or 27-gauge short
Operator position	8 or 9 o'clock, right-handed 4 or 3 o'clock, left-handed
Penetration site	Height of the mucobuccal fold above the apex of the target tooth (Fig. T8.2) **Fig. T8.2** Penetration site. (Dental Hygiene Procedures Videos, St Louis, Saunders/Elsevier; 2015.)
Landmarks	Mucobuccal fold Crown of tooth Root contour of tooth
Syringe orientation	Parallel to the long axis of the tooth (Fig. T8.2)
Hand rests	Patient's chin Forefinger or wrist of operator's opposite hand (Fig. 43.31)
Deposition site	Apical region of the target tooth
Penetration depth	Approximately 5 mm or one-quarter of a short needle
Aspiration	Aspirate on arrival and then rotate syringe one-quarter turn and reaspirate
Amount of anesthetic to be deposited	0.6 mL or one-third of a cartridge
Length of time to deposit	Approximately 30 seconds

Potential Problems	Technique Tips
Anesthetic deposition below apex of target tooth, resulting in insufficient pulpal anesthesia	Increase depth of penetration so the needle is at the apical region of the target tooth
Needle too far from bone and solution is deposited into buccal tissue	Redirect needle closer to periosteum
Dense bone may cover apices Most often occurs on permanent maxillary first molars in children because the apex is located under the dense zygomatic bone May occur on central incisors where the apex lies beneath the nose	Administer a nerve block
Pain on insertion with the needle against the periosteum	Withdraw the needle and reinsert farther away (laterally) from the periosteum

TABLE 43.9   Anterior Superior Alveolar (ASA) Nerve Block

Nerves Anesthetized	Anterior Superior Alveolar
Areas anesthetized	Pulpal tissue of the following maxillary teeth unilaterally (Fig. T9.1): Central incisor Lateral incisor Canine Facial tissues and periodontium of these same teeth
	 Fig. T9.1 Areas anesthetized with the anterior superior nerve block and syringe orientation. (Dental Hygiene Procedures Videos, St Louis, 2015, Saunders/Elsevier.)
Needle gauge and length	25-gauge or 27-gauge short
Operator position	8 or 9 o'clock, right-handed 4 or 3 o'clock, left-handed
Penetration site	Height of the mucobuccal fold just mesial to the canine eminence (Fig. T9.2)
	 Fig. T9.2 Penetration site for the anterior superior nerve block. (Dental Hygiene Procedures Videos, St Louis, 2015, Saunders/Elsevier.)
Landmarks	Mucobuccal fold Canine and canine eminence
Syringe orientation	Parallel to the long axis of the canine
Hand rests	Patient's chin Forefinger or wrist of operator's opposite hand (Fig. 43.31)
Deposition site	Apical region of the canine
Penetration depth	Approximately 5 mm or one-quarter of a short needle
Aspiration	Aspirate on arrival and then rotate syringe one-quarter turn and reaspirate
Amount of anesthetic to be deposited	0.9–1.2 mL or one-half to two-thirds of a cartridge
Length of time to deposit	Approximately 30–40 seconds

Potential Problems	Technique Tips
Anesthetic deposition below apex of target tooth, resulting in insufficient pulpal anesthesia	Increase depth of penetration so the needle is at the apical region of the canine
Needle too far from bone and solution is deposited into buccal tissue	Redirect needle closer to periosteum
Pain on insertion with the needle against the periosteum	Withdraw the needle and reinsert farther away (laterally) from the periosteum
Persistent sensitivity at mesial surface of central incisor resulting from cross innervations	Infiltrate contralateral central incisor

TABLE 43.10   Middle Superior Alveolar (MSA) Nerve Block

Nerves Anesthetized	Middle Superior Alveolar
Areas anesthetized	Pulpal tissue of the following maxillary teeth unilaterally (Fig. T10.1): First premolar Second premolar Mesial buccal root of first molar Buccal tissues and periodontium of these same teeth

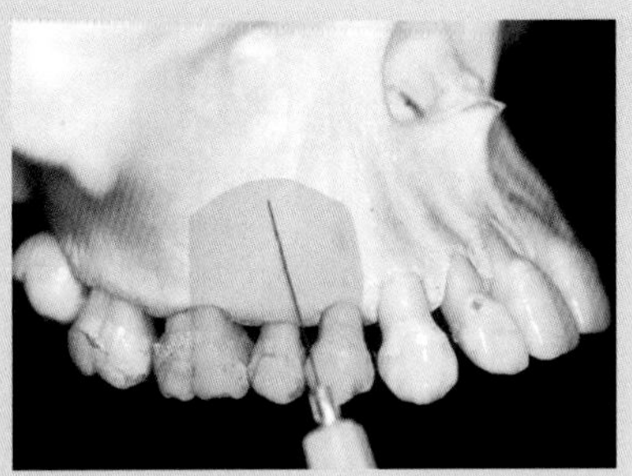

Fig. T10.1 Area anesthetized by a middle superior alveolar nerve block. (Dental Hygiene Procedures Videos, St Louis, 2015, Saunders/Elsevier.)

Needle gauge and length	25-gauge or 27-gauge short
Operator position	8 or 9 o'clock, right-handed 4 or 3 o'clock, left-handed
Penetration site	Height of the mucobuccal fold above second premolar (Fig. T10.2)

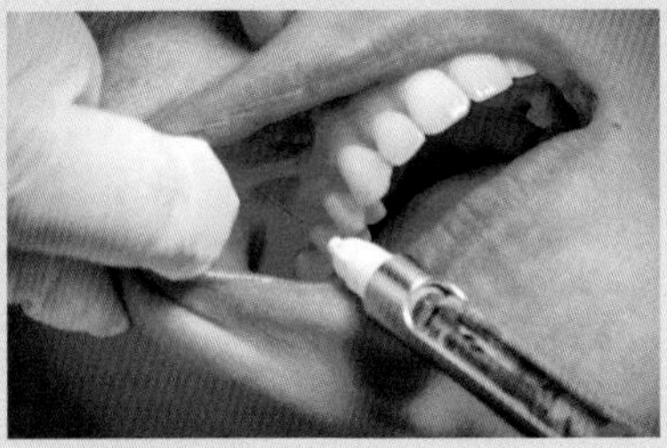

Fig. T10.2 Needle penetration between maxillary premolars and syringe orientation for the MSA nerve block. (From Logothetis D. Local Anesthesia for the Dental Hygienist. 3rd ed. Elsevier; 2022.)

Landmarks	Mucobuccal fold at apex of second premolar
Syringe orientation	Parallel to the long axis of the second premolar (closer to vertical than in the anterior maxilla) (Fig. T10.2)
Hand rests	Patient's chin Patient's cheek Forefinger or wrist of operator's opposite hand (Fig. 43.31)
Deposition site	Above the apical region of the second premolar
Penetration depth	Approximately 5 mm or one-quarter of a short needle
Aspiration	Aspirate on arrival and then rotate syringe one-quarter turn and reaspirate
Amount of anesthetic to be deposited	0.9–1.2 mL or one-half to two-thirds of a cartridge
Length of time to deposit	Approximately 30–40 seconds

Potential Problems	Technique Tips
Anesthetic deposition below apex of target tooth, resulting in insufficient pulpal anesthesia	Increase depth of penetration so the needle is at the apical region of the second premolar
Needle too far from bone, and solution is deposited into buccal tissue	Redirect needle closer to periosteum
Pain on insertion with the needle against the periosteum	Withdraw the needle and reinsert farther away (laterally) from the periosteum
Dense bone of the zygomatic arch at the injection site prevents diffusion of anesthetic solution	Administer an infraorbital block instead of the MSA block
Buccal frenum present at preferred penetration site	Penetrate slightly mesial to the frenum

TABLE 43.11	Infraorbital (IO) Nerve Block
Nerves anesthetized	Infraorbital Anterior superior alveolar Middle superior alveolar Inferior palpebral Lateral nasal Superior labial
Areas anesthetized	Pulpal tissue of the following maxillary teeth unilaterally: Central incisor Lateral incisor Canine First premolar Second premolar Mesial buccal root of first molar Buccal periodontal tissues and bone of these same teeth Lower eyelid Lateral aspect of the nose Upper lip (Fig. T11.1) 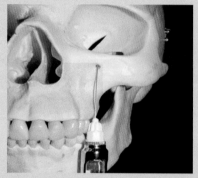 **Fig. T11.1** Area anesthetized and syringe orientation for the infraorbital (IO) block. (Dental Hygiene Procedures Videos, St Louis, 2015, Saunders/Elsevier.)
Needle gauge and length	25-gauge or 27-gauge short or long (for child or small adult, use short)
Operator position	8 or 9 o'clock, right-handed 4 or 3 o'clock, left-handed
Penetration site	Height of the mucobuccal fold above first premolar (Fig. T11.2) 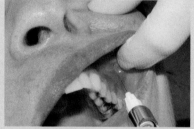 **Fig. T11.2** IO penetration site. (From Logothetis D. *Local Anesthesia for the Dental Hygienist.* 3rd ed. Elsevier; 2022.)

TABLE 43.11   Infraorbital (IO) Nerve Block—cont'd

Landmarks	Infraorbital notch Infraorbital ridge Infraorbital foramen Mucobuccal fold First premolar (Figs. T11.3, T11.4)

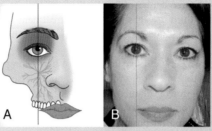

Fig. T11.3 Landmarks for the IO injection. (Dental Hygiene Procedures Videos, St Louis, 2015, Saunders/Elsevier.)

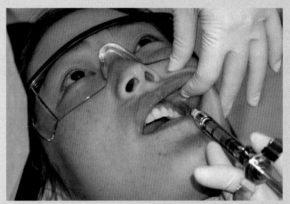

Fig. T11.4 Using a finger over the foramen, lift the lip and hold the tissues in the mucobuccal fold taut. (From F. O'Brien Photography.)

Syringe orientation	Parallel to the long axis of the first premolar; follow the angle (Fig. T11.4)
Hand rests	Patient's chin Patient's cheek Forefinger or wrist of operator's opposite hand (Fig. T11.4)
Deposition site	Upper rim of the infraorbital foramen; the needle should gently contact bone before deposition (Fig. T11.1)
Penetration depth	16 mm or three-quarters of a short needle or one-half of a long needle
Aspiration	Aspirate on arrival and then rotate syringe one-quarter and reaspirate
Amount of anesthetic to be deposited	0.9–1.2 mL or one-half to two-thirds of a cartridge
Length of time to deposit	Approximately 30–40 seconds

Technique Notes

1. Locate the infraorbital foramen. With your forefinger, palpate across the zygomatic arch; the foramen lies at the area of concavity directly below the medial border of the patient's iris when the patient gazes straight ahead.
2. Maintain finger pressure over the foramen throughout the injection and for 1 to 2 minutes after deposition. This will aid in directing the needle to the foramen and assist in directing the anesthetic solution to the foramen.

Potential Problems	Technique Tips
Needle contacting bone below the infraorbital foramen; anesthesia of the lower eyelid, nose, or upper lip, with little or no pulpal anesthesia	Keep needle in line with the infraorbital foramen during penetration; line the syringe up with your finger over the foramen

area of soft tissue with no bony landmarks (hence no bone contact), it is a comfortable injection for the patient (Table 43.12).

Complete pulpal anesthesia is obtained in the first, second, and third molars (first molar in at least 72% of persons).[1,4] Dissection studies reveal, however, that the MSA nerve, when present, may supply sensory innervation to the mesiobuccal root of the first molar, therefore necessitating a supraperiosteal injection, an MSA nerve block, or an IO nerve block to anesthetize the remainder of this tooth. Furthermore, if access is difficult or if the third molar is missing and treatment is limited to only the first and second molars, supraperiosteal injections may be substituted.

Other considerations are safety and needle length. When a long 25-gauge needle is used for this injection, problems have been associated with the needle length due to the increased risk of hematoma formation. There are no anatomic safety features to prevent inadvertently inserting the needle too far posteriorly into the pterygoid plexus of veins and the facial artery, thereby causing a hematoma. Therefore, to minimize the risk of hematoma formation after the PSA nerve block, a short 25-gauge or 27-gauge needle is recommended. Although depth of insertion with the long needle is 16 mm, or one-half of its length, the short needle is inserted three-fourths of

its length. Thus, the risk of overinsertion and hematoma formation decreases when a short needle is used. Regardless of the needle length used, multiple aspirations and slow anesthetic deposition are imperative to ensure a safe injection.

Table 43.12 and the Evolve Video Resource provide the essential criteria for the PSA nerve block. Of particular significance to this injection is the syringe orientation of 45 degrees to the maxillary occlusal plane and 45 degrees to the midsagittal plane. This angulation, maintained throughout the injection, advances the needle around the maxillary tuberosity to reach the deposition site.

INJECTION TECHNIQUES FOR THE PALATAL HARD AND SOFT TISSUES

When dental hygiene care involves the hard and soft tissues of the palate, such as during therapeutic scaling, root planing, and soft tissue curettage procedures, anesthesia of the palatal tissue may be needed. Unfortunately, for many patients these injections are traumatic, but palatal injections need not be painful if appropriate techniques are followed. Especially important to facilitate comfort during palatal injections are the following tasks:

TABLE 43.12	Posterior Superior Alveolar (PSA) Nerve Block	
Nerves Anesthetized	**Posterior Superior Alveolar**	
Areas anesthetized	Pulpal tissue of the following maxillary teeth unilaterally: First molar distal buccal root Second molar Third molar Buccal tissues and periodontium of these same teeth (Fig. T12.1) **Fig. T12.1** Areas anesthetized and needle at the target area for a posterior superior alveolar nerve block. (Dental Hygiene Procedures Videos, St Louis, 2015, Saunders/Elsevier.)	
Needle gauge and length	25-gauge or 27-gauge short	
Operator position	8 or 9 o'clock, right-handed 4 or 3 o'clock, left-handed	
Penetration site	Height of the mucobuccal fold posterior and superior to the second molar (Fig. T12.2) **Fig. T12.2** Penetration site for the PSA. (Dental Hygiene Procedures Videos, St Louis, 2015, Saunders/Elsevier.)	
Landmarks	Mucobuccal fold Maxillary tuberosity Maxillary occlusal plane Midsagittal plane Maxillary molars (Fig. T12.1)	

TABLE 43.12   Posterior Superior Alveolar (PSA) Nerve Block—cont'd

Nerves Anesthetized	Posterior Superior Alveolar
Syringe orientation	45° to the maxillary occlusal plane and 45° to the midsagittal plane (Fig. T12.3A–D)

Fig. T12.3 (A) Forty-five degrees to the maxillary occlusal plane. (B) Forty-five degrees to the midsagittal plane. (C) Orientation of syringe and hand rest for the left PSA. (D) Orientation of syringe and hand rest for right PSA. (Dental Hygiene Procedures Videos, St Louis, 2015, Saunders/Elsevier. Courtesy of F. O'Brian Photography.)

Hand rests	Forefinger or thumb of opposite hand as it retracts patient's buccal tissue (Fig. T12.3C right side and Fig. T12.3D left side)
Deposition site	Posterior and superior to the posterior border of the maxilla at the PSA nerve foramina (Fig. T12.1)
Penetration depth	16 mm or three-quarters of a short needle
Aspiration*	Aspirate on arrival; rotate syringe one-quarter turn toward operator; reaspirate; rotate back one-quarter to original plane; aspirate
Amount of anesthetic to be deposited	0.9–1.8 mL or one-half to one cartridge
Length of time to deposit	Approximately 30–60 seconds

Technique Notes

Owing to the high vascularity of the deposition site for the PSA, a triple aspiration is recommended to ensure that the needle bevel is not against the interior wall of a vessel, thus providing a false-negative aspiration (see Step 20 in Procedure 43.4). To aspirate in multiple planes, perform a single aspiration as usual, then rotate the body of the syringe toward you slightly, reaspirate, then rotate the body of the syringe back to the original position and perform a final aspiration. If all three aspiration tests are negative, it is safe to administer the anesthetic solution. After the initial triple aspiration, it is recommended to do a single aspiration after each quarter of the cartridge has been deposited.

Potential Problems	Technique Tips
Bone is contacted when the angle of needle is too great in reference to the midsagittal plane	Withdraw the needle and bring the syringe closer to the midline
Mandibular anesthesia: the mandibular division of the trigeminal nerve is lateral to the PSA nerves	Review landmarks and syringe orientation so as not to deposit lateral to the PSA nerves

- Provide pressure anesthesia with a cotton swab at the penetration site both before (see Fig. T13.2A in Table 43.13) and during (see Fig. T13.2B in Table 43.13) the injection because topical anesthetics have limited value on keratinized tissues such as the palate.
- Deposit the solution slowly to avoid tearing the palatal tissue, which is dense and firmly attached to the bone.
- Be confident that you, the dental hygienist, will administer the injection with minimal patient discomfort.
- Use a triple injection technique whenever possible when administering the NP nerve block to minimize patient discomfort.

Injection techniques used to anesthetize the palatal hard and soft tissues are the GP, NP, and AMSA.

Greater Palatine Nerve Block

The GP nerve block is used to anesthetize the hard and soft palatal tissues overlying the molars and premolars; no pulpal anesthesia is obtained (see Fig. T13.1 in Table 43.13). This nerve block provides anesthesia to a large area, thereby minimizing the number of needle penetrations and total amount of anesthetic solution needed; however, the GP nerve can be blocked at any point after it emerges from the foramen and passes anteriorly between the hard and soft tissues. As a result, anesthesia is obtained only anterior to the injection site. For example, if treatment is limited to the first molar and premolars, the injection site should be slightly posterior to the first molar along the GP nerve path. This practice ensures that the areas to be treated are

TABLE 43.13   Greater Palatine (GP) Nerve Block

Nerves Anesthetized	Greater Palatine
Areas anesthetized	Hard palate and overlying soft tissue unilaterally from the maxillary third molar to the first premolar (Fig. T13.1)

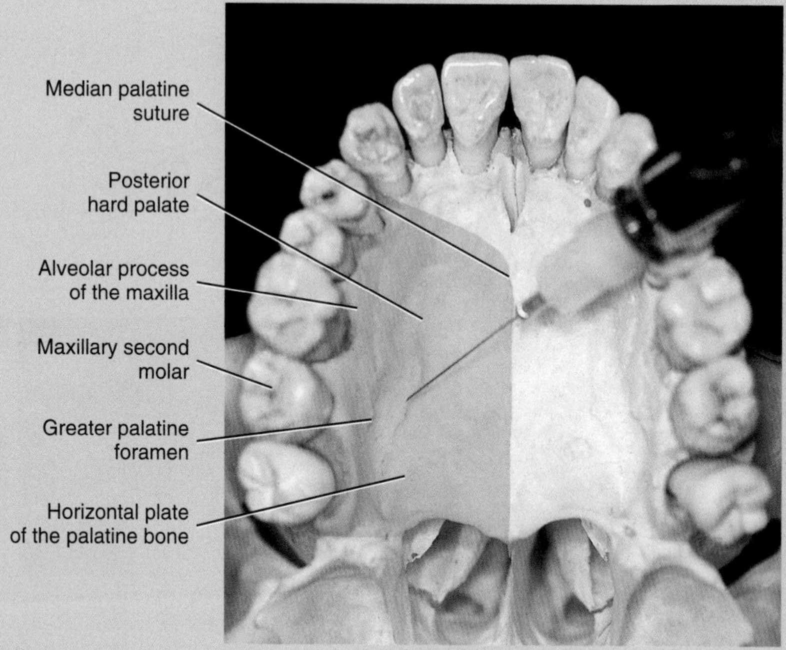

- Median palatine suture
- Posterior hard palate
- Alveolar process of the maxilla
- Maxillary second molar
- Greater palatine foramen
- Horizontal plate of the palatine bone

Fig. T13.1 Area anesthetized and deposition site with the greater palatine nerve block. (Courtesy of Margaret J. Fehrenbach, RDH, MS.)

Needle gauge and length	25-gauge or 27-gauge short
Operator position	8 or 9 o'clock, right-handed 4 or 3 o'clock, left-handed
Penetration site	Just anterior to the greater palatine foramen (Fig. T13.2A)

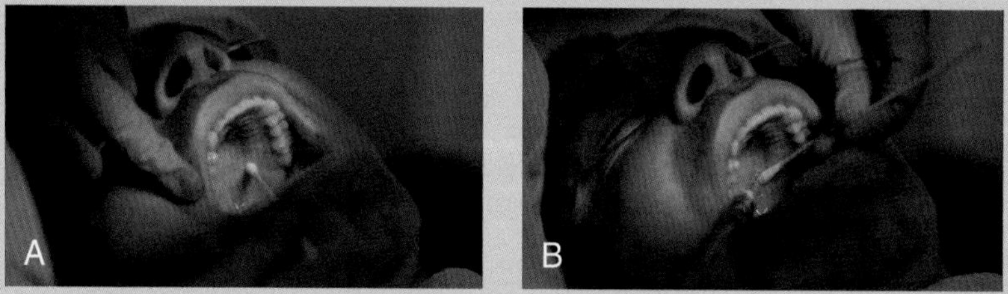

Fig. T13.2 (A) A cotton swab is pressed against the hard palate at the junction of the maxillary alveolar process and palatal bone. (B) Penetration site is slightly anterior to the cotton tip applicator. The barrel of the syringe is stabilized by the corner of the mouth and the teeth. (From Dental Hygiene Procedures Videos, Saunders; 2015.)

Landmarks	Greater palatine foramen Junction of alveolar process and palatine bone Maxillary second molar
Syringe orientation	Approaches from opposite the side being injected with the needle at a right angle to the penetration site (Figs. T13.2B, T13.3)

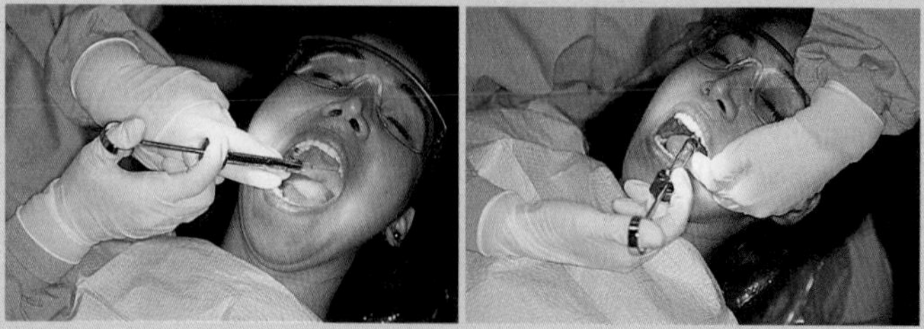

Fig. T13.3 Hand rests for a greater palatine nerve block. (Courtesy of F. O'Brien Photography.)

TABLE 43.13 Greater Palatine (GP) Nerve Block—cont'd

Nerves Anesthetized	Greater Palatine
Hand rests	Back of opposite hand Corner of patient's mouth (Fig. T13.3)
Deposition site	Just anterior to the greater palatine nerve foramen (Fig. T13.1)
Penetration depth	Approximately 4–5 mm or until gentle contact with bone
Aspiration	Aspirate on arrival and then rotate syringe one-quarter and reaspirate
Amount of anesthetic to be deposited	0.45mL-0.6mL or one quarter to one third of a cartridge; determine by development of blanching of palatal tissues
Length of time to deposit	Approximately 20–30 seconds

Technique Notes

1. To locate the greater palatine foramen, palpate the posterior palate with a cotton-tipped applicator or your forefinger at the junction of the hard palate and the alveolar process near the second molar until a depression is felt.
2. Topical anesthetics have very limited action on keratinized tissue such as the palate.
   To ensure patient comfort, pressure anesthesia with a cotton-tipped applicator is recommended for a minimum of 1 minute before injection and throughout deposition (Fig. 13.2A)

Potential Problems	Technique Tips
Deposition of the anesthetic solution too far anterior of the foramen, resulting in inadequate anesthesia	Move the needle posteriorly
Inadequate anesthesia of the first molar resulting from cross innervation from the nasopalatine nerve	Infiltrate palate in area of first molar

anesthetized, but that the posterior region of the palate is not unnecessarily anesthetized.

Table 43.13 and Evolve Video Resources provide the criteria pertinent to the administration of a GP nerve block and include suggestions for locating the GP foramen and maximizing patient comfort.

Nasopalatine Nerve Block

The NP nerve block anesthetizes the palatal hard and soft tissues from canine to canine. As with the GP nerve block, a minimal number of needle penetrations and a small amount of anesthetic solution are needed to anesthetize a wide area. Because the soft tissue is dense, firmly attached to the bone, and very sensitive, however, this nerve block is potentially the most uncomfortable of all the injections unless the protocol for an atraumatic injection is closely followed.

Two techniques are available for giving this injection. The first involves only one needle penetration on the lateral side of the incisive papilla (see Fig. T14.2C in Table 43.14). The second technique includes giving two or three sequential injections, one supraperiosteal injection between the maxillary central incisors, followed by a second penetration into the papilla between the maxillary central incisors. In some cases, these two injections provide sufficient pain control for dental hygiene care. If not, an injection is made into the partially anesthetized palatal tissues on the lateral side of the incisive papilla to complete the NP nerve block (see Fig. T14.3A–C in Table 43.14).

Each approach is acceptable, and dental hygienists should select the procedure they feel most comfortable with and that provides the most atraumatic injection possible for the patient. Table 43.14 and Evolve Video Resource provide the criteria pertinent to the administration of an NP nerve block.

Anterior Middle Superior Alveolar Nerve Block

The AMSA is an injection that involves innervation of several nerves: the ASA, MSA, GP, and NP nerves.[3] Therefore, dental hygienists may consider this block when desiring to anesthetize a large area when treating upper quadrants. The AMSA injection will affect the pulps of the maxillary anterior teeth and premolars and their associated facial

tissues, periodontium, and palatal soft tissues to the midline of the palate. This injection should also affect the palatal gingiva of the molars, but not the pulps.[8] The advantage of the AMSA is that one injection takes the place of administering four separate ASA, MSA, NP, and GP injections. In addition, the upper lip and upper face are not anesthetized, which are important factors when assessing the patient's smile line for cosmetic dentistry procedures. It is important to note, however, in order to have complete anesthesia of an upper quadrant, the dental hygienist will also need to perform the PSA injection to anesthetize the pulps and buccal tissues of the molars and the associated periodontium.

The effectiveness of the AMSA varies. Studies show that a successful method of performing this block is to use a C-CLAD.[8] Clinicians may have success using a manual syringe and the recommended 27-gauge short needle; however, use of the standard syringe and needle may challenge the clinician to adequately penetrate the thicker tissue lining of the hard palate, which is necessary for anesthetic diffusion through the pores of the bony hard palate (see Fig. T15.3 in Table 43.15).[8] As the volume of anesthetic solution increases, so does the risk of ischemia (tissue sloughing). In addition, the duration and hemostatic control of the anesthetic is not always reliable.[3] Therefore, if left without a computer-controlled device, the clinician should question whether it is better to use a standard syringe to perform the AMSA or choose to administer traditional nerve blocks. The latter involve more injections but are more clinically effective because they provide longer, deeper levels of anesthesia and hemostatic control. Table 43.15 provides the essential criteria for the AMSA nerve block.

MANDIBULAR ANESTHESIA INJECTION TECHNIQUES

The dense bone of the mandible that covers the apices of the teeth eliminates the possibility of supraperiosteal injections into the posterior teeth. In addition, because of mandibular bone density, anesthetic solution must be deposited within 1 mm of the target nerve to obtain pulpal anesthesia.

TABLE 43.14 Nasopalatine (NP) Nerve Block

Nerves Anesthetized	Nasopalatine
Areas anesthetized	Hard palate and overlying soft tissue bilaterally from the maxillary canine to canine (Fig. T14.1)

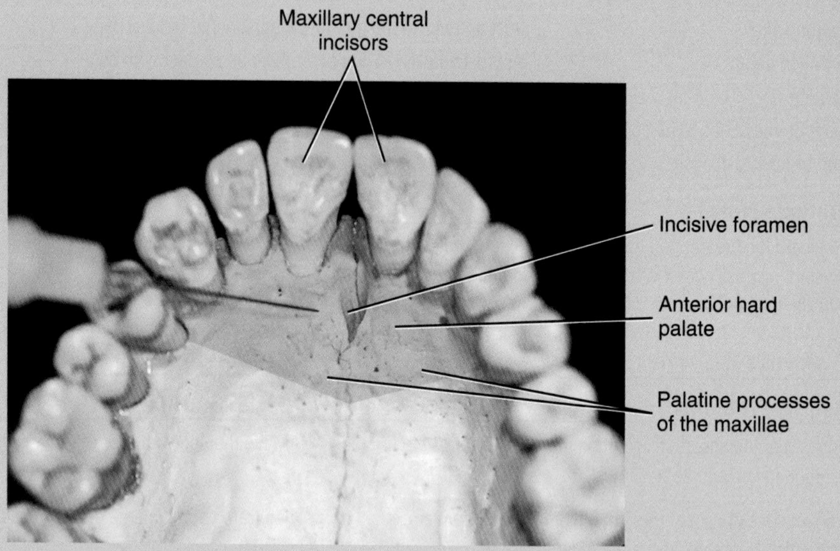

Fig. T14.1 Area anesthetized and deposition site for the nasopalatine nerve block. (Courtesy of Margaret J. Fehrenbach, RDH, MS.)

Needle gauge and length	25-gauge or 27-gauge short
Operator position	8 or 9 o'clock, right-handed 4 or 3 o'clock, left-handed
Penetration site	Just lateral to posterior portion of the incisive papilla (Fig. T14.2A–B)

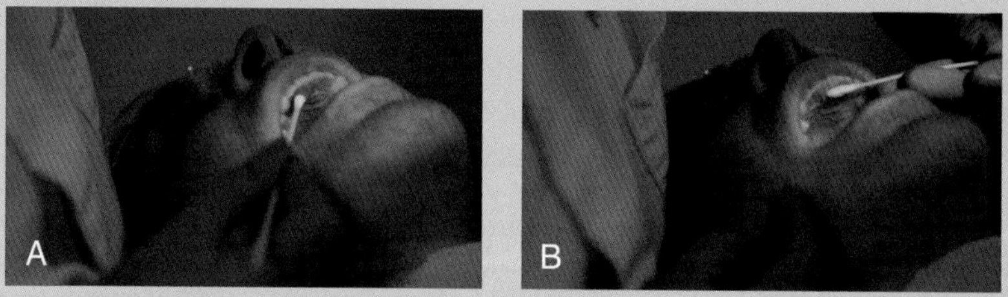

Fig. T14.2 (A) Topical application for 1 to 2 minutes at the penetration site. (B) Pressure anesthesia for 1 to 2 minutes with cotton tip applicator. Confirm presence of blanching. (Dental Hygiene Procedures Videos, St Louis, 2015, Saunders/Elsevier.)

Landmarks	Central incisors Incisive papilla
Syringe orientation	Approaches from canine or premolar region at a 45° angle to the incisive papilla (Fig. T14.3D)
Hand rests	Finger of opposite hand Syringe can be stabilized against the corner of the patient's mouth (Fig. T14.3D)
Deposition site	Incisive foramen beneath incisive papilla (Fig. T14.1)
Penetration depth	Approximately 4–5 mm or until gentle contact with bone
Aspiration	Aspirate on arrival and then rotate syringe one-quarter turn and reaspirate
Amount of anesthetic to be deposited	0.45 mL, or one-quarter of a cartridge; determine by development of blanching of palatal tissues
Length of time to deposit	Approximately 20–30 seconds

Technique Notes

1. Topical anesthetics have very limited action on keratinized tissue such as the palate. To ensure patient comfort, pressure anesthesia with a cotton-tipped applicator is recommended for a minimum of 1 minute before injection and throughout deposition (Figs. T14.2A–B).

TABLE 43.14 Nasopalatine (NP) Nerve Block—cont'd

Nerves Anesthetized	Nasopalatine

2. For greatest patient comfort, the nasopalatine nerve block is best administered in a triple injection sequence as follows: infiltration of a central incisor, papillary infiltration of teeth 8 and 9, and then the nasopalatine. Each injection anesthetizes the area of the subsequent injection, resulting in an atraumatic procedure for the patient (Figs. T14.3A–D).

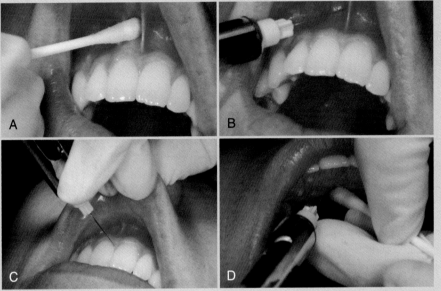

Fig. T14.3 (A) Topical anesthetic is applied to mucosa of the frenum. (B) First injection into the labial frenum. (C) Use a finger of the opposite hand to stabilize the syringe during the second injection into the intended papilla between the central incisors. (D) Pressure is maintained until the deposition of solution is completed. Needle penetration is just lateral to the incisive papilla. (From Malamed SF. *Handbook of Local Anesthesia.* 7th ed. Elsevier; 2020.)

Potential Problems	Technique Tips
Unilateral anesthesia due to deposition of anesthetic solution to one side of incisive foramen	Reinsert the needle until it is directly over the incisive foramen
Inadequate anesthesia of canine or first premolar due to cross innervation from the greater palatine nerve	Infiltrate the palate at the area of the canine or first premolar

TABLE 43.15 Anterior Middle Superior Alveolar Nerve Block (AMSA)

Nerves anesthetized	Anterior superior alveolar Middle superior alveolar Nasopalatine Greater palatine
Area anesthetized	Pulpal tissue of the following maxillary teeth unilaterally: Central incisor Lateral incisor Canine First premolar Second premolar Mesial root of the first molar Gingival tissue of the following maxillary area unilaterally: Buccal gingiva of the above teeth Palatal gingiva from the midline to the free gingival margin on the above teeth, including the gingiva of the molars (Fig. T15.1)

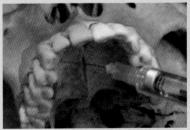

Fig. T15.1 Areas anesthetized, syringe orientation, and deposition site for the AMSA injection. (From Fehrenbach MJ, Herring SW. *Illustrated Anatomy of the Head and Neck.* 6th ed. Elsevier; 2021.)

Continued

TABLE 43.15   Anterior Middle Superior Alveolar Nerve Block (AMSA)—cont'd

Needle gauge and length	C-CLAD with 30-gauge short needle or a 27-gauge short needle
Operator position	8 or 9 o'clock, right-handed 4 or 3 o'clock, left-handed
Penetration site	The halfway point of an imaginary line on a horizontal plane from the interproximal premolar contact area and the midline of the hard palate (Fig. T15.2A)

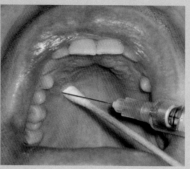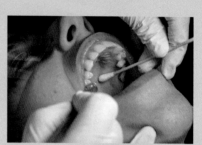

Fig. T15.2 (A) Penetration site for the right AMSA injection. (B) Syringe orientation and hand rest for left AMSA. (From Logothetis D. *Local Anesthesia for the Dental Hygienist*. 3rd ed. Elsevier; 2022.)

Landmarks	Midpalatal suture Contact point between premolars
Syringe orientation	45° angle to the palate (Fig. T15.2A)
Hand rests	Pinky finger on patient's chin (Fig. T15.2B) *or* Syringe barrel resting on index finger of the other hand holding the cotton tip applicator *or* Corner of mouth and teeth in the area (Fig. T15.2B)
Deposition site	Bony surface of the palate or pores in the maxilla of the hard palate (Fig. T15.3)

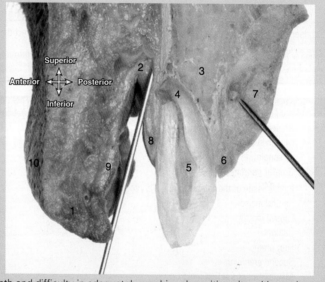

Fig. T15.3 Depicts depth and difficulty in adequately reaching deposition site with regular needle. The thickness of the palatal tissue presents an obstacle to reliable effectiveness of anesthesia, and thus the C-CLAD is recommended and should be considered the standard of care. (From Logan BM, Reynold PA, Hutching RT. *McMinn's Color Atlas of Head and Neck Anatomy*. 4th ed. London: Elsevier; 2010.)

Penetration depth	Approximately 4–7 mm or until gentle contact with bone
Aspiration	Aspirate on arrival and then rotate syringe one-quarter turn and reaspirate
Amount of anesthetic to be deposited	1.4–1.8 mL or until blanching of palatal tissue occurs
Length of time to deposit	Approximately 0.5 mL/min (C-CLAD approximately 4 minutes)

TABLE 43.15   Anterior Middle Superior Alveolar Nerve Block (AMSA)—cont'd

Potential Problems	Technique Tips
Palatal ulcer due to rapid, excessive administration of vasoconstrictor Dense tissue may cause the solution to squirt back into the mouth, resulting in unpleasant taste Unreliable duration and hemostatic control of the anesthetic	For maximum patient effectiveness and comfort, the use of the C-CLAD is preferred when administering this injection Consider alternative injections such as the ASA, MSA, GP, and NP

The injection techniques available to anesthetize the mandibular teeth and hard and soft tissues include the IANB, buccal, mental, incisive, and Gow-Gates (GG) nerve blocks. Of these, only the IANB, GG, and incisive nerve blocks cause pulpal anesthesia.

Inferior Alveolar Nerve Block

The IANB is often employed when dental hygiene care involves the mandible. The biggest advantage is that one penetration anesthetizes the entire quadrant, with the exception of the facial soft tissue over the molars. The disadvantage, however, may be due to the success rate of the IANB being slightly lower (15% to 20%) than that of other injections.[1,3] Reasons for lack of success are as follows:

- The anatomic variations with regard to the height of the mandibular foramen on the medial side of the ramus
- Accessory innervation by means of the mylohyoid nerve or a bifid inferior alveolar nerve
- The considerable depth of soft tissue penetration needed to reach the nerve

In addition, the IANB has the highest rate of positive aspiration of all the intraoral injections.[1] Table 43.16 describes the criteria essential for administering the IANB. It is important to carefully follow the guidelines regarding the landmarks for the penetration and deposition sites to ensure a successful injection and minimize or eliminate complications. To determine the height of the injection, place the index finger or thumb of the nondominant hand in the coronoid notch (see Fig. T16.3 in Table 43.16). An imaginary line extends posteriorly from the fingertip in the coronoid notch to the deepest part of the pterygomandibular raphe, determining the height of injection. This imaginary line should be parallel with the occlusal plane of the mandibular molar teeth and usually lies 6 to 10 mm above the occlusal plane (see Fig. T16.3B in Table 43.16).

To locate the pterygomandibular triangle, roll the index finger or thumb of your nondominant hand from the coronoid notch to locate the internal oblique ridge (see Fig. T16.3A–B in Table 43.16). The point of needle penetration is between the internal oblique ridge and the pterygomandibular raphe in the pterygomandibular triangle. The syringe barrel is placed in the corner of the mouth on the contralateral side over the premolars (see Fig. T16.5 in Table 43.16).

Appropriate care planning is important when the mandible is anesthetized. Bilateral IANBs should be avoided. Such procedures produce anesthesia of the patient's entire tongue and lingual soft tissues, resulting in an inability to swallow and enunciate, and a lack of sensation. Thus, anesthetizing the entire mandible creates a high risk of patient self-injury to the soft tissues and is not recommended. The optimal care plan is to anesthetize only the right side or only the left side at one appointment. Another alternative is to administer the IANB to the side that requires the most treatment (particularly involving lingual tissue)

or has the greatest number of teeth and administer the incisive nerve block (see below) on the opposite side. Because the incisive nerve block does not provide pain control to the lingual tissues, a lingual nerve block or lingual intraseptals may be given, if necessary. The deliberate deposition of anesthetic solution to anesthetize the lingual nerve is unnecessary because solution deposited for the IANB diffuses and anesthetizes the lingual nerve; however, a separate technique for a lingual nerve block is described in the Technique Notes of Table 43.16 in the event that deliberate anesthetic solution deposition of the lingual tissue is needed. Whenever a bifid inferior alveolar nerve exists, a second mandibular foramen located more inferiorly may present a problem resulting in insufficient anesthesia. Injecting solution below the normal landmark can correct the situation. See Box 43.7 for patient education and communication tips regarding what to expect with local anesthesia and postoperative care.

Buccal Nerve Block

The buccal nerve block, which anesthetizes the long buccal sensory nerve, provides pain control to the soft tissues buccal to the mandibular molars. This injection, along with the IA and lingual nerve blocks, anesthetizes the entire quadrant in which it is given. If dental hygiene care involves manipulation of the buccal tissues of the molars, such as therapeutic scaling, root planing, and soft tissue curettage, this injection is indicated. If treatment does not include these tissues, however, the dental hygienist may simply forgo this injection. Unlike the other injections needed to anesthetize the mandible, the buccal nerve block is easy to administer (see Fig. T17.2 in Table 43.17) and has a high success rate. Table 43.17 and the Evolve Video Resource describe technique for the buccal nerve block.

Mental Nerve Block and Incisive Nerve Block

The procedures for these two nerve blocks are essentially the same except for one additional step of applying gentle pressure (discussed below) for the incisive nerve block. Both nerve blocks are terminal branches of the inferior alveolar nerve and are located at the mental foramen at or near the premolar apices.

The mental nerve exits the mental foramen and innervates the facial soft tissues anterior to the foramen, the lower lip, and the chin on the side of the injection. Because of the easy access to the anatomic landmarks, the mental nerve block is simple to administer, has a high success rate, and is usually atraumatic (see Fig. T18.2 in Table 43.18). Although this injection has limited application in restorative dentistry, it may be used more commonly by dental hygienists doing gingival curettage and debridement in the anterior portion of the mandible. The mental nerve block does not provide pain control to the lingual tissues, so lingual infiltrations may be needed. Local infiltrations can be

TABLE 43.16   Inferior Alveolar Nerve Block (IANB)

Nerves anesthetized	Inferior alveolar Incisive Mental Lingual
Areas anesthetized	Mandibular teeth unilaterally to midline Body of mandible Inferior portion of the ramus Facial tissue anterior to the first molar Lower lip to midline All lingual gingival tissue unilaterally to midline Anterior two-thirds of the tongue unilaterally to midline Floor of the mouth unilaterally (Fig. T16.1) 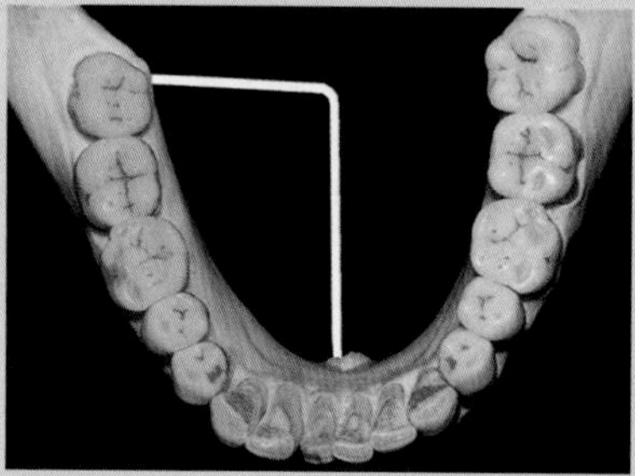

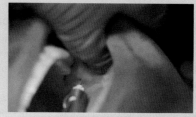

Fig. T16.1 Areas anesthetized for the inferior alveolar and lingual. (Dental Hygiene Procedures Videos, St Louis, 2015, Saunders/Elsevier.)

Needle gauge and length	25-gauge or 27-gauge long
Operator position	8 or 9 o'clock, right-handed 4 or 3 o'clock, left-handed
Penetration site	Middle of the pterygomandibular triangle (formed by the pterygomandibular raphe medially and the internal oblique ridge laterally) at the height of the coronoid notch, 6–10 mm above the mandibular occlusal plane (Fig. T16.2)

Fig. T16.2 Penetration site for the IA and lingual. (Dental Hygiene Procedures Videos, St Louis, 2015, Saunders/Elsevier.)

Landmarks	Anterior border of the ramus External oblique ridge Coronoid notch Internal oblique ridge Pterygomandibular raphe (fold) Pterygomandibular triangle Mandibular foramen Lingula Mandibular occlusal plane (Figs. T16.3A–B) 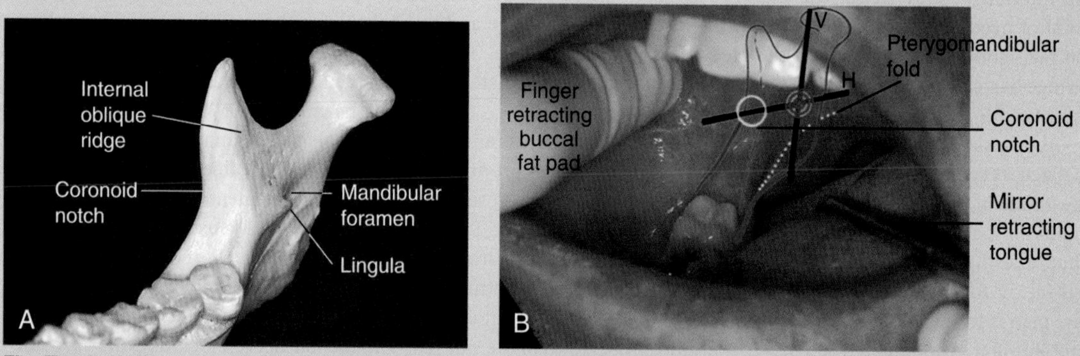

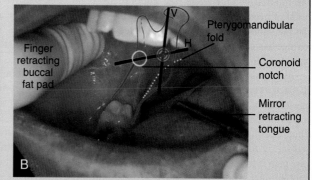

Fig. T16.3 (A–B) Landmarks on the mandible for the IANB. ([B] Dental Hygiene Procedures Videos, St Louis, 2015, Saunders/Elsevier.)

TABLE 43.16   Inferior Alveolar Nerve Block (IANB)—cont'd

Syringe orientation	Approaches from contralateral premolar area, parallel to the occlusal plane (Fig. T16.4)

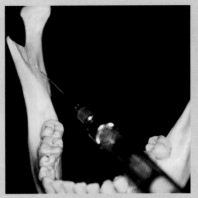

Fig. T16.4 Syringe orientation for the IANB. (Dental Hygiene Procedures Videos, St Louis, 2015, Saunders/Elsevier.)

Hand rests	Small finger on patient's chin (Fig. T16.5)

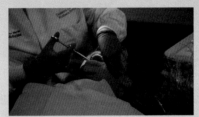

Fig. T16.5 Hand rests for the IANB. (Dental Hygiene Procedures Videos, St Louis, 2015, Saunders/Elsevier.)

Deposition site	Superior to the mandibular foramen
Penetration depth	Approximately 20–25 mm or two-thirds to three-quarters of long needle (withdraw 1 mm before deposition) until bone is gently contacted (Fig. T16.2)
Aspiration*	Aspirate on arrival; rotate syringe one-quarter turn toward operator; reaspirate; rotate back one-quarter turn to original plane; aspirate
Amount of anesthetic to be deposited	1.5 mL or three-quarters of a cartridge (save 0.3 mL or one-eighth of cartridge for the buccal nerve block)
Length of time to deposit	60–90 seconds

Technique Notes

1. To locate the pterygomandibular triangle, place your thumb or index finger on the greatest depression on the anterior border of the ramus; this is the coronoid notch. Roll your finger medially to locate the internal oblique ridge. The point of penetration is between the internal oblique ridge and the pterygomandibular raphe (in the pterygomandibular triangle), 6–10 mm above the mandibular occlusal plane (Figs. T16.3A–B and T16.4). While inserting, advancing, and withdrawing the needle, it is important to place the thumb or index finger on the internal oblique ridge and at the same time, grasp the posterior border of the mandible with the remainder of your hand. This technique provides stabilization and control in the event the patient moves unexpectedly during the procedure.

2. *Owing to the high vascularity of the deposition site for the IANB, a triple aspiration is recommended to ensure that the needle bevel is not against the interior wall of a vessel, thus providing a false-negative aspiration (see Step 20 in Procedure 43.4). To aspirate in multiple planes, perform a single aspiration as usual, rotate the body of the syringe toward you slightly and reaspirate, then rotate the body of the syringe back to the original position and perform a final aspiration. If all three aspiration tests are negative, it is safe to administer the anesthetic solution. After the initial triple aspiration, it is recommended to do a single aspiration after each quarter of the cartridge has been deposited.

3. If bone is contacted prematurely, before half of the needle length has entered the tissues, it is likely that the needle is too far anterior and has contacted the lingula, which covers the mandibular foramen (Fig. T16.6A). To correct, withdraw the needle halfway but do not remove from the tissues. Bring the body of the syringe over the mandibular anterior teeth and reinsert past the depth previously penetrated. Redirect the body of the syringe back over the contralateral premolars and continue to penetrate until bone is contacted (Fig. T16.6B).

4. If bone is not contacted and the penetration depth is nearing the hub of the needle, it is likely that the needle is too far posterior (Fig. T16.7A). To correct, withdraw the needle halfway but do not remove it from the tissues. Redirect the syringe further over the contralateral molars and continue insertion until bone is contacted (Fig. T16.7B).

Continued

TABLE 43.16 Inferior Alveolar Nerve Block (IANB)—cont'd

5. In the rare event that lingual soft tissue anesthesia is inadequate, a separate lingual nerve block injection can be administered. Insert the needle one-third to one-half its length at the IANB penetration site, aspirate, and deposit one-quarter to one-third of a cartridge (0.45 mL) for 10–15 seconds to anesthetize the lingual nerve.

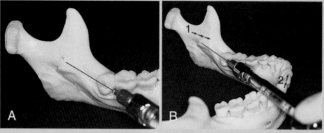

Fig. T16.6 (A) Premature bone contact on the lingula. (B) Path of syringe orientation to correct for premature contact of bone.

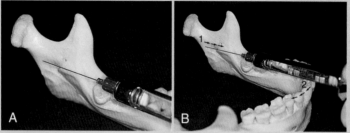

Fig. T16.7 (A) The needle is too far posterior; no bone is contacted. (B) Path of syringe orientation to correct needle position.

Potential Problems	Technique Tips
Deposition of anesthetic below the mandibular foramen	Reinject at a higher penetration site
Deposition of anesthetic too far anterior on the ramus, indicated by early bone contact, with less than one-half the needle length inserted	See Technique Note 3
Radiographic detection of bifid IA nerve or mylohyoid innervation, resulting in incomplete pulpal anesthesia of the molars (often mesial root of the first molar) or incisors. It is theorized that the mylohyoid nerve, which is not blocked by the IA, provides accessory innervations to these areas.	For bifid IA nerve, deposit volume of solution inferior to normal IANB landmark. For mylohyoid nerve, use a 27-gauge long needle, direct syringe from opposite corner of mouth, and penetrate the apical region of the tooth just distal to the unanesthetized tooth. Advance 3–5 mm and deposit 0.6 mL or one-third of a cartridge over 20 seconds (Fig. T16.8).

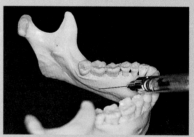

Fig. T16.8 Direct the needle tip below the apical region of the tooth immediately posterior to the tooth in question.

Incomplete anesthesia of the central or lateral incisors. May be due to cross innervation from the opposite side inferior alveolar nerve.	Using a 27-gauge short needle, infiltrate the mucobuccal fold and advance to the apical region of the unanesthetized tooth. Deposit 0.6 mL or one-third of a cartridge over 20 seconds (Fig. T16.9).

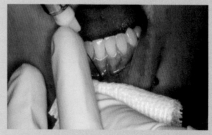

Fig. T16.9 Local infiltration of the mandibular incisors.

Patient Education Example: Informing patient about expected inferior alveolar nerve block anesthetic sensations and postoperative instructions.

"Christopher, it is important that you know ahead of time what to expect after you have received the local anesthetic. Typically, the lower lip is the first area to tingle, and then you may notice half of your tongue will begin to feel numb. These are good signs that the anesthetic is taking effect. Before I start scaling, I will test your teeth to make sure they are numb as well. You can expect the numbness to last approximately 1 to 3 hours after the appointment, but this varies from patient to patient (scenario assumes 1 cartridge of lidocaine with 2% + epinephrine 1 : 100,000 is used). When we are done, please avoid eating and drinking until all the feeling in your mouth returns to normal. If you need to eat or drink, carefully chew on the side that is not numb and only drink room-temperature beverages. This will help you prevent any mouth injuries."

accomplished readily by inserting a 27-gauge short needle through the interdental papilla on both the mesial and distal aspects on the tooth being treated. Because the buccal soft tissues are already anesthetized, the needle penetration is atraumatic.

The incisive nerve innervates the teeth anterior to the foramen. The incisive nerve block may be the injection of choice in instances where treatment is targeted to the lower anterior teeth including bicuspids; therefore, it does not need to be a separate injection if the treatment plan necessitates an IANB injection. It is not necessary to enter into the mental foramen with the needle to affect the incisive nerve. Anesthesia is obtained easily and safely by depositing the solution outside the foramen and then using the additional step of applying pressure over the site to direct the anesthetic into the foramen, thus anesthetizing the teeth in this area.

Table 43.18 and the Evolve Video Resource present the criteria necessary for administration of both nerve blocks and suggestions for locating the mental foramen.

TABLE 43.17 Buccal Nerve Block (Long Buccal)

Nerves anesthetized	Buccal
Areas anesthetized	Soft tissues buccal to the mandibular molars unilaterally (Fig. T17.1)

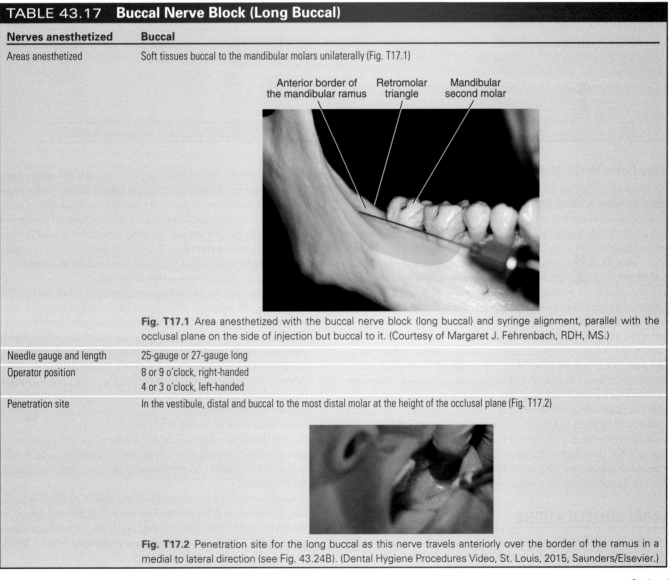

Fig. T17.1 Area anesthetized with the buccal nerve block (long buccal) and syringe alignment, parallel with the occlusal plane on the side of injection but buccal to it. (Courtesy of Margaret J. Fehrenbach, RDH, MS.)

Needle gauge and length	25-gauge or 27-gauge long
Operator position	8 or 9 o'clock, right-handed 4 or 3 o'clock, left-handed
Penetration site	In the vestibule, distal and buccal to the most distal molar at the height of the occlusal plane (Fig. T17.2)

Fig. T17.2 Penetration site for the long buccal as this nerve travels anteriorly over the border of the ramus in a medial to lateral direction (see Fig. 43.24B). (Dental Hygiene Procedures Video, St. Louis, 2015, Saunders/Elsevier.)

Continued

TABLE 43.17   Buccal Nerve Block (Long Buccal)—cont'd

Nerves anesthetized	Buccal
Landmarks	Mandibular molars
	Buccal vestibule
	Mucobuccal fold
Syringe orientation	Parallel to the mandibular occlusal plane on the buccal side of the teeth (Fig. T17.2)
Hand rests	Patient's cheek or chin
	Back of operator's opposite hand (Fig. T17.3)

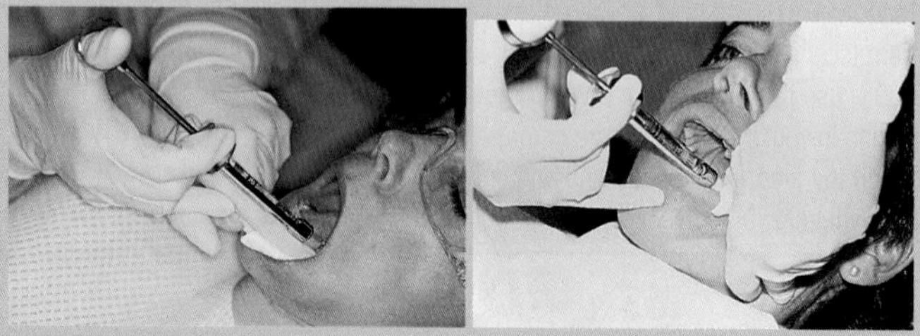

Fig. T17.3 Hand rests for the buccal nerve block. (Courtesy of F. O'Brien Photography.)

Deposition site	Buccal nerve as it passes over the anterior border of the ramus (Figs. 43.23B, T17.1)
Penetration depth	Approximately 2–4 mm until bone is gently contacted
Aspiration	Aspirate on arrival and then rotate syringe one-quarter turn and reaspirate
Amount of anesthetic to be deposited	0.3 mL or one-eighth of a cartridge
Length of time to deposit	Approximately 10 seconds

Technique Notes

The buccal nerve block can be administered immediately after the IANB; therefore the penetration sites can be prepared simultaneously with topical anesthetic.

Gow-Gates Nerve Block

An alternative injection for mandibular anesthesia is the GG injection, a true mandibular block, because the entire mandibular division of the sensory nerves of the trigeminal nerve or V₃ is anesthetized.[8] With the GG block, the IA, lingual, mental, incisive, mylohyoid, auriculotemporal, and long buccal nerves (approximately 75% of the time) are affected. This means all the mandibular teeth in a quadrant and the associated periodontium, lingual gingiva, and facial gingiva of the premolars and anterior teeth to the midline, and possibly the buccal periodontium and gingiva of the mandibular molars are anesthetized. The benefit of the GG block is the administration of one injection that covers a wide range of soft tissue and pulps of the mandibular teeth in a quadrant. The advantages of the GG are its higher success rate for mandibular anesthesia; its inclusion of the mylohyoid nerve, whose accessory innervation is also anesthetized; and a decreased risk of positive aspirations.[1] Therefore, patients who repeatedly fail to achieve anesthesia or clinical effectiveness with the IANB due to the variation of anatomy (differences in height of mandibular foramen and depth of penetration through soft tissues) or accessory innervation could benefit from the GG injection. A disadvantage of a GG block is that the patient's mouth must remain open for 2 minutes post injection. Table 43.19 and Evolve Video Resource provide the criteria pertinent to the administration of a GG nerve block.

LOCAL COMPLICATIONS

Despite careful preanesthetic patient assessment and adherence to the recommended procedures for LA administration, the following local complications may develop.

Needle Breakage

The introduction of disposable stainless steel needles has significantly reduced the incidence of needle breakage; however, virtually all needle breaks are preventable. When breakage does occur, it is primarily caused by a sudden, unexpected movement by the patient during needle insertion or by poor injection technique.[1] If a needle does break during insertion and can be retrieved without surgical intervention, no emergency exists. Those needles that are not retrieved most often remain in place and become encased by scar tissue. Leaving the needle in the tissue often produces fewer difficulties than the surgery required for its removal.

To prevent needle breakage, do the following:

- Inform the patient about the local anesthesia procedure both before and during the injection. Effective communication helps the individual anticipate the dental hygienist's actions and control anxiety.
- Use long, large-gauge needles (e.g., 25-gauge) when penetrating significant tissue depth. These are less likely to break than smaller needles.
- Never bend the needle because it weakens the metal.
- Advance the needle slowly. A forceful contact with bone may break the needle or may precipitate a quick movement by the patient because of associated pain.
- Never force a needle against firm resistance such as bone.
- Do not change the direction of the needle while it is almost completely within the tissues. If it is necessary to redirect the needle, first withdraw almost completely out of the tissue and then modify the direction.
- A needle should not be inserted into the tissues all the way to the hub. This juncture at the needle shaft and hub is the weakest part of the needle and is vulnerable to breakage. If needle breakage occurs at this point, a portion of the shaft must be exposed in order for the needle to be retrieved without surgery.

When a needle breaks, do the following:

- Remain calm; do not panic.
- Instruct the patient not to move. Do not remove your hand from the patient's mouth, and keep the patient's mouth open. If possible, place a bite block in the patient's mouth.

TABLE 43.18 Mental and Incisive Nerve Blocks

Nerves Anesthetized	Mental And Incisive (Terminal Branches Of Inferior Alveolar Nerve)
Areas anesthetized	Mental: facial soft tissues unilaterally from the mental foramen anterior to midline Lower lip Skin of chin (Fig. T18.1) Incisive: same as above with the addition of mandibular second premolar to central incisor unilaterally.

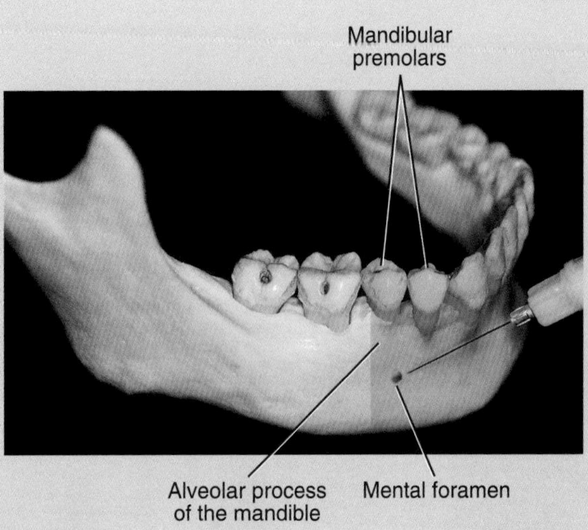

Fig. T18.1 Area anesthetized with the mental and/or the incisive nerve block and deposition site. (Courtesy of Margaret J. Fehrenbach, RDH, MS.)

Needle gauge and length	25-gauge or 27-gauge short
Operator position	8 or 9 o'clock or 11 or 1 o'clock, right-handed 4 or 3 o'clock or 1 or 11 o'clock, left-handed
Penetration site	Mucobuccal fold directly over the mental foramen (Fig. T18.2)

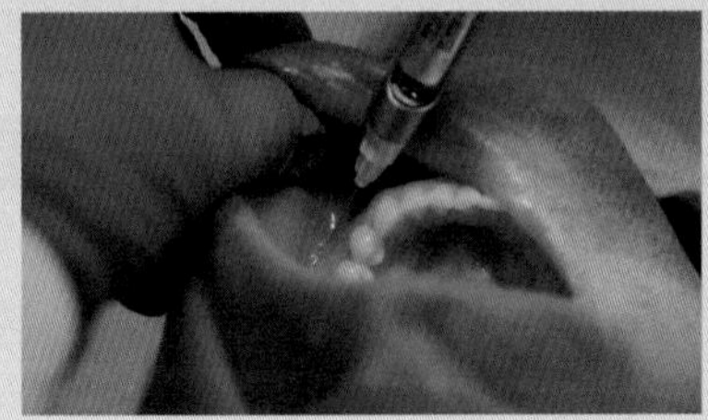

Fig. T18.2 Mental nerve block needle penetration site. (Dental Hygiene Procedures Videos, St Louis, 2015, Saunders/Elsevier.)

Landmarks	Mucobuccal fold Mandibular premolars Mental foramen
Syringe orientation	Directed toward the mental foramen with needle in recommended horizontal position (Fig. T18.2)
Hand rests	Patient's chin Back of operator's opposite hand or wrist (Fig. T18.3)

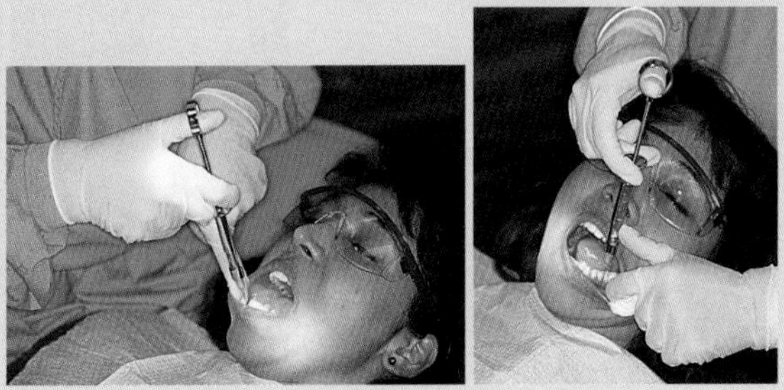

Fig. T18.3 Hand rests for the mental and incisive nerve blocks. When possible, hold the arms close to the body to increase stabilization. (Courtesy of F. O'Brien Photography.)

Continued

TABLE 43.18 Mental and Incisive Nerve Blocks—cont'd

Nerves Anesthetized	Mental And Incisive (Terminal Branches Of Inferior Alveolar Nerve)
Deposition site	Anterior to the mental foramen, between the apices of the premolars (Fig. T18.1)
Penetration depth	Approximately 5 mm or one-quarter of a short needle (do not enter the mental foramen)
Aspiration	Aspirate on arrival and then rotate syringe one-quarter turn and reaspirate
Amount of anesthetic to be deposited	0.6 mL or one-third of a cartridge
Length of time to deposit	Approximately 20–30 seconds

Technique Notes

1. To locate the mental foramen, place your forefinger in the mucobuccal fold against the body of the mandible near the first molar. Palpate anteriorly until a depression is felt or the bone feels irregular. This is the mental foramen, which is most often found between the apices of the first and second premolars (Fig. T18.4).
2. Use radiographs to assist you in finding the mental foramen (Fig. T18.5).
3. If the tissue balloons, stop the deposition, withdraw the needle, and gently massage the area.
4. Incisive Block Injection: maintain pressure or massage over the mental foramen with your finger for 1–2 minutes after the injection. This aids the flow of solution into the foramen, providing the pulpal anesthesia (Fig. T18.6).

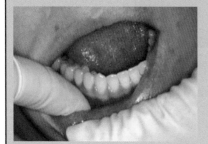

Fig. T18.4 Locate the mental nerve foramen by palpating the vestibule at the premolars.

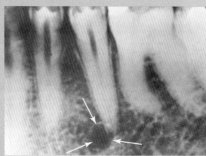

Fig. T18.5 Radiographs can assist in locating the mental foramen.

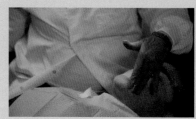

Fig. T18.6 Massage the area for 1 to 2 minutes to aid pulpal anesthesia. (Dental Hygiene Procedures Videos, St Louis, 2015, Saunders/Elsevier.)

TABLE 43.19 Gow-Gates Nerve Block (GG)

Nerves anesthetized	Inferior alveolar Mental Incisive Lingual Auriculotemporal Buccal Mylohyoid
Area anesthetized	Pulpal anesthesia of the mandibular teeth to the midline, buccal, and lingual gingiva on the side of the injection, anterior two-thirds of the tongue and adjacent floor of the mouth, body of the mandible and the inferior portion of the ramus, skin of the cheek, and temporal region (Fig. T19.1)

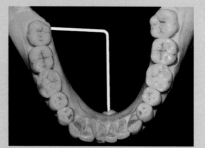

Fig. T19.1 Areas anesthetized with the Gow-Gates nerve block. (Dental Hygiene Procedures Videos, St Louis, 2015, Saunders/Elsevier.)

Needle gauge and length	27-gauge long
Operator position	8 o'clock (R GG), 10 o'clock (L GG), right-handed 4 o'clock (L GG), 2 o'clock (R GG), left-handed

TABLE 43.19   Gow-Gates Nerve Block (GG)—cont'd

Penetration site	Immediately distal to the maxillary second molar at the height of the tip of the mesiolingual cusp (Fig. T19.2)

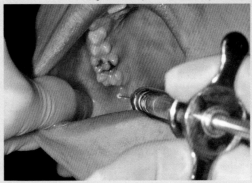

Fig. T19.2 Penetration site for the Gow-Gates. (Courtesy of Margaret J. Fehrenbach, RDH, MS.)

Landmarks	Extraoral: Tragus of ear, intertragic notch of ear, corner of the open mouth (Figs. T19.3A–B) Intraoral: Mesiolingual (mesiopalatal) cusp of the maxillary second molar (Fig. T19.3C)

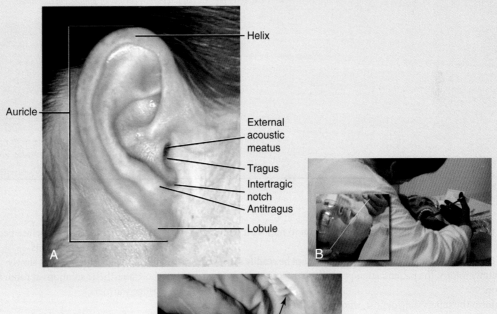

Fig. T19.3 (A) The tragus and intertragic notch serve as extraoral landmarks. (B) An imaginary extraoral line connects the corner of the mouth and the intertragic notch to determine needle pathway. Pinky on chin for hand rest for right GG is shown. (C) The distal palatal cusp of the second molar is an intraoral landmark for the GG penetration site. (Dental Hygiene Procedures Videos, St Louis, 2015, Saunders/Elsevier.)

Syringe orientation	Barrel placed in the corner of the mouth of the opposite side and directed toward the site of the injection (Fig. T19.4)

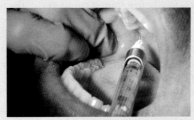

Fig. T19.4 Penetration depth of needle and syringe orientation for right GG. (Dental Hygiene Procedures Videos, St Louis, 2015, Saunders/Elsevier.)

Continued

TABLE 43.19	**Gow-Gates Nerve Block (GG)—cont'd**
Hand rests	Pinky finger of injection hand on chin or cheek
	Barrel of syringe resting on the corner of the mouth (Fig. T19.3B)
Deposition site	When bone (neck of the condyle) is contacted by the needle
Penetration depth	25 mm or three-fourths of the needle (Fig. T19.4)
Aspiration	Aspirate on arrival and then rotate syringe one-quarter turn and reaspirate
Amount of anesthetic to be deposited	1.8 mL or 1 total cartridge
Length of time to deposit	60–90 seconds

Technique Notes

1. Aspiration in only two planes is needed because deposition site is less vascular.
2. This injection is used when a patient has a history of unsuccessful inferior alveolar nerve block anesthesia.

Potential Problems	Technique Tips
Hematoma	<2% incidence
Trismus	Deposit solution slowly
Temporary paralysis of the cranial nerves	Do not deposit solution *unless* bone has been contacted
Additional clinical experience may be needed for clinical effectiveness	Patient to keep mouth open for 2 minutes post injection (use of a bite block may be helpful) (Fig. T19.5)
	Extraoral and intraoral anatomy review of deposition site area

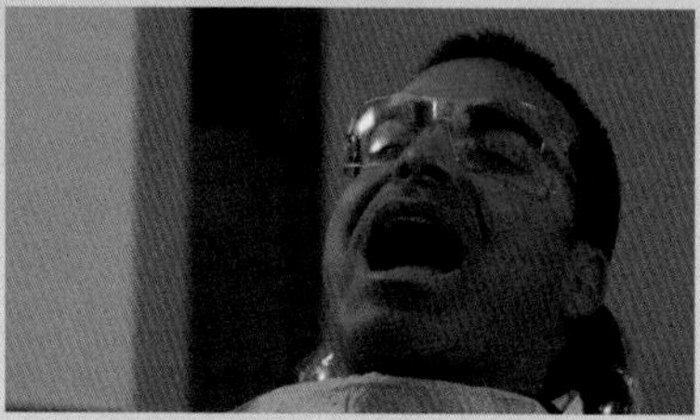

Fig. T19.5 With the mouth kept open, the condyle is in a more frontal position and gives the anesthetic better access to the mandibular nerve. (Dental Hygiene Procedures Videos, St Louis, 2015, Saunders/Elsevier.)

- If the needle fragment is protruding, attempt to remove it with cotton pliers or a hemostat.
  If the needle fragment is not visible and cannot be readily retrieved:
- Calmly inform the patient; attempt to alleviate fears and apprehension.
- Inform the supervising dentist, who may refer the patient to an oral and maxillofacial surgeon for consultation and removal.
- Document the incident and the patient's response in the patient's chart. Keep the remaining needle fragment. Inform your insurance carrier immediately.

Pain During the Injection

Pain during LA agent administration may be attributed to several factors: a careless injection technique and callous attitude toward the patient, a dull needle from multiple injections, a barbed needle from hitting bone, or rapid deposition of the anesthetic solution. It is not possible to ensure that every injection is totally free from discomfort because patients' reactions vary; however, the dental hygienist should take every precaution to prevent pain during the injection or prevent its recurrence.

To prevent pain during injection, do the following:

- Adhere to the proper techniques of administration as described in Procedure 43.4 and Tables 43.8 to 43.19.
- For anxious patients, depositing a few drops as the needle advances is an option.
- Use sharp disposable needles.
- Apply topical anesthetic before needle insertion.
- Use sterile anesthetic agents.
- Inject the anesthetic agent slowly.
- Store anesthetic solutions at room temperature and avoid using cartridge warmers.

Burning During the Injection

A burning sensation reported by the patient during deposition of the LA agent may be caused by an LA with a vasopressor that is more acidic than the tissue in which it is deposited. The burning sensation, which lasts only a few seconds, disappears as anesthesia develops. A more acute burning may occur, however, if the LA solution is contaminated from improper storage of the cartridge in a chemical disinfectant; if the cartridge is overheated in a cartridge warmer; if the expiration date of the solution has lapsed; or if the solution is deposited too rapidly, particularly on the palate. When burning occurs as a result of these factors, the tissue is damaged and subsequent postanesthetic trismus, edema, or possible paresthesia may develop.

To prevent burning during the injection, do the following:

- Store the cartridges in a dark place at room temperature in the original container. Avoid storing cartridges in chemical disinfectants or using cartridge warmers.
- Check the expiration date of each cartridge before use. Anesthetic solution that has exceeded the expiration date should be discarded.
- Inject the anesthetic solution slowly.

Most often, burning during an injection is a temporary condition and needs no specific treatment.

Hematoma

A **hematoma** is a swelling and discoloration of the tissue resulting from the effusion of blood into the extravascular spaces (Fig. 43.32). Hematomas occur subsequent to an inadvertent puncture of a blood vessel, particularly an artery, during LA administration. They appear most often after the PSA injections, followed by IANB and mental/incisive nerve blocks, because the tissues associated with these injections are less dense and readily accommodate large volumes of blood. Bleeding continues until extravascular pressure exceeds intravascular pressure or until clotting occurs. A hematoma is less likely to develop after a palatal injection because of the density of the tissue in this area.

A hematoma that ensues after a PSA nerve block is the largest and most visible. The bleeding occurs in the infratemporal fossa, and swelling and discoloration appear on the side of the face. Clinical manifestations of a hematoma following an IANB include intraoral tissue discoloration and swelling on the lingual aspect of the ramus. Other than the bruise, which may or may not be visible extraorally, a hematoma may be accompanied by trismus and pain.

To prevent a hematoma, do the following:
- Be attentive to anatomic detail involved in each injection.
- Modify the injection technique as indicated by the patient's anatomy. For example, the depth of needle penetration for a PSA nerve block may be shallower for a patient with small anatomic features.
- Use a short needle for the PSA nerve block to minimize the risk of overinsertion and the potential for hematoma formation.
- Minimize the number of needle insertions.
- Observe the appropriate techniques for LA administration.

Management includes the following:
- If swelling appears, immediately apply direct pressure to the site of the bleeding for at least 2 minutes. For an IANB, the pressure point is the medial side of the ramus. For the mental or incisive nerve block, pressure is applied over the mental foramen. If hematoma formation follows an IO nerve block, the pressure point is the skin over the IO foramen. Unfortunately, it is difficult to apply pressure directly to the site of bleeding after a PSA nerve block because the vessels are located posterior, superior, and medial to the maxillary tuberosity. Pressure may be applied to the tissues of the mucofacial fold as far distally as the patient can tolerate.
- Apply ice to the region when hematoma formation begins. Ice constricts the blood vessels, minimizes the size of the hematoma, and acts as an analgesic.
- Inform the patient about the possibility of soreness and movement limitation. If soreness develops, analgesics may be taken. Beginning

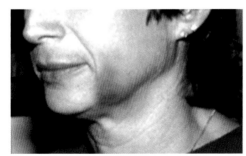

Fig. 43.32 Hematoma resulting from administration of left mental block.

the next day, warm, moist towels may be applied to the affected region for 20 minutes every hour. This warm, moist towel application provides comfort and helps blood resorption. Heat therapy should not commence for at least 4 to 6 hours after hematoma formation, however. Before this time, heat may produce further vasodilation and an even larger hematoma.
- Advise the patient that the swelling and discoloration will gradually disappear over 7 to 14 days.
- Dismiss the patient when the bleeding has stopped. Avoid further dental hygiene care in the area until signs and symptoms of the hematoma have disappeared. Document the incident and the patient's response in the patient's chart.

Facial Nerve Paralysis

Facial paralysis is a loss of motor function of the facial expression muscles. Unilateral facial nerve paralysis occurs when the LA solution is inadvertently deposited into the parotid gland, located on the posterior border of the ramus, during an IANB.

Motor function loss is temporary and subsides in a few hours; however, during this time, the patient is unable to control these muscles and the face appears lopsided. It also may be impossible for the patient to voluntarily close the eye on the affected side. Fortunately, the corneal reflex is functional, and tears continue to lubricate the eye.

To prevent facial nerve paralysis, do the following:
- Adhere to the techniques recommended for the IANB.
- Make sure the needle contacts bone (medial aspect of the ramus) before deposition of the LA solution.
- If bone is not contacted, withdraw the needle almost entirely out of the tissue, bring the barrel of the syringe more posterior (thereby directing the needle more anterior), and readvance the needle until bone is contacted.

Following these steps precludes solution deposition into the parotid gland.

Within a short time after anesthetic solution deposition into the parotid gland, the patient senses a weakening of the facial muscles on the affected side. The inferior alveolar nerve is not anesthetized. Management includes the following:
- Reassure the patient. Explain that the paralysis lasts only a few hours and resolves with no residual effects.
- Instruct the patient to remove contact lenses.
- Ask the patient to close the eyelid manually to keep the cornea lubricated. Advise patient to wear an eye patch.
- There are no contraindications to proceeding with treatment at this time, but it may be advisable to reschedule the patient.
- Document the incident and the patient's response in the patient's chart.[1]

PARESTHESIA

Prolonged anesthesia or paresthesia is a condition wherein the patient experiences numbness for many hours or days after an LA injection. Paresthesia may be the result of irritation to the nerve after injection of an anesthetic agent that has been contaminated with alcohol or a disinfectant. The ensuing edema places pressure on the nerve, leading to paresthesia. Persistent anesthesia also may result from trauma to the nerve sheath caused by the needle contacting the nerve during an injection. Patients often report the sensation of an electric shock when this occurs. Finally, hemorrhage into or around the neural sheath may create pressure and subsequent paresthesia.

A complication of paresthesia is the patient anticipating a biting, thermal, or chemical injury from the diminished sensation in the area.

To prevent paresthesia, do the following:

- Store dental cartridges properly. Avoid placing cartridges in disinfectants.
- Follow the proper injection protocol as recommended in Procedure 43.4 and Tables 43.8 to 43.19.

Most often, paresthesia involves the lingual nerve or the inferior alveolar nerve. The sensory deficit usually is minimal and rarely is accompanied by permanent nerve damage. Fortunately, most incidents resolve within 8 weeks. Recommendations for the management of a patient with paresthesia are as follows:

- Reassure the patient. The patient usually contacts the dental office the day after treatment to report continuing numbness. Explain that paresthesia after LA administration is not uncommon.
- Arrange for an examination of the patient by the dentist, who will determine the location and extent of paresthesia. Explain to the patient that paresthesia often continues for 2 months and may last longer.
- Arrange to have the patient examined every 2 months until cessation of the paresthesia. Consultation with an oral and maxillofacial surgeon is advisable if paresthesia persists after 12 months or sooner if the patient and dentist consider it appropriate.
- Record the incident, conversations with the patient, and all clinical findings in the patient's chart. Inform your liability carrier of the circumstances.
- Dental and dental hygiene care may continue. Avoid injecting into the area of the traumatized nerve and employ alternative pain control techniques.[1]

Trismus

Trismus, a spasm of the mastication muscles that results in soreness and difficulty opening the mouth, most often occurs as a result of trauma to the muscles in the infratemporal space after intraoral injections. This trauma may be the result of multiple needle insertions, administration of an anesthetic solution contaminated with a disinfectant, injection of large amounts of LA solution into a restricted area causing distention of the tissues, hemorrhage that leads to muscle dysfunction as the blood is resorbed, or a low-grade infection.

To prevent trismus, do the following:

- Store the LA cartridges properly. Avoid immersing the cartridges in a disinfectant.
- Use sharp, sterile, disposable needles.
- Follow appropriate infection control protocol. Needles that become contaminated should be replaced.
- Use minimal effective amounts of LA solution and deposit the solution slowly.
- Adhere to the recommended techniques of LA administration as outlined in Procedure 43.4 and Tables 43.8 to 43.19. Observe anatomic landmarks and strive to improve administration techniques. Each of these recommendations facilitates atraumatic injections and prevents repeated needle insertions.

Patients often complain of soreness and difficulty in opening the mouth the day after the administration of an inferior alveolar or a posterior superior nerve block. Recommendations for management of patients with trismus follow:

- Arrange for an examination of the patient by the dentist.
- Start heat therapy immediately. Place moist, hot towels on the affected area for 20 minutes every hour. Analgesics may be recommended to manage the discomfort. Codeine and muscle relaxants may be prescribed by the dentist if needed.
- Direct the patient to open and close and move the mandible from side to side (lateral) for 5 minutes every 3 to 4 hours. This exercise may be accomplished by chewing gum.

- Continue heat therapy, analgesics, and exercise until the patient is symptom-free. Improvement is often reported within 48 hours, and symptoms diminish gradually over several days.
- If symptoms continue after 48 hours, the possibility of an infection exists. Antibiotic therapy (prescribed by the dentist) should be added to the recommended care regimen.
- If severe pain and dysfunction continue despite therapy, referral to an oral and maxillofacial surgeon for consultation is appropriate.
- Record the incident, conversations with the patient, the results of clinical examinations, and care recommended in the patient's chart.
- Avoid elective dental hygiene care until symptoms resolve and the patient is more comfortable.[1]

Infection

Infection from LA administration occurs rarely with the introduction of sterile disposable needles and glass cartridges; however, postinjection infection may be precipitated by contamination of the needle before the injection, improper handling of the local anesthesia armamentarium, or improper tissue preparation before the injection. When a contaminated needle or LA solution is introduced into the deeper tissues, infection may occur. If infection is not recognized and treated, trismus may ensue.

To prevent infection, do the following:

- Use sterile disposable needles.
- Sheath the needle before use and resheath it after use to prevent it from coming in contact with nonsterile surfaces.
- Use appropriate infection control protocol when handling the anesthetic cartridges. Store the cartridges in their original container, and, if necessary, wipe the cartridge diaphragm with a disinfectant before syringe assembly.
- To reduce microorganisms at the penetration site, wipe the tissue with gauze and apply a topical antiseptic before the initial needle insertion.

When infection occurs, the patient often reports pain and dysfunction, similar to trismus, a few days after dental hygiene care. At this point, signs and symptoms of infection often are not obvious, and immediate treatment includes procedures for managing trismus (e.g., heat therapy, physiotherapy, analgesics, and muscle relaxants). If the patient does not respond to therapy within 3 days, an infection most likely exists, and antibiotic therapy should be prescribed by the dentist or physician. Document the recommended therapy and patient progress in the patient record.

Edema

Edema, a swelling of the tissues, is a clinical sign of a complication. It may be caused by trauma during the injection, administration of contaminated solutions, hemorrhage, an infection, or an allergic response. Most often, edema manifests as localized pain and dysfunction. In the most severe case, edema precipitated by an allergic response may produce airway obstruction and represents a life-threatening emergency.

To prevent edema, do the following:

- Follow appropriate infection control protocol when storing and handling components of the local anesthesia armamentarium.
- Observe the guidelines for administering atraumatic injections, as described in Procedure 43.4.
- Conduct an adequate preanesthetic patient assessment before LA administration.

The course and treatment of edema depend on its cause.[1] When produced by the administration of a contaminated anesthetic solution or traumatic injection, edema usually subsides in 1 to 3 days without treatment. Analgesics may be recommended. If edema is caused by hemorrhage, the tissue appears discolored and should be managed in the same manner as a hematoma. Resolution of the edema may take 7 to 14 days as the blood is resorbed into the tissues. Edema produced by infection often becomes progressively worse. If the pain and dysfunction do not subside in 3 days, antibiotic therapy may be instituted by the dentist or physician. The treatment of edema caused by an allergic reaction depends on the degree and location of the tissue swelling. If there is no airway obstruction, treatment involves the administration of intramuscular and oral antihistamines and consultation with an allergist or physician. If the edema occurs in an area where it compromises the airway, the recommendations outlined in the section on systemic complications should be followed.

Tissue Sloughing

Surface layers of epithelium may be lost because of tissue irritation caused by the application of topical anesthetic for an extended period or a patient's heightened sensitivity to the LA. A sterile abscess (see Fig. 43.2), a form of tissue sloughing most frequently occurring on the hard palate, may develop after prolonged ischemia induced by the inclusion of a vasoconstrictor in the LA agent.

To prevent tissue sloughing, do the following:
- Use topical anesthetics appropriately. Apply a limited amount of topical anesthetic to the tissue for 1 to 2 minutes to minimize irritation and maximize effectiveness.
- When using vasoconstrictors for hemostasis, avoid using high concentrations such as epinephrine 1:50,000 as it is likely to cause prolonged ischemia leading to a sterile abscess.

Tissue sloughing usually requires no treatment and disappears within a few days. A sterile abscess resolves in 7 to 10 days. Analgesics may be recommended for discomfort, and topical ointment can be applied to minimize irritation. Document the progress and response of the patient in the patient's record.

Soft Tissue Trauma

Lip, tongue, or cheek trauma results when the patient inadvertently chews or bites these tissues while they are still anesthetized. Trauma—most often observed in children or in mentally or physically disabled individuals—may lead to swelling and significant discomfort when the anesthesia subsides.

To prevent soft tissue trauma, do the following:
- Select an LA agent with appropriate duration for the length of the dental hygiene appointment.
- Warn the patient not to eat, drink, or test the anesthetized area by biting until normal sensation has returned. The patient's guardian also should be advised of the potential for injury.
- If anesthesia is still present on dismissal, place a cotton roll between the teeth and soft tissues. The cotton roll can be held in position with dental floss wrapped around the teeth.
- Warning stickers may be placed on children to serve as a reminder to the child and the guardian to be careful.

Management of soft tissue trauma includes the following:
- Coat the lip with petrolatum to minimize irritation and discomfort.
- Recommend warm saline rinses to help decrease swelling.
- Recommend analgesics for pain.
- If infection occurs, the dentist or physician may prescribe antibiotic therapy.

Postanesthetic Intraoral Lesions

Intraoral lesions, such as those from aphthous stomatitis or herpes simplex virus, may develop after the administration of local anesthesia or trauma to the intraoral tissues. Aphthous stomatitis occurs on tissue not attached to bone, such as the mucofacial fold or inner lip. Herpes simplex virus lesions may develop intraorally on tissues attached

to bone, such as the hard palate, or extraorally. Trauma to the area by a needle or any equipment used during the dental hygiene care appointment may activate herpetic recurrence.

Preventing the development of postanesthetic intraoral lesions is impossible in susceptible patients; however, minimizing trauma during procedures for LA administration is advisable.

Approximately 2 days after the dental hygiene care appointment, the patient reports ulcerations and intense pain, usually near the injection site(s). If the discomfort is tolerable, no management is necessary. If the pain is acute, topical anesthetic solutions or protective pastes, such as Orabase, may provide relief. The lesions last for 7 to 10 days. Reassure the patient and document the occurrence of the lesion in the patient's record.

SYSTEMIC COMPLICATIONS

Patient assessment is a key factor in preventing systemic complications associated with LA administration. It is estimated that a comprehensive health assessment will prevent approximately 90% of potentially life-threatening situations.[4] The remaining 10% occur despite all preventive efforts.

The dental hygienist should be able to recognize the signs and symptoms of an adverse drug reaction and properly manage the emergency that may develop. To be adequately prepared for an emergency, the dental hygienist, as well as all members of the oral health team, should be able to recognize and manage medical emergencies, monitor vital signs, administer oxygen, and perform basic life support procedures. By establishing an airway and performing basic cardiopulmonary resuscitation, the dental hygienist administers care to reverse the emergency or to sustain the patient until advanced life support systems arrive (see Chapter 11).

Local Anesthetic Overdose

A drug overdose reaction or toxic reaction is defined as those signs and symptoms that result from overly high blood levels of a drug in various organs and tissues.[1] Normally, the drug is continually absorbed from its site of administration. Concurrently, the drug is being removed from the blood as it undergoes redistribution and biotransformation. When this equilibrium exists, high blood levels of the drug seldom occur. If this equilibrium is altered, however, the elevation of the blood level of the drug may be sufficient to produce an overdose reaction.

Many factors influence the rate at which an LA drug level is elevated and the length of time it remains elevated. The presence of one or more of these factors predisposes the patient to the development of an overdose reaction. These factors are divided into predisposing patient factors and drug factors. Patient factors modify the response of an individual to the usual drug dosage. Drug factors involve the drug and its site of administration. Table 43.20 describes how each of these factors influences the potential for an overdose reaction.

Causes and Prevention

High blood levels of LAs may occur in one or more of the following ways:
- Biotransformation of the anesthetic is unusually slow.
- Elimination of the anesthetic from the body through the kidneys is unusually slow.
- The total dose administered is too large.
- Absorption of the anesthetic from the site of injection is unusually rapid.
- The anesthetic is inadvertently administered intravascularly.[1]

The first two potential causes of an overdose, delayed biotransformation and elimination of the anesthetic agent, relate to the health of the patient. Therefore, it is imperative that the dental hygienist carefully

TABLE 43.20 Predisposing Factors to Local Anesthetic Overdose Reaction

Predisposing Factors	Causative Factors
Patient Factors	
Age	Biotransformation may not be fully developed in younger age groups and may be diminished in older age groups
Body weight	Lower body weight increases risk
Genetics	Genetic deficiencies may alter response to certain drugs (e.g., atypical plasma cholinesterase)
Disease	Presence of disease may affect the ability of the body to biotransform the drug into an inactive substance (e.g., hepatic or renal dysfunction, cardiovascular disease)
Mental attitude and environment	Psychologic attitude affects response to stimulation; anxiety decreases seizure threshold
Gender	Very slight risk increases during pregnancy
Drug Factors	
Vasoactivity	Vasodilation increases risk
Drug dose	Higher dose increases risk
Route of administration	Intravascular route increases risk
Rate of injection	Rapid injection increases risk
Vascularity of injection site	Increased vascularity increases risk
Presence of vasoconstrictors	Presence decreases risk
Other medications	Concomitant medications may influence LA drug levels

Adapted from Malamed SF. *Medical Emergencies in the Dental Office.* 7th ed. Mosby; 2015.

assess the patient's health status, obtain medical consultation if necessary, and modify the dental hygiene care plan as indicated to prevent drug-related complications.

Biotransformation and elimination of the anesthetic. Ester anesthetics are biotransformed primarily in the blood by the enzyme pseudocholinesterase, which causes the drug to undergo hydrolysis to paraaminobenzoic acid (PABA). Patients with a familial history of atypical pseudocholinesterase may be unable to detoxify ester anesthetic agents at the usual rate. As a result, high blood levels of anesthetic may develop. Amide anesthetics may be administered to these individuals without an increased risk of overdose.

Biotransformation of amide anesthetics occurs mostly in the liver. Articaine would be an exception because biotransformation occurs in both the plasma and the liver.[3] A history of liver disease may indicate some hepatic dysfunction, and the ability of the liver to biotransform amide anesthetics may be compromised. Patients with a history of liver disease who are ambulatory may still receive amide LAs, but only small amounts should be injected because average amounts may produce an overdose reaction. In addition, articaine, an amide with ester characteristics, would be an appropriate choice—because its biotransformation occurs in both the plasma and the liver, its elimination is more than twice as fast as all other amide agents, resulting in a decreased risk of systemic toxicity.[1]

Both ester and amide anesthetics are eliminated to some degree through the kidneys. Renal dysfunction may delay elimination of

the LA from the blood, precipitating accumulated levels of LA and increased potential for an overdose. Those patients who have significant renal impairment or who require renal dialysis should receive the minimal amount of LA needed for effective pain control.

Excessive total dose of anesthetic. If an excessive total dose of LA is administered to a patient, toxic effects develop. Responses to drugs vary considerably, but guidelines exist for the dental hygienist to calculate MRDs of LA agents based on body weight. The dental hygienist also needs to factor in the patient's age and physical status and adjust the dose accordingly. A more detailed discussion can be found under the earlier section on MRDs of LAs.

Rapid absorption of anesthetic into the circulation. The addition of a vasoconstricting drug in the LA solution reduces the systemic toxicity of the anesthetic agent by slowing its absorption, minimizing the potential for an overdose reaction, and increasing patient safety. Therefore, unless specifically contraindicated because of health status or limited duration of dental hygiene care, LA solutions containing a vasoconstrictor should be employed.

Topical anesthetic agents applied to the oral mucosa are absorbed rapidly into the circulation. The concentration of these topical agents is much greater than that of injectable anesthetic solutions. When small amounts are used in a localized area, there is little chance of complications developing. If topical anesthetic agents are applied over a large area such as a quadrant or the entire arch, a significant increase in blood level may occur, precipitating an overdose reaction.[1] To prevent complications with topical anesthetics, it is recommended to limit the area of application and avoid topical anesthetic aerosol sprays because of lack of dosage control and sterility concerns.

Intravascular injection. The introduction of an LA solution directly into the bloodstream via an intravascular injection (intravenous or intraarterial) may produce an overdose response. An intravascular injection may result with any intraoral injection; however, it is more likely to occur during a nerve block, particularly an inferior alveolar, mental, incisive, or PSA nerve block.

Fortunately, an overdose reaction from an intravascular injection can be prevented by having a complete knowledge of the anatomic features of the area to be anesthetized and by adhering to careful injection technique. This includes using an aspirating syringe, using a 25-gauge or 27-gauge needle, aspirating in two planes before deposition, and injecting slowly—which is the most significant factor, even more important than aspiration.[1]

Clinical Manifestations and Management

The onset, intensity, and duration of an LA toxic reaction may vary depending on the original cause of the overdose. Table 43.21 compares the various patterns of LA overdose reactions.

Table 43.22 describes the clinical signs and symptoms that may occur during an overdose reaction (with minimal to moderate and moderate to high blood levels of anesthetic) and the procedures for managing an LA overdose response. Management of an overdose response depends on the severity of the reaction. Most often, the reaction is mild and transitory, with little or no specific treatment need.[1] A severe or longer-duration reaction necessitates prompt recognition and immediate care.

Epinephrine Overdose

Although several vasoconstrictors are currently used in oral healthcare, epinephrine is the most potent and most widely employed. Consequently, overdose reactions occur more often with epinephrine than with other vasopressor agents because the latter agents are weaker and are used less frequently.

TABLE 43.21   Comparison of Forms of Local Anesthetic Overdose

Factors Related to Overdose	Rapid Intravascular	Too Large a Total Dose	Rapid Absorption	Slow Biotransformation	Slow Elimination
Likelihood of occurrence	Common	Most common	Likely with "high normal" doses if no vasoconstrictors are used	Uncommon	Least common
Onset of signs and symptoms	Most rapid (seconds); intraarterial faster than intravenous	3–5 minutes	3–5 minutes	10–30 minutes	10 minutes to several hours
Intensity of signs and symptoms	Usually most intense	Gradual onset with increased intensity; may prove quite severe		Gradual onset with slow increase in intensity of symptoms	
Duration of signs and symptoms	2–3 minutes	Usually 5–30 minutes; depends on dose and ability to metabolize or excrete		Potentially longest duration because of inability to metabolize or excrete agents	
Primary prevention	Aspirate, slow injection	Administer minimal doses	Use vasoconstrictor; limit topical anesthetic use or use nonabsorbed type (base)	Adequate pretreatment physical assessment of patient	
Drug groups	Amides and esters	Amides; esters only rarely	Amides; esters only rarely	Amides and esters	Amides and esters

From Malamed SF. *Medical Emergencies in the Dental Office.* 7th ed. Mosby; 2015.

TABLE 43.22   Clinical Manifestations and Management of an LA Overdose Reaction

Signs and Symptoms	Management
Minimal to Moderate Blood Levels (Mild Overdose Reaction) Confusion Talkativeness Apprehension Excitedness Lightheadedness Dizziness Ringing in ears (tinnitus) Headache Slurred speech Generalized stutter Muscular twitching and tremor of face and extremities Blurred vision, unable to focus Numbness of perioral tissues Flushed or chilled feeling Drowsiness, disorientation Elevated blood pressure Elevated heart rate Elevated respiratory rate Loss of consciousness	Step 1: Terminate procedure Step 2: Reassure patient Step 3: Position patient comfortably Step 4: Provide basic life support as indicated Step 5: Administer oxygen as needed Step 6: Monitor vital signs Step 7: Summon medical assistance if needed Step 8: Allow patient to recover, then discharge
Moderate to High Blood Levels (Severe Overdose Reaction) Tonic-clonic seizure, followed by: Central nervous system depression Depressed blood pressure, heart rate, and respiratory rate Unconsciousness	Step 1: Terminate procedure Step 2: Position patient supine, legs elevated Step 3: Summon medical assistance Step 4: Manage seizure—protect patient from injury Step 5: Provide basic life support as indicated Step 6: Administer oxygen Step 7: Monitor vital signs Step 8: EMS/DDS administers an anticonvulsant (prolonged seizure) as needed Step 9: EMS transports patient to hospital after stabilization

EMS, Emergency medical services.
Some data from Malamed SF. *Medical Emergencies in the Dental Office.* 7th ed. Mosby; 2015.

Causes and Prevention

An epinephrine overdose reaction may develop if concentrations of epinephrine greater than 1:100,000 are administered. Some authorities state that a lesser concentration of 1:250,000 epinephrine provides adequate duration of action for dental procedures and minimal toxicity. Therefore, the use of a 1:50,000 concentration of epinephrine for pain control is unwarranted. The only benefit this concentration may have over lesser concentrations is its ability to control bleeding. If epinephrine is to be used for hemostasis, only small quantities of solution need to be infiltrated into the immediate area. Overdose reactions under these circumstances are rare. Therefore, to avoid an epinephrine overdose reaction, it is recommended that the dental hygienist use the lowest effective concentration of epinephrine needed to produce the desired effect and carefully observe dosage guidelines (see Table 43.2).

Patients with cardiovascular disease have a greater potential for epinephrine overdose. An increased workload may precipitate further cardiac distress on an already compromised CVS. Therefore, the total dose of vasoconstrictor must be reduced to avoid systemic complications.

An intravascular injection may also produce an epinephrine overdose reaction.[1] Recommendations for prevention of an intravascular injection may be found in the preceding section on LA overdose.

Clinical Manifestations and Management

Clinically, the signs and symptoms of epinephrine toxicity resemble the fight-or-flight response. Table 43.23 identifies signs and symptoms of an epinephrine overdose reaction and procedures for management. Most cases of epinephrine overdose are of short duration and need little or no definitive management. If a prolonged reaction occurs, however, the dental hygienist must be prepared to respond accordingly. Use critical thinking to analyze the legal, ethical, and safety issues concerning epinephrine overdose and the situation the dental hygienist encounters in Box 43.8.

Allergy

Allergic reactions are the result of an antigen-antibody response to a specific agent. Exposure to an initial dose of a medication causes an immunologic response. The drug acts as an antigen, prompting antibodies to be produced. As a result, administration of a subsequent dose causes the patient to develop an allergic response to the drug, its chemical preservative, or a metabolite. Once patients manifest a specific drug allergy, they remain allergic to that drug indefinitely.

Causes

Allergic reactions to amide-type LAs are extremely rare. As a result of their nonallergenic nature, amides are now used almost exclusively for pain control during dental and dental hygiene procedures.

Allergic responses to other contents of the dental cartridge have been demonstrated. Reports of allergy to sodium bisulfite and metabisulfite are numerous.[1,3] Beware of the confusion between sulfite preservatives in dental cartridges and sulfa-containing medications such as antibiotics. Both can cause allergic reactions in patients, but they are not chemically related.[3] Bisulfites are incorporated in all dental cartridges containing a vasoconstrictor; however, they are not included in cartridges that contain no vasopressor. These agents are also sprayed on fruits and vegetables to prevent discoloration. A patient with a history of bisulfite allergy (e.g., allergic induced or intrinsic, as opposed to nonallergic/extrinsic or stress induced) or asthmatic patients with a known allergy should alert the dental hygienist to the possibility of a similar reaction if an LA containing a vasoconstrictor is administered. See the earlier section on preanesthetic patient assessment and allergies for further discussion.

Prevention

The preanesthetic patient assessment is the primary measure for prevention of an allergic reaction. A patient who has multiple allergies (e.g., asthma, hay fever, allergy to foods) has an increased potential for allergic reactions to medications.[4] Thus, the dental hygienist must proceed cautiously when considering administration of LAs to these patients.

If the patient reports that they have experienced an allergic reaction to LAs, it is important that the dental hygienist assume that the patient is truly allergic to the LA in question until proven otherwise. Unfortunately, any adverse drug reaction is often labeled an allergy by patients when in fact overdose reactions occur much more frequently than allergic reactions.[4] Thus, it is imperative for the dental hygienist to seek as much information as possible from the patient so that the exact nature of the reaction can be determined. A dialogue history is used, whereby the dental hygienist asks the patient a series of questions to ascertain the validity of the allergy (Box 43.9).[4] It is important that the anesthetic agent or any closely related agent to which the patient claims to be allergic not be used until the allergy is disproved.

After the dialogue history, if questions remain about the cause of the reaction, the dental hygienist should consult with the dentist and the patient's physician, and referral for allergy testing should be considered.

TABLE 43.23   Clinical Manifestations and Management of a Patient With an Epinephrine Overdose Reaction

Signs and Symptoms	Management
Fear, anxiety	Step 1: Terminate procedure
Tenseness	Step 2: Position patient upright
Restlessness	Step 3: Provide basic life support as indicated
Throbbing headache	Step 4: Reassure patient
Tremor	Step 5: Monitor vital signs
Perspiration	Step 6: Summon medical assistance if needed
Weakness	Step 7: Administer oxygen if needed
Dizziness	Step 8: Allow patient to recover, then discharge
Pallor	
Respiratory difficulty	
Palpitations	
Sharp elevation in blood pressure, primarily systolic	
Elevated heart rate	
Cardiac dysrhythmias	

Some data from Malamed SF. *Medical Emergencies in the Dental Office.* 7th ed. Mosby; 2015.

BOX 43.8 Legal, Ethical, and Safety Issues

Scenario:

Patient Name: David O'Brien

Patient Profile: Male, 68 years of age, and recently widowed

Chief Complaint: "My gums itch and bleed whenever I brush my teeth. I wish I could do something for my dry mouth and bad breath."

Medical History: BP: 140/90; hospitalized 6 months ago when he was treated for a heart attack

Dental History: Last cleaning was approximately 5 years ago

Social History: Limited alcohol drinker, nonsmoker

Periodontal Assessment: Patient requires quadrant scaling with local anesthesia to allow for comfortable periodontal therapy treatment

Treatment Plan: Four quadrants of scaling with lidocaine 1:100,000 + epinephrine

Through no fault of her own, the dental hygienist is 15 minutes behind schedule and feels pressured to seat this next patient before he starts to complain to the receptionist. In her haste, she forgets to ask her patient for an update on his medical history and only takes the blood pressure.

What are the legal, ethical, and safety issues that the hygienist needs to consider?

Local anesthetics used for the purpose of hemostatic and pain control help with reducing patient anxiety and improving patient comfort during the appointment. However, patients with cardiovascular disease have a greater potential for epinephrine overdose; vasopressors are relative contraindications. The risk versus the benefit of using a low concentration of epinephrine should be considered and the patient's physician should be consulted (see Chapter 48 on patients with cardiovascular disease). The hygienist always needs to take the time to review the medical history to avoid the legal, ethical, and safety ramifications that may result because of negligence and pressure to satisfy patients.

BOX 43.9 Dialogue With Patient to Evaluate an Alleged Allergic Reaction to a Local Anesthetic

- Describe exactly what occurred.
- What treatment was given?
- What position were you in during the injection?
- What was the time sequence of events?
- What drug was used?
- What amount of drug was administered?
- Did the drug contain a vasoconstrictor?
- Were you taking any other medications at the time of the incident?
- What is the name and address of the doctor (dentist, physician, hospital) who was treating you when the reaction occurred?

Adapted from Malamed SF. *Handbook of Local Anesthesia.* 7th ed. Elsevier; 2020.

Dental hygiene care requiring LAs (topical or injectable) should be delayed until an evaluation of the patient is complete. Dental hygiene procedures not requiring anesthesia may be performed in the interim.

For patients who have a confirmed allergy to LAs, management varies according to the nature of the allergy. Table 43.7 lists alternative drugs that may be employed in place of agents that cause an allergic response.

Clinical Manifestations and Management

The amount of time that elapses between exposure to an allergenic agent and manifestation of signs and symptoms is important. As a rule, the more rapid the onset of signs and symptoms after exposure, the more severe the ultimate reaction.[4] Conversely, the greater the time between exposure and onset of signs and symptoms, the less severe the reaction. This time factor helps the dental hygienist determine the appropriate management of the reaction.

The most common allergic reaction associated with LAs is a dermatologic reaction. A skin reaction that appears alone or after a considerable lapse of time (60 minutes or more) is usually not life-threatening; however, if a skin reaction develops rapidly, it may be the first indication of an ensuing generalized reaction.

An allergic reaction may manifest solely in the respiratory tract or may accompany other systemic responses. In slowly evolving generalized allergic reactions, respiratory distress follows skin and gastrointestinal reactions but occurs before cardiovascular signs and symptoms.

Generalized anaphylaxis is the most life-threatening allergic reaction. Most reactions develop quickly, reaching maximum intensity within 5 to 30 minutes of exposure, although delayed responses have been reported.[4]

Table 43.24 describes the signs and symptoms and the management of patients with dermatologic and respiratory reactions and generalized anaphylaxis. Reaction types are further defined as delayed or immediate.

TRENDS THAT PROMOTE PATIENTS' FREEDOM FROM PAIN

Patients will often comment that receiving an intraoral injection stings or burns. This happens because of the acidic nature of the anesthetic solution. For example, an LA with a vasoconstrictor has a pH of approximately 3.5.[1] The body's pH is approximately 7.4. Before this acidic solution can cross the nerve membrane to block the nerve conduction, it must buffer itself to a level above 7.35, which can take up to 10 minutes.[1] A buffering agent added to a local anesthesia is one trend used in dentistry. A buffer is a basic pH (sodium bicarbonate) added to highly acidic LA solutions to raise the pH. Buffering systems are available using a penlike device to be used at chairside, resulting in reduction of patient pain and faster onset of analgesia.[1,3]

Another issue that concerns patients is the long duration of soft tissue anesthesia (STA) or numbness of the lips, cheeks, and tongue. The STA can last long after the patient has left the dental office and can interrupt normal daily activities such as eating, drinking, and speaking. For certain patients, this lack of sensation is awkward or embarrassing and in some instances, causes self-inflicted injury. A vasodilator reversal agent, phentolamine mesylate, is sometimes used to reverse the long duration of STA or numbness after dental care. Children and patients with special needs may benefit because of the risk of self-inflicted injuries caused by not being able to control numb lips, cheeks, and tongue or understand postoperative instructions. A dose of the reversal agent is administered through injection and based on an equal ratio to the amount of LA plus vasoconstrictor that was given; however, the maximum dosage is two cartridges. Using this reversal agent has the potential of reducing the time of STA significantly.[1,3]

A nasal spray LA is another product that has been used in patients undergoing nasal surgery but can certainly have implications for dental hygiene care. Patients receiving the intranasal LA reported that their maxillary teeth felt different. This type of anesthesia could particularly be useful for needle-phobic patients and in cosmetic dentistry. Because the combined 3% tetracaine with the vasoconstrictor oxymetazoline is an ester-type anesthetic, the dental hygienist should use caution for its various contraindications.[1,3,9]

Another trend for future applications in dentistry is a biologic technique known as optogenetics which uses both genetics and light to

TABLE 43.24   Clinical Manifestations and Management of an Allergic Reaction

Type of Allergic Response	Signs and Symptoms	Management
Delayed		
Skin	Erythema Urticaria (hives) Pruritus (itching) Angioedema (localized swelling of extremities, lips, tongue, pharynx, larynx)	Administer antihistamine Obtain medical consultation
Respiration	Bronchospasm Distress Dyspnea Wheezing Perspiration Flushing Cyanosis Tachycardia Anxiety	Step 1: Terminate procedure Step 2: Position patient semierect Step 3: Reassure patient Step 4: Provide basic life support as indicated Step 5: Summon medical assistance if needed Step 6: Administer epinephrine Step 7: Monitor vital signs Step 8: Administer antihistamine Step 9: Allow patient to recover, then discharge
Laryngeal edema	Swelling of vocal apparatus and subsequent obstruction of airway Respiratory distress Exaggerated chest movements High-pitched sound to no sound Cyanosis Loss of consciousness	Step 1: Terminate procedure Step 2: Position patient supine Step 3: Summon medical assistance Step 4: Administer epinephrine Step 5: Maintain airway Step 6: Administer oxygen Additional drug management: antihistamine, corticosteroid Additional step: Cricothyrotomy if needed Step 7: Transfer patient to hospital
Immediate Anaphylaxis		
Skin	Pruritus (itching) Flushing Urticaria (face and upper chest) Feeling of hair standing on end Conjunctivitis, vasomotor rhinitis	Step 1: Terminate procedure Step 2: Position patient supine, legs elevated Step 3: Provide basic life support as indicated Step 4: Summon medical assistance Step 5: Administer epinephrine Step 6: Administer oxygen Step 7: Monitor vital signs Additional drug management: antihistamine, corticosteroid Step 8: Transport patient to hospital
Gastrointestinal or genitourinary	Abdominal cramps Nausea, vomiting Diarrhea	Same as management of anaphylaxis related to skin
Respiratory	Substernal tightness or chest pain Cough, wheezing Dyspnea Cyanosis of mucous membranes, nail beds Laryngeal edema	Same as management of anaphylaxis related to skin
Cardiovascular	Pallor Lightheadedness Palpitations, tachycardia Hypotension Cardiac dysrhythmias Unconsciousness Cardiac arrest	Same as management of anaphylaxis related to skin

Modified from Little JW, Falace DA, Miller CS, Rhodus NL: *Dental Management of the Medically Compromised Patient*. 9th ed. Elsevier; 2018.

control neuroactivity. Light-activated compounds are targeted at precise areas needing treatment, thereby minimizing or avoiding unnecessary STA and modulating a patient's discomfort. Although very early in development, this technique may have promise for a new means of managing pain, thus meeting the patient's needs to include wholesome facial image and freedom from stress and fear in addition to freedom from pain.[1]

Visit the website at http://evolve.elsevier.com/Pieren/Hygiene for competency forms, suggested readings, glossary, and related websites.

KEY CONCEPTS

- Local anesthesia is the temporary loss of sensation in a circumscribed area brought about by the reduction of nerve membrane permeability to sodium ions. When sodium ions are blocked, the nerve cell cannot depolarize, stopping transmission of a stimulus to the brain.
- LA agents are classified chemically as either amides or esters, which differ in how they are metabolized: esters are metabolized in the blood by pseudocholinesterase, and amides are metabolized primarily in the liver with the exception of articaine.
- LA agents produce vasodilation. For the maximum anesthetic effect, vasoconstrictors are often combined with LAs to slow down absorption, reduce hemorrhage, and increase the length of time the anesthesia is effective.
- Many LA drugs are available. The clinician must choose the best agent for the circumstances, considering each of the following: the health of the patient, medications taken by the patient, possible patient allergies, the amount of time anesthesia is desired, the areas being anesthetized, the planned procedure and injections, the patient's past response to anesthesia, and the possible need for hemostasis.
- There is a maximum amount of LA agent and vasoconstrictor that can safely be administered to a patient at one time. This amount varies with the patient's weight, health status, and age, and with the specific agent administered.
- A thorough health history evaluation before LA delivery is crucial. Many medications influence a patient's response to local anesthesia. There are also several systemic conditions that require modifications of LA delivery, such as pregnancy, hyperthyroidism, liver dysfunction, renal dysfunction, allergies to sulfites that are found in cartridges to preserve vasoconstrictors, atypical plasma cholinesterase, methemoglobinemia, and malignant hyperthermia.
- Medications that are excreted through the kidneys may be retained in the body of the diabetic patient with kidney disease, causing toxic effects. When LA agents are administered, minimal use of vasoconstrictors is required because epinephrine is capable of raising blood glucose. A medical consult is appropriate.
- The local anesthesia armamentarium includes a syringe, a needle, LA agent, topical anesthetic agent, cotton-tipped applicators, gauze, cotton forceps or hemostat, a needle recapping device, and a mouth mirror.
- Oral anesthetic procedures involve the maxillary and mandibular branches of cranial nerve V, the trigeminal nerve.
- There are three categories of local anesthesia procedures: local infiltration, field block (supraperiosteal), and nerve block. These differ in the relationship between the area anesthetized and the area of delivery of the anesthetic agent, and in the scope of the area anesthetized; nerve blocks are delivered further from the treatment site and anesthetize a larger area when compared with field blocks (supraperiosteal), which are delivered directly at the apex of the target tooth and anesthetize only one to two teeth.
- The attitude and demeanor of the clinician have a significant impact on the comfort of the patient and the overall success of the LA injection.
- Local anesthesia procedures for maxillary anesthesia include papillary, anterior superior alveolar field block, middle superior alveolar field block, infraorbital nerve block, posterior superior alveolar nerve block, greater palatine nerve block, nasopalatine nerve block, and the anterior middle superior alveolar nerve block.
- Local anesthesia procedures for mandibular anesthesia include the inferior alveolar nerve block, buccal nerve block, mental nerve block, incisive nerve block, and Gow-Gates nerve block.
- LA delivery has the potential to cause both local and systemic complications. Potential local complications include needle breakage, pain during injection, burning during injection, hematoma, facial nerve paralysis, paresthesia, trismus, infection, edema, tissue sloughing, soft tissue trauma, and postanesthetic intraoral lesions. Potential systemic complications include LA overdose, epinephrine overdose, and allergy. Most of these potential complications can be avoided with proper preanesthetic patient assessment, careful selection of anesthetic agent, conscientious delivery techniques, and proper postoperative instructions.

ACKNOWLEDGMENT

The authors acknowledge Renee Hannebrink, Gwen Essex, Michele Darby, Margaret Walsh, and Elena Ortega for their past contributions to this chapter.

REFERENCES

1. Malamed SF. *Handbook of Local Anesthesia*. 7th ed. Elsevier; 2020.
2. Arua S, Ngwu CC, Agbo EE, Silas H, Ucheka PI. The roles of dental therapists as frontline clinicians. *Orapua Literature Reviews*. 2021;1(1):OR005.
3. Logothetis D. *Local Anesthesia for the Dental Hygienist*. 3rd ed. Elsevier; 2022.
4. Malamed SF. *Medical Emergencies in the Dental Office*. 8th ed. Elsevier; 2023.
5. Babak B, Hersh E, Hilario M, Alvarez K, Mc Laughlin B. True allergy to amide local anesthetics: a review and case presentation. *Anesth Prog*. 2018 Summer;65(2):119–123.
6. Oraqix. Product information available from DENTSPLY Pharmaceuticals, York, PA. Available at: www.dentsplydental.com.
7. US Department of Labor—Occupational Safety & Health Administration. Standard Interpretation Re: 1910.1030. Available at: http://www.osha.gov/pls/oshaweb/owadisp.show_document?p_table=INTERPRETATIONS&p_id=25618.
8. Fehrenbach M, Herring S. *Illustrated Anatomy of the Head and Neck*. 6th ed. Elsevier; 2021.
9. Ciancio S, Marberger A, Ayoub F, et al. Comparison of 3 intranasal mists for anesthetizing maxillary teeth in adults: a randomized, double-masked, multicenter phase 3 clinical trial. *J Am Dent Assoc*. 2016;147(5):339–347.e1.

44

Nitrous Oxide–Oxygen Sedation

Anthony S. Carroccia and Ann Brunick

PROFESSIONAL OPPORTUNITIES

Dental professionals must strive to deliver comprehensive and appropriate care to patients while ensuring they are as comfortable as possible. The dental hygienist, with the knowledge of nitrous oxide–oxygen (N_2O-O_2) sedation, will have a distinct advantage in achieving this goal. The competent provider using this evidence-based method can minimize pain and anxiety for a large number of patients.

COMPETENCIES

1. Determine whether administration of N_2O-O_2 sedation is appropriate, based on the indications and contraindications for its use.
2. Provide information for patients about the advantages and disadvantages of N_2O-O_2 sedation for patient introduction to the procedure.
3. Recognize the signs and symptoms associated with safe and effective administration of N_2O-O_2 sedation.
4. Discuss equipment associated with N_2O-O_2 sedation, ensure patient and provider safety by monitoring the many safety features associated with N_2O-O_2 sedation equipment, and describe various delivery styles for sedation.
5. Describe administration and monitoring of N_2O-O_2 sedation, recognize potential complications that may occur during N_2O-O_2 sedation, and acknowledge appropriate response measures.

INTRODUCTION TO SEDATION AND NITROUS OXIDE

Dental anxiety affects millions of people.[1] There is fear of the unknown with a dental problem, the corrective measures, the costs, and, arguably the most crucial, the pain. Every dental team member must strive to deliver oral healthcare as comfortably as possible. The most common and familiar way to achieve this goal is through local anesthesia. A helpful adjunct to local anesthesia is sedation.

Sedation is the reduction of anxiety or agitation typically by administering sedative drugs. It can be classified in many ways. One such classification is according to the route of administration. Sedation can be introduced through the oral route and the intravenous route. A common dental sedation route is inhalation, historically accomplished with nitrous oxide and oxygen.[1]

Today, the route is not considered as important as the depth of sedation. Therefore in-office dental sedation is classified as minimal, moderate, or deep. **Minimal sedation** is best defined as a minimally depressed level of consciousness, produced by a pharmacologic method that retains the patient's ability to independently and continuously maintain an airway and respond *normally* to tactile stimulation and verbal commands. Although cognitive function and coordination

may be modestly impaired, ventilatory and cardiovascular functions are unaffected.[2]

Moderate sedation is a drug-induced depression of consciousness, during which patients respond *purposefully* to verbal commands, either alone or accompanied by light tactile stimulation. No interventions are required to maintain a patient's airway; spontaneous ventilation is adequate and cardiovascular function is usually maintained.[2] N_2O-O_2 sedation combined with any synergistic sedative drug renders a patient in the category of moderate sedation.

Deep sedation is a drug-induced depression of consciousness during which patients are not aroused easily, but they will respond to painful or repeated stimulation. The ability to maintain ventilatory function can be compromised.[2]

Nitrous oxide, when used in combination with other sedative agent(s), may produce minimal, moderate, or deep sedation, or even general anesthesia. If more than one oral drug is administered to achieve the desired sedation effect, with or without the concurrent use of nitrous oxide, the patient is considered in moderate sedation.[2] In other words, the addition of nitrous oxide to other sedatives will make the sedation deeper. Careful and constant monitoring is always required with any level of in-office sedation. One of the primary advantages of using N_2O-O_2 as a sedative is its ability to be titrated. **Titration** is best defined as the administration of incremental doses of an intravenous or inhalation drug over time until a desired effect is reached.[2]

Environmental or room air is comprised primarily of (~78%) nitrogen gas, which is of no benefit for respiration. The second most common gas is oxygen (~21%), which humans need for respiration, whereas the other ~1% contains trace gases. Nitrous oxide is a colorless, slightly sweet-smelling gas. The body prefers nitrous oxide more than either atmospheric nitrogen or oxygen individually. The relative insolubility of this gas explains why the onset is so much faster than other anesthetic gases. Although nitrous oxide is a good analgesic, it is a weak general anesthetic. Nitrous oxide is a central nervous system depressant. Its application promotes increased pain tolerance and decreases stress, both of which are beneficial during a dental appointment, especially for anxious or fearful patients. Although the exact mechanism of action is unknown, several nerve receptors are implicated, which may explain why it has the effects it does. It is acceptable to reassure patients that they are doing well while they are receiving N_2O-O_2 sedation.

Patients sedated with N_2O-O_2 or other pharmacologic agents should be classified by their health history and in accordance with the American Society of Anesthesiologists (ASA) Physical Status Classification System. An ASA I patient is healthy, whereas a person with a mild systemic disease that is controlled, such as hypertension, would be considered an ASA II patient. The ASA III patient has a severe systemic disease. An example would be a patient with diabetes and elevated blood glucose. An ASA IV classification is used disease is a constant threat to life. The ASA Physical Status Classification System is a valuable assessment tool in cooperation with the comprehensive health history.[2]

INDICATIONS

N_2O-O_2 sedation is indicated in the following situations:

- Pain management
- Anxiety relief
- Assistance with hypersensitive gag response
- Assistance for lengthy procedures

Pain and Anxiety

Anxiety is best defined by the International Association for the Study of Pain as a nonspecific feeling of apprehension, worry, uneasiness, or dread, the source of which may be vague or unknown. It is a normal reaction when a person's body, lifestyle, values, or loved ones are threatened.[3] Anxious patients are quite concerned about dental treatment; therefore, good communication and listening skills are necessary. The use of N_2O-O_2 sedation can be beneficial for a successful appointment.

For children, anxiety can also be a concern, and unruly or fidgeting children can test a practitioner's patience. N_2O-O_2 sedation can help soothe the child and allay the fear and anxiety to get treatment completed in a timely fashion.

Nitrous oxide is not a replacement for local anesthesia; however, it can make the injection process more comfortable. In rare cases, patients have a true allergy to some dental local anesthetic drugs; therefore N_2O-O_2 sedation for minor procedures normally warranting local anesthesia could be better than no pharmacologic assistance at all.

The patient who has controlled cardiovascular disease or hypertension is typically a candidate for N_2O-O_2 sedation. The vasodilation that nitrous oxide induces relaxes the great vessels and helps the heart not work as hard in a potentially stressful environment. Together with the increased oxygen that is respired beyond room air, it is easy to see why these patients are well served by this adjunct.

Gag Response

Some patients have a hyperactive gag response and/or reflex. The use of N_2O-O_2 sedation can help offset the gag response as the patient's gag reflex relaxes. Useful examples for its use are for patients who have difficulty taking radiographs or tolerating periodontal debridement in the molar areas.

Lengthy Procedures

Sedation helps patients with challenges in sitting for great lengths of time, such as individuals with back or leg problems. Due to the amnesic properties, time can pass with less repercussion of restlessness.[3]

RELATIVE CONTRAINDICATIONS TO USE

Very few true contraindications exist with N_2O-O_2 sedation. However, it is important to realize this adjunct is not appropriate for everyone. The following conditions and situations would warrant postponement or refrainment:

- Pregnancy
- Claustrophobia
- Cystic fibrosis
- Chronic obstructive pulmonary diseases
- Upper respiratory infections
- Pneumoencephalography
- Language or consent

- Drug or alcohol abuse
- Recent eye or ear surgeries

Pregnancy

There are some health professionals who assert nitrous oxide may be the only sedative to use during pregnancy; many more believe it is imperative to avoid its use. Regardless, in the first trimester, no drugs are recommended. In the third trimester, there is a concern with low oxygen tension and levels of homocysteine. Any time N_2O-O_2 sedation is considered for a pregnant woman, a medical consult is warranted. Paradoxically, nitrous oxide is a drug that can be administered for labor and delivery assistance.

All dental and dental hygiene care providers, especially if pregnant, should minimize exposure to nitrous oxide. The clinical work environment can be tested for trace waste anesthetic gas. It is vital to follow all of the best practice guidelines to protect pregnancy and fertility. Many offices do not allow dental team members to work with nitrous oxide during pregnancy.

Claustrophobia

Patients with this condition are already not fond of dental professionals in their personal space. They may be unable to tolerate this type of sedation primarily because of the need to wear a traditional nasal hood. However, new nasal hoods that are less intrusive are available and may prove to be a more viable option.

Cystic Fibrosis

A patient with cystic fibrosis may incur bullae or bubblelike cavities filled with air in the lungs. This situation may be exacerbated with nitrous oxide due to the expansive nature of the gas. Medical consultation in these instances is advised, though usage of nitrous oxide is likely not to be recommended.

Chronic Obstructive Pulmonary Diseases

Chronic obstructive pulmonary diseases include emphysema and chronic bronchitis. Patients with these conditions use less oxygen naturally as a sequela of their condition. Giving such a patient more than the normal amount of oxygen could cause the body to think it does not need to respire, thus initiating a respiratory crisis such as **dyspnea**, difficulty breathing, or **apnea**, which is not breathing at all. Consultation with the patient's medical team is advised.

Upper Respiratory Infections and Issues

Patients with a cold or flu typically cannot breathe well through their nasal passages, so the N_2O-O_2 induction will be improbable. A sinus infection may be problematic as well because the pharmacodynamic nature of nitrous oxide will increase the pressure in the bone-bound sinus cavities. A deviated septum could also pose a problem for certain delivery styles that introduce the medical gases only on one side of the nose.

Pneumoencephalography

Pneumoencephalography refers to a procedure during which a patient's cerebrospinal fluid is displaced with gas to better visualize the spine and/or brain.[3] If a patient needs dental treatment after such an event, N_2O-O_2 sedation is contraindicated.

Language or Consent

If the patient is unable to give verbal informed consent to treatment because of mental capacity reasons or language barriers, the proper protocol should be to discuss the situation with the caregiver or arrange for translation services. The ethical principle of autonomy must always be observed. Care must be taken to ensure the patient understands the intent and actions of the procedure and is able to alert the practitioner if adverse symptoms occur.

Drug or Alcohol Abuse

Patients who are addicted to drugs or alcohol present challenges to dental providers. Some may come to a clinic seeking prescriptions. Nitrous oxide could significantly potentiate any drug or drugs already in a patient's system. Practitioners must also be vigilant about the security of the nitrous oxide supply.

Recent Eye or Ear Surgeries

The use of halogenated gases for vitreoretinal surgery poses a contraindication for N_2O-O_2 sedation for such a time as determined by the ophthalmologist. Some ear surgeries can be problematic as pressure could build in the tympanic cavity. Again, a medical consultation is advised as to the length of time needed to postpone N_2O-O_2 sedation. Some patients express symptoms of slight hearing changes while N_2O-O_2 sedation is being administered; these changes are temporary.

CAUTIOUS USE OF NITROUS OXIDE–OXYGEN SEDATION

A category of conditions exists in which the dental hygienist should proceed with careful reflection, medical consultation, and meticulous observation of the patient if N_2O-O_2 sedation is considered to be used. These conditions include the following:

- Psychoses
- Bleomycin sulfate
- Vitamin B_{12} deficiency

Psychoses

Although many psychiatric medications do not have a serious contraindicated reaction, issues may manifest in other ways. The manifestation of antipsychotic drugs and N_2O-O_2 sedation may be unpredictable. It is best to refrain from its use, especially when a cocktail of antipsychotic drugs is prescribed.[1]

Bleomycin Sulfate

The cancer drug bleomycin sulfate has significance for dental inhalation sedation. This drug is most likely encountered as part of a combination therapy for patients who have been diagnosed with lymphomas, testicular cancer, and certain squamous cell carcinomas, including head and neck cancer and other malignancies. Patients who are taking the medication solely or in an antineoplastic combination should not receive 100% oxygen. Additional health concerns can occur with hyperoxygenation, an especially important consideration for induction and recovery with N_2O-O_2 sedation. A medical consultation is recommended prior to administration.

Vitamin B_{12} Deficiency

Methotrexate is an antimetabolite and an antifolate drug often used to treat lupus, rheumatoid arthritis, eczema, and other autoimmune diseases. Patients taking this medication can have issues with low vitamin B_{12} or cobalamin levels. This situation is similar to the earlier contraindication of pregnancy and folic acid as it affects the enzyme methionine synthase.

There are some rare genetic issues that could present a warning to the dental professional considering using N_2O-O_2 sedation. Such conditions include but are not limited to methylenetetrahydrofolate reductase deficiency, hyperhomocysteinemia reductase deficiency, and dihydropteridine reductase deficiency. The literature describes negative complications associated with a vitamin B_{12} deficiency and nitrous oxide abuse and/or chronic exposure.[3] Medical consultation is advised, and vitamin B_{12} supplementation may be prescribed prior to sedation or general anesthesia.

Advantages of Nitrous Oxide–Oxygen Sedation

There are many advantages to using N_2O-O_2 sedation:

- It works well with local anesthetics.
- It is cost effective for the patient in contrast to other sedation modalities.
- Rapid **induction** and **emergence** (onset and recovery) exists, which eliminates the need for surgical centers, expensive monitoring, or highly trained personnel.
- This sedation typically does not require a companion to transport the patient. After careful evaluation of recovery, patients are usually dismissed and function as normal.
- Its administration is allowed by hygienists with proper training and appropriate supervision in most states.[4]
- The patient is awake and responsive, with cardiac and respiratory functions intact.
- The perception of time is decreased due to the amnestic effect.
- The margin of safety and a nearly 200-year history show that the morbidity and mortality rates are virtually nonexistent for N_2O-O_2 sedation alone and when used appropriately in a dental setting.

Disadvantages of Nitrous Oxide–Oxygen Sedation

No drug is without its potential pitfalls; however, the disadvantages are minimal for this type of sedation.

- There are very few patients for whom N_2O-O_2 sedation will not work; however, some patients will have difficulty relaxing or fighting through the effects. Individuals with challenging behavior problems may need another type of sedation in addition to or in lieu of N_2O-O_2 sedation.
- Some patients experience nausea, dizziness, and other uncomfortable symptoms. These reactions are usually associated with either sedating more deeply than intended or rapid induction. Decreasing the concentration of nitrous oxide administered or discontinuing administration, depending on the severity, typically alleviates these issues.

SIGNS AND SYMPTOMS OF NITROUS OXIDE–OXYGEN SEDATION

Signs of N_2O-O_2 sedation are those responses that the clinician objectively observes in the patient that are due to the action or lack of action. The following normal signs are observed by the dental hygienist administering or monitoring a patient undergoing N_2O-O_2 sedation, although it is unlikely that all signs will occur simultaneously in all patients (Box 44.1):

- The patient will be awake and responsive.
- Normal reactions to perceived painful experiences are lessened or diminished.
- Pupil reactions are normal; however, the Verrill sign, which is the half-closed appearance of the eyelids or a slow blink rate (Fig. 44.1), may be observed. The inability to keep the eyes open is a sign of a sedation that is deeper than intended and that can easily be remedied by decreasing the nitrous oxide concentration. The patient may lacrimate or have tears in their eyes but not cry.
- Vital signs are constant and consistent, showing physiologic stability.
- The feet will cease to be upward and parallel. Often, they will separate or open, falling to the sides (Fig. 44.2).

BOX 44.1 Signs of Nitrous Oxide and Oxygen Sedation

- Awake patient
- Lessened pain reaction
- Relaxed appearance
- Normal eye reaction and pupil size
- Normal respiration rate, blood pressure, and pulse
- Minimal movement of limbs
- Flushing of skin
- Perspiration
- Lacrimation
- Lessened gagging or coughing
- Infrequent and slow speech

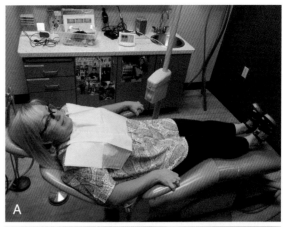

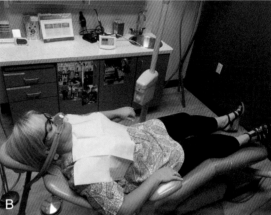

Fig. 44.2 (A) Patient before N₂O-O₂ sedation shows tension in her raised shoulders, eyes wide open, grabbing of the arm rests, and feet that are flexed, parallel, and pointed up. (B) Patient with N₂O-O₂ sedation showing signs of a good sedation with relaxed shoulders, face, and hands and with feet separated apart and fallen. (Courtesy Dr. Anthony Carroccia.)

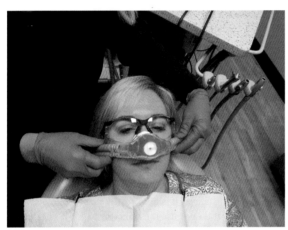

Fig. 44.1 Patient with N₂O-O₂ sedation showing Verrill sign of the eyes and a slight smile. (Courtesy Dr. Anthony Carroccia.)

- The lips will curl into a slight smile. The patient will appear content (see Fig. 44.1).
- Some patients may show peripheral perspiration or blotches of redness on the face and neck due to vasodilation of the superficial blood vessels.
- The shoulders will be relaxed and away from the neck (see Fig. 44.2).
- Hypersensitive gag response will be decreased.

A symptom is something experienced and reported by the patient to the dental professional and can be a subjective finding. The following is a list of the subjective symptoms that may be reported (Box 44.2):

- Acceptance to the procedures (e.g., local anesthetic injection) that are about to occur suggests physical and mental relaxation.
- The patient may report being unaware of time passing or have a slight anterograde amnesia of the procedure.
- Warmth may be experienced as being uncomfortable or comfortable to the patient.
- The patient may ask the provider to repeat things that have been said as they may say that sounds are distant or muffled.
- The patient may report tingling in the extremities or that their limbs feel slightly heavy.
- The patient may report that their lips tingle or feel numb, causing them to ask if their mouth is numbed already.

EQUIPMENT

The armamentarium for inhalation sedation can be divided into a few major categories—cylinders, gas machines, and delivery style.

BOX 44.2 Symptoms of Nitrous Oxide–Oxygen Sedation

- Mental and physical relaxation
- Indifference to surroundings and passage of time
- Lessened pain awareness
- Lightweight sensations or heavy feeling in extremities
- Drowsiness
- Warmth
- Tingling or numbness
- Sounds that seem distant

Cylinders

Cylinders are tanks that store the medical gases, and certain protocols exist for the care of cylinders. Each cylinder must be colored in accordance with the gas contained within. Every cylinder must have a label stating the contents and when the tank was last inspected, which must be within 5 to 10 years, dependent upon the gas. Cylinders must be secured in an upright position with a strap or chain, and tanks are not to be located near heat sources (Fig. 44.3). They should also never be near grease, oil, or any other lubricant in any manner; such a medium may contribute to combustion. It is suggested that the valves on tanks be opened halfway prior to use. A cylinder that is completely opened may have a stick or catch that makes the provider think it is closed when

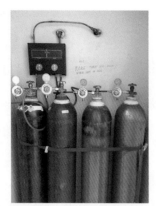

Fig. 44.3 G and H cylinders stored upright and secured and attached to a manifold. (Courtesy Dr. Anthony Carroccia.)

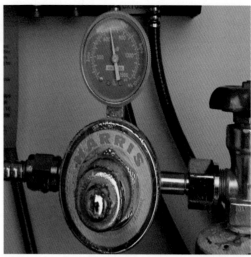

Fig. 44.5 A regulator attached to a nitrous oxide cylinder exhibits condensation. (Courtesy Dr. Anthony Carroccia.)

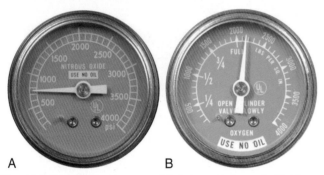

Fig. 44.4 Pressure gauges on an inhalation sedation unit. (A) Nitrous oxide pressure gauge for nitrous oxide cylinder. (B) Oxygen pressure gauge for oxygen cylinder. Note color coding of blue for nitrous oxide and green for oxygen. (Courtesy Dr. Mark Dellinges and Cory Price.)

in actuality, it is open. The cylinder valves should be closed promptly after use or at the end of the day when it is certain that no other dental care providers in the office need the gases. Tanks for portable N_2O-O_2 sedation units are smaller, size E; the cylinders for central units are size G for nitrous oxide and size H for oxygen.

In the United States, oxygen is in a green-colored tank. In many other nations, it is white, white with green shoulders, or white with a green cross. The amount of compressed gas in the cylinder will be accurately reflected on the pressure gauge. When the tank is full, it reads as such. The needle on the gauge will always correspond to the remaining oxygen in the cylinder (Fig. 44.4).

Nitrous oxide is in a blue cylinder in the United States. The contents of a full cylinder are approximately 95% liquid and 5% actual gas. The gas, being the lighter state of matter, is at the top, closest to the regulator. As nitrous oxide is used, more liquid is vaporized. The vaporization process often leaves the nitrous oxide cylinder cool to touch, and it may even exhibit frost. In the presence of humidity, condensation on the cylinder or regulator may be seen (Fig. 44.5), although this does not represent a leak. The needle on the nitrous oxide gauge will show it is full until the tank only has a minimal amount of liquid remaining (Fig. 44.6). At that time, the dial on the gauge will begin to drop. Therefore the gauge does not accurately reflect what is remaining in the tank.

Gas Machines

The gas machines for N_2O-O_2 sedation generally come in several variations of two major forms: portable and central (Fig. 44.7). Some variations include cabinet-installed or enclosed portable machines, and the mounting systems vary as well. Mounts include a flush mount, a chair

mount, wall arms, a mobile stand, and an undermount slide. Factors to consider when deciding on different modalities include ergonomics, usage, costs, and operatory space.

Regardless of the machine and mount, all machines have common parts. Attached to the tanks are regulators or pressure-reducing valves. These regulators act as a funnel for the gas coming from the tank into the line for use. The reservoir bag is an air bladder that usually holds 3 L of gas. The oxygen flush button, when depressed, will fill the reservoir bag with 100% oxygen. This high concentration and flow can be used in emergent circumstances. It is noteworthy that certain delivery styles recent to the market do not use the reservoir bag. All systems must be connected to a scavenging system or vacuum for minimizing environmental trace gas contamination.

Flowmeters have a gauge that shows the flow of gas being delivered in liters. Either a ball floating in a tube or a digital display is associated with numeric values (Fig. 44.8). The sum of oxygen and nitrous oxide flow indicates the total flow. The amount of flow should correspond with the patient's **minute volume**. Some systems retain the established minute volume as gases are introduced or decreased, whereas others must be manually adjusted. Corrective decreases in flow rate are required as nitrous oxide is introduced. The opposite is true when the nitrous oxide is terminated; the oxygen will need to be elevated. It is important to note that the nitrous oxide is expressed in a percentage of the flow rate. Today's equipment will not allow for more than 70% nitrous oxide to be given. Moreover, machines will not permit less than 30% oxygen being delivered at any time as a separate safety feature. These features are designed to ensure that the patient is as safe as possible.

Delivery Systems

A nasal hood is the most common delivery system for an ambulatory dental office setting. There are several varieties of nasal hoods and tubing. Each must have the ability to scavenge trace gas. Some companies have a variety of sizes; some offer a variety of scents. The use of an unscavenged nitrous oxide system is not permitted. Some options from manufacturers allow for autoclaving and reusing nasal hoods, whereas others are for single-patient use and intended to be disposed of.

Some delivery systems have a singular hood (Fig. 44.9). Such systems are connected to a vacuum line by tubes and a circular plastic attachment to the hood itself. Double-hood or hood-in-hood systems are available as well (Fig. 44.10). These systems incorporate an outer hood to eliminate waste gases following the expiration of gases.

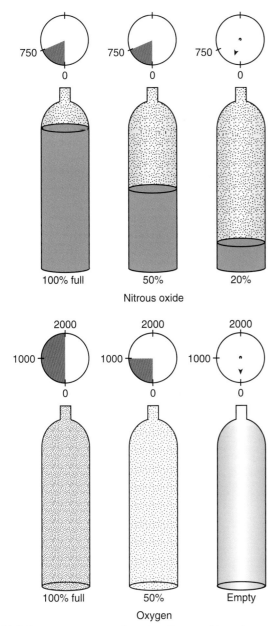

Fig. 44.6 Pressure gauge readings for nitrous oxide and oxygen cylinders. (From Clark MS, Brunick AL. *Handbook of Nitrous Oxide and Oxygen Sedation.* 5th ed. Mosby; 2019.)

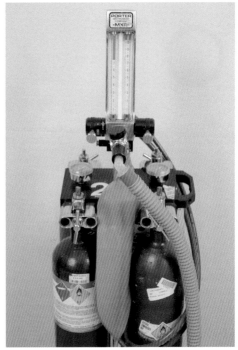

Fig. 44.7 A portable gas machine with a green cylinder containing oxygen and a blue cylinder containing nitrous oxide, stored directly on the gas machine. (Courtesy Dr. Mark Dellinges.)

Cannula systems have been introduced to the market, advocating minimal tubing and smaller profiles to eliminate dead space, increase comfort, and promote better access for delivery of patient care (Fig. 44.11). These single-use hoods and disposable systems allow gases to enter on one side and be scavenged on the other. These systems do not use a reservoir bag.

SAFETY MEASURES

Many safety measures have been introduced throughout this chapter; several more exist. Among those discussed are color coding, labels, maximum nitrous oxide flow, scavenger vacuum systems, minimum oxygen percentage, and the oxygen flush button. The portable systems using size E cylinders have another safety feature that prevents delivering 100% nitrous oxide by accidently switching the tanks. This safety measure is called the Pin Index Safety System. Each gas cylinder has a pin combination unique to that gas (Fig. 44.12). The pins must fit precisely into the cylinder stem valve before it can be opened. This safety measure is similar to a lock-and-key system in a door knob. The G and H cylinders have their own version of this in the geometry of their threaded stem valves. A Diameter Index Safety System (Fig. 44.13) ensures hoses cannot be crossed when attaching them to manifolds or flowmeters. These connections vary in both width and length.

Centrally plumbed systems have other safety measures. Copper pipes that lead from the manifold or multicylinder connection unit have different diameters for each type of gas. The size of the copper pipe for oxygen is one-half inch, as it is the most important gas, whereas the copper pipe size for nitrous oxide is three-eighths inch. Visual inspection can be performed to be certain that the lines are not erroneously switched. The manifold must be connected to an alarm system. The alarm system will alert the dental team with light and sound when the tanks are nearing empty (Fig. 44.14). It may also alert the office team if the pressure is too excessive.

A recent safety measure that may be used with N_2O-O_2 sedation is **capnography**. This measure requires a special monitor similar to those seen in surgical centers or hospitals. Instead of watching the reservoir bag for its motions of ebb and flow, the monitor visualizes the patient's exhaled carbon dioxide in wave form (Fig. 44.15). This feature allows for continuous assessment of the depth and frequency of each respiratory cycle. By watching the reservoir bag alone, the dental care provider may not be alerted to hyperventilation, hypoxia, airway obstructions, and other emergencies as quickly as with a capnometer. Emergency measures can be taken sooner if capnography is available.

Capnography is different than pulse oximetry. Pulse oximetry is used in moderate and deeper sedations. It tells the clinical team about the status of blood oxygenation. There is a slight time delay in the machine's report to actual time. Therefore capnography gives a faster indication of a crisis as it shows true respiration. Since each device monitors different things, it is not uncommon to see a sedation-oriented practice using both. Neither device is required for minimal sedation.[2]

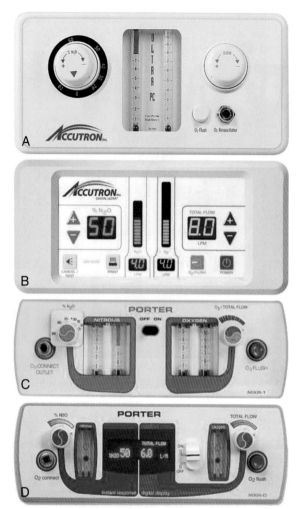

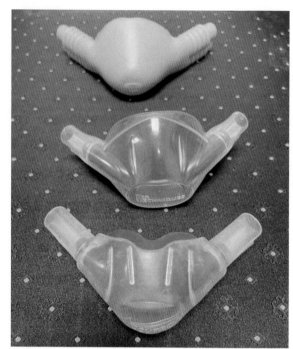

Fig. 44.10 Double-hood systems from top to bottom: Porter autoclavable, Air Techniques FlowStar, Accutron ClearView. (Courtesy Dr. Anthony Carroccia.)

Fig. 44.8 (A) Accutron traditional flowmeter. (B) Accutron digital flowmeter. (C) Porter traditional flowmeter. (D) Porter digital flowmeter.

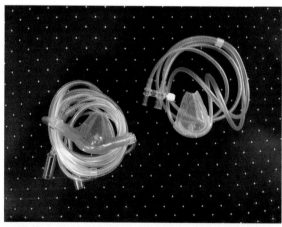

Fig. 44.11 Cannula hood systems: Accutron Axess and Porter Silhouette. (Courtesy Dr. Anthony Carroccia.)

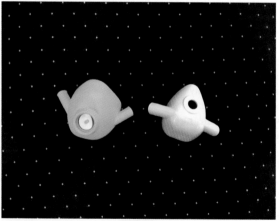

Fig. 44.9 Single-hood systems: Accutron Personal Inhaler Plus and Porter Matrx Dynomite. (Courtesy Dr. Anthony Carroccia.)

Measures are in place to make N_2O-O_2 sedation safe for both the patient and the operator. Well-fitting scavenging hoods that draw the waste anesthetic gas to the suction are an example of how to protect the operator by reducing exposure to this occupational hazard. Evidence indicates that chronic exposure to high levels of nitrous oxide can result in reproductive health issues in animals. Chronic exposure to high levels of nitrous oxide has been linked to concerns associated with vitamin B_{12} deficiency and neurologic deficits such as loss of psychomotor ability and an uncoordinated gait. In addition, blood disorders such as leukopenia and some forms of anemia can occur with chronic overexposure to nitrous oxide as well. For these reasons, it is important to minimize the mouth breathing and conversation of the patient during N_2O-O_2 sedation and ensure all equipment is connected properly with no leaks. The positioning of sweep fans to improve air circulation in the operatory and to disperse the waste anesthetic gas to the outside may be recommended. Regular inspection of hoods, hoses, bags, tanks, and flowmeters is highly encouraged. Dental personnel can also wear a dosimetry badge similar to a radiation badge to document exposure (Fig. 44.16). Exposure levels established by the American Conference of Governmental Industrial Hygienists (ACGIH) and the National Institute for Occupational Safety and Health (NIOSH) are 50 parts per million (ppm) or less for dental office personnel.

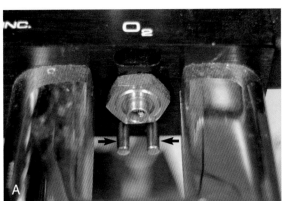
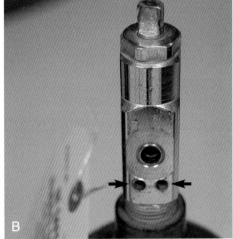

Fig. 44.12 (A) Pins *(arrows)* that are located on the yoke of the gas machine are aligned to permit attachment of only one specific type of compressed gas, either oxygen or nitrous oxide, but not both. (B) Oxygen cylinder head with holes *(arrows)* placed at a specific distance apart to fit the prongs on the yoke designed to hold oxygen cylinder. (Courtesy Dr. Mark Dellinges.)

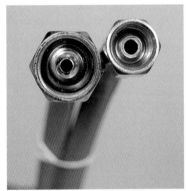

Fig. 44.13 Diameter Index Safety System. Diameter and threading of nitrous oxide coupling *(left)* differ from those of oxygen coupling *(right)*, thus preventing accidental attachments to wrong side of inhalation unit. (Courtesy Dr. Mark Dellinges and Cory Price.)

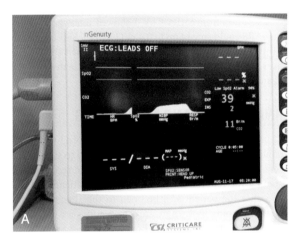

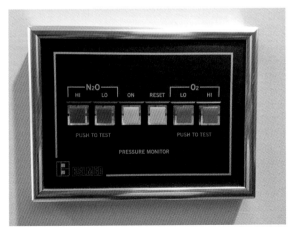

Fig. 44.14 Nitrous oxide and oxygen alarm panel. (Courtesy Dr. Anthony Carroccia.)

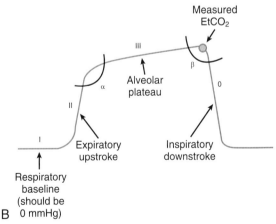

Fig. 44.15 (A) Capnometer for capnography. (B) Capnogram wave form of capnography. *EtCO₂*, End-tidal carbon dioxide. ([A] Courtesy Dr. Anthony Carroccia.)

SARS-CoV-2, or COVID-19, is one of the newer challenges to dentistry. This disease is an airborne coronavirus hazard, and generation of aerosols places clinical dental teams at risk. Aerosols are generated by ultrasonic instruments as well as handpieces and polishing equipment.

Much is still being learned about the short-term and long-term issues of prevention, infection, vaccination, and recovery. Questions may arise about disinfection of nitrous oxide and oxygen tubing systems. If cannula-based delivery styles are being used, they are disposable. Other nasal hoods are for single-patient use and can be discarded. One

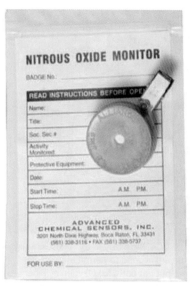

Fig. 44.16 Nitrous Oxide Dosimeter Badge.

system is autoclavable. The tubing is considered a semicritical instrument. Hui's studies from SARS-CoV-1 showed that when respiring at 4 L/min, SARS could spread up to 0.4 m (15.75 inches) inside the tubing.[5-7] This means that the tubing should be detached and cleaned per the office's specifications in accordance with the Centers for Disease Control and Prevention (CDC) specifications.

ADMINISTRATION AND MONITORING

The technique of administering and monitoring N_2O-O_2 sedation is not complicated. Prudent observation is the secret to success. Observation entails communicating with the patient, and recognizing signs and listening for reports of symptoms by the patients. Confidence is key because the patient will be open to the suggestion that the appointment is going well. There are four sections for consideration: the preparation, administration, recovery, and postoperative phases (Procedure 44.1).

Preparation Phase

The preparation phase involves the patient and the armamentarium. At the beginning of any dental appointment, it is important to review the medical history, discuss any concerns with the patient, and seek consultation if needed. Informed consent for the use of N_2O-O_2 sedation includes a discussion of what is intended, expected experiences, and answers to any questions about the risks, benefits, or complications associated with N_2O-O_2 sedation (Box 44.3). Consent is obtained and client education is provided before the procedure so the patient is alert and can interact as needed (Box 44.4).

Preparation of equipment includes ensuring the equipment is properly assembled, all connections are secure, and the vacuum or suction line is on. It is recommended that vacuum or scavenger lines run at 45 liters per minute (L/min) and are vented to the outdoors. The hoses and bag require regular inspection for punctures, tears, or rips, and should be replaced, if indicated. Preoperative vital signs are recommended for every patient. Next, the best-sized nasal hood is selected for the patient. It should fit close to the skin (Fig. 44.17). If the nasal hood cannot fit closely, gauze is useful (Fig. 44.18; see also Fig. 44.1).

Administration Phase

The administration phase begins when the cylinders are opened and the manifold alarm system is activated if using a central system. The

---

PROCEDURE 44.1 Administration and Monitoring of Nitrous Oxide–Oxygen Sedation

1. Open tanks and turn on vacuum line. Check connections and equipment.
2. Review patient's health history for any contraindications.
3. Discuss risks, benefits, and complications with the patient. Obtain the patient's consent.
4. Obtain and record the patient's vital signs
5. Select hood, and attach to hoses.
6. Initiate flow of 100% oxygen.
    a. Adults: initially set at ~6 L/min; children: initially set at ~4 L/min.
    b. Securely place nasal hood on patient. Gauze under the hood and on the bridge of the nose may need to be placed.
7. Determine minute volume. Fill the reservoir bag ⅔ full with oxygen by pressing the flush button.
    a. Decrease the flow if the bag overfills.
    b. Increase the flow if it empties.
8. Begin nitrous oxide administration with 10% to 20% flow rate. Maintain the established minute volume.
9. Add nitrous oxide in 5% to 10% increments and wait a few minutes to evaluate effect (see Table 44.1).
10. Accomplish dental procedures when appropriate sedation is achieved.
11. Terminate the nitrous oxide flow and correct the minute volume with 100% oxygen.
12. Sit the patient up at least halfway; leave the patient on oxygen for at least 5 minutes.
13. Reassess emotional and physical state; compare with when the patient was seated. Make sure the patient is alert and oriented.
14. Check and record the vital signs. Ensure readings are similar to preoperative values.
15. Dismiss the patient.
16. Record the data:
    a. Preoperative and postoperative vital signs
    b. Times sedation began and ended
    c. Maximum concentration of nitrous oxide delivered and oxygenation time
    d. Complications, if any, and corrective actions taken
17. Discard the disposables; clean, disinfect, and/or sterilize other components.

---

reservoir bag should be filled about two-thirds full by depressing the oxygen flush button. A good rule of thumb for the initial flow rate of oxygen is 6 L/min for the average adult and 4 L/min for a child. To ensure patient comfort and adequate flow, it is necessary to observe the reservoir bag after placing the nasal hood on the patient with the oxygen flowing. A bag that is deflated indicates the patient is breathing deeply or heavily enough to warrant an increase in the flow rate. Conversely, if the bag is distended, the problem may be an occlusion of the line or the rate is too great; a decrease in the flow rate is required (Fig. 44.19). Once the proper flow rate has been established, nitrous oxide can be introduced as oxygen is reduced, thus keeping the flow rate constant. The initial introduction of nitrous oxide may be up to 20%. After each increase in the percentage of nitrous oxide, a few minutes should pass to evaluate the effect (see Boxes 44.1 and 44.2). Approximately 3 to 5 minutes are required by the brain to process each dose. Add increments of 5% to 10% nitrous oxide, adjusting the flow rate and waiting a few minutes to observe the patient's response, until the proper signs and symptoms are observed (Table 44.1). It may be necessary to reduce the nitrous oxide concentration to help the patient feel more comfortable if a deeper level than intended was reached or if the patient seems to need less drug once relaxed.

- The dental hygienist has the legal responsibility to practice within the scope authorized by state law concerning N_2O-O_2 sedation administration.
- Informed consent is required prior to N_2O-O_2 sedation.
- The dental hygienist must evaluate the patient's health history carefully to determine suitability for N_2O-O_2 sedation.
- The dental hygienist is responsible for protecting the patient while they are under the influence of N_2O-O_2 sedation during dental hygiene care.
- The dental hygienist must document completely the provision of N_2O-O_2 sedation in the patient's record.

BOX 44.4 **Patient Education Tips**

- Explain what N_2O-O_2 sedation is and what it does.
- Explain the sensations that will be experienced, and describe them in positive terms (e.g., warmth, tingling).
- Explain that patients are in control and responsive at all times. If they feel they are receiving too much sedation, they simply need to alert the hygienist so that the nitrous oxide will be decreased and the oxygen increased.

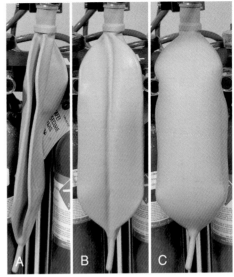

Fig. 44.19 (A) Deflated reservoir bag usually indicates either a leak around the mask or a deficient minute volume. (B) Partially inflated reservoir bag usually indicates adequate seal and minute volume. (C) Distended reservoir bag indicates either an overly large minute volume or occluded breathing tubes. (Courtesy Dr. Mark Dellinges and Cory Price.)

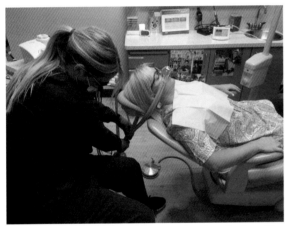

Fig. 44.17 The hood is tightened by adjusting the slip ring. (Courtesy Dr. Anthony Carroccia.)

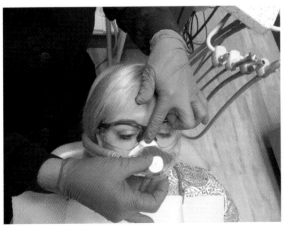

Fig. 44.18 A folded 2 × 2 gauze is placed under the hood and over the bridge of the nose to prevent leaks. (Courtesy Dr. Anthony Carroccia.)

The equilibrium point of both gases is noteworthy. Most patients will attain an appropriate level of sedation with less than 50% nitrous oxide. Once the 50% marker is reached, care must be taken as exceeding this amount, especially with a child, is considered moderate sedation by definition.[8] A smaller percentage of patients require more nitrous oxide; however, the decision to exceed 50% nitrous oxide should be carefully considered.

The amount of nitrous oxide needed for sedation is not an exact science. It will vary from patient to patient and can vary for an individual from one appointment to the next.[1] Often, the disposition of the patient is an influential factor. During the titration, the reservoir bag or capnograph, if available, is watched for proper flow rate and respirations. It is not uncommon to need minor adjustments as the appointment transpires. A dental hygienist may choose to briefly increase the nitrous oxide when an injection is given or during periodontal debridement of deeper pockets and then reduce the anesthetic gas when procedures less likely to cause discomfort are performed.

Recovery Phase

The recovery phase is the reverse of induction. The reversal must include the return of the patient's original emotional and physiologic state. As the gases are inhaled for effect, they will also be exhaled. Nitrous oxide is neither metabolized by the liver nor excreted by the kidneys. Placing the patient on 100% oxygen will saturate the respiratory system with oxygen. Since the body prefers nitrous oxide to oxygen, this competition is often necessary. Furthermore, since the sedation can occur within minutes, so can the emergence. It is recommended that the patient receive 100% oxygen postoperatively for a minimum of 5 minutes. This time is usually sufficient for a patient to return to a normal state. There are exceptions as some patients may require more oxygenation time. Assessment is also accomplished by asking the patient how they feel. Preoperative vital signs are retaken and compared with postoperative vital signs. Postoperative values should be similar to the earlier values. Patients may report being cold, or shivering could be witnessed. This response is a direct result of the vasoconstriction of the vessels as the nitrous oxide and its vasodilation exits the body. Patients

TABLE 44.1   Percent of Nitrous Oxide Administered

Nitrous Oxide (Liters per Minute)	OXYGEN (LITERS PER MINUTE)									
	1	2	3	4	5	6	7	8	9	10
1	50	33	25	20	17	14	13	11	10	9
2	67	50	40	33	29	25	22	20	18	17
3		60	50	43	38	33	30	27	25	23
4		67	57	50	44	40	36	33	31	29
5			63	56	50	45	42	38	36	33
6			67	60	55	50	46	43	40	38
7			70	64	58	54	50	47	44	41
8				67	62	57	53	50	47	44
9				69	64	60	56	53	50	47
10					67	63	59	56	53	50

Greater than 70% nitrous oxide administered exceeds amount able to be delivered by sedation machine.

should be alert and oriented. Only after the clinician is confident that the patient has returned to a normal physiologic and emotional disposition should the patient be dismissed.

Postoperative Phase

After the patient has been dismissed, the operatory is disinfected, instruments are sterilized, and documentation occurs. First, disposable sundries and single-use nasal hoods are discarded, and hoses and bag are disinfected because they are noncritical instruments. Items are sterilized if necessary. The clinician should be cognizant of all standard precautions.

Documentation of the procedures done is mandatory to be considered fully completed. An undocumented procedure is considered as if it did not happen (see Chapter 24 on Dental Hygiene Care Plan, Evaluation, and Documentation). A review of the health history, medications, ASA classification, and vital signs should be noted. It is important to list the times the administration began and ended. The maximum percentage of nitrous oxide administered must also be recorded and is likely required by state law. If there were any complications or side effects, those should be listed in addition to the corrective measures taken. The record should also reflect that the patient was alert, oriented after administration of a minimum of 5 minutes of 100% oxygen, and then dismissed. Finally, the record should be initialed or signed by the dental professional responsible for administering N_2O-O_2 sedation. See Box 44.5 for scenarios to apply principles important to the administration of N_2O-O_2 sedation.

COMPLICATIONS

All dental procedures have risks that could lead to complications. Nitrous oxide is a drug and should be respected as such. Risks and

BOX 44.5   Critical Thinking Scenario A

Complete the following critical thinking scenarios, applying the information learned in this chapter.

Scenario 1. You have an energetic 6-year-old boy present for his biannual dental appointment. You discuss the treatment plan with the parent and obtain consent to continue with an oral examination, oral prophylaxis, fluoride treatment, and sealants on the first molars. As you begin, you find he has difficulty keeping his mouth open, his attention span is short, and he has a highly responsive gag reflex.
- Practice obtaining informed consent from the parent and acceptance from the child for N_2O-O_2 sedation.

Scenario 2. An adult new to your dental practice indicates she has not had regular dental care during her life and thus says the appointments she did have were often to resolve complicated issues associated with pain and anxiety. Describe how N_2O-O_2 sedation could assist her.
- Role play a description of what can be expected with N_2O-O_2 sedation, and indicate the risks, benefits, and complications.

Scenario 3. You have established that your 40-year-old patient is anxious because he explains that he has not seen a dentist in over 5 years after a bad experience. He is worried he will have a lot of problems and he does not have dental insurance. He admits he is not good about his oral hygiene routine and has noticed sensitive and bleeding gums. He consents to using N_2O-O_2 sedation for his appointment today.
- What steps would you need to take for preparation, administration, emergence, and documentation that are associated with the procedure?

complications associated with N_2O-O_2 sedation are not severe or frequent.

Nausea is the most common complication, but it happens infrequently. Nausea may result for many various reasons. It could be from anxiety or from a heavy meal ingested shortly before the dental appointment. Children are more predisposed to nausea than adults. The incidence of vomiting is 0.5% or 1 in 200 patients, and most vomiting occurs as a result of sedating the patient more deeply than intended.[3] If a patient indicates nausea, lower the nitrous oxide concentration, and place the patient immediately on 100% oxygen. This change alone may help alleviate the feeling. If vomiting occurs, have the patient turn to the side and use a wastebasket while being ready with suction. It is important to avoid aspiration of the vomitus into the lungs to prevent an emergency situation.

CONCLUSION

The use of N_2O-O_2 sedation administration and monitoring is a positive way, when indicated, to assist the patient through the dental hygiene appointment. N_2O-O_2 sedation is relatively easy to learn and has a wide safety index. The complications are exceptionally rare and their administration is quite manageable in the dental office. Educating dental hygienists about this technique will enable them to offer their patients a positive adjunct to their care to improve their experience and potentially influence the frequency of preventive and periodontal maintenance appointments essential to their health and well-being.

KEY CONCEPTS

- Delivery of nitrous oxide in combination with oxygen is an inhalation method of sedation known as N_2O-O_2 sedation. It relaxes individuals who are mildly apprehensive about the dental or dental hygiene experience and provides some pain control for procedures that are only slightly or moderately painful.
- Minimal sedation (<50% nitrous oxide) is often appropriate for most dental hygiene procedures.
- Subjective symptoms of N_2O-O_2 sedation include heaviness of limbs, lightweight sensation, tingling, decreased fear, decreased pain memory, comfortable state, feeling of warmth, and decreased awareness of time passage.
- Objective signs of a desired level of N_2O-O_2 sedation are Verrill sign, normal eye reaction and pupil size, normal blood pressure and pulse, ability to answer questions, and relaxation of hands, fingers, and mandible.
- Relative contraindications to N_2O-O_2 sedation include breathing difficulties or nasal obstruction, communication difficulties, pregnancy, chronic obstructive pulmonary diseases, negative past experiences, fear of sedation, and emotional instability.
- N_2O-O_2 sedation may be particularly useful for clients with a history of hypersensitive gag reflex or an inability to endure lengthy procedures.
- Nausea during or after N_2O-O_2 exposure may occur with a sedation level that is deeper than intended or during rapid induction of the nitrous oxide delivery.
- After the administration of N_2O-O_2 sedation, 100% oxygen should be given for a minimum of 5 minutes and until the patient is oriented and feeling normal before the client is released.
- When adjusting the proportions of nitrous oxide and oxygen to achieve the desired level of sedation, the clinician should ensure each adjustment is at the rate of 0.5 to 1 L/min nitrous oxide depending upon the minute volume or approximately 5% to 10%; allow at least 1 minute and up to 5 minutes to pass between incremental dose delivery.
- A scavenger system incorporated into the N_2O-O_2 units removes nitrous oxide that is exhaled through the mask.
- The effects of chronic exposure to high levels of trace amounts of nitrous oxide may include spontaneous abortion, birth defects, vitamin B_{12} deficiency, and neurologic signs such as loss of psychomotor ability and an uncoordinated gait.
- Informed consent is required prior to N_2O-O_2 sedation.
- To reduce exposure to trace amounts of nitrous oxide, the dental hygienist uses a scavenging mask system, ensures office air flow, discourages unnecessary patient talking, and regularly checks all the equipment for leaks.
- Before the mask is placed on the patient, minute volume is established with oxygen.
- Thorough documentation of informed consent, concentration and length of time of N_2O-O_2 administration, adverse patient reactions and their resolutions, and emergence using 100% oxygen for at least 5 minutes is required.

REFERENCES

1. Malamed SF. *Sedation: A Guide to Patient Management*. Mosby; 2017:6.
2. American Dental Association. *Guidelines for the Use of Sedation and General Anesthesia by Dentists. Adopted by the House of Delegates*; 2016. Available at: https://www.ada.org/-/media/project/ada-organization/ada/ada-org/files/resources/research/oral-health-topics/ada_sedation_use_guidelines.pdf?rev=b8b34313071d416a99182e8b37add4dd&hash=06A52EC1C4BA50BEA9ABAA5C3A6DD095. Accessed May 5, 2022.
3. Clark MS, Brunick AL. *Handbook of Nitrous Oxide and Oxygen Sedation*. Elsevier; 2019:5.
4. American Dental Hygienists Association. Nitrous oxide. 35 states. Updated March 2021. Available at: https://adha.org/resources-docs/7522_Nitrous_Oxide_by_State.pdf; 2021. Accessed May 5, 2022.
5. Hui DS. SARS: lessons learnt in Hong Kong. *J Thorac Dis*. 2013;5(S2):S-122–S-126.
6. Hui DS, Ip M, Tang JW, et al. Airflows around oxygen masks – a potential source of infection?. *Chest*. 2006;130:822–826. American College of Chest Physicians.
7. James T. Infection control in dental anesthesiology: a time for preliminary reconsideration of current practices. *Anesth Prog*. 2020;67:109–120.
8. American Academy of Pediatric Dentistry and American Academy of Pediatrics. *Guideline for Monitoring and Management of Pediatric Patients before, during, and after Sedation for Diagnostic and Therapeutic Procedures; Update*; 2019. Available at: http://www.aapd.org/media/Policies_Guidelines/G_Sedation1.pdf. Accessed May 5, 2022.

45

Children and Adolescents

Denise C. McKinney

PROFESSIONAL OPPORTUNITIES

Dental hygienists have the expertise to promote early oral health prevention through increasing oral health literacy and interprofessional collaboration and delivering evidence-based dental hygiene care to children and adolescents.

COMPETENCIES

1. Recognize the need for interprofessional collaborative practice to meet the health and oral health needs of children.
2. Promote oral health literacy among nonclinical and clinical primary care team members and caregivers.
3. Advocate for a healthy oral life span among children and adolescents.
4. Discuss fluoride consumption and therapy, including water fluoridation and fluoride toxicity.
5. Employ the Decayed, Missing, Filled Teeth (DMFT) and Decayed, Missing, Filled Surfaces (DMFS) indices to quantify clinical observations in children and adolescents.
6. Appreciate behavioral management strategies for pediatric patients during a dental care visit.

◗ EVOLVE VIDEO RESOURCE

The following video procedure and technique demonstrations are available for viewing on Evolve (http://evolve.elsevier.com/Pieren/hygiene/):
- Applying Fluoride Professionally Using the Paint-On Technique
- Applying Fluoride Professionally Using the Tray Technique

INTRODUCTION

The trajectory of a child's oral health is multidimensional and interconnected with familial characteristics, the environment, social norms, beliefs, and resources. During the developmental stages and into adulthood, parents and/or caregivers establish the oral health regimen and are advocates for their child's well-being. Therefore caregivers must be properly educated on the appropriate oral health behaviors to institute for themselves and their children. Oral healthcare professionals have a responsibility to provide oral health education, evidence-based information, and best practices that promote healthy oral behaviors for caregivers and nonclinical and clinical team members. Using an

interprofessional approach and methods to increase oral health literacy are means to improve the likelihood that necessary measures will be taken to protect children and adolescents from preventable diseases. Strategies for caries management by risk assessment are discussed in Chapter 19.

INTERPROFESSIONAL COLLABORATION

Using an interprofessional approach increases the opportunity for caregivers to obtain preventive dental services for their child. In the earlier stages of life, health professionals such as midwives, obstetricians, pediatricians, primary care providers, social workers, and personnel from the Supplemental Nutrition Women, Infant, and Children (WIC) program have more frequent interactions with caregivers and children and are well positioned to promote the importance of a dental visit by age 12 months. This interprofessional collaboration allows for a seamless transition with the oral healthcare team.

Interprofessional education (IPE) and interprofessional collaboration (IPC) are the foundation for improving patient health outcomes. **Interprofessional education** is "when students from two or more professions learn about, from and with each other to enable effective collaboration and improve health outcomes" (p.13).[1] **Collaborative practice** occurs when "multiple health workers from different professional backgrounds provide comprehensive services by working together with patients, their families, carers, and communities to deliver the highest quality of care across settings" (p.13).[1] The disparities in the prevalence of dental caries among children and adolescents are unwavering and require a collaborative approach among health professionals, caregivers, and stakeholders. Through collaborative efforts, caregivers and children can be properly educated on preventive strategies to reduce children's dental caries risk (Fig. 45.1).

The oral health literacy of the caregiver impacts oral health outcomes and quality of life for the child. **Oral health literacy (OHL)** is "the degree to which a person is able to get, evaluate, understand, and use oral health information and services to make good decisions about health" (p.1).[2] Some caregivers require customized communication to assist them in making suitable healthcare decisions. Dental hygienists often need to consider the caregiver's OHL as well as their **social determinants of health (SDOH)** when providing oral health education. The SDOH are "conditions in the environments where people are born, live, learn, work, play, worship, and age that affect a wide range of health, functioning, and quality-of-life outcomes and risks."[3] Early

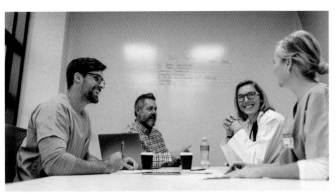

Fig. 45.1 Interprofessional collaboration. (Copyright iStock.com.)

communication about oral health prevention such as during pregnancy (see Chapter 46) can minimize dental caries risk.

EARLY CHILDHOOD CARIES

Dental caries, or "cavities," remains a public health crisis for infants, children, and adolescents, impacting both primary and permanent teeth. In children younger than 71 months, **early childhood caries (ECC)** is "the presence of one or more decayed (non-cavitated or cavitated lesion), missing (due to caries), or filled tooth surface in a primary tooth."[4] The Fisher-Owens et al. model (Fig. 45.2) explains the complexity of early childhood caries, which can be attributed to the host (child), microflora, substrate (diet), environment (child-level, family-level, and community-level influences), and time.[5] At the microlevel

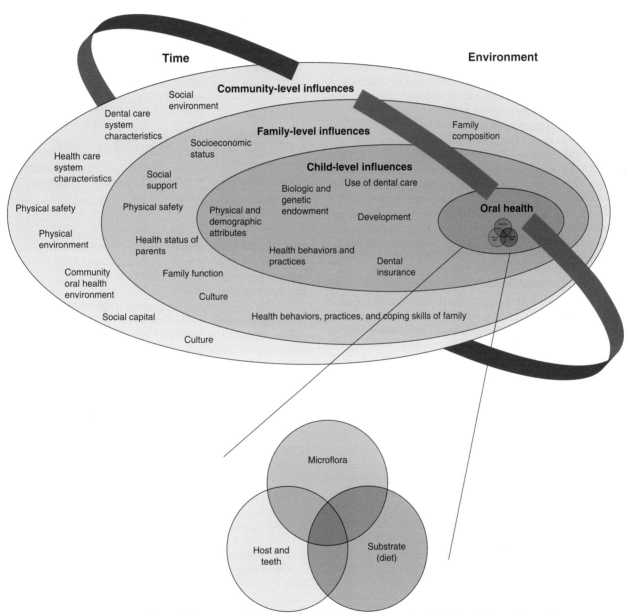

Fig. 45.2 Fisher-Owen: Influences on Children's Oral Health. A conceptual model. (Adapted from Keyes PH. Int Dent J . 1962;12:443– 464; and the concentric oval design was adapted from the National Committee on Vital and Health Statistics. Shaping a Health Statistics Vision for the 21st Century . Washington, DC: Department of Health and Human Services Data Council, Centers for Disease Control and Prevention, National Center for Health Statistics; 2002:viii.)

BOX 45.1   Decay Susceptibility During Primary Tooth Development[6]

Age	Teeth Impacted
1 year	Maxillary central and lateral incisors
2 years	Maxillary central incisors followed by mandibular first molars
3 years	Mandibular second molars and maxillary central incisors
4 years	Mandibular second molars
5 years	Mandibular second molars, mandibular first molars, maxillary second molars and maxillary central incisors

prolonged and repeated exposure to dietary free sugars found in sugar-sweetened beverages (SSBs), milk-based sweetened drinks, and foods should be avoided at certain ages and limited to mealtimes where age appropriate.[6] Nocturnal and frequent feedings to include human milk beyond 12 months of age may increase the risk of dental caries.[7] Further, among children >12 months, caregivers should closely monitor dietary intake, habits, bottle feeding, and oral health practices to minimize dental caries risk. During this stage of development, the maxillary anterior teeth are the most susceptible to dental caries in children aged 1 year.[6] The susceptibility of teeth impacted by dental caries increases with age and the eruption pattern (Box 45.1).[6]

Early prevention is essential to reducing dental caries throughout the lifetime and can be effective if started during pregnancy through the child's second birthday.[6] The American Academy of Pediatric Dentistry (AAPD) recommends that children have a **dental home** no later than 12 months of age in order to assist children and their families to establish good oral health throughout the lifespan.[8] A dental home is "the ongoing relationship between the dentist and the patient, inclusive of all aspects of oral health care delivered in a comprehensive, continuously accessible, coordinated, and family-centered way" (p.15).[8]

Enamel Developmental Defects

Enamel developmental defects (EDDs) are deviations in the enamel that are influenced by several factors (e.g., genetic and environmental) that occur during development (amelogenesis).[9] The visible enamel appearance of EDDs is characterized as hypoplasia, hypomineralization/hypocalcification, hypomaturation, opacity, and diffuse or demarcated opacities.[9] Due to the degree of irregularities in the enamel associated with some EDDs, plaque formulation occurs and, if not properly removed, increases the risk of dental caries. Thus children with an EDD have an increased risk for developing dental caries in the primary dentition.[10]

INFANT ORAL CARE

Prior to infancy, during embryonic development, oral structures begin to form in the third and fourth weeks.[11] Eruption of the first primary (deciduous) tooth, located in the mandibular anterior portion of the mouth, known as the central incisors, occurs at around 5 to 8 months (Fig. 45.3).[12] Around 20 to 30 months the eruption of all 20 primary teeth has occurred. Thus it is common for girls to obtain full eruption of the primary dentition earlier than boys.[11] Delays in tooth eruption may be related to oral space (a single tooth prohibiting eruption), endocrine (hypothyroidism, hypopituitarism, calcium or phosphorus metabolism disorders), familial (parathyroid hormone 1 receptor [PTH1R] gene), or genetic (e.g., Down syndrome, ectodermal dysplasias, rickets) factors.[11] If no signs of eruption around 12 to 18 months, diagnostic assessments and referral should occur. Eruption of

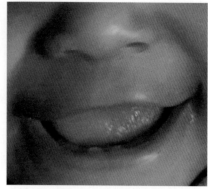

Fig. 45.3 Eruption of mandibular anterior teeth. (Courtesy of Chawntile Rasheed, BSDH, MS [parent] and Aspen Rasheed [child].)

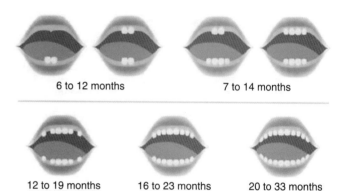

Fig. 45.4 Primary dentition. (From https://dentagama.com/news/primary-dentition.)

primary teeth is symmetrical (mandibular anterior teeth prior to maxillary anterior teeth). The primary teeth include central incisors, lateral incisors, canines, first molars, and second molars. This is known as the **primary dentition** (Fig. 45.4).[11]

During the eruption of the primary teeth, infants and toddlers can become uncomfortable. Oral healthcare providers have an important role to remain current with the symptoms associated with teething, and resources available to assist caregivers in managing symptoms. Symptoms include but are not limited to increased biting, drooling, gum rubbing, sucking, irritability, wakefulness, ear rubbing, facial rash, decreased appetite for solid foods, and mild temperature elevation[13,14] (Fig. 45.5, teething aid).

Caregivers can alleviate their child's pain by doing the following:[13]
- Regularly checking the teeth and mouth
- Rubbing clean fingers around the gingiva; using solid teething toys (e.g., avoiding loose or small teething toys, teething necklaces, or toys that can cause choking)
- Providing the child with clean cool items to chew on (e.g., clean spoons, pacifiers, teething rings, washcloths)
- Offering whole frozen fruit (e.g., bananas) or bagels for the child to chew with the child seated in a highchair
- Avoiding using teething gels or liquids

Client education tips (birth to 1 year of age) are presented in Box 45.2.

Bacterial and Viral Transmissions to Children
Dental Caries

Children are most susceptible to the inoculation of *Streptococcus mutans* through transmission from the mother (**vertical transmission**).[15] This process occurs through saliva that is passed from mother

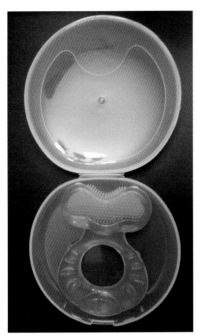

Fig 45.5 Teething device. (Courtesy of Chawntile Rasheed, BSDH, MS.)

BOX 45.2 Patient or Client (Caregiver) Education Tips

Infants (Birth to 1 Year of Age)

- Before teeth begin to erupt, thoroughly clean the infant's gums after each feeding with a water-soaked infant washcloth or gauze pad to stimulate the gum tissue and remove food. When the baby's teeth begin to erupt, brush them gently with a small, soft-bristled toothbrush.
- As solid foods are introduced to the infant, ensure that healthy foods and snacks (e.g., fruits and vegetables) are consumed and avoid juice or other carbohydrate-dense liquids.[37]
- Encourage children to drink from a cup as they approach their first birthday; wean children from bottle at 12 to 14 months of age.
- Instead of soothing a baby with a bottle, rely on strategies such as cuddling, patting, talking, singing, reading, or playing.
- Cleaning a child's teeth after ingestion of sugar-containing medication can prevent dental caries formation.
- Schedule regular dental hygiene appointments starting at the eruption of the first primary tooth or no later than 12 months. The oral health professional checks for cavities in the primary teeth and monitors developmental problems as well as helps to create a positive experience that may alleviate fear at future visits.
- Fluoride varnish can be used on very young children who are at moderate to high risk of early childhood caries.

BOX 45.3 Patient or Client Education Tips

Preventing Transmission of Bacteria Associated With Caries

- Recommend that caregivers seek preventive dental care at least every 6 months and follow the recommendations of their oral healthcare provider.
- Give babies a clean pacifier. Do not give them pacifiers that have been dipped in sugar, honey, syrup, juice, soda, or other sugary substances.
- Avoid "cleaning" a pacifier in another person's such as the parent's or caregiver's mouth. This practice can infect a baby's mouth with bacterial pathogens that cause dental caries and periodontal disease or other viral infections (vertical transmission of disease from parent or caregiver to infant).
- Avoid sharing eating utensils with an infant. Infectious *Streptococcus mutans*, the initiator of the caries disease process, can be transferred from the parent's or caregiver's mouth to the baby's mouth.
- Dental caries can develop as early as 11 months of age. The danger of infecting an infant's teeth is increased when the parents or caregivers dental caries themselves (vertical transmission of disease).

---

to child. In addition, **horizontal transmission**, which occurs between family members or peers, places the child at risk for dental caries.[15] The modes of transmission may include sharing eating utensils, testing food, and sharing toothbrushes.[6,15] Furthermore, caregivers should be aware of their dental caries and oral health status and obtain a dental visit at least twice a year or as recommended by the oral healthcare provider. See Box 45.3 for client education tips to prevent transmission of bacteria associated with dental caries.

Herpetic Infections

An infection prevalent in infants and young children under age 5 years is primary herpetic gingivostomatitis (herpes simplex virus [HSV]-1).[16] Some of the symptoms of HSV-1 in infants include fever, crying, oral pain, and an unwillingness to eat or drink.[16] Gingivae appear intensely red and painful, with blisters on the tongue and lips. Children can be infected with this herpes virus by sharing toys, washcloths, towels, or toothbrushes with others who may be infected (home or daycare setting). Parents with herpetic lip sores can infect their babies by mouth kissing. If a child is in daycare, toys, rattles, and sleeping mats should be wiped and cleaned at least twice a day with a diluted bleach solution to prevent transfer of pathogenic microorganisms.

TODDLER TO PRESCHOOL (1 TO 5 YEARS) ORAL HEALTH

By age 1 year old, a dental home should be established and the child should have received their first dental visit. It is imperative that caregivers receive age-appropriate anticipatory guidance at each dental visit. This anticipatory guidance should include dietary habits, homecare, fluoride intake, age-appropriate injury prevention, counsel on nonnutritive oral habits and nontrauma prevention, and growth and development.[17] Caregivers should be cautioned about the dental caries risk associated with frequent snacking on cariogenic foods and beverages throughout the day (see Chapter 19 and Fig. 45.6). During the toddler and early-childhood stages, oral hygiene care is the caregivers' responsibility until the child understands and has the ability to perform such tasks independently.[17] Caregivers should monitor the eruption and

exfoliation patterns of the child's dentition and discuss any areas of concern. The oral health professional should provide literature at each visit that reflects the stages of development. In addition, oral healthcare professionals, along with primary care providers, must advise parents to schedule preventive oral care appointments for the child at least twice a year.

During the toddler and preschool stages, children are susceptible to dental trauma in the primary dentition. Specifically, among children aged 2 to 3 years, due to increased mobility and coordination development, the maxillary incisors are the most impacted.[18] Therefore age-appropriate injury prevention counseling should be discussed during dental appointments and well-child visits.[17] Preventive counseling should include car seat safety, open water, stairs, sharp objects, hazardous items (e.g., medications, household cleaners), and the dangers of open outlets and accessible home electrical cords.[19] In addition

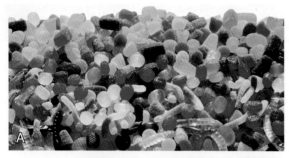

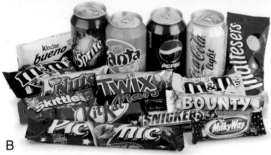

Fig. 45.6 (A–B) Cariogenic beverages and snacks. ([A] Copyright iStock.com. [B] iStock.com/Samohin.)

to avoiding trauma-related events, nonnutritive oral habits such as thumb sucking, pacifier habits, bruxism, and tongue thrust should be discussed, as these habits impact palate and occlusion.[17] Through an interprofessional approach and streamlined referral system, nonnutritive habits and safety risks can be minimized. Box 45.4 outlines client education tips for toddler and preschool children's oral health. See also the Critical Thinking Exercise on providing dental hygiene care for children ages 2 to 3 years.

CRITICAL THINKING EXERCISE

Dental Hygiene Care Provided for Children 2 to 3 Years of Age

Scenario 1: Sarah and her 2-year-old daughter, Mae, arrive for Mae's first dental visit. Mae is very anxious and nervous when she comes through the dental office door. The mother is soothing and bribing Mae with fruit snacks and a sippy cup that contains juice. After reviewing the medical and dental history with Sarah, the oral health assessment and examination is performed. Based on the data collected from the assessments, it is determined that Mae is considered high risk for dental caries.

1. What specific anticipatory guidance is needed for Sarah?
2. How would you explain to Sarah that Mae is at high risk for dental caries?
3. Would you need to consult with Mae's pediatrician?

STRATEGIES TO DECREASE INCIDENCE OF EARLY CHILDHOOD CARIES AND TO PROMOTE HEALTHY ORAL CARE FOR LIFE

For children 1 to 5 years of age, fluoridated mouth rinses are avoided, as swallowing can cause fluorosis or toxicity. Fluoride can be consumed in the community water supplies, some bottled waters, and some foods (USDA National Fluoride Database of Selected Beverages and Foods; https://www.ars.usda.gov/ARSUserFiles/80400525/Data/Fluoride/F02.pdf). The parent or caregiver should be advised to teach the child to expectorate (spit out) the toothpaste while supervised. Using a small

---

BOX 45.4   Patient or Client Education Tips

Toddler and Preschool Children's Oral Health
- Thumb- or finger-sucking is a soothing mechanism, and most children stop this habit between age 2 and 4 years. Consult with an oral healthcare provider if the habit is prolonged or shifting in teeth occurs.[38]
- Avoid frequent snacking or eating between meals and cariogenic-conducive behaviors.
- Preventive dental visits should occur at least twice a year.
- Close all outlets that are not in use.
- Avoid leaving cords plugged into outlets that are not in used. Keep electrical cords out of reach or sight of the child.

---

amount (a smear or pea-sized amount of toothpaste, based on age) of fluoridated toothpaste inhibits decay and minimizes the chance of developing fluorosis when used after 2 to 3 years of age. The dental hygienist provides recommendations for preventive self-care practices as follows:

- When a child is 2 or 3 years old, begin to teach proper brushing techniques. Remember that parents or caregivers need to follow up with brushing and gentle flossing until age 6 or when the child has the dexterity to do it alone.
- Keep dentifrices and oral rinses away from children to avoid accidental ingestion.
- Candies and gums should be given only to children who can manage these supplements properly and should be supervised by an adult to avoid choking hazards. When given to a child, xylitol-containing candies or gums are preferable to those containing sugar.
- Encourage the child to discuss any fears about dental visits and together, read a book or watch a video about a dental visit.

SCHOOL-AGE (6 TO 11 YEARS) CHILDREN AND ORAL HEALTH

An oral examination should occur prior to matriculation into public school. In states such as California, there is legislation that requires children to have an oral health assessment completed by a licensed dental professional before or within the first year of matriculation in public school.[20] The oral health risk assessment tool (OHRT) is available for use by oral health professionals or primary care providers (Fig. 45.7). Additionally, the caries assessment management by risk assessment (CAMBRA®) is a detailed evidenced-based screening tool that can be used in a clinical setting by oral healthcare professionals (discussed in detail in Chapter 19).

As the child enters primary school, the primary teeth will begin to exfoliate. The mandibular central incisors are the first primary teeth to exfoliate, around 6 to 7 years.[12] In addition, eruption of the first permanent molars occurs before or around the same age. The placement of dental sealants is recommended to protect the occlusal surfaces of permanent molars.[17] (Fig. 45.8 and Chapter 35). This primary prevention method is recommended because of anatomic grooves or pits and fissures on the occlusal surfaces that can trap food debris, thus increasing the presence of bacterial biofilm and dental caries risk. Children and adolescents who receive sealants on noncavitated pit-and-fissure occlusal surfaces have a reduced dental caries risk. Hence this primary preventive measure should be recommended to caregivers once the eruption of permanent molars occurs.

Sports Involvement

Dental and facial traumas are common sports-related injuries among children and adults. Most sport-related injuries involve the maxilla;

Oral Health Risk Assessment Tool

The American Academy of Pediatrics (AAP) has developed this tool to aid in the implementation of oral health risk assessment during health supervision visits. This tool has been subsequently reviewed and endorsed by the National Interprofessional Initiative on Oral Health.

Instructions for Use

This tool is intended for documenting caries risk of the child, however, two risk factors are based on the mother or primary caregiver's oral health. All other factors and findings should be documented based on the child.

The child is at an absolute high risk for caries if any risk factors or clinical findings, marked with a α sign, are documented yes. In the absence of α risk factors or clinical findings, the clinician may determine the child is at high risk of caries based on one or more positive responses to other risk factors or clinical findings. Answering yes to protective factors should be taken into account with risk factors/clinical findings in determining low versus high risk.

Patient Name:_____ Date of Birth:_____ Date:_____

Visit: ☐6 month ☐9 month ☐12 month ☐15 month ☐18 month ☐24 month ☐30 month ☐3 year
☐4 year ☐5 year ☐6 year ☐Other_____

RISK FACTORS	PROTECTIVE FACTORS	CLINICAL FINDINGS
α Mother or primary caregiver had active decay in the past 12 months ☐Yes ☐No	● Existing dental home ☐Yes ☐No	α White spots or visible decalcifications in the past 12 months ☐Yes ☐No
● Mother or primary caregiver does not have a dentist ☐Yes ☐No	● Drinks fluoridated water or takes fluoride supplements ☐Yes ☐No	α Obvious decay ☐Yes ☐No
	● Fluoride varnish in the last 6 months ☐Yes ☐No	α Restorations (fillings) present ☐Yes ☐No
● Continual bottle/sippy cup use with fluid other than water ☐Yes ☐No	● Has teeth brushed twice daily ☐Yes ☐No	● Visible plaque accumulation ☐Yes ☐No
● Frequent snacking ☐Yes ☐No		● Gingivitis (swollen/bleeding gums) ☐Yes ☐No
● Special health care needs ☐Yes ☐No		● Teeth present ☐Yes ☐No
● Medicaid eligible ☐Yes ☐No		● Healthy teeth ☐Yes ☐No

ASSESSMENT/PLAN

Caries Risk:
☐Low ☐High

Completed:
☐Anticipatory Guidance
☐Fluoride Varnish
☐Dental Referral

Self Management Goals:
☐Regular dental visits   ☐Wean off bottle   ☐Healthy snacks
☐Dental treatment for parents   ☐Less/No juice   ☐Less/No junk food or candy
☐Brush twice daily   ☐Only water in sippy cup   ☐No soda
☐Use fluoride toothpaste   ☐Drink tap water   ☐Xylitol

Treatment of High Risk Children

If appropriate, high-risk children should receive professionally applied fluoride varnish and have their teeth brushed twice daily with an age-appropriate amount of fluoridated toothpaste. Referral to a pediatric dentist or a dentist comfortable caring for children should be made with follow-up to ensure that the child is being cared for in the dental home.

Adapted from Ramos-Gomez FJ, Crystal YO, Ng MW, Crall JJ, Featherstone JD. Pediatric dental care: prevention and management protocols based on caries risk assessment. *J Calif Dent Assoc.* 2010;38(10):746–761; American Academy of Pediatrics Section on Pediatric Dentistry and Oral Health. Preventive oral health intervention for pediatricians. *Pediatrics.* 2003; 122(6):1387–1394; and American Academy of Pediatrics Section of Pediatric Dentistry. Oral health risk assessment timing and establishment of the dental home. *Pediatrics.* 2003;111(5):1113–1116.

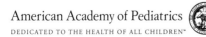

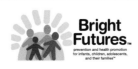

American Academy of Pediatrics
DEDICATED TO THE HEALTH OF ALL CHILDREN™

Bright Futures.
prevention and health promotion for infants, children, adolescents, and their families™

National *Interprofessional Initiative* on Oral Health *engaging clinicians eradicating dental disease*

Fig. 45.7 Oral Health Risk Assessment Tool—American Academy of Pediatrics. (Reprinted with permission from the American Academy of Pediatrics Oral_Health_Assessment_Tool.pdf (smilesforlifeoralhealth.org), accessed September 27, 2023.)

Continued

Oral Health Risk Assessment Tool Guidance

Timing of Risk Assessment

The Bright Futures/AAP "Recommendations for Preventive Pediatric Health Care," (ie, Periodicity Schedule) recommends all children receive a risk assessment at the 6- and 9-month visits. For the 12-, 18-, 24-, 30-month, and the 3- and 6-year visits, risk assessment should continue if a dental home has not been established. View the Bright Futures/AAP Periodicity Schedule—http://brightfutures. aap.org/clinical_practice.html.

Risk Factors

Maternal Oral Health

Studies have shown that children with mothers or primary caregivers who have had active decay in the past 12 months are at greater risk to develop caries. **This child is high risk.**

Maternal Access to Dental Care

Studies have shown that children with mothers or primary caregivers who do not have a regular source of dental care are at a greater risk to develop caries. A follow-up question may be if the child has a dentist.

Continual Bottle/Sippy Cup Use

Children who drink juice, soda, and other liquids that are not water, from a bottle or sippy cup continually throughout the day or at night are at an increased risk of caries. The frequent intake of sugar does not allow for the acid it produces to be neutralized or washed away by saliva. Parents of children with this risk factor need to be counseled on how to reduce the frequency of sugar-containing beverages in the child's diet.

Frequent Snacking

Children who snack frequently are at an increased risk of caries. The frequent intake of sugar/refined carbohydrates does not allow for the acid it produces to be neutralized or washed away by saliva. Parents of children with this risk factor need to be counseled on how to reduce frequent snacking and choose healthy snacks such as cheese, vegetables, and fruit.

Special Health Care Needs

Children with special health care needs are at an increased risk for caries due to their diet, xerostomia (dryness of the mouth, sometimes due to asthma or allergy medication use), difficulty performing oral hygiene, seizures, gastroesophageal reflux disease and vomiting, attention deficit hyperactivity disorder, and gingival hyperplasia or overcrowding of teeth. Premature babies also may experience enamel hypoplasia.

Protective Factors

Dental Home

According to the American Academy of Pediatric Dentistry (AAPD), the dental home is oral health care for the child that is delivered in a comprehensive, continuously accessible, coordinated and family-centered way by a licensed dentist. The AAP and the AAPD recommend that a dental home be established by age 1. Communication between the dental and medical homes should be ongoing to appropriately coordinate care for the child. If a dental home is not available, the primary care clinician should continue to do oral health risk assessment at every well-child visit.

Fluoridated Water/Supplements

Drinking fluoridated water provides a child with systemic and topical fluoride exposure, a proven caries reduction intervention. Fluoride supplements may be prescribed by the primary care clinician or dentist if needed. View fluoride resources on the Oral Health Practice Tools Web Page http://aap.org/oralhealth/PracticeTools.html.

Fluoride Varnish in the Last 6 Months

Applying fluoride varnish provides a child with highly concentrated fluoride to protect against caries. Fluoride varnish may be professionally applied and is now recommended by the United States Preventive Services Task Force as a preventive service in the primary care setting for all children through age 5 http://www.uspreventiveservicestaskforce.org/Page/Topic/recommendation-summary/dental-caries-in-children-from-birth-through-age-5-years-screening. For online fluoride varnish training, access the Caries Risk Assessment, Fluoride Varnish, and Counseling Module in the Smiles for Life National Oral Health Curriculum, www.smilesforlifeoralhealth.org.

Tooth Brushing and Oral Hygiene

Primary care clinicians can reinforce good oral hygiene by teaching parents and children simple practices. Infants should have their mouths cleaned after feedings with a wet soft washcloth. Once teeth erupt it is recommended that children have their teeth brushed twice a day. For children under the age of 3 (until 3rd birthday) it is appropriate to recommend brushing with a smear (grain of rice amount) of fluoridated toothpaste twice per day. Children 3 years of age and older should use a pea-sized amount of fluoridated toothpaste twice a day. View the AAP Clinical Report on the use of fluoride in the primary care setting for more information http://pediatrics.aappublications.org/content/early/2014/08/19/peds.2014-1699.

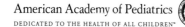 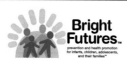 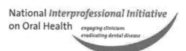

Fig. 45.7, cont'd

Clinical Findings

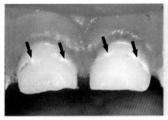

ⓐ White Spots/Decalcifications
This child is high risk.
White spot decalcifications present—immediately place the child in the high-risk category.

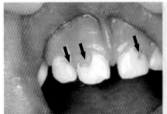

ⓐ Obvious Decay
This child is high risk.
Obvious decay present—immediately place the child in the high-risk category.

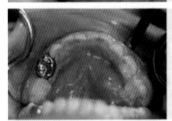

ⓐ Restorations (Fillings) Present
This child is high risk.
Restorations (Fillings) present—immediately place the child in the high-risk category.

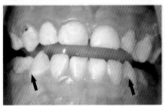

Visible Plaque Accumulation
Plaque is the soft and sticky substance that accumulates on the teeth from food debris and bacteria. Primary care clinicians can teach parents how to remove plaque from the child's teeth by brushing and flossing.

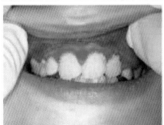

Gingivitis
Gingivitis is the inflamation of the gums. Primary care clinicians can teach parents good oral hygiene skills to reduce the inflammation.

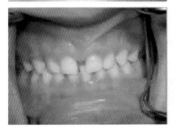

Healthy Teeth
Children with healthy teeth have no signs of early childhood caries and no other clinical findings. They are also experiencing normal tooth and mouth development and spacing.

For more information about the AAP's oral health activities email oralhealth@aap.org or visit www.aap.org/oralhealth.

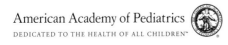

American Academy of Pediatrics
DEDICATED TO THE HEALTH OF ALL CHILDREN™

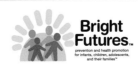

Bright Futures™
prevention and health promotion for infants, children, adolescents, and their families™

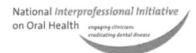

National *Interprofessional Initiative* on Oral Health *engaging clinicians eradicating dental disease*

Fig. 45.7, cont'd

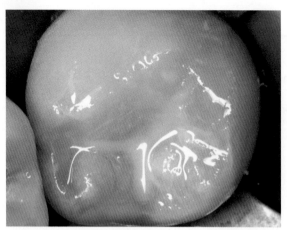

Fig. 45.8 Pit and fissure sealant placed on a molar. (From Simonsen R. From prevention to therapy: minimal intervention with sealants and resin restorative materials. *J Dentistry*. 2011;39:S27.)

therefore, the use of properly fitted mouthguards is a preventive measure to ensure the oral cavity and soft tissues are protected during recreational activities and organized sports. Oral health professionals should discuss sports involvement during dental visits and recommend mouthguards as needed. The most protective mouthguards are properly fitted and custom made, as this ensures proper fit for the patient. Other types of mouth guards include boil and bite and stock (readymade);[21] these styles can be purchased over the counter (see Chapter 38). The Academy of Sports Dentistry (ASD) encourages the use of a properly fitted custom mouthguard in all collision and contact sports.[22]

Dental hygienists teach their clients and their parents or caregivers the following:

- Obtain preventive dental services at minimum twice a year and prior to matriculation to school.
- Ensure that the child has a properly fitted mouthguard for any recreational or organized sport.
- Inquire about dental sealants once the first permanent molars erupt, around 6 to 7 years of age.

ADOLESCENT STAGES (12 TO 17 YEARS) AND ORAL HEALTH

Adolescents have distinctive needs during the ages of 12 to 17 years. During this time, adolescents are susceptible to potential high caries incidence; traumatic injury; periodontal disease; poor nutritional habits; a esthetic appearance and desire; orthodontic and restorative care; exposure to tobacco, drugs, and alcohol; and social and psychologic needs.[23] The use of e-cigarettes or vaping has become more prevalent among children, teens, and young adults. In general, the product is unsafe for all ages, still contains some form of nicotine, and increases the chances for an individual to smoke cigarettes.[24] In order to assist clients and their caregivers through this developmental period, a current and accurate medical and social history should be obtained at each visit. During the earlier ages of adolescence, the remaining primary teeth exfoliate, and the eruption of premolars and molars occurs. Third molars tend to erupt during late adolescence to adulthood (17 to 30 years).[12] As with the previous life stages, the same measures should be followed into the adolescent years—for example, established dental home, scheduled preventive dental visits, fluoride therapy, self-care education, dietary counseling, and anticipatory guidance.

Puberty and Menses

Puberty and menses are marked by the development of secondary sex characteristics throughout the body and increased estrogen level. The bacteria associated with increased estrogen levels (*Prevotella* species and *Tannerella forsythensis*) have been implicated in periodontal disease. Irregular ovulations usually occur for the first 1 to 2 years before the start of menstruation. Endogenous sex steroid hormone gingival disease, which includes puberty-associated gingivitis and menstrual cycle gingivitis, may occur as estrogen and progesterone levels rise. These gingival diseases are classified as plaque-induced gingival diseases modified by systemic factors (see Chapter 20). The body reacts to bacterial challenges differently, depending on the integrity of the immune system. The host response appears to be altered in the presence of increased sex steroid hormones, suggesting an effect of these hormones on the immune system. Swollen, erythematous gingival tissues may be present, as well as herpes labialis and aphthous ulcers, prolonged hemorrhage after oral surgery, and swollen salivary glands. Minor increases in tooth mobility may be seen, along with an increase in gingival exudate. These transient changes are attributed to peak levels of estrogen and progesterone.

Although sex steroid hormone effects may be transient, irreversible oral damage could result if proper self-care is lacking. Dental hygiene preventive strategies during puberty and menses include stressing optimal oral hygiene via increased frequency and duration of toothbrushing with an extra-soft toothbrush or a power toothbrush and meticulous interdental cleaning (see Chapters 24 and 25). Therapeutic modalities include topical corticosteroids; frequent periodontal debridement, scaling, and root planing; antimicrobial mouth rinses; fluoride rinses, gels, and varnish; and use of xylitol products. Painful oral manifestations of puberty and menses, although disconcerting and uncomfortable, can be managed with topical viscous lidocaine, Orahesive, or Zilactin-B, and OTC systemic analgesics such as aspirin, ibuprofen, or acetaminophen.

HUMAN PAPILLOMAVIRUS

The **human papillomavirus (HPV)** is a common sexually transmitted infection in the United States affecting teens and young adults.[25] In 2018, there were an estimated 43 million HPV infections among late teens and young adults.[25] There are over 100 variants of HPV, of which 13 are noted to cause cancer. However, in the United States, HPV16 has been linked to oropharyngeal squamous cell cancer (HPV-OPC).[23] Primary prevention through vaccination is recommended for this virus for all preteen (aged 11 or 12 years; or as early as aged 9 years) boys and girls and adults through aged 26 years.[25]

CRITICAL THINKING EXERCISE

Scenario 2: Molly, a 14-year-old female patient, has recently moved to a community where the drinking water contains suboptimal fluoridation. Through anticipatory guidance to the caregiver, this information is provided. In addition, recommendations are provided to the caregiver to ensure Molly receives optimal fluoride for her age. These recommendations include purchasing bottled water with fluoride, using an OTC fluoride toothpaste, and receiving professional fluoride during recare dental visits. The caregiver explains her philosophy, which is against fluoride and products that contain fluoride.

1. What information can be shared with Molly's caregiver regarding the role of fluoride in reducing dental caries risk?
2. Is there an interprofessional approach that can be used to explain the relationship between fluoride and dental caries?

FLUORIDE CONSUMPTION AND THERAPY

Water Fluoridation

Community water fluoridation within localities began in the mid-1940s.[26] The fluoride mineral occurs naturally on earth and is released from rocks into the soil, water, and air.[26] All forms of water contain varying levels of fluoride, and the US Public Health Service regulates the level. If not optimal, municipalities often add fluoride to the water supply to attain optimal levels for health. The Public Health Service recommends an optimal fluoride concentration of 0.7 mg/L be used in drinking water to protect the teeth against dental caries while also minimizing dental fluorosis (Fig. 45.9).[27] The use of water fluoridation is a cost-effective mechanism that benefits all individuals regardless of sociodemographic background.[26-27] By 2030, the United States has a national goal for 77% of US citizens to have access to a fluoridated water supply that will prevent dental caries.[26]

Fluoride Supplements

While most communities in the United States have water fluoridation, there are some communities without a water fluoridation system. When there is no or suboptimal exposure to fluoride, health and oral healthcare providers can recommend fluoride supplements.[28] A caries risk assessment (Chapter 19), in addition to an assessment of fluoride concentration in primary drinking sources, dietary fluoride sources, and age of the child should be considered prior to prescribing supplements.[28] The supplements recommended when the fluoride concentration in drinking water is below optimal level are presented in Fig. 45.10.

Dietary fluoride supplements in the United States are prescribed and available in tablets, drops, or lozenges.[28] The Centers for Disease Control and Prevention and state public health webpages can be used to identify fluoride concentration in community drinking water.

Dental hygienists are responsible for advising parents or caregivers about water fluoridation and fluoride supplements as follows:

- Determine if the water supply that serves the patient's or caregiver's home is fluoridated adequately. The local or district public health department can be contacted regarding this testing service, and a sample can be taken to the appropriate agency or office.

- If there is an inadequate amount of fluoride resulting from filtration or lack of fluoride in the water, then discuss supplemental options with the parent. Fluoride also is found in OTC mouth rinses, foods, beverages, and a few bottled waters; however, many brands of bottled water have no fluoride. Parents and caregivers should be advised to check whether the bottled water given to the child has fluoride. Explain to the parent or caregiver the benefits of consuming water from a fluoridated system.
See fluoride toxicity (Box 45.5).

Topical Fluoride Gels and Varnish

Professionally applied in-office acidulated phosphate fluoride (APF) gels and foams are still used in dental settings, while fluoride varnish has become more widely used among professionals. The American Dental Association (ADA) Council on Scientific Affairs published evidence-based clinical recommendations for clients who have an elevated risk for dental caries, which include 2.26% fluoride varnish or 1.23% APF gel (3-6 months), or a prescription-strength, home-use 0.5% fluoride gel or paste (twice daily) or 0.09% fluoride mouth rinse (weekly) for those aged 6 to 18 years. Additionally, for children aged <6 years, 2.26% fluoride varnish (3 to 6 months) is recommended.[29] See Chapter 19 for information about indications for and effectiveness of fluoride varnishes and home-use fluoride mouth rinses in children and adolescents.

Acidulated phosphate fluoride gels with a fluoride concentration of 1.23% or 12,300 ppm benefit children and adolescents in reducing the incidence of dental caries in primary and permanent teeth.[29] (Fig. 45.11). See Procedure 45.1 for professional application of APF gels using a tray method. Caution should be used when filling the fluoride tray with a fluoride gel or foam. In addition, the manufacturer's guidelines should be followed, in addition to suction to reduce the risk of excessive ingestion, which can cause gastrointestinal irritation and nausea.

Fluoride varnish is used for caries prevention in the clinical setting, school sealant programs, community health clinics, public health programs, and primary care provider settings. Its application does not require dental equipment, and it is an effective modality for caries prevention in children and adolescents. Procedure 45.2 outlines armamentarium and steps for professionally applied fluoride varnish.

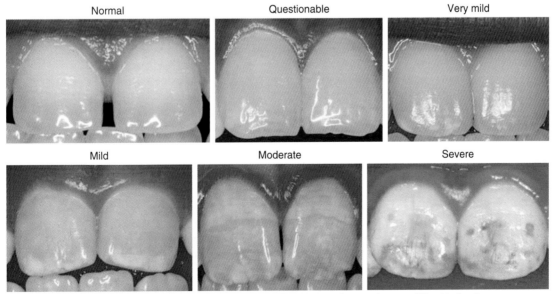

Fig. 45.9 Dental fluorosis. (From Carey CM. Focus on fluorides: update on the use of fluoride for the prevention of dental caries. *J Evid Based Dent Pract.* 2014;14:95–102.)

Silver Diamine Fluoride

Silver diamine fluoride (SDF) was approved by the US Food Drug and Administration (FDA) in 2014 for dental use in treating hypersensitivity.[30] The American Academy of Pediatric Dentistry (AAPD) Clinical Practice Guidelines currently provide a conditional recommendation in support of using 38% SDF for cavitated primary teeth along with dental caries management.[31] The SDF application is available in liquid and gel form. Once the application is painted onto the cavitated lesions, the area is permanently stained black.[31-32] While SDF esthetically is undesirable, other factors to consider include the following: there is a contraindication for individuals with a silver allergy, the treatment does not cure dental caries, reapplication of the product is needed for unrestored dental caries, and the success of treatment depends on oral hygiene and maintaining dental visits. Some advantages of this treatment method include reduced hypersensitivity, inexpensive, no discomfort during application, easy application of product, and the ability to be completed during one visit.[32]

EPIDEMIOLOGIC INDICES FOR ASSESSING DENTAL CARIES PREVALENCE AND INCIDENCE

There are several indices available for quantifying clinical observations of dental caries lesions. The Decayed, Missing, Filled Teeth (DMFT) is a well-established and documented index used to measure dental caries in epidemiologic research.[33] This index quantifies health status and clinical observations among primary and permanent dentition. In addition to the DMFT, the Decayed, Missing, Filled Surfaces (DMFS) has also been used to quantify dental caries incidence among populations.

DMFT/dmft

The DMFT is used for permanent dentition, whereas the dmft is used for primary dentition. The DMFT is expressed in the total number of teeth decayed, missing, or filled in an individual. Decayed teeth (D) include the following: carious tooth, recurrent decay in a restored tooth (to include defective), crown missing with roots remaining, temporary restoration, and a filled tooth surface with remaining decay in another surface.[34] For M, missing teeth, only teeth missing due to decay or disease are counted; teeth that are unerupted, congenitally missing, supernumerary, or removed for reasons other than dental caries are not counted in the index. In addition, only teeth filled (F) due to caries are counted; restorations for trauma, hypoplasia, sealants, erosion, bridge abutments, or with root canals are not counted.[34] When a carious lesion(s) and a restoration are present on the same tooth, the tooth is recorded as decayed (D). The individual score is a sum of D + M + F, ranging from 0 to 28 or 32, depending on whether the third molars are used.[35] When obtaining the DMFT of a population or sample, the equation is expressed as an average obtained by adding together the number of decayed, missing, and filled teeth and dividing them by the number of subjects in a sample.[34-35] Similar to the DMFT, the same principles apply to the dmft index. The dmft index in primary dentition is expressed as number of affected teeth. Individual scores for pediatric patients range from 0 to 20.[34]

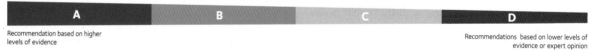

Dietary Fluoride Supplements: Evidence-based Clinical Recommendations[1]

Levels of evidence and strength of recommendations: Each recommendation is based on the best available evidence. Lower levels of evidence do not mean the recommendation should not be applied for patient treatment.

Correlate these colors with the text and table below.

A	B	C	D

Recommendation based on higher levels of evidence

Recommendations based on lower levels of evidence or expert opinion

Practitioners are encouraged to evaluate all potential fluoride sources and conduct a caries risk assessment before prescribing fluoride supplements.

For children at **low caries risk**, dietary fluoride supplements are **not** **recommended** and other sources of fluoride should be considered as a caries preventive intervention. **(D)**
For children at **high caries risk**, dietary fluoride supplements are **recommended** according to the schedule presented in the following table. **(D)**
When fluoride supplements are prescribed, they should be **taken daily** to maximize the caries prevention benefit. **(D)**

ADA dietary fluoride supplement schedule for children at high caries risk			
Age (Years)	Fluoride Concentration in Drinking Water (ppm)*		
	<0.3	0.3-0.6	>0.6
Birth to 6 months	None **(D)**	None **(D)**	None **(D)**
6 months to 3 years	0.25 mg/day **(B)**	None **(D)**	None **(D)**
3 to 6 years	0.50 mg/day **(B)**	0.25 mg/day **(B)**	None **(D)**
6 to 16 years	1.0 mg/day **(B)**	0.50 mg/day **(B)**	None **(D)**

*1.0 ppm = 1 mg/liter

Fig. 45.10 American Dental Association (ADA). Dietary Fluoride Supplements for Caries Prevention Clinical Practice Guideline (2010). (Courtesy of American Dental Association.)

Making a shared decision

Determine balance between need for caries prevention and risk of fluorosis

The Clinician

&

The Patient

Fluoride Exposure
Consider all sources of fluoride intake including bottled water.

Contact local, county and/or state health departments about local water fluoride content or test water sample.

Caries Prevention
Repeat caries risk assessment at frequent intervals because risk status can change.

Caries risk assessment tools are available for dentists* and physicians.**

Comply with prescription
Use dietary fluoride supplements as directed to maximize the caries prevention benefit
Chew tablets or suck lozenges for 1–2 minutes before swallowing to maximize topical effect
For infants, supplements are available as a liquid and used with a dropper

ADA American Dental Association®
America's leading advocate for oral health

*American Dental Association. Caries Risk Assessment Form (0–6 years). http://www.ada.org/sections/professionalResources/docs/topics_caries_under6.doc.
*American Dental Association. Caries Risk Assessment Form (patients over 6 years). http://www.ada.org/sections/professionalResources/docs/topics_caries_over6.doc.
*American Academy of Pediatric Dentistry. Policy on use of a caries-risk assessment tool (CAT) for infants, children and adolescents Oral Health Policies Reference Manual; 2006. http://www.aapd.org/media/Policies_Guidelines/P_CariesRiskAssess.pdf.
*Featherstone JD, Domejean-Orliaguet S, Jenson L, Wolff M, Young DA. Caries risk assessment in practice for age 6 through adult. J Calif Dent Assoc 2007;35(10):703-7, 10-3.
*Ramos-Gomez FJ, Crall J, Gansky SA, Slayton RL, Featherstone JD. Caries risk assessment appropriate for the age 1 visit (infants and toddlers). J Calif Dent Assoc 2007;35(10):687-702.
**Bright Futures in Practice: Oral Health Pocket Guide. http://www.mchoralhealth.org/PocketGuide/tables1.html

Fig. 45.10, cont'd

BOX 45.5 Fluoride Toxicity

- Fluoride toxicity occurs when the consumption surpasses the optimal level or the prescribed intake by a provider.
- Acute fluoride toxicity for children and adults occurs when the dose range is 5 to 8 mg/kg body weight and may involve systems such as the gastrointestinal irritation (common) (nausea, vomiting, abdominal pain, diarrhea, weakness, and hypocalcemia), which may lead to muscle tetany. Additional symptoms include hypotension, respiratory, pupil changes, hyperkalemia, cardiac, renal, and metabolic system a result of these impacted cardiac systems. Changes in the renal and metabolic systems as a result of mixed renal and metabolic acidosis due to renal and respiratory failure, may lead to coma, convulsion and to the latter end death.[39]
- Chronic fluoride toxicity occurs based on the dose and duration as well as the health or function of other body systems. These symptoms may include dental and skeletal fluorosis, gastrointestinal, renal, and muscular problems, central nervous system problems, and to the latter end, birth defects and cancer.[39]

DMFS/dmfs

The DMFS/dmfs applies similar principles to the DMFT/dmft, except "tooth surfaces" are accounted for rather than individual teeth. Therefore an assessment for each tooth surface using the DMF/dmf principles is applied. For posterior teeth, five surfaces are used, namely the mesial, distal, buccal, lingual, and occlusal surface, and for anterior teeth, four surfaces are measured, as there is no occlusal surface. Individual scores will range from 0 to 128, or 148 if third molars are used.[34] When using

the dmfs index for primary dentition, scores will range from 0 to 88 surfaces.[34] Note that in primary dentition, the decayed, filled, teeth, or surface (dft/dfs) has been used because of the inability to discern if a tooth is missing due to exfoliation or extraction due to dental caries.[34]

BEHAVIORAL MANAGEMENT OF PEDIATRIC PATIENTS DURING DENTAL HYGIENE CARE

The AAPD developed a guideline for healthcare providers and parents about influences on behavior of children as pediatric dental patients, with suggestions for behavioral techniques to use in contemporary dental practices. Both nonpharmacologic and pharmacologic techniques are described for alleviating anxiety and nurturing positive attitudes for safe and high-quality oral healthcare. Selection of techniques needs to be tailored to each individual patient and the skills of the clinician.[36] Many factors influence the behaviors of children and adolescents during oral healthcare, including special needs, fears or situational anxiety, previous negative or painful dental treatment, and parenting practices. In addition, cultural sensitivity by the clinician is important, as cultural, linguistic, and language factors may play a role. Qualified interpreters may be needed for families without English language proficiency. Communication is key, and the AAPD guideline presents detailed information on several useful techniques. The guideline describes in detail and provides examples of positive reinforcement, nonverbal communication, show-tell-do, ask-tell-ask, teach back, and motivational interviewing (Chapter 5) and other behavior guidance techniques that can reflect the oral health professional's caring and engaging in a patient/parent-centered approach (Box 45.6) includes legal, ethical, and safety considerations for pediatric patient care).

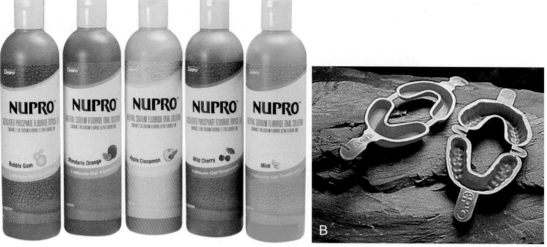

Fig. 45.11 (A) Professionally administered APF fluoride gel. (Courtesy DENTSPLY Sirona, York, PA.) (B) Professionally administered fluoride gel tray. (From Bird D, Robinson D. *Modern Dental Assisting*. 12th ed. Elsevier; 2018; (From Clark C, Kent KA, Jackson RD. Open mouth, open mind: expanding the role of primary care nurse practitioners. *J Pediatr Health Care*. 2016;30(5):480. Copyright ©2015 National Association of Pediatric Nurse Practitioners.)

PROCEDURE 45.1 Professionally Applied Topical Fluoride Using the Tray Technique for In-Office Fluoride Treatment (Gel or Foam)

Equipment
Mouth mirror
Cotton forceps
Fluoride tray(s)
Cotton rolls
1.23% acidulated phosphate fluoride (APF) or 2.0% sodium fluoride gel
Air syringe
Timer
Saliva ejector
2 × 2 gauze
Tissues
2-oz cup
Personal protective barriers and equipment barriers

Steps
1. Assemble equipment

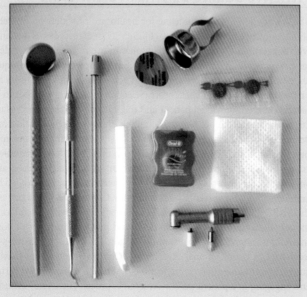

2. Seat patient in upright position. Reiterate benefits and obtain informed consent.

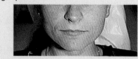

3. Try tray of appropriate size. Complete dentition must be covered, including areas of recession.

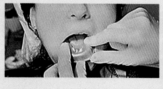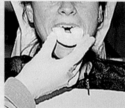

4. Load fluoride gel into trays for maxillary and mandibular teeth: 2 mL maximum per tray for small children; 4 mL maximum per tray for large children (>44 lb), 2.5 mL maximum per tray for adults.

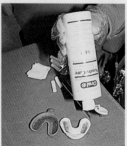

5. Dry teeth with air syringe.

PROCEDURE 45.1 Professionally Applied Topical Fluoride Using the Tray Technique for In-Office Fluoride Treatment (Gel or Foam)—cont'd

6. Insert both trays in mouth.

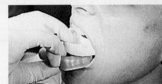

7. Press tray against teeth; ask patient to close mouth and bite gently on trays or cotton rolls.

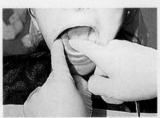

8. Place saliva ejector over mandibular tray. Set timer for 4 minutes. Never leave patient unattended during procedure.

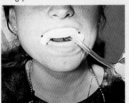

9. Tilt chin down to remove trays.

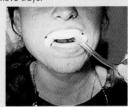

10. Ask patient to expectorate; suction excess fluoride from the mouth with saliva ejector.

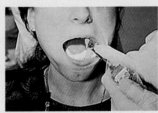

11. Instruct patient not to eat, drink, or rinse for 30 minutes.
12. Record service in patient's chart under "services rendered"; e.g., "Applied topical APF fluoride gel to existing teeth for 4 minutes. Used stock trays to apply approximately 2 to 2.5 mL of 1.23% APF (insert brand name). Patient assented and parent or caregiver consented to procedure; no complications or adverse reactions during treatment. Patient instructed not to eat or drink for 30 minutes."

PROCEDURE 45.2 Professionally Applied Sodium Fluoride Varnish Using the Paint-On Technique

Equipment
Mouth mirror
5% sodium fluoride varnish (unit dosage)
Cotton-tip applicators or syringe applicator
Paper cup
Personal protective barriers and equipment barriers

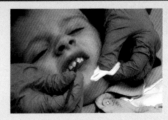

Steps
1. Select unit dose fluoride varnish product; gather equipment and supplies for application.
2. Provide patient with information about procedure; reiterate benefits. Obtain informed consent.
3. Unless an oral prophylaxis has been performed at the same appointment, have patient cleanse teeth with toothbrush.
4. Recline patient for ergonomic access to oral cavity.
5. Wipe application area with gauze or cotton rolls and insert a saliva ejector. Can be applied in the presence of saliva and without a saliva ejector.
6. Using a cotton-tip, brush, or applicator, apply 0.3 to 0.5 mL of varnish (unit dose) to clinical crown of teeth: application time is 1 to 3 minutes.

7. Dental floss may be used to draw the varnish interproximally.
8. Allow patient to rinse on completion of procedure.
9. Remind patient to avoid eating hard foods, drinking hot or alcoholic beverages, brushing, and flossing until the next day, or at least for 4 to 6 hours after application. Drink through a straw for the first few hours after application.
10. Record service in patient's record under "Services Rendered," e.g., "Applied 0.3 mL of 5% (22,600 ppm) sodium fluoride varnish (insert brand name) per tooth. Patient consented to this procedure; no complications or adverse reactions during treatment. Patient instructed to keep varnish on the teeth for at least 4 to 6 hours or preferably until the next day. Patient told to drink through a straw and avoid hard foods, alcoholic and hot beverages, brushing, and flossing until preferably the next day to prolong the varnish treatment. Varnish can be removed the next day with toothbrushing and interdental cleaning."

BOX 45.6 Legal, Ethical, and Safety Considerations

Pediatric Dental Hygiene Care

- Dental hygienists must engage both the parent or caregiver and the child in informed consent or assent, respectively, as well as in client education and self-care recommendations.
- Report suspected abuse or neglect to the proper authorities: child protective services as mandated by law (Chapter 58).
- Take a complete health history, monitor and record vital signs, and ask specific questions about drugs, herbs, vitamins, fluoride, and other supplements. The safety of most natural or herbal remedies is unknown because it is not controlled by the US Food and Drug Administration (FDA) (Chapters 13, 14, and 15).
- Conduct a comprehensive oral assessment including a caries risk assessment (Chapter 19).
- Follow the AAPD guidelines for behavior guidance for the pediatric dental patient.
- Document informed consent, client education, all treatment provided, and important observations about the child's behavior, including any complications and how they were addressed.

KEY CONCEPTS

- When possible, use an interprofessional approach to discuss health and oral health preventive measures with caregivers.
- Increasing oral health literacy among caregivers will decrease risk for oral diseases among children.
- Collaborate with medical colleagues to ensure that comprehensive preventive care is maintained through childhood and adolescence.
- Discuss age-appropriate anticipatory guidance with the caregiver at each dental appointment.
- Remain current with fluoridation levels in local communities.
- Apply topical fluoride for caries prevention using evidence-based recommendations.
- Use the DMFT/dmft, DMFS/dmfs to quantify clinical findings in individual patients and populations.

REFERENCES

1. World Health Organization. Framework for Action on Interprofessional Education & Collaboration. Available at: http://apps.who.int/iris/bitstream/10665/70185/1/WHO_HRH_HPN_10.3_eng.pdf. Updated 2010. Accessed June 7, 2022.
2. Brush Up on Oral Health. Available at: https://eclkc.ohs.acf.hhs.gov/sites/default/files/pdf/00341-improving-oral-health-literacy.pdf; U.S. Department of Health and Human Services, Administration for Children and Families. Office of Head Start, National Center on Health, Behavioral Health, and Safety. n.d. Accessed June 7, 2022.
3. Healthy People 2030. Social Determinants of Health. Available at: https://health.gov/healthypeople/objectives-and-data/social-determinants-health. U.S. Department of Health and Human Services, Office of Disease Prevention and Health Promotion. n.d. Accessed June 8, 2022.
4. Definition of early childhood caries (ECC). *American Academy of Pediatric Dentistry*; 2008. Available at: https://www.aapd.org/assets/1/7/d_ecc.pdf. Accessed June 8, 2022.
5. Fisher-Owens SA, Gansky SA, Platt LJ, et al. Influences on children's oral health: a conceptual model. *Pediatrics*. 2007;120(3):e510–e520. https://doi.org/10.1542/peds.2006-3084.
6. WHO expert consultation on public health intervention against early childhood caries. *Report of a Meeting, Bangkok, Thailand, 26–28 January 2016*. World Health Organization; 2017. Available at: https://www.who.int/publications/i/item/who-expert-consultation-on-public-health-intervention-against-early-childhood-caries. Accessed November 28, 2022.
7. Tham R, Bowatte G, Dharmage SC, et al. Breastfeeding and the risk of dental caries: a systematic review and meta-analysis. *Acta Paediatrc*. 2015;104:62–84. https://doi.org/10.1111/apa.13118.
8. American Academy of Pediatric Dentistry. Definition of Dental home. *The Reference Manual of Pediatric Dentistry*. American Academy of Pediatric Dentistry; 2021:15.
9. Seow W. Developmental defects of enamel and dentine: challenges for basic science research and clinical management. *Aust Dent J*. 2014;59:143–154. https://doi.org/10.1111/adj.12104.
10. Costa FS, Silveira ER, Pinto GS, et al. Developmental defects of enamel and dental caries in the primary dentition: a systematic review and meta-analysis. *J Dent*. 2017;60:1–7.
11. Clark M, Krol D. Protecting all children's teeth (PACT): dental development. *MedEdPORTAL*. 2014;10:9684. Available at: https://doi.org/10.15766/mep_2374-8265.9684.
12. Dental growth and development. *The Reference Manual of Pediatric Dentistry*. [Internet]. Available at: www.aapd.org/globalassets/media/policies_guidelines/r_dentalgrowth.pdf. n.d. Accessed November 28, 2022.
13. *Healthy Habits for Happy Smiles: Helping Your Baby with Teething Pain*. National Center on Early Childhood Health and Wellness; 2016.
14. Macknin ML, Piedmonte M, Jacobs J, et al. Symptoms associated with infant teething: a prospective study. *Pediatrics*. 2000;105(4):747–752.
15. Berkowitz RJ. Mutans streptococci: acquisition and transmission. *Pediatr Dent*. 2006;28(2):106–198.
16. Aslanova M, Ali R, Zito PM. Herpetic Gingivostomatitis. In: *StatPearls* [Internet]. StatPearls Publishing. Available at: https://www.ncbi.nlm.nih.gov/books/NBK526068/. Updated 2021. Accessed June 23, 2022.
17. American Academy of Pediatric Dentistry. *Periodicity of Examination, Preventive Dental Services, Anticipatory Guidance/Counseling, and Oral Treatment for Infants, Children, and Adolescents*. The Reference Manual of Pediatric Dentistry. American Academy of Pediatric Dentistry; 2021:241–251.
18. Guideline on management of acute dental trauma. [Internet]. *Reference Manual, Clinical Guidelines*. American Academy of Pediatric Dentistry. Available at: https://www.aapd.org/assets/1/7/g_trauma.pdf. Updated 2010. Accessed December 16, 2022.
19. Centers for Disease Control and Prevention. Positive parenting tips. [Internet]. National Center on Birth Defects and Developmental Disabilities, Centers for Disease Control and Prevention. Available at: https://www.cdc.gov/ncbddd/childdevelopment/positiveparenting/toddlers.html. Updated 2022. Accessed July 20, 2022.
20. California Dental Association. *Kindergarten Oral Health Requirement*. California Dental Association; 2022.
21. American Dental Association. Athletic Mouth Protectors (Mouthguards). [Internet]. Available at: https://www.ada.org/resources/research/science-and-research-institute/oral-health-topics/athletic-mouth-protectors-mouthguards. Updated 2019. Accessed December 14, 2022.
22. Academy for Sports Dentistry. Academy for Ports Dentistry Position Statement on the Use of Mouthguards and Other Appliance for the Prevention of Concussion and Enhancement of Strength and Performance. Available at: http://www.academyforsportsdentistry.org/index.php?option=com_content&view=article&id=51:position-statements&catid=20:site-content&Itemid=111. Updated 2019. Accessed July 20, 2022.
23. National Institutes of Health. *Oral Health in America: Advances and Challenges*. US Department of Health and Human Services, National Institutes of Health, National Institute of Dental and Craniofacial Research; 2021.
24. Centers for Disease Control and Prevention. *About Electronic Cigarettes (E-Cigarettes)*. Office of Smoking and Health, National Center for Chronic Disease Prevention and Health Promotion; 2022. Available at: https://www.cdc.gov/tobacco/basic_information/e-cigarettes/about-e-cigarettes.html. Accessed July 20, 2022.
25. Centers for Disease Control and Prevention. *Genital HPV Infection-Basic Fact Sheet*. Division of STD Prevention, National Center for HIV, Viral

Hepatitis, STD, and TB Prevention, Centers for Disease Control and Prevention. Available at: https://www.cdc.gov/std/HPV/STDFact-HPV.htm. Updated 2022. Accessed July 14, 2022.

26. Centers for Disease Control and Prevention. *Water Fluoridation Basics.* Division of Oral Health, National Center for Chronic Disease Prevention and Health Promotion. Available at: https://www.cdc.gov/fluoridation/basics/index.htm. Accessed July 20, 2022. Updated 2021.

27. U.S. Department of Health and Human Services Federal Panel on Community Water Fluoridation. U.S. Public Health Service recommendation for fluoride concentration in drinking water for the prevention of dental caries. *Public Health Rep.* 2015;130(4):318–331.

28. Association of State & Territorial Dental Directors. *Fluoride Supplement Policy Statement.* Association of State and Territorial Dental Directors (ASTDD); 2013. Available at: https://www.astdd.org/docs/fluoride-supplement-policy-statement-january-28-2013.pdf. Accessed December 14, 2022.

29. Weyant R, Tracy SL, Anselmo T, et al. Topical fluoride for caries prevention. *J Amer Dent Assoc.* 2013;144(11):1279–1290.

30. U.S. Department of Health and Human Services. *Product Classification.* U.S. Food & Drug Administration. Available at: https://www.accessdata.fda.gov/scripts/cdrh/cfdocs/cfpmn/pmn.cfm?ID=K102973. Accessed July 27, 2022. Updated 2022.

31. Crystal YO, Marghalani AA, Ureles SD, et al. Use of silver diamine fluoride for dental caries management in children and adolescents, including those with special health care needs. *Pediatr Dent.* 2017;39(5):E135–E145.

32. Silver diamine fluoride. *Policy and Summary;* 2021. Available at: www.aapd.org/globalassets/media/policy-center/sdf.factsheet.pdf. Accessed July 27, 2022.

33. World Health Organization. *Oral Health Surveys: Basic Methods.* 5th ed. 2013. Available at: https://www.who.int/publications/i/item/9789241548649. Accessed July 27, 2022.

34. Community. Lec. 6: Indices Used for Dental Caries Assessment. Available at: www.uoanbar.edu.iq/eStoreImages/Bank/10672.pdf. n.d. Accessed July 28, 2022.

35. Khamis AH. Re-visiting the Decay, Missing, Filled Teeth (DMFT) index with a mathematical modeling concept. *J Epidemiol.* 2016;6:6–12.

36. American Academy of Pediatric Dentistry. *Behavior Guidance for the Pediatric Dental Patient.* The Reference Manual of Pediatric Dentistry. American Academy of Pediatric Dentistry; 2021:306–324.

37. American Academy of Pediatrics. *Infant Food and Feeding;* 2021. [Internet]. Available at: www.aap.org/en/patient-care/healthy-active-living-for-families/infant-food-and-feeding/. Accessed November 29, 2022.

38. American Dental Association. Mouthhealthy. *Thumbsucking;* 2022. [Internet]. Available at: https://www.mouthhealthy.org/all-topics-a-z/thumbsucking/. Accessed November 29, 2022.

39. Ullah R, Zafar MS, Shahani N. Potential fluoride toxicity from oral medicaments: a review. *Iran J Basic Med Sci.* 2017;20(8):841–848. https://doi.org/10.22038/IJBMS.2017.9104.

46

Pregnancy and Oral Health

Katy Battani and Alice M. Horowitz

PROFESSIONAL OPPORTUNITIES

Dental hygienists play a critical role in educating and providing oral healthcare to pregnant women. Physiologic changes during pregnancy may increase a woman's susceptibility to certain oral conditions. Pregnancy provides a "teachable moment" for the dental hygienist to counsel women about positive oral hygiene and nutrition behaviors for herself and preventive strategies to avert early childhood caries (ECC) for her future child. Dental providers should work in collaboration with prenatal healthcare providers to ensure optimal oral health of pregnant women before and after delivery.

COMPETENCIES

1. Explain and classify the current state of evidence regarding maternal periodontal disease and adverse birth outcomes. Additionally, discuss potential oral manifestations during pregnancy.
2. Describe oral disease prevention and health behaviors during pregnancy, including professional oral healthcare during pregnancy and the prevention of ECC for infants.
3. Discuss the impact of low health literacy on the oral health of pregnant women and infants.
4. Describe healthcare provider guidelines on oral healthcare during pregnancy, including national priorities.
5. Collaborate interprofessionally with nondental providers in fostering the importance of oral health for pregnant women.
6. Discuss various community programs that serve pregnant women.

INTRODUCTION

Oral health is an important component of a healthy pregnancy and should be maintained or improved during the **prenatal** period, defined as occurring or existing before birth. Pregnancy is divided into three trimesters, roughly 3 months per trimester (Table 46.1). A woman's estimated due date is calculated by counting 40 weeks from the first day of her last menstrual period. **Organogenesis**, or the formation of the organs, occurs during the first 10 weeks of pregnancy; for an environmental factor to be considered a teratogen, exposure must occur during this time period. Pregnancy is an opportune time for women to adopt healthy behaviors, including those related to oral hygiene practices, nutrition, and routine professional oral healthcare. Dental

hygienists play a key role in providing oral healthcare to pregnant women as well as education about oral changes that may occur during pregnancy and ways to prevent and treat oral diseases. It is important for dental hygienists to assure women that oral healthcare during all trimesters of pregnancy is safe (including dental radiographs with proper shielding) for both themselves and their developing fetuses.

Research has clearly demonstrated how to prevent dental caries. Application of primary prevention strategies by the dental hygienist to avert **ECC**—the presence of one or more decayed (noncavitated or cavitated lesions), missing due to caries, or filled tooth surfaces in any primary tooth in a child under the age of 6 years—for the woman's future child is also essential during pregnancy. Timely delivery of educational messages, skills, and preventive therapies to pregnant women can prevent or reduce the incidence of ECC, prevent the need for dental rehabilitation under general anesthesia, and improve the oral health of children.[1] *Mutans streptococci* (MS) may be transmitted vertically from primary caregiver to child through saliva, affected by frequency and amount of exposure. Infants whose mothers have high levels of MS as a result of untreated dental caries are at greater risk for acquiring the organisms earlier than children whose mothers have low levels; thus, pregnant women should have all carious lesions restored prior to delivery to reduce MS levels.[2] Horizontal transmission also can occur, which involves the transfer of MS from another family member or another child (i.e., in a daycare setting). See Chapters 19 and 45 for more information on ECC and severe ECC.

Although reported figures on the prevalence of periodontitis in pregnancy vary, an estimated 42% of US adults 30 years and older have this inflammatory condition, which is characterized by destruction of bone and soft tissue that support the teeth.[3] Since the first report suggesting a potential link between maternal periodontal infection and delivery of preterm and low birth weight infants in 1996, many researchers have examined this association. Systematic reviews have found associations between periodontitis and adverse pregnancy outcomes.[4,5] However, a 2017 Cochrane review found that when pregnant women with periodontal disease who received periodontal treatment were compared to those who did not receive periodontal treatment, (1) there was no evidence that treatment of periodontal disease reduced the number of babies born before 37 weeks of pregnancy and (2) there may be fewer babies born weighing less than 2500 g (5.5 lb).[6] It is important to note that the quality of the evidence for both findings was considered low and that it was unclear if one periodontal treatment was better than another in preventing adverse birth outcomes.[6] While evidence showing a cause-and-effect relationship is lacking between periodontal disease and adverse pregnancy outcomes, oral healthcare during pregnancy has repeatedly been shown to be safe. Thus, women should not avoid oral healthcare during pregnancy or postpone it until after delivery; rather, women should seek oral healthcare and practice good oral hygiene and nutrition behaviors to ensure a healthy mouth that is free of infection. This care is not only essential for the woman's oral and systemic health but is also critical to reduce her child's risk for ECC.

TABLE 46.1	Trimesters of Pregnancy
Trimester	**Time Period**
First	First day of last menstrual period to 13 weeks
Second	14 weeks to 27 weeks
Third	28 weeks to 40 weeks

Medical, dental, and social service professionals and community-based programs that serve pregnant women play a critical role in informing women that oral healthcare during pregnancy is important and safe during all trimesters of pregnancy for both the woman and developing fetus. Access to oral healthcare is affected by many factors including a woman's level of income, health literacy, insurance coverage, trust in the healthcare system, and education level. Availability of transportation, child care, and dental providers to deliver care are also key factors that influence utilization of care by pregnant women. Assisting women with determining Medicaid eligibility, finding a dentist, scheduling appointments, and obtaining child care and transportation help improve access and attainment of oral healthcare during pregnancy, especially for disadvantaged and low income populations.

ORAL MANIFESTATIONS DURING PREGNANCY

Physiological changes during pregnancy may result in changes in the oral cavity. These conditions are listed in Table 46.2. It is important that the dental hygienist be knowledgeable about these conditions to adequately assess and address them with pregnant patients. In addition to providing clinical services to pregnant women, dental hygienists should reinforce the importance of comprehensive oral health behaviors during pregnancy to prevent or reduce the severity of these conditions.

TABLE 46.2 Oral Manifestations During Pregnancy	
Pregnancy gingivitis	An increased inflammatory response to bacterial plaque during pregnancy causes signs of gingivitis in most women, with the anterior teeth affected more than the posterior teeth. These signs are exacerbated by poor plaque control and mouth breathing. Pregnancy gingivitis typically peaks during the third trimester. Women who have gingivitis before pregnancy are more prone to exacerbation during pregnancy. 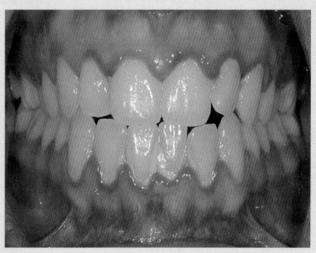 Pregnancy gingivitis
Benign oral gingival lesions (known as pyogenic granuloma, granuloma gravidarum, or epulis of pregnancy; pregnancy tumors)	In approximately 5% of pregnancies, a highly vascularized, hyperplastic, and often pedunculated lesion up to 2 cm in diameter may appear, usually on the anterior gingiva. These lesions may result from a heightened inflammatory response to oral pathogens and usually regress after pregnancy. Excision is rarely necessary but may be needed if there is severe pain, bleeding, or interference with mastication. 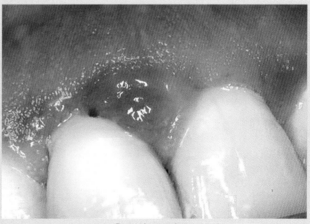 Pyogenic granuloma
Tooth mobility	Increased tooth mobility has been associated with microbial shifts from aerobic to anaerobic bacteria. These shifts are accompanied by increased inflammation in the attachment apparatus as well as mineral disturbances in the lamina dura. This condition appears to reverse after pregnancy.

Continued

TABLE 46.2   Oral Manifestations During Pregnancy—cont'd

Tooth erosion

Erosion of tooth enamel may be more common because of increased exposure to gastric acid from vomiting secondary to morning sickness, hyperemesis gravidarum, or gastric reflux during late pregnancy.

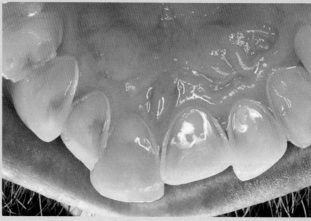

Enamel erosion

Dental caries

An increase in dental caries has been associated with frequent carbohydrate loading and consumption of sugary drinks during pregnancy. Decreased attention to oral hygiene care during pregnancy may also increase dental caries risk.

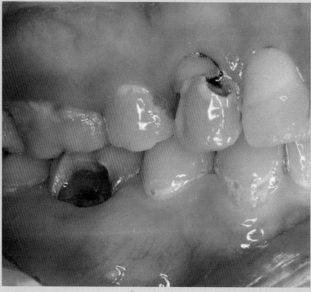

Dental caries

Periodontitis

Untreated gingivitis can progress to periodontitis, which is characterized by a progressive and irreversible loss of alveolar bone and other tissues surrounding the teeth.

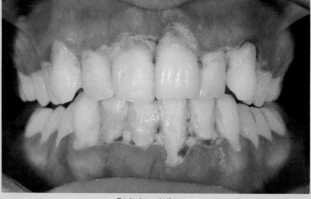

Periodontal disease

Data from Oral health care during pregnancy and through the lifespan. Committee Opinion No. 569. American College of Obstetricians and Gynecologists. *Obstet Gynecol.* 2013;122:417–422. Available at: https://www.acog.org/-/media/Committee-Opinions/Committee-on-Health-Care-for-Underserved-Women/co569.pdf?dmc=1&ts=20171117T1737486115.

ORAL DISEASE PREVENTION AND HEALTH BEHAVIORS DURING PREGNANCY

Oral Hygiene for Pregnant Women

Personal oral healthcare during pregnancy is essentially the same as for any other adult. The best way to prevent dental caries is to drink optimally fluoridated water (see Chapter 45). Adults and children benefit from this public health measure.[7] Drinking tap water is especially beneficial for dental caries prevention when it is optimally fluoridated at 0.7 ppm (0.7 milligrams of fluoride per liter of water). Drinking bottled water is not recommended because it can contain inconsistent and suboptimal amounts of fluoride and expose the consumer to more plastic. Positively, most water filters sold commercially do not remove fluoride. Drinking water rather than sugar-sweetened beverages is better for oral and overall health.

An important regimen for **gravid** (pregnant) women is brushing teeth with fluoride-containing toothpaste twice a day and flossing (interdental cleaning) once a day (see Chapters 24 and 25). Women may experience pregnancy gingivitis that is most likely due to hormonal changes and inadequate oral hygiene practices; however, it can be prevented or reversed with thorough plaque control via brushing and flossing in conjunction with professional dental hygiene preventive services. Gingivitis may be exacerbated if a woman has this condition prior to becoming pregnant. Thus, the dental hygienist should explain and ensure understanding of these important oral hygiene behaviors, even with established pregnant patients and those who have good oral hygiene practices. See Box 46.1, Advice for Pregnant Women.

In addition to drinking fluoridated tap water and using fluoride-containing toothpaste to prevent dental caries, gravid women should consume a varied and balanced diet and limit consumption of sugar-containing foods and drinks between meals. This dietary restriction can be challenging as women may crave certain sweetened foods and drinks and may snack between meals to mitigate nausea. The dental hygienist should complete a comprehensive diet analysis, recommend healthy food and drink options (see Chapter 36), and encourage women to take prenatal supplements as directed by their prenatal healthcare provider. Gravid women should avoid consuming raw meat and certain high-mercury fish, as mercury can be harmful to the developing brain and nervous system (Fig. 46.1).

BOX 46.1 Advice for Pregnant Women

- Get early prenatal care
- Get early dental care
- Enroll in prenatal classes
- Drink tap water, especially if it is optimally fluoridated
- Brush twice a day with fluoride-containing toothpaste
- Floss or interdental cleaning daily
- Eat a well-balanced diet, including supplements as prescribed by obstetrician
- Select nutritious snacks and avoid those that increase caries risk and unwanted weight gain
- Adapt to the proper weight for your pregnancy, whether that is to gain, lose, or maintain weight
- Exercise regularly with physician's approval
- Avoid alcohol, all tobacco products, and illicit drugs, and limit caffeine
- Avoid hot tubs and saunas
- Avoid individuals with infections
- If you vomit, rinse your mouth with one teaspoon of baking soda in a cup of water and avoid toothbrushing for about an hour

---

Professional Oral Healthcare During Pregnancy

Oral healthcare is eminently safe and important during pregnancy. As with all patients, the dental hygienist should take a thorough medical and oral health history with pregnant women (see Chapter 13) and should ask for and document estimated delivery dates. The dental hygienist should consult with other prenatal healthcare providers as necessary regarding comorbid conditions that could affect management of oral health problems such as diabetes, hypertension, pulmonary or cardiac disease, and bleeding disorders. If a pregnant woman has diabetes prior to becoming pregnant and it is poorly controlled during her first trimester, the developing baby's organs, such as the brain, heart, kidneys, and lungs, which start forming during the first 8 weeks of pregnancy, may be affected. High blood glucose levels can be harmful during this period and can increase the baby's risk of birth defects, such as heart defects or defects of the brain or spine.[8]

Gestational diabetes develops during pregnancy (it is not present prior to pregnancy), usually around the 24th week of gestation. The prevalence of gestational diabetes is as high as 9.2%.[9] Hormones from the placenta during pregnancy can block the action of the mother's insulin, which results in insulin resistance. This blockage makes it harder for the mother's body to use insulin, which may lead to needing more insulin than normal to transfer glucose from the bloodstream to cells to be converted into energy. If glucose accumulates in the blood at high levels, hyperglycemia occurs, which can affect the developing baby. The glucose crosses the placenta, which increases the baby's glucose levels, causing the baby's pancreas to make extra insulin to remove the blood glucose. This extra energy is stored as fat because the energy is in excess of what the baby needs to grow and develop. Fat storage can lead to macrosomia, or a "large" baby, and can increase a child's risk for obesity and type 2 diabetes in the future as an adult. At birth, babies may have very low blood glucose levels due to extra insulin made by the baby's pancreas. Low blood glucose levels can result in an increased risk of breathing problems.[10] It is important for the dental hygienist to assess a pregnant woman's diabetes control and to explain the bidirectional relationship between oral health and diabetes to pregnant patients (see Chapter 21). Consulting with the pregnant woman's prenatal healthcare provider about her diabetes control and management is critical to improving oral health and pregnancy outcomes.

Dental hygienists should also assess over-the-counter and prescription drug, herb, and supplement use by pregnant women. In 2015, the US Food and Drug Administration (FDA) released its new "Pregnancy and Lactation Labeling Rule" (PLLR). The PLLR removed the pregnancy letter categories (A, B, C, D, and X) and requires drug labels to be updated when information becomes outdated. The Pregnancy section now includes information organized into three subheadings: Risk Summary, Clinical Considerations, and Data. This information includes potential risks to the developing fetus (including an assessment of risk), known dosing alterations during pregnancy, effects of timing and duration of exposure during pregnancy, maternal adverse reactions, effects of the drug on labor or delivery, and information on pregnancy exposure registry for the drug, if one exists. Information described in the Risk Summary will include an assessment, characterization, and summary of known risks to the developing fetus.[11] For more information, see Chapter 15.

Unfortunately, for a variety of reasons, many pregnant women with low incomes do not have access to dental providers to obtain care. Depending on the state in which they reside, women who are insured by Medicaid (a state- and federal-funded program of financial assistance designed for those unable to afford healthcare services) may or may not have dental benefits. Some of the barriers to oral healthcare

Advice About Eating Fish

What Pregnant Women & Parents Should Know

Fish and other protein-rich foods have nutrients that can help your child's growth and development.

For women of childbearing age (about 16-49 years old), especially pregnant and breastfeeding women, and for parents and caregivers of young children.

- Eat 2 to 3 servings of fish a week from the "Best Choices" list OR 1 serving from the "Good Choices" list.
- Eat a variety of fish.
- Serve 1 to 2 servings of fish a week to children, starting at age 2.
- If you eat fish caught by family or friends, check for fish advisories. If there is no advisory, eat only one serving and no other fish that week.*

Use this chart!

You can use this chart to help you choose which fish to eat, and how often to eat them, based on their mercury levels. The "Best Choices" have the lowest levels of mercury.

What is a serving?

To find out, use the palm of your hand!

 For an adult 4 ounces

 For children, ages 4 to 7 2 ounces

Best Choices EAT 2 TO 3 SERVINGS A WEEK OR Good Choices EAT 1 SERVING A WEEK

Best Choices			Good Choices		
Anchovy	Herring	Scallop	Bluefish	Monkfish	Tilefish (Atlantic Ocean)
Atlantic croaker	Lobster, American and spiny	Shad	Buffalofish	Rockfish	Tuna, albacore/ white tuna, canned and fresh/frozen
Atlantic mackerel	Mullet	Shrimp	Carp	Sablefish	
Black sea bass	Oyster	Skate	Chilean sea bass/ Patagonian toothfish	Sheepshead	Tuna, yellowfin
Butterfish	Pacific chub mackerel	Smelt	Grouper	Snapper	Weakfish/seatrout
Catfish		Sole	Halibut	Spanish mackerel	White croaker/ Pacific croaker
Clam	Perch, freshwater and ocean	Squid	Mahi mahi/ dolphinfish	Striped bass (ocean)	
Cod	Pickerel	Tilapia			
Crab	Plaice	Trout, freshwater			
Crawfish	Pollock	Tuna, canned light (includes skipjack)			
Flounder	Salmon	Whitefish			
Haddock	Sardine	Whiting			
Hake					

Choices to Avoid HIGHEST MERCURY LEVELS

King mackerel	Shark	Tilefish (Gulf of Mexico)
Marlin	Swordfish	Tuna, bigeye
Orange roughy		

*Some fish caught by family and friends, such as larger carp, catfish, trout and perch, are more likely to have fish advisories due to mercury or other contaminants. State advisories will tell you how often you can safely eat those fish.

www.FDA.gov/fishadvice
www.EPA.gov/fishadvice

EPA United States Environmental Protection Agency

FDA U.S. FOOD & DRUG ADMINISTRATION

THIS ADVICE REFERS TO FISH AND SHELLFISH COLLECTIVELY AS "FISH." / ADVICE UPDATED JANUARY 2017

Fig. 46.1 Advice about eating fish. (From US Food and Drug Administration. Eating Fish: What Pregnant Women and Parents Should Know. Available at: https://www.fda.gov/Food/ResourcesForYou/Consumers/ucm393070.htm. November 29, 2017.)

BOX 46.2 Barriers to Care for Low-Income Gravid Women

- Low level of oral health literacy
- Cannot afford dental fees/copayments
- Do not understand the impact of oral health on general health
- Difficulty in finding dentists who accept Medicaid and/or pregnant women
- Office hours are not convenient for those who work
- Obstetricians and nurse-midwives often do not urge gravid women to seek dental care
- Fear of going to dentist because of past experience
- Uncertainty about whether dental care is safe during pregnancy for woman and fetus
- Lack of transportation
- Lack of child care

BOX 46.3 Positioning of Pregnant Women in the Dental Chair

- Keep the woman's head at a higher level than her feet.
- Place the woman in a semireclining position as tolerated and allow frequent position changes.
- Place a small pillow under the right hip or have the woman turn slightly to the left as needed to avoid dizziness or nausea resulting from hypotension.

with morning nausea. Positioning pregnant women appropriately in the dental chair to ensure comfort is essential (Box 46.3). The woman's head should always be higher than her feet, and frequent position changes should be accommodated as necessary. A small pillow can be placed under her right hip, or the woman can turn slightly to the left as needed to avoid dizziness or nausea resulting from hypotension.[12]

Oral Hygiene for Infants

It is imperative that dental hygienists inform pregnant women, parents, and caregivers that dental caries is preventable and teach preventive strategies to keep children free of dental caries. Dental hygienists also are responsible for ensuring understanding of this concept and

during pregnancy, especially for women with low incomes, are shown in Box 46.2.

When providing oral healthcare to pregnant women, it is best to schedule them in the afternoon during the first trimester and early part of the second trimester. This scheduling approach may avert bouts confirming that parents and caregivers have the necessary skills to do so. Appropriate oral hygiene practices for the infant should begin as soon as the child returns from the hospital or place of delivery. Many references suggest that caregivers begin oral hygiene when the first tooth arrives. This recommendation is too late to establish appropriate behaviors on the part of the caregiver and the infant. It is best to begin soon after birth. Dental hygienists should teach pregnant women, new mothers, and other caregivers how to clean an infant's mouth using a clean, damp infant washcloth. The dual purposes are to disrupt bacterial plaque and get the infant and mother accustomed to the procedure. When the first tooth erupts, begin using a tiny smear (size of a grain of rice) of fluoride-containing toothpaste to brush the child's teeth (Fig. 46.2). Equally important is to teach caregivers how to "lift the lip" of the infant to look for white spot lesions along the gingival margin once a month and what to do if there is discoloration of the teeth. A suggestion to help caregivers remember to "lift the lip" is to do it on the infant's birth date each month. See Box 46.4 for strategies to decrease ECC through the infant's second year of life and Box 46.5

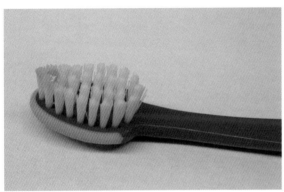

Fig. 46.2 Toothpaste amount: smear.

BOX 46.4 Strategies to Decrease Early Childhood Caries, Birth to Year 2

- Determine whether patient's water supply is optimally fluoridated.
- If the tap water is not optimally fluoridated, discuss prescriptions for dietary fluoride drops or tablets, or use of bottled water, like Nursery Water, which is optimally fluoridated and available in gallon containers.
- Begin cleaning infant's mouth daily as soon as mother and infant are home from hospital/birthing center.
- This is to establish habit for mother and infant. Do not wait until the first tooth erupts to begin cleaning infant's mouth.
- When first tooth erupts at about 6 to 8 months, brush with smear of fluoride toothpaste.
- Never put child to bed with a bottle.
- At about 8 to 10 months, begin lifting baby's lip to check for white spots: white lines along the gum line.
- White spots are noncavitated dental caries that can be healed with fluoride.
- Take child to dentist at once if white spots are observed.
- Wean infant from bottle by 12 to 14 months.
- Avoid frequent consumption of foods and drinks containing sugar.
- No juice during the first year of life.
- Ask doctor about fluoride varnish.
- Brush teeth twice a day with fluoride toothpaste.

for a critical thinking scenario to practice oral health education with a pregnant patient.

The Role of Health Literacy in Oral Health of Pregnant Women and Their Children

Health literacy has been defined in two dimensions, personal and organizational health literacy. *Healthy People 2030* defines personal health literacy as "the degree to which individuals have the ability to find, understand, and use information and services to inform health-related decisions and actions for themselves and others" and organizational health literacy as "the degree to which organizations equitably enable individuals to find, understand, and use information and services to inform health-related decisions and actions for themselves and others."[13]

The word *individuals* in the definition of personal health literacy includes patients as well as healthcare providers and policy makers. Supporting individual patients' capacity means providers must communicate clearly and health facilities must be patient-friendly and easy to navigate as noted in the definition of organizational health literacy. Oral health literacy is especially important because often, oral health is not considered an integral part of overall health. It is important for dental hygienists to understand and internalize that oral health and well-being are not determined by the health system alone. Oral health literacy is the nexus of creating better communication and education to increase primary and secondary preventive regimens. Low levels of health literacy negatively impact oral health outcomes.[14] When pregnant women do not understand the importance of oral health for their overall health and well-being and that oral healthcare during pregnancy is safe and recommended, it is unlikely that they will obtain care. Similarly, if a mother does not understand her role in preventing ECC, it is unlikely that she will clean her infant's mouth, avoid bedtime bottle feeding, or lift the infant's lip once a month to check for early carious lesions and then take corrective action. For patients to adhere to educational instructions, they must understand them; thus, always use the **Teach Back Method**, a communication method used by healthcare providers to confirm whether a patient or caregiver understands what is being explained to them. If a patient understands, they are able to explain or "teach back" the information accurately to the provider. See the Critical Thinking Scenario in Box 46.5 to practice patient education and communication with a pregnant patient/mother.

BOX 46.5 Critical Thinking Scenario A

You are a dental hygienist practicing in an optimally fluoridated community. Mrs. Brown, who is pregnant in her early second trimester, comes in for her routine dental hygiene appointment. Mrs. Brown explains to you that her 4-year-old child just had eight cavities filled and four silver crowns placed on her canines by a pediatric dentist. It was a 3-hour-long procedure done under general anesthesia, costing thousands of dollars. Mrs. Brown says, "I keep tearing up because I can't help but blame myself. This is our second child that has needed such extensive work and after the first time it happened, I swore I would make sure to brush all the kids' teeth morning and night and floss … now I'll have four silver crowns every day reminding me that I didn't do it and of my failures as a parent." Upon clinical examination, Mrs. Brown has poor plaque control, two active caries lesions, and gingivitis.

What oral health education and recommendations would you provide to Mrs. Brown for herself and for her children, including for the child she is expecting? What communication techniques could be used to ensure Mrs. Brown understands the information you share with her?

HEALTHCARE PROVIDER GUIDELINES

In 2012, building on the development of several state healthcare provider guidance documents on oral healthcare during pregnancy, the American College of Obstetricians and Gynecologists (ACOG), in partnership with the American Dental Association (ADA) and other organizations, issued *Oral Health Care During Pregnancy: A National Consensus Statement*. This document includes practice guidance for both prenatal and oral healthcare providers as well as educational material for pregnant women. In 2013, the ACOG released a Committee Opinion titled *Oral Health Care During Pregnancy and Through the Lifespan*, and in 2016, the American Academy of Pediatric Dentistry released *Guideline on Perinatal and Infant Oral Health Care*. These documents provide practice guidance and resources for medical and dental providers regarding the safety of oral healthcare during pregnancy, including the use of dental radiographs (Box 46.6) and indications, contraindications, and special considerations about specific pharmacologic agents (Table 46.3). These documents continue to be updated as new evidence-based information and recommendations become available. See the Critical Thinking Scenario in Box 46.7 to practice dental hygiene treatment planning and patient and prenatal provider communication. See Box 46.8 for legal, ethical, and safety issues related to oral healthcare for pregnant patients.

National Priorities

Oral healthcare utilization by pregnant women is one of the 15 Maternal and Child Health (MCH) National Performance Measures (NPM) for the State Title V Block Grant program (Table 46.4), which aims to improve the health and well-being of women (particularly mothers) and children throughout the nation (Box 46.9).[15] NPMs reflect short- and medium-term outcomes of health behaviors and healthcare access/quality measures.

Beginning in 2015, the oral health NPM changed from the percentage of third-grade children who have received protective dental sealants on at least one permanent tooth to a two-part measure focused on (1) the percentage of women who had a dental visit during pregnancy and (2) the percentage of children and adolescents ages 1 to 17 who had a preventive dental visit in the last year. This change broadened the population beyond third-grade children and made oral health during pregnancy a top MCH priority.

Healthy People 2030

Healthy People is a national initiative that began in 1979 with overarching health goals and national health objectives. HP2030

BOX 46.6 ALARA Principle: Limiting Radiation Exposure for All People

Dental radiographs account for approximately 2.5% of the effective dose received from medical radiographs and fluoroscopies. Even though radiation exposure from dental radiographs is low, it is the dentist's responsibility to follow the ALARA Principle (As Low as Reasonably Achievable) to minimize the patient's exposure once a decision to obtain radiographs is made.

Examples of good radiologic practice include:

- Use of the fastest image receptor compatible with the diagnostic task (F-speed film or digital)
- Collimation of the beam to the size of the receptor whenever feasible
- Proper film exposure and processing techniques
- Use of protective aprons and thyroid collars when appropriate
- Limiting the number of images obtained to the minimum necessary to obtain essential diagnostic information.

TABLE 46.3 Pharmacologic Considerations for Pregnant Women[a]

Pharmaceutical Agent	Indications, Contraindications, and Special Considerations
Analgesics	
• Acetaminophen • Acetaminophen with codeine, hydrocodone, or oxycodone • Codeine • Meperidine • Morphine	May be used during pregnancy. Oral pain can often be managed with nonopioid medication. If opioids are used, prescribe the lowest dose for the shortest duration (usually less than 3 days) and avoid issuing refills to reduce risk for dependency.
• Aspirin • Ibuprofen • Naproxen	First trimester: avoid use. Second trimester: • 13 weeks up to 20 weeks: may use for short duration, 48 to 72 hours. • 20 weeks up to 27 weeks: limit use. Third trimester: avoid use.
Antibiotics	
• Amoxicillin • Cephalosporins • Clindamycin • Metronidazole • Penicillin	May be used during pregnancy.
• Ciprofloxacin • Clarithromycin • Levofloxacin • Moxifloxacin	Avoid during pregnancy.
• Tetracycline	Never use during pregnancy.
Anesthetics[b]	
Local anesthetics with epinephrine (e.g., bupivacaine, lidocaine, mepivacaine)	May be used during pregnancy.
Nitrous oxide (30%)	May be used during pregnancy when topical or local anesthetics are inadequate. Pregnant women require lower levels of nitrous oxide to achieve sedation; consult with prenatal care health professional.
Antimicrobials[c]	
• Cetylpyridinium chloride mouth rinse • Chlorhexidine mouth rinse • Xylitol	May be used during pregnancy.

[a]The pharmacologic agents listed in this table are to be used only for indicated medical conditions and with appropriate supervision.
[b]Consult with a prenatal care health professional before using intravenous sedation or general anesthesia. Limit duration of exposure to less than 3 hours in pregnant women in the third trimester.
[c]Use alcohol-free products during pregnancy.
From Oral Health Care During Pregnancy: A National Consensus Statement—Summary of an Expert Workgroup Meeting © 2012 by the National Maternal and Child Oral Health Resource Center, Georgetown University. Table updated 2022. Courtesy of the National Maternal and Child Oral Health Resource Center. Available at https://www.mchoralhealth.org/PDFs/OralHealthPregnancyPharmacological.pdf.

BOX 46.7 Critical Thinking Scenario B

Ms. G is a 19-year-old low-income woman who presented to a dental school clinic. She is 28 weeks pregnant but did not learn of her pregnancy until the 22nd week. She has seen a nurse-midwife for an initial prenatal visit at a local community health center. She is Spanish speaking but speaks broken English (her boyfriend was with her to help translate). She presented with a chief complaint of "My gum hurts and it hurts to eat," which turned out to be localized pain from a large pyogenic granuloma on the gingiva above teeth Nos. 11 and 12. She has Medicaid insurance and reports having had her "teeth cleaned" 3 months ago, but her radiographs show bone loss and heavy subgingival calculus. She grew up in Guatemala, a country that has limited access to dental care.

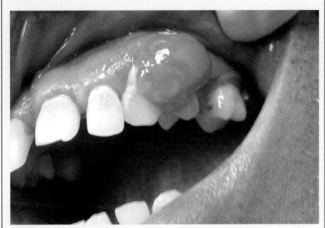

Large pyogenic granuloma.

Describe your treatment plan for Ms. G, including how you would sequence her care plan. What education would you provide and how would you provide it to ensure that she and her partner understand? How and what would you communicate with her prenatal care provider?

BOX 46.8 Legal, Ethical, and Safety Issues

You are working as a newly hired dental hygienist in a group practice with multiple dentists and dental hygienists. You find that some of the dentists refuse to treat pregnant women and that it is office policy to schedule pregnant women for dental hygiene care only during the second trimester of pregnancy. The dental practice accepts Medicaid insurance, and in your state, Medicaid covers dental services for pregnant women but only during pregnancy. Women lose their dental coverage once they deliver.

Discuss the legal, ethical, and safety issues regarding this situation, including how you could use the ADHA Code of Ethics to guide you (see Chapter 7). How would you address this situation with your dental colleagues? What information and resources could you share with them?

As a dental hygienist, how could you promote the importance and safety of oral healthcare during pregnancy for women in the practice and in your community?

US Preventive Services Task Force

The US Preventive Services Task Force began in 1984 and consists of an independent panel of volunteer experts in given fields of prevention and evidence-based medicine and dentistry. A panel's recommendations are based on rigorous reviews of peer-reviewed publications and are assigned a letter grade of A, B, C, or D, or an I statement (Table 46.5). The recommendation relevant to this topic is Prevention of Dental Caries in Children Younger than 5 Years: Screening and Interventions as shown in Table 46.6.

American Public Health Association Policy Statement

In October 2020, the American Public Health Association (APHA) Governing Council approved the APHA Oral Health Section's policy statement, Improving Access to Dental Care for Pregnant Women through Education, Integration of Health Services, Insurance Coverage, an Appropriate Dental Workforce, and Research.[16] The policy statement describes the public health problem, opposing arguments, and evidence-based strategies and action steps to address the problem at federal, state, and local levels. The policy statement was disseminated to stakeholders throughout the country to encourage them to use the policy statement to learn about and advocate for improved access to dental care for pregnant women.

CENTERS FOR MEDICARE AND MEDICAID SERVICES

In June 2022, the White House released a *Blueprint for Addressing the Maternal Health Crisis*, which describes the administration's approach to improving maternal health and addressing inequities in maternal health outcomes.[17] The blueprint identifies opportunities to enhance maternity care delivered to enrollees in Medicare, Medicaid, the Children's Health Insurance Program, and the Health Insurance Marketplace—specifically, through a focus on driving improvements in access to and quality of care during pregnancy, childbirth, and the postpartum period. Centers for Medicare and Medicaid Services (CMS) identified five key gaps in maternity care related to its programs (i.e., coverage and access to care, data, quality of care, workforce, and social supports). Unfortunately, across income and education level, people of color are far more likely to die from pregnancy-related complications, and, in some cases, Black, American Indian, and Alaska Native people are up to five times more likely to die due to pregnancy-related causes than their White peers.[17]

INTERPROFESSIONAL COLLABORATION AND PRACTICE

Most healthcare providers are not trained to practice as part of integrated teams. Especially lacking is collaboration between medicine and dentistry. Interprofessional collaboration in dentistry is an emerging and long-overdue practice because oral health is an integral part of overall health. Another emerging healthcare trend relates to government policies that promote prevention and keeping people healthy rather than providing treatment. Although these latter changes have not impacted dentistry as much as medicine, they are on the horizon to enhance health and the patient experience and to decrease costs, also known as the Triple Aim (Fig. 46.3).[18]

Medical providers often lack knowledge about the importance and safety of oral healthcare during pregnancy and the relationship between oral health and general health.[19] This lack of information for medical providers is a missed opportunity to educate their gravid patients and connect them with necessary dental providers. Similarly,

contains no specific oral health objectives focused on pregnant women or oral healthcare during pregnancy; however, objectives in two topic areas are pertinent. In the Oral Health topic area, relevant objectives include those shown in Box 46.10. It is equally as important for dental hygienists to be aware of objectives in the Health Communication and Health Information Technology topic areas shown in Box 46.11.

TABLE 46.4 Title V National Performance Measures[15]

Number	Priority Area	Population Domain
1	Well-Woman Visit	Women/Maternal Health
2	Low-Risk Cesarean Delivery	Women/Maternal Health
3	Risk-Appropriate Perinatal Care	Perinatal/Infant Health
4	Breastfeeding	Perinatal/Infant Health
5	Safe Sleep	Perinatal/Infant Health
6	Developmental Screening	Child Health
7	Injury Hospitalization	Child Health and/or Adolescent Health
8	Physical Activity	Child Health and/or Adolescent Health
9	Bullying	Adolescent Health
10	Adolescent Well-Visit	Adolescent Health
11	Medical Home	Children with Special Healthcare Needs
12	Transition	Children with Special Healthcare Needs
13 • NPM 13.1: Percent of women who had a dental visit during pregnancy • NPM 13.2: Percent of children ages 1 through 17 who had a preventive dental visit in the past year	Preventive Dental Visit	Cross-Cutting/Life Course
14	Smoking	Cross-Cutting/Life Course
15	Adequate Insurance	Cross-Cutting/Life Course

BOX 46.9 Goals of Title V of the Social Security Act

Title V funds are distributed to grantees from 59 states and jurisdictions. The funds seek to provide:
- Access to quality care, especially for people with low incomes or limited availability of care
- Assistance in the reduction of infant mortality
- Access to comprehensive prenatal and postnatal care for women, especially low-income and at-risk pregnant women
- An increase in health assessments and followup diagnostic and treatment services
- Access to preventive and child care services as well as rehabilitative services for certain children
- Family-centered, community-based systems of coordinated care for children with special healthcare needs
- Toll-free hotlines and assistance in applying for services to pregnant women with infants and children who are eligible for Title XIX (Medicaid)

From: httpsfs://www.mchoralhealth.org/titlevbg/index.php.

dental providers should also always confirm with their gravid patients that they have a prenatal healthcare provider and are obtaining routine prenatal care.

Pregnancy is an ideal time for interprofessional collaboration because of the impact of pregnancy on the woman's oral health. Thus, dental hygienists' working with obstetricians, family medicine physicians, nurses, nurse-midwives, social service professionals, and others is essential for optimal health for gravid women. For example, there may be opportunities for dental hygienists to teach or contribute to prenatal class education offered by medical group practices, community health centers, local health departments, birthing centers, and hospitals. Additionally, dental hygienists could be embedded in medical clinics and private practices. Further, by working with pediatricians

and family medicine physicians, additional collaboration can take place to prevent ECC.

In addition to lack of training on both sides of the medical-dental equation, a major barrier to interprofessional collaboration is that most electronic health record (EHR) systems do not have fully integrated medical and dental records that are compatible with one another. However, this issue is being addressed by some EHR companies, and such compatibility is most likely found in health maintenance organizations and federally qualified health centers.

Critical Thinking Scenario

See the Critical Thinking Scenario in Box 46.12 about educating prenatal providers on the importance of oral health during pregnancy.

COMMUNITY PROGRAMS THAT SERVE PREGNANT WOMEN

Community programs that serve pregnant women largely focus on women and children with low incomes and provide a variety of services. These programs often need assistance regarding oral health of pregnant women and their children, thus providing opportunities for dental hygienists to practice and research.

Special Supplemental Nutritional Program for Women, Infants, and Children

One of the largest of these programs is the US Department of Agriculture's Special Supplemental Nutritional Program for Women, Infants and Children, known as **WIC**. WIC provides grants to states for nutritious supplemental foods, referrals for healthcare services, nutrition education, and breastfeeding education for pregnant women, infants, and children through age 5 with low incomes who are at nutritional risk.[20] WIC programs can be located in a variety of settings, including city or county health departments, hospitals, schools, mobile clinics, migrant health centers and camps, and Indian Health Service facilities.

BOX 46.10 Oral Conditions 2030 Objectives

General
- Reduce the proportion of adults with active or untreated tooth decay
- Increase the proportion of oral and pharyngeal cancers detected at the earliest stage
- Increase use of the oral healthcare system

Adolescents
- Reduce the proportion of children and adolescents with lifetime tooth decay
- Reduce the proportion of children and adolescents with active and untreated tooth decay

Healthcare Access and Quality
- Reduce the proportion of people who cannot get the dental care they need when they need it
- Increase the proportion of people with dental insurance

Health Policy
- Increase the proportion of people whose water systems have the recommended amount of fluoride

Nutrition and Healthy Eating
- Reduce consumption of added sugars by people aged 2 years and over

Older Adults
- Reduce the proportion of older adults with untreated root surface decay
- Reduce the proportion of adults aged 45 years and over who have lost all their teeth
- Reduce the proportion of adults aged 45 years and over with moderate and severe periodontitis

Preventive Care
- Increase the proportion of low-income youth who have a preventive dental visit

- Increase the proportion of children and adolescents who have dental sealants on 1 or more molars

Public Health Infrastructure
- Increase the number of states and DC that have an oral and craniofacial health surveillance system
- Reduce the proportion of children and adolescents who have dental caries experience in their primary or permanent teeth
- Reduce the proportion of children aged 3 to 5 years with dental caries experience in their primary teeth
- Reduce the proportion of adults with untreated dental decay
- Reduce the proportion of adults aged 35 to 44 years with untreated dental decay
- Reduce the proportion of adults who have ever had a permanent tooth extracted because of dental caries or periodontal disease
- Increase the proportion of children, adolescents, and adults who used the oral healthcare system in the past year
- Increase the proportion of low-income children and adolescents who received any preventive dental service during the past year
- Increase the proportion of Federally Qualified Health Centers (FQHCs) that have an oral healthcare program
- Increase the proportion of local health departments that have oral health prevention or care programs
- Increase the proportion of patients who receive oral health services at FQHCs each year
- Increase the proportion of adults who receive preventive interventions in dental offices
- Increase the proportion of adults who received information from a dentist or dental hygienist focusing on reducing tobacco use or on smoking cessation in the past year
- Increase the number of states and DC that have a system for recording and referring infants and children with cleft lips and cleft palates to craniofacial anomaly rehabilitative teams

BOX 46.11 Health Communication and Health Information Technology

- Improve the health literacy of the population
- Increase the proportion of persons who report their healthcare provider always gave them easy to understand instructions about what to do to take care of their illness or health condition
- Increase the proportion of persons who report their healthcare providers always asked them to describe how they will follow the instructions
- Increase the proportion of persons who report their healthcare providers always explained things so they could understand them

WIC began as a pilot program in 1972 and became permanent in 1974. Most state WIC programs provide vouchers or credit card–like cards that participants use in stores that are authorized to accept WIC vouchers or cards. There are approximately 46,000 authorized merchants nationwide. There are both positive and negative limitations on what can be purchased—for example, participants can purchase fruit and/or vegetable juice or juice blends (must be 100% juice) which often contain high amounts of sugar, but they cannot purchase fluoride toothpaste or toothbrushes.

WIC has demonstrated its effectiveness by improving the health of pregnant women, new mothers, and their children. To qualify for WIC,

an applicant must be a pregnant woman, be a postpartum woman (up to 1 year if breastfeeding and 6 months if not breastfeeding), be an infant, or be a child younger than 5 years of age, be at nutritional risk, and have a family income at or below 185 percent of the US poverty level or participate in the Supplemental Nutrition Assistance Program (SNAP), Medicaid, or Temporary Assistance for Needy Families (TANF).[21] WIC served about 6.2 million participants each month in fiscal year 2021, including an estimated 43 percent of all infants in the United States.[21]

Depending on the state, WIC programs provide educational sessions and materials, primarily on nutrition, need for prenatal care, and breastfeeding practices. Some state WIC programs include educational information about the oral health of pregnant women and their infants, and some use educational materials developed by their state's Office or Division of Oral Health. Some WIC programs also have dental hygienists at WIC sites to educate pregnant women and mothers about oral health and to provide risk assessment, oral screenings, fluoride applications, and case management services. This is an excellent opportunity for dental hygienists who are interested in working with pregnant women, mothers, and young children to provide oral healthcare in a nontraditional setting and collaborate with WIC staff.

Early Head Start and Head Start Programs

Head Start and Early Head Start are federally sponsored programs of the Agency for Children and Families, Health Resources and

TABLE 46.5   US Preventive Services Task Force Grade Definitions

Grade	Definition	Suggestions for Practice
A	The USPSTF recommends the service. There is high certainty that the net benefit is substantial.	Offer or provide this service.
B	The USPSTF recommends the service. There is high certainty that the net benefit is moderate or there is moderate certainty that the net benefit is moderate to substantial.	Offer or provide this service.
C	The USPSTF recommends selectively offering or providing this service to individual patients based on professional judgment and patient preferences. There is at least moderate certainty that the net benefit is small.	Offer or provide this service for selected patients depending on individual circumstances.
D	The USPSTF recommends against the service. There is moderate or high certainty that the service has no net benefit or that the harms outweigh the benefits.	Discourage the use of this service.
I Statement	The USPSTF concludes that the current evidence is insufficient to assess the balance of benefits and harms of the service. Evidence is lacking, of poor quality, or conflicting, and the balance of benefits and harms cannot be determined.	Read the clinical considerations section of USPSTF Recommendation Statement. If the service is offered, patients should understand the uncertainty about the balance of benefits and harms.

Grade Definitions. US Preventive Services Task Force. November 2017. https://www.uspreventiveservicestaskforce.org/Page/Name/grade-definitions.

TABLE 46.6   Final Recommendation Statement

Prevention of Dental Caries in Children Younger Than 5 Years: Screening and Interventions
USPSTF, Released December 2021
Summary of Recommendations and Evidence

Population	Recommendation	Grade
Children younger than 5 years	The USPSTF recommends that primary care clinicians prescribe oral fluoride supplementation starting at age 6 months for children whose water supply is deficient in fluoride.	B
Children younger than 5 years	The USPSTF recommends that primary care clinicians apply fluoride varnish to the primary teeth of all infants and children starting at the age of primary tooth eruption.	B
Children younger than 5 years	The USPSTF concludes that the current evidence is insufficient to assess the balance of benefits and harms of routine screening examinations for dental caries performed by primary care clinicians in children younger than 5 years.	I

From *Final Recommendation Statement: Prevention of Dental Caries in Children Younger Than 5 Years: Screening and Interventions.* US Preventive Services Task Force. December 2021. https://www.uspreventiveservicestaskforce.org/uspstf/recommendation/prevention-of-dental-caries-in-children-younger-than-age-5-years-screening-and-interventions1.

Service Administration (ACF, HRSA) for low-income pregnant women, infants, and toddlers. Head Start provides services to more than 1 million children each year in all states and territories. It began more than 50 years ago and was originally developed for 3- and 4-year-olds.[22] From the beginning, oral health was included in Head Start. Head Start is designed to provide comprehensive early childhood education to low-income families to help ensure that children are healthy and ready for school. Early Head Start programs are available to families until a child turns 3 years old and can transition into Head Start or another preschool program. All programs include early learning, health (including oral health), and family support.

Early Head Start and Head Start programs are located in schools, child care centers, family care centers, farm worker camps, and tribal communities. Some Early Head Start programs provide home visiting services in which the teacher goes to the home to provide lessons and assistance. Dental hygienists often work with Head Start programs, staff, and families by providing oral health education and topical fluoride applications for children.

Home Visiting Programs

The Maternal, Infant and Early Childhood Home Visiting Program (MIECHV) is a program sponsored by the Maternal and Child Health Bureau of HRSA. Home visiting programs focus on the improvement of MCH by preventing child abuse and neglect, educating about positive parenting, and promoting child development and school readiness.[23] These programs also focus on improved family economic self-sufficiency and reduction in crime and domestic violence. At this time, there is relatively little oral health content included in-home visits. However, this is an area of need and potential for dental hygienists who are interested in home visiting programs.

Other Programs

Different organizations such as churches, the United Way, and other civic groups hold community baby showers for all, but especially for low-income pregnant women and their families. This is an excellent opportunity to provide oral health education for women and their infants and families. Dental hygienists can play a major role in providing health education and oral health resources, such as toothbrushes,

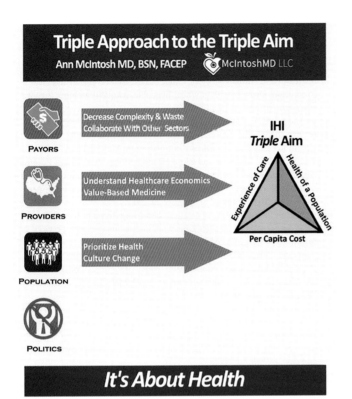

Fig. 46.3 Triple Aim. (Courtesy Ann McIntosh MD; McIntoshMD, Sustainable healthcare solutions.)

BOX 46.12 Critical Thinking Scenario C

You are a public health dental hygienist trying to organize an oral health session to be included in a prenatal class provided by a local hospital. Your presentation urges pregnant women to complete all dental care prior to delivery to help ensure their oral health and that of their infants and teaches the women how to care for their infants' mouths. The CEO of the hospital has asked you to speak with a group of obstetricians who have privileges at the hospital because one of them has voiced concerns about the safety of gravid women having dental treatment.

What would you do to prepare yourself for the meeting with the obstetricians? What information would you provide them and what would you ask them to do to facilitate women obtaining oral healthcare during pregnancy?

---

fluoride toothpaste, and floss, for women and their families at these venues.

Boxes for Babies is a relatively new concept in the United States, but it has been a practice in Finland for nearly 75 years. The boxes are a safe, inexpensive place for newborns to sleep and are provided free by the Finnish government, which points out that the box is the reason Finland has one of the lowest infant mortality rates globally. Baby boxes usually also provide bedding and a selection of clothes and products for use in the first few months of life. None of the baby boxes, globally, provide tips for keeping infant caries-free, nor do they include an infant washcloth or other supplies for disrupting plaque on the baby's gums. Providing appropriate information for agencies to include in these boxes or advocating for its inclusion are examples of how dental hygienists can become involved in their communities.

KEY CONCEPTS

- Both adults and children benefit from drinking fluoridated water. Gravid women should drink fluoridated water, brush their teeth with fluoride toothpaste twice daily, and clean interdentally once a day.
- Dental hygienists should teach pregnant women about oral hygiene, nutrition behaviors, and the prevention of oral diseases, and work collaboratively with prenatal healthcare providers to ensure optimal health of women before and after delivery.
- Essential care includes primary prevention strategies by the dental hygienist to avert ECC, including education about the transmissibility of dental caries–causing bacteria between the mother or caregiver and the child and ensuring restoration of all caries before the child's birth.
- While evidence showing a cause-and-effect relationship is lacking between periodontal disease and adverse pregnancy outcomes, oral healthcare during pregnancy has repeatedly been shown to be safe during all trimesters.
- Women should seek oral healthcare during pregnancy because it is essential for the woman's oral and systemic health and critical to reducing her child's risk for ECC.
- Medical and dental healthcare providers and community programs should address barriers to oral healthcare during pregnancy, including how and where to find oral healthcare providers, cost of care, availability of dental benefit coverage, transportation, child care, safety concerns, and fear.
- Oral manifestations that may occur during pregnancy include hormone-related gingivitis, benign oral lesions, tooth mobility, tooth erosion, periodontitis, and dental caries.
- It is important for the dental hygienist to assess a pregnant woman's diabetes control and to explain the bidirectional relationship between oral health and diabetes to pregnant patients.
- Dental hygienists should assess the dosage and safety of all medications, herbs, and supplements taken by pregnant women.
- Appointments during early afternoon are recommended for oral healthcare during the first trimester and early second trimester.
- Appropriate oral hygiene practices for the infant should begin as soon as the child returns from the hospital or place of delivery.
- Improving oral health literacy of pregnant women is essential to increasing awareness of the need for oral healthcare and education during pregnancy.
- Always use the Teach Back Method, a communication method used by healthcare providers to confirm whether a patient or caregiver understands what is being explained to them.
- Dental hygienists should consult current practice guidelines for providing oral healthcare for pregnant women to deliver evidence-based care.

ONLINE RESOURCES

Videos on oral cleaning of an infant's mouth, patient-provider knee-to-knee dental examination, and the teach-back communication method are available for viewing on Evolve (http://evolve.elsevier.com/Pieren/hygiene/).

Healthy Mouths for You and Your Baby (11:49)
English: https://www.youtube.com/watch?v=ycTettc04YI
(The English-language video with Spanish and Korean subtitles can be viewed by clicking on the "Settings" tool [gear on the bottom right of YouTube video] → "Subtitles" → "Auto-translate" and then choosing the desired language for subtitles.)
Healthy Mouths for You and Your Baby (2-minute video clips) (2:10)
English: https://go.umd.edu/healthymouths
Spanish subtitles: https://go.umd.edu/bocassanas

Brushing Toddlers Teeth (2:18)
English: https://www.youtube.com/watch?v=eW2SlJenJNg
Lift the Lip to Prevent Dental Decay (2:24)
English: https://www.youtube.com/watch?v=80DDOcsZOIc
Spanish subtitles: https://www.youtube.com/watch?v=LpwqqrAnIfw

REFERENCES

1. American Academy of Pediatric Dentistry. Policy on Early Childhood Caries: Classifications, Consequences, and Preventive Strategies. *American Academy of Pediatric Dentistry*; 2016. Available at: http://www.aapd.org/media/Policies_Guidelines/P_ECCClassifications.pdf.

2. American Academy of Pediatric Dentistry. Perinatal and infant oral healthcare. *American Academy of Pediatric Dentistry*. 2016;39(6):208–212. Available at: http://www.aapd.org/media/Policies_Guidelines/BP_PerinatalOralHealthCare.pdf.

3. Eke P, Thornton-Evans G, Wei L, Borgnakke W, Dye B, Genco R. Periodontitis in US adults: national health and nutrition examination Survey 2009–2014. *J Am Dent Assoc*. 2018;149(7):576–586.

4. Corbella S, Taschieri S, Del Fabbro M, et al. Adverse pregnancy outcomes and periodontitis: a systematic review and meta-analysis exploring potential association. *Quintessence Int*. 2016;47:193–204.

5. Daalderop LA, Wieland BL, Tomsin K, et al. Periodontal disease and pregnancy outcomes: overview of systematic reviews. *J Dent Res*. 2017;20(10):1–18.

6. Iheozor-Ejiofor Z, Middleton P, Esposito M, et al. Treating gum disease to prevent adverse birth outcomes in pregnant women. *Cochrane Database Syst Rev*. 2017;11(6):CD005297. Available at: http://www.cochrane.org/CD005297/ORAL_treating-gum-disease-prevent-adverse-birth-outcomes-pregnant-women. Accessed November 12, 2017. Published June 12, 2017.

7. O'Mullane DM, Baez RJ, Jones S, et al. Fluoride and oral health. *Comm Dent Health*. 2016;33:69–99.

8. The National Institute of Diabetes and Digestive and Kidney Diseases Health Information Center; 2017. Available at: https://www.niddk.nih.gov/health-information/diabetes/diabetes-pregnancy. Accessed November 19, 2017.

9. DeSisto CL, Kim SY, Sharma AJ. Prevalence estimates of gestational diabetes mellitus in the United States, pregnancy risk assessment Monitoring system (PRAMS), 2007–2010. *Prev Chronic Dis*. 2014;11:130415. Available at:https://doi.org/10.5888/pcd11.130415.

10. American Diabetes Association. What Is Gestational Diabetes? 2016. Available at: http://www.diabetes.org/diabetes-basics/gestational/what-is-gestational-diabetes.html. Accessed November 19, 2017.

11. U.S. Food and Drug Administration. *Pregnancy and Lactation Labeling*; 2016. Available at: https://www.fda.gov/Drugs/DevelopmentApprovalProcess/DevelopmentResources/Labeling/ucm093307.htm. Accessed November 10, 2017.

12. Oral Health Care During Pregnancy Expert Workgroup. *Oral Health Care during Pregnancy: A National Consensus Statement*. Washington, DC: National Maternal and Child Oral Health Resource Center; 2012.

13. "Healthy People 2030 Building a healthier future for all." U.S. Department of Health and Human Services. Office of Disease Prevention and Health Promotion. https://health.gov/healthypeople. Available at: https://www.cdc.gov/nchs/healthy_people/hp2010.htm. Accessed July 1, 2022.

14. Jones M, Lee JY, Rozier RG. Oral health literacy among adult patients seeking dental care. *J Am Dent Assoc*. 2007;138(9):1199–1208.

15. Health Resources and Services Administration: Maternal and Child Health. Title V Maternal and Child Health Services Block Grant Program. Available at: https://mchb.hrsa.gov/maternal-child-health-initiatives/title-v-maternal-and-child-health-services-block-grant-program. Published December 2016. Accessed September 29, 2017.

16. American Public Health Association. *Improving Access to Dental Care for Pregnant Women through Education, Integration of Health Services, Insurance Coverage, an Appropriate Dental Workforce, and Research*. American Public Health Association; 2021. https://www.apha.org/Policies-and-Advocacy/PublicHealth-Policy-Statements/Policy-Database/2021/01/12/ImprovingAccess-to-Dental-Care-for-Pregnant-Women. Accessed June 30, 2022.

17. White House Blueprint for Addressing the Maternal Health Crisis. Available at: https://www.whitehouse.gov/wp-content/uploads/2022/06/Maternal-Health-Blueprint.pdf. Published June 2022. Accessed November 21, 2022.

18. Berwick DM, Nolan TW, Whittington JW. The triple aim: care, health, and cost. *Health Aff*. 2008;273:759–769.

19. Weatherspoon DJ, Horowitz AM, Kleinman DV. Maryland physicians' knowledge, opinions and practices related to dental caries etiology and prevention in children. *Pediatr Dent*. 2016;38(1):61–67.

20. U.S. Department of Agriculture. Women, Infants, and Children. Available at: https://www.fns.usda.gov/wic/women-infants-and-children-wic. Published August 15, 2017. Accessed August 31, 2017.

21. U.S. Department of Agriculture. Women, Infants, and Children. Available at: https://www.ers.usda.gov/topics/food-nutrition-assistance/wic-program/. Published August 10, 2022. Accessed November 21, 2022.

22. U.S. Department of Health and Human Services. *Head Start Programs. Administration for Children and Families: Office of Heath Start*; June 15, 2017. Available at: https://www.acf.hhs.gov/ohs/about/head-start. Accessed September 29, 2017.

23. Health Resources and Services Administration: Maternal and Child Health. *Home Visiting*; June 2017. https://mchb.hrsa.gov/maternal-child-health-initiatives/home-visiting-overview. Accessed September 29, 2017.

47

The Older Adult

Joan I. Gluch

PROFESSIONAL DEVELOPMENT OPPORTUNITIES

Given the demographic projections in the United States and worldwide for the increase in the elderly population, as well as the significant disparities in frequency of dental visits and prevalence of oral diseases among the elderly, dental hygienists will need the requisite knowledge and skills to provide customized, competent dental hygiene care for the increasing elderly population in both clinical practice and the public health setting. This chapter provides the foundational knowledge for dental hygienists to gain competency in customizing dental hygiene care and public health programs for older adults with a wide range of complex medical, dental, and related psychosocial issues in aging.

COMPETENCIES

1. Explain and apply demographic characteristics of the aging population, including oral health disparities, to gain an increased understanding of best practices in customizing dental hygiene care for the older adult.
2. Define "geriatrics," discuss healthcare for older adults, and provide the rationale for performing a health assessment of an older person that includes a functional appraisal in addition to a review of health, dental, and personal histories.
3. Describe how health promotion, including the *Healthy People 2030* initiatives, contributes to an increase in the overall well-being and health, including oral health, of older adults
4. Describe and apply various theories of aging to the dental hygiene process of care.
5. Differentiate age-related health changes from those health and oral health conditions that occur as a result of acute or chronic diseases or medications in the elderly.
6. Customize each step in the process of dental hygiene care for elderly patients in light of their complex medical, dental, and related psychosocial issues.
7. Discuss the public health role of the dental hygienist in treating older adults in both the community-based and institutional settings.

INTRODUCTION

Dental hygienists face many challenges when they provide care for older adults because of the varied biologic, psychologic, and social needs within this population. Older adults are a heterogeneous group owing to their lifetime of unique experiences. Life at any given moment is the result of physiologic capabilities, environmental variables, psychosocial factors, and a sense of one's own skills and alternatives. Therefore, dental hygienists should assess the healthcare needs of each older adult individually, without prior assumptions based on preconceived stereotypes or myths. The health status of older adults represents the entire continuum of healthy to severely ill individuals. Working with older adults demands that dental hygienists understand the complex medical, social, and psychologic needs of their older patients and the coordination of multiple levels of healthcare necessary when working with the elderly.

DEMOGRAPHIC ASPECTS OF AGING

Throughout the world, and most notably in the United States, we are experiencing considerable growth in the older adult population. Between 2010 and 2019, the number of US individuals 65 years and older increased by 14.4 million (34.2%) for a total of 54.1 million older adults, as compared to the modest increase of 3% for those under 65 during the same time period.[1,2] In 2019, the elderly in the United States represented 16% of the population, and the US Census Bureau projects the increase in the number of US older adults to continue with 80.8 million older adults in 2040 who will comprise 21.6% of the US population.[1,2] The US aging trends mirror the world total population, with 1 in 10 people in the world over the age of 65 in 2022, with older adults projected to make up 1 in 6 people in world population in 2050.[3]

Researchers explain the rise in numbers of elderly as due to increases in life expectancy, not an increase in the overall life span. Life expectancy is the average number of years lived by any group of individuals born in the same period and is computed at birth or a specific time point. Life span is the maximal length of life potentially possible in a species: the age beyond which no one can expect to live.

Individuals born in 1900 had a life expectancy of 47.3 years, which increased to 78.7 years for those born in 2010. For those born in 2021, provisional life expectancy is 79.1 years for females and 73.2 years for males.[4] An increased number of deaths due to COVID-19, unintentional injuries, and heart disease in 2020 and 2021 has resulted in projected slowed rate in life expectancy after a succession of life expectancy increases since 2010.[4] For example, in 2021, those individuals who survived to age 65 can expect to live an average of 18.3 more years, and individuals who lived to age 80 can expect to live an average of 8.6 more years.[5] Life expectancy rates for older adults have increased because more people are surviving young life (infant and childhood mortality have declined), fertility rates have decreased, and medical care and technology have improved. However, recent changes in life expectancy rates in 2021 can be explained by increases in death due to COVID-19, as well as unintentional injuries, heart diseases, and chronic liver disease.[5]

In addition, the number of people who reach age 65 years in a given year depends heavily on the number of births 65 years earlier. By 2030, all of the "baby boomers" will be 65 years and over, so there will be a "boom" of older adults increasing at a rate greater than the total population. For example, the population age 65 and over will increase from 13% (43 million) in 2010 to 70 million, about 20% of the total population in 2030, reflecting the aging of the baby boom generation.[1,5]

Other demographic changes in the older adult population that affect healthcare include the following.[6]

- The older adult population is becoming more racially and ethnically diverse. In 2018, older individuals from minority population groups represented 22% of the elderly population. Future projections predict an increase of the minority population to 42% of elderly over the age of 65 in 2060.
- Elderly females outnumber males, and in 2018, females accounted for 56% over the population over the age of 65 and for 64% of the population age 85 and over. However, because life expectancy rates for males are rising, the population differences for males and females will narrow, based on predictions for future years. For example, in 2020, the sex ratio among adults age 65 and older is 81 males for 100 females and is projected to increase to 86 males to 100 females in 2060.
- The older adult population varies geographically and is concentrated in certain states. Maine, Florida, West Virginia, Vermont, and Delaware have the highest population of elderly as a percent of their states' population, all at 20% or higher. Changes in population composition and proportion of older adults will have a major impact on our society, on healthcare, and on services provided by federal, state, and local governments.

HEALTHCARE FOR OLDER ADULTS

Geriatrics is the branch of medicine concerned with the illnesses of old age and their treatment. **Gerontology** is the scientific study of the factors affecting the normal aging process and the effects of aging, especially in relation to quality-of-life issues. Although commonly used, these terms are not interchangeable. A gerontologist is an individual who investigates numerous factors that affect the process of aging. Gerontologists have divided study of the older population into several categories based on age: young-old (65 to 74 years), middle-old (75 to 84 years), and old-old (85-plus years). Some sociologists have classified those between the ages of 55 and 64 years as the "new-old" and those older than 95 years as the "very old." Although these age categories are helpful to categorize elderly patients, two important facts exist: (1) characterizations of age should include assessment of functional ability in addition to chronologic age, and (2) the majority of older adults perform at a relative level of independent function. **Chronologic age** refers to age as measured by calendar time since birth, whereas **functional age** describes the capability to maintain activity.[7]

Health assessment of older persons should include a functional appraisal in addition to a review of health, dental, and personal histories.[8] The items generally included within a functional assessment are divided into **activities of daily living** (ADLs) and **instrumental activities of daily living** (IADLs). ADLs are those abilities fundamental to independent living, such as bathing, dressing, brushing teeth, toileting, feeding, and continence. IADLs represent tasks requiring complex skills and include using the telephone, preparing meals, and managing money.[8] In 2014, the National Health Interview survey found that limitations in both ADL and IADL increased with age. For adults over the age of 75, 10.6% required assistance with ADLs and 18.8% required assistance with IADLs.[9]

The World Health Organization (WHO) uses the term "functional ability" as an essential part of their definition of healthy aging as "the process of developing and maintaining the functional ability that enables wellbeing in older age." WHO further explains functional abilities as the interaction between the individual's mental and physical capabilities with their home and community environmental supports to maintain abilities to support healthy aging.[10]

Knowledge of a patient's functional abilities helps the dental hygienist customize dental hygiene care, especially in recommending appropriate and realistic preventive homecare routines. In addition, knowledge of functional abilities allows the dental team to identify resources and supports necessary to provide the most appropriate level to ensure optimum quality of life.

Functional assessment becomes important because patterns of illness and disease have changed over the past century. Although acute conditions were predominant during the early 1900s, in 2018, most US adults over the age of 65 reported at least one chronic condition, with hypertension, arthritis, heart diseases, cancer, and diabetes cited as the most common chronic conditions.[6]

AGING AND HEALTH PROMOTION

The US trend of greater numbers and proportion of elderly with chronic disease has occurred at the same time as another important US trend: preventing disease and promoting health. From a federal perspective, the *Healthy People 2030* initiatives are designed to increase the overall well-being and health of the nation. Focus areas, goals, and specific objectives in the *Healthy People 2030* report provide a concrete baseline from which to plan programs, set priorities, and evaluate progress in meeting health objectives and increasing health status.[11] The dental hygienist can provide appropriate wellness information and reinforce positive lifestyle habits as customized dental hygiene care from the perspective of improving quality of life.

On the positive side, research indicates that older adults, on average, take better care of their health than does the general population. For example, older adults are less likely than younger adults to drink alcohol, be overweight, smoke, or report that stress affects their health adversely.[1]

However, as compared to younger individuals, older adults have a greater number of chronic health problems, are less likely to engage in regular physical exercise, are more likely to fall, and are more likely to be hospitalized for infectious diseases. Dental hygienists should emphasize health promotion activities for their elderly patients as part of the wellness component of the medical care activities.[11]

Since 2000, adults 65 and older have increased their dental visits, from 38.3% in 2000 to 43.3% of adults 65 and older visiting the dentist in 2016. The increase in proportion of older adults visiting the dentist is due to the continued availability for some retirees of employer-based private dental insurance, and also due to the inclusion of optional dental services in some Medicare Advantage plans. In 2016, 68.7% of elders with insurance had a dental visit, with only 37.5% of uninsured older adults visiting the dentist.[12] Dental visits also vary by income because in 2016, 61.3% of elderly with incomes greater than 400% of the federal poverty level had dental visits as compared with 24.4% of elderly with incomes below the federal poverty level.[12] While the percentage of older adults with dental visits is increasing, significant disparities exist related to insurance coverage and income. Impetus for including dental benefits in Medicare has been increasing to ensure necessary dental care for seniors; however, recent legislative attempts in 2022 to ensure a dental benefit in Medicare were not successful, despite the clear need for equitable access to dental care.

WHY AND HOW PEOPLE AGE

No single theory can explain why and how people age. Rather, an intermingling of social, psychologic, biologic, environmental, physiologic, and lifestyle factors contributes to the aging process, either in accelerating or in retarding its progress, and produces a different course for each individual.[13] Aging is a progressive yet fluid process, with each factor affecting the others. Understanding the theories of aging—those that have validity and those that contribute to stereotypes—enables the dental hygienist to understand their patients and plan dental hygiene care to maximize quality of life.

Social Theories of Aging

Social science researchers looking at aging use an interdisciplinary perspective to focus on social, psychologic, and environmental factors that affect the lives of older persons.[13] Dental hygienists, when planning care, must be aware of and consider the dynamic social processes that influence each older patient.

Physiologic Aspects of Aging

Senescence is the term that describes the normal physiologic process of growing old.[13] The fact that everyone, given time, eventually experiences physical changes in all of the body systems makes aging universal. Physical changes that occur are normal for all people, and they take place at various rates and depend on accompanying circumstances (e.g., environmental, psychosocial, lifestyle, and biologic factors) in an individual's life. Typically, normal age changes have been studied in collaboration with pathologic or disease conditions, leading to the misconception that all age changes indicate illness or disease. For example, research has shown that no decrease in salivary production occurs in healthy older adults. Diminished salivary flow is, instead, a byproduct of medications or disease, not part of the normal aging process.

Biologic Theories of Aging

Most theorists agree that a unifying theory does not yet exist that explains the mechanics and causes underlying the biologic phenomenon of aging.[13] A search for a universal factor or factors is complicated by the fact that signs of aging do not appear in all individuals at the same chronologic age. Biologic theories can be divided into three major categories, including program theories, damage theories, and a combination of these two theoretical types. Program theories view aging as a sequential, deliberate biological deterioration over time as a predetermined sequence through the life span. Damage theories describe a series of randomly occurring events that accumulate over time to explain the loss of function and disease in aging. Most recently, theorists have combined components of both program hypotheses and damage error hypotheses to more fully explain the aging process. Each hypothesis generated provides a clue to the aging process, yet many unanswered questions remain.[13]

ORAL HEALTH IN THE ELDERLY

As with other physiologic alterations in the body, the distinction between age-related oral changes and those that are disease induced is not always clear or conclusive.[14] Disease, consequences of disease, and use of medications often manifest oral changes and pathology independent of the aging process.

Age-Related Tooth Changes

With age, teeth undergo several changes, including alterations in the enamel, cementum, dentin, and pulp. Enamel becomes darker in color because of lifetime consumption of stain-producing foods and drinks and the formation of secondary dentin. The enamel surface develops numerous cracks (acquired lamellae) and obtains a translucent appearance. Arrested dental caries in older adults often appears as a brownish-black discoloration because of lifelong uptake of stain in enamel lamellae.[14]

Cementum undergoes compositional changes in aging, including an increase in fluoride and magnesium content. Deposition of

cementum at the apical end and bifurcated areas of the roots compensates for coronal enamel tooth wear. This secondary cementum normally is deposited slowly and continuously throughout life.[14]

Dentin shows two independent changes: secondary dentin formation and obturation of dentinal tubules (dentin sclerosis). As a result, the vitality of the dentin is decreased greatly, and aged dentin may become entirely insensitive and impermeable.[14]

The pulp undergoes the same changes that occur in similar tissues elsewhere in the body: pulpal blood supply decreases, the number of cells decreases, and the number of fibers increases in aged adults. Because pulp calcifications increase with advancing age, the size of the pulp chamber is reduced. Pulp calcifications appear to form in erupted and unerupted teeth.

Tooth wear due to erosion and attrition is common in the elderly as a result of a lifetime of habits and dietary factors. Erosion is caused by tooth exposure to dietary acids and acid reflux, shown in Fig. 47.1 Occlusal attrition often smooths the occlusal area, which reduces microbial accumulation in the fissure. These fissures may appear slightly sticky on probing, but they may not need restoring. Therefore, clinicians should avoid vigorous instrumentation in order to prevent mechanical damage to the porous part of the fissure enamel. The attrition present in older individuals is often so severe that dentin exposures appear on the incisal and occlusal surfaces.[15]

Many of today's older adults may have used a stiff toothbrush and abrasive toothpaste in the past. Consequently, tooth abrasion, especially in the cervical area and on root surfaces, may be evident (Fig. 47.2). Abrasion, although common among older adults, is the result of a physiochemical process rather than a result of aging. Although modern dentifrices are not abrasive enough to damage intact enamel, they can cause remarkable wear of cementum and dentin if the toothbrush is used incorrectly or with too much pressure. Dental hygienists can assist individuals in maintaining a biologically sound dentition and freedom from pain through appropriate oral hygiene educational instructions.

Tooth Loss

In the past century, perhaps the most significant change in older adults' oral status has been the decline in total tooth loss, also known as **edentulousness**. In those 65 years and older, edentulousness declined from approximately 50% in 1960 to 24% in 2002 and to 13% in 2021.[16] Tooth loss is greater among those in poverty: 34% of older adults living below the poverty line are edentulous, as compared with 11% of their peers above the poverty line. Non-Hispanic Black older adults are twice as

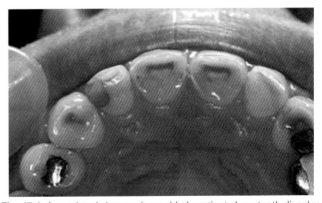

Fig. 47.1 Age-related changes in an elderly patient show tooth discoloration, staining, and erosion due to chronic acid reflux. (From Bartlett D. A new look at erosive tooth wear in elderly people. *J Am Dent Assoc.* 2007;138:S21.)

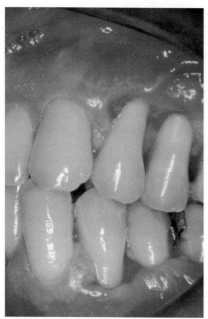

Fig. 47.2 Root abrasion and gingival trauma due to overzealous tooth-brushing habit. (From Newman M, Takei H, Perry K, eds. *Carranza's Clinical Periodontology.* 12th ed. Saunders; 2015.)

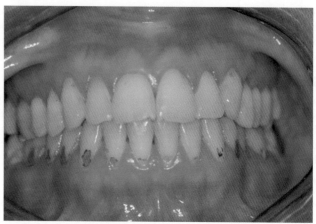

Fig. 47.3 Root caries seen at the cervical region of the teeth in patients with xerostomia. (From Jensen SB, Vissink A. Salivary gland dysfunction and xerostomia in Sjögren's syndrome. *Oral Maxillofac Surg Clin.* 2014;26(1):35.)

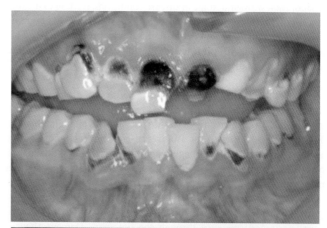

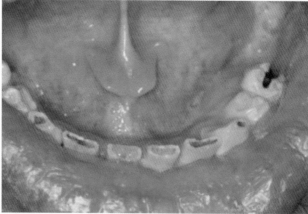

Fig. 47.4 Rampant dental caries seen in an elderly patient. (From Davis M, Ortner P, Feyer P, Zimmerman C. *Supportive Oncology.* Saunders; 2011.)

likely (31%) to be edentulous as Mexican American (17%) older adults and non-Hispanic White adults (15%).[16] Although rates of total tooth loss have decreased, older adults have on average 20.7 teeth, with those older adults living in poverty with fewer teeth than those with incomes above the federal poverty guidelines (17.6 teeth vs. 22.2 teeth).[16]

Dental Caries

Throughout their lifetime, 96% of all older adults have experienced dental caries, and 1 in 6 older adults currently have untreated tooth decay. Disparities exist based on poverty status and race/ethnicity, with non-Hispanic Black (29%) and Mexican American (36%) older adults more than two times more likely to have untreated decay than non-Hispanic White (14%) elders. Elders living in poverty were at least three times more likely to have untreated tooth decay than those elders above the poverty line (33% vs 10%).[16]

Root caries is common, seen in one in six elders because of local oral factors and factors related to aging (Fig. 47.3). Local factors include exposed root surfaces and tooth longevity, and factors related to aging include changes in salivary quantity and composition, and inability to complete thorough oral hygiene because of disabilities, diminished chewing abilities, and chronic health conditions.[15] Predictors of caries include the presence of elevated amounts of caries-related bacteria, presence of plaque biofilm, presence of restored coronal and root decay, xerostomia, and gingival recession.[15] Severe root caries can develop rapidly in the absence of adequate oral hygiene and in the presence of xerostomia, suboptimal periodontal health, and ingestion of fermentable carbohydrates (Fig. 47.4).

Caries prevention with the older adult includes four interrelated factors:
- Daily mechanical removal and chemical control of biofilm in a thorough manner
- Reduction of sugars and refined carbohydrates
- Use of topical fluoride, amorphous calcium phosphate, antibacterial agents, and salivary replacement therapy to address xerostomia
- Use of 38% silver diamine fluoride as noninvasive treatment for dental caries

Older adults may not be able to complete thorough oral hygiene every day independently because of sensory and neuromuscular changes commonly seen in aging (see the critical thinking scenario in Box 47.1 and Chapters 59 [Disability and Healthcare], 60 [Intellectually and Developmentally Challenged], and 62 [Neurologic Disabilities]). Use of adaptive devices, such as power toothbrushes and modifications in toothbrush handle size, width, and grip, assists older adults in

BOX 47.1 Critical Thinking Scenario

Instant Aging as a Dental Patient

This activity asks participants to simulate what it is like to be an older dental patient in their office. This exercise provides a good opportunity to learn what older patients may be experiencing and provides insight for participants regarding sensory changes in aging. Clinicians should work in groups of two, alternating the role of patient and dental hygienist. Partners are asked to complete tasks while they have simulated several sensory deprivations that older individuals may experience.

Task A: Partner 1 wears glasses with a thin film of oil or lubricant to inhibit clear vision. In addition, partner 1 tapes the fingers of both hands to make fine motor tasks difficult. Partner 1 completes a health history form and/or other office forms for a new patient. After the forms are completed (a brief time limit should be imposed), partner 1 walks unassisted back to the treatment room and fills out additional forms in the dental chair.

Task B: Partner 2 wears earplugs or uses cotton or wax ear protectors to limit hearing. In addition, this partner uses an Ace bandage or shoulder harness to restrict shoulder movement. Partner 2 walks unassisted to the treatment room and completes a brief written form in the dental chair. Partner 2 demonstrates brushing and flossing technique and should be asked to describe the technique and answer questions about the performance.

Debriefing Discussion: After the simulated dental appointments are completed, participants discuss their experiences in completing routine dental tasks with some sensory impairments. Although this is only a simulation, partners are encouraged to discuss how this simulation is related to the experiences of their older patients. Partners should complete an "environmental audit" of their dental offices to assess how difficult their office environment is for the older individual to negotiate, based on the environmental considerations discussed in this chapter. Hearing, vision, and motor skill impairments pose significant obstacles even when the environment is optimal for older adults. By adopting the perspective of the patient with some sensorimotor deficits, partners may be able to identify difficulties for older patients and make changes to provide care in a more sensitive, appropriate manner.

thorough biofilm removal. Dental hygienists should involve caregivers in providing routine and thorough oral hygiene with older adults as needed. Antimicrobial toothpastes and mouth rinses will also assist older adults in reduction of pathogenic bacteria. Poor dietary practices involving the overconsumption of soft, retentive carbohydrates and frequent snacking are often common among older adults and are complicated by salivary changes and diminished chewing abilities that may promote dental decay.[16]

Aggressive caries prevention and management must include caries risk assessment (Chapter 19) and frequent and liberal use of topical fluoride products for home use and professional application of a range of fluoride products. In addition to daily use of a stannous fluoride toothpaste, many older adults find sodium fluoride rinses easy to use and helpful in caries reduction. As an alternative, many older adults prefer the use of stannous fluoride dentifrice or sodium fluoride gel applied directly to the root surfaces. For high caries risk, 5000 ppm (1.1%) sodium fluoride applied with a toothbrush or small interproximal brush or applied in a preformed mouth tray is recommended. Professionally applied sodium fluoride varnish has been shown to be an effective caries-preventive agent for coronal and root caries in the elderly.

Since many older adults have chronic medical conditions that may limit dental care, caries management may include interim therapeutic restorations using glass ionomer materials and/or silver diamine fluoride has been shown to be an effective and affordable caries management strategy, especially for older adults in a homebound or institutionalized setting. Applied directly to root and/or coronal caries, silver

diamine fluoride requires no tooth removal and minimal training and support equipment to safely deliver conservative caries management.[16]

Xerostomia

Xerostomia is a common side effect of many prescription and over-the-counter medications, such as antihypertensives, antipsychotics, antidepressants, muscle relaxants, antihistamines, and laxatives. Xerostomia can also be due to salivary gland blockage, dysfunction, and disease. Many systemic diseases, most notably Sjögren syndrome, diminish saliva as well. Saliva provides a source of minerals for enamel remineralization to reduce and repair dental decay. Saliva also plays an important role in proper function of the oral cavity because it lubricates the oral mucosa, assisting speech and swallowing, and facilitates the retention of oral appliances.[15] Diminished salivary flow can alter taste, contribute to plaque formation and dental caries, and cause the oral mucosa to appear dry and inflamed. For edentulous persons, denture retention, comfort, and ability to chew and speak may become difficult when less saliva is present.[15]

Management of xerostomia should include palliative care, such as saliva substitutes, oral lubricants, xylitol-containing mints or chewing gum, mouth rinses, and frequent water intake, although the evidence is weak from systematic reviews on xerostomia management. Attempts to stimulate salivary flow can also include medications, such as cevimeline (Evoxac) or systemic pilocarpine tablets (Salagen).[15]

Patients with xerostomia should return for frequent recall, assessment, and management of caries status because the presence of xerostomia places them in an extremely high risk category for caries. All of the following caries-prevention efforts are essential for the older adult to control root and coronal caries associated with xerostomia.[15]

- Daily and thorough brushing with fluoride dentifrice and thorough interproximal plaque removal through flossing and/or use of interdental aids
- Use of fluoride rinses, gel, or paste depending on patients' preferences and providers' judgment
- Frequent use of salivary substitute and dry mouth products
- Nutritional counseling
- Antimicrobial use (e.g., 0.12% chlorhexidine mouth rinses)
- Use of amorphous calcium and phosphate pastes
- Frequent professional debridement
- Frequent professional application of topical fluoride
- Use of xylitol-containing products

Periodontal Diseases and Changes

Contemporary research indicates that the effect of age on the progression of periodontitis is negligible when risk factors are controlled and patients maintain good oral hygiene.[16] However, the concept of **immunosenescence** refers to the greater susceptibility to periodontal infection in the elderly from the repeated immune system challenges throughout life.[16] Thus, the cumulative effect of prolonged microbial challenges contributes to the aging of the periodontium and the greater susceptibility and presence of periodontal disease. Not surprisingly, studies confirm an association between increased age and increased recession, loss of attachment, and higher prevalence of gingival inflammation.[16]

Age-Related Changes

As individuals age, numerous morphologic, biochemical, and metabolic changes are observed in the periodontium with aging. The overall significance of these factors as they affect susceptibility and periodontal disease progression is unclear; however, in the absence of clinical signs of disease, these changes in the periodontal structures attributable to aging alone are therapeutically insignificant.[15]

Gingival epithelium shows evidence of a thinning of the epithelium, diminished keratinization, and increased cellular density. Older individuals often display a reduction in cellular elements and an increase in fibrous intercellular substance in the gingival connective tissue. There is a reduced number of nerves in the gingiva and increased evidence of nerve degeneration with increasing age, along with arteriosclerotic changes in gingival vessels.[15] The periodontal ligament shows evidence of diminished cellular function and increases in calcification and arteriosclerosis with advancing age. There is an increase in alveolar bone porosity and a decrease in cortical width with aging, but this increased porosity is not related to the presence of teeth and does not lead to crestal resorption. Research shows that crestal bone loss with aging is minimal in healthy persons.[15]

Pathology-Induced Changes

In 2018, Eke reported that 42.2% of US adults over age 30 have periodontitis. A distinct age difference exists, with 59.8% of adults 65 years and older and 29.5% of those ages 30 to 44 years showing signs of periodontitis.[16] Many reasons exist for the greater prevalence of periodontitis among the elderly, including an increase in local oral risk factors, increased prevalence of systemic diseases (diabetes, cardiovascular diseases), tobacco use, immunosenescence, and lack of routine professional dental visits. Dental hygienists should provide aggressive treatment to prevent and control periodontal diseases in older adults. More frequent dental hygiene care visits provide the opportunity to instruct the older adult in proper oral hygiene, especially in the use of powered toothbrushes, and the use of antimicrobial agents to control gingivitis, such as stannous fluoride dentifrice and/or essential oil mouth rinse. Use of 0.12% chlorhexidine gluconate also is indicated for older patients who need an additional level of microbial control.[16]

Most common in elderly females, osteoporosis decreases bone mass and increases bone porosity, frequently affecting the alveolar bone.[16] Reductions in bone metabolism and healing capacities influence the quality of bone and periodontal treatment prognosis. Alveolar bone quality can significantly affect the older adult's risk and prognosis for periodontal diseases, as well as the ability to wear oral prosthetics and achieve proper mastication. Dental hygienists should monitor patients with osteoporosis and those taking antiresorptive agents such as bisphosphonate drugs to reduce the incidence of osteoporosis-related bone fractures. Dental hygiene care should proceed in a conservative manner based on the patient's dental needs and health status.

Oral Mucosal Changes
Age-Related Changes

In the absence of disease, the oral mucosal status of older adults is comparable to that of younger adults, suggesting that aging alone does not lead to changes in the oral mucosa.[14,15]

Pathology-Induced Changes

Some mucosal alterations are a result of systemic factors (e.g., xerostomia) and are not related to aging. Systemic disease and medication use cause some older adults to have changes in their oral mucosa, including atrophy of epithelium and connective tissues with a decrease in vascularity.

Oral mucosa, especially lips, may appear dry and drawn due to dehydration and loss of elasticity within the tissues. Angular cheilitis, commonly evidenced among the aged, clinically appears as fissuring at the angles of the mouth, with cracks, erythema, and ulcerations (Fig. 47.5). Moistness from drooling, deficiency of vitamin B$_2$ (riboflavin), and infection with *Candida albicans* are the causative factors associated with this condition.[17]

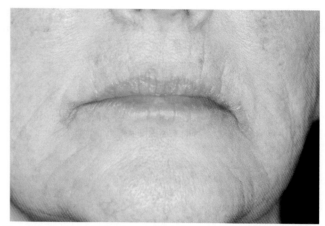

Fig. 47.5 Angular cheilitis in an elderly female. (From Waring E, Villa A. Oral manifestations of immunodeficiencies and transplantation medicine. *Atlas Oral Maxillofac Surg Clin North Am.* 2017;25:105.)

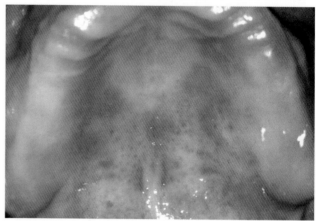

Fig. 47.6 Chronic atrophic candidiasis. (From Radović K, Ilić J, Roganović J, et al. Denture stomatitis and salivary vascular endothelial growth factor in immediate complete denture wearers with type 2 diabetes. *J Prosthet Dent.* 2014;111:373.)

Ill-fitting dentures and/or poor denture hygiene also can result in mucosal irritation and infection, including denture stomatitis or candidiasis and denture-induced fibrous hyperplasia. "Denture sore mouth" reflects a commonly seen condition also known as chronic atrophic candidiasis, present in as many as 65% of older individuals who wear dentures (Fig. 47.6). Chronic atrophic candidiasis is associated with poor prosthesis fit, which leads to chronic trauma, and retention of the denture during sleeping hours, which promotes bacterial and fungal growth. The signs of denture-induced fibrous hyperplasia include single or multiple elongated folds near the border of ill-fitting dentures.[15] Dental hygienists should educate clients and their caregivers as cotherapists regarding proper denture oral hygiene and denture wearing patterns, especially to alert them to the early signs of bacterial/fungal infections for prompt referral and treatment (see Chapter 41).

Traditionally, oral cancer has been most prevalent in males over 50 who use tobacco and report heavy alcohol use. However, in the past 10 years, the profile of oral cancer has changed, based on the prevalence of oropharyngeal squamous cell cancer (OPC) caused by the human papillomavirus (HPV). OPC has doubled in the past 25 years, with males having 3.5 times more OPC than females.[16] Despite the changing profile, all older adults should receive a thorough soft tissue oral examination at each visit so the dental hygienist can carefully evaluate any early mucosal changes that may indicate precancerous or cancerous lesions and provide early referrals for prompt evaluation and treatment (Chapter 16). The low utilization rate of dental care for older individuals represents a concern since they are at high risk for oral cancer and may not receive the oral examinations to diagnose the condition in an early state until symptoms appear.[16]

Tongue Changes
Age-Related Changes
Changes in the tongue may include a decrease in the number and sensitivity of papillae. Combined with a decline in the sense of smell, some foods have less appeal and nutritional needs may not be met. Sublingual varicosities are customary findings among the aged; however, they are not problematic. Clinically, they appear as deep red or bluish-black dilated vessels on either side of the midline on the ventral surface of the tongue.[17]

Pathology-Induced Changes
Because of nutritional factors, older adults frequently have anemia due to iron deficiencies. Atrophic glossitis is a symptom of this condition, and the tongue appears smooth, shiny, and denuded (Fig. 47.7). Often, individuals complain of a burning sensation. In addition, the tongue often increases in size in edentulous mouths or as a result of disease (e.g., pernicious anemia).[17] The dental hygienist can assist the individual by recommending an oral lubricant to reduce discomfort and by providing dietary counseling.[17]

Salivary Gland Changes
Research has shown that reductions in salivary flow are not a result of the normal aging process. Rather, decreases in salivary flow usually are attributed to systemic disease, radiation therapy, tumors, or medications that cause temporary or permanent xerostomia.[17] Signs and symptoms of salivary reduction should be evaluated carefully to determine the cause. In the absence of medications, possible underlying diseases and salivary gland tumors should be investigated.

Sjögren Syndrome
Sjögren syndrome is an autoimmune disorder of the salivary glands, occurring most frequently in postmenopausal females (Chapter 53). Approximately 60% of people with this disorder are older than 50 years. Clinically, the oral mucosa is extremely dry and saliva is ropy. Initially, the tongue shows marked atrophy of the papillae, and later, the surface becomes smooth and lobulated.[17] To meet the need for mucous membrane integrity, persons with Sjögren syndrome should be instructed to use saliva substitutes and products for dry mouth. For

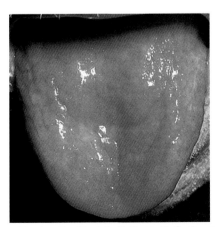

Fig. 47.7 Atrophic glossitis. (Epstein O, Perkin G, Cookson J, et al, eds. *Clinical Examination*. 4th ed. Mosby; 2008.)

dentate individuals, fluoride therapies may be recommended to help meet the need for a sound dentition.[17]

Drug-Induced Oral Changes
Approximately one-third of all prescription and over-the-counter drugs are used by older adults, even though these individuals account for only 13% of the population. **Polypharmacy** is the term to describe the common practice of prescribing multiple drugs to patients to manage their many medical conditions.[16] On average, most older adults take more than three therapeutic agents, and the institutionalized elderly use five to seven drugs at the same time. Older clients are more likely to experience adverse reactions because of physiologic changes in the heart, liver, and kidney, and also because of the increased exposure and potential for interaction of prescription and over-the-counter medications. Medications most frequently used by older adults include analgesics, diuretics, oral hypoglycemics, antihypertensives, antidepressants, and sedatives. Multiple medical problems, along with multiple drug use, can lead to a high rate of adverse drug reactions. Many drugs produce oral changes in the mouth because of side effects or as a consequence of the actions of the drug.[16] Dental hygienists play an especially important role in identifying medication use and potential side effects, educating patients about side effects, and referring patients to their physicians for further evaluation.

Drug-Induced Gingival Enlargement
Persons taking anticonvulsants such as phenytoin may exhibit gingival hyperplasia as a side effect (see Chapter 15—Pharmacological History).[17] Adequate plaque control, particularly if started before the administration of drugs such as phenytoin, may reduce the magnitude of gingival enlargement. Patients with prescribed cardiovascular drugs (nifedipine) and immunosuppressants (cyclosporine) may exhibit gingival enlargement as well.[17]

DENTAL HYGIENE PROCESS OF CARE WITH OLDER ADULTS
Assessment and Dental Hygiene Diagnoses
Dental hygienists begin their assessment of overall physical factors by observing the older adult in the reception area. It is important to observe gait and balance because some elderly persons may require assistance to the treatment area, especially those who appear unsteady or who have severe visual impairments. Sufficient space in the dental operatory should accommodate easy access for the patient to the dental chair and room for patient's wheelchair to ensure safety during dental hygiene care (see Chapter 59). For most procedures, it is preferable to keep the patient in the wheelchair and use a portable or swivel head rest for stability and comfort.

Impairments in vision and hearing commonly seen in older adults may necessitate providing assistance in completing any written forms in the office (see Chapter 60). Large-print health history forms allow visually impaired patients to complete the form independently, although it may be more effective and efficient to interview the patient to obtain the needed information. Hearing-impaired older patients should be addressed directly, with the face mask removed and background music or other noise eliminated, especially if patients are using hearing aids. Older adults accompanied by others should be addressed directly, not the family member or caregiver. By speaking directly to the elderly patient, dental hygienists create a respectful, independent environment.

The health history should include the patient's personal, medical, and dental background (see Chapter 13), especially since many social determinants of health greatly influence care with older adults (see

Chapter 4). Personal history, for example, may show that a patient is widowed and lives alone, has a reduced income, and has limited access to transportation, all of which affect the ability to receive dental care.

When reviewing the health history, dental hygienists should also include questions about mental health since the CDC estimates that 20% of individuals 55 years or older experience anxiety, depression, and/or cognitive impairment.[18] Dental hygienists are in an optimal position to detect early changes in mood and/or cognitive functioning during dental hygiene care appointments and should initiate discussions with families for additional social support and medical evaluation as needed. Recent research regarding the association between specific periodontal pathogens and Alzheimer disease points to the critical role that brain health discussions play during periodontal care especially among the elderly.[19]

Dental hygienists should question their older patients regarding their use of prescription and over-the-counter medications, especially because many older individuals take multiple medications and frequently experience side effects, and consult with the patient's physician if there is doubt regarding treatment (see Chapter 15). Vital signs, including respiration, pulse, blood pressure, and temperature (if indicated), should be evaluated and recorded.

The extraoral examination can reveal abnormalities in the skin of the face and neck, lymph nodes, salivary glands, and underlying muscles (see Chapter 16). The mandible is examined for movement, and the temporomandibular joint should be palpated for crepitation, tenderness, or limitations in movement. A patient with arthritis may not be able to open their mouth fully.

Lips are evaluated for signs of angular cheilitis, muscle inelasticity, and presence of lesions (Fig. 47.5). A complete dental charting and periodontal assessment are part of every dental history to provide documentation for reevaluation. The saliva quantity and quality are assessed to ascertain if saliva substitutes should be recommended.

Radiographs and other diagnostic aids such as study models are used as indicated and appropriate. A referral for biopsy may be indicated for suspicious lesions.

Oral hygiene status, including plaque biofilm distribution, calculus, and stains, is assessed. Assessment of the patient's ability to perform oral hygiene practices is essential. The older person's homecare practices generally should be modified rather than attempts being made to change long-term habits completely. Physical changes such as arthritis and impaired vision may affect the patient's ability to carry out oral hygiene recommendations.

If the patient's vision and dexterity permit, they are instructed to perform self-assessments of plaque control methods and oral soft tissue examination. Periodic evaluation of oral hygiene and other self-care measures can be accomplished by using disclosing solution or gingival and plaque indices. Individuals are advised to conduct an oral self-examination monthly to look for lesions that are painless and do not heal within 2 weeks.

The older patient's nutritional status should be evaluated because of the many physiologic and psychosocial complexities that have been documented regarding dietary patterns for the elderly. Dental hygienists should ask patients for a 1-day diet diary as part of the health history information to detect any deficiencies in food intake and related patterns that affect oral health and nutrition. For example, older adults may avoid eating nutritious foods because of decreased oral function or because they are unable or unwilling to cook a full meal because they live alone or cannot shop at the usual location. Merely asking an older adult to describe their typical diet often sheds light on multiple issues that affect nutrition and health.

Dental hygienists plan and implement care based on the dental hygiene diagnosis, type and severity of chronic conditions, cognitive abilities and attitudes of the older adult, level of self-care, expectations,

and financial ability. Short morning appointments are recommended because many older adults have a lower stress tolerance and tire more easily than younger people. A written note of the date and time of each appointment should be provided to help remind the patient and assist caregivers when necessary. See Chapter 22 – Dental Hygiene Diagnosis, where the human needs model and the Oral Health-related Quality of Life Model are used in the development of a dental hygiene diagnosis.

Planning

Dental hygiene care planning for older adults is often more complex than for younger persons because the vast majority have at least one chronic condition, and many have complex dental and periodontal conditions.[15] Also, normal aging alterations may create a compromised oral situation. Individual considerations guide treatment modalities in collaboration with the dental hygienist, dentist, and, at times, the physician and physical and occupational therapists.

The individual's and their family's attitudes toward oral health affect care planning and outcomes. Many older adults view oral problems as an inevitable part of aging, and some older adults do not use dental services as frequently as recommended or do so only when dental emergencies occur.

Planning considerations for care with older individuals include:

- *Appointment time.* Short morning appointments are best for older adults because they are physically strongest in the morning. Because many cannot sit for long periods, however, 2 hours should be the limit, including transportation time.
- *Accessibility and transportation to the dental office.* Parking lots, ramps, and doorways must accommodate wheelchairs. Legally, the Americans with Disabilities Act of 1993 mandates access to all public facilities. Elderly individuals may depend on transportation from family or agencies that may complicate arrival time as well.
- *Legal considerations.* The elderly patient may not be capable of providing informed consent. In such cases, written permission from the individual's physician, family, or facility should be obtained before care is provided. See Box 47.2 for legal, ethical, and safety considerations related to dental hygiene care for the older adult.
- *Multiple health conditions and drug therapies.* Many elderly individuals have a multitude of chronic health conditions. Consultation with the physician may be necessary.
- *Communication with long-term care facilities.* Most facilities require that documentation of care provided and followup instructions be forwarded to the facility for their records for each appointment.

BOX 47.2   Legal, Ethical, and Safety Issues

- Complete and document informed consent for care as well as a thorough medical, personal, and dental history and oral examination with each patient. As necessary, discuss and document treatment with family and/or caregivers.
- Evaluate the patient's health history and use of medications, and refer the patient to their physician for consultation when indicated.
- Explain the results of consultation with the older adult, and document conversations and the physician's recommendations in the patient's dental record.
- Involve older adults in treatment decisions.
- Treat older adults with dignity and respect.
- Provide written instruction that can be read easily by older patients and/or caregivers, and reinforce instructions verbally.
- Provide aggressive oral health prevention programs for caries and periodontal diseases.
- Ensure that the dental office facility is wheelchair accessible based on guidelines from the Americans with Disabilities Act.
- Provide care without discrimination.

Implementation

During instrumentation, as little trauma as possible to the gingiva is required because of reduction in healing capabilities. Loss of elasticity of the lips and oral mucosa and xerostomia may make retraction of oral tissues uncomfortable. More frequent periodontal maintenance therapy visits may be required for older adults with a history of periodontal disease, and care may need to be sequenced to allow for short appointment times. Individuals who receive antibiotic premedication need to have as much care as possible at one time; however, the person's medical condition may make lengthy appointments difficult.

Specific and customized client education including oral hygiene instruction is provided to older adults to ensure that they have the knowledge and skills necessary to removal plaque biofilm thoroughly (Box 47.3). Antimicrobial products, such as stannous fluoride dentifrice, essential oil mouth rinse, or 0.12% chlorhexidine mouth rinse, are recommended when necessary to supplement mechanical plaque biofilm removal. Recommendations for improving the adequacy of the diet with regard to food choices are provided, with specific directions for limiting refined carbohydrate foods and limiting cariogenic snacking.

Home use of topical fluoride products has been advocated for all older individuals with teeth. In addition to using a fluoride dentifrice, patients can use a daily nonprescription 0.05% sodium fluoride rinse, especially if they notice decreased quality and quantity of saliva. Because many older patients have difficulty rinsing their mouths, a fluoride gel applied by a toothbrush may be easier to use, especially in reaching susceptible proximal and root surfaces. Patients who have undergone head and neck radiation therapy, who have severe xerostomia, or who have rampant caries can use the tray method to apply the fluoride gel for 5 minutes twice a day. The tray method of application is best completed with an unflavored fluoride product because of the frequency and intensity of the application.

For individuals with xerostomia, self-applied and professionally applied topical fluoride is recommended to promote remineralization (see Chapter 19). Calcium and phosphate remineralizing products can also be used. Saliva substitutes that coat the mucosa and teeth to keep them moist are recommended to reduce enamel solubility and the accumulation of plaque biofilm. Saliva substitutes can be used without limit on the frequency of use and come in liquid, gel, or spray formulations that are distributed through the mouth with the tongue. Several over-the-counter products are available, with many containing fluoride and xylitol.

Exposed root surfaces are susceptible to dental caries, and professionally applied and home-applied topical fluoride products are recommended to help meet the need for a biologically sound dentition. The role of plaque biofilm and diet in relation to dental caries formation must be stressed. A desensitization treatment and dentifrice also may be recommended to help ensure freedom from pain if root surfaces are sensitive.

At the completion of the appointment, dental hygienists should return the dental chair to an upright position slowly. It is important to allow the patient to sit up for a short time before dismissal to avoid any problems with postural hypotension. The dental hygienist should pay close attention to see if the patient needs assistance out of the chair. Postoperative instructions are reviewed and a written copy provided as indicated.

The reader is referred to Chapter 23—Dental Hygiene Care Plan, Evaluation, and Documentation, where both the human needs and oral health-related quality of life models are used to guide the dental hygienist through this important aspect of care.

See the Critical Thinking Exercise below to apply principles of assessment, dental hygiene diagnosis, planning, and implementation to a clinical case.

BOX 47.3 Patient or Client Education Tips

- Explain the differences between normal physiologic changes seen in aging and pathologic changes in the oral cavity.
- Communicate a wellness philosophy of care to maximize health in light of many chronic conditions experienced among the elderly.
- Select and explain health promotion strategies based on older adults' needs.
- Assess the patient's level of oral health literacy and customize instructions appropriate for each patient.
- Encourage compliance with all medication and medical regimens.
- Relate patient's health status to any modifications necessary for dental hygiene care.
- Adapt oral hygiene instructions to any functional limitations and oral health conditions.
- Explain the development and prevention of dental caries and periodontal diseases.
- Provide nutritional counseling regarding the reduction of refined carbohydrates, limitation of cariogenic snacking, and adequacy of dietary intake.
- Recommend the use of topical and professional fluorides to prevent dental decay.
- Recommend the use of oral hygiene products and antimicrobial agents by the patient to prevent and control periodontal diseases.
- Assist with tobacco cessation efforts.
- Explain the importance of oral cancer prevention and early detection.
- Provide education regarding drug-induced changes in the oral cavity.
- Explain methods to identify and manage xerostomia.
- Instruct family caregivers regarding appropriate oral assessment and oral hygiene care.

CRITICAL THINKING EXERCISE

Dental Hygiene Care for an Older Patient

Profile: Mrs. F., age 77, returns for a dental hygiene visit on her regular 6-month maintenance schedule.

Chief Complaint: "I have a removable partial denture to replace my lower back teeth that I don't wear because it makes my mouth feel dry and taste bad. Also, I have a large freckle on my left cheek that has grown in the past several months."

Social History: Mrs. F. has been widowed for 3 years and is active with her church and the families of her two daughters who live nearby.

Health History: Mrs. F. has had a history of angina for the past 6 years and takes 50 mg atenolol (Tenormin) once a day to prevent angina attacks.

Dental History: Mrs. F. has a history of regular dental visits and has all of her teeth, with the exception of the four mandibular molars. Oral examination reveals a flat, brown, elongated lesion approximately 10 mm long and 6 mm wide on the center of her left cheek. Mrs. F. denies any pain or exudate from this lesion. Dental examination reveals no areas of decay and recession with no evidence of periodontal disease.

Oral Health Behavior Assessment: Good oral hygiene. Uses a power toothbrush and flosses daily.

Supplemental Notes: During dental hygiene care, Mrs. F. states that she thinks her teeth are too short and ugly and asks you if she is too old to get "caps" on her teeth to improve her appearance.

1. What are the dental hygiene diagnoses for this patient (see Chapter 22)?
2. Develop a dental hygiene care plan for this patient that includes goals and interventions (see Chapter 23).
3. What patient education issues should be addressed, especially in terms of health literacy?
4. What factors could be contributing to this patient's dry mouth?
5. Are there any contraindications to this patient's care?
6. What measures should be taken during treatment to prevent an angina attack?

Evaluation

After care has been completed, older patients need to be reevaluated more frequently and more carefully because of the many physiologic changes, chronic conditions, and pathologic changes frequently seen in this age group. Dental hygienists must be aware that health status can change quickly with an older patient and that even small changes may be significant, especially in relation to cardiovascular and cognitive changes. Often a dental hygienist may be the first to notice cognitive declines over a series of appointments or at the recall visit. These qualitative perceptions that "something is not quite right" about the older patient should be discussed with the patient, relatives, and/or caregivers, and referrals for further medical evaluation provided.

Dental hygienists should allow a longer time to assess results of soft tissue debridement because of a slower and decreased potential for tissue healing, and provide additional care when necessary. Quantitative evaluation of health status through bleeding and plaque indices and pocket depth recording is essential to document healing and plan new interventions with older patients.

More frequent maintenance intervals are recommended for older patients to evaluate any changes in functional abilities to complete oral hygiene, any nutritional changes, and the occurrence of new disease. Dental hygienists should not assume that older adults still have the same functional abilities, even after a 3-month period. For example, patients with musculoskeletal disorders frequently note varying functional abilities and may need more assistance with oral hygiene at times. In addition, patients may be taking new medications and may alter their nutritional patterns because of the unpleasant taste or increased xerostomia experienced with a different medication. These older adults are at extreme risk for caries and need more aggressive caries management. More frequent visits for dental hygiene care provide opportunity to assess patients' oral health and to recommend preventive and therapeutic interventions specific to the patient's needs.

Documentation

All components of the process of care are interrelated and depend on ongoing assessments and evaluation of treatment outcomes to determine the need for change in the dental hygiene care plan. Thus, it is critical to document ongoing patient progress in the dental record to provide documentation for reevaluation. Documenting the patient's health status during active therapy and over a lifetime of regular maintenance care is the best defense against a patient's accusation of negligence. It is important to provide and document informed consent with all older patients. When necessary, discuss and document treatment with family and/or caregivers.

ROLE OF THE DENTAL HYGIENIST IN COMMUNITY AND INSTITUTIONAL SETTINGS

Institutionalized elderly make up approximately 4.5% of the elderly population in 2020. Partially due to COVID-19, the percentage of homebound, semidependent elderly increased to 13% in 2020 and signals a heightened risk of social isolation, having unmet care needs (including oral health) and high mortality.[20] Individuals who are functionally dependent are more likely to be edentulous and may not have used dental services for several years.

Several factors explain this neglect. First, individuals who are in a long-term care facility (LTCF) or are homebound may not be able to care for themselves. They may have numerous complicated and interrelated problems, and dental care may not be a priority for them or for their caregivers. In addition, dental professionals historically have not been active in providing services because of their own attitudes toward treating the frail elderly, low financial return, and state practice acts that limit dentists and dental hygienists' ability to work in LTCFs or with

the homebound.[16] The number of dental hygienists providing direct preventive and therapeutic services in these settings has increased in the past decade as laws are changing to expand the scope of practice to serve this population in many states (Fig. 47.8).[16]

For older adults, provision of routine dental services is not included under Medicare benefits. Dental benefits and eligibility for low-income Medicaid public insurance vary by state; however, preventive dental care for elderly patients is usually not a priority. Given the high dental needs of the homebound or institutionalized elderly, dental hygienists' services are needed, and dental hygienists must advocate for and establish systems to provide care (Box 47.4).

ON-SITE DENTAL AND DENTAL HYGIENE PROGRAMS

Providing care in an LTCF, a senior day center, or a patient's home has several advantages, including care for the frail elderly in a comfortable, familiar setting without the transportation disruptions and requirements. There are three options that dental professionals can use when providing care in an LTCF, senior day center, or with homebound clients. Many facilities have space to build dental operatories, which may be more common in a larger LTCF and provide a more comfortable permanent arrangement for dental professionals and patients. However, for smaller LTCFs, dedicated permanent space may not be available, and the use of portable dental equipment set up in a conference room or other space allows the provision of dental care as needed for clients. As a third option, mobile dental vehicles provide "dental offices on wheels," with dental laboratories and other amenities to customize care with older adults. Whichever option is selected, it is important to educate the family and/or caregivers about appropriate daily oral hygiene regimens and follow-up care to dental treatment for the client.[16]

Dental hygienists serve in an important capacity to provide care with the institutionalized and homebound elderly. In 2021, 42 states permitted direct access to dental hygiene services, which means that dental hygienists provide dental hygiene care without the specific authorization or supervision of a dentist.[21] Direct-access dental hygienists complete the following activities:

- Providing clinical dental hygiene care in the patient's home, the LTCF, a senior day center, or when the patient is transported to the clinical facility.

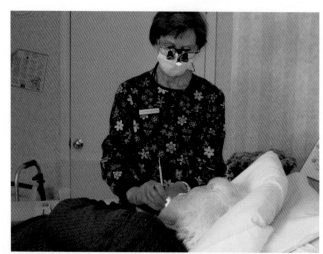

Fig. 47.8 Dental hygienist providing care to a patient in a nursing home. (Brown EJ. Dental hygienist providers in long term care: meeting the need. *Journal of Evidence Based Practice.* 2016;16(Supplement):77–83).

BOX 47.4 Visit a Senior Community Center

Most communities provide a variety of services to older adults who currently are living in the community but who may need some assistance with meals, social activities, healthcare, or housing to function in an independent manner for as long as possible.

In this learning activity, participants should contact the director of a local senior center and request to visit and/or volunteer at the center at least twice. Visits to these senior centers provide an interesting window into the daily life of older adults, especially if participants have little experience with older individuals. The centers generally emphasize a philosophy of wellness and provide a wide range of activities to encourage participation by members, such as arts and craft projects, discussion groups, and scheduled trips to social and cultural events.

Those who visit a senior center should keep a diary regarding the activities the seniors completed on the days on which they visited and should participate actively in the events scheduled for the day. For example, learners may wish to volunteer to share a craft activity with the older adults, lead an exercise or dance class, or call bingo for the session. During the visits, the participants should speak with as many seniors as possible to learn about their daily activities, why they participate in the center activities, and which activities and functions of the center they use most frequently. These informal discussions generally are welcomed by the older adults, who view these sessions as a chance to advise and guide younger individuals about the needs of older adults. In addition, these visits provide participants with the opportunity to understand the wide range of abilities these older individuals possess, even in light of chronic and disabling conditions. By observing and sharing activities, participants can view the active and varied nature of the seniors in their daily activities and gain an understanding of the challenges older adults face each day.

- Providing in-service education programs for staff and/or family members
- Marking dentures for identification
- Giving fluoride applications
- Developing individual care plans with the interprofessional team
- Ensuring availability of oral hygiene supplies and quality assurance for daily oral care programs with residents

Interprofessional Collaboration

When providing care in a senior day center or long-term care facility, dental hygienists work as integral members of the healthcare team in assessing needs and providing care to increase quality of life. Nursing and social services staff members should be encouraged to refer elderly individuals to the dental office or consulting dentist if they detect unusual signs, such as swelling or discoloration, or if they hear a verbal complaint. The Brief Oral Health Status Examination (BOHSE) is a tool to evaluate oral health of patients systematically at the entrance to the care facility and routinely during care.[22] Dental hygienists can develop and implement in-service education programs to ensure that staff members have the knowledge and skill necessary to complete thorough oral assessments and daily oral hygiene care.

For homebound individuals, establishment of a prevention program using visiting nurses or home healthcare workers is needed when family members are not available. Dental hygienists can collaborate with local agencies, dental and dental hygiene associations, and dental hygiene educational institutions to develop oral screening, referral, and preventive programs for homebound elderly people.

KEY CONCEPTS

- Older adults are a heterogeneous group, and there is tremendous variability in the physical, psychosocial, and environmental issues within this age group. Functional age, rather than chronologic age, is the best measure to use when providing care to older adults.
- Current demographic reports and projections indicate a significant rise in the number and proportion of older adults in the United States.
- The older adult population is becoming more racially and ethnically diverse. Elderly females outnumber elderly men. Older adults are concentrated in certain states and are not distributed evenly in the population.
- There is not one accepted theory to explain how and why we age. Multiple social and biologic theories of aging have been proposed and complement each other to shed light on the aging process.
- There are normal physiologic changes in most body systems that occur as individuals age. These normal changes should not be confused with pathologic changes caused by disease; however, distinctions between normal aging and pathologic conditions are sometimes difficult to discern.
- Most older adults have at least one chronic condition, and the most common chronic conditions are arthritis, hypertension and heart disease, cancer, diabetes, and stroke. Evaluate mental status regarding dementia.
- Older adults develop coronal and root caries at a rate higher than the adult population; however, the rate of edentulousness (total tooth loss) among the elderly has decreased since 1960 and is projected to continue to decrease in future years.
- Caries prevention and control strategies for older adults must stress daily removal of plaque biofilm, reduction of refined carbohydrates, and daily use of topical fluorides, salivary substitutes, and calcium and phosphate products, especially when xerostomia is present.
- A small but significant number of older adults have advanced periodontitis, and there is a higher degree of loss of attachment and prevalence of gingivitis among older adults.
- Prevention and control of periodontal diseases should include daily removal of plaque biofilm, use of antimicrobial agents, and more frequent visits for professional debridement and evaluation.
- A small percentage of older adults either reside in long-term care facilities or are homebound and confined to their homes. These individuals have a higher prevalence of dental disease and a lower use rate of dental care than the adult population in general.
- Dental hygienists can work with nursing staff in long-term care facilities, with caregivers, and with homebound individuals in a variety of roles to improve the oral health status of elderly patients.

REFERENCES

1. US Census Bureau. *65 and Older Population Grows Rapidly as Baby Boomers Age*; June 25, 2020. https://www.census.gov/newsroom/press-releases/2020/65-older-population-grows.html. Accessed November 7, 2022.
2. *Administration for Community Living, US Department of Health and Human Services*; 2020. Profile of Older Americans, May 2021. https://acl.gov/sites/default/files/Profile%20of%20OA/2020ProfileOlderAmericans_RevisedFinal.pdf. Accessed November 7, 2022.
3. *World Population Ageing 2019*. New York: United Nations; 2019. https://www.un.org/en/development/desa/population/publications/pdf/ageing/WorldPopulationAgeing2019-Highlights.pdf. Accessed November 7, 2022.
4. Crimmins EM. Lifespan and healthspan: past, present and promise. *Gerontol*. 2015;55(6):901–911.
5. Arias E, Tejada-Vera B, Kochanek KD, Ahmad FB. *Provisional Life Expectancy Estimates for 2021. NVSS Vital Statistics Rapid Release, Report 23*; 2022. https://www.cdc.gov/nchs/data/vsrr/vsrr023.pdf. Accessed November 7, 2022.

6. Federal Interagency Forum on Aging-Related Statistics. *Older Americans 2020: Key Indicators of Well-Being*. U.S. Government Printing Office; 2020. https://agingstats.gov/docs/LatestReport/OA20_508_10142020.pdf. Accessed November 7, 2022.

7. Soto-Perez-de-Celis E, Li D, Yuan Y, Lau YM, Hurria A. Functional versus chronological age: geriatric assessments to guide decision making in older patients with cancer. *Lancet Oncol*. 2018;19(6):e305–e316.

8. Lee H, Oh B, Kim S, Lee K. ADL/IADL dependencies and unmet healthcare needs in older persons: a nationwide survey. *Arch Gerontol Geriatr*. 2021;96:104458.

9. QuickStats. Percentage of adults with activity limitations, by age group and type of limitation—national health interview survey, United States, 2014. *MMWR Morb Mortal Wkly Rep*. 2016;65:14. https://doi.org/10.15585/mmwr.mm6501a6external icon. Accessed November 7, 2022.

10. World Health Organization, Healthy Ageing and Functional Ability 2020. https://www.who.int/news-room/questions-and-answers/item/healthy-ageing-and-functional-ability. Accessed February 17, 2023.

11. Older Adults, Healthy People 2030. https://health.gov/healthypeople/objectives-and-data/browse-objectives/older-adults. Accessed November 7, 2022.

12. Yarbrough C, Vujicic M. Oral health trends for older Americans. *JADA*. 2019;150(8):2019.

13. Da Costa JP, Vitorino R, Silva G, Vogel C, Duarte A, Rocha-Santos T. A synopsis on aging – theories, mechanisms and future prospects. *Ageing Res Rev*. 2016;29:90–112.

14. Carvalho TS, Lussi A. Age-related morphological, histological and functional changes in teeth. *J Oral Rehabil*. 2017;44:291–298.

15. Razak PA, Jose Richard JM, Thankachan RP, Abdul Hafiz KA, Kumar KN, Sameer KM. Geriatric oral health: a review article. *J Int Oral Health*. 2014;6(6):110–116.

16. Oral Health in America. *Advances and Challenges*. Bethesda, MD: US Department of Health and Human Services, National Institutes of Health, National Institute of Dental and Craniofacial Research; 2021. https://www.nidcr.nih.gov/sites/default/files/2021-12/Oral-Health-in-America-Advances-and-Challenges.pdf.

17. Little JW, Falace DA, Miller CS, et al. *Dental Management of the Medically Compromised Patient*. 9th ed. Mosby; 2017.

18. Centers for Disease Control and Prevention and National Association of Chronic Disease Directors. *The State of Mental Health and Aging in America Issue Brief 1: What Do the Data Tell Us?* National Association of Chronic Disease Directors; 2008.

19. Beydoun MA, Beydoun HA, Hossain S, El-Hajj ZW, Weiss J, Zonderman AB. Clinical and bacterial markers of periodontitis and their association with incident all-cause and Alzheimer's Disease dementia in a large national study. *J Alzheimers Dis*. 2020;75(1):157–172.

20. Ankuda CK, Leff B, Ritchie CS. Association of COVID-19 pandemic with the prevalence of homebound older adults in the United States, 2011–2020. *JAMA Intern Med*. 2021;181(12):1658–1660.

21. American Dental Hygienists Association. Direct Access. https://www.adha.org/resources-docs/ADHA_Direct_Access_Map_6-2021.pdf. Accessed November 7, 2022.

22. Kayser-Jones J, Bird WF, Paul SM, et al. An instrument to assess the oral health status of nursing home residents. *Gerontol*. 1995;35(6):814–824.

48

Cardiovascular Disease

Laura Mueller-Joseph and Marleen Azzam

PROFESSIONAL DEVELOPMENT OPPORTUNITIES

Cardiovascular disease includes many different types of commonly occurring heart disease. Thus, dental hygienists frequently treat patients with heart disease. Knowledge of cardiovascular disease allows dental care providers to use best practices to educate, manage, and provide dental hygiene care to patients with this disease status.

COMPETENCIES

1. Apply knowledge of cardiovascular disease and its risk factors while critically evaluating the relationship between cardiovascular diseases and periodontal disease.
2. Distinguish the etiology, risk factors, signs, symptoms, and medical and dental hygiene care of patients with hypertensive cardiovascular disease, history of angina or myocardial infarction, coronary heart disease, congestive heart failure, congenital heart disease, valvular heart defects, and rheumatic heart disease.
3. Identify the types of cardiovascular surgery and their implications for dental hygiene treatment.
4. Discuss oral manifestations of cardiovascular medications.
5. Understand implications of developing a dental hygiene diagnosis and care plan for a patient with cardiovascular disease, including comprehensive preventive and therapeutic dental hygiene services as well as the management of cardiac emergencies.

INTRODUCTION

Patients with cardiovascular disease have a unique set of health concerns that may or may not directly influence dental hygiene care. These patients are considered individuals with special needs and, depending on their situation, dental hygiene care plans may have to be altered to ensure optimal treatment outcomes. Normal cardiovascular structure and physiology establish the baseline for the discussion of cardiac pathology (Fig. 48.1).

Cardiovascular disease (CVD), an alteration of the heart and/or blood vessels that impairs function, is the leading cause of death, responsible for 32% of all deaths or 17.9 million people worldwide each year.[1] Furthermore, cardiovascular comorbidities are typical in patients with SARS-CoV-2. Research shows that patients with SARS-CoV-2 are at an increased risk for a comprehensive assortment of cardiovascular disorders including but not limited to dysrhythmias, ischemic and nonischemic heart disease, pericarditis, myocarditis, and heart failure.[2] Therefore, prevention through management of CVD risk factors

remains important. Risk factors associated with poor cardiovascular health are listed in Table 48.1.

The American Heart Association notes that periodontal disease and heart disease share common risk factors such as diabetes mellitus, smoking, increasing age, and poor socioeconomic conditions; however, the association between these two diseases appears to go beyond their common risk factors.[3,4] Research suggests that the systemic inflammatory or immune response to periodontal infection may increase cardiovascular risk.[3,4] The current position of the American Heart Association and the American Dental Association is that although periodontal disease and heart health have an association, additional research is needed to determine if a direct causal relationship exists.[3,4] Changing risk-related behaviors remains key in decreasing the risk and prevalence of heart disease in the population (see Table 48.1).

There are many types of cardiovascular disease. Four of the main types of CVD include coronary heart disease, strokes and TIAs (transient ischemic attacks), peripheral arterial disease, and aortic disease.[5] The following will outline various types of cardiovascular diseases and discuss their etiology, risk factors, disease process, prevention, and medical treatment. In many cases, these diseases and their treatment warrant special considerations for dental hygiene care. The role of the dental hygienist in providing person-centered care, where healthcare providers work collaboratively with patients and other healthcare providers to do what is in the best interest of the patient's health and well-being, will also be addressed.

HYPERTENSIVE CARDIOVASCULAR DISEASE

Most individuals with hypertension, also termed "silent killer," are unsuspecting of the problem as it may have no warning signs or symptoms.[6] For this reason, it is essential that blood pressure is assessed routinely.[6] Sustained elevated blood pressure may affect several organ systems like the heart, the kidneys, the brain, and the eyes. Chronic elevation through either the hypertension being undiagnosed or poor medical compliance places the patient at increased risk for cardiovascular disease. **Hypertensive cardiovascular disease** (HCD) or **hypertension** is a persistent elevation of the blood pressures ≥130 to 139 mm Hg systolic or ≥80 to 89 mm Hg diastolic (stage 1), and ≥140 mm Hg systolic or ≥90 mm Hg diastolic (stage 2) (see Chapter 14). Individuals with systolic and diastolic blood pressure readings in different categories should be designated to the higher category.[7] Nearly half of people with high blood pressure (45.6%) do not have it under control.[8] High blood pressure is a substantial single risk factor for TIA and stroke.[9] Many individuals with diagnosed hypertension are not treated or are

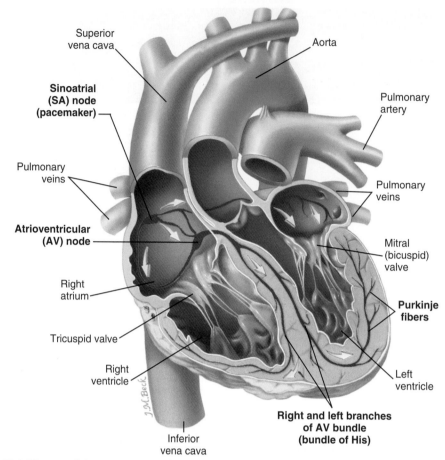

Fig. 48.1 Diagram of the heart. (From Patton KT, Thibodeau GA. *Anatomy and Physiology.* 8th ed. Mosby; 2013.)

treated inadequately, leaving the condition uncontrolled and the person at risk for other serious diseases.

Etiology

Hypertension is not considered a disease but rather a physical finding or symptom. A sustained elevated blood pressure affects the condition of the heart, with increased risk of CVD, end-stage renal disease, atherosclerosis, and potentially resulting in congestive heart failure (CHF), myocardial infarction (MI), cerebrovascular accident (stroke), and kidney failure.[7,8]

Risk Factors

Risk factors for hypertension include family history, race, stress, obesity, a high dietary intake of saturated fats or sodium, use of tobacco or oral contraceptives, fast-paced lifestyle, and age (over age 40). Hypertension is three times more common in obese persons than in normal-weight persons. There is a higher incidence of hypertension among African Americans than American Whites.

Disease Process

The two major types of hypertension are as follows:
- Primary hypertension (essential idiopathic hypertension), with no known cause, is the most common type, characterized by a gradual onset or an abrupt onset of short duration.
- Secondary hypertension is the result of an existing disease of the cardiovascular system, renal system, adrenal glands, or neurologic system. Because hypertension usually follows a chronic course, patients with this condition may be asymptomatic. Early clinical

signs and symptoms are occipital headaches, vision changes, ringing ears, dizziness, and weakness of the hands and feet. As the condition persists, advanced signs and symptoms can include hemorrhages, enlargement of the left ventricle, CHF, angina pectoris, and renal failure. The dental hygienist refers patients for medical diagnosis if a hypertensive disorder is suspected.

Prevention

Blood pressure screening is part of the assessment protocol for all dental patients and typically performed by the dental hygienist prior to dental hygiene treatment. Blood pressure measurement identifies individuals with elevated readings, possibly indicating undiagnosed heart disease or hypertensive heart disease (see Chapter 14). Early identification of hypertensive patients minimizes the occurrence of medical emergencies, helps meet the patient's human need for protection from health risks, and may be lifesaving for undiagnosed individuals.

Medical Treatment

Treatment of hypertension aims at lifestyle changes to reduce risk factors, antihypertensive drug therapy, and/or correction of the underlying medical condition in the case of secondary hypertension. The goal is to reduce and maintain the diastolic pressure level at 89 mm Hg or lower. Some patients need only to watch their dietary consumption of sodium and saturated fats; others must reduce their daily stress level and alter their lifestyle (see Table 48.1). When a patient needs drug therapy, periodic monitoring is essential. Some drugs may stabilize the condition temporarily and then an elevation can occur, indicating that an alternative drug is needed.

TABLE 48.1 Risk Factors for Cardiovascular Disease

Factors	Examples
Nonmodifiable Risk Factors: Personal Factors	
Genetic predisposition or family history	Family members have cardiovascular disease; congenital abnormality
Age	Prevalence increases in both males and females ages >35
Race	Blacks and Whites are more likely to have cardiovascular disease than Hispanics or Asians or Pacific Islanders
Gender	Coronary heart disease incidence rate is higher in males than females
Disease Patterns	
History of anorexia nervosa or bulimia	Females are at increased risk of developing coronary heart disease if they have (had) an eating disorder
Past use of fen-phen (fenfluramine and phentermine)	May damage heart valves if used longer than 2 months
Modifiable Risk Factors	
Personality traits (type A personality)	Hard-driving, competitive individuals who worry excessively about deadlines and consistently overwork
Professional stresses	Occupations that impose tremendous responsibility
Oral contraceptive use	Females <40 years of age who take oral contraceptives
Tobacco use	Smoking and use of smokeless tobacco increase risk of coronary heart disease
Alcohol use	Moderate to heavy consumption of alcohol elevates the risk of high blood pressure, heart attack, and stroke
Sedentary occupation and lifestyle	Lack of exercise promotes mental depression and obesity
Diet high in calories, cholesterol, fat, and sodium	Overeating and consuming fatty foods promote obesity, lipid abnormalities, diabetes, metabolic syndrome; high-sodium diet promotes hypertension
Hypertension	Individuals with systolic readings between 130 to 139 and diastolic readings between 80 to 89 have a 67% increased risk of myocardial infarction
Obesity	Weight 30% or more above that considered standard for an individual of a certain height and build
Lipid abnormalities	Serum cholesterol >200 mg/100 mL or fasting triglycerides of >250 mg/100 mL; abnormal level of C-reactive protein
Diabetes mellitus	Fasting blood sugar of >120 mg/dL or a routine blood sugar level of ≥180 mg/dL increases risk
Periodontal disease	Periodontal disease increases chronic systemic inflammation, possibly increasing risk of fatal cardiovascular disease

Drugs used for hypertension vary in their method of action, as follows:

- Diuretics—promote renal excretion of water and sodium ions
- Sympatholytic agents—modify sympathetic nerve activity
- Vasodilators—increase blood vessel size and facilitate blood flow

Patients receiving hypertensive drug therapy may experience fatigue, gastrointestinal disturbances, nausea, diarrhea, cramps, xerostomia, orthostatic hypotension with dizziness, and/or depression (Table 48.2).

Dental Hygiene Care

If an individual's hypertension is uncontrolled, treatment is postponed until the disorder is regulated. If the patient is being treated with antihypertensive agents and if clinical blood pressure evaluations are within normal limits, care can continue; however, stress and anxiety reduction strategies and local anesthetic drug modification will reduce the risk for medical emergencies. Drug considerations for local anesthetic use in patients with hypertensive heart disease are based on the careful use of vasopressors (such as epinephrine), which constrict blood vessels, concentrate the anesthetic in the desired area, and prevent its dissipation. A vasopressor side effect is elevation in blood pressure. A slight elevation in blood pressure normally is harmless; however, with vasopressors, hypertensive individuals have increased risk of a cerebrovascular accident, MI, or CHF. Therefore anesthetic agents with vasopressors are avoided or used with caution and in reduced amounts in patients with a history of hypertension (see Chapter 43). The risk versus benefit of using a low concentration of epinephrine to local anesthetic agent

is considered. See Box 48.1 for a Critical Thinking Scenario based on hypertension.

Appointment guidelines include the following:

- Care plan considerations for individuals with controlled hypertension focus on stress reduction strategies (see Chapters 11 and 44) and local anesthetic drug modification to reduce potential for medical emergencies (as discussed in previous section). Box 48.2 displays cases based on initial blood pressure measurement and family history information. Each situation demonstrates appropriate dental hygiene care modifications to meet a specific human need, or in the case of the Oral Health-Related Quality of Life model of care, to increase quality of life. Refer to Chapters 2, 22, and 23 that support the use of the Human Needs and Oral Health-Related Quality of Life theories for the development of dental hygiene diagnoses and care plans.

See Box 48.3 for a discussion of legal, ethical, and safety issues in the treatment of patients with cardiovascular disease.

CORONARY HEART DISEASE

Coronary heart disease (CHD) (coronary artery disease or ischemic heart disease) is the most common heart disease, resulting from insufficient blood flow from the coronary arteries into the heart or myocardium. Disorders associated with this condition are arteriosclerotic heart disease, angina pectoris, coronary insufficiency, and MI. Certain patients will be prescribed aspirin combined with another antiplatelet drug; this is known as dual antiplatelet therapy.[10]

TABLE 48.2   Commonly Prescribed Cardiovascular Medication

Brand Name	Generic Name	Indications for Use	Oral Implications
Glycosides			
Lanoxin	Digoxin	Congestive heart failure (CHF)	Excessive salivation, sensitive gag reflex
Farxiga	Dapagliflozin		
Diuretics			
Diuril	Chlorothiazide	CHF, hypertension	Decreased salivary flow
Midamor	Amiloride		
Lasix	Furosemide		
Aldactone	Spironolactone		
Beta Blockers			
Tenormin	Atenolol	Hypertension, angina	Xerostomia
Inderal	Propranolol		
Lopressor	Metoprolol		
Zebeta	Bisoprolol		
Calcium Channel Blockers			
Cardizem	Diltiazem	Hypertension, angina	Decreased salivary flow, gingival enlargement
Procardia	Nifedipine		
Calan	Verapamil		
Vascor	Bepridil		
Norvasc, Lotrel	Amlodipine		
ACE (Angiotensin-Converting Enzyme) Inhibitors			
Capoten	Captopril	Hypertension	Xerostomia, taste impairment, oral ulceration
Vasotec	Enalapril		
Zestril	Lisinopril		
Lotensin	Benazepril		
Vasodilators			
Nitroglycerin	Nitroglycerin	Angina	Burning under tongue
Angiotensin II Receptor Inhibitors			
Avapro	Irbesartan	Hypertension	Xerostomia, taste impairment, oral ulceration
Losartan	Cozaar		
Diovan	Valsartan		
Micardis	Telmisartan		
Anticoagulants			
Lovenox	Enoxaparin	Angina, stent placement, after myocardial infarction (MI)	Increased bleeding
Coumadin	Warfarin		
Calciparine	Heparin		
Xarelto	Rivaroxaban		
Eliquis	Apixaban		
Antiplatelet Agents			
Aspirin	Acetylsalicylic acid	Angina, after MI	Decreases blood clotting
Ticlopidine	Ticlid		
Clopidogrel	Plavix		
Dual Antiplatelet Therapy (DAPT)			
Persantine	Dipyridamole	Stent placement, after MI	Decreases blood clotting
Effient	Prasugrel		
Brilinta	Ticagrelor		
Angiotensin-Receptor Neprilysin Inhibitors (ARNIs)			
Entresto	Sacubitril/valsartan	CHF	Xerostomia

Etiology

The major cause of coronary heart disease is **atherosclerosis,** a narrowing of the lumen of the coronary arteries, thereby reducing blood flow volume. Narrowing of the lumen is caused by fibrofatty deposits containing lipids and cholesterol. Deposits thicken with time and eventually can occlude the vessel (Fig. 48.2). Atherosclerosis usually develops in high-flow, high-pressure arteries and has been linked to many risk factors. Other causes of coronary heart disease are congenital abnormalities of the arteries and changes in the arteries because of infection, autoimmune disorders, and coronary embolism (blood clot).

Risk Factors

Coronary heart disease is influenced by systemic risk factors such as age, gender, race, diet, lifestyle, and environment. Individuals who are obese, anorectic, bulimic, physically inactive, or who smoke increase their coronary heart disease risk (see Table 48.1).

BOX 48.1 Critical Thinking Scenario A

Hypertension

While taking the vital signs of patient L., age 45, the dental hygienist obtains a blood pressure reading of 144/90 mm Hg. The dental hygienist waits 10 minutes, retakes the blood pressure, and obtains the same reading. Patient L. is surprised that their blood pressure is being taken at the dental office and that the blood pressure reading is high. Patient L. then mentions that they smoke a pack of cigarettes a day and the last time the patient had gone for their annual physical to their physician was 3 years ago. Patient L. stated they have not been to their physician because the patient does not have time, placing the blame on their busy and fast-paced lifestyle.

1. Should the dental hygienist continue with dental hygiene care for this patient at this moment? Why or why not?
2. Based on the assessment findings of this patient, what patient education could be given?
3. Should this patient consult with their primary care physician?

- *Age.* Being older than 40 is associated with coronary heart disease. Pathologic changes in the arteries are noticeable with age, usually producing disease symptoms.
- *Gender.* Males are four times more likely to suffer from coronary heart disease than females up to age 40; after age 40, the prevalence of coronary heart disease among females and males is the same. Females younger than 40 years old are at an increased risk for developing coronary heart disease if they are taking oral contraceptives or have a history of anorexia nervosa or bulimia.
- *Race.* White males and non-White females are at a higher risk for coronary heart disease than non-White males and White females. Researchers are trying to determine the genetic factors involved; however, a familial connection is suspected.
- *Diet.* Populations in which a low-cholesterol, low-fat diet is consumed have little coronary heart disease; populations in which the diet consists of foods rich in cholesterol and saturated fat have a very high rate of coronary heart disease.
- *Environment.* Coronary heart disease is seven times more prevalent in North America than in South America, and urban populations are at a higher risk than rural dwellers. Stressful life situations increase an individual's chance of developing coronary heart disease at an early age.
- *Tobacco use.* Cigarette smoking and use of smokeless tobacco increases an individual's chance of developing coronary heart disease at an early age.

In addition, research supports an association between inflammation in the body and coronary heart disease. C-reactive protein (CRP) levels are used to determine systemic inflammation associated with disease including an individual's risk for cardiovascular disease. Elevated levels of CRP are key markers of atherosclerosis. Studies have correlated increased CRP levels with the presence of periodontitis.[11] This finding supports other studies that suggest the presence of periodontitis increases one's risk for CVD.[3,4] Although the exact link is unclear, evidence suggests that a relationship exists. Further research is needed to determine a causal relationship whereby periodontal disease would be considered a direct risk factor.

Disease Process

Basic manifestations of coronary heart disease are angina pectoris, MI, and sudden death.

BOX 48.2 Patients with Various Hypertensive Conditions and Appropriate Dental Hygiene Actions

Patient With No History of Hypertension, Elevated Blood Pressure

During assessment, the patient reports no history or symptoms of hypertension; however, a blood pressure reading of 144/90 mm Hg was obtained. One dental hygiene diagnosis may be an unmet need for protection from health risks caused by a potential for heart attack or stroke as evidenced by an elevated blood pressure of 144/90 mm Hg. The dental hygienist should repeat blood pressure measurements during the assessment phase, approximately 5 to 10 minutes apart. If after repeated measurements the diastolic pressure is still greater than 90 mm Hg, the appointment should be limited to assessment and planning; no treatment is implemented. The patient should be educated that tobacco use is a risk factor for hypertension. The patient must be referred to the physician of record for medical consultation and diagnosis. If the patient is diagnosed as nonhypertensive by the physician, it can be inferred that dental care anxiety causes the elevated blood pressure. Blood pressure must be monitored at each appointment thereafter and strategies implemented to minimize stress.

Patient Under Treatment for Hypertension

During assessment, the patient indicates that they are hypertensive and under a physician's care. At each visit, the hygienist obtains information on the patient's medications and verifies that the prescribed medication has been taken. The patient may have fear or stress; therefore stress reduction protocol is needed, and the care plan includes the administration of nitrous oxide–oxygen analgesia to reduce patient anxiety. At each visit, the patient's blood pressure is monitored, periodically remeasured, and recorded.

Patient Noncompliant with Hypertension Treatment

Patient indicates that they are hypertensive and have discontinued their recommended medication because it is too expensive. Rather, they take the medication irregularly, based on symptoms. This patient has uncontrolled hypertension and a need for protection from health risks. Dental hygiene care is stopped after assessment and should not resume until the hypertension is stabilized. The patient is referred to the physician of record for further medical evaluation and treatment. Although dental hygiene care is postponed, the remaining appointment time can facilitate protection from health risks via educational strategies directed toward the importance of controlling hypertension, information about the oral inflammation and systemic inflammation link, and possible lethal effects if hypertension is uncontrolled. Throughout the appointment, the blood pressure is monitored and recorded periodically.

Client With Hypertension and Acute Symptoms

During assessment, the patient demonstrates hypertension with diastolic readings greater than 120 mm Hg and symptoms (e.g., headache, dizziness, restlessness, decreased level of consciousness, blurred vision, palpitations) indicative of hypertensive cardiovascular disease (HCD). To meet the human need for protection from health risks, the patient is referred to the physician of record for immediate medical consultation and evaluation. Dental hygiene care is delayed until the HCD is controlled. Because hypertension can be related to anxiety and stress, the dental hygienist must determine if the patient needs stress management and, if so, can reduce apprehension associated with therapy (e.g., encourage the patient to express fears and concerns, involve patient in goal setting and care planning, explain procedures completely, obtain informed consent, demonstrate humanistic behaviors, and discuss apprehensions directly).

BOX 48.3 Legal, Ethical, and Safety Issues

Dental Hygiene Care for Cardiac Patients and Potential Medical Emergencies[11]

A cardiovascular medical emergency or "incident" may subject the practitioner to liability for causing additional harm (even death) resulting from negligent care and treatment, or the occurrence of an inherent risk (e.g., infection) following such treatment.

If a client reports a cardiac condition that requires antibiotic premedication to prevent infective endocarditis (per American Heart Association guidelines) and the patient is not premedicated, the practitioner may be liable for morbidity and mortality that develops after treatment.

If a client with CVD develops chest pain and begins to feel nauseated and sweat profusely, the provider should (1) stop dental hygiene care; (2) alert the dentist; and (3) together with the dentist, manage the immediate emergency situation, which may include use of the automated external defibrillator and Basic Life Support.

Medical emergency situations must be prevented and properly managed or a malpractice suit could arise.

Angina Pectoris

Angina pectoris is the direct result of inadequate oxygen flow to the myocardium, manifested clinically as a burning, squeezing, or crushing tightness in the chest that radiates to the left arm, neck, and shoulder blade. The person typically clenches a fist over the chest or rubs the left arm when describing the pain. When sudden attacks of angina pectoris follow physical exertion, emotional excitement, or exposure to cold, and the symptoms are relieved by administration of nitroglycerin, they are classified as stable angina. Conversely, unstable angina may occur at rest or during sleep, and pain is of longer duration and not relieved readily with nitroglycerin.

Medical treatment for angina pectoris has two goals: reduce myocardial oxygen demand and increase oxygen supply. Therapy consists primarily of physical rest to decrease oxygen demand and the administration of nitrates, such as nitroglycerin, to provide more oxygen. Nitroglycerin (glyceryl trinitrate) is a vasodilator that increases blood flow (oxygen supply) by expanding the arteries. Administration can be sublingual for immediate absorption, or by nitroglycerin pads and patches for time-released medication absorbed by the skin and into the

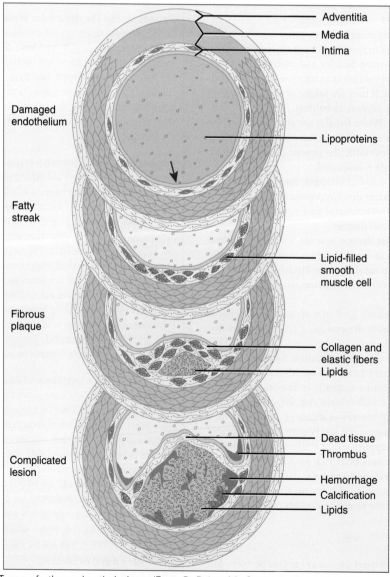

Fig. 48.2 Types of atherosclerotic lesions. (From DeBakey M, Grotto A. *The Living Heart.* David McKay; 1977.)

bloodstream; an overdose can cause headache. Obstructive lesions that do not respond to drug therapy may necessitate surgery.

Myocardial Infarction

Myocardial infarction, the second manifestation of coronary heart disease, is a reduction of blood flow through one of the coronary arteries, resulting in an infarct. An infarct is an area of tissue that undergoes necrosis because of the elimination of blood flow. An MI is also known as a heart attack, coronary occlusion, and coronary thrombosis. Symptoms associated with MI are similar to those experienced with angina pectoris; however, the pain usually persists for 12 or more hours and begins as a feeling of indigestion. Other manifestations include a feeling of fatigue, nausea, vomiting, and shortness of breath.

Medical treatment includes combination therapy to reduce cardiac workloads and increase cardiac output. Cardiac workload reduction therapies include bed rest, morphine for pain reduction and sedation, and oxygen if necessary. To increase cardiac output, therapy for the control and reduction of cardiac dysrhythmias is recommended (e.g., antiarrhythmic drugs, possibly a cardiac pacemaker). Nitroglycerin can relieve chest pain and increase cardiac output by intensifying the blood flow and redistributing blood to the affected myocardial tissue. Anticoagulants may be used to thin the blood in an effort to increase blood flow and reduce the possibility of another MI. Coronary stents, another medical management option, are often used to dilate narrow arteries to increase blood flow and reduce the occurrence of a myocardial infarction.

Sudden Death

Sudden death, the last manifestation of coronary heart disease, occurs during the first 24 to 48 hours after the onset of symptoms. Most sudden cardiovascular deaths are caused by ventricular fibrillation. For example, ventricular fibrillation results in ventricular standstill (cardiac arrest) if insufficient blood is pumped into the coronary arteries to supply the myocardium with oxygen. Biologic death results when oxygen delivery to the brain is inadequate for 4 to 6 minutes. Therefore, the use of an **automated external defibrillator** (AED) (also known as *precordial shock*) is followed by cardiopulmonary resuscitation (CPR) to maintain enough blood oxygen to sustain life. Transportation to the hospital for emergency medical care is necessary.

Prevention

Lifestyle behaviors associated with the prevention of coronary heart disease are as follows:
- Regular medical checkups
- Healthy diet (e.g., reduction in saturated fat and cholesterol; increases in whole grains, fruits, and vegetables)
- Regular physical exercise
- Stress management
- Avoidance of tobacco
- High blood pressure control
- Prevention of periodontal disease
- Knowledge of the warning signs of a heart attack

Factors associated with coronary heart disease must be taken into consideration when providing nutritional counseling to improve a patient's oral health. In facilitating the individual's human need for protection from health risks, the dental hygienist recognizes the importance of dietary choices related to coronary heart disease and incorporates that knowledge into the nutritional education session (see Chapter 36).

Given that periodontal disease is a risk factor for coronary heart disease, patients need this information to make sound decisions about their oral health. Therefore, client education should emphasize the link between oral disease and systemic disease. By stressing the importance of oral disease prevention, the dental hygienist promotes active self-care by the client as a cotherapist—for example, teaching self-care behaviors to maintain oral wellness, encouraging active participation in formulating goals for care, establishing frequent periodontal maintenance or preventive care appointments, and facilitating choices and client decision making.

Dental Hygiene Care

Patients with coronary heart disease are susceptible to angina pectoris and MI.

Angina Pectoris

The patient with angina pectoris should be treated in a stress-free environment to meet the human need for protection from health risks and freedom from stress. Considerations associated with angina pectoris include identification of the patient's condition and frequency of angina attacks. Health history interview questions to ascertain the stability of the patient's angina are as follows:
1. Do you have chest pain on exertion? At rest?
2. How frequent are your attacks?
3. Is your chest pain relieved promptly with nitroglycerin?
4. How long are your periods of discomfort?
    a. If patients report that their angina has worsened and the painful episodes occur more frequently and not only during exertion, their condition is classified as unstable angina. These patients should be referred to their physician of record, and dental hygiene care should be postponed.
    b. For patients with stable angina, appointments should be short and preferably scheduled for the morning. The atmosphere should be friendly and conducive to relaxation. If the patient becomes fatigued or develops significant changes in pulse rate or rhythm, termination of the appointment is suggested.
5. Before care for a patient with a history of angina pectoris is initiated, the patient's supply of nitroglycerin should be placed within reach of the dental hygienist. Potency of nitroglycerin is lost after 6 months outside of a sealed container; consequently, fresh supplies should be available in the oral care environment. If an emergency develops, dental hygiene treatment is stopped; the patient is placed in an upright position, reassured, and given nitroglycerin sublingually. Emergency medical services (EMS) should be activated if the patient continues to experience pain after administration of nitroglycerin (see Chapter 11). Vital signs must be monitored and recorded on the patient's record.

Myocardial Infarction

Patients who have a history of MI with no complications do not require care plan modifications. However, if the MI has occurred within the past 30 days, dental hygiene therapy should be postponed until the individual is 30 days or more postinfarction with no complications and no other risk factors or ischemic symptoms such as chest pain, shortness of breath, dizziness, or fatigue. The patient's medical status and dental hygiene treatment plan require medical consultation if symptoms, risk factors, or complications persist. It is imperative to assess a patient's functional capacity, which is the patient's capability to physically function to perform daily tasks. Patients should value the importance of physical function and wellness after an MI. Exercise training is the primary therapy to improve functional capacity. It is important for individuals with a history of MI to prioritize exercise so they can perform daily living activities (climbing stairs) to minimize vulnerability and disabilities.[9]

Drugs used to treat MI are anticoagulants, digitalis, and antihypertensive agents. These drugs necessitate care plan alterations. Anticoagulant drugs increase bleeding time and may have to be altered several days before care that involves invasive tissue manipulation. Some cardiologists believe that it is more dangerous to take the individual off the anticoagulant than it is to keep the individual on the drug and provide care; therefore, confirmation from the patient's cardiologist is recommended.

Digitalis, a glycoside, is a drug that increases the contractility of the heart. Improvement in force makes the heart more efficient as a pump, increasing its volume in relation to cardiac output. The most commonly prescribed digitalis drug is digoxin (e.g., Lanoxin).

Oral health professionals may detect early signs of digitalis toxicity in patients (i.e., anorexia, nausea, vomiting, neurologic abnormalities, and facial pain). If digitalis toxicity is not detected early, cardiac irregularities can develop (e.g., arrhythmias can progress to ventricular fibrillation and sudden death).

Antihypertensive agents used to control MIs are similar to those used to control hypertension. These agents do not influence the care plan unless the underlying condition is uncontrolled.

Patients with coronary heart disease may experience fear, depression, and disturbances in body image, associated with a change in lifestyle (e.g., dietary restrictions, exercise, and maintaining low stress). The patient's psychologic condition also may influence oral health.

Emergency situations associated with MI should be managed by an emergency medical team. Oral health professionals are responsible for monitoring vital signs, administering nitroglycerin, and performing AED and CPR if the patient experiences cardiac arrest. Certification in basic life support (BLS) should be maintained by all oral health professionals (see Chapter 11).

See Box 48.4 relating to angina pectoris and Box 48.5 for education tips for patients with cardiovascular disease and those on anticoagulant medication.

BOX 48.4 Critical Thinking Scenario B

Angina Pectoris

Patient S., age 45, states in their medical history that they are on anticoagulant therapy.

What further interview questions should the dental hygienist ask prior to treatment? After further questioning and discovering that patient S.'s previous INR levels were 3, how should the dental hygienist proceed with the dental hygiene appointment and any future appointments?

BOX 48.5 Patient or Client Education Tips

Anticoagulant Medication

Explain that reducing gingival inflammation and oral biofilm is important when taking anticoagulant medication. Explain that periodontal disease may increase one's risk for coronary heart disease.

Lifestyle Changes

Discuss how some forms of cardiovascular disease are preventable by lifestyle changes such as following a low-sodium, low-fat, low-cholesterol diet that is rich in fruits, vegetables, and whole grains; getting daily exercise; performing stress management; and not using tobacco.

Infective Endocarditis

Explain that prophylactic antibiotic premedication must be taken 1 hour before the scheduled appointment to achieve optimal blood levels and to reduce the possibility of infective endocarditis (IE) in persons with the highest categories of risk for IE (see Chapter 13). Explain that oral health maintenance reduces self-induced and professionally induced transient bacteremias (prevention of IE).

Appointment guidelines for an individual with coronary heart disease include the following:

- Ask questions when taking the health history related to functional capacity.
- Clarify the stability of the client's angina or symptoms after 30 days following MI. If uncontrolled, do not treat. If stable, continue treatment with caution.
- Schedule short morning appointments to help control environmental stress.
- Use adequate pain control modalities, including nitrous oxide–oxygen analgesia to reduce stress if no contraindications exist.
- Select interventions that address the patient's lifestyle changes and periodontal disease status.

Cardiac Dysrhythmias and Arrhythmias

Cardiac dysrhythmias and **arrhythmias**, terms used interchangeably, are dysfunctions of heart rate and rhythm that manifest as heart palpitations. Dysrhythmias may develop in normal and diseased hearts. In healthy hearts, arrhythmia may be associated with physical and emotional stresses (e.g., exercise, emotional shock) and usually subsides in direct response to stimulus reduction. Diseased hearts develop dysrhythmias directly associated with the CVD present, most commonly valvular heart disease, arteriosclerotic heart disease, or coronary artery disease. In some cases, a cardiac dysrhythmia may develop in response to drug toxicities and electrolyte imbalances.

Etiology

Dysfunction of heart rate and rhythm arises from disturbances in nerve impulses and is categorized according to the part of the heart in which it originates. Common dysrhythmias include bradycardia, tachycardia, atrial fibrillation, premature ventricular contractions (PVCs), ventricular fibrillation, and heart block.

Cardiac dysrhythmias are medically diagnosed using an electrocardiogram (ECG) and/or a Holter monitoring system. **Electrocardiography**, a graphic tracing of the heart's electrical activity, determines heart rate, rhythm, and size. Each dysrhythmia is associated with a specific graphic pattern indicating a definitive medical diagnosis.

Risk Factors

See Table 48.1.

Bradycardia

Bradycardia is defined as slowness of the heartbeat as evidenced by a decline in the pulse rate to less than 60 beats per minute (BPM). This normally occurs during sleep or in physically fit athletes; however, severe bradycardia can lead to fainting and convulsions. If a patient has an episode of bradycardia following a normal pulse rate of 80 BPM, emergency medical treatment is necessary. This individual may be encountering the initial symptoms of an acute MI. Emergency medical treatment would include discontinuing the dental hygiene appointment, administrating oxygen, and activating EMS.

Tachycardia

Increased heartbeat, termed **tachycardia**, is associated with an abnormally high heart rate, usually greater than 100 BPM. Tachycardia can increase risk of developing angina pectoris, acute heart failure, pulmonary edema, and MI if not controlled. These conditions are related directly to the amount of work the heart is doing and decreased cardiac output. Treatment consists of antiarrhythmic drug therapy to control tachycardia and reduce potential for recurrence.

Atrial Fibrillation

Atrial fibrillation, a condition of rapid, uneven contractions in the upper chambers of the heart (atrium), is the result of inconsistent impulses through the atrioventricular (AV) node transmitted to the ventricles at irregular intervals. The lower chambers (ventricles) cannot contract in response to the impulses and the contractions become irregular, with a decreased amount of blood pumped through the body. During assessment, the pulse rate may appear consistent with periods of irregular beats. Atrial fibrillation may contribute to the formation of a thrombosis, leading to a stroke or TIAs (transient ischemic attacks).[9]

Medical treatment targets the causative factors, not the condition itself. CHF, mitral valve stenosis, and hyperthyroidism may be linked to atrial fibrillation.

Premature Ventricular Contractions

PVCs are identified easily as pauses in an otherwise normal heart rhythm. The pause develops from an abnormal focus of the ventricle, allowing the ventricle to be at a refractory (resting) period when the impulse for contraction arrives. The feeling of the heart skipping a beat is PVC; these increase with age and are associated with fatigue, emotional stress, and excessive use of coffee, alcohol, or tobacco.

Recognition of PVCs has significance in the patient with CVD. If five or more PVCs are detected during a 60-second pulse examination, medical consultation is recommended strongly. Individuals who are distressed and have five or more detectable PVCs per minute may be undergoing an acute MI or ventricular fibrillation. As with other medical emergencies related to heart disease, emergency medical treatment would include discontinuing the dental hygiene appointment, administrating oxygen, and activating EMS.

Ventricular Fibrillation

Ventricular fibrillation, one of the most lethal dysrhythmias, is characterized as an advanced stage of ventricular tachycardia with rapid impulse formation and irregular impulse transmission. The heart rate is rapid and disordered and has no rhythm. Immediate medical treatment for ventricular fibrillation is urgent, requiring the use of an AED (precordial shock) to halt the dysrhythmia, followed by CPR. Electric current at the time of shock depolarizes the entire myocardium, allowing the cardiac impulses to gain control of the heart rate and rhythm. This depolarization should reestablish cardiac regulation. The person then is placed on drug therapy to maintain regulation of cardiac rate and rhythm. Without immediate medical attention (advanced cardiac life support), blood pressure falls to zero, resulting in unconsciousness; death may occur within 4 minutes.

Heart Block

Heart block is a dysrhythmia caused by the blocking of impulses from the atria to the ventricles at the AV node; it is an interference with the electrical impulses controlling the heart muscle. Each of the three forms of heart block is dangerous; however, third-degree heart block presents the greatest danger of cardiac arrest. The three forms are as follows:

- First-degree heart block—usually associated with coronary artery disease or digitalis drug therapy. The individual usually is asymptomatic with a normal heart rate and rhythm.
- Second-degree heart block—atrial and ventricular rates are disordered; impulses from the AV node are fully blocked in irregular patterns.
- Third-degree heart block—blocking of all impulses from the atria at the AV node, resulting in atrial and ventricular dissociation. The ventricles begin beating in response to their biologic pacemaker cells, producing an independent heartbeat from the atrium.

Medical Treatment

There are various methods of treatment to regulate a patient's heartbeat, depending on their specific case and condition.

The **cardiac pacemaker**, an intracardiac device, is an electronic stimulator used to send electrical currents to the myocardium to control or maintain heart rate. Two types of pacemakers that control one or both of the heart chambers include temporary pacemakers used in emergency situations and permanent pacemakers inserted transvenously into the body. Some pacemakers have fixed-rate pacing, while others operate only when needed to stimulate ventricular contraction.

Pacemakers vary in their sensitivity to electrical interference that may alter or stop their function. Newer models, bipolar and shielded to protect against interference, do not require any special consideration during dental hygiene care. When in doubt, consult the patient's cardiologist.

Cardioversion is another form of medical treatment used to reinstate a regular heart rhythm. There are two types of cardioversion:

1. Pharmacologic (chemical) cardioversion—when the physician provides the patient with medication to reinstate a regular heartbeat.[12] The specific type of medication varies based on the patient's type of abnormal heart rhythm as well as consideration of any other underlying medical problems.
2. Electrical cardioversion—sending an electrical shock to the heart.[12]

Patients who have nonemergency or elective cardioversion treatment typically schedule an appointment to have their treatment performed in a clinic or hospital. If the patient has atrial fibrillation, they may be placed on anticoagulant medication two to three weeks prior to their cardioversion appointment to prevent blood clots.[12] It is imperative to know that defibrillation is used in emergency situations for individuals who suffer sudden life-threatening arrhythmias (see Chapter 11).

An **implantable cardioverter defibrillator (ICD)** is useful in preventing sudden death in patients with known sustained ventricular tachycardia or fibrillation. An ICD is a battery-powered device placed under the skin that keeps track of the heart rate. Thin wires connect the ICD to the heart. If an abnormal heart rhythm is detected, the device will deliver an electric shock to restore a normal heartbeat if the heart is beating chaotically and too fast. Newer-generation ICDs may have a dual function that includes the ability to serve as a pacemaker.[10] The pacemaker feature would stimulate the heart to beat if the heart rate is detected to be too slow. Modern ICDs have built-in features to protect them from most types of interference produced by other electrical devices encountered in daily routines; however, individuals with ICDs must still be aware of their surroundings and the devices that may interfere.[10] Dental ultrasonic scalers pose little to no risk to ICDs; however, it is important that the dental hygiene provider be made aware of any implanted device.[13]

Dental Hygiene Care

During assessment, the dental hygienist determines the type of pacemaker a patient has and whether it is shielded from electrical interference. Dental devices that apply an electrical current directly to the patient (e.g., ultrasonic scaling systems, equipment for iontophoresis in desensitization, pulp testers, power toothbrushes, and electrosurgery equipment) are likely to cause interference in unshielded pacemakers. Use of such equipment, even in the proximity of the patient with an unshielded pacemaker, is contraindicated. Instead, nonelectrical alternatives to avoid functional interference are used (e.g., hand-activated instruments, tooth desensitization with a nonelectronic technique, and pulp testing performed by tooth percussion). Additional pacemaker protection can be accomplished for older, unshielded pacemakers by placing a lead apron on the patient as a barrier to interrupt electrical interference generated by dental equipment such as the air-abrasive system, low- or high-speed handpiece, and computerized periodontal probe. Care should be taken in an open clinical setting where electrical dental equipment may be used for an adjacent patient.

The latest cardiac devices have improved shielding and may be less prone to interference, allowing for the use of some dental devises. When considering dental device use on these patients, piezoelectric dental instruments may be safer than magnetostrictive types. In addition to manufacturer recommendations, the dental hygienist should consult with the patient's cardiologist to determine if certain dental devices are safe to use.

Prophylactic antibiotics before dental hygiene care are not recommended after pacemaker implantation to prevent IE.

Care plan development for the individual with a cardiac pacemaker also can be affected by the drugs used to treat the underlying medical condition—anticoagulants and antihypertensive agents. Monitoring and assessment of drug therapy provide information necessary to modify treatment.

If the cardiac pacemaker fails or malfunctions during the dental hygiene appointment, the patient may experience difficulty breathing; dizziness; a change in the pulse rate; swelling of the legs, ankles, arms, and wrists; and/or chest pain. When this situation arises, do the following:

1. Turn off all sources of electrical interference.
2. Activate EMS.
3. Prepare to administer basic life support (BLS) (see Chapter 11).

For patients undergoing a cardioversion procedure, special consideration by the dental hygienist is needed to check if the patient was placed on any new medications such as anticoagulants. Consultation with the patient's cardiologist is recommended to ensure that dental hygiene treatment is not contraindicated.

See Box 48.6 for a Critical Thinking Scenario related to arrhythmia. Appointment guidelines include the following:

- Although uncommon, older, unshielded pacemakers can be affected by electrical interference in the oral healthcare setting.
- Use a lead apron to interrupt electrical interference generated by dental equipment.
- Use manual rather than mechanized procedures to avoid electrical interference created by dental equipment.
- Monitor patient and be prepared to administer BLS (see Chapter 11).

Peripheral Arterial Disease

Congestive heart failure (disease of the heart muscle) is a syndrome characterized by myocardial dysfunction that leads to diminished cardiac output or abnormal circulatory congestion. The weakened heart develops compensatory mechanisms to continue to function (i.e., tachycardia, ventricular dilation, and enlargement of the heart muscle).

CHF can occur as two independent failures (left-sided and right-sided heart failure); however, because the heart functions as a closed unit, both pumps must be functioning properly or the heart's efficiency is diminished.

Etiology

Causative factors associated with CHF are arteriosclerotic heart disease, hypertensive CVD, valvular heart disease, pericarditis, circulatory overload, and coronary heart disease. These factors contribute to the gradual failure of the heart by reducing the inflow of blood to the heart, increasing the inflow to the lungs, obstructing the outflow of blood from the heart, or damaging the heart muscle itself.

Risk Factors
See Table 48.1.

Disease Process

Patients who have left-sided heart failure have difficulty receiving oxygenated blood from the lungs, resulting in increased fluid and blood in the lungs, causing dyspnea on exertion, shortness of breath on lying supine, cough, and expectoration. These patients tend to require extra pillows to sleep and cannot be placed in a supine position.

Right-sided heart failure is associated with the blood return from the body, resulting in systemic venous congestion and peripheral edema. Patients with right-sided heart failure have foot and ankle edema and often complain of cold hands and feet.

Medical Treatment

CHF treatment is related directly to the removal of the cause. Usually, the corrective therapy associated with the underlying disease eliminates the presence of CHF. Some patients require additional methods of rehabilitation, such as dietary control, reduced physical activity, and drug therapy (e.g., diuretics to reduce salt and water retention and digitalis to strengthen myocardial contractility, or new drug combinations to reduce strain on the heart).

Dental Hygiene Care

Individuals with CHF who are monitored closely by a physician do not require a change in conventional dental hygiene care; however, factors associated with the cause of CHF should be considered in the care plan. Alterations are based on the causative factors (e.g., hypertension, valvular heart disease, coronary heart disease, and MI) in association with the individual's current medical status.

Patients taking digitalis are prone to nausea and vomiting during dental procedures. Therefore, procedures that may promote gagging should be performed with extra care. In addition, the dental hygienist should be aware of any underlying heart conditions that are responsible for CHF. These conditions must be evaluated and appropriate precautions taken.

Alterations in the care plan for a patient with left-sided CHF are related to stress reduction. Patient positioning must be upright to support breathing. Actions should be taken to minimize distress, and instructions should reinforce the need for a reduced-sodium diet to alleviate fluid retention.

If an emergency arises, medical assistance should be obtained. The patient is usually conscious with difficulty breathing. The following treatment is recommended:

1. Position the person upright to facilitate breathing.
2. Administer oxygen if necessary.
3. Monitor vital signs.

See Box 48.7 for a Critical Thinking Scenario related to heart failure. Appointment guidelines include the following:

- Position patient upright to decrease collection of fluid in the lungs.
- Limit ultrasonic instrumentation use or use high-speed suction to avoid unnecessary fluid accumulation in the throat. This fluid reduction minimizes patient anxiety and facilitates breathing.
- Recommend nutritional counseling to decrease sodium intake and alleviate fluid retention.

CONGENITAL HEART DISEASE

Congenital heart disease is an abnormality of the heart's structure and function caused by abnormal or disordered heart development before birth. Commonly observed congenital heart malformations are ventricular septal defect, atrial septal defect, and patent ductus arteriosus.

Etiology

The cause of congenital heart disease is generally unknown; however, genetic and environmental factors may impair intrauterine development. Genetic conditions, related to heredity, are apparent in some situations. Environmental factors are based on the mother's health—for example, rubella (German measles) and drug addiction have produced delayed fetal development and growth retardation associated with the cardiovascular structure.

Disease Process and Medical Treatment

Congenital heart disease is the result of various heart defects that dictate the disease process.

Ventricular Septal Defect

A ventricular septal defect—a shunt (opening) in the septum between the ventricles—allows oxygenated blood from the left ventricle to flow into the right ventricle (Fig. 48.3). Small defects that close spontaneously or are correctable by surgery have a good prognosis. Larger defects that are left untreated or are irreparable usually result in death from secondary cardiovascular complications. The ventricular septal defect can be detected by a characteristic heart murmur audible at birth, followed by medical tests to confirm a diagnosis.

Clinical manifestations vary with the size of the defect, infant age, and the effect of the deviated blood passage on the cardiovascular structure. Large ventricular septal defects cause hypertrophy of the ventricles, resulting in CHF.

Atrial Septal Defect

The atrial septal defect—a shunt (opening) between the left and right atria—is responsible for approximately 10% of congenital heart defects. The blood volume overload eventually causes the right atrium to enlarge and the right ventricle to dilate (Fig. 48.4).

Usually the patient is asymptomatic and the defect goes undetected; however, in adults, clinical symptoms can become more pronounced. The patient is fatigued easily and short of breath after mild exertion. Treatment includes cardiovascular repair surgery, observance of developing atrial arrhythmias, and monitoring of vital signs.

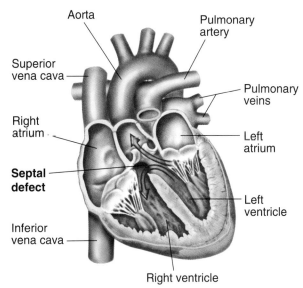

Fig. 48.3 Ventricular septal defect. (From Bleck E, Nagel D. *Physically Handicapped Children: A Medical Atlas for Teachers.* 2nd ed. Allyn & Bacon; 1982.)

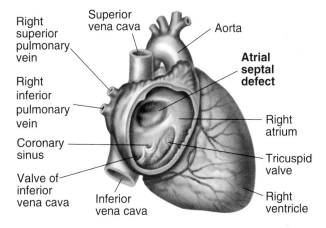

Fig. 48.4 Atrial septal defect. (From Bleck E, Nagel D. *Physically Handicapped Children: A Medical Atlas for Teachers.* 2nd ed. Allyn & Bacon; 1982.)

Patent Ductus Arteriosus

Patent ductus arteriosus is the most common congenital heart defect found in adults. During development, the fetal heart contains a blood vessel called the *ductus arteriosus.* This vessel connects the pulmonary artery to the descending aorta. Normally, after birth, the vessel closes. If the vessel fails to close, a congenital heart defect forms. Failure to close is more common in premature births; however, it also occurs in full-term births. Treatment includes drug therapy, catheter-based procedures, and surgery to close the defect. Untreated shunting of blood in a patent ductus arteriosus defect is from the aorta to the pulmonary artery (Fig. 48.5). This type of blood flow results in the recirculation of oxygenated blood through the lungs, creating increased workload on the left side of the heart, which can result in CHF. If the condition is left untreated, severe obstructive pulmonary vascular disease may develop.

Clinical manifestations include respiratory distress, susceptibility to respiratory tract infections, and slow motor development. Treatment consists of surgical correction and elimination of symptoms associated with secondary complications.

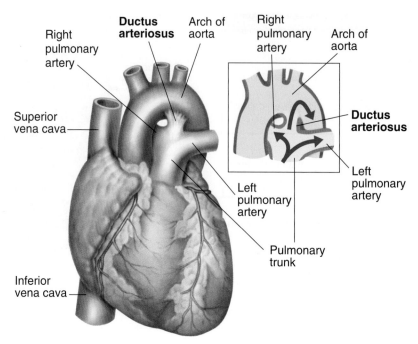

Fig. 48.5 Patent ductus arteriosus defect. (From Bleck E, Nagel D. *Handicapped Children: A Medical Atlas for Teachers.* 2nd ed. Allyn & Bacon; 1982.)

Tetralogy of Fallot

Tetralogy of Fallot is a rare and complex congenital heart defect generally associated with cyanosis. The defect is composed of four congenital abnormalities: ventricular septal defect, pulmonary stenosis, right ventricular hypertrophy, and malposition of the aorta. The blood shunts right to left through the ventricular septal defect, permitting unoxygenated blood to mix with oxygenated blood, resulting in cyanosis. Treatment includes measures to relieve cyanosis, and palliative and corrective surgery.

Dental Hygiene Care

The individual with congenital heart disease does not require extensive alterations in care. However, the American Heart Association recommends prophylactic antibiotics before dental hygiene procedures to prevent IE in persons with residual defects following repair, with unrepaired cyanotic congenital heart defects including palliative shunts, and during the first 6 months after surgery to correct congenital defects. Secondary concerns focus on the management of cardiovascular complications, such as CHF and cardiac dysrhythmias, should they result from the congenital defect.

Dental hygiene care includes physician consultation to confirm drugs prescribed and current medical status, prophylactic antibiotic medication to prevent IE, and assessment of symptoms secondary to the disease that may require treatment alteration. If the individual develops CHF, then care plan considerations should follow those outlined.

See Box 48.8, a Critical Thinking Scenario related to congenital heart defects.

VALVULAR HEART DEFECTS

Valvular heart defects (VHDs) result in cardiovascular damage from malfunctioning heart valves such as the mitral valve, the aortic valve, or the tricuspid valve (see Fig. 48.1). **Mitral valve prolapse** (MVP) is one of the most frequently occurring VHDs. When the left ventricle pumps

---

> **BOX 48.8 Critical Thinking Scenario E**
>
> **Congenital Heart Defects**
> Patient L. conveys that they have a history of recurrent infective endocarditis and shared that they may need cardiac valve replacement surgery.
> 1. Based on what the patient stated, the dental hygienist should consult with patient's physician to confirm what other information?
> 2. What does the American Heart Association recommend in regard to treating patients with infective endocarditis?

blood to the aorta, the mitral valve flops backward (prolapses) into the left atrium, resulting in MVP. Other names for MVP are "floppy mitral valve syndrome" and the "click murmur syndrome," referring to the sound the valve makes when it flops backward (Fig. 48.6). Most patients with heart murmurs related to MVP require no alteration in dental hygiene care, although a thorough patient history can identify VHDs that require modifications—for example, when valves have been replaced.

Etiology

VHDs commonly are associated with rheumatic fever but also may be caused by congenital abnormalities or may develop after IE.

Disease Process

Valvular malfunction can occur by **stenosis**, an incomplete opening of the valve, or regurgitation, a backflow of blood through the valve because of incomplete closure. When malfunction occurs, the left ventricle hypertrophies to compensate for the increased amount of blood. This, in turn, can cause the left atrium to hypertrophy, leading to pulmonary congestion and right ventricular failure. If the condition is left untreated, the person ultimately develops congestive heart failure (CHF).

Echocardiography uses ultrasonic waves to detect heart size, valvular function, and other structural deformities. The echocardiogram

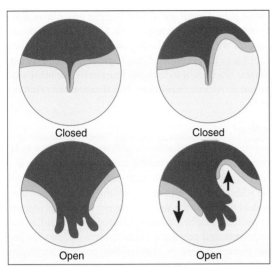

Fig. 48.6 Diagram of a normal (*left*) and a prolapsed (*right*) mitral valve. (Courtesy of Mid-Island Hospital, Bethpage, New York.)

BOX 48.9 Critical Thinking Scenario F

Valvular Heart Defect
Patient A. states that they have atrial fibrillation and reports that they are taking Eliquis.
1. The dental hygienist proceeds to consult Patient A.'s physician. What specific questions should the dental hygienist ask regarding the client's current health and medication status?
2. What dental hygiene care plan modifications should be made?

is the record produced by the evaluation and used by the physician to diagnosis VHD.

Medical Treatment

Some patients with VHD take anticoagulant medications, depending on the underlying cardiac condition that caused the defect. Corrective surgery is performed for most VHDs. If the valve cannot be repaired, prosthetic valves are available to replace defective valves, in most cases. For individuals with MVP, surgical treatment is not usually necessary unless it is aimed at alleviating symptoms such as palpitations, chest pain, nervousness, shortness of breath, and dizziness. Medications are given to control chest pain, slow the heart rate, reduce palpitations, and/or lower anxiety.

Dental Hygiene Care

To protect the patient from health risks, frequent continued care appointments and meticulous daily oral biofilm control are necessary. Good oral health maintenance reduces the possibility of developing a self-induced bacteremia from toothbrushing or interdental cleaning. In cases in which defective valves are replaced with prosthetic valves, prophylactic antibiotic is required before dental hygiene care (see Chapter 13). See Box 48.9 for a Critical Thinking Scenario based on valvular heart defects.

Appointment guidelines for patients who take anticoagulant medications include the following:
- VHDs require care plan modifications only if the patient has an underlying cardiovascular condition or is on anticoagulant drug therapy. The frequently prescribed anticoagulants—heparin, warfarin (Coumadin), and indanedione derivatives—affect the dental hygiene care plan if periodontal debridement procedures are indicated or if the gingiva bleeds spontaneously.

- Consultation with the patient's physician is recommended to validate the patient's current health and medication status. When the patient is taking anticoagulant medication, the dental hygienist or dentist consults with the patient's physician to determine if a dose reduction should be made or if it is safer to maintain the prescribed dosage and use treatment precautions to minimize hemorrhage. In many cases, no adjustment is needed or recommended because it takes a long time to regain good control of the condition requiring these medications.
- If indicated, reduction in medication dosage should increase the prothrombin time by 2 seconds.
- Normal prothrombin time varies between 11 and 14 seconds.
- Optimal prothrombin time for dental hygiene therapy in persons taking anticoagulants should be less than 20 seconds on the day of the scheduled procedure.[14] For laboratory consistency, the international normalized ratio (INR) is used to document bleeding time. When the INR value is used, the normal range is less than 1.5, and routine care can be performed when the INR is 2 to 3.[14]

Treatment of a patient on anticoagulant medication includes the following steps:
- Consult the patient's physician to verify prothrombin time or INR.
- Debride one area at a time to manage bleeding.
- Begin in the least inflamed area so bleeding will be minimal.
- Periodically check for clotting; discontinue therapy if there is a long delay in clotting.
- Emphasize importance of daily oral biofilm control for reduction of disease and associated bleeding during professional treatment.

RHEUMATIC HEART DISEASE

Rheumatic heart disease (RHD) is the cardiac manifestation of rheumatic fever. Persons with a history of rheumatic fever often have valvular heart damage that is affected detrimentally by bacteremia (microorganisms in the bloodstream), often occurring during dental hygiene care. Persons with a history of RHD are not at high risk for IE, and prophylactic antibiotic premedication before dental hygiene care is not required.

Etiology

Rheumatic fever is an acute or chronic systemic inflammatory process characterized by attacks of fever, polyarthritis, and carditis. The last eventually may result in permanent valvular heart damage.

Risk Factors

Persons who have had a beta-hemolytic streptococcal pharyngeal infection (strep throat) may develop rheumatic fever within 2 to 3 weeks after initial infection. People with a history of rheumatic fever are predisposed to RHD because of the involvement of the heart muscles, resulting in cardiac valve damage.

Disease Process

The most destructive effect of rheumatic fever is carditis, an inflammation of the cardiac muscle that is found in most individuals exhibiting signs and symptoms of rheumatic fever. Carditis may affect the endocardium, myocardium, pericardium, or heart valves. Valvular damage is responsible for the familiar organic (nonfunctional) heart murmur associated with rheumatic fever and RHD. The **heart murmur** is an irregularity of the auditory heartbeat caused by a turbulent flow of blood through a valve that has failed to close. Valves most commonly affected are the mitral valve and the aortic valve. Damaged valves are susceptible to infection that may lead to IE. Many heart murmurs are innocent, also called functional. This type is not associated with

RHD; therefore, innocent murmurs do not require alterations in dental hygiene care.

Prevention

RHD prevention requires early diagnosis and treatment of streptococcal pharyngeal infections that may lead to rheumatic fever. Patients need to be informed of the importance of early medical diagnosis and treatment for prevention of this disease.

Dental Hygiene Care

According to the American Heart Association's Guidelines for the Prevention of Infective Endocarditis, prophylactic antibiotics prior to dental care are not required for clients with RHD.[15] To protect patients from health risks, the care plan must include meticulous oral biofilm control. Good oral health maintenance by the client reduces the possibility of developing a self-inflicted bacteremia during toothbrushing or interdental cleaning.

Appointment guidelines include the following:
- Frequent continued-care intervals to maintain good oral health
- Patient-centered homecare instruction to maintain optimal oral health practice
- Preprocedural antimicrobial rinse before tissue manipulation to reduce severity of bacteremia

Infective Endocarditis

Infective or bacterial endocarditis is an infection of the endocardium, heart valves, or cardiac prosthesis resulting from microbial invasion.

Etiology

IE, caused by the formation of a bacteremia (microorganisms in the bloodstream), is characterized in most cases by vegetative growths of *Staphylococcus aureus, Staphylococcus epidermidis, Streptococcus viridans,* and, the most prevalent, alpha-hemolytic streptococci on heart valves or endocardial lining. Although staphylococci and streptococci are found in the majority of cases, yeast, fungi, and viruses also have been identified—hence the term *infective* rather than *bacterial.* If untreated, endocarditis is usually fatal; with proper antibiotic treatment, recovery is possible.

Risk Factors

During **invasive dental or dental hygiene therapy** (defined as procedures that involve manipulation of oral soft tissues, manipulation of the periapical area of teeth, or oral mucosa perforation), a transient bacteremia is produced. Tissue trauma from instrumentation coupled with periodontal disease status determines the severity of the bacteremia. In addition, a patient may create a self-induced bacteremia during mastication and daily oral hygiene care. Those at risk for IE include patients with a previous history of endocarditis, prosthetic heart valves, or serious congenital heart conditions, and heart transplant patients who develop a problem with a heart valve.[15]

Disease Process

There are two types of IE considered when classifying IE, given as follows:
- Acute bacterial endocarditis (ABE) is a severe infection with a rapid course of action usually caused by pathogenic microorganisms, such as *S. aureus* and *S. epidermidis,* capable of producing widespread disease.
- Subacute bacterial endocarditis (SBE) is a slow-moving infection with nonspecific clinical features. Affected persons usually exhibit a continuous low-grade fever, marked weakness, fatigue, weight loss,

and joint pain. Dental and dental hygiene procedures that manipulate soft tissue may be responsible for the development of SBE in patients with previous heart conditions that make them more susceptible to it. As endocarditis progresses, the circulating microorganisms attach to the damaged heart valves or other susceptible areas and proliferate in colonies. This invasion can result in cardiac failure.

Prevention

Patients with conditions that increase their susceptibility to IE—such as previous IE; unrepaired cyanotic congenital heart disease (CHD); completely repaired congenital heart defect with prosthetic material or device within the first 6 months after the procedure; repaired CHD with residual defects at the site, or adjacent to the site, of a prosthetic patch or prosthetic device; cardiac valvulopathy in cardiac transplantation recipients; and prosthetic cardiac valves—all require preventive antibiotic therapy before procedures that produce bacteremias (see Chapter 11).[15]

Dental Hygiene Care

The following steps help prevent IE in patients with these conditions:
- Identify high-risk individuals via the health history and patient questioning.
- Ensure that the patient with underlying cardiac conditions associated with the highest risk of adverse outcome from infective endocarditis according to the American Heart Association took the prescribed antibiotic prophylaxis medication 1 hour before procedures that produce bacteremias so that optimal blood levels are established.
- Have the patient use a preprocedural antimicrobial rinse before tissue manipulation.
- Prevent unnecessary trauma during intraoral procedures to reduce severity of bacteremia.
- Help each client as a cotherapist maintain optimal oral health and daily oral biofilm control to minimize self-induced bacteremias.
- Encourage patients to schedule continued-care visits as needed.
  See Box 48.3 related to a patient with infective endocarditis and Box 48.5 for client education and motivation tips.

Appointment guidelines include the following:
- When a patient is taking the prescribed prophylactic antibiotic regimen, appointment scheduling is affected. It is not in the patient's best interest to prolong treatment procedures. If periodontal debridement or scaling and root planing (SRP) is indicated, appointments should be scheduled in longer periods and as close together as possible. The interval between antibiotic coverage should be 9 to 14 days. If a patient has periodontitis, a care plan may divide invasive procedures (periodontal debridement or SRP) into an organized sequence that allows for 9- to 14-day periods between prophylactic antibiotic premedication. Considering the Dental Hygiene Human Needs Theory, the human need for protection from health risks is met by dividing the invasive treatment appointments into two separate intervals with a lag time between the appointments (see Box 48.4).
- See Box 48.3 for a discussion of legal, ethical, and safety issues.

CARDIOVASCULAR SURGERY (INTERVENTIONS)

Open-heart surgery is necessary for complex procedures that require direct visualization of the heart (e.g., heart transplants, some heart valve replacements, and coronary bypass surgery). Open-heart surgery always is performed with the use of a heart-lung machine that completely controls cardiopulmonary function, enabling surgeons to operate for long periods without interfering with the individual's metabolic needs. Closed-heart surgery usually is associated with cardiac catheterization.

Types of Cardiovascular Surgery
Angioplasty

The most common type of closed-heart surgery, **angioplasty** (also known as *percutaneous coronary intervention* [PCI]), involves the use of a catheter (a long, slender tube) with a tiny balloon at the end that is inserted into the coronary artery. Specifically, the balloon is inserted into places where the artery narrows, is inflated to flatten fatty deposits, and is deflated to allow the increased blood flow to compress and redistribute the atherosclerotic lesion. This procedure is used in individuals who have a small atherosclerotic lesion constricting blood flow. If the lesion cannot be corrected by the angioplasty procedure, bypass surgery may be necessary.

Coronary Stent

The coronary stent is a device made of meshlike metal used to open narrow arteries. Placed in conjunction with PCI procedures, the stent maintains the lumen opening in the arteries, allowing blood to flow freely, thereby reducing angina and potential myocardial infarctions.

Coronary Bypass Surgery

Coronary bypass surgery, a common procedure to replace blocked arteries, is performed by removing part of a leg vein or chest artery and then grafting it onto the coronary artery, thereby creating a new passageway for the blood. This type of surgery can be done for more than one artery at a time and is named accordingly (double bypass, triple bypass). The benefits of coronary bypass surgery include relief from angina, increased tolerance to exercise, improved quality of life, and extended life span. A person who has had bypass surgery has no contraindications to dental hygiene therapy.

Valvular Defect Repair

Valvular defect repair or replacement is performed frequently. Persons with artificial cardiac valves are at high risk for infections and IE and must be prescribed prophylactic antibiotics before dental hygiene care (see Box 48.9 and Chapter 11).

Heart Transplantation

Heart transplantation is a viable option for individuals with end-stage heart disease for which no other therapeutic intervention is considered effective. Although many hospitals perform cardiac transplantation, the dilemma is finding donors. Future goals and implications of heart transplantation include the development of a safe, reliable, permanent, totally implantable artificial heart device that allows a recipient to carry out normal activities. The development of such a device may increase availability of this lifesaving procedure for eligible recipients who at this time await donors.

Dental Hygiene Considerations When Treating a Patient Who Has Had Heart Surgery
Patient Who Has Had Closed-Heart Surgery

No contraindications are associated with dental or dental hygiene treatment unless the individual is taking anticoagulant medication. As in all cardiac-associated situations, consultation with the patient's cardiologist is recommended.

Patient After Open-Heart Surgery

No dental hygiene procedures relate uniquely to the individual who has had cardiovascular surgery. When in doubt, the cardiologist is consulted; however, prosthetic valvular heart replacements and those cardiac surgeries that make the patient susceptible to infection require prophylactic antibiotic premedication.

Complications from dental hygiene care observed in patients who have had cardiovascular surgery are associated with the drug therapy used rather than the surgery itself. Most postsurgical patients are placed on medication to increase healing, suppress immune response, reduce infection, and/or decrease clot formation. Careful evaluation of drug contraindications and reactions is necessary.

Patient Who Has Had a Heart Transplant

A major concern of the heart transplant patient is infection and transplant rejection. Before care, consultation with the patient's cardiologist is highly recommended to determine if additional premedication is indicated. Most transplant patients are on long-term preventive antibiotic therapy to control systemic bacteremias. They also are placed on immunosuppressant medications such as cyclosporine (Sandimmune) to reduce the possibility of rejection.

DENTAL HYGIENE CONSIDERATION OF ORAL MANIFESTATIONS OF CARDIOVASCULAR MEDICATIONS

Some medications used in CVD therapy have a profound effect on the oral cavity (see Chapter 15 and Table 48.2). These medications typically include those that treat hypertension or CHD or are used for stabilization after heart transplant. Persons taking cardiovascular medications should seek regular dental hygiene care and maintain excellent oral biofilm control to balance their increased vulnerability to dental and periodontal diseases.

Most medications for the treatment of hypertension cause xerostomia, increasing the individual's risk for dental caries and periodontal disease. Individuals with exposed root surfaces are at risk for root surface caries and dentinal hypersensitivity. Self-administered fluoride therapy, reduced frequency of sugar intake in diet, use of saliva substitutes or salivary stimulants, and buffering mouth rinses should be part of the individual's daily self-care regimen, depending on degree of dry mouth. Some calcium channel blockers alter taste perception, cause drug-influenced gingival enlargement, and create salivary gland pain. Immunosuppressants used for the stabilization of heart transplants increase the individual's risk for developing periodontal disease or may exaggerate a preexisting condition, leading to an unmet need in skin and mucous membrane integrity.

Another dental hygiene diagnosis to consider is a need for protection from health risks and impact on quality of life because immunosuppressants increase risk for developing opportunistic infections such as candidiasis, herpes simplex, herpes zoster, necrotizing ulcerative gingivitis, and drug-influenced gingival enlargement. Refer to Chapters 22 and 23 for the development of dental hygiene diagnosis and care plans. In addition to regular professional dental hygiene care, these individuals should use an antimicrobial mouth rinse for 30 seconds twice daily as part of their self-care regimen to reduce oral disease risk.

Persons with a history of heart attack or cerebrovascular accident are placed on blood thinners (anticoagulants) to increase blood flow. The side effects are prolonged bleeding and spontaneous oral bleeding in the presence of infection. These individuals must maintain a healthy periodontium to reduce periodontal disease risk.

See Box 48.10 for a Critical Thinking Scenario related to medication.

PREVENTING AND MANAGING CARDIAC EMERGENCIES

The individual with a CVD or cardiovascular symptom or defect is considered high risk—one whose life may be threatened by daily activities. These patients have a need for protection from health risks because of their increased potential for an emergency. The most common physical pain encountered is chest pain accompanied by difficulty breathing. If the patient complains of physical pain that cannot be alleviated, EMS should be activated or 9-1-1 called.

For individuals with angina pectoris, hypertension, previous MI, or CHF, the risk for life-threatening medical emergencies rises as a result

of an increase in fear and stress. It is important to assess past responses in oral healthcare situations and to monitor the patient's reactions to dental hygiene procedures. Muscular tension, perspiration, and verbal cues indicate a potential emergency, and the patient's need for protection from health risks must be met.

Individuals with CVD may not take responsibility for their oral health. Understandably, these individuals fail to relate their life-threatening medical condition to oral disease; however, by increasing a patient's awareness that periodontal disease and the systemic condition are linked, the dental hygienist may change the patient's value system and oral health behavior and improve systemic health. Accurate assessment of the patient's personal beliefs, behaviors, and values can identify motivators (needs) that may lead to the patient's commitment to therapeutic goals and priorities. Table 48.3 illustrates sample dental hygiene diagnoses for a patient with coronary heart disease.

Planning prevents emergencies and ensures that patient needs are the focus of therapeutic interventions. When a care plan is developed, attention is given to drug therapies to ensure that no contraindications are present and that side effects are identified (see Table 48.2). Tables 48.4 and 48.5 can be used when developing care plans for patients with a CVD.

BOX 48.10   Critical Thinking Scenario G

Medication

A patient is on medication for the treatment of hypertension and complains of having a dry mouth and hypersensitivity.

1. Explain to the patient the effects of xerostomia in the oral cavity.
2. What homecare recommendations should be given to meet this client's specific needs?

TABLE 48.3   Sample Dental Hygiene Diagnoses—Patient With Coronary Heart Disease

Dental Hygiene Diagnosis	Related to	As Evidenced by
Protection from health risks: potential for myocardial infarction	Stress Anxiety Recent life-threatening medical diagnosis	Chest, jaw, neck, throat, interscapular area, and left arm pain Agitation
Responsibility for oral health	Low value ascribed to oral health	Lack of interest in performing daily oral self-care
Potential for health risks: potential for infection	History of infective endocarditis	Condition indicated on health history questionnaire
Biologically sound and functional dentition	Drug therapy (diuretics) taken by patient	Xerostomia Root caries
Biologically sound and functional dentition (nutrition)	Dietary restrictions of cholesterol, saturated fat, and sodium	Obesity, high LDL cholesterol or lipid blood values

LDL, Low-density lipid.

TABLE 48.4   Quick Reference—Signs, Symptoms, and Treatment of Individuals With Cardiovascular Disease

Disease	Signs and Symptoms	Medical and Surgical Treatment
Rheumatic heart disease	Carditis, polyarthritis, chorea, erythema marginatum, subcutaneous nodules, fever	Bed rest and medications associated with manifestations
Infective endocarditis	Initial high fever, cardiac decompensation, heart murmur	Antibiotic therapy
Valvular heart defects	Fatigue, shortness of breath, and pulmonary edema If defects are left untreated, congestive heart failure will develop	Valvular repair or replacement with prosthetic heart valve
Mitral valve prolapse	Palpitations, chest pain, nervousness, shortness of breath, dizziness	Treatment is not always necessary; aimed at alleviating symptoms
Cardiac dysrhythmias and arrhythmias	Bradycardia: pulse rate <60 beats per minute (BPM) Tachycardia: pulse rate >150 BPM	Antiarrhythmic drug therapy or cardiac pacemaker
Hypertension	Headache, fatigue, diminished exercise tolerance, shortness of breath	Antihypertension drug therapy; dietary control of sodium
Coronary (ischemic) heart disease	Angina pectoris, discomfort in jaw, neck, throat, interscapular area, and left arm	Bed rest; administration of nitroglycerin
Congestive heart failure	Fatigue, weakness, dyspnea, cough, anorexia	Treatment directed at the underlying cause
Congenital heart disease	Dependent on type of defect	Surgery to correct defect

TABLE 48.5 Quick Reference—Dental Hygiene Care Implications for Individuals With Cardiovascular Disease

Disease	Implications for Dental Hygiene Care	Dental Hygiene Actions
Rheumatic heart disease	Special attention to oral self-care practices; self-inflicted bacteremias may occur when oral disease is present.	Careful manipulation of soft tissues during instrumentation; ADA-accepted antibacterial mouth rinse to reduce transient bacteremia.
Infective endocarditis	Patient susceptible to reinfection with transient bacteremia. Prophylactic antibiotic premedication is indicated for invasive dental hygiene procedures.	Careful manipulation of soft tissue; antibacterial mouth rinse to reduce transient bacteremia.
Valvular heart defects	Infective endocarditis may occur after dental hygiene procedures that cause transient bacteremias. Patients receiving anticoagulant medication may have a prolonged bleeding time.	If anticoagulant medication is being used and scaling procedures are planned, dosage of anticoagulant medication should be discussed with patient's cardiologist.
Mitral valve prolapse	Special attention to oral self-care practices because self-inflicted bacteremias may occur when oral disease is present.	Careful manipulation of soft tissues during instrumentation and preprocedural antimicrobial rinsing to reduce transient bacteremia.
Cardiac dysrhythmias and arrhythmias	Electrical interference can cause an unshielded pacemaker to malfunction.	Use of electrical dental equipment is contraindicated.
Hypertension	Stress and anxiety about treatment may increase blood pressure.	Use stress reduction strategies; if blood pressure is uncontrolled, dental hygiene care is contraindicated.
Coronary (ischemic) heart disease	Stress and anxiety about treatment may precipitate angina.	Have nitroglycerin available during treatment. Implement stress reduction strategies; create atmosphere conducive to relaxation.
Congestive heart failure	None if person is under appropriate medical care.	Keep patient in upright position to decrease lung fluid.

BOX 48.11 Basic Steps in a Cardiac Emergency

Make certain patient is comfortable; loosen restricting garments, elevate head slightly, provide reassurance.

Angina Pectoris
- Immediately administer nitroglycerin sublingually and 100% oxygen with a face mask or nasal cannula to prevent disease transmission.*
- Monitor vital signs.

Myocardial Infarction
- Call 9-1-1 and activate EMS.
- Have patient transferred to an emergency facility as soon as possible.
- Apply automated external defibrillator and/or administer cardiopulmonary resuscitation if necessary.
- Stay with the patient until the physician or emergency medical technician takes over.

*Note: An overdose of nitroglycerin can cause headache.

TABLE 48.6 Sample Evaluation of Dental Hygiene Interventions

Patient Goals	Evaluation Measures	Expected Outcomes
Complete invasive dental hygiene therapy (scaling and root debridement) so that antibiotic coverage occurs with a 9- to 14-day interval between coverage	Appointments scheduled 9 to 14 days apart	No drug resistance occurring. Hard and soft deposits removed
By 9/13, reduce gingival bleeding by 90%	Document clinical outcomes using bleeding on probing	Minimal to no gingival bleeding on probing
By 12/13, reduce periodontal probing depths	Document clinical outcomes using periodontal probing depths and clinical attachment levels	Periodontal probing depths reduced by at least 1 mm. Clinical attachment levels stable

Implementation of care takes into consideration the possibility of a medical emergency (see Chapter 11). The most life-threatening emergency situation is cardiac arrest. Emergency situations require the following steps:
1. Contact EMS or call 9-1-1.
2. Monitor vital signs and state of consciousness.
3. Administer oxygen.
4. Provide BLS.

Other medical emergencies associated with CVD are attacks of angina pectoris and MI. Box 48.3 and Box 48.11 list actions to be taken.

Oral care professionals evaluate the patient's current health status in light of the established patient goals. By reviewing assessment data, dental hygiene diagnoses, care plan, and interventions used, practitioners can determine where less than desirable outcomes occurred and modify care as necessary. Table 48.6 illustrates an evaluation of dental hygiene interventions.

Finally, it is important to document in the dental record all components of the dental hygiene process of care. This documentation includes the objective, complete, concise, and accurate recording of all collected data, treatment planned and provided, consultations sought, recommendations made, and all other information relevant to patient care and treatment. Doing so meets ethical and legal standards and ensures continuity of care by subsequent healthcare providers.[16]

See Boxes 48.3 and 48.5.

KEY CONCEPTS

- Review health history, dental history, cultural history, pharmacologic history, and risk factors for systemic and oral disease as a standard of care; consult with patient's physician or cardiologist as required.
- Periodontal disease may contribute to one's risk for developing cardiovascular disease (CVD) (e.g., the inflammatory process increases risk for thrombosis development).
- The practitioner must follow the *Prevention of Infective Endocarditis* guidelines from the American Heart Association and strive to maintain the oral health of patients with cardiovascular disease.
- Hypertension can be detected by measuring blood pressure as part of the dental hygiene assessment.
- Unstable angina pectoris indicates that a patient has increasing chest pain at rest and during sleep. Patients with unstable angina are at risk for a possible medical emergency and should not be treated in the dental setting until medical clearance is obtained.
- The drug of choice for a patient experiencing angina is nitroglycerin, usually administered sublingually. Too much nitroglycerin can cause headache.
- Dental hygiene care should be postponed if a patient has had a myocardial infarction within 30 days of the scheduled appointment or if ischemic symptoms persist.
- Cardiac dysrhythmias and arrhythmias are dysfunctions of the heart rate and rhythm and may be detected when assessing the patient's pulse rate.
- Unshielded cardiac pacemakers may be susceptible to interference generated by some dental equipment (e.g., ultrasonic scalers, pulp testers, equipment for iontophoresis in desensitization, air-abrasion systems, computerized periodontal probes, low- or high-speed handpieces).
- Patients with congestive heart failure have difficulty breathing in a supine position.
- Patients with a history of CVD can be given local anesthetic agents that contain epinephrine at the minimally safe dose.
- Anticoagulant medications increase bleeding time. Patients taking such medications need a medical consultation and prothrombin time values within the range of normal before dental hygiene care is performed.
- Patients taking immunosuppressant medication for a heart transplant and calcium channel blockers for hypertension are at risk for drug-influenced gingival enlargement.
- Prevention of CVD requires healthy lifestyles (i.e., reduction in saturated fat, cholesterol, and sodium intake; increased exercise; decreased stress; no tobacco use; and control of hypertension).

REFERENCES

1. World Health Organization. Cardiovascular Disease. Available at: https://www.who.int/health-topics/cardiovascular-diseases#tab=tab_1. Published 2021. Accessed April 18, 2022.
2. Abbasi J. The COVID heart-one year after SARS-CoV-2 infection, patients have an array of increased cardiovascular risks. *JAMA.* 2022;327(12):1113–1114. https://doi.org/10.1001/jama.2022.2411.
3. Stewart R, West M. Increasing evidence for an association between periodontitis and cardiovascular disease. *Circulation.* 2016;133:549–551. Available at: http://circ.ahajournals.org/content/133/6/549. Accessed April 19, 2022. Published January 13, 2016.
4. American Dental Association. Oral-Systemic Health. Available at: https://www.ada.org/resources/research/science-and-research-institute/oral-health-topics/oral-systemic-health. Updated December 23, 2021. Accessed April 18, 2022.
5. NHS. Cardiovascular Disease. Available at: https://www.nhs.uk/conditions/cardiovascular-disease/. Updated April 22, 2022. Accessed November 14, 2022.
6. Hypertension. World Health Organization. https://www.who.int/news-room/fact-sheets/detail/hypertension#:~:text=Hypertension%20is%20called%20a%20%22silent,blood%20pressure%20is%20measured%20regularly. Published August 25, 2021. Accessed November 26, 2022.
7. Benjamin EJ, Blaha MJ, Chiuve SE, et al. Heart disease and stroke statistics-2017 update: a report from the American Heart Association. Circulation. https://www.ncbi.nlm.nih.gov/pmc/articles/PMC5408160/. Published March 7, 2017. Accessed April 23, 2022.
8. Whelton PK, Carey RM, Aronow WS, et al. ACC/AHA/AAPA/ABC/ACPM/AGS/APHA/ASH/ASPC/NMA/PCNA guideline for the prevention, detection, evaluation, and management of high blood pressure in adults: a report of the American College of Cardiology/American Heart Association task force on clinical practice guidelines. *Hypertension.* 2017;71:e13–e115.
9. Are you at risk of stroke? Stroke Association. https://www.stroke.org.uk/what-is-stroke/are-you-at-risk-of-stroke. Published March 11, 2022. Accessed November 26, 2022.
10. HeartorgCardiac Medications At-a-Glance. Cardiac Medications. Available at: https://www.heart.org/en/health-topics/heart-attack/treatment-of-a-heart-attack/cardiac-medications. Updated January15, 2020. Accessed November 14, 2022.
11. Podzimek S, Mysak J, Janatova T, et al. C-reactive protein in peripheral blood of patients with chronic and aggressive periodontitis, gingivitis, and gingival recessions. *Mediators Inflamm.* 2015;2015:564858. Available at: https://www.hindawi.com/journals/mi/2015/564858/. Accessed July 30, 2017. Published June 2, 2015.
12. American Heart Association. Cardioversion. Available at: https://www.heart.org/en/health-topics/arrhythmia/prevention--treatment-of-arrhythmia/cardioversion. Accessed November 14, 2022 Updated September 30, 2016.
13. Heartorg. Implantable Cardioverter Defibrillator (ICD). Implantable Cardioverter Defibrillator (ICD). Available at: https://www.heart.org/en/health-topics/arrhythmia/prevention--treatment-of-arrhythmia/implantable-cardioverter-defibrillator-icd. Updated September 30, 2016. Accessed November 14, 2022.
14. Pickett FA, Gurenlian JAR. *Preventing Medical Emergencies: Use of the Medical History.* 3rd ed. Lippincott Williams & Wilkins; 2014.
15. Heartorg. Infective Endocarditis. Available at: https://www.heart.org/en/health-topics/infective-endocarditis. Updated March 4, 2021. Accessed November 14, 2022.
16. Beemsterboer P. *Ethics and Law in Dental Hygiene.* 3rd ed. Saunders/Elsevier; 2010.

49

Diabetes

Amber W. Hunt

PROFESSIONAL DEVELOPMENT OPPORTUNITIES

With patient-centered and coordinated care, the dental hygienist can improve the quality of life of the person with diabetes and those at risk for developing diabetes. The bidirectional relationship between diabetes and periodontal disease is supported by consistent and robust evidence, and dental hygienists can have a positive impact on both conditions.

COMPETENCIES

1. Differentiate between prediabetes, type 1 and type 2 diabetes, and gestational diabetes in terms of prevalence, characteristics, pathophysiology, and potential complications.
2. Discuss the two-way relationship between diabetes and periodontal disease. In addition, provide client education regarding self-monitoring, lifestyle changes, and pharmacological therapy to engage patients with diabetes as cotherapists in management of diabetes and oral care.
3. Plan dental hygiene care, including all steps in the process of care, for a person with diabetes and periodontal disease, and collaborate interprofessionally with a patient's primary healthcare provider.
4. Recognize a diabetic emergency and take appropriate action for management.
5. Assist patients at risk for diabetes in preventing diabetes and recommend referral for screening.

INTRODUCTION

Diabetes (or diabetes mellitus), which is one of the most widespread diseases, affects approximately 37.3 million adults and children in the United States, about 11.3% of the population.[1] Of these individuals, more than 8.5 million are unaware of their diabetes.[1] The prevalence of diagnosed and undiagnosed cases is increasing substantially with increasing obesity. Current estimates project at least one in three people will develop diabetes in their lifetime.[1] Individuals with poorly controlled diabetes face shortened life spans and a high probability of developing acute and chronic health complications.

Diabetes is actually a group of disorders characterized by **hyperglycemia** (high levels of blood glucose) resulting from defects in insulin production, how insulin works, or both. Chronic hyperglycemia damages the nerves (**neuropathy**), eyes, kidneys, heart, and blood vessels (**microangiopathy**). The dental hygienist plays a key role in managing oral disease in persons with diabetes and thus has the potential to impact metabolic control (Box 49.1).

PREDIABETES

Prediabetes is a condition that precedes type 2 diabetes when people have blood glucose levels that are higher than normal but below diagnostic levels. Approximately 38% of the US adult population has diagnosed prediabetes.[1] Prediabetes is also called **impaired glucose tolerance** and **impaired fasting glucose**, other terms that refer to metabolic stages somewhere between normal glucose homeostasis and diabetes (Fig. 49.1). People with prediabetes are at high risk for developing diabetes and cardiovascular disease. Impaired glucose tolerance and impaired fasting glucose are associated with abdominal obesity; high triglyceride levels, low high-density lipoprotein (i.e., "good cholesterol") levels, or both; and hypertension. Individuals who are at high risk for developing diabetes can use a variety of interventions to delay and often prevent diabetes. Interventions that have been shown to prevent type 2 diabetes include the following:

- Increasing physical activity to include 150 minutes per week of moderate activity, such as brisk walking
- Targeting a 7% weight reduction
- Reinforcing behaviors with followup counseling
- Adding metformin therapy for those with body mass indices of more than 35 kg/m² who are less than 60 years old and for those females with prior gestational diabetes; see Oral Hypoglycemic Agents later in this chapter for more information.
- Obtaining annual monitoring

Prediabetes has no symptoms, so it is important for the dental hygienist to know the risk factors, ask questions, refer patients for screening, and encourage patients to make healthy behavior changes.

CLASSIFICATION OF DIABETES

Classification of diabetes is important for understanding treatment considerations (Box 49.2). The four major clinical types of diabetes are as follows:[2]

- Type 1 diabetes (Table 49.1)
- Type 2 diabetes (see Table 49.1)
- Gestational diabetes mellitus
- Other specific types

Type 1 Diabetes

Type 1 diabetes is a condition characterized by high blood glucose levels caused by a total lack of insulin. This type involves about 5% of the adult diabetic population. It commonly presents during childhood and adolescence, but it can strike at any age. People who develop type 1 diabetes are rarely obese due to **diabetic ketoacidosis** (DKA, a buildup of acids in the blood). To survive, people with type 1 diabetes require regular lifelong administration of insulin via injection or pump. The

BOX 49.1 The Dental Hygienist's Role in the Care of a Person With Diabetes

- Conduct periodontal risk assessment.
- Determine the need for comanagement.
- Monitor the pharmacologic history for drug interactions with glucose control.
- Minimize potential risks for emergencies.
- Detect undiagnosed and uncontrolled diabetes and refer.
- Modify dental hygiene care plan on the basis of patient needs.
- Monitor the outcomes of dental hygiene care (evaluation).

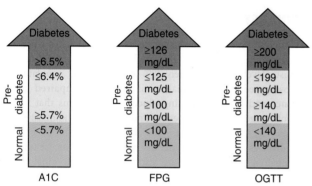

Note: A random blood glucose test of ≥200 mg/dL at any time of the day with symptoms of diabetes is diagnosed as diabetes.

Fig. 49.1 The figure demonstrates the progression from normal to a diagnosis of prediabetes and from prediabetes to a diagnosis of diabetes. Prediabetes and diabetes can be identified using any one of three tests: glycosylated hemoglobin A1c (A1C), fasting plasma glucose (FPG), or oral glucose tolerance test (OGTT). These tests each have distinct diagnostic thresholds for the diagnosis. (Data from the American Diabetes Association. Available at: https://www.diabetes.org/diabetes/a1c/diagnosis. Accessed July 26, 2022.)

BOX 49.2 Diabetes

Prediabetes
- Metabolic stage intermediate between normal glucose homeostasis and diabetes; indicates relatively high risk for development of diabetes

Type 1 Diabetes
- Results from beta-cell destruction in pancreas, usually leading to defective insulin production
  A. Autoimmune
  B. Idiopathic

Type 2 Diabetes
- Progressive loss of beta-cell insulin secretion, frequently with insulin resistance (the body cannot use the insulin it makes).

Other Specific Types
- Other types of diabetes associated with certain conditions or syndromes: pancreatic disease, endocrine diseases, infections, chemical- or drug-induced disease, genetic defects, genetic syndromes, insulin-receptor abnormalities, and others

Gestational Diabetes Mellitus
- Any degree of glucose intolerance with onset or first recognition during pregnancy

disease results when the body's immune system attacks and destroys the insulin-producing beta cells in the pancreas. Genetic predisposition related to the presence of certain human leukocyte antigens that influence immune activity directed against islet cells is essential for type 1 diabetes. Research studies suggest a genetic origin associated with type 1 and type 2 diabetes. The role of genetics is stronger in type 1 diabetes than in type 2 diabetes. Environmental factors, which are still poorly defined, likely play a causative role in genetically predisposed individuals. Autoimmune reactions and environmental factors (e.g., viral infections) have been demonstrated in research. Twin studies reveal that if one twin develops type 1 diabetes, the other twin will develop the disease in approximately 50% of cases.[3]

Type 2 Diabetes

Type 2 diabetes, which is the most common form of diabetes, results from a lack of insulin or the body's inability to use insulin efficiently. Type 2 diabetes is preventable. People with type 2 diabetes constitute approximately 90% to 95% of the diabetic population. Of the undiagnosed, the vast majority have type 2 diabetes. The risk of developing type 2 diabetes increases with obesity, age, lack of physical activity, history of gestational diabetes mellitus, hypertension, and **dyslipidemia** (i.e., abnormal amounts of blood lipids). The frequency of type 2 diabetes varies with racial and ethnic groups. Ketoacidosis seldom occurs in individuals with type 2 diabetes, but when present, it is associated with infection. Type 2 diabetes usually goes undiagnosed for years because hyperglycemia develops gradually without classic symptoms. It is estimated that people have type 2 diabetes for 10 years before they are clinically diagnosed. Nevertheless, the risk of developing **macrovascular** and **microvascular complications** (i.e., problems in the large and small blood vessels) is high. Unlike type 1 diabetes, symptoms may be gradual, and weight loss is uncommon (see Table 49.1).

Persons with type 2 diabetes often respond to weight reduction, dietary management, exercise, and oral hypoglycemic medications. Persons with type 2 diabetes may require insulin therapy to achieve good control or during illness, which is an important distinction between insulin-dependent and insulin-treated individuals.

Type 2 diabetes is predominantly genetically inherited, and it has no association with autoimmune beta-cell destruction. In studies, when one identical twin develops type 2 diabetes, the other twin has a 100% chance of developing the disease.[3] Obesity has a major role in the development of type 2 diabetes, but further research is needed to determine if it is a cause.

Gestational Diabetes Mellitus

Gestational diabetes mellitus (GDM) occurs in 7.8% of pregnancies in the United States.[4] Clinical characteristics include glucose intolerance that has its onset or is recognized during pregnancy. Therefore diabetic females who become pregnant do not fall into the GDM classification. High-risk individuals include those with the following conditions:
- Marked obesity
- Previous GDM
- Strong family history of diabetes
- **Glucosuria** (i.e., glucose in the urine)

Even in the nondiabetic individual, normal pregnancy affects both fetal and maternal metabolism and exerts a diabetogenic effect. GDM generally reverts after birth because the condition is a consequence of the normal antiinsulin effects of pregnancy hormones and the diversion of natural glucose to the fetus.

GDM increases the risk of perinatal morbidity and mortality. Maternal complications include an increased rate of cesarean delivery and chronic hypertension. Furthermore, approximately 50% of females with a history of GDM will develop type 2 diabetes.[5] Six weeks or more

TABLE 49.1 Characteristics of Type 1 and Type 2 Diabetes Mellitus

Factor	Type 1	Type 2
Age at onset	Usually young but may occur at any age	Usually in persons >40 years old but may occur at any age
Type of onset	Usually abrupt	Gradual and subtle
Genetic susceptibility	Human leukocyte antigen–related DR3, DR4, and others	Frequent genetic background; not related to human leukocyte antigen
Environmental factors	Viruses, toxins, autoimmune stimulation	Obesity
Islet-cell antibody	Present at outset	Not observed
Endogenous insulin	Minimal or absent	Stimulated response is adequate but with delayed secretion or reduced but not absent
Nutritional status	Thin, catabolic state	Obese or may be normal
Symptoms	Thirst, polyuria, polyphagia, fatigue	Frequently none or mild
Ketosis	Prone at onset or during insulin deficiency	Resistant except during infection or stress
Control of diabetes	Often difficult, with wide glucose fluctuation	Variable; helped by dietary adherence
Dietary management	Essential	Essential; may suffice for glycemic control
Insulin	Required for all	Required for about 40%
Sulfonylurea	Not efficacious	Efficacious
Vascular and neurologic complications	Seen in majority after ≥5 years of diabetes	Frequent

after pregnancy ends, the female with GDM should be reclassified as having one of the following:

- Diabetes
- Prediabetes
- Normal glucose regulation

Other Specific Types of Diabetes

The category of other specific types of diabetes is heterogeneous in nature and includes diabetes in which the causative relationship is known, such as diabetes associated with certain conditions and syndromes (e.g., genetic defects of the beta cells, pancreatic disease, endocrine disease, chemical-induced agents, and genetic syndromes).

PATHOPHYSIOLOGY OF DIABETES

To use glucose, the pancreas must produce insulin. A person with diabetes produces too little insulin or has an inability to use insulin (Fig. 49.2). **Insulin**, which is an anabolic hormone (i.e., it is used to build up the body), stimulates the entry of glucose into the cell and enhances fat storage. Without insulin, glucose remains in the bloodstream (hyperglycemia) rather than being stored or used by cells to produce energy.

Insulin Deprivation

The net effect of insulin deficiency is a rise in blood glucose concentration (**hyperglycemia**). Without insulin, the glucose derived from a meal cannot be used or stored. When the blood glucose level rises to more than 150 mg/dL, the kidney tubules become incapable of resorption. Glucose appears in the urine (glucosuria), taking with it a large amount of fluid, thereby raising the volume of urine (**polyuria**) and necessitating frequent urination. Dehydration follows, leading to excessive thirst (**polydipsia**). **Diabetic ketoacidosis** (DKA) may follow hyperglycemia when blood glucose levels rise to more than 400 mg/dL (Box 49.3). Defective carbohydrate metabolism, which the body interprets as energy starvation, causes the excessive ingestion of food (**polyphagia**) and necessitates the use of fats and proteins (hyperglycemia progressively glycates body proteins) to satisfy energy requirements. Keto acids and ketone bodies (acetone) are produced as a result of the catabolism of fatty acids (**lipolysis**). Ketones accumulate in the tissues, are excreted in the urine (**ketonuria**), and circulate in the blood

(**ketonemia**). Without treatment, this process causes a drop in the pH of the blood and leads to seizures. Untreated DKA can lead to diabetic coma and death.

Clinical Signs and Symptoms

Diabetes is characterized by hyperglycemia. In type 1 diabetes, the predominant problem is impaired insulin production; in type 2 diabetes, the predominant problem is the inability to use the insulin produced by the body. However, a considerable overlap exists with regard to the clinical features of the two forms of diabetes. The deficiency of insulin action leads to defects in the metabolism of carbohydrates, protein, and lipids. In clinical practice, the suspicion of diabetes is gleaned from the patient's history and physical findings (Box 49.4).

Indicators of probable diabetes (i.e., the cardinal signs of diabetes) include the following:

- Polydipsia
- Polyuria
- Polyphagia
- Unexplained weight loss
- Weakness

Symptoms of marked hyperglycemia also include **polyphagia** (eating extreme amounts of food) and blurred vision. Impairment of growth and susceptibility to certain infections may also accompany chronic hyperglycemia. Family histories of diabetes, obesity, GDM, premature atherosclerosis, or neuropathic disorders also are indications of probable diabetes. Sleep disorders are also a risk factor for type 2 diabetes.[6] Furthermore, sleep disturbances may impede meeting glycemic targets among people with type 1 and type 2 diabetes.[6] Dental hygienists should consider screening for sleep disorders and refer to a sleep specialist as indicated. Dental hygienists aware of indications and risk factors can refer potentially undiagnosed patients for testing (Boxes 49.5 and 49.6).

Chronic Complications

People with both types of diabetes show a tendency for severe, multisystem, long-term complications (Table 49.2), including the following:

- Microvascular and macrovascular disease
- Diabetic retinopathy with potential vision loss
- Nephropathy leading to renal failure

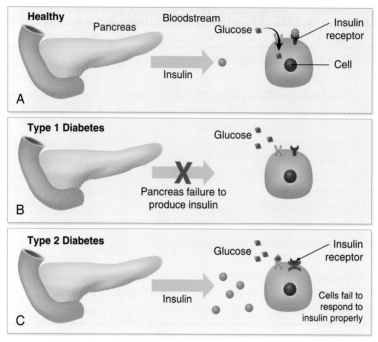

Fig. 49.2 Pancreas and Insulin Activity in Health, Type 1 Diabetes, and Type 2 Diabetes. (A) When the pancreas is healthy, it produces insulin and excretes it into the bloodstream. Insulin binds to the insulin receptor on the cell and stimulates the entry of glucose into the cell. (B) In type 1 diabetes, the pancreas does not produce insulin and there is no entry of glucose into the cell. (C) In type 2 diabetes, too little insulin is produced or the cell has an inability to use insulin and there is no entry of glucose into the cell. (Modified from: iStock.com/ttsz.)

BOX 49.3 Signs and Symptoms of Ketoacidosis

Common Cardinal Symptoms
"Fruity" acetone breath
Frequent urination
Excessive thirst
Unusual hunger
Weight loss
Weakness
Nausea
Dry skin and mucous membranes
Flushed facial appearance
Abdominal tenderness
Rapid, deep breathing
Depressed sensory perception

Other Symptoms
Recurrence of bedwetting
Repeated skin infections
Malaise
Drowsiness
Headache
Marked irritability

BOX 49.4 Warning Signs of Diabetes

Type 1 diabetes is characterized by the sudden appearance of the following:
• Frequent urination
• Unusual thirst
• Extreme hunger
• Unusual weight loss
• Irritability
• Extreme fatigue
• Blurred vision
• Very dry skin
  Type 2 diabetes is characterized by its slow onset; it includes any of the type 1 symptoms, in addition to the following:
• Cuts and bruises that are slow to heal
• Tingling or numbness in the hands and feet
• Recurring or hard-to-heal skin, gingival, or bladder infections

Data from the American Diabetes Association. *Diabetes Symptoms.* Available at: http://www.diabetes.org/diabetes-basics/symptoms/?loc=DropDownDB-symptoms. Accessed July 30, 2022.

• Peripheral neuropathy with risk of foot ulcers, amputation, and neuropathic joint disease
• Autonomic neuropathy causing gastrointestinal, genitourinary, and cardiovascular symptoms as well as sexual dysfunction
• Periodontal disease
Mechanisms thought to cause tissue damage in people with diabetes involve alterations in the host immunoinflammatory response, including altered function of immune cells (i.e., neutrophils, monocytes, and macrophages); elevated levels of tumor necrosis factor-alpha; alterations in connective tissue metabolism; and the glycation of tissue proteins forming advanced glycation end products.[7] Individuals with diabetes have an increased incidence of atherosclerotic, cardiovascular, peripheral vascular, and cerebrovascular disease (see Chapter 48—Cardiovascular Disease). Hypertension, abnormalities in lipoprotein metabolism, and periodontal disease are found in people with diabetes (See Chapter 20—Periodontal Assessment and Charting, and Chapter 21—Oral-Systemic Health Connection). There is not enough data to determine whether diabetes is a risk factor COVID-19; however, diabetes is a risk factor for some of the worst

BOX 49.5 Type 2 Diabetes: Risk Factors and Criteria for the Testing of Asymptomatic Undiagnosed Adults[2]

Testing for diabetes should be considered in the following situations:
- At age 35 years for all people; if results are normal, testing should be repeated at 3-year intervals.
- At a younger age or more frequently for adults who are overweight (i.e., body mass index of ≥25 kg/m²) with one or more risk factors:
  - Physical inactivity
  - First-degree relative with diabetes
  - Member of a high-risk ethnic population (e.g., African American, Latino, Native American, Asian American, Pacific Islander)
  - Delivered a baby weighing >9 lb or diagnosed with gestational diabetes mellitus
  - Hypertensive (≥130/80 mm Hg or receiving therapy for hypertension)
  - High-density lipoprotein cholesterol level of <35 mg/dL (0.90 mmol/L) and/or triglyceride level of >250 mg/dL (2.82 mmol/L)
  - Polycystic ovary syndrome
  - A1c level of ≥5.7%, impaired glucose tolerance, or impaired fasting glucose on previous testing
  - History of cardiovascular disease
- Those with prediabetes should be tested annually.

BOX 49.6 Type 2 Diabetes in Children: Risk Factors and Criteria for Testing[2]

- Overweight or obese (body mass index of ≥85th percentile) plus one or more of the following risk factors:
  - Family history of type 2 diabetes in a parent, sibling, grandparent, aunt, uncle, niece, or nephew
  - Native American, African American, Latino, Asian American, or Pacific Islander race or ethnicity
  - Hypertension, dyslipidemia, polycystic ovary syndrome, or infants with low birthweight for gestational age
  - Mother who had gestational diabetes while pregnant with the child
- Age at initiation of testing: 10 years or at onset of puberty, if puberty occurs at a younger age
- Frequency of testing: every 3 years

TABLE 49.2 Complications of Diabetes Mellitus

Affected Area	Complications and Results
Eyes	Retinopathy Blindness Cataracts Glaucoma
Kidneys	Glomerulonephritis Chronic dialysis Nephrosclerosis Kidney transplant Pyelonephritis
Mouth	Gingivitis Dental caries Periodontitis
Reproductive system	Sexual dysfunction Stillbirths Miscarriages Babies with high birthweights Congenital defects Neonatal deaths
Skin	Xanthoma diabeticorum Pruritus Furunculosis Limited joint mobility
Vascular system	Atherosclerosis Stroke Microangiopathy Heart disease Large-vessel disease Hypertension Myocardial infarction
Peripheral nerves	Earliest recognized complication Erectile dysfunction Somatic neuropathy Autonomic neuropathy Slowed digestion in stomach Impaired sensation in feet and hands Carpal tunnel syndrome Lower-extremity amputations

COVID-19 outcomes, including hospitalization and death.[8] The emotional and social impact of diabetes and the demands of therapy cause significant unmet human needs in individuals with diabetes and their families. All complications affect patients with both type 1 and type 2 diabetes, although clinical consequences differ greatly. Generally, kidney and eye diseases predominate with type 1 diabetes, atherosclerotic disease predominates with type 2 disease, and neuropathy occurs with both types (see Table 49.2).

Diabetes and Periodontal Disease: A Two-Way Relationship

For more information about this topic, see Modifiable Risk Factors in Chapter 20 and Diabetes sections in Chapter 21.

Periodontal disease is the sixth most common complication of diabetes. Diabetes is a systemic risk factor for periodontitis and patients with diabetes have a 24% increase in the incidence of periodontal disease when compared to people without diabetes.[9] For patients with periodontitis, the risk of developing diabetes is elevated by 26%.[9] A systematic review specifically studying persons with type 1 diabetes,

found they were more than twice as likely to develop periodontitis compared to the general population.[10] Several meta-analyses confirm that periodontal therapy can result in reduced glycated hemoglobin (A1c) levels. Reduced systemic inflammation seems to be an important determinant in the relationship. Inflammation is the factor common to both diabetes and periodontal disease. In fact, evidence supports an increased risk for diabetes onset in patients with severe periodontitis.[7]

Diabetes is a risk factor that may modify the periodontitis grade of the patient.[11] After primary criteria is initially used for determining periodontitis grade, the patient's HbA1c level can then shift the grade score higher.[9] Since Grade A or slow rate of progression indicates normoglycemic/no diagnosis of diabetes, patients with periodontitis and diabetes with an HbA1c less than 7% would be given a grade score of Grade B or moderate rate of progression at a minimum. However, a HBA1c level of 7% or greater may shift the grade to a Grade C or rapid rate of progression.

DISEASE MANAGEMENT

As dental hygienists, we are expected to remain current in our knowledge of evidence-based practice (EPP) in order to provide the most up-to-date care for our patients (see Chapter 3). At the time of writing this chapter, the *Standards of Care in Diabetes—2023* were released.[6] This is a perfect example of why continuing education is so critical to the practice of dental hygiene. As the Standards note, diabetes care is rapidly changing based on new research, technology, and treatments that ultimately have the impact to improve the health and quality of life of people with diabetes.

Social Determinants of Health

The social determinants of health should be incorporated into diabetes management to help achieve health equity for all populations (See Chapter 4—Community Health).

Glycemic Control: Self-Monitoring of Blood Glucose and A1c

The most important aspect of the **control of diabetes** is the self-monitoring of blood glucose with small automated devices. The frequency of self-monitoring is highly individualized. Monitoring requires placing a small drop of blood on a reagent strip, which is then inserted into a meter. The meter measures glucose concentration and displays a value of glucose in milligrams per deciliter (mg/dL) of blood.

The hemoglobin A1c test (also known as HbA1c or A1c) is used by the patient and healthcare providers to monitor overall glycemic control. The test often is prescribed by a primary healthcare provider and completed at the office or clinic or at a laboratory. With the increasing prevalence of diabetes and the potential serious complications of the disease, home testing of HbA1c should be an integral part of diabetes management; however, home testing of HbA1c does not replace daily monitoring of blood glucose, as the tests have different purposes. Blood glucose testing examines a current blood sugar (glucose) level that can be affected by recent dietary intake, whereas HbA1c examines longer-term average blood glucose control over the past 2 to 3 months. Regular professional monitoring of A1c is important. When using an at-home testing device, it should be approved by the Food and Drug Association for the most reliable results. Even so, the home use tests will not always produce accurate results. If a reading is significantly different from the previous professional testing result, the patient should repeat the test in 1 hour or consult with their health professional. Hemoglobin A is made during the 120-day life span of a red blood cell. Blood glucose attaches to hemoglobin A and is used as a record of blood glucose levels over the prior 3 months. In addition, the A1c test is the preferred test for prediabetes. An A1c level between 5.7% and 6.4% indicates prediabetes; 6.5% or greater indicates diabetes. Abnormal A1c levels correlate with glucose intolerance and the development of diabetic complications. Thus, early diagnosis and good control are very important. Recommendations for A1c levels and blood measurements in patients with diabetes are presented in Box 49.7.

Lifestyle Changes

Diet remains the hallmark of diabetes therapy, despite advances in insulin formulations, insulin delivery systems, and oral medications. Diabetic diets are designed to provide appropriate quantities of healthy food at regular intervals, to supply daily caloric requirements to help with achieving or maintaining desirable body weight, and to reduce fat intake to correct an unfavorable lipid profile that is conducive to hypertension and cardiovascular disease. Patients also should be advised to try to limit carbohydrates with added sugars or those with refined grains, such as white bread and white rice, and instead eat

---

BOX 49.7   Glycemic Control: Summary of Recommendations for Adults With Diabetes[17]

A1c	<7.0%
Pre-meal glucose	80 to 130 mg/dL
Peak postmeal glucose*	<180 mg/dL

Key Concepts for Setting Glycemic Goals
- Goals should be individualized.
- Children, pregnant females and elderly patients require special considerations.
- More or less intense glycemic goals may be appropriate for certain individuals.

* Post-meal glucose measurements should be made 1 to 2 hours after the beginning of the meal, which is generally when the peak level occurs in persons with diabetes.
American Diabetes Association. Glycemic targets: Standards of care in diabetes-2023. *Diabetes Care.* 2023;46(suppl 1):S97-S110. https://www.cdc.gov/diabetes/managing/manage-blood-sugar.html

---

carbohydrates from fruit, vegetables, whole grains, beans, and low-fat or nonfat milk. This advice can be provided for caries prevention as well as metabolic control.

With type 2 diabetes, a reduction in hyperglycemia is correlated with weight loss. For people with type 2 diabetes who are overweight or obese, 5% weight loss is associated with benefits for glycemic control.[6] However, higher weight loss goals such as 15% may be appropriate for maximum effect.[6] With type 1 diabetes, nutritional strategies involve monitoring the percentages of carbohydrate (i.e., 55% to 60% of total calories) and protein (i.e., 12% to 20% of total calories) intake (see Chapter 36—Nutritional Counseling). Meal planning for people with diabetes is based on the food exchange system of the American Diabetes Association.[12] Additionally, referring patients with diabetes to a registered dietitian for nutritional therapy may be beneficial for improving their HbA1c level. Research shows people with type 2 diabetes who apply healthy behavior interventions provided by a registered dietitian improve their glycemic control.[13]

Physical activity is essential for diabetes control. Exercise is associated with a decrease in hyperglycemia and increased sensitivity to insulin in people with diabetes. Lifestyle changes improve the control of blood glucose, prevent diabetes in some cases, and may decrease cardiovascular complications. Tobacco use prevention or cessation counseling is essential. Adults with diabetes who drink alcohol should do so in moderation (maximum of one drink a day for females and two drinks a day for males).

Pharmacologic Therapy: Type 1 and Type 2
Insulin Therapy

More than 20 different insulins are sold in the United States.[14] Approximately 15% of people with diabetes (either type 1 or type 2) use insulin only to control hyperglycemia; 52% use oral medications only, 14% use a combination of insulin and oral medications, and 19% do not take either insulin or oral medication.[15] Persons with type 1 diabetes have essentially no pancreatic insulin, are unresponsive to oral sulfonylurea hypoglycemic agents, and are prone to ketosis; therefore, they are dependent on lifelong exogenous insulin administration. For patients with type 2 diabetes who are not achieving glycemic goals, insulin therapy should not be delayed. Human insulin and insulin analogs are categorized by their speed of onset, their peak effect, and their duration; they are available in mixture preparations as follows:

- Rapid-acting
- Short-acting

TABLE 49.3   Types of Insulin

Insulin Classification	Types	Onset of Action	Peak Effect (hr)	Duration (hr)
Rapid-acting	Insulin aspart (Fiasp, NovoLog) Insulin glulisine (Apidra) Insulin lispro (Admelog, Humalog, Lyumjev)	15 minutes	1-2	2-4
Rapid-acting inhaled	Technosphere insulin-inhalation system (Afrezza)	12-15 minutes	30 minutes	3
Regular or short-acting	Human Regular (Humulin R, Novolin R, Velosulin R)	30 minutes	2-3	3-6
Intermediate-acting	Neutral protamine Hagedorn (NPH) (Humulin N, Novolin N, ReliOn)	2-4 hours	4-12	12-18
Long-acting	degludec (Tresiba) detemir (Levemir) glargine (Basaglar, Lantus)	Several hours	None	Up to 24
Ultralong-acting	Glargine U-300 (Toujeo)	6 hours	None	36 or more

Source: https://diabetes.org/healthy-living/medication-treatments/insulin-other-injectables/insulin-basics. Accessed September 18, 2023.

- Intermediate-acting
- Long-acting
- Ultralong-acting

Insulin may be injected subcutaneously with an insulin syringe or a penlike device. Insulin pumps are widely used to deliver a programmed steady drip of insulin (i.e., a basal rate) under the skin 24 hours a day. The push of a button on the pump delivers a bolus dose to respond to the number of carbohydrate grams consumed at a meal. Numerous new products are awaiting approval from the US Food and Drug Administration (FDA). Table 49.3 illustrates insulin types that may be used alone or in combination. Dosages, frequency, and times of administration are highly individualized.

Oral Hypoglycemic Agents

Oral hypoglycemic agents are only used in the treatment of type 2 diabetes. Metformin therapy is started by a primary care provider or an endocrinologist upon diagnosis of type 2 diabetes. Generally, oral hypoglycemic agents stimulate the pancreas to secrete more insulin, increase the body's response to insulin, slow glucose digestion, or decrease glucose production by the liver as follows:

- **Metformin** (biguanide [Glucophage]) decreases the amount of glucose secreted by the liver, decreases intestinal glucose absorption, and increases insulin action. Hypoglycemia is not a side effect. Metformin, if not contraindicated and if tolerated, is the preferred initial pharmacologic agent for type 2 diabetes. Metformin is contraindicated for people with reduced kidney function.
- **Sulfonylureas** (glyburide [Glynase, Micronase, and Diabeta]; glipizide [Glucotrol]); glimepiride [Amaryl]) increase insulin secretion. Hypoglycemia is a side effect. Weight gain is a disadvantage.
- Meglitinides (repaglinide [Prandin]; nateglinide [Starlix]) increase insulin secretion in the presence of glucose. These drugs are taken before each meal.
- Thiazolidinedione (TZD) (pioglitazone [Actos]) makes the body more sensitive to insulin.
- Dipeptidyl peptidase-4 (DPP-4) inhibitors (sitagliptin [Januvia]; saxagliptin [Onglyza]; linagliptin [Tradjenta]) reduce glucagon secretion and increase insulin secretion. A potential side effect is the increased incidence of heart failure.
- Alpha-glucosidase inhibitors (acarbose [Precose]; miglitol [Glyset]) inhibit enzymes in the small intestines that are responsible for carbohydrate digestion, thus delaying absorption. These are not often used because of frequent dosing and gastrointestinal side effects.
- Bile acid sequestrants (BASs) (colesevelam [Welchol]) bind to bile acids in the digestive tract and increase the conversion of cholesterol

into bile, which helps lower cholesterol and blood glucose levels. Possible side effects are constipation and flatulence.

- Dopamine-2 agonists (bromocriptine [Cycloset and Parlodel]) help decrease blood glucose after meals.
- Sodium-glucose transporter 2 (SGLT2) inhibitors (canagliflozin [Invokana], dapagliflozin [Farxiga], and empagliflozin [Jardiance]) block resorption of glucose in the kidneys. Potential side effects are yeast and urinary tract infections.

Injectable Agents for Type 2 Diabetes

The following are injectable agents for the treatment of type 2 diabetes:

- Glucagon-like peptide-1 receptor agonist (GLP-1 RA) Exenatide (Byetta) and liraglutide (Victoza), derived from the saliva of the Gila monster, stimulates the incretin effect (increased insulin response), which is diminished in patients with type 2 diabetes.
- Amylin mimetics (pramlintide [Symlin]) are analogs of human amylin, which modulates gastric emptying. Pramlintide is also approved for patients with type 1 diabetes, but it requires an additional injection.
- Insulin + GLP-1 RA (insulin glargine/lixisenatide [Soliqua]), insulin degludec/liraglutide [Xultophy]; insulin helps glucose enter the cells and the GLP-1 RA helps release insulin with blood glucose is high.

Other Medications

Many people with diabetes are also treated with anticoagulant/antiplatelet drugs, antihypertensive drugs, or lipid-lowering medications.

DENTAL HYGIENE PROCESS OF CARE

Diabetes care is constantly changing as new research emerges to improve the health of people with diabetes. Therefore it is important for dental hygienists to stay up to date on the latest research evidence to incorporate into evidence-based decision making (see Chapter 3—Evidence-Based Decision Making). The American Diabetes Association provides clinical practice guidelines that are updated annually or more frequently if new evidence indicates need for a more immediate update.[16]

Well-controlled diabetes occurs when the patient's blood glucose is within the normal range as a result of a careful balance of medication, diet, and exercise. A blood glucose concentration of 80 to 130 mg/dL is the target range for nonpregnant adults with diabetes.[17] Patients with well-controlled diabetes can be treated safely, provided that their daily routine is not affected. People with well-controlled diabetes have a reduced incidence of dental caries. It is important for dental hygienists to know that only about 50% of people with type 2 diabetes attain an A1c level of less than 7%.[18]

Infections of any type can cause a profound disturbance of glycemic control that potentially leads to ketoacidosis and diabetic coma. When infection is present, counterregulatory hormone secretion increases (specifically cortisol and glucagon), thereby leading to hyperglycemia and increased ketogenesis. Infection is the most common precipitating factor for severe ketoacidosis. In the patient with poorly controlled diabetes, phagocytic function is impaired and resistance to infection is decreased. The prevention of oral diseases and infections is critical to the patient's diabetic control, and poor diabetic control may aggravate the oral disease status.

Several unmet human needs relate to dental hygiene care for individuals with diabetes. For example, emotional stress induced by a dental appointment causes the release of epinephrine, which mobilizes glucose from glycogen stored in the liver. Stress, therefore, can contribute to a hyperglycemic condition becoming ketoacidotic. Periods of waiting and treatment time should be minimized to reduce stress. Good diabetic control also can enhance an individual's quality of life.

Diabetes among people who undertake intensive regimens of multiple insulin injections and the daily self-monitoring of blood glucose may abruptly become uncontrolled as a result of an active periodontal infection. It is important to complete an assessment for signs of periodontal infection prior to referring patients with possible undiagnosed or uncontrolled diabetes, or high blood glucose or HbA1c values so that the medical care provider is aware of the coexisting infection.

Assessment
Health History

When obtaining a patient's health history, the dental hygienist questions the patient about the signs and symptoms of ketoacidosis (see Boxes 49.3 and 49.4) to determine whether an **undiagnosed diabetic** condition is present. When the patient presents without a diabetes diagnosis but with known risk factors for type 2 diabetes (see Boxes 49.5 and 49.6) and periodontitis, they should be informed about their risk for having prediabetes or diabetes, assessed using a point-of-care A1c test approved by the US FDA,[2] and/or referred to a primary healthcare provider for testing and followup. The administration of the American Diabetes Association's Diabetes Risk Test is recommended to assist with early diagnosis. In addition, the CDC recommends that dental offices administer the chairside A1c test or use a blood glucose self-monitoring device to screen patients who are at risk for prediabetes. When a patient's results confirm higher than normal ranges, refer them to a physician. Among the aging population, classic symptoms do not usually manifest. Rather, clinical findings are related to chronic complications of the disease, such as vascular disorders or neuropathic syndromes.

When the person is a **known diabetic**, the patient and health history interview should address the following:
- Type of diabetes
- Methods used to control diabetes (e.g., medications, diet, exercise, weight loss)
- Medication schedule and dosages
- Date and results of the last A1c test
- Frequency of self-monitoring of blood glucose
- Fasting blood glucose levels
- Results of self-monitoring (i.e., trends as well as those of the day of the appointment)
- Blood glucose levels 2 hours after meals
- Date of the last hypoglycemia episode

- Date of onset of diabetes
- Regularity of appointments with a physician
- Six complications of diabetes

The decision to continue the comprehensive assessment, consult with a physician, or defer treatment and refer the patient to a physician should be made on the basis of the patient's responses to questions during the health history and pharmacologic assessment (Boxes 49.8, 49.9, and 49.10).

Oral Assessment

Intraoral findings may reveal the following conditions that are more common in patients with poorly controlled diabetes (Table 49.4):

BOX 49.8 Levels of Blood Glucose for Care Planning

- <70 mg/dL: Too low; hypoglycemia. Provide 15 mg of carbohydrates and wait 15 minutes. If condition continues, check with a physician. Risk for emergency situations.*
- Indicates that dental hygiene care should not be provided at these blood glucose levels.
- 70 to 79 mg/dL: Monitor at least once during dental hygiene care appointment to prevent an emergency.
- 80 to 149 mg/dL: Normal levels.
- 150 to 200 mg/dL: Higher levels. Monitor infections, insulin intake, stress, and food intake.
- >200 mg/dL: Too high; tendency toward hyperglycemia. Check with physician. Risk for emergency situations.*

* Indicates that dental hygiene care should not be provided at these blood glucose levels.

BOX 49.9 When to Refer to a Physician

Refer the patient to a physician for diagnosis and treatment when the patient has the following:
- Cardinal signs of diabetes (see Box 49.3)
- Symptoms that suggest diabetes
- Estimated fasting blood glucose level ≥126 mg/mL
- 2-Hour postmeal blood glucose level ≥200 mg/mL
- Long period since patient was last seen by a physician
- Frequent episodes of hypoglycemia
- Diagnosed diabetes plus signs and symptoms of diabetes (not controlled)
- Type 1 diabetes with extreme hyperglycemia and hypoglycemia
- An infection anywhere in the body

Adapted from Little JW, Falace DA, Miller CS, Rhodus NL. *Dental Management of the Medically Compromised Patient.* 9th ed. Elsevier; 2017.

BOX 49.10 When to Consult With the Patient's Physician

When the patient has the following:
- Type 1 or 2 diabetes; determine level of control
- Complications such as renal disease or cardiovascular disease
- Prescribed insulin
- Lapses in good medical management
- Indications for extensive periodontal or oral-maxillofacial surgery

Adapted from Little JW, Falace DA, Miller CS, Rhodus NL. *Dental Management of the Medically Compromised Patient.* 9th ed. Elsevier; 2017.

- Cheilosis
- Xerostomia
- Increased levels of cariogenic microorganisms
- Glossodynia (burning mouth)
- Enlarged salivary glands
- Increased glucose in the saliva
- Fungal infections such as candidiasis (thrush)
- Dental caries
- Periodontal disease

The International Diabetes Federation and European Federation of Periodontology jointly published a comprehensive review of diabetes and periodontal disease.[7] The prevalence and severity of periodontal disease increase in individuals with both type 1 and type 2 forms of diabetes as compared with individuals without diabetes. Poorer glycemic control as measured by HbA1c level is linked with poorer periodontal status and periodontal treatment results in patients with type 2 diabetes.[7] The presence of hyperglycemia contributes to enhanced periodontal inflammation and alveolar bone loss in patients with diabetes. Hyperglycemia progressively leads to an increase of proinflammatory **cytokines** such as tumor necrosis factor-alpha, interleukin 6, and others that destroy connective tissue and bone. The chronic increased cytokine levels augment inflammatory tissue destruction. The control of hyperglycemia reduces the level of proinflammatory cytokines. Glycemic control is an integral part of the control of periodontal disease in individuals with diabetes.[7]

Uncontrolled diabetes increases dental caries risk as a result of reduced saliva secretion and increased glucose in saliva. Other oral complications associated with diabetes may affect nutrition by

TABLE 49.4 Oral Complications of Diabetes

Clinical Signs and Symptoms	Pathophysiology
Salivary and Oral Changes	
Xerostomia	Increased fluid loss
Bilateral asymptomatic parotid gland swelling with increased salivary viscosity	Increased fatty acid deposition Increased salivary glucose levels Compensatory hypertrophy as a result of a decrease in saliva production
Increased dental caries, especially in the cervical region	Secondary to xerostomia and salivary glucose levels
Unexplained odontalgia and percussion sensitivity (acute pulpitis)	Pulpal arteritis from microangiopathies
Lingual erosion of anterior teeth*	Complications of anorexia nervosa and bulimia
Periodontal Changes	
Periodontal disease	Induction and accumulation of advanced glycation end products
Tooth mobility	Loss of attachment associated with poor glycemic control
Rapidly progressive pocket formation	Degenerative vascular changes
Gingival bleeding	Microangiopathies Local factors
Subgingival polyps	Cause unknown
Infection and Wound Healing	
Slow wound healing (including periapical lesions after endodontics) and increased susceptibility to infection	Hyperglycemia reduces phagocytic activity Ketoacidosis may delay chemotaxis of granulocytes Vascular changes lead to decreased blood flow Abnormal collagen production
Oral ulcers refractory to therapy, especially in association with a prosthesis	Microangiopathies Neuropathies
Irritation fibromas	Altered wound healing
Increased incidence and prolonged healing of dry socket	Degenerative vascular changes Postextraction infection
Tongue Changes	
Glossodynia (also referred to as burning mouth syndrome)	Neuropathic complications Xerostomia Candidiasis
Median rhomboid glossitis (glossal central papillary atrophy)	*Candida albicans*
Other Changes	
Opportunistic infections: *Candida albicans* and mucormycosis	Repeated use of antibiotics Compromised immune system
Acetone or diabetic breath (seen when the person is close to a diabetic coma)	Ketoacidotic state
Increased incidence of lichen planus (as high as 30%)	Compromised immune system

*Although this is not a complication of diabetes per se, this pattern is seen when the person wants to maintain the weight-loss aspect of diabetes while ignoring or tolerating the hyperglycemic side effects. The patient may not be taking proper insulin doses and may not be truthful when asked about this.

causing the person to select foods that are easy to chew but nutritionally inadequate.

For children and adolescents diagnosed with diabetes, an annual oral exam for early signs of periodontal involvement is recommended starting at the age of 6 years.

Diagnosis and Planning

A dental hygiene care plan focuses on the patient's unmet human needs in the instance of the Human Needs Model, and on the biopsychosocial variables collected using the Oral Health-Related Quality of Life Model (see Chapters 22 and 23). The use of these models for developing a dental hygiene diagnosis and subsequent care plan assists the clinician in managing risks of potential diabetic emergencies, thereby protecting the patient from health risks while maintaining quality of life. Persons with diabetes may not be under good glycemic control, so it is important to check blood glucose levels (see Box 49.8). Appointments should be brief to minimize anxiety and stress and to avoid interference with medication and eating schedules. Morning appointments are ideal because most people with diabetes are best controlled at this time. Two hours after breakfast is best for appointments to avoid the peak action time of medication. Regular (short-acting) insulin, which is often taken in the morning or at each meal, peaks within 2 to 3 hours after the injection. Oral hypoglycemic agents do not cause peaks.

Periodontal debridement is postponed for people with uncontrolled diabetes (i.e., blood glucose levels of <70 mg/dL or >200 mg/dL) until glycemic control is improved.[19] After an assessment for oral infection, periodontal disease, and dental caries to identify possible interactions with glycemic control that need to be reported, patients should be referred to the primary healthcare provider of record for systemic evaluation. Dental hygiene care should not begin until the diabetic condition is controlled. The short-term risk for infections in persons with diabetes has been shown to increase with average blood glucose levels of 200 to 230 mg/dL.[19] When care is planned, interventions are likely to include the following:

- Health status monitoring
- Emphasis on self-care and oral biofilm control

- Preventive and nonsurgical periodontal interventions
- Nutritional and dietary analysis (see Chapter 36)
- Fluoride and chlorhexidine therapies (see Chapter 19)
- Salivary replacement therapy as needed
- A longer initial appointment, a reevaluation appointment, and frequent periodontal maintenance intervals
- Collaboration with the patient's primary healthcare provider and a certified diabetes educator or nutritionist (see Box 49.5)

See Box 49.11 for patient or client education tips. A Critical Thinking Exercise and a sample dental hygiene care plan are shown in the accompanying box.

BOX 49.11 Patient or Client Education Tips

- Emphasize that patients with diabetes are at increased risk for periodontitis.[7]
- Relate the greater risk of infection and increased healing times of the patient with diabetes to the need for oral biofilm control.
- Inform the patient with diabetes and periodontal disease that their glycemic control may be more difficult and that they are at higher risk for other complications such as cardiovascular and kidney disease.[7]
- Teach the use of daily subgingival irrigation for the target delivery of an antimicrobial agent or the twice-daily use of an American Dental Association (ADA)–accepted antimicrobial mouth rinse; the use of an antiplaque and antigingivitis dentifrice; the use of caries-control products (e.g., fluoride mouth rinse, xylitol mints and chewing gum, calcium- and phosphorus-based products); and the use of saliva replacement therapy (e.g., artificial saliva, sucking on ice chips, xylitol gum and mints).
- Discuss the maintenance of dentition for chewing healthy foods and the fact that diet and nutrition are essential to diabetes control.
- Emphasize that individuals with diabetes may not tolerate dentures because of their oral conditions.
- Stress meticulous daily oral biofilm removal as a method to control oral disease progression and diabetes. Oral health contributes significantly to long-term systemic health in the patient with diabetes.

CRITICAL THINKING EXERCISE

Read the following scenario and dental hygiene care plan, and then answer the questions that follow.

Patient Case With Diabetes

Venessa Johnson is a 40-year-old executive assistant secretary who is employed full-time at a large university. She has had type 1 diabetes for 20 years. Venessa has been using an insulin pump for 2 years, and this drug delivery modality has greatly lowered her blood glucose levels. Her 24-hour blood sugar test results average 180 mL/dL, and her 3-month A1c level was 8%. Venessa walks the family dog at a fast pace every evening for 30 minutes. She is embarrassed that she has not been careful about eating a nutritionally balanced diet for the last year and a half. During Venessa's examination, the dental hygienist notes a low risk for dental caries and generalized moderate gingival inflammation and bleeding on probing, with localized 4- and 5-mm pocket depths in the molar areas.

- What changes would you make, if any, to the following dental hygiene care plan?
- What emergency would you prepare for when treating this patient? What steps would you take to prevent this emergency?
- **Develop a detailed self-care plan for this patient before reviewing the sample care plan that follows and compare the two.***

Dental Hygiene Diagnosis	Goal or Expected Behavior
Unmet need for conceptualization and problem solving	By 12/1, patient explains the role of oral biofilm in causing periodontal disease.
Unmet need for responsibility for oral health	By 12/1, patient verbalizes the role of oral infection in glycemic control.
Unmet need for skin and mucous membrane integrity	By 1/1, patient decreases bleeding points by 75%.
	By 1/1, patient reports improvement in hyperglycemia through the control of periodontal disease.

Dental Hygiene Interventions

1. Present "bleeding gums" as an indicator of a bacterial infection that further complicates glycemic control; explain diabetes as a risk factor for periodontal disease.
2. Demonstrate oral biofilm control measures.
3. Discuss antimicrobial agents for the control of plaque and inflammation and the technique for their application.
4. Scale and root debride with ultrasonic and hand instrumentation.
5. Consult with the dentist regarding possible systemic doxycycline therapy.

CRITICAL THINKING EXERCISE—cont'd

6. Monitor the patient's oral health behavior through frequent evaluation.
7. Schedule followup evaluation.

Evaluative Statements

1. Patient explains the two-way relationship of diabetic control and periodontal infection. Goal met.
2. Patient demonstrates oral health behavior congruent with the maintenance of glycemic control. Goal met.
3. Patient decreases gingival bleeding by 75% to enhance glycemic control. Goal met.

Dental Hygiene Diagnosis	Goal or Expected Behavior
• Periodontitis with active inflammation	By 2/1, patient verbalizes the need for adequate nutrition.
• In the context of human needs theory, unmet need for skin and mucous membrane integrity of the head and neck	By 2/1, patient participates in dietary counseling.
• Undernutrition and increased frequency of carbohydrate consumption	By 4/1, patient increases nutrients in the diet.

Dental Hygiene Interventions

1. Relate nutritional needs for diabetes control and integrity of the periodontium.
2. Relate the frequency of eating to the need for oral biofilm control.
3. Relate the importance of a healthy dentition and periodontium to optimal diet consumption and glycemic control.
4. Design oral biofilm control measures that are consistent with the patient's frequency of carbohydrate consumption.
5. Refer the patient to a certified diabetes educator for dietary prescription and meal planning.

Evaluative Statements

1. Patient reports normal blood glucose levels and 1% point reduction in A1c level. Goal met.
2. Patient indicates compliance with individual dietary prescription and meal plan. Goal met.

* Chapters 22 and 23 walk the reader through Case Study 22.1 (patient is a 27-year-old recently diagnosed with type 2 diabetes) using both the Human Needs Model and the Oral Health-Related Quality of Life Model.

Implementation

Periodontal Debridement and Preventive Interventions

The mechanical removal of hard and soft deposits and bacterial toxins from tooth crown and root surfaces is critical to the prevention of periodontal infection in people with diabetes and has been shown to improve diabetic control in people with type 2 diabetes, in combination with sustained effective homecare.

Severe periodontitis is associated with poor glycemic control and increased A1c; therefore severe periodontitis may be a risk factor in the onset of diabetes. Thorough periodontal therapy is indicated in patients with diabetes and periodontitis to enhance control of both diseases.

Increased glucose in gingival crevicular fluid may result in the proliferation of oral microflora, thus increasing periodontal disease and dental caries risk. The short-term (i.e., 3 to 4 months) response to nonsurgical periodontal therapy in probing depths, bleeding on probing, attachment levels, and subgingival microbiota in patients with diabetes appears to be equivalent to the response seen in patients without diabetes; however, patients with poorly controlled diabetes have more rapid clinical attachment loss and a compromised long-term response. Five years after nonsurgical periodontal therapy and surgical periodontal treatment in combination with regular periodontal maintenance therapy, patients with diabetes who were well controlled had clinical attachment levels similar to those of patients without diabetes.[7] In patients with diabetes, the addition of professionally administered controlled-release local antimicrobials as an adjunct to scaling and root planing (see Chapter 27) may lead to additional benefits in probing depth reduction and clinical attachment loss gain, especially in deep sites and patients with well-controlled diabetes.

A patient with well-controlled diabetes with no evidence of infection does not require prophylactic antibiotic premedication. In fact, antibiotic use in patients with diabetes may lead to oral or systemic fungal infections. If an acute or purulent infection is present either preoperatively or postoperatively, antibiotic therapy is mandatory. Prophylactic antibiotics before periodontal instrumentation should be considered for the patient with uncontrolled diabetes after consultation with the patient's physician.

Diabetic microangiopathy causes blindness and kidney disease. Therefore a patient who reports eye disorders may also have kidney disease. Medications that are excreted by the kidney may be retained in the body of the patient with diabetes who also has kidney disease, thereby causing toxic effects. When local anesthetic agents are administered, the minimal use of vasoconstrictors is required because epinephrine is capable of raising blood glucose.

Evaluation and Documentation

The periodontal tissues of the patient with well-controlled diabetes respond positively to nonsurgical periodontal therapy. However, delayed healing may indicate hyperglycemia, which decreases the normal healing actions of leukocyte phagocytosis, chemotaxis, and adherence properties. Frequent oral assessments, periodontal maintenance, the evaluation of the patient's response to dental hygiene care, and the monitoring of diabetic control with current A1c test results are recommended.

It is a legal requirement of all healthcare providers to accurately record in the patient's record all data collected, the treatment planned, services provided, and recommendations and other information related to patient care and treatment. All relevant information and interactions between the patient and the practitioner need to be recorded objectively to enhance interprofessional communication and to promote risk management. See Box 49.12.

DIABETIC EMERGENCIES (SEE CHAPTER 11)

Individuals with uncontrolled diabetes have an increased risk of the following medical emergencies:

- Coma
- Hypoglycemia
- Ketoacidotic hyperglycemia
- Nonketotic hyperosmolar hyperglycemia
- Lactic acidosis
- Uremia
- Nondiabetic coma
- Infection
- Myocardial infarction
- Stroke
- Emergency surgery

The occurrence of stupor or coma in patients with diabetes results from several causes. For example, the diabetic condition may be undiagnosed, or the person with type 1 disease may not have followed the

BOX 49.12   Legal, Ethical, and Safety Issues and Interprofessional Collaboration

- Monitor diabetic glycemic status at each appointment.
- Be prepared to manage a diabetic medical emergency should one arise.
- Inform patients that their role in control of diabetes and periodontal disease are related to one another and to self-care.
- Document and record all assessment data, care planned, appropriate therapeutic and preventive therapy, and discussion with the patient and other healthcare providers.
- Collaborate with the patient's primary healthcare provider or endocrinologist when infection is present, signs of blood tests monitoring metabolic control are abnormal, or healing is delayed after periodontal instrumentation.
- Collaborate with a certified diabetes educator, health education consultant, nutritionist, or staff at hospital-based diabetes management centers.
- Dental hygienists can collaborate with diabetes management centers, for example, by sharing their expertise in the area of oral disease prevention and by providing patient education, oral health screenings, and referrals.

required insulin regimen. Stress, infection, and an increased level of activity contribute to an emergency situation.

Hypoglycemia (Box 49.13)

Hypoglycemia (i.e., a blood glucose concentration of <70 mg/dL) is the most common metabolic emergency in persons with type 1 diabetes (Table 49.5); it results from an excess of insulin and a glucose deficiency in the body. A blood glucose concentration of 80 to 130 mg/dL is the target range for nonpregnant adults with diabetes.[17] Each year, severe episodes affect approximately 20% of diabetic individuals; minor episodes occur every 2 weeks on average in each insulin-treated person. In patients with type 2 disease who are treated with sulfonylurea agents, hypoglycemia is more common than is generally recognized, and it may be severe, especially among older persons treated with longer-acting agents. Alterations in dental hygiene care for older adults with diabetes are outlined in Box 49.14. Hypoglycemia signs and symptoms result from a lack of glucose in the brain and compensation by the nervous system for this lack (see Box 49.13). Main causes of hypoglycemia in persons with type 1 disease are listed in Table 49.6.

Individuals with diabetes can manage mild hypoglycemia themselves by ingesting glucose, sweet drinks, or milk. Between 10 and 20 g of glucose (i.e., about the amount in an 8-ounce glass of 2% fat milk, a 4-ounce glass of orange juice, 3 pieces of hard candy, or 8 Life Savers candies) is generally adequate, although many persons take considerably more because they fear prolonged hypoglycemia. More severe hypoglycemia can also be treated via the oral ingestion of carbohydrates, but another person may have to administer the carbohydrates. If the victim is unconscious, treatment requires intravenous dextrose solution or an intramuscular injection of 0.5 mg to 1.0 mg glucagon; this should be followed on awakening by oral complex carbohydrates with a protein source (e.g., a small meat or cheese sandwich, cottage cheese and fruit).

Hyperglycemic Ketoacidotic Coma (Diabetic Coma) (Box 49.15)

Diabetic deaths caused by hyperglycemia ketoacidotic coma currently represent 1% of adults with type 1 diabetes and are higher among younger individuals. Prevention is the best treatment; however, emergency treatment requires hospitalization.

Coma that results from absolute lack of insulin is found in persons with acute-onset type 1 diabetes in whom diagnosis was unknown or delayed and in individuals with known diabetes who discontinued or

BOX 49.13   Identification and Treatment of Hypoglycemia in the Dental Office

Signs and Symptoms of Hypoglycemia
Shakiness
Anxiety
Sweating
Hunger
Dizziness
Confusion
Irritability
Tachycardia
Pale skin
Blood glucose level of less than 70 mg/dL
Loss of consciousness, seizure, or coma (in severe cases)

General Principles
Treatment for hypoglycemia should be initiated as soon as possible, and staff members should not wait for laboratory results or for a response from a physician.

If the blood glucose levels are extremely low (e.g., less than 40 mg/dL), a transfer for medical evaluation may be needed, as blood should be drawn and sent to the laboratory for accurate blood glucose level measurement because the precision of glucometers is low at extremely low blood glucose levels.

Conscious Hypoglycemic Patient
Treat with 15 g of simple carbohydrates
- 4 ounces of regular fruit juice
- 3 to 4 glucose tablets or gel tube
Hard candies, jelly beans, or gumdrops (check package equivalence to 15 g carbohydrates)
Repeat finger-stick glucose test in 15 minutes.

If the blood glucose level is more than 70 mg/dL, the patient should be asked to eat a meal if it is close to mealtime. If it is not close to mealtime, a mixed snack that includes carbohydrates, proteins, and fat (e.g., peanut butter and jelly sandwich or graham crackers with peanut butter, or milk and crackers) should be given to maintain the blood glucose level. A pure carbohydrate snack will cause the patient to revert back to hypoglycemia quickly. Proteins and carbohydrates in the snack provide sustained glucose release.

If the blood glucose level is less than 70 mg/dL, repeat treatment of 15 g of simple carbohydrates and check the blood glucose level in 15 minutes. Continue this protocol until the blood glucose level is higher than 70 mg/dL and then follow with a mixed snack.

Ask the patient to discuss the hypoglycemia with the physician who is managing their diabetes.

Unconscious Hypoglycemic Patient or Patient Unable to Consume Oral Carbohydrate
Call EMS.

With Intravenous Access
Administer 10 to 25 g of 50% dextrose immediately; it will be followed by quick recovery.
Notify patient's physician immediately.

Without Intravenous Access
Apply glucose gel inside the mouth in a semiobtundent patient or treat with 1 mg of glucagon intramuscularly or subcutaneously; the patient should regain consciousness in 15 to 20 minutes.
Repeat the blood glucose test in 15 minutes.
Establish intravenous access and notify the patient's physician immediately.

Thome, J. Byon, D. Addressing hypoglycemic emergencies. *US Pharm.* 2018;43(10):HS2–HS6.

TABLE 49.5 Hypoglycemia Compared With Hyperglycemia

Signs and Symptoms	Hypoglycemia (<70 mg/dL)	Hyperglycemia (400–600 mg/dL)
Onset	Rapid (minutes)	Slow (days to weeks)
Thirst	Absent	Increased
Nausea and vomiting	Absent	Frequent
Vision	Double	Dim
Respirations	Normal	Difficult; hyperventilation
Skin	Moist, pale	Hot, dry, flushed
Tremors	Frequent	Absent
Blood pressure	Normal	Hypotension

decreased their insulin dose for some reason. Coma from a temporary lack of insulin may be caused by infection or stressful situations in which there is an increase in the secretion of antiinsulin hormones (i.e., glucagon, cortisol, and catecholamine; see Box 49.15). Infection is the most common precipitating factor, and it is present in more than 50% of all persons with DKA coma.

A series of biochemical events explains the basis of severe ketoacidosis, the signs and symptoms of which are presented in Table 49.7. Clear guidelines for maintaining control should be provided to the diabetic patient with infection to resolve the infection early (Box 49.16).

Diabetic ketoacidosis treatment requires hospitalization to restore the disturbed metabolic fluid and electrolyte state to normal. Fluid rehydration (i.e., salt and water), insulin, potassium, broad-spectrum antibiotic therapy, and the treatment of precipitating factors are the main elements of diabetic coma treatment.

BOX 49.14 Alterations in the Dental Hygiene Care of Older Adults With Diabetes

Potential Risks Related to Dental Hygiene Care

In older adult with controlled diabetes:
- Infection
- Poor wound healing

In older adult being treated with insulin:
- Insulin reaction

In older adult with poorly controlled diabetes:
- Early onset of complications related to cardiovascular system, eyes, kidneys, nervous system, angina, myocardial infarction, cerebrovascular accident, renal failure, peripheral neuropathy, blindness, hypertension, or congestive heart failure

Prevention of Medical Complications

Detection via the following:
- Health history
- Clinical findings
- Screening blood sugar
- Referral for medical diagnosis

Older adult receiving insulin:
- Prevent insulin reaction.
- Advise older adults to eat normal meals before appointments.
- Schedule appointments in the morning or the midmorning.
- Advise older adults to inform you of any symptoms of insulin reactions when they first occur.
- Have sugar in some form to give if an insulin reaction occurs.
- Older adults with diabetes who are being treated with insulin and who develop oral infections may require an increase in insulin dosage; consult

with a physician, in addition to performing local and systemic aggressive management of infection (Box 49.14).

Drug considerations:
- Insulin: insulin reaction
- Hypoglycemic agents: on rare occasions, aplastic anemia and similar conditions may occur
- In severe diabetics, avoid general anesthesia.

Dental Hygiene Care Plan Modifications

For older patients with well-controlled diabetes, no alteration of dental hygiene care plan is indicated unless complications of diabetes are present, such as the following:
- Hypertension
- Congestive heart failure
- Myocardial infarction
- Angina
- Renal failure

Oral Complications
- Accelerated periodontal disease
- Periodontal abscesses
- Oral ulcerations and opportunistic infections
- Numbness, burning, or pain in the oral tissues
- Xerostomia
- Glossodynia
- Prolonged healing

Data from Little JW, Falace DA, Rhodus NL. *Dental Management of the Medically Compromised Patient.* 9th ed. Mosby; 2017. Box prepared by Pamela P. Brangan.

TABLE 49.6   Causes of Hypoglycemia in Individuals With Type 1 Diabetes Mellitus

Factor	Cause
Insulin	Inappropriate insulin regimens
	Day-to-day variability in absorption
	Insulin antibodies
	Inappropriate site rotation
	Factitious hypoglycemia
	Renal failure
Food	Delayed intake
	Decreased intake
Exercise	Increased energy requirements
	Increased insulin absorption
Other	Impaired counterregulation
	Liver disease
	Hypoendocrine states
	Alcohol
	Potentiating drugs
	Hypoglycemic unawareness (absence of signs and symptoms, long-standing diabetes, autonomic neuropathy)

BOX 49.15   Causes of Hyperglycemic Ketoacidotic Coma

Absolute Insulin Deficiency
- Newly diagnosed type 1 diabetes with beta-cell depletion
- Incorrect insulin dose (omitted or decreased)

Relative Insulin Deficiency
- Stress states
- Infection
- Myocardial infarction
- Trauma
- Cerebrovascular accident

Drugs and Endocrine Disorders
- Steroids
- Adrenergic agonists
- Hyperthyroidism
- Pheochromocytoma
- Thiazide diuretics

TABLE 49.7   Features of Severe Diabetic Ketoacidosis

Features	Possible Causes
Symptoms	
Thirst	Dehydration
Polyuria	Hyperglycemia, osmotic diuresis
Fatigue	Dehydration, protein loss
Weight loss	Dehydration, protein loss, catabolism*
Anorexia	Depression*
Nausea, vomiting	Ketones,* gastric stasis, ileus
Abdominal pain	Gastric stasis,* ileus, electrolyte deficiency*
Muscle cramps	Potassium deficiency*
Signs	
Hyperventilation	Acidemia
Dehydration	Osmotic diuresis, vomiting
Tachycardia	Dehydration
Hypotension	Dehydration, acidemia
Warm, dry skin	Acidemia (peripheral vasodilation)
Hypothermia	Acidemia-induced peripheral vasodilation (when infection is present)
Impaired consciousness or coma	Hyperosmolality
Ketotic breath	Hyperketonemia (acetone)

*Indicates speculated or unknown cause.

BOX 49.16   Guidelines for Maintaining Glycemic Control in Persons With Diabetes

- Perform frequent self-monitoring of blood glucose (at least eight times per day)
- Obtain a regular A1c test twice a year if glycemic control is good, four times a year if treatment or control has changed.
- If not eating normally, replace carbohydrate content of meals and snacks with sugar-containing drinks or milk; ensure adequate fluid intake (2 to 3 L/day).
- If two preceding blood tests show a glucose level of >200 mg/dL (11.1 mmol/L), contact the physician.
- Test for urine ketones if the blood glucose level is >300 mg/dL.
- If vomiting occurs or if the blood glucose level is >300 mg/dL in the presence of positive ketones for >24 hours, call for urgent medical advice.

Risk for infection following treatment has been shown to increase with blood glucose levels of 200 to 230 mg/dL, which is considered a contraindication to safe treatment.

KEY CONCEPTS

- Many people with diabetes do not know that they have the disease.
- Type 2 diabetes can be prevented or delayed with actions taken by the individual who is at risk. Dental hygienists can make a difference and resources are available to help.
- Type 1 diabetes involves about 5% of the diabetic population. These individuals need to take insulin injections or use an insulin pump.
- The presence of certain human leukocyte antigens creates a genetic predisposition for the autoimmune cause of type 1 diabetes.
- Type 2 diabetes affects about 90% to 95% of patients with diabetes. These individuals usually respond well to weight reduction, dietary management, exercise, and oral medications.
- Insulin resistance or a defect in insulin secretion is the cause of type 2 diabetes. The risk of developing type 2 diabetes increases with obesity, age, inactivity, history of gestational diabetes mellitus (GDM), hypertension, and dyslipidemia.
- GDM occurs in 7.8% of pregnancies. Those who are at high risk include females with obesity, a family history of diabetes, or previous GDM.
- GDM usually disappears after birth because the condition is a consequence of the normal anti-insulin effects of pregnancy hormones and the diversion of natural glucose to the fetus.
- Without insulin, glucose remains in the blood (hyperglycemia) rather than being stored or used by the cells to produce energy. The suspicion of diabetes is gleaned from a history of symptoms: glucosuria, polyuria, polydipsia, weight loss, polyphagia, and blurred vision.
- Diabetes causes severe multisystem, long-term complications. Kidney and eye diseases predominate with type 1 diabetes; atherosclerosis predominates with type 2; peripheral nerve disease occurs with both.
- Hypoglycemia, which is the most common emergency in persons with type 1 diabetes, results from insulin excess and glucose deficiency.
- Hyperglycemic ketoacidosis requires hospitalization to correct fluid and electrolyte imbalances.
- Infection is the most common precipitating factor of hyperglycemic ketoacidosis.
- Well-controlled diabetes occurs when the individual's blood glucose level is within the normal range as a result of a careful balance of medication, diet, and exercise.
- Emotional stress (which can be induced in the oral healthcare setting) causes a release of epinephrine, which mobilizes glucose in the body, thereby contributing to a hyperglycemic condition becoming diabetic ketoacidosis (DKA).
- The strict application of oral care protocols increases the chances of achieving good clinical outcomes for individuals with diabetes.
- Dental hygiene care should not be provided when blood glucose levels are less than 70 mg/dL or more than 200 mg/dL.
- When administering local anesthetics, it is recommended to use the lowest dose and lowest concentration of a vasoconstrictor that produces the desired effect, because epinephrine is an insulin antagonist that is capable of raising the blood glucose level. Monitor the patient for signs of hyperglycemia.
- A patient with well-controlled diabetes with no evidence of infection does not require prophylactic antibiotic premedication.

ACKNOWLEDGMENT

The author acknowledges Deborah Blythe Bauman for past contributions to this chapter.

REFERENCES

1. Centers for Disease Control and Prevention. National Diabetes Statistics Report website. Available at: https://www.cdc.gov/diabetes/data/statistics-report/index.html. Accessed July 19, 2022.
2. American Diabetes Association. Classification and diagnosis of diabetes: standards of care in diabetes-2023. *Diabetes Care*. 2023;46(suppl 1):S19–S40.
3. Skyler J, Bakris G, Bonifacio E, et al. Differentiation of diabetes by pathophysiology, natural history, and prognosis. *Diabetes*. 2017;66(2):241–255.
4. Gregory ECW, Ely DM. Trends and characteristics in gestational diabetes: United States, 2016–2020. *Natl Vital Stat Rep*. 2022;71(3).
5. Centers for Disease Control and Prevention. Gestational Diabetes. Available at: https://www.cdc.gov/diabetes/basics/gestational.html. Accessed July 21, 2022.
6. American Diabetes Association. Facilitating positive health behaviors and well-being to improve health outcomes: standards of care in diabetes—2023. *Diabetes Care*. 2023;46(suppl 1):S68–S96.
7. Sanz M, Ceriello A, Buysschaert M, et al. Scientific evidence on the links between periodontal diseases and diabetes: consensus report and guidelines of the joint workshop on periodontal diseases and diabetes by the International Diabetes Federation and the European Federation of Periodontology. *J Clin Periodontol*. 2018;45:138–149.
8. American Diabetes Association. Comprehensive medical evaluation and assessment of comorbidities: standards of care in diabetes—2023. *Diabetes Care*. 2023;46(suppl 1):S49–S67.
9. Stöhr J, Barbaresko J, Neuenschwander M, et al. Bidirectional association between periodontal disease and diabetes mellitus: a systematic review and meta-analysis of cohort studies. *Sci Rep*. 2021;11(1):13686. https://doi.org/10.1038/s41598-021-93062-6.
10. Dicembrini I, Serni L, Monami M, et al. Type 1 diabetes and periodontitis: prevalence and periodontal destruction—a systematic review. *Acta Diabetol*. 2020;57(12):1405–1412. https://doi.org/10.1007/s00592-020-01531-7.
11. Tonetti MS, Greenwell H, Kornman KS. Staging and grading of periodontitis: framework and proposal of a new classification and case definition. *J Periodontol*. 2018;89(suppl 1):S159–S172. https://doi.org/10.1002/JPER.18-0006.
12. American Diabetes Association. The Diabetic Exchange List (Exchange Diet). Available at: https://diabetesed.net/page/_files/THE-DIABETIC-EXCHANGE-LIST.pdf. Accessed December 15, 2022.
13. Dobrow L, Estrada I, Burkholder-Cooley N, Miklavcic J. Potential effectiveness of registered dietitian nutritionists in healthy behavior interventions for managing type 2 diabetes in older adults: a systematic review. *Front Nutr*. 2022;8:737410. https://doi.org/10.3389/fnut.2021.737410.
14. American Diabetes Association. Insulin & Other Injectables. Available at: https://www.diabetes.org/healthy-living/medication-treatments/insulin-other-injectables. Accessed July 31, 2022.
15. American Diabetes Association. Fast Facts: Data and Statistics about Diabetes. Available at: https://professional.diabetes.org/sites/professional.diabetes.org/files/media/sci_2020_diabetes_fast_facts_sheet_final.pdf. Accessed July 27, 2022.
16. American Diabetes Association. Practice Guidelines Resources. Available at: https://professional.diabetes.org/content-page/practice-guidelines-resources. Accessed December 15, 2022.
17. American Diabetes Association. Glycemic targets: standards of care in diabetes-2023. *Diabetes Care*. 2023;46(suppl 1):S97–S110.
18. Fang M, Wang D, Coresh J, Selvin E. Trends in diabetes treatment and control in U.S. adults, 1999–2018. *N Engl J Med*. 2021;384:2219–2228.
19. Little JW, Falace DA, Miller CS, et al. *Dental Management of the Medically Compromised Patient*. 9th ed. Elsevier; 2018.

50

Cancer

Joan M. Davis and Matthew Greaves

PROFESSIONAL OPPORTUNITIES

Dental hygienists encounter patients with cancer or a history of cancer on a regular basis. The dental hygienist must understand cancer risk factors, treatments, oral complications of treatment, and how the dental hygienist can provide oral healthcare before, during, and following cancer treatment as a part of the interprofessional healthcare team.

COMPETENCIES

1. Explain the incidence of cancer and oral cancer, as well as the risk factors and common signs and symptoms.
2. Describe various forms of cancer therapy.
3. Discuss various oral complications from cancer treatment, including complications specific to chemotherapy, the rationale for bisphosphonate use, and the potential for osteonecrosis.
4. Explain the dental hygiene process of care for patients with cancer before, during, and after cancer therapy in collaboration with the interprofessional oncology team.

INTRODUCTION

Dental hygienists must be prepared to provide care for patients who have recently been diagnosed with cancer, are about to receive treatment, or are cancer survivors. In the United States, there are more than 1.9 million new cancer cases each year and an estimated 18.5 million cancer survivors.[1] A well-prepared dental hygienist will need to understand the oral, physical, and psychologic issues surrounding a patient who is currently battling cancer or who has survived it.

Cancer is not a single disease but rather, a broad classification of more than 100 types of diseases. A malignant neoplasm, or cancer, is the abnormal and unrestricted growth of cells that destroy surrounding healthy tissue and can **metastasize**, or spread, to distant sites. In contrast, a benign neoplasm or benign tumor usually grows slowly, does not invade surrounding tissue, and is encapsulated. The treatment of cancer is known as oncology and often involves extensive collaboration among multiple healthcare, dental, and social service professionals.

CANCER

Incidence

To many people, a cancer diagnosis evokes immediate fear of suffering and death. Fortunately, there has been a 32% drop in cancer deaths attributed primarily to a reduction in smoking and improvements in early detection and treatment.[2] Fig. 50.1 lists the leading types of new cancer cases and deaths according to the American Cancer Society

2022 estimates. Of the estimated 609,360 deaths annually from cancer, 130,180 deaths are caused by cigarette smoking. Health behavior changes, including discontinuing all tobacco products, good nutrition, increased physical activity, regular protection from the sun, and certain vaccinations, could reduce the estimated 805,600 new cancer cases by 42%. Of the new cancer cases each year, approximately 87% occur in people who are 55 years and older.[3] Health disparities, or limited access to preventive and healthcare services, continue to have a negative impact on cancer incidence, prevalence, morbidity, and mortality for some members of racial and ethnic minority groups (Table 50.1).[4] Other factors such as geographic location, income, education level, and a higher incidence of negative health behaviors can also disproportionately affect cancer prevention, detection, and treatment.

Risk Factors

Carcinogenic, or cancer-causing, influences may be environmental, behavioral, viral, or genetic, resulting in potential genetic damage and abnormal cell growth. The US National Cancer Institute clearly implicates tobacco use (primarily smoked) as the single major cause of preventable cancer deaths (see Chapter 37).[4] Other environmental carcinogenic agents include excessive alcohol use, chemical exposure, radon, radiation, sunlight, and asbestos. There is also evidence that certain viruses and bacteria (e.g., hepatitis B virus, human immunodeficiency virus, and *Helicobacter pylori*) may be associated with the development of cancers, especially cancers of the liver, nasopharynx, cervix, and lymphatic system.[3] In recent years, the human papillomavirus (HPV) has been identified as the primary causative agent for oropharyngeal and cervical cancers.

Common Signs and Symptoms

During the early stages, most cancers exhibit no symptoms. Box 50.1 lists the most common presenting signs and symptoms of early cancers.

> ### BOX 50.1 Early Signs and Symptoms of Cancer
>
> - Changes in bowel or bladder habits
> - A sore that does not heal
> - Unusual bleeding or discharge
> - Thickening or a lump in the breast or elsewhere
> - Indigestion or difficulty swallowing
> - Obvious changes in a wart or mole
> - Nagging cough or hoarseness

From the American Cancer Society. Cancer Facts and Figures 2022. https://www.cancer.org/content/dam/cancer-org/research/cancer-facts-and-statistics/annual-cancer-facts-and-figures/2022/2022-cancer-facts-and-figures.pdf. Accessed July 8, 2022.

Male

Prostate	268,490	27%
Lung & bronchus	117,910	12%
Colon & rectum	80,690	8%
Urinary bladder	61,700	6%
Melanoma of the skin	57,180	6%
Kidney & renal pelvis	50,290	5%
Non-Hodgkin lymphoma	44,120	4%
Oral cavity & pharynx	38,700	4%
Leukemia	35,810	4%
Pancreas	32,970	3%
All sites	**983,160**	

Female

Breast	287,850	31%
Lung & bronchus	118,830	13%
Colon & rectum	70,340	8%
Uterine corpus	65,950	7%
Melanoma of the skin	42,600	5%
Non-Hodgkin lymphoma	36,350	4%
Thyroid	31,940	3%
Pancreas	29,240	3%
Kidney & renal pelvis	28,710	3%
Leukemia	24,840	3%
All sites	**934,870**	

Estimated New Cases

Male

Lung & bronchus	68,820	21%
Prostate	34,500	11%
Colon & rectum	28,400	9%
Pancreas	25,970	8%
Liver & intrahepatic bile duct	20,420	6%
Leukemia	14,020	4%
Esophagus	13,250	4%
Urinary bladder	12,120	4%
Non-Hodgkin lymphoma	11,700	4%
Brain & other nervous system	10,710	3%
All sites	**322,090**	

Female

Lung & bronchus	61,360	21%
Breast	43,250	15%
Colon & rectum	24,180	8%
Pancreas	23,860	8%
Ovary	12,810	4%
Uterine corpus	12,550	4%
Liver & intrahepatic bile duct	10,100	4%
Leukemia	9,980	3%
Non-Hodgkin lymphoma	8,550	3%
Brain & other nervous system	7,570	3%
All sites	**287,270**	

Estimated Deaths

Estimates are rounded to the nearest 10, and cases exclude basal cell and squamous cell skin cancers and in situ carcinoma except urinary bladder. Estimates do not include Puerto Rico or other US territories. Ranking is based on modeled projections and may differ from the most recent observed data.

©2022, American Cancer Society, Inc., Surveillance and Health Equity Science

Fig. 50.1 Leading Sites of New Cancer Cases and Deaths—2022 Estimates (American Cancer Society incidence and deaths by site and sex, 2022 estimates). (From the American Cancer Society. *Cancer Facts and Figures 2022*. Available at: https://www.cancer.org/content/dam/cancer-org/research/cancer-facts-and-statistics/annual-cancer-facts-and-figures/2022/2022-cancer-facts-and-figures.pdf. Accessed July 8, 2022.)

TABLE 50.1   Examples of Cancer Disparities in the United States

Breast Cancer	Kidney Cancer	Liver Cancer	Prostate Cancer	Cervical Cancer
Despite having similar rates of breast cancer, Black/African American females are more likely than White females to die of the disease.	American Indians/Alaska Natives have higher death rates from kidney cancer than any other racial/ethnic group.	Rates of liver cancer are higher among American Indians/Alaska Natives and Asian and Pacific Islanders than those of other racial/ethnic groups.	Black/African American males are twice as likely as White males to die of prostate cancer and continue to have the highest prostate cancer mortality among all US population groups.	Hispanic/Latino and Black/African-American females have higher rates of cervical cancer than females of other racial/ethnic groups, with Black/African American females having the highest rates of death from the disease.

From US Department of Health and Human Services, National Institutes of Health, National Cancer Institute. *Cancer Disparities*. Available at: https://www.cancer.gov/about-cancer/understanding/disparities. Accessed July 8, 2022.

Pain is not often a symptom during the early stages of cancer. A person who has one of the seven common signs of cancer for more than 2 weeks should see a doctor promptly. The **prognosis**, or likely outcome, for a specific cancer is highly variable and depends on the stage (the size of the lesion, whether it has spread to other parts of the body, and the location of the disease when first diagnosed), as well as on genetics and personal health habits. Early detection is a key to survival.

Oral Cavity and Pharyngeal Cancer Incidence and Risk Factors

Oral cancer is a general term that refers to malignant lesions found in the oral tissue. Oral cavity cancers are in the anterior part of the mouth and include the lips, tongue, gingiva, hard palate, and oral cavity. **Oropharyngeal** (sometimes called head and neck) cancers are found in the posterior part of the mouth and include the back third or base of

---

BOX 50.2   Common Signs of Oral Cavity and Pharynx Cancer

- A swelling, lump, growth, or area of induration or hardness anywhere in or about the mouth or neck that is usually painless
- Erythroplakia patch (velvety, deep red)
- Leukoplakia patch (white or red-and-white patch)
- Any sore (ulcer, irritation) that does not heal after 2 weeks
- Ear pain
- Coughing up blood
- Difficulty swallowing or persistent hoarseness

BOX 50.3   Oral Cavity and Pharynx Cancer Risk Factors

- Use of tobacco products (primarily smoked)
- HPV infection of the mouth and throat
- Excessive use of alcohol
- A diet low in fruits and vegetables

From the American Cancer Society. Cancer Facts and Figures 2022. https://www.cancer.org/content/dam/cancer-org/research/cancer-facts-and-statistics/annual-cancer-facts-and-figures/2022/2022-cancer-facts-and-figures.pdf. Accessed July 8, 2022.

---

the tongue, soft palate, lingual and palatine tonsils, and the posterior pharyngeal wall. The American Cancer Society estimates that approximately 54,000 new cases (38,700 males and 15,300 females) of oral cavity and pharyngeal cancer will be diagnosed in the United States in 2022. The incidence rates have seen an increase of approximately 1% per year, primarily among non-Hispanic Whites, associated with HPV-related infections.[3]

It is estimated that 9 of every 10 oral malignancies are squamous cell carcinomas, which often manifest as a painless swelling or lump in the oral cavity or the pharynx and larynx area (Box 50.2). The median age of a person with newly diagnosed oral cancer is 62 years. Of the estimated newly diagnosed US cases in 2022, 7,870 males and 3360 females are expected to die from these cancers. The overall 5-year relative survival rate for oral and pharyngeal cancer is 69% for Whites and 51% for African Americans.[3]

Specific oral cancer risk factors include the use of all tobacco products (i.e., cigarettes, cigars, pipes, smokeless tobacco, and betel quid), excessive alcohol use, age, sun exposure, and a diet low in fruits and vegetables (Box 50.3). Cigarette smokers have approximately 10 times the chance of developing squamous cell carcinoma as compared with people who have never smoked.[5] The risk of developing any type of cancer increases with both the amount and duration of tobacco product use. The US National Institute of Dental and Craniofacial Research reports that persons with a small, localized oral squamous cell cancer lesion have an 83% 5-year survival rate as compared with only a 28% rate among those whose cancer has metastasized to other parts of the body (distant).[6]

The HPV–Oropharyngeal/Head and Neck Cancer Connection

HPV is the most common sexually transmitted infection in the United States and has been identified as a causative agent for almost all cervical cancers, as well as many cancers found in the genital and oropharyngeal area. More than 200 subtypes of HPV have been identified. HPV 16 and 18 are considered carcinogens and pose a high risk in the

---

BOX 50.4   Legal, Ethical, and Safety Issues

You have a 17-year-old patient with a cauliflower-like lesion in the mouth. Consider your ethical responsibilities to the patient. How would the ADHA ethical principles apply to this patient?

---

development of cancerous lesions. The subtypes of HPV that can cause genital warts, a cauliflower-like benign lesion, have not been shown to go on to cause oral cancer.[7]

Of special concern to the dental hygienist is the role high-risk HPV types have in the development of oropharyngeal/head and neck cancers affecting the back of the throat, the base of the tongue, and the tonsil area. While oral cavity cancer has declined overall in the United States, the prevalence of HPV-related oropharyngeal cancers has seen a dramatic increase, going from 16% between 1984 and 1989 to 72% during 2000 to 2004 with approximately 85% to 96% of oropharyngeal cancers caused by HPV-16 infections.[8] Due to the difficulty accessing the oropharyngeal area, it is unclear whether traditional oral cancer screening is effective in identifying this head and neck cancer (see Chapter 16).

The *Gardasil 9* (Merck) vaccine has been shown to be highly effective in preventing HPV 16, 18, 31, 33, 45, 52, and 58 infections, as well as the two HPV viruses that cause most genital warts. The CDC recommends routine vaccination at age 11 or 12 years and the Advisory Committee on Immunization Practices recommends those up to 26 years be vaccinated if inadequately vaccinated in the past.[9] As oral health professionals, we have an ethical obligation to assess whether 11- to 12-year-old females and males have been vaccinated for HPV. Then, as difficult as it may be, the dental professional needs to have a conversation with the youth and parent/guardian (if the patient is a minor) regarding the use of the HPV vaccination to help prevent head and neck cancer. Finally, we need to consider the dental hygienist's role in discussing the use of abstinence, dental dams, and condoms to prevent the transmission of this and other highly communicable sexually transmitted diseases (Box 50.4).

Suspicious Oral Lesion Assessment

The most common sites for oral-cavity squamous cell carcinomas are the lateral borders and ventral surfaces of the tongue and the floor of the mouth. Current American Dental Association Council on Scientific Affairs evidence-based recommendations (see Online Resources box) should be followed for screening protocol for any of the signs and symptoms that persist for more than 2 weeks after the removal of potentially irritating factors. A benign or malignant tumor can be confirmed only by performing a surgical biopsy, the surgical removal of all or part of the lesion, and microscopic evaluation.

CANCER THERAPY

Forms of Cancer Therapy

The choice of cancer treatment is dependent on the type, location, and stage of the cancer as well as the health, age, and treatment preferences of the patient. Advancements in the development of innovative and highly effective therapies have provided more treatment options, often leading to better treatment outcomes. Cancer treatment is increasingly tailored to the individual and may include one or more of the following: transoral laser microsurgery (TLMS), transoral robotic surgery (TORS), traditional surgery, radiotherapy therapy, chemotherapy, immunotherapy, targeted therapy, hormone therapy, stem cell transplant, and precision medicine.[10] The goal of cancer treatment is to remove or destroy the malignant cells, allowing the body to heal.

Surgery involves the physical removal of a cancerous tumor from the body using a scalpel, cryosurgery (extreme cold), lasers (intense beams of light), hyperthermia (extreme heat—an experimental treatment), or photodynamic therapy (the use of drugs to sensitize cells to a specific type of light). Surgery is the treatment of choice for solid tumors that are isolated in one region, such as oral cancer lesions. It may be used as the only form of treatment or a component of multiple cancer treatments to improve outcome. Side effects may include latent pain, numbness, and loss of motion.

Radiation therapy, or radiotherapy, involves a high dose of targeted radiation to kill or shrink tumors by damaging the DNA, rendering the cancer cells unable to reproduce leading to cell death. There are two main types of radiation therapy. External-beam radiation therapy is an external beam of radiation aimed at specific part of the body affected by a cancerous tumor, including oral/head and neck cancers. Internal radiation therapy, or brachytherapy, involves ribbons or capsules containing a radiation source being placed *in* the body near the tumor. Because both healthy and cancerous cells are affected by radiation therapy, patients often experience side effects including fatigue, hair loss, and skin changes. Oral cavity and head and neck cancer radiation therapy can result in osteoradionecrosis, xerostomia, difficulty swallowing, and **mucositis** (mucosal edema, inflammation, and ulcerations).

Chemotherapy is the use of toxic drugs to stop or slow the growth of quickly dividing cancer cells. Cancer drugs can be administered in many ways, including by mouth as pills or liquids, intravenously, by muscular injection, or as a cream rubbed on the skin. Combinations of chemotherapeutic agents have resulted in significant improvements in the cure rates of some cancers. These chemotherapeutic agents often impair bone marrow function, leading to **myelosuppression**: the suppression of the red blood cells, white blood cells, and platelets. Chemotherapy may be used in combination with surgery, radiation, or newer therapies to destroy rapidly dividing cancer cells, thus increasing the chance of a positive outcome.

If a semipermanent catheter or port is surgically inserted to administer chemotherapy, a medical consult with the oncologist may be warranted prior to any dental care because of the possible risk of bacterial endocarditis. Chemotherapy has numerous side effects, including fatigue, diarrhea, nausea, vomiting, constipation, oral infection, mucositis, and pain.

Immunotherapy, using antibody drugs, is an innovative group of cancer therapies that do not directly kill cells but rather, use the patient's own immune system to destroy the cancer cells. Antibody drugs are designed to alter cell receptors, or mark cancer cells, allowing the patient's own antibodies to identify and destroy the malignant cells. Adaptive cell transfer boosts the natural ability of T cells to effectively attach to the cancer cells. The use of cytokines, a normal part of the body's immune system, is another method used to boost the body's own immune response to cancer. The advancement of immunotherapy in the treatment of head and neck cancers, known for their immune suppressive activity, has shown positive results and continues to evolve. Side effects from immunotherapy include skin reactions at the injection site and flulike symptoms including fever, weakness, fatigue, and headache.

Targeted therapy acts by interfering with cellular proteins that support cancerous tumor growth and metastasis. Targeted therapies include the following: boosting the immune system, altering the cancer cell's signals to divide, preventing cells from signaling the body to create a blood supply needed to support cancer cell growth, and altering signals within the cancer cell leading to cell death. This therapy may be more effective when used in combination with chemotherapy and radiation therapy, as cancer cells can become resistant with targeted therapy alone. Side effects include diarrhea, liver dysfunction, and mucositis.

Hormone therapy slows or stops the growth of tumors that depend on hormones, such as breast or prostate cancer, by preventing the production or normal functioning of hormones. A tumor treated with hormone therapy will often shrink, thus increasing the success of surgery or other types of therapy and lessening the chances of the cancer returning. Side effects include hot flashes, weakened bones, nausea, and fatigue.

Stem cell transplantation, sometimes referred to as a bone marrow transplant (BMT), is the placement of the healthy bone marrow into the bone cavity of the cancer patient to restore blood-forming stem cells following chemotherapy or radiation therapy. Several cancers, especially hematologic diseases, are treated with chemotherapy followed by stem cell transplantation, including aplastic anemia, leukemia, lymphoma, neuroblastoma, and immunodeficiency diseases. An immunologic reaction that can occur where the donor's white blood cells react against the host tissue antigens is called **graft-versus-host disease (GVHD)**. This reaction can occur within a few weeks of stem cell transplantation and may include oral mucositis, salivary gland dysfunction or xerostomia (dry mouth), esophageal and vaginal strictures, pulmonary insufficiency, intestinal problems, and chronic liver disease. Viral infections, including herpes simplex virus and fungal infections, are common. See the critical thinking scenario in Box 50.5.

Precision medicine, or personalized medicine, is an approach to cancer therapy based on a genetic assessment of the patient's disease. Scientists and oncologists knew that individuals' responses to cancer therapy varied but did not understand why. Researchers have recently discovered that cancerous tumors contain genetic changes that signal the cancerous cells to grow and spread. Though in the experimental stages, the goal of precision medicine is to identify the tumor's genetic deviations and use target therapy or precision medicine to stop the cancer from growing, spreading, or reccurring.

BOX 50.5 Critical Thinking Scenario A

Profile: Ms. H. is a 23-year-old female who has undergone chemotherapy and radiation for Hodgkin lymphoma. The cancer has not gone into remission.

Chief Complaint: "I have been referred by my oncology team for a dental evaluation and treatment before the next phase of my cancer therapy."

Social History: She is single and has moved back in with her family after the cancer diagnosis.

Health History: She is scheduled for an allogeneic bone marrow transplant. Prior to the transplant, she will receive total body irradiation and chemotherapy. She will enter the bone marrow transplant unit in 3 weeks.

Dental History: She had no dental support during her previous cancer treatment. Her dental evaluation reveals a sensitive maxillary premolar with a large carious lesion and a radiolucent periapical lesion, several areas of mild demineralization, moderate plaque and calculus, and chapped lips. No other gross caries or periodontal disease is evident. There are no impacted teeth or bony lesions detected by radiographs. She has numerous painful oral lesions and is finding it difficult to eat.

Oral Health Behavior Assessment: The patient reports that she tries to brush her teeth once a day, but her mouth is very sore. She does not use any interdental cleaning devices.

Supplemental Notes: She appears motivated to improve her oral hygiene care but is very discouraged over her cancer and how tired the treatments make her.

1. Using the interprofessional collaborative model, explain how the oral health team would actively work with the oncology team to provide the best possible care for this patient.

2. Develop a dental hygiene care plan to be implemented before the bone marrow transplant.

ORAL COMPLICATIONS RELATED TO CANCER THERAPY

Oral side effects from cancer treatment (Box 50.6) can directly affect the patient's ability to complete cancer therapy. Patients experiencing oral pain may not be able to eat or swallow, leading to a weakened state and lowered immune response. Oral pain could be so debilitating that

---

BOX 50.6   Oral Complications of Various Cancer Therapies

- Oral mucositis
- Neurotoxicity
- Infection
- Bleeding or hemorrhage
- Xerostomia or salivary gland dysfunction
- Dental caries or demineralization
- Altered tooth development

Adapted from the US Department of Health and Human Services, National Institutes of Health. Oral Complications of Cancer Treatment: What the Dental Team Can Do, 2009. https://www.nidcr.nih.gov/sites/default/files/2017-09/oral-complications-cancer-oncology-team.pdf. Accessed September 28, 2022.
National Cancer Institute. Oral Complications of Chemotherapy and Head/Neck Radiation (PDQ®)–Health Professional Version. https://www.cancer.gov/about-cancer/treatment/side-effects/mouth-throat/oral-complications-hp-pdq. Accessed September 28, 2022.

---

the patient may choose a less effective dose of cancer therapy, or even delay or stop scheduled treatments altogether. Dental hygienists play a key role in the prevention and management of oral complications (Table 50.2). Early intervention can increase chances of survival and a better quality of life. The US National Institutes of Health formally recognizes the essential role that dentists and dental hygienists play in the overall care of the cancer patient.[10]

Oral mucositis is a common and painful side effect for those undergoing chemotherapy (40%), oral radiation therapy (100%), and stem cell transplant therapy (80%).[10] Though mucositis is a dynamic process, it can be divided into five stages: initiation, primary, damaged response, signal amplification, ulceration, and healing. Mucosal ulcerations from cancer therapy are alike in their clinical presentation (Fig. 50.2). The gingival tissues are particularly vulnerable to mucositis due to the rapid turnover of the epithelial tissues and microtraumas caused by eating, brushing, and poorly fitting dental appliances. In a healthy individual, oral tissues undergo continuous healing and restoration. During cancer therapy, healthy and cancerous cells are damaged, leaving the rapidly turning-over cells with the greatest destruction. Mucositis can increase the risk of oral and systemic infection as well as unpleasant odors, difficulty in talking, and nutritional deficiencies. Gradual resolution of mucositis can be expected once the cancer therapy has been completed.

Box 50.7 summarizes ways to help patients with mouth pain caused by oral mucositis. Meticulous oral hygiene care and a well-hydrated mouth during cancer therapy can possibly prevent or reduce the severity of mucosal ulceration and the risk for oral infection. Toothbrushes

---

TABLE 50.2   Management of Oral Manifestations of Cancer Therapies

Manifestation	Prevention	Palliative Measures and Management	Dental Hygiene Care Guidelines
Mucositis or stomatitis (related to direct effects of radiation therapy and cytotoxic chemotherapy)	These conditions are caused by the toxicity of the cancer therapy Early onset and severity can be minimized by consistent hydration and excellent bacterial plaque control Gentle tooth and gingival brushing with extrasoft toothbrush Discontinue toothpastes with strong, irritating flavoring agents and replace with baking soda and water paste Discontinue alcohol-based rinses, full-strength peroxide, and irritating foods	Increased hydration with water, saliva substitutes, ice chips, or sugar-free popsicles Cool mist humidifiers may be helpful, especially in dry environments Baking soda and water solutions (1 tsp of baking soda, one-half tsp of salt, and 16 oz. of water*) may be used as rinses or placed in a disposable irrigation bag (let the solution flow through the mouth to gently rinse) Topical anesthetics	Do not schedule dental hygiene procedures while the patient is experiencing oral ulcerations and pain
Salivary gland dysfunction or xerostomia (related to direct radiation damage to salivary gland tissue and possible indirect effect of chemotherapeutic agents) Salivary gland dysfunction is permanent after radiation therapy, whereas function usually returns after chemotherapy	Eliminate use of products with alcohol and irritating agents Diminish caffeine intake Discontinue tobacco use Humidify air with cool mist humidifier Consult with oncologist for salivary gland stimulant prescription	Suggest over-the-counter saliva substitutes (see recommendations for patients with xerostomia) Stimulate functional salivary gland tissue by chewing xylitol gum or a wax bolus Consult physician for salivary gland stimulant prescription Lubricate the lips with balm or cream (not pure petrolatum) Increase hydration with water, ice chips, and high-moisture foods Thin foods with liquids Recommend the use of a cool mist humidifier, especially while patient is sleeping Suggest baking soda and water rinsing for ropy saliva (see recommendations for patients with mucositis)	To prevent rampant caries, encourage improved oral hygiene measures, a diet low in sucrose, and fluoride supplementation (e.g., the daily use of 1.1% neutral-pH sodium fluoride gels for 5 to 10 minutes in customized fluoride trays for home use)

TABLE 50.2 Management of Oral Manifestations of Cancer Therapies—cont'd

Manifestation	Prevention	Palliative Measures and Management	Dental Hygiene Care Guidelines
Infection: fungal, viral, and bacterial (related to chemotherapy-induced immunosuppression) Oral infections may not cause typical signs and symptoms Candidiasis is common during radiation therapy	Frequent and consistent oral hydration with water, ices, and saliva substitutes Increase bacterial plaque control Oral infections may be unrelenting when the patient is severely immunosuppressed during chemotherapy	Oral microbiologic culturing and assessment Alert oncologist at first signs of oral infection Encourage use of antifungals that are sugar-free	Do not proceed with dental hygiene procedures while a patient has an acute oral infection Schedule dental hygiene procedures when the patient's absolute neutrophil count is >1000/mm³ If the patient has a central venous catheter, the American Heart Association antibiotic prophylactic protocol should be followed for invasive dental hygiene procedures, including dental prophylaxis
Bleeding (related to chemotherapy-induced myelosuppression)	Bleeding is not preventable, but bacterial plaque can exacerbate the complication if not consistently removed	Refer to oncologist for management	Dental hygiene procedures should be delayed until the patient has a platelet count of >50,000/mm³ or a blood transfusion
Rampant dental caries or demineralization (related to therapy-induced salivary gland dysfunction)	Bacterial plaque control Frequent oral hydration with water, ices, and saliva substitutes Professional application of silver diamine fluoride (SDF) Daily 5- to 10-minute application of 1.1% sodium fluoride gel in custom gel carriers (soft vinyl trays adapted to extend beyond the cervical line of the teeth) or topical fluoride In-office application of fluoride varnish to exposed cementum Dietary guidelines to discourage frequent snacking on cariogenic foods, sugared beverages, or acidic beverages (i.e., diet sodas with citric or phosphoric acid) If there is evidence of dental decay despite daily fluoride application, place patient on 2-week chlorhexidine regimen and in-office fluoride varnish application	Same as prevention measures	Encourage the participation of patient when planning oral hygiene homecare and ensure strict adherence by frequent monitoring Establish a 2- to 3-month continued-care interval until the patient demonstrates the ability to care for their teeth and the acute side effects of therapy have resolved
Trismus or temporomandibular disorder (related to the direct effect of radiation on the muscles of mastication or the temporomandibular joint)	Daily exercise for muscles of mastication: instruct the patient to open and close the mouth 20 times without causing pain to the temporomandibular joint; this should be repeated 3 times a day	Same as prevention measures Instruct patient to encourage further opening of the mouth by placing increasing numbers of tongue blades between posterior teeth for several minutes a day Therabite could also support jaw movement: https://www.atosmedical.us/product/therabite-jaw-motion-rehabilitation-system/	Dental hygiene procedures may need to be altered for patients with trismus to avoid exacerbating the associated pain (e.g., shortened appointments or sedation)
Soft tissue necrosis and osteoradionecrosis (related to the direct effect of radiation on tissue and bone) Tissue becomes hypovascular, hypoxic, and hypocellular; damage to the bone and soft tissue is permanent	All teeth within the field of radiation that have a poor lifelong prognosis should be extracted 14 to 21 days before the initiation of radiation therapy Avoid all surgical insult to irradiated bone throughout the patient's lifetime	Referral to an oral surgeon for possible hyperbaric oxygen therapy and surgical management of the necrotic tissue and bone	Establish a frequent and regular dental hygiene continued-care interval to ensure the prevention of periodontal disease and adherence to the oral hygiene homecare protocol

*The specific formulation for sodium bicarbonate and saline solutions may vary based on desired effect and the source of the formula. Most protocols use topical, frequent (every 4–6 hours) rinsing with approximately 0.9% saline.

should be extra soft, possibly further softened in hot water. Toothpastes with strong flavoring agents should be temporarily discontinued and replaced with a nonirritating paste made from baking soda and water.

If toothbrushing becomes impossible due to painful tissues, the teeth, gingiva, and tongue may be swabbed with gauze that has been moistened in warm water. Glycerin swabs are not effective and should be

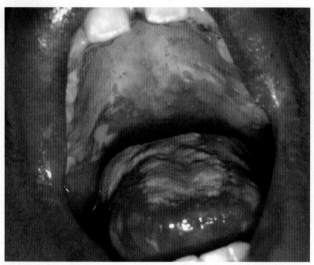

Fig. 50.2 Radiation mucositis. (From Napeñas JJ. Intraoral pain disorders. *Dent Clin North Am.* 2013;57(3):429.)

BOX 50.7 Management of Oral Mucositis

- Early detection and treatment of oral infection
- Good oral hygiene, including tongue brushing, to prevent further infection
- Frequent irrigation with one-fourth tsp of baking soda, one-fourth tsp of salt, and 32 oz. of water (1 qt)
- Frequent rinsing with sodium bicarbonate mouth rinses and nonalcoholic mouth rinses (e.g., Biotene or Spry Alcohol-Free mouthwash)
- Daily cleaning of dentures and changing of soaking solution; removal of dentures while sleeping
- Use of prescribed topical anesthetics with caution to avoid anesthetizing the soft palate, which could cause food aspiration; excessive use may potentiate mucositis
- Use of over-the-counter or prescribed systemic analgesics if necessary
- Avoidance of irritating or rough-textured foods
- Use of perioral moisturizers as directed by the radiation oncologist

Adapted from the US Department of Health and Human Services, National Institutes of Dental and Craniofacial Research. https://www.nidcr.nih.gov/health-info/cancer-treatments. Accessed September 28, 2022.
Centers for Disease Control and Prevention. Oral Mucositis Staging: Mucositis. https://www.cdc.gov/nchs/ppt/icd9/att_mucositis_sep05.ppt. Accessed September 28, 2022.

---

avoided. Dental flossing should be continued as long as possible and resumed as soon as the mucositis resolves.

Commercial mouthwashes with alcohol or phenol should be avoided because of their drying and/or irritating effects. Alcohol-free chlorhexidine rinse has been shown to aid in the prevention and reduction of symptoms associated with oral mucositis. The US National Cancer Institute recommends swishing with bland rinses such as a 0.9% normal saline and/or sodium bicarbonate solutions, such as one-fourth tsp salt, one-fourth tsp baking soda, 1 quart of warm water, then rinse with plain warm water three or four times a day.[10,11] In addition to the soothing, bland rinses, topical anesthetics (sprays and gels), coating agents (antacid solutions), and cellulose film–forming covering agents (Table 50.3) can provide temporary relief. All patients, especially children and their parents, should be cautioned that topical anesthetic agents may anesthetize the soft palate and the epiglottis, potentially causing aspiration of food. Some patients may require systemic analgesics and occasionally narcotics to control mucositis pain. See the Critical Thinking Scenario in Box 50.8.

Oral infection can result from bone marrow suppression, or myelosuppression, caused by cancer therapies including chemotherapy, radiation therapy, or immunotherapy. During these periods, the patient is at risk for developing localized or systemic fungal, viral, and bacterial infections. These infections may increase the risk of developing septicemia and the risk of death in patients with profound immunosuppression.[10-12] The fungal organism *Candida albicans* is most often implicated in the development of cancer-related oral infection.

Antibiotic prophylaxis before dental treatment may be required to prevent bacterial endocarditis if the patient has an implanted central venous catheter chemotherapy port. Although no data are currently available to document the absolute need for prophylactic antibiotics in this patient population, it is recommended that the oncology team be consulted prior to dental care.

Patients with dentures or partials should be evaluated frequently during cancer therapy to minimize potential trauma due to ill-fitting appliances. Oral tissues may change significantly during chemotherapy because of edema, inflammation, ulceration, or weight loss. Patients should be advised to remove the appliance if trauma or pain is experienced and to seek dental care to avoid further trauma. Early detection and the treatment of any oral infection is imperative to prevent the worsening of mucositis that may lead to the interruption of cancer therapy.

Salivary gland dysfunction occurs when a cancer therapy damages the salivary glands, resulting in xerostomia (dryness of the mouth), ropy saliva, or the absence of saliva. Although chemotherapy or immunotherapy patients may experience xerostomia, salivary gland exposure to head and neck radiation therapy is unavoidable. During treatment, the glands are near the lymphatic system and cannot be shielded or protected. Ionizing radiation causes fibrosis and atrophy of the salivary gland tissue, leading to a change in salivary flow within the first week of radiation therapy. Because the irradiated salivary glands are permanently damaged, the change in both the quality and the quantity of saliva often does not improve. The lack of adequate saliva increases the risk of caries, infection, bleeding, loss of the ability to speak, and **dysphagia**, or difficulty chewing or swallowing food. Patients who report salivary dysfunction should be offered **palliative** measures, relieving discomfort without directly treating the condition. In addition, the lips should be lubricated with a moisturizing lip balm or cream that is recommended by the radiation oncologist (Box 50.9).

Alteration or loss of taste can occur with chemotherapy, radiation therapy, or other modes of cancer therapy. When the tongue is in the field of radiation therapy, the patient experiences partial or full taste loss. The loss of taste is a significant side effect of radiation therapy. Patients complain that all food tastes like mush or straw and must force themselves to eat to maintain their nutritional status (Box 50.10). Healthcare providers may notice patients' shift towards softer, processed foods due to relative ease in chewing and increased ability to provide convenient and more flavored food options in the presence of decreased or altered taste. These dietary changes can lead to increased plaque formation and likelihood of tooth decay. For many, taste returns a few months after the completion of radiation therapy but may be altered from its preradiation status.

Complications Specific to Chemotherapy

Neurotoxicity, damage to nervous tissue caused by toxic substances, may occur with chemotherapeutic agents that are derived from plant alkaloids (e.g., vincristine) and are toxic to not only cancer cells but also healthy nerve tissue. As a result, a patient may report severe, deep, and often bilateral odontogenic-like pain. When no dental pathology can be found, nerve damage from the cancer drug may be the cause. The pain often subsides within a few days after the administration of the chemotherapeutic agent.

Hemorrhage during chemotherapy may be the result of thrombocytopenia (the reduction of platelets) due to myelosuppression. Patients with platelet counts of less than 75,000/mm^3 may experience oral hemorrhaging (bleeding) during invasive dental and dental hygiene procedures.[10,12] If at all possible, dental and dental hygiene care should be completed prior to chemotherapy. If dental care is required during chemotherapy, the attending oncologist should be consulted regarding the status of the patient's blood counts. The patient should also be warned that trauma from improper toothbrushing or a poorly fitting dental prosthesis may cause bleeding when platelet levels are low.

Bisphosphonates and Medication-Related Osteonecrosis of the Jaw

Patients diagnosed with multiple myeloma, breast, thyroid, lung, or prostate cancer may experience metastatic lesions or tumors that spread to the bones. Cancerous bone lesions can lead to extreme pain, potential bone fractures, and hypercalcemia, excess calcium in the blood. To lessen these conditions, oncologists may administer bisphosphonates, a class of drugs that inhibit the ability of osteoclasts to resorb, suppressing bone turnover. As a result, bisphosphonates

stabilize the skeletal matrix and reduce the formation of solid cancerous tumors and potential bone fractures. The **half-life** of bisphosphonates, or the time required for a medication to lose half of the initial effect in the body, can last as long as 10 or more years following administration.[13] In addition, bisphosphonates can be prescribed in pill form (e.g., alendronate sodium [Fosamax], risedronate sodium [Actonel], ibandronate sodium [Boniva]) to treat osteoporosis and Paget disease of the bone. They act by slowing bone loss while increasing bone density.

Less than 5% of cancer patients receiving intravenously administered bisphosphonate and to a lesser extent the drug in pill form develop a condition called medication-related osteonecrosis of the jaw (MRONJ).[13] This often painful intraoral or extraoral lesion may resemble an osteoradionecrosis lesion caused by radiation treatment. MRONJ presents as an irregular ulceration with exposed necrotic bone (Fig. 50.3). Bisphosphonate-related bone death in the mandible or maxilla is believed to occur because of conditions that are unique to the oral cavity. The mouth, unlike the rest of the body, is constantly being assaulted with small traumas through mastication, ill-fitting appliances, and oral infections (e.g., periodontitis or apical abscesses) that are bathed in microbe-laden saliva and plaque.

TABLE 50.3 Oral Hygiene Products Used During Cancer Therapy

Product	Description	Indication, Rationale, or Use	Precautions
Toothbrushes	Several are available with extrasoft or super-soft bristles, such as Rx Ultra Suave (PHB, Inc, www.phbdirect.com); Biotene SuperSoft (Laclede, Inc, www.laclede.com); Colgate Extrasoft (www.colgatetotal.com/Toothbrushes); and Oral-B Sensi Soft (https://oralb.com/en-us/products/toothbrushes/manual-toothbrushes/). A child-sized brush may be helpful for patients with limited mouth opening. Some brushes are available with suctioning capabilities. (Possible alternative: sponge toothbrushes only when a regular toothbrush is not feasible)	Plaque biofilm removal should be performed after meals when patients are not severely compromised from surgery, chemotherapy, or bone marrow transplantation. The tongue must also be brushed, especially by patients who are receiving soft or liquid diets.	Beware of inexpensive, hospital-supplied, hard, unpolished, bristled toothbrushes. The benefits versus the risks of brushing may need to be assessed for patients with severely compromised conditions.
Floss	Unwaxed or waxed versions are available.	Flossing is important for plaque biofilm removal at least once per day.	Assess the patient's dexterity and assist if necessary. Discontinue only when the patient is at high risk for bleeding and bacteremia.
Dentifrices	Commercial dentifrices without strong flavoring agents can be used. Paste made from baking soda and water is an alternative.	These help with plaque biofilm removal.	Strong flavoring agents may intensify mucositis. Fully rinse baking soda residue from the oral cavity.
Gauze	Gauze is another alternative to a toothbrush. Use 2 × 2 or 4 × 4 squares.	Gauze is used to cleanse the oral cavity only when toothbrushing is not possible as a result of pain associated with ulcerated tissues or when toothbrushing precipitates bleeding. Moisten the gauze in water, saline 0.9% (1 tsp of sodium chloride to 16 oz. of water), or baking soda solution. Wrap the gauze around the finger and cleanse the teeth, tongue, and tissues.	Gauze does not adequately remove plaque biofilm.
Baking soda and saline rinse	This is a mucolytic cleansing solution made up of one-half tsp of baking soda, one-fourth tsp of salt, and 16 oz. of water.	An alkaline soothing rinse is used to cleanse the mouth every 2 to 4 hours for patients with mucositis, xerostomia, or thick secretions, or after emesis. It may be used in an irrigation bag to assist with the rinsing of a painful mouth. Rinse the mouth with plain water after use.	This mixture has a high sodium content. Instruct the patient not to swallow the solution. This is not to be used by patients on sodium-restricted diets.

Continued

TABLE 50.3   Oral Hygiene Products Used During Cancer Therapy—cont'd

Product	Description	Indication, Rationale, or Use	Precautions
Topical anesthetics	These palliative agents include over-the-counter products such as alcohol-free Benadryl mixed in equal parts with a coating agent such as Maalox to create a rinse. Other agents that are helpful are topical Orabase and benzocaine (www.colgateprofessional.com), which are available over the counter at most pharmacies.	They are used to control the pain associated with mucosal ulcerations.	Topical anesthetics may decrease the gag reflex, thereby resulting in the aspiration of food. Over-the-counter agents or rinses may not provide adequate relief from severe oral ulcerations. The patient's oncologist may prescribe analgesics or narcotics.
Saliva replacement and xerostomia palliation	Saliva substitutes include over-the-counter rinses and gels such as Oral Balance Gel (Laclede, Inc, www.laclede.com), and Moi-Stir (Kingswood Labs, www.kingswood-labs.com/moistir.html). Dietary guidelines should encourage the intake of high-moisture foods, oily foods, and sugar- and acid-free foods. Saliva stimulants include pharmacologic prescription drugs (pilocarpine or cevimeline) for the systemic stimulation of functional salivary gland tissue and mechanical stimulation with xylitol-containing chewing gum or candy.	They are used for the palliation of xerostomia and dysphagia.	Patients may find saliva substitutes to be unacceptable in taste and too expensive. Patients should be discouraged from using tobacco products, consuming excessive alcohol, and using alcohol-containing mouthwash because these products promote dry mouth or may be irritating.
Chlorhexidine gluconate 0.12%	This is a bactericidal mouth rinse.	These are prophylactic or therapeutic mouth rinses that are used to reduce plaque biofilm and oral microbes. Rinse for 30 seconds with 1 capful twice daily.	Products that are available in the United States are prepared with alcohol and may be irritating. This agent should be used only when mechanical plaque control is inadequate. It may cause staining of the teeth, which is removable with dental prophylaxis. It may also alter taste perception.
Commercial mouthwashes	These should be heavily diluted with water.	They may serve as mouth fresheners.	Most commercial mouthwashes have a high concentration of alcohol or phenol, which may be drying and irritating to tissues unless diluted heavily with water. Flavoring agents may intensify mucositis. Alcohol-free mouthwashes are available (i.e., Biotene, Pro-Health, and Clear Choice).

BOX 50.8   Critical Thinking Scenario B

A patient is undergoing chemotherapy for breast cancer and has been referred to your office by the oncology treatment team to help relieve mucositis pain. Create a dental hygiene care plan, stating specific professional and homecare strategies.

Bone containing bisphosphonates does not have the ability to go through the normal healing process of breaking down and remodeling. If traumatized, the bone may become necrotic and subsequently form lesions. Typical symptoms include loose teeth, pain, discharge, swelling, a heavy feeling, and numbness. Management strategies that can prevent MRONJ include completing any needed oral surgery for the patient prior to cancer therapy, continuing cancer treatment, and supporting oral and bone health before, during, and after cancer treatment.[14] The patient must be informed by the oral health and oncology team of the potential risks associated with the use of both oral and intravenous bisphosphonates. Careful assessment and consideration for the potential development of MRONJ should be undertaken prior to any invasive dental procedure throughout the patient's lifetime.

BOX 50.9   Recommendations for Patients With Xerostomia

- Carry bottled water; sip it often.
- Use liquids to soften or thin foods.
- Use xylitol gum or xylitol hard candies to help stimulate saliva flow.
- Use over-the-counter saliva substitutes.
- Rinse frequently with one-fourth tsp of baking soda, one-eighth tsp of salt, and 8 oz. of water.
- Let ice chips melt in the mouth.
- Suck on sugar-free frozen pops.
- Humidify rooms with cool mist humidifiers.
- Avoid highly seasoned foods, tobacco, and the drying effects of alcohol and alcohol-containing products.
- Ask the dentist or oncologist to prescribe a saliva stimulant.
- Lubricate lips with a moisturizing lip balm or cream rather than with pure petrolatum.

Adapted from the National Institutes of Dental and Craniofacial Research. Cancer Treatments & Oral Health. https://www.nidcr.nih.gov/health-info/cancer-treatments. Accessed September 28, 2022; https://www.cancer.gov/about-cancer/treatment/side-effects/appetite-loss/nutrition-pdq. Accessed November 28, 2023.

Patients experiencing alteration or loss of taste should be assured that taste dysfunction is a normal radiation side effect and that taste will most likely return several months after treatment. The use of nutritional liquid substitutes or referral for nutritional counseling may be necessary to avoid weight loss and medical complications. If patients do not maintain adequate nutrition during the treatment process, a stomach tube may be surgically placed for liquid feeding.

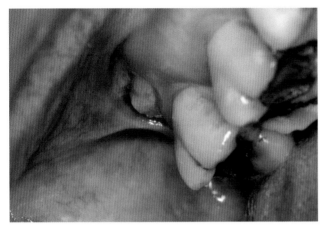

Fig. 50.3 Bisphosphonate-related osteonecrosis of the maxilla. (From Regezi J, Sciubba J, Jordan R. *Oral Pathology.* 7th ed. Saunders; 2017.)

Complications Specific to Head and Neck Radiation Therapy

Within the first week of radiation therapy, the patient often experiences acute or short-term side effects (e.g., loss of taste, dry mouth). Other complications may not become evident until later during radiation therapy. These complications are summarized in Box 50.11.

Radiation-Related Caries

Enamel demineralization (the loss of minerals without decay) and/or rapid decay (Fig. 50.4) are a result of changes in both the quality and the quantity of saliva after cancer treatment. The decreased salivary flow limits the availability of both calcium and phosphate in the saliva, which prevents the natural remineralization of the tooth structure and the buffering of acids produced by cariogenic bacteria in the plaque biofilm. Rampant caries and tooth demineralization usually begin within the first year after radiation therapy unless intensive oral hygiene and preventive measures are instituted. Compounding the problem, radiation therapy damages the soft tissue, making it dry and friable (crumbly). As a result, patients may change to a soft, high-carbohydrate diet, thereby adding to the risk of rampant dental decay.

Prior to oral cavity or head and neck radiation therapy, patients should be referred to their dentist for treatment. Custom fluoride trays should be made from a soft vinyl material and extend slightly beyond the cervical line of the teeth to include full coverage of all teeth. The tray edges must be smooth and nonirritating to the patient's oral tissues. Patients should be instructed to first brush and floss their teeth and then to place a thin ribbon of the 1.1% neutral-pH sodium fluoride gel in each of the trays, which must be left in place for 5 to 10 minutes. Patients should not rinse their mouths or eat anything for 30 minutes. If severe mucositis prevents fluoride application with trays, the patient is encouraged to use nonalcoholic and bland fluoride rinses to increase the hydration of tissues. Daily fluoride gel applications should resume

Acute
- Xerostomia
- Loss of taste
- Mucositis
- Dysphagia
- Secondary infection
- Trismus
- Impaired nutrition (from xerostomia, pain, and dysphagia)
- Hearing loss
- Fatigue

Chronic
- Xerostomia or salivary gland dysfunction
- Alterations in sense of taste as compared with preradiation status
- Telangiectasia and friable mucosa
- Continued fungal infections caused by the lack of saliva
- Osteoradionecrosis or soft tissue necrosis
- Rampant caries
- Muscle fibrosis, temporomandibular disorder, and trismus
- Altered tooth and jaw development in children

National Cancer Institute. Oral Complications of Chemotherapy and Head/Neck Radiation (PDQ®)–Health Professional Version. https://www.cancer.gov/about-cancer/treatment/side-effects/mouth-throat/oral-complications-hp-pdq. Accessed September 28, 2022.

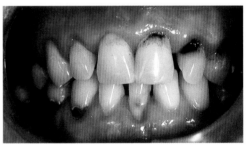

Fig. 50.4 Clinical appearance of radiation caries. (Courtesy of Dr. Jonathan A. Ship.)

as soon as the mucositis resolves. In addition, assessment of sugar, acidic juice, energy drinks, and soda pop (diet soda included) intake should be an integral part of pretherapy dental hygiene care.

Soft Tissue Necrosis and Osteoradionecrosis

Radiation therapy in the oral cavity and head and neck area may irreversibly injure the vascularity of soft tissue and bone. This damage results in the bone's decreased ability to heal if traumatized and increases the susceptibility to infection.[12] *Osteoradionecrosis* (ORN) is irradiated bone that becomes devitalized, is exposed, and does not heal for at least 2 months' time. There is a higher risk of osteoradionecrosis as the dose of radiation and the volume of irradiated bone and tissue increase. Nonhealing soft tissue or bone may become secondarily infected, resulting in intolerable pain and jaw fracture. The mandible appears to be more susceptible than the maxilla because of its dense bone and limited blood supply. Cancer survivors who have oral surgery, dental trauma, or infection in close proximity to irradiated tissue and bone are at the greatest risk for developing ORN. The best management is the prevention of osteoradionecrosis by undergoing dental

Profile: Ms. G. is a 45-year-old female with a soft palate lesion and a large mass in the right side of her neck. A biopsy reveals squamous cell carcinoma. She is scheduled for surgery followed by unilateral radiation therapy to the right posterior mandible and maxilla and the lateral neck.

Chief Complaint: "I have been referred by my oncology team for a dental evaluation and dental hygiene care before starting my cancer therapy."

Dental History: Her pretherapy radiographic and clinical oral and dental evaluation reveals no dental caries, generalized gingivitis, and moderate plaque, calculus, and tobacco staining.

Social History: The patient has recently moved to the area, is single, and has a full-time job.

Health History: The patient has been diagnosed with squamous cell carcinoma of the soft palate. She currently takes no medications, and her blood pressure is within normal limits.

Oral Health Behavior Assessment: Ms. G. states that she brushes her teeth once a day, that she does not use floss, and that she visits her dentist every year. She takes over-the-counter antacids, chewable vitamin C, and Aspergum for her sore throat. She has smoked one pack a day for 25 years.

Supplemental Notes: She has dental insurance, she demonstrates sincere interest in and motivation to maintain her teeth, and she is very interested in tobacco cessation interventions.

1. Using the interprofessional collaborative model, explain how the oral health team would actively work with the oncology team to provide the best possible care for this patient.
2. What procedures will be included in the dental treatment plan before surgery and radiation therapy?
3. Develop a dental hygiene care plan to be implemented before, during, and after radiation therapy.
4. What measures do you suggest for relieving this patient's anticipated xerostomia and the pain associated with mucositis?
5. What dental hygiene interventions and recall schedule are appropriate for this patient after radiation therapy?
6. What are the signs and symptoms of osteoradionecrosis?

evaluation and treatment before radiation therapy. Following radiation therapy, the patient should seek out regular preventive oral healthcare and continue careful oral hygiene to minimize disease. See the Critical Thinking Scenario in Box 50.12.

Trismus

Trismus, the limited ability to open the mouth, may result from a loss of elasticity of the masticatory muscles or the temporomandibular joint ligaments after a high dose of radiation. This condition can result in significant discomfort and interfere with eating, talking, and posttreatment dental examinations. Trismus usually occurs within 3 months after therapy and remains a lifelong problem. The patient receiving radiation therapy to the mastication muscles should be placed on an exercise program to prevent trismus. The jaw should be exercised three times a day by opening and closing the mouth 20 times as wide as possible without causing pain.

Altered Tooth and Jaw Development

The latent effects of oral cavity radiation therapy on children vary with the radiation dose, the area exposed, and the child's stage of growth and development. Radiation therapy has the potential to alter or arrest craniofacial growth and tooth development. Older children may experience only slightly altered root development. Younger children may experience gross malformation of the dentition and may suffer significant skeletal deformities.

Complications Due to Surgical Treatment of Oral Cancer

Acute physical complications after head and neck cancer surgery may include infection, airway obstruction, fistula formation, and necrosis in the surgical site; impairment of swallowing, hearing, vision, smell, and speech; and compromised nutritional status. Long-term complications include speech impairment, malnutrition from the inability to swallow foods, drooling, malocclusion, temporomandibular disorders, facial deformity, and chronic pain in the shoulder muscles.

Rehabilitation following oral cancer surgery depends on the extent of the actual surgery. An interprofessional team approach is needed to address the many and varied complications a patient may experience. The role of the dental hygienist includes regular assessment of oral health conditions and oral cancer examination. Informing the patient how to perform self-oral cancer examinations between appointments would also be appropriate.

INTERPROFESSIONAL COLLABORATIVE CANCER CARE

Cancer diagnosis, treatment, and recovery involves an extensive team of professionals to effectively meet the many needs of the cancer patient and their family. Interprofessional collaborative practice (ICP), defined as communication and decision-making activities by different disciplines to improve patient outcomes, provides the most comprehensive and safest care possible. According to the American Cancer Society, more than 60 different professionals could potentially make up the ICP team of a cancer patient, including a medical oncologist, dietitian, case manager, pharmacist, chaplain, genetic counselor, home health nurse, occupational therapist, hematologist, palliative care specialist, pathologist, patient navigator, and psychologist. The dental hygienist plays a key role in preventing and/or minimizing many of the oral complications associated with cancer treatment, including rampant caries, periodontitis, xerostomia, and mucositis. Open and continuous collaboration among the ICP oncology team members maximizes the patient's chances to achieve the best possible outcome.

The **Dental Hygiene Process of Care/ADPIE** model provides the basis for all dental hygiene care, including the creation of a comprehensive oral health plan for cancer patients. In collaboration with the ICP oncology team, the dentist and dental hygienist should assess the oral health and needs of the patient, diagnose/describe the anticipated conditions that may develop during and after cancer therapy, plan or create a detailed treatment plan, implement needed oral healthcare, evaluate the adequacy of the planned and implemented treatment, and ensure documentation of all care provided. The dental hygiene care plan should reflect the overall personalized oncology care plan, including pretherapy, during therapy, posttherapy, and throughout the survivor's life.

Oral Healthcare Before Cancer Therapy

Prior to the start of any therapy, newly diagnosed cancer patients should obtain a comprehensive oral health exam and any required dental treatment. Oral surgical procedures should be performed at least 7 days before periods of immunosuppression and 14 to 21 days before the initiation of radiation therapy involving the oral cavity and the salivary glands. All carious lesions with favorable restorative prognosis should be repaired and sources of infection and irritation removed prior to any cancer therapy. The fabrication of new dental prostheses should be delayed until several months after head and neck radiation therapy ends, when all acute side effects of radiation have been resolved (Box 50.13).

BOX 50.13 Benefits of Good Oral Hygiene Care Before, During, and After Cancer Therapy

- Reduces the risk and severity of oral complications
- Improves the likelihood that patient will tolerate optimal doses of cancer treatment
- Prevents oral infections that could lead to potentially fatal systemic infections
- Prevents or minimizes complications that can compromise nutrition
- Prevents or reduces oral pain
- Prevents or reduces the incidence of bone necrosis in patients undergoing radiation
- Preserves oral health
- Improves quality of life

Adapted from the US Department of Health and Human Services, National Institutes of Health. *Oral Complications of Cancer Treatment: What the Dental Team Can Do,* 2009. https://www.nidcr.nih.gov/sites/default/files/2017-09/oral-complications-cancer-dental-team.pdf. Accessed September 28, 2022.

Psychosocial Issues

Patients may feel scared, anxious about the upcoming cancer therapy, and overwhelmed by the sheer amount of information they must attend to. The oral health team should make every effort to listen, accept the patient's feelings, and provide a supportive, nonjudgmental environment. The patient is a "person living with cancer," not a "cancer case."

Oral Hygiene Instruction and Self-Care

Comprehensive oral hygiene instructions should be presented prior to cancer therapy to lessen treatment complications. If a patient is scheduled for therapy that will significantly compromise the oral tissues, initial instruction is given verbally and in print regarding methods for cleansing the mouth, in addition to any preventive and palliative products recommended (see Table 50.3). Gentle tooth and gingival brushing can continue during cancer therapy.

Tobacco and Alcohol Cessation Counseling

It is imperative that all members of the oncology/oral healthcare team strongly encourage the patient to stop using tobacco products and to limit excessive alcohol intake during cancer therapy. Referral to the state or national tobacco cessation Quitline (1-800-QUITNOW), a local tobacco treatment program, or a cessation support group can support cessation efforts. Quitting tobacco products is highly recommended to support the best possible outcome for the patient (see Chapter 37).

Nutritional Counseling

A patient's nutritional status affects their overall response to cancer therapy and psychological well-being. The nutritionist on the oncology team assumes primary responsibility for monitoring the patient's nutritional status and providing counseling regarding diet selection. The dental hygienist consults with the nutritionist and educates the patient about diet selection and dietary habits to promote a clean and healthy oral environment and to reduce caries development.

Dental Hygiene Instrumentation

Dental hygiene instrumentation may need to be altered to accommodate the patient's physical condition related to recent surgery, disease manifestations, and the status of the patient's blood counts and clotting factors. The oncology team should be consulted regarding the safest time to schedule an appointment and the need for antibiotic prophylaxis before dental hygiene instrumentation. Overall, dental hygiene care promotes a clean and well-hydrated oral environment, promotes control of periodontal disease, and reduces the risk of oral infection, caries, and bacteremia.

Fluoride Therapy

When the patient is scheduled for radiation therapy to the salivary glands or total body irradiation for BMT, custom fluoride gel trays are fabricated for daily application of a 1.1% neutral-pH sodium fluoride gel to prevent rampant dental caries. Patients who complain of a dry mouth during chemotherapy require at least a daily fluoride rinse and possibly a 1.1% sodium fluoride toothpaste or gel.

Oral Healthcare During Cancer Therapy

Once cancer therapy has begun, oral assessment and dental hygiene care should continue in collaboration with the oncology team. Assessment of the immune status and any therapy-related conditions such as mucositis, xerostomia, dysphagia, or oral candidiasis that may be present, triggering recommended treatment, should be conducted. Meticulous oral care should once again be stressed to minimize oral complications to cancer therapy.

Management of Oral Complications

Patients with mouth pain may benefit by using topical anesthetic or coating agents before eating (see Table 50.3). In addition, patients with oral ulcerations or dry mouth may find it helpful to eat foods that are high in moisture, thin their food with liquids, and take frequent sips of water while eating. Irritating, hot, spicy, or acidic foods should be avoided. Table 50.2 summarizes dental hygiene interventions that may prevent or improve the oral complications associated with radiation therapy and chemotherapy.

Nutritional Counseling

The side effects of cancer therapy often result in a high risk for dental caries. Patients may be placed on a soft and bland diet or a high-carbohydrate liquid diet because of recent oral surgery or therapy-induced mucositis. They may also be encouraged to eat small, frequent meals and snacks to increase their caloric intake and to counteract nausea and vomiting. The dental hygienist must recognize the complications that frequent snacking places on patients' ability to maintain appropriate oral hygiene and be prepared to educate patients accordingly. With a team approach to care, oral health and nutritional professionals need to work closely together when creating a nutritional plan.

Oral Healthcare After Cancer Therapy

Following cancer therapy, the dental hygienist continues to have an important role in patient care. Continued education and frequent contact and support are essential. The dental hygienist must not only assess the oral condition but understand the side effects of the specific cancer therapies and provide personalized care.

After Chemotherapy

At the completion of chemotherapy, most of the associated oral manifestations resolve on their own. With full bone marrow recovery, conditions associated with acute cytotoxicity, immunosuppression, and thrombocytopenia disappear. After long and intensive chemotherapy, some patients take months to recover fully and experience chronic oral infections such as candidiasis and herpetic infections. Continual assistance with oral hygiene and a health-promoting diet is necessary to prevent infections.

After Stem Cell Transplantation

After patients are released from a transplant unit, they may remain susceptible to infections for several months as a result of immunosuppressive therapy. Ongoing monitoring and care should be given to those who continue to experience xerostomia, predisposing them to an altered oral flora, infections, trauma, and rampant dental caries. Patients with GVHD may experience additional complications that involve thinned and friable mucosa and mucosal lesions. The dental hygienist should assist the patient with establishing consistent and effective oral hygiene methods that do not create additional trauma and irritation. Elective dental procedures should be delayed until the patient has full hematologic function, which is sometimes up to a year or more after the completion of cancer treatment.

After Radiation Therapy

Following oral cavity radiation therapy, frequent dental and dental hygiene maintenance visits are essential because of permanent salivary gland and bone damage. Patients are at permanent risk for the development of rampant radiation caries, tooth demineralization, and osteoradionecrosis. Lifelong daily use of the custom fluoride trays is highly recommended, using a 1.1% neutral-pH sodium fluoride gel for 5 to 10 minutes followed by 30 minutes of abstinence from food and water. If there is evidence of dental decay despite compliance with daily fluoride applications, the patient should be placed on a 2-week chlorhexidine regimen to decrease cariogenic bacteria and then scheduled for in-office fluoride varnish applications. A daily remineralizing gel application may also be necessary in addition to the daily fluoride gel application.

If trismus occurs, the patient should be instructed to place tongue blades between the teeth for several minutes each day, gradually increasing the number of blades until adequate opening is achieved. This strategy may be painful and requires patience and perseverance.

The key to providing compassionate, competent dental hygiene care for cancer patients and survivors is to establish a working relationship with the interprofessional oncology team during all stages of care.

KEY CONCEPTS

- Cancer is a term that defines a wide variety of malignant processes and is estimated to kill more than 600,000 Americans a year, with approximately one-third caused by cigarette smoking.
- There remains a cancer disparity based on race/ethnicity and rural and urban population groups.
- Though oral cavity cancers have decreased over the past several years, oropharyngeal/head and neck cancers have increased due to the human papillomavirus (HPV) in young adults.
- Innovative cancer therapies have focused on personalized medicine, looking at numerous patient-specific components such as immunotherapy or genetic therapy when designing cancer therapy. Patients may receive single or combination therapies, including surgery, chemotherapy, radiation therapy, hormone therapy, or bone marrow or blood stem cell transplantation.
- Oral mucositis is a common oral complication caused by many cancer therapies and is experienced by approximately 40% to 100% of persons undergoing care. Meticulous oral hygiene care can lessen the severity of oral lesions.
- Preexisting oral or dental pathology can adversely affect the individual who is undergoing cancer therapy and should be treated prior to cancer treatment.
- Medication-related osteonecrosis of the jaw (MRONJ) can occur years after administration because of bisphosphonate half-life. Therefore all dental and periodontal therapy should be completed prior to administration.
- Head and neck cancer radiation treatment results in permanent oral complications that need to be managed during and after radiation therapy.
- Cancer treatment is multifaceted and requires numerous health and social service professionals to support a positive patient outcome. Comprehensive care includes the dental hygienist working closely with the interprofessional oncology team at all stages of care.

ACKNOWLEDGMENT

The author acknowledges Gerry J. Barker for her past contributions to this chapter.

ONLINE RESOURCES

American Dental Association Council on Scientific Affairs. *Evidence-based clinical recommendations regarding screening for oral squamous cell carcinomas.* Available at: http://jada.ada.org/article/S0002-8177(14)61524-5/fulltext?dgcid=PromoSpots_EBDsite_oral-cancer. Accessed September 28, 2022.

Centers for Disease Control and Prevention. *Cancer prevention and control.* Available at: https://www.cdc.gov/cancer/index.htm. Accessed September 28, 2022.

National Institute of Dental and Craniofacial Research (NIDCR). *Oral cancer.* https://www.nidcr.nih.gov/health-info/oral-cancer. Accessed September 28, 2022.

REFERENCES

1. U.S. Department of Health and Human Services, National Cancer Institute, Division of Cancer Control & Population Sciences. Statistics. Available at: https://cancercontrol.cancer.gov/ocs/statistics. Accessed July 8, 2022.
2. Siegel RL, Miller KD, Fuchs HE, Jemal A. Cancer statistics, 2022. *CA Cancer J Clin.* 2022;72(11):7–33. https://doi.org/10.3322/caac.21708. https://acsjournals.onlinelibrary.wiley.com/doi/epdf/10.3322/caac.21708. Accessed July 8, 2022.
3. American Cancer Society. *Cancer Facts and Figures*; 2022. Available at:https://www.cancer.org/research/cancer-facts-statistics/all-cancer-facts-figures/cancer-facts-figures-2022.html . Accessed July 8, 2022.
4. U.S. Department of Health and Human Services, National Institute of Health, National Cancer Institute. *Cancer Disparities.* Available at: https://www.cancer.gov/about-cancer/understanding/disparities. Accessed July 8, 2022.
5. Sturgis EM, Cincirpini PM. Trends in head and neck cancer incidence in relation to smoking prevalence: an emerging epidemic of human papillomavirus-associated cancers? *Cancer.* 2007;110(7):1429–1435.
6. U.S. Department of Health and Human Services, National Institute of Health, National Institute of Dental and Craniofacial Research. Oral Cancer 5-Year Survival Rates by Race, Gender, and Stage of Diagnosis. Available at: https://www.nidcr.nih.gov/research/data-statistics/oral-cancer/survival-rates. Accessed July 8, 2022.
7. Centers for Disease Control and Prevention. *Human Papillomavirus.* Available at: https://www.cdc.gov/vaccines/pubs/pinkbook/hpv.html. Accessed August 28, 2022.
8. Lechner M, Liu J, Masterson L, et al. HPV-associated oropharyngeal cancer: epidemiology, molecular biology and clinical management. *Nat Rev Clin Oncol.* 2022;19:306–327. https://doi.org/10.1038/s41571-022-00603-7.
9. Centers for Disease Control and Prevention. *Human Papillomavirus (HPV) Vaccination Information for Clinicians.* Available at: https://www.cdc.gov/vaccines/vpd/hpv/hcp/index.html. Accessed Aug 28, 2022.
10. U.S. Department of Health and Human Services, National Institute of Health, National Cancer Institute. *Types of Cancer Treatment.* Available at: https://www.cancer.gov/about-cancer/treatment/types. Accessed July 13, 2022.
11. U.S. Department of Health and Human Services, National Institutes of Health. *Oral Complications of Cancer Treatment: What the Dental Team Can Do*; 2009. Available at: https://www.nidcr.nih.gov/sites/default/files/2017-09/oral-complications-cancer-oncology-team.pdf. Accessed September 28, 2022.
12. U.S. Department of Health and Human Services, National Institute of Health, National Cancer Institute. *Oral Complications of Chemotherapy and Head/Neck Radiation (PDQ)—Health Professional Version.* Updated

July 14, 2021. Available at: https://www.cancer.gov/about-cancer/treatment/side-effects/mouth-throat/oral-complications-hp-pdq. Accessed July 8, 2022.

13. Ruggiero SL, Dodson TB, Aghaloo TJ, et al. American Association of Oral and Maxillofacial Surgeons position paper on medication-related osteonecrosis of the jaw—2022 Update. *J Oral Maxillofac Surg.* 2022;80(5):920943. https://doi.org/101016/j.joms.2022.02.008. Epub 2022, Feb 21 https://pubmed.ncbi.nlm.nih.gov/35300956/.

14. Poxieitner P, Engelhardt M, Schmeizeisen R, et al. The prevention of medication-related osteonecrosis of the jaw. *Disch Arstebl Int.* 2017;114:63–69.

51

HIV and Oral Health

Helene Bednarsh, David A. Reznik, Herve Y. Sroussi, and Uhlee (Yuri) Oh

PROFESSIONAL OPPORTUNITIES

The dental hygienist may often be the first in the oral healthcare team to see signs and symptoms of human immunodeficiency virus (HIV) disease; therefore, it is critical to have an index of suspicion when noting lesions or conditions in the oral cavity. The importance of understanding the patient from all perspectives, including their medical and dental histories, is critical to providing safe and effective care. People with HIV (PWH) are not unlike other medically complex patients with chronic conditions that require medical-dental collaboration. As stated in the first-ever Surgeon General's Report on Oral Health, people are not healthy without sound oral health. Recently, the FDI World Dental Federation approved a new definition of oral health: "Oral health is multifaceted and includes the ability to speak, smile, smell, taste, touch, chew, swallow and convey a range of emotions through facial expression with confidence and without pain, discomfort, and disease of the craniofacial complex." This definition applies to all patients, but particularly those who may be impacted by medical comorbidities that, either on their own or as a result of treatment, may fall outside this definition.

COMPETENCIES

1. Discuss the history of human immunodeficiency virus (HIV) in relation to the current status of HIV and AIDS.
2. Describe HIV modes of transmission, HIV latency and immune status, and pharmaceutical management for PWH.
3. Elucidate why people with weakened immune systems may be more vulnerable to an opportunistic infection (OI) and describe the epidemiology of HIV infection and AIDS.
4. Explain the concept of the HIV continuum.
5. Describe the dental hygiene process of care for PWH, including systemic health and oral health considerations.
6. Discuss the risk of HIV infection among healthcare workers and mechanisms to prevent transmission in the dental office.
7. Understand the national HIV/AIDS strategy inclusive of the plan to end the HIV epidemic in the United States.

HUMAN IMMUNODEFICIENCY VIRUS

There have been many advancements in HIV over the past four decades in the areas of diagnosis, treatment, understanding oral implications, and policies. This chapter reviews basic information on HIV infection, treatment considerations for PWH, diagnosis and treatment of oral manifestations, and the role of the oral healthcare team in Ending the HIV Epidemic (EHE).

HIV INFECTION

What is now known as HIV was first reported by the US Centers for Disease Control and Prevention (CDC) in June and July 1981 as opportunistic illnesses most commonly seen in older immunocompromised individuals began presenting in one of the first groups affected by the disease, men who have sex with men (MSM).[1] However, as more was learned, new associated complications were included to better characterize HIV and the more advanced state of HIV infection, acquired immunodeficiency syndrome (AIDS). It should be noted that oral/mucosal candidiasis was observed and documented in the first cases of HIV infection, well before the disease and its etiology were better defined. Oral health is an important component of HIV disease, and it was recognized as such from the early days of what would become a pandemic of considerable proportion.

Oral healthcare professionals should understand the history of HIV but more importantly, what they, as integral members of the healthcare team, can do to positively impact the health of PWH and the overall course of the pandemic. Oral health is integral to general health, and it is of particular importance for PWH.[2] By some estimates, more than 90% of HIV-infected patients will have at least one HIV-related oral manifestation in the course of their disease.[3]

The natural history of HIV disease and the trajectory of the pandemic has morphed significantly from what it was in its early years. Preventive measures fueled by educational efforts and significant pharmaceutical breakthroughs, most notably the use of HIV-specific protease inhibitors (PIs) and integrase inhibitors in combination with other antiretrovirals, have resulted in a considerable improvement of the overall disease prognosis. A significant decrease in AIDS mortality first became apparent in 1996, the year after the first PI was introduced.[4] PIs and other more recent pharmaceutical innovations (i.e., integrase inhibitors, long-acting injectables) have made it possible to change the course of HIV disease to a more chronic medical condition. Despite this progress, concerns regarding access to care, complications and morbidities associated with treatment modalities, and stubborn new infection rates have remained pertinent to this day.[4] Increased life expectancy in PWH receiving treatment is enhanced among those who are retained in care and achieve viral suppression.[5]

This disappointing HIV treatment continuum potentially has a significant deleterious effect on our ability to decrease rates of new infections as undiagnosed or untreated PWH are more likely to infect others.[6] On the other hand, successful viral suppression (VL < 50 copies/mL) prevents sexual transmission of HIV, otherwise known as U=U (undetectable = untransmissible). To better contribute to the overall effort to contain the spread of HIV, the role of oral healthcare workers must include recognition of possible signs and symptoms of HIV infection, implementation of rapid HIV screening programs or referral to testing sites, client education, linking patients to care, and assisting patients with retention in care when necessary.

Oral health for PWH and the role of oral healthcare providers have been discussed in the National HIV/AIDS Strategy (NHAS), The *2020 Surgeon General's Report Oral Health in America: Advances and Challenges*, and the updated EHE reports.[7-9] The consensus is that oral healthcare is vital to PWH and that the role of oral health should be expanded to include early HIV screening and linkage to confirmatory testing and care. PWH are among groups identified as not having enough access to care and are less likely to have had a dental visit in the past 2 years due to several barriers such as financial, stigma, and competing priorities.

The strategy in EHE is to reduce the number of new infections, improve health outcomes, and reduce disparities and inequities by integrating healthcare for PWH. There are four pillars to this initiative: diagnose, treat, prevent, and respond.[9] It specifically notes the importance of educated oral health teams in terms of identifying PWH. Screening and testing within dental facilities can impact positively diagnosis and interprofessional collaboration, and it is vital to the other pillars.

Natural Course of HIV Infection

There are several mechanisms by which HIV can be transmitted, but the most significant is through the exchange of bodily fluids such as blood and semen. For HIV to infect a host, several steps must occur for the HIV to successfully go through its life cycle (Fig. 51.1). The eight stages of the HIV life cycle are: (1) binding, (2) fusion, (3) reverse transcription, (4) integration, (5) replication, (6) assembly, (7) budding, and (8) maturation.

Although the disease was first recognized among MSM, from the early days HIV was observed in heterosexual populations, intravenous drug users, and those receiving blood products.

Today, HIV has become a worldwide pandemic. In 2020, an estimated 37.7 million people were living with HIV (including 1.7 million children), with a majority of affected individuals living in Eastern and Southern Africa.[10] Of the estimated 1.2 million Americans living with diagnosed or undiagnosed HIV infection, 87% are diagnosed, and about half of all Americans living with HIV are successfully controlling the virus through treatment, according to the CDC.[11] Diagnosing even some of those people, starting them on antiretroviral drugs, and keeping them in treatment could have a large and immediate impact on transmission of the virus. "If all the people with HIV who either don't know they have the virus or are not receiving HIV clinical services were receiving care and treatment, we could expect a 90 percent reduction in new HIV infections in the United States," according to Jonathan Mermin, as director of the National Center for HIV/AIDS Viral Hepatitis, STD and TB Prevention at the CDC; he later noted, "That is a goal worth striving for."[12]

HIV includes two closely related viruses, HIV-1 and HIV-2. The former is the more common of the two viruses, and it is predominant in most of the world, including the United States. HIV-2 is primarily found in West Africa and it is more closely related to the simian immunodeficiency virus. HIV-1 is known to have at least nine subtypes or clades, identified on the basis of genetic sequencing.[13]

To understand each stage of the HIV life cycle, it helps to first imagine what HIV looks like.

The HIV **virion** or virus particle is composed of a core of ribonucleic acid (RNA) encapsulated within a lipid coating (Fig. 51.2). A serologic marker on the coating binds to receptor sites on **CD4+ T lymphocytes**, a type of white blood cell that is important for cell-mediated immunity. CD4+ T lymphocytes do not have **cytotoxicity**, or the ability to kill a cell, but they do play an important role in activating cytotoxic T

lymphocytes. The virus infects by fusing with the cell membrane of the CD4+ T lymphocyte and entering the cell, where it releases its RNA. HIV is called a **retrovirus** because, once it is within the cell, it uses the enzyme **reverse transcriptase** to convert viral RNA into deoxyribonucleic acid (DNA). This process is the reverse of what typically occurs in animal cells (i.e., the conversion of DNA into RNA).

After the viral RNA is released into the host cell and then changed into DNA, it can integrate into the host cell's genome. This process effectively allows HIV to "hijack" the host cell so that it produces more HIV viruses and creates long-lasting viral reservoirs. When activated, the infected cell will synthesize viral proteins, create more HIV virions, and kill or weaken the host immune cell. The HIV virions produced can then circulate and infect other cells of the immune system.[14] The resultant destruction of immune cells, including CD4+ T lymphocytes and macrophages, weakens the host immune system. The characteristic immunodeficiency occurs when the virus suppresses the immune response, which is the body's natural defense against invasion by an organism.

If left untreated, HIV infection leads to a gradually diminishing **immune response** as a result of the depletion of CD4+ T lymphocytes. The weakened immune response makes the host susceptible to opportunistic infections and malignancies.[14] This explanation of the disease process is a simplified description of complex and multifactorial immunologic phenomena and is intended to present the general idea of how the virus replicates within and harms the human body.

HIV TRANSMISSION

HIV is transmitted through contact with bodily fluids such as semen, vaginal secretions, breast milk, infected blood products, and injection drug use (IDU). Sexual contact is the primary source of infection among MSM, whereas IDUs are at high risk as a result of sharing blood-contaminated needles. HIV-positive mothers may transmit the virus to their fetuses during pregnancy, at birth, or when breastfeeding the infant. However, it must be noted that near elimination of mother-to-child transmission is a recognized benefit of medical advances when the mother is treated before giving birth. With all of the knowledge gained on how to prevent mother-to-child transmission of HIV, these transmissions still occur far too frequently in the United States.

Acute HIV Infection

Acute HIV infection syndrome occurs 6 to 56 days after exposure. Manifestations of initial infection vary but may include some or all of the following prodromal signs and symptoms:

- Fever
- Lymphadenopathy (lymph node enlargement)
- Headache
- Malaise
- Rash
- Pharyngitis (sore throat)
- Myalgia (aching muscles)
- Arthralgia (aching joints)

There are considerable variations in the presentation of acute HIV infection, but it has been reported that most persons who are undergoing HIV **seroconversion** (i.e., the acquisition of the HIV-specific antibodies in the blood serum) are often ill enough to seek medical attention. It is also important to note that some people are infected with HIV and seroconvert but have a mild clinical disease associated with this early phase. They remain unsuspicious of their HIV infection, so it is impossible to rule out HIV infection solely on the basis of an acute phase. The CDC recommends that all adults and adolescents aged 13 to 64 be tested at least once for HIV.[15] Individuals at risk for the

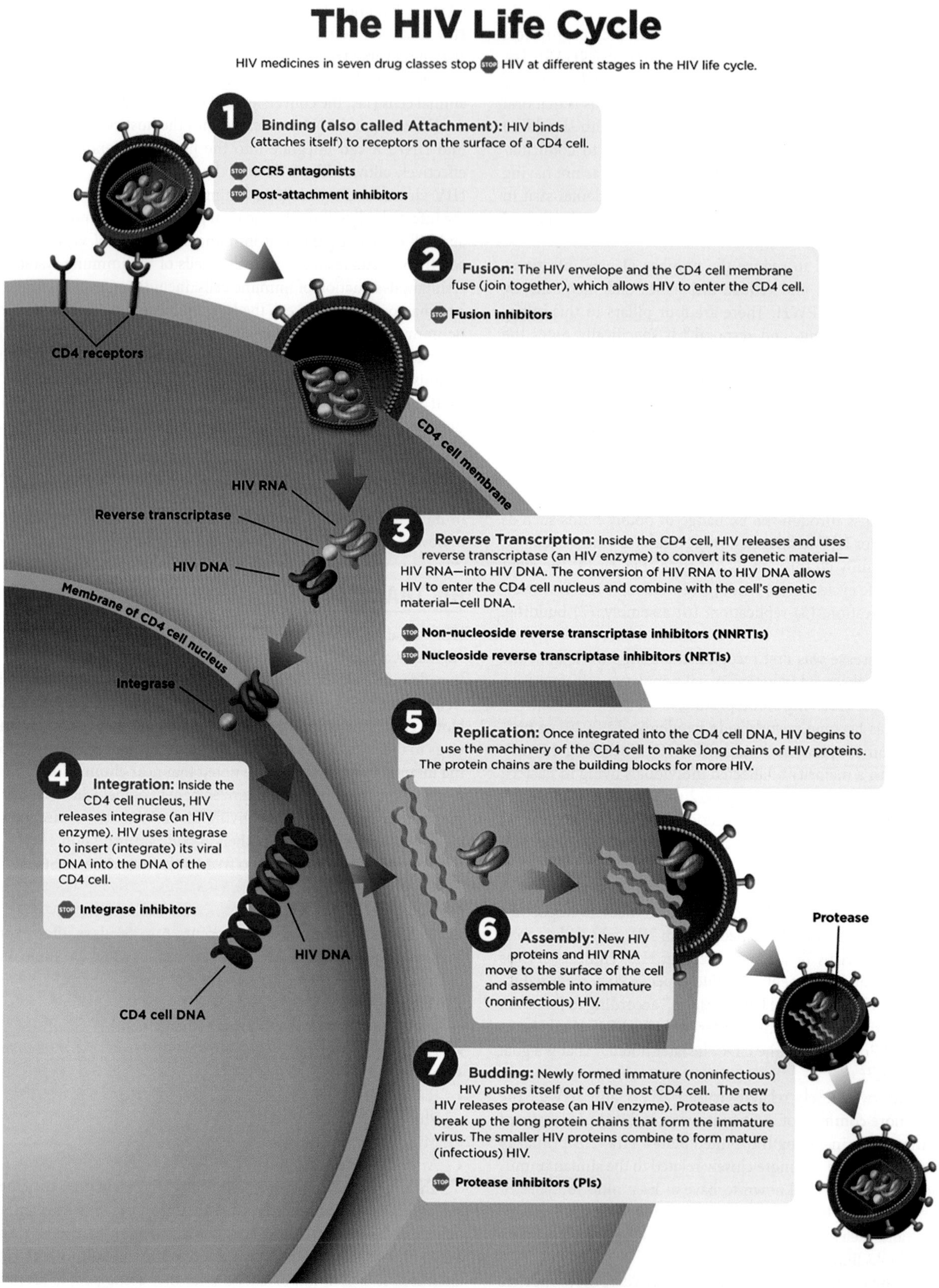

The HIV Life Cycle

HIV medicines in seven drug classes stop 🛑 HIV at different stages in the HIV life cycle.

1   **Binding (also called Attachment):** HIV binds (attaches itself) to receptors on the surface of a CD4 cell.

🛑 **CCR5 antagonists**

🛑 **Post-attachment inhibitors**

2   **Fusion:** The HIV envelope and the CD4 cell membrane fuse (join together), which allows HIV to enter the CD4 cell.

🛑 **Fusion inhibitors**

CD4 receptors

CD4 cell membrane

HIV RNA

Reverse transcriptase

HIV DNA

3   **Reverse Transcription:** Inside the CD4 cell, HIV releases and uses reverse transcriptase (an HIV enzyme) to convert its genetic material—HIV RNA—into HIV DNA. The conversion of HIV RNA to HIV DNA allows HIV to enter the CD4 cell nucleus and combine with the cell's genetic material—cell DNA.

🛑 **Non-nucleoside reverse transcriptase inhibitors (NNRTIs)**

🛑 **Nucleoside reverse transcriptase inhibitors (NRTIs)**

Membrane of CD4 cell nucleus

Integrase

5   **Replication:** Once integrated into the CD4 cell DNA, HIV begins to use the machinery of the CD4 cell to make long chains of HIV proteins. The protein chains are the building blocks for more HIV.

4   **Integration:** Inside the CD4 cell nucleus, HIV releases integrase (an HIV enzyme). HIV uses integrase to insert (integrate) its viral DNA into the DNA of the CD4 cell.

🛑 **Integrase inhibitors**

HIV DNA

CD4 cell DNA

Protease

6   **Assembly:** New HIV proteins and HIV RNA move to the surface of the cell and assemble into immature (noninfectious) HIV.

7   **Budding:** Newly formed immature (noninfectious) HIV pushes itself out of the host CD4 cell. The new HIV releases protease (an HIV enzyme). Protease acts to break up the long protein chains that form the immature virus. The smaller HIV proteins combine to form mature (infectious) HIV.

🛑 **Protease inhibitors (PIs)**

Fig. 51.1 The HIV life cycle. (From US Department of Health and Human Services. Understanding HIV/AIDS. The HIV Life Cycle. Updated March 21, 2018. Available at: https://aidsinfo.nih.gov/understanding-hiv-aids/infographics/7/hiv-life-cycle. Accessed June 29, 2018.)

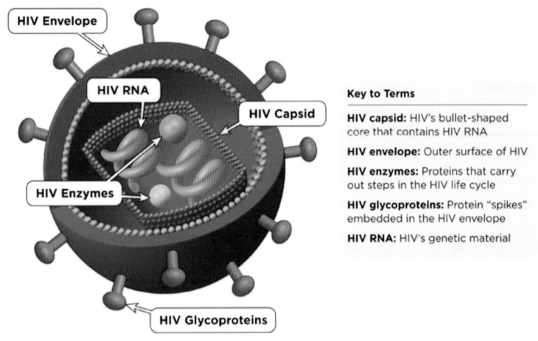

Key to Terms

HIV capsid: HIV's bullet-shaped core that contains HIV RNA

HIV envelope: Outer surface of HIV

HIV enzymes: Proteins that carry out steps in the HIV life cycle

HIV glycoproteins: Protein "spikes" embedded in the HIV envelope

HIV RNA: HIV's genetic material

Fig. 51.2 The HIV virion. (From US Department of Health and Human Services. Aids Info: Fact Sheets: The HIV Life Cycle. Updated August 18, 2017. Available at: https://aidsinfo.nih.gov/understanding-hiv-aids/fact-sheets/19/73/the-hiv-life-cycle. Accessed June 29, 2018.)

virus, including sexually active MSM, are encouraged to test more frequently. Acute HIV infection is also characterized by **primary viremia** or the initial spike in the viral levels in the bloodstream.

HIV Latency and Immune Status

When primary viremia is suppressed by the body's initial immune response, an asymptomatic period follows that may last for a variable period of time that ranges from months to years. Even though symptoms are not present during this latency period, the virus is present and replicating. On average, this asymptomatic period has been reported to lead to the loss of approximately 10% of CD4+ T lymphocytes per year in infected individuals.[14]

Depending on the health status of the human host, HIV infection can remain latent for several years before any clinical signs or symptoms are noted. Only when diseases called AIDS-defining illnesses become apparent is the HIV-infected individual classified as having stage 3 HIV infection or AIDS. The CDC categorization of HIV/AIDS is based on the lowest documented CD4+ T lymphocyte cell count (Table 51.1) and the presence of certain OIs.

The current classification system for HIV progression includes categories for asymptomatic infection, symptomatic infection, and AIDS-defining conditions.[16] The classification system and case definitions are presented in (Table 51.2). The CDC also performs annual surveillance studies to document the prevalence of HIV/AIDS in the United States on the basis of these classification criteria.

MEDICATION THERAPY

The first medications that were used to control HIV infection were developed in the 1980s. The drugs used to inhibit the replication of HIV target key steps in its life cycle. HIV is an RNA virus, which means that its replication requires reverse transcribing its RNA into DNA. The first drugs approved by the Food and Drug Administration (FDA) were accordingly targeting the reverse transcriptase enzyme that enables this process. This first class of drugs can be divided into nucleoside

analogue reverse transcriptase inhibitors (NRTIs) (i.e., AZT, 3TC, d4T) and nonnucleoside analogue reverse transcriptase inhibitors (NNRTIs) (i.e., delavirdine, nevirapine, efavirenz, rilpivirine).

Currently, several classes of HIV-targeting medications approved by the FDA are prescribed. PIs, such as indinavir or saquinavir, introduced in 1995, profoundly and positively affected the course of the disease. Integrase inhibitors such as raltegravir, first approved in 2009, and dolutegravir are a component of many standard drug regimens used today. The fusion inhibitor enfuvirtide was approved in 2003 by the US FDA and was used in salvage therapy. It is rarely used today because of cost, inconvenience in its use, and poor safety profile. The chemokine receptor antagonist (CCR5 antagonists) maraviroc, approved in 2007, is a component of antiretroviral therapy or ART. In addition, a new type of attachment inhibitor, fostemsavir, has been studied in research trials for heavily experienced patients who have significant resistance profiles. The long-acting injectable HIV treatment Cabenuva has been approved by the US FDA as an additional treatment option. Injectable treatments are long lasting, reduce the burden of taking daily medication, and further assist people with HIV to adhere to their treatment regime. Hygienists are encouraged to discuss with their patients their current health status including pharmaceutical management plan and consult with their treating physician(s) and/or other member(s) of their medical care team (with consent) if any questions or concerns arise.

Viral resistance to most of the different drugs and classes mentioned has been described. What is more, HIV-targeting medications work better in combination and are prescribed as such; thus, standard therapy includes drugs from more than one of the classes described. Taking multiple medications at different times of the day, some with food and some without, was a barrier to adherence and made HIV treatment complicated and less efficient. This is not true today, as once-daily pills containing several medications are available. For example, Stribild, a commonly prescribed regimen to be taken once daily, is a combination of elvitegravir (integrase inhibitor), cobicistat (boosting agent), tenofovir (NRTI), and emtricitabine (NRTI).

TABLE 51.1   HIV Infection Stage* Based on Age-Specific CD4 Count or Percentage

| | AGE ON DATE OF CD4+ T-LYMPHOCYTE TEST | | | | | |
| | <1 year | | 1 to 5 years | | ≥6 years | |
Stage	Cells/μL	%	Cells/μL	%	Cells/μL	%
1	≥1500	≥34	≥1000	≥30	≥500	≥26
2	750–1499	26–33	500–999	22–29	200–499	14–25
3	<750	<26	<500	<22	<200	<14

*The stage is based primarily on the CD4 cell count; the CD4 cell count takes precedence over the CD4 percentage, and the percentage is considered only if the count is missing. If a stage 3–defining opportunistic illness has been diagnosed, then the stage is 3, regardless of CD4 test results. From Centers for Disease Control and Prevention. Revised surveillance case definition for HIV infection—United States, 2014. *MMWR* 2014;63(No. RR-3):1–10.

TABLE 51.2   Classification System by Clinical Categories (A to C) and Levels of CD4+ T Cells for HIV Infection and AIDS in Adults

| | CLINICAL CATEGORIES | | |
CD4+ T Cell Categories	A: Asymptomatic Acute (Primary) HIV	B: Symptomatic (No C Conditions) HIV	C: AIDS Indicator
500 cells/mm³	A1	B1	C1
200 to 499 cells/mm³	A2	B2	C2
<200 cells/mm³	A3	B3	C3

Centers for Disease Control and Prevention. AIDS and Opportunistic Infections. HIV. Updated May 20, 2021. https://www.cdc.gov/hiv/basics/livingwithhiv/opportunisticinfections.html. Accessed July 26, 2022.

Other indications for the use of HIV-targeting medications include reducing the risk of vertical transmission during birth. The seminal clinical HIV prevention trial HPTN 076 provided evidence that HIV vertical transmission could be reduced dramatically through treatment with zidovudine (an NRTI) during pregnancy. Zidovudine (also known as AZT) was originally given as a **monotherapy** (i.e., treatment with just one drug) to treat HIV-infected patients. Monotherapy resulted in resistance mutations and eventually made the drugs ineffective for the suppression of viral replication. The resistance observed with single-agent treatment has led to the use of multiple drugs as discussed. These multidrug regimens are referred to as **combination active antiretroviral therapy (cART)**. Such treatment has for a long time been considered the standard of care, and it is now referred to simply as ART.

Today's HIV regimens are all better tolerated and easier to manage compared to earlier regimens. They are recommended for everyone diagnosed with HIV to preserve the immune system and improve health outcomes. Test and treat are key efforts to preserve immune function and reduce the viral burden to prevent sexual transmission. There are side effects associated with ART that are managed by a primary care provider. Drug holidays (i.e., breaks in treatment) have been shown to be detrimental to patients and are not commonly used. A patient may report taking medications to reduce the impact of side effects. Adherence is critical to avoid drug resistance and other complications. ART used as a daily treatment for HIV:

- Does not cure HIV
- Targets HIV at various stages in its life cycle
- Reduces the amount of circulating HIV
- Helps protect the immune system
- Improves quality of life
- Reduces the risk of transmission

HIV/AIDS-RELATED OPPORTUNISTIC INFECTIONS

People with weakened immune systems may be more vulnerable to an OI. These infections can be the result of exposure to a variety of pathogens and may be treated prophylactically to prevent an OI or therapeutically to resolve one. For example, oral mucosal and vaginal candidiasis are common OIs, treated with antifungal agents. Similar to the recommendations made for the general population, the CDC recommends PWH receive immunizations for vaccine-preventable diseases such as chicken pox, polio, COVID-19, and influenza. The patient's primary care provider would be the overseer of these.[17]

EPIDEMIOLOGY OF HIV INFECTION AND AIDS

As of 2008, all 50 states, the District of Columbia, and six US-dependent areas had instituted the confidential name-based reporting of HIV. For these reporting areas, the CDC estimates that at the end of 2019, the total estimated number of people who were more than 13 years old living with HIV was approximately 1.2 million.[11] Precise estimates of HIV incidence are not known because the new infection rate is difficult to track. However, the CDC estimates that approximately 36,940 new HIV infections occurred in 2019.[11] Overall, the infection rate has been decreasing since 1997, but the absolute number of cases or prevalence continues to increase in part due to improved prognosis and longevity in PWH.

Racial and ethnic minorities make up a disproportionately large percentage of the population of PWH (Fig. 51.3). On the basis of the ongoing racial disparities seen in the HIV incidence rate, these prevalence trends are likely to continue. African Americans represent 40% of people with HIV while only making up 13% of the US population, whereas 29% of people with HIV were White and 25% were Hispanic/

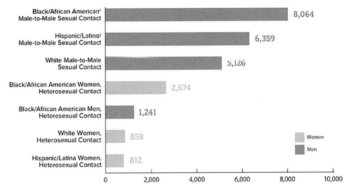

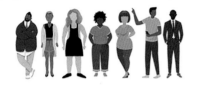

Gay and bisexual men are the population most affected by HIV.

Data for 2020 should be interpreted with caution due to the impact of the COVID-19 pandemic on access to HIV testing, care-related services, and case surveillance activities in state and local jurisdictions

NOTE: Subpopulations representing 2% or less of all people who received an HIV diagnosis in 2020 are not represented in this chart.

* Among people aged 13 and older.

† Black refers to people having origins in any of the Black racial groups of Africa. African American is a term often used for people of African descent with ancestry in North America.
‡ Hispanic/Latino people can be of any race.

Source: CDC. Diagnoses of HIV infection in the United States and dependent areas, 2020. *HIV Surveillance Report* 2022;33.

Fig. 51.3 New HIV diagnoses in the United States for the most affected subpopulations in the US and Dependent Areas, 2019. (Note: Subpopulations representing 2% or less of HIV diagnoses are not reflected in this chart.). (From Centers for Disease Control and Prevention: HIV in the United States: At a Glance. Available at: https://www.cdc.gov/hiv/images/basics/statistics/infographics/cdc-hiv-statistics-diagnoses-subpopulations-1200x630.png.)

Latino.[18] Furthermore, the incidence of HIV infections among Black females is 11 times that of White females and four times that of Latina females. Asian, Native American/Alaska Native, and Native Hawaiian/other Pacific Islander have less than a 2% prevalence rate.[18] It is thought that multiple factors contribute to these racial disparities, including same-race partner selection, limited access to HIV testing and care services, stigma, sexual power imbalances, and the social disruption caused by poverty. Current data are available online regarding the prevalence of HIV/AIDS cases among high-risk groups; these are updated regularly.

HIV and Aging

As previously stated, HIV is considered a chronic disease. The CDC reports that thousands of people aged 50 and older are diagnosed with HIV each year in the United States and estimates that approximately 50% of all PWH are over the age of 50.[18] These older PWH are not immune to known age-associated comorbidities such as cardiovascular disease, diabetes, and non-AIDS-defining malignancies. In addition, problems associated with poor bone density and its pharmaceutical management (i.e., bisphosphonate and RANKL inhibitors) may potentially impact dental treatment. Oral healthcare providers may at times consult with the primary care providers to provide safe and effective care.

Despite the well-documented aging of the population of PWH, healthcare providers still do not routinely consider HIV when treating older patients. This occurs despite guidelines that recommend HIV screening through age 64.[19] Providers may be reluctant to take a sexual history of older adults and may sometimes erroneously attribute HIV symptoms to age-related issues, such as heart disease. Given these findings, the CDC recommends that everyone aged 13 to 64 be tested at least once for HIV infection.

THE HIV CARE CONTINUUM

The AIDS Cascade was introduced in 2011, commonly referred to as the HIV Care Continuum (Fig. 51.4).[20–22] This tool is important to effectively measure the progress in reducing HIV transmission and improving access to and retention in care. Timely linkage and retention in care positively affect health outcomes and are linked with high rates of viral suppression. In 2019, of the estimated 1.2 million Americans living with HIV infection, 87% were diagnosed, and about 66% of all Americans living with HIV were controlling the virus through antiviral treatment.[22] The HIV care continuum is characterized as follows:

1. The first stage is testing and diagnosis; however, 14% are unaware of their infection.
2. Knowing one's status is the first step on the path to controlling HIV infection.
3. Next is to connect with medical care and begin an ART regimen.
4. Retention in care and adherence to treatment follows to get to the next stage.
5. Viral suppression is the next stage; an undetectable viral load is significant in reducing the potential transmission to others and for quality of life.

As illustrated in this Care Continuum, the oral healthcare team can play an important role in controlling the epidemic, as they have many unique opportunities to collaborate with medical and support teams to ensure that patients are linked to medical care, are retained in care, and adhere to their prescribed regimens. The oral health teams can also contribute to first pillar of the continuum by improving screening and testing for HIV among their patients. This can be accomplished through providing rapid testing chairside. In the absence of testing in a dental facility and per AMA recommendation, all patients should be asked to be tested at least once in their lifetime and referred to the appropriate testing facilities.

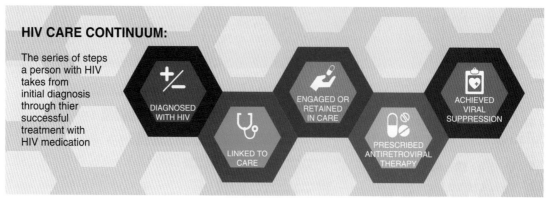

HIV CARE CONTINUUM:

The series of steps a person with HIV takes from initial diagnosis through thier successful treatment with HIV medication

DIAGNOSED WITH HIV

LINKED TO CARE

ENGAGED OR RETAINED IN CARE

PRESCRIBED ANTIRETROVIRAL THERAPY

ACHIEVED VIRAL SUPPRESSION

Fig. 51.4 HIV Care Continuum, U.S., 2014, Overall and by Age, Race/Ethnicity, Transmission Route, and Sex. (Adapted from U.S. Department of Health & Human Services. HIV Care Continuum. Updated December 30, 2016. Available at: https://www.hiv.gov/federal-response/policies-issues/hiv-aids-care-continuum.)

For someone living with HIV, during a medical history intake or update, dental hygienists can determine if a person is linked to medical care, retained in care, on ART, and adhering to treatment. The absence of any of these indicators of appropriate care provides an opportunity to discuss the importance of routine medical and oral healthcare and advise the patient to see their primary care provider. The medical team should be reinforcing the importance of routine oral healthcare and question their patients on their past dental visits. If a patient does not have a dental provider, a referral to one should be made.

THE DENTAL HYGIENE PROCESS OF CARE IN PATIENTS WITH HIV

As oral healthcare providers, dental hygienists have an ethical responsibility to be aware of the various health issues affecting their patients. Dental hygienists should offer information and education to patients so that they can live healthier and more productive lives.

A dental hygienist's clinical care delivery is determined by state or provincial laws and regulations. Preventive clinical and educational services are most common, as are therapeutic services for gingival and periodontal conditions. A thorough assessment of clinical findings should be performed and a care plan should be developed based on identified conditions rather than the HIV serostatus of the patient (Box 51.1).

Infection Control and Risk of HIV Infection Among Healthcare Workers

It is important to follow standard precautions when providing oral healthcare services to all patients (see Chapter 10). Healthcare workers are at risk for occupational exposure to HIV infection (as well as to other blood-borne pathogens) as a result of their work-related contact with contaminated blood and bodily fluids; however, this risk is very low. Of the documented transmissions of HIV in healthcare settings tracked since 1999, none have occurred in dental healthcare workers.[23] Prospective studies of healthcare workers occupationally exposed to HIV have estimated the risk of acquiring HIV infection through an occupational exposure to be approximately 0.23%; in other words, the vast majority of occupational exposures do not result in HIV infection.[24] The risk of transmission by other routes (e.g., exposure through the eye, nose, or mouth) is even lower at approximately 0.1%.[24]

The proper use of personal protective equipment (PPE), such as gloves and eyewear, along with safety devices to prevent injuries from sharp medical devices, can help minimize the risk of exposure

BOX 51.1   Legal, Ethical, and Safety Issues

- The dental hygienist has an ethical and legal responsibility to care for PWH. To withhold treatment or provide treatment in a manner outside the norm of the practice is discriminatory under most state laws and under the Americans with Disabilities Act of 1990.
- Treatment is necessary and effective for PWH.
- The provision of oral healthcare is based on an individual's needs and treatment plan and not on any bloodborne serostatus.

to HIV. When workers are exposed, the CDC recommends immediate treatment with a short course of antiretroviral drugs to prevent infection. The Exposure Control Manual in oral healthcare settings should include a section on postexposure management. In addition, there should be a designated provider who has been identified as capable of managing an exposure. Management of an exposure is considered an urgent medical concern and should not be delayed. If indicated, ART should be initiated as soon as possible, ideally within 2 hours. Postexposure ART must be started within 72 hours to be effective. Postexposure prophylaxis should be taken for 28 days.

Health History Assessment

When conducting the patient interview, the dental hygienist must be particularly sensitive to the patient's health history and pharmacologic history, as well as observations of clinical conditions associated with HIV infection. All health history questions should be reviewed and discussed with the patient.

The patient's current medication regimen (as part of the medical history), including antiretroviral drugs and any prophylactic antimicrobials to prevent opportunistic infections, should also be noted. While validating the health history and during the interview, the patient may report recent hospital stays for conditions associated with HIV status, as listed in Table 51.3. Throughout the assessment, it is imperative to build trust with the patient by reaffirming professional confidentiality and explaining the medical importance of gathering personal health information.

HIV Preexposure Prophylaxis (PrEP)

In 2021, the CDC published a clinical practice guideline recommending the use of PrEP to reduce transmission to HIV-negative individuals at high risk of exposure. This is accomplished by prescribing a once-a-day ART regimen that with proper adherence, reduces the risk of transmission by over 92%.[25]

TABLE 51.3 AIDS-Defining Conditions and Diagnostic Criteria

Candidiasis of the bronchi, trachea, lungs, or esophagus

Invasive cervical cancer

Disseminated or extrapulmonary coccidioidomycosis

Extrapulmonary cryptococcosis

Chronic intestinal cryptosporidiosis (>1 month in duration)

Cytomegalovirus disease other than of the liver, spleen, or nodes

Cytomegalovirus retinitis with loss of vision

HIV-related encephalopathy

Herpes simplex with chronic ulcer(s) (>1 month in duration) or bronchitis, pneumonitis, or esophagitis

Disseminated or extrapulmonary histoplasmosis

Chronic intestinal isosporiasis (>1 month in duration)

Kaposi sarcoma, either intraoral or extraoral

Lymphoma (Burkitt, immunoblastic, or primary brain)

Mycobacterium avium complex or *Mycobacterium kansasii* (disseminated or extrapulmonary)

Mycobacterium tuberculosis (pulmonary or extrapulmonary)

Pneumocystis jirovecii (formerly *Pneumocystis carinii*) pneumonia

Recurrent pneumonia

Progressive multifocal leukoencephalopathy

Recurrent salmonella septicemia

Toxoplasmosis involving the brain

HIV-related wasting syndrome

Centers for Disease Control and Prevention. AIDS and Opportunistic Infections. HIV. Updated May 20, 2021. https://www.cdc.gov/hiv/basics/livingwithhiv/opportunisticinfections.html. Accessed July 26, 2022.

Oral health professionals should be aware that individuals on PrEP:
1. Are HIV negative but have a high potential for exposure to the virus
2. Are on HIV antiviral, which greatly reduces their risk of HIV infection when adhering to their prophylactic regimen
3. Should receive routine dental care as determined by their oral health needs

It is important to reiterate that a person taking PrEP may indicate an HIV-associated medication on their medical history but check negative for HIV status because the medication is being taken as a preventive measure, not as a therapeutic regimen.

Extraoral and Intraoral Examination

Extraoral assessments of PWH may reveal purplish-red nodules on the skin that are indicative of Kaposi sarcoma. Intraorally, no oral lesions have been identified as only being associated with HIV. PWH have a higher risk than the general population of having oral lesions that are fungal, bacterial, viral, neoplastic, or idiopathic. Intraoral conditions may include signs and symptoms associated with candidiasis, oral hairy leukoplakia, Kaposi sarcoma lesions, oral warts secondary to HPV, and/or necrotizing forms of periodontal disease. They may also present with xerostomia as a side effect of medications or glandular conditions that reduce salivary flow. Such clients should always be referred to a dentist or a physician for further evaluation.

Fungal Infections

Oral candidiasis is the most commonly seen manifestation and can be found not just in PWH but also in patients using steroid inhalers for asthma, undergoing chemotherapy, presenting with uncontrolled diabetes, or using broad-spectrum antibiotics. Pseudomembranous candidiasis, erythematous candidiasis, and angular cheilitis are examples of mucosal disease caused by an overgrowth of *Candida albicans*.

Candidiasis is by no means unique to the HIV-infected population, and its presence is not necessarily indicative of HIV/AIDS.
- **Pseudomembranous candidiasis** (thrush) appears as soft, yellow-white, curdlike plaques on the oral tissues that, when wiped away, leave red, tender, and bleeding patches of mucosa. These plaques occur most frequently on the hard and soft palate, the labial and buccal mucosa, and the oropharynx (Fig. 51.5).
- **Erythematous candidiasis** appears as smooth, red, denuded patches on the tongue or red patches on the buccal or palatal mucosa. Erythematous candidiasis is caused by the same organisms that cause the pseudomembranous form. These lesions are less obvious and more easily missed than white patches; however, patients may complain of burning notably when eating salty or spicy foods or drinking acidic beverages. These fungal infections can be associated with acrylic appliances, so appliances must be treated as well as the candidiasis (Fig. 51.6).
- **Angular cheilitis** appears as redness, cracks, crusting, or fissures at the commissures of the lips. The lesions are moderately painful and eroded (Fig. 51.7).

Bacterial Infections

Necrotizing ulcerative periodontitis (NUP) is characterized by severe pain described as deep jaw pain, fetid odor, bleeding, and loose teeth with rapid loss of bone and soft tissue (Fig. 51.8). Ulcerations may be present. This condition can be associated with severe immune suppression and is not isolated to PWH.

Viral Infections

Human papillomavirus (HPV) is commonly found in the general population. This virus has many subtypes, some of which are associated with the formation of oral warts, which may be singular or multifocal (Fig. 51.9). These warts may cause aesthetic and functional problems. An increase in oral warts may occur in PWH receiving antiretroviral therapy. Recurrence is common after treatment. Other HPV types are known to be oncogenic, among them HPV16, which is the one overwhelmingly associated with oropharyngeal cancer. Most HPV-related cancer on the head and neck regions are in the posterior oropharynx in the tonsillar and posterior (nonoral) tongue. Cancer of the oral cavity proper is rarely related to HPV infection or etiology.

Herpes simplex virus, also known as HSV, is an infection that causes herpetic lesions (Fig. 51.10). Many individuals have been exposed to primary herpetic infections that are either clinical or subclinical in nature at some time during their lives. HSV is found on keratinized tissue or the vermilion border of the lip as shallow ulcerations. The recurrence of herpes appears to be related to the breakdown in local immune activity or alterations in local inflammatory mediators that allow the herpesvirus to become active again. In general, HSV lesions heal within 1 to 2 weeks and are not related to secondary infections. More severe lesions or longer healing time can be related to immunosuppression. Pain that may be associated with oropharyngeal herpes lesions can significantly restrict the patient's intake of food, thereby compromising adequate nutrition.

Hairy leukoplakia presents as a white corrugated lesion on the lateral border of the tongue and is associated with the Epstein-Barr virus (Fig. 51.11). It cannot be wiped off like white lesions associated with candidiasis. It is usually painless and does not require treatment.

Neoplastic Lesions

Kaposi sarcoma is a malignant lesion that appears as flat, red, or purple to dark purple macules or raised ulcerations that may present in PWH (Fig. 51.12). Biopsy confirmation is indicated. Kaposi sarcoma has several associated causative factors, most notably a viral infection with

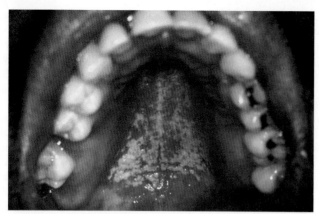

Fig. 51.5 Pseudomembranous candidiasis in an individual with AIDS, manifested as white-yellow curdlike plaques on the palate. (From Reznik D. Screening for infectious diseases in the dental setting. *Dent Clin North Am.* 2012;56(4):809.)

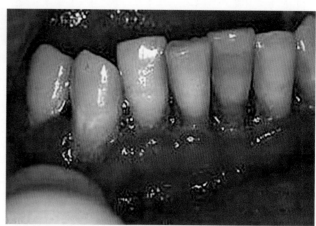

Fig. 51.8 Necrotizing ulcerative periodontitis in an individual with AIDS showing color change, necrosis, and sloughing of the periodontal tissues. (Copyright 1996–2000 David Reznik, DDS. All rights reserved. Available HIVdent. Oral manifestation: picture gallery. http://www.hivdent.org/_picturegallery_/_picturegallery.htm.)

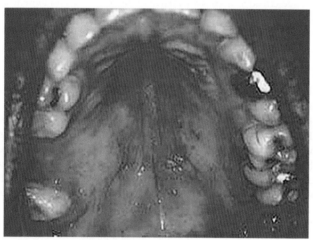

Fig. 51.6 Erythematous candidiasis. (Copyright 1996–2000 David Reznik, DDS. All rights reserved. Available HIVdent. Oral manifestation: picture gallery. http://www.hivdent.org/_picturegallery_/_picturegallery.htm.)

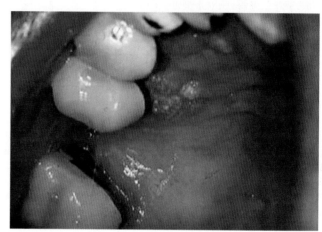

Fig. 51.9 Human papillomavirus (HPV) intraoral lesion. (Copyright 1996–2007 HIVdent.org. All rights reserved. Available HIVdent. Oral manifestation: picture gallery. http://www.hivdent.org/_picturegallery_/_picturegallery.htm.)

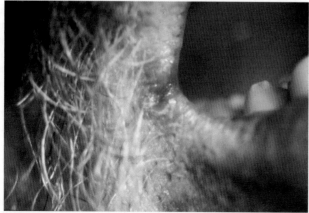

Fig. 51.7 Angular cheilitis. (Copyright 1996–2007 HIVdent.org. All rights reserved. Available HIVdent. Oral manifestation: picture gallery. http://www.hivdent.org/_picturegallery_/_picturegallery.htm.)

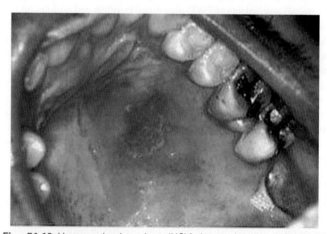

Fig. 51.10 Herpes simplex virus (HSV) intraoral lesion. (Copyright 1996–2007 HIVdent.org. All rights reserved. Available HIVdent. Oral manifestation: picture gallery. http://www.hivdent.org/_picturegallery_/_picturegallery.htm.)

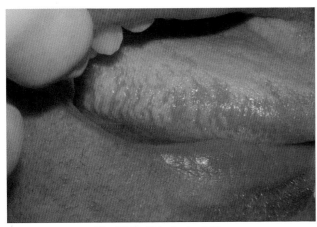

Fig. 51.11 Hairy leukoplakia.

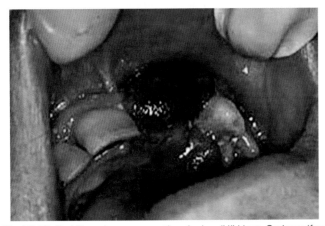

Fig. 51.12 Oral Kaposi sarcoma on the gingiva. (HIVdent. Oral manifestation: picture gallery. http://www.hivdent.org/_picturegallery_/_picturegallery.htm.)

human herpesvirus-8 and alterations in the immune system. It may appear on the skin of the extremities as well as internal organs. These lesions may also appear anywhere in the oral cavity and, depending on their position, may cause problems with phonation, swallowing, or breathing. Since the advent of ART, Kaposi sarcoma is less frequently seen but is still the most common oral cancer noted among individuals with untreated or unmanaged HIV.[26]

Squamous cell carcinoma is the most common type of oral cancer in the general population, accounting for about 90% of all oral cancers.[27] As with other neoplasms, a biopsy confirmation is indicated before treatment such as excision and chemotherapy or radiation. Other neoplasms may involve lymph nodes, salivary glands, or metastasis from a primary carcinoma. Diagnosis by biopsy is indicated to determine treatment.

Idiopathic Lesions

Aphthous ulcers are characterized by a halo appearance of inflammation and a gray or yellow cover over the ulcer. They occur on nonkeratinized tissue such as buccal/labial mucosa, maxillary/mandibular vestibules, and the posterior oropharynx. They are very painful.

Diagnosis and Planning of Dental Hygiene Care

As previously mentioned, the dental hygiene care plan for PWH should not be driven by the HIV serostatus of the patient (Box 51.1). The care plan should include, independently of HIV status, oral health education, oral biofilm control, periodontal debridement when indicated, the provision of posttreatment instructions, the evaluation of care, and

continued care. Dental hygiene care must be integrated with overall dental treatment (Box 51.2). Once an individualized care plan has been formulated, it is implemented in accordance with the goals and priorities established by the patient and the oral healthcare team.

Implementation of Periodontal Debridement

Generally, PWH present with oral needs similar to those of the HIV-negative population and require routine dental prophylaxis. As seen in other patients, they can have gingivitis, periodontitis, xerostomia, dental caries, etc., or they can simply have healthy, well-maintained oral tissues. The etiology of such oral diseases in PWH is similar in people living without HIV. It is unethical and discriminatory to withhold any known procedure based solely on HIV status.

- PWH presenting with xerostomia should be treated in the same manner as in other patients, such as encouraging drinking more water; avoiding caffeine, tobacco, vaping, and alcohol; and incorporating saliva-stimulating agents, topical fluorides, or diet modifications to reduce the risk of dental caries.
- For those presenting with fungal infections that result from *Candida* infection, treatment involves a variety of topical or systemic antifungal drugs. These may be prescribed by a dentist or primary care provider. Topical applications of nystatin or clotrimazole are commonly used to treat mild to moderate candida infections. In more severe cases, patients may require systemic administration of antifungal medications, such as fluconazole.
- HPV lesions may be cancer causing or benign. However, it is important to note infection with multiple types of HPV, some cancer causing, may coexist, so close monitoring of all HPV lesions and a comprehensive soft tissue oral exam should be indicated at each visit.
- Due to the contagious nature of HSV, elective dental treatment should be postponed for patients presenting with active HSV lesions until the lesion has healed.[28] HSV is treated with antiviral therapy.
- Patients presenting with aphthous ulcers are treated not only to resolve the ulcer but also to manage the pain. Treatments may include topical analgesics/antiinflammatory agents (e.g., 20% benzocaine pastes, benzydamine hydrochloride mouthrinses), antimicrobials (e.g., 0.12% chlorhexidine mouthrinse), and topical corticosteroid agents (e.g., dexamethasone elixir).[29–30]
- For neoplastic lesions such as Kaposi sarcoma (KS) lesions and oral squamous cell carcinoma, a biopsy, consultation with the patient's physician/primary care provider, and referral are necessary. Oral KS lesions are treated with systemic chemotherapy. Dental hygienists and dentists are sometimes hesitant to manipulate gingival tissue for fear of harming nearby KS lesions or causing significant bleeding. However, periodontal care must be provided; in some cases, tumor reduction is achieved with nonsurgical periodontal therapy. Oral biofilm removal and periodontal debridement are essential to maximizing the effects of periodontal therapy and may help to reduce the size of the tumor before tumor-specific therapy.

- During periodontal debridement, the use of powered instruments is not prohibited. Aerosols are not among the modes of transmission of HIV.
- The most appropriate treatment for those presenting with necrotizing ulcerative periodontitis (NUP) should be prompt and aggressive control of the microbial challenge and local irritants. The initial treatment of NUP should involve systemic antibiotic therapy, local debridement of tissues, nutritional counseling, and pain management. NUP is a marker of severe immune deterioration and should involve medical/dental collaboration.[31] In addition, periodontal surgery may be required to remove necrotized tissues, including bone. Local irrigation of the gingiva and affected tissues with 0.12% chlorhexidine gluconate also has been recommended. Disposable syringes with blunt needles or cotton swabs are required to adequately flush the affected tissues. Persons who are being treated for NUP require frequent monitoring and evaluation. Postoperative care requires good mechanical oral biofilm control and twice-daily 0.12% chlorhexidine rinses for chemical oral biofilm control throughout the mouth. Patients must be informed about the possible side effects of chlorhexidine, including staining of the teeth, discoloration of the oral mucosa, calculus accumulation, and altered taste sensation. Antibiotics such as metronidazole to control oral anaerobic pathogens often are prescribed.

Evaluation

After comprehensive dental hygiene care has been provided, the dental hygienist should evaluate the patient to ensure that the established goals have been met. Evaluation should take place at appropriate intervals. After initial therapy, reevaluation should occur in about 4 weeks. This allows time for the healing of the connective tissue so that the patient can be probed and assessed accurately. Recall intervals thereafter should follow the same guidelines as used for patients who are HIV negative. Appropriate care intervals provide opportunities to assess the patient's oral health, self-care practices, and nutrition for optimal long-term outcomes. The evaluation phase of the dental hygiene process of care also provides the opportunity to identify other human needs related to oral health and disease that may require attention. As with all patients, the process of care for patients with HIV occurs on a continuum.

The former Surgeon General Regina Benjamin, in a special issue of *Public Health Reports*, noted that, "While good oral health is important to the well-being of all population groups, it is especially critical for PWH. Inadequate oral healthcare can undermine HIV treatment and diminish quality of life, yet many individuals living with HIV are not receiving the necessary oral healthcare that would optimize their treatment."[32]

CONCLUDING STATEMENT

Providing healthcare to all, including PWH, is both an ethical and legal duty of all healthcare providers, including dentists and dental hygienists. Delivering oral care for PWH does not require any advanced skills and does not necessitate, per se, a modification of the treatment or special precautionary measures that would not be taken for all patients. There is no evidence to support the assertion that the dental and periodontal diseases seen in PWH are intrinsically different from the diseases observed in HIV-seronegative patients. The oral treatments rendered are also identical to the ones used in all patients.

The standard of care mandates that PWH be evaluated for their health status as any patient would be and not triaged or treated differently based on their HIV status. Although it is true that PWH are more likely to suffer from certain ailments such as the dental, periodontal, or mucosal consequences of hyposalivation or from OIs due to defective

immunity, oral examination including that of soft tissues is not different in PWH from that conducted on all patients. The mucosal lesions seen in PWH are also seen in HIV-seronegative patients, albeit at lower incidence rates. Accordingly, the oral examination of PWH can be conducted by any hygienist and dentist, and it must include a soft tissue examination as performed for all patients.

The care of PWH has historically suffered from stigmatization and nonevidence-based deviations from what the standard of care would mandate. It is important for healthcare workers including hygienists to base their care of PWH on scientific evidence. That evidence tells us that HIV status is not intrinsically a reason for refusal of care, treatment modification, or additional precautionary measures to protect the healthcare workers or the patient (see Box 51.1).

KEY CONCEPTS

- HIV infection is a disease that may severely suppress the host's immune response.
- U=U. Evidence supports the fact that virally suppressed PWH (Undetectable) do not infect their sexual partners (Untransmittable)
- HIV is a chronic, treatable condition.
- The risk of acquiring HIV infection from providing dental hygiene care to infected individuals is extremely low when appropriate infection control protocols are followed.
- Standard precautions must be used as they are for treating all patients.
- Most periodontal disease in HIV-positive individuals is indistinguishable from disease patterns seen in HIV-negative clients.
- There are no oral lesions associated only with HIV. The appearance of an oral manifestation related to HIV should be evaluated and, with consent, discussed with the patient's primary care or infectious disease physician.
- There is no evidence-based reason for antibiotic prophylaxis for a patient based solely on their HIV status.
- In the event of an occupational injury, have in place a postexposure protocol that involves local expertise. If local expertise is not available, call (888) 448-4911, 9 AM to 2 AM EST, 7 days a week for a telephone consultation and get timely answers for postexposure management. Get rapid, expert guidance in managing healthcare worker exposures to HIV and hepatitis B and C. Find immediate recommendations on when and how to initiate PEP through an online Quick Guide for urgent PEP decision making, or from experienced clinicians on the telephone consultation service.

ACKNOWLEDGMENT

The authors acknowledge Dorothy A. Perry, Devan Darby Bartels, and Saran Rai for their past contributions to this chapter.

REFERENCES

1. Leveton LB, Sox Jr HC, Stoto MA. *HIV and the Blood Supply: An Analysis of Crisis Decisionmaking*. National Academies Press (US); 1995.
2. U.S. Department of Health and Human Services. *Oral Health in America: A Report of the Surgeon General–Executive Summary*. U.S. Department of Health and Human Services, National Institute of Dental and Craniofacial Research, National Institutes of Health; 2000.
3. Saini R. Oral lesions: a true clinical indicator in human immunodeficiency virus. *J Nat Sci Biol Med*. 2011;2(2):145–150.
4. Quinn TC. HIV epidemiology and the effects of antiviral therapy on long-term consequences. *AIDS*. 2008;22(suppl 3):S7–S12.
5. Hsieh YH, Kelen GD, Laeyendecker O, et al. HIV care continuum for HIV-infected emergency department patients in an inner-city academic emergency department. *Ann Emerg Med*. 2015;66(1):69–78.

6. Escudero DJ, Lurie MN, Mayer KH, et al. The risk of HIV transmission at each step of the HIV care continuum among people who inject drugs: a modeling study. *BMC Publ Health*. 2017;17(1):614.

7. The White House Office of National AIDS Policy. *National HIV/AIDS Strategy for the United States 2022–2025*. The White House; 2021.

8. U.S. Department of Health and Human Services. *Oral Health in America: Advances and Challenges*. U.S. Department of Health and Human Services, National Institute of Dental and Craniofacial Research, National Institutes of Health; 2021.

9. Health Resources and Services Administration. *HIV/AIDS Bureau. Ending the HIV Epidemic in the U.S. Initiative Data Report 2020*. Division of Policy and Data, HRSA, U.S. Department of Health and Human Services; 2021.

10. World Health Organization. HIV/AIDS. The Global Health Observatory. Updated July 2021. https://www.who.int/data/gho/data/themes/hiv-aids#:~:text=Global%20situation%20and%20trends%3A&text=Globally%2C%2037.7%20million%20%5B30.2%E2%80%93,considerably%20between%20countries%20and%20regions. Accessed July 26, 2022.

11. Centers for Disease Control and Prevention. *HIV Surveillance Report, 2020*. Division of HIV Prevention, National Center for HIV, Viral Hepatitis, STD, and TB Prevention, Centers for Disease Control and Prevention (CDC), U.S. Department of Health and Human Services; 2022. Report No. 33.

12. Bernstein L. We could cut the HIV transmission rate by more than 90 percent, CDC says. The Washington Post. Published February 23, 2015. https://www.washingtonpost.com/news/to-your-health/wp/2015/02/23/we-could-cut-the-hiv-transmission-rate-by-more-than-90-percent-cdc-says/?utm_term=.71ab9bfcc8b0. Accessed July 26, 2022.

13. Kandathil AJ, Ramalingam S, Kannangai R, et al. Molecular epidemiology of HIV. *Indian J Med Res*. 2005;121:333.

14. Boswell SL, Fuller JD. Pathogenesis and natural history. In: Libman H, Makadon HJ, eds. *HIV. American College of Physicians*. American Society of Internal Medicine; 2000.

15. Center for Disease Control and Prevention. Which STD Tests Should I Get? Sexually Transmitted Diseases (STDs). Updated December 14, 2021. https://www.cdc.gov/std/prevention/screeningreccs.htm. Accessed July 26, 2022.

16. Centers for Disease Control and Prevention: 1993 Revised Classification System for HIV Infection and Expanded Surveillance Case for AIDS Among Adolescents and Adults. *MMWR (Morb Mortal Wkly Rep)*. Published December 18, 1992. http://www.cdc.gov/mmwr/preview/mmwrhtml/00018871.htm. Accessed July 26, 2022.

17. Centers for Disease Control and Prevention. AIDS and Opportunistic Infections. HIV. Updated May 20, 2021. https://www.cdc.gov/hiv/basics/livingwithhiv/opportunisticinfections.html. Accessed July 26, 2022.

18. Centers for Disease Control and Prevention. *Estimated HIV incidence and prevalence in the United States, 2015–2019*. Division of HIV/AIDS prevention, National Center for HIV/AIDS, viral hepatitis, STD, and TB prevention, Centers for disease control and prevention (CDC), U.S. Department of Health and Human Services; 2021. HIV Surveillance Supplemental Report Volume 26, No. 1.

19. U.S. Department of Health & Human Services. Should You Get Tested for HIV? HIV.gov. Updated June 15, 2020. https://www.hiv.gov/hiv-basics/hiv-testing/learn-about-hiv-testing/who-should-get-tested#:~:text=CDC%20recommends%20that%20everyone%20between%20the%20ages%20of,with%20someone%20whose%20sexual%20history%20they%20don%E2%80%99t%20know. Accessed July 26, 2022.

20. Gardner EM, McLees MP, Steiner JF, et al. The spectrum of engagement in HIV care and its relevance to test-and-treat strategies for prevention of HIV infection. *Clin Infect Dis*. 2011;52(6):793–800.

21. Centers for Disease Control and Prevention. Understanding the HIV Care Continuum. Published July 2019. https://www.cdc.gov/hiv/pdf/library/factsheets/cdc-hiv-care-continuum.pdf. Accessed July 26, 2022.

22. U.S Department of Health and Human Services. What Is the HIV Care Continuum? HIV.gov. Updated July 1, 2022. https://www.hiv.gov/federal-response/policies-issues/hiv-aids-care-continuum. Accessed July 26, 2022.

23. Joyce MP, Kuhar D, Brooks JT. Notes from the field: occupationally acquired HIV infection among health care workers—United States, 1985–2013. *MMWR (Morb Mortal Wkly Rep)*. 2015;63(53):1245–1246.

24. Bell DM. Occupational risk of human immunodeficiency virus infection in healthcare workers: an overview. *Am J Med*. 1997;102(suppl 5B):9.

25. Centers for Disease Control and Prevention. US Public Health Service: Preexposure Prophylaxis for the Prevention of HIV Infection in the United States—2021 Update: A Clinical Practice Guideline. Published 2021. https://www.cdc.gov/hiv/pdf/risk/prep/cdc-hiv-prep-guidelines-2021.pdf. Accessed July 26, 2022.

26. U.S. Department of Veterans Affairs. Kaposi sarcoma. HIV. https://www.hiv.va.gov/patient/diagnosis/OI-Kaposi-sarcoma.asp. Accessed July 26, 2022.

27. American Association of Oral and Maxillofacial Surgeons. Oral Cancer Symptoms and Types. Oral, Head and Neck Pathology. Updated March 2020. https://myoms.org/what-we-do/oral-head-and-neck-pathology/oral-cancer-symptoms-types/. Accessed July 26, 2022.

28. Miller CS. Subject: Dental Care for the Patient with an Oral Herpetic Lesion. The American Academy of Oral Medicine. Published November 25, 2014. Updated January 2, 2016. https://www.aaom.com/index.php?option=com_content&view=article&id=161:clinical-practice-statement--dental-care-for-the-patient-with-an-oral-herpetic-lesion&catid=24:clinical-practice-statement. Accessed July 26, 2022.

29. Clark D. How do I manage a patient with aphthous ulcers? *J Can Dent Assoc*. 2013;79:d48.

30. Staines K, Greenwood M. Aphthous ulcers (recurrent). *BMJ Clin Evid*. 2015;2015:1303.

31. Glick M, Muzyka BC, Salkin LM, Lurie D. Necrotizing ulcerative periodontitis: a marker for immune deterioration and a predictor for the diagnosis of AIDS. *J Periodontol*. 1994;65(5):393–397.

32. Benjamin RM. Oral health care for people living with HIV/AIDS. *Public Health Rep*. 2012;127(suppl 2):1–2.

52

Palliative Dental Hygiene Oral Care

L. Lynda McKeown, Carolyn Weiss, Heather Woodbeck, Ruth Bushby, and Susan Raynak

PROFESSIONAL OPPORTUNITIES

Dental hygienists and other oral health professionals contribute to persons' oral/dental health through all ages and abilities. They need to be important members of the palliative care teams in all healthcare settings. Sadly, the role of the dental hygienist is often overlooked. Oral care of persons in the palliative and end-of-life stages is frequently inadequate.

Older persons are a growing demographic group in society in almost every country in the world.[1] As the population ages, persons are likely to develop frailties. Increasing physical and cognitive defects lead to dependence on others. Oral self-care can become difficult, providing an opportunity for dental hygienists. **Palliative dental hygiene oral care** is provided when a person becomes dependent. Palliative dental hygiene focuses on reducing the severity of oral/dental symptoms, preventing pain, and maintaining cleanliness and comfort in the mouth to end of life.

As professionals, dental hygienists are committed to maintaining competence in supporting the evolving and diverse health needs of the public. With the aging population, providing palliative dental hygiene oral care is a wide-open field for dental hygienists. Being competent in providing palliative dental hygiene oral care is an opportunity to apply the full scope of dental hygiene practice by implementing noninvasive techniques. Integration of dental hygienists as a collaborative partner in palliative care is paramount to help maintain persons' dignity and wellbeing throughout all stages of life.

COMPETENCIES

1. Discuss palliative care and explain palliative dental hygiene oral care.
2. Describe the role of the dental hygienist and appropriate palliative dental hygiene oral care practices in any setting.
3. Advocate for inclusion of dental hygienists as an essential healthcare provider in legislation across the healthcare system.
4. Apply the dental hygiene process of care to persons who are palliative and/or at the end of life.
5. Recognize the signs of aging, frailty, and oral complications manifested in the mouth during the process of dying and death.
6. Integrate strategies of palliative dental hygiene oral care used to accommodate increasing oral frailty, disability, and interprofessional collaboration.
7. Integrate an approach that respects the person's choices and values in the palliative and end-of-life stages.
8. Evaluate the impact of palliative dental hygiene oral care on the person.

PALLIATIVE AND END-OF-LIFE CARE

Palliative care is defined as "the active holistic care of individuals across all ages with serious health-related suffering (SHS). Suffering is health related when it is associated with illness or injury of any kind. Health-related suffering is serious when it cannot be relieved without medical intervention and when it compromises physical, social, spiritual, and/or emotional functioning."[2,3] End-of-life oral care is considered to be the subset of palliative oral care that occurs as the person is in the process of actively dying.[4]

Palliative medical care begins after a person of any age is diagnosed with a life-limiting situation, such as cancer, cognitive, neurological, developmental, cardiovascular, respiratory, and/or any other chronic condition that prevents people from doing their own oral self-care. The dental hygienist's role is important in all phases of palliative care. It can be delivered in the home as well as in long-term and acute care facilities. Challenges in doing one's oral care can last for many years, so dental hygienists can have long-term relationships with their palliative oral care clients.

Internationally, researchers developed frameworks for palliative care approaches. The guiding principles in the Canadian Framework for Palliative Care (Box 52.1) describes the principles that embody person and family-centered care: "... the person and their family members at the centre of health care and services. Person-and family-centered care respects and empowers individuals to be genuine partners with health-care providers for their health."[5] Dental hygienists need to demonstrate the effective use of palliative care principles (Box 52.1) used in the palliative stages.

PALLIATIVE DENTAL HYGIENE ORAL CARE

Palliative dental hygiene oral care is the concept of providing compassion, support, and care for persons' oral health as they progress through their chronic illness and disability so that they may live as fully and comfortably as possible until the end of life. Advanced care planning is a way to help people think through and talk about their values and wishes in relation to their future healthcare. Dental hygienists need to encourage people to plan ahead for their oral/dental care. There comes a point when for the sake of oral cleanliness and comfort for the person—palliative dental hygiene oral care is the rational choice.

Typically, but not exclusively, physical and cognitive deficits accumulate with aging. Dental hygienists need to recognize how these changes impact oral care. Frailties may directly or indirectly affect the health of the mouth and may determine the choice of dental hygiene therapies. These therapeutic services include treatments such as **noninvasive debridement** and interim stabilization therapy, but not necessarily traditional debridement. Noninvasive debridement involves removal of any soft deposit, biofilm, plaque, food particles, and pathogens that may cause inflammation and strain the body's ability to fight infection, from all areas of teeth and gum interface and embrasures using **oral physiotherapy tools,** not scalers, curettes, or ultrasonic or aerosol generation tools. Oral physiology tools include brushes for all surfaces (occlusal, buccal and lingual), floss, stimulators, and tongue cleaners.

BOX 52.1 Ten Guiding Principles for Palliative Care

1. Palliative care is person- and family-centered care.
2. Death, dying, grief, and bereavement are a normal part of life.
3. Caregivers are both providers and recipients of care.
4. Palliative care is integrated and holistic.
5. Access to palliative care is equitable
6. Palliative care recognizes and values diversity.
7. Palliative care services are valued, understood, and adequately resourced.
8. Palliative care is high quality and evidence based.
9. Palliative care improves quality of life.
10. Palliative care is a shared responsibility.

Adapted from Health Canada: Framework on Palliative Care in Canada. December 4, 2018. Available at: https://www.canada.ca/en/health-canada/services/health-care-system/reports-publications/palliative-care/framework-palliative-care-canada.html.

BOX 52.2 Impacts of Increased Frailty on Oral Health

Increased Frailty > Risks (Rockwood)	Impact on Oral Health and Oral Healthcare (MacEntee/Donnelly)
Medications	• Xerostomia/salivary hypofunction
Cognitive status (e.g., demented, delirious)	• Hypertenacious oral biofilm
	• Elevated risk of caries from
Emotional status (e.g., depressed, anxious, fatigued)	inadequate buffering capacity of saliva
Communication (speech, vision, hearing)	• Elevated risk of mucositis, gingivitis, and candidiasis
Strength-manual dexterity	• Difficulty expressing complaints
Balance	• Resistance to oral care and treatments
Nutrition (weight, appetite)	
Activities of daily living (feeding, bathing, dressing, toileting)	• Disregard/disinterest in oral care
	• Inability to follow treatment regimens
Mobility	• Impaired ability to perform oral hygiene
Social support and engagements	• Intolerance to dentures
	• Difficulty seeking oral care and treatments
	• Limited financial and social resources for oral care

Adapted from Dalhousie University. Rockwood's Clinical Frailty Scale. Available at: https://www.frailtytoolkit.org/rockwood and MacEntee MI, Donnelly LR. Oral health and the frailty syndrome. *Periodontol 2000.* 2016 Oct;72(1):135–141. https://doi.org/10.1111/prd.12134. PMID: 27501496.

Aging is a global phenomenon (see Chapter 47). It is anticipated that one in six people in the world will be aged 65 years or over by 2050.[1] According to a recent census, the population 85 and older is one of the fastest growing age demographics and is expected to triple by 2046.[1] Aging is a process usually accompanied by increased frailty. It is a condition that manifests throughout the body, including the mouth. Frailties such as arthritis, cognitive and physical deficits, and diminished sight and hearing can impact a person's oral hygiene.

Frailties in the mouth can include age-related loss of mucosal elasticity, submucosal tissue, and tactile sensitivity. Within the pulp of the vital teeth, there is a decrease in the number of blood vessels and cells, with an increase in secondary dentine deposits, often leading to dying and death of teeth (see Box 52.2).

Frailties in the mouth are often overlooked. The clinical signs and symptoms are usually not recognized by non–oral health professionals. Oral health and oral healthcare can be severely compromised by frailty in people who cannot attend to their personal hygiene or receive assistance from a caregiver.[6]

Mobility issues such reliance on others for transportation and accumulating physical and cognitive frailties add to a person's challenge accessing oral care. Dental hygienists with mobile practices provide oral care services where the person lives. Onsite dental hygiene services help a person maintain a comfortable clean mouth through increasing aging and frailties to end of life.

Another challenge in palliative dental hygiene oral care is lack of funding. Those who are most in need of care—seniors and people with functional disabilities—tend to have minimal access to dental care insurance coverage. Government-based oral health programs are usually quite limited in services. Dental insurance programs do not have the appropriate billing codes to reimburse the therapeutic services provided by a dental hygienist. People and their families may not value or believe that oral care is important for their overall health. When funding is a problem, oral care can become a low priority.

- A huge impediment is the general lack of knowledge, experience, and expertise on the importance of oral care. Policy decisions about mouth care are usually made by physicians and nurses. Rarely are dental hygienists included in any policy deliberation.
- Direct care staff who are assigned the daily task of mouth care in residential care facilities have minimal relevant education and lack competency to provide effective oral care. Therefore a dental hygienist is the appropriate healthcare professional to lead the health team in providing oral care. The profession of dental hygiene

must be prepared to provide appropriate therapies for persons with frailty, aging, and oral manifestations to end of life.

People residing in long-term care or those experiencing long hospitalizations are especially at risk for oral problems as they are frail and dependent on others for personal care needs. Systemic health breakdown and multiple prescription and nonprescription medications can cause xerostomia and impact oral health. Diets high in refined sugars and carbohydrates contribute to dental caries. The pattern of offering food continuously throughout the day means the mouth is always somewhat acidic (see Chapter 19). As well, medications are often crushed and put into sugar-laden products without doing oral care afterward. With onset of dementia, a person is less likely to select nutritious foods and/or to keep mouth, teeth, and dentures clean. The result may be dental caries, gingival wounds, mucositis, and/or candidiasis.

Other factors including stress, lack of social support, and many other emotional factors play a significant role in general and oral health. Lack of accessibility to appropriate professional oral care and resources such as oral hygiene tools contribute to diseases of mouth. Care staff may have limited competency to assist with daily oral hygiene. Persons may exhibit resistive behaviors and refuse to have oral care. It can be difficult for the persons with physical impairments and/or cognitive dysfunction to accept appropriate care and treatment.

ORAL COMPLICATIONS

Xerostomia (See Chapters 41, 47, 50, and 53)

There are multiple causes of **xerostomia** (see Box 52.3). Medications are generally prescribed for physical and cognitive disabilities. These pharmaceuticals disturb the buffering capacity of saliva which is

| BOX 52.3 | Causes of Xerostomia |

BOX 52.3   Causes of Xerostomia

Medications
- Anticholinergic drugs
- Antihistamines
- Antihypertensives

Conditions or diseases
- Radiation therapy
- Sjögren syndrome
- Diabetes mellitus
- HIV/AIDS
- Mumps
- Parotid agenesis
- Diarrhea, vomiting, hemorrhage
- Calculi (mineral deposits that block the salivary glands
- Reduced fluid intake

Radiation therapy

Chemotherapy

required to neutralize the salivary pH caused by acidogenic bacteria. Frequent exposure to acidic pH increases the risk of dental caries.[7]

Dental hygienists recognize saliva's contributions to oral and systemic health.[7] Tube feeding, masks, inhalers, and respiratory therapy medications tend to dry out mucous membranes. Oxygen administration in particular causes dry mouth. Continuous positive airway pressure (CPAP) masks for sleep apnea can be drying for oral tissues. Cancer chemotherapy, radiation therapy, and surgery to the head and neck are all risk factors for xerostomia and salivary gland hypofunction. Alcohol use, including alcohol in mouthwashes, increases the risk for xerostomia. Dental hygienists must assess for evidence of dry mouth in order to prevent tooth decay and oral wounds.[7]

In order to manage xerostomia, dental hygienists may work with dietitians and direct care staff to optimize oral hydration. Water should be the fluid of choice. Caffeine and alcohol dry the mouth, worsening xerostomia, and ideally should be avoided in high-risk persons. Sweetened fluids such as juice, pop, and sugary hot drinks create an acidic environment and can contribute to carious lesions. Food supplement drinks high in sugar should be avoided, if possible, as these supplements cause imbalances in the oral ecosystem that promote rapid tooth decay and oral wounds in a dry mouth. The diabetic versions of supplement drinks are a better choice. Provide water to all persons at the end of a meal and after a snack. At a minimum, rinse or wipe the mouth with water after eating to clear food debris (see Table 52.1).

Mucositis (see Chapter 50)

Mucositis is a condition that commonly occurs in patients receiving palliative care, especially those undergoing cancer chemotherapy and radiation treatment. Chemotherapy affects the oral cavity by reducing the mitosis rate in the oral tissues. In patients receiving cancer therapy, mucositis can be extremely widespread and painful. Mucositis can cause a burning, tingling sensation, followed by generalized pain and discomfort that hinders the person's ability to talk, eat, and swallow. Secondary infections of the weakened mucosa can be virulent and painful causing interruption to cancer therapy.[6]

In chronic mucositis, the oral mucosa thins and loses elasticity with age. The mucosa shows signs of frictional keratosis when subjected to chronic trauma. The mucosa may show signs of atrophy in persons with diabetes, hypertension, gastrointestinal disease, and malnutrition.[6]

Dental hygiene therapies for mucositis focus on keeping the mouth clean and hydrated (see Table 52.1).

ORAL CANDIDIASIS

Oral candidiasis is the most common fungal infection in humans with a high incidence among clients in palliative care (see Table 52.1).

Candida albicans, a natural oral cavity inhabitant, is the organism responsible for most cases of candidiasis. Although there are many predisposing factors to oral candidiasis, the main cause is an imbalance in oral flora and host immunity (see Box 52.4). Oral candidiasis symptoms include pain, bleeding, burning mouth, inability to taste food, malnutrition, and impaired quality of life.

There are four clinical types of candidiasis; each clinical type of oral candidiasis can occur in combination or independently of one another. **Hyperplastic candidiasis** presents as elevated white-yellow patches, similar to pseudomembranous candidiasis, only it cannot be wiped off. **Erythematous candidiasis** appears as red lesions, usually on the hard palate and dorsal surface of the tongue.

The type most commonly seen by dental hygienists is **pseudomembranous candidiasis or "thrush."** It presents clinically as white or yellowish patches on the tongue, buccal mucosa, hard palate, soft palate, and oral pharynx. The patches can be easily wiped off leaving inflamed and bleeding tissue. Candidiasis may manifest as **angular cheilitis**. It can present as white and red fissures at the commissures of the mouth. Angular cheilitis is common in denture wearers, as well as those with folic acid, iron, riboflavin (vitamin B_2), thiamine, and cobalamin (vitamin B_{12}) deficiencies (see Chapters 41 and 51).

If left untreated, oral candidiasis can progress systemically and increase mortality. Candidiasis is frequently seen in the mouth at the end of life. An alarming amount of candidiasis in the last days is often a sign that death is imminent.

The dental hygienist's role is to maintain function and comfort in and around the mouth. A referral to a health professional for an antifungal agent may be necessary (see Table 52.1).

DYSPHAGIA

Dysphagia is a common condition in elderly in which there is difficulty swallowing food and/or fluids.[7] It is caused by weakening of muscles associated with swallowing. Xerostomia may exacerbate swallowing dysfunction and can lead to dehydration, malnutrition, and weight loss. Dysphagia is a major risk factor for airway obstruction and aspiration pneumonia (see Box 52.5). Low salivary flow, associated with dysphagia, can lead to aspiration pneumonia from inhaling gramnegative anaerobes that originate in the mouth.

Aspiration pneumonia is a major problem that can lead to hospitalization, decreased quality of life, and death. Evidence suggests that effective mechanical removal of food debris and biofilm can reduce the incidence of aspiration pneumonia in at-risk children and frail elders.[8,9] Denture wearing during the night may double the risk of aspiration pneumonia and should be discouraged in geriatric patients.[9]

Dysphagia, postural difficulties, defects in hand-to-mouth coordination, and cognitive behavioral problems all contribute to difficulty eating for many frail persons. Dysphagia is often seen in persons with Parkinson disease, stroke, advanced dementia, and head and neck cancers (see Table 52.1).[10]

Dental hygienists working with persons with dysphagia need to be aware of pocketing of food, risk of airway obstruction, and aspiration pneumonia. Proper positioning during daily routines of oral hygiene care is important when reducing oral bacterial pathogens. The use of chlorhexidine gluconate solution (0.12%) has been shown to reduce the risk of aspiration pneumonia in geriatric persons.[11,12] Dietary modifications or postural changes may help improve swallowing abilities and safety. Dental hygienists may collaborate with the speech-language pathologist and/or a dietitian, who both assess clinical swallowing (see Box 52.5).

TABLE 52.1 Common Oral Complications

Assessment/Observation	Signs and Symptoms	Dental Hygiene Interventions
Mucositis and ulcerations 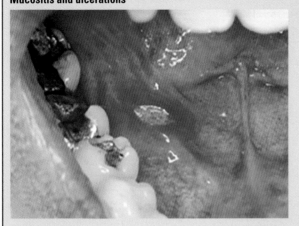 Oral ulceration (From Ibsen OAC, Phelan JA. *Oral Pathology for the Dental Hygienist*. 6th ed. Saunders; 2013.)	• Red, swollen tissue • Yellow membrane-covered • Burning, pain, and general discomfort reported by client	• Consistent hydration • Proper oral hygiene • Daily denture cleaning; remove dentures while sleeping • Avoid spicy foods, alcohol, and tobacco use • Soothing baking soda, saline, and water rinse • Physician-prescribed topical anesthetics with caution to avoid aspiration • Use of perioral moisturizers as directed by physician • Prescribed pharmaceutical mouthwash, i.e., Mayo Clinic "magic" mouthwash containing combined ingredients such as antihistamines, antifungals, topical anesthetics, and antibiotics
Oral candidiasis 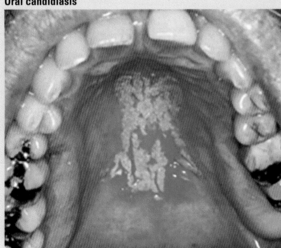 Oral candidiasis. (From Ibsen OAC, Phelan JA. *Oral Pathology for the Dental Hygienist*. 6th ed. Saunders; 2013.)	• **Pseudomembranous candidiasis**: white plaques that wipe off, with red, inflamed tissue underneath • **Erythematous candidiasis**: red lesions, usually on the hard palate and tongue • **Hyperplastic candidiasis**: white-yellow patches that cannot be wiped off	• Proper oral hygiene • Daily denture care; dentures out overnight • Saline rinses • Mouth moisturizer • Prescribed topical and/or systemic antifungal agents (see Box 52.6) • Do not eat or drink for 20 minutes after topical treatment • Replace denture container and toothbrush • Treat dentures for oral candidiasis (see Box 52.7)
Angular Cheilitis 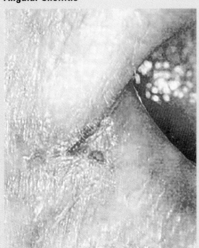 Photo credit: David Banting. Used with permission.	• **Angular cheilitis**: White and red fissures at the corners of the mouth • Symptoms: pain, bleeding, burning mouth, inability to taste food, malnutrition (vitamin B riboflavin deficiency), and impaired quality of life • Inadequate vertical dimension in occlusion resulting in overclosure of teeth	• See DH interventions above and referral to physician or dietitian for nutritional deficiency • Moisturize lips with a nonpetroleum-based product

Continued

TABLE 52.1 Common Oral Complications—cont'd

Xerostomia (dry mouth) 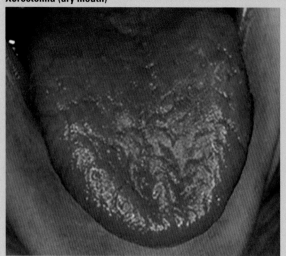 This patient has severe xerostomia. The tongue filiform papillae are lacking. (From Ibsen OAC, Phelan JA. *Oral Pathology for the Dental Hygienist.* 6th ed. Saunders; 2013.)	• Dryness of mucous membranes • Dryness of lips • No pool of saliva on floor of mouth • Difficulty chewing and swallowing • Difficulty speaking • Fissured tongue	• Proper oral hygiene • Maintain hydration • Avoid use of products containing alcohol, lemon, glycerin, and petroleum • Consult with physician about minimizing use of prescriptions associated with salivary hypofunction • Use nonalcohol fluoride mouthwash • Swab water-soluble lubricants throughout mouth • Use baking soda and saline rinse every 1 to 3 hours for 1 week • Increase hydration with water, ice chips and/or sugar-free ice pops, sugar-free gum, high-moisture foods, or water sprayed from pump dispenser • Use over-the-counter saliva substitutes • Apply water-based lubricants to lips • Ask physician or dentist to prescribe saliva stimulant
Dysphagia	• Difficulty swallowing food or liquids • Drooling • Sensation of food getting stuck in the throat or chest	• Maintain adequate hydration • Elevate the head of the bed to at least a 30° angle • Head in neutral to slightly downward position • Provide appropriate oral hygiene • Avoid toothpaste with any detergent or surfactant, such as sodium lauryl sulfate • Use "dip and brush" with fluoridated or chlorhexidine rinse

Adapted from PDQ Supportive and Palliative Care Editorial Board. *PDQ Oral Complications of Chemotherapy and Head/Neck Radiation.* National Cancer Institute. Updated December 16, 2016. Available at: https://www.cancer.gov/about-cancer/treatment/side-effects/mouth-throat/oral-complications-hp-pdq. Accessed July 25, 2022; Millsop JW, Fazel N. Oral candidiasis. *Clin Dermatol.* 2016;34(4):487.

BOX 52.4 Predisposing Factors for Oral Candidiasis

Local Factors
- Poor oral hygiene
- Xerostomia
- Wearing dentures
- Overclosure of mouth, drooling
- Tissue trauma
- Smoking tobacco

Medical Factors
- Immunosuppression
- Corticosteroids, including inhalers
- Broad-spectrum antibiotics
- Diabetes
- HIV/AIDS
- Cancer chemotherapy
- Head and neck radiation
- Poor nutritional status

Data from Centers for Disease Control and Prevention. Oropharyngeal/Esophageal Candidiasis ("Thrush"). Available at: https://www.cdc.gov/fungal/diseases/candidiasis/thrush/. Accessed July 25, 2022.

BOX 52.5 Aspiration Pneumonia

- Aspiration of oral and throat secretions is the main cause of pneumonia.
- Pneumonia is the leading cause of death in personal care homes.
- A correlation has been shown between aspiration pneumonia and the following:
  - Swallowing disorders
  - Impaired cough reflex sensitivity
  - Compromised health
  - Poor management of oral secretions
  - Dependence for feeding
  - Recent antibiotic therapy
  - Periodontal disease
  - Poor dental plaque control
  - Dry mouth
  - Having natural teeth, especially with untreated dental caries
  - Nightly denture wearing

Data from DiBardino DM, Wunderink RG. Aspiration pneumonia: a review of modern trends. *J Crit Care.* 2015;30(1):40.

PALLIATIVE DENTAL HYGIENE ORAL CARE SCENARIO

Frailty to End of Life—Bruna's Story

Bruna's story shows how frailty and oral health are connected. The story illustrates how palliative dental hygiene oral care is initiated when a person's frailties increase and they are unable to sustain oral self-care. They progress from needing assistance to being completely dependent for oral care. Preventive dental hygiene procedures and noninvasive therapies are initiated to keep a person comfortable and clean.

BOX 52.6 Antifungal Agents for the Treatment of Oral Candidiasis

Topical Antifungal Agents (First Route)
- Gentian violet
  - Solution: 1.5 mL of 0.5% twice daily
  - *Side effects*: Skin irritation, oral ulcers, purple staining of clothes and skin
- Nystatin
  - Cream and ointment: Apply three to four times daily
  - Suspension: 100 U four times daily
  - Lozenge: 100,000 U a maximum of 5 times daily for 7 to 14 days
  - *Side effects*: Nausea and vomiting, skin irritation
- Amphotericin B
  - Cream, ointment, lotion: Apply three to four times daily for a maximum of 7 to 14 days
  - Suspension: 100 mg/mL
  - *Side effects*: Not absorbed from the gut
- Miconazole 2%
  - Cream and ointment: Twice daily for 2 to 3 weeks
  - Gel: Three to 4 times daily for 2 to 3 weeks
  - Lacquer: Apply 1 g once weekly to dentures for 3 weeks
  - *Side effects*: Skin irritation, burning sensation, maceration
- Clotrimazole 1%
  - Solution: Three to 4 times daily for 2 to 3 weeks
  - Cream: Two to 3 times daily for 2 to 3 weeks
  - Troche: 10 mg 5 times daily for 2 weeks
  - *Side effects*: Skin irritation, nausea, and vomiting
- Ketoconazole 2%
  - Cream: Two to 3 times daily for 14 to 28 days (for treatment of angular cheilitis)
  - *Side effects*: Skin irritation, headache

Systemic Antifungal Agents (Second Route)
- Fluconazole
  - Capsule: 200 mg loading dose; 50 to 200 mg daily thereafter for 7 to 14 days
  - *Side effects*: Pregnancy risk, gastrointestinal disturbance, hepatotoxicity, medication interactions
- Posaconazole
  - Suspension: 100 mg twice daily on the first day, then 100 mg daily thereafter for 13 days
  - *Side effects*: Pregnancy risk, gastrointestinal upset, neutropenia
- Itraconazole
  - Capsule: 100 to 200 mg daily for 2 weeks
  - *Side effects*: Pregnancy risk, gastrointestinal disturbance, hepatic dysfunction, dizziness and headache

Data from Millsop JW, Fazel N. Oral candidiasis. *Clin Dermatol.* 2016;34(4):487.

BOX 52.7 Denture Treatment for Oral Candidiasis

- Thoroughly clean with denture brush and nonabrasive cleanser
- Oral health professionals should remove heavy deposits using an ultrasonic instrument
- Disinfect each day along with treatment
- Change solution daily
- Store in well-identified container overnight in solutions of:
  - Water or mouth rinse
  - Water + antifungal agent
  - Diluted sodium hypochlorite
  - Chlorhexidine solution

Data from Yarborough A, Cooper L, Duqum I, et al. Evidence regarding the treatment of denture stomatitis. *J Prosthodont.* 2016;25(4):288.

arthritis, osteoporosis, and seizure disorder. She took several medications for her various medical conditions, but these did not affect dental hygiene care. Bruna had no known allergies. Bruna had no dental insurance. The public trustee was assigned the responsibility of managing her finances, which covered dental treatment and dental hygiene home visits. Initially, Bruna was able to visit her dentist and have teeth repaired/restored (see Figs. 52.1 and 52.2).

When it became too difficult for her to go to the dentist for oral care, the dental office linked her with a mobile dental hygienist, who provided noninvasive debridement every 2 weeks in a comfortable chair in Bruna's home.

As her cognitive and physical functions declined, Bruna became more frail and had to move into a long-term care home. As her frailty increased, she required even more professional dental hygiene care. Bruna's brother, Peter, who was her power of attorney for health care, requested dental hygienist visits be increased to once a week. Debris from teeth, gums, and tissues was removed using noninvasive debridement.

Although she walked into long-term care independently, Bruna's health continued to decline. Through the palliative stage, she came to need a walker, then a wheelchair, and was finally confined to her bed. In the last year of her life, Bruna developed dysphagia. The dietitian modified her diet to a pureed texture and honey-fluid consistency because chewing and swallowing became a challenge.

In spite of her frailty and less-than-picture-perfect mouth (see Fig. 52.3), Bruna remained pleasant, joking, and smiling with staff and visitors. She became more frail and less communicative. She died when she was 88 years old. It was 6 years after the first professional dental hygiene onsite visit and 6 days after the last dental hygiene visit. Her favorite personal support worker (healthcare aide) stayed by her side while she passed, speaking to her in glowing terms of the life she lived. She shed a tear as she closed her eyes and died.

Bruna's story demonstrates how persons are unique and adaptable and learn to cope with oral health deficits within his/her living environment. When executive function of the brain declines and physical barriers increase, oral self-care becomes impossible. Yet, frail elders living in long-term care have natural teeth, expensive, complex restorations, and prosthetics that require professional daily care to maintain cleanliness and comfort.

THE ROLE OF THE DENTAL HYGIENIST ETHICAL AND LEGAL OBLIGATIONS

The dental hygienist applies dental hygiene theory and uses full scope of practice for palliative dental hygiene oral care while working where

Bruna was an engaging and quick-witted 82-year-old woman when a palliative care dental hygienist came into her life. Bruna led an active, busy life. After a tough childhood that included losing her mother at age 10 years and time in an orphanage, she built a successful career as a pediatric nurse. Though a brain injury disrupted her PhD studies, dancing was her passion. Bruna never married but was close to her older brother, Peter, who rescued her from the orphanage.

Years after retiring, Bruna needed some help with activities of daily living and moved to an assisted living complex. Her medical conditions included benign hypertension, unspecified dementia, unspecified

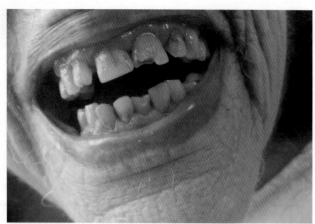

Fig. 52.1 Left central incisor defect. (Courtesy of Lynda McKeown.)

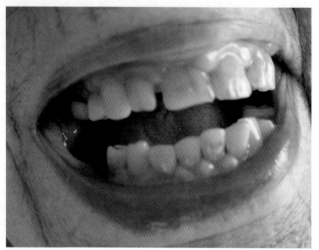

Fig. 52.2 Left central incisor restored in the dentist office. (Courtesy of Lynda McKeown.)

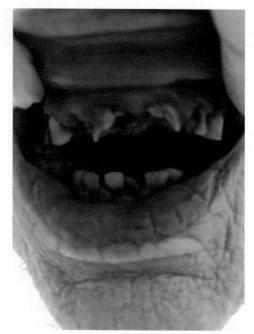

Fig. 52.3 Asymptomatic oral decline near end of life. (Courtesy of Lynda McKeown.)

BOX 52.8 Interprofessional Education Opportunity for the Dental Hygienist

- Encourage interprofessional care teams to include dental hygienists as primary oral health care providers to assess oral/dental condition on admission and provide routine noninvasive debridement of debris.
- Provide education to direct care providers who are usually responsible for daily oral care of persons in all settings.
- Dental hygienists' expertise can be shared through interprofessional education to teach nurses and other health providers about the importance of effective mouth care and its links to overall health.
- Interprofessional educational sessions between dental hygienists and other healthcare professionals are an opportunity to share knowledge, expertise, and best practices.
- Promote professional interdependence and collaboration.

---

the person lives. It is the responsibility of dental hygienists to adhere to standards of practice, ethics, and regulations set out by their professional regulatory body when providing care.

Palliative dental hygiene care is more than an adjunct to medical palliative care. Dental hygienists have the educational background and expertise needed to contribute greatly to the palliative care team. Currently, in long-term care homes, nursing staff are responsible for oral/dental assessments and constructing oral care plans. Nursing staff oversee and assign mouth care, which is an activity of daily living, to direct care staff.

Dental hygienists are the ideal oral health professional to support persons as their dependency increases. Most personal aides and support workers lack knowledge and experience about the mouth and oral care. There is seldom a dental hygienist on staff to guide oral assessments, direct oral care plans, and support daily oral care. As the person's ability to perform oral self-care declines, it is the dental hygienist who is educated and trained to recognize the effects of aging, increased frailties, and changing conditions of the mouth (see Box 52.8).

The COVID-19 pandemic highlighted existing issues. The devastating reality of oral care's low priority in long-term care homes became evident. One case study reported how a lack of oral care during a COVID-19 outbreak caused infection and complete loss of teeth within a few months. The Canadian Armed Forces identified poor mouth care issues in their report on conditions in Ontario long-term care homes.[13]

Despite this shocking evidence, dental hygienists are generally not identified as essential workers in long-term care facilities. It is important that dental hygienists be included in the circle of care. Dental hygienists must work with professional associations to advocate for and encourage support of legislative changes, enabling the profession to work in all healthcare settings in communities.

THE DENTAL HYGIENE PROCESS OF CARE FOR PALLIATIVE DENTAL HYGIENE ORAL CARE

Consent

For the dental hygienist, palliative dental hygiene oral care often brings with it the challenge of obtaining informed consent for assessment and treatment. As a person declines and moves from independence to requiring full assistance, the responsibility and consent for oral care shifts from the person to the family or substitute decision maker (SDM) or power of attorney (POA). With the increasing focus on privacy and confidentiality, explicit consent for oral care is required in many jurisdictions, especially for persons who live in residential facilities or whose cognitive abilities are failing.

Obtaining consent can be difficult and time consuming as the dental hygienist is required to seek the appropriate legal power of attorney. It is critical to determine who is the person's POA. Consent for the initial assessment by the dental hygienist is usually granted by the person's power of attorney for healthcare. However, ongoing consent from the person is required for each procedure. Courses such as the Gentle Persuasive Approach can prepare the dental hygienist to work with persons with cognitive impairment and responsive behaviors in order to gain ongoing consent.[14]

Communication

Effective communication plays a key role in oral care. Dental hygienists providing palliative dental hygiene oral care require the ability to communicate with healthcare managers and nursing and all staff members associated with the person's daily activities of living. Skillful communication is necessary to advocate for policy change when speaking with senior authorities in organizational hierarchies of residential facilities and with various government departments.

On an individual level, it is important to establish a trusting relationship with all persons (see Box 60.2—Strategies for Establishing a Trusting Relationship). The Gentle Persuasive Approach and other methods can prepare dental hygienists for communicating, responding respectfully, and confidently to behaviors associated with dementia.[14] Understanding how to support persons who lack capacity will grow in importance as population ages with increasing levels of frailty and dependency.[6]

The dental hygienist discusses and clarifies relevant issues with the person, POA, and/or family caregivers after a thorough review of the person's medications, medical issues, cognitive level, diet, and prior treatment that might impact oral health. The rationale and recommendations for palliative dental hygiene care are communicated to families and caregivers.

A variety of educational tools on palliative oral self-care may include print, audio-visual or online resources, demonstration, and verbal instruction. Dental hygienists need time and training to develop effective communication and education skills.

Assessment (see Chapters 13 and 16)

A consistent oral assessment can reduce the risk of oral problems developing. It is key to evaluate oral dental changes and other potential oral issues. During palliative dental hygiene, the oral health assessment process may be adapted to the practice setting. In the institutional setting, previous documentation related to oral health must be reviewed. When necessary, a family member or primary caregiver should be present at the assessment to discuss any questions and concerns regarding the person's oral care needs.

The Dental Hygiene Human Needs and the Oral Health Quality of Life models are both applicable to the provision of palliative dental hygiene oral care (see Chapters 2 and 22). The assessment process includes appraising a person's overall health including their frailties. It is important to assess frail persons carefully, as often they have an unhealthy mouth and teeth, due to visual and cognitive impairment, loss of manual dexterity, and/or depression. Limited income and transportation issues can make dental treatment unattainable, unaffordable, and unreasonable.[15]

Prior to oral/dental assessment, the dental hygienist must access the person's clinical records pertaining to their oral health. An in-depth review includes the person's medical history, medications, behaviors, oral dental assessments, including if applicable the most recent Resident Assessment Instrument Minimum Data Set (RAI-MDS) oral/dental section, nutrition chewing and swallowing assessment, and the person's oral care plan. RAI-MDS is an internationally recognized assessment tool that is used in numerous healthcare settings—home care, complex continuing care, and residential facilities (see Fig. 52.4).

In the review process, the dental hygienist assesses potential oral health risks.

- Is the person on nutritional supplements that are high in sugar?
- Are high-sugar drinks the main fluids provided?
- Are the person's medications being crushed and mixed with sweetened products such as applesauce or yogurt?
- Is the person on a soft, pureed diet?
- How often are the person's teeth exposed to refined carbohydrates?

It is important for dental hygienists to assess the person's ability to perform self-care. Responsibility for oral health shifts from one person to other caregivers as aging and frailties increase. When the person becomes dependent for toileting and eating assistance, they likely will require assistance with oral care. Decline in function affects all aspects of care.

The assessment continues with examining the extraoral structures of the head and neck to determine the integrity of the face, head, neck, and lips. Next, proceed intraorally to assess the buccal mucosa, tongue,

Section I. Oral/dental status

1.	Oral status and disease prevention	Debris (Soft, easily movable substances) present in mouth prior to going to bed at night	a.
		Has dentures or removable bridge	b.
		Some/all natural teeth lost–does not have or does not use dentures (or partial plates)	c.
		Broken, loose, or carious teeth	d.
		Inflamed gums (gingiva); swollen or bleeding gums; oral abcesses; ulcers or rashes	e.
		Daily cleaning of teeth/dentures or daily mouth care–by resident or staff	f.
		None of above	g.

Fig. 52.4 Oral/Dental Section L of Minimum Data Set (MDS)—Version 2.0 Resident Assessment Instrument (RAI) for Nursing Home Resident Assessment and Care Screening. Available from: https://www.cms.gov/Medicare/Quality-Initiatives-Patient-Assessment-Instruments/NursingHomeQualityInits/downloads/MDS-20MDSAllForms.pdf.

palate, floor of mouth, and gingiva (see Chapter 16). It is common to find abundant debris in a mouth, which contributes to caries and gingival inflammation. Table 52.2 describes levels of debris (see Fig. 52.5A & B).

DENTAL HYGIENE DIAGNOSIS (SEE CHAPTER 22)

The diagnosis phase is ongoing and ever-changing, depending on the person. Identification of the conditions and needs is critical to determine the best care plan to maintain the person's oral comfort and quality of life. It relies on the expertise of the dental hygienist.

Planning (See Chapter 23)

Palliative dental hygiene oral care is introduced to keep the mouth clean and comfortable, manage disease, preserve the tooth structure, minimize inflammation, and maintain integrity of the mucous membranes. Pain management and maintenance of hydration may be high priorities. Set goals accordingly. For restorative treatment needs, a goal would be to refer the person to an oral health professional for further evaluation.

A discussion about the person's goals of care, as well as the risks and benefits of potential treatment options, is necessary to help the person and/or the POA to make decisions. A systematic approach to discussing goals of care should be used by dental hygienists to promote person-centered decision making and palliative dental hygiene oral care planning.

Dental hygienists work with the healthcare team and family to establish a treatment plan that meets the needs of the person. A traditional dental hygiene schedule in office, with therapy two to three visits a year, is insufficient and inadequate to keep the mouth clean

for dependent persons. Depending on the person's requirements and financial means, dental hygiene palliative care may be done every week or two times per month. Many requirements regarding mouth care are beyond the scope and role of personal support workers and healthcare aides. Dental hygienists are the appropriate professional to inform staff, the person, and their family member/POA of the need for dental hygiene care (see Box 52.9).

Implementation

Depending on the dental hygienist's assessment, diagnoses, and oral care plan, dental hygiene interventions are introduced to meet the person's overall goals of care, human need deficits, and oral health quality of life. Dental hygienists must also acknowledge the legal and ethical issues related to palliative oral care prior to implementing dental hygiene interventions.

Oral care is provided where a person resides, in their environment. The dental hygienist provides care where the person is most comfortable, be it at the bedside, wheelchair, or other (see Fig. 52.6). This approach requires the dental hygienist to be flexible and creative while ensuring that the person is comfortable and cooperative. The dental hygienist must do their best to use good body mechanics and ergonomic principles while adapting to the person's needs. For people with cognitive impairments, the bathroom mirror may be problematic, as they often do not recognize themselves and become disturbed by the unfamiliar image facing them. Other distractions, such as music, can help to set a positive atmosphere. For children, incorporating play into the oral care therapy can be effective.

Start by applying a nonpetroleum moisturizer to dry lips. To maintain the integrity of the mucous membrane, start by sanitizing the

TABLE 52.2   Index of Debris

Definition	Healthy	Unhealthy	Level	Criterion
DEBRIS: any soft deposit present; biofilm, plaque, food particles, anything that needs to be and can be removed with oral physiotherapy tools (brushes, floss, interproximal and tongue cleaners)—consistently and daily	No soft easily removed substances—food or plaque in mouth or on dentures	Easily removed substances • food/plaque in mouth • on dentures	None 0 Minimal 1 Moderate 2 Substantial 3 Abundant 4	No debris present Debris along gumline Debris not covering more than one-third of teeth and tissue surface Debris covers one-third to two-thirds of teeth and tissue surfaces Debris covers greater than two-thirds teeth and tissue surfaces

Adapted from Lynda McKeown to define the levels of debris based on the Resident Assessment Instrument—Minimum Data Set RAI-MDS definition.

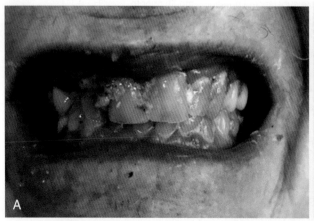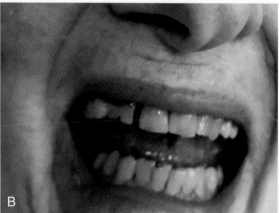

Fig. 52.5 (A) Picture showing substantial debris - 3. (B) After palliative dental hygiene oral care. (Courtesy of Lynda McKeown.)

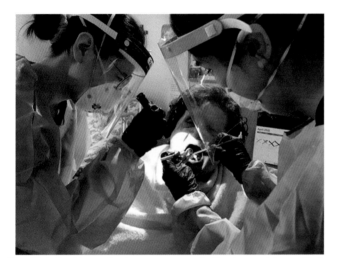

Fig. 52.6 Resident of a long-term care facility is receiving palliative dental hygiene oral care by dental hygiene students while sitting in her wheelchair. (Courtesy of Lynda McKeown.)

mouth with antimicrobial rinse to remove initial debris (Antimicrobial—Chlorhexidine, see Chapter 19). The dental hygienist can safely use an untreated, disposable sponge swab to remove large amounts of loose debris. Avoid lemon glycerin swabs as these are drying. Use caution as the sponge of the swab can be bitten off and become a choking hazard.

Usually, **oral physiotherapy tools** are sufficient to remove remaining debris (see Fig. 52.7). These are kept with the person's oral care supplies. No aerosols are required. All the oral care is done with hand instrumentation. Toothpaste is contraindicated because it requires the person to spit and is a choking hazard. In the 'dip and brush' technique, oral physiotherapy tools are dipped into the chlorhexidine rinse as they are being used to effectively remove debris and biofilm.

For a person who has difficulty keeping their mouth open, the two-toothbrush technique can be used. With this technique, the handle of one toothbrush is used as a mouth prop while the other brush is the working tool (see Fig. 52.8) showing two toothbrush technique.

The next step is to apply therapies to the teeth that are asymptomatic and no longer biologically sound to help maintain tooth integrity (see Chapters 19 and 39). To prevent, reverse, and arrest carious lesions, apply Interim Stabilization Therapy (IST). These therapies may include silver diamine fluoride (SDF), zinc oxide and fluoride (Coltosol F), and glass ionomers (Fuji GC IX) (see Fig. 52.9). If there is a dentist of record and the tooth is salvageable, collaboration is recommended.

When working with palliative persons, it is not always necessary to remove calculus. A risk-benefit analysis must be done to determine if calculus removal will cause more harm than good. For example, in a person whose healing ability is compromised, calculus removal can cause an unstable tissue response. For persons with unpredictable behaviors, it can be a safety hazard to use a sharp instrument in the mouth. If calculus is to be removed, manual curettes are used. The dental hygienist must ensure proper transport for reprocessing the instruments and ensure adherence to dental hygiene regulatory requirements.

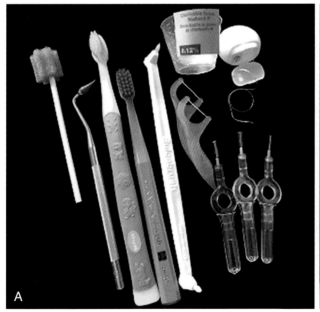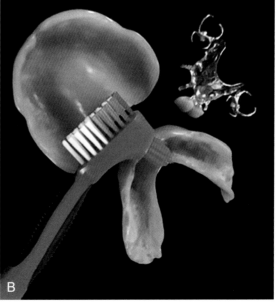

Fig. 52.7 (A) Oral physiotherapy tools. (B) Denture brush for prosthetics. (Courtesy of Lynda McKeown.)

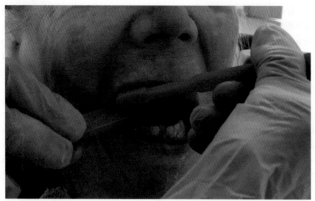

Fig. 52.8 Handle of one brush used as mouth prop to keep the mouth open, with a second brush used for debridement. (Courtesy of Lynda McKeown.)

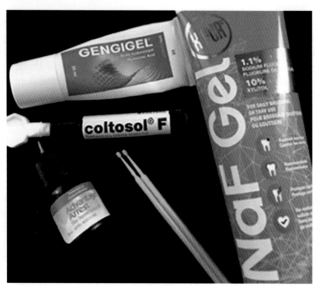

Fig. 52.9 Interim Stabilization Therapies (IST). (Courtesy of Lynda McKeown.)

Evaluation of Care and Documentation (See Chapter 23)

The physical and cognitive abilities of dependent persons will change throughout the process of palliative dental hygiene care. It is important to continually evaluate and modify the care plan and adjust goals and outcomes accordingly. This may include evaluating whether the education of persons, families, and staff has been effective.

Document utilizing a chronological account of services in accordance with Standards for Clinical Dental Hygiene Practice (see Table 23.5). Documentation should include the Dental Hygiene process of care, as well as discussions with family and caregivers. A copy of the oral/dental assessment and recommendations for the oral care plan is left with the facility.

CONCLUSION

The dental hygienist as a member of the healthcare team provides insight, professional oral healthcare, and training to all caregivers, including family members. The dental hygienist's dental hygiene diagnosis, planning, appropriate interventions, evaluation, and documentation of care. The dental hygienist recognizes when the person's increasing physical frailty and cognitive and physical decline requires need for palliative dental hygiene oral care. Dying is inevitable and

death is not curable. Palliative dental hygiene oral care enhances a person's health and wellbeing to the end of life. Pathways to providing preventive oral health services will gain momentum as dental hygienists become an integral part of healthcare teams for palliative care in all settings.

BOX 52.10 Critical Thinking Scenario

Referring back to Palliative Dental Hygiene Oral Care Scenario, Bruna's story, and Figs. 52.1–52.5. Apply the knowledge learned from this chapter.
1. Discuss ethical and legal considerations during Bruna's palliative dental hygiene care.
2. What health risks may exist in the facility that contributed to Bruna's oral decline?
3. What are the signs of aging, frailty, and oral complications manifested in Bruna's mouth?
4. What is the main palliative dental hygiene oral care priority for Bruna?
5. Develop a dental hygiene care plan for Bruna that includes goals and interventions.
6. Discuss dental hygiene palliative care and how it applies to Bruna.
7. What can dental hygiene organizations do to improve mouth care for persons like Bruna?

KEY CONCEPTS

- Palliative dental hygiene oral care focuses on providing a comfortable, clean mouth and professional assistance to reduce symptoms and to maintain oral health in people who have physical and/or cognitive limitations, through the stages of increasing frailty to dying and death.
- Consistent, ongoing oral health assessments are used to evaluate changes in the mouth and update oral care plans. Referrals to appropriate professionals are made when required.
- Dental hygienists can provide a range of specific, therapeutic interventions that support the provision of daily oral care.
- Dental hygienists need to be acknowledged as essential healthcare providers in legislation for long-term care, residential, hospice care, and other settings.
- Dental hygienists provide insight, education, and training to caregivers about the oral cavity, its proper care, and the importance of the oral microbiome to all body systems.
- Interprofessional collaboration of dental hygienists with healthcare providers can help to apply oral care best practices throughout the palliative stage to end of life.
- Dental hygienists must develop their knowledge base regarding death and dying to most effectively treat a person to the end of life.
- See Box 52.10 for Critical Thinking Activity.

ACKNOWLEDGMENTS

With thanks to dental hygiene student Ashlee Cooke for her valuable input and the past contributions of Elizabeth Couch and Margaret M. Walsh.

REFERENCES

1. United Nations, Department of Economic and Social Affairs, Population Division. World Population Ageing 2019: Highlights (ST/ESA/SER.A/430). https://www.un.org/development/desa/pd/sites/

www.un.org.development.desa.pd/files/files/documents/2020/Jan/worldpopulationageing2019-highlights.pdf#:~:text=Population ageing is a global phenomenon: Virtually every, projected to double to 1.5 billion in 2050 Accessed July 26, 2022.

2. Serious health-related suffering (SHS). IAHPC Pallipedia. https://pallipedia.org/serious-health-related-suffering-shs/. Accessed June 30, 2022.

3. Radbruch L, De Lima L, Knaul F, et al. Redefining palliative care-a new consensus-based definition. *J Pain Symptom Manage*. 2020;60(4):754–764. https://doi.org/10.1016/j.jpainsymman.2020.04.027.

4. Registered Nurses' Association of Ontario. *A Palliative Approach to Care in the Last 12 Months of Life*. Registered Nurses' Association of Ontario; 2020. https://rnao.ca/sites/rnao-ca/files/bpg/PALLATIVE_CARE_FINAL_WEB_2.pdf. Accessed June 30, 2022.

5. Nurses' Association of Ontario R. *Person- and Family-Centred Care*. Registered Nurses' Association of Ontario; 2015:74. https://rnao.ca/sites/rnao-ca/files/FINAL_Web_Version_0.pdf. Accessed June 30, 2022.

6. MacEntee MI, Donnelly LR. Oral health and the frailty syndrome. *Periodontol 2000*. 2016;72(1):135–141. https://doi.org/10.1111/prd.12134. PMID: 27501496.

7. Woodbeck H, Greenhorn P, McKeown L, Weiss C, Peachman-Faust T. Xerostomia: it's a desert in there- dry mouth and wounds. *Wound Care Canada Journal*. 2021. Summer issue https://www.woundscanada.ca/docman/public/wound-care-canada-magazine/wcc-2021-v20-n1/2149-wcc-summer-2021-v19n1-final-p-72-81-xerostomia/file. Accessed July 26, 2022.

8. CDHO. Vignette Pneumonia. https://cdho.org/wp-content/uploads/2023/10/Vignette_Pneumonia.pdf. Accessed July 26, 2022.

9. Müller F. Oral hygiene reduces the mortality from aspiration pneumonia in frail elders. *J Dent Res*. 2015;94(3 Suppl):14S–16S. https://doi.org/10.1177/0022034514552494. https://www.ncbi.nlm.nih.gov/pmc/articles/PMC4541086/.

10. Carr M, McKeown L, MacEntee M. Oral health, dysphagia, and aspiration pneumonia. In: MacEntee ML, ed. *Oral Health Care and the Frail Elder*. Blackwell publishing; 2011.

11. Scannapieco FA, Shay K. Oral health disparities in older adults: oral bacteria, inflammation, and aspiration pneumonia. *Dent Clin North Am*. 2014;58(4):771–782.

12. Hua F, Xie H, Worthington HV, et al. Oral hygiene care for critically ill patients to prevent ventilator-associated pneumonia. *Cochrane Database Syst Rev*. 2016;10:CD008367.

13. *National Standards for Long-Term Care: Addressing Oral Health for Overall Health*. A Discussion Paper from the Canadian Dental Hygienists Association; 2021. *https://files.cdha.ca/Profession/Policy/National_standards_for_long- term_care_Nov2021.pdf*. Accessed July 26, 2022.

14. Tabamo J, Hung L, Bohl D, Hillier N, Martin J. Gentle persuasive approaches in dementia care: building staff confidence and efficacy. *Innovation in Aging*. 2017;1(suppl 1):165–166. https://doi.org/10.1093/geroni/igx004.645. Published 2017 Jun 30.

15. Frenkel H, Matthews D, Nitschke I. *Prevention of oral diseases for a dependent populationOral Health Care and the Frail Elder A Clinical Perspective*. ; 2011. https://doi.org/10.1002/9781118786789.ch12.

53

Autoimmune Diseases

Leciel Bono

PROFESSIONAL DEVELOPMENT OPPORTUNITIES

Dental hygienists encounter patients with one or more autoimmune diseases on a regular basis. The diseases themselves and related medication management can adversely affect the oral cavity and have a significant impact on quality of life. Dental hygienists are important advocates for affected individuals, recommending interventions that improve patient function and oral health.

COMPETENCIES

1. Explain immune dysfunction.
2. Describe the pathophysiology of autoimmune diseases.
3. Describe pharmacologic considerations for autoimmune diseases.
4. Implement the dental hygiene process of care for patients presenting with autoimmune diseases, including:
   - Recognize the systemic and oral manifestations of common autoimmune diseases.
   - Develop a dental hygiene care plan appropriate for persons with autoimmune disease.
   - Deliver dental hygiene services safely and effectively for patients with autoimmune disease.

IMMUNE DYSFUNCTION

The human immune system exhibits **self-tolerance**, which is the unique ability to recognize the difference between "self" and "foreign" antigens. This ability to discriminate between one's own antigens and nonself (typically microbial) antigens is known as **immunologic tolerance**. When innate mechanisms that normally prevent the immune system from attacking self-antigens fail, activated T cells and antibodies begin to attack the individual's own tissues, a process known as **autoimmunity**. Conditions associated with autoimmunity collectively are called autoimmune diseases.[1]

Understanding how self-antigens induce tolerance is important, because these same mechanisms may be applied to interventions that prevent or control unwanted immune reactions.[1] For example, many of the interventions developed to treat autoimmune diseases target specific cells or mediators that modulate immune function. Other examples include series of injections given to an individual to desensitize the person after exposure to an allergen, or immunosuppressive medications used to prevent organ rejection in transplant recipients.[1]

There are two primary factors necessary for the development of autoimmunity. First, an individual inherits genes creating a genetic predisposition for developing an autoimmune disease that increase susceptibility and contribute to failure of self-tolerance. Multiple genes predispose to autoimmune disease, the most important of which are major histocompatibility complex (MHC) genes that encode cytokines and are recognized by T lymphocytes for antigen processing. Second,

one or more environmental triggers initiate activation of autoantibodies. Triggers frequently include infection, fever, or severe trauma.

The manifestation of many autoimmune diseases is often preceded by an infection.[2] An infection triggers a local immune response, causing the release of cytokines and chemical stimulators that activate self-reactive T cells, producing an immune attack against self-antigens. Infections also injure tissues and release antigens that normally are not seen by the immune system or are ignored. The presence of these antigens can initiate an autoimmune reaction. Seasonal patterns of infections also correlate with onset of autoimmune disease or disease flareup, such as flares in systemic lupus erythematosus observed with Epstein-Barr virus in winter, or type 1 diabetes mellitus onset preceded by infection with Coxsackievirus in late summer.[2] There is emerging evidence that a variety of other environmental factors contribute to autoimmunity, including low levels of vitamin D, exposure to UV radiation, and fluctuations in melatonin.[2,3]

PATHOPHYSIOLOGY OF AUTOIMMUNE DISEASES

Autoantibodies against self-antigens associated with autoimmune diseases bind to self-antigens in tissues or form immune complexes with circulating self-antigens. The tissue destruction observed with autoimmune diseases generally occurs in one of two ways. First, bound antibodies deposit in tissues that express self-antigens, which is usually in a specific tissue or organ. Second, immune complexes deposit in blood vessels, resulting in systemic involvement, manifesting as vasculitis, and joint and kidney damage.

However, autoantibodies also can cause disease without directly causing tissue injury. Some autoantibodies inhibit receptor function on cells, as in myasthenia gravis, where acetylcholine receptors are inhibited and neuromuscular transmission fails, causing paralysis of the muscles of the head and neck. Other antibodies stimulate receptors that normally would be stimulated by a hormone. This is evident in hyperthyroidism, where antibodies stimulate thyroid cells directly.

Several common characteristics of autoimmune disease may be observed. Patients often exhibit cluster disorders presenting with more than one autoimmune disease. Because antibodies can travel throughout the body, patients usually experience multisystem organ involvement that may not be explained or diagnosed easily. Signs and symptoms of this involvement are nondescript and often present as fatigue, joint pain, muscle aches, sleep disorders, and anemia. Some patients experience psychiatric difficulties, most commonly depression and frustration, as a consequence of numerous consultations with multiple healthcare providers without receiving definitive diagnosis or treatment recommendations for lengthy periods of time. The result is that patients live with diminished quality of life and ongoing health challenges, including compromised oral health.

There are more than 100 different types of autoimmune diseases, affecting more than 50 million people. Examples of the more common

TABLE 53.1 Examples of Autoimmune Diseases

Autoimmune Disease	Definition
Adrenal insufficiency	Primary condition is known as Addison disease, which is caused by destruction of the adrenal glands from infections, cancer, or chronic use of steroid hormones Secondary adrenal insufficiency is caused most often by chronic use of steroids Adrenal crisis is a life-threatening condition caused by acute adrenal suppression
Cicatricial pemphigoid	A benign, chronic blistering disease affecting the oral and genital mucosa, conjunctiva of the eye, skin; characterized by healing of lesions with scarring
Fibromyalgia	A widespread musculoskeletal disorder characterized by pain in the muscles, ligaments, and joints, and fatigue. Has a frequent comorbidity with other autoimmune conditions including chronic fatigue syndrome, rheumatoid arthritis, systemic lupus erythematosus, and hypothyroidism
Hyperthyroidism	Also known as thyrotoxicosis, an excess of thyroxine (T4) and triiodothyronine (T3) in the bloodstream, affecting the body's metabolic rate. Primary is used to designate hyperthyroidism arising from an intrinsic thyroid abnormality. Secondary is used to designate that arising from processes outside of the thyroid, such as TSH-secreting pituitary tumor.
Hypothyroidism	Structural or functional derangement that interferes with the production of thyroid hormone (e.g., autoimmune thyroiditis, congenital hypothyroidism, iatrogenic hypothyroidism—surgical or radiation-induced ablation)
Multiple sclerosis	The most common autoimmune disease affecting the nervous system, characterized by demyelination of nerves in the central nervous system because of chronic inflammation
Myasthenia gravis	A chronic autoimmune disease that affects the neuromuscular system, representing a decrease in acetylcholine receptors in muscle fibers, resulting in progressive fatigability and abnormality of skeletal muscles
Pemphigus vulgaris	A progressive, severe disease affecting the skin and mucous membranes characterized by bullae that rupture and form painful ulcers
Pernicious anemia	Failure of the stomach to produce intrinsic factor and lack of cobalamin, or vitamin B_{12}
Psoriasis	Chronic inflammatory dermatosis characterized by well-demarcated pink to salmon-colored plaques covered by loosely adherent silver-white scales on the surface of lesions; approximately 15% is associated with arthritis (psoriatic arthritis)
Rheumatoid arthritis	A chronic inflammatory condition principally attacking the joints and producing a nonsuppurative proliferative and inflammatory synovitis characterized by pain, swelling, stiffness, and loss of function
Scleroderma	A chronic disease of connective tissue secondary to vascular injury and progressive interstitial and perivascular fibrosis of the skin and multiple organs; better known as systemic sclerosis
Sjögren syndrome	A triad of keratoconjunctivitis sicca, xerostomia, and connective tissue disorder manifesting as a wide spectrum of severity; includes primary and secondary forms
Systemic lupus erythematosus	A disease in which injury is caused mainly by deposition of immune complexes and binding of antibodies to various cells and tissues; affects major organ systems; characterized by periods of remissions and exacerbations

types of autoimmune diseases appear in Table 53.1.[4] Omitted from this chapter are specific details concerning three particular autoimmune diseases (immune-mediated diabetes mellitus, rheumatic heart disease, and acquired immunodeficiency syndrome) because these conditions are discussed in other chapters of this text. A description of signs and symptoms reflecting major system involvement of various autoimmune diseases is found in Table 53.2.[4]

PHARMACOLOGIC CONSIDERATIONS

Management of autoimmune diseases typically includes pharmacotherapy beginning with antiinflammatory medications and progressing to immunosuppressive drugs. The goals of medication therapy used to treat autoimmune diseases include reduced pain, improved function, slowed rate of disease progression, and limiting tissue destruction. Many autoimmune conditions are treated with drugs that reduce inflammation using corticosteroids and anticytokine therapies. Because activated T cells mediate organ-specific autoimmune diseases, immunosuppressive drugs also are used to inhibit T cell responses. Drugs used to treat rheumatoid arthritis provide a classic model for understanding pharmacologic management of autoimmune diseases, which are described further here. A variety of classes of medications

may be indicated for patient management, a list of which is found in Box 53.1.[4]

Nonsteroidal antiinflammatory drugs (NSAIDs) block the synthesis of prostaglandins by inhibiting the enzyme cyclooxygenase, which reduces the formation of inflammatory mediators that create swelling, fever, and pain. NSAIDs are categorized as either salicylates (e.g., aspirin) or nonsalicylates. Aspirin and other salicylates are standard first-line agents for treatment of rheumatoid arthritis and provide relief from pain, swelling, and fever. Prevention of joint and tissue damage often necessitates the addition of a disease-modifying antirheumatic drug (DMARD). Large doses of salicylates and NSAIDs often are required for pain relief, which may not be tolerated in some individuals. Although acetaminophen has potency and efficacy similar to that of aspirin, it has no antiinflammatory activity, and thus its usefulness is limited.

DMARDs are a wide range of compounds used for the treatment of rheumatoid arthritis and osteoarthritis, either in conjunction with NSAIDs or in patients who have not responded to cyclooxygenase-2 (COX-2) inhibitors. DMARDs slow the course of joint disease and help to prevent further destruction but have a relatively slow onset of action. Patients may need to take these drugs for up to 4 months before seeing an effect.[4–6]

TABLE 53.2	Signs and Symptoms of Major System Involvement of Autoimmune Diseases
System	**Features**
Constitutional	Fatigue, fever in the absence of infection, weight loss/gain, difficulty sleeping, cold or heat intolerance
Musculoskeletal	Arthralgia, myalgia, arthritis, joint pain and swelling, loss of joint range of motion, carpal tunnel syndrome, flexion contractures, muscle weakness, diaphoresis, tremors, warm/flushed skin
Skin	Photosensitivity, diffuse rash, skin lesions or nodules, mucous membrane lesions, purpura, alopecia, Raynaud phenomenon, urticaria, vasculitis, skin pigment changes, skin tightness and induration, telangiectasis, calcinosis, edema, thin/fine hair, soft or brittle nails
Renal	Hematuria, proteinuria, casts, nephritic syndrome, renal crisis or failure
Gastrointestinal	Nausea, vomiting, gastroparesis, abdominal pain, peritonitis with or without ascites, hepatomegaly, pancreatitis, gastroesophageal reflux disease, dysphagia, dyspepsia, diarrhea alternating with constipation, candidiasis, primary biliary cirrhosis, malabsorption, diverticula
Pulmonary	Pleurisy, pleural effusion, chest pain, shortness of breath, pulmonary parenchyma, pulmonary hypertension, cough from restrictive lung disease
Cardiovascular	Pericarditis, noninfective endocarditis, myocarditis, chest pain, arrhythmia, valve abnormalities, myocardial infarction, congestive heart failure, myocardial fibrosis, palpitations, bradycardia, tachycardia
Reticuloendothelial	Lymphadenopathy, splenomegaly, hepatomegaly
Hematologic/vascular	Anemia, autoimmune thrombocytopenia purpura or thrombocytopenia as a consequence of antiphospholipid antibody syndrome, leukopenia with lymphoma, Raynaud phenomenon, ulcerations of digits, ischemic resorption of digits, gangrene of digits, lips, nose, and ears
Ocular	Anterior uveitis, iridocyclitis, retinal vasculitis, central retinal artery occlusion, central retinal vein occlusion, ischemic optic neuropathy, xerostomia with keratoconjunctivitis sicca, retinopathy, blindness, edema of eyelids
Neuropsychiatric	Cerebrovascular accidents, seizure, organic effective disorders, personality disorder, psychosis, coma, vascular or migraine headaches, organic brain syndrome, dementia, cranial neuropathies, peripheral neuropathies, depression, facial pain, nervousness and anxiety, slowed mental acuity
Ear, nose, and throat	Earaches, chronic cough, aberrant voice with nasal tone, dysphagia, gangrene
Oral	Tooth mobility, sicca syndrome, widened periodontal ligaments, microstomia, anterior open bite, resorption of mandible, xerostomia, delayed/early eruption of teeth, salivary gland enlargement, temporomandibular joint swelling, preauricular pain, decreased mobility, locking, crepitus, stomatitis, loss of taste, hyperkeratosis, secondary infection of candidiasis, petechial ecchymosis, bleeding, drug-induced gingival enlargement, gangrene of lips, impaired lip movement, soft palate weakness, tremor of tongue, thickened tongue
Endocrine	Erectile dysfunction, vaginal dryness, dyspareunia, menstrual irregularity, xerostomia, xerophthalmia, miscarriages, goiter, osteoporosis

Methotrexate is an immunosuppressant that produces antirheumatic effects within 6 weeks of initiating treatment. It is used alone or in combination with other DMARDs. It is the drug of choice for severe rheumatoid arthritis or psoriatic arthritis, and for cases that are unresponsive to NSAIDs. It has a faster onset of action than other DMARDs, often providing relief within 6 weeks after initiating treatment.[4–6]

Interleukin-1β and tumor necrosis factor-α are proinflammatory cytokines that stimulate synovial cells to proliferate and synthesize collagenase, which degrades cartilage, stimulates bone resorption, and inhibits proteoglycan synthesis. Anticytokine therapies are used to block these unwanted effects and also provide some antiinflammatory effects. These drugs are used in patients with severe rheumatoid arthritis who are unresponsive to other DMARDs, and in those with other autoimmune conditions that affect connective tissue and bones. Examples of these drugs include etanercept, infliximab, adalimumab, and anakinra.[4–6]

New emerging oral medications known as Janus kinase (JAK) inhibitors are part of the targeted small molecule treatment therapies used to treat rheumatoid arthritis known as tsDMARDs.[7] The JAK inhibitors suppress intracellular signaling mediated by cytokines involved in rheumatoid arthritis and many other autoimmune disease processes. Tofacitinib, baricitinib, upadacitinib, peficitinib, and filgotinib are the current medications approved by various agencies in this category and have demonstrated favorable results with a rapid onset by initiating direct analgesic effects and by decreasing joint inflammation. JAK inhibitors are also being considered for other autoimmune diseases including systemic lupus erythematosus, spondyloarthritis, psoriasis, atopic dermatitis, and inflammatory bowel disease.[7]

Penicillamine depresses circulating immunoglobulin M (IgM) rheumatoid factor and depresses T-cell activity. Antimalarial agents impair complement-dependent antigen-antibody reactions and typically are used in combination with aspirin and steroids, especially for patients with rheumatoid arthritis who are unresponsive to NSAIDs. Antimalarial agents slow the progression of erosive bone lesions and may induce remission. Agents include chloroquine and hydroxychloroquine. Gold compounds inhibit mononuclear phagocyte maturation and function and may suppress cellular immunity.[4]

Azathioprine and cyclophosphamide are immunosuppressive drugs used to treat a variety of autoimmune conditions but most often are used for refractory cases of rheumatoid arthritis. Cyclosporine is an immunosuppressant agent that inhibits the production of interleukin-2 by helper T cells and reduces the production and release of other lymphokines in response to an antigenic stimulus.[4]

Dental hygienists must be aware that the drugs used to treat autoimmune diseases produce numerous adverse effects, and patients may present with signs and symptoms that reflect their drug treatment and their disease. Each patient requires a comprehensive pharmacologic history review to determine the impact of drug therapy on the dental hygiene process of care. Chapter 15 contains detailed information about the pharmacologic history review.

BOX 53.1 Medications Used to Treat Autoimmune Diseases[4,7]

Antiinflammatory Agents
Salicylates (aspirin, sulfasalazine)
NSAIDs
COX-2 inhibitors
Corticosteroids:
  Prednisone
  Prednisolone

DMARDs (Disease-Modifying Antirheumatic Drugs)
Immune modulators:
  Methotrexate
  Leflunomide
Anticytokine therapies:
  Etanercept
  Infliximab
  Adalimumab
  Anakinra
Janus kinase inhibitors:
  Tofacitinib
  Baricitinib
  Upadacitinib
  Peficitinib
  Filgotinib
Antimalarials:
  Chloroquine
  Hydroxychloroquine
Penicillamine
Gold compounds:
  Aurothioglucose
  Auranofin
  Gold sodium thiomalate
Immunosuppressants:
  Azathioprine
  Cyclophosphamide
  Cyclosporine

COX-2, Cyclooxygenase-2; *NSAID,* nonsteroidal antiinflammatory drug.

BOX 53.2 Complications With Chronic Use of Corticosteroid Medications[4]

Insomnia
Peptic ulceration
Osteoporosis
Cataract formation
Glaucoma
Growth suppression
Delayed wound healing
Psychosis
Weight gain

Salicylates, NSAIDs, and COX-2 inhibitors are associated with adverse bleeding events, including bruising, gastrointestinal hemorrhage, and gingival bleeding. All of the DMARDs described earlier have known toxicities, making compliance difficult and requiring regular monitoring by the physician. Patients often experience general fatigue and malaise, which can be difficult to differentiate from symptoms of the autoimmune disease. Dermatologic problems including skin lesions, rashes, and hair loss are common, as is delayed wound healing. Lesions may occur on the oral mucosa, including the appearance of bluish-black pigmentation. Immunosuppressive drugs may cause gingival enlargement. Patients may experience severe hematologic effects, including alterations in red and white blood cell counts and altered cell function. Because DMARDs alter the immune response, patients become susceptible to infections, such as pneumonia, and may experience a reactivation of latent viruses, leading to diseases such as hepatitis, tuberculosis, and herpetic infections such as shingles. Rarely, immune modulators may promote the development of cancers.[4]

Many patients are treated with corticosteroids for their antiinflammatory effects and for suppression of the immune response. It is this suppressive activity that results in the desired as well as undesired effects of corticosteroids. Adverse reactions are proportional to dose, frequency, time of administration, and duration of treatment. Multiple adverse events associated with steroids limit their long-term use. Complications associated with chronic steroid use are listed in Box 53.2.[4]

Patients undergoing chronic corticosteroid therapy are at risk for candidiasis, the most common oral side effect of these medications, which is related directly to their xerostomic effect. They also may exhibit poor wound healing after dental hygiene therapy. Oral infections may be masked because of the antiinflammatory effects of these medications. Chronic dry mouth increases risks for a variety of oral complications that require dental hygiene interventions.

Adrenal Insufficiency and Adrenal Crisis

Regulation of cortisol secretion is controlled by the hypothalamic-pituitary-adrenal axis. Virtually any type of stress, whether physical or psychologic, causes an immediate increase of pituitary secretion of adrenocorticotropic hormone (ACTH), which stimulates the adrenal cortex to produce and secrete cortisol. Surgery is one of the greatest stressors that produce this response.[4]

Chronic use of corticosteroids suppresses the body's own production and release of cortisol, resulting in secondary, or medication-induced, adrenal insufficiency. The danger is that when the patient is physically (infection, surgery) and/or psychologically (fear, anxiety, pain) stressed, the patient will not be able to produce an adequate amount of their own cortisol, known as the stress response, placing them at risk for decreased cardiac output, hypoglycemia, and circulatory shock.[4] One method used to minimize this suppression is to administer hydrocortisone on alternating days, with higher doses used to maintain adequate serum levels while still allowing the body to secrete its own cortisone on opposing days.

Dental professionals must determine whether patients on chronic corticosteroid therapy require steroid supplementation before treatment. Other than for major surgical procedures, most patients do not require supplementation for general or routine dental and dental hygiene procedures. Even for minor surgeries, patients taking their medications at their usual dose within 2 hours of the procedure should have enough exogenous and endogenous steroids to handle the procedure. Further, local anesthesia and conscious sedation lower the stress response to pain, which helps to eliminate the need for supplementation.[4]

Adrenal crisis is a rare, life-threatening condition caused by acute adrenal suppression. It does not commonly occur with secondary adrenal insufficiency. Four factors contribute to the risk of adrenal crisis during oral surgery: the extent and severity of the surgery, medications used, health status of the patient, and the degree of pain control. Adrenal crisis leads to circulatory collapse and death if not treated promptly. Treatment of adrenal crisis requires hospitalization and interventions including intravenous injections of hydrocortisone, glucose, fluids, and electrolyte replacement.[4] Dental professionals must recognize the signs

PROCEDURE 53.1 Implementation of a Stress Reduction Protocol[4]

Steps	Rationale
Schedule patients for dental procedures, especially surgical procedures, first thing in the morning.	Cortisol levels are highest in the morning, which helps to ensure patient safety by minimizing risks for adrenal crisis.
Use measures to minimize pain and anxiety.	Use of local anesthetics, nitrous oxide sedation, and antianxiety medications helps to minimize exogenous stress from pain and fear associated with dental procedures.
Monitor the patient's vital signs before the procedure, during the perioperative period, and before dismissing the patient.	Monitoring the patient's blood pressure is essential to detect a drop in pressure, an important sign of adrenal crisis. During this crisis, the patient may exhibit a weak pulse, temperature changes, and difficulty breathing. Regular monitoring of vital signs helps to ensure early detection of this potential medical emergency so that the patient can be treated and maintained safely.
Respond appropriately to a drop in blood pressure.	A blood pressure reading below 100/60 indicates hypotension and immediate action must be taken to ensure patient safety. The patient should be positioned with the feet elevated above the height of the head, with fluid replacement, administration of vasopressors, and treatment of hypoglycemia given as needed; 100 mg of hydrocortisone is administered by IV and the patient then is transported to the hospital.

BOX 53.3 Signs and Symptoms of Adrenal Crisis[4]

Sunken eyes	Myalgias
Profuse sweating	Arthralgias
Hypotension	Hyponatremia
Weak pulse	Eosinophilia
Dyspnea	Hypothermia
Cyanosis	Severe hypotension
Nausea/vomiting	Hypoglycemia
Headache	Circulatory collapse (shock)
Dehydration	Death
Fever	

BOX 53.4 Legal, Ethical, and Safety Issues

The dental hygienist thoroughly updates the patient's health, dental, and pharmacologic histories, and documents any updates or changes in health status at each visit. If concern exists that the patient is at risk for harm by proceeding with care, the dental hygienist must inform the dentist and patient and make a prompt referral to the physician of record.

and symptoms of adrenal crisis listed in Box 53.3. Implementation of a stress reduction protocol in patients with adrenal suppression can minimize the risk for adrenal crisis during dental treatment (Procedure 53.1).[4]

DENTAL HYGIENE PROCESS OF CARE

Autoimmune diseases are multifaceted and present challenges to general and oral healthcare professionals. Given the nature of these diseases, patients may present with multiple needs that affect dental hygiene care. Using the dental hygiene process of care ensures adequate planning for the delivery of safe and comprehensive oral care.

Assessment

During the assessment phase, it is of utmost importance to obtain a thorough health, oral, and pharmacologic history from the patient to identify conditions that warrant referral for medical evaluation. The clinician must be able to determine if the need for medical care supersedes the need for oral care, whether it is safe to provide treatment, and what the patient will be able to tolerate in terms of appointment scheduling and procedures. Oral care may have to be deferred until additional medical evaluation and/or treatment is provided. Box 53.4 considers these ethical and safety issues.

In some cases, patients report signs and symptoms that may reflect autoimmune disease characteristics without having received a definitive diagnosis. Upon completion of the health history, the dental hygienist can use a risk assessment tool to assist with the identification of autoimmune characteristics, referrals needed, and considerations or modifications necessary to provide dental hygiene treatment. Table 53.3 presents an example of a risk assessment tool for suspected and confirmed autoimmune diseases. This risk assessment tool is to be completed after reviewing the health history when suspecting an autoimmune condition. The clinician should ask all questions of the patient and make treatment modifications and referrals based on responses and clinical examination findings.

In addition, individuals with chronic conditions such as autoimmune diseases may experience changes that impact oral health-related quality of life (OHRQL). OHRQL can be defined as a multidimensional concept that demonstrates one's comfort in managing daily activities of living such as eating and sleeping and satisfaction with oral health. It also encompasses social interactions and self-esteem, psychological and social factors, and pain and discomfort. Dental hygiene practitioners can measure OHRQL through two scales, the modified Oral Health Impact Profile (OHIP) and the Mouth Handicap in Systemic Sclerosis scale (MHISS). Comparisons can be made in a patient's quality of life using these assessments at different appointments and as their autoimmune disease progresses or treatment regimen changes.

Diagnosis

The dental hygiene diagnosis depends largely on the signs observed by the clinician and the symptoms reported by the patient during the assessment phase. Objective and subjective assessment findings are used to identify key diagnoses and are summarized to support proposed treatment. Patients with autoimmune diseases will likely present with multiple dental hygiene diagnoses. The dental hygiene student should determine those needs that can be improved through the delivery of dental hygiene interventions and identify referrals needed for further dental care and those within other health care disciplines based on those dental hygiene diagnoses. Figs. 53.1 through 53.12 illustrate clinical signs of autoimmune diseases.[8]

TABLE 53.3 Risk Assessment Tool for Autoimmune Diseases

Questions	Notes	Dental Hygiene Treatment Modifications and Referrals
How would you describe your overall health?		
Have you had any changes in your health within the last year? (Examples: significant weight loss or gain, chronic or frequent colds, flulike symptoms)		
Have you experienced any of the following: infection, fever, illness, stress, trauma, or motor vehicle accident?		
Have you had any changes to your activities of daily living? (Examples: less active, more difficulty performing routine duties such as laundry, grocery shopping, work, school, sleeping, loss of interest in activities/hobbies, frustration with inability to perform routine tasks, loss of motivation for eating or cooking)		
Have your medications changed since your last visit or are you using your medications differently since last time? (Examples: new medications, increasing frequency of use, taking more NSAIDs, self-medication with drugs and alcohol, use of antidepressants)		
Have you noticed changes in eating behaviors? (Examples: less interested in food, increased eating for comfort, uninterested in or difficulty with eating out with friends)		
Signs and symptoms suggesting autoimmune condition (Examples: fatigue, arthralgia, myalgia, xerostomia, rash, GERD, anemia, shortness of breath, chest pain, lymphadenopathy, arrhythmia, goiter, salivary gland enlargement)		
Assess need for prophylactic antibiotics		
Assess vital signs		
Assess potential for infection		
Assess potential for medical emergency		
Assess need for supportive or assistive devices		

GERD, Gastroesophageal reflux disease; *NSAIDs*, nonsteroidal antiinflammatory drugs.

Planning

The planning phase may be complicated by the physical demands on the patient and medical attention needed at the time of dental hygiene care. Shorter appointments may be necessary to accommodate patients with joint pain, stiffness, swelling, shortness of breath, and other manifestations that may affect their ability to sit for long periods of time. Assistive and supportive devices needed to provide comfort for the patient during the dental hygiene appointment should be discussed in advance and included as part of preparation for treatment.

Consultation with the patient's physician to establish goals and communication is helpful to determine how to coordinate dental hygiene care with concurrent medical care in a safe manner. Regular physician evaluation and reporting of those findings to the oral healthcare team are important to maintaining coordinated, comprehensive healthcare (Boxes 53.5 and 53.6). Dental hygienists have an opportunity to serve as an advocate for those who require physical and psychological support when recognizing that needs are not being met by the current medical system.

In planning for individualized treatment for each patient presenting with autoimmune diseases, it is important to consider specific interventions that may be necessary. Patients may have unusual oral complaints or manifestations of autoimmune disease that require attention to comprehensive care. Consultation with the patient's physician may be necessary to complete the planning process to ensure patient safety. For example, a patient who presents with multiple sclerosis should be scheduled for treatment during periods of remission and may need steroid supplementation. Depending on the medications being used to treat rheumatoid arthritis, the dental hygienist may have to evaluate

blood work such as bleeding time and platelet function before beginning periodontal debridement. For those individuals who present with systemic lupus erythematosus who have a history of low white blood cell counts from taking immunosuppressants, additional blood assays are needed to determine whether it is safe to proceed with planned treatment and if antibiotic premedication is needed before treatment. The American Academy of Orthopedic Surgeons' Appropriate Use Criteria should be consulted to determine the need for antibiotic premedication for individuals with rheumatoid arthritis who have undergone joint replacement surgery.[9,10] In other instances, depending on the medications used and level of xerostomia, an antifungal therapy for secondary candidiasis may have to be prescribed. Recognizing these special care considerations in the planning process assists the dental hygienist in meeting the multiple needs of the patient. Table 53.4 provides an overview of oral manifestations of autoimmune diseases accompanied by respective dental hygiene interventions to facilitate the planning process.[4,11-13]

Examples of planning goals may be the following:
- "Patient will report a decrease in oral discomfort at next appointment."
- "Patient will report greater ability to tolerate time frame of appointment with assistance from use of supportive devices and stabilization techniques."
- "Patient will report improved sense of safety maneuvering within the dental hygiene operatory setting."
- "Ease of breathing will be monitored throughout appointment for patients with myasthenia gravis to ensure adequate airway exchange."[14]
- "Avoid administering local anesthesia with epinephrine to patients with uncontrolled hyperthyroidism to minimize risk of thyroid storm."[15]

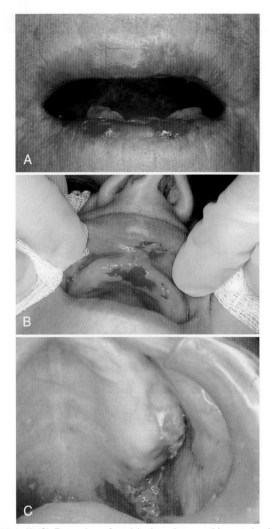

Fig. 53.1 (A–C) Examples of oral lesions in pemphigus vulgaris. ([A] From Ibsen OAC, Phelan JA. *Oral Pathology for the Dental Hygienist.* 6th ed. Saunders; 2014. [B] Courtesy Dr. Fariba Younai. [C] Courtesy Dr. Sidney Eisig.)

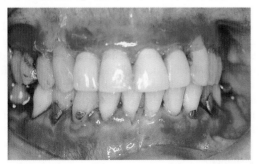

Fig. 53.2 Cicatricial pemphigoid (desquamative gingivitis). (Courtesy Dr. Victor M. Sternberg.)

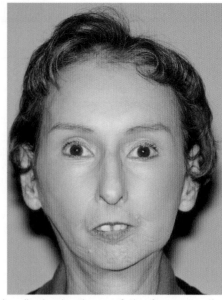

Fig. 53.3 Localized scleroderma of the face presenting a scarlike appearance (coup de sabre).

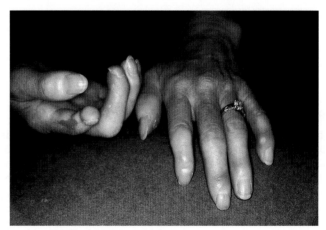

Fig. 53.4 Clawlike finger position characteristic of systemic sclerosis. (From Regezi JA, Sciubba JJ, Jordan RCK. *Oral Pathology: Clinical Pathologic Correlations.* 7th ed. Elsevier; 2017.)

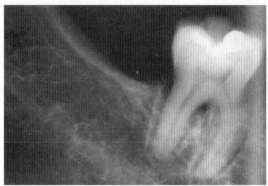

Fig. 53.5 Widening of the periodontal ligament space characteristic of systemic sclerosis.

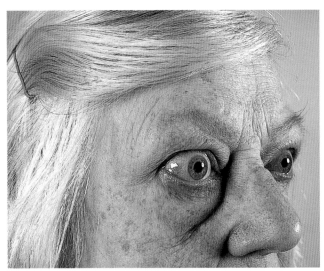

Fig. 53.6 Pernicious anemia symptoms observed in a 38 year old female including premature graying of hair and yellowing of the skin and eyes (caused by jaundice). (From Little JW, Falace DA, Miller CS, et al. *Little and Falace's Dental Management of the Medically Compromised Patient.* 8th ed. Elsevier; 2012.)

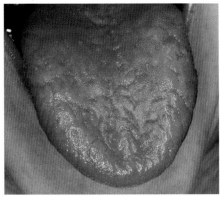

Fig. 53.7 Sjögren syndrome. This individual had severe xerostomia. The filiform papillae are lacking. (From Ibsen OAC, Phelan JA. *Oral Pathology for the Dental Hygienist.* 6th ed. Saunders; 2013.)

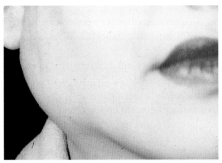

Fig. 53.8 Enlargement of parotid gland in Sjögren syndrome. (Courtesy Dr. Donald M. Cohen and Dr. Indraneel Bhattacharyya.)

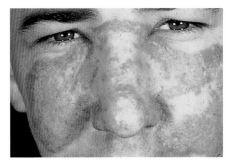

Fig. 53.9 Malar rash seen in systemic lupus erythematosus. (Courtesy Dr. Donald M. Cohen and Dr. Indraneel Bhattacharyya.)

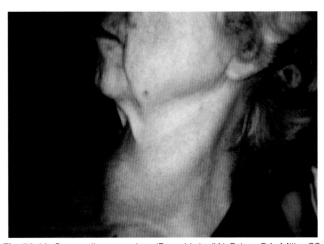

Fig. 53.10 Graves disease goiter. (From Little JW, Falace DA, Miller CS, Rhodus NL. *Little and Falace's Dental Management of the Medically Compromised Patient.* 8th ed. Elsevier; 2012.)

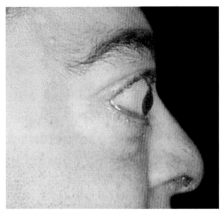

Fig. 53.11 Exophthalmos of Graves disease. (From Stein HA, Stein RM, Freeman MI. *The Ophthalmic Assistant: A Text for Allied and Associated Ophthalmic Personnel.* 9th ed. Elsevier; 2013.)

Further, the clinician should review the potential for a medical emergency to occur given the patient's condition and medications taken. Preparing in advance to prevent and/or manage a medical emergency is advised.

Implementation

Implementation includes the administration of dental hygiene interventions to minimize oral infections and restore oral health, prevent future disease, and educate patients. Patients must understand the relationship between their autoimmune condition, medical management, and oral care. Some patients may require further care with an oral specialist if mucosal lesions are not responding to initial treatment protocols. Others may need more definitive periodontal treatment. In these instances, referrals to an oral pathologist, oral surgeon, or periodontist are warranted.

Patient education must include disease pathophysiology, effects on the oral cavity, palliative treatments for oral discomfort, and preventive oral therapies where appropriate. Table 53.4 lists common oral

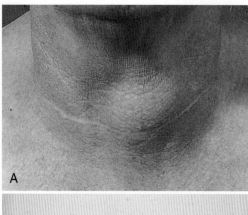

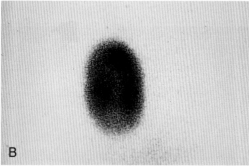

Fig. 53.12 (A) Toxic adenoma of the thyroid gland causing hyperthyroidism. (B) Toxic adenoma in the right thyroid demonstrated with the use of Tc-pertechnetate scanning. (From Forbes CD, Jackson WF. *Color Atlas and Text of Clinical Medicine.* 3rd ed. Mosby; 2003.)

BOX 53.5 Compliance With Professional Recommendations

Dental hygienists must explain to their patients that strict adherence to the physician and dental professional recommendations help to ensure that adequate care is rendered. Patients must not self-medicate, stop medications, or ignore preventive practices recommended by the healthcare team.

BOX 53.6 Critical Thinking Scenario

Patient: Mrs. T.

Profile: Mrs. T, age 56, has been presenting to the same dentist and dental hygienist on a regular basis for the past 10 years. She has valued the relationship she has had with her oral care providers and feels that she has good oral health. She trusts them to offer her good products and to manage her oral health and that of her family well.

Chief Complaint: "My mouth gets sores all the time and it makes it difficult to eat."

Health History: Mrs. T reports that she avoids toothpaste, spicy foods, cinnamon, and soft drinks due to the strong flavoring. Also noted is that Mrs. T has a mucous membrane covering part of her right eye.

Social History: Mrs. T is married with three children; however, she has recently become an empty nester. She reports drinking an occasional alcoholic beverage but has never smoked or used drugs.

Dental History: Mrs. T presents with generalized desquamative gingivitis. The gingival tissues are friable, leaving an erythematous, ulcerated surface. Moderate biofilm is present.

There is no evidence of periodontal disease. Demineralization of the buccal/facial surfaces of the teeth is present.

Oral Health Behavior Assessment: Mrs. T is highly motivated; however, her painful gingival tissues make home care challenging. She reports using a manual soft toothbrush twice per day if her gingival tissues are not red and ulcerated, rinsing with saltwater and a fluoride mouth rinse, and flossing three times per week if her tissues allow it. She reports that she will often avoid toothpaste because the flavoring agents bother her.

Supplemental Notes: Mrs. T presents with conjunctiva of the right eye. She occasionally reports that she experiences dysphagia when the sores in her mouth are present in her esophagus.

1. Use the assessment data to arrive at a dental hygiene diagnosis, set the patient goals, and plan dental hygiene interventions.
2. What connections can the dental hygienist make between the chief complaint, health history, and supplemental notes?
3. What referrals would you make to support Mrs. T's systemic and oral health?

---

manifestations and dental hygiene interventions for numerous autoimmune conditions.[4,11–17] The dental hygienist should consider recommending products and oral devices that will provide the best possible results for biofilm, caries, and xerostomia management.[4] Patients presenting with disease- or drug-induced fungal and viral infections require definitive treatment with antifungal and antiviral medications. Patients with medication-induced oral lesions may require agents for topical pain control (Box 53.7).[4] Table 53.5 provides examples of oral health product considerations based on clinical indications.[4] In addition, patients should be taught to perform an oral self-examination so that they can identify changes that are occurring and seek immediate treatment. Teaching patients to be attentive to their oral health and aggressive in seeking additional evaluation may help avoid long-term adverse effects from their health condition or medication management.

Evaluation

Patients with autoimmune disease must be placed on 2- to 3-month maintenance intervals because of their compromised immune system. Furthermore, it is important that after initial therapy is completed, an evaluation appointment be scheduled to assess host response to dental hygiene care, to determine if additional treatment is needed, and to reinforce self-care.

At each subsequent appointment, the patient's overall health, as well as oral health, is reassessed. OHRQL can be reassessed at this time as well. Continued communication between the dental hygienist, dentist, and physician is extremely important when changes are made in planned professional care.

The diagnostic statements and goals are used to guide clinical decisions regarding appropriate dental hygiene interventions so that oral health can be achieved. Whether signs and symptoms first documented are still evident at the evaluation appointment determines if the goals were met, partially met, or not met. Further treatment and referral may be necessary, depending on outcomes.

Documentation

The final step in the dental hygiene process of care is to document the process and outcomes of each appointment. The practitioner should report the extent to which goals were met and factors influencing outcomes. Proposed future treatment, referrals, and patient response to dental hygiene care should be recorded. Any adverse reactions or emergency situations during the provision of care should be noted, including details of the event or situation, vital signs, emergency assistance required, treatment provided, and family members and/or healthcare professionals contacted. This information must be shared with the dentist and physician of record.

TABLE 53.4 Oral Manifestations With Dental Hygiene Interventions

Autoimmune Disease	Oral Manifestation(s)	Dental Hygiene Interventions
Cicatricial pemphigoid	Vesicles or bullae that rupture, leaving large areas of superficial, ulcerated, and denuded mucosa; lesions are painful and may persist for weeks or months if untreated	Physician consult if difficulty with speaking or breathing Treat lesions with topical or systemic corticosteroids Topical pain control for lesions as needed Protect eyes if ocular involvement
Fibromyalgia	Temporomandibular joint (TMJ) dysfunction Pain in face and head Xerostomia	Referral to physician for evaluation Caries risk reduction: fluorides, remineralization therapy, xylitol Salivary replacement therapy Consult for TMJ and jaw pain
Hyperthyroidism	Mild tremor in tongue Osteoporosis in bones of skull, axial and peripheral skeleton Children: premature loss of deciduous teeth, with accelerated tooth eruption and faster development of jaw Adults: marked loss of alveolar process, diffuse demineralization of mandible Rapidly progressive periodontal disease Lingual thyroid tissue appears on posterior dorsal region of tongue, below area of foramen cecum	Inspect thyroid gland carefully; note enlargement, presence of nodules, pain and tenderness on palpation Avoid overpalpation of gland; risk for thyroid storm More sensitive to pain; require more anesthesia More sensitive to catecholamines; limit vasoconstrictor; avoid if uncontrolled hyperthyroidism More tolerant to centrally acting drugs; require higher doses of sedatives and analgesics Manage stress, anxiety, and infections to minimize risk of thyroid storm; monitor vital signs
Hypothyroidism	Children: enlarged tongue, delayed eruption patterns, malocclusion Adults: hoarse voice, enlarged tongue, swelling of facial features	More sensitive to central nervous system depressants; lower dose of opiates and sedatives
Multiple sclerosis	Oral manifestations occur in 2% to 3% of population Paresthesia Difficulty with speech Orofacial numbness Trigeminal neuralgia Drug-induced xerostomia	Schedule short morning appointments Treat during periods of remission: avoid treatment during active disease period Steroid supplementation may be needed Provide assistance with ambulation, transfer to dental chair Caries risk reduction: fluorides, remineralization therapy, xylitol Salivary replacement therapy Patient education: augmentation of oral hygiene regimen in cases of limited manual dexterity; modify oral hygiene devices or use power devices
Myasthenia gravis	Drooping eyelids and double vision Muscle weakness in face, head, and neck Difficulty chewing, swallowing Difficulty wearing dentures Soft palate weakness Impaired lip movement Altered voice with nasal tone	Patient education: assist patient with "feel" of oral hygiene aids in mouth if visual impairments Use hands to support lower jaw during mastication Consult with physician for supportive device for lower jaw between meals to prevent spontaneous dropping Consult for implant-supported dentures Schedule short, early morning appointments Use rubber dam, evacuation, and mouth props during appointments Consider nitrous oxide–oxygen sedation to reduce stress and anxiety Consult before prescribing antibiotics and muscle relaxants because some antibiotics have muscle relaxant properties Monitor ease of breathing
Pemphigus vulgaris	Superficial, "ragged" erosions and ulcerations, haphazard distribution; most common areas are palate, labial mucosa, buccal mucosa, ventral surface of the tongue, and gingiva	Consultation with physician for early diagnosis Monitor patient for long-term effects of treatment with corticosteroids and immunosuppressants
Pernicious anemia	Painful, red, burning tongue with atrophy of papillae Oral ulcerations	Topical pain control for oral lesions and sore tongue
Psoriasis	Oral manifestations are rare Oral lesions appear as white or red plaques, mixed red and white lesions, pustules, vesicles, or ulcerations Geographic tongue may occur	Consult with dermatologist as needed for oral lesions Topical pain control if lesions become symptomatic

TABLE 53.4 Oral Manifestations With Dental Hygiene Interventions—cont'd

Autoimmune Disease	Oral Manifestation(s)	Dental Hygiene Interventions
Rheumatoid arthritis	TMJ involvement (75% of cases) Limited or difficulty opening of the mouth Drug-induced gingival bleeding Drug-induced oral mucosal lesions	Patient education; risk of TMJ involvement; regular panoramic radiographs to assess mandibular condylar wear and TMJ Soft diet Moist heat or ice Consultation for occlusal appliance Patient education: augmentation of oral hygiene regimen in cases of limited manual dexterity Determine if premedication is indicated before treatment using AAOS appropriate use criteria Evaluate bleeding time, platelet function Blood studies if taking immunosuppressants Pain control for drug-induced oral lesions Shorter appointments for comfort if difficulty sitting Use supportive devices to maintain patient comfort in the dental chair
Scleroderma	Radiographically: widened periodontal ligament spaces; osseous destruction of TMJ, mandibular angle, coronoid process, or condyle Jaw fractures late in disease process Microstomia Limited opening of the mouth Xerostomia Loss of attached gingival mucosa and generalized recession Firm, hypomobile tongue; difficulty with speech and swallowing Anterior open bite	Patient education: augmentation of oral hygiene regimen in cases of limited manual dexterity; modify oral hygiene devices or use power devices Semireclined position if gastrointestinal problems Nutritional counseling Caries risk reduction: fluorides, remineralization therapy, xylitol Antimicrobial mouth rinses Salivary replacement therapies Isometric exercises to maintain mobility of muscles of face and neck and to improve mouth opening
Sjögren syndrome	Erythematous oral mucosa Enlarged salivary glands, especially parotids Severe xerostomia Difficulty swallowing Altered taste Difficulty wearing dentures Fissured tongue; atrophy of papillae Candidiasis, often erythematous form Caries, cervical most common Periodontal disease	Referral to physician or ophthalmologist if necessary Patient education: daily fluoride application at home to prevent xerostomia-induced dental caries Daily fluoride regimen, remineralization therapy Xylitol gum and candy to stimulate salivary flow and therapeutic doses to interfere with *Streptococcus mutans* Nutritional counseling Use of artificial tears and saliva Salivary stimulants Salivary replacement therapy Antifungal therapy for secondary candidiasis Hydration Avoid spicy or acidic foods
Systemic lupus erythematosus (SLE)	Oral lesions (5% to 25% of patients) Location of lesions: palate, buccal mucosa, gingiva May appear lichenoid; may look nonspecific or granulomatous Ulceration, pain, erythema, hyperkeratosis Xerostomia Taste alteration Oral mucosal pain Candidiasis Periodontal disease	Referral to physician for consultation because of complex medical history Possible antibiotic premedication if history of pericarditis or noninfective endocarditis, or low white blood cell count from immunosuppressants Consult for need for supplemental steroids Antifungal therapy as needed Topical pain control for oral lesions Monitor nutrition if taste alteration Caries prevention: fluorides, remineralization therapy, xylitol Salivary stimulant or replacement therapies Avoid spicy foods Patient education: meticulous oral hygiene; avoid excessive sun exposure Schedule shorter appointments
Chronic cutaneous lupus erythematosus (CCLE)	Painful lesions are practically identical to lesions of erosive lichen planus	Referral to dermatologist or physician if necessary Patient education: avoid exposure to acidic or salty foods if painful intraoral lesions are present; avoid excessive sun exposure

BOX 53.7 Agents for Topical Pain Control[4]

Over-the-Counter Products

Benzocaine 10% ointment

Lidocaine 2.5% ointment

Tetracaine hydrochloride 1% ointment

Diphenhydramine elixir

Benzocaine, gelatin, pectin, and sodium carboxymethylcellulose adhesive oral paste

Diphenhydramine elixir added in equal amounts to Maalox, Mylanta, or Kaopectate

Prescription Products

2% Viscous lidocaine mouth rinse

Sucralfate (Carafate) prepared as a 1 g/15 mL suspension for rinsing

Diphenhydramine elixir added in equal amounts to Maalox, Mylanta, or Kaopectate and 2% lidocaine mouth rinse

Amlexanox oral paste 5%

TABLE 53.5 Oral Health Product Considerations

Product Category	Indications
Fluorides	Caries risk reduction Hypersensitivity
Nonfluoride remineralization therapies	Caries risk reduction Hypersensitivity
Xylitol	Caries risk reduction
Salivary stimulants (pilocarpine, cevimeline)	Oral disease risk reduction Salivary hypofunction and xerostomia Improved comfort and function
Salivary substitutes	Oral disease risk reduction Salivary hypofunction and xerostomia Improved comfort and function
Antimicrobial agents (chlorhexidine, essential oils, triclosan,* cetylpyridinium chloride)	Oral disease risk reduction Halitosis
Mechanical devices (power brushes, oral irrigators, interdental aids)	Biofilm removal and oral cleansing Salivary stimulation

*Triclosan is only available in some countries.

KEY CONCEPTS

- The incidence of encountering individuals with autoimmune diseases in the oral care environment increases as the percentage of aging persons increases.
- The dental hygienist screens for and recognizes typical signs, symptoms, and manifestations of autoimmune diseases.
- Some autoimmune diseases affect the head and neck area only, whereas others can affect multiple organ systems of the body.
- Autoimmune diseases compromise patient's immune systems, which puts them at risk for oral diseases and systemic infections.
- Some autoimmune diseases can be managed effectively with medication.
- The dental hygienist consults appropriate use criteria to minimize unnecessary use of antibiotics for premedication in patients with prosthetic joint replacement.[9,10]
- Scleroderma and rheumatoid arthritis may affect a patient's ability to perform adequate oral self-care measures.
- Chronic xerostomia places an individual at extreme risk for dental caries. Professional and daily self-applied topical fluoride applications, use of remineralization therapies, antimicrobials, antiseptics, xylitol, and salivary substitutes may help manage xerostomia and caries risk in those with Sjögren syndrome and others with chronic dry mouth (see Chapters 19 and 27).
- Referral and consultation with the patient's physician are essential to providing optimum dental hygiene care to patients with autoimmune disease.

ACKNOWLEDGMENT

The author acknowledges JoAnn R. Gurenlian and Ann Eshenaur Spolarich for their past contributions to this chapter.

REFERENCES

1. Laxminarayana D. Is tolerance broken in autoimmunity? *Clin Med Insights Pathol.* 2017;10:1179555717712716.
2. Watad A, Azrielant S, Bragazzi NL, et al. Seasonality and autoimmune diseases: the contribution of the four seasons to the mosaic of autoimmunity. *J Autoimmun.* 2017:pii:S0896-8411(17)30313-X.
3. Lin J, Liu J, Davies ML, et al. Level and rheumatoid arthritis disease activity: review and meta-analysis. *PLoS One.* 2016;11(1):e0146351.
4. DeRossi SS, Ciarrocca KN. Autoimmune and connective tissue diseases. In: Patton LL, Glick M, eds. *The ADA Practical Guide to Patients with Medical Conditions.* 2nd ed. Wiley Blackwell; 2016.
5. Carsons SE, Vivino FB, Parke A, et al. Treatment guidelines for rheumatologic manifestations of Sjögren's syndrome: use of biologic agents, management of fatigue, and inflammatory musculoskeletal pain. *Arthritis Care Res.* 2017;69(4):517–527.
6. Alam J, Jantan I, Bukhari SNA. Rheumatoid arthritis: recent advances on its etiology, role of cytokines and pharmacotherapy. *Biomed Pharmacother.* 2017;92:615–633.
7. Toth L, Juhasz MF, Szabo L, et al. Janus kinase inhibitors improve disease activity and patient-reported outcomes in rheumatoid arthritis: a systemic review and meta-analysis of 24,135 patients. *Int J Mol Sci.* 2022;23(3):1246. https://doi.org/10.3390/ijms23031246.
8. Regezi JA, Sciubba JJ, Jordan RCK. *Oral Pathology: Clinical Pathologic Correlations.* 7th ed. Elsevier; 2017.
9. American Dental Association-Appointed members of the Expert Writing and Voting Panels contributing to the development of American Academy of Orthopedic surgeons appropriate Use criteria. American dental association guidance for utilizing appropriate use criteria in the management of the care of patients with orthopedic implants undergoing dental procedures. *J Am Dent Assoc.* 2017;148(2):57–59.
10. American Academy of Orthopedic Surgeons. Ortho guidelines. Appropriate use criteria. Management of patients with orthopaedic implants undergoing dental procedures. Published September 23, 2016. Available at: https://www.aaos.org/globalassets/quality-and-practice-resources/dental/auc-patients-with-orthopaedic-implants-dental-procedures.pdf. Accessed November 2, 2022.
11. Zhang GQ, Meng Y. Oral and craniofacial manifestations of multiple sclerosis: implications for the oral health care provider. *Eur Rev Med Pharmacol Sci.* 2015;19(23):4610–4620.
12. Magliocca KR, Fitzpatrick SG. Autoimmune disease manifestations in the oral cavity. *Surg Pathol Clin.* 2017;10(1):57–88.
13. Taylor J, McMillan R, Shephard M, et al. World Workshop on Oral Medicine VI: a systematic review of the treatment of mucous membrane pemphigoid. *Oral Surg Oral Med Oral Pathol Oral Radiol.* 2015;120:161–171.
14. Tamburrini A, Tacconi F, Barlattani A, et al. An update on myasthenia gravis, challenging disease for the dental profession. *J Oral Sci.* 2015;57(3):161–168.
15. Burch HB, Cooper DS. Management of Graves disease: a review. *JAMA.* 2015;314(23):2544–2554.
16. Huang WJ, Chen WW, Zhang X. Multiple sclerosis: pathology, diagnosis and treatments. *Exp Ther Med.* 2017;13(6):3163–3166.
17. Saccuccu M, Di Carlo G, Bossu M, et al. Autoimmune diseases and their manifestations on oral cavity: diagnosis and clinical management. *J Immunol Res.* 2018;2018:6061825. https://doi.org/10.1155/2018/6061825.

54

Organ Transplantation and Renal Disease

Sandra D'Amato-Palumbo

PROFESSIONAL OPPORTUNITIES

An increasing number of individuals are either currently wait listed for a solid organ transplant or have received a solid organ transplant. Once individuals are added to the national organ transplant waiting list, they may receive an organ rather quickly or they may wait many years. The most affected potential end-stage organ disease candidates are those waiting for a kidney, followed by those needing a liver, heart, lung, and pancreas. To provide effective oral care to these special needs patient populations, dental hygienists must be able to develop and apply individualized dental hygiene care plans, especially for patients presenting with end-stage organ disease, solid organ transplantation, and renal disease.

COMPETENCIES

1. Explain the concept of solid organ transplantation, discuss the indications for organ transplantation, and describe the role that the United Network for Organ Sharing (UNOS) plays in organ transplantation.
2. Determine specialized dental management considerations of patients' oral health needs before solid organ transplantation and after transplantation.
3. Discuss the world-recognized Kidney Disease Outcomes Quality Initiative (K/DOQI), as well as compare and contrast chronic kidney disease and end-stage renal disease.
4. Discuss dialysis treatment modalities.
5. Describe various secondary medical conditions that could develop with kidney disease and dialysis and relate these conditions to overall oral care.
6. Discuss the need for interprofessional communication among members of the transplant patient's medical healthcare team.

INTRODUCTION

End-stage organ disease eventually leads to permanent and complete failure of an organ's function. Examples of end-stage organ failure are congestive heart failure, chronic obstructive pulmonary disease, or chronic renal failure. With end-stage kidney (renal) disease, kidneys shut down and the patient then requires dialysis. With end-stage heart disease, the heart functions very poorly and may need mechanical support or transplantation in order for the patient to survive. Considered a major cause of death worldwide, end-stage organ disease affects individuals regardless of socioeconomic status or age, which creates the need for organ transplantation to sustain one's quality of life.

SOLID ORGAN TRANSPLANTATION

Solid organ transplant refers to the surgical placement of a viable, functioning organ, such as a heart, liver, kidney, pancreas, lung, small bowel, or bone marrow, into an appropriate patient (**recipient**) ailing from end-stage organ disease.

The organ donation process involves a donation either from a living person or from a deceased person (donation after brain death or cardiovascular death). The organ can be donated from an identical twin to another twin (syngeneic), from one living relative to another (allogeneic), between unrelated individuals (xenograft), or from cadaver organs. Living donors potentially can donate one of two kidneys; one of two lobes of a liver (cells in the remaining lobe of the liver grow or regenerate until the liver is almost its original size in the donor and recipient); or a lung or part of a lung; part of the pancreas; or part of the intestines (parts do not regenerate but fully function in the donor and recipient).[1] Transplantation of cadaver organs yields the largest pool of organs; however, it is the poorest match of these combinations.

Several decades ago, organ transplantation was still a relatively new progressive procedure in medicine. In recent years, though, clinical advances, greater numbers of organ donors, changing reimbursement structures, complex administrative models such as the United Network for Organ Sharing, and strict government regulations have led to improved healthcare outcomes for individuals receiving organ transplants.[2] Major medical advances in organ transplantation have occurred because of effective immunosuppressant drugs, such as cyclosporine, tacrolimus, steroids, azathioprine, mycophenolate mofetil, and sirolimus.

Indications for organ transplantation are specific to the organ involved. Many diseases can lead to organ failure, including heart disease, diabetes, hepatitis, cystic fibrosis, and cirrhosis. Injury and birth defects may also cause organ failure. Common etiologies for heart transplantation are cardiomyopathy or severe coronary artery disease. In adults, liver transplantation is indicated for patients who suffer from cirrhosis of the liver, chronic hepatitis, hepatic organ failure, and metabolic disorders. Common reasons for kidney transplantation include bilateral chronic kidney disease, end-stage renal failure, and transplantation of the pancreas for patients with severe diabetes mellitus who are also receiving a kidney transplant.

Regardless of the etiology, organ involved, or comorbidities, major medical complications associated with organ transplantation can result in hypertension, diabetes mellitus, excessive bleeding, anemia, osteoporosis, adrenal crisis, severe immunosuppression, infection, delayed healing, tumors, rejection of the transplanted organ or graft failure, death, retransplantation of the heart, liver, or bone marrow, cancers, adrenal crisis, and possibly other complications.[3] Although acute organ rejection is a relatively rare occurrence in today's world of advanced medicine, sepsis and chronic rejection continue to threaten the medical stability of the organ transplant recipient.[3]

UNITED NETWORK FOR ORGAN SHARING

The **United Network for Organ Sharing (UNOS)** is a nonprofit scientific and educational organization that maintains the nation's only

Organ Procurement and Transplantation Network (OPTN). The organ transplant waiting list includes persons who have a medical need and qualify medically to benefit from organ transplantation. UNOS manages the OPTN, establishes organ donation policies and procedures, facilitates organ matching and placement, and maintains the national database of organ transplant candidates and donors. Although waiting periods can vary greatly, oral healthcare providers can determine average waiting times for specific hospitals and geographic areas. For example, the average renal patient waiting for a deceased donor kidney usually waits at least 2 years before receiving a transplant. Recipients who are fortunate enough to receive a direct donation from a related or nonrelated living donor can expect to have virtually no waiting time. With this information, a dental hygiene care plan can be developed for the patient in the pretransplant waiting phase to avoid postoperative complications from poor oral health and hygiene.

MANAGING ORAL HEALTH FOR PRETRANSPLANTATION AND POSTTRANSPLANTATION PATIENTS

As medical treatment for end-stage organ disease advances, dental hygienists are likely to provide oral healthcare treatment to patients living with dialysis, solid organ transplant candidates, and solid organ transplant recipients. Because of the complexities and variations of care for these medically compromised patients, it is important to work closely with the patient's (medical) transplant team, which cannot be overemphasized. However, dental hygienists often discover variations in patient care across hospitals and across organs transplanted. The National Institutes of Health—National Institute of Dental and Craniofacial Research provides the dental team with practical treatment guidelines for managing a patient's oral health before and after organ and stem cell transplantation.

Managing Oral Health Before Transplantation

When formulating the patient's dental/dental hygiene care plan, consider the following care plan guidelines for the pretransplant recipient:
- Obtain the patient's health history, including vital signs; perform a noninvasive, extraoral, and intraoral clinical assessment; perform a dentition, periodontal (without periodontal probing), and nutritional assessment; obtain radiographs; and provide homecare instructions.
- Consult with the patient's transplant team regarding the patient's overall medical status to establish whether the patient is able to tolerate dental/dental hygiene treatment. Postpone treatment when necessary.
- Consider current standards and evidence-based decision making about the timing of implementing dental/dental hygiene treatment.
- Consider the need for antibiotic prophylaxis to prevent systemic infection from invasive dental or dental hygiene treatment. Unless advised otherwise by the physician, the American Heart Association's standard regimen to prevent endocarditis is an accepted option.
- Consider the need to assess the patient's bleeding potential with appropriate laboratory tests, including taking precautions to limit bleeding and the need to ensure appropriate selection, dosage, and administration of drugs, especially drugs used for management of dental pain and treatment of oral infections.
- Pretransplant patients may be taking multiple medications, such as anticoagulants, beta-blockers, calcium channel blockers, diuretics, and others.

- Address possible systemic/oral side effects of medications, such as xerostomia, gingival hyperplasia, and bleeding.
- Determine the need to refer the patient to dental providers for care outside of the dental hygiene scope of practice (active dental disease and oral infection; prescribing of medications; removing nonrestorable teeth; and adjustment of dental prostheses, all strongly advised to be addressed to reduce the likelihood of posttransplant infection).
- Emphasize the importance of oral health and proper oral self-care to minimize bacteremia and to prevent oral and dental problems after transplantation.[4]

Managing Oral Health After Transplantation

When formulating a patient's dental/dental hygiene care plan after an organ or bone marrow transplantation, consider the following care plan guidelines for the transplant recipient:
- Patients who receive organ or stem cell transplants should avoid dental treatment for up to 6 months, except for emergency dental treatment. Once the graft stabilizes (which is typically within a 3- to 6-month period after the transplant procedure), obtain medical clearance from the transplant team so that the patient can be treated in the dental office with proper precautions and considerations.
- During the consultation with the patient's physician, determine the patient's medical stability and ascertain whether the patient can tolerate treatment. Evidence-based decision making needs to address whether the patient requires antibiotic prophylaxis, especially in patients with suppressed immune systems or for those patients who show signs of transplant rejection, or to determine if prophylactic coverage is indicated to prevent infective endocarditis.
- Consult with the patient's physician to discuss medication considerations for the following:
  - Immunosuppressive drugs can potentially cause gingival hyperplasia, poor and slow healing, drug-induced liver disease, and interactions with commonly prescribed medications.
  - Immunosuppression may result in an increased risk for bacterial, viral, or fungal infections.
  - Anticoagulant medications may contribute to excessive bleeding problems; thus assess the patient's bleeding potential with appropriate laboratory tests. Consider the use of hemostatic agents/precautions to limit bleeding.
  - Patients taking steroids are at risk for acute adrenal crisis (a life-threatening condition associated with high doses or long-term use of steroids).
- Identify and treat (when appropriate) bacterial, viral (e.g., herpes simplex virus), and fungal infections.
- Address new dental disease(s).
- Contact the patient's treating physician immediately if the patient's blood pressure exceeds acceptable guidelines, discontinue treatment, and refer the patient for a medical consultation.
- Recommend twice-daily antimicrobial mouth rinses, saliva substitutes, xylitol-containing products, and/or fluoride rinses, when appropriate.
- Educate the patient about necessary professional oral care, including:
  - Proper oral self-care
  - Frequent oral debridement
  - Frequent oral hygiene counseling
- Provide regular screening for oral, head, and neck cancer. Organ transplant recipients have an increased incidence of squamous and basal cell carcinomas.
- Consult with the patient's treating physician to discuss appropriate selection, dosage, and administration of prescribed medications and drugs and to ensure the safety of prescribed and over-the-counter medications.[4]

Box 54.1 presents patient or client education tips for solid organ transplant candidates and recipients.

Gingival Enlargement

The discovery of the drug cyclosporine provided a breakthrough in solid organ transplantation. Cyclosporine, however, increases the risk of **nephrotoxicity** and damage to kidney cells caused by a toxic agent, such as a drug. Most transplant recipients are treated with a trio of immunosuppression medications (cyclosporine, prednisone, and mycophenolate mofetil). Because even prednisone can cause long-term complications of bone metabolism and adrenal crisis, the pursuit of immunosuppressive therapy with minimal side effects continues. In addition, a wide variety of prescription and common over-the-counter medications are nephrotoxic to transplant recipients. Even common herbs can cause disruption in cyclosporine levels, endangering a patient's delicate balance of immunosuppression. Therefore the dental team *always* must consult the patient's medical team to ensure the safety of medications prescribed, including over-the-counter medications.

The literature is replete with instances of drug-influenced gingival enlargement in solid organ transplant recipients. Gingival enlargement, also known as gingival overgrowth, is another adverse side effect associated with immunosuppressive therapy. Gingival enlargement may occur due to sensitivity to cyclosporine and may be exacerbated by poor oral hygiene. Although modifications in immunosuppressive therapy may be explored when gingival enlargement is a concern, transplant physicians are often reluctant to alter the immunosuppressive therapy when the patient's medical condition is stable. Drug-influenced gingival enlargement has been associated with the immunosuppressive medication tacrolimus.[5]

Gingival enlargement should be prevented, if possible. Meticulous daily oral self-care should emphasize optimal oral biofilm removal to avoid infection and inflammation and frequent oral debridement appointments (3- to 4-month continued-care intervals) by the dental hygienist to reduce gingival enlargement risk. The dental hygienist always must be aware that immunosuppressive therapy can mask inflammation.

See the Critical Thinking Scenario in Box 54.2.

Infection

Immunosuppressive therapy is at its most aggressive level in transplant recipients immediately after transplant surgery. In the months after surgery, the patient's immunosuppressive therapy gradually is reduced and then maintained at a level that balances the threat of rejection and infection. Any infection (such as vascular or catheter infections, pneumonia, cellulitis, or periodontal abscess) can be reactivated or exacerbated in the immediate postoperative period during the introduction of immunosuppressive therapy or afterward, depending on the overall state of immunosuppression.[6] When providing care, oral healthcare

providers should educate patients about the potential risk dental infections play in organ rejection and infection.

Infective Endocarditis and Invasive Dental Procedures

The need for antibiotic prophylaxis for invasive dental procedures in patients who have undergone solid organ transplants remains controversial. Although surveys of transplant survivors demonstrate opposing views, the majority of medical providers usually recommend antibiotic prophylaxis because the bacteremia arising from invasive dental procedures represents a significant risk in the immunocompromised patient, particularly during the 6-month period after transplantation. The American Heart Association, the K/DOQI, and the Kidney Disease: Improving Global Outcomes (KDIGO) initiative do not directly address this issue of care in their guidelines. Extreme variations within the transplant population make universal recommendations inappropriate. Therefore, solid organ transplant recipients should be evaluated individually for risk of infection, and necessary medical and dental consultations should determine the following:

- If or when the person can receive routine dental care
- Transplant recipient's medical stability
- Comorbidities present (e.g., diabetes mellitus, hypertension, cardiovascular disease)
- Medical management of the recipient; concerns during the pretransplant and/or posttransplant phase
- Pharmacologic history

Candidiasis and Viral Infections

Patients taking immunosuppressive therapy often experience candidiasis or recurrence of herpetic infections in the oral cavity. Employing interprofessional practice, the oral healthcare provider should collaborate with the transplant team to determine appropriate treatment for such patients.

Malignancies

Organ transplant recipients have an increased incidence of squamous and basal cell carcinomas. Therefore, frequent screening of the skin and oropharyngeal area is indicated. Liver transplant recipients with a history of tobacco use and/or alcoholism are at particular risk for oropharyngeal cancer.

RENAL DISEASE

Although nearly 107,000 solid organ transplant adult candidates were wait-listed with UNOS in 2021, only 41,355 transplants were performed in that year (Fig. 54.1).[7] Of those 41,355 transplants, 24,670 were kidney transplants alone, which was by far the largest population of recipients by organ type.[7] Because patients with end-stage renal disease can use dialysis as a bridge to transplantation, the fact that kidney transplants can be provided by a living donor (not only by a deceased donor) and deceased kidneys have a 48-hour window (a significantly greater amount of time compared with heart, liver, lung, and other organs), an increased number of kidney transplant recipients and candidates exist, compared with other potential end-stage organ disease candidates.

See Box 54.3 for educational resources on kidney transplantation and dialysis.

Kidney Disease Outcomes Quality Initiative

The world-recognized **Kidney Disease Outcomes Quality Initiative (K/DOQI)** publishes evidence-based clinical practice guidelines for all stages of kidney disease and its associated complications, including:
- Acute kidney injury
- Anemia in chronic kidney disease (CKD)

- Diagnosis, evaluation, and treatment of mineral and bone disorder in CKD
- Management of blood pressure and lipids (cholesterol and triglycerides) in CKD
- Evaluation, classification, and stratification of CKD
- Evaluation of laboratory measurements for clinical assessment of kidney disease
- Diabetes and CKD
- Glomerulonephritis (a disease that causes inflammation of the glomeruli or the kidney's filtering units)
- Hemodialysis and peritoneal dialysis adequacy and vascular access
- Prevention, diagnosis, evaluation, and treatment of hepatitis C in CKD
- Nutrition in CKD and chronic renal failure
- Care of kidney transplant recipients[8]

Kidney Disease: Improving Global Outcomes

Because kidney-related medical outcomes in the United States surpass those in other countries, the K/DOQI implemented in the United States is part of a larger global initiative by the National Kidney Foundation

> **BOX 54.3 Kidney Transplantation and Dialysis Educational Videos**
>
> Access information about:
> - Kidney transplantation by viewing a video at https://www.kidney.org/atoz/atozTopic_Transplantation
> - Hemodialysis by viewing a video at https://www.youtube.com/watch?v=-JgXaIRCLV1I
> - Peritoneal dialysis by viewing a video at https://www.youtube.com/watch?v=kBX4bD10MXM
> - Hemodialysis and what patients need to know at https://www.kidney.org/sites/default/files/11-50-0214_hemodialysis.pdf

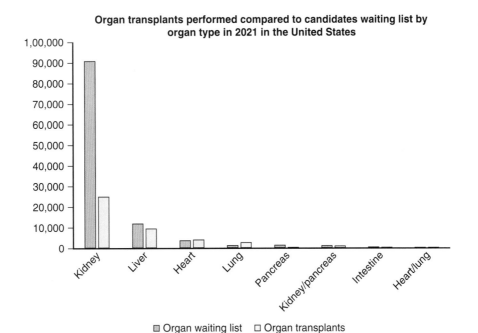

Fig. 54.1 U.S. solid organ transplant data for 2021. (Data from United Network for Organ Sharing, Richmond, VA.)

(NKF). This initiative, titled Kidney Disease: Improving Global Outcomes (KDIGO), has increased the efficiency of using available expertise, guidelines, and resources in improving global outcomes of kidney disease and avoids duplication of efforts in other countries.[9]

Renal Physiology

Kidneys perform three essential bodily functions: excretion of nitrogenous waste products; regulation of fluid volume, composition, and acid-base balance of plasma; and synthesis of hormones necessary for erythrocyte production, bone metabolism, and maintenance of blood pressure.[10] Under normal physiologic conditions, blood is filtered through a complex series of tubules and glomerular capillaries inside the nephron, which is the functional part of the kidney (Fig. 54.2).[3]

When kidney function declines, wastes and excess fluids begin to accumulate; hypertension and anemia often develop. As a result, **chronic renal failure or CKD** causes a gradual loss of the ability of the kidneys to remove wastes, concentrate urine, and conserve electrolytes. Table 54.1 presents the systemic (clinical) manifestations caused by CKD, according to multiple body systems.[3] Table 54.2 presents the extra- and intraoral manifestations and complications of end-stage renal disease with dental hygiene and dental treatment considerations (Fig. 54.3).[3,11]

Some people do not notice early signs or symptoms, and many individuals are not diagnosed until there is irreversible, bilateral damage to the kidneys (Fig. 54.4). The most accurate means of measuring renal function and the extent of kidney damage (CKD) is the blood laboratory test called the **glomerular filtration rate** (GFR), an expression of the quality of glomerular filtrate created each minute in the renal nephrons. The National Kidney Foundation defines the five-stage classification system for CKD based on the GFR.[8] The GFR determines stages of CKD as follows:

- Stage 1: Renal damage with normal GFR (GFR ≥90). Renal damage may occur before a reduction in GFR. The primary treatment goals are to delay the progression of CKD and reduce the risk of cardiovascular disease.
- Stage 2: Renal damage with mild decrease in GFR (GFR 60 to 89). The treatment goals are to delay the progression of CKD and reduce the risk of cardiovascular disease.
- Stage 3: Moderate decrease in GFR (GFR 30 to 59). Anemia and bone metabolism disorders become more common. CKD is defined by kidney damage or GFR <60.
- Stage 4: Severe reduction in GFR (GFR 15 to 29).

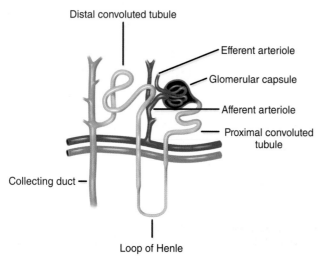

Distal convoluted tubule

Efferent arteriole

Glomerular capsule

Afferent arteriole

Proximal convoluted tubule

Collecting duct

Loop of Henle

Fig. 54.2 The nephron. (Courtesy of Matt Hazzard, University of Kentucky.)

- Stage 5: End-stage renal disease or kidney failure (GFR <15). The patient is unable to maintain essential life functions unless dialysis is initiated. (http://kidneyfoundation.cachefly.net/professionals/KDOQI/guidelines_ckd/p4_class_g1.htm).

Preventive treatment to delay (or avoid) end-stage renal disease includes the pharmacologic use of angiotensin-converting enzyme (ACE) inhibitors and angiotensin receptor blockers (ARBs).

Chronic Kidney Disease

The NKF estimates that 37 million, or 15%, of American adults have CKD. Ninety percent of people with kidney damage or mildly reduced kidney function are not aware of having CKD. It is estimated that CKD is more common in females and in non-Hispanic Blacks than in non-Hispanic Whites.[12]

TABLE 54.1	Clinical Manifestations Caused by Chronic Renal Disease (CKD)
Body Systems	**Clinical Manifestations**
Cardiovascular	• Hypertension • Congestive heart failure • Cardiomyopathy • Pericarditis • Atherosclerosis
Gastrointestinal	• Anorexia or loss of appetite • Nausea and vomiting • Peptic ulcer and bleeding of the intestine • Hepatitis • Pericarditis that results in chest pain
Neuromuscular	• Fatigue and weakness • Drowsiness leading to coma • Headaches • Vision disturbances that interfere with normal sight • Sensory disturbances that result in peripheral neuropathy • Seizures or coma • Muscle spasms
Dermatologic	• Pruritus or itchiness • Bruising or ecchymosis • Hyperpigmentation • Pallor • Uremic frost
Hematologic	• Bleeding • Anemia • Lymphopenia • Leukopenia • Hypersplenism
Immunologic	• Risk of infections (bacterial, viral, fungal)
Metabolic/Endocrine	• Polyuria (excessive urination) and excessive thirst • Nocturia (excessive urination at night) • Glycosuria (excessive glucose in the urine) • Metabolic acidosis • Elevated serum urea, creatine, lipids, and uric acid • Electrolyte disturbances • Secondary hyperparathyroidism

Adapted from Little JW, Falace DA, Miller CS, et al. *Dental Management of the Medically Compromised Patient.* 9th ed. Mosby Elsevier; 2018.

TABLE 54.2 Complications of End-Stage Renal Disease

Oral Manifestations	Description	Dental Treatment Considerations
Pallor of the oral mucosa	Pale appearance of the oral mucosa results from anemia.	Observed and documented during the intraoral clinical assessment
Xerostomia (dry mouth)	Reduction in salivary flow results in dry mouth, caries, gingival disease, and viral and fungal infections.	Xerostomia: recommend saliva substitutes/moisturizing agents (oral mouth rinses, oral sprays, gels, or lozenges) that are alcohol-free, contain xylitol, contain carboxymethyl cellulose or hydroxyethyl cellulose Caries: determine the need for fluoride therapy, including type, strength, and frequency of use based on oral risk factors (xerostomia, diet, medications, other).
Red-orange pigmentation of the cheeks and oral mucosa	Pruritus (severe itching of skin), dryness of the skin, and deposition of carotene-like pigmentation result from decreased renal filtration.	Observed and documented during the intraoral clinical assessment
Dysgeusia	Altered or metallic taste sensation; saliva may exhibit a characteristic ammonia-like odor resulting from a high urea content.	Observed and documented during the intraoral clinical assessment
Bacterial, viral, and fungal infections	Fungal infections (candidiasis) are more frequent, resulting from reduction or lack of salivary flow and/or systemic immunosuppression.	Treat oral infections using appropriate interventions to reduce risk for systemic complications and to restore oral health
Petechiae and ecchymoses, and gingival bleeding	Bleeding tendencies observed on the oral mucosa, soft palate, borders of the tongue, and gingiva, resulting from thrombocytopenia, infection, medication use, and use of anticoagulants such as heparin.	Observed and documented during the extraoral and intraoral assessment. Consider ordering screening tests to assess risk for bleeding. Consider using hemostatic agents for hemostasis and clot retention. Consult with the patient's nephrologist as needed to discuss appropriate timing of the invasive procedure.
Dentition abnormalities of children	Enamel hypoplasia and a red-brownish discoloration of the teeth occur in children. Delayed or altered eruption pattern occurs. Dental pulps may appear narrowed.	Observed and documented during the intraoral clinical assessment
Dental erosion of lingual surfaces	Erosion of teeth is associated with regurgitation and persistent vomiting from high levels of uremia.	Systemic fluoride supplements are contraindicated in patients with chronic renal insufficiency and renal failure.
Uremic stomatitis	Two forms: Erythemopultaceous-type features dry, erythematous burning and painful oral mucosa that is covered with thick gray exudates; the ulcerative form is characterized by mucosal ulcerations.	Management of oral ulcerations includes topical over-the-counter products with benzocaine that help to alleviate painful ulcerations; 0.12% chlorhexidine gluconate mouth rinses; prescription-strength anesthetic and analgesic preparations are also recommended.
White patches or uremic frost	Crystallized or powderlike urea deposits that can be found on the skin or oral mucosa, resulting from excretion of nitrogenous compounds in the sweat; observed in severe uremia	Observed and documented during clinical assessment
Osseous changes of the maxilla and mandible	Loss of lamina dura, demineralized bone characterized as "ground glass" in appearance, and localized radiolucent lesions (central giant cell granulomas) may appear.	Observed and documented during the radiographic survey
Infection or inflammation of the periodontium (periodontal or endodontic abscesses, periodontitis)	Periodontal inflammation may be more severe than for normal biofilm-induced gingivitis. Periodontal attachment loss may result from poor oral hygiene/lack of biofilm removal.	Prevention of acute periodontal infections and/or management of chronic periodontal conditions can be achieved by reducing biofilm levels through optimal oral hygiene care and use of therapeutic antimicrobial mouth rinses; however, an exaggerated inflammatory response associated with alterations in host defense mechanisms may be linked to severe renal disease.
Increase in calculus formation	Dental calculus formation arises from uremic status and duration of renal disease.	Observed and recorded during the extraoral and intraoral clinical assessment. Instruct patient on proper oral hygiene and recommend appropriate OTC dental products.

Adapted from Little JW, Miller CS, Nelson LR. Dental Management of the Medically Compromised Patient. 9th ed. Mosby Elsevier; 2018; Ursula R, Eshenaur Spolarich A, Pwint Han P. A Comprehensive Oral Preventive Care Protocol for Caring for the Renal Transplant Population. Available at: https://jdh.adha.org/content/90/2/88. Accessed June 22, 2022.

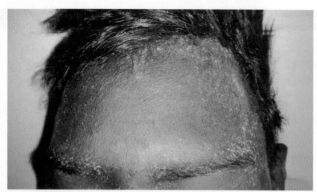

Fig. 54.3 Uremic frost. (From Mathur M, D'Souza AVL, Malhotra V, et al. Uremic frost. *Clin Kidney J.* 2014;7:418.)

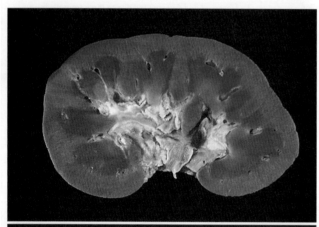

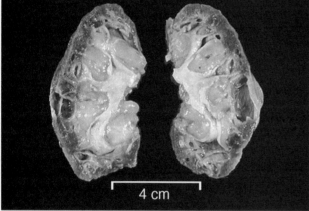

4 cm

Fig. 54.4 Gross renal anatomy. (From Klatt EC. *Robbins and Cotran Atlas of Pathology.* 3rd ed. Saunders; 2015.)

Several systemic factors increase the risk of developing CKD. Adults with diabetes mellitus, high blood pressure, or both have a higher risk of developing CKD than individuals without these diseases. Other contributing risk factors for developing CKD include cardiovascular disease, obesity, a family history of kidney failure, and being age 60 or older.

Patients with CKD may suffer from the following systemic conditions:

- Anemia or a lowered number of erythrocytes (red blood cells), causing fatigue and weakness
- Infections because of a weakened immune system
- Low calcium levels and high phosphorus levels in the blood, causing bone problems

- High potassium levels in the blood (hyperkalemia), causing an irregular heartbeat/pulse
- Loss of appetite or reduction in food intake
- Excess fluids in the body causing high blood pressure, swelling (edema) in the legs, or shortness of breath because of fluid in the lungs (pulmonary edema)
- Depression or lower quality of life
- Premature death, likely due to heart disease and stroke[12]

End-Stage Renal Disease

When the kidneys stop functioning (kidney failure or **end-stage renal disease** [ESRD]), dialysis or a solid organ kidney transplant is needed to sustain one's life. Diabetes mellitus and hypertension are the most prevalent causes of ESRD. Not all patients with kidney disease progress to ESRD but in some patients, kidney disease may progress to ESRD, even with proper treatment.

Dialysis is a treatment method of cleaning and filtering wastes and toxins from the blood when the kidneys lose their function in ESRD. In addition to cleansing wastes from the blood, dialysis:

- Removes salt and extra water to prevent them from building up in the body
- Maintains a safe balance of certain chemicals in the blood, such as potassium, sodium, and bicarbonate
- Helps to control blood pressure
  With ESRD, medical treatment modalities include the following:
- In-center hemodialysis
- Home hemodialysis
- Peritoneal dialysis
- Renal transplantation

Dialysis Treatment Modalities

In **hemodialysis,** the patient's blood (a few ounces at a time) is cleansed with a special filter called an artificial kidney or a dialyzer. A vascular surgeon creates the dialysis access (vascular access, fistula, or graft), usually in the forearm (Fig. 54.5). During each dialysis treatment session, a large intravenous cannula is inserted into the vascular access. Patients are connected to the hemodialysis machine at the vascular access site, and the patient's blood is passed through the dialyzer, filtered, or cleaned, and returned back to the patient (Fig. 54.6). Hemodialysis treatments may be performed in a dialysis center by trained medical personnel (typically three times a week for a prescribed period for each treatment session) or in the home with a special home hemodialysis machine and supplies, where the patient is assisted by family members or friend as a care partner. See Box 54.4.

No dialysis treatment modality is considered medically superior to another; however, the success of treatment is complex and often is geared toward compliance, convenience to the patient, and acceptable clinical outcomes obtained by the treatment modality. For instance, senior citizens living unassisted often are placed at an in-center hemodialysis because of the lack of a treatment partner (often a spouse, caretaker, or friend) to ensure safety in connection with home hemodialysis treatment. Furthermore, although renal transplantation is not a cure for ESRD, it provides a less restricted lifestyle than required with dialysis treatment; therefore many (although not all) patients seek consideration for the National Solid Organ Transplantation Waiting List.

Medical considerations and modifications in the dental hygiene care plan for the patient receiving hemodialysis treatments are as follows:

- Consult with and obtain medical clearance from the nephrologist (a physician who deals with the diagnosis and management of kidney disease) to do the following:
  - Confirm that the patient is medically stable to receive dental treatment.

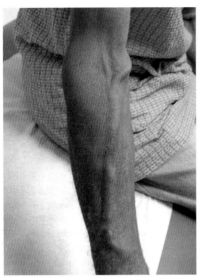

Fig. 54.5 Hemodialysis access (fistula).

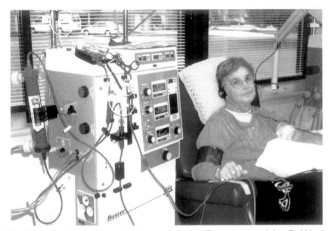

Fig. 54.6 Patient undergoing hemodialysis. (From Ignatavicius D, Workman ML. *Medical-Surgical Nursing: Patient-Centered Collaborative Care.* 6th ed. Saunders; 2010.)

- Determine if antibiotic prophylaxis is indicated to prevent either infection of the dialysis access or infective endocarditis (IE). For patients who do not have known cardiovascular risk factors and/or other comorbidities (e.g., altered host defenses, altered cardiac output and mechanical stresses, and bacterial infection), the American Heart Association Guidelines, confirmed by the 2021 scientific statement, do not include a recommendation for antibiotic prophylaxis prior to invasive dental procedures on patients with intravascular access devices.
- *Do not take blood pressure readings in the dialysis access arm* (this could cause the access to become occluded or infected and may delay or compromise dialysis therapy). Dialysis access is a patient's lifeline and must be protected at all costs.
- Avoid invasive dental treatment on the same day as dialysis treatment because of coagulation complications associated with the use of heparin (blood anticoagulant therapy) administered during dialysis therapy. Additionally, hemodialysis tends to exacerbate bleeding tendencies because it causes physical destruction of platelets. Thus, when a high risk of excessive gingival bleeding is expected, review laboratory screening test results: partial thromboplastin time (aPTT) and platelet count when hemostasis and clot retention are critical.[3]

- Use hemostatic precautions/agents to address coagulation and limit bleeding.

Peritoneal dialysis (PD), like hemodialysis, filters the blood of the person living with ESRD. However, this treatment modality uses the person's own peritoneal lining to filter the blood. A surgeon places a specialized catheter into the person's abdomen, giving access to the peritoneal lining; the patient then uses this catheter to inject a prescribed dialysate solution into the person's peritoneal lining. This fluid contains dextrose, salt, and other minerals dissolved in water. These ingredients create a chemical exchange that allows the patient's waste products and extra body fluid to pass from the patient's blood, through the peritoneal filter, and into the dialysis solution. After a prescribed period of time, the waste-filled solution is drained from the patient's abdomen and immediately replaced with fresh solution, and the dialysis process of filtering the blood begins again.

PD is offered in-center in select dialysis centers but usually is chosen by patients for its flexibility of self-administered, at-home treatment, and its elimination of an intravenous cannula in a vascular access three times per week in exchange for daily dialysis performed through an abdominal catheter. Neither hemodialysis nor peritoneal dialysis is considered medically superior; rather, treatment is prescribed typically based on the patient's needs and abilities and which treatment modality seems to work best for their clinical needs.

The two primary forms of PD are as follows:
- **Continual ambulatory peritoneal dialysis (CAPD):** Dialysate solution is delivered manually to the abdominal catheter for dialysis treatment without the use of a machine. With CAPD, the solution is removed and replaced during prescribed intervals throughout the day by the patient. As the word *ambulatory* suggests, the person can walk around freely while the dialysis process is being performed within the peritoneal cavity. Because no equipment is used in the process, there is no need to use electricity.
- **Continuous cyclic-assisted peritoneal dialysis (CCPD):** Dialysate solution is delivered to the abdominal catheter via a peritoneal dialysis machine. Unlike CAPD, during CCPD, the solution is removed and replaced during the evening/night at prescribed intervals, usually while the patient sleeps. Although it does require electricity to operate, it is convenient because it allows a machine to exchange solutions during sleep and frees up valuable time during the day.

Alterations in the dental hygiene care plan for patients living with PD treatments are as follows:

- Consult with and obtain medical clearance from the patient's nephrologist to accomplish the following:
  - Confirm that the patient is medically stable to receive dental treatment. (Oral healthcare appointments may have to be delayed if heparin was used within the last 24-hour period during PD treatment.)
  - Determine if prophylactic antibiotic premedication is indicated to prevent infection of the PD dialysis access, infective endocarditis, or unless other comorbidities.
- Unless patients have comorbidities or evidence-based conditions that indicate antibiotic treatment per the American Heart Association Guidelines (2021) or the American Academy of Orthopedic Surgeons guidelines, PD patients usually do not require prophylactic antibiotic premedication based on PD status alone. However, cardiovascular complications (the most prevalent cause of mortality) are extremely common within the hemodialysis and PD population. With that in mind, all patients should be evaluated individually for antibiotic prophylaxis based on their risk factors.
- Consider the function of compromised organs and how the malfunction of any organs will affect body systems (e.g., secondary hypertension and diabetes mellitus).

Box 54.5 presents educational resources for kidney transplantation and dialysis patients.

Secondary Medical Conditions

Regardless of the cause or treatment modality chosen, ESRD patients are also prone to secondary diabetes and hypertension that may be complications considered in the process of care. **Secondary medical conditions** are not part of the original etiology of disease but rather a complication developed because of a disease or condition. For instance, although the primary cause of ESRD may be diabetes mellitus owing to a cascade of complications (e.g., fluid retention, anemia), the patient may develop secondary hypertension. Furthermore, a patient living with ESRD with the initial etiology of hypertension also can develop secondary diabetes. In addition to secondary hypertension and secondary diabetes mellitus, secondary anemia, hyperparathyroidism, and malnutrition are serious conditions to manage in persons receiving dialysis therapy.

Cardiovascular disease and inflammation. Persons with renal disease have a greater risk of cardiovascular disease than persons without renal disease. Regardless of the stage of CKD, inflammation plays an important role in clinical outcomes of medical (and also dental) treatment.[13,14]

BOX 54.5   Kidney Transplantation and Dialysis Patient Educational Resources From the National Kidney Foundation

Access information about:

- Kidney transplantation by viewing a video at https://www.kidney.org/atoz/atozTopic_Transplantation
- Hemodialysis and what patients need to know at https://www.kidney.org/sites/default/files/11-50-0214_hemodialysis.pdf
- Hemodialysis by viewing a video at https://www.youtube.com/watch?v=-JgXalRCLV1I*
- Peritoneal dialysis by viewing a video at https://www.youtube.com/watch?v=kBX4bD10MXM*

* Source: National Kidney Foundation. Published on March 27, 2014.

Anemia. With normal, healthy renal function, the kidneys produce the hormone **erythropoietin** (EPO), which stimulates bone marrow to produce red blood cells, essential in delivering oxygen throughout the body. Diseased kidneys fail to make enough EPO, which results in **anemia** (the reduction of the mass of circulating red blood cells) and less oxygen distributed throughout the body.

Anemia is not a disease but rather a symptom of other illnesses. Anemia may be present in the early stages of renal disease and worsens as renal disease progresses. Nearly all people living with end-stage renal failure (less than 10% renal function) have anemia. Additional factors that contribute to anemia in people with ESRD include iron deficiency, shortened red blood cell life span, hypothyroidism, secondary hyperthyroidism, blood loss, and acute and chronic inflammation. Oral manifestations of anemia include pallor of the oral mucosa, glossitis (an early sign of folate or vitamin B_{12} deficiency), recurrent aphthous ulcers, candidiasis, and angular stomatitis (cheilitis). Fatigue and increased risk of infection are common systemic complications of anemia and likely affect a person's ability to perform home oral hygiene. Furthermore, anemia also may contribute to cardiovascular complications.

According to K/DOQI and KDIGO guidelines, persons living with kidney disease are considered anemic when hemoglobin levels are less than 11 g/dL or hematocrit levels fall below 33%. Anemia treatment for those with chronic kidney disease may include a genetically engineered form of the EPO hormone, iron supplements, and/or folate supplements.

Mineral and bone disorder. A serious complication of chronic kidney disease characterized by excessive secretion of parathyroid hormone (PTH) is known as **mineral and bone disorder** (formerly referred to as **secondary hyperparathyroidism**). As renal disease progresses, the kidneys lose their ability to excrete phosphorus from the body and produce the active form of vitamin D necessary in bone metabolism. These changes result in decreased serum calcium. In response, to reestablish balance, increases in PTH result, causing hypercalcemia. This impediment in bone metabolism is recognized for causing greater potential complications and calcifications within the body's vascular system and organs.

Persons with mineral and bone disorders must limit phosphorus intake. In addition, vitamin D supplements and medications known as *phosphorus binders* may be prescribed to reduce absorption of phosphorus. A renal dietitian (available for consultation at almost all in-center dialysis and transplant centers) works with the nephrologist and patient to plan a kidney-friendly diet (see the discussion about nutrition in the following section).

Oral manifestations of mineral and bone disorders may include areas of abnormal calcium leaching from osseous structures and calcium deposits on and in teeth, soft tissues, vasculature, and/or organs. In addition to detecting dental calculus on radiographs, calcium deposits may be detected on panoramic radiographs as calcifications in the carotid arteries. Periapical radiographs may show narrowing or obliteration of the pulp chamber. Other osseous findings include the triad of loss of lamina dura, loss of trabecular pattern (demineralized bone) which assumes a *ground glass* appearance, and expansile radiolucent osseous lesions (central giant cell granulomas, also called brown tumors). Early diagnosis and management of mineral and bone metabolism disorders are essential for positive medical outcomes. Dental radiographs may help screen patients with CKD for calcifications because of their high diagnostic potential.[3,15]

Nutrition

To offset complications associated with CKD, patients typically are prescribed a **renal diet** that restricts fluid and sodium intake (owing to decreased renal output, excess body fluid, and hypertension) and limits dietary phosphorus and potassium. The dental hygienist should collaborate with the patient's renal dietitian when counseling the patient on recommended dental products that may be ingested. The dietitian can provide guidance specially designed for the patient's exact needs. The National Kidney Foundation website (https://www.kidney.org/nutrition) is a valuable resource for accessing a kidney-friendly diet. Diets can vary greatly; however, such factors as the stage of disease, etiology, compliance with medications and dietary restrictions, and comorbidities can affect variations in dietary needs. It is always best to consult with the renal dietitian to develop a plan tailored toward a specific patient's dietary needs.

Fluid restrictions result in reduced salivary flow, which interferes with the cleansing role of saliva. Consequently, patients receiving dialysis treatment and experiencing xerostomia commonly have increased deposits of dental calculus and oral candidiasis. Uremia compounds the dental calculus problem.

Because dialysis treatment removes varying amounts of protein during the procedure, dialysis patients routinely have their albumin levels measured and monitored. Albumin is a laboratory test that is an excellent indicator of protein intake. Dietary allowances for dialysis patients may be higher in protein to compensate for protein loss, aid in tissue healing, and avoid infection. Patients who have CKD stages 1 through 4 are typically on lower amounts of protein. After organ transplantation, patients often return to normal dietary intake of protein.

Salivary pH and Xerostomia

As kidney disease progresses, nitrogenous materials accumulate in the body, producing a condition known as **uremia**, thus altering the pH of blood and saliva. Whether uremia is a protective factor or a risk factor for dental caries remains unclear. Nevertheless, an increased risk of caries in this population can be correlated to poor oral hygiene, reduced saliva production, drug therapy or parotid infection causing dry mouth, other debilitating conditions and diseases, and/or an increase in the number of cariogenic bacteria. Moreover, when reduced caries prevalence was reported in ESRD patients, it was likely attributed to the protective effect of metabolism of urea in saliva, inhibiting bacterial growth and neutralizing bacterial acids.[16,17]

Also, nearly 50% of adults with CKD/ESRD suffer from dry mouth (xerostomia), which is possibly caused by restriction in fluid intake; adverse effects of drug therapy (primarily antihypertensive medications); salivary gland hypofunction causing a low salivary flow rate; and mouth breathing secondary to lung perfusion problems (reduced blood flow to the lungs).[18,19]

From a care plan perspective, dental professionals can recommend the following oral hygiene products, prescription drugs, salivary stimulants, and other alternative therapies that can alleviate dry mouth:
- Gustatory (taste) stimulation (sugar-free candies)
- Mechanical stimulation (power toothbrush, xylitol-containing chewing gum or lozenges)
- Food such as apples, carrots, celery, etc.
- Pharmacologic stimulation (drugs that require a prescription such as pilocarpine HCl or cevimeline HCl)
- Over-the-counter salivary substitutes
- Chewing on ice chips
- Sleeping with a humidifier to aid in moisturizing the oral and nasopharyngeal passages.[20,21]

Again, the dental hygienist should consult with the renal dietitian to be sure that all oral self-care recommendations and products are within the patient's prescribed renal diet and medical treatment plan.

Periodontal Disease

At best, a moderate relationship exists between periodontal disease and renal insufficiency.[6] The risk for periodontal disease appears to be significantly increased in individuals with severe renal disease or in

---

> ## BOX 54.6 Critical Thinking Scenario C
>
> *Patient:* Mrs. T. is a 60-year-old retired public school teacher with end-stage renal disease. She is on in-center hemodialysis; however, she desires a less-restrictive lifestyle without dialysis.
>
> *Chief Complaint:* "I would like to get on the waiting list for a new kidney, but I've been told by my dialysis center that I need a dental clearance first."
>
> *Social History:* Mrs. T. has been on in-center hemodialysis for 3 years. She has a low energy level but does have a daughter and grandchildren who live next door and help her when necessary.
>
> *Dental History:* Mrs. T. has a history of regular dental visits before she started dialysis but has not had a professional oral debridement since she started dialysis 3 years ago. Her oral hygiene is poor and her gingival tissue bleeds easily upon homecare. Oral assessment findings reveal heavy supragingival oral biofilm and dental calculus deposits generalized throughout the mouth, spontaneous gingival bleeding, candidiasis, and a uremic mouth odor. Dental examination does not reveal active carious lesions.
>
> *Oral Self-Care Assessment:* Poor oral hygiene, xerostomia, use of a manual toothbrush once daily, with no interdental or tongue cleaning.
>
> *Supplemental Notes:* Mrs. T. wants to be listed on the organ transplant waiting list.
>
> 1. What are the primary concerns for this patient?
> 2. If the patient receives an organ transplant, what are the long-term concerns?
> 3. Develop a dental hygiene care plan including an appointment schedule for this patient that includes the dental hygiene diagnoses and patient goals.
> 4. Develop a treatment plan that accommodates a Monday-Wednesday-Friday (afternoons) in-center dialysis schedule.
> 5. What factors may be contributing to this patient's xerostomia and candidiasis? What interventions can be suggested?
> 6. Identify special precautions and/or care plan modifications for safe, high-quality care.

those patients receiving hemodialysis. The reasons for this risk include increased levels of calculus formation on teeth, patients' noncompliance or improper oral hygiene procedures, and exaggerated inflammatory response associated with alterations in host defense mechanisms. Secondary hyperthyroidism may contribute to accelerated bone loss in the presence of periodontal disease. Although individuals with successful kidney transplants may not be more susceptible to periodontal disease compared to the general population, frequent 3- to 4-month continued-care interval appointments are recommended.[20] See Box 54.6 for a Critical Thinking Scenario and Box 54.7 for a discussion of legal, ethical, and safety issues.

Interprofessional Collaboration

The **nephrology team** usually includes the following members:
- Nephrologist
- Nephrology nurse
- Renal dietitian
- Nephrology social worker
- Patient care technician
- Pretransplant and posttransplant coordinators

In the pretransplant phase, the dental hygienist likely communicates solely with the pretransplant coordinator on the renal transplant team. In most instances, this is a registered nurse or physician's assistant. The pretransplant coordinator is responsible for coordinating all required preoperative appointments for the transplant candidate.

In the posttransplant phase, the patient receives care at a transplant center or returns to a primary healthcare provider if a transplant center is not located nearby. The dental hygienist should consult with the patient's current healthcare provider to determine the patient's medical stability and precautions during dental hygiene care.

BOX 54.7 Legal, Ethical, and Safety Issues

- Medical consultation is required to evaluate the patient's medical stability, use of medications, and necessary precautions before invasive dental treatment.
- Document results from the medical consultation, including medical provider's recommendations and conversation with the patient or caregiver.
- Obtain and document informed consent from all patients.
- Involve the patient in the decision-making process.
- Apply evidence-based information when developing the dental hygiene care plan.
- Treat patients with dignity, respect, and empathy.
- Provide oral and written instructions that can be read easily by patients who may have impaired eyesight or hearing.
- Provide definitive instructions and interventions to prevent dental caries, periodontal disease, soft-tissue infection, xerostomia, and fungal infections.

A reliable bridge to transplantation does not yet exist for liver, heart, and lung transplant candidates. Therefore, they are often in more critical condition and treated in a hospital setting. In this situation, oral healthcare providers consult directly with the patient's medical specialist.

KEY CONCEPTS

- Patients awaiting solid organ transplantation outnumber the actual number of transplants performed each year.
- The most common pre–solid organ transplant recipient is a patient living with end-stage renal disease who is most likely receiving dialysis therapy.
- When assessing a patient who is on renal dialysis, do not take blood pressure readings in the dialysis access arm because doing so could cause the access to become occluded or infected.
- Avoid dental treatment if and when dialysis treatment is performed on the same day because of coagulation complications associated with the use of heparin (blood anticoagulant therapy) administered during dialysis therapy.
- When treating patients on dialysis, consult with and obtain clearance from the nephrologist to confirm that the patient is medically stable to receive dental treatment and to determine whether prophylactic antibiotic premedication is indicated to prevent either infection of the dialysis access or infective endocarditis.
- Among solid organ transplant centers, K/DOQI, or KDIGO, there is no one standard pretransplant or posttransplant dental care protocol. Because of extreme variations in medical conditions and other variables, professional oral healthcare must be tailored to each individual patient.
- The need for antibiotic prophylaxis for invasive dental procedures in patients who have undergone solid organ transplants remains controversial. Patients should be evaluated on an individual basis.
- The K/DOQI and the KDIGO are globally recognized guidelines that address care for medical issues for all stages and aspects of renal disease.
- In persons with mineral and bone disorder, calcium deposits may be visible on panoramic radiographs as calcifications in the carotid arteries, on periapical radiographs as narrowing of the pulp chamber or abnormal calcifications in soft tissues, or as a radiolucent osseous lesion (known as a *brown tumor*). Other radiographic manifestations include loss of the lamina dura, loss of trabecular pattern, and bone density changes.
- Good oral health and effective daily oral biofilm control are important for minimizing the risk of self-induced bacteremias.
- Thorough oral cancer screenings should be performed on a frequent basis.
- The dental hygienist should consult with the patient's renal dietitian to be sure that all oral self-care recommendations and products are within the patient's prescribed renal diet and medical treatment plan.

ACKNOWLEDGMENT

The author acknowledges Cheryl Thomas for her past contributions to this chapter.

REFERENCES

1. The living donation process. U.S. Department of Health & Human Services. Last Reviewed April 2021. https://organdonor.gov/about/process/living-donation.html. Accessed June 18, 2022.
2. 5 keys to a successful organ transplant program. HealthLeaders Media. Published June 2, 2016. http://www.healthleadersmedia.com/leadership/5-keys-successful-organ-transplant-program#. Accessed June 18, 2022.
3. Little JW, Miller CS, Nelson LR. *Dental Management of the Medically Compromised Patient*. 9th ed. Mosby Elsevier; 2018.
4. Dental management of the organ or stem cell transplant patient. National Institute of Dental and Craniofacial Research. Published July 2016. https://catalog.nidcr.nih.gov/catalog/dental-management-organ-or-stem-cell-transplant-patient. Accessed July 5, 2022.
5. Nappalli D, Lingappa A. Oral manifestations in transplant patients. *Dent Res J (Isfahan)*. 2015;12(3):199–208. Available at: https://www-ncbi-nlm-nih-gov.p.atsu.edu/pmc/articles/PMC4432601/.
6. Danovitch GM. *Handbook of Kidney Transplantation*. 6th ed. Wolters Kluwer; 2017.
7. Transplant trends. United Network for Organ Sharing. https://unos.org/data/transplant-trends/#transplants_by_organ_type+year+2017. Accessed June 20, 2022.
8. NKF-KDOQI guidelines. National Kidney Foundation. https://www.kidney.org/professionals/guidelines/guidelines. Accessed June 22, 2022.
9. We're on a mission. KDIGO. https://kdigo.org/mission/. Accessed June 22, 2022.
10. How your kidneys work. National Kidney Foundation. http://www.kidney.org/kidneydisease/howkidneyswrk.cfm. Accessed June 22, 2022.
11. Ursula R, Eshenaur Spolarich A, Pwint Han P. A comprehensive oral preventive care protocol for caring for the renal transplant population. *J Dent Hyg*. 2016;90(2):88–99. https://jdh.adha.org/content/jdenthyg/90/2/88.full.pdf.
12. *National Chronic Kidney Disease Fact Sheet*. U.S. Department of Health and Human Services, Centers for Disease Control and Prevention; 2017. https://www.cdc.gov/diabetes/pubs/pdf/kidney_factsheet.pdf. Accessed June 22, 2022.
13. Jankowski J, Floege J, Fliser D, Böhm M, Marx N. Cardiovascular disease in chronic kidney disease. *Circ J*. 2021;143(11):1157–1172. https://www.ncbi.nlm.nih.gov/pmc/articles/PMC7969169/.
14. Kumar S, Bogle R, Banerjee D. Why do young people with chronic kidney disease die early? *World J Nephrol*. 2014;3(4):143–155. https://doi.org/10.5527/wjn.v3.i4.143.
15. Parthiban J, Aarthi Nisha V, Asokan GS, et al. Oral manifestations in a renal osteodystrophy patient – a case report with review of literature. *J Clin Diagn Res*. 2014;8(8):ZD28–ZD30. https://doi.org/10.7860/JCDR/2014/8879.4722.
16. Ruospo M, Palmer SC, Jonathan JC, et al. Prevalence and severity of oral disease in adults with chronic kidney disease: a systematic review of observational studies. *Nephrol Dial Transplant*. 2014;29(2):364–375. https://doi.org/10.1093/ndt/gft401.
17. Kaushik A, Reddy SS, Umesh L, et al. Oral and salivary changes among renal patients undergoing hemodialysis: a cross-sectional study. *Indian J Nephrol*. 2013;23(2):125–129. https://doi.org/10.4103/0971-4065.109421.
18. Honarmand M, Farhad-Mollashahi L, Nakhaee A, et al. Oral manifestation and salivary changes in renal patients undergoing hemodialysis. *J Clin Exp Dent*. 2017;9(2). https://doi.org/10.4317/jced.53215. e207–e210.
19. Gupta M, Gupta M, Abhishek. Oral conditions in renal disorders and treatment considerations – a review for pediatric dentist. *Saudi Dent J*. 2015;27(3):113–119. https://www.ncbi.nlm.nih.gov/pmc/articles/PMC4501439/.
20. DeLong L, Burkhart N. *General and Oral Pathology for the Dental Hygienist*. 3rd ed. Lippincott Williams & Wilkins; 2019.
21. Nappalli D, Lingappa A. Oral manifestations in transplant patients. *Dent Res J (Isfahan)*. 2015;12(3):199–208. https://www.ncbi.nlm.nih.gov/pmc/articles/PMC4432601/.

55

Respiratory Diseases

Sarah Ostrander and Curtis Aumiller

PROFESSIONAL OPPORTUNITIES

Becoming knowledgeable about respiratory diseases will help the dental hygienist properly develop and adapt dental hygiene treatment plans and promote oral health for patient safety. Knowledge of respiratory conditions, treatment regimens, and prevention will enhance the role of the dental hygienist in all practice settings, particularly for elderly, infirm, or intubated patients. Knowledge of sleep-related breathing disorders will enrich the interprofessional role of the dental hygienist in the treatment of these disorders.

COMPETENCIES

1. Discuss the etiology, risk factors, signs and symptoms, and related medications associated with asthma and chronic obstructive pulmonary disease (COPD) as they relate to the process of dental hygiene care. Develop a dental hygiene care plan applicable to a person with either asthma or COPD, addressing adaptations needed for the specific respiratory disease.
2. Discuss the etiology, risk factors, signs and symptoms, and related medications of tuberculosis as they relate to the process of dental hygiene care. Develop a dental hygiene care plan applicable to a person with tuberculosis, addressing adaptations needed for the disease.
3. Discuss the etiology and types of pneumonia as they relate to the process of dental hygiene care. Develop a dental hygiene care plan applicable to a person with pneumonia, and relate the role of a dental hygienist to caring for the infirmed or intubated patient, as well as educate other healthcare providers involved in oral care to prevent pneumonia.
4. Apply knowledge of sleep-related breathing disorders to assessment, care planning, and treatment implementation by dental hygienists and other oral healthcare providers.

INTRODUCTION

Respiratory diseases are common among the general population and can compromise dental and dental hygiene care. To properly manage this group of patients, it is important for dental hygienists to understand respiratory diseases, medications used in their treatment, their link with periodontal health and oral hygiene, and their implications for dental hygiene care.

The most frequently encountered respiratory diseases are asthma and chronic obstructive pulmonary disease (COPD). In addition, tuberculosis, a disease that has affected humankind for centuries, continues to be a worldwide problem. The incidence of multidrug-resistant strains of tuberculosis continues to pose infection control and treatment challenges to healthcare providers.[1] The unknown long-term

effects of SARS-CoV-2 (COVID-19) may also present a new challenge to the dental professional as new drug therapies and new discoveries regarding long COVID emerge in the coming years.

Dental professionals who treat patients in long-term care facilities must be educated about the proper oral care of intubated/tracheostomy and infirmed patients and its critical role in preventing pneumonia. As dental professionals engage in interdisciplinary roles with medical professionals, dental hygienists should be knowledgeable about implications for assessment and dental hygiene care of patients with sleep-related breathing disorders (Box 55.1).

RESPIRATORY DISEASES

Asthma

Asthma is a chronic inflammatory respiratory disease characterized by an increased responsiveness of the bronchial airways to various stimuli. Management of the asthma patient depends on assessment of the individual's severity level, degree of control, and responsiveness to treatment. Asthma severity is classified as intermittent or persistent (mild, moderate, or severe) based on current impairment of quality of life and risk for future exacerbations and/or lung damage. These classifications are determined by clinical tests as well as the occurrence of airflow obstruction symptoms in relation to environmental factors, exercise, and nighttime sleep disturbances.[2]

Etiology

Various substances or environmental factors can precipitate an asthma attack, including specific antigens such as pollen, ragweed, molds, foods, dyes, flavorings, latex, cockroaches, and house dust mites. Chemical irritants such as smoke (from tobacco or burning wood and/or grass), scents, and house sprays may trigger an asthma attack. Other nonallergic stimulators—respiratory infections, environmental pollutants and irritants, exercise, cold air, and emotional stress—also can cause an attack. Generalized narrowing of bronchi and bronchioles caused by mucosal inflammation, increased secretions, and smooth muscle contraction produces asthmatic symptoms (Fig. 55.1).[3,4]

Signs and Symptoms

Clinical manifestations of asthma include periodic wheezing, **dyspnea** (difficulty in breathing), coughing, and chest tightness. These and other signs and symptoms are listed in Box 55.2. The onset of an asthma attack usually begins with mild wheezing and coughing, progressing to increased difficulty in breathing. As the attack develops, the individual may experience a sense of pressure or tightness in the chest and a feeling of suffocation. Blood pressure and heart rate may increase slightly during an attack.[3] A severe asthma attack that does not respond to treatment with an adequate dose of commonly used bronchodilators is referred to as **status asthmaticus**. This condition may produce bronchospasms for hours or days without remission, often requiring hospitalization, and it can lead to death.

Implications for Dental Hygiene Care

To prevent an acute asthmatic attack and to address the unique needs of the asthmatic patient, the dental hygienist does the following:

BOX 55.1 **Patient or Client Education Tips**

Patients With Respiratory Diseases
Asthma
- Explain that rinsing the mouth with water and expectorating after using an inhaled corticosteroid decreases the risk of oral candidiasis and dental caries.
- Explain that if the patient experiences xerostomia and/or an unpleasant taste after inhalant therapy, the use of xylitol-containing chewing gum or mints will increase salivary flow, minimizing the risks of dental caries and gingivitis.

COPD
- Proper management of dental hygiene care for patients with COPD will help prevent an exacerbation during treatment.

Tuberculosis
- Patients with active tuberculosis should delay elective dental treatment but when necessary, should be treated in a hospital setting to minimize risk of disease transmission to personnel or other patients.

COPD, Chronic obstructive pulmonary disease.

- Assesses the frequency, conditions and time of onset, and type—intermittent or persistent (mild, moderate, or severe)—of asthmatic attacks experienced; their management, including the type of medication used and precipitating factors; and whether a previous attack has warranted emergency treatment.[3]
- Seeks a medical consultation in cases of persistent severe asthma or when reported symptoms suggest poorly controlled asthma. Documents if the patient is taking systemic corticosteroids, such as prednisone, for chronic asthma. Ensures compliance with the usual

---

BOX 55.2 **Signs and Symptoms of an Acute Asthmatic Attack**

- Wheezing
- Cough
- Nasal flaring
- Dyspnea
- Feeling of pressure or tightness in the chest
- Need to stand, sit upright, or lean forward
- Increased anxiety and apprehension
- Perspiration
- Respiratory rate of more than 30 rpm
- Increased pulse rate of more than 120 bpm
- Rise in blood pressure (particularly in severe attacks)
- Confusion
- Agitation
- Cyanosis

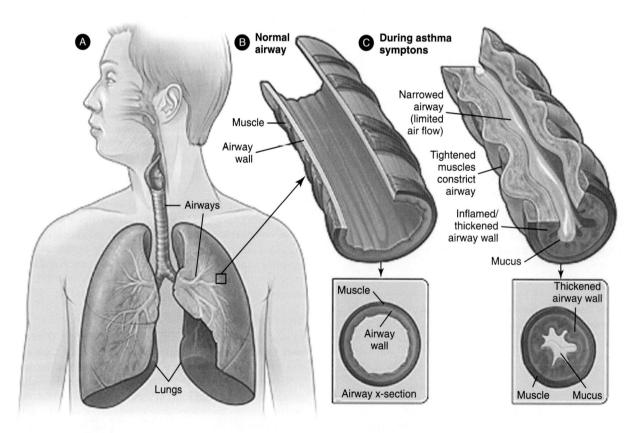

Fig. 55.1 (A) The location of the lungs and airways in the body. (B) A cross section of a normal airway. (C) A cross section of an airway during asthma symptoms. (From National Heart, Lung, and Blood Institute; National Institutes of Health; U.S. Department of Health and Human Services.)

regular dose of prednisone on the day of a particularly stressful dental appointment.
- Notes the precipitating factors (including allergies) reported by the patient and avoids these factors during professional care.
- Instructs patients to bring the medical inhalers prescribed by the physician to every appointment for use in case of an acute attack or prophylactically when chronic moderate to severe disease is present.

- Notes that some medications used by patients with asthma cause xerostomia (dry mouth) and unpleasant taste sensation after inhalation use. Consequently, the patient with asthma may be more prone to dental caries and gingivitis. Children in particular may increase their sucrose intake to combat the unpleasant taste from the inhalant. Table 55.1 describes drugs commonly used in the treatment of asthma and other respiratory conditions.

TABLE 55.1 Drugs Commonly Used in the Treatment of Respiratory Diseases

Action	Indication	Generic Name (Brand Name)	Drug Classification	Adverse Reactions and Dental Drug Implications
Antiinflammatory agents	Inhibit release by inflammatory cells of agents that trigger asthma; taken on a daily basis to achieve and maintain control of asthma	Beclomethasone dipropionate (Beclovent) Fluticasone (Flovent, Flonase, Arnuity Elipta)	Inhaled synthetic corticosteroids	Cough, hoarseness; oral candidiasis, unpleasant taste, xerostomia
Antiinflammatory agents	Used to speed resolution of airway obstruction and reduce rate of recurrence of symptoms of chronic obstructive pulmonary disease (COPD)	Methylprednisolone, prednisolone (Deltasone, Meticorten) Budesonide (Pulmicort, Rhinocort)	Systemic (oral) corticosteroids	Hyperglycemia, osteoporosis, fluid retention Suppresses adrenal gland; slower healing, infection more likely, symptoms may be masked
Bronchodilators (Beta₂-Adrenergic)	Temporarily dilate or relax the muscles surrounding the bronchial tubes that tighten during an asthma attack	Albuterol (Ventolin, Proventil) Levalbuterol (Xopenex)	Short-acting inhaled beta₂-adrenergic agonists	Nervousness, xerostomia, throat irritation, fast or irregular heartbeat
Bronchodilators (Beta₂-Adrenergic)	Relax bronchial smooth muscles and inhibit release of mast cell inhibitors in COPD patients	Arformoterol Olodaterol (Striverdi Respimat) Salmeterol (Serevent Diskus)	Long-acting beta₂-adrenergic agonists	Nervousness, xerostomia, throat irritation, fast or irregular heartbeat
Anticholinergics and Antimuscarinic	Provide maintenance regulation of airway smooth muscle tone; may be used instead of beta₂-adrenergic agonists when not well tolerated by patient. Used primarily in COPD patients	Ipratropium bromide (Atrovent) Tiotropium bromide (Spiriva) Aclidinium bromide (Tudorza Pressair) Umeclidinium (Incruse Elipta)	Anticholinergic, long-acting bronchodilator	Nervousness, xerostomia, headache, cough
Oral sustained-release tablet or capsule	Used as adjunct to inhaled corticosteroids for prevention of nighttime symptoms; relaxes smooth muscles of respiratory system in COPD patients.	Theophylline (Theo-Dur, Slo-Bid)	Methylxanthine	Gastric reflux, headache, tachycardia, insomnia, nausea, trembling, nervousness Erythromycin may increase levels of theophylline
Nonsteroidal preventive therapy (leukotriene modifiers)	Long-term control and prevention of symptoms in cases of mild persistent asthma in those 12 years of age or older	Zafirlukast Zileuton Montelukast (Singulair)	Selective leukotriene receptor antagonist	Nausea, central nervous system depression, increase in liver function test results, myalgia, headache Erythromycin lowers zafirlukast levels; aspirin raises zafirlukast levels
Combined Medications				
Antiinflammatory agents and bronchodilator	Indicated for use in asthma patients	Fluticasone and salmeterol (Advair) Mometasone furoate and formoterol (Dulera) Fluticasone and Vilanterol (Breo Elipta)		Same possible side effects as each drug individually
Antiinflammatory agents and bronchodilator	Indicated for use in COPD patients	Budesonide and formoterol (Symbicort)		
Anticholinergic and long-acting beta₂-agonist	Indicated for use in COPD patients	Umeclidinium and vilanterol (Anoro Elipta) Tiotropium bromide and olodaterol (Stiolto Respimat)		Same possible side effects as each drug individually
Bronchodilators	Indicated for use in COPD patients	Albuterol and ipratropium bromide (Combivent)		Same possible side effects as each drug individually

Data from Centerwatch.com. Available at: https://www.centerwatch.com/directories/1067-fda-approved-drugs/topic/109-pulmonary-respiratory-diseases.

TABLE 55.2   Drugs That Are Contraindicated or Used Cautiously for the Individual With Asthma

Drugs	Rationale
Aspirin-containing medications	Ingestion of aspirin is associated with precipitating attacks in some patients
Nonsteroidal antiinflammatory drugs (NSAIDs)	Ingestion of NSAIDs may precipitate asthma attack in some individuals
Barbiturates and narcotics	Association of these drugs with precipitation of asthma attacks
Erythromycin and ciprofloxacin in patients taking theophylline	May result in toxic blood level of theophylline

TABLE 55.3   Techniques to Be Avoided or Used Cautiously in Individuals With Certain Respiratory Diseases

Disease	Techniques Contraindicated or Used With Precautions	Rationale
Asthma	Use of air polisher (contraindicated with poorly controlled asthma) Use of power-driven polisher (use cautiously)	Aerosols created by air polisher may precipitate asthma attack Polisher may exacerbate existing breathing problems
Chronic obstructive pulmonary disease	Avoid use of dental dam Use of power-driven polisher (use cautiously) Nitrous oxide–oxygen analgesia (contraindicated)	Dental dam may cause more breathing difficulties Polisher may exacerbate existing breathing problems May produce cessation of respiration (apnea) if levels are too high
Clinically active tuberculosis	No treatment is provided on an outpatient basis for patients with active tuberculosis	Risk of transmission requires isolation room with special administrative, environmental, and respiratory controls

- Instructs the patient to avoid drugs listed in Table 55.2 such as aspirin-containing medications, nonsteroidal antiinflammatory drugs, barbiturates, and narcotics because they can precipitate an attack.
- Uses preprocedural antimicrobial rinse and high-speed suction to reduce contaminated dental aerosols that may be inhaled when using an ultrasonic scaler or any aerosol-producing equipment. Note: All patients should receive a preprocedural antimicrobial rinse prior to treatment.
- Considers using a local anesthetic agent without epinephrine or levonordefrin because some patients with asthma are sensitive to the sulfite preservatives present in these anesthetic solutions.[3]
- Conveys a calm, caring, and compassionate attitude to relax the patient, making the oral care environment as stress-free as possible because anxiety can induce an asthmatic attack in many people, particularly children.
- Uses nitrous oxide-oxygen analgesia and/or small doses of diazepam, as prescribed by the dentist, to reduce stress if indicated (see Chapter 44).[3]
- Evaluates children carefully for malocclusion; many children with asthma are mouth breathers, and a correlation has been observed between higher palatal vaults, greater overjets, posterior crossbite incidence, and mouth breathing in children.[5]
- Observes any asthmatic symptoms during and after dental procedures because decreased lung function can be triggered by anxiety, supine positioning, tooth enamel dust, and aerosols commonly created by dental procedures (Table 55.3).
- Takes prompt action to manage symptoms of an acute asthmatic episode (Procedure 55.1).[3]
- Sets goals with the patient to achieve meticulous self-care and optimal fluoride benefits to combat negative effects of medication and mouth breathing on oral health.
- Considers the legal, ethical, and safety issues associated with asthma as listed in Box 55.3; see Box 55.4.

Chronic Obstructive Pulmonary Disease

Chronic obstructive pulmonary disease (COPD) as defined by the Global Initiative for Chronic Obstructive Lung Disease is "a

PROCEDURE 55.1   Management of Acute Asthma

1. Recognize symptoms.
2. Terminate the dental procedure and remove all materials from the patient's mouth immediately.
3. Activate office emergency protocol.
4. Place the patient in a comfortable position as soon as signs are apparent—usually sitting upright—while trying to calm patient and allay apprehension.
5. Assess ABCs (airway, breathing, circulation) and perform basic life support as needed.
6. Provide definitive care:
   a. Administer bronchodilator (patient's prescribed medication preferred).
   b. If attack persists, administer oxygen.
   c. Call for emergency assistance if bronchodilators fail to resolve bronchospasm.
   d. Administration of parenteral drugs (epinephrine) by dentist if necessary (available in preloaded syringe).
7. Continue dental care or discharge of the patient: alone, escorted, or with emergency personnel, depending on severity of attack.

Adapted from *Malamed SF. Medical Emergencies in the Dental Office.* 7th ed. Elsevier; 2015.

common, preventable and treatable disease that is characterized by persistent respiratory symptoms and airflow limitation that is due to airway and/or alveolar abnormalities usually caused by significant exposure to noxious particles or gases."[6] COPD, a leading cause of death and chronic disease worldwide, often is associated with periods of acute exacerbations of symptoms. Often, COPD can be directly related to tobacco smoking; however, in some cases outdoor, indoor, and occupational air pollution can be identified as major risk factors. Because many individuals often experience other significant nonpulmonary conditions (weight loss, musculoskeletal disease, cardiovascular disease, osteoporosis, anemia, metabolic syndrome, and diabetes) associated with COPD, the severity of the disease may be affected.[6]

BOX 55.3 Legal, Ethical, and Safety Issues

Clients With Asthma, COPD, and Other Respiratory Diseases

- It is critical for dental hygienists to properly assess patients' history of asthma. Proper documentation of asthma attack triggers, severity, medications, and past treatment will help prevent an asthmatic episode during treatment.
- Acute asthma attacks may occur before, during, and after dental procedures. Dental hygienists must be knowledgeable in the management of such an attack. Avoidance of precipitating factors is the best risk management strategy.
- Patients reporting a history of asthma must have their bronchodilators at each dental appointment for immediate administration if necessary.
- Proper management of dental hygiene care for patients with COPD will help prevent an exacerbation during treatment.
- Patients with active tuberculosis should defer elective dental treatment but when necessary should be treated in a hospital setting to minimize risk of disease transmission to personnel or other patients.
- To prevent nosocomial pneumonia, hospitals and long-term healthcare facilities should make oral care a priority and provide in-service programs to properly educate staff members.

COPD, Chronic obstructive pulmonary disease.

BOX 55.4 Critical Thinking Exercise A

Asthma Patient

Patient: Mr. G.

Profile: A 5 ft., 10 in., 18-year-old White male weighing 175 lb, presents for dental hygiene care.

Chief Complaint: "My gums bleed, particularly around my upper front teeth, and I have a dry mouth most of the time, which is very uncomfortable."

Health History: Patient's vital signs: blood pressure: 112/64 mm Hg, pulse rate: 70 bpm, and respiration rate: 14 rpm. Patient reports history of asthma for past 10 years, exacerbated by exposure to cats, pollens, and dust. He currently sees a physician for acne and is being treated with doxycycline 100 mg daily as well as Proventil 90 mcg aerosol inhaler (two puffs as needed for asthma attack).

Dental History: Suspected carious lesions on occlusal surfaces of teeth 2, 3, 15, and 31.

Gingival evaluation reveals slight gingival enlargement and rolled margins throughout with moderately enlarged, erythematous gingiva and bulbous papillae in the maxillary anterior facial region. Pocket depths 3 mm or less throughout, except in maxillary anterior and posterior molar regions, where some 4- to 5-mm pockets are noted.

Oral Health Behavior Assessment: Patient brushes twice daily but does not floss. Moderate biofilm is noted throughout on the gingival third of teeth and interproximal surfaces.

Supplemental Notes: He smokes one pack of cigarettes per week.

1. What are the dental hygiene diagnoses for this patient?
2. Develop a dental hygiene care plan for this patient that includes goals and interventions.
3. What patient education issues should be addressed?
4. What factors could be affecting this patient's periodontal health?
5. Are there any contraindications to this patient's care?
6. What measures should be taken during treatment to prevent an asthmatic attack?

The characteristic airflow limitation of COPD is the result of a combination of small airway diseases. While multiple disorders can cause COPD, historically the primary causes have been chronic bronchitis and emphysema.[6] **Emphysema** has become a pathologic term to describe the overinflation, called hyperinflation, of lungs and irreversible destruction of structures in the lungs known as **alveoli** or air sacs. This overinflation is caused by a breakdown of the walls of the alveoli, resulting in decreased respiratory function and often dyspnea.[6] Emphysema describes just one of the structural irregularities characterized by COPD. More prevalent among older males emphysema is rapidly increasing among females primarily because of tobacco use.[6] Although chronic bronchitis and emphysema can be described individually, they often coexist and represent the irreversible progression of the disease. Because of the progressive nature of COPD, quality of life is compromised greatly in severe cases.[6]

Bronchitis is an inflammation of the lining of the bronchial tubes. These tubes or bronchi connecting the trachea with the lungs become inflamed and/or infected. As a result, less air is able to flow to and from the lungs, and heavy mucus or phlegm is expectorated.[6] **Chronic bronchitis** is associated with the presence of a mucus-producing cough with expectoration for at least 3 months of the year for more than 2 consecutive years, without other underlying disease to explain the cough.[7] Smokers may dismiss symptoms of chronic bronchitis as a "smoker's cough" and avoid medical care. Consequently, the individual may be in danger of developing serious respiratory problems or heart failure. Chronic bronchitis is consistently more prevalent in females than in males and can affect people of all ages but is usually higher in those more than 45 years old.[8] With **spirometry** (common pulmonary test used to measure lung function), COPD can be classified into four levels: stage I, mild; stage II, moderate; stage III, severe; and stage IV, very severe.[6]

Etiology of COPD

Cigarette smoking has been identified as the major risk factor in COPD. Air pollutants and industrial dust and fumes may contribute to COPD.[7,8] In some parts of the world, air pollutants may be a primary risk factor for COPD.[6] Underlying respiratory disease, severe respiratory infection in early childhood, underdeveloped lungs (during gestation and childhood), and genetic tendencies can be risk factors for COPD.[6]

Emphysema also can have a genetic predisposition known as alpha-1 antitrypsin deficiency or what is commonly called alpha-1.[9] Alpha-1 occurs in about 1 of every 50 cases of emphysema. **Alpha-1 antitrypsin** is a blood protein produced in the liver that helps to protect the lungs from the enzyme elastase. Elastase is found in white blood cells (WBCs) and helps to kill invading bacteria and neutralize small particles that are inhaled into the lungs. When WBCs are destroyed, the elastase is released into the bloodstream. Alpha-1 antitrypsin inactivates the elastase so that it can be excreted by the body. However, if an individual has low alpha-1 antitrypsin levels, the elastase attacks and destroys the elastic tissues of the lungs, which leads to emphysema. Alpha-1 antitrypsin deficiency can be diagnosed with a blood test, and many patients do not have any other predisposing factors that would lead to such severe emphysema.[7]

Signs and Symptoms of Chronic Obstructive Pulmonary Disease

Chronic bronchitis symptoms appear gradually but intensify in individuals who smoke or when atmospheric concentrations of sulfur dioxide and other air pollutants increase. A cough producing large amounts of sputum may linger for several weeks after a winter cold seems to be cured. With time, upper respiratory infections become more serious, and coughing and expectoration of phlegm continue for longer periods after each episode.[8] Dyspnea (difficulty breathing) initially is mild and is brought on only by exercise or exertion. Eventually, breathing difficulty becomes more frequent and is brought on with less

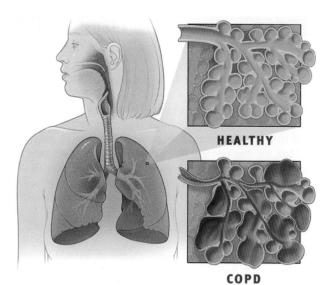

Fig. 55.2 Comparing healthy lungs and lungs with chronic obstructive pulmonary disease (COPD). The elasticity of airways and sacs in healthy lungs allows air to move quickly in and out of lungs. The airways and sacs in lungs with COPD lack the elasticity to allow lungs to retain their original shape. These airways lack support and become enlarged and lined with mucus, thereby making breathing more difficult. (From NHLBI Health Information Center. Available at: https://www.nhlbi.nih.gov/health/copd.)

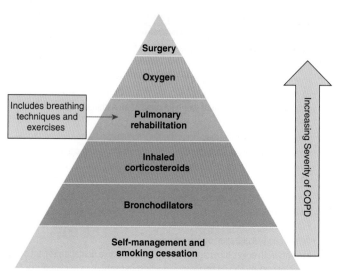

Fig. 55.3 Chronic obstructive pulmonary disease (COPD) is a progressive disease but with early diagnosis, may progress slowly. Providers must monitor COPD clients carefully, ensuring that treatment is appropriate for the level of disease. Self-management and smoking cessation are foundational in COPD management. (Adapted from NHLBI Health Information Center. Available at: https://www.nhlbi.nih.gov/health/copd.)

effort. At this point, other symptoms of respiratory failure are evident.[3] As the disease progresses and becomes more obstructive, there may be evidence of prolonged expiration and wheezing. Acute attacks of breathing distress with rapid, labored breathing, intensive coughing, and bluish skin can occur; hence, the term **blue bloater** has been used to describe an individual with these signs.[7] As seen in Fig. 55.2, COPD damages the airways and sacs in the lungs by reducing their elasticity, thereby making breathing more difficult.

Emphysema can be localized or generalized. Individuals with localized emphysema may have no symptoms. At the early stage, in most cases, symptoms of chronic bronchitis with cough and expectoration predominate. As with chronic bronchitis, dyspnea occurs only with exertion but gradually, over time, intensifies in severity and frequency. Some individuals may experience rapid progression of dyspnea and disability, and others experience a slower progression. Chronic coughing with expectoration, wheezing, recurrent respiratory infection, and fatigue also may be present. In later stages, severe dyspnea, cyanosis, and other signs of respiratory failure may be evident.[3] As with chronic bronchitis, individuals may experience periods of exacerbation of symptoms usually related to infections or other complications.

Physical findings may be normal in cases of mild or localized emphysema. However, in more advanced cases there is usually weight loss and a "barrel-chest" appearance.[6] The patient may appear short of breath and use accessory respiratory muscles. Many may find it easier to breathe in a sitting position, bent over and resting their elbows on their thighs. Usually, the expiration phase of ventilation is prolonged, and the patient may be breathing against pursed lips. With some individuals, wheezing may be heard on expiration. In advanced stages of emphysema, cyanosis may be evident along with other signs of respiratory failure such as a change in mental state, headache, weakness, digital clubbing, and muscle tremor or twitching.[3]

Management of COPD

The management of COPD includes the following components:[8]
1. Assess and monitor disease

2. Reduce risk factors
3. Manage stable COPD
4. Manage exacerbations of COPD

As shown in Fig. 55.3, treatment options begin with self-management, education, and avoidance of risk factors, especially smoking. Relieving symptoms and improving overall health through exercise, nutritional counseling, and treatment of complications as part of pulmonary rehabilitation can greatly improve the quality of life for these individuals.[8,9]

Drugs Commonly Used in the Treatment of COPD

Although there is no cure for COPD and medications cannot alter disease progression, they can improve airflow, relieve symptoms, and enhance the quality of life.[8] Antibiotics often are prescribed during the acute attack of symptoms (exacerbation), particularly if there is a bacterial infection present. Bronchodilators, such as those used by people with asthma, have been used commonly as treatment. These drugs, particularly the beta$_2$-agonists, are fast acting and, in addition to relaxing the bronchial tubes, improve mucus clearance.[8] See Table 55.3 for more details.

Advanced cases of COPD often are treated with the addition of more medications as the disease state progresses. Treatment is individualized and monitored based on the response to therapy and side effects reported during treatment. A long-acting beta$_2$-agonist, along with an anticholinergic or antimuscarinic, may be followed by a methylxanthine as an add-on therapy for patients who have insufficient relief of symptoms. An inhaled glucocorticosteroid or combinations of medications in one inhaler also may be effective. At this stage, many individuals are also on long-term oxygen therapy at home. Surgical removal of one lung or part of a lung may be indicated for some individuals.

Implications for Dental Hygiene Care

Poor oral health has been associated with COPD, particularly during periods of exacerbation. To meet the specialized needs of the individual with COPD, the dental hygienist does the following:

- Seats the patient in a semisupine or upright chair position.
- Plans short appointments or provides short breaks to decrease stress if the patient does not tolerate sitting in a dental chair for long periods of time.
- Assesses severity, frequency of symptoms, and conditions that exacerbate symptoms.
- Assesses the patient's signs, symptoms, and self-reporting of acute respiratory infection and reappoints if present.
- Reviews the health history for evidence of concurrent heart disease; takes appropriate precautions if heart disease is present (see Chapter 48).
- Assesses for ineffective salivary flow related to medication-induced xerostomia and the use of supplemental oxygen and/or other devices intended to improve ventilation.
- If applicable, advises patient to stop smoking and set goals with the patient to initiate a smoking cessation program (see Chapter 37).
- Monitors periodontal status; the patient is at increased risk for disease if they smoke (see Chapter 20).
- Is especially observant of the potential for oral lesions if the patient is a smoker.
- Is especially observant of the potential for oral candidiasis if the patient is on inhaled corticosteroids.
- Avoids use of dental dams if possible because this may further obstruct ventilation.
- When needed, cautiously uses dental materials with a powder component (alginate or powdered gloves) because they may worsen the patient's airway obstruction if inhaled.
- Avoids or minimizes the use of a power-driven polisher, particularly an air polisher (see Table 55.3).
- Uses preprocedural antimicrobial rinse and high-speed suction to reduce contaminated dental aerosols that may be inhaled when using an ultrasonic scaler.
- Avoids nitrous oxide–oxygen inhalation sedation with emphysema (see Table 55.3).
- Suggests low-dose oral diazepam or other benzodiazepine, as prescribed by the dentist, if needed to reduce stress.
- Ensures that patients taking systemic corticosteroids have taken the usual dose on day of appointment, particularly for stressful dental procedures.
- Instructs the patient to consult their physician regarding herbal and drug interactions and use of alcohol if the patient is taking theophylline.[8]
- See Box 55.3 for legal, ethical, and safety issues related to dental hygiene care for patients with COPD and other respiratory diseases. See Box 55.5 for a Critical Thinking Exercise related to patients with COPD.

Tuberculosis

Tuberculosis (TB), an airborne communicable disease, affects primarily the lungs but also can attack other organs and tissues.[10] TB is one of the oldest diseases known to strike humans and still remains one of the most widespread ailments in the world.[1] Although epidemiologic data show a decline in disease incidence among Americans and in many parts of the world, the number of new cases each year continues to present challenges to many nations in their efforts to significantly reduce or eliminate the disease. The continued high incidence of global TB cases has been attributed to adverse social and economic conditions, international travel, and migration of individuals who have TB, and to the human immunodeficiency virus (HIV) epidemic. The suppressed immune system of HIV patients and those who are immunosuppressed from use of medications makes these individuals susceptible to opportunistic diseases such as TB, pneumonia, and other fungal, bacterial, and viral lung infections.[1,10]

BOX 55.5 Critical Thinking Exercise B

COPD Patient

A new patient arrives for her dental appointment. The dental hygienist notices that the patient is short of breath upon walking to the chair and breathes through pursed lips. The patient verbally gives the dental hygienist a list of the medications that she takes on a daily basis. The patient says that she uses an inhaler called Spiriva once a day. When questioned further, the patient is unsure of the exact name of the condition she has been diagnosed with.

1. Based on this medication, what respiratory disease might this patient have?
2. What other physical signs and symptoms might give a more definitive indication that the patient has this respiratory disorder?
3. Develop a treatment plan based on this patient's condition, noting any modifications needed to prevent an exacerbation of her condition.

COPD, Chronic obstructive pulmonary disease.

Etiology of TB

TB is caused by the bacterium *Mycobacterium tuberculosis.* Close contact with persons having TB increases the incidence of disease transmission to others including healthcare providers. See Box 55.6 for a list of population groups that are at greatest risk for contracting TB.

Signs and Symptoms of TB

The diagnosis of TB is made via an evaluation of several assessments, including a medical history, physical examination, Mantoux tuberculin skin test, commonly called a TST or *PPD* (purified protein derivative), chest radiograph, sputum culture, and review of clinical symptoms. If TB is diagnosed, testing for drug resistance follows. TB is usually a chronic infection with various clinical manifestations, depending on the stage and duration of the disease.[10] Persons with primary pulmonary TB infection or latent tuberculosis infection (LTBI) often have no clinical evidence of the disease. They test positive on a tuberculin skin test but do not have active TB and are not infectious. When symptoms of active TB infection are present, they are usually mild and include a low-grade fever, listlessness, loss of appetite, malaise, and occasional cough. The most common obvious symptom of active TB is a chronic cough. Other signs of disease progression include fever, night sweats, weight loss, central pulmonary necrosis (death of lung tissue), and **cavitation** (hollow spaces in the lungs).[7]

Treatment of TB

Treatment of TB depends on whether an individual has active TB or only LTBI. Those persons who test positive for TB but do not have the disease may be treated with a preventive therapy. This treatment usually involves a daily dose of isoniazid (also called INH) or rifampin for 4 to 9 months.[10] Treatment for individuals with active TB may include a short hospital stay, along with the concurrent administration of several drugs prescribed for at least 18 months if in the past and at least 9 months if recently treated. Multidrug-resistant TB is a dangerous form of TB often resulting from low patient compliance or inadequate treatment. A treatment referred to as "directly observed therapy," which involves observing patients as they take each dose of medication, has successfully remedied this problem in some cases. Patients on a TB drug therapy regimen must be vigilant about taking medication as it has been prescribed, even if symptoms have subsided (Box 55.7).[10]

Prevention of TB

Although the prevalence of TB in the United States is very low, international travel can increase the chances of exposure. High-risk populations previously noted should minimize exposure to known TB patients, particularly in crowded, enclosed environments such as hospitals or other healthcare settings.

Bacille Calmette-Guérin (BCG) is a vaccine for TB offered to high-risk populations, mainly for children in countries with a high prevalence of TB. It is rarely recommended in the United States because of the relatively low risk of contracting the disease. However, further research is being conducted to develop more effective vaccines, especially for adults.[1] A positive PPD test will always result for those who receive the vaccine.

Implications for Dental Hygiene Care

When considering treatment options for the individual with a history of TB, the dental professional addresses the major concern: the risk of disease transmission.[1] TB may be transmitted from patients to dental professionals; conversely, if the clinician is infected, patients and other staff members may contract the disease. To prevent disease transmission and meet the needs of the patient with a history of TB, the dental hygienist does the following:

- Uses standard infection control precautions, keeping in mind that many patients with infectious diseases such as TB may not be identified during assessments.[10]
- Recognizes signs and symptoms of TB when assessing the patient's health history, informs the dentist, and refers for medical evaluation.
- Questions patients who report a history of TB, or a positive result from a skin test for TB, concerning dates and results of chest radiographs, sputum cultures, and physical examinations by their physicians, as well as treatment regimens, compliance, and followup evaluation.
- Determines the type of tuberculosis reported and the current health status of the individual.

- Consults with a physician to determine if it is safe to treat the patient outside of a hospital setting; a patient with active tuberculosis should be treated in a hospital setting under strict infection control conditions (see Box 55.2). Aerosol-producing devices should not be used.[10]
- Instructs the patient with suspected or confirmed TB to observe strict respiratory hygiene and cough etiquette protocols; patients should be kept in the dental setting no longer than is absolutely necessary.[10]

Pneumonia

Pneumonia is an inflammation of the gas-exchanging units of the lungs caused by microorganisms such as bacteria, fungi, and viruses as well as the aspiration of irritating chemicals.[11] Pneumonia can be broadly categorized into two types: **community-acquired pneumonia** (CAP) and **nosocomial pneumonia**.[11] CAP is most often associated with pathogens that normally reside on the oropharyngeal mucosa.

Etiology of Pneumonia

Bacterial infections are the cause of over 50% of CAP cases. Viruses account for almost 40%, and mixed bacterial and viral infections account for 11% of CAP.[11] Organisms that cause these types of pneumonia are *Streptococcus pneumoniae* (most commonly), *Haemophilus influenzae*, *Pseudomonas aeruginosa*, methicillin-resistant *Staphylococcus aureus* (MRSA), Enterobacteriaceae (e.g., *Klebsiella pneumoniae*), *Moraxella catarrhalis*, *Mycoplasma pneumoniae*, *Chlamydophila pneumoniae*, *Coxiella burnetii*, *Chlamydophila psittaci*, and *Legionella pneumophila*, as well as respiratory viruses.[11] Common risk factors for CAP include COPD, alcohol abuse, cystic fibrosis, neurologic impairment, HIV/AIDS, travel, time of year, animal exposure, IV drug use, postinfluenza, and frequent use of antibiotics. Clinical signs and symptoms include rapid onset of shaking chills, moderate to high fever, flulike symptoms, dry or productive cough, runny nose, and general ill feeling. The symptoms will vary depending on the organism that is afflicting the patient. Dental professionals should note any of these symptoms and inquire if the patient has any of the common risk factors. If the patient does have these symptoms and risk factors, the dental procedure should be rescheduled and the patient referred to his/her family physician.

Nosocomial pneumonia can be broken down into three major subcategories, hospital-acquired pneumonia (HAP), ventilator-associated pneumonia (VAP), and healthcare-associated pneumonia (HCAP).[11] HCAP refers to pneumonia in nonhospitalized patients with recent healthcare exposure. Nosocomial pneumonia is caused by a very different spectrum of organisms. These organisms are not normally found in the oropharynx but enter this region from the environment. These organisms more commonly are multidrug resistant and can rapidly develop resistance to antibiotics. Improper methods of handwashing, gloving, and the use of contaminated equipment by healthcare workers in a clinical setting contribute greatly to the transmission of nosocomial pneumonia. Nosocomial pneumonia frequently prolongs hospital stays, increases healthcare costs, and causes death, especially in the elderly and the immunocompromised.

Aspiration pneumonia is another type of pneumonia most often associated with the elderly, particularly those who are considered frail and who suffer from other conditions that may hamper their ability to swallow.[12] Aspiration of oral microorganisms that have been associated with aspiration pneumonia can occur from inhaling food, drink, vomit, or saliva from the mouth into the lungs. This can occur at any time but may occur in healthcare settings, such as a dental facility, long-term care facility, or hospital setting. Elderly patients and those with **dysphagia** (difficulty in swallowing) are especially prone to aspiration pneumonia. Proper oral care has been shown to help prevent aspiration pneumonia.[12]

Ventilator-associated pneumonia (VAP) is a type of pneumonia that is diagnosed when a patient free of pneumonia on hospital admission has been intubated and mechanically ventilated for at least 48 hours.[13] Risk factors for VAP include long duration of mechanical ventilation, advanced age, depressed level of consciousness, preexisting lung disease, immune suppression, and malnutrition. Common microbes include *H. influenzae* and *S. pneumoniae*. Biofilm is thought to develop on the endotracheal tube and migrate to the lower airway, thereby introducing the pathogens to the respiratory tract.[14]

Because of the presence of the oral endotracheal tube, oral gastric tubes, bite blocks, and the adhesive tape that secures such devices, proper oral hygiene care for intubated patients may be challenging. This restricted access to the oral cavity may result in delays in performing tasks such as toothbrushing or the substitution of oral swabs, which have been shown to be less effective than toothbrushing in removing oral pathogens. The concern that toothbrushing may contribute to increased intracranial pressure has been another reason cited by critical care nurses in the neurosurgical field for their reluctance to perform consistent toothbrushing for intubated patients.[15]

Prevention of Pneumonia

Proper oral care for elderly, infirm, and intubated patients is critical in the prevention of pneumonia among these population groups. Chronically ill patients who are hospitalized or in nursing homes often are unable to carry out proper oral self-care. The lack of attention to oral self-care results in an increase in amounts and complexity of dental plaque biofilm. Researchers have concluded that the teeth and periodontium may serve as reservoirs for respiratory infection.[15] Health professionals caring for patients in hospital and long-term care settings must be educated in preventive oral care procedures. See Box 55.8 for oral care recommendations to prevent both community-acquired and nosocomial pneumonia in elderly, infirm, and/or intubated patients. Protocols for oral care with intubated patients are often nonexistent or can vary greatly between facilities. Even when present, some protocols are used inconsistently and are not made a priority by healthcare team members.[16] The availability of VAP prevention oral care kits should make oral care of the intubated patient more convenient and standardized. See Fig. 55.4 for an example of a VAP prevention oral care kit.

Postacute COVID-19 Syndrome

With the onset of COVID-19, healthcare is learning to cope with a new disease and the problems that can be associated with that disease. Postacute COVID-19 syndrome (PACS) is sometimes referred to as long COVID.[17] Many patients who have been afflicted with COVID-19 suffer from lingering effects known as PACS. This disorder is just now in its infancy and will require years of research. Most patients are complaining of fatigue, brain fog, headache, dyspnea, stress, and dehydration. With the onset of this new syndrome, the dental professional needs to be aware that a patient could be experiencing symptoms and side effects similar to other respiratory diseases.[17] This should be documented and education given regarding oral hygiene as with any other respiratory disorder. Remember that the patient may not have asthma or COPD but can still have a reaction to dental procedures as if they had one of those diseases.

Implications for Dental Hygiene Care

Proper biofilm control by traditional brushing and flossing techniques is ideal. However, modifications individualized for the patient's needs, as described in Chapter 47, such as the use of modified toothbrushes,

BOX 55.8 Oral Care Recommendations to Prevent Pneumonia in Elderly, Infirm, and Intubated/Tracheostomy Patients

- Remove and clean dentures daily; refrain from wearing while sleeping.
- Brush after meals to disrupt bacterial plaque; floss or use interdental cleaner once per day.
- For ventilated patients:[17]
  - Pooling of secretions should be minimized through regular drainage and suction.
  - Subglottic suction endotracheal tubes should be utilized if possible.
  - Patient's head should be elevated 30° to 45°.
  - Brush teeth twice a day.
  - Use foam swab with chlorhexidine rinse or gel to debride oral cavity every 2 to 4 hours. Commercially prepared oral care kits are available for ease of use by healthcare team members.[12] See Fig. 55.4.
- Emphasize importance of proper oral care to family members and/or caregivers. Ensure access to oral care products.

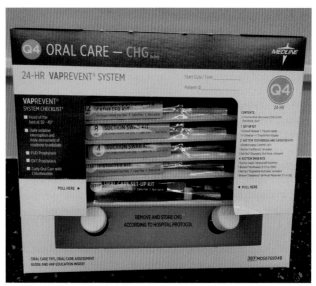

Fig. 55.4 Oral care kits are commercially available for use of the intubated patient. They often include toothbrushes, oral swabs, chlorhexidine gluconate, and oral gel specifically designed for the intubated patient. Recommendations for a daily regimen are also included in this specific kit. (© Medline Industries, Inc. 2018.)

interdental aids, and mouth rinses, may improve the patient's ability to remove bacterial biofilm. For those who are infirm and/or physically disabled, nursing staff must be knowledgeable and vigilant in oral care practices. Family members of those in long-term care facilities should be encouraged to make oral care a priority with their loved ones. See Box 55.3 for legal, ethical, and safety issues related to nosocomial pneumonia.

Interprofessional Role of the Dental Hygienist

The interprofessional role of the dental hygienist can be used in the future with respect to the oral care of elderly, infirm, and intubated patients. As ongoing research provides more evidence for the link between oral health and systemic health, the collaborative care of these patients will include dental professionals. In-service education programs for nursing staff members and, in some states, direct patient care

are increasing the dental hygienist's opportunities to be a part of the overall healthcare team.[15]

Sleep-Related Breathing Disorders

The term *sleep-related breathing disorders* refers to a range of breathing abnormalities, from chronic or habitual snoring to various types of sleep apnea. **Obstructive sleep apnea** (OSA) is a condition that involves the partial or complete collapse of the upper airway while breathing during sleep. OSA is characterized by loud snoring and periods of breathing cessation or awakening with a choking sensation. OSA causes a decrease in arterial oxygen, which often results in daytime sleepiness, fatigue, irritability, and a general reduction in quality of life.[18] Dental hygienists should identify and discuss the oral manifestations as listed in Box 55.9 that may result from OSA. Because of the additional stress placed on the heart during apnea episodes, OSA has been associated with metabolic, cardiovascular, and respiratory disorders.[18]

Etiology of Sleep-Related Breathing Disorders

Apnea (the cessation of breathing) during sleep is most often caused by excess weight and obesity, which is associated with oral tissues. When asleep, the muscles of the mouth and throat are relaxed and allow the soft tissue to block the airway either partially or completely. Other contributing factors include nasal congestion, smoking, and excessive alcohol use.[18] In children, enlarged tonsils are the major causative factor. However, a tumor or birth defects involving the tongue or mandible may be contributing factors because of the size and/or position of the tongue and decreased muscle tone often found in these patients.[18]

Signs and Symptoms of Obstructive Sleep Apnea

Signs and symptoms of OSA include the following:

- Loud chronic snoring or snoring followed by periods of silence that may indicate an apnea event
- Awakening occurring with sounds of snorting, gasping, and choking
- Quality of life changes that may involve physical, psychologic, and occupational limitations including social interaction

---

BOX 55.9   Oral Manifestations Associated With Obstructive Sleep Apnea (OSA)[18]

- Extraoral features including retrognathic mandible, often accompanied by Class II malocclusion; increased anterior height resulting in long-looking face; and decreased nasal passage size
- Bruxism while sleeping that can result in notable attrition, possibly leading to exposed dentin, abfraction, or tooth fracture
- Anterior wear due to positioning of the mandible forward in an attempt to open airway
- Enlarged tongue with scalloped borders
- Acid erosion on lingual surfaces of teeth due to acid reflux, which may occur when patient attempts to breathe during OSA events
- Enlarged tonsils, edema, and erythema of the soft palate and surrounding structures that may indicate snoring and OSA
- Red and edematous gingival tissues, particularly in anterior teeth, may be a sign of mouth breathing due to sleep-related breathing disorder
- Constricted maxillary and mandibular arches can crowd the tongue and may result in the tongue being more posterior in the mouth, further blocking the airway when the patient is relaxed during sleep
- Abnormal enlargement of the tonsils, along with constricted arches, particularly in children, often contributes to a sleep-related breathing disorder

Adapted from Heinrich R, Elliott E. Sleep apnea for dentists: an overview of signs, symptoms, consequences, and treatment. *Dent Econ.* 2017;107(7):73–80. [serial online], Dentistry & Oral Sciences Source, Ipswich, MA. Accessed August 15, 2017.

- Other symptoms related to decreased oxygen levels and sleep disturbances include headache, xerostomia, and depression.

See Box 55.9 for oral manifestations of sleep-related disorders.

Treatment of Sleep-Related Breathing Disorders

Individuals identified with OSA are most commonly treated with the use of a continuous positive airway pressure (CPAP) or bilevel positive airway pressure (BiPAP) device that opens up the airway during sleep. The device consists of a mask that covers both the nose and the mouth and is connected to a ventilating machine.[7] Although shown to be effective in many cases, the cumbersome nature of the device and sometimes ill-fitting masks often result in noncompliance. Despite humidification of most devices, patients often complain of nighttime dryness of oral tissues. Other modes of treatment include oral appliances, surgery, and behavior modification. Dental hygienists who are educated about the signs and symptoms of OSA and other sleep-related disorders can assess for the condition, relate the oral manifestations to the patient, and make proper referrals for treatment.[19]

Implications for Dental Hygiene Care

When assessing and treating a patient with a suspected sleep-related disorder, the dental hygienist does the following:

- Assesses for and records any extraoral and/or intraoral signs and symptoms of a sleep-related disorder. See Box 55.9.
- Further questions the patient regarding sleep habits and any medical intervention previously discussed. If no current treatment, they make a proper referral.
- Encourages patient to be compliant with physician's or other healthcare provider's recommendations for treatment.
- If being treated with CPAP or BiPAP devices, encourages patients to ensure proper humidification and care of the device.
- Identifies signs of xerostomia or other oral manifestations and educates patients about conditions that may result.

KEY CONCEPTS

- Asthma is a respiratory disease characterized by an increased responsiveness of the airways to various stimuli, which causes periodic wheezing, dyspnea, coughing, and chest tightness.
- An asthma attack may be triggered by allergens, anxiety, cold air, or exercise, or no apparent irritant may be involved.
- Many asthma medications have side effects, including oral candidiasis and xerostomia.
- Two major diseases that can contribute to chronic obstructive pulmonary disease (COPD) are emphysema and chronic bronchitis.
- COPD is caused most often by cigarette smoking, but the presence of the genetic predisposition of alpha-1 antitrypsin deficiency and chronic exposure to occupational and environmental pollutants are also risk factors associated with COPD.
- The major risk associated with treating patients with active tuberculosis is disease transmission; patients with active tuberculosis should be treated in a hospital setting only for emergency dental care.
- Patient compliance problems during lengthy drug therapy for tuberculosis have contributed to the problem of multidrug-resistant strains of tuberculosis.
- Effective daily oral hygiene care reduces the amount of oral bacteria available for aspiration into the lungs and may prevent respiratory tract infections such as pneumonia, particularly among intubated and infirm patients.
- The increased prevalence of obstructive sleep apnea diagnoses has heightened awareness of the condition and the role of the dental practitioner in its treatment.

ACKNOWLEDGMENT

The authors acknowledge Joan Gugino Ellison for past contributions to this chapter.

REFERENCES

1. Schwartz NG, Price SF, Pratt R, et al. Tuberculosis—United States, 2019. *MMWR Morb Mortal Wkly Rep*. 2020;69:286–289. Available at: https://www.ncbi.nlm.nih.gov/pmc/articles/PMC7739979/. Accessed May 22, 2022.

2. National Heart, Lung, and Blood Institute, National Asthma Education and Prevention Program Expert Panel. *Expert Panel Report 3 (EPR3): Guidelines for the Diagnosis and Management of Asthma. Asthma Management Guidelines: Focused Updates*; 2020. Updated February 1, 2021. Published August, 2007. Available at: https://www.nhlbi.nih.gov/health-topics/asthma-management-guidelines-2020-updates. Accessed May 22, 2022.

3. Malamed SF. Asthma. In: Malamed SF, ed. *Medical Emergencies in the Dental Office*. Mosby; 2015:213–231.

4. American Lung Association. *Learning about Asthma*; 2020. Available at: http://www.lung.org/lung-health-and-diseases/lung-disease-lookup/asthma/. Accessed May 22, 2022.

5. Tanaka L, Dezan C, Chadi S, et al. The influence of asthma onset and severity on malocclusion prevalence in children and adolescents. *Dent Press J Orthod*. 2012;17(1):50–51. ([serial online], Available at: http://www.scielo.br/scielo.php?script=sci_arttext&pid=S2176-94512012000100007. Accessed December 5, 2022.

6. Global Initiative for Chronic Obstructive Lung Disease. *Global Strategy for the Diagnosis, Management and Prevention of Chronic Obstructive Pulmonary Disease (2022 Report)*. Available at: http://goldcopd.org. Accessed May 22, 2022.

7. Des Jardins TR, Burton GG. *Clinical Manifestations and Assessment of Respiratory Disease*. Mosby; 2020.

8. Centers for Disease Control and Prevention, National Center for Health Statistics. *Chronic Obstructive Pulmonary Disease (COPD) Includes: Chronic Bronchitis and Emphysema*. Updated February 1, 2022. Available at: https://www.cdc.gov/nchs/fastats/copd.htm Accessed May 22, 2022.

9. National Heart Lung and Blood Institute. *Diseases and Conditions Index*. Available at: https://www.nhlbi.nih.gov/health/health-topics/topics/copd/. Accessed May 22, 2022.

10. Centers for Disease Control and Prevention. *Basic TB Facts*. Available at: https://www.cdc.gov/tb/topic/basics/default.htm. Accessed May 22, 2022.

11. Hess DR, MacIntyre NR, Mishoe SC, et al. *Respiratory Care, Principles and Practice*. Jones & Bartlett; 2021.

12. Kanzigg LA, Hunt L. Oral health and hospital-acquired pneumonia in elderly patients: a review of the literature. *J Dent Hyg*. 2016;90:15–21.

13. Centers for Disease Control and Prevention. *Pneumonia (Ventilator-Associated [VAP] and Non-ventilator-associated Pneumonia [PNEU]) Event*; 2022. Available at: https://www.cdc.gov/nhsn/PDFs/pscManual/6pscVAPcurrent.pdf. Accessed May 22, 2022.

14. Chang DW. *Clinical Application of Mechanical Ventilation*. Delmar Cengage; 2014.

15. Prendergast V, Kleiman C. Interprofessional practice: translating evidence-based oral care to hospital care. *J Dent Hyg*. 2015;89(suppl 1):33–35.

16. Muller F. Oral hygiene reduces the mortality from aspiration pneumonia in frail. *Elders J Dent Res*. 2015;94(3 suppl):14S–16S.

17. Tabacof L, Tosto-Mancuso J, Wood J, et al. Post acute Covid-19 syndrome negatively impacts physical function, cognition, health-related quality of life, and participation. *Am J Phys Med Rehabil*. 2022;101:48–52. https://doi.org/10.1097/PHM.0000000000001910. PMID: 34686631. PMCID: PMC8667685.

18. Heinrich R, Elliott E. Sleep apnea for dentists: an overview of signs, symptoms, consequences, and treatment. *Dent Econ*. 2017;107(7):73–80. [serial online], Dentistry & Oral Sciences Source, Ipswich, MA. Accessed August 15, 2017.

19. Kornegay EC, Brame JL. Obstructive sleep apnea and the role of dental hygienists. *J Dent Hyg*. 2015;89(5):286–292.

56

Substance Use Disorders

Margaret Lemaster

PROFESSIONAL OPPORTUNITIES

Substance misuse, abuse, and associated mental health disorders continue to be an ongoing worldwide health problem, affecting all socioeconomic groups. It is inevitable that the dental hygienist will encounter patients with current or past addictions. These patients will present for dental treatment, whether it be due to an acute dental issue or a desire for comprehensive oral care. By assisting patients to seek help and maintain optimal oral health during rehabilitation, dental hygienists may contribute to their overall health and well-being.

COMPETENCIES

1. Describe concepts of substance misuse and use disorders and mental illness.
2. Discuss concepts of illicit and over-the-counter drug use, including drug schedules, club drugs, marijuana, and the opioid crisis in the United States.
3. Explain which medical treatments are used for various substance misuse and abuses.
4. Analyze the dental hygiene process of care related to patients with substance use disorders and those in recovery.
5. Discuss why dental professionals may be at risk for substance use disorders.

CONCEPTS OF SUBSTANCE USE DISORDERS

Substance misuse is a pattern of self-administered drugs or alcohol use that may lead to addiction. **Substance use disorder** (SUD) is the repeated misuse of drugs or alcohol. For the purpose of this chapter, while references to SUD may include the concept of misuse of a substance for its unintended purpose, substance misuse, and SUD are not identical beyond the context of this discussion.

The Substance Abuse and Mental Health Services Administration's (SAMHSA's) 2020 National Survey on Drug Use and Health (NSDUH) reports that approximately 40.3 million people aged 18 or older had a substance use disorder in the past year.[1] Research demonstrates that about half of the individuals who experience SUD will also experience a co-occurring **mental illness.**[1] A co-occurring disorder is the coexistence of both an SUD and a mental health disorder; however, one condition does not necessarily cause the other (see Fig. 56.1).

Any mental illness (AMI) is defined as having had a diagnosable mental disorder (excluding developmental disorders and substance use disorders) within the past year. Disorders include depression, attention-deficit hyperactivity disorder (ADHD), bipolar disorder, personality disorders, and schizophrenia.[2,3] **Serious mental illness** (SMI) is defined as an adult over age 18 having a diagnosable mental, behavior, or emotional disorder that causes serious functional impairment that substantially interferes with or limits one or more major life activities within the last year. According to the National Institute of Mental Health, serious mental illness is relatively rare, affecting only 5% of the population over 18. Serious mental illness includes schizophrenia, the subset of major depression called "severe, major depression," and the subset of bipolar disorder classified as "severe."

In this chapter, a *substance* is a psychoactive compound with the potential to cause health problems, substance misuse, substance use disorders, and addiction. These substances affect the central nervous system and the perceptions of the environment through chemical changes. Note that the effects of nicotine on oral health and overall health are not addressed in this chapter. See Chapter 37, Tobacco Cessation, for more information on tobacco, vaping, and related nicotine use disorders.

SUDs include the use of natural and synthetic substances as well as psychoactive drugs used by those with substance misuse or abuse issues. These substances can be divided into three major categories: alcohol, illicit drugs (including misuse of prescription drugs), and over-the-counter drugs (see Table 56.1 and Box 56.1).

Alcohol and drug misuse, SUDs, AMI, and SMI affect millions of Americans.[4] (See Box 56.1.) They may be temporary and of low severity, but they may also result in serious, enduring, and costly consequences. (See Table 56.2.) SUD affects the individual, the family, and the community. Alcohol, drug, and/or otherwise impaired drivers cause a significant number of deadly automobile accidents annually. In 2020, almost two-thirds of drivers involved in serious injury or fatal crashes tested positive for at least one active drug, including alcohol, marijuana, or opioids. According to the 2018 NSDUH, 20.5 million people aged 16 or older drove under the influence of alcohol in the past year and 12.6 million drove under the influence of illicit drugs.[5]

In 2021, most drug-related emergency department visits involved alcohol (39.33%), followed by opioids (14.07%), methamphetamine (11.02%), marijuana (10.78%), and cocaine (4.71%).[6]

Patients who are dependent on alcohol or drugs or are in treatment for an SUD present the dental hygienist with complex issues related to preventive oral healthcare. Poor oral health is common as SUDs directly affect oral health: xerostomia, increased caries rate, enamel erosion, periodontal disease, bruxism, and poor self-care. Additionally, similar oral health symptoms occur in those with SMI and AMI. Such patients must be identified so they may be treated safely. To do this, dental hygienists must understand basic concepts and causes associated with SUD, related mental illnesses, and associated medical treatments (see Box 56.2).

Addiction, Dependence, Withdrawal, Tolerance, and Relapse

Addiction is the prolonged, repeated misuse or abuse of any substance—a chronic and compulsive need to use drugs despite causing the user physical and emotional harm. Prolonged misuse or abuse can produce changes to the brain that can lead to an SUD that

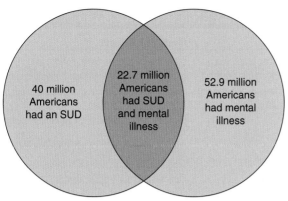

Fig. 56.1 Statistics on SUDs and AMI. (Statistics on SUDs and AMI (SAMHSA 2020) (From samhsa.gov).)

TABLE 56.1	Examples of Abused Substances
Substance Category	**Examples of Abused Substances**
Alcohol	• Beer • Wine • Malt liquor • Distilled spirits
Illicit Drugs	• Cocaine, including crack • Heroin • Hallucinogens, including LSD, PCP, Ecstasy, peyote, mescaline, psilocybin • Methamphetamines, including crystal meth • Marijuana, including hashish • Synthetic drugs, including K2, Spice, and "bath salts" • Prescription-type medications that are misused for nonmedical purposes • Pain relievers—synthetic, semisynthetic, and nonsynthetic opioid medications, including fentanyl, codeine, oxycodone, hydrocodone, and tramadol products • Tranquilizers, including benzodiazepines, meprobamate products, and muscle relaxants • Stimulants and methamphetamine, including amphetamine, dextroamphetamine, and phentermine products; mazindol products; and methylphenidate or dexmethylphenidate products • Sedatives, including temazepam, flurazepam, or triazolam and any barbiturates
Over-the-Counter Drugs	• Cough and cold medicines • Inhalants, including amyl nitrite, cleaning fluids, gasoline and lighter gases, anesthetics, solvents, spray paint, nitrous oxide • Tobacco products including vaping (see Chapter 37)

significantly impairs health and function and may require special treatment. Addiction disorders can range from mild to severe. The specific substances being used and how they enter the body influence additional medical conditions experienced by chemically dependent patients. For example, patients with a history of intravenous drug

use have a higher incidence of HIV infection and hepatitis B, C, and D. Injection methods place the user at risk for hepatitis, septicemia, abscesses, and HIV infection.

Long-term alcohol use may result in liver, heart, kidney, and pancreas damage. Years of alcohol abuse may damage the reproductive system and cause permanent brain damage and a lack of muscle coordination. Alcohol use during pregnancy may lead to disorders such as fetal alcohol spectrum disorders (FASDs). The systemic impact of drug addiction can include cardiovascular disease, stroke, cancer, HIV/AIDS infection, hepatitis, and lung disease, especially after prolonged use.

Child abuse, neglect, and intimate partner and sexual violence are often directly related to parents, caregivers, spouses, or partners with substance abuse issues. Suicide attempts and fatalities and overdoses are also tied to SUDs. Because addiction often results in criminal behavior to finance a drug habit, substance abusers are often viewed as morally weak or corrupt individuals who willingly engage in self-destructive behaviors that affect themselves and everyone around them.

Psychological dependence refers to the cognitive and emotional aspects of addictive behaviors or the withdrawal process from addictive substances. Psychological dependence is rooted in the belief that the substance is needed to maintain a state of well-being. **Physiological dependence** results from a biologic alteration in the user's brain from consistent long-term drug use. A person who has developed physiological dependence on a drug will go through symptoms of drug **withdrawal** when the drug use ceases, which may include vomiting, diarrhea, rapid pulse, sweating, anxiety, convulsions, severe cramps, high blood pressure, and severe headaches.

Another aspect of physiological dependence is the development of drug **tolerance,** whereby an increasingly larger dose is required to produce the same physiological or psychological effect obtained earlier with smaller doses. Nicotine, opiates, alcohol, psychedelics, central nervous system (CNS) stimulants, and sedative-hypnotics all require increased doses to establish the same "high" or euphoric feeling that the user experienced with first use. If the drug dosage is not increased, the effects of the drug are diminished, and withdrawal symptoms occur. **Relapse** is a return to heavy and frequent substance use that existed before treatment or commitment to behavioral change.

CONCEPTS OF ALCOHOL MISUSE AND ABUSE

Alcohol is the most pervasive sensory-altering substance used in the United States, and it is associated with a significant number of oral health/overall health-related diseases and deaths. (See Box 56.3.) Alcohol reduces anxiety by causing intoxication and sensory alterations. Excessive alcohol use can also lead to risk-taking behavior, including driving while impaired. Alcohol use disorder (AUD) is an impaired ability to stop alcohol use regardless of undesirable social, occupational, or health consequences. AUD has also been known as alcohol abuse, alcohol dependence, alcohol addiction, and the colloquial term, alcoholism.[7]

TABLE 56.2	**Drug Categories of Abused Substances and Their Effects on the Body**		
Hallucinogens	**Short-Term Use**	**Long-Term Use**	**Systemic Effects**
Cannabinoids Marijuana Hashish Sinsemilla	Relaxation; euphoria; confusion; poor coordination; red, bloodshot eyes; intense hunger or thirst; difficulty with concentration, memory, and learning; distorted perception of sights, sounds, time, and touch; difficulty with problem solving	Increases risk of lung cancer, bronchitis, and emphysema—smoking one joint of marijuana has the same effect as smoking 14 to 16 cigarettes; weakens immune system	Dilated pupils, tachycardia, peripheral vasodilation, bronchial hyperactivity, insomnia, impaired short-term memory, disruption in testosterone secretion. Decreases nausea and pressure behind the eyes; sometimes taken by cancer and glaucoma patients to alleviate symptoms Chronic use can result in withdrawal symptoms Can cause thrombocytopenia if injected intravenously
LSD (lysergic acid diethylamide)	Causes sensory distortions and illusions, extreme emotions from euphoria to panic, unpredictable reactions	Acute anxiety, fear of loss of control, paranoia, delusions of grandeur	Increased heart rate and blood pressure, hyperthermia; prolonged psychotic reaction or severe depression, mental flashbacks to sensations experienced while taking LSD can occur
PCP (phencyclidine)	Sensory deprivation, reduces inhibitions, deadens pain, mild depression	Combative behavior, inability to speak, confusion, agitation, paranoia, amnesia	Extremely high blood pressure, cardiovascular instability, respiratory depression, catatonia, coma, convulsions, seizures. Retained in fat cells for several months after use and can be released during exercise, during fasting, or when under stress, causing flashbacks.
Inhalants	**Short-Term Use**	**Long-Term Use**	**Systemic Effects**
Volatile solvents Airplane glue Rubber cement Spray paint Hair spray Paint thinner Spot remover Gasoline	Reduced inhibitions, impulsiveness, excitement, irritability, euphoria, dizziness, slurred speech, drowsiness	Confusion, delirium, psychomotor dysfunction, emotional instability, impaired thinking	Brain, liver, kidney, nervous system, bone marrow, and lung disorders as a result of the effect of the solvent or ingredients in the solvent Respiratory arrest, cardiac arrhythmia, asphyxia, suicide
Volatile nitrites Room deodorizers Amyl nitrite	Relaxation of all smooth muscles, altered consciousness, enhanced sexual pleasure	Increased blood flow to the brain resulting in headaches, dizziness and giddiness, vomiting, shock, and loss of consciousness	Nitrite poisoning; damage to the nervous system; impaired perception, reasoning, and memory; dementia; defective muscular coordination
Anesthetics Nitrous oxide	Giddiness, profound laughter, euphoria	Addiction, loss of consciousness, frostbite of the nose and vocal cords from direct inhalation out of a pressurized tank	Peripheral nerve damage, frozen lung tissue, brain cell damage due to oxygen deprivation
Alcohol	**Short-Term Use**	**Long-Term Use**	**Systemic Effects**
	Feeling of well-being, loss of inhibitions, slowed reactions, intoxication, slurred speech, sedation, unconsciousness Especially dangerous when used with other central nervous system depressants or narcotics	Addiction, increased risk of oral cancer and breast cancer, malnutrition, inflammation of the stomach, hepatitis and other liver damage, alcohol amnestic disorder, dementia	Cognitive impairment; cardiovascular impairment; cirrhosis of the liver; damage to kidney, central nervous system, and gastrointestinal tract

---

BOX 56.2   DH Scope of Practice

Although the scope of dental practice does not include the diagnosis or treatment of SUDs or mental illnesses, dental hygienists should recognize the signs, symptoms, and impact these disorders have on oral health to enable them to develop an appropriate treatment plan and implement suitable preventive oral healthcare therapies.

BOX 56.3   National Survey on Drug Use and Health

Recent data from the National Survey on Drug Use and Health (NSDUH) reveals that there were approximately 29.9 million people in the United States who had an AUD. This equates to 1 in 13 adults over the age of 18 and an estimated 7.7 million adolescents aged 12 to 17.

Alcohol impacts or contributes to more than 200 illnesses that include liver disorders, cancers, and injuries.[2] Almost 100,000 people in the United States die every year from alcohol-related causes, making alcohol one of the leading causes of preventable death. Most of these deaths result from chronic heavy alcohol abuse and injuries experienced while intoxicated. Studies confirmed dose-response associations between alcohol consumption and cancers of the oral cavity, pharynx, larynx, esophagus, colon, rectum, liver, and breast,[8] and these cancers may originate with relatively low amounts of alcohol consumption (see Box 56.4).

Oral healthcare providers need to be aware that individuals who drink heavily have five times the risk of developing esophageal and head and neck cancers compared to people who drink only occasionally or not at all.[8] Additionally, the risk for developing oral cancers increases exponentially when the individuals are also heavy smokers.

Previous research suggested cardiovascular benefits when consuming small amounts of alcohol, especially red wines, but recent and more robust studies found no health benefits of alcohol consumption on cardiovascular or other outcomes,[9] and there are no safe drinking amounts of alcohol (see Box 56.5).

CONCEPTS OF ILLICIT AND OVER-THE-COUNTER SUBSTANCE USE

Illicit drugs are a variety of drugs that are used for nonmedical purposes and are illegal to manufacture, use, or sell. They include cocaine, heroin, amphetamines, and hallucinogens. Illicit drugs are often highly addictive and create serious health and safety risks. The use of illicit drugs often begins with youthful experimentation or curiosity.

If misused, many **over-the-counter (OTC) drugs**, those that are available for purchase without a prescription, have psychoactive or mind-altering properties that can lead to serious medical and mental health conditions. These harmful effects become more complex when combined with alcohol or illicit drugs. Common misused OTC drugs are dextromethorphan (found in cough syrups) and pseudoephedrine (found in cold medicines).

Drug Schedules

The Controlled Substances Act (CSA) is a law that regulates legal and illegal substances in the United States. Under the CSA, substances are classified into five categories or **schedules** according to a drug's danger and potential for addiction. The addiction potential is the most important factor in scheduling a drug. Schedule I drugs, such as heroin, have a high potential for abuse and a high potential to create severe psychological and/or physical dependence. As the drug schedule number increases, the abuse potential decreases (see Table 56.3).

Club Drugs

Club drugs are a group of psychoactive drugs that act on the central nervous system and cause changes in mood, awareness, and behavior. The collection of club drugs used by adolescents and young adults includes substances classified as dissociative anesthetics, hallucinogens, and/or inhalants. Club drugs are popular among nightclub attendees, raves, and all-night dance parties. Stimulant club drugs help the user stay awake all night and cause hallucinatory effects and intense feelings of elation, well-being, and sensory awareness. Sedative club drugs ease "coming down" from the high. The National Institute on Drug Abuse identified dextromethorphan (DXM), flunitrazepam (Rohypnol), gamma-hydroxybutyrate (GHB), inhalants, ketamine, lysergic acid diethylamide (LSD), methylenedioxymethamphetamine (MDMA), phencyclidine, *Salvia divinorum* (salvia), synthetic cannabinoids, and/or synthetic cathinones (bath salts) as club drugs. Rohypnol, GHB, and ketamine are also considered predatory or date rape drugs (see Table 56.4).[10]

Marijuana

After tobacco and alcohol, marijuana is the most commonly used addictive drug.[11] Over 48 million people used marijuana at least once and almost 12 million young adults used marijuana in the past year.[11] According to a 2021 survey, almost 31% of senior high students used marijuana in some form daily. In addition, the number of youths and young adults who believe regular marijuana use is risky is decreasing.[12]

Recent research estimated that approximately 3 in 10 people who use marijuana have marijuana use disorder. For people who begin using marijuana before age 18, the risk of developing marijuana use disorder is even greater.[13] Marijuana use directly affects the brain, specifically the parts of the brain responsible for memory, learning, attention, decision making, coordination, emotion, and reaction time. Infants, children, and teens (who still have developing brains) are especially susceptible to the adverse effects of marijuana. Long-term or frequent marijuana use has been linked to increased risk of psychosis or schizophrenia in some users. Using marijuana during pregnancy may increase the person's risk for pregnancy complications. Pregnant and breastfeeding women should avoid marijuana.

As marijuana laws are changing, so too is the drug itself, with average potency more than doubling over the past decade. The mode of marijuana use is also changing: in addition to smoking, consuming edible forms such as baked goods and candies, using vaporizing devices, and using high-potency extracts and oils (e.g., "dabbing") are becoming increasingly common.[8] Because these products and methods are unregulated even in states that have legalized marijuana use, users may not have accurate information about dosage or potency, which may lead to serious consequences such as hospitalizations for psychosis and other overdose-related symptoms.[6] Marijuana use can impair driving and is linked to roughly two times the accident risk. The risk is greater when marijuana is used in combination with alcohol or other drugs. Research suggests, however, that there is potential therapeutic value of marijuana use in positively affecting several health conditions, such as pain, nausea, epilepsy, obesity, addiction, and autoimmune disorders.

TABLE 56.3   Drug Schedules

Drug Schedule	Definition	Drug Examples
I	Drugs with no currently accepted medical use and a high potential for abuse. These drugs are considered dangerous.	Heroin Lysergic acid diethylamide (LSD) Marijuana (cannabis) 3,4-Methylenedioxymethamphetamine (Ecstasy) Methaqualone Peyote
II	Drugs with a high potential for abuse, with use potentially leading to severe psychological or physical dependence. These drugs are also considered dangerous.	Combination products with less than 15 mg of hydrocodone per dosage unit (Vicodin), cocaine, methamphetamine, methadone, hydromorphone (Dilaudid), meperidine (Demerol), oxycodone (OxyContin), fentanyl, Dexedrine, Adderall, and Ritalin
III	Drugs with a moderate to low potential for physical and psychological dependence.	Products containing less than 90 mg of codeine per dosage unit (Tylenol with codeine), ketamine, anabolic steroids, testosterone
IV	Drugs with a low potential for abuse and low risk of dependence	Xanax, Soma, Darvon, Darvocet, Valium, Ativan, Talwin, Ambien, Tramadol
V	Drugs with lower potential for abuse than Schedule IV and consist of preparations containing limited quantities of certain narcotics. Schedule V drugs are generally used for antidiarrheal, antitussive, and analgesic purposes.	Cough preparations with less than 200 mg of codeine or per 100 mL (Robitussin AC), Lomotil, Motofen, Lyrica, Parepectolin

TABLE 56.4   Club Drugs

Drug Name	Also Known As
Methylenedioxymethamphetamine (MDMA)	Ecstasy, XTC, X, E, Adam, Molly, Hug Beans, Love Drug
Gamma-hydroxybutyrate (GHB)	G, Liquid Ecstasy, and Soap
Ketamine	Special K, K, Vitamin K, Jet
Rohypnol	Roofies
Methamphetamine	Speed, Ice, Chalk, Meth, Crystal, Crank, Glass
Lysergic acid diethylamide (LSD)	Acid, Blotter, Dots

Synthetic marijuana, also known as Spice or K2, is an herbal mixture laced with synthetic chemicals similar to THC, the main active ingredient in marijuana. These mixtures are wrongly perceived as a safe alternative to marijuana.

Opioid Crisis in the United States

Opioid abuse has become a public health crisis in the United States. **Opioid** analgesic pain relievers are now the most prescribed class of medications in the United States, with almost 142 million prescriptions written in 2020. Opioid drug overdose deaths also occur as a result of the illicit manufacturing and distribution of synthetic opioids, such as fentanyl, and the illegal diversion of prescription opioids. Illicit fentanyl is often combined with heroin or counterfeit prescription drugs or sold as heroin and may be contributing to drug overdose deaths. The increase in prescriptions of opioid pain relievers has been accompanied by dramatic increases in the number of emergency department visits due to opioid overdose (see Fig. 56.2) and rates of overdose deaths associated with opioids.

CAUSES OF SUBSTANCE MISUSE AND SUDS

Physiological Factors

After a drug enters the body (see Box 56.6), it is carried by the bloodstream to the central nervous system (the brain and spinal cord) within 10 to 15 seconds. When a drug crosses the blood-brain barrier, it can affect all parts of the body by interfering with the information sent to the CNS by the autonomic nervous system and the peripheral nervous system. The autonomic nervous system controls involuntary functions such as circulation, digestion, and respiration, and it helps the body to establish a stable internal environment. The peripheral nervous system transmits messages between the external environment and the CNS. The CNS is responsible for formulating decisions similar to that of computer. As the CNS receives messages from the autonomic nervous system and the peripheral nervous system, it analyzes those messages and sends a response to the correct body system—muscular, skeletal, circulatory, nervous, respiratory, digestive, excretory, endocrine, or reproductive—to react to the stimuli. Psychoactive drugs alter the information sent to the brain and disrupt the messages sent back to the body, interrupting cognitive thought and logic.

Neurotransmitters

Neurotransmitters are chemicals produced within the neuron that allow neurons to communicate with each other throughout the body. They enable the brain to provide many diverse functions through the process of chemical synaptic transmission. These endogenous chemicals are necessary for everyday life and are essential to the functions of complex neurological performance.[14]

Many psychoactive drugs interfere with the method that neurons use to send, receive, and process signals through neurotransmitters. The chemical structure of some drugs such as marijuana and heroin trigger neurons and mirror natural transmitters present in the brain. This allows the drugs to latch onto and set the neurons in motion. Although these drugs closely imitate the brain's own chemistry, they do not activate neurons in the same way as a natural neurotransmitter. Normal function of the neurotransmitters is disrupted, and abnormal messages are sent. CNS depressants increases activity of gamma-aminobutyric acid (GABA), a chemical that inhibits brain activity. Sometimes this is a desirable effect. This action causes drowsiness and calming effects, thereby dulling and weakening the pain signal. This effect is desirable if a physician prescribes morphine to alleviate pain in a person with a terminal illness. Heroin attaches itself to certain receptor sites in the emotional center of the brain and induces a sensation of pleasure or reward;

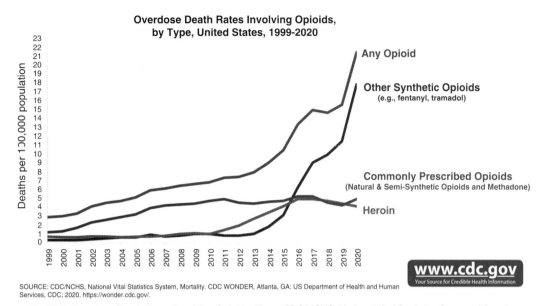

Overdose Death Rates Involving Opioids, by Type, United States, 1999-2020

SOURCE: CDC/NCHS, National Vital Statistics System, Mortality. CDC WONDER, Atlanta, GA: US Department of Health and Human Services, CDC; 2020. https://wonder.cdc.gov/.

Fig. 56.2 Overdose Death Rates Involving Opioids. (From CDC/NCHS, National Vital Statistics System, Mortality, CDC WONDER, Atlanta, GA: US Department of Health and Human Services, CDC; 2020. https://wonder.cdc.gov/.)

BOX 56.6   How Substances Enter the Body

- Direct contact with skin or mucous membranes, including vaginally or rectally
- Oral ingestion
- Snorted through the nose
- Placed sublingually
- Placed against oral mucosa
- Injected either directly into the bloodstream (intravenously), into a muscle (muscling), or under the skin (skin popping).

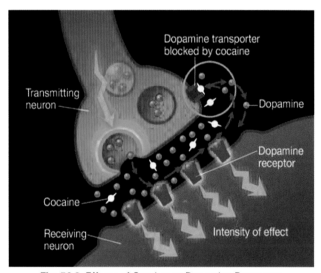

Fig. 56.3 Effects of Cocaine on Dopamine Receptors.

---

however, it also attaches itself to the area of the brain that controls respiration and can slow it down to a dangerous level. CNS stimulants such as cocaine force the release of large amounts of neurotransmitters such as epinephrine and dopamine, which can create, stimulate, and exaggerate messages to and from the CNS. Psychedelic drugs will confuse neurotransmitters by exaggerating and distorting messages and by creating visual and auditory images in the brain. Studies show that brain images are altered when methamphetamine, alcohol, nicotine, or cocaine are present in the body. All addictive drugs deplete the brain's receptors for dopamine (see Fig. 56.3).

Endorphins are hormones released by the hypothalamus and pituitary glands that relieve both pain and create a general feeling of well-being. The level of endorphins in the human body varies from person to person. Individuals who have lower levels of endorphins may be more likely to have depression or other AMI. The term "endorphins" comes from endogenous morphine: endogenous being produced in the body and morphine referring to the opioid painkiller whose actions they imitate. Endorphin and enkephalin neurotransmitters have an opiate-like effect on the brain, thereby causing the individual to experience a feeling of well-being.

Genetic Factors

Researchers have not yet been able to isolate the specific gene responsible for substance abuse, but it is believed that several modified genes may contribute to addiction. Genes that interfere with serotonin metabolism and that affect the serotonin-dopamine balance in the

brain have been implicated in a multitude of mental health disorders. Such disorders include alcoholism, drug addiction, depression, suicide, aggressive behaviors, antisocial borderline personality disorder, phobias, panic attacks, eating disorders, and attention-deficit/hyperactivity disorder.

Additionally, individuals who are born with the inability to produce sufficient quantities of endorphins and enkephalin can have a genetic predisposition toward opiate and alcohol addiction. Additionally, they are often codiagnosed with mental health disorders and may look for alternative means to adjust their moods.

Environmental Factors

Friends and social media influence addictive behaviors and SUDs, but the greatest environmental influence is family dynamics. Early family life experiences, interactions, parenting styles, and levels of supervision highly contribute to the development of later mental health difficulties and SUDs. It is important that children develop strategies to cope with stress during the early formative years of life. When these strategies are dysfunctional or maladjusted in younger years, they can lead to risky or self-destructive behaviors during the teen and young adult years.

Although substance abuse prevention programs for youth are found in schools, the media, and the community, they are insufficient by themselves. Without parental supervision, consistent discipline, and dedicated family relationships, community programs are not as effective.

Families play an important role in determining how children respond to the temptation to use alcohol, cigarettes, and illegal drugs. Substance abuse by one family member affects all members of the family in some way. Family members feel many of the emotions experienced by the addict, although they tend to suppress their feelings. Often their confidence and self-esteem are diminished, they experience depression, and one-third become chemically dependent themselves (Fig. 56.4).

COVID-19 Impact on SUDs and Mental Health

The COVID-19 pandemic adversely impacted adults by exacerbating use of alcohol or drugs among people who had used drugs before the pandemic. Additionally, those who were diagnosed with mental health and substance use disorders also saw a rise in substance use. During the pandemic, about 4 in 10 adults reported symptoms of anxiety or depressive disorder.[13]

TREATMENT OF SUBSTANCE MISUSE

Behavioral Treatment

It is often stated that substance abusers must "hit rock bottom" in their lives before they willingly seek help. Reaching rock bottom often means that they are unemployed and lack emotional support from friends and family. The most effective treatments for substance abuse occur when the abuser is motivated to seek medical intervention, behavioral changes, and social reinforcement, although treatment does not need to be voluntary to be effective. Court-appointed treatments and sanctions or enticements provided by family or employers can also result in effective treatment.

No single treatment is appropriate for all individuals. Effective treatment addresses multiple needs of the individual, including medical, psychological, social, vocational, and legal issues that the substance abuser must manage. Remaining in treatment for an adequate amount of time is critical to success. Most patients realize significant improvement by the end of 3 months in treatment. Individual or group counseling and other behavioral therapies are needed to help the patient develop skills to resist drug use. Recovery from a substance addiction can be a long-term process and frequently requires multiple treatments. Participation in self-help support programs such as Alcoholics Anonymous or Narcotics Anonymous during and after treatment often helps the individual to maintain abstinence.

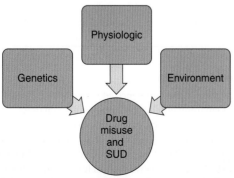

Fig. 56.4 Causes of Substance Misuse and SUDs.

Pharmacologic Treatment

Treatment for substance addiction may involve drug therapy. The use of pharmacology and psychotherapy together in the treatment of SUDs can greatly improve relapsing and facilitating longer periods of abstinence.

Pharmacological medications have three objectives:
1) Management of acute withdrawal syndromes through detoxification
2) Attenuation of cravings and urges to use illicit drugs
3) Prevention of relapse to compulsive drug use

Drugs that are usually prescribed to treat the symptoms of depression and anxiety disorders are often used to treat patients with addictive behavior disorders. Preventing self-harm and treatment retention can also be enhanced by the use of agonist therapies such as methadone and buprenorphine (see Table 56.5).

IMPLICATIONS FOR THE DENTAL HYGIENE PROCESS OF CARE

Despite increased awareness about addiction through public health efforts, the number of patients with a history of substance abuse has been consistently growing. Oral healthcare providers can expect to see an increase in patients who misuse alcohol and illicit substances.

Chemically dependent patients must be identified so that they can be treated safely. Extra caution must be taken to minimize drug interactions and adverse effects while providing care; however, substance abuse treatment is not within the scope of dental hygiene practice. It is helpful if oral healthcare settings develop simple protocols for referrals for patients with SUDs and have a list of community resources available. Brochures about specific programs can be provided, or the patient can be given the telephone number of the National Council on Alcohol and Drug Dependence (see Box 56.7).

Assessment

Only about 10% of patients who have an SUD are identified by healthcare providers; however, several visits over time for dental hygiene services may reveal behaviors that can be confirmed by a well-focused health history and a thorough extraoral and intraoral examination.

Health History

In the health history interview, the dental hygienist identifies all current medications the patient is taking to avoid possible drug interactions between a prescribed or an abused substance and medications offered in the oral health setting. Such interactions may pose a life-threatening situation for the patient.

TABLE 56.5 **Pharmacologic Agents Used in the Treatment of SUD**	
Substance	**Purpose**
Alcohol	
Acamprosate	Decreases cravings and urges for alcohol
Disulfiram (Antabuse)	Blocks the metabolism of alcohol
Naltrexone (Trexan)	Decreases or eliminates cravings for alcohol
Opioids	
Buprenorphine	Suppresses and reduces cravings for opioids
Methadone	Reduces opioid cravings and withdrawal and blocks the effects of opioids
Naltrexone	Blocks the euphoric and sedative effects of opioids
Naloxone	Prevents opioid overdose; naloxone reverses the toxic effects of the overdose

BOX 56.7 Patient Education Information

1. Discuss the risk of negative interactions between local anesthetics and the misused or abused substance.
2. Describe how the misused or abused substance affects oral and general health. Inform patients that antibiotic premedication before dental hygiene care may be necessary to prevent infective endocarditis or to manage an immunocompromised status.
3. Stress the need for routine professional care, optimal self-care, and proper nutrition. Identify oral manifestations of SUD/AUD and malnutrition in the patient's own mouth.
4. Tailor biofilm removal techniques specific to the patient's abilities.
5. Recommend nonalcoholic antimicrobial mouth rinses and fluoride rinses for alcoholics.
6. Inform patients with AUD that alcohol is a risk factor for oral cancer.
7. Inform patients with a history of AUD on Antabuse that over-the-counter and prescription mouth rinses (antibacterial and fluoride) may contain up to 30% alcohol and should be avoided.

BOX 56.8 Red Flags for Suspicion of SUDs

- Unreliable; frequently misses appointments
- Careless in appearance and hygiene
- Lapses in memory and/or concentration
- Alcohol on breath
- Speech is slurred; appearance of intoxication
- Needle marks on arm
- Rapid mood swings (within minutes)
- Frequently requests written excuses from work
- Frequently requests specific medication for pain
- Calls the dental office and complains of severe pain and requests that a prescription for pain medication be given without making an appointment with the dentist
- High tolerance to sedatives and analgesics
- Pupils are abnormally dilated or constricted

Questions about substances used and routes of administration should appear on dental office health history forms. When reviewing the patient's responses and when interacting with the patient, the dental hygienist looks for signs of substance abuse. If the dental hygienist suspects the patient may be dependent on a substance, that information should be recorded in the patient's dental record. Specific objective observations, patient behavior, and assessment findings such as pupil changes or needle marks should be recorded using objective terminology.

Patients are often reluctant to reveal alcohol or drug use because of the social stigma associated with substance abuse. Also, many substance abusers are in denial and will not admit to any type of dependence when asked. Chronic drinkers, in particular, are often overlooked in the dental setting. However, the astute dental hygienist recognizes signs and symptoms of dependence and discusses the possibility of a substance abuse problem with the patient in a nonjudgmental manner. Recognition of a drug abuse problem by a healthcare professional may prompt the abuser to seek help. It is essential that patients understand that the reason for obtaining information is to protect them from health risks and that all information will remain confidential.

When abuse is suspected, it is recommended that the dental hygienist ask the following questions:
1. Have you ever felt the need to cut down on your drinking or drug use?
2. Have you ever felt bad or guilty about your drinking or drug use?
3. Have you ever used drugs or had a drink first thing in the morning as an eye-opener to steady your nerves or to feel normal?

If the patient answers "yes" to two or more of these questions, then the dental hygienist should strongly suspect abuse and consider how to motivate the patient to seek treatment. It is necessary to determine if the patient "self-medicated" for the dental appointment. If the patient used any form of drugs or alcohol before the appointment, then the care plan for that day may need to be modified or canceled to avoid any drug interactions and/or drug-associated behavioral problems.

Extraoral Examination
The general appearance of patients can alert the dental hygienist to the possibility of substance abuse. Do they look substantially older than their stated age, have a disheveled appearance, have poor personal hygiene, insist on wearing sunglasses, and wear long sleeves even in hot weather (perhaps to cover needle marks)? Are alcohol or other odors detected on their breath? Do they appear to be lethargic or intoxicated without the accompanying odor of alcohol? Do they experience tremors? Look at patients' eyes for signs of substance abuse (see Box 56.8).

Needle marks in the antecubital fossae and forearms or bruises and increased pigmentation over veins caused by multiple injections observed during the taking of a blood pressure reading may indicate illicit drug use. Subcutaneous "popping" of heroin can cause skin abscesses. Crack abusers will often have burns and scars on the thumb of the dominant hand from repeated use of a disposable lighter. Multiple healed and healing burns or abrasions may be the result of physical trauma experienced while the patient was under the influence of alcohol or drugs. Snorting or inhaling substances can burn nasal passages, cause nosebleeds, and significantly damage nasal structures. Often, patients continually sniff their noses and use handkerchiefs or tissues.

The patient's behavior and speech should be watched for signs of confusion, disorientation, lethargy, lack of concentration, or memory impairment. Extreme depression or agitation may indicate a drug overdose.

Tremors of the hands, tongue, and eyelids may be signs of alcohol withdrawal. Other extraoral signs of AUD include the following:
1. Redness of facial skin and spider petechiae on the nose from dilated blood vessels
2. Yellowish facial skin from jaundice due to liver disease
3. Facial trauma due to falls when intoxicated
4. Angular cheilitis due to vitamin B deficiency
5. Red or swollen eyes

Intraoral Examination
Placement of drugs directly in the vestibule or sublingually may cause localized tissue necrosis. Gingival lesions may be caused by cocaine placement. Alcohol and drug abusers often crave sweets. Consequently, large dark areas of buccal cervical caries from ingesting large quantities of carbohydrates may be present. Methadone abusers develop "meth mouth" (Fig. 56.5), a condition that results in rampant caries and evidence of advanced periodontal disease.

Other oral manifestations associated with substance abuse include oral candidiasis as a result of immunosuppression, **glossodynia** (pain in the tongue) from malnutrition, and immunosuppression because of a secondary addiction to alcohol. Cocaine users tend to have severe bruxism, causing flat cuspal planes on premolars and molars. Because the substance abuser's body is burdened by drug use, tissue healing is affected (see Tables 56.6 and 56.7).

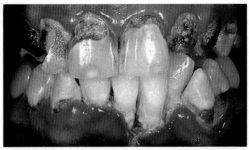

Fig. 56.5 "Meth Mouth." (Courtesy Dr. Stephen Wagner.)

Dental Hygiene Diagnosis and Care Planning

Substance abuse must be addressed in care planning. People who are deeply immersed in drug abuse will probably seek dental care only when they are in severe pain. Because the pain sensation can be diminished by the use of drugs, the dental problem is usually in an advanced state. Substance-abusing patients may request the use of nitrous oxide sedation for treatment and specific medication for pain. It is important that oral care professionals have knowledge of the type and amount of drugs patients have taken before planning any pain control or other care (see the Critical Thinking Scenarios in Box 56.9).

TABLE 56.6   Additional Assessment Findings Associated With SUD and AUD

Abused Substance	Oral Findings	Treatment Considerations
Methamphetamines	Xerostomia, increased caries, bruxism (extreme tooth wear in Ecstasy users) leading to trismus. "Meth mouth" induces excessive clenching and bruxism, osteonecrosis of mandible	Drugs can increase bleeding and interfere with coagulation. Chronic abusers should have blood tests before surgery or periodontal treatment. Abusers generally have poor oral hygiene with rampant caries. Treatment should be deferred for a minimum of 6 hours after the last administration of methamphetamine, and local anesthetic containing a vasoconstrictor should not be used when the patient is intoxicated to avoid a hypertensive crisis.
Alcohol	Tooth erosion from sugar in alcohol or regurgitation, sialosis, xerostomia, stomatitis due to nutritional deficiencies and anemia, orofacial injuries from accidents or violence, severe infections due to immunosuppression, poor oral hygiene, gingival bleeding on probing, coated tongue, glossitis due to nutritional deficiency, attrition related to bruxism, erosion related to vomiting, broken teeth due to accidents while intoxicated, cervical buccal caries Predisposition to oropharyngeal cancer Predisposition to periodontal disease	Increased dosage of drugs for anesthesia and sedation. Increase in bleeding after surgery. Increased healing time due to immunosuppression.
Cocaine	Placement of cocaine in maxillary premolar area to test the purity of a drug sample can cause localized gingival and alveolar bone necrosis. Increased caries from carbohydrates added to cocaine as filler. Bruxism, clenching, and noncarious tooth wear are a common finding. Gingival erosions and ulcerative lesions may be present. Chronic sinusitis, epistaxis, and nasal crusting are frequent adverse effects. Long-term intranasal use can lead to perforations of the hard palate and nasal septum. Recurrent chronic maxillary sinusitis, burns, blisters, and sores; use of the powder form intraorally causes a substantial decrease in saliva pH, creating an opportunity for caries-causing bacteria.	Possible spontaneous gingival bleeding from thrombocytopenia. Critical life-threatening interaction between cocaine and anesthetics containing epinephrine. Defer dental treatment for 6 to 24 hours after the last administration of cocaine.
Opiates and opioids (heroin, morphine, methadone)	Salivary hypofunction causing xerostomia, caries, burning mouth, and taste impairment; opioids induce a preference for sweet foods; poor oral hygiene, and nutritional deficiencies that contribute to oral health complications. Methadone treatment for opiate addiction is a sugary syrup taken orally, which may cause an increase in caries.	Increased possibility of hepatitis, HIV infection from drug injection. Poor pain tolerance. Increased possibility of bacterial endocarditis in scaling procedures. Increased bleeding from thrombocytopenia. Interactions between opioids and dentally prescribed medications.
Barbiturates and benzodiazepines	Xerostomia, lesions on oral mucosa in the area of drug use	Tolerance to sedative drugs
Cannabis (marijuana)	Leukoplakia and increased incidence of lingual carcinoma; gingival enlargement. Cannabis stomatitis, leukoedema of the buccal mucosa and hyperkeratosis. Periodontitis can be present in young adults due to frequent marijuana use.	Interaction between cannabis and anesthetics containing epinephrine Abusers generally have poor oral and periodontal health. Cannabis-intoxicated patients may experience acute anxiety and dysphoria during treatment. Local anesthetic containing epinephrine may prolong tachycardia following an acute dose of cannabis. Chronic smokers of cannabis have increased risk of developing oral leukoplakia and oral cancer, oral candidiasis, and other oral infections.
LSD, PCP	Orofacial injuries experienced while "tripping." Bruxism resulting in trismus.	Flashback that may cause panic attacks can occur owing to a stressful dental environment. Respiratory depression if opioids are prescribed.
Inhalants	"Glue-sniffer's rash," erythema around the labial borders, oral frostbite.	Anesthetic toxicity is increased; sensitization to epinephrine can occur; increased risk of seizures.

TABLE 56.7 Precautions When Treating Patients With SUD and AUD

Drug	Precautions
Alcohol	Alcoholism may result in liver disease. Prior to dental surgery, a medical consult is recommended to establish the ability of the patient to control bleeding.
Cocaine, Ecstasy, and methamphetamines	Anesthetics containing epinephrine should be avoided due to a systemic increase in blood pressure that usually follows use.
Cannabis (marijuana)	Use of local anesthetic containing epinephrine can cause prolonged tachycardia.
Opioids	Do not prescribe opioids analgesics in suspected abusers of any drug. Consult with the patient's interprofessional team concerning pain management prior to treating pain-producing procedures.

Patients in recovery programs, however, may seek long-neglected dental treatment as part of their attempt to achieve total body health. It is under these circumstances that the dental hygienist will most probably be providing care. Recovering addicts may be extremely cautious or anxious about taking any type of medication, making it difficult to control pain during scaling and root debriding procedures. Some chemically dependent patients also may experience a tolerance to sedatives and analgesics. For patients recovering from substance abuse, pain control should be coordinated with the patient's appropriate interprofessional licensed specialist (see Box 56.10). In addition, chemically dependent patients can experience emotional anxiety or instability and may be able to tolerate only short appointments. For this reason, the use of multiple short (20-minute) appointments may be necessary.

After a thorough assessment and consultation with the patient's primary care provider, if indicated, complete diagnostic statements are formulated by the dental hygienist based on identified human need deficits. Once the diagnostic statements are complete, patient goals are set. Care planning priorities include setting realistic goals with the patient to improve oral self-care and to enable the patient to undergo periodontal scaling and root debridement with a minimum of discomfort. Also, because malnutrition is clearly associated with substance abuse, dietary analysis, nutritional counseling, or referral to a registered dietician may be indicated. With the patient's permission, consultation with interprofessional team members aids the dental hygienist in planning effective care (see Box 56.11).

Implementation

Because good oral health and a pleasant smile add to an individual's self-esteem, receiving necessary dental hygiene care may have a significant positive impact on recovery from substance abuse. A discussion concerning referral for treatment of substance abuse should be initiated as soon as possible.

Appointments

Patients with SUDs, AMI, and SMI may experience emotional instability or take no responsibility for their behavior. As a result, they may not keep scheduled appointments. If the patient arrives too late for an appointment, the appointment should be canceled. If the patient fails to come to an appointment, all remaining appointments should be canceled. Failure to keep appointments should not

BOX 56.9 Critical Thinking Scenarios

Case 1

Mr. S., age 24, was scheduled for routine dental hygiene care. This is his first-ever dental appointment for preventive care. His last dental appointment was for extraction of teeth 2 and 15. He has a history of asthma, smokes a pack of cigarettes a day, and is currently taking 5 mg of prednisone twice a day. He reports that he took part in a drug and alcohol rehabilitation program 1 year ago. His girlfriend has suggested he "do something about his teeth." His chief complaint is that his teeth are discolored, are sensitive to cold, and are "soft" and decay easily; he also states that his mouth feels dry. Intraorally, his clinical gingival attachment loss ranges from 3 to 7 mm, with bleeding on probing in the mandibular anterior teeth. His gingiva appears pale except on the mandibular anterior, where the gingival margins are magenta. The tissues are edematous and have rolled gingival margins. The tissue consistency is spongy and the interdental papillae are blunted. There is inadequate attached gingiva on the facial and lingual areas of teeth 3 and 14 and the mandibular anterior teeth. He has heavy subgingival and supragingival calculus on the mandibular anterior teeth and generalized interproximal nodules throughout the mouth. He has a class 2 AAP periodontal classification. Eight carious lesions are identified. He brushes his teeth once a day using a medium-bristle toothbrush and uses no other dental aids. His community water is not fluoridated. His diet includes no milk or vegetables, and he eats two king-size chocolate candy bars daily. He is aware that the status of his oral health is poor.

1. What are the dental hygiene diagnoses for this patient?
2. Develop a dental hygiene care plan including goals and interventions for this patient.
3. What patient education issues should be addressed?
4. What factors could be contributing to this patient's periodontal health?
5. Are there any contraindications to this patient's care?

Case 2

Ms. B., age 20, is a new patient for dental hygiene care. She completed the health and dental history form when she arrived for the appointment. After reviewing the health history, the dental hygienist noted that Ms. B. answered "yes" to the question regarding drug or alcohol addiction. The dental hygienist asked for further clarification. Ms. B. told the dental hygienist that she had been released from a drug and alcohol addiction program 1 year ago. Ms. B. had been sent to the treatment program for her cocaine use as an alternative to jail. The dental hygienist asked if Ms. B. had been able to abstain from using cocaine since she left the program. She encouraged Ms. B. to be totally honest in her response and stressed that if Ms. B. was currently using cocaine, it could cause a life-threatening situation if she were to receive a dental anesthetic. Ms. B. confided that dental appointments always caused her great anxiety and that she did self-medicate before coming to her appointment.

1. What may happen as a result of the patient's drug use before the dental hygiene appointment?
2. Should the dental hygienist proceed with care, and if so, what care should be rendered?
3. What are the moral and ethical issues in this situation?

be reinforced as acceptable behavior. Because of potential unreliability and to provide additional incentive to show up for care, payment should be received in advance of treatment. Esthetic restorations should be treated last to ensure that patients show up for all necessary treatment.

It is unethical to abandon patients once they are accepted for treatment in a dental practice. If a patient continually fails to keep scheduled treatment appointments, the dental office may dismiss the patient from the practice by written notification. Legal guidelines dictate that the patient must be assured, in writing, that emergency dental treatment

---

BOX 56.10   Interprofessional Providers Who Cotreat Dental Patients With SUD/AUD

- Physician
- Nurse practitioner
- Physician assistant
- Social worker
- Physical therapist
- Occupational therapist
- Pharmacist
- Speech-language pathologist

BOX 56.11   Legal, Ethical, and Safety Issues

Patients' personal, social, and health history forms must be kept confidential

1. Patient behavior, assessment findings, professional recommendations, referrals, and treatment should be recorded in the patient's permanent record. Personal opinions and judgmental statements are inappropriate.
2. Some states have parental notification laws that direct healthcare professionals to reveal knowledge of any medical or psychological conditions found during an examination to a minor's parent or legal guardian. Knowledge of the statutes in the legal jurisdiction is important so that confidential information about minors is managed correctly.
3. Keep prescription pads out of sight and medications locked in a place unknown to patients.
4. Dentists should never write a prescription for a pain medication without knowing the patient's history and without first examining the patient.
5. With approval from patients being treated for substance misuse, contact their primary care physician and/or mental health professional when planning oral care.
6. Reduce the patient's anxiety level by keeping appointments short and comfortable.
7. Perform only those procedures the patient can easily tolerate.
8. Keep oral care products containing alcohol in a secure place away from persons with a history of alcohol misuse.
9. Do not render treatment that may cause an interaction between a misused substance and dental anesthetics or other drugs offered as part of healthcare.
10. Continue to encourage patients to seek help for substance abuse if they have been through a treatment program and have relapsed.
11. Identifying dental patients who are chemically dependent is important; however, substance misuse treatment is not within the scope of dental hygiene practice.

---

will be provided for a length of time sufficient to obtain a new dentist of record, usually 30 days or more from receipt of the dismissal letter. When the patient makes a request in writing, all dental records must be forwarded to the new dentist, along with notification of what services are still needed.

Pain and Anxiety Control

Adequate pain and anxiety control is a necessity when treating the patient with an SUD because unrelieved pain may trigger a relapse. Local anesthetics with vasoconstrictors can increase cardiovascular risks and cerebral hemorrhage in substance users. Cocaine abusers experience convulsions with the use of lidocaine. Using Oraqix (a combination of lidocaine/prilocaine 2.5%/2.5% gel supplied in cartridges) can also increase the risks due to the absorption of significant amounts of vasoconstrictors. It is recommended that dental professionals consult with the patient's primary care physician or interprofessional team members to mutually coordinate and plan treatment that includes conscious sedation for dental procedures.

The use of long-acting local anesthetics for periodontal therapy should be considered to reduce the overall amount of anesthetics. Long-acting anesthetics such as 0.5% bupivacaine with 1:200,000 epinephrine could delay the onset and reduce the intensity of postoperative pain, though bupivacaine has also been shown to cause severe toxicity including cardiovascular arrest. Levobupivacaine and ropivacaine may be safer alternatives for long-acting anesthetics.

For postoperative pain, nonsteroidal antiinflammatory medications (NSAIDs) are recommended because all other pain medications are potentially addictive. Studies have shown that combining ibuprofen and acetaminophen was just as effective as some opioids (oxycodone, hydrocodone, or codeine) at relieving moderate to severe pain.[15,16] If the dentist feels that narcotic analgesics or sedative hypnotics for postoperative pain are indicated, patients with an SUD require a higher dose than nonsubstance-abusing patients, and a limited number of doses should be prescribed. Analgesic depressants may be indicated unless the patient is taking other illicit depressants at the same time. Anesthesia and pain control may be difficult to achieve for heroin-addicted patients who are in a methadone treatment program because they have developed a tolerance to the analgesic and euphoric effects of their daily methadone dose. Consultation with the patient's physician/interprofessional team is necessary to determine the best method to alleviate patient discomfort.

Control of patient anxiety also can help alleviate the patient's perception of pain. Pain perception has both physical and psychological components. If the patient trusts the clinician, emotional distress can be minimized, reducing the perception of pain. A dental hygienist with excellent communication skills and empathy can help dispel the patient's anxiety.

Some patients with an SUD may see dental treatment as an opportunity to obtain prescriptions for abused substances. Consequently, they often will exaggerate their response to pain in an effort to obtain a prescription for a strong pain control medication. Prescription pads should be kept out of sight and inaccessible to patients. Pain medication in the dental office should be locked in a place unknown to patients. Drug-seeking patients often call the dental office, complain that they are in severe pain, and request that a prescription for pain medication be given to them without making an appointment with the doctor. Dental offices should maintain a policy of prescribing medications only after the dentist has evaluated the patient.

Dental Hygiene Care

Because short (20-minute) appointments are suggested, the dental hygienist may be able to complete only limited treatment at each appointment. If there is a need for prophylactic antibiotic premedication, the dental hygienist ensures that the patient has taken premedication as directed. If a patient identifies a history of intravenous drug use, the need for prophylactic antibiotic premedication must be considered for the following reasons:

1. Many intravenous drug users develop venous thrombosis and organic valvular heart disease.
2. Damage to the tricuspid valve between the right atrium and ventricle is often associated with substance abuse.
3. Intravenous drug use can result in endocarditis caused by *Staphylococcus aureus* found on nonsterile needles.

Consequently, all patients with a history of intravenous drug abuse should be evaluated by their physician before dental or dental hygiene care to determine if any of these conditions exist, indicating the need for antibiotic premedication.

General supragingival and subgingival debridement, which will enable the patient to initiate adequate homecare, may be all that the patient will tolerate in a short appointment. Such treatment would allow the dentist to place needed restorations in a state of improved gingival health. This improved tissue response is especially important when cervical restorations are placed because inflamed gingival margins can interfere with the placement of restorative materials.

The patient's response to the initial scaling visit will dictate further appointment planning. The patient may be able to tolerate quadrant scaling and root debridement so that optimum treatment for periodontal disease may be provided. Confirmation from the patient's physician that there is no immunosuppression or kidney or liver damage should be sought before aggressive nonsurgical or surgical periodontal therapy is undertaken. The use of an ultrasonic scaling instrument is indicated to reduce the incidence of a transient bacteremia.

It is best to postpone definitive scaling and root debridement until a later time if the patient is unable or unwilling to comply with treatment. In this case, a short, 2- or 3-month continued-care interval is indicated. Once patients have progressed further with recovery from addiction, they may be more tolerant of dental hygiene care.

Oral Health Instruction

Lack of oral hygiene is common among those with SUDs. Oral health instruction should begin with basic toothbrushing instructions and encouragement to practice toothbrushing daily. Once daily toothbrushing techniques have been mastered or a power toothbrush has been recommended and demonstrated, interdental oral physiotherapy aids can be introduced. The choice of aid will depend on the patient's physical and mental capabilities and the type of embrasures present. If the patient is incapable of the fine motor skills necessary to manipulate dental floss, other aids should be suggested. Interdental wooden stimulators, interproximal brushes, or a power floss aid may be easier for the patient to use. If patients are frustrated by an inability to master a technique, they will most likely do nothing. The patient in addiction recovery has already been required to make numerous behavioral changes and may see a complex oral hygiene regimen as an additional burden.

Suggesting a daily fluoride rinse regimen is appropriate, especially if the patient has a moderate to high caries risk. Use of fluoride therapy is also important for heroin addicts enrolled in a methadone program: the daily methadone dose is administered as a sugary syrup. Antimicrobial rinses to control gingivitis may also be recommended. For alcoholics, it is important to recommend products that do not contain alcohol to avoid contributing to the negative health effects they experience from their alcohol use. Even very small amounts of alcohol ingested by a patient taking disulfiram or similar alcohol-sensitizing drugs can cause an emergency. Therefore alcohol-free fluoride mouth rinses and antimicrobial mouth rinses are recommended for homecare and for preprocedural rinses. Xerostomia may be a result of antidepressant medications prescribed for the patient. Suggest that the patient sip water frequently during the day or use xylitol-containing gums or mints to reduce the effects of dry mouth.

The dental hygienist may also suggest that the patient eat a well-balanced diet and limit cariogenic foods to encourage both oral and general health. Positive reinforcement and encouragement should be given to patients for any improvement in their oral hygiene.

Evaluation

The outcomes of dental hygiene care can serve as positive reinforcement for a healthier lifestyle for those patients in recovery. If evaluation of dental hygiene care occurs 6 to 8 weeks after initial debridement, patients may be further along in their recovery and may be more receptive to additional periodontal therapy, if needed. For those patients who are not in recovery, the evaluation of dental hygiene care provides another opportunity to encourage patients to seek help for their substance abuse. The initial recall or continued-care interval should be 3 months after treatment. This is especially important if there was extensive periodontal therapy complicated by immunosuppression.

DENTAL PROFESSIONALS AND SUBSTANCE USE DISORDERS

AUD, SUD, AMI, and SMI are widespread in American culture, and dental professionals are not exempt from addiction. In fact, the prevalence of substance abuse among professionals may be the same or higher than in the general population. Dental professionals can self-prescribe medications; they have the opportunity for easy access to abuse drugs. Many states have begun monitoring prescription-writing habits of dentists.

Why Professionals Are at Risk for Chemical Dependence

Healthcare professionals are usually required to have high academic grades to be admitted to a professional educational program. Once accepted, professional education requires hours of instruction to reach competence. Students enrolled in healthcare educational programs are usually competitive, overworked, narrowly specialized, self-sacrificing, and grade conscious.

Dental and dental hygiene students have their work continually criticized by faculty. Trying to prove one's competence can easily lead to little sleep, an unbalanced and emotionally unrewarding lifestyle, physical and emotional exhaustion, stress and anxiety, irritability, and depression. Completion of a professional program often requires students to become "self-denying," and their personal lives become of secondary importance to their education. This situation can lead to emotional conflicts within themselves and their families. Often students will use stimulants to enhance their performance at school or alcohol on the weekend to relieve stress. This cycle often continues once the student has become a practicing professional.

Although taught to recognize symptoms of chemical dependence in patients, health professionals rarely recognize addiction in themselves. Most are convinced that they are in control of their substance abuse and can stop whenever they choose. Chemical dependence may be the underlying cause of licensure suspension or malpractice.

Many state dental associations sponsor educational programs and workshops on addiction within the profession. Diversion from the court system to a treatment program is available to addicted professionals unless they have engaged in unethical treatment by causing harm to patients or violating major criminal laws. Health and well-being committees of state dental associations help colleagues with addiction problems. Confidentiality is ensured, and referrals may be made anonymously. The committees may contract for services through the state medical society and provide appropriate referrals, posttreatment follow-up, monitoring, and advocacy.

Many professionals decide that it is time to stop drug abuse when they are faced with the loss of their professional license. Some seek help through residential or outpatient formal recovery programs, and others seek help through self-help programs. Dental support groups such as Caduceus meetings, which are modeled on the principles of Alcoholics Anonymous, may also provide psychological support for professionals in recovery.

KEY CONCEPTS

- Substance use disorders are chronic, cyclic diseases that affect millions of people in the United States, including oral healthcare professionals.
- Substance addiction is a compulsive use of a substance despite adverse medical and social consequences.
- Psychological and physical dependence on drugs and genetic predisposition are the reasons people continue substance abuse.
- Tolerance to alcohol and drugs creates the need for continued increases in the amounts used to gain the same effect.
- Dental hygienists need to identify chemically dependent patients for the following reasons:
  - Avoid interactions between drugs offered at the dental office, such as local anesthetics or nitrous oxide–oxygen analgesia, and abused substances
  - Determine the need for antibiotic premedication before beginning dental hygiene care
  - Recognize increased risk of immunosuppression, heart disease, liver disease, human immunodeficiency virus, and hepatitis B, C, and D
  - Recognize drug-seeking behavior of patients with a history of misuse
  - Modify care plans
- Addictive behaviors are the result of genetic, environmental, psychological, and physiological factors.
- Culture, ethnicity, poverty, behavioral problems, child abuse, peer rejection, and environment can be risk factors for SUDs.
- Opioid abuse is a crisis in the United States.
- Drugs affect the transmission of messages among the central, autonomic, and peripheral nervous systems by interfering with neurotransmission. Key neurotransmitters include dopamine, serotonin, and endorphins.
- With the legalization of marijuana in several US states, marijuana use has increased exponentially.
- Specific extraoral and intraoral findings are associated with the specific type of substances that are misused or abused.
- The American Dental Association encourages treatment rather than punishment of oral care professionals who seek help for substance abuse.

REFERENCES

1. Substance Abuse and Mental Health Services Administration. *Key Substance Use and Mental Health Indicators in the United States: Results from the 2020 National Survey on Drug Use and Health (HHS Publication No. PEP21-07-01-003, NSDUH Series H-56)*. Center for Behavioral Health Statistics and Quality, Substance Abuse and Mental Health Services Administration; 2021. Retrieved from https://www.samhsa.gov/data/. Accessed June 30, 2022.
2. Ross S, Peselow E. Co-occurring psychotic and addictive disorders: neurobiology and diagnosis. *Clin Neuropharmacol.* 2012;35(5):235–243. https://doi.org/10.1097/WNF.0b013e318261e193.
3. Kelly TM, Daley DC. Integrated treatment of substance use and psychiatric disorders. *Soc Work Public Health.* 2013;28(0):388–406. https://doi.org/10.1080/19371918.2013.774673.
4. Substance Abuse and Mental Health Services Administration. *Key Substance Use and Mental Health Indicators in the United States: Results from the 2020 National Survey on Drug Use and Health (HHS Publication No. PEP21-07-01-003, NSDUH Series H-56)*. Center for Behavioral Health Statistics and Quality, Substance Abuse and Mental Health Services Administration; 2021. Retrieved from https://www.samhsa.gov/data/. Accessed July 6, 2022.
5. Center for Behavioral Health Statistics and Quality. *Results from the 2018 National Survey on Drug Use and Health: Detailed Tables.* SAMHSA; 2019. https://www.samhsa.gov/data/report/2018-nsduh-detailed-tables. Accessed June 9, 2022.
6. Substance Abuse and Mental Health Services Administration. *Preliminary Findings from Drug-Related Emergency Department Visits, 2021; Drug Abuse Warning Network (HHS Publication No. PEP22-07-03-001).* Center for Behavioral Health Statistics and Quality, Substance Abuse and Mental Health Services Administration; 2022. Retrieved from https://www.samhsa.gov/data/. Accessed June 12, 2022
7. Substance Abuse and Mental Health Services Administration (SAMHSA), Center for Behavioral Health Statistics and Quality. 2019 National Survey on Drug Use and Health. Table 5.4A—Alcohol Use Disorder in Past Year Among Persons Aged 12 or Older, by Age Group and Demographic Characteristics: Numbers in Thousands, 2018 and 2019. https://www.samhsa.gov/data/sites/default/files/reports/rpt29394/NSDUHDetailedTabs2019/NSDUHDetTabsSect5pe2019.htm?s=5.4&#tab5-4a. Accessed June 15, 2022.
8. Bagnardi V, Rota M, Botteri E, et al. Alcohol consumption and site-specific cancer risk: a comprehensive dose-response meta-analysis. *Br J Cancer.* 2015 Feb 3;112(3):580–593. PMCID: PMC4453639.
9. GBD 2016 Alcohol Collaborators. Alcohol use and burden for 195 countries and territories, 1990–2016: a systematic analysis for the Global Burden of Disease Study 2016. *Lancet.* 2018 Sep 22;392(10152):1015–1035.
10. National Institute on Drug Abuse. Drugs of Abuse. Available at: https://nida.nih.gov/. Accessed May 1, 2022.
11. Substance Abuse Center for Behavioral Health Statistics and Quality. Results from the 2018 National Survey on Drug Use and Health: Detailed Tables. SAMHSA. https://www.samhsa.gov/data/report/2018-nsduh-detailed-tables. Accessed June 20, 2022.
12. Johnston L, O'Malley P, Miech R, Bachman J, Schulenberg J. *Monitoring the Future National Survey Results on Drug Use: 1975-2015: Overview: Key Findings on Adolescent Drug Use.* Institute for Social Research, The University of Michigan; 2015.
13. 2020 National Survey on Drug Use and Health (NSDUH). SAMHSA Available at: https://www.samhsa.gov/data/release/2020-national-survey-drug-use-and-health-nsduh-releases. Accessed July 1, 2022.
14. Rizo J. Mechanism of neurotransmitter release coming into focus. *Protein Sci.* 2018;27(8):1364–1391.
15. Moore PA, Hersh EV. Combining ibuprofen and acetaminophen for acute pain management after third-molar extractions: translating clinical research to dental practice. *J Am Dent Assoc.* 2013;144(8):898–908. https://doi.org/10.14219/jada.archive.2013.0207. PMID: 23904576 https://pubmed.ncbi.nlm.nih.gov/23904576/. Accessed July 12, 2022.
16. Chang AK, Bijur PE, Esses D, Barnaby DP, Baer J. Effect of a single dose of oral opioid and nonopioid analgesics on acute extremity pain in the emergency department: a randomized clinical trial. *JAMA.* 2017;318(17):1661–1667. https://doi.org/10.1001/jama.2017.16190. PMID: 29114833; PMCID: PMC5818795 https://pubmed.ncbi.nlm.nih.gov/29114833/. Accessed July 12, 2022.

Eating Disorders

Lorraine Glassford and Laura L. MacDonald

PROFESSIONAL OPPORTUNITIES

One of the many roles required of a dental hygienist is to serve as a patient advocate. When a dental hygienist encounters a patient with an eating disorder, the dental hygienist has a responsibility to advocate for that patient. For example, dental hygienists can enable access to needed healthcare, facilitate honest disclosure about the disorder and the behaviors associated with it, promote healthy thinking and being, and help the patient obtain and maintain good oral and general health.

COMPETENCIES

1. Describe the diagnosis and epidemiology of both anorexia nervosa and bulimia nervosa.
2. Discuss oral and overall health effects of anorexia nervosa and bulimia nervosa.
3. Develop a dental hygiene care plan for a patient with an eating disorder that includes (a) engaging the patient in a dialogue of disclosure of an eating disorder, (b) assessing oral health needs, (c) planning for reduction of harm and promotion of oral health, (d) implementing dental hygiene interventions, and (e) evaluating outcomes of care.
4. Discuss the need for interprofessional collaboration for patient-centered care of a patient with an eating disorder.
5. List resources available to help patients with eating disorders.

INTRODUCTION

Eating disorders affect all of us in some way or another—either one personally has experienced an eating disorder or knows someone who has or is recovering from one. Eating is a fundamental human need; we need to eat to survive. What happens when eating, the act and thought of eating is the key barrier to being able to eat? The dental hygienist needs to know and respect that eating disorders are categorized as mental health disorders.[1]

This chapter focuses on two eating disorders, anorexia nervosa and bulimia nervosa. However, the dental hygienist should be aware that there are other eating disorders such as binge eating disorder, avoidant/restrictive food intake disorder (neophobia), and other disorders that fall under a category called *other specified feeding or eating disorders*, including night eating syndrome. To understand anorexia nervosa and bulimia nervosa is to realize that both are reflective of a complex interrelationship among biological, genetic, environmental, temporal, physiological, psychodevelopmental, neurochemical, and sociocultural factors.[1-4] The dental hygienist must stay abreast of clinical practice guidelines for eating disorders as these inform health professionals about best practices.

Although mental health counseling and the treatment of eating disorders are outside the scope of dental hygiene practice, the dental hygienist, as a primary healthcare provider, is ethically responsible to help the patient access healthcare. Eating disorders are a challenge for all—the patient, the patient's family and friends, healthcare professionals, and society. The challenge arises from the very nature of the illness, which includes the following: comorbidity with other mental health and medical conditions, insidious onset, secretive behaviors, and manipulation of the person's way of thinking about their body, eating habits, and personal health and wellness. When a person is diagnosed with an eating disorder, they can be so deeply engaged in the thinking associated with the disorder and the resultant body and mental dysfunction that the restructuring of thought to healthy habits and mindset is challenging to manage, often requiring many years for recovery. When a dental hygienist suspects that a patient has an eating disorder, the hygienist must address it and become a person in the patient's life who enables recovery from the illness rather than one who hesitates and vacillates, saying, "I should have…" or "I would have, but…," as illustrated in Box 57.1. The time to take action is now. The longer the eating disorder grips a patient, the more difficulty the patient may have fighting the illness and repossessing their life.

Regardless of whether the dental hygienist is using the Dental Hygiene Human Needs Conceptual (DH HNC) Model or the Oral Health-Related Quality of Life (OHRQL) Model to understand the role the dental hygienist plays with persons with eating disorders, the dental hygienist may find it challenging to identify the patient's needs, given the tendency for nondisclosure of this mental illness. From a DH HNC Model perspective, the dental hygienist in Box 57.1 missed the opportunity to help the patient reveal or disclose her illness by evading inquiry about the weight loss, which would have been related to a human need for protection from health risks. From an OHRQL Model perspective, the dental hygienist would have explored the patient's views on her health and relationship to weight loss with the intent of discovering the impact of the illness on the patient's oral health and quality of life. Importantly, the dental hygienist seeks to understand the patient's needs.

Because eating disorders are complex in terms of both cause and treatment, care is enhanced by a patient-centered collaborative practice approach involving many health professionals, such as specially trained psychologists for individual and family therapy; psychiatrists and social workers; physicians and nurses with experience with eating disorders; nutritionists and exercise therapists for education and the reorientation of eating and exercise habits; and the oral healthcare team for the support and treatment of oral manifestations of the illness (Fig. 57.1). The dental hygienist's collaboration with other health professionals as part of the patient's healthcare team is vital. For example, the dental hygienist informs the healthcare team about oral conditions; manages oral health risk and harm reduction; and reinforces consistent messages regarding recovery from the illness and participates in a team approach to care (Box 57.2).

When Phillip, the dental receptionist, comes into Sandra Hamm's dental hygiene room, he says, "Have you noticed how skinny Linda Pham is getting?"

"Yes, 2 months ago when she had her braces removed, she looked great," replies Sandra. "I did notice her weight loss when I walked by the reception area. It looks like she has lost at least 20 pounds. She's a waif of a figure now." Sandra makes a mental note to ask Linda about her weight loss during her dental hygiene appointment. Sandra suspects a possible eating disorder. Sandra has known Linda for most of Linda's 20 years, but she feels uncomfortable asking Linda such questions. Throughout the appointment, it becomes evident to Sandra that Linda is not behaving like herself. She is evasive when answering questions about her health history. By the end of the appointment, Sandra has not asked Linda about the weight loss and decides that perhaps it is none of her business.

A few months pass, and Linda's father arrives for his dental hygiene appointment. He discloses to Sandra that Linda has been hospitalized for anorexia nervosa. He apologizes for his own oral health state, saying, "All our attention has been centered on Linda. She nearly died from malnutrition. We've been busy with doctor appointments, family therapy sessions, and group support, and we've been just plain occupied with strategizing to support her as she recovers from this illness."

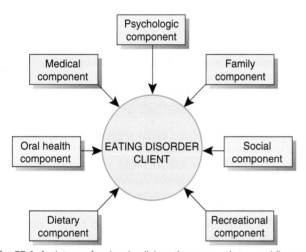

Fig. 57.1 An interprofessional collaboration approach to providing care to individuals with eating disorders.

A dental hygienist may be the first health professional to identify the oral and physical manifestations characteristic of eating disorders. Purging-type eating disorders, in particular, tend to result in tooth sensitivity. Pain is a driver to seek help; however, for the person with bulimia nervosa, it may be a cry for help for tooth sensitivity and not for the disorder itself. Whether the dental hygienist is coming to know the patient's needs, such as a human need for sound dentition and freedom from pain and/or stress or revealing functional status as per the OHRQL Model, the patient will likely be reluctant to acknowledge the gravity of the eating disorder and carefully protect the disorder as if it is a secret due to the nature of the illness (Box 57.3).

ANOREXIA NERVOSA

Anorexia nervosa is a mental illness.[1] The term *anorexia* literally means "loss of appetite." However, the patient with anorexia nervosa suppresses and denies the sensation of hunger. It is suspected that some

"Jayden, are you ready to have your parents come into the room?" asks Dr. Beckham, Jayden's psychiatrist.

"Oh, whatever. Let's just get this over with! I'm fine. You all are just overreacting. They're going to freak with your diagnosis of bulimia. I hate this! I wish everyone would just leave me alone. I'm 17 years old!" shouts Jayden back to Dr. Beckham and the healthcare team, Sally Friesen (social worker), Marlee Ford (nutritionist), and Darcy MacAlroy (nurse and case manager).

After team meetings with Jayden Black over the course of several appointments, Jayden has been informed that their behavior is consistent with that of a person with bulimia nervosa, a mental illness. Darcy invites Mr. and Mrs. Black into the conference room. Jayden does not even look at them; instead, they noticeably sit with their body in a closed position. Dr. Beckham welcomes them and informs them that Jayden is ready to discuss some behaviors that explain why they brought them to the eating disorder clinic program in the first place a couple of weeks ago.

Jayden begins to cry. "Mom, Dad, I'm so ashamed. I can barely say it, but for the last 7 months, I've forced myself to throw up five times a day. At first, I only did it once a day, and then I just kept doing it. Dr. Beckham says I have bulimia. Inside I know I do, and I am so embarrassed because I think it's disgusting. I can't seem to stop. I'm ready for help. I can't stop doing this on my own."

Mrs. Black replies, "We're all about helping you fight this illness. We'll fight it with you. You can count on us. Admitting you have bulimia is a great first step."

About 2 months ago, Mrs. Black began suspecting that Jayden had an eating disorder. Jayden was excusing themself from the supper table and disappearing. Further, Jayden was complaining about sensitive teeth. When Mrs. Black gently asked if Jayden was experiencing any issues with eating, Jayden denied any problem. In the end, Mrs. and Mr. Black persuaded Jayden to see Dr. Beckham, which Jayden did after initially being very reluctant and dismissive of the idea. Their healthcare team strongly recommended Jayden see their dental hygienist regarding ways to lessen the tooth sensitivity while they recovered and, in addition, that the dental team become part of the healthcare team—this required Jayden's consent. Their dental hygiene appointment is booked for next week.

"My dental hygienist was the first person to help me disclose that I had bulimia nervosa. When he looked in my mouth, he saw signs of erosion and asked me about them. It was how he asked me, his tone of voice—calm, kind, empathetic—that enabled me to be truthful with him. I had never ever spoken the words aloud before when I said them to him, 'I throw up. I throw up many times a day and have been doing this for a couple of years. I think I have bulimia.' My dental hygienist helped me contact an eating disorder clinic, and I am now on my way to recovery."

From a DH HNC Model perspective, the dental hygienist helped the patient reveal a deficit in the human need for freedom from stress, sound dentition, and possibly freedom from pain. The dental hygiene care plan could address these deficits via actions, such as using prevention measures like fluoride therapy to strengthen tooth enamel, engaging in interprofessional collaboration to promote a multidisciplinary team approach to helping the patient recover from the illness, and promoting the patient's health by way of kindness and presence that health is achievable. The OHRQL Model would recognize the patient's need via symptom status and general quality of life.

OHRQL, Oral Health-Related Quality of Life.

people have a brief episode of the disorder and recover on their own, but people in whom the course of illness is severe will require help to recover from it.

Diagnosis

There are three diagnostic criteria for anorexia nervosa, with two specified types: restricting type or binge eating and purging type. The criteria involve the following: (1) restriction of eating relative to required nutritional needs, resulting in significantly low body weight; (2) intense fear of being fat or of gaining weight that interferes with weight gain; and (3) lack of recognition of health challenges related to the restrictions and thought processes alongside a distorted view of the shape of one's body.[1] Anorexia nervosa diagnosis also includes activity state and severity, such as partial and/or full remission, which is determined by the presence and/or absence of the previously listed criteria, and mild to extreme severity, which is based on body mass index (BMI). During an anorexia nervosa episode, persons with the **restricting type** achieve weight loss through dieting, fasting, or excessive exercise. By comparison, persons with the **binge eating and purging type** may engage in purging behaviors such as self-induced vomiting or the misuse of laxatives, diuretics, or enemas in addition to binge eating. Patients with anorexia nervosa may demonstrate the distortion of their body image by verbalizing how they feel or think about appearance in relation to "being fat" when they are thin or underweight.

Epidemiologic Factors

Anorexia nervosa is seen during adolescence and young adulthood, although it can appear in adulthood. It is more prevalent in females than males, with a crude mortality rate of 5% per decade.[1] Anorexia can be seen across culturally and socially diverse populations. The course is variable, ranging from a single episode, a relapse, or a chronic course running several years to remission and recovery. Table 57.1 outlines the primary symptoms of anorexia nervosa.

Psychological, emotional, and mental health challenges that are comorbid with eating disorders include major depression and anxiety disorders, substance abuse, self-injurious behavior, and restricted affect and capacity for insight. There are many medical problems associated with anorexia nervosa involving many systems, including cardiovascular, hematopoietic, gastrointestinal, and endocrine systems (Table 57.2). Thus a person with anorexia nervosa becomes medically and psychiatrically compromised. Box 57.4 shows the role that the dental hygienist may be asked to play with respect to an eating disorder and a comorbid condition, in this case, the use of street drugs. The dental hygienist's holistic approach to oral health recognizes the oral health–systemic health link and understands that upsetting one body system affects whole-body wellness.

BULIMIA NERVOSA

Bulimia nervosa is a mental health illness.[1] Unlike people with anorexia nervosa, those with bulimia nervosa are often able to maintain a body weight within a normal range for their body type. However, they are unduly focused on body shape and weight and express a general dissatisfaction with their body image. The term *bulimia* literally means "ox hunger," which refers to the abnormal craving for food characteristic of the illness.

Diagnosis

Bulimia nervosa is characterized by repeated binge eating. There are two specific types of bulimia nervosa—bingeing/purging type and restricting type, each with five diagnostic criteria: (1) eating significantly more food than what would be considered normal amounts at

TABLE 57.1	Primary Symptoms of Anorexia Nervosa and Bulimia Nervosa
Anorexia Nervosa	**Bulimia Nervosa**
• Resistance or refusal to maintain a minimally normal body weight for age and height • Weight loss primarily due to reductions in food consumption, even after significant weight loss • Intense fear of weight gain or being "fat," although underweight • Weight loss viewed as evidence of self-control • Denial of seriousness of medical implications; lack of insight • Loss of menstrual periods in females after puberty	• Regular intake of large amounts of food accompanied by a sense of loss of control over eating behavior • Regular use of inappropriate compensatory behaviors such as self-induced vomiting, laxative, or diuretic abuse, fasting, or obsessive or compulsive exercise • Extreme concern with body weight and shape

Data from the *Diagnostic and Statistical Manual of Mental Disorders*. 5th ed. Text Revision (Copyright © 2022). American Psychiatric Association.

TABLE 57.2	Examples of Medical and Health Consequences of Anorexia Nervosa and Bulimia Nervosa
Anorexia Nervosa	**Bulimia Nervosa**
• Associated with depressive symptoms and social dysfunction and suicide risk • Leukopenia and mild anemia and other metabolite disturbances • Dehydration and its results (e.g., renal failure) • Signs and symptoms of starvation; emaciation • Amenorrhea • Constipation, cold intolerance, lethargy, and excessive energy • Hypotension, hypertension, and bradycardia • Dry skin and hair loss • Lanugo (growth of a downy layer of hair)	• Increased frequency of depressive symptoms and mood disorders • Associated with the use of stimulants and alcohol • Fluid and electrolyte imbalances, which can lead to serious medical problems • Dental decay and eroded enamel • Salivary gland enlargement • Calloused fingers (from digitally inducing purge) • Dependency on laxatives, if used on a chronic basis • Esophageal tears, gastric rupture, and cardiac arrhythmias—rare but potentially fatal

Data from the *Diagnostic and Statistical Manual of Mental Disorders*. 5th ed. Text Revision (Copyright © 2022). American Psychiatric Association.

a certain point in time and doing so without control over eating; (2) purging behaviors to offset the binge, such as self-induced vomiting, the use of laxatives or diuretics, excessive exercising, fasting, and enemas; (3) the bingeing and purging behaviors occur approximately once a week for a minimum of 3 months; (4) the individual's sense of worth is dependent on their body weight and shape; and (5) the disturbance does not occur excessively during episodes of anorexia nervosa.[1] The difference between the bingeing/purging type and restricting type is how and what the person does to offset the binge. If the individual engages in self-induced vomiting or the misuse of laxatives, diuretics, or enemas, the condition is the **bingeing/purging type**. If they use another type of inappropriate compensatory behavior to prevent weight gain (e.g., excessive exercise, fasting) but does not regularly vomit or misuse laxatives, the condition is the **restricting type**.

Epidemiologic Factors

Bulimia nervosa is more common than anorexia nervosa. Onset generally occurs during the late teenage years and young adulthood, but it can be seen in adulthood. Prevalence is higher among females than males. The crude mortality rate is 2% per decade.[1]

It appears that sociocultural factors impact the development of bulimia nervosa. Although high-risk populations include people involved in activities in which weight and body image are associated with the activity, such as dance and sports, bulimia nervosa is prevalent in the general population and can be seen across culturally and socially diverse populations.[5–7]

The course and outcome of bulimia nervosa are variable, but the condition may be chronic or intermittent, with periods of remission. It has a comorbid association with other mental health conditions. Because bulimia nervosa is a secretive illness and the affected person can maintain a normal body weight, it can go on for a very long time without ever being disclosed or diagnosed. It may be chronic with periods of quiescence and relapse; therefore recovery can occur but may require diligence, professional assistance, and, at times, pharmaceutical interventions (e.g., antidepressants) (Box 57.5).

Table 57.1 lists the primary symptoms of bulimia nervosa, and Table 57.2 lists some medical complications associated with the disorder. Persons may develop cardiac problems such as arrhythmias, gastrointestinal problems (e.g., gastroesophageal reflux disease), esophagitis, irritable bowel syndrome, and fluid and electrolyte abnormalities. It is rare to develop gastrointestinal abnormalities, although esophageal tears or gastric ruptures can occur and are potentially life-threatening. Bulimia nervosa is associated with anxiety and mood disorders, particularly major depressive disorders, dysthymic disorder, self-injurious behavior, substance abuse, and personality disorders. The person may seek professional help because of the tooth sensitivity associated with perimylolysis, so the dental hygienist may be the first health professional to help the patient begin the journey to recovery.

HEALTH EFFECTS OF ANOREXIA NERVOSA AND BULIMIA NERVOSA

The effects of anorexia nervosa and bulimia nervosa on an individual's psychosocial and physiological well-being are significant.[1–4] From a patient-centered approach, anorexia nervosa can be thought of as an eclipsing of the person's thinking by the eating disorder; in other words, the person's identity is centered on the eating disorder.[8] Recovery or fighting against the condition is like fighting against one's sense of self or identity. Box 57.6 illustrates the possessiveness of anorexia nervosa over the individual. People with bulimia nervosa report an overwhelming sense of lack of control with food; they are driven to consume and purge food, as described in Box 57.7. The treatment is challenging for both anorexia nervosa and bulimia nervosa, and the recovery period can be lengthy. The dental hygienist must be vigilant to support recovery. They must be empathetic in helping the patient prevent oral implications and deterioration and in enabling oral rehabilitation and reconstruction.

Psychosocial Dimension

In the individual with anorexia nervosa, body image distortion and obsession with food restriction results in self-starvation. Keep in mind that the "self" aspect of "self-starvation" is an illness in thinking and not truly self-guidance. Patients with anorexia nervosa report that control of food and perfectionist behaviors bring feelings of being more competent and more in control of their lives—this is part of the illness.

In bulimia nervosa, low self-esteem and subsequent feelings of inadequacy are reinforced by the guilt and embarrassment associated with the binge and purge behavior. However, the behavior becomes self-reinforcing because achievement and maintenance of a lower weight drives the binge-purge cycle. Persons with bulimia nervosa obsess about their body image. They may appear quite successful in the management of their lives; however, underlying the facade are feelings associated with anxiety, guilt, and dysphoria.

Impaired psychological development and the associated distortion of attitudes in the patient with an eating disorder provide the foundation for continued dysfunction and the progression of the disorder. Those with bulimia nervosa may eventually seek help as a result of tooth sensitivity or a change in the appearance of their teeth. However, persons with eating disorders do not necessarily seek professional assistance on their own and may resist recommendations and offers of help from family members and friends. From a DH HNC Model perspective, for example, the dental hygienist would

BOX 57.6 Critical Thinking Scenario F

BOX 57.6   Critical Thinking Scenario F

Clare, a 22-year-old female patient, said the following to Dianne, her dental hygienist, "Annie (anorexia nervosa) was my best friend. Annie and I saw nurse Joan as an enemy. During my initial days in treatment for anorexia nervosa, she was always telling me Annie was lying to me, that her voice telling me, 'I am so fat and I must not eat' was all based on the deceitful nature of the illness. It wasn't until I began to hear Annie's voice as separate from my own that I started to believe what nurse Joan and my healthcare team were saying to me; Annie was my enemy, not them." Clare told Dianne that she learned through treatment to call her anorexia nervosa "Annie." Personifying anorexia nervosa enabled her to find her own identity as separate from the illness. Her recovery from the condition began when she could do this. It was a long, hard, and intense journey that consumed 7 years of her life.

BOX 57.7   Critical Thinking Scenario G

"When I was 21, I discovered by chance that I could throw up all I had eaten and I wouldn't gain weight," said Amanda, a 23-year-old patient, to Janet, a dental hygienist. Amanda added, "I was an active university student with good friends, okay grades, and this ever-present worry about weight gain."

Janet asked, "Amanda, do you still throw up? Your teeth are showing very slight erosion. Do they hurt? Are they sensitive? Sometimes a person who vomits regularly develops enamel erosion. I'm just seeing some slight evidence of this on your teeth."

Amanda replied, "Well, this is so embarrassing; I do feel ashamed—even mortified—that I even got into this, but I did, and to answer your question, I haven't vomited for a while, and when I do, it's just when I feel too full. I'm better about not eating until I feel too full."

Janet nodded and said, "I'm glad you told me this. It is important to know for your oral health. Let's work on a plan. Have you sought help for this behavior?"

understand that a key role is to help the patient with the human need for conceptualization and problem solving. From the OHRQL Model perspective, the key role is to facilitate the patient's understanding of health perceptions.

Physiological Responses

Many body systems are at risk for disruption as a result of an eating disorder. The body as a systemic whole is affected, thereby requiring the dental hygienist to consider the oral systemic outcomes of eating disorders. In anorexia nervosa, restricted food intake and resulting undernutrition impair the individual's overall functioning and health. A common physiological effect of anorexia nervosa behavior is hormonal abnormalities. Among females a prolonged decrease in estrogen, along with a decreased body fat level, may contribute to amenorrhea and decreased bone density (i.e., osteoporosis). Osteoporosis may be evident in the jaw and facial bones. The cardiovascular, gastrointestinal, renal, and hematologic systems may be compromised in patients with anorexia nervosa. Vital statistics in the patient will likely reveal low pulse rates, decreased blood pressure, and reduced left ventricular output. The patient may not openly complain about physiological symptoms such as constipation; however, a comprehensive health history may identify abnormal function such as this gastrointestinal disturbance. If a person is constipated, they may be dehydrated; dehydration is evident in salivary flow and quality and affects oral health. A person with pale skin or general fatigue may be experiencing hematologic changes and electrolyte imbalances that result in the immune system not functioning optimally. This affects the body's ability to prevent and withstand infection (e.g., oral candidiasis). Conducting a health

history is about differentiating normal from abnormal and then following through to improve the diagnosis and resulting care.

The repeated binge and purge cycle in the patient with bulimia nervosa and the purge subtype of anorexia nervosa may result in dangerous complications that, if left untreated, can become life-threatening. Excessive vomiting and diuretic and laxative abuse lead to dehydration and electrolyte imbalance. Ipecac syrup used by some to induce vomiting after a binge period is particularly dangerous. Ipecac syrup contains emetine, which can destroy heart muscle fibers. Chronic ipecac ingestion and absorption can lead to fatal myocardial dysfunction. In addition, repeated binge eating and vomiting can cause gastric dilation, esophagitis, esophageal tears, or esophageal rupture. Although uncommon, these physiological responses are life-threatening.

Other General Physical Findings

Whether viewed from a DH HNC Model perspective or an OHRQL Model viewpoint, there are general physical findings that the dental hygienist must consider when treating a person with an eating disorder. As an eating disorder progresses, general physical characteristics become evident as a result of the disorder. The dental hygienist must look for these signs during the assessment phase. Two common physical findings for persons with anorexia nervosa during the more developed stages of the disorder are lanugo and "feeling cold." Lanugo is a fine, downy hair that is usually found on the lower half of the face and upper body. Dry skin and hair and decreased scalp hair are predictable findings as the eating disorder progresses. Patients might even report losing hair or that they no longer brush the hair because it is "falling out." Hypothermia and increased sensitivity to cold may be evidenced by the patient wearing inappropriately warm clothing when environmental temperatures are moderate. The dental hygienist needs to be aware of these presentations and gently engage the patient in a discussion about them.

The dental hygienist may suspect that a patient is engaging in oral purging if they notice calloused knuckles. Persons who orally purge using their fingers may have calloused knuckles from the repetitive friction of the teeth riding over the fingers during the digital stimulation used to induce vomiting. Although it is common to use one's own fingers to create the urge to vomit, other objects are used as well (e.g., spoons). These objects, in addition to the fingers, can traumatize the palate and other soft tissues of the mouth. During the intraoral examination, the dental hygienist needs to look for lesions and bruises, because these may be clues that a person is orally purging.

Oral Health Implications

Intraoral and extraoral manifestations of eating disorders occur, particularly with bulimia nervosa and the binge and purge subtype of anorexia nervosa (Table 57.3).[9–16] The patient with an eating disorder may exhibit one or more of these manifestations, yet some may exhibit none of them. Many of these signs are seen only after the person has had the disorder for some time. Early identification and prompt intervention for an eating disorder are not likely to occur in the dental hygiene practice, given the secretive and nondisclosing nature of a patient with an eating disorder. It is more likely that the dental hygienist will notice oral changes in the patient who has an established eating disorder and then look to employ tertiary prevention interventions. After conducting a comprehensive health history and oral assessment in a nonjudgmental, respectful environment, the dental hygienist acts to promote prompt intervention to lessen the disorder's effect on the oral cavity and on the person's overall health and wellness.

Parotid Enlargement

Extraorally, parotid enlargement has been observed with both anorexia nervosa and bulimia nervosa. This enlargement is noninflammatory in

TABLE 57.3 Potential Effects of Eating Disorders on the Oral and Perioral Tissues

Effects on Oral and Perioral Tissues*	Anorexia Nervosa, Restricting Type	Bulimia Nervosa and Binge-and-Purge Anorexia Nervosa
Parotid enlargement	No	Yes
Diminished taste acuity	Yes	Yes
Dehydration and xerostomia or reduced salivary flow	Yes	Yes
Enamel erosion (perimylolysis)	No	Yes
Intraoral trauma (e.g., palatal abrasion, palatal hematoma)	No	Yes
Increased risk of dental caries (given xerostomia and/or exposed dentin)	?*	?*
Periodontal disease	?*	?*
Other comorbid disorders (e.g., self-injurious behavior)	Yes	Yes
Oral side effects of medications (e.g., antidepressants)	Yes	Yes
Oral health–systemic health issues (e.g., esophageal reflux disease, yeast infection)	Yes	Yes

*Evidence in the literature is inconclusive regarding dental caries and periodontal disease in direct relationship with eating disorders. Both may occur as a result of xerostomia, exposed dentin, poor oral hygiene, and other known risk factors that are general to these two dental diseases.

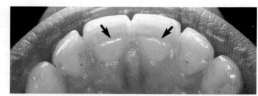

Fig. 57.2 Perimylolysis on the maxillary incisors *(arrows)* as a result of the habitual vomiting associated with bulimia nervosa. (Courtesy J. Charbonneau, August 2017.)

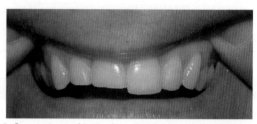

Fig. 57.3 Comparison of loss of vertical height of teeth 7 and 8 versus teeth 9 and 10. Vertical height is restored with resin restorations. Height loss was due to the regular vomiting of a patient with bulimia nervosa. (Courtesy J. Charbonneau, August 2017.)

nature. It gives the jaw an enlarged appearance that subsides with abstinence from self-induced vomiting. Palpation will reveal the enlargement to be soft and generally painless. Patients with parotid gland enlargement may express concern about the unesthetic appearance of the enlargement. If the individual understands that the enlargement usually decreases when the eating disorder behaviors are brought under control, this understanding may increase their motivation for following through with psychological and medical care.

Diminished Taste Acuity

Although it will not be obvious from the intraoral examination, diminished **taste acuity** has been reported by patients with eating disorders. This alteration in taste sensation is thought to result from malnutrition (i.e., specifically trace metal deficiency) or hormonal abnormalities. Changes in hormonal levels have been shown to decrease the sensations of taste and smell.

Dehydration and Xerostomia

Xerostomia (dry mouth), dry chapped lips, and commissure lesions resembling angular cheilitis may occur if the patient is dehydrated from vomiting, diuretic or laxative abuse, or antidepressant medications used to treat eating disorders. Little is known about the salivary factors for persons with eating disorders; however, it appears that salivary differences exist, such as lower salivary pH levels, different proteolytic enzymes, and lessened salivary flow rates.[17–18] **Ghrelin** is a hormone produced in the stomach that signals the brain to indicate hunger. Ghrelin increases the appetite and thus regulates food intake and body weight. Because ghrelin is found in saliva, it is hoped that studying ghrelin could improve an understanding of the development

of eating disorders and potentially aid in future treatment.[19] Further investigation is needed to understand the cause and effect relationships of these salivary differences, as well as to determine if salivary testing might aid in identifying periods of activity of the secretive illness.

Perimylolysis or Enamel Erosion

Perimylolysis (also spelled as *perimylosis*) or enamel erosion is the most common dental finding in the patient who orally purges (Figs. 57.2 through 57.6). The gastric acids are thought to result in the erosion of tooth surfaces. Initially, the maxillary anterior teeth are involved, but over time, the posterior teeth experience the same erosion. Subsequent mechanical erosion occurs when the tongue or toothbrush moves against the teeth. Slight pitting is evident on the incisal surfaces of the anterior teeth, and a cupping appearance may be present on the cusps of the posterior teeth. This dished-out appearance should be differentiated from the typical flattened appearance that occurs with abrasion. As perimylolysis progresses, the teeth exhibit a loss of normal anatomic features, such as developmental grooves and pits and rounded margins. Enamel loss occurs both vertically and horizontally and may become so extensive that complete enamel loss is evident with dentinal exposure. A loss of lingual and incisal enamel on the anterior teeth weakens the tooth structure, thereby making these teeth susceptible to chipping. An open bite may form as a result of vertical height loss of the anterior teeth. The teeth can appear translucent, in some areas more so than others. Enamel loss around amalgam restorations results in a raised-island appearance of the amalgam. Unless the vertical and horizontal dimensions of the teeth are measured and documented via the use of dental erosion indices or study casts as part of a routine clinical examination, early perimylolysis is difficult for practitioners to identify because tooth structure loss usually is subtle. The longer the duration of the illness, the more damage is done to the dentition.

Dentinal Hypersensitivity

Perimylolysis may eventually result in dentinal exposure and associated tooth sensitivity. Patients who purge their food may complain of tooth sensitivity, which often is their chief reason for seeking dental and/or dental hygiene care.

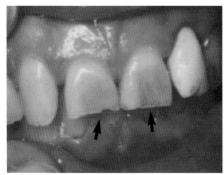

Fig. 57.4 Thinning and chipping of incisal third of teeth 8 and 9 *(arrows)* in a person with bulimia nervosa. (Courtesy S. Isaac, August 2017.)

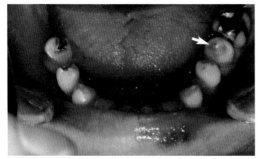

Fig. 57.5 Perimylolysis and resin loss on tooth 20 *(arrow)*; lip lesions caused by oral purging. (Courtesy S. Isaac, August 2017.)

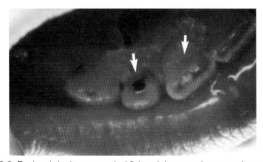

Fig. 57.6 Perimylolysis on tooth 10 involving amalgam and on tooth 9 lingual surface *(arrows)*. (Courtesy S. Isaac, 2017.)

Dental Caries

Decreased salivary flow along with disturbed dietary patterns may predispose the patient to an increased dental caries rate. Not all studies support the theory that individuals with eating disorders have an increased dental caries prevalence. However, evidence suggests that persons with bulimia nervosa may be prone to caries as a result of their high carbohydrate intake, changes in their oral pH levels, decreased saliva quantity and quality, and the use of antidepressants or other medications associated with a diminished salivary flow rate. Xerostomia can also result from illicit drug use, which is a potential coexisting condition among patients with eating disorders.[1]

Periodontal Disease

Eating disorders place the patient at risk for periodontal disease due to a number of factors. First, nutritionally deprived persons, including patients with eating disorders, are at an increased risk for periodontal disease. Second, malnutrition inhibits the body's ability to properly maintain itself, not only in the oral cavity but also in the heart and other body organs. Third, prescribed medications or other drugs taken in connection with the eating disorder may contribute to xerostomia, which exacerbates dental biofilm growth. Fourth, depression, combined with an eating disorder, may result in apathy toward oral hygiene habits, thus increasing the risk of periodontal disease.

Intraoral Trauma

Intraoral trauma may be evident in the patient who orally purges or regurgitates the stomach contents. In addition, the oral soft tissues may be fragile because of nutritional deficiencies. Findings may include the presence of traumatic lesions such as ulcerations or hematomas on the hard and soft palates, as well as cheek and lip bites.

DENTAL HYGIENE PROCESS OF CARE FOR PATIENTS WITH EATING DISORDERS

The secrecy and shame associated with eating disorders may cause patients to avoid dental and dental hygiene care until oral manifestations appear. These oral manifestations result in the dental hygienist's involvement in care at a secondary and tertiary prevention level (see Chapter 4). From a primary prevention and health promotion perspective, the dental hygienist and the oral healthcare team can ensure that the practice promotes healthy lifestyle messaging and establishes an environment in which all patients feel safe to disclose their health and lifestyle information. The secondary prevention measures include screening for eating disorders or for the patient's susceptibility to an eating disorder, harm reduction by preventing further damage to the oral structures, and referring patients for care and interprofessional collaborative practice. All of these measures are aimed at prompt intervention to address the eating disorder to lessen disability. Tertiary prevention measures take place during and after recovery as continued eating disorder behaviors destroy reconstructed dentition, which is very costly for the patient. Open dialogue regarding dental rehabilitation or reconstruction during active illness must occur between the dental provider and the patient to ensure informed consent.

For individuals with eating disorders who have not been diagnosed, the dental hygienist may be the first health professional who identifies the need for a referral to the healthcare team. A working knowledge of organizations and individuals within the patient's community who specialize in caring for individuals with eating disorders allows the dental hygienist to guide the patient to appropriate care. This knowledge can be obtained by contacting credible national mental health organizations or eating disorder treatment facilities within the community. The national organizations may not be in the immediate geographic locale, but they are generally knowledgeable about available support throughout the area. Creating a formal referral protocol with eating disorder treatment centers or with healthcare professionals and eating disorder specialists is important for the oral healthcare team. Health professionals who are actively treating patients with eating disorders often need oral healthcare professionals to whom they can refer patients who are experiencing oral problems. A liaison between the oral healthcare team and other healthcare team members will open the door for comprehensive patient care through referrals and interprofessional collaboration.

Evidence that oral healthcare professionals have a low comfort level when dealing with sensitive issues such as addressing or asking a patient about an eating disorder led to the development of a framework to better enable oral health clinician communication with patients pertaining to eating disorders.[20] The *Evaluate, Assess, Treat* framework is based on motivational interviewing, and it has been proposed as a means for engaging in the active secondary prevention measures for eating disorders.

TABLE 57.4 Assessment of Patient With a Suspected or Previously Diagnosed Eating Disorder

Component	Assessment Technique
Health History	
Physical appearance and gait: skin, build, hair, and pallor	Observation
Vital signs: blood pressure, heart rate, and body temperature	Objective measurement
Systemic disease: current and past status	Interview, collaborative consultation
Systems review (e.g., bowel movements, postural hypertension)	Interview, collaborative consultation
Medications: drug names, doses, duration, and purpose	Interview, collaborative consultation
Substance abuse: alcohol, nonprescription medications, and street drugs	Interview
Physical activity: frequency and duration	Interview
Dietary habits: cariogenicity of diet and general healthy eating habits	Interview, dietary analysis for dental caries control and general healthy eating habits
Oral homecare: routine, products, and techniques	Interview, observation
Extraoral Assessment	
Salivary and lymph glands	Palpation
Temporomandibular joint	Palpation, auscultation
Skin: color, moisture, facial hair (lanugo), and lesions	Observation
Perioral structures: commissure lesions, lip integrity, and trauma	Observation
Hands (calloused knuckles)	Observation
Intraoral Assessment	
Soft tissue: mucous membranes, palatal tissue, tongue, floor of mouth, and throat	Observation, palpation
Salivary flow rate and pH level	Observation, salivary flow rate measure, pH test
Dental caries and tooth color	Observation, radiographic assessment, manual assessment
Tooth wear: presence or absence, location, appearance (rounded margins, cupped, thinned, abraded), and open bite	Observation, comparative study model
Periodontal tissues	Observation, radiographic assessment, manual assessment
Oral hygiene	Observation, manual dexterity assessment

Dental Hygiene Assessment

The dental hygiene assessment provides the opportunity to reveal an eating disorder through a thorough and patient-centered health history and potential for oral manifestations (Table 57.4). In the patient with a diagnosed eating disorder, historical information regarding the course and treatment of the eating disorder, past medical and dental and dental hygiene care and treatment interventions, and the current status of the oral environment are necessary to provide appropriate dental hygiene care. This evaluation should clearly depict the extent to which the eating disorder relates to associated behaviors, the patient's current status regarding psychotherapy or other supportive care, and the current physical and oral findings. In addition, intraoral photographs, dental erosion indices, and study models help establish a baseline for followup assessment of objective clinical observations of enamel erosion. When the clinician observes deviations from normal in a patient assessment that are suggestive of an eating disorder, followup questions are needed.[21] The validated SCOFF questionnaire (Box 57.8) is an assessment tool to consider.[22] There are other possible explanations for dental erosion other than an eating disorder (Box 57.9). Potential causes for some observed oral manifestations are as follows:

- Commissure lesions and dry, chapped lips are typical findings of an eating disorder; however, they may also result from other illnesses that cause dehydration or undernutrition. Usually, however, patients who have been ill and who subsequently have dehydration willingly convey this information on questioning.
- Dental erosion, which is the most common oral finding in patients with bulimia nervosa and the binge and purge subtype of anorexia

BOX 57.8 SCOFF Questionnaire* for Screening Eating Disorders

1. Do you make yourself **s**ick because you feel uncomfortably full?
2. Do you worry you have lost **c**ontrol over how much you eat?
3. Have you recently lost more than **o**ne stone (14 pounds) in a 3-month period?
4. Do you believe yourself to be **f**at when others say you are too thin?
5. Would you say that **f**ood dominates your life?

*One point for every "yes"; a score of 2 points indicates a likely case of anorexia nervosa.
Reprinted with permission (August 2017) from Hill LS, Reid F, Morgan JF, Lacey JH. SCOFF, the development of an eating disorder screening questionnaire. *Int J Eat Disord.* 2010;43:344–351.

nervosa, has also been associated with vomiting as a result of gastric disturbances (e.g., gastroesophageal reflux disease) and other conditions.

- Intraoral trauma may result from an accident or it may be evidence of self-mutilation that is indicative of psychological problems other than eating disorders.

During the assessment of a patient with a suspected eating disorder, it is imperative that the dental hygienist gather specific information in a professional and nonjudgmental manner. Avoid drawing premature conclusions regarding the presence of an eating disorder without adequate assessment, which would place the patient and clinician in an unnecessary and uncomfortable position.

BOX 57.9 Possible Causes for Oral Findings Commonly Associated With Patients Who Have Eating Disorders

Perimylolysis and Erosion
- High citric acid fruit or fruit juice intake
- Antabuse therapy for alcoholism
- Habitual eating of or sucking on vitamin C tablets or sweet-and-sour candies
- Intake of medications that contain hydrochloric acid
- Exposure to industrial acids

Parotid Enlargement
- Salivary neoplasms
- Inflammatory diseases (e.g., mumps, infectious mononucleosis, tuberculosis, sarcoidosis, histoplasmosis)
- Metabolic disturbances (e.g., malnutrition, alcoholic cirrhosis, diabetes mellitus)
- Autoimmune diseases (e.g., Sjögren syndrome)
- Parotid duct obstruction
- Acquired immunodeficiency syndrome

Xerostomia
- Medications (e.g., antihypertensives, antidepressants, antipsychotics, antihistamines)
- Systemic diseases (e.g., diabetes, Sjögren syndrome)
- Side effect of radiation therapy for cancer of the head and neck area
- Dehydration from recent flulike illnesses or high fever

Commissure Lesions
- Loss of vertical dimension or overclosure
- Vitamin B deficiency
- Yeast infection

Dental Hygiene Diagnosis

Dental hygiene diagnoses can be accomplished using objective and subjective findings to determine deficits in the DH HNC Model or OHRQL Model issues related to dental hygiene care. The actual diagnosis of the eating disorder is not a function of members of the oral healthcare team; a diagnosis is determined through a thorough psychological evaluation. A patient usually exhibits several human needs deficits that arise directly or indirectly from the eating disorder. For example, the repeated binge eating of carbohydrates followed by vomiting may result in a deficit related to a biologically sound dentition as evidenced by perimylolysis (enamel erosion) and potentially increased signs of dental caries. Dehydration from vomiting or diuretic or laxative abuse may also result in a deficit relating to the integrity of the soft tissue, as evidenced by dry, chapped lips and commissure lesions similar to angular cheilitis. It is essential that the dental hygienist consider all possible reasons for these deficits so that appropriate care may follow. Examples of dental hygiene diagnoses based on the DH HNC Model are presented in Table 57.5.

Planning

The dental hygiene care planning phase for the patient who is suspected of having an eating disorder includes the following:
- Phase 1: Referral of the patient to medical and psychological treatment providers.
- Phase 2: Roles and responsibilities of the oral healthcare team as part of the patient's interprofessional collaborative healthcare team.
- Phase 3: Management and support of oral health during and after eating disorder treatment.

Oral healthcare team members must recognize their limitations when treating patients with these disorders. Either palliative or definitive oral, dental, and dental hygiene treatment may be necessary. However, initially, the primary role of the oral healthcare team treating the patient with a suspected eating disorder is to refer the patient to eating disorder specialists. Such specialists can

TABLE 57.5 Example of Dental Hygiene Human Needs Diagnoses for Patients With Eating Disorders

Dental Hygiene Diagnosis Deficit	Due or Related to	As Evidenced by
Wholesome facial image	Self-induced vomiting Excessive diet soda intake Bruxing habits Salivary gland hypertrophy from binge-purge behavior	Patient expression of dissatisfaction with tooth discoloration, loss of tooth structure, open bite, visible dental caries, parotid gland enlargement
Freedom from pain	Frequent vomiting Diminished saliva flow rate from diuretic or laxative abuse	Oral discomfort from exposed dentin from enamel erosion, dental caries, dehydration of oral tissues
Integrity of skin and mucous membranes	Laxative or diuretic abuse and vomiting Use of fingers and other objects to orally purge	Dehydration of oral environment Self-induced trauma during purging, self-abusive behavior Dry skin or hair
Protection from health risks	Self-starvation Anemia or alteration in body metabolism Decreased cardiac function	Dry skin or hair Enlarged parotid glands Bradycardia, low blood pressure, low body temperature, thin, pale
Freedom from fear and stress	Low or endangered self-esteem Need for acceptance by others Feelings of guilt Fear of being found out	Lack of willingness to communicate fully, denial of or providing false explanations for oral manifestations, fatigued
Responsibility for oral health	Lack of self-control Feelings of unworthiness	Lack of ownership of problems, impaired self-care, self-inflicted oral trauma

help patients with the psychological- and medical-related aspects of their eating disorders. Establishing a caring and nonjudgmental environment based on mutual trust is necessary to successfully achieve a referral.

Patient involvement in the setting of goals is essential. Dental hygiene goals must be set with the following characteristics:

- Specific and measurable outcomes, including target dates for achievement
- Based on the dental hygiene diagnoses
- Realistic
- Measurable by both the patient and the healthcare professional

A sample dental hygiene care plan based on the DH HNC Model for a patient with an eating disorder is shown in Table 57.6.

Implementation

Confirming the presence of an eating disorder with a patient may be uncomfortable for the dental hygienist given the sensitivity of the illness itself. Setting the stage and employing an empathetic, caring approach facilitates the dialogue between the patient and the dental hygienist. Box 57.10 outlines strategies for engaging the patient. If dental erosion is the most apparent oral finding, asking questions that eliminate other reasons for erosion allows the clinician to gain valuable information

---

TABLE 57.6   Example Items for Dental Hygiene Human Needs Care Plan for Patient With Bulimia Nervosa*

Human Need Deficit	Dental Hygiene Goal	Dental Hygiene Intervention	Evaluative Statement
Freedom from pain	By 2/28/25, patient will have oral function with no discomfort.	Emphasize abstinence from oral purging. Use a professional fluoride varnish and offer a home fluoride therapy regimen (neutral sodium fluoride gel or rinse; dentifrice). Use a nonabrasive desensitizing dentifrice. Advise patient to avoid toothbrushing for at least 30 minutes after purging.	Patient follows professional and home fluoride therapy programs and uses desensitizing dentifrice. Patient reports abstinence or attempted abstinence from oral purging. Patient avoids toothbrushing after oral purging.
Sound dentition	By 8/1/24, patient will have reduced risk of further loss of tooth structure. By 8/1/24, patient will not exhibit further loss of tooth structure.	Use both professional and home fluoride therapies. Demonstrate dental plaque control measures. Refer patient to a dentist for palliative or dental reconstruction and rehabilitation of damaged teeth.	See previous statements, in addition to the following: Patient complies with recommended oral hygiene regimen; there is no evidence of progressive enamel loss (perimylolysis). Patient is in the care of a dentist regarding dental palliative care, rehabilitation, and reconstruction needs.
Responsibility for oral health	By 8/1/24, patient will participate in the treatment of bulimia by attending all health professional appointments, including oral health appointments. By 8/1/24, patient will communicate openly with dental hygienist and participate in the management of oral conditions.	Consult with the healthcare team or refer the patient for care (e.g., eating disorder program, physician, psychologist, dietitian). Recommend that the patient consent to collaboration between the oral healthcare team and the eating disorder program or healthcare team. Explain the risks of vomiting to the hard oral tissues (e.g., removal of tooth structure, sensitivity, risk of trauma). Schedule frequent dental hygiene and dental appointments during active bulimia periods.	Patient complies with eating disorder healthcare team or program recommendations. Patient provides written consent for interprofessional health collaboration for patient-centered care. Coordinate with healthcare team after dental or dental hygiene appointments and vice versa when appropriate (e.g., if patient is experiencing a period of bulimic activity). Patient states risks of vomiting to oral health. Patient self-initiates dental hygiene or dental appointments during active bulimia periods and attends scheduled appointments.
	By 2/2/24, patient will participate in the management of oral conditions by using oral self-care skills. By 2/2/24, patient will self-monitor oral health.	Involve the patient in the design of oral self-care skills and monitoring that coordinate with a concomitant eating disorder therapeutic program.	Patient demonstrates successful use of oral self-care skills; there is no evidence of perimylolysis, palatal trauma, or dental disease.
Wholesome facial image	By 11/15/24, patient will participate in an active eating disorder program for 2 years. By 12/30/24, patient will verbalize that the mouth looks and feels better.	Collaborate with the patient's healthcare team, which includes the oral healthcare team. Refer the patient to a dentist for rehabilitation and reconstruction of the dentition. Provide education regarding the patient's expressed dissatisfaction with the oral condition.	Patient is compliant with oral and healthcare team treatment recommendations and therapeutic program. Patient has realistic expectations of dental treatment outcomes. Patient states that the mouth looks and feels better.

*Respect and honor each patient as an individual with personal needs.

while desensitizing the patient to the more direct questions to follow. The discussion should be conducted by asking direct questions while maintaining eye contact.

Few patients openly admit to having an eating disorder when questioned about it. Many have become quite accomplished at denial and can maintain that position in the oral healthcare environment. However, most patients with eating disorders experience discomfort when confronted with objective information that they have attempted to hide. The dental hygienist should be aware of nonverbal clues, such as the avoidance of eye contact by the patient. These clues are usually indications that the clinician is on the right track with the questions, even if the patient verbally responds negatively.

Individuals with eating disorders commonly react to initial discussions with various emotions. Two common responses are denial accompanied by tears and outright anger. It is important for the dental hygienist to maintain a professional demeanor during emotional outbursts and to reinforce the observation that the patient's oral, physical, or health history findings are consistent with an eating disorder and seem to have no other causative explanation. Some patients are relieved that someone is helping and are receptive to suggestions for referral to an eating disorder specialist. Persistence on the part of the oral

healthcare team when no other explanations can be identified for the oral findings of a patient who is unable to disclose an eating disorder is crucial, because untreated eating disorders can be life-threatening. Ethically, failing to refer a patient with the signs and symptoms of an eating disorder to an eating disorder specialist or another appropriate healthcare professional neglects the dental hygienist's professional responsibility as a healthcare provider.

Phase 1: Referral of the Patient to Medical and Psychological Treatment Providers

Suggesting that the patient make an appointment with an identified eating disorder specialist or treatment center for an evaluation is a less-threatening approach than making a definitive statement that the patient has an eating disorder. Many patients are receptive to having the dental hygienist initiate a consultation appointment for them at an eating disorder treatment center; Box 57.11 provides referral suggestions. Others prefer to take the referral information with them to initiate the consultation appointment on their own. It is important that the patient assumes personal responsibility for attending a consultation appointment. Followup contact is necessary to promote the patient taking action.

The dental hygienist must thoroughly document discussions and decisions regarding referral for evaluation in the patient's permanent dental record. This documentation permits subsequent patient evaluation and monitoring at future appointments. In addition, it legally documents that the discussion took place and that the oral healthcare team is offering help to the patient.

Phase 2: Roles and Responsibilities of the Oral Healthcare Team as Part of the Patient's Interprofessional Collaborative Healthcare Team

Recovery from an eating disorder and the success of oral healthcare interventions to lessen resultant oral disabilities and to rehabilitate the dentition is largely determined by the patient's ability to learn through psychological therapy to manage the thinking and behaviors associated with the eating disorder. For this reason, open dialogue among

---

BOX 57.10 Suggestions for Confronting a Person With a Suspected Eating Disorder

Setting
- Use a private setting to ensure patient confidentiality.
- Be proactive. Establish an interprofessional collaborative practice for patient-centered care.
- Create a climate of calmness, acceptance, and nonjudgment.
- Ensure confidentiality within the collaborative healthcare team.

Approach
- Do no harm. Know your limitations; professionally refer and collaborate with others for patient-centered care.
- Focus on the illness rather than the person. Remember that the illness possesses the person's thinking. Separate the disorder from the person.
- Be firm, formal, objective, and concerned. Keep in mind that eating disorder behavior is associated with low self-esteem, depression, and emotional problems.
- Anticipate patient resistance and defensiveness. Recognize patient sympathy-evoking tactics or manipulation; these are part of the illness.
- Focus on observed signs and symptoms and concern for the patient's health.
- Ask if the patient engages in specific behaviors associated with the disorder (e.g., "Do you vomit after eating sometimes?" "Do you restrict the amount of food that you usually eat?" "Have you ever heard of bulimia and anorexia?").
- Empower the patient to seek help and, if they are already engaged in an eating disorder program, to comply with it. Instill hope.
- Gain patient consent for interprofessional collaboration.
- Be informed about issues that the patient is experiencing that may impact oral health and likewise, keep the healthcare team apprised of oral issues that impact health and recovery.
- Know that eating disorders are complex mental disorders that are often comorbid with other psychiatric disorders such as substance abuse, self-injurious behaviors, anxiety, and depression. Know to look for signs and symptoms of these disorders and those of an eating disorder.
- Tell the patient that you are ethically obligated to intervene if you believe the patient may harm him or herself or others.
- Value harm reduction, knowing that patients with eating disorders can have a long road to recovery.

BOX 57.11 Referring a Person With a Suspected Eating Disorder

Refer the Individual
- Have an established collaboration with an eating disorder program or healthcare professional.
- Meet the patient's human need for conceptualization and problem solving. Give specific information about resources for professional evaluation and offer support.
- Enable and empower the patient to access eating disorder programming or help.

Collaborate With the Professional Person to Whom You Are Referring the Patient
- Inform the counselor or therapist of the referral.
- Discuss the symptoms and signs of concern, including the oral ones.
- Discuss areas of difficulty with confrontation and referral, as well as the appropriateness of the referral.

Followup and Support
- Recognize that seemingly small accomplishments may be major to the patient.
- Expect periods of recurrence of eating disorder behaviors. Harm reduction is paramount.
- Support recovery, not the illness.

all health providers prevents segmented care planning and permits an integrated approach to patient care. Many persons with bulimia nervosa and binge and purge anorexia nervosa have extensive dental erosion that requires significant dental reconstruction. A lack of coordination among healthcare providers may mean dental failure if the reconstruction is completed before the patient has made adequate progress with the eating disorder. For example, a dental hygienist must collaborate with an orthodontist or an implant provider.[23–24] The use of a signed release form allows oral healthcare professionals to contact and collaborate with the eating disorder healthcare providers and is recommended when a patient with an eating disorder is in active care. A sample release form is shown in Fig. 57.7.

Professional collaboration between the oral healthcare team and the eating disorder team permits the oral healthcare team to have a better understanding of the patient's specific psychological issues and increases the success rate of all dental hygiene and dental interventions. The patient is often confronting significant personal issues during psychological therapy; these may influence the timing and ultimate success of definitive oral, dental, and dental hygiene care. Without a dialogue between the oral healthcare team and the eating disorder team, oral healthcare professionals may make treatment decisions that fail to address the comprehensive oral healthcare needs of the patient. If patients are aware that all healthcare providers are working together for their care, then they are less likely to claim that "all is well" to have their short-term desires met. Given the nature of these conditions, it is not uncommon for patients with eating disorders to attempt to manipulate healthcare providers during therapy. Dental hygienists and dentists must maintain a collaborative interprofessional approach to healthcare for maximal success for patients with an eating disorder.

Phase 3: Management and Support of Oral Healthcare During and After Eating Disorder Treatment

The implementation of individualized education and preventive strategies to support a healthy oral environment is a primary focus of this phase of the dental hygiene process, such as the patient understanding the effects of eating disorder behaviors on oral health and providing self-care strategies to lessen associated problems. However, in general, continued research is needed to better understand how eating disorders affect oral health and what interventions are effective for lessening the adverse oral health effects.

From an evidence-based practice perspective, most eating disorder care is based on tradition and shared experience. However, metaanalysis and a systematic review inform us of the relationship between eating disorders and poor oral health.[9] It is from this body of knowledge that the dental hygienist provides the patient with information to promote patient knowledge and decision-making during and after eating disorder care. The dental hygienist needs to educate the patient about the following oral health issues related to eating disorders: (1) perimylolysis, (2) effect of diet on oral health, (3) oral self-care, and (4) pain management during and after periodontal debridement and instrumentation. Box 57.12 provides an overview of issues for patient oral health education. These issues may not be relevant for all patients since education is individualized and uses a patient-centered approach.

Perimylolysis. Education for patients with perimylolysis aims to eliminate pain, maintain and fortify existing tooth structure, and prevent further erosion. The following oral harm reduction interventions have been suggested:

- Knowing that the low pH level of stomach contents is associated with the chemical dissolution of tooth enamel and the importance of saliva in oral health
- Rinsing immediately after an oral purge with a pH-neutralizing solution

---

CONSENT FORM

I hereby give consent for my dentist and dental hygienist to contact all healthcare providers and therapists involved in the treatment of my eating disorder. I understand that coordination of care among these health professionals is in my best interests. In addition, I understand that all consultation and discussion among these individuals will be held in strict confidence.

Client Signature   Date

Witness   Date

Fig. 57.7 Sample patient consent form.

BOX 57.12 Example of Oral Health Education Issues for the Patient With an Eating Disorder

- Cause of observed oral signs and symptoms of eating disorder behaviors
- Effect of eating disorder behaviors on oral health
- Connection of oral health with systemic health
- Discussion of patient-specific current oral status
- Informing the patient of potential progression of oral problems
- Discussion of oral health harm reduction strategies:
  - Abstinence from oral purging
  - Effect of diet and nutrients on dental and oral health
    - Frequency of ingestion
    - Types of foods and drinks consumed
- Toothbrush abrasion on teeth with perimylolysis
- Neutralizing oral pH level immediately after an oral purge
- Benefits of fluoride therapy
- Benefits of dental sensitivity therapy
- Role of saliva in oral health

- Self-applying daily fluoride therapy
- Desensitizing dentinal hypersensitivity with either professionally applied or over-the-counter agents
- Waiting 30 to 40 minutes after oral purging before toothbrushing to lessen the mechanical abrasion of an eroded tooth surface
- Avoiding abrasive prophylaxis

One suggestion with no evidence of its effectiveness is the use of a mouthguard fabrication to provide tooth coverage during vomiting episodes.

Effect of diet on oral health. Individuals with eating disorders commonly have eating behaviors that are not conducive to oral health. For example, foods that contain simple carbohydrates such as cookies, cake, and other sweets are common binge foods. It is important for the dental hygienist to counsel the patient about the effects of repeated binge eating, frequent sucrose intake, and the excessive intake of carbonated drinks and sports drinks due to their low pH levels. The continual consumption of low-pH diet beverages in the presence of diminished salivary flow enhances dental erosion and accompanying dentinal hypersensitivity. By adequately assessing eating habits in relation to oral health, the dental hygienist can provide appropriate preventive education and treatment. The dental hygienist, as part of the eating disorder healthcare team, promotes healthy eating and lifestyle.

Oral self-care. Dental hygiene patient education is specific to oral care but, in general, dental hygiene recommendations are to lessen the acidity of the oral cavity; to maintain a wet mouth; to effectively remove dental plaque biofilm without damage to the tooth and surrounding tissues; to remineralize the dentition to protect and restore it; to prevent soft tissue lesions; and to comply with dental and dental hygiene appointments. Patients need to be informed about the following ways that they can reduce harm to their oral cavities:

- *Rehydrating the mouth with salivary substitutes, frequent sips of water, ice chips (let melt), and sugar-free gum.* For the person with an eating disorder, such as anorexia nervosa, this may be a formidable challenge during acute phases because the person is hypersensitive to the prospect of water retention and hence "feeling fat." Further, ice chips may not be tolerable for a person with dentinal sensitivity.
- *Not toothbrushing after a purge due to the mechanical abrasion of the already chemically assaulted tooth structure.* The patient should neutralize the acidity in the mouth by promptly rinsing with a neutralizing solution such as sodium bicarbonate (1 tsp in 8 oz of water), slightly alkaline mineral water, or magnesium hydroxide (milk of magnesia) solutions. The toothbrush, itself should be soft and used with a gentle touch so as to not further destroy enamel crystals.
- *Using desensitizing fluoridated dentifrices and mouthrinses to provide additional benefit for exposed dentin from erosion.*
- *Employing a home fluoride therapy regimen in addition to professional fluoride therapies to remineralize fragile dentition.* The daily use of neutral sodium fluoride gel (administered either with a custom-fabricated tray or by brushing) or a sodium fluoride mouth rinse provides protection while strengthening enamel to prevent additional erosion. Critical to the oral cavity integrity is the reestablishment of a normal pH level; therefore the fluoride product must have a low pH level.
- *Using a fabricated mouthguard for home fluoride application.*
- *Realizing the staining potential of certain agents, such as coffee, red wine, and tobacco products.*

These strategies aim to meet the patient's human needs for the integrity of the skin and mucous membranes of the head and neck and a biologically sound and functional dentition.

Pain management during and after periodontal debridement and instrumentation. During periodontal debridement and instrumentation, appropriate pain management techniques are used to protect sensitive hard and soft tissues. Maintaining a moist, clean environment by frequent rinsing of the oral cavity during instrumentation increases comfort, especially if the individual has xerostomia. Consider the effect of rubber-cup prophylaxis on eroded dentition and if it should be done at all, given the damaged tooth structure. Many polishing pastes are abrasive to dentin and should be avoided. Avoid polishing the teeth if the individual does not have extrinsic stains or if the dental hypersensitivity impedes patient comfort during stain removal. Dental hygiene care and necessary palliative treatment of discomfort (e.g., the use of desensitization treatments) must be scheduled for both periods of quiescence and those of activity of the eating disorder.

Evaluation

The evaluation of dental hygiene care for a patient with an eating disorder consists of the following two parts:

- An objective evaluation that is based on mutual goals previously established by the dental hygienist and the patient to determine whether the goals have been met, partially met, or unmet
- A subjective evaluation by the patient

Objective Evaluation

For an objective evaluation, the dental hygienist compares baseline findings involving plaque biofilm accumulation, periodontal status, dental caries, enamel erosion, salivary flow rate and quality, dentinal hypersensitivity, and oral tissues obtained at each subsequent appointment in terms of established goals. Many changes that occur over time are subtle and defy detection unless accurate measures are taken for comparison. It is important for the dental hygienist to use objective measurements to monitor the oral impact of the disorder and its associated comorbidities. The comparison of objective measures (e.g., oral dental erosion indices, photographs, study models, salivary flow, quality data) provides information for the dental hygiene continued care plan.

Subjective Evaluation

The patient's subjective evaluation provides additional information for the dental hygiene continued care plan. The successful treatment of eating disorders requires intensive therapy, followed by many years of maintenance. It is common for patients who have successfully controlled eating disorder behaviors for several weeks or months to relapse during the recovery phase. Awareness and verbal acknowledgment of this during the dental hygiene continued care plan evaluation permits patients to share honestly about areas of progress and distress. The oral health findings can then be used in conjunction with observations from other attending health professionals to guide subsequent care.

On occasion, objective and subjective evaluations conflict with each other. A patient with previously documented dental erosion may report that binge and purge episodes have been under control for six months and seemingly want to opt out of continued eating disorder care. The dental hygienist should consider the nature of the eating disorder and question whether the patient's statement is a reflection of the thinking influenced by the eating disorder. The comparison of the current dental status with intraoral photographs and diagnostic models obtained six months previously may indicate that the erosion is progressive. The dental hygienist becomes instrumental in encouraging the patient to continue with eating disorder therapy by acknowledging the relapse period as being consistent with recovery.

Continual evaluation of the patient's oral health status and the status of psychological therapy is one of the most critical functions of the dental hygienist when managing an individual with an eating disorder. At several points during the dental hygiene process of care, the clinician may need to reassess the patient's condition, revise care goals, plan alternative strategies, implement these strategies, and reevaluate the outcome. The dynamic nature of the dental hygiene process of care for patients with an eating disorder creates a challenge for the professional dental hygienist.

EATING DISORDER TREATMENT: INTERPROFESSIONAL COLLABORATION

The treatment for a person with an eating disorder involves many health professionals and interventions in addition to family and social support.[3] With informed consent from the patient, health professionals can collaborate for patient-centered care to learn about the perspectives of care and the needs of the patient that are outside the individual health professional's scope of practice. Such collaboration enhances the quality of care and improves patient outcomes. Importantly, the dental hygienist must advocate and contribute to interprofessional education around eating disorders and oral health education so the healthcare team can provide holistic care that includes the client's perspective.[25-30]

An interprofessional healthcare plan for a person with an eating disorder may be as follows:

- *Inpatient, outpatient, day program, and hospitalization treatment settings:* These settings are determined on the basis of the severity of the patient's eating disorder and their responsiveness to recommendations.
- *Psychotherapy such as cognitive behavioral therapy, interpersonal psychotherapy, group therapy, and family or caregiver therapy:* Given that the eating disorder is a disorder related to thinking, value is placed on helping the patient think about the eating disorder as a separate entity from themselves.
- *Nutritional treatment planning by dietitians with the patient and, if applicable, the patient's family:* Nutritional treatment is aimed at weight restoration and an understanding of what constitutes a balanced healthy dietary lifestyle. By restoring weight, the mind is better able to respond to cognitive therapy. A starved or nutritionally deprived brain does not function optimally.
- *A physical education therapist:* After a healthy weight is achieved, a physical education therapist may begin discussions with the individual to help establish a healthy approach to physical fitness. Persons with anorexia nervosa often overexercise to burn calories, so the reintroduction of physical activity occurs later during the recovery plan.
- *Possible psychopharmacologic treatment determined by the team and the patient:* Appropriate medications may include antidepressants and antianxiolytics. Little evidence exists to support medication use as a single treatment for eating disorders. Usually, medication is for the treatment of comorbid conditions associated with the eating disorder. These medications have the potential side effect of dry mouth. Supplemental drug treatment may be provided (e.g., hormone and nutrient replacement).
- *Prevention of oral health risks, particularly with bulimia nervosa and purging-type anorexia nervosa:* Interprofessional patient-centered collaboration is of great value to understanding which oral health interventions may be of benefit to recovery and which ones may inhibit it. For example, reconstructing the patient's dentition during active illness may be viewed by the healthcare team as enabling the continuation of oral purging because the dental concerns of the patient have been temporarily addressed while the eating disorder still possesses the patient. There is a need to coordinate nonemergency restorative and prosthetic dental care with psychological therapy (Box 57.13).

EATING DISORDER RESOURCES

There are many myths and misunderstandings that surround eating disorders. As critical thinkers and patient advocates, dental hygienists follow an evidence-based, best-practice philosophy that guides dental hygiene practice. Valuable information about eating disorders is available online through credible organizations and associations such as the National Eating Disorders Association (NEDA, United States https://www.nationaleatingdisorders.org), the National Eating Disorder Information Centre (NEDIC, Canada http://nedic.ca), the National Association of Anorexia Nervosa and Associated Disorders (ANAD, United States http://www.anad.org), the King's College/London Institute of Psychiatry (IoP, England https://www.kcl.ac.uk/ioppn/depts/pm/research/eatingdisorders/index.aspx), and Beating Eating Disorders (beat, United Kingdom http://beatingeatingdisorders.com). Each association has resource listings for professional and personal help that the dental hygienist can share with patients (Box 57.14).

BOX 57.13 Patient or Client Education Tips

- Inform the patient that help is available and that harm reduction and recovery are possible.
- Explain the need for referral and the interprofessional collaboration of the healthcare team for comprehensive care.
- Ensure that the patient knows about health resources that are available for people with eating disorders.
- Explain the effect of the eating disorder on the oral tissues.
- Promote self-care strategies to prevent or control oral manifestations associated with the eating disorder.
- At a community level, provide educational materials that address oral health and eating disorders in both the dental hygiene practice and other healthcare settings.

BOX 57.14 Legal, Ethical, and Safety Issues

- Oral healthcare team members must recognize their limitations with regard to treating patients with eating disorders. The primary role of the oral healthcare team is to refer the patient with a suspected eating disorder to specialists who treat the psychological and medical aspects of eating disorders.
- Documentation of objective and subjective findings and recommendations, as well as decisions regarding referral for evaluation in the patient's permanent dental record, are part of the patient's confidential healthcare record.
- Failure to recommend a patient who has an eating disorder for referral for subsequent psychological evaluation is neglecting the hygienist's professional responsibility as a healthcare provider. Keep in mind that comorbid conditions may necessitate referral as well. Following up after the referral is also important.
- All information related to a patient's eating disorder is confidential. The dental practitioner requires the patient's consent to refer the patient to medical and psychological therapy systems.
- Use of a signed release form allows oral healthcare professionals to contact and collaborate with the eating disorder treatment team.

KEY CONCEPTS

- Eating disorders are complex mental health illnesses with comorbid associations with other mental health conditions.
- Eating disorders impact the individual's health and wellness and can be life-threatening.
- Eating disorders affect oral health and can result in the destruction of the dentition.
- Dental hygienists practice in a professional and nonjudgmental manner that enables patient disclosure of an eating disorder.
- Dental hygienists must be proactive and have eating disorder information readily available.
- Dental hygienists must have the courage and integrity to openly communicate with a patient regarding objective and subjective observations of an eating disorder.
- Screening for signs of eating disorders and employing evidence-based dental hygiene interventions are part of the professional role of the dental hygiene clinician.
- It is critical to promote health and wellness through interprofessional collaborative practice for the treatment of eating disorders.

ACKNOWLEDGMENT

The authors acknowledge Karen B. Williams for her past contributions to this chapter.

REFERENCES

1. American Psychiatric Association. *Diagnostic and Statistical Manual of Mental Disorders.* 5th ed. American Psychiatric Association; 2022. text revision.
2. National Institute for Health and Care Excellence, NICE guideline. *Eating Disorders: Recognition and Treatment.* National Institute for Clinical Excellence; 2017. From www.nice.org.uk/guidance/ng69. Accessed June 2022.
3. National Eating Disorders Association. National Eating Disorders Association Website. Available at: www.nationaleatingdisorders.org. Accessed June 2022.
4. Monteleone AM, Castellini G, Volpe U, et al. Neuroendocrinology and brain imaging of reward in eating disorders: a possible key to the treatment of anorexia nervosa and bulimia nervosa. *Prog Neuro-Psychopharmacol Biol Psychiatry.* 2018;80(Pt B):132–142.
5. Mathisen F, Sundgot-Borgen C, Anstensrud B, Sundgot-Borgen J. Mental health, eating behaviour and injuries in professional dance students. *Res Dance Educ.* 2022;23(1):108–125. https://doi.org/10.1080/14647893.2021.1993171.
6. Mancine RP, Gusfa DW, Moshrefi A, Kennedy SF. Prevalence of disordered eating in athletes categorized by emphasis on leanness and activity type – a systematic review. *J Eat Disord.* 2020;8(1):47. https://doi.org/10.1186/s40337-020-00323-2.
7. Smolak L, Murnen SK, Ruble AE. Female athletes and eating problems: a meta-analysis. *Int J Eat Disord.* 2000;27(4):371–380. https://doi.org/10.1002/(SICI)1098-108X(200005)27:4<371::AID-EAT1>3.0.CO;2-Y.
8. Espindola C, Blay S. Anorexia nervosa treatment from the patient perspective: a metasynthesis of qualitative studies. *Ann Clin Psychiatry.* 2009;21:38.
9. Kisely S, Baghaie H, Lalloo R, et al. Association between poor oral health and eating disorders: systematic review and meta-analysis. *Br J Psychiatry.* 2015;207(4):299–305.
10. Monda M, Costacurta M, Maffei L, Docimo R. Oral manifestations of eating disorders in adolescent patients. A review. *Eur J Paediatr Dent.* 2021;22(2):155–158. https://doi.org/10.23804/ejpd.2021.22.02.13.
11. Pallier A, Karimova A, Boillot A, et al. Dental and periodontal health in adults with eating disorders: a case-control study. *J Dent.* 2019;84:55–59. https://doi.org/10.1016/j.jdent.2019.03.005.
12. Panico R, Piemonte E, Lazos J, Gilligan G, Zampini A, Lanfranchi H. Oral mucosal lesions in anorexia nervosa, bulimia nervosa and EDNOS. *J Psychiatr Res.* 2018;96:178–182. https://doi.org/10.1016/j.jpsychires.2017.09.022.
13. Lourenco M, Azevedo A, Brandao I, Gomes PS. Orofacial manifestations in outpatients with anorexia nervosa and bulimia nervosa focusing on the vomiting behavior. *Clin Oral Invest.* 2018;22(5):1915–1922. https://doi.org/10.1007/s00784-017-2284-y.
14. Rosten A, Newton T. The impact of bulimia nervosa on oral health: a review of the literature. *Br Dent J.* 2017;223(7):533–539. https://doi.org/10.1038/sj.bdj.2017.837.
15. Brandt LMT, Fernandes LHF, Aragao AS, et al. Relationship between risk behavior for eating disorders and dental caries and dental erosion. *Sci World J.* 2017;2017:1656417. https://doi.org/10.1155/2017/1656417.
16. Holmes SR, Sabel A, Gaudiani JL, et al. Management of oropharyngeal dysphagia in patients with severe anorexia nervosa: a large retrospective review. *Int J Eat Disord.* 2016:159–166.
17. Johansson AK, Norring C, Unell L, et al. Eating disorders and biochemical composition of saliva: a retrospective matched case-control study. *Eur J Oral Sci.* 2015;158:64.
18. Paszynska E, Schlueter N, Slopien A, et al. Salivary enzyme activity in anorexic persons—a controlled clinical trial. *Clin Oral Investig.* 2015;19(8):1981–1989.
19. Yagi T, Ueda H, Amitani H, et al. The role of ghrelin, salivary secretions, and dental care in eating disorders. *Nutrients.* 2012:967–989.
20. DeBate RD, Cragun D, Gallentine AA, et al. Evaluate, assess, treat: development and evaluation of the EAT framework to increase effective communication regarding sensitive oral-systemic health issues. *Eur J Dent Educ.* 2012;16:232.
21. Range H, Pallier A, Ali A, Huas C, Colon P, Godart N. Risk factors for oral health in Anorexia Nervosa: comparison of a self-report questionnaire and a face-to-face interview. *Int J Environ Res Publ Health.* 2021;18(8). https://doi.org/10.3390/ijerph18084212.
22. Hill LS, Reid F, Morgan JF, et al. SCOFF, the development of an eating disorder screening questionnaire. *Int J Eat Disord.* 2010;43:344.
23. Smorthit K, Sawbridge D, Fitzgerald R. Eating disorders and the orthodontist: diagnosis, considerations, and referral. *J Orthod.* 2021;48(3):313–322. https://doi.org/10.1177/1465312521993491.
24. Turhani D, Ohlmeier KH, Sutter W, Kielbassa AM. Undesirable course of an oral implant rehabilitation in a patient with a long history of bulimia nervosa: case report and review of the literature. *Quintessence Int.* 2019;50(1):68–79. https://doi.org/10.3290/j.qi.a41367.
25. Patterson-Norrie T, Ramjan L, Sousa MS, Sank L, George A. Eating disorders and oral health: a scoping review on the role of dietitians. *J Eat Disord.* 2020;8. https://doi.org/10.1186/s40337-020-00325-0.
26. Johnson LB, Boyd LD, Rainchuso L, Rothman A, Mayer B. Eating disorder professionals' perceptions of oral health knowledge. *Int J Dent Hyg.* 2017;15(3):164–171. https://doi.org/10.1111/idh.12183.0.
27. Bassiouny MA, Tweddale E. Oral health considerations in anorexia and bulimia nervosa. 2. Multidisciplinary management and personalized dental care. *Gen Dent.* 2017;65(5):24–31.
28. Yodogawa T, Nerome Y, Tokunaga J, Hatano H, Marutani M. Effects of food neophobia and oral health on the nutritional status of community-dwelling older adults. *BMC Geriatr.* 2022;22(1):334. https://doi.org/10.1186/s12877-022-03013-7.
29. Kavitha PR, Vivek P, Hegde AM. Eating disorders and their implications on oral health–role of dentists. *J Clin Pediatr Dent.* 2011;36(2):155–160. https://doi.org/10.17796/jcpd.36.2.3785414p682843wj.
30. Silverstein LS, Haggerty C, Sams L, Phillips C, Roberts MW. Impact of an oral health education intervention among a group of patients with eating disorders (anorexia nervosa and bulimia nervosa). *J Eat Disord.* 2019;7:29. https://doi.org/10.1186/s40337-019-0259-x.

58

Child Abuse and Neglect and Family Violence

Sheryl L. Syme and Susan Camardese

PROFESSIONAL DEVELOPMENT OPPORTUNITIES

Human abuse and neglect is a public health problem affecting individuals from every segment of the population. The unimaginable trauma resulting from abuse and neglect has long-lasting effects on victims across the lifespan. Dental hygienists are mandated reporters for child abuse and neglect, vulnerable adult abuse, and victims of human trafficking. Dental hygienists encounter victims in all practice and community settings and are professionally responsible for recognizing the signs and symptoms of abuse and neglect occurring in family violence and human trafficking situations. Dental hygienists should be familiar with their state's definitions of abuse and neglect, along with the reporting requirements and social support services for maltreated children, adults, and trafficked human victims.

COMPETENCIES

1. Apply knowledge of indicators of abuse and neglect in clinical patient care and utilize social support and public health resources to report and assist victims of family violence and human trafficking.
2. Incorporate assessment of abuse and neglect among child, adult, elderly, vulnerable adults, and victims of human trafficking as a routine part of the dental hygiene visit.
3. Collaborate with interprofessional healthcare providers in the education, early detection, and early intervention for victims of child maltreatment, intimate partner violence, elder and vulnerable adult abuse and neglect, and human trafficking.
4. Assume primary prevention and advocacy roles in educating patients, communities, and professional colleagues in health, law, and social support services regarding dental findings associated with abuse and neglect.
5. Explain the links between child maltreatment and intimate partner violence and bullying and the power and control demonstrated by perpetrators of family violence and neglect and human trafficking.

INTRODUCTION

Family violence extends across a wide range of individuals affected by acts including emotional, financial, physical, and sexual abuse. Family members can also suffer from neglect which impacts their emotional, physical, and cognitive development and/or quality of life. Victims of family violence and neglect suffer serious educational, health, social, psychopathological, and financial consequences. Family violence not only traumatizes[1] the victim but presents harm for others who witness and are left to cope with the deleterious outcomes of the abuse and neglect of family members.[2] Adverse childhood experiences (ACEs) include abuse, neglect, and potentially traumatic events that occur before age 18 that affect health across the lifetime.[3] Examples of ACEs are:

- experiencing violence, abuse, or neglect
- witnessing domestic or community violence
- multiple deaths and traumatic loss
- racism over time

Social determinants of health and aspects of a child's environment where they live, learn, work, and play can undermine their sense of safety, stability, and bonding, such as growing up in a household with:

- an impaired caregiver, substance use disorder
- a family member with mental health problems
- unsafe conditions
- instability due to parental separation or household members being incarcerated.
- poverty

Dental hygienists are uniquely positioned to identify signs and symptoms of abuse and neglect and recognize medical and dental history disclosures suspicious of maltreatment of children, adolescents, adults, elderly, and vulnerable adults. Detection of injuries and trauma to the head, face, neck, and oral cavity from acts of family violence and human trafficking (HT) and knowing the ethical and legal procedures for reporting suspicious findings to the appropriate social support agencies are crucial professional responsibilities of dental hygienists. The frequency of dental hygiene care visits provides the opportunity to develop close and trusting patient-provider relationships and to obtain detailed health, dental, and social histories, and conduct thorough extra- and intraoral clinical assessments. Identifying early signs and symptoms of maltreatment and knowing the proper, safe, and legal interventions available for victim reporting may save victims from further maltreatment and even death. Abusers may avoid visiting the same physician but return to the same oral healthcare professional when seeking treatment for victims of perpetrated abuse and neglect. Therefore, even greater professional responsibilities align for dental hygienists to detect changes in patient well-being, healthy and dysfunctional family relationships, and even the most subtle changes in patients' behaviors, health, and signs and symptoms resulting from the trauma and victimization occurring in their lives.

Maltreatment is the term used to define abuse and neglect of human victims. Legislation in every state and US territory as well in most countries mandate the reporting of suspected maltreatment of children, vulnerable adults, and trafficked victims to local jurisdictions' child and adult protective services agencies and law enforcement, respectively.[4] State and international laws differ regarding reporting adult victims of intimate partner violence (IPV) and elder abuse and neglect. Although craniofacial and neck injuries are commonly present in abused individuals, oral healthcare professionals may be missing the connection to family violence and HT and the opportunity to refer victims to and make timely reports to the proper authorities.[5] Dental hygienists must be able to identify signs and symptoms of abuse and neglect and reporting procedures to support victims of child maltreatment, family violence, and HT.

ABUSE AND NEGLECT

Abuse includes the most serious harm committed against human victims that can be physical, sexual, emotional, or verbal, or any combination of types. **Neglect** is any act of omission from parents, caretakers, or those responsible for another individual, which may include failure to provide adequate care, support, nutrition, and health or hygiene needs. Neglect also encompasses the failure to follow through with filling prescriptions and other prescribed therapies by those responsible for the medical, social, psychological, and emotional well-being of individuals under their care, and in the case of children, failure to provide for their educational needs as required by law.

Mid-Atlantic Prevent Abuse and Neglect through Dental Awareness (Mid-Atlantic P.A.N.D.A.) is an educational resource and awareness program created to promote an atmosphere of understanding in dentistry and other professional communities to increase the prevention of abuse and neglect through early identification and appropriate intervention for victims.[6] The educational focus is on child abuse and neglect, IPV, vulnerable adults, HT, and bullying. The emphasis of the program is for oral healthcare professionals to recognize, refer, and report their findings to appropriate local social support service agencies and law enforcement to address the specific needs of victims for safety, comfort, health and dental care interventions, and protection from further abuse and neglect.

CHILD MALTREATMENT

Child abuse and neglect has far-reaching economic, health, psychological, and social impacts on its victims, families, and communities. Although the federal government originally enacted key legislation, the **Child Abuse Prevention and Treatment Act** (CAPTA: P.L. 93-247) of 1974, to acknowledge concerns about physical abuse of children, most occurrences of maltreatment today are child neglect. Neglect may present risk to the child's health, safety, and well-being resulting from failure to provide food, clothing, shelter, medical care, or supervision. CAPTA defines abuse and neglect of children and youth below the age of 18 years. Each state is then responsible for establishing its own definitions within the minimum standards set by federal legislation.

Additionally, CAPTA provides grant monies to states and nonprofit organizations to support prevention, data collection and evaluation, interventions, research, and prosecutions regarding child abuse and neglect. In 1980, CAPTA began using the term *child maltreatment* for abuse and neglect. In 1988, the Child Maltreatment Report Series was established to collect and publish child maltreatment information and statistics annually for each state and the District of Columbia. The Child Abuse Prevention and Treatment Act (CAPTA; 42 U.S.C. §5101) as amended by the CAPTA Reauthorization Act of 2010,[7,8] broadly defined child abuse and neglect as follows:

- any recent act or failure to act on the part of a parent or caretaker that results in death, serious physical or emotional harm, sexual abuse, or exploitation; or
- an act or failure to act that presents an imminent risk of serious harm

The CAPTA Reauthorization Act of 2010 extended the law through 2015 and amended it in 2015, 2016, 2018, and 2019. In 2015, the federal definitions of child abuse and neglect and sexual abuse were amended by the Justice for Victims of Trafficking Act to identify children who are victims of sex trafficking or other forms of trafficking. The CAPTA Reauthorization Act of 2021 strengthens states' services to strengthen families and better distinguish neglect from circumstances associated with financial stress, address racial bias in overrepresentation of families of color and of low income in the Child Protective Services (CPS)

system, and protect children at highest risk of child abuse and neglect. The Comprehensive Addiction and Recovery Act of 2016 provided a requirement for CPS to report the number of infants with prenatal substance exposure as amended in CAPTA. This is relevant to dental hygienists regarding assessing and advocating for patients to be alcohol- and substance- free during pregnancy and to be knowledgeable about **fetal alcohol spectrum disorders**.

CURRENT PREVALENCE

Child maltreatment is a global public health problem. Worldwide, 300 million or nearly 3 in 4 children aged 2 to 4 years of age regularly are subjected to physical and/or psychological violence perpetrated by parents and caregivers.[9] Globally, 1 in 5 females and 1 in 13 males report they suffered from sexual abuse as a child before age 18. United States national and state child abuse and neglect statistics are based on data collected by CPS agencies and reported to the National Child Abuse and Neglect Data System (NCANDS). NCANDS is a national data collection and analysis program of state child abuse and neglect information based on data received from the 50 states, the District of Columbia, and the Commonwealth of Puerto Rico. The data are collected from states and analyzed by the Children's Bureau in the Administration on Children, Youth and Families, the Administration for Children and Families within the US Department of Health and Human Services. NCANDS data are used for the yearly Child Maltreatment report series.

Data published in the Child Maltreatment 2020 report are different compared to previous years because of the COVID-19 pandemic.[10] State, country, and territorial lockdown restrictions, including closure of recreational venues, afterschool programs, and schools converting to virtual instruction to prevent the spread of COVID-19, made it difficult for the typically largest group of child abuse and neglect reporters, educational personnel, to observe maltreatment and submit reports of suspected maltreatment. For 2020, in the professional reporters' category, legal and law enforcement personnel (20.9%), education personnel (17.2%), and medical personnel (11.6%) submitted the majority (66.7%) of reports of alleged child abuse and neglect. Nonprofessionals, including friends, neighbors, and relatives, submitted 17% of the reports and unclassified sources submitted the remaining reports (16.3%) as reported in the United States in 2022 by Administration for Children and Families, Administration on Children, Youth and Families, Children's Bureau.[10] Similarly, the COVID-19 pandemic impacted child protection services and the safety net for violence prevention resulting in similar underreporting as a result of social distancing, quarantining, and continued school closures in Australia, Brazil, Canada, Colombia, Germany, Israel, and South Africa.[11] In 2021, twice as many children were living in countries with complex emergencies. Those countries hardest hit with situations of human fragility and war/conflict, and civil unrest experienced concomitant threats to child safety such as poverty, loss of parental livelihoods, violence along migration routes, and, increasingly, violence in the virtual world. The conundrum of underreporting and disruption of health, social, and child protection services occurring during the COVID-19 pandemic and increased risk of violence against children, child marriages, child labor, trafficking, and family separation as a result of complex worldwide emergencies compounded by caregiver sickness and death due to COVID-19 placed the most vulnerable children at risk of multiple safety and rights violations.

In 2020, US CPS agencies received 3.9 million referrals alleging child maltreatment. Nationally, there were 618,000 child victims of abuse and neglect. The national victim rate is 8.4 victims per 1000 children in the population. The highest victimization rate occurs among children younger than 1 year old (25.1 per 1,000 children of the same

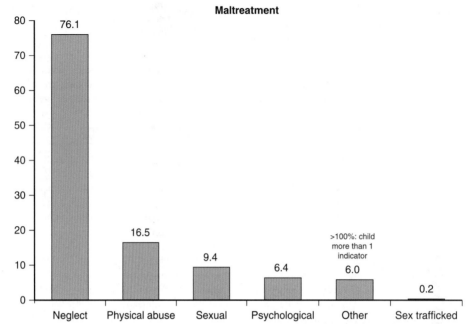

Fig. 58.1 Types of child maltreatment victims. (From US Department of Health & Human Services, Administration for Children and Families, Administration on Children, Youth and Families, Children's Bureau. Child Maltreatment 2020; 2022. Available at: https://https://www.acf.hhs.gov/cb/data-research/child-maltreatment.)

age). Young females have a higher victimization rate (8.9 per 1000) compared to young males (7.9 per 1000). The victimization rate of American Indian or Alaska Native children is highest at 15.5 per 1000, and second highest among African American children (13.2 per 1000 children of the same race or ethnicity).[10]

Neglect continues to be the most common type of maltreatment. In 2020, 76.1% of victims were neglected, 16.5% physically abused, 9.4% sexually abused, and 0.2% sex trafficked (Fig. 58.1). Many of the reported children suffered multiple forms of maltreatment, and many were subjects of repeated reports, indicating that abuse and neglect were not isolated episodes. Often, the abuse and neglect escalates into violence and trauma inflicted on the victims. In 2020, 1750 children died from abuse and neglect in the United States. Of those fatalities, 68% were younger than age 3 and nearly one-half (46.4%) of the child fatalities were younger than 1 year old. Young males continue to have a higher child fatality rate than young females. The decreased numbers of victims and child fatalities from the prior year may be the result of school lockdowns during the pandemic and less educator personnel allegation reports, yet child welfare advocates are optimistic that significant progress is being made in reducing child maltreatment victimization.

CHILD MALTREATMENT TYPES

Child maltreatment includes all types of abuse and neglect of a child under the age of 18 years by a parent or caregiver or another person who frequently encounters a child in their vocation or employment role (e.g., clergy, coach, teacher). In the familial type, the cycle of child maltreatment can be intergenerational in some families; in other words, maltreated children are at high risk for maltreating their children.[12] Child maltreatment victim types are recorded as medical neglect, neglect encompassing physical and educational neglect or supervision acts of omissions preventing a child's basic needs from being met, psychological maltreatment, sex trafficking, and "Other." Some victims' maltreatment type is tabulated as "Unknown" in the Child Maltreatment 2020 report. NCANDS added sex trafficking as a new maltreatment type and states began reporting this data in 2018.

In 2018, states also began reporting infants with prenatal substance exposures to NCANDS under the code of "Other" maltreatment. Types of child maltreatment are found in Table 58.1. Children with special needs may have a higher victimization risk for maltreatment than children without special needs.[13]

Common indicators of abuse and neglect are found in Table 58.2.

Physical Abuse

Physical abuse is the use of physical force, such as hitting, kicking, punching, beating, stabbing, biting, pushing, shoving, throwing, pulling, dragging, dropping, shaking, strangling or choking, smothering, burning, scalding, poisoning, or other physical acts that harm or have the potential to harm or injure children.[10,14] "Those who don't cruise rarely bruise" is a pediatric proverb referring to the **sentinel findings** of bruising, frenum tears, intraoral injury, and subconjunctival hemorrhage on the face or torso of nonambulatory infants that should raise suspicions.[15] Other physical abuse findings may include imprints or marks made by objects used by the perpetrators of abuse that may leave *tattoo* effects on the victim's skin. The victim's skin can reveal pattern bruises that mirror the object of abuse left by belt buckles, ropes, and looped cords, as well as linear markings from skin compressed between the perpetrator's fingers during an open-handed slap or strike. Skin injuries are the most common sign of physical abuse, and minor forms of skin injuries, unless detected early, may lead to more serious outcomes, including death. Other red flags of physical abuse include inappropriate seasonal clothing worn to cover trauma inflicted to the arms and legs, uncorrelated explanations, and reports of injuries inconsistent with the child's developmental stage, and evidence of repeated injuries. Formerly, bruises were assigned a uniform age based on color, but more recent evidence suggests great variation in the color and healing of bruises from one person to another; therefore multiple-colored bruises are no longer diagnostic of inflicted physical injuries.

Other indicators of abuse include welts, bite marks, burns, fractures, lacerations, abrasions, head injuries, and delay of treatment. **Abusive head trauma** has replaced the term shaken baby syndrome since neuropathological symptoms formerly associated with the act

TABLE 58.1   Types of Child Maltreatment

Category	Description
Neglect	Deprivation of adequate food, water, clothing, shelter, medical care (medical neglect), or supervision, including failure to educate a child as required by law
Physical abuse	When a child is deliberately physically injured or put at risk of harm by another person
Sexual abuse	Use of sex to hurt, degrade, dominate, humiliate, and gain power over the victim
Psychologic abuse	Emotional and psychological abuse destroys the child's self-esteem and includes verbal abuse, excessive demands on the child's performance, and withholding of love and affection.
Other	States may code "other" in their reports if the maltreatment does not fit into any other NCANDS categories. "Other" maltreatment types include threatened abuse and neglect, infants born and affected by maternal substance abuse resulting from prenatal drug exposure or withdrawal symptoms to an illegal or a legal substance, including healthcare providers involved in delivery or care of infants reporting infants born with fetal alcohol spectrum disorder.
Sex trafficking	The recruitment, harboring, transportation, provision, or obtaining of a person for the purpose of a commercial sex act. NCANDS provides the provision to states to report any sex trafficking victim under age 24 years.

TABLE 58.2   Indicators of Abuse and Neglect in Patients

Type of Abuse	Indicators
Physical abuse	Unexplained injuries such as bruises, broken bones (fractures), or burns
	Injuries nonmatching to explanation or are noncompatible with child's developmental age
	Multiple bruises on face, lips, arms, legs
	Bruising on nonbony protuberances*
	Shaped or patterned injuries or bruises such as belt or belt buckle marks, iron burns, hand slap or finger markings, rope burns
	Cigarette burns
	Scalding injuries (glovelike or socklike immersion burns)
	Broken nose
	Black eyes
	Inappropriate seasonal dress (long sleeves in the summer to cover bruises)
	Cuts or lacerations, especially on face or neck
	Oral trauma including the following:
	Torn frenum
	Avulsed teeth
	Discolored teeth (resulting from pulpal necrosis), indicator of past traumatic injury
	Fractured teeth
	Gingival abrasions
	Burns from scalding liquids or hot utensils
	Oral lacerations resulting from forced feeding
	Trauma to the corners of the mouth (may indicate the use of gags)
	Gingival contusions
	Petechiae or bruising (may indicate forced oral sex)
	Palatal lesions and scars
Neglect	Poor hygiene
	Rampant caries, early childhood caries
	Unmet medical or dental needs
	Lack of regularity of dental hygiene appointments
	Poor or no parental supervision
	Delay in seeking treatment
	Failure to follow through with needed care
Sexual abuse	Petechiae on soft palate (may be a sign of forced oral sex)
	Venereal warts (condyloma acuminatum) on lips, tongue, palate, or gingivae
	Venereal disease (in prepuberty)
	Itching of genitalia
	Difficulty in walking or sitting
Emotional maltreatment	Withdrawn or fatigued
	Record of suicide attempts
	Parent or caregiver:
	Constantly blames or berates child
	Is unconcerned about child
	Overtly rejects child

*Normal childhood injuries tend to occur on skin covering bony protuberances (e.g., knees, elbows). Bruises caused by abuse often are found on nonbony areas (e.g., arms, legs, neck).

of shaking infants can also be attributed to blunt force trauma to the head and hypoxic-ischemic (smothering) means. Abusive head trauma is the leading cause of serious or fatal brain injuries occurring in children under the age of 2 years.[16] Other typical sites for inflicted injuries of abuse are the buttocks and lower back, genitals and inner thighs, cheeks, ears, lip and labial frenum, neck, arms, and hands. Because craniofacial, head, face, and neck injuries occur in more than one-half of child abuse cases, dental professionals should be knowledgeable of dentofacial trauma associated with abuse.[17–18] Notably, tongue, lip, gingiva, buccal and alveolar mucosa, palatal and frenum lacerations, contusions, or burns; facial bone fractures; jaw fractures or displacement; tooth fractures; discolored teeth from pulpal necrosis; avulsed teeth (Fig. 58.2); and nonvital teeth warrant further assessment of suspected abuse. Aside from blows to the face and head, aggressive or forced feeding with utensils, bottles, cups, hands, or fingers, or scalding liquids or caustic substances cause many oral injuries associated with abuse.[19] Restraints applied to the mouth, such as gags and ties, may produce bruised, irritated, scarred, or leathery conditions at the corners of the mouth from the continuous rubbing, stretching, or scratching of the skin.

Bite Marks

Children exhibiting fresh or healed bite marks in an elliptical or oval shape with indentations consistent with the human adult arch form and with an interchained distance (i.e., distance of the canine cusp tips) greater than 3.0 cm that may be accompanied without abrasions, contusions, or lacerations, should arouse suspicion of an adult human bite rather than one inflicted by an animal or another child.[18] A human bite mark compresses the victim's flesh, producing abrasions, ecchymoses, and lacerations, whereas dogs or other carnivorous animals tend to tear into flesh, causing irregular breaks and tears to the skin of those

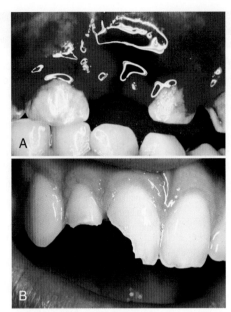

Fig. 58.2 (A) Tooth avulsion in a child as a consequence of being punched in the mouth. (B) Tooth fracture of central and lateral incisors as a consequence of a beating when the child landed against a chest of drawers. (Courtesy Dr. Lynn Douglas Mouden, founder of P.A.N.D.A. [Prevention of Abuse and Neglect through Dental Awareness].)

they attack. Human adult perpetrators may be identified by the DNA present in oral epithelial cells deposited from bite marks as detected by forensic odontologists and experts trained in bite mark identification and fabrication of bite models.[18] Adults who bite children inflict pain as punishment or inappropriately act in response to the inability to control a child's behavioral, eating, or emotional responses.

Caregiver-Fabricated Illness in a Child

Caregiver-fabricated illness in a child—also referred to as Munchausen syndrome by proxy, pediatric condition falsification, factitious disorder by proxy, or medical child abuse—is a type of child maltreatment caused by a primary or secondary adult caregiver who falsifies and subjects a child to unnecessary and potentially harmful medical care by providing either misinformation to a medical provider, fabricating symptoms, coaching the child or others to misrepresent the illness, or inducing illness in the child, resulting in diagnoses, the need for medications, procedures, or attention from healthcare clinicians.[14,18] The caregiver often seeks care for the child from different medical providers and healthcare facilities in attempts to fragment continuity of treatment, prevent discovery, and continue gaining the desired attention from the medical community for their own misaligned psychologic needs. An adult perpetrator may falsify conditions of the child because of a traumatic event, attempt to transfer their own real or fantasy sickly behaviors to the child, keep the child dependent, and/or seek regard as a devoted parent to fulfill a psychologic need for medical attention, fabricate false reports of child maltreatment, or for unknown reasons. Inconsistent stories, implausible histories, reports or findings of illness or injuries occurring only in the caregiver's presence, discrepancies in the condition's clinical presentation with the history provided by the caregiver, increasing symptomology and exaggerated nonrelated symptoms, and suspicious multiple infections all are indicators of fabricated illness in the child. In the parent or caregiver, exhibition of unstable adult behaviors, focus on an undiagnosed illness, refusal of recommended interventions in lieu of dangerous or controversial treatments unsubstantiated through evidence-based medicine, requests for medications solely on the basis of the caregiver's history, and siblings with

common histories of the disorder, who in some cases may have died under suspicious circumstances, are all red flags for the healthcare provider.[14,18] Similarly, oral healthcare providers may be targeted by perpetrators who request walk-in, urgent, or emergency dental care and resistance to establish a dental home for the child, who may exhibit unusual or real oral symptoms and peculiar real or alleged dental conditions. Excessive healthcare evaluations and treatments are the mechanisms of abuse that can result in lingering and escalating physical and mental harm to the child while appeasing the caregiver's psychological need for attention.

Sexual Abuse

CAPTA[7] defines sexual abuse as:

"...the employment, use, persuasion, inducement, enticement, or coercion of any child to engage in, or assist any other person to engage in, any sexually explicit conduct or simulation of such conduct for the purpose of producing a visual depiction of such conduct; or the rape, and in cases of caretaker or inter-familial relationships, statutory rape, molestation, prostitution, or other form of sexual exploitation of children or incest with children."

Most victims and perpetrators know each other. Disclosures of sexual abuse by verbal children are most often made to a nonprofessional individual.[14] Long-term symptoms include anxiety, fear, or posttraumatic stress disorder (PTSD), and in some cases, arrested development.

Although the oropharyngeal area is a common site of sexual abuse in children, oral injuries or infections may not be visible. However, some oral signs of sexual abuse are condyloma acuminatum (venereal warts), which appear as a cauliflower-like growth on the lips, palate, gingiva, or tongue (Fig. 58.3). In addition, syphilis may emerge as an ulcerated chancre or mucous patch. Pharyngeal, oral, and perioral gonorrhea when appearing in prepubertal children are pathognomonic of sexual abuse.[18] Herpes can manifest as gingivostomatitis (Fig. 58.4A,B,C). Human papillomavirus (HPV) is recognized as another possible sign of child sexual abuse associated with the formation of oral warts. Palatal petechiae could be a sign of forced oral sex (Fig. 58.5).

When sexual abuse is suspected, all observations should be documented, and a complete patient history is obtained from the parents or caregivers separately from the child. This documentation allows for a determination of the child's safety and information to report immediately to the local **Child Protective Services (CPS)** agency.

Psychological Maltreatment

Psychological maltreatment refers to a repeated pattern or extreme occurrence(s) of caregiving behavior that jeopardizes the psychological and nurturing needs of the child. When a child is constantly criticized or belittled or not provided with love or guidance, serious harm occurs to the child's development and self-esteem. Children who have key developmental processes disrupted as a result of emotional maltreatment will experience mental well-being changes such as anxiety, low mood, aggression, deficits in social skills, and poor interrelationships and suffer negative long-term educational outcomes such as attention problems, poor reading ability, and failure to be enrolled in and complete high school or be employed.[20] Parental emotional abuse is a risk factor for serious mental health problems and more severe PTSD symptoms in children and adolescents experiencing trauma from other types of child maltreatment.[21] Behavioral and emotional signs of psychological maltreatment include antisocial conduct, expressions of aggression, disruptive behavior, or anger, rage, or unusual anxiety or fear.

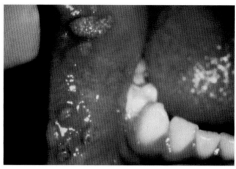

Fig. 58.3 Indicator of oral sexual abuse. Condylomas, venereal warts transmitted to the oral cavity through sexual abuse. (Courtesy Dr. Lynn Douglas Mouden, founder of P.A.N.D.A. [Prevention of Abuse and Neglect through Dental Awareness].)

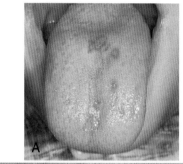

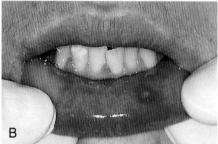

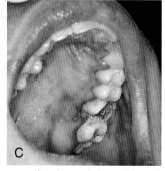

Fig. 58.4 (A) Indicators of oral sexual abuse. Herpetic gingivostomatitis in a child. (B and C) Herpetic gingivostomatitis in an adolescent.

Bullying

Bullying is the use of force or coercion to abuse or intimidate others. Nationally, nearly 15% of youths have been electronically bullied and 19% have been bullied on school property.[22] Youths who grow up without familial or nonfamilial role models to guide, teach, advise, and provide emotional support to them in nurturing relationships and are in unstable and unsafe environments are more likely to bully others or be bullied. Bullies and victims of bullying are more likely to be exposed to violence at home. The aggressive behavior of bullying is defined by

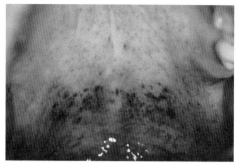

Fig. 58.5 Indicator of oral sexual abuse. Palatal petechiae may indicate forced oral sex.

repetition of the harmful behavior, the intentionality of acts, and the imbalance of social or physical power. It can include verbal harassment or threat, or physical assault directed repeatedly toward particular victims, perhaps on the grounds of race, religion, gender, sexuality, appearance, or ability. It may be in person or electronic. Bullying is an extremely prevalent public health problem and it does not happen in isolation. Bullying continues in a variety of settings, including schools; cyberspace via computers, cell phones, and other devices; and the workplace.

Neglect

Neglect is typically a failure by the parent or caregiver to provide for basic physical, educational, or emotional needs. It may include deprivation of adequate food, clothing, shelter, healthcare, psychological support, and other needs or supervision. The manifestations of dental neglect include poor oral hygiene, untreated dental disease (e.g., rampant dental caries, pain, infection, bleeding, trauma), and a caregiver's willful failure to ensure continuity of care after being alerted to the child's oral health needs (Fig. 58.6). Nurturing caretakers would not hesitate to seek immediate medical or dental treatment for an injured child. Perpetrators, on the other hand, are typically less forthcoming about the nature of nonaccidental injuries and are more likely to delay seeking treatment intentionally for the child because they fear discovery.

The American Academy of Pediatric Dentistry defines dental neglect as the willful failure to seek and follow through with treatment to ensure oral health.[23] Parents and caregivers with adequate oral health literacy with a willful failure to seek care must be distinguished from those without knowledge of the need for the child's oral care when identifying the need to report to CPS. Social determinants of health such as living in poverty, being among a socially marginalized population, and geographic constraints limiting access to dental care perpetuate as barriers to preventive oral healthcare and is a global challenge.[24] Poor oral health literacy and/or lack of access to oral healthcare may contribute to dental neglect, presenting a conundrum for oral health professionals worldwide.

Indicators of Child Maltreatment

The abused child may present warning signs of abuse, such as repeated injuries and/or inappropriate behavior or a neglected appearance. The patient may confide in the caregiver, complain of hunger or thirst, or display a lack of interest in the surroundings. Abuse victims may exhibit passive or withdrawn behavior, poor self-image, sexual acting out, depression, anxiety disorders, substance and alcohol abuse, eating disorders, hostility, lack of cooperation, self-destructive or self-abusive behavior, suicidal thoughts, social or academic problems, and/or a reluctance to return to a waiting adult. The victim's abuser may monitor interactions, answer questions directed to the patient, seem overly solicitous, refuse to leave the treatment area, or display hostility. Caregiver alcohol and drug abuse and intimate partner violence (IPV)

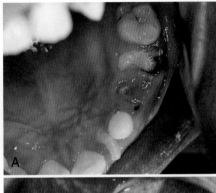
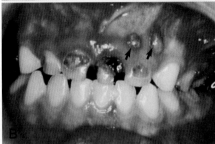

Fig. 58.6 (A) Dental neglect. Rampant dental caries destroyed primary maxillary molar to the root. (B) Dental neglect. Multiple paruli caused by rampant tooth decay. (Courtesy Dr. Lynn Douglas Mouden, founder of P.A.N.D.A. [Prevention of Abuse and Neglect through Dental Awareness].)

in the home are risk factors for child maltreatment.[3,10] Caregivers with substance abuse dependency are not necessarily the adults perpetrating the child maltreatment but may be so impaired in judgment that they expose children to unstable living conditions and other adults who maltreat them. For children with the caregiver risk factor of domestic violence, the caregiver could be the perpetrator of, the victim of, or a witness to domestic violence.

The goal of good parenting is enabling a child to grow up with feelings of satisfaction, security, and self-respect. An abused child may not experience these positive feelings because they are growing up in nonnurturing environments. Overly critical or strict parents and extremely isolated families are other warning signs of nonnurturing environments. In addition, exposure to harsh punishment and physical discipline that causes deliberate pain in response to undesired child behaviors is related to more severe child maltreatment or revictimization in IPV in the future.[3] Understanding that traumatic adverse childhood experiences (ACEs) directly affect adolescent and adult long-term health emphasizes the need for a trauma-informed care early intervention for maltreated children.

Abuse Versus Findings Mistaken for Abuse

Physical findings mistaken for abuse may be of accidental, genetic, acquired, infectious, or cultural origin. Healthcare providers use their professional judgment and clinical skill to assess the location, size, shape, and mode of injuries. Accidental injuries normally heal at the same time, whereas repeated injuries from abuse are in various stages of healing. Accidental injuries also normally occur over bony protuberances such as knees and elbows, whereas injuries from abuse often occur on surfaces away from bony protuberances such as the neck, head, trunk, buttocks, hands, and upper arms.

In addition, several genetic conditions have manifestations that mimic the signs of physical abuse such as the following:

- **Sturge-Weber syndrome (encephalotrigeminal angiomatosis)** is a rare disorder that is present at birth. A child with this condition has a port-wine stain birthmark (usually on the face) and nervous system problems.
- **Ehlers-Danlos syndrome (EDS)** is a group of inherited connective tissue disorders marked by extremely loose joints, hyperelastic skin that bruises easily, and easily damaged blood vessels. Symptoms of EDS include fragile and stretchy skin and easy scarring and poor wound healing.
- **Idiopathic thrombocytopenic purpura (ITP)** (immune thrombocytopenic purpura) is a bleeding disorder in which the immune system destroys platelets, which are necessary for normal blood clotting. Persons with ITP have too few platelets in the blood, which can manifest as easy bruising, nosebleeds, hemorrhaging in the mouth, and bleeding into the skin causing characteristic red, pinpointed spots (petechial skin rash).

Human immunodeficiency virus (HIV) and hemophilia are acquired medical conditions that have skin conditions that may mirror injuries from physical abuse. Infectious skin conditions such as eczema, dermatitis, or impetigo may be mistaken as abuse. Cultural practices such as cupping, coining, or scraping (gua sha) used in some families to alleviate illness may cause unintentional injuries to the child. In some cultures, it is believed that the use of cups warmed by a flame placed on the back of a child with respiratory illness will draw out the infections. The suction created by the cup-to-skin contact on the back leaves markings that appear to be the result of inflicted child abuse. Additionally, since copper is believed to be a healing metal and a copper coin is rubbed in various directions on the back of a sick child, it is thought that it helps to draw out illness. The rubbing produces various red markings on the child's back that resemble abuse. Scraping, performed with a kitchen spoon rubbed over the back for up to 30 minutes, is a traditional home remedy based in some cultures to relieve respiratory problems. The scraped skin may look alarming but is reported to be not painful. See Case 1 in Box 58.3 (Critical Thinking Scenarios), which pertains to a medical condition mistaken for child abuse.

Assessment

All patients are assessed for health history and physical, behavioral, and oral findings. Documentation procedures are consistent among all dental hygiene patients. Collaboration with physicians, social workers, and other interdisciplinary healthcare providers may be needed to manage the physical, psychological, and social consequences of maltreated individuals. Suspected cases of child maltreatment may warrant taking separate child and adult histories (stories) to elicit the nature of the observed injury.

- Do child and adult histories match?
- Is there consistency with the injury, timeline, and explanation?
- Have other similar injuries occurred to the child and/or other household members?

Determine whether to discuss your suspicions with an adult on the basis of the child's safety. Parents and caregivers should be approached separately, always in private, without the child or others present. Because there may be a suspicion of child maltreatment, there may be a lack of awareness by the adult who brought the child. Remind the adult that you are concerned about the welfare of the child and the well-being of all your patients. Effective statements, if you decide to talk with the adult, include the following:

- "Because I care about children and I care about your child …"
- "I am concerned about your situation …"
- "In my practice, I care about my patients' overall health and well-being …"

Based on the interviewed adult's response:

- If the adult's response or attitude seems suspicious and you are not sure, you may consult with other healthcare providers or contact CPS.

- If you feel the child may be in danger, contact CPS.
- If the histories (stories) match, all is fine.

Box 58.1 provides other patient or client education tips.

Documentation

Documentation includes text, photographs, and other pertinent information or data that serve as an official and legal record of present and past dental or dental hygiene care. Separate the facts from opinion. Box 58.2 includes related legal, ethical, and safety issues.

If child maltreatment is suspected, the following documentation should be included:

- Record all clinical and behavioral findings.
- Document all conversations that transpired during the appointment.
- Use full names.
- Use quotes for verbal statements associated with the person.
- Record the reason for seeking treatment (or the reason for delaying treatment).
- Obtain the usual consent for clinical photographic and or radiographic needs.
- Document the report made to local CPS agency.

FAMILY VIOLENCE AND IPV

There is an association between child maltreatment and **intimate partner violence** (IPV).[3] Victims of child maltreatment are at risk of being victimized by IPV, including adolescent dating violence. Long-range health, psychological, and social implications in children have been attributed to IPV exposure. Emotional and behavioral problems including mood and anxiety disorders, PTSD, substance abuse, and school-related problems in children and adolescents also can result from exposure to IPV. They also might mistreat their own children or intimate partners in the future. Clearly, abuse and neglect have far-reaching negative risks for the health, well-being, and longevity of its traumatized victims.

Intimate Partner Violence

The power and control tactics used in bullying overlap with those in IPV, a possible indicator that bullying could be a precursor to IPV. Both bullying and IPV involve an aggressor exerting power over an individual perceived to be weaker. Stalking and cyberstalking of victims commonly occur in both IPV and bullying. IPV is a pattern of abusive behavior used by a current or former partner or spouse to gain or maintain power and control over another intimate partner. It can occur in heterosexual or same-sex couples and dating relationships and does not require sexual intimacy.[25] IPV occurs in all demographic groups. A substantial proportion of female and male adults in the United States have had at least one experience of sexual violence, stalking, or IPV over their lifetimes, many occurring before age 18 years. An estimated 71.1% of females and 58.8% of males were under age 25 when they first encountered sexual violence, physical violence, or stalking by an intimate partner.[26] Physical violence can result in lacerations, broken or fractured bones, head trauma, sexually transmitted infections, chronic pain syndromes, irritable bowel syndrome, urinary tract infections, and unintended pregnancies as a consequence of sexual violence. Mental health consequences include risk of depression, mood and anxiety disorders, PTSD, suicide, poor self-esteem and memory loss, chronic headaches, and concussions resulting from battery to the head.

Pregnancy, Reproduction, and Intimate Partner Violence

Rates of IPV during pregnancy are alarmingly high. Mental health and physical impacts of IPV are magnified in pregnancy with the risk of poor pregnancy outcomes such as preterm birth, low birth weight, decreased gestational age, and miscarriage. Reproductive coercion is a common aspect of IPV and includes the abusive partner controlling reproductive or sexual health (e.g., refusal to use birth control, destroying contraceptive measures), fear of condom negotiation, coerced abortions or forced pregnancy continuation, or intentionally getting the partner pregnant to control the victim.[27] In many US cities, suicide and violent homicide are the leading causes of pregnancy-associated deaths. Intimate partner homicides of pregnant females by a current or former intimate partner most commonly occur in the early stages of pregnancy.

Patient Screening and Education Tools

Routinely ask about IPV always in private, and document disclosures. Always assess the safety of the patient and refer them to local resources for assistance in leaving the abusive relationship. Examples of screening questions are the following:

- "Do you feel safe at home?"
- "Because intimate partner violence is so common, we are asking all our patients these questions because we know health is affected by this."
- "Has your partner ever threatened, hit, slapped, choked, or harmed you?"

Victims of IPV having one previous nonfatal strangulation are seven times more likely to die by homicide than those who have not experienced nonfatal strangulation. Victims of strangulation have a higher risk for loss of consciousness, miscarriage, other IPV injuries, and homicide. If adults deny any issues, you may jeopardize their safety if you pursue the line of questioning. If a patient discloses information, the oral health professional should reassure the patient by using such phrases as, "It is not your fault, help is available, and I can give you information if you like." If the patient denies abuse but you suspect IPV, your response may be, "I'm concerned. There is help available for you. I have information if you would like." You should never put yourself or the patient in jeopardy by forcing the issue if the patient does not feel safe pursuing or receiving further information at the time.

IPV is rampant, yet not all states have mandatory requirements for reporting it. Many states do, however, encompass IPV reporting requirements under laws requiring the reporting of injuries resulting from violent criminal acts, deadly weapons, or moving vessels. Oral health professionals should check their state's legislative policies for reporting responsibilities.

ELDER AND VULNERABLE ADULT ABUSE AND NEGLECT

Elder abuse is a growing international problem, with different manifestations in various countries and cultures. Definitions in state and international laws vary for older and vulnerable adult maltreatment. Distinctions are made between the abuse and neglect of elder adults by family members and professionals and, in addition, when self-neglect is occurring. **Elder abuse** is a broad term encompassing abuse, neglect, and exploitation of an older adult person who is targeted because of age or dependency on others. It also includes contractor scams and self-neglect.

Domestic elder adult abuse generally refers to any form of maltreatment of an elderly person by someone (e.g., spouse, sibling, child, friend, caregiver) who has a close or special relationship with them. Institutional elder abuse occurs in residential facilities (e.g., nursing homes, foster homes, group homes, boarding and long-term care facilities). Perpetrators of institutional abuse usually are staff, professionals, or caregivers who are paid to provide care and protection.

Elder adult maltreatment can occur in cognitively intact individuals, as well as persons with other nonhealth vulnerabilities. Most reports of older adult maltreatment involve neglect. The vulnerability to severe neglect is highest when the older person's care needs increase, functional impairment is greater, household incomes are lower, and the need for assistive resources rises.

Elder adult maltreatment is a pervasive public health problem that includes the following:
- Physical abuse
- Financial abuse, financial exploitation, and financial neglect
- Emotional abuse
- Sexual abuse
- Neglect
- Abandonment

Older adult neglect includes failure of caregivers to provide: (1) protection from health and safety hazards, such as withholding medical devices and medications, and (2) basic needs such as personal hygiene, clothing, shelter, or nutrition, and the failure to follow up with medical and dental care.

Self-neglect is a unique and serious phenomenon and, as such, is generally separated from the general discussion of older adult maltreatment. **Self-neglect** is the harm or the potential for harm created by a person's own behaviors rather than resulting from others' actions. Self-neglect is the result of the older adult's failure to address their own self-care needs.

As life expectancy increases, the number of maltreated older adults is also likely to rise. Not all older adults are vulnerable. Conversely, not all **vulnerable adults** are older adults. Vulnerable adults are individuals older than age 18 years who have a substantial mental or functional impairment that limits their ability for self-care without the assistance and oversight of another person. Often, because of social isolation and limited mobility, visits to medical or dental professionals are the only contact that older or vulnerable adults have outside of the home. This places the responsibility of identifying maltreatment in the hands of healthcare professionals. Similar to IPV, maltreated older adult victims' dependency, loneliness, self-blame, guilt, fear of abandonment or retaliation by perpetrators, and feelings of hopelessness, despair, or shame often make them reluctant to report the perpetrating family member, spouse, child, close caretaker, or person trusted by others. Currently, there are no standards for how professionals should screen older patients for possible abuse. However, reporting abuse and neglect of vulnerable adults is mandated in every state.

HUMAN TRAFFICKING

HT is a major global public health problem occurring both domestically in the United States and internationally. It is a devastating crime against humanity in which humans are treated as merchandise and bought and sold by traffickers seeking to profit from the exploitation of their victims. The Trafficking Victims Protection Reauthorization (TVPR) Act of 2017 (PL115-427) amended the Trafficking Victims Protection Act of 2000 (PL106-386) to modify criteria for determining whether countries are meeting minimum guidelines for combating HT. **Human trafficking** in the United States is defined as (1) sex trafficking, in which a victim is induced by force, fraud, or coercion into a commercial sex act or in which the person who is induced to perform the commercial sex act is under 18 years of age; and (2) recruiting, harboring, transporting, supplying, or obtaining a person for labor or services through the use of force, fraud, or coercion for the purpose of involuntary service, bondage, or slavery.[28] The exploitation of humans for profit is the defining element of HT, rather than the physical transport of victims from one area to another. People can be trafficked within their own country, including the United States, and it does not have to involve movement or crossing borders to be considered trafficking. HT is often confused with human smuggling. The difference is that human smuggling is frequently the result of a consensual agreement between the smuggled individual and the transporter, after which the relationship ends when the desired destination is reached. In contrast, the trafficked individual may reach a target destination, but the relationship with the trafficker continues and movement is controlled for the trafficker's ongoing personal profit from the victims' repeated labor or commercial sex servitude. In addition, if movement does occur in an HT situation, it may be just the beginning of the crime and a means to engage the victim in ongoing labor and commercial sex services. Traffickers also disorient victims by moving them to unknown places, which enables their isolation from family, friends, and the public in an effort to keep trafficked individuals under control and unable to reach out to familiar social supportive networks. The personal identification papers of a victim often are kept in the possession of the trafficker for control and prevention of escape. Limiting community connectivity ensures that any contact with the public is superficial in nature and prevents the victim from being recognized, forming relationships, or building or reestablishing social supports, and continues the trafficker's cycle of exploitative intentions. See Case Study 2 in Box 58.3 (Critical Thinking Scenarios), which pertains to a victim of HT.

General and Oral Health Issues

HT victims are subjected to physical and/or psychological coercion and, as such, experience a range of physical, sexual, and mental health issues that are often advanced by the injuries sustained from violence, trauma, and/or infections of the head and neck, dental and oral facial tissues, gynecologic and genital organs, and malnutrition. The health problems experienced by labor trafficking victims may include loss of body parts, head injuries, persistent cough, lacerations, skin damage, weight loss, exhaustion, and dizziness. Sex trafficking victims may specifically experience headaches, memory problems, insomnia, gynecologic and reproductive problems, substance abuse and addiction, sexually transmitted diseases (STDs) and oral lesions associated with STDs, and multiple pregnancies, forced abortions, and adoptions. Often, the trafficked individual has other neglected health issues, such as uncontrolled asthma, hypertension, diabetes, malnutrition, obesity or underweight, substance abuse, skin infections, caries, periodontal disease, and noncompliance with medical and dental health prescribed therapies. Therefore medical and dental healthcare providers are often

BOX 58.3 Critical Thinking Scenarios

Case 1

Mary is now 32 years old but starting at a young age she went to many hospital emergency departments (EDs) for various injuries sustained at home and school. It began with a falling incident that also dislocated her shoulder. Her mother, Becky, accompanied her to the ED. Upon arrival, Mary was separated from her mother. Becky was taken into a separate room and questioned about the injury. Becky later learned that Mary was asked if anyone in her family had caused this injury. This was only one of many visits to ED departments with the same scenario.

As time went on during childhood, Mary had other injuries that were questioned such as broken thumbs, dislocated hips, knees, and the inability to walk and control her bladder. Each injury required an ED visit with the same questions posed to both Mary and her parents.

At a regular dental visit, the dental staff thought it was odd that Mary was in a wheelchair and unable to walk. She was there 6 months ago without a wheelchair. She was a young teen and did not appear to have any physical marks. Also, her health history did not reveal any medical conditions. When her father insisted he had to stay in the room with her, this seemed to be a red flag. Mary needed new dental radiographs, so her father agreed to leave the room. The dental hygienist then questioned Mary in such a way that Mary perceived that they thought her father was the cause of her inability to walk and perhaps abused her. Her father was also questioned about the change in her health status by the dentist. Mary dispelled their theory with an explanation of her medical journey to find out why she had all of these issues. Her father also explained that he wanted to be close to Mary because of her inability to walk and to make sure she was comfortable. He also shared with the dentist that Mary did not have any health issues at this time.

Mary's parents thought she was clumsy. They could not find any other reason because she was an active child and teen. Trying to find out why this was happening to her, her parents took her to many doctors at prestigious medical institutions in several different states.

At one institution, her parents were told that she was a drug addict and was feigning her injuries to get drugs. Her mother told the doctor the pain medications she was given were untouched because she did not like how the medications made her feel when she took them. Mary also asked her parents not to fill the prescriptions for pain medications any more.

At 18, Mary was also accused of injuring herself and was recommended for psychiatric evaluation. Mary thought it was her fault. Unbeknownst to her parents, she committed herself for evaluation. After a week at the psychiatric hospital, it was determined that Mary was "normal" and the doctor who said she was self-inflicting her injuries was incorrect.

Both Mary and her parents were very confused and did not know how to find out why Mary was having all of the injuries. Her father said, "We had thousands of ED and doctor visits and they all seem to think that we, her parents, were to blame, or Mary was self-inflicting the injuries for attention." At their wits' end, Mary and her parents made one last attempt to find answers. They scheduled an evaluation appointment at another medical educational institution that a friend has suggested. It was here that she finally received a diagnosis of EDS: Ehlers-Danlos syndrome.

Mary has had many surgeries and doctor appointments that are related to her EDS. She has a positive attitude and has great family support as she continues her health journey.

Discussion of Case 1: There are several signs that this could have been a case of inflicted abuse. The unexplained injuries and the change in mobility from one appointment to another and taking the child to multiple health centers could raise suspicions of abuse. However, the family dynamics indicated nurturing and concerned parents who promptly brought their daughter in for treatment and followed through with her care and safety. Additionally, the parents and child were separated and histories were obtained which seemed to match that the injuries were random and accidental. Mary was able to provide a full history of all the events she had experienced, with no indication of the injuries involving any other person. The child's behavior provided no indication she feared her parents nor that there were any unusual relationships within the family. A comprehensive medical, dental, and social history renders this case nonreportable since behaviors, history, and physical injuries were relayed by both the patient and the parents in a caring and concerned manner, with timely and appropriate medical attention for Mary's injuries.

Case Study 2:

An embassy worker brings a young lady to a dental office in an upscale neighborhood in Washington, D.C. The person who brings her is well known to the dental office because he has brought or referred several patients to the office from his country. He does not have any information about her health, and the young lady does not speak English. She cannot fill out any of the office dental forms on her own, so the man who brought her agrees to interpret and fill out the forms for her. He said she was 21 years old and was in the United States to go to school. It appears that he asks her the questions on the health questionnaire so that she can provide the needed information on her dental and health history background. The man conveys that he wants the best dental work for her, such as porcelain crowns, veneers, and tooth whitening, among other services, and that money is no object. He says he can pay in cash for the dental work. He wants her to regain her smile. The young lady is shy and very reserved and only responds to the man who brought her to the dental office. She does not smile, and the man explains that it is because of her teeth. She is, however, very compliant with whatever the dental team requests or asks her to do. The dental team was happy to help this young lady and make her smile again. Radiographs and a dental examination were conducted, and a treatment plan was presented with her restorative and dental hygiene needs. The treatment plan included quadrant scaling and root planing before beginning any restorative work, oral hygiene instructions (with assistance of the man who agreed to interpret at the current and future visits), topical prescription fluoride gel for daily home use, veneers for teeth 8 and 9, and several posterior restorations for carious teeth. During the initial scaling and root planing appointment, it appeared the young lady had not had any prior dental care and did not know how to use a toothbrush or dental floss. It was unclear if she had yet been able to fill the prescription for fluoride. For each appointment, the man who brought her stayed in the operatory. He explained that he needed to be there to help with communicating about the dental treatment in her language. At times, he was very helpful in explaining what was being done and what she needed to do. After several appointments, the young lady seemed to be satisfied and actually smiled. The man who attended each dental appointment also seemed very pleased. When treatment was complete, they left the office satisfied and he said they would return for the recommended 3-month maintenance visit and an examination.

Discussion of Case 2: This scenario seemed to be a success story for the dental team in that they were able to help someone who had never received professional oral care and appeared to exhibit a better self-image upon completion of the recommended treatment. They were surprised, however, when Federal Bureau of Investigation (FBI) agents visited the office a few weeks later, showed the dental team members a picture of the young lady, and questioned the dentist, dental assistant, and dental hygienist about her and the man in attendance for her dental appointments. The FBI agents shared that the man who accompanied this young lady was a known sex trafficker and that he used his status at the embassy to bring victims to the United States to traffic for commercial sex in an extensive multiple-state sex trafficking operation. The young lady was actually under 18 years of age. The dental team did not know anything was amiss until the visit from the FBI agents. The dental team did not know much about human trafficking and did not think that it would ever occur in their practice. The FBI agents suggested education would be a good start.

Continued

BOX 58.3   Critical Thinking Scenarios—cont'd

- What would be some of the questions that the dental team members should have asked during the initial presentation by the embassy worker with the young lady?
- What legal or other connection did the man have to this young lady that warranted his extensive financing and oversight of her dental treatment? Did his involvement as a nonfamily member seem unusual?
- What questions would you ask about the young lady's family?
- Did the young lady have any identification papers or a passport that could provide more information than conveyed by the man, including verification of her name, country of residence, and date of birth?
- Was there anything about the young lady's appearance that may have resulted in doubt that she was 21 years of age as reported by the embassy worker?

- Could the young lady actually comprehend treatment options and could she agree to the treatment plan? Was informed consent possible with the man interpreting for her?
- Did the man's discussion of the young lady's purpose for being in the United States for college attendance seem plausible or warrant any additional questions that might have shed light on how and why she arrived?
- Perhaps asking more questions might have exposed some discrepancies in the man's stories. What other red flags can you spot in this case scenario?
- How can you avoid what happened with the multiple oversights that occurred with this dental team?
- Are you knowledgeable about human trafficking cases in your hometown and the local resources available to assist victims?

---

the few professionals to interact with victims while they are still being trafficked.

Although trafficked individuals often exhibit physical injuries from inflicted violent blows to the head and face, resulting in jaw and teeth fractures and dislocations of the temporomandibular joint, traffickers are primarily interested in seeking cosmetic dental services when they bring the trafficked victims for care at later stages of the disease progression. Often, the ongoing deprivation of dental care and dental hygiene products has had a profound effect on the victim's oral health, yet the trafficker's primary concern is making the victim more attractive to clients for the ultimate purpose of increasing sales and profit from increased client demand. Victims rarely self-identify and report their victimization because of the extensive power and control and the psychologic entrapment techniques used against them by traffickers; consequently, identification is difficult for professionals providing medical and dental healthcare. The rate of dentists and other healthcare providers identifying victims while they are being trafficked in the United States has been poor; therefore increased interdisciplinary training and education of healthcare professionals is warranted.

Clinical Interventions

Dental professionals should be alert to the possible indicators that a trafficked individual might exhibit, warranting followup communication without the presence of the victim's attendant. Refusal to leave the room and allow the patient to interact alone with the healthcare provider is a cardinal red flag; the third-party attendant is more concerned about being revealed as a trafficker or abuser than doing what is best for the individual's healthcare needs. In addition, the third party's denial of interpreter service offers, in contradiction to professional recommendations, is another sign that the trafficker is not concerned with the victim's health needs. Dental hygienists should not inquire about trafficking-specific details, make promises to the patient, divulge their personal address, or offer to harbor the trafficked person. Rather, dental hygienists can follow up their suspicions of trafficking by asking screening questions that identify their interest in aiding the victim without conveying judgment of the individual or the situation. The National Institute of Justice offers a screening tool for identifying trafficking victims and is available on the Human Trafficking website.[29] Since trauma and fear are constants in the lives of trafficked individuals, it is imperative that a trauma-informed approach, building trust and demonstrating sensitivity, is used during the screening process.

All dental professionals are mandated to report maltreatment of minors under the age of 18 years, vulnerable adults regardless of consent, and victims of HT. Reports of suspected HT should be made to local law enforcement, antitrafficking hotlines in each country, or if the situation occurs in the United States, to federal law enforcement. The National Human Trafficking Hotline or text line, operated by Polaris and supported by the Administration for Children and Families, can be reached 24/7 and is available in over 200 languages to get help or connect with local services. If victims are in immediate danger, contact 9-1-1 or the local police. Dental professionals should not force the trafficked adult to report and should be aware that resistance to offers of help may stem from the victim's fear of trafficker retaliation and threatened harm to either the victim or the victim's family if the crime is reported or there is an attempt to leave the situation.

REPORTING ABUSE AND NEGLECT

Dental hygienists and dentists are mandated reporters for child abuse and neglect, vulnerable adult abuse, and victims of HT. State-established **immunity** laws protect reporters from civil law or criminal penalties resulting from filing a confidential report of suspected abuse and/or neglect.

Each state has its own reporting mechanisms for suspected abuse and/or neglect. For example, suspected child abuse or neglect can be reported to CPS, but the mechanisms for reporting suspected IPV and older or vulnerable adult abuse can vary. Some states have dedicated family violence or adult protective services, but regardless of the state or type of abuse suspected, oral health professionals always may report suspected abuse as an emergency by dialing 9-1-1.

Oral healthcare professionals do not gather evidence to build an abuse or neglect case if they suspect abuse; rather, their duty is to report their suspicions to the appropriate authority and document their observations in the patient record. As a legal document, the patient record must document objectively all findings and disclosures made by the client.

For a complete list of definitions and reporting hotlines for child victims, visit the website for US Department of Health & Human Services, Administration for Children & Families:

https://www.childwelfare.gov/topics/responding/reporting/how/

CPS and law enforcement have the expertise and resources to investigate such reports. CPS is the designated agency that receives child maltreatment reports, investigates cases, and provides intervention and treatment services to children and families when child maltreatment has occurred. Frequently, this agency is located within governmental social service agencies, such as the Department of Social Services.

Adult Protective Services are agencies to help elder adults and those unable to provide for or care for their daily needs. These agencies serve people who are in danger of being mistreated or neglected, are unable to protect themselves, and/or have no one to assist them. Mandated reporting by oral health professionals varies among states for elder adults and victims of domestic violence. Refer to your state licensing board for reporting requirements.

Additional abuse and neglect resources are listed in Box 58.4

BOX 58.4 Abuse and Neglect Resources

- Family Violence Prevention Fund, (800) 595-4889
- National Health Resource Center on Domestic Violence, (888) 792-2873
- National Center on Elder Abuse, (855) 500-3537
- National Coalition Against Domestic Violence, (303) 839-1852
- National Human Trafficking Resource Center, (888) 373-7888
- Text message "HELP" or "INFO" to 233733 (Befree)
- Homeland Security Investigations Human Trafficking Tip Line, 1-866-2423
- European Freedom Network (find your country's antitrafficking hotline): https://www.europeanfreedomnetwork.org/hotline/

KEY CONCEPTS

- Dental hygienists should be especially aware of physical abuse, because many physical signs of abuse occur on the neck and craniofacial regions.
- Legislation in all 50 states mandates that dentists and dental hygienists report suspicions of child, vulnerable adult abuse and neglect, and human trafficking to child and adult protective services agencies and law enforcement, respectively.
- Failure of a mandated reporter to report suspected child abuse or neglect is a misdemeanor in most states, punishable by a fine and/or imprisonment.
- The Justice for Victims Act of 2015 changed the CAPTA definition of child abuse to include child sex trafficking.
- Parents or caregivers of abused children often change physicians, but they will more than likely return to visit their child's dentist.
- Neglect accounts for most of all reported cases of maltreatment in the United States.
- Because the patient's dental hygiene care record is a legal document, the dental hygienist should record all indicators of abuse or neglect accurately and clearly.
- Given a relationship of trust and rapport, patients may disclose information to dental hygienists pertaining to abuse and neglect.
- Oral healthcare professionals do not diagnose or investigate incidents of suspected abuse and neglect. Rather, they should report suspected cases of child and vulnerable adult abuse or neglect to the proper authorities.
- Abusers use power and control tactics in bullying and intimate partner violence.
- Intimate partner violence and homicide during pregnancy is highly prevalent.
- Strangulation in intimate partner violence has a high risk for homicide.
- Human traffickers exploit victims through ongoing sex or labor servitude and often withhold healthcare and dental care.
- Most trafficked individuals do not self-disclose that they are trafficked.

REFERENCES

1. Zeanah CH, Humphreys KL. Child abuse and neglect. *J Am Acad Child Adolesc Psychiatry.* 2018;57(9):637–644.
2. U.S. Department of Justice. Office of Justice programs. *Family Violence. Special Feature.* August 14, 2020. Updated October 8, 2021 https://www.ojp.gov/feature/family-violence/overview. Accessed July 25, 2022.
3. Goddard A. Adverse childhood experiences and trauma-informed care. *J Pediatric Health Care.* 2021;35(2):145–155.
4. *Responding to Child Maltreatment: A Clinical Handbook for Health Professionals.* World Health Organization; 2022. License: CC BY-NC-SA3.0 IGO.
5. Singh V, Lehi G. Child abuse and the role of a dentist in its identification, prevention and protection: a literature review. *Dent Res J.* 2020;17(3):167–173.
6. Mid-Atlantic P.A.N.D.A. Coalition. Prevent Abuse and Neglect Through Dental Awareness. [Internet]; Available at: https://midatlanticpanda.org/. Accessed July 25, 2022.
7. U.S. Department of Health & Human Services, Administration for Children and Families, Administration on Children, Youth and Families, Children's Bureau. Child Abuse Prevention and Treatment Act (CAPTA) amended by P.L. 111-320, the CAPTA reauthorization act of 2010. December 20, 2010. Available at: https://www.congress.gov/111/plaws/publ320/PLAW-111publ320.pdf. Accessed July 25, 2022.
8. U.S. Department of Health and Human Services, Administration for Children and Families, Children's Bureau. Child welfare information Gateway. *What is Child Abuse and Neglect? Recognizing the Signs and Symptoms.* 2019. https://www.childwelfare.gov/pubPDFs/whatiscan.pdf. Accessed July 25, 2022.
9. World Health Organization. *Child Maltreatment;* 2020. https://www.who.int/news-room/fact-sheets/detail/child-maltreatment.
10. U.S. Department of Health & Human Services. *Administration for Children and Families, Administration on Children, Youth and Families.* Children's Bureau. Child Maltreatment 2020; 2022. Available from: https://www.acf.hhs.gov/cb/data-research/child-maltreatment. Accessed July 25, 2022.
11. Katz I, Katz C, Andresen S, et al. Child maltreatment reports and Child Protection Service responses during COVID-19: knowledge exchange among Australia, Brazil, Canada, Colombia, Germany, Israel, and South Africa. *Child Abuse Negl.* 2021;116(Pt 2):105078.
12. Afifi TO, Mota N, Sareen J, et al. The relationship between harsh physical punishment and child maltreatment in childhood and intimate partner violence in adulthood. *BMC Publ Health.* 2017;17(1):493–502.
13. Traisman E. Recognizing maltreatment in children with special needs. *Pediatr Ann.* 2016;45:e273–e277.
14. Jackson AM, Kissoon N, Greene C. Aspects of abuse: recognizing and responding to child maltreatment. *Curr Probl Pediatr Adolesc Health Care.* 2015;45(3):58–70.
15. Sugar NF, Taylor JA, Feldman KW. Bruises in infants and toddlers: those who don't cruise rarely bruise. *Arch Pediatr Adolesc Med.* 1999;153:399–403.
16. Hinds T, Shalaby-Rana E, Jackson AM, et al. Aspects of abuse: abusive head trauma. *Curr Probl Pediatr Adolesc Health Care.* 2015;45(3):71–79.
17. Kaur H, Vinod KS, Singh H, Arya L, Verma P, Singh B. Child maltreatment: Cross-sectional survey of general dentists. *J Forensic Dent Sci.* 2017;9(1):24–30.
18. Fisher-Owens SA, Lukefahr JL, Tate AR. Oral and dental aspects of child abuse and neglect. *Pediatr Dent.* 2017;39(4):278–283.
19. Costacurta M, Benavoli D, Arcudi G, et al. Oral and dental signs of child abuse and neglect. *Oral Implantol.* 2015;8(2–3):68–73.
20. Strathearn L, Giannotti M, Mills R, Kisely S, Najman J, Abajobir A. Long-term cognitive, psychological, and health outcomes associated with child abuse and neglect. *Pediatrics.* 2020;146(4):e20200438.
21. Hoeboer C, de Roos C, van Son GE, Spinhoven P, Elzinga B. The effect of parental emotional abuse on the severity and treatment of PTSD symptoms in children and adolescents. *Child Abuse Negl.* 2021;111:104775.
22. Kann L, McManus T, Harris WA, et al. Youth risk behavior surveillance – United States, 2017. *MMWR Surveill Summ.* 2018;67(8):1–114.

23. American Academy of Pediatric Dentistry. *Definition of dental neglect. The Reference Manual of Pediatric Dentistry*. American Academy of Pediatric Dentistry; 2021:16. www.aapd.org/policies/. Accessed July 25, 2022.

24. Peres MA, Macpherson LMD, Weyant RJ, et al. Oral diseases: a global public health challenge [published correction appears in *Lancet*. 2019 Sep21;394(10203):1010]. Lancet. 2019;394(10194):249–260.

25. Messinger AM, Birmingham RS, DeKeseredy WS. Perceptions of same-gender and different-gender intimate partner cyber-monitoring. *J Interpers Violence*. 2021;36(7–8):NP4315–NP4335.

26. Smith SG, Zhang X, Basile KC, et al. *The National Intimate Partner and Sexual Violence Survey (NISVS): 2015 Data Brief – Updated Release.*

National Center for Injury Prevention and Control, Centers for Disease Control and Prevention; 2018.

27. Fay KE, Yee LM. Birth outcomes among women affected by reproductive coercion. *J Midwifery Wom Health*. 2020;65(5):627–633.

28. United States Department of State. *Trafficking in Persons Report*; 2022. Available at: https://www.state.gov/reports/2022-trafficking-in-persons-report/. Accessed July 25, 2022. Published July 2022.

29. National Institute of Justice. "A Screening Tool for Identifying Trafficking Victims," September 19, 2016, nij.ojp.Gov: Available at:https://nij.ojp.gov/topics/articles/screening-tool-identifying-trafficking-victims. Accessed July 27, 2022.

59

Disability and Healthcare

Tracye A. Moore, Adrien Gupton, and Cynthia C. Gadbury-Amyot

PROFESSIONAL OPPORTUNITIES

Dental hygienists have the responsibility to both understand and provide quality care to patients with disabilities. No one is alike. People with disabilities are not handicapped; they are genuinely special. That is why disabilities are special needs. Dental hygienists can improve the quality of life of these individuals by caring for their oral health needs and helping them prevent dental disease requiring treatment that is more complex.

COMPETENCIES

By the end of this chapter, the reader will be able to:
1. Define "disability" and acquire knowledge about major developments or circumstances affecting patients with disabilities.
2. Distinguish different classifications for patients with disabilities.
3. Consider and recommend means to address healthcare barriers, assistive devices, and oral self-care devices for patients with disabilities. Provide oral self-care education to patients with disabilities and their caregivers.
4. Explain how to use protective stabilization and patient-positioning techniques throughout the delivery of professional care.
5. Care for patients in wheelchairs and recommend opportunities to advocate for patients with disabilities.

INTRODUCTION

Disability is part of the human condition as almost everyone experiences temporary or permanent degrees of disability in life through changes in their health or in the environment. Over the years, different terms have been used in an attempt to describe people with disabilities, including special needs, impaired, and handicapped. The term *handicap ped* is criticized in literature and in practice as it is insensitive; therefore people should refrain from using the term *handicapped*.

DEFINING DISABILITY

An individual with a **disability** was defined by the Americans with Disabilities Act (ADA) of 1990 as a "person who has a physical or mental impairment that substantially limits one or more major life activities, a person who has a history or record of such an impairment, or a person who is perceived by others as having such an impairment."[1] **Major life**

activities are those that the average person can perform with little or no difficulty (e.g., self-care, walking, hearing, seeing, breathing, standing, speaking, sitting, learning, thinking, interacting with others).[1] The ADA Amendment Act of 2008 further broadened the scope of major life activities to include the operation of major bodily functions like circulation, reproduction, and individual organs.

It is critical to recognize that people with disabilities represent a diverse spectrum of individuals with different needs. Common misconceptions about individuals with disabilities include that they are sick, dependent on others, debilitated, or live in institutions. In reality, most of these individuals are capable of living in the community either alone or with assistance. Disabilities can be hidden or apparent on observation. Even people with the same type of disability function in their own way. Disability affects approximately 61 million or nearly 1 in 4 (26%) people in the United States living in communities. Disability affects more than 1 billion people worldwide.[2-3]

Social and Political Context

Over the years, several national health policies, such as the Rehabilitation Act of 1973, the ADA, the Olmstead Decision of 1999, the New Freedom Initiative of 2001, and the Patient Protection and Affordable Care Act, often shortened to the Affordable Care Act (ACA) of 2010, have been developed to protect people with disabilities. Section 504 of the Rehabilitation Act of 1973 and the ADA achieved the most significant outcomes in removing barriers for people with disabilities by guaranteeing that discrimination would not affect a qualified person's ability to acquire education, employment, social services, or healthcare because of his or her disability. The Patient Bill of Rights under the ACA protects patients with disabilities against discriminatory practices by health insurance companies. Under the ACA, patients with disabilities are no longer denied health coverage due to preexisting health conditions. Healthcare reform continues to be a highly debated topic in national policies.

People-first language is the recommended approach used to speak appropriately and respectfully to or about most individuals with a disability. People-first language focuses on the person first and not the disability, thus preventing the dehumanization of people with disabilities. In essence, a person's disability or adaptive equipment should follow the person's name. For example, when referring to a person with a disability, refer to the person first by saying, "a person with a disability" rather than "a disabled person." (Table 59.1 provides additional examples of the people-first approach).

TABLE 59.1   People-First Language

People-First Language	Language to Avoid
Person with a disability	Disabled, handicapped person
Person without a disability	Normal person, healthy person
Person with an intellectual, cognitive, or developmental disability	Slow, simple, moronic, defective, afflicted, special person
Person with an emotional or behavior disability Person with a mental health or a psychiatric disability	Insane, crazy, psycho, maniac, nuts
Person who is blind or visually impaired	Blind person
Person who uses a wheelchair	Confined or restricted to a wheelchair, wheelchair bound
Person with a physical disability	Crippled, lame, deformed, invalid, spastic
Person with cerebral palsy	Cerebral palsy victim
Person of short stature	Midget

Source: Centers for Disease Control and Prevention: Communicating With and About People With Disabilities, 2022.

BOX 59.1   Legal, Ethical, and Safety Issues in Healthcare for Persons With Disabilities

- If the adult patient is ambulatory, high functioning, and without cognitive impairment, consent to speak with other caregivers and providers as well as permission to proceed with care must be obtained directly from the patient.
- If the patient is a minor or has cognitive impairment, consent is obtained from parents, legal guardians, or caregivers.
- Patients are active participants in all conversations with caregivers who attend the appointment. Healthcare professionals should include and be sensitive to the patient's needs and preferences in rendering healthcare.
- Patients are at an increased risk for being victims of violence, abuse, and/or neglect. Healthcare professionals are obligated to report suspected cases of abuse and neglect to the proper authorities (see Chapter 58 on child abuse and neglect and family violence).
- Maintain original copies of written correspondence from other healthcare professionals in the patient's chart.

Healthcare Context

Patients With Special Healthcare Needs

Patients with **special healthcare needs** (SHCN) include a broad spectrum of "physical, developmental, mental, sensory, behavioral, cognitive, or emotional impairment or limiting condition that requires comprehensive medical management, health care intervention, and/or use of specialized services of programs."[4] People with disabilities have increasingly less access to healthcare services and often experience high unmet healthcare needs. Demand for rehabilitation-related healthcare services continues to rise because of population-related changes, including an aging society and more people living with disease and/or injury. Fortunately, advancements in evidence-based healthcare have reduced the development of several health conditions that affect patients with disabilities, thereby contributing to overall improved health-related quality of life (HRQOL).

Dental hygienists need to apply critical thinking skills when seeking informed consent from patients who have disabilities. In some instances, the clinician must defer to the patient's parent or legal guardian to obtain necessary consent to render healthcare services. Box 59.1 summarizes some of the legal, ethical, and safety issues in healthcare for dental hygienists to consider while caring for persons with disabilities.

CLASSIFICATION OF DISABILITIES

Dimensions of Disabilities

Disabilities are classified into three primary dimensions: (1) impairments, (2) activity limitations, and (3) participation restrictions.[5] Impairments can occur because of a pathologic condition, accident, or disease and may include any loss or abnormality in function, which may or may not be permanent. For example, impairments include the loss of a limb or body organ or a broken limb or hip. An activity limitation is difficulty in performing activities. For example, activity limitations include having difficulty with basic activities of daily living because of a medical condition. A participation restriction is the inability to engage in everyday life activities for reasons that may not be under the patient's control. For example, participation restriction includes a working-age person with a severe health condition; consequently, the person may have a hard time finding work because of a lack of reasonable accommodations by the employer or be denied access to employment because of discrimination.[5]

Disability Adjusted Life Years

Disability also includes social factors such as the impact the environment has on the patient's ability to function in society. **Disability adjusted life years** (DALYs) refer to the sum or years of potential life lost due to premature mortality and the years of productive life lost due to a disability.[6] One DALY can be estimated as 1 lost year of healthy life. DALY is a common metric used to measure the gap, either at the individual or population level, between current health status and the ideal health status.[6]

International Classification of Functioning, Disability, and Health

There is no universal approach to organizing various categories of disabilities. The International Classification of Functioning, Disability and Health (ICF) provides a standard language and framework for the description of health and health-related states; in particular, the ICF model (Table 59.2) aims to shift the model of health from an exclusive medical model to a more inclusive biopsychosocial model of human functioning and disability[7] (Fig. 1). The Dental Hygiene Human Needs Conceptual Model applies well when working with individuals with disabilities, as it considers eight human needs for all clients and thus broadens the view of dental hygiene care beyond the traditional medical model. Likewise, the Oral Health-Related Quality of Life Conceptual Model provides a framework for looking at the complex interrelationship between health and disease, and its biological, psychological, and social consequences for the individual experiencing it (see Chapter 2).

Disability and function are a result of complex interactions between health conditions and contextual factors, which include both environmental and personal factors. Environmental factors include social attitudes, architectural characteristics, legal and social structures, and climate, whereas personal factors include sex, gender, age, coping styles, social background, education, profession, experience, behavior patterns, and character.[5] Clustering disabilities by stage of exposure or by similar impairments (Table 59.3) is particularly useful when studying a group of disabilities or when attempting to classify the condition of a patient with an oral pathologic condition associated with a known disorder.

TABLE 59.2 International Classification of Functioning, Disability, and Health Components and Domains

Bodily Functions:
- Mental functions
- Sensory functions and pain
- Voice and speech functions
- Functions of the diverse human systems (e.g., cardiovascular, respiratory, reproductive, metabolic)

Activities and Participation:
- Learning and applying knowledge
- General tasks and demands
- Communication
- Mobility
- Self-care
- Domestic life
- Interpersonal interactions and relationships
- Major life areas
- Community, social, and civic life

Bodily Structures:
- Eye, ear, and related structures
- Structures involved in voice and speech
- Structures of the diverse human systems (e.g., cardiovascular, respiratory, reproductive, metabolic)

Contextual Factors:
- Products and technology
- Natural environmental and human-made changes to environment
- Support and relationships
- Attitudes
- Services, systems, and policies

Source: World Health Organization: International Classification of Functioning, Disability and Health (ICF) Framework, 2023.

Stage of Exposure to Disability

- **Congenital disabilities** refer to an irregularity present at birth, which may or may not be traceable to genetic factors.
- **Acquired disabilities** refer to disabilities present after birth, which can be traceable to disease or trauma.
- **Developmental disabilities** refer to a group of conditions with impairment in physical, learning, language, or behavioral areas. Developmental disabilities are diagnosed before the age of 22 years; they may affect day-to-day functioning and can last indefinitely.
- **Age-associated disabilities** refer to disabilities with people typically over the age of 65 years. As people age, they are at a higher risk for developing chronic diseases, which may result in disability. Chronic diseases include cancer, diabetes, cardiovascular disease, arthritis, osteoporosis, and chronic obstructive pulmonary disease. Cognitive impairments, such as dementia and Alzheimer disease and physical deterioration also can cause an older individual to become disabled.
- **Military service disabilities** refer to members who have served in the United States military who are injured or ill because of a service-connected disability. Military veterans have disabilities ranging from limb amputation(s), eye injuries, and hearing loss to neuralgia, traumatic brain injury, and cancer.[8]

ADDRESSING BARRIERS TO HEALTHCARE

Globally, patients with disabilities experience health inequities. Morbidity and mortality rates are higher in patients with disabilities compared to the general population. Barriers to quality healthcare among this aggregate include the lack of training of healthcare providers, patient communication, fear and embarrassment, and access to healthcare, which is the most common barrier.[9] Addressing barriers to healthcare for patients with disabilities requires a multidisciplinary and interprofessional delivery model.

TABLE 59.3 Clustering Disabilities by Impairments

Classification of Disabilities	Characteristics
Developmental Disabilities	Attention-deficit/hyperactivity disorder, autism spectrum disorder, cerebral palsy, fetal alcohol spectrum disorders, intellectual disabilities, muscular dystrophies, Tourette syndrome, hearing loss and vision impairment
Medical Disabilities	
Cardiovascular-related diseases	Angina, artificial heart valve, congenital heart defects, hypertension, hypotension, rheumatic heart disease, congestive heart disease, heart failure
Orthopedic-related disorders	Fibromyalgia, gout, lupus, scleroderma, osteoarthritis, osteoporosis, osteopenia, rheumatoid arthritis, osteogenesis imperfecta
Autoimmune-related diseases	HIV, AIDS, mononucleosis, MRSA, sexually transmitted infections
Pulmonary-related diseases	Asthma, chronic bronchitis, chronic obstructive pulmonary disease, sleep apnea, tuberculosis, pneumonia
Endocrinologic-related diseases	Adrenal gland disorder, diabetes, hyperglycemia, hypoglycemia, hyperthyroidism, hypothyroidism, dialysis, renal failure
Oncologic-related diseases	Oral cancer, systemic cancer
Hematologic-related diseases	Anemia, deep vein thrombosis, hemophilia, leukemia, lymphoma, sickle cell diseases, thalassemia, multiple myeloma
Gastrointestinal- and/or eating-related diseases	GERD, cirrhosis, Crohn disease, hepatitis, jaundice, anorexia nervosa, bulimia nervosa
Mental Health and Psychiatric Disabilities	
Neurologic conditions	Epilepsy, migraine headaches, multiple sclerosis, neuritis, paralysis, fainting, cardiovascular accident (stroke)
Psychiatric conditions	Anxiety, depression, PTSD
Degenerative nervous system disorders	Alzheimer disease, Parkinson disease, Huntington's disease, cerebellar ataxias, multiple sclerosis, myasthenia gravis, neurofibromatosis, Creutzfeldt-Jakob disease.

AIDS, Acquired immunodeficiency syndrome; *GERD,* gastroesophageal reflux disease; *HIV,* human immunodeficiency virus; *MRSA,* methicillin-resistant *Staphylococcus aureus*; *PTSD,* posttraumatic stress disorder.

Health Policy and Programmatic Barriers

People with disabilities experience significant disadvantages when it comes to health. Adults with disabilities are three times more likely to have heart disease, stroke, diabetes, or cancer than adults without disabilities. Adults with disabilities are more likely than adults without disabilities to be current smokers, and females with disabilities are less likely than females without disabilities to have received a breast cancer X-ray test (mammogram) during the past 2 years.[2] People with disabilities have unique risk factors affecting their HRQOL (Figure 59.1). Affordability of healthcare services continues to be among the primary reasons why people with disabilities do not receive needed healthcare services.[7] Public healthcare funds often fail to cover the costs of

Bio-psycho-social model of functioning, disability and health

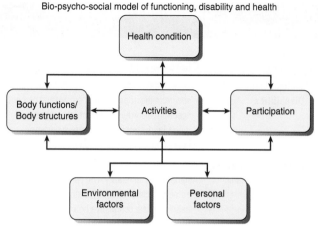

Fig. 59.1 The Integrative Bio-Psycho-Social Model of the International Classification of Functioning, Disability and Health [ICF]). (Modified from WHO's International Classification of Functioning, Disability and Health [ICF] 2001.)

everyone's needs, forcing many people with disabilities to prioritize their spending, often at the expense of basic needs. Many people with disabilities in the United States rely on federal and state support to assist in covering daily expenses. Governmental agencies can improve health outcomes for people with disabilities by improving their access to quality and affordable healthcare services.

Evidence indicates that people with disabilities are significantly less likely to be employed, compared with people without disabilities.[10] People with disabilities who are able to work often earn lower wages, and unemployment rates remain relatively high. All employers in the United States are required to provide reasonable accommodations to qualified individuals with disabilities. Reasonable accommodations refer to any modifications to a job- or work-related environment that enables a qualified applicant or employee with a disability to participate in the application process or to perform essential job functions.[1]

Disability Inclusion

Disability inclusion allows for people with disabilities to take advantage of the benefits of the same health promotion and prevention activities experienced by people who do not have a disability. Examples of these activities include education and counseling programs that promote physical activity and improve nutrition or reduce the use of tobacco, alcohol, or drugs; blood pressure and cholesterol assessment during annual health exams; and screening for illnesses such as cancer, diabetes, and heart disease. Including people with disabilities in these activities begins with identifying and eliminating barriers to their participation.[11]

Health Insurance and Expenditures

For many people with disabilities who are on a limited income without health insurance, healthcare services are out-of-pocket expenses and thus sought on a crisis basis (i.e., for emergencies or pain control). People with disabilities often have health insurance policies that either do not sufficiently meet their healthcare needs or lack coverage for the healthcare services associated with their disability, such as oral healthcare. Many healthcare institutions and dental offices struggle with providing convenient appointments and accessible medical equipment for patients with disabilities. For people with disabilities living in an institution, limited medical and/or dental services may be provided with costs either often passed onto the family or paid

by governmental funds. If a person with severe disabilities becomes institutionalized, costs to the family may drain personal financial resources. Therefore many families that care for people with severe disabilities often elect to provide care at home rather than at institutions because long-term institutionalized care is far too great of a financial burden.

Attitudinal and Communication Barriers

The attitudes of people at the individual, societal, and professional levels are among the most significant barriers, and these attitudes exacerbate other barriers.[4] Examples of attitudinal barriers include stereotyping, stigma, prejudice, and discrimination. Some people may perceive a disability as something needing prevention or cure or as inability to contribute in society. Others may think that disabilities occur because of a personal tragedy or as a punishment for wrongdoing. People with disabilities are more likely to experience discrimination and denial of necessary healthcare services.

A major complaint that people with disabilities have is finding healthcare professionals who are willing or sufficiently trained to care for their SHCN.[4] Some healthcare professionals choose not to treat patients with disabilities because Medicare and Medicaid reimbursements are often not equivalent to the fee schedules typically charged. In addition, treating individuals with SHCN often requires extra time; therefore the time needed and the income from treating others is lost.

Some healthcare professionals' fear of interacting with patients with disabilities and conflicting personal values about disabilities are reasons why healthcare professionals avoid caring for patients with disabilities. Moreover, many healthcare providers are unaware of the relationship between oral health and overall system health and fail to prioritize the oral healthcare needs of patients with disabilities. Advanced training, education, and continuing education should integrate these aspects of health and the unique needs of these patients as part of interprofessional education efforts.[4] Unfortunately, because of inadequate training on caring for patients with disabilities, many healthcare professionals do not feel qualified to care for these patients.

Healthcare Interventions

People with disabilities can also experience hearing-, speaking-, reading-, writing-, and/or understanding-related impairments. Dental hygienists should adapt their communication methods to the needs of their patients with disabilities. For example, a clinician can use larger-sized printed health promotion messages for patients with visual impairments, educational videos that include captioning and support oral communication with manual interpretation (i.e., American Sign Language) for patients with auditory impairments, and/or basic vocabulary when communicating for patients with cognitive impairments.[4]

Physical and Transportation Barriers

People with disabilities have been excluded from everyday activities such as going to various stores, neighborhood restaurants, and movie theaters due to an inability to access these places. The ADA prohibits discrimination against people with disabilities, including physical barriers in business establishments, regardless of the size or age of the business; in particular, the ADA mandates that all public facilities contain a barrier-free design.[1]

Public Accommodations

Public accommodations (i.e., businesses providing goods or services to the public) extend to various healthcare facilities including medical and dental offices. In addition, people who own, lease, sublet, or operate

BOX 59.2 Legal, Ethical, and Safety Issues Related to Discrimination of Persons With Disabilities

- Healthcare professionals and associated institutions cannot discriminate in any form against people with disabilities in places of public accommodation (e.g., medical and dental establishments, hospitals).
- Healthcare professionals have a duty to communicate with all patients effectively. The ADA requires healthcare professionals to have alternative forms of communication, including auxiliary aids and services for patients with disabilities.

ADA, Americans with Disabilities Act.

TABLE 59.4 Examples of Assistive Devices and Technologies

Category	Examples of Devices
Mobility	Walking sticks, crutches, canes, walkers, manual and powered wheelchairs, scooters Artificial leg or hand, leg or hand splint, clubfoot brace Corner chair, supportive seat, standing frame, toilet frame Arjo Sara Stedy®
Vision	Eyeglasses, magnifier White cane, GPS-based navigation device Braille systems for reading and writing, screen reader for computers, audiobook player
Hearing	Headphones, hearing aids Amplified telephone, hearing loop
Communication	Communication cards with texts, letters, symbols, or pictures Enhanced communication devices with recorded or synthetic speech
Cognition	Task lists, picture schedule and calendar, picture-based instructions Timer, manual or automatic reminder, smartphone with adapted task lists, schedules, calendars, and audio recorder Adapted therapeutic learning systems

GPS, Global Positioning System.
Source: World Health Organization and United Nations International Children's Emergency Fund (UNICEF): Assistive Technology for Children with Disabilities: Creating Opportunities for Education, Inclusion, and Participation, 2015.

places of public accommodation in existing buildings are responsible for ensuring the removal of all barriers. A facility that is barrier free enables a person to function independently within and outside of the home environment.[1] For example, a building that contains elevators and accessible restrooms is not truly barrier-free if there are no ramps or electronically operated doors to gain entrance. A dental office may be accessible; however, equipment in the hallways or operatories serves as barriers to independent movement by patients. Dental hygienists can clear a path for individuals with disabilities before seating their patients in the treatment room. Specific building codes and architectural standards for a barrier-free facility are available from federal and state resources. Refer to Box 59.2 for legal, ethical, and safety issues related to discriminating against persons with disabilities.

Transportation barriers often interfere with a person's ability to be successfully independent and function in society. All too often, people with disabilities have long distances to travel to a healthcare facility that is qualified and willing to treat them. Public transportation, such as subways, buses, rail systems, and airplanes, provide limited assistance to people with disabilities, despite federal regulations that require modifications for greater access. Interpreting the schedule, finding the exact fare, waiting at a boarding stop during inclement weather, boarding the right vehicle, and tracking the number of stops can be extremely difficult for someone with impairments.

As a result, many people with disabilities choose not to use mass transportation and would rather stay home than risk traveling. People with visual or cognitive impairments often cannot drive themselves and therefore lack access to convenient transportation options. Reliance on others for transportation to and from the home may not be convenient for the person with disabilities or for the driver. This reliance on others for transportation often places an added burden on family members or associated caregivers. These factors might affect an individual's ability to schedule a followup appointment for dental hygiene care or a recare or periodontal maintenance appointment in advance in offices where the staff members schedule these appointments at the end of an appointment with the dental hygienist. Arrangements for a followup telephone call or electronic communication can help these individuals adhere to regular appointments for preventive or nonsurgical periodontal therapy. Prevention of conditions requiring extensive dental care can save money and spare treatment challenges in the future.

ASSISTIVE DEVICES

Patients with disabilities may require assistive devices or tools to achieve independence in daily functions and communications. **Assistive devices** are tools and/or technologies that primarily maintain or improve an individual's functioning and independence to facilitate participation and enhance overall well-being.[12] Examples of assistive devices (Table 59.4) include mobility aids, visual and auditory aids, communication aids, and cognitive aids. Many assistive devices are readily available through pharmacies and other specialty stores.

Integrating Assistive Technology

Electronic devices, such as smartphones, tablets, and other technologies, are integrating into education and rehabilitation programs for patients with disabilities. Unfortunately, assistive devices result in additional costs for people with disabilities and can increase financial and access-related barriers. The demand for rehabilitation products and services is increasing worldwide, particularly with aging demographics and the consequences of disease and injury.[12] Dental hygienists should be familiar with these assistive devices; their use may affect patient goals and decisions in healthcare.

Mobility Assistive Equipment

Several devices are available for patients who experience challenges with ambulation or mobility. Mobility assistive equipment (MAE) or mobility aids either replace unilateral or bilateral function, significantly increase mobility for ambulation, or support people with disabilities as they move from one point to another. Examples of MAE include walking sticks, crutches, canes, walkers, wheelchairs, scooters, prosthetics, and orthoses, among others.

A prosthetic device is any assistive device that helps replace, correct, or support a particular body part or function. Prosthetic devices can include a wide array of assistive devices such as artificial limbs, pacemakers, hearing aids, dentures, and implants. Prosthetic devices may be fitted permanently through surgical implantation or may be removable and worn only when needed for functional or cosmetic purposes. Patients with removable devices, such as those designed for the loss of facial structure, may feel more comfortable when the prosthesis is in place; therefore removal should occur only during assessment or when indicated during dental hygiene care. (Refer to Chapter 41 on fixed and removable dental prostheses.) The focus of this chapter is assistive devices for patients with disabilities. See the Critical Thinking Exercise designed to enhance the dental hygienist's appreciation of patients with various disabilities.

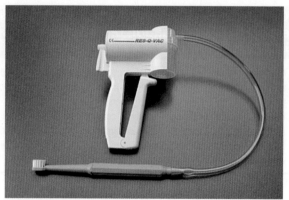

Fig. 59.2 Plak-Vac Oral Suction Toothbrush. (Copyright 2010 Trademark Medical Corporation.)

CRITICAL THINKING EXERCISE TO ENHANCE APPRECIATION OF PATIENTS WITH DISABILITIES

- Assume the role of an impaired person for several hours and complete a set of exercises designed to enhance your appreciation of patients with various disabilities.
- Randomly draw from a list that includes hearing and visual impairments, inability to speak, blindness, and limited mobility (arm, leg, both legs). Assemble equipment and assistive devices for use during these activities (e.g., canes, dark glasses, safety glasses coated with petroleum jelly, ear plugs, crutches, wheelchairs, splints, slings, shoe lifts). Consult a physical therapist or physical therapy student for assistance.
- While assuming the role of a person who is impaired, students should complete a health history form in the clinical setting, ride in elevators, and visit another building to retrieve a newspaper or beverage, obtain signatures from faculty in other departments, or purchase supplies from the campus bookstore.
- After completing these exercises, discuss the experiences. (Take extreme caution and care to plan activities that will not place the student in danger while "impaired." Students should not cross roadways or other high-traffic areas to prevent accidental injury. Consider pairing students who are severely "impaired" with a classmate for assistance or for safety. Always inform campus officials when students will be completing this exercise to help ensure student safety and participation by others.)

ORAL SELF-CARE DEVICES

Although many assistive devices help in the function of basic activities, few assistive devices help patients carry out oral self-care behaviors. Patients with disabilities, including those in a hospital or extended care facility, may benefit from specialized toothbrushes such as the Plak-Vac Oral Suction Toothbrush, a uniquely designed toothbrush that can be connected either to a bedside or portable suction device (Fig. 59.2). Assistive oral self-care devices ideally should adapt to the patient's needs, skill level, and functional status.

Patient Assessment

Dental hygienists assess the extent of a patient's physical and mental impairment before using assistive oral self-care devices.

- **Range of motion:** Evaluate the patient's ability to reach the oral cavity with arms and hands. Range of motion indicates the required length of the assistive device to accommodate the patient's physical limitations in reaching the mouth. For example, patients with muscular impairments may only be able to reach halfway across their body and elevate their arm only to heart level. Patients in this scenario would be unable to reach the mouth and would need a customized assistive device to improve their ability to reach all aspects of the oral cavity.

- **Grip strength:** Patients with neuromuscular impairments may have trouble holding an assistive device that is too narrow or too small. Strategies to assess grip strength include having the patient grasp various sizes of foam cylinders and retain finger closure for an extended length of time.

- **Skill level:** Watching patients simulate or actually brush their teeth is useful to assess a patient's skill level. Patients should be prompted to perform skills such as reaching into the upper right quadrant, brushing their tongue, cleaning lingual surfaces, and brushing the facial surfaces of their anterior teeth. It is important for dental hygienists to note what a patient is capable of performing with relative ease and which behaviors present difficulty or confusion.

- **Cognitive application:** Evaluate this ability during the skill level assessment phase by asking questions to determine whether the patient is capable of responding accurately to verbal commands and instructions. For example, patients who have intellectual impairment may have difficulty in producing a response on command and may require an assistive device such as a powered toothbrush that helps them accomplish the brushing task with little effort.

These assessment measures work well with patients who are physically and mentally capable of learning self-care techniques; however, some patients may not move their upper extremities at all and therefore must rely on a primary caregiver to perform daily care. Caregiver interviews are important to assess their willingness to provide daily oral care, determine the existing skill level of the caregiver, provide instruction as appropriate, and address related concerns.

Customizing Oral Self-Care Assistive Devices: An Interprofessional Opportunity

Customized oral self-care assistive devices are helpful for patients with significant limitations in range of motion, grip strength, skill level, and/or cognitive application. The occupational therapist and the dental hygienist should work together to create these customized oral self-care assistive devices while also providing training for the patient and/or caregiver to maintain the devices thereafter. A wide variety of equipment is readily available and accessible to patients and their caregivers to use in customizing oral self-care assistive devices.

To assist patients with limited range of motion, attach plastic rulers and rods, available from most hardware stores, to toothbrushes and floss holders with heavy electrical tape. Angle the existing plastic handle of the toothbrush against the curve of the arches. To assist the patient with limitations in grip strength, supplement the toothbrush handle with a variety of materials to fit the patient's finger closure capability. Bicycle grips, styrofoam molds, and crafted compounds as alternative handles greatly improve the patient's ability to hold the toothbrush

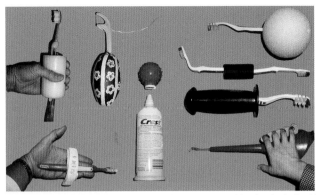

Fig. 59.3 Customized oral care aids for persons with physical disabilities. (Courtesy Kathleen Muzzin, Texas A&M College of Dentistry, Caruth School of Dental Hygiene, Dallas, TX.)

BOX 59.3 Ideal Design Characteristics for Customized Oral Self-Care Assistive Devices

- Lightweight and easy to use
- Readily available and accessible
- Inexpensive and easily constructed
- Interchangeable and water-resistant parts

(Fig. 59.3). Patients with poor dexterity and coordination and/or a limited gripping ability may benefit from power toothbrushes with larger handles. Box 59.3 offers considerations on ideal design characteristics that dental hygienists and occupational therapists (interprofessional collaboration opportunity) can keep in mind when designing customized self-care assistive devices for patients with disabilities. Refer to the Critical Thinking Exercise on designing oral self-care assistive devices.

CRITICAL THINKING EXERCISE ON DESIGNING ORAL SELF-CARE ASSISTIVE DEVICES

Design oral self-care devices for the following patient conditions:
- Inability to grasp and hold
- Inability to raise the arm and hand
- Inability to move the forearm in a back-and-forth motion.

PROTECTIVE STABILIZATION AND PATIENT POSITIONING

Understanding Protective Stabilization

Patients with disabilities frequently have problems with support and balance; therefore the dental hygienist should conduct a physical assessment before delivering clinical care to determine the need for adaptations to treat the patient in a safe and effective manner. A variety of behavior guidance techniques, including protective stabilization, can improve patient safety and access to the oral cavity while providing dental hygiene services to patients with SHCN. **Protective stabilization** refers to "any manual method, physical or mechanical device, material, or equipment that immobilizes or reduces the ability of a patient to move his or her arms, legs, body, or head freely."[13]

- *Active stabilization* involves physical immobilization by another person, such as the parent, caregiver, or healthcare professional.

- *Passive stabilization* involves using an immobilization device, such as a papoose.

Protective stabilization should, to the extent possible, be person centered and conducted in a fashion that maintains the patient's privacy and dignity. Protective stabilization should be provided in the least restrictive manner possible. Staff should be trained in the safe, efficacious employment of any devices, techniques, or protocols.[13]

Regulatory Considerations

Protective stabilization is an advanced practice in healthcare delivery and is subject to increased regulation. When indicated, dental hygienists should first use the least restrictive technique and then evaluate the need for more restrictive immobilization techniques. Ideal qualities of immobilization devices include ease of use, appropriately sized for the patient, soft and contoured to minimize potential injury to the patient, specifically designed for patient stabilization, and ability to be disinfected.[13]

Both sufficient didactic and hands-on education is needed to ensure safe and effective implementation of protective stabilization. When correctly executed, protective stabilization can aid in the delivery of quality dental hygiene services; however, the inappropriate use of protective stabilization can lead to potential consequences, including harm to the patient and violation of patient's rights. Unnecessary use of physical restraints has been associated with increased risk for bruising, respiratory compromise, aspiration pneumonia, and cellulitis from limb restraint.[14]

Indications for protective stabilization include the following:
- A patient requires immediate diagnosis and/or urgent limited treatment and cannot cooperate because of medical, physical, or behavioral conditions.
- Emergent care is needed and uncontrolled movements risk the safety of the patient, staff members, parent, caregiver, or dental hygienist without the use of protective stabilization.
- A previously cooperative patient quickly becomes uncooperative during the appointment; protective stabilization is needed to protect the patient's safety and help expedite the completion of treatment.
- A sedated patient may become uncooperative during treatment.
- A patient may experience uncontrolled movements that would be harmful or significantly interfere with the quality of care.

Contraindications for protective stabilization include the following:
- Cooperative nonsedated patients
- Patients who cannot be immobilized safely due to associated medical, psychologic, or physical conditions
- Patients with a history of physical or psychologic trauma due to restraint (unless no other alternatives are available)
- Patients with nonemergent treatment needs to accomplish full mouth or multiple quadrant dental rehabilitation

Informed Consent

Protective stabilization requires informed consent. Patient records must include documentation of informed consent and explicit details regarding the patient's care (Box 59.4). Dental hygienists must explain the indications, benefits, and associated risks of protective stabilization, as well as alternative approaches to care (e.g., deferral of treatment, sedation, general anesthesia).[14] Certain jurisdictions mandate written consent; therefore it is necessary for the healthcare professional to be aware of applicable statutes. Refer to Box 59.5 to learn about the legal, ethical, and safety issues related to protective stabilization needed to provide safe and comfortable dental hygiene services.

BOX 59.4 Documenting Protective Stabilization

The patient's record must include:
- Indication for protective stabilization
- Type of protective stabilization used
- Informed consent for protective stabilization
- Rationale for parent or caregiver exclusion during protective stabilization (if applicable)
- Duration of the application of protective stabilization
- Behavior evaluation and rating during stabilization
- Any untoward outcomes, such as skin markings
- Management implications for future appointments

Source: The American Academy of Pediatric Dentistry (AAPD), 2013.

BOX 59.5 Legal, Ethical, and Safety Issues Related to Protective Stabilization During the Delivery of Healthcare

- Healthcare professionals should uphold professional ethics and use minimally restrictive techniques on patients who require immobilization.
- Healthcare professionals should thoroughly discuss indications, benefits and risks, and alternatives to care, as well as obtain written informed consent before immobilization.
- Healthcare professionals should complete advanced formal education before using protective stabilization.

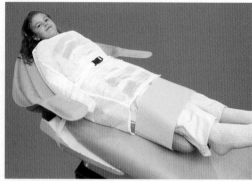

Fig. 59.4 Papoose boards used for protective stabilization. (Courtesy Specialized Care Co., Hampton, NH.)

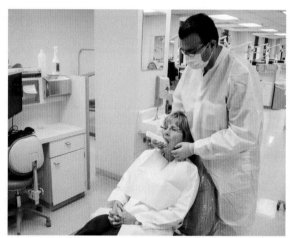

Fig. 59.5 Clinician using the Open Wide disposable mouth prop on an adult. (Courtesy Faizan Kabani and Kathleen Muzzin, Texas A&M College of Dentistry, Caruth School of Dental Hygiene, Dallas, TX.)

Using Protective Stabilization

Patients with neuromuscular impairments, such as tremors, muscle spasms, or hyperactive responses, may require a stabilization device. Dental hygienists can place pillows or rolled towels underneath the knees and neck of the patient to prevent muscle spasms and to provide additional support during care. Similarly, patients with aggressive behavioral tendencies may benefit from the use of medical immobilization devices, such as papoose boards (Fig. 59.4).

Mouth props are helpful in preventing trauma from biting, particularly when patients lack behavioral or motor control. Mouth props come in various designs and strengths (Fig. 59.5). When indicated, begin by using the soft mouth prop and if necessary, upgrade to using harder strength mouth props (Fig. 59.6). Ideally, the assisting healthcare professional, not the primary healthcare professional, should use mouth props during oral healthcare delivery. The appropriate use of a mouth prop requires careful technique, with special attention toward preventing the patient from biting their lip once the mouth prop is introduced into the patient's mouth. Minimize trauma by using a double fulcrum (Fig. 59.7). Before using the mouth prop, dental hygienists should inspect the oral cavity for mobile teeth. The presence of mobile teeth increases aspiration-related risks, particularly if the mouth prop inadvertently dislodges a mobile tooth when being used. A chest X-ray image is indicated to rule out aspiration if a mobile tooth dislodges in the oral cavity and remains unaccounted for during care. Refer to Procedure 59.1 for a demonstration of proper techniques using mouth props.

Use protective stabilization devices with caution for patients who are prone to seizures; in particular, remove immobilization devices quickly in the event of a seizure onset. In patients with whom cooperation is near impossible, it may be necessary to use immobilization devices at every visit to render safe and effective oral healthcare services. To prevent injuries during patient care, a caregiver or assisting healthcare professional may hold the patient's arms and legs in a comfortable position. In the case of

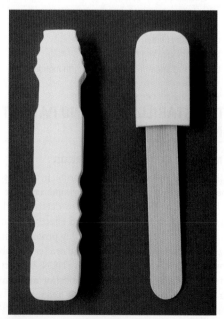

Fig. 59.6 Different types of mouth props. Soft mouth prop *(left)* and medium mouth prop *(right)*. (Courtesy Faizan Kabani, Texas A&M College of Dentistry, Caruth School of Dental Hygiene, Dallas, TX.)

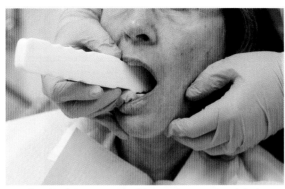

Fig. 59.7 Double fulcrum used with mouth props to minimize trauma. (Courtesy Faizan Kabani and Kathleen Muzzin, Texas A&M College of Dentistry, Caruth School of Dental Hygiene, Dallas, TX.)

PROCEDURE 59.1 Proper Use of Mouth Prop and Establishing a Double Fulcrum

Steps

1. Hold the mouth prop using the hand opposite to the half of the mouth receiving treatment. For example, if the dental hygienist intends to provide treatment on the right half of the mouth, then hold the mouth prop with the left hand and vice versa.
2. Gently pull the patient's lower lip forward using the index finger and thumb of the available hand. This step is essential in preventing the patient from inadvertently biting the lip when the mouth prop is inserted into the mouth.
3. Gently insert the smaller end of the mouth prop horizontally into the patient's mouth while continuing to protect the lower lip from biting trauma.

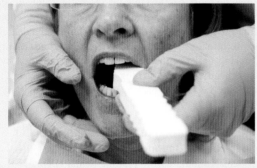

Gently insert smaller end of the mouth prop horizontally into the patient's mouth while continuing to protect the lower lip from a biting trauma. (Courtesy Faizan Kabani and Kathleen Muzzin, Texas A&M College of Dentistry, Caruth School of Dental Hygiene, Dallas, TX)

4. Carefully turn the mouth prop from a horizontal to a vertical position to help open the patient's mouth. Be sure to use the mouth prop only between the patient's posterior teeth, which are built to withstand biting pressure.
5. Place the ring finger of the hand holding the mouth prop on the gingiva buccal to the mandibular anterior sextant. The ring finger establishes the first fulcrum and prevents the lower lip from biting trauma.
6. Place the pinky finger of the hand that is holding the mouth prop on the patient's chin. The pinky finger establishes the second fulcrum and assists in stabilizing the mouth prop (see Fig. 59.6).

a child who may be difficult to keep still in the dental chair, the child can lie on top of the parent or caregiver, with the parent or caregiver's arms around the child's body. Make an effort to discontinue this practice early in the course of care after conducting behavioral guidance techniques, as well as trust- and rapport-building exercises with the child (Table 59.5).

TABLE 59.5 Basic Behavioral Guidance Techniques

Basic Techniques	Description
Positive previsit imagery	Show the patient positive images of dentistry and dental treatment in the waiting area before the dental appointment.
Direct observation	Show the patient a video or permit the patient to observe a cooperative young patient undergoing dental treatment.
Tell-show-do	The tell-show-do technique involves verbally explaining the procedures in phrases appropriate to the developmental level of the patient (tell); demonstrating for the patient visual, auditory, olfactory, and tactile aspects of the procedure in a carefully defined, nonthreatening setting (show); and then, without deviating from the explanation and demonstration, showing the completion of the procedure (do).
Ask-tell-ask	The ask-tell-ask technique involves inquiring about the patient's visit and feelings toward or about any planned procedures (ask); explaining the procedures through demonstrations and nonthreatening language appropriate to the cognitive level of the patient (tell); and again inquiring if the patient understands and how they feel about the impending treatment (ask).
Voice control	Provides deliberate alterations of voice volume, tone, or pace to influence and direct the patient's behavior. The use of an assertive voice may be considered aversive to some patients who are unfamiliar with this technique.
Nonverbal communication	Reinforcement and guidance of behavior are provided through appropriate contact, posture, facial expression, and body language.
Positive reinforcement and descriptive praise	Positive reinforcement rewards desired behaviors, thereby strengthening the likelihood of a recurrence of those behaviors. Social reinforcement includes positive voice modulation, facial expression, and verbal praise. Descriptive praise emphasizes specific cooperative behaviors, such as, "Thank you for sitting still," rather than a generalized praise, such as, "Good job." Nonsocial reinforcement includes tokens and toys.
Distraction	Distraction involves diverting the patient's attention from what may be perceived as an unpleasant procedure. Giving the patient a short break during a stressful procedure can be an effective use of distraction before considering more advanced behavioral guidance techniques.
Memory restructuring	Memory restructuring is a behavioral approach during which memories associated with a negative or difficult event (e.g., first dental visit, local anesthesia, extraction) are restructured into positive memories using information suggested after the event has taken place. Restructuring involves four components: (1) visual reminders; (2) positive reinforcement through verbalization; (3) concrete examples to encode sensory details; and (4) sense of accomplishment.
Parental presence or absence	The presence or absence of the parent sometimes can be used to gain cooperation for treatment. Dental hygienists must consider the parents' desires and wishes and be open to a paradigm shift in their own thinking.

Source: The American Academy of Pediatric Dentistry (AAPD): Guidelines on Behavior Guidance for the Pediatric Dental Patient, 2015.

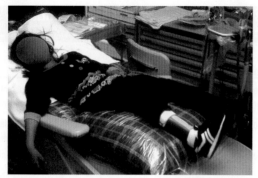

Fig. 59.8 Beanbags help support limbs of patients with physical disabilities.

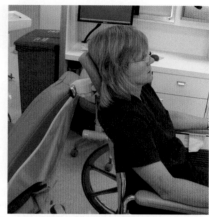

Fig. 59.9 Wheelchair positioned so that the head is leaning against the back of the dental chair's headrest. (Courtesy Kathleen Muzzin, Texas A&M College of Dentistry, Caruth School of Dental Hygiene, Dallas, TX.)

Dental hygienists may need to provide additional head support and stabilization for the patient during care. By sitting at the 12 o'clock position, the clinician can wrap their nondominant arm around the patient's head and firmly under the patient's chin for stabilization. Placing small pillows, neck rolls, or a rolled bath sheet on either side of the patient's head provides additional support.

Beanbag chairs placed in the dental chair can provide additional support for patients with unstable joints and limbs (Fig. 59.8). Headrests, solid backrests, seatbelts, chest straps, lateral trunk supports, and hip guides on wheelchairs help keep the patient positioned correctly. Cushions and/or beanbags are helpful with patients with physical impairments, such as paralysis, to provide additional support and to minimize pressure injuries.

Patient Positioning

Many patients with disabilities are at an increased risk for aspiration. To reduce aspiration risk, the dental hygienist should place the patient in a sitting position or in as close to an upright position as possible, using a semiinclined position to prevent aspiration of materials, fluids, or instruments. Rubber dam isolation can also help prevent aspiration of dental materials; however, routine use is not recommended for patients with significant dysphagia, compromised airway, and those who are aggressive or uncooperative. It is helpful to maintain adequate suctioning with the aid of other healthcare professionals, particularly when increased salivation or fluids are present.

Dental hygienists should also limit the use of water or other fluids in the oral cavity for patients with an increased aspiration risk. One alternative method to using the air-water syringe is to use wet gauze as towelettes to cleanse the oral cavity of debris. Dental hygienists can also recommend caregivers apply a dentifrice or other topical agents when the patient is sitting in the supine position. The patient with neuromuscular or behavioral impairments may use an ingestible dentifrice as a safe alternative.

CARING FOR PATIENTS IN WHEELCHAIRS

In most cases, the patient is one of the best sources for learning how to best approach positioning and movement. Some patients who use wheelchairs are able to transfer themselves independently, whereas others may need assistance. Dental hygienists first assess the patient's needs by asking about the patient's preferred transfer method, the patient's ability to help in the transfer, the need for specialized assistive transfer devices, and the probability of neuromuscular spasms. Next, dental hygienists inquire regarding the use of assistive bowel and bladder devices (e.g., catheters, collecting bags) and take precautionary

steps to prevent dislodgement during a transfer. A damaged catheter can result in inadequate bladder drainage and toxic waste accumulation and could trigger an emergency. A consultation with the patient's physician about specific medical concerns before any transfer is attempted is recommended.

Ideally, patients should receive care in the dental chair; however, some patients in a wheelchair may be too tired or weak to transfer into the dental chair or may require specialized positioning that only the wheelchair can provide. Some MAE, such as power wheelchairs, have seat functions that recline or tilt for adequate positioning and may be more comfortable for the patient. Ideally, patients in a wheelchair should be cared for in an operatory wide enough for positioning the patient either alongside or behind the dental chair. Patients who remain in the wheelchair may need additional head support during oral healthcare, which can be obtained by using the portable headrest or by turning the wheelchair around so that the patient's head is leaning back against the dental chair's headrest (Fig. 59.9).

Guidelines on Preparing for Wheelchair Transfer
Preparing the Dental Operatory

Dental hygienists should ensure that the dental operatory is conducive to a safe and effective wheelchair transfer. Preparation includes removing the dental chair armrest and relocating equipment such as hoses, foot controls, operatory lights, and bracket tables from the transfer path. Dental hygienists should position the wheelchair near the dental chair and adjust the dental chair's position to either the same height as the wheelchair or a slightly lower plane.[15] Transferring patients from a higher to a lower plane accommodates for weight and minimizes the strength necessary to transfer the patient safely and successfully.

Preparing for the Transfer

Many patients who use wheelchairs have experienced physical rehabilitation therapy and may be accustomed to transfer techniques, particularly if patients independently transfer themselves at home. Some patients have the ability to assist with the transfer but may be unfamiliar with the actual steps involved. Others may perceive that they have the physical strength and skills necessary to assist with the transfer when actually they do not possess these abilities. Misconceptions may be dangerous if transfers occur without verifying whether the patient's

BOX 59.6   Guidelines for the Dental Hygienists' Safety During Patient Transfers

- The dental hygienist should not attempt to transfer a patient alone. Although the one-person transfer technique requires only one person, an additional person should be available to provide assistance when needed. The presence of an additional person reduces the risk for falling or injury during a transfer.
- One person should not attempt to transfer a patient who is very tall or heavy, especially if the patient has minimal upper body strength. These patients have a much greater likelihood of falling and injury because of their lack of coordination and balance.
- Dental hygienists should perform transfers with feet separated for good balance and knees bent to protect against back strain. Lifting procedures should be performed with the legs while keeping the back straight and slightly bent forward at the waist to prevent muscular back injury.

When lifting and transferring the patient, the dental hygienist should not twist the back; twisting increases the risk for severe muscular back strain and injury. Rather, healthcare professionals should use the *stand-pivot-sit* method and lift with the legs.

perceptions and abilities are correct. Dental hygienists should use good judgment and ergonomics when performing patient transfers (Box 59.6).

The patient's level of coordination and balance can assist in determining the need for assistance with the transfer process. Assistance may be required from another healthcare professional or dental team member. The patient's willingness to transfer is essential for the dental hygienist to know, particularly if the patient depends on the hygienist to some extent during the transfer. An uncooperative patient who overestimates or underestimates their abilities or a patient who resists transfer attempts poses significant management challenges, as well as increased risks for injury to the patient and healthcare professional.

Before beginning the transfer procedure, the dental hygienist should explain the steps in chronological order to help reduce the patient's fear. If the patient expects to assist with the transfer, reiterate to the patient exactly how and when to provide assistance. Performing a simulation is helpful before the actual transfer, especially for patients new to transfers. Introduce the patient to any specialized armamentarium used in the transfer, such as transfer belts and/or sliding boards.

A. Transfer belts are straps secured around the patient's waist and provide a designated location for dental hygienists to hold the patient in the event that the patient begins to fall during the transfer process. Transfer belts are particularly useful in patients who have minimal upper body strength.

B. Sliding boards assist patients with favorable upper body strength by helping the patient slide out of the wheelchair, across the board, and into the dental chair. One end of the sliding board is placed underneath the patient, and the other end is laid across the dental chair. Position the wheelchair close to the dental chair, and remove the arms to both chairs to accommodate the sliding board. Sliding boards also are useful with patients who are overweight or those who otherwise find it too difficult for only one person to move safely. Transfer belts are an added precaution during a sliding board transfer.

C. The use of MAE, such as the Arjo Sara Steady®, can be used in the dental setting to transfer a patient from the wheelchair to the dental chair. This device is typically used in hospital settings, nursing homes, or other healthcare facilities to transfer patients who have

the ability to stand unaided or who can stand with minimal assistance. However, the Sara Steady can be used in the dental setting to quickly and easily transport or transfer patients from one sitting position to another e.g. from the wheelchair to the dental chair.[16] A demonstration video can be found at: https://www.youtube.com/watch?v=3qlVrYG6zgU

Wheelchair Transfers in the Dental Operatory

Transferring From Wheelchair to Dental Chair. At the beginning of the appointment, the patient should transfer from the wheelchair into the dental chair, when possible. Before the transfer, dental hygienists should ensure that the wheelchair locks into position and the dental chair should be even with or at a lower plane than the wheelchair to minimize the risk for falls and injury. Dental hygienists should check the nearby area for any sharp edges, hazards, obstacles, or cords that could cause injury during the transfer. Dental hygienists should also transfer any special padding underneath the patient in the wheelchair to the dental chair to help with patient comfort throughout the appointment.

Procedure 59.2 describes transferring the patient from the wheelchair to the dental chair using a one-person lift. Assistance may be required from another healthcare professional (Procedure 59.3), or the dental hygienists can use a transfer belt or sliding board. If the patient cannot be moved to the dental chair, then dental treatment can be completed with the patient in the wheelchair and the provider standing (Fig. 59.10). Refer to Box 59.7 for the legal, ethical, and safety issues related to wheelchair transfers. (See associated Competency Forms for one-person and assisted wheelchair transfers on Evolve.)

Transferring From Dental Chair to Wheelchair. At the end of the appointment, the patient should be transferred from the dental chair back into the wheelchair. Similar safety guidelines apply when moving the patient, including making sure the wheelchair is locked into position. The dental chair should be at a slightly higher plane than the wheelchair to minimize the risk for falls and injury, and padding should be transferred.[15]

Transfer techniques require practice, especially for those dental hygienists who perform transfers infrequently. Refer to the Critical Thinking Exercise on practicing wheelchair transfers. Dental hygienists unfamiliar with providing care for patients in wheelchairs have an opportunity to work interprofessionally with rehabilitation therapists to learn more about transfers and, in turn, help rehabilitation professionals learn more about the importance of regular oral hygiene care for patients with disabilities. Transfer techniques enable dental hygienists to care for patients who may otherwise not receive oral care.

CRITICAL THINKING EXERCISE ON PRACTICING WHEELCHAIR TRANSFERS

Form groups of three to practice wheelchair transfers and patient positioning and stabilization techniques. Alternate the roles of the patient and the dental hygiene care providers. Practical exercises should include one-person and two-person lifts and, when possible, a sliding board. Consider consulting rehabilitation therapists for collaborative learning.

Complications in Wheelchair Transfers
Muscular Paroxysms

Patients undergoing wheelchair transfers are at an increased risk for experiencing muscular paroxysms or muscle spasms. Dental hygienists involved in moving patients should be prepared to protect the patient

PROCEDURE 59.2   **Transferring a Patient From a Wheelchair to Dental Chair Using a One-Person Lift**

Steps

1. Position the transfer belt around patient's waist just below the ribcage.

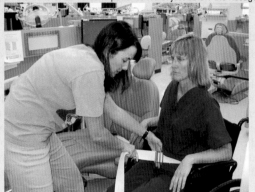

Transfer belt is placed around the patient's waist and below the ribcage.

2. Insert your hands underneath the patient's thighs, and gently slide the patient forward in the wheelchair seat so that the patient's buttocks are positioned on the front portion of seat. Place the sliding board under the patient so that one end of the board is underneath the patient's thighs and the other end lies across the dental chair.

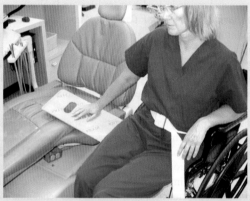

One end of the sliding board is placed under the patient and the other end is laid across the dental chair. (Courtesy Kathleen Muzzin, Texas A&M College of Dentistry, Caruth School of Dental Hygiene, Dallas, TX; and Bobi Robles, Baylor Institute for Rehabilitation, Dallas, TX.)

3. Place the patient's feet together and hold them in place on either side by your feet. Close your knees or thighs on the patient's knees, thus supporting and

stabilizing the patient's leg, which allows the patient to bear some of their own weight during the lift.

4. Place the patient's arms on their lap or on the side of the wheelchair; instruct the patient to rest their head over your shoulder and to look in the opposite direction of the transfer.

5. Grasp the patient around the waist and hold the transfer belt securely between both hands. If there is no transfer belt available, use an overlapping wrist grasp for greater stability.

6. With the patient in position and looking away from the transfer, rock gently backward onto your heels and, using your leg muscles, lift the patient off the seat. The patient is now resting against you, the operator.

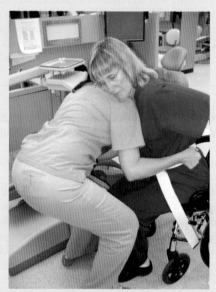

Patient's hands are placed on the side of the wheelchair and the head is positioned on the operator's shoulder, opposite the direction of the transfer. Patient is lifted off the wheelchair and transferred to the dental chair. (Courtesy Kathleen Muzzin, Texas A&M College of Dentistry, Caruth School of Dental Hygiene, Dallas, TX; and Bobi Robles, Baylor Institute for Rehabilitation, Dallas, TX.)

7. Pivot on your foot closer to the dental chair and maneuver the patient over the seat of the dental chair. Complete the procedure in a smooth motion.

8. Lower the patient onto the dental chair by bending at your knees. Do not release the transfer belt around patient until the patient is placed securely into the chair.

9. Release one hand to lift the patient's legs onto chair while still supporting the patient with the other hand. Reposition the armrest of the dental chair for patient safety.

from injury in the event that muscle spasms occur. Spasms can affect multiple types of muscles in the body and can exacerbate other health conditions or vice versa. The use of supportive pillows or beanbags can reduce muscular paroxysms induced by movement.[15] Increased anxiety levels can also contribute to spasms; therefore dental hygienists should engage in stress reduction protocols with patients prior to wheelchair transfers.

Pressure Injury

People who use wheelchairs and those who have areas of insensate skin are prone to pressure injuries, which are damages to the skin and underlying soft tissue. Pressure injuries typically occur on body sites such as buttocks, shoulders, back, heels of the feet, and sacral tissues. Pressure injuries can appear as intact skin or an open-faced ulceration, which may be painful. If left untreated, pressure injuries

PROCEDURE 59.3 Transferring a Patient From Wheelchair to Dental Chair Using a Two-Person Lift

Steps

1. The first operator stands behind the patient and reaches around the patient's torso underneath the armpits. The operator crosses their arms in front of the patient and grasps the patient's hands at the wrists with the opposite hands (i.e., right over left, left over right). The operator slides their arms down so they are positioned under the patient's ribcage on the abdomen. The stronger and/or taller operator is behind the patient.

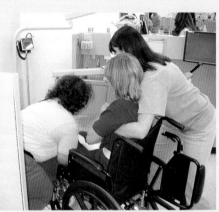

During the two-person transfer, the first operator stands behind the wheelchair and the second operator is positioned at the patient's thighs. (Courtesy Kathleen Muzzin, Texas A&M College of Dentistry, Caruth School of Dental Hygiene, Dallas, TX; and Bobi Robles, Baylor Institute for Rehabilitation, Dallas, TX.)

2. The second operator is positioned on the far side of the wheelchair at the patient's knees or thighs. Bending at the knees, the operator slides one arm

underneath the patient's thighs (approximately midway point) while the other arm is placed slightly above the knees.

3. Both operators lift the patient at a prearranged signal—"1, 2, 3, lift." One person coordinates the lift, preferably one who is supporting the patient's torso (i.e., the operator who is lifting the most weight). Lift the patient in one smooth motion and place them into the dental chair.

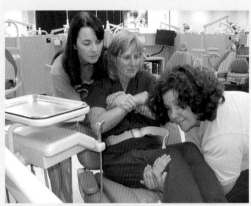

The operator who is supporting the patient's torso coordinates the lift, lifts the patient in one smooth motion, and places the patient in the dental chair. (Courtesy Kathleen Muzzin, Texas A&M College of Dentistry, Caruth School of Dental Hygiene, Dallas, TX; and Bobi Robles, Baylor Institute for Rehabilitation, Dallas, TX.)

4. The operator holding the legs releases the grasp on the patient and repositions the patient in chair. The other operator does not release the patient until the patient is stabilized and then replaces the arm of the dental chair.

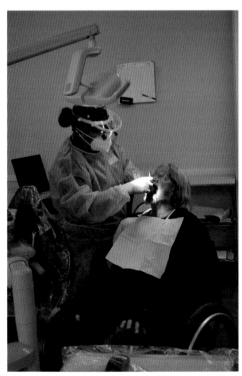

Fig. 59.10 Providing dental care in a wheelchair for a patient who cannot be moved to the dental chair. (Courtesy of Trayce Moore, Northern Arizona University, Dental Hygiene.)

BOX 59.7 Legal, Ethical, and Safety Issues Related to Wheelchair Transfers During Healthcare

• Healthcare professionals should ensure patient stability during wheelchair transfer and positioning. Closely attend to all patients undergoing wheelchair transfers to prevent the risk for falling and injury.
• Healthcare professionals should protect their patients from complications in wheelchair transfers, including using beanbags and pillows to redistribute pressure to prevent seizures and pressure injuries.

can gradually worsen. Dental hygienists should discuss the presence of pressure injuries during the health history review with the patient, avoid positioning the patient on body areas with pressure injuries, and continue to assist in repositioning the patient approximately every 20 minutes to prevent pressure injuries. Monitor the changes in the patient's skin, and discuss the findings with the patient's physician.

Health Promotion and Advocacy

Dental hygienists support and care for patients with disabilities by promoting them as valuable, contributing members of society. Opportunities to advocate for patients with disabilities include actively participating in organized efforts to improve access to care (e.g., participating on councils, on local boards, and in area support groups; holding leadership positions in organizations; initiating community programs; contributing to lay and professional communities via speaking engagements and publications).

KEY CONCEPTS

- Disability is a universal part of the human condition, with almost everyone experiencing degrees of disability in life through either changes in their health or in the environment.
- Using the term *handicap* is discontinued because of its negative connotations.
- The people-first language is the recommended approach because it focuses on the person first, not the disability.
- Access to healthcare, education, and employment opportunities is essential to achieve an acceptable quality of life and to maintain as much independence as possible.
- Assistive devices help achieve independence in daily function and communication.
- Dental hygienists should assess the extent of a patient's range of motion, grip strength, skill level, and cognitive ability to learn using self-care techniques.
- Protective stabilization, when used correctly, can facilitate the delivery of quality healthcare services, whereas inappropriate use of protective stabilization can lead to potential consequences, including harm to the patient and violation of the patient's rights.
- Dental hygienists should place the patient with disabilities in as much of an upright position as possible during care to minimize the risk for aspiration of dental materials, fluids, or instruments.
- Dental hygienists should first assess the patient's needs by asking about the patient's preferred wheelchair transfer method, the patient's ability to help in the transfer, the need for specialized assistive transfer devices, and the probability of neuromuscular spasms.
- Dental hygienists should use good judgment and ergonomics when participating in patient transfers, including transferring patients from a higher to a lower plane.
- Dental hygienists should protect their patients from complications in wheelchair transfers, including using beanbags and pillows to redistribute pressure to prevent muscular paroxysms and pressure injuries.

ACKNOWLEDGMENTS

The authors acknowledge Faizan Kabani, Ann Spolarich, and Kathleen Muzzin for their past contributions to this chapter.

EVOLVE RESOURCES

Please visit http://evolve.elsevier.com/Pieren/hygiene/ for additional practice and study support tools.

REFERENCES

1. U.S. Department of Justice. *Introduction to the ADA*; 2023. Available at: https://www.ada.gov/topics/intro-to-ada/. Accessed January 30, 2023.
2. Centers for Disease Control and Prevention. *Disability Impacts All of Us*; 2022. Available at: https://www.cdc.gov/ncbddd/disabilityandhealth/infographic-disability-impacts-all.html#:~:text=61%20million%20adults%20in%20the,Graphic%20of%20the%20United%20States. Accessed January 30, 2023.
3. The World Bank. *Disability Inclusion*; 2022. Available at: https://www.worldbank.org/en/topic/disability. Accessed January 30, 2023.
4. American Academy of Pediatric Dentistry. Guideline on management of dental patients with special healthcare needs. *Pediatr Dent*. 2021. Available at: https://www.aapd.org/media/Policies_Guidelines/BP_SHCN.pdf. Accessed January 30, 2023.
5. Centers for Disease Control and Prevention. *Disability and Health Overview*; 2020. Available at: https://www.cdc.gov/ncbddd/disabilityandhealth/disability.html. Accessed January 30, 2023.
6. World Health Organization. *Global Health Estimates: Life Expectancy and Leading Causes of Death and Disability*; 2023. Available at: https://www.who.int/data/gho/data/themes/mortality-and-global-health-estimates. Accessed January 30, 2023.
7. World Health Organization. *International Classification of Functioning, Disability and Health (ICF)*; 2023. Available at: https://www.who.int/standards/classifications/international-classification-of-functioning-disability-and-health. Accessed January 30, 2023.
8. Goss B. *Most Common Disabilities for Army, Navy, Airforce, Marines*; 2021. Available at: https://www.militaryveteranlawyer.com/most-common-disabilities-for-army-navy-air-force-marines/. Accessed January 30, 2023.
9. Doherty AJ, Atherton H, Boland P, et al. *Barriers and Facilitators to Primary Health Care for People with Intellectual Disabilities And/or Autism; an Integrative Review*. National Library of Medicine/National Institute of Health; 2020. Available at: Barriers and facilitators to primary health care for people with intellectual disabilities and/or autism: an integrative review - PMC nih.gov. Accessed January 30, 2023.
10. U.S. Department of Labor Bureau of Labor Statistics. *Persons with a Disability: Labor Force Characteristic*; 2021. Available at: https://www.bls.gov/news.release/pdf/disabl.pdf. Accessed January 30, 2023.
11. Centers for Disease Control and Prevention. *Disability and Health. Disability and Health Promotion; Disability Inclusion*; 2020. Available at: https://www.cdc.gov/ncbddd/disabilityandhealth/disability-inclusion.html.
12. World Health Organization. *Assistive Technology*; 2018. Available at: https://www.who.int/news-room/fact-sheets/detail/assistive-technology. Accessed January 30, 2023.
13. American Academy of Pediatric Dentistry. *Use of Protective Stabilization for Pediatric Dental Patients. The Reference Manual of Pediatr Dent*; 2021:325–331. Available at: https://www.aapd.org/media/Policies_Guidelines/BP_Protective.pdf.
14. Wong A, Perlman SP, Waldman HB, Rader R. Guidelines for medical immobilization/protective stabilization for your practice. *Compendium AEGIS Dental Network*. 2022;43:7. Available at: https://www.aegisdentalnetwork.com/adn/cced/2022/07/guidelines-for-medical-immobilization-protective-stabilization-for-your-practice.
15. National Institute of Dental and Craniofacial Research. *Developmental Disabilities and Oral Health*. Retrieved from Wheelchair Transfer: A Healthcare Provider's Guide; 2014. Available at: https://www.nidcr.nih.gov/sites/default/files/2017-09/wheelchair-transfer-provider-guide.pdf. Accessed January 30, 2023.
16. Sara A. *Stedy® Compact Instructions for Use*; 2022. Available at: https://www.arjo.com/globalassets/localisation/au-site/pdf/rental-ifu-pdf/sara-stedy-ifu-001-12325-en-rev.-5.pdf. Accessed January 30, 2023.

60

Intellectually and Developmentally Challenged

Ann Michelle Bruhn

PROFESSIONAL OPPORTUNITIES

Dental hygienists treat patients with a wide variety of intellectual and developmental disabilities. Patients with intellectual and developmental challenges can display mild to severe intellectual disability and/or physical limitations leading to difficulty receiving dental hygiene care. Dental professionals with the knowledge and skills to communicate and provide educational interventions will be the most successful in providing dental hygiene treatment.

COMPETENCIES

1. List and describe the levels of intellectual disabilities (IDs) and relate general characteristics and individual needs and abilities of patients within each category of intellectual disabilities to modifications recommended for self-care education.
2. Plan alterations in dental hygiene care based on common medical conditions and intellectual disabilities associated with Down syndrome and other intellectual or developmental conditions.
3. Discuss general theories and characteristics of autism spectrum disorder (ASD).
4. Select and use effective instructional strategies to manage communication barriers with apatient who has ASD.
5. Value educational interventions for a patient with intellectual disabilities, Down syndrome, and ASD, and discuss the legal and ethical aspects of treating patients with developmental and/or physical challenges.

INTRODUCTION

Developmental disabilities are lifelong severe chronic disabilities that can be cognitive, physical, or both, and present before the age of 21 years. An **intellectual disability (ID)** is a type of developmental disability that must occur before the age of 18 years and be characterized by limitations in adaptive functioning in at least two of the following skill areas: communication, self-care, home living, social or interpersonal skills, use of community resources, self-direction, functional academic skills, work, leisure, health, and safety. Individuals who are intellectually and developmentally disabled usually have an intelligence quotient (IQ) of less than 70; however, the Diagnostic and Statistical Manual of Mental Disorders (DSM-5) implements impairments in conceptual, social, and practical domains versus IQ cutoffs to determine severity level.[1] In general, the average IQ is between 81 and 108, with only a small fraction, 1% to 3%, of the world population diagnosed with ID.[2,3] Individuals with ID experience inequality in receiving healthcare, with access to professional dental care as one of the largest barriers. The American Association on Intellectual and Developmental Disabilities is the overarching organization in support of persons with IDs and a leader in innovation and research for persons living with ID.[4]

LEVELS OF INTELLECTUAL DISABILITIES

IDs are categorized as mild, moderate, severe, or profound, as follows:

- *Mild ID (IQ of approximately 50 to 69).* This group represents the largest population with IDs (approximately 85%). These individuals are designated as educable and able to acquire some academic skills, and they typically live either independently or in supervised settings. Persons with mild ID can learn simple skills in detail, but their attention spans and memories are short. For patients with mild ID, dental hygienists need to explain and demonstrate oral hygiene instructions and teach activities instead of concepts. Patients with mild ID require public recognition, praise, and rewards for their progress.
- *Moderate ID (IQ of approximately 36 to 49).* These persons can learn self-care behaviors, social adjustment, and economic usefulness, but they acquire very few academic skills past the second-grade level. Poor hand and finger coordination may be evident; consequently, dental hygienists need to teach patients only fundamental skills via the show-and-tell method. Additional skills may be taught, depending on progress. Every successful step performed during therapy and oral hygiene instruction should be rewarded with tangible and verbal praise. Oral hygiene instructions are reviewed at each appointment because of the patient's short memory and attention span. Individuals typically live in group settings, where a primary caregiver can supervise the daily regimen to ensure that self-care behaviors are practiced.
- *Severe ID (IQ of approximately 20 to 35).* These individuals can be trained in elementary self-care skills; thus, the individual can acquire some oral care behaviors with supervision. These patients learn by habit training (i.e., repeating procedures and movements continuously), so they can grasp the procedures. It is important to set realistic goals and to include the caregiver when teaching oral hygiene behaviors. These individuals typically reside at home with their families or in group homes. Depending on the environment, successfully performed skills should be rewarded by the dental hygienist or the caregiver (Table 60.1).
- *Profound ID (IQ of less than 20).* People with this level of ID are incapable of total self-care, social skills, or economic work skills and require continual supervision and care from the primary caregiver. Some self-care may be achievable in a highly structured environment when appropriate training is provided by the caregiver. The caregiver is responsible for the patient's general and oral hygiene care. Thus, the dental hygienist provides education about the daily oral care regimen to caregivers to assist them with their own oral self-care, as well as the patient's care. The caretaker's task is challenging and oral care may not be a top priority.

TABLE 60.1	Rewards That Can Be Used to Reinforce Positive Behavior for Patients With Intellectual Disabilities
Types of Rewards	**Examples of Rewards**
Social rewards	Attention, smiles, hugs, praise, and other signs of approval and affection
Activity rewards	Any activity that the person enjoys, such as watching television, playing a game, or going to a party
Material rewards	An item that the person can use, play with, wear, or consume, such as toys, money, food, or clothing

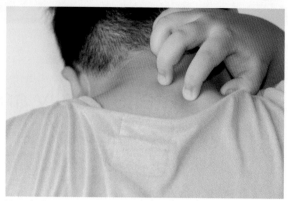

Fig. 60.1 Self-injurious behavior in a person with intellectual and developmental disabilities. (Copyright istock.com.)

ETIOLOGIC FACTORS

IDs can stem from genetic biologic factors (e.g., chromosomal and genetic disturbances), nongenetic biologic and nutritional factors (e.g., prenatal, perinatal, or postnatal causes), and psychosocial factors (e.g., inadequate caregiving environment, lack of stimulation). The cause can also be unknown.

Genetic

Genetic biologic factors include disorders that are evident at conception. In approximately 15% of affected persons, the ID falls into this category, which includes chromosomal disturbances (10%) such as **Down syndrome** and metabolic disorders such as in **phenylketonuria** (5%), which causes an abnormal accumulation of phenylalanine that is toxic to the brain. Other examples of genetic ID include fragile X syndrome and Prader-Willi syndrome. Fragile X is the most common type of ID due to genetic factors and includes changes in a gene called fragile X messenger ribonucleoprotein, which causes a higher presence of social anxiety.[4] Prader-Willi syndrome occurs from deletion of part of chromosome 15 and causes ID along with behavior issues and short stature.[4]

Nongenetic Biologic and Nutritional Factors

The causes of nongenetic biologic IDs are grouped as prenatal, perinatal, and postnatal causes. Approximately 32% of IDs occur during the prenatal period, 11% occur during the perinatal period, and 4% occur during the postnatal period. Prenatal causes include infections such as rubella, toxoplasmosis, syphilis, cytomegalovirus infection, and human immunodeficiency virus (HIV) infection; maternal-fetal blood incompatibilities; drug and alcohol consumption (i.e., fetal alcohol spectrum disorder, which occurs with exposure to alcohol before birth); maternal-fetal irradiation; poor nutrition; and chronic maternal health problems, such as hypertension and diabetes; as well as dental-related signs, such as Hutchinson incisors, mulberry molars, and microdontia. The term *perinatal* refers to the time immediately before, during, and after birth. Premature birth, **hypoxemia** (i.e., low oxygen in the brain due to intracranial hemorrhage), head trauma, infection (e.g., HIV, herpes), and **kernicterus** (i.e., toxic accumulation of bilirubin in the brain) are perinatal causes of IDs. With advances in medicine, the occurrence of an ID as a result of perinatal causes is rare. Postnatal factors include brain infections (e.g., encephalitis, meningitis), cerebral trauma (e.g., head injury, brain tumor, accident), poison, environmental toxins, and dietary protein deficiency.

Psychosocial Factors

Psychosocial causes include an environment that is void of sensory and intellectual stimulation during the growth and development phases. Severe developmental delays were found in the cognitive and social development of a representative sample of Romanian orphans ages 23

to 50 months with limited resources to include caregivers due to poor conditions in the Ceausescu regime at the time. Out of the 24 children studied, 20 had cognitive and social functioning less than half of their age, which were not linked to other factors such as age, amount of time spent at the orphanage, or birthweight. Future research is needed to further understand interventions that may assist those impacted by ID from psychosocial factors.

GENERAL CHARACTERISTICS OF PERSONS WITH INTELLECTUAL DISABILITIES

Although common traits are associated with various ID levels, overgeneralization and stereotypic expectations are avoided; instead, individual needs, abilities, and circumstances are assessed. Persons with an ID typically have the following characteristics:

- **Health-related abilities**—Common traits include less physical stamina and delayed physical development and speech, in addition to physical challenges such as poor motor coordination, vision, and hearing. Individuals may be overweight or underweight as a result of environmental factors such as inadequate parental or institutional care, or genetic and metabolic factors such as phenylketonuria. They may also have poor oral health because of nutritional deficiency, limited self-care capabilities, barriers to care, and limited access to care.

- **Mental and motor abilities**—Individuals demonstrate short memories; an inability to concentrate or to see differences or likenesses between objects; limited speech; and a lack of adaptive, associative, or organizational skills. Success usually occurs from concrete rather than abstract experiences; therefore, these persons are more adept with manual skills than academic skills. Depending on the ID level, patients in this group may be able to render their own oral self-care, and this should be encouraged.

- **Social and emotional abilities**—Persons are followers rather than leaders (i.e., they tend to imitate others) and exhibit behavioral problems to gain attention or release emotion, which may be destructive (e.g., aggressiveness directed toward others, property destruction, self-injury). These individuals have an awareness of not fitting in and can become discouraged easily. Criticism is not taken positively and there is an inability to learn through experience.

- **Self-injurious behavior (SIB)**—SIBs include head banging, self-biting, self-striking, and bruxism (Fig. 60.1). SIB has been viewed as an early developmental stress response that disappears in typically developing children, but it remains in patients with IDs. SIBs can intimidate caregivers to the point that the patient's demands are met. If the patient is allowed this power, they become difficult to manage.

Oral Manifestations

Tooth anomalies and delayed eruption patterns are usually present as a result of developmental abnormalities (Box 60.1). Tooth surface abrasion from bruxism, which is linked to anxiety and emotional distress, has also been observed. Consequences of bruxism can include dental attrition, functional problems such as temporomandibular joint disorders, and eventually sensitivity and pain. Wear is usually seen in the incisors and canines and increases with age. By the time these individuals are 30 to 49 years old, wear becomes so significant that restorative measures may be needed. Bruxism may be the result of a lack of personal contact, or it may be a type of self-stimulation. Before treatment can be given for these problems, assessment must be completed to determine the origin and chronicity of the behavior. Periodontal disease and untreated dental caries are more common and are attributed to risk factors such as a lack of professional care and knowledge to treat patients with ID, a lack of funds to support or to access care, host susceptibility, poor oral hygiene, and caregivers, oral health knowledge.[5] Research shows a prevalence of 32% of individuals with ID experiencing dental caries, and 80% periodontitis.[2] These persons usually depend on others to facilitate their access to oral healthcare and many barriers exist for caregivers to include access to care of special facilities equipped for individuals with ID,

BOX 60.1 Some Oral Manifestations Observed in Patients With Intellectual Disabilities

- Self-biting
- Bruxism
- Thick, flaccid lips
- Microdontia
- Malocclusion
- Delayed tooth eruption
- Dental attrition and sensitivity
- Temporomandibular joint disorder
- Periodontal disease
- Heavy oral biofilm accumulation

dental professionals' knowledge and ability to treat individuals with ID, and cost of such care.[2]

MANAGEMENT OF PATIENTS WITH INTELLECTUAL DISABILITIES

A significant gap remains today regarding caregivers' knowledge of when and how to manage the oral health of patients with ID due to the heterogeneous nature of the population and various life stages.[5] Since caregivers are essential to oral healthcare for patients with ID, dental hygienists can play a significant role in educating caregivers to provide adequate oral home care for technique along with the need for promoting independence.[2] Research assessing caregivers experiences indicated many felt limited or not able to provide oral hygiene care at home for individuals with ID. Regular reminders and/or use of reminder charts by caregivers for oral homecare may be beneficial for those with ID. Research has shown educational support and strategies as successful interventions for caregivers of those with ID.[5] In addition, regular professional dental hygiene treatment is vital to optimal oral health—management techniques throughout the dental hygiene process of care increase the likelihood of a successful visit.[6] Dental professionals should have increased knowledge through courses and trainings on the use of sensory-adapted environments, which have been shown to increase treatment acceptance for patients with ID. During assessment, the dental hygienist collects data about the patient's skills of daily living (e.g., toilet training, oral hygiene regimen, eating habits, dressing). To prevent SIBs (self-injurious behaviors), the dental hygienist initiates fact finding with the caregiver to identify SIB triggers and antecedents. Nonverbal and verbal cues of emotional distress must be observed and acknowledged immediately to avoid SIBs. The most commonly used behavioral treatment is **differential reinforcement** of another behavior. The goal of this treatment is to reinforce any behavior other than the SIB. For example, if the patient strikes themselves in the mouth, then the hygienist gives the patient something to assemble or hold with their hands or lets the patient hold a cotton roll or mirror until it is needed. Strategies for managing SIB are listed in Table 60.2.

Factors to consider include diet and ability to chew, self-care potential, interests, level of cooperation, and barriers to care, as well as the parents' and caregivers' interests, values, and level of

TABLE 60.2 Strategies for Managing Self-Injurious Behaviors

Strategy	Definition	Examples
Differential reinforcement	Reinforcement of any behavior other than the self-injurious behavior (SIB)	Draw interest away from the SIB: "Can you sing a song for me about your teeth?"
Positive reinforcement	Reinforcement to get a person to repeat a desired behavior	Offer verbal praise: "You really did well"; "Good job"; "You brush your teeth so well, I want to see you doing this again."
Ignoring unwanted behavior	Refusing to take notice of the SIB	Consciously ignore the negative behavior.
Positive reinforcement of wanted behavior	Reinforcement when the wanted behavior is directly addressed	Offer verbal praise: "You really cleaned those back teeth well, so I will give you a prize."
Psychoactive medication	Medication that alters one's psychologic state	Examples include neuroleptics, antidepressants, and psychostimulants.
Restraint	Physical confinement of a person	Papoose board or Velcro straps are used.
Counseling	Professional guidance of a person using psychologic methods	Offer support, positive reinforcement, and trust.
Application of consequences after behavior	Punishment after the unwanted behavior for reinforcement	Apply a time-out period or do not offer a reward after treatment.
Overcorrection	Correction requiring duties above and beyond addressing the specific unwanted behavior	Joe colored on the wall, so he should clean more of the wall than where he colored.

cooperation. Fig. 60.2 provides a sample dental hygiene care plan. Oral irrigators, interdental cleaning aids, and disclosing tablets can be used by patients with mild ID. Patients with moderate ID require repetitive training, but they can usually manipulate a power toothbrush. For patients with severe ID, emphasis is on as much self-care as possible, with the caregiver following up to achieve daily oral biofilm control. Normally, these patients are limited to a push-pull stroke, and they often isolate brushing to one side. Patients with profound ID depend on caregivers for oral cleansing. Emphasis is on the acceptance of oral hygiene procedures, which is accomplished through nonverbal communication and desensitization techniques. When working with patients with severe and profound ID, the use of a toothbrush designed for a suction attachment can prevent aspiration (see Chapter 59, Fig. 59.2). It is important to note that research shows those with severe and profound ID may require professional care under general anesthesia; however, this option can come at a high cost to caregivers.[2,5]

Communication may be a challenge if the patient also has visual or hearing limitations (Chapter 59). Visual cues work best for persons with hearing impairments, and tactile and auditory cues are

Dental Hygiene Diagnosis Based on Legal Scope of Practice	Dental Hygiene Diagnosis Based on Human Needs Model	Due to or Related to	As Evidenced by	Dental Hygiene Care Plan Goals	Evaluative Statements
Dental caries (to be confirmed by dental diagnosis or to be restored) High caries risk	Biologically Sound and Functional Dentition	Inadequate oral care by caregiver Inadequate self-care Lack of resources	Signs of caries, defective restorations, and missing teeth	Reduce caries index score and sugar in diet Seek dental treatment for caries and defective restorations Use 5000 ppm fluoride dentifrice and 0.12% chlorohexidine mouth rinse to eliminate *Streptococcus mutans* infections	Reduced caries index score at 3-month continued-care interval Completed restorative treatment by 3-month continued-care interval
Plaque-induced gingivitis	Skin and Mucous Membrane Integrity of the Head and Neck	Inadequate oral care by caregiver Inadequate self-care Lack of resources	Presence of numerous gingival bleeding points Attachment loss of 4–7 mm	Decrease gingival bleeding by 50% Stop progression of attachment loss Find additional resources to enable patient to receive needed care (e.g., Medicaid program)	Decreased gingival bleeding on probing by 50% Attachment loss remains stable Patient enrolled in Medicaid program
Possible emergency caries lesions; possible need for endodontics (pending dental diagnosis)	Freedom from Head and Neck Pain	Inadequate care by caregiver Inadequate self-care	Signs of caries Verbal indicators of pain	Seek dental treatment for pain relief and caries	All carious lesions restored No evidence of oral pain
Poor self-care and oral hygiene skills	Responsibility for Oral Health	Impaired mental ability Impaired motor coordination Low value placed on oral health	Presence of plaque, bleeding, and caries Reports no previous dental care and fails to report to appointments	Demonstrate self-care by the patient with followup by caregiver Seek dental care Verbalizes a commitment to having a healthy mouth	Performs oral hygiene with minimal supervision Reports for scheduled dental visits Verbalizes that she likes the way her teeth feel and look
Low oral health literacy	Conceptualization and Problem Solving	Knowledge deficiency in oral disease risk factors	Inability to verbalize that oral biofilm contributes to bleeding gums and tooth decay	Patient and caregiver verbalize the relationship between biofilm, bleeding gums, and caries	Patient and caregiver verbalize the role of plaque in oral disease Patient and caregiver use disclosing agent to evaluate oral hygiene

Dental Hygiene Interventions

- Assess Jill's mental level, functional level, and oral health knowledge and skill level.
- Provide education on dental disease.
- Provide education to Jill and the caregiver on toothbrushing (power toothbrush due to limited psychomotor skills) and flossing (by caregiver); power interdental cleaner.
- Communicate importance of at-home fluoride therapy for dental caries control.
- Provide periodontal debridement and prescribe a high concentration fluoride dentifrice and 0.12% chlorhexidine gluconate antimicrobial rinse to control *Streptococcus mutans* infection (prescription written by dentist or dental hygienist as defined by law).
- Teach Jill and caregiver to evaluate their oral hygiene for progress (i.e., less bleeding points, use of disclosing agent).
- Apply pit and fissure sealants.
- Apply fluoride varnish 4x per year.
- Provide nutritional assessment and counseling, including use of xylitol gum and mints to control caries.
- Introduce procedures slowly based on Jill's mental age.
- Provide rewards for oral health and healthy behavior.
- Use techniques for establishing a trusting relationship.
- At 3-month continued-care interval, reevaluate the homecare.
- Restore caries within the scope of practice and refer to dentist for restorative procedures, possible endodontics.

Fig. 60.2 Sample dental hygiene care plan; client with intellectual and developmental disabilities.

BOX 60.2 Strategies for Establishing a Trusting Relationship

- Familiarize the patient with their surroundings and have the caregiver rehearse the patient for the appointment.
- Schedule a time for the healthcare team to meet the patient; alleviate anxieties by getting to know the patient and by allowing the patient to get to know the team.
- Keep the first appointment short, nonthreatening, and fun.
- Give explanations slowly, with one instruction at a time.
- Use a tell-show-do technique when teaching; teach one technique at each appointment to avoid overwhelming the patient.
- Validate the patient's understanding (e.g., ask the patient to perform the self-care behavior [brushing, interdental cleaning, and mouth rinsing, among others]).
- Reward the patient often for positive behavior (e.g., use verbal positive reinforcement such as "Good job"; offer tangible reinforcement such as a toy, a special outing arranged by the caregiver, or public recognition such as a certificate that can be displayed in the patient's home or work setting).
- Provide handouts and pictures that have been designed at the appropriate level of reading comprehension for home use.

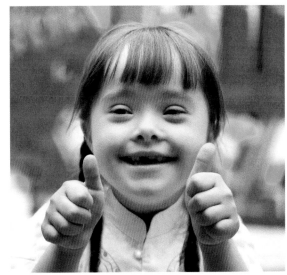

Fig. 60.3 Facial characteristics of a child with Down syndrome. (Copyright istock.com.)

used for patients who are visually impaired. A hypersensitive gag reflex may be managed by placing the patient in a semisupine position and eliminating the use of toothpaste to reduce gagging and to provide better visualization for the caregiver. Dental professionals and caregivers may need to use a mouth prop to allow for access during oral care. If problems arise (e.g., crying, frustration), the dental hygienist or home caregiver repeats an earlier achievement level to meet the need for freedom from fear and stress. Effective communication leads to a trusting relationship which, in turn, allows the oral healthcare experience to be successful for both the patient and the clinician. Approaches to forming this trusting relationship are listed in Box 60.2.

DOWN SYNDROME[6,7]

Down syndrome, which is the most common and frequently observed chromosomal abnormality in the human race, occurs among individuals of all socioeconomic levels, geographic regions, ethnic groups, and cultures. Down syndrome occurs in 1 out of approximately every 772 live births; therefore 5100 babies are diagnosed with Down syndrome each year in the United States.[7] Worldwide, cases have increased to 1,579,784 in 2019 from 1,257,110 in 1990 according to the Global Burden of Disease database in 2019.[8] These individuals are at increased risk for congenital heart defects, respiratory and hearing problems, Alzheimer disease, childhood leukemia, and thyroid conditions. Because many of these conditions are treatable, the life expectancy of an individual with Down syndrome is approximately 60 years of age.

Etiologic Factors

Down syndrome results from a genetic etiology as stated above. An abnormality in the number of chromosomes (i.e., three rather than two copies of the chromosome 21) is responsible for the specific physical characteristics and mental deficiencies observed in persons with Down syndrome. The following three manifestations of chromosomal abnormality can also occur:

1. Trisomy 21 is the failure of a pair of number 21 chromosomes to segregate (nondisjunction) during the formation of either an egg or a sperm before conception. It has no known cause and occurs in approximately 95% of people with Down syndrome. Incidence is correlated with increased maternal age; however, more recently, because of the high fertility rates in younger women, 51% of people with Down syndrome are born to mothers under the age of 35 years.
2. Translocation occurs when a piece of chromosome in pair 21 breaks off and attaches to another chromosome, usually chromosome 14. Translocation occurs in approximately 3% of children with Down syndrome.
3. Mosaicism occurs in only 2% of children with Down syndrome; it is a result of an error in one of the first cell divisions that occurs shortly after conception.

GENERAL CHARACTERISTICS OF PERSONS WITH DOWN SYNDROME

Approximately 50 specific physical characteristics have been reported in persons with Down syndrome; however, not every person with Down syndrome exhibits all characteristics. When these characteristics are present, they may occur in various degrees. The most common characteristics follow:

- The person's head usually appears small; it is shortened in its anterior-to-posterior diameter (i.e., from the forehead to the crown).
- The eyes have an upward slant and prominent epicanthal folds, the folds of skin that extend from the root of the nose to the median end of the eyebrow. The iris of the eye is speckled with marks called Brushfield spots.
- The nose is recessed and reduced in size, the nostrils are upturned, and the nasal bridge is depressed. Deviations in the nasal septum also are common. Because of the flat nasal bridge and the underdevelopment of the midfacial region, the face appears flat. This flat facial profile is the most frequently observed characteristic of Down syndrome.

Fig. 60.3 depicts the facial features of a child with Down syndrome. The ears may appear small and abnormal in structure and contour, which results in a round or square appearance, and the hands may appear short and broad, with nails that are hyperconvex. Persons with Down syndrome tend to be short and overweight. Despite IQ limitations in the range of 20 to 85, most children with Down syndrome develop into happy and, in some cases, self-reliant individuals.

Medical Considerations

The life expectancies of persons with Down syndrome can be lengthened by high-quality healthcare, healthy lifestyle behaviors, stimulating home environments, and positive support structures from family, friends, employers, and the community. Individuals with this condition may have various medical conditions that affect the process of care (Table 60.3). Knowledge of potential health problems, care modifications, and available community resources, as well as the use of a collaborative approach, are required to meet the patient's oral health and wellness needs. Specific support organizations may not be in the patient's immediate geographic location, but they can supply

TABLE 60.3	Medical and Dental Hygiene Considerations for Patients With Down Syndrome*		
Concern	**Clinical Expression**	**When Seen**	**Dental Hygiene Care Implications and Management Issues**
Hypotonia	Reduced muscle tone Increased range-of-joint movement Motor function problems	Throughout life Improvement with maturity	Addressing the patient's comfort while they are in the dental chair is important. Limited neck movement and pain may be observed. Motor function problems can make oral care difficult. Patient may exhibit spastic movements. Considerations should be made with patient positioning. Alterations in oral hygiene aids may be necessary.
Delayed growth	Typically at or near the third percentile of the general population	Throughout life	Evaluate mental age. Offer nutritional assessment and counseling. During assessment, delays in tooth development and facial growth may be observed.
Intellectual and developmental delays	Some global delay, degree varies Specific processing problems Specific expressive language delay	First year; monitor throughout life	Assess patient's mental age to appropriately plan oral care instruction. Use the caregiver to communicate with the patient as needed.
Hearing deficits	Otitis media Small ear canals Conductive impairment	Assess by 6 months Review annually	May need to speak clearly and use visual aids. Obtain a thorough health history to identify hearing problems. Involve the caregiver to determine what mode of communication will work best.
Eye disease	Refractive errors Strabismus Cataracts Tear duct abnormalities Amblyopia Nystagmus	Eye examination during early months of life Regular followup	Tactile communication is important. Assist the patient to prevent injury. Obtain a thorough health history to identify ocular problems. Involve the caregiver to determine the severity of a problem. When giving oral care instruction, be in clear view. Adjust the instruction to the patient's need (e.g., do not expect patient to see small anatomy on a radiograph). Avoid glare of the dental light in the patient's eyes.
Cervical spine problems	Atlantoaxial instability Skeletal cervical anomalies Possible spinal cord compression	Radiographic examination by 3 years of age	May require shorter appointments for comfort. Help the patient with walking to the treatment area as needed. Place the patient in a comfortable position for treatment.
Thyroid disease	Hypothyroidism (rarely hyperthyroidism) Decreased growth and activity	Some congenital; most during second decade of life or later Check by 1 year of age; repeat throughout life	Be cognizant of room temperature for patient comfort; the patient may be cold and require a blanket. Assess pharmacologic history. Create a low-stress environment. Stress good oral hygiene to prevent infection. Gingiva may appear spongy and the tongue may be swollen.
Obesity	Excessive weight gain	Especially when 2 to 4 years old, 12 to 13 years old, and during adult life	May require a large blood pressure cuff. Offer nutritional counseling. If the patient is in a group home, consider doing in-house services. May have an exaggerated inflammatory response.
Seizure disorder	Primarily generalized tonic-clonic (grand mal) seizures In addition, myoclonic seizures and hypsarrhythmia	Any time	Assess pharmacologic history. Minimize stress. Avoid flashing dental light into the patient's eyes. Avoid stress-inducing situations. Dental sealants and fluoride are beneficial. If gingival enlargement is present, more frequent continued care may be needed.

TABLE 60.3 Medical and Dental Hygiene Considerations for Patients With Down Syndrome*—cont'd

Concern	Clinical Expression	When Seen	Dental Hygiene Care Implications and Management Issues
Emotional problems	Inappropriate behavior Depression	Middle to late childhood and adulthood	Praise the patient to build self-esteem and cooperation. Treat the patient with respect. Assess the patient's frame of mind via the caregiver or healthcare decision maker before appointment, and validate during the appointment. Assess pharmacologic history.
Premature senescence	Behavioral changes and functional losses	Fifth decade of life and beyond	Evaluate mental age. Treat the patient with respect and concern. Assess the patient's frame of mind with the caregiver before the appointment. Assess pharmacologic history.

*This information also applies to patients with variable occurrences of congenital gastrointestinal anomalies such as Hirschsprung disease (an extreme dilation of the colon), imperforate anus, duodenal obstruction, and tracheoesophageal fistula, as well as other conditions such as celiac disease, leukemia, Alzheimer disease, attention-deficit/hyperactivity disorder, autism spectrum disorders, hepatitis B carrier state, keratoconus (conical protrusion of the center of the cornea), dry skin, hip dysplasia, diabetes, and mitral valve prolapse.

information and referrals. An Internet search, using such terms as Social Services, Disabilities, or Intellectual and Developmental Disabilities, can be used to identify local assistance.

Congenital Heart Disease[9]

Congenital heart disease is the most common and serious medical condition among persons with Down syndrome. Most cardiovascular malformations associated with Down syndrome are acutely or chronically life-threatening. Cardiac problems are present in 40% to 60% of children with Down syndrome, and heart defects are the major cause of high mortality during the first 2 years of the infant's life.

Atrioventricular septal defects, ventricular septal defects, atrial septal defects, patent ductus arteriosus, and tetralogy of Fallot are common in the population of patients with Down syndrome with congenital heart disease. The most common congenital heart defects detected by echocardiogram are the atrioventricular septal defects. Endocardial cushions are ridges in the developing fetal heart. Pulmonary artery hypertension is another condition in patients with Down syndrome and is characterized by the constriction of the blood vessels of the lungs. This condition causes back pressure and right ventricle overload. Pulmonary artery hypertension is often a consequence of the increased flow to the lungs caused by the heart defects.

Medical intervention depends on the severity of symptoms. When providing care, it is imperative to obtain a detailed health and pharmacologic history to determine any cardiac abnormalities that may be present. The dental hygienist needs to provide a prescription for prophylactic antibiotic premedication and oral health instruction for the patient and caregiver as appropriate when indicated prior to dental hygiene care. See Chapters 11 and 48 for a complete discussion of prophylactic antibiotic premedication for cardiac conditions associated with the highest risk of adverse outcomes from valvular cardiovascular disease and a history of endocarditis.

Orthopedic Concerns

Orthopedic problems in these patients are usually a result of hypotonia (low muscle tone) and low bone mass.[10]

Atlantoaxial instability, which is found in 10% to 20% of younger individuals with Down syndrome, is characterized by an abnormal increase in mobility within the joint between the first two cervical (neck) vertebrae, thereby placing the person at risk for spinal cord compression and injury. Most persons with Down syndrome have no symptoms of atlantoaxial instability, but if signs or symptoms are present (e.g., easily fatigued, difficulty walking, neck pain, abnormal gait, extremity weakness, spasticity, limited neck movement, torticollis [head tilt], lack of coordination or clumsiness, sensory deficits, hyperreflexia), they are related to spinal cord compression.

Scoliosis (curvature of the spine), which is frequently detected among individuals with Down syndrome, is usually mild. Persons with Down syndrome usually have excessive external hip rotation and abduction. As a result, a wide-angled gait and widespread legs when sitting are evident. Persons with mild scoliosis may not be aware that they have a spinal problem, but it is still important to ensure patient comfort during care.

Other Disorders[10]

Endocrine disorders involving the thyroid, adrenal, or pituitary glands are common among persons with Down syndrome. As many as 24% of older individuals with Down syndrome have thyroid disorders, with hypothyroidism being the most common and a higher incidence of congenital hypothyroidism. Classic symptoms of hypothyroidism include delayed growth, short stature, obesity, lethargy, and dry skin. Evidence suggests that individuals with one endocrine autoimmune disorder (e.g., thyroiditis) are at increased risk for developing a second disorder (e.g., type 1 diabetes mellitus). Type I diabetes tends to be diagnosed earlier from birth when compared to persons without Down syndrome.[7] (See Chapter 53 for information regarding autoimmune disorders.)

Ear, nose, and throat problems are common in persons with Down syndrome as a result of associated anatomic predispositions. Hearing loss that is usually mild to moderate is often caused by persistent fluid in the middle ear and chronic ear infections. Other disorders include chronic rhinitis and sinusitis.

Eye disease affects persons with Down syndrome. Cataracts, tear duct abnormalities, strabismus, amblyopia, and nystagmus are known to occur and should be treated by an ophthalmologist.

Seizure activity in infants and young children with Down syndrome occurs at the same rate as it does in the general population; however, at

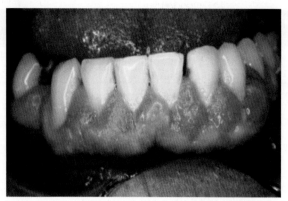

Fig. 60.4 Mild drug-influenced gingivitis associated with Dilantin (phenytoin) therapy for seizure control in a person with Down syndrome. (Neville B, Damm D, Allen C, Chi A. *Oral and Maxillofacial Pathology.* 4th ed. Saunders; 2016.)

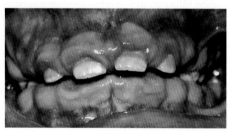

Fig. 60.5 Severe drug-influenced gingivitis associated with Dilantin (phenytoin) therapy for seizure control in a person with Down syndrome. (Courtesy Dr. F.T. McIver, Department of Pediatric Dentistry, University of North Carolina School of Dentistry, Chapel Hill, NC.)

> **BOX 60.3 Some Oral Manifestations Observed in Persons With Down Syndrome**
>
> - Underdeveloped maxilla
> - Narrow palate with broadened alveolar ridges
> - Congenitally missing teeth
> - Malocclusion
> - Enamel hypoplasia
> - High rate of tooth loss caused by periodontal disease
> - Shortened roots
> - Enlarged tonsils and adenoids
> - Mouth open with protruding tongue
> - Fissured tongue
> - Enlarged circumvallate papillae on tongue
> - Microdontia
> - Tetracycline tooth staining
> - Periodontal diseases
> - Heavy oral biofilm accumulation

the age of 20 to 30 years, generalized tonic-clonic seizures (i.e., grand mal seizures) are seen more frequently in persons with Down syndrome. Seizures may take the form of staring spells, momentary lapses of attention, jerking of the arms and legs, or loss of consciousness. Gingival enlargement caused by medications that are taken to control seizure activity is of particular significance (Figs. 60.4 and 60.5). Effective oral biofilm control reduces the extent of drug-influenced gingival enlargement, so daily self-care must be effective before some seizure-control medications are used.

Adults with Down syndrome often demonstrate neuropathologic changes similar to those of individuals diagnosed with Alzheimer disease. The anatomic changes of those with Alzheimer disease appear to be almost universal among adults with Down syndrome who are older than 40 years of age, most of whom do not show behavioral signs of Alzheimer disease. The relationship between Alzheimer disease and Down syndrome is under investigation.

Oral Manifestations (Box 60.3)
Tongue

A person with Down syndrome often has an open mouth and a protruding tongue. The tongue seems enlarged as a result of an underdeveloped maxilla, mandibular prognathism, a narrow palate with broadened alveolar ridges, and enlarged tonsils and adenoids, all of which create a small oral cavity space. Tongue fissures and enlarged circumvallate papillae are observed in 37% to 60% of persons with Down syndrome. Therefore, good daily oral hygiene—including tongue brushing and the use of an American Dental Association–accepted antimicrobial dentifrice and mouth rinse to reduce oral biofilm, gingivitis, and halitosis—is requisite. The cooperation level of the patient

must be considered when recommending daily oral care regimens and products.

Sleep Apnea

Approximately 45% of persons with Down syndrome also have obstructive sleep apnea as a result of their flattened midfaces, their narrowed nasopharyngeal areas, the low tone of the muscles of their upper airways, and their enlarged tongues, tonsils, and adenoids. There are many problems associated with obstructive sleep apnea in these patients. In children with obstructive sleep apnea and heart disease, the low blood oxygenation level causes an increase in the blood pressure of the lungs as the body tries to get more oxygen. This pulmonary hypertension can cause the right side of the heart to become enlarged, thereby causing cardiac complications. Children with Down syndrome may also have larger than usual soft palates that usually do not create obstructions but tend to cause snoring. When a child sleeps, their brain goes to sleep in different stages. The child appears to sleep well, but the brain never actually gets the rest it needs to function at peak performance. A sleep study is required to diagnose obstructive sleep apnea, and treatment ranges from occlusal repositioning appliances to continuous positive airway pressure with or without surgical correction. Adenotonsillectomy in children with Down syndrome and obstructive sleep apnea has been helpful in some cases.

Tooth Morphologic Manifestations

The teeth of these patients may be small (microdontia), with maxillary teeth generally more affected in size than mandibular teeth. All teeth except for the maxillary first molars and the mandibular incisors are reduced in size; although the roots are shortened, root formation is complete.[11] The most frequently affected permanent teeth in the maxillary arch are the second molars (52%), the lateral incisors (42%), the canines (41%), the first molars (40%), and the central incisors (35%). In the mandibular arch, the first and second premolars are most commonly affected (63% and 48%, respectively). Tetracycline staining and hypoplastic enamel may be evident as a result of the significant number of early childhood infections requiring antibiotic therapy experienced by persons with Down syndrome.

Missing Teeth and Malocclusion

Congenitally missing teeth and delayed eruption occur in persons with Down syndrome at a significantly higher rate than in the general population. The increased incidence of congenitally missing perma-nent teeth (25% to 50%) is probably related to ectodermal dysplasia, local inflammation that damages the tooth germ, or other medical infections. The most frequently missing permanent teeth in persons with Down syndrome are mandibular second premolars (3.4%) and lateral incisors (2.2%). Within each quadrant, it is more common to find the most posterior tooth missing than the most anterior tooth. Malocclusion also is seen frequently, with mandibular overjet and pos-terior crossbite occurring in virtually all persons with Down syndrome. The correction of malocclusion is usually not indicated. If crossbites are corrected, an earlier tissue breakdown may occur as a result of the underdeveloped maxilla and its relation to the basal bone. The lingual movement of the mandibular teeth is difficult because of the tendency of persons with Down syndrome to have large, protruding tongues.

As a result of an increase in the number of persons with Down syndrome working and living in the community, dental professionals have observed an increase in patients with Down syndrome seeking extensive dental care. With most individuals who are working and functioning, there is an increase in self-esteem and self-image. Health-care professionals assess the patient to determine their tolerance for extensive treatment. Patients with Down syndrome are given the same treatment options as patients without Down syndrome, and care plans are adapted to conditions related to the syndrome. Overall the goal is to provide comprehensive care. A recent study on the perception of children with Down syndrome's oral health–related quality of life by caregivers revealed difficulty speaking, tooth decay, and toothache as affecting oral health–related quality of life related to performing daily activities, emotional well-being, and social relationships.[12]

Periodontal Disease

Individuals with Down syndrome have a high incidence of periodon-tal disease; this is a function of the associated immunodeficiency and impaired host defense rather than poor oral hygiene alone. Periodontal disease may begin as early as the age of 6 years in these individuals, and by adulthood nearly all people with Down syndrome are affected. Fig. 60.6A and C depict a patient with Down syndrome with gingival inflammation and enamel hypoplasia. Fig. 60.6B shows the more severe periodontal problems that can occur in patients with Down syndrome.

Periodontal disease is more common among individuals living in institutions when compared with individuals living in the community. This finding may be the result of the lack of education given to the healthcare providers in these institutions, diet, and inadequate daily oral health behavior. In individuals with Down syndrome living in the community, the level of oral hygiene practiced and the extra care given by their caregivers may be sufficient to slow disease progression.

Management of Patients With Down Syndrome

The maintenance of optimal oral hygiene is very difficult for persons with Down syndrome. Tooth loss attributed to the high prevalence of periodontal disease in this population occurs in about 50% of individu-als with Down syndrome. Therefore, dental hygienists educate caregiv-ers and stress the importance of close supervision during oral hygiene procedures and dietary habits that promote health and wellness. If oral healthcare professionals can incorporate effective oral self-care as part of the patient's daily routine, gingival and periodontal conditions may be prevented or controlled.

Generally, persons with Down syndrome are content and affection-ate, but they can become aggressive if they are confused or disoriented. Although their speech patterns are somewhat hindered, most adults with this condition speak intelligently, with a husky quality of voice. It is important to assess the patient's intellectual level by observing behavioral patterns, evaluating responses during conversation, and questioning the caregiver. The patient may not comprehend the need for care or that it is beneficial. Everything related to care should be introduced slowly, explained, and shown, if possible. Some patients with Down syndrome with higher IQs (i.e., those with mild and slightly moderate IDs) can participate, and they appreciate the attention given to them during care.

If patients are unmanageable, it is usually because of fear, a previ-ous traumatic dental experience, or cognitive limitations that do not allow them to comprehend the procedure. Preoperative medications and general anesthesia can be prescribed and administered by the den-tist if necessary. When care requires a general anesthetic agent, a thor-ough health history review is imperative, and all possible needs should be met while the person is anesthetized. A sample dental hygiene care plan for the patient with Down syndrome is presented in Fig. 60.7.

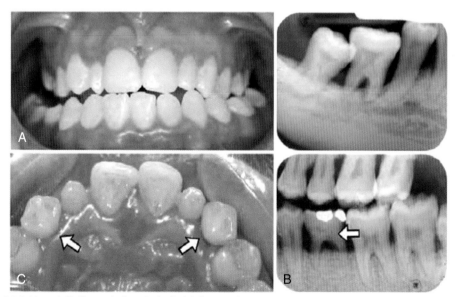

Fig. 60.6 (A and C) Plaque-induced gingival inflammation and enamel hypoplasia *(arrows)* in an individual with Down syndrome. (B) Severe periodontal disease *(arrow)* in a person with Down syndrome. (From Cheng RHW, Yiu CKY, Leung WK. Oral health in individuals with Down syndrome. In Dey S, ed. *Prenatal Diagnosis and Screening for Down Syndrome,* Rijeka, Croatia, 2011, InTech.)

Dental Hygiene Diagnosis Based on Legal Scope of Practice	Dental Hygiene Diagnosis Using Human Needs Model	Due to or Related to	As Evidenced by	Dental Hygiene Care Plan Goal	Evaluative Statements
Dental caries (to be confirmed by dental diagnosis or to be restored) High caries risk	Biologically Sound and Functional Dentition	Inadequate home care and diet	Signs of caries at gingival margin	Reduce caries index score and sugar in diet Seek dental treatment for caries and defective restorations Use 5000 ppm fluoride dentifrice and 0.12% chlorhexidine mouth rinse to reduce *Streptococcus mutans*	No evidence of caries activity in 6-month period
Plaque-induced gingivitis	Skin and Mucous Membrane Integrity of the Head and Neck	Inadequate daily home care	Numerous gingival bleeding points	Performance of successful oral hygiene by the caregiver and patient (power toothbrush 2x per day; antimicrobial dentifrice or mouth rinse; tongue cleaning)	Demonstrates successful oral hygiene at 3-month continued-care interval Decrease gingival bleeding points by 50%
Dental fear and anxiety	Freedom from Fear and Stress	Fear of dental chair	Patient will not sit in the chair while it is moving	Adjust normal chair position; patient able to relax and sit in chair without disruptive behavior	Demonstrates comfort with the dental setting
Poor oral hygiene skills and self-care	Responsibility for Oral Health	Lack of caregiver supervision Too much autonomy for self-care by the client Skill deficiency	Biofilm accumulation Signs of caries Coated tongue	Reduce deposit accumulation by next continued-care interval Decrease plaque index score by 1 point by next appointment Patient cleans his own teeth, then caregiver follows up Both caregiver and patient demonstrate effective oral hygiene techniques	Demonstrates improved oral self-care
Low oral health literacy	Conceptualization and Problem Solving	Oral disease knowledge deficiency of caregiver	Inability to explain disease process and risk	Caregiver can: • Explain disease process and risk factors • See a difference in James' gingival tissues • Verbalize the value of oral disease	Patient and caregiver report that they evaluate oral hygiene and oral health at least 1x per month in the home environment

Dental Hygiene Interventions
- Address concerns with the medication:
  - Zyprexa: Monitor vital signs
  - Assess salivary flow
  - Begin with patient in semisupine position; have him sit upright for 2 minutes before standing
- Conduct nutritional counseling for caries control (include use of xylitol gum and mints).
- Discuss value of daily fluoride for caries control.
- Assess need and apply dental sealants if indicated.
- Instructions for caregiver:
  - Disease risk factors; protective factors
  - Use of oral hygiene devices
  - Techniques for success: how to look for improvements in the deposits and tissue
  - Importance of frequent continued-care intervals
- Place dental chair in semisupine position, then have James get into the chair. Introduce procedures slowly based on James's mental age.
- Give patient and caregiver positive reinforcement. Use techniques for forming trusting relationships.
- Complete periodontal debridement and apply fluoride varnish. Place pit and fissure sealants.
- At 3-month continued-care interval, reevaluate the home care.
- Modify plan if needed. Keep open communication between caregiver and healthcare providers. Complete or refer to dentist for restorative procedures.

Fig. 60.7 Sample dental hygiene care plan for a patient with Down syndrome.

AUTISM SPECTRUM DISORDERS[13–19]

Autism spectrum disorders (ASDs) cover a wide spectrum of neurodevelopmental disorders that affect how a person interacts, communicates, relates, plays, imagines, and learns. Stereotypic body movements such as rocking, spinning, sniffing, hand clapping, and swaying, as well as a range of behaviors including hyperactivity, a short attention span, impulsivity, and aggressiveness, are evident. Research suggests that 16% to 18% of those with Down syndrome also have ASD.

The Center for Disease Control's (CDC's) Autism and Developmental Disabilities Monitoring Network (ADDM) has found that the prevalence of ASDs is 1 in every 44 eight-year-old children in the United States. Males have an approximately four times higher incidence of ASDs than females. About one-third of children with ASD are found to also have ID. Currently the CDC is conducting and funding research called the Study to Explore Early Development (SEED), which is one

of the largest multiyear studies assessing risk factors and behaviors on ASD. Given the prevalence of ASDs, dental hygienists are likely to care for individuals with these disorders. The cause of ASD may be multifactorial. Several theories exist, including those related to psychogenic, genetic, biochemical, and neurophysiologic deficits; however, no single theory has been completely accepted. ASDs include the following:

- *Autistic disorder (classic autism):* Autistic disorder is the most severe form of ASD; the person has difficulty talking and relating to others and the environment, and they display compulsive and ritualistic behaviors.
- *Asperger syndrome:* Asperger syndrome is a mild form of autism characterized by impairment in social interactions without significant problems in language, cognitive ability, or age-appropriate developmental skills. Affected individuals are socially awkward; they do not understand the use of gestures, they lack empathy, they avoid eye contact, and they seem unengaged.

- *Rett syndrome:* Rett syndrome is rare form of autism and is found almost exclusively in females, appearing between 6 and 18 months after a period of normal development. It is characterized by poor head growth, a regression of mental and social development, a lack of response to parents, the avoidance of social contact, and excessive hand (e.g., wringing, clapping, washing) and foot activity.
- *Childhood disintegrative disorder:* This form of autism develops in children who initially seem normal. After at least 2 years of normal development, an affected child exhibits a dramatic loss of vocabulary, language, motor, and social skills. They experiencs the failure to make friends, loss of bowel and bladder control, and seizures.
- *Pervasive developmental disorder not otherwise specified (PDD-NOS):* In this atypical form of autism, some but not all of the classic signs are observed; therefore, it does not meet the criteria for a specific diagnosis. This condition is characterized by varying degrees of impairment in communication skills and social interactions, sensitivities to sights and sounds, and restricted, repetitive, and stereotypic behavior patterns.

Treatment

The care of patients with ASD is consistent with the theory held by the healthcare provider with the goal to reduce symptoms and increase daily quality of life and functioning. Early treatment for ASD is critical to provide therapies and intervention to assist in reduction of difficulties related to ASD symptoms. Types of treatment include psychotherapy, dietary intervention, educational intervention, speech and language therapy, occupational therapy, social-relational approaches, complementary and alternative treatments, special education, medications, and behavioral therapy. The most common form of behavioral therapy is called **Applied Behavior Analysis** (ABA), which promotes desired behaviors and discourages undesired behaviors with a goal of increased skill sets. Medications can help associated symptoms of ASD, but there is not a medication that can treat all ASD symptoms currently. The most commonly prescribed medications include stimulants such as methylphenidate (Ritalin); tranquilizers such as thioridazine or diphenhydramine; anticonvulsants such as phenytoin and carbamazepine; and risperidone, an antipsychotic medication, to improve behavior.

GENERAL CHARACTERISTICS OF PERSONS WITH AUTISM SPECTRUM DISORDER

From the beginning of life, children with ASD are unable to relate in an ordinary manner to people and situations, and they desire an extreme aloneness that ignores, disregards, and shuts out anything that comes from outside of themselves. Children with ASD are sometimes described as being self-sufficient, living life in a shell, happiest when alone, acting as if people were not there, and giving the impression of silent wisdom. The child has an all-powerful need for being left undisturbed. Everything and anything that changes their external environment is looked at as an intrusion. ASD symptoms can be realized by 18 months of age; typically, by age 2, a reliable diagnosis by a medical professional can be made. The first characteristic sign of ASD is few or no big smiles or other warm, joyful, engaging expressions by 6 months of age. Many children with ASD come from highly intelligent families. According to the Diagnostic and Statistical Manual of Mental Disorders (DSM-5), for a person to be diagnosed with ASD, developmental monitoring can assist in assessing for delays or abnormal functioning within (1) communication and interaction with others, (2) restricted interests and repetitive behaviors, or (3) symptoms that affect their ability to function in school, work, and other areas of life. The CDC has developed materials along with a Milestone Tracker app or checklist for caregivers and professionals to record developmental monitoring and determine when screening may

be necessary. Autism Speaks, an ASD advocacy organization, has developed the M-CHAT (Modified Checklist for Autism in Toddlers) to assist in determining signs and symptoms of ASD. The American Academy of Pediatrics (AAP) recommends children be screened for ASD during their 18- and 24-month well visit checks. Persons with ASD are usually normal physically, although ASD may occur along with other conditions such as metabolic disturbances (e.g., phenylketonuria, Tay-Sachs disease), Down syndrome, and epilepsy. Some individuals with ASD acquire skill in fine muscle coordination, whereas others have a poor gait or poor gross motor performance.

Communication and Relationship Behaviors

Children with ASD are usually devoid of speech or have abnormal language. Their language consists primarily of naming nouns and adjectives that identify objects and indicating colors and numbers that represent nothing specific. This type of language is referred to as *excellent rote memory*. Language becomes a valueless or grossly distorted memory exercise with no use for communication. In other words, children with ASD meaninglessly imitate what they hear (**echolalia**). When sentences are formed, they are mostly repetitions of word combinations that have been heard. For the child with ASD, words become inflexible and cannot be used with any other reference but the original acquired meaning. Children with ASD repeat and use personal pronouns just as they are heard. For example, if a child with ASD desires milk, they may say, "Are you ready for your milk?" Children with ASD slowly learn to speak of themselves in the first person and of the person addressed in the second person; this occurs around the age of 6 years. It has also been noted that children with ASD avoid eye-to-eye contact, facial expressions, and any other form of nonverbal communication.

Children with ASD are more interested in objects than people because objects rarely change in appearance or position. The sameness of objects does not threaten the child, thereby allowing them to have undisturbed power and control. Despair and confusion can be caused by minor changes in routine, everyday tasks, and furniture arrangement. Children with ASD are not afraid of people but rather of the objects that they acquire. For example, a child with ASD fears a pin pricking the body, not of the person doing the pricking. Dental hygienists should try to alleviate a fear of dental instruments by explaining each procedure and the use of each instrument. The children are not interested in surrounding conversation. When addressed, children with ASD respond quickly to "get it over with" so that they can continue their activity, or they may not respond at all. Family members derive the same response as a casual acquaintance. Similarly, children with ASD are very interested in pictures of people but not in the people themselves. The pictures of people cannot disturb their environment.

Progress

By the age of 5 or 6 years, language becomes more communicative because the child with ASD has experienced several patterns. Food is accepted, noises and motions are tolerated, and panic tantrums subside. The children also experience increased contact with people, especially people who satisfy their needs, answer their questions, and help them do things (e.g., reading). By the age of 6 or 8 years, children with ASD play alongside other children (this is known as *parallel play*) but never with a group. They also acquire reading skills quickly at this age. As children with ASD grow older, several changes begin to occur. They are still in their world of aloneness and sameness, but they emerge from solitude to varying degrees. Some people are accepted into their life because they finally compromise and gradually extend feelers into a world to which they have been total strangers. Other behaviors exhibited by persons with ASD at various ages are shown in Table 60.4. Only a small percentage of patients with ASD will live and work independently.

TABLE 60.4 **Possible Behaviors Exhibited by People With Autism Spectrum Disorder**

Age Period	Response to Environment	Social and Play Skills	Language Communication Skills	Feeding and Eating	Motor Development
Infancy	Good: Infant is quiet and placid, seldom cries, and is fascinated by lights. Irritable: Infant screams and may be quiet only with vigorous rocking or car rides. Fights washing, dressing, and feedings. Is stiff and hard to cuddle. Rocks body, bangs head.	Is unresponsive to parents' presence. Reacts with a poor response to social games. Makes little eye contact. Does not reach or point. Has no interest in baby toys. May enjoy rough play.	Ignores speech. Ignores loud sounds. Is fascinated with soft sounds. Has decreased verbalizations.	Has poor sucking. Refuses to eat lumpy foods. Does not cry when hungry.	Is on schedule or uneven. May bypass a motor stage, such as creeping.
Toddler	Has self-stimulating behaviors, rocking, head banging. Has irregular sleep patterns. Resists changes in routine. Is disturbed in response to stimuli; is fascinated with some sounds. Uses touch, taste, and smell to extremes. Ignores objects of usual childhood interest. Zeroes in on details. Uses peripheral vision. Recognizes parents by outline rather than by features. Does not respond to painful stimuli.	Has an inappropriate use of an attachment to objects. Play is stereotypic, repetitive. May be extremely passive. May be destructive, aggressive, and self-injurious. Is difficult to manage. Has frequent tantrums.	Is unresponsive to voice, tone, or name. Echolalia: Is delayed or immediate. Screams. Leads adult by the arm. Responds to simple commands.	Likes pureed foods. Will eat only a limited variety of foods. Does not recognize foods in other forms, such as a banana without the peel.	Is a prolonged cruiser. Tiptoe walks. May be normal. May be hyperactive.
Preschool age	Toddler responses continue.	Is aloof and expressionless. Delays toilet training. Is more affectionate. Displays socially embarrassing behaviors. Tantrums continue. Stereotypic, repetitive play continues. Passivity may continue.	Echolalia may develop. Meaningful speech is produced with effort. Has poor pronunciation and voice control. Is unable to understand most speech. Can understand short, concrete sentences. Is confused with pronouns, similar-sounding words, and word order. Uses and understands limited gestures.	Food jags occur.	May be normal. May jump, spin, and flap arms and hands. May be graceful or clumsy. Fine-motor ability may differ from gross-motor proficiency. Has difficulty with copying movements. May walk with elbows bent, hands together, and wrists dropped. Hyperactivity may continue.
School years	Behaviors (tantrums) decrease. Sleep irregularities may continue. Continues to have disturbances in response to stimuli.	Displays increased affection. Displays increased social skills. May help with simple household chores.	Language skills may increase. Same problems seen as a preschooler may continue.	Food jags continue. May begin trying new foods.	Displays increased motor skills. Has an unusual walk. Splinter skills may develop. May pace, jump, spin.
Adulthood	Same responses as seen during the school years may continue.	Displays increased affection. Displays increased social skills.	Language skills continue to increase.	Diet broadens. Food jags continue.	Motor skills continue to increase. Is relatively self-sufficient.

MANAGEMENT OF PATIENTS WITH AUTISM SPECTRUM DISORDERS

Persons with ASD exhibit no specific oral findings, although particular circumstances may increase the risk and prevalence of caries and periodontal disease. Infants with ASD may find eating difficult and may result in vomiting. Their unsuccessful struggle against the intrusion of food leads to a limited selection of food choices. If food selection includes regular sucrose intake, dental caries may be a major concern. Oral care may have been neglected as a result of language difficulties, anxiety, and a lack of social contact. Depending on the level of cooperation, dental sealant therapy should also be considered. Persons with ASD may also have epilepsy, thereby requiring medication that produces drug-influenced gingival enlargement, especially when the individual has poor oral biofilm control. Psychotropic medications may be used as adjuncts to other treatments, thereby causing decreased salivation. The patient may benefit from a saliva substitute, daily therapeutic doses of xylitol-containing products, fluoride varnish therapy, and at-home fluoride therapy.

Individuals with ASD often have nutritional needs as a result of dietary fixation, preferences for soft or sweet foods that require little chewing, a lack of tongue coordination, or pouching their food (i.e., holding food in their cheeks) rather than swallowing. Thus these persons may have heavy accumulations of materia alba, food debris, and oral biofilm. Because of these behaviors, nutritional counseling and rigorous plaque control interventions may be needed.

The management of patients with ASD incorporates three approaches: (1) communication techniques, (2) behavioral modification, and (3) pharmacologic therapies. To choose the best approach, the dental hygienist interviews the caregiver to gather information about the patient's uniqueness, behaviors, and communication and social skills.

Communication includes the caregiver, patient, and dental professional. A patient with ASD may require conditioning before dental hygiene care, especially prior to the first visit, due to foreign sounds, smells, and sights in the dental environment. Sensory overload is common in children with ASD and can lead to inappropriate behaviors such as aggression, emotional outbursts, and SIBs. To accomplish this goal, the caregiver is encouraged to bring the patient to the office to familiarize them with the new environment and upcoming care. Technologies such as instructional video clips on electronic screen media can also assist the child with ASD to become familiar with the dental visit.[17] Children with ASD can repetitively watch videos of what will happen during the visit in preparation for the actual appointment day, which reduces the anxiety surrounding a new environment. It may also be helpful for the video clips to have images of the child and dental professionals treating the patient to provide familiar faces. Patients with ASD must be able to pay attention to the videos for at least 10 to 26 seconds to have an impact on increasing communication and reducing fears related to the unknown. Mobile applications can benefit patients with mild forms of ASD in the dental environment. Applications downloaded to mobile devices such as smartphones are customizable for step-by-step training on dental hygiene care and can be used before or during the dental visit.

Rehearsals at home can be advantageous. The caregiver practices commands that the dental professional may use, such as "Hands down," "Open your mouth," and "Look at me." Picture cards using the Picture Exchange Communication System (PECS), along with social stories read prior to the dental visit can be very beneficial to practice at home for increased communication in children with more severe forms of ASD. Children with ASD can select the appropriate card that expresses their feelings or needs while understanding what takes place during a dental hygiene appointment using a social story.[17] The reception area should be quiet, with as few people as possible. The patient should not wait for extended periods because of the possibility of heightened fear and stress. The dental hygienist keeps procedures short and organized.

Pharmacologic therapies and behavior modifications are needed if all other methods fail. A behavioral approach is used to reinforce desired behaviors and to decrease unwanted behaviors. **Behavior modification** techniques consist of telling, showing, and doing, as well as immediate and frequent positive and negative reinforcement used with short, clear commands (Box 60.4). Caregivers are encouraged to be present during treatment, particularly if immobilization is needed for behavior control. Holding the patient's hands down, the use of a papoose board [indicated only when a safe working environment is not attainable] and mouth props) can be used if needed (Chapter 59). If the patient needs to return, the appointments should remain on the same day of the week, at the same time, and with the same dental professionals. The procedure and routine should remain constant as much as possible. The most commonly prescribed medications include nitrous oxide–oxygen analgesia, diazepam, hydroxyzine, chloral hydrate, meperidine, and promethazine. Pharmacologic therapies may be administered in various combinations and doses, depending on individual needs. Fig. 60.8 provides a sample dental hygiene care plan for a patient with ASD. The dental hygienist should remain current on ASD research and best management strategies and techniques for patients with ASD.

PATIENT EDUCATION AND MOTIVATION

When developing oral self-care behaviors for patients with IDs, Down syndrome, and ASD, the dental hygienist teaches at a level that is congruent with the individual's **mental age** (i.e., age reflected by the level of functioning) rather than their **chronologic age** (i.e., true age based on the date of birth). Patient education might involve only the patient or the caregiver or both. After the treatment plan has been designed, the hygienist begins instructions with familiar activities, praises small accomplishments, and uses a gentle but firm demeanor. Extra instructional time may be required for conveying new information. Successful teaching methods include the use of a show-tell-do technique and modeling.

A consistent challenge that these patients face is brushing long enough; therefore, an egg timer or a power toothbrush with a built-in timer could be used to lengthen brushing time. In general,

---

BOX 60.4   Steps in Behavioral Modification for Individuals With Autism Spectrum Disorders

- Use extensive positive social reinforcement to put the patient at ease.
- Use a very simple and suitable reward system (e.g., the patient could be given a toy if good behavior is exhibited throughout the appointment), and explain the system to the patient. If the patient is an adult, a trip to a favorite restaurant may be appropriate.
- Give constant positive social reinforcement throughout each appointment.
- Provide precise verbal praise immediately after each desired behavior.
- Give instructions in a reassuring manner with each desired behavior.
- Do not discuss dental treatment that is needed during dental hygiene care.
- Points earned for desired behavior always entitle the person to a prize at the end.
- Conclude each session with excessive praise.

Dental Hygiene Diagnosis Based on Legal Scope of Practice	Dental Hygiene Diagnosis Based on Human Needs	Due to or Related to	As Evidenced by	Dental Hygiene Care Plan Goal	Evaluative Statements
Dental caries (to be confirmed by dental diagnosis or restored) High caries risk Acquired tooth defects/abrasion	Biologically Sound and Functional Dentition	Inadequate home care Inadequate diet Inadequate fluoride Harmful toothbrushing technique	Signs of dental caries Signs of cervical abrasion	Complete restorative care for caries and defective restorations Reduce caries index score and sugar in diet Use 5000 ppm fluoride gel; 0.12% chlorohexidine mouth rinse to reduce *Streptococcus mutans* Use power toothbrush	Decrease plaque index score by 1 point Report of noncariogenic snacks and include xylitol mints or gum No additional abrasion evident
Plaque-induced gingivitis Xerostomia or dry mouth or reduced salivary flow	Skin and Mucous Membrane Integrity of the Head and Neck	Medication (Zoloft) Inadequate home care	Signs of xerostomia Supragingival soft and hard deposits Inflamed gingiva	Use of saliva substitutes, xylitol gum and mints, and fluoride Caregiver and patient to demonstrate use of power toothbrush; and antimicrobial and moisturizing mouth rinses	Less xerostomia observed and reported Reduction of deposit accumulation at continued-care visit
Dental fear and anxiety	Freedom from Fear and Stress	Sensitivity to high-pitched noise Patient unsure of environment	Verbal and nonverbal indicators of stress Tapping and well thought-out, deliberate walking	Respond positively to the use of equipment that typically causes unpleasant sensation in the ears Decrease behaviors that interfere with treatment	Patient appears comfortable and cooperative during care Tapping and deliberate walking behaviors decreased by 50%
Poor oral hygiene	Responsibility for Oral Health	Lack of caregiver supervision Too much patient autonomy for self-care Skill deficiency	Biofilm accumulation Signs of supragingival deposits	Decreased biofilm accumulation by 50% at continued-care appointment Caregiver reports that patient cleans his own mouth daily and that it is followed up by caregiver Caregiver and patient demonstrate appropriate oral hygiene techniques	Plaque index score decreases by 50%
Low oral health literacy	Conceptualization and Problem Solving	Knowledge deficiency of caregiver and client	Inability to explain disease process and risk factors	Caregiver can: • Explain disease process, risk factors, and protective factors • See a difference in patient's gingival tissues	Caregiver verbalizes that a difference is observed in Ben's oral health as a result of homecare

Dental Hygiene Interventions
• Addresses concerns with medication Zoloft:
 ▪ Monitor vital signs
 ▪ Assess salivary flow
 ▪ Consider semisupine position; have patient sit upright for 2 minutes before standing
• Conduct nutritional counseling.
• Instructions for caregiver:
 ▪ Disease risk factors/protective factors
 ▪ Rationale for plaque index
 ▪ Use of oral hygiene devices; use power toothbrush
 ▪ Techniques for successful patient care management; avoid equipment with high-pitched noises
 ▪ How to look for improvements in the gum tissue (i.e., bleeding points, tongue cleanliness)
 ▪ Importance of frequent continued-care appointments
• Communicate the value of at-home fluoride therapy for caries control.
• Discuss use of xylitol mints or gum, frequent water, and saliva substitutes for xerostomia.
• Give verbal commands for desired behavior. Allow Ben time to process request and wait for response.
• Incorporate behavior modification techniques and techniques for forming a trusting relationship.
• Give Ben positive reinforcement for appropriate behavior.
• Implement instructional video clips, electronic media, Picture Exchange Communication System, or social stories during visits; recommend use at home with caregiver.
• Complete periodontal debridement and apply fluoride varnish; place pit and fissure sealants.
• Complete or refer to dentist for restorative procedures.
• After 3 months, reevaluate home care and oral health status.
 ▪ Modify care plan if needed; maintain communication between caregiver and other healthcare providers.

Fig. 60.8 Sample dental hygiene care plan for a patient with autism spectrum disorder.

the toothbrush handle should be longer to facilitate reaching the posterior areas; the brush head size should be selected on the basis of the patient's oral cavity size and their ability to open their mouth. Existing toothbrushes can be altered according to need (e.g., motor ability, grip problems; see Chapter 59). Power toothbrushes are ideal for patients with grip problems and limited fine-motor control. Power toothbrushes enable persons with minimal motor control to perform oral self-care independently, thereby facilitating the human need for responsibility for oral health and enhancing oral health-related quality of life. If persons can perform their own self-care, they own the task and are likely to perform the behavior regularly.

Interdental cleaning may be extremely difficult for patients and caregivers, but some is better than none. Interdental cleaning devices with long handles are recommended to protect fingers from inadvertent or intentional biting and to reach posterior areas. Holders must be easy to thread and to use to ensure compliance. Oral irrigators are not generally recommended for this population except to deliver prescribed antimicrobial agents. The use of 0.12% chlorhexidine gluconate mouth rinse is commonly prescribed for patients with disabilities to help control oral biofilm and gingivitis. It can be administered via an oral irrigator, a spray, or a swab. (Note that chlorhexidine is absorbed through the gastrointestinal system; therefore, no harm is caused by swallowing a small amount of the agent.) Other agents may be indicated, including the American Dental Association–accepted antimicrobial mouth rinses, sodium fluoride gels and mouth rinses, povidone-iodine (Betadine) mouth rinses, and similar products. These products are often less expensive and do not stain teeth or alter taste as much as 0.12% chlorhexidine gluconate. The use of an antimicrobial fluoride dentifrice twice daily is also recommended. If cooperation is high, home fluoride application is commonly done with a toothbrush after toothbrushing. Substitute therapeutic doses of xylitol gum and mints for candy and for behavior modification.

Clear and concise oral hygiene instructions must be presented to the patient with an ID, Down syndrome, or ASD and to the primary caregiver. Many persons with IDs, Down syndrome, or ASDs learn better from visual rather than auditory teaching; therefore, instruction should include pictures, models, and diagrams. If written instructions are necessary, pictures underneath the written instructions are helpful due to possible limitations in emergent literacy skills, especially for preschool-aged children with IDs, Down syndrome, or ASDs.[19] It is important to communicate directly with the patient to determine motivation, skill, and cooperation levels; however, verbal and written instructions should be given to the caregiver for reference if needed. Box 60.5 provides the practice interventions that are needed to achieve patient goals and therapeutic outcomes in a school-based setting for patients with developmental and/or physical disabilities. Ensuring that the patient and caregiver both have the knowledge and equipment to perform effective daily oral hygiene for patients with cognitive and/or physical challenges is most important to optimal oral health (Box 60.6).

LEGAL AND ETHICAL ASPECTS OF TREATING PATIENTS WITH DEVELOPMENTAL AND/OR PHYSICAL CHALLENGES

During the provision of health services in places of public accommodation, discrimination against persons with disabilities and those with whom they associate is illegal and unethical. Many dental practices do not treat patients with disabilities on the basis of a lack of knowledge and experience, a lack of equipment, and inadequate compensation. Many disabled persons rely on government-funded sources for income and financing healthcare; therefore, access to care is a problem. Box 60.7 offers a summary of the legal, ethical, and safety issues to consider when treating patients with developmental or intellectual challenges.

BOX 60.5 Critical Thinking Scenario

- Visit a school for severely and profoundly intellectually disabled persons. On the basis of your observations and discussions with the teachers, what would you do to improve the oral health status of these students? What recommendations would you have for the teachers?
- Read each of the dental hygiene care plans (see Figs. 60.2, 60.7, and 60.8). Use these to plan a series of appointments to address the diagnosed problems. Are other interventions needed to achieve patient goals and therapeutic outcomes? Assuming that the goals are met, what future goals might move these patients to higher levels of oral health and wellness?

BOX 60.6 Patient or Client Education Tips

- When toothbrushes are chosen, the handle should be long and the brush size should be selected based on the client's ability to open the mouth and the size of the oral cavity.
- Power toothbrushes are excellent for individuals with limited fine-motor control (see Chapters 24 and 59).
- Floss holders are recommended to reach posterior areas and to protect the fingers from inadvertent or intentional biting (see Chapter 25).
- When formulating a care plan for a client with an ID, the dental hygienist must be empathetic and realistic, especially if a caregiver is responsible for the client's daily care.
- When planning oral hygiene interventions for clients with severe or profound IDs, the caregiver should be included. Clients with severe IDs can learn by habit training but need followup by the caregiver.

BOX 60.7 Legal, Ethical, and Safety Issues to Consider for Patients With Developmental or Intellectual Disabilities

- The American Dental Hygienists' Association Code of Ethics states that patients should be treated without discrimination. Dental hygienists who are ill prepared to treat patients with disabilities should seek continuing education opportunities or refer these patients to ensure that high-quality care can be rendered.
- Depending on legal guardianship, the clinician must defer to the patient's legal parent or guardian to obtain necessary consent to render healthcare services.
- Healthcare professionals have an ethical obligation to communicate with all patients effectively. Effective communication may include alterations in communication and self-care instructions for patients with IDs.
- Care plans are adapted to the individual's conditions, but overall the goal is to provide beneficent, comprehensive care.
- Dental hygienists should strive to provide oral self-care instructions to allow as much autonomy as possible for the patient with intellectual disabilities while ensuring safety of all recommendations.

KEY CONCEPTS

- Causes of intellectual disabilities (IDs) are grouped as prenatal, perinatal, and postnatal causes.
- The level of an ID determines if the patient is capable of giving informed consent for care. Consultation with the patient's physician, social worker, or caregiver (i.e., healthcare decision maker) is necessary.
- Persons with an ID may have poor oral health as a result of heightened susceptibility to infection, malnutrition, limited self-care capabilities, economic barriers to care, and limited access to care.
- Oral manifestations observed in patients with an ID often coincide with a specific type of syndrome.
- The lips of patients with an ID are sometimes larger than those of the general population, and tooth anomalies such as microdontia and delayed eruption patterns are usually present as a result of developmental abnormalities. Tooth surface attrition from bruxism is often seen as a result of anxiety or stress.
- The prevalence of periodontal disease among individuals with IDs is attributed to a lack of professional care, a lack of funds to support care, an increased susceptibility, and poor oral hygiene.
- Down syndrome is the most common and frequently observed chromosomal abnormality in humans.
- Congenital heart disease is the most common and serious medical condition among persons with Down syndrome; therefore, the dental hygienist must determine the need for treatment alterations, possibly including prophylactic antibiotic premedication, based on current guidelines.
- Individuals with Down syndrome have a high incidence of periodontal disease.
- Autism spectrum disorder (ASD) includes autistic disorder, Asperger syndrome, Rett syndrome, and pervasive developmental disorder not otherwise specified, all of which are characterized by varying degrees of impairment in communication skills and social interactions and restricted, repetitive, and stereotypic patterns of behavior.
- Body movements such as rocking are characteristically observed in some persons with ASD.
- Patients with ASD may take psychotropic medications that decrease salivation; therefore, saliva substitutes and therapeutic doses of xylitol-containing products may be prescribed for daily use.
- Patients with mild IDs are educable; therefore, oral hygiene instructions should be explained and demonstrated with the use of activities rather than concepts.
- Patients with moderate IDs should be taught fundamental skills by employing the show-and-tell method.
- Behavior modification is the recommended technique when working with persons with ASD.
- When developing oral hygiene skills in a patient with an ID, teach at a level that is based on the patient's mental age rather than their chronologic age.
- When educating patients with IDs, their cognitive and physical limitations and abilities; level of periodontal health and caries risk; level of deposit accumulation, medications, and diet; and their ability to cooperate should be assessed.
- The dental hygienist chooses toothbrushes and interdental or supplemental oral hygiene aids based on oral conditions and intellectual abilities of each patient with an ID. Caregivers are engaged in oral self-care instruction as indicated by the individual patient's abilities and intellectual functioning.
- When formulating a care plan for a patient with an ID, the dental hygienist must be empathetic and realistic, especially if a caregiver is responsible for the patient's daily care.

ACKNOWLEDGMENTS

The author acknowledges Ginger B. Mann, Michele L. Darby, and Kelly M. Schulz for their past contributions to this chapter.

REFERENCES

1. American Psychiatric Association. Available at: https://www.psychiatry.org/Patients-Families/Intellectual-Disability/What-is-Intellectual-Disability. Accessed January 12, 2023.
2. Hassona Y, Aljafari A, Atef A, Abdalfattah L, Hosey MT. Failure on all fronts: qualitative analysis of the oral health care experience in individuals with intellectual disability. *Spec Care Dentist*. 2021;41(2):235–243. https://doi.org/10.1111/scd.12550.
3. Lynn R, Meisenberg G. National IQs Calculated and Validated for 108 Nations. *Intelligence*. 2010;38.
4. American Association of Intellectual and Developmental Disabilities. Available at: www.aaidd.org/about-aaidd#.UmSFWha_Oa4. Accessed July 21, 2022.
5. Wilson NJ, Lin Z, Villarosa A, et al. Countering the poor oral health of people with intellectual and developmental disability: a scoping literature review. *BMC Publ Health*. 2019;19:1530. https://doi.org/10.1186/s12889-019-7863-1.
6. National Institute of Dental and Craniofacial Research. Developmental Disabilities and Oral Health. Available at: https://www.nidcr.nih.gov/health-info/developmental-disabilities. Last reviewed Oct 2020. Accessed July 21, 2022.
7. National Down Syndrome Society. *National Down Syndrome Society Website*; 2022. Available at: http://www.ndss.org. Accessed July 21, 2022.
8. Chen L, Wang L, Wang Y, et al. Global, regional, and national burden and trends of Down Syndrome from 1990 to 2019. *Front Genet*. 2022:13.
9. The National Association for Child Development. Congenital Heart Disease in Children with Down Syndrome. 1986–2017. Available at: http://downsyndrome.nacd.org/heart_disease.php. Accessed July 21, 2022.
10. Whooten R, Schmitt J, Schwartz J. Endocrine manifestations of down syndrome. *Curr Opin Endocrinol Diabetes Obes*. 2018;25(1).
11. Marques J, Silva PG, Pereira KF, et al. The incidence of tooth abnormalities in Down's syndrome patients by digital radiographic evaluation. *Braz J Surg Clin Res*. 2016;14:2.
12. Al Jameel AH, Watt RG, Tsakos G, Daly B. Down Syndrome and oral health: mothers' perception on their children's oral health and its impact. *J Patient Rep Outcomes*. 2020;4(45).
13. Centers for Disease Control and Prevention. About Autism. Available at: www.cdc.gov/ncbddd/autism. Accessed July 21, 2022 Updated May, 2022.
14. Autism speaks. Autism Speaks Website. Available at: www.autismspeaks.org. Accessed July 21, 2022.
15. National Institute of Mental Health: Autism Spectrum Disorder. Available at: https://www.nimh.nih.gov/health/publications/autism-spectrum-disorder - part_6152. Accessed July 21, 2022.
16. Raposa KA, Perlman SP. *Treating the Dental Patient with a Developmental Disorder*. Wiley-Blackwell; 2012.
17. Elmore JL, Bruhn AM, Bobzien JL. Interventions for the reduction of dental anxiety and corresponding behavioral deficits in children with autism spectrum disorder. *J Dent Hyg*. 2016;90:2.
18. National Institute of Neurological Disorders and Stroke. Autism Spectrum Disorder Fact Sheet. Available at: https://www.ninds.nih.gov/health-information/patient-caregiver-education/fact-sheets/autism-spectrum-disorder-fact-sheet?search-term=autism%20spectrum%20disorder. Accessed July 21, 2022.
19. Westerveld MF, Paynter J, Trembath D, et al. The emergent literacy skills of preschool children with autism spectrum disorder. *J Autism Dev Disord*. 2017;47:424–438.

61

Orofacial Clefts

Joanna L. Harris-Worelds

PROFESSIONAL DEVELOPMENT OPPORTUNITIES

In practice, dental hygienists encounter patients with an orofacial cleft in various stages of treatment. In addition, dental hygienists are well positioned to participate in interprofessional healthcare teams to address the needs of these individuals and their caregivers. Knowledge of oral conditions, developmental processes, risks and benefits of treatment, and preventive interventions allows dental hygienists to provide evidence-based care and education to patients with orofacial clefts.

COMPETENCIES

1. Discuss the incidence, prevalence, and etiology of orofacial clefts, and differentiate between the types of treatment indicated for lip and palatal clefts.
2. Educate patients and caregivers about the risks and oral complications for patients with orofacial clefts.
3. Describe the dental hygienist's role in planning individualized dental hygiene care to address the prevention and treatment of oral health conditions and challenges associated with cleft lip and palate.
4. Discuss the importance of interprofessional collaboration to address the multitude of needs of a patient with orofacial clefts or the patient's caregiver.

INTRODUCTION

Failure of the lip and palate tissues to close during embryonic development creates **orofacial clefts**. Orofacial clefts, one of the most common craniofacial anomalies and congenital (birth) defects, have the following characteristics:
- They result from a malformation, a deformation, or a disruption in one or more parts of the body.
- They are present at birth.
- They have serious adverse effects on health, development, or functional ability.

These congenital anomalies are categorized into two groups: cleft palate only and cleft lip with or without cleft palate.

INCIDENCE AND PREVALENCE

Orofacial clefts are the third most prevalent congenital disability in the United States, affecting approximately 6000 infants annually.[1] One in 1000 infants is affected by an orofacial cleft; clefts affecting the lip with palate (1 in 1563 infants) and palate only (1 in 1687 infants) are more common than cleft lip only (1 in 2807 infants).[1] The condition has the highest prevalence among non-Hispanic American Indians or Alaska Natives, followed by Hispanics, non-Hispanic Whites, and non-Hispanic Asians or Pacific Islanders.[1] African Americans or Blacks have the lowest prevalence of orofacial clefts among all racial and ethnic groups.[1] Orofacial clefts are more predominant among male infants than female infants.[2] Regarding the type of orofacial cleft, males are more likely to exhibit an orofacial cleft involving both the lip and the palate. There is a female predominance for only cleft palate without cleft lip.[2-4]

ETIOLOGIC FACTORS

Orofacial classifications divide clefts into two groups: nonsyndromic (isolated) clefts (the patient has no other related health problems) and syndromic (clefts associated with other congenital disorders or syndromes).[3] A **syndrome** is a group of symptoms characterizing a disease, disorder, or condition. Clefts are associated with more than 500 syndromes, but most of these syndromes are rare.[3] Orofacial clefts more commonly occur as Pierre Robin sequence, which is not a syndrome but a specific presentation of three distinct characteristics: cleft palate, **micrognathia** (small mandible), and **glossoptosis** (airway obstruction caused by tongue displacement).

Etiologic factors for nonsyndromic orofacial clefts, or those not associated with syndromes, are not entirely understood. Clefts may result from inherited or endogenous (internal) factors, environmental or exogenous (external) factors, or interactions between multifactorial causes.[3,5] Genetics plays a significant role in nonsyndromic orofacial cleft development. Identification of over two dozen gene variants, genetic mutations, and chromosomal abnormalities elevates the inherited (endogenous) risk of orofacial clefts.[3] Risk can arise within a family; however, inherited risk depends on how many family members have clefts, how closely they are related, the race and sex of the affected individuals, and the type of cleft.[4]

Environmental (exogenous) factors include teratogens, which seem to be strongly associated with nonsyndromic orofacial clefts. A **teratogen** is an agent or substance that can cause congenital abnormalities in a developing embryo or fetus. Several known teratogens increasing the risk for orofacial clefts are maternal smoking, maternal alcohol consumption, nutritional deficiencies such as lack of folic acid or zinc, pregestational or gestational diabetes, maternal obesity, and certain drugs ingested during pregnancy, especially vasoactive or anticonvulsant medications.[2,3,5] Although the preventative extent folic acid has in reducing cleft development remains inconclusive, a multivitamin high in folic acid is recommended for women of childbearing age to reduce neural tube defects. Additional environmental factors elevating cleft risk involve maternal indicators of lower socioeconomic status, such as using the Special Supplemental Nutrition Program for Women, Infants, and Children (WIC) or being a Medicaid recipient.[2] Two environmental factors identified as protective and thus reducing the risk of orofacial clefts are maternal education level of bachelor's degree or higher and early prenatal care.[2]

TYPES OF OROFACIAL CLEFTS

Embryologic Factors

Development of the lip and palate occurs during the early to middle portion of the first trimester of pregnancy. A cleft is a split or fissure (schisis) involving the soft and/or hard tissues that do not fuse during embryonic development. **Cheiloschisis**, a cleft of the upper lip, begins during the fifth week of fetal development; it is complete by the tenth week of pregnancy. At this time, the fusion of the medial nasal and maxillary processes (prominences) forms the philtrum (Fig. 61.1). **Palatoschisis**, a cleft of the palate, may occur at any time during the development of the palate and at different locations and in different structures of the palate.

The palate begins to form at the end of the fifth week of fetal development; it is complete by the twelfth week of pregnancy. Comprising the median palatine process are the median nasal process and the maxillary processes. It fuses with the lateral palatine processes—internal aspects of the maxillary process—or shelves to form the secondary palate. During palatal development, the lateral palatine processes in the maxilla are positioned downward initially and then elevated horizontally for fusion with each other. Failure to fuse might be attributed to the shelves' late horizontal movement, rupture after fusion, or other factors, such as micrognathia and **macroglossia** (enlarged tongue), which can block or affect the movement of the shelves.[5] Palatal development progresses from the anterior to the posterior or from the primary palate to the uvula (Fig. 61.2).[5]

Location of Clefts

Orofacial clefts may or may not simultaneously involve the lip and palate. Clefts may be unilateral or bilateral (Fig. 61.3). The severity of the cleft will vary, depending on the extent of the lack of fusion between the hard and soft structures. The depth of tissue involvement is referred to as incomplete or complete. The extent of palatal clefts also varies, involving the anterior palate, posterior palate, or both (Fig. 61.4). Severity ranges from least severe, which is an incomplete unilateral cleft lip, to most severe, which is a complete bilateral cleft lip and cleft palate. Table 61.1 provides orofacial cleft types, locations, and illustrations.

TREATMENT

Cleft lip and cleft palate are treatable congenital disorders; however, the extent of treatment varies with the type and severity of the cleft. Cleft lip repair (cheiloplasty) occurs within the first 12 months, often between 3 and 6 months of age. Closure of a cleft palate (palatoplasty) transpires between 9 and 18 months of age.[6,7] For certain types of clefts, a surgeon may utilize elastomeric taping to help decrease cleft lip width or a nasoalveolar molding (NAM) appliance to reshape the nose and primary palate bone for a more favorable surgical outcome.[7] Surgical intervention usually follows the "rule of 10" to determine when a healthy baby can undergo surgery for an elective procedure (i.e., 10 weeks of age, 10 lb. in weight, and hemoglobin value greater than 10 g/dL).[7] Although early orofacial cleft treatments help speech development, these surgeries can affect subsequent facial growth and development. Cosmetic surgery, reconstructive surgery, or **orthognathic surgery**—which involves corrective surgery of the jaw and face to alter the relationship of the teeth and supporting bones, sometimes in conjunction with orthodontic treatment—may be indicated as secondary surgeries after the primary orofacial cleft surgery if maxillary deficiency, malocclusion, and lip and nasal deformities

result.[6] Specific treatments for orofacial clefts can be found in oral and maxillofacial surgery textbooks.

Interprofessional Collaboration

A multidisciplinary or interprofessional team works to manage an orofacial cleft: a plastic surgeon, a pediatrician, a pediatric dentist, an orthodontist, a speech-language pathologist, a psychologist, an otolaryngologist, a social worker, an oral and maxillofacial surgeon, a geneticist, an audiologist, a prosthodontist, and a sociologist.[5–7] Table 61.2 explains the problems associated with a facial cleft, the corrective therapy, the specialists involved, and the rationale for specialist involvement. Dental hygienists also participate in interprofessional collaborations for clients with orofacial clefts (Box 61.1).

COMPLICATIONS

Individuals with orofacial clefts can experience feeding difficulties as infants, malocclusion, nasal deformities, and problems with hearing and speech. Feeding problems most often are associated with a cleft palate.[8,9] Infants with a cleft palate have difficulty producing the negative pressure needed to suck milk from a bottle or breast. The infant's sucking and swallowing reflexes are normal; however, their musculature is underdeveloped or not properly oriented for effective sucking.[7] Nasal regurgitation, long feeding times, and difficulty coordinating swallowing and breathing occur. Excessive inhalation of air necessitates frequent burping. Interventions such as a squeezable bottle or syringe improve feeding as opposed to using a rigid bottle or spoon.[8]

In children with orofacial clefts, the most common problem is middle ear infection from a lack of ventilation from the eustachian tubes because palatal muscles control the opening of these tubes. Retrognathia and glossoptosis worsen ventilation obstruction. Without ventilation, fluid accumulates in the middle ear, and bacteria from the nasopharynx multiply to cause acute infections. Chronic ear infections can result in hearing impairments from permanent damage to the auditory sensory nerves if the problem is not addressed.[5]

Hearing problems contribute significantly to speech disorders common in persons with orofacial clefts. Individuals with an orofacial cleft have normal or close to normal speech; however, those with a cleft palate may have speech delays as closure occurs later than cleft lip repairs. The development of speech is directly impacted by when orofacial clefts are repaired. During speech, the muscles of the soft palate elevate and draw it posteriorly to the pharyngeal wall for closure to prevent air from escaping through the nose (Fig. 61.5). If closure does not occur, it is called **velopharyngeal dysfunction** (VPD). VPD, which allows air to escape into the nasal cavity, may cause a patient to have hypernasal speech. The goal of treatment is to eliminate VPD as early as possible to help a child develop normal speech patterns. Treatment may involve surgery, a special speech device that may also function as an **obturator** which closes the palate, speech therapy, or a combination of these approaches (see Figs. 61.6 and 61.7).[5]

Malocclusion is especially likely in individuals with cleft palates. Class III malocclusion is most common. Malocclusion can result from missing teeth or stunted maxillary growth. Maxillary growth is constricted due to scar tissue formation after primary surgeries to correct orofacial clefts. Other dental problems that may be present are congenitally missing teeth and supernumerary teeth. Because of the location of the cleft, the lateral incisor and the canine may be absent or severely displaced. Teeth may also be morphologically deformed, hypoplastic, or hypomineralized. Nasal architecture can also be deformed if a cleft involving the lip extends into the floor of the nose.[5–7]

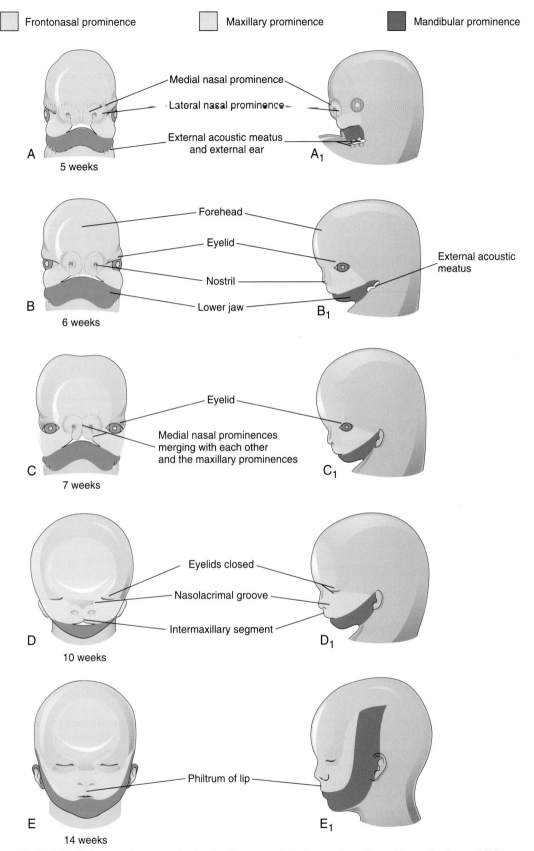

Fig. 61.1 (A–E) Progressive stages in the development of the human face. (From Moore KL, Persaud TVN, Torchia MG. *The Developing Human: Clinically Oriented Embryology.* 10th ed. Elsevier; 2016.)

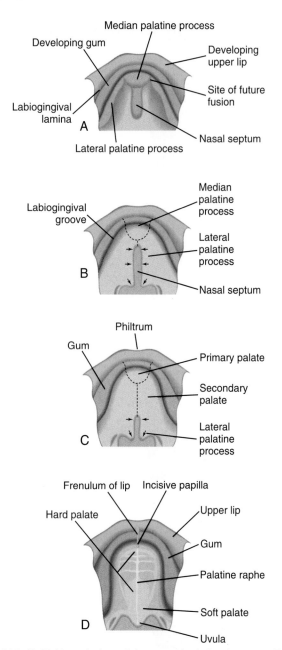

Fig. 61.2 (A–D) Ventral view of human palatal development. (From Moore KL, Persaud TVN, Torchia MG. *The Developing Human: Clinically Oriented Embryology*. 10th ed. Elsevier; 2016.)

DENTAL HYGIENISTS' ROLE

Caries Risk and Prevention

Dental hygiene care for a patient with cleft lip, cleft palate, or both is crucial during childhood because caries risk is high. Children with orofacial clefts have significantly higher decayed surfaces than children without clefts. Caries prevalence is more evident in the primary dentition among patients with orofacial clefts, particularly the maxillary incisors, the teeth adjacent to the cleft, and the molars.[10] Patients with a cleft palate have a higher caries risk because of a longer oral clearance time for foods, more fermentable sugars from starches, longer bottle-feeding time, decreased salivary flow, mouth breathing, and the tenacious nature of nasal fluid, which promotes the adherence of oral biofilm.[10] Other parental factors contributing to increased caries risk include insufficient dietary counseling, reduced oral health knowledge,

the trauma of coping with a child with a cleft, and poor accessibility of the toothbrush around the cleft area.[4]

Patients with an orofacial cleft may also undergo treatments, such as orthodontic treatment to correct malocclusion or wearing an intraoral appliance to correct speech dysfunction, which increases caries risk. More surface irregularities with orthodontics and intraoral appliances (obturators) retain food and biofilm (Chapter 40). Treatment appliances and soft foods increase substrate retention, thereby increasing acid production and caries risk.

Orofacial clefts presence significantly increases the risk for higher dental biofilm accumulation, gingivitis, and periodontitis.[11] Also, intraoral appliances may contribute to an increased risk for periodontal disease. Chronic tissue irritation from ill-fitting prostheses can increase gingival inflammation, leading to hyperplastic tissue response, and the mechanical rubbing against the natural dentition may lead to recessed gingiva. Additional complications from wearing prostheses may occur (Chapter 41).

With the risk of demineralization in patients with orofacial clefts, the hygienist is well positioned to provide evidence-based prevention recommendations to decrease caries risk. Preventive measures include patient and parental dietary counseling, frequent hygiene recall, fluoride therapy, and dental sealants (Chapters 19 and 35). Dietary counseling must emphasize decreasing or limiting cariogenic foods and beverages and provide healthier nutritional choices and behaviors to reduce caries risk (Chapter 36). Children with orofacial clefts could benefit from more frequent hygiene appointments, such as every 3 or 4 months. Increased recall intervals aid the hygienist in performing additional oral health and risk assessments, reinforcing oral hygiene homecare, providing professional biofilm reduction, and applying topical fluoride therapy, such as varnish (Chapter 19). In addition, systemic fluoride therapy, such as supplemental tablets and drops, may be indicated as enamel disturbances are possible during tooth development with orofacial clefts (Chapter 45). Box 61.2 provides legal, ethical, and safety issues to be considered when providing dental hygiene care for patients with orofacial clefts.

Oral Hygiene Care

The Fones technique of toothbrushing and the sulcular toothbrushing technique is most appropriate for children (Chapter 24). A power toothbrush and a small brush head size are helpful because toothbrushing may be inadequate, and teeth may be difficult to access due to less elasticity of the surgically repaired lip, the anatomy of the cleft, and the fear of brushing around the cleft area. In addition, the crowding of the dentition restricts the toothbrush and the self-cleaning ability of the mouth. Patients with orofacial clefts must also clean interdentally daily to remove biofilm and food debris. Caregivers responsible for children's oral hygiene should be educated about the importance of daily food debris and oral biofilm removal.

Oral hygiene instructions also need to address the care of intraoral speech prostheses and obturators (Figs. 61.6 and 61.7). These appliances can retain replacement teeth. Daily care for these appliances is similar to the care of partial and complete dentures (Box 61.3; Chapter 41).

Interaction With Patients and Caregivers

Effective communication, education, and emotional awareness with patients with orofacial clefts and their caregivers is an essential role of the dental hygienist. Individuals with orofacial clefts often experience hearing problems and speech disorders. Similar to patients with sensory disorders, the hygienist may encounter communication challenges, for example, difficulty understanding hypernasal speech and verbally explaining procedures (see Chapters 59 and 60 for

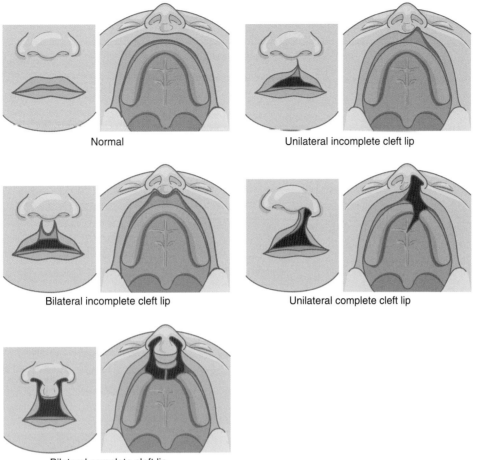

Fig. 61.3 Types of facial clefts (frontal view). (A) Normal. (B) Unilateral cleft lip. (C) Bilateral cleft lip. (Modified from *Cleft Palate and Craniofacial Conditions: A Comprehensive Guide to Clinical Management.* 4th ed. by Ann W. Kummer; 2020.)

Normal

Unilateral incomplete cleft lip

Bilateral incomplete cleft lip

Unilateral complete cleft lip

Bilateral complete cleft lip
and anterior (primary) palate

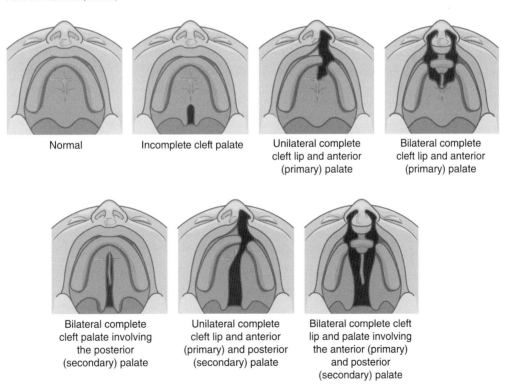

Normal

Incomplete cleft palate

Unilateral complete
cleft lip and anterior
(primary) palate

Bilateral complete
cleft lip and anterior
(primary) palate

Bilateral complete
cleft palate involving
the posterior
(secondary) palate

Unilateral complete
cleft lip and anterior
(primary) and posterior
(secondary) palate

Bilateral complete cleft
lip and palate involving
the anterior (primary)
and posterior
(secondary) palate

Fig. 61.4 Palatal clefts (ventral view). (A) Normal. (B) Cleft of lip and alveolus. (C) Cleft of lip and primary palate. (D) Unilateral cleft lip and palate. (E) Bilateral cleft lip and primary palate. (F) Bilateral cleft lip and palate. (G) Cleft palate only. (Modified from *Cleft Palate and Craniofacial Conditions. A Comprehensive Guide to Clinical Management.* 4th ed. by Ann W. Kummer; 2020.)

TABLE 61.1 Orofacial Cleft Embryology

Cleft Location	Description	Type of Cleft	Figure
Incomplete cleft lip	Notch of any depth that involves the philtrum; does not invade hard structures or the nostrils	Incomplete unilateral cleft lip	(From Fonseca RJ, Marciani RD, Turvey TA. *Oral and Maxillofacial Surgery*. 2nd ed. Saunders; 2009.)
Unilateral or bilateral cleft lip	Lack of fusion of the median nasal and maxillary processes is observed.	Incomplete bilateral cleft lip	(From Fonseca RJ, Marciani RD, Turvey TA. *Oral and Maxillofacial Surgery*. 2nd ed. Saunders; 2009.)
Complete cleft lip	Involves the alveolar bone and primary palate; extends into the nostrils.	Complete unilateral cleft lip	(Courtesy Dr. John B. Mulliken, Children's Hospital Boston, Harvard Medical School, Boston, Massachusetts.)
		Complete bilateral cleft lip	(Courtesy Dr. John B. Mulliken, Children's Hospital Boston, Harvard Medical School, Boston, Massachusetts.)

TABLE 61.1   Orofacial Cleft Embryology—cont'd

Cleft Location	Description	Type of Cleft	Figure
Complete cleft palate	Involves the anterior (primary) palate; is anterior to the incisive foramen and posterior (secondary) palate; extends posterior to the incisive foramen and involves the hard and soft palate	Complete unilateral palate	 (Courtesy Dr. John B. Mulliken, Children's Hospital Boston, Harvard Medical School, Boston, Massachusetts.)
Unilateral or bilateral cleft palate	Lack of fusion between one of the two lateral palatine processes; the nasal septum is observed.	Complete bilateral cleft palate	 (Courtesy Dr. John B. Mulliken, Children's Hospital Boston, Harvard Medical School, Boston, Massachusetts.)
		Cleft palate only	 (From Hupp JR, Ellis E, Tucker M. *Contemporary Oral and Maxillofacial Surgery*. 6th ed. Mosby–Elsevier; 2014.)

Continued

TABLE 61.1　Orofacial Cleft Embryology—cont'd

Cleft Location	Description	Type of Cleft	Figure
Incomplete cleft palate	Cleft of the uvula is observed	Bifid uvula	 (From Hupp JR, Ellis E, Tucker M. *Contemporary Oral and Maxillofacial Surgery.* 6th ed. Mosby–Elsevier; 2014.)
	Lacks muscle or bone fusion, yet soft tissue is present	Submucosal cleft	 (From Neville BW, Damm DD, Allen CM, Chi AC. *Oral and Maxillofacial Pathology.* 4th ed 4. Saunders; 2016.)

TABLE 61.2　Multidisciplinary Team Approach

Problem	Therapy	Specialist	Reason
Orofacial cleft	Surgery	Oral and maxillofacial surgeon Plastic surgeon	Perform lip and palatal repair and closure.
	Screening and evaluation	Geneticist or genetic counselor	Diagnose a syndrome. Establish risk for future pregnancies.
Feeding	Squeeze bottles rather than rigid bottles Nipples: soft, elongated, cross-cut opening	Pediatrician	Promote easier feeding for the infant. Ensure adequate nourishment.
Ears or hearing	Antibiotics Pressure equalization tube placement	Otolaryngologist	Reduce ear infections (otitis media). Address lack of fluid drainage.
	Hearing aid	Audiologist	Perform hearing tests to determine hearing impairments.
Speech	Surgery	Oral and maxillofacial surgeon	Correct velopharyngeal dysfunction. Reduce hypernasal speech.
	Speech therapy	Speech pathologist	Retrain or develop articulation skills.
	Nonsurgical appliances	Prosthodontist	Fabricate prostheses (obturators): speech bulb or palatal lift.
Malocclusion	Orthognathic surgery	Oral and maxillofacial surgeon	Correct function and appearance of jaws.
	Orthodontic treatment	Orthodontist	Align dentition.
Missing teeth	Fixed bridge Denture or partial denture Implants	General dentist or pediatric dentist Prosthodontist	Improve esthetics. Maximize functionality of dentition.
Supernumerary teeth	Retention or extraction	General dentist or pediatric dentist	Assist or interfere with prostheses. Existence aids in maintaining alveolar bone.
Nasal deformity	Surgery	Oral and maxillofacial surgeon Plastic surgeon	Modify esthetics to obtain symmetry. Refine nasal breathing.
Learning, emotional, or behavioral disorders	Screening and evaluation	Psychologist Sociologist	Provide counseling and guidance for specific problems. Improve performance.
Biofilm retention	Hygiene assessment	Dental hygienist	Provide prosthetic appliance care instructions. Modify toothbrushing techniques. Provide product recommendations and use.

Data from Kummer AW. *Cleft Palate and Craniofacial Conditions: A Comprehensive Guide to Clinical Management.* 4th ed. 2020, Jones & Bartlett Learning. Parameters for evaluation and treatment of patients with cleft lip/palate or other craniofacial differences. American Cleft Palate-Craniofacial Association website. Published January 2018. Geneser MK, Allareddy V. Cleft lip and palate. In: Nowak AJ, Christensen JR, Mabry TR, et al. (eds). *Pediatric Dentistry: Infancy Through Adolescence.* 6th ed. 2019; Elsevier.

BOX 61.1 Dental Hygienists' Participation in Interprofessional Collaborations

In addition to delivering clinical dental hygiene services, dental hygienists can participate in interprofessional teams by providing oral screenings and examinations, risk assessment and management, and oral health education to support groups for patients and caregivers. Dental hygienists can offer professional continuing education opportunities for groups of other healthcare providers involved in the treatment of individuals with cleft lip and palate to enhance their awareness of the risk factors for oral diseases, prevention of caries and periodontal diseases, oral hygiene methods recommended for their patients with orofacial clefts, and the importance of frequent oral healthcare visits.

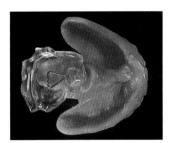

Fig. 61.7 Prosthetic appliance: palatal obturator (extraoral view). (Courtesy of Dr. Charles Babbush.)

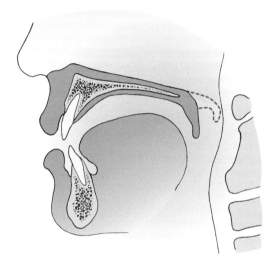

Fig. 61.5 Upward and backward movement of the soft palate during normal speech. Soft palate contact with the posterior pharyngeal wall is shown. (From Hupp JR, Ellis E, Tucker MR. *Contemporary Oral and Maxillofacial Surgery.* 6th ed. Mosby–Elsevier; 2014.)

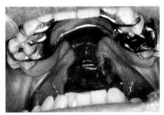

Fig. 61.6 Prosthetic appliance: speech bulb (intraoral view). (From Hupp JR, Ellis E, Tucker MR. *Contemporary Oral and Maxillofacial Surgery.* 6th ed. Mosby–Elsevier; 2014.)

BOX 61.2 Legal, Ethical, and Safety Issues

Dental hygienists should consider the following legal, ethical, and safety issues when caring for patients with orofacial clefts.
- An interprofessional healthcare team approach provides the most beneficial, comprehensive care for individuals with orofacial clefts as these patients have specialized healthcare needs. Coordinate dental hygiene services with members of the cleft palate team.
- For the safety of patients with orofacial clefts, look for signs of physical abuse during the oral examination. Note findings in the patient's chart and report any suspected abuse to Child Protective Services as required by law. Abuse is more common in children with developmental disabilities and often exhibits oral trauma.
- Autonomous care requires choices for patients, and providing information helps them make informed choices.
- Educating patients and caregivers experiencing orofacial cleft complications about fluoride application and dietary counseling is essential to prevent and reduce caries risk and thus reduce the high healthcare costs associated with this condition.

BOX 61.3 Critical Thinking Scenario A

Oral Appliance

A 3-year-old girl arrives with her mother for her first dental appointment in your office. The health history interview reveals a history of ear infections, hearing problems, and speech difficulties. During followup questioning, the mother states that these problems are associated with the child's having been born with a cleft palate. The mother indicates that the child will have corrective surgery next year and is currently wearing an obturator. What instructions would you give the caregiver about obturator cleaning and care? What are appropriate oral hygiene instructions for the patient and caregiver? About what other complications involving cleft palates would you educate the caregiver?

further discussion on hearing deficits). Managing these challenges with focused listening, slowed speech, clear articulation, and use of visible hand gestures or facial expressions can aid interactions between the patient and hygienist.

When interacting with parents or caregivers of children born with an orofacial cleft, the hygienist should offer appropriate education, anticipatory guidance, support, and compassion. Early prenatal diagnosis of orofacial clefts during an ultrasound aids the parent or caregiver in planning care for a child born with a facial congenital defect. A cleft diagnosis may elicit emotional responses such as disbelief, confusion, fear, shock, grief, guilt, sadness, and anxiety.[9] Whether the parents share the child's diagnosis before or after birth, the hygienist

should be able to provide education regarding potential dental complications, feeding difficulties, and timing and frequency of hygiene care, and reinforce the building of a relationship with a multidisciplinary treatment team (Box 61.4). As the child grows, the hygienist needs to help the parents or caregivers adapt to the changing dental needs of the child with an orofacial cleft, such as product recommendations and their use. Often healthcare professionals offer parents or caregivers the opportunities to lead conversations, display their feelings, voice their concerns, and ask questions. Appropriate healthcare, including special psychologic support, also may lead to improvement in quality of life for families with children with cleft lip and palate.[6,9] The dental hygienists' role is summarized in Box 61.5.

BOX 61.4 Critical Thinking Scenario B

Educational Knowledge

A 33-year-old female patient of record arrives for her 6-month dental hygiene appointment. She has her 2-month-old infant in a car carrier with a light blanket draped over the child. As you bring the patient and infant into the treatment area, you ask to see the child. The mother becomes visibly upset and states that her baby has a birth defect—a cleft lip and palate. How would you react to the situation? What questions would you ask the patient to determine her current knowledge about her infant's congenital disability? What resources and dental hygiene information could you give the patient?

BOX 61.5 Patient or Client Education Tips

Dental Hygienists' Role in Orofacial Clefts
- Explain the contributory factors of nonsyndromic clefts.
- Discuss the role of embryologic factors in the development of facial clefts.
- Explain the roles of specialists in addressing orofacial cleft complications.
- Individualize oral hygiene instructions for orofacial clefts, malocclusion, missing teeth, and prostheses.
- Provide evidence-based prevention recommendations and nutritional counseling to reduce the risk of caries.
- Communicate effectively with clients with orofacial clefts, including patients, caregivers, families, and community groups.
- Offer guidance and support to caregivers who are learning how to care for a child with an orofacial cleft.

KEY CONCEPTS

- Orofacial clefts are a common congenital disability that the dental hygienist will encounter during practice; corrective cleft treatment is likely to be completed in industrialized nations.
- Interprofessional collaboration is important when providing oral healthcare interventions for patients with orofacial clefts.
- High risk for caries and periodontal disease are common in individuals with orofacial clefts; thus, risk assessment and preventive interventions are essential.
- Caregivers must be educated about the importance of regular dental hygiene care and preventive interventions.

REFERENCES

1. Mai CT, Isenburg JL, Canfield MA, et al. National population–based estimates for major birth defects, 2010–2014. *Birth Defects Res.* 2019;111(18):1420–1435. https://doi.org/10.1002/bdr2.1589.
2. Vu GH, Warden C, Zimmerman CE, et al. Poverty and risk of cleft lip and palate: an analysis of United States birth data. *Plast Reconstr Surg.* 2021;149(1):169–182. https://doi.org/10.1097/PRS.0000000000008636.
3. Nasreddine G, El Hajj J, Ghassibe-Sabbagh M. Orofacial clefts embryology, classification, epidemiology, and genetics. *Mutat Res.* 2021;787:108373. https://doi.org/10.1016/j.mrrev.2021.108373.
4. Silva CM, Moraes Pereira MC, Queiroz TB, Neves LT. Family history in non-syndromic orofacial clefts: is there a pattern? *Oral Dis.* 2021:1–10. [early view]00, https://doi.org/10.1111/odi.13942.
5. Kummer AW. *Cleft Palate and Craniofacial Conditions: A Comprehensive Guide to Clinical Management.* 4th ed. Jones & Bartlett Learning; 2020.
6. Parameters for Evaluation and Treatment of Patients with Cleft Lip/Palate or Other Craniofacial Differences. American Cleft Palate-Craniofacial Association. https://journals.sagepub.com/doi/full/10.1177/1055665617739564. Published January 2018. Accessed August 1, 2022.
7. Geneser MK, Allareddy V. Cleft lip and palate. In: Nowak AJ, Christensen JR, Mabry TR, et al., eds. *Pediatric Dentistry: Infancy through Adolescence.* 6th ed. Elsevier; 2019:77–89.
8. Penny C, McGuire C, Bezuhly M. A systematic review of feeding interventions for infants with cleft palate. *Cleft Palate Craniofac J.* 2021. https://doi.org/10.1177/10556656211051216. [online ahead of print]00:1–10.
9. Hlongwa P, Rispel LC. "People look and ask lots of questions": caregivers' perceptions of healthcare provision and support for children born with cleft lip and palate. *BMC Publ Health.* 2018;18(506):1–10. https://doi.org/10.1186/s12889-018-5421-x.
10. Grewcock RE, Innes NPT, Mossey PA, Robertson MD. Caries in children with and without orofacial clefting: a systematic review and meta-analysis. *Oral Dis.* 2022;28(5):1400–1411. https://doi.org/10.1111/odi.14183.
11. Marzouk T, Youssef M, Tsigarida A, et al. Association between oral clefts and periodontal clinical measures: a meta-analysis. *Int J Paediatr Dent.* 2021;32(4):558–575. https://doi.org/10.1111/ipd.12934.

62

Neurologic Disabilities

Suzanne Smith and Ruth Palich

PROFESSIONAL OPPORTUNITIES

The dental hygienist must learn how to effectively manage the patient with neurologic disabilities through the incorporation of treatment modifications into an individualized care plan that will result in the enhancement of the patient's oral and overall well-being.

COMPETENCIES

1. Explain features, symptoms, and considerations for patient management and oral self-care of various dysfunctions of the motor system, including tremors, Parkinson disease, cerebral palsy, multiple sclerosis, amyotrophic lateral sclerosis, and Huntington disease.
2. Explain features, symptoms, and considerations for patient management and oral self-care of various dysfunctions of the central nervous system, including traumatic brain injury and posttraumatic stress disorder, spinal cord injury, seizures, and epilepsy.
3. Explain features, symptoms, and considerations for patient management and oral self-care of various peripheral neuropathies, including facial neuropathy (Bell palsy) and trigeminal neuralgia.
4. Explain features, symptoms, and considerations for patient management and oral self-care of various disorders of higher cortical function, including dementia and Alzheimer disease (AD).
5. Explain features, symptoms, and considerations for patient management and oral self-care of cerebrovascular accidents (strokes).
6. Apply knowledge of neurologic disabilities to dental hygiene practice and interprofessional collaboration.

INTRODUCTION

The nervous system makes each individual unique. It senses and evaluates the internal and external environment, controls one's body, and is responsible for a person's abilities, intellect, and personality. These characteristics are the result of complex interactions within the nervous system, and any structural damage or physiologic change to a component of this system may cause functional loss and a variety of neurologic deficits.

Persons with neurologic disorders present unique challenges for the clinician to deliver comprehensive dental hygiene care. The dental hygienist must be knowledgeable about the specific condition, its clinical symptoms, considerations for provision of dental hygiene services, and oral self-care instructions. Decision making about patient care must be based on the best available scientific evidence in conjunction with the clinical expertise of the practitioner and input from the patient and/or caregiver (see Chapter 3). The incidence and prevalence of the neurologic diseases and conditions discussed in this chapter are listed in Table 62.1. See Box 62.1 for legal, ethical, and safety issues related to patients with neurologic disabilities and Box 62.2 for a discussion of the use of marijuana in treatment of neurologic disorders.

DYSFUNCTIONS OF THE MOTOR SYSTEM

Anatomy of the Nervous System

Motor actions require the integration of several central nervous system (CNS) and peripheral nervous system (PNS) components. The CNS is composed of the brain and the spinal cord (Table 62.2), and the PNS is composed of the spinal, cranial, and autonomic nerves and ganglia. Several brain regions are involved in voluntary movement control and in motor responses to sensory stimuli, particularly the motor region (frontal lobe) of the cerebral cortex, the cerebellum, and the basal ganglia. The outline of the CNS in Table 62.2 and the diagram of the brain in Fig. 62.1 demonstrate the relationship of these specific regions to other components of the CNS. The basal ganglia are clusters of neuron cell bodies (gray matter) embedded deep within the CNS forebrain and midbrain.

Disorders affecting cells of the cerebellum and basal ganglia, which project to the motor regions of the cerebral cortex, disturb movements and produce abnormalities of muscle tone, abnormal posturing, and tremors. There may be **hyperkinesia** (increase in movement), **hypokinesia** (lessening of muscular movement), a decrease in associated movements (e.g., arm swing when walking), or abnormal involuntary movements. Degenerative, metabolic, or vascular diseases; toxins; infections; trauma; or neoplasms (tumor, abnormal growth) may cause these abnormalities.

Tremors

Tremors are involuntary rhythmic repetitions or oscillations of movement at regular intervals. Tremors are classified by whether they occur during rest or action and are further categorized according to frequency, amplitude, and body part affected. They are most common in middle-aged and older adults, and they occur for a variety of reasons. Diseases or syndromes, such as Parkinson disease (PD), drugs and toxins, genetics, and certain situational triggers, like stress and anxiety, have all been implicated in individuals with tremors.[1] Generally speaking, tremors can affect nearly any body part but may be specific to its type. Rest tremors are classified as such because they occur when the muscles are at rest. This type of tremor is often seen in PD. One example is the pill=rolling tremor involving the thumb and forefinger that is commonly seen in these individuals. Rest tremors associated with PD can cause movement in other parts of the body, most notably the chin, lips, and jaw, and will require modifications to dental treatment.

Action tremors occur when the muscles of a limb are contracting. Essential tremor disorder falls into the category of action tremors and is the most common, with over 7 million people diagnosed in the United States.[2] Individuals with essential tremor disorder may

TABLE 62.1 Prevalence and Incidence of Common Neurologic Disabilities

Disorder	Prevalence	Incidence
Alzheimer disease and other dementias	6.5 million people	4 out of every 1,000 per year for people age 65 to 74. Incidence increases with age.
Amyotrophic lateral sclerosis (ALS)	16,000	5,000 per year
Bell palsy	No data available	23 to 25 per 100,000 annually; 40,000
Cerebral palsy	760,000 people	3 per 1,000 births
Epilepsy	3.4 million people; 1.2% of the US population	150,000 diagnosed yearly; 48 per 100,000
Huntington disease	41,000	75,000 will develop the disease due to abnormal gene
Multiple sclerosis (MS)	1 million people	2.1 per 100,000 typically diagnosed between ages 20 and 50 years
Parkinson disease	930,000 people	60,000 per year
Spinal cord injury (SCI)	291,000	54 cases per 1 million or 17,730 new SCI cases
Stroke	No data available	795,000 per year
Traumatic brain injury (TBI) and posttraumatic stress disorder (PTSD)	12 million (PTSD)	2.9 million or 823.7 per 100,000 (TBI)
Trigeminal neuralgia	No consensus in the literature	12 per 100,000 annually

Sources:

Alzheimer disease: Alzheimer's Association. 2022 Alzheimer's Disease Facts and Figures.
ALS: https://www.als.org/understanding-als.
Bell's palsy: Gagyor I, et al. "Antiviral Treatment for Bell's Palsy (Idiopathic Facial Paralysis), 2019.
Cerebral palsy: https://www.birthinjuryhelpcenter.org/cerebral-palsy-statistics.html
Epilepsy: https://www.epilepsy.com/what-is-epilepsy/understanding-seizures/who-gets-epilepsy
Huntington disease: https://www.genome.gov/Genetic-Disorders/Huntingtons-Disease
MS: https://www.nationalmssociety.org/What-is-MS/Who-Gets-MS and https://www.verywellhealth.com/multiple-sclerosis-ms-prevalence-and-incidence-5210305
Parkinson disease: https://www.parkinson.org/understanding-parkinsons/statistics/Prevalence-Project and https://parkinsonsnewstoday.com/parkinsons-disease-statistics/
PTSD: https://www.ptsd.va.gov/understand/common/common_adults.asp
SCI: https://www.nscisc.uab.edu/Public/Facts%20and%20Figures%202019%20-%20Final.pdf
Stroke: https://www.cdc.gov/stroke/facts.htm
TBI: https://www.cdc.gov/traumaticbraininjury/pdf/TBI-surveillance-report-2016-2017-508.pdf
TBI: https://www.cdc.gov/traumaticbraininjury/pdf/tbi_report_to_congress_epi_and_rehab-a.pdf
TN: Porto De Toledo I, et al. Prevalence of trigeminal neuralgia. A systematic review. *JADA*. 2016;147(70).

BOX 62.1 Legal, Ethical, and Safety Issues

Patients With Neurologic Disabilities

- In planning new construction or remodeling office space and/or surrounding areas, such as parking lots, consideration must be given to following the Americans with Disabilities Act of 1990 (see Box 62.4).
- Patients with severe neurologic disabilities may not be able to receive care in a traditional office setting. In some states, dental hygienists are permitted to treat patients in alternative settings, such as long-term care facilities, hospitals, specialized schools and workshops, and mobile dental units. When considering alternative practice settings, dental hygienists should always consult the dental practice act of the state in which they practice.
- Evolving legislation, such as regarding the use of medical marijuana, has the potential to impact patients with neurologic disabilities and quality of life. Dental healthcare professionals should be knowledgeable about such practices and be prepared to modify patient care as needed. See Box 62.2 for a discussion on the use of medical marijuana.

BOX 62.2 Legal, Ethical, and Safety Issues

Medical Marijuana

A growing body of research discusses the use of medical marijuana to treat symptoms of certain disabilities, such as spasticity in patients with multiple sclerosis, seizures in patients with epilepsy, and patients who suffer from fibromyalgia and chronic pain. Although marijuana is an illegal substance under federal law, many US states have approved the use of marijuana for medical and recreational purposes. Dental hygienists need to consider the treatment implications and both systemic and oral adverse effects of medicinal and recreational marijuana use. The dental hygienist must complete a comprehensive medical history that includes reviewing the patient's medications and use of other substances, such as cannabinoids. Consideration should also be given to any potential cognitive impairment of the patient, which may preclude a valid informed consent and present an ethical and legal problem.

Points to consider:

- How does medicinal marijuana use differ from recreational use?
- How is medicinal marijuana prescribed, dispensed, and administered?
- What are ways to screen individuals who are suspected of using recreational drugs?
- What are some oral manifestations of smoking marijuana?
- What are some systemic effects of marijuana use?
- Discuss the impact of marijuana on obtaining a valid informed consent.

TABLE 62.2 Overview of the Major Subdivisions of the Central Nervous System

Structure	Primary Function(s)
Brain	
Cerebral Hemispheres	
Lobes	
Frontal lobe	Voluntary motor control, including speech
Parietal lobe	Somatic sensations
Occipital lobe	Vision
Temporal lobe	Hearing, memory
Limbic lobe	Drives, emotions, memory
Basal ganglia	Motor control
Diencephalon	
Thalamus	Reciprocal connections with cerebral cortex
Hypothalamus	Integrative control of autonomic functions
Subthalamus	Motor control
Cerebellum	Control of range and force of movement and acquisition of motor skills
Brainstem	
Midbrain	Control of motor and sensory functions; substantia nigra
Pons	Motor relay from hemispheres to cerebellum
Medulla	Control of vital autonomic functions
Spinal Cord	Integration of sensory and motor information from body and control of body movements

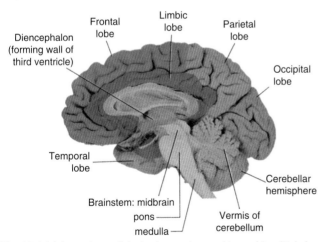

Fig. 62.1 Major regions of the brain, as observed in a midsagittal view. Lobes of the cerebral cortex, diencephalon, brainstem, and cerebellum are illustrated; the regions of the basal ganglia are not evident in this view. (From Nolte J. *The Human Brain.* 6th ed. Mosby; 2009.)

experience involvement of their hands, legs, head, neck, and voice.[1] As with any tremor disorder, special considerations must be made to treat the patient safely and effectively. Dental management for patients with PD and tremors is further discussed in the next section.

Parkinson Disease

Parkinson disease is a chronic progressive neurodegenerative disorder of the motor system, resulting from the loss of dopamine-producing neurons. It is more common in middle and old age, with the majority

of people diagnosed with PD over age 60, although an early onset form of the disease begins before the age of 50. The incidence of PD is higher among males than females.[3]

Pathologically, the disorder is characterized by the progressive loss of dopamine-synthesizing neurons in the substantia nigra of the midbrain of the brainstem (see Fig. 62.1). Dopamine is released from axons that originate from the cell bodies in the substantia nigra and terminate in the basal ganglia, where it serves as a neurotransmitter. A deficiency of dopamine at this site interferes with the conduction of nerve impulses related to muscle activity.

A specific cause for the destruction of dopamine-producing neurons has not been determined. Many studies have shown the disease results from a combination of genetic susceptibility and exposure to one or more environmental factors that trigger the disease. Currently, there is a growing body of research that postulates a possible relationship between neuroinflammation and gut health, specifically how bowel inflammation contributes to the destruction and death of the dopaminergic neurons that produce dopamine.[4] Research has shown that prior to being diagnosed with PD, patients experienced nonmotor symptoms related to the gastrointestinal tract, such as constipation, bloating, and abdominal pain that lasted throughout the course of the disease.[5] It is the alteration of the gut microbiota as a biomarker for PD that has triggered a great deal of interest and could eventually be used for earlier diagnosis for patients with PD.

There is currently no cure for PD. Once diagnosed, patients usually deteriorate progressively over the course of the disease. The most effective treatment is dopamine replacement in the CNS through the use of the medication levodopa, which is converted to dopamine. Most individuals significantly improve on levodopa therapy, although there is some debate over when to use it. Because of its unpleasant peripheral side effects (e.g., nausea, vomiting, low blood pressure), levodopa is almost always given in combination with carbidopa. Carbidopa is a medication that is used to prevent nausea and enhance the effect of levodopa. Levodopa-carbidopa can be given as a pill, a capsule, in gel form, or through an inhaler.[6]

Clinical Symptoms

The cardinal manifestations of PD are rigidity, **akinesia** (impaired muscle movement), and tremor. However, tremor absence does not exclude the diagnosis of the disease. The tremor is rhythmic, is seen most commonly at rest, usually involves primarily the hands, and has been given the name pill-rolling tremor. The tremor usually stops during intended movements. Muscle rigidity is felt in all passive movements. Akinesia or **bradykinesia** (movement slowness) leads to an expressionless face, infrequent blinking, and posture and gait disturbances, such as the characteristic short, shuffling steps (Fig. 62.2). Other symptoms include a low audible monotone voice and progressive difficulty with writing.

Patients with PD often have great difficulty rising from a sitting position and trying to turn from one side to the other in the recumbent position. They usually stand in a slightly stooped posture with the arms flexed. When attempting to walk, they may have great difficulty getting started and, when they finally succeed, steps are short and arm swing is decreased or absent. When these patients turn, the normal fluid movements become replaced by turning the body as a whole, and they may have difficulty stopping immediately. Depression and anxiety are common and impaired cognitive function may be present.

One of the first noticeable signs of PD is a lack of facial expression and animation, also known as "masked face." The characteristic tremors also occur in the tongue, lips, and neck. Common manifestations are the "fly-catcher" tongue, tongue thrusting, and lip pursing. In the

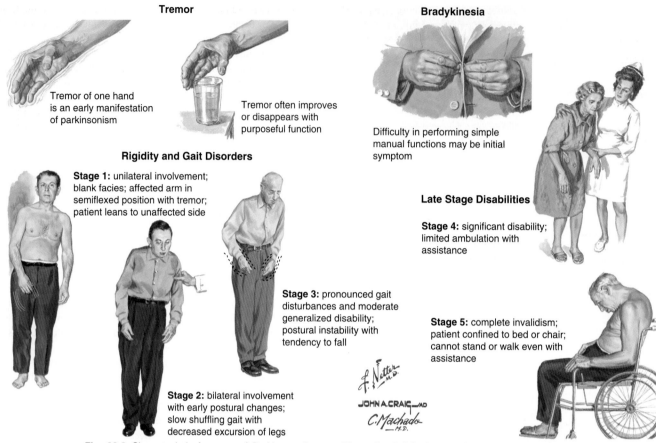

Fig. 62.2 Characteristic features of Parkinson disease. (From Small BS, Chaves C, Jayashri Srinivasan J. *Netter's Neurology.* Available from: Pageburstls, 3rd ed. Elsevier Limited (UK); 2019.)

later stages of the disease, the muscles used in swallowing may work less efficiently, causing **dysphagia** (impaired swallowing) and drooling. The muscles of mastication and orofacial function are impaired as the disease progresses; therefore, food and saliva may collect in the mouth and the back of the throat, which can cause choking and drooling. Conversely, xerostomia can result from medications. Some patients may also experience burning mouth syndrome, a pulsating, burning pain involving the anterior tongue, hard palate, lip, and alveolar ridge.

Considerations for Provision of Clinical Dental Hygiene Services and Oral Self-Care Instructions

The patient's involuntary muscle movements create a safety concern for the clinician and, in severe cases, it may be necessary to refer the patient for treatment under general anesthesia. If the patient can be treated in an office setting, extra appointment time may be needed. Additionally, appointments should be scheduled when medications taken for PD are most effective, usually 60 to 90 minutes after a meal as most medications are taken with food.[7] The patient may be susceptible to orthostatic hypotension and dizziness caused by low blood pressure induced by medications taken for PD. Therefore, the clinician should monitor vital signs, including blood pressure, and be cautious when adjusting the patient's chair and dismissing the patient. Dysphagia and impaired gag reflex are not uncommon in patients as PD progresses. To prevent choking or aspiration pneumonia, the use of high-volume evacuation and elevated chair position should be considered, while powered instrumentation and air polishing should be

limited.[7] Xerostomia is another common side effect of the medications prescribed for PD and can result in an increase in the risk for caries. The dental hygienist should consider recommending the use of sealants and fluorides to the patient or caregiver as needed. Recommendations regarding xerostomia are outlined in Box 62.3.

In the early disease stages, individuals may be able to maintain their own oral self-care, but their dexterity level must be continually assessed. As tremors and postural instability become more pronounced, it can be increasingly difficult for patients to perform their own oral self-care, and they may become more dependent on their caregivers (see Chapter 59). Patients and caregivers may find that brushing the teeth with a specially adapted manual or power toothbrush and using other adaptive aids and devices may be helpful.

Cerebral Palsy

Cerebral palsy (CP) is a chronic, nonprogressive neuromuscular disorder caused by damage to motor areas of the immature brain, affecting primarily the ability to control posture and movement. It is the second most common neurologic impairment in childhood following intellectual and developmental disability. Although CP affects muscle movement, it is not caused by problems in muscles or nerves but by abnormalities inside the brain that disrupt the brain's ability to control movement and posture.

Risk factors for CP are divided into those occurring prior to birth and those occurring after birth. Common risk factors occurring prior to birth include malformation of the central nervous system, maternal diabetes, maternal bleeding, prolonged rupture of the amniotic membranes, carrying multiple fetuses, maternal infections, exposure to toxic substances, and blood type incompatibility. Common risk factors for cases occurring during or after birth include hypoxic-ischemic encephalopathy (HIE) or lack of oxygen to the brain, complicated delivery, premature birth, low birth weight, neonatal blood infections, seizures, jaundice, injury, and not receiving proper immunizations [8,9] CP is most prevalent in males, especially in those born prematurely. Some children die in infancy, but most grow to adulthood. The main causes of death are lung and heart disease. Many types of therapy are used to help a patient reach optimum capabilities: physical and occupational therapy, speech and language therapy, biofeedback, orthopedic devices, and medications.

Clinical Symptoms

The symptoms of CP vary from mild, with only an awkwardness of movement or difficulty with fine motor skills, to severe, which may incapacitate the person completely. There may be associated conditions such as hearing and vision problems, communication problems, impairment of other senses, **epilepsy**, and intellectual and developmental challenges. CP is classified into four broad categories according to the type of movement disorder and subdivided based on the number of limbs involved: monoplegia affects one limb; diplegia, two limbs and usually both legs; triplegia, three limbs; and quadriplegia, four limbs. Hemiplegia affects both limbs on one side of the body.

The types of movement disorders are classified on the basis of motor activity and the part of the brain that was damaged (see Table. 62.3)[8]:

- *Spastic:* Most CP patients are of the **spastic** type, characterized by **spasticity** in the muscles leading to stiffness, resistance to movement, and contractures (loss of joint motion) (Fig. 62.3). The

sudden, involuntary muscle contractions or spasms result from damage to the motor area (frontal lobe) of the cerebral cortex.
- *Athetoid or Dyskinetic:* Characterized by slow, writhing, uncontrolled movements that usually affect the hands, feet, arms, or legs, and sometimes the face, causing drooling and grimacing. The movements may increase with emotional stress and disappear during sleep. Children with CP may have dysarthria (difficulties with articulation) caused by problems in speech muscle coordination. People often think that children with CP have a mental or emotional problem because of their awkward movements. However, this form of CP usually involves only the motor centers, resulting from damage to the basal ganglia.
- *Ataxic:* Associated with problems in balance, coordination, and depth perception, caused by damage to the cerebellum. The affected patients have poor coordination, walk with a wide-based gait, and may have difficulty with quick or precise movements.
- *Mixed Forms:* Spastic-athetoid type involves a combination of symptoms.

Most oral clinical findings in CP patients are related to disturbances of the oral musculature. Abnormal functioning of the tongue, lips, and cheeks can make oral clearance of food difficult, which often requires the consumption of a soft, carbohydrate-rich diet. Those who have an associated convulsive disorder may be being treated with the medication phenytoin and therefore are susceptible to gingival overgrowth, which is discussed later in this chapter.

Fractures of the maxillary anterior teeth are common because of the uncoordinated ambulation and seizures that lead to frequent falls and the lack of lip protection for the protrusive teeth. Signs of attrition and

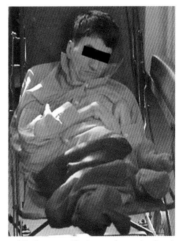

Fig. 62.3 A man with the spastic type of cerebral palsy. The spasticity of his antigravity muscles has caused his limbs to assume a severe flexed posture. (From Porter SR, Scully C, Gleeson P. *Medicine and Surgery for Dentistry.* 2nd ed. Churchill Livingstone; 1999.)

BOX 62.3 Xerostomia Therapy Protocol

Do:
- Sip on water (preferably fluoridated)
- Use saliva substitutes (sprays, lubricants, or mouth rinses)
- Chew gum or suck on mints sweetened with xylitol as needed
- Supplement with fluoride
  - Over-the-counter mouth rinse
  - Prescription paste/gel
  - Professionally applied varnish
- Use alcohol-free mouth rinses
- Use a humidifier to keep room air moist

Don't:
- Sip on sugar-sweetened beverages or those with acidic ingredients
- Drink alcoholic or caffeinated beverages
- Suck on hard candy or mints sweetened with sugar
- Use tobacco products

TABLE 62.3 Parts of the Brain Affected in Major Types of Cerebral Palsy

Type	Area of Brain Affected	Symptom
Spastic	Frontal lobe of cerebral cortex	Muscle stiffness and spasticity
Athetoid or dyskinetic	Basal ganglia	Uncontrolled movements that may affect hands feet, arms, or legs; may vary between hypertonia and hypotonia; facial grimacing and drooling
Ataxic	Cerebellum	Poor balance and coordination; difficulty with precise movements
Mixed forms	Multiple areas affected	Combination of symptoms according to area of brain affected; most common is spastic-dyskinetic

Adapted from United Cerebral Palsy of Minnesota. Available at https://ucpmn.org/.

bruxism can result from severe involuntary grinding of the teeth. The teeth of children with congenital CP may exhibit enamel hypoplasia. This enamel defect may be related to the stage of tooth development during the time of cerebral injury. Malocclusion commonly results from the abnormal functioning of the facial, masticatory, and lingual musculature, in conjunction with oral habits such as tongue thrusting, mouth breathing, and faulty swallowing. Drooling, caused by dysphagia and hypotonic lip muscles, frequently is observed.

Gastroesophageal reflux disease (GERD) is common in patients with CP and can contribute to dental erosion. The occurrence of GERD in patients with CP is estimated to be as high as 75%, especially when severe gross motor disabilities are present.[9] Enamel erosion, occurring on its own or in conjunction with GERD, is frequently seen on upper and lower posterior teeth and upper incisors. Bruxism is also a common finding in patients with CP. The occurrence of bruxism may be related to several factors, including GERD, sleep disorders, motor and cognitive deficits, abnormal proprioception of the periodontium, dopamine function, and involuntary movements.[10,11]

Patients with CP have a higher risk of developing periodontal infections due to the decreased ability to perform oral self-care measures. Additionally, if the patient requires antiseizure medication, such as phenytoin, gingival enlargement may contribute to the patient's poor periodontal condition. Studies also relate CP with a higher incidence of caries, especially in patients with severe motor and cognitive deficits.[10]

Considerations for Provision of Clinical Dental Hygiene Services and Oral Self-Care Instructions

When considering dental hygiene care and oral self-care instructions, clear communication with the patient and caregiver is critical. Understanding the needs and capabilities of the patient and caregivers will allow the clinician to make appropriate recommendations for dental hygiene care in the treatment setting and at home. In consultation with the caregiver, it is important for the clinician to assess the patient's ability to communicate, whether the patient is apprehensive or fearful of dental treatment, and if the patient can be treated effectively in an office setting or if sedation and anesthesia in a specialty or hospital setting are needed. If the patient with CP is uncooperative and/or the patient's involuntary muscle movements create a safety concern for the patient and clinician, sedation may be necessary.[10] The clinician should consider scheduling an initial visit where no treatment is performed. Instead, the clinician makes a preliminary assessment of the patient and attempts to establish rapport with the patient and caregiver.

If the patient can be treated in an office setting, positioning and careful adjustment of the chair must be considered. Abnormal muscle responses or reflexes often are triggered by changing the patient's head or neck position in the dental chair. The clinician can help control the tonic labyrinthine and asymmetric tonic reflexes, as indicated in Table 62.4. Informing the patient when lowering, raising, or tilting the dental chair may also help to prevent a startled reflex.

If the patient uses a supportive wheelchair, treatment can be given with the patient in the wheelchair reclined for patient comfort and clinician accessibility. A finger guard can be worn or a ligated mouth prop can be used in order to prevent injury to the clinician. Caution must be exercised when using sharp instruments to prevent trauma to the patient and clinician.[10] Stabilization of the patient is another point to consider. Assistance may be needed from the caregiver or a member of the dental team to help stabilize the patient's head and neck. In some situations, restraints must be used to care for the patient safely. The use of restraints requires additional training by the dental team and protocols in place to obtain informed consent from the patient and/or caregiver.

Recommendations for oral self-care at home should be based on the patient's dexterity level and the patient's ability to follow through with oral self-care instructions, as well as the level of support from caregivers. If a patient with CP is unable to perform oral self-care, it is imperative that the caregiver be knowledgeable and competent in maintaining oral health for the patient. Therefore the caregiver should be included in all communication regarding the patient's oral health status, treatment recommendations, and instructions for home care, with appropriate considerations for consent. Written instructions should be given to patients and/or caregivers for home reference.

A specially adapted manual toothbrush or power toothbrush, as well as a flossing aid or device, can be suggested. Fluoride or chlorhexidine rinses can be recommended, but rinsing may have to be monitored by a caregiver. Many oral medications given to children for conditions associated with CP contain sucrose, so it is important that the oral cavity be rinsed with water after medication is given.[12] Saliva substitutes can be recommended for medication-induced xerostomia. Pit and fissure sealants should be considered for caries prevention.

Multiple Sclerosis

Multiple sclerosis (MS) is an autoimmune CNS disorder in which there is myelin sheath destruction of specific axons causing multiple neurologic symptoms that accrue over time. MS is the most common

TABLE 62.4	**Reflex Responses of Cerebral Palsy Conditions and Their Management**		
Condition	**Tonic Labyrinthine Reflex**	**Asymmetric Tonic Neck Reflex**	**Startle Reflex**
Stimuli	Tilting head backward so neck loses support	Turning head to one side, away from midline	Surprising stimuli, such as lights, movement, noises
Response	Body into full extension	Arm and leg on face side extend	Strong, uncontrolled movements of whole body
	Arms and legs extend and stiffen	Opposite arm and leg flex	
Prevention	Keep head supported and flexed	Use rear operating position	Minimize stimuli
	Maintain chair in upright position	Stabilize head in midline position	Warn patient of any changes in chair position, noises from dental equipment, using overhead lights
	Hands folded at midline		
Management	Bring arms forward	Place face in midline	Minimize movements, lights, and sounds
	Separate legs	Help flex extended arm and leg	Communicate with patient
	Massage shoulders		

Adapted from DeBiase CB. Treating the patient with cerebral palsy. *Dent Hyg News.* 1987;5:13.

Adapted from Practical Oral Care for People with Cerebral Palsy. Available at: https://www.nidcr.nih.gov/sites/default/files/2017-09/practical-oral-care-cerebral-palsy.pdf.

progressive and disabling neurologic condition affecting younger adults. It typically begins in early adulthood, with a majority of diagnoses occurring between ages 20 and 50. Females are affected more frequently, as much as three times more than males. MS is more common in the cold and temperate climates of the higher latitudes, predominantly affecting individuals of northern European ancestry.[13]

There are four classifications of MS: Clinically Isolated Syndrome, Relapsing-remitting MS (RRMS), Secondary progressive MS, and Primary progressive MS. Relapsing-remitting MS is the most common form, with over 85% of patients being diagnosed initially with RRMS.[13] Evidence suggests that MS is caused by a combination of genetic and environmental factors. Susceptibility to MS may be inherited, and all of the identified genes have been associated with immune functions. Deficiency of vitamin D is now known to be a risk factor, possibly because those who live in higher latitudes receive less sunlight intensity—those with decreased exposure to sunlight increase their susceptibility to a vitamin D deficiency, which increases the risk of MS.[13] Additionally, studies are revealing a potential relationship between obesity, especially at a young age, and increased susceptibility to MS. Research suggested a 41% increase in the odds of developing MS when a person's Body Mass Index (BMI) moves from overweight to obese.[14] The adoption of healthy lifestyle behaviors may decrease the risk of developing MS.[15] Individuals who have comorbidities as well as those who are current or past smokers have an increased risk of developing MS.[15] Epstein-Barr virus (EBV) has also been widely implicated as a leading cause of MS, with the risk of developing MS increasing more than 30% when compared to individuals who have not been diagnosed with EBV.[16] Conversely, higher income levels may act as a "protective factor" from developing MS.[15]

The main disease characteristic is the presence of numerous demyelinated nerve axons in the brain and spinal cord. The myelin sheath's lipid composition provides axon insulation, so the sheath degeneration interferes with nerve impulse transmission. Current theories favor an immunologic pathogenesis of MS, with or without the presence of a triggering infectious agent. Demyelination results from autoimmune-related inflammation, involving the action of macrophages, lymphocytes, cytokines, antimyelin antibodies, or a combination of these agents. No two individuals with MS are exactly alike, and the clinical manifestations in a particular individual are related to the lesion distribution within the CNS. Lesions may be found virtually anywhere within the white matter regions, named for the white appearance of the myelinated axons located there. The cerebral hemispheres, brainstem, cerebellum, and spinal cord are particularly vulnerable (see Fig. 62.1 and Table 62.2). The affected areas consist of discrete demyelinated plaques that range in size from a few millimeters to several centimeters and are often around the lateral brain ventricles (Fig. 62.4). The natural progression of MS is unpredictable. In most MS patients, the disease is initially relapsing and remitting, and after several years, there is a transition to a slow and relentless chronic progression. In some patients, the disease maintains a relapsing-remitting course, and in others, the course is benign, with the patient having only one or two mild exacerbations and no permanent functional disability.

Trauma, infection, and surgery have been associated with worsening of MS. Fever, heavy physical exertion, hot weather, hot showers or baths, and exposure to sunlight may cause a transient and reversible worsening of existing symptoms. The management of MS includes treating the acute exacerbation with medications, such as steroids, and preventing and treating associated medical and psychologic complications with medications appropriate for the symptoms. Currently, there are many medications that are approved by the US Food and Drug Administration (FDA) to manage symptoms, treat relapses, and

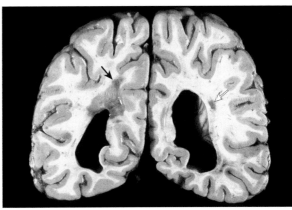

Fig. 62.4 Coronal section of the brain of a patient who had multiple sclerosis. Note the large demyelinated plaque over the left ventricle *(black arrow)* and a smaller demyelinated plaque lateral to the right ventricle *(white arrow)*. (From Little JW, et al. *Dental Management of the Medically Compromised Patient.* Available from: Pageburstls 9th ed. Elsevier Health Sciences [US]; 2018.)

modify the course of the disease. These medications can be injected, infused, or taken orally.[13] Additionally, many patients with MS take medications for bladder control, sexual function, bowel irregularity, depression, pain, and fatigue.

Clinical Symptoms

Motor symptoms are common and include muscular weakness and spasticity caused by lesions on nerve fibers from the cerebral motor cortex to the spinal cord motor neurons. Lesions in the cerebellar white matter or cerebellar pathways may produce prominent gait and ataxia (extremity incoordination) and a halting or scanning quality of speech. Severe upper extremity intention tremor may make the simplest self-care tasks impossible, and severe gait ataxia may prevent effective ambulation, even when muscular strength is adequate.

Visual disturbances (e.g., impaired visual acuity, impaired color vision, visual field deficits, double vision, optic neuritis, and pain in or behind the eye) are common and may be the first symptoms. Other sensory symptoms include numbness, tingling, impairment of temperature sensation, abnormal sense of limb position, and pain. Bladder, bowel, and sexual dysfunction can also result from the nerve conduction disturbance. Severe fatigue complaints are common, and exhaustion after an ordinary day's activities may be disabling.

Patients with MS generally rate their overall oral health as being fair to poor, with higher rates of oral dryness, toothache, tooth sensitivity, orofacial pain, and taste sensation.[17] Patients with MS exhibit extraoral complications. They often experience facial pain, temporomandibular joint and muscle dysfunction, and sometimes trigeminal neuralgia (see discussion later in this chapter). With progression of MS, as the patient loses muscular coordination, oral hygiene care is difficult, and the involvement of the tongue and facial muscles interferes with the self-cleansing mechanisms in the oral cavity. Medications for symptoms of MS may induce xerostomia or gingival enlargement.

Considerations for Provision of Clinical Dental Hygiene Services and Oral Self-Care Instructions

Relapses in disease symptoms may be stimulated by various types of infections. Frequent dental hygiene appointments help prevent oral infections and thus prevent exacerbations of the disease process. Short appointments scheduled in the morning may minimize fatigue, and a comfortable, quiet, relaxed environment should be provided to reduce stress. The patient may be sensitive to heat, so the room temperature must be kept cool. Patients may have incontinence problems, so frequent bathroom breaks may be needed.

Disturbances in the MS patient's visual acuity must be considered in discussions of oral health maintenance. Because of the patient's limited dexterity, power or modified toothbrushes and other powered devices, such as a water flosser or irrigator, may be easier for the patient to use. Recommendations for xerostomia are outlined in Box 62.3. Patients may have a slow response to instructions; using visual aids in the office and providing written instructions for the patient and caregiver to take home may enhance patient compliance.

Amyotrophic Lateral Sclerosis

Amyotrophic lateral sclerosis (ALS), also known as Lou Gehrig disease, is a progressive neurodegenerative disease that affects the cells in the nervous system, particularly motor neurons of the brain and spinal cord. The condition causes a lack of muscle nourishment that leads to muscle atrophy (wasting away). This "progressive degeneration" refers to the cell death of the motor neurons, which debilitates the brain's ability to initiate and control muscle movements. As these nerve cells degenerate, sclerosis (scarring and hardening) in the brain and spinal cord region occurs. Sclerosis then affects the nerve cells that signal and control muscle movements such as those involved with speech, eating, movement of limbs, swallowing, and walking. Sclerosis can ultimately lead to loss of breathing and resultant death.

There are two types of ALS, sporadic and familial. Sporadic ALS is the most common (90% to 95% of cases) and generally affects those individuals who are 55 to 65 years of age. The cause is unknown because there are no known risk factors, such as a family history of ALS. Familial ALS (5% to 10% of cases) is inherited from a parent. Researchers have identified mutations in several genes that can cause ALS. White and non-Hispanic males are at higher risk than females of any other ethnicity.[18]

No cure exists for ALS, but research is ongoing. Radicava, Rilutek, Tiglutik, Exservan, and Nuedexta are medications approved by the FDA to slow the progression of ALS.[18,19] Previously approved for IV administration, an oral form of Radicava has been most recently approved by the FDA. Palliative care (see Chapter 52), providing relief from the symptoms to promote comfort, is delivered upon diagnosis. The type of palliative care needed will depend on the patient's current symptoms and needs. An interprofessional approach is required to enhance the patient's quality of life. This may include professionals in physical therapy, social workers, respiratory therapists, psychologists, speech therapists, and homecare, and/or hospice workers. A variety of medications can be prescribed for symptoms such as muscle twitches, muscle cramps, depression/anxiety, bronchial secretions, pain, constipation, GERD, or insomnia. Antidepressants and antianxiety medications are prescribed because a person with ALS retains their mental capabilities, such as reasoning, remembering, understanding, and problem solving. Thus psychologic disorders are very common at all stages of the disease.

Clinical Symptoms

Symptoms will vary from person to person, depending on the stage of the disease. Typically, once a person is diagnosed, the disease progresses quickly and leads to a life expectancy of 3 to 5 years due to respiratory complications. However, some individuals will live longer and may experience a slower progression of the disease. Early onset of ALS presents with muscle weakness and stiffness and can progress into a wasting and paralysis of muscles of the limbs and trunk. Range of motion (ROM) is reduced, making it difficult to sit or stand for long periods of time, to change positions frequently, or to walk fluently. Fine motor skills such as speech, swallowing, writing, facial expression, or

overall use of hands and feet become increasingly difficult. With progression of muscle loss, inability to breathe leads a person to depend on a ventilator for survival. Those with ALS may use a cane, walker, or wheelchair for mobility purposes. Box 62.4 provides information regarding compliance with the Americans With Disabilities Act of 1990 (ADA).

BOX 62.4 The Americans with Disabilities Act of 1990 (ADA)

The Americans with Disabilities Act of 1990 (ADA) is a federal civil rights law that prohibits discrimination and ensures equal opportunity for persons with disabilities to participate in mainstream American life, which includes employment, the purchase of goods and services, and participation in state and local government programs and services.

Implications for the Dental Healthcare Setting
The ADA bans discrimination against a person with a documented disability who is seeking:
* Employment
* Access to services

Building and office design includes:
* Parking, sidewalks, and ramps
* Accessible doorways (width, threshold height, and ease of opening)
* Elevators, if applicable
* Wide aisles/hallways and handrails
* Reception room, treatment area, and restroom design (furniture style, lighting, and room for navigation of wheelchairs and transfers)
* Floors (removal of deep pile carpeting and/or rugs and plants that may restrict mobility)
* Consideration of counter, telephone, drinking fountain, mirror, and paper towel dispenser height

Auxiliary aids and services must be provided when needed to communicate:
* You are encouraged to consult with the disabled individual regarding the preferred form of communication; a free telephone relay service is available by dialing 7-1-1
* A surcharge may not be imposed on disabled patients for the cost of auxiliary aids and services

Service animals must generally be permitted:
* In all public areas
* Only dogs are recognized as service animals as of March 15, 2011

Exceptions:
* Services may be denied or referred if reasonable accommodations cannot be made and there is a direct threat to the health or safety of others
* Discrimination based on an individual's current use of illegal drugs is not prohibited
* Provision of an auxiliary aid or service is not required if it is proven to result in an "undue burden" due to a significant difficulty or expense or if it would fundamentally alter the nature of the services provided

ADA definitions of disability include individuals who:
* Have a physical or mental impairment that substantially limits one or more major life activities
* Have a history or record of such impairment
* Are perceived by others as having such an impairment

Staff training is a necessary and often overlooked component in the successful provision of the ADA requirements. The Americans with Disabilities Act defines service animals; however, definitions may vary at the state and local levels. Additional information may be obtained from the relevant state attorney general's office. For more information, refer to https://www.ada.gov/service_animals_2010.htm.

Source: www.ada.gov (accessed July 12, 2022).

Considerations for Provision of Clinical Dental Hygiene Services and Oral Self-Care Instructions

Xerostomia is a very common side effect of the various medications prescribed to patients with ALS. Lack of muscle control in the face and oral cavity can increase the likelihood of the mouth being open for long periods of time, which can also lead to xerostomia. However, some patients may exhibit **sialorrhea** (excessive saliva). This condition is due not to an increase in saliva production but instead to the inability to manage normal saliva production. Excessive saliva in the patient's oral cavity can be annoying and embarrassing for the patient and can make dental treatment difficult.

The oral health status of patients with ALS has been shown to be poor overall for reasons such as diminished manual dexterity and poor oral clearance.[20] Further, aspiration pneumonia is a leading cause of death for ALS patients. Therefore, treating patients with ALS requires special consideration. The patient will need to be placed in a semisupine or upright position to prevent aspiration. If the patient uses a supportive wheelchair, it can be tilted back slightly for clinician accessibility. Control of excessive saliva can be obtained with the use of an assistant and high-volume evacuator (HVE). As mentioned previously, dysphagia is a common symptom of ALS, so the use of ultrasonic instrumentation and air polishing may be contraindicated. Shorter appointments and frequent breaks may be necessary.

It is also important to be aware that the patient may have a sensitive gag reflex, which can be triggered during intraoral radiograph exposure, dental hygiene procedures, and medicament applications. Difficulty speaking can be cumbersome while trying to communicate, and it is recommended that the patient bring someone with them during the appointment to facilitate conversation. Managing some of the above conditions is part of the palliative care that is performed by dental professionals as part of a team-oriented approach to creating a care plan for patients with ALS.

Modified brushing techniques and auxiliary aids are part of oral self-care instruction for ALS patients. The loss of muscle control can make brushing and interdental care very difficult. In all stages of the disease, modified and power toothbrushes, interdental aids, tongue scrapers, fluoride treatments, and frequent preventive care appointments are beneficial. Patients with late-stage ALS are often unable to communicate and perform oral self-care independently; however, it is important for the dental team to understand that they may still fully comprehend instructions. Therefore, the caregiver should be educated on home care instructions, and conversation should be directed to both the patient and the caregiver.

Huntington Disease

Huntington disease (HD) is a rare, highly complex neurodegenerative disorder resulting from the degeneration of neurons within the basal ganglia, the area deep in the brain that controls movement. HD also affects the cortex of the brain, which controls many things including thought, perception, cognition, and memory. HD is characterized by decline of intellectual capacity, emotional disturbances, and rapid, jerky involuntary movements called chorea. HD affects males and females of all races and ethnicities in every country around the world. Currently, there are approximately 41,000 individuals living with HD in the United States, with many more at risk of developing the disease.[21]

HD is inherited through a mutation on the huntingtin gene on chromosome 4 associated with deoxyribonucleic acid (DNA) that is passed from parent to child. This mutation is a minute pattern of DNA in which three nucleotides, cytosine, adenine, and guanine (CAG), abnormally repeat dozens of times. Through the generations, repetitions of CAG may expand even further, putting an individual at higher

risk for developing the disease earlier in life.[22] Each child of a parent with HD has a 50% chance of developing the disease. If the child has not inherited the mutated gene, they will never develop the disease and cannot pass it on to the next generation.

Clinical Symptoms

The symptoms of HD usually begin to occur during middle age—often between ages 30 and 50—although HD has been diagnosed at a young age (juvenile HD) and after age 55.[21] The symptoms can include changes in personality, mood swings, and depression, as well as impaired thinking and judgment, slurred speech, dysphagia, weight loss, and chorea. Although the progression of the disease varies between individuals, HD generally occurs in three stages: early, middle, and late. The early stage starts as minor changes in physical coordination and possible chorea. Impaired thinking, depression, and irritability also become apparent. The affected individual is not able to maintain the same level of activity as in the past.

During the middle stage, the patient's movements become more difficult to control, and chorea may become more pronounced. Difficulties with speech, eating, swallowing, and walking may necessitate speech, occupational, or physical therapy for the patient. Encouraging patients with HD to keep active and exercise is crucial to helping the patient feel better physically and mentally. Medications such as tetrabenazine and antipsychotic drugs are given to help control choreic movements, along with antidepressants to combat symptoms of depression. In some cases, antipsychotic medications are given to control delusions, hallucinations, and uncontrolled violent outbursts.

The late stage of HD is characterized by the patient's inability to speak or walk, although some individuals may still be able to understand language, communicate emotion, and recognize family and friends. Chorea may be severe or, in some cases, cease altogether. Around-the-clock care is required for the patient, and proper nutrition and hydration is of the utmost importance. Choking also becomes a major concern for the patient and caregiver, and swallowing therapy may be necessary. Patients with HD are at high risk for swallowing impairment and severe dysphagia.[22] It is common for patients with HD to die from secondary complications, such as choking, injuries sustained from falls, or pneumonia.

HD is fatal and, at present, no cure is available. Because of the complexity of this disease, an interprofessional approach, including primary care physicians, dietitians, therapists, counselors, social workers, and oral health professionals, is essential to the quality and continuity of care. Treatment consists of managing the symptoms of HD, usually with medications. However, many of the drugs that are available have debilitating side effects, and it can be difficult for the patient and caregiver to distinguish a symptom of HD from a response to medication. Research on this disease gained momentum in the late 20th century in the fields of molecular genetics, neurobiology, psychology, and psychiatry, and research efforts are continuing.

Considerations for Provision of Clinical Dental Hygiene Services and Oral Self-Care Instructions

Xerostomia associated with antidepressant and antipsychotic medications used to treat the symptoms of HD is very common in these patients. The reduction of salivary flow can lead to higher incidence of caries, not to mention the discomfort associated with dry mouth. Saliva substitutes, xylitol, and fluoride can provide protection from caries. However, as HD progresses and patients have difficulty with swallowing, oral health professionals should use caution when recommending oral care products for home use, as these could become choking hazards. As the patient's functional ability declines, it is imperative that the dental team be prepared to provide appropriate care.

Patients may present with various oral conditions associated with HD, including dysphagia, poor oral and pharyngeal clearance, rigidity of the mandible, and lingual chorea. Additionally, oral and facial trauma resulting from frequent falls and injuries, severe bruxism, and low tolerance for dental prostheses has been noted.[23] Poor biofilm control, increased caries, increased gingival and periodontal disease, and tooth loss were also found in patients with HD.[22] Patients with HD will require treatment modifications during the dental visit as the disease worsens. Clinicians may need to help with transfers if the patient uses a wheelchair (see Chapter 59). Positioning the back of the patient chair in a semisupine or upright position and using pillows, rolled blankets, or cushions will help stabilize and relax the patient. Limiting or discontinuing the use of powered instrumentation may be indicated to prevent difficulty swallowing and reduce the risk of choking. Assistance by other team members with suctioning, retraction, and stabilization may be necessary. During the early and middle stages of HD, local anesthesia can be used for restorative care. However, as the disease progresses, intravenous sedation or general sedation will be necessary for most treatment.

Providing oral self-care instructions with emphasis on prevention to patients with HD and their caregivers is important during all stages of the disease. Dental hygienists should consider the wide array of dental care devices, manual and powered, when making recommendations to the patient and/or caregiver. Toothbrushes that clean the buccal and lingual surfaces simultaneously, such as the Collis curve toothbrush, are recommended. The use of weighted wrist cuffs or weighted handles may help to control the chorea and increase stability for the patient.[23] Dental hygienists should consider the patient's dexterity and customize a care plan to meet the patient's current needs. Because of the degree of motor impairment and the difficulty performing adequate homecare, patients with HD should have frequent dental visits, as often as necessary, to maintain good oral health and preserve the natural dentition for as long as possible. Many patients with HD do not receive the healthcare services, including oral health services, that are necessary to maintain health-related quality of life.[24,25] An approach that includes an interdisciplinary and multidisciplinary team is imperative, and the dental hygienist plays a key role in offering care and guidance to the patient and caregivers. When compared to patients without HD, those patients with the disease have an impaired oral health status.[24] A thorough preventive oral health program should be implemented as soon as HD is diagnosed to prevent oral disease and potentially harmful sequelae.

DYSFUNCTIONS OF THE CENTRAL NERVOUS SYSTEM

Traumatic Brain Injury and Posttraumatic Stress Disorder

Traumatic brain injury (TBI) is an acquired brain injury that occurs when an external force disrupts the normal function of the brain. The acute phase of TBI may be caused by the force of an explosive blast or a blow or jolt to the head resulting in a closed injury. It may also be caused by a penetrating, open injury of the head. Postconcussive symptoms may not occur until a few days after the initial injury, and a chronic phase may follow due to an inflammatory response. Postconcussion syndrome (PCS) is a long-term consequence of TBI in which symptoms may persist for longer than a year. Another chronic condition is a delayed neurodegenerative disorder known as chronic traumatic encephalopathy (CTE), which has been identified in the postmortem brains of individuals with repetitive brain injuries.[26]

The gold standard for diagnosis of TBI is the clinical interview, which judges difficulties with learning, memory, concentration, and

problem solving.[27] TBI severity is then classified as mild (includes concussion), moderate, or severe, depending upon the extent of the damage to the brain. Factors affecting classification include the score on an injury indicator scale, such as the Glasgow Coma Scale (GCS), with additional consideration of the duration of altered mental state or loss of consciousness and duration of posttraumatic amnesia. The results of brain imaging procedures, such as computed tomography (CT) scans, can also contribute to the classification of TBI.[26,28]

Surveillance reporting by the Centers for Disease Control and Prevention (CDC) has established key findings related to TBI. Some common causes are blows to the head from or against an object, such as in sports injuries, assault, and military service.[29] The most common causes of TBI hospitalization are unintentional falls and motor vehicle accidents (MVAs), whereas suicide and unintentional falls were the most common causes of TBI-related death.[29] The age group most often affected are adults aged 75 years and older. Males have significantly higher rates as compared to females, and the racial/ethnic group with the highest rates are American Indian/Alaska Native.[29]

Psychiatric disorders, including **posttraumatic stress disorder (PTSD)**, frequently occur following a traumatic brain injury. PTSD is a disorder that develops following either a physical or emotional trauma. It shares many of the same symptoms as TBI and also manifests as intrusion symptoms of upsetting memories, nightmares, and flashbacks. Avoidance behaviors and guilt may also be present. When both TBI and PTSD are diagnosed concurrently, there are increased neuropsychiatric complications, health risks, and cognitive impairments.[30,31]

Clinical Symptoms

Clinical symptoms can cause a lower functional outcome as well as a decreased quality of life. Cognitive impairment is characteristic of TBI.[28] Cognitive elements may include slowed information processing, attention problems, and confusion. Behavioral changes may be demonstrated as irritability, emotional instability, and hyperactivity. Common physical manifestations are motor and sensory impairment as well as somatic symptoms (e.g., headache, fatigue, sleep disturbance, dizziness, nausea, and chronic pain).[26,28] The differentiation of symptoms for TBI and PTSD is often difficult; a need exists to include treatment for PTSD following TBI to improve patient outcomes.[27]

Considerations for Provision of Clinical Dental Hygiene Services and Oral Self-Care Instructions

Specific protocols for patient management depend not only on the extent of the injury but also on the health of the individual before the injury, access to appropriate healthcare, family and social support, and the therapies involved. Treatments for TBI and PTSD are individualized and may include a variety of psychotherapy and pharmaceutical mechanisms. Cognitive behavioral therapy (CBT), in particular, is effective for improving cognition in the treatment of TBI, and it is effective for reducing anxiety symptoms in both TBI and PTSD. Prescribed drugs may include antidepressants, antipsychotics, and other medications.[31] The use of stem cell therapy is currently being studied and may offer new options for TBI and PTSD recovery in the future.[30]

TBI and PTSD may create challenges with daily tasks, including oral self-care. It is important for the healthcare provider to establish the patient's mental capabilities and communication skills. There may also be behavioral complications, physical disabilities, and medication-related concerns present.[32] Furthermore, involvement of family members and/or caregivers may be required not only to help provide stress relief and strengthen coping abilities but also to participate in decisions regarding a care plan and for the provision of oral self-care measures. Medication use increases the potential occurrence of xerostomia, which elevates the patient's risk level for dental caries and periodontal disease (see Box 62.3). Measures should be employed to avoid a decline in oral health. The patient and/or caregivers should be instructed on proper methods of daily toothbrushing, interdental care, and selection of a nonalcohol-containing mouth rinse. Regular continuing care appointments are important, and the healthcare professional should learn appropriate skills and techniques to meet the unique oral healthcare needs of TBI and PTSD patients.[32]

Spinal Cord Injury

The spinal cord is a part of the CNS and is secondary to the brain in complexity. It lies within the vertebral column and serves three basic functions: to conduct sensory impulses from the PNS to the brain; to conduct motor impulses from the brain to muscles and glands; and to serve as a reflex center. There are 31 pairs of spinal nerves that arise along the spinal cord. These nerve pairs are numbered according to the level at which they emerge from the spinal column. The most superior are 8 cervical pairs, followed by 12 thoracic pairs, 5 lumbar pairs, 5 sacral pairs, and finally 1 coccygeal pair, which is the most inferior. All spinal nerves are referred to as mixed nerves because they contain both sensory and motor axons. Spinal cord dysfunction may be of traumatic (injury) or nontraumatic (inflammation or infection) origin and may cause permanent changes in strength, sensation, and other body functions below the site of the injury.

Spinal cord injury (SCI) is caused primarily by MVAs but also may be caused by falls, acts of violence, sports and recreation accidents (especially diving), and diseases. Risk factors for SCI are male gender (about 80%), 16 to 30 years of age (more than 50%) or over 65 years of age, alcohol use (about 25%), engaging in risky behavior (diving in shallow water or playing sports without the proper gear), or having certain diseases, such as cancer, arthritis, osteoporosis, and inflammation/infections of the spinal cord or disk degeneration of the spine. The effects experienced from SCI will correspond to the level of the spinal nerves affected and extend inferiorly. The lowest level of the spinal cord that functions normally is referred to as the *neurologic level*. The severity of the injury to those nerves is also a factor and is referred to as the *completeness*. A complete injury indicates the loss of almost all sensation and all ability to control movement below the SCI. An incomplete injury retains some sensory and motor function below the affected area. Injuries may also be described as paraplegia, which describes involvement of the trunk, legs, and pelvic organs, or tetraplegia (also

termed quadriplegia), which is more extensive and also involves the arms and hands.[33]

Clinical Symptoms

Assessment of SCI describes the neurologic level and the completeness of the injury. The extent of motor function at various levels and the person's potential for independence are indicated in Table 62.5. Signs and symptoms may include loss of movement, loss of or altered sensation (temperature and touch), loss of bowel or bladder control, exaggerated reflex activities or spasms, changes in sexual function, sexual sensitivity and fertility, pain or an intense stinging sensation caused by damage to the nerve fibers in the spinal cord, and difficulty breathing, coughing, or clearing secretions from the lungs.[33]

Considerations for Provision of Clinical Dental Hygiene Services and Oral Self-Care Instructions

Individuals with SCI face physical, financial, psychological, and social barriers to dental care. The oral clinical findings, subsequent special considerations for dental hygiene care, and oral self-care instructions depend on the neurologic level and completeness of SCI. Adaptations for persons with disabilities are described in Chapter 59. Patients using wheelchairs may be treated more easily in their wheelchairs, in either a reclined or an upright position. Transferring patients from their wheelchairs increases the risk of serious accidents or other complications.

The SCI population experiences all of the risk factors for the development of oral diseases as are experienced by the general population, as well as some issues unique to this group. Use of both smoking and smokeless tobacco is common in people with SCI and is a risk factor for periodontal disease, recession, and root caries. Impaired mobility and environmental barriers impede the completion of self-care measures independently. Scheduling and transportation to dental appointments are likely to require the assistance of a caregiver. Furthermore, for tetraplegic patients, the mouth and teeth play a critical role in performing a variety of tasks. The use of mouth-held appliances for driving and controlling devices, such as a mouthstick, may cause trauma to the hard and soft oral tissues as well as harboring microorganisms (Fig. 62.5). The widespread use of antidepressants and anticholinergic agents can cause xerostomia and increase the risk of oral diseases. Last, depression can reduce patient motivation to perform self-care and seek professional care.

TABLE 62.5 Functional Significance of Spinal Cord Lesions

Level	Intact Sensation and Motor Ability	Deficit[a]	Functional Potential and Independence	Required Aids
C4	Head and upper neck	1, 2, 3, 4	None	WC, ventilator, tracheotomy
C5	Lateral upper arm[b]	1, 2, 3, 4	Minimal	Electric WC
C6	Lateral forearm and hand[b]	1, 2, 3, 4	Sitting, eating with devices	Manual WC, hand splints
C7	Middle finger[b]	1, 2, 3, 4	Personal self-care with devices	Manual WC
C8–T1	Medial hand and forearm[b]	1, 2, 3, 4	Personal self-care, WC self-transfers	Manual WC
T1–T6	Upper trunk[b]	2, 3, 4, 5	Complete, WC self-transfers	Manual WC, leg braces
T11–L2	Torso, anterior thigh[b]	3, 5	Complete, limited walking	Manual WC, leg braces
L4–L5	Medial and lateral leg, dorsal foot[b]	3, 5	Complete	Foot braces, crutches
S2–S4	Posterior thigh, calf, lateral foot[b]	4, 6	Complete	Catheter
S5	Complete except ring around anus	None	Complete	None

[a]1, Quadriplegia; 2, impaired respiration; 3, some reflex control of pelvic organs (bowel, bladder), sexual function; 4, impaired autonomic reflexes, poor thermoregulation, orthostatic hypotension; 5, paraplegia; 6, lack of control of pelvic organs.
[b]Plus regions at preceding levels.
WC, Wheelchair.

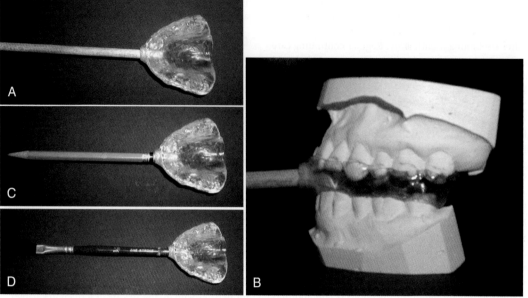

Fig. 62.5 Mouthsticks. (A) Custom-fabricated mouthstick for persons with tetraplegia. (B) Mouthstick is fabricated so that the biting forces are equally distributed across the maxillary arch. (C–D) Hole on anterior surface of mouth guard can also hold a pencil or a paintbrush. (Courtesy of Kathleen Muzzin, Texas A&M University, Baylor College of Dentistry, Caruth School of Dental Hygiene, Dallas, Texas.)

Studies have shown that people with SCI are often unaware of their oral health needs. A lack of routine oral self-care measures such as toothbrushing, interdental care, and mouth rinsing may also be due to personal attitudes, time spent dealing with other health issues, depressive mood, or reliance on a caregiver. Recommendations can be summarized by emphasizing the need to educate and encourage the SCI population and/or caregivers to consistently seek preventive and therapeutic oral healthcare. More specific recommendations include mouthstick hygiene, biofilm control, healthy diet, and the use of fluoride and sealants. If xerostomia is present, recommendations for care are outlined in Box 62.3. Finally, power toothbrushes or adaptations to manual toothbrushes are modifications that will make oral self-care possible.

Seizures

A **seizure** is a sudden, uncontrolled burst of electrical activity in the brain that causes a temporary interruption of communication between neurons. This alteration in cerebral function has a typical duration of 30 seconds to 2 minutes. It is considered to be a medical emergency if it lasts 5 minutes or longer.[34,35]

Seizures are common and every person has the potential to have a seizure. Some identified causes include a high fever, lack of sleep, flashing lights, low blood sodium, drug use (prescription or illegal), head trauma, cardiovascular disorders, autoimmune disorders, brain tumor, alcohol use, COVID-19 virus infection, and metabolic imbalances. Many times, the specific cause cannot be identified.[34,35]

There are three major classifications for seizure types. They are focal onset, generalized onset, or unknown onset. Focal seizures are caused by abnormal electrical activity in one area of the brain, whereas generalized seizures involve diffuse areas of the brain. A spectrum of symptoms may range from mild to severe and may be described as motor or nonmotor (alterations in a person's emotions and/or level of consciousness). A diagnosis of epilepsy is related to two or more seizures occurring at least 24 hours apart with unknown onset.[34–36]

Epilepsy

Epilepsy is a seizure disorder in which the excessive abnormal neuronal discharges from cerebral function disturbances are recurrent and unprovoked. The specific underlying brain dysfunction causing the seizure disorder is not a temporary medical condition.[37] Worldwide, epilepsy is ranked as the fourth most common neurological disorder.[35]

Clinical Symptoms

Within the three major classifications, there are many types of seizures. The most common ones are described here.[36]

- **Generalized Onset Seizures** affect both sides of the brain and may be tonic-clonic, absence, or atonic. **Tonic-clonic seizures** (formerly called grand mal) are the most common type and can be divided into several phases, beginning with vague prodromal symptoms (aura) that occur hours to days before the convulsion. A series of brief, bilateral muscle contractions may precede the tonic phase. Tonic (stiffening) contractions begin in the trunk and progress, including contraction of abdominal muscles, producing forced expiration across the vocal cords and causing the characteristic cry or groan (Fig. 62.6). In the clonic (convulsion) phase, the arms and legs bend and relax as the tonic contractions alternate with loss of muscle tone, causing rhythmic jerking of all four extremities, until contractions cease (Fig. 62.7). The face may begin to turn blue if breathing is affected. Autonomic dysfunction (loss of bowel and bladder control) often occurs during the tonic and clonic phases. Persons experiencing seizures may bite the tongue or break bones as a result of the violence of the jerking during the clonic phase. Afterward the individual may enter a deep sleep or experience headaches, muscle aches, and stiffness. The duration is usually 1 to 3 minutes. Call 911 if the seizure lasts longer than 5 minutes or if there are three seizures in a row without the individual regaining consciousness between them. This is called **Status Epilepticus** and is a life-threatening medical emergency that can lead to irreversible neurologic damage. **Absence seizures** (formerly called petit mal) are common in children 4 to 14 years of age and consist of brief

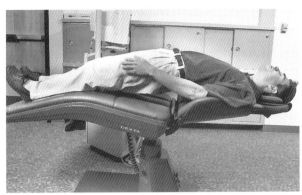

Fig. 62.6 A patient during the tonic phase of a generalized tonic-clonic seizure (grand mal). Note the extensor rigidity of the extremities and trunk. (Adapted from Malamed SF. *Medical Emergencies in the Dental Office.* 7th ed. Mosby; 2015.)

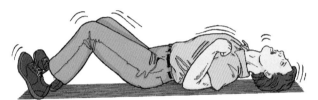

Fig. 62.7 Diagrammatic representation of the violent flexor contractions of the clonic phase of a generalized tonic-clonic seizure (grand mal). (From Malamed SF. *Medical Emergencies in the Dental Office.* 6th ed. Mosby; 2007.)

episodes of an altered state of consciousness or staring into space. Changes in muscle tone may include eyelid blinking, lip smacking, or hand motions. The duration is usually 10 to 20 seconds, recovery is immediate, and there is no recollection of the seizure.[36]

- **Focal Onset Seizure** is a term that depicts the origin of the seizure in one area of the brain more accurately than using the term "partial." These can be further divided into Focal Onset Aware Seizures or Focal Onset Impaired Awareness Seizures.[36]
- **Unknown Onset Seizures** describe a seizure when the beginning is not known by the individual or it is not witnessed by anyone. It may be classified as focal or generalized when more information is learned.[36]

Seizures and epilepsy themselves do not produce oral changes, but the accidents resulting during the seizures and the medications used to treat the condition may have negative effects. Scarring of the lips, buccal mucosa, and especially the tongue may be indicative of past injury to the oral cavity during a seizure. Teeth also may have been fractured from the forceful biting that frequently occurs during a tonic-clonic seizure (Fig. 62.8).

Pharmacologic therapies are effective in preventing seizures, and several are available (see Box 62.5). However, phenytoin may cause severe gingival enlargement or overgrowth (Fig. 62.9). The drug alters the metabolism of the gingival fibroblasts so that the cells produce excessive amounts of collagen. This drug-influenced gingival enlargement, which occurs in approximately half of these patients, may be disfiguring and may interfere with mastication and speech. See the critical thinking scenario in Box 62.6.

Considerations for Provision of Clinical Dental Hygiene Services and Oral Self-Care Instructions

Major considerations in managing patients with epilepsy are prevention of seizures in the dental chair and preparation for managing seizures if they occur. When a patient responds positively to seizures on a

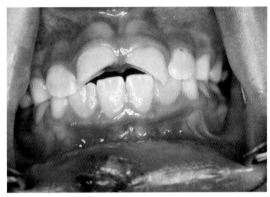

Fig. 62.8 Fractured teeth and lacerated lower lip sustained during a grand mal seizure. (From Little JW, et al. *Dental Management of the Medically Compromised Patient.* Available from: Pageburstls. 9th ed. Elsevier Health Sciences [US]; 2018.)

BOX 62.5 **Medications Used to Treat Seizures**
Carbamazepine (Carbatrol; Tegretol)
Phenytoin (Dilantin; Phenytek)
Valproic acid (Depakene)
Oxcarbazepine (Oxtellar; Trileptal)
Lamotrigine (Lamictal)
Gabapentin (Gralise; Neurontin)
Topiramate (Topamax)
Phenobarbital
Zonisamide (Zonegran)

Adapted and used with permission of Mayo Foundation for Medical Education and Research. All rights reserved.

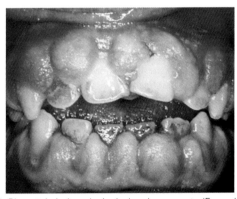

Fig. 62.9 Phenytoin-induced gingival enlargement. (From Little JW, et al. *Dental Management of the Medically Compromised Patient.* Available from: Pageburstls. 9th ed. Elsevier Health Sciences [US]; 2018.)

BOX 62.6   **Critical Thinking Scenario**
A new patient is scheduled for an initial exam. The health history form reveals the patient has a history of seizure activity and takes medication, but does not list what medicines are taken. What types of questions should you ask to further understand your patient's condition? What actions should you take before beginning any invasive clinical procedures? The patient is unsure as to why the history of seizure activity is relevant to dental hygiene care and seems agitated by your questions. You know that they needs to understand why it is important for you to learn about this condition. What information can you share with your patient to help persuade them to comply with your request for information about their seizure history?

health history form, further information should be obtained. Examples of questions are listed in Chapter 13. Based on the patient's responses, treatment may need to be postponed to prevent triggering a seizure in the dental chair. Nitrous oxide and oxygen sedation is known to elicit seizures in patients with epilepsy, so it is not recommended for them. Likewise, fatigue can induce seizures, so appointments should be made early in the day. Despite all preventive measures, seizures may still occur. Management focuses on preventing injury and maintaining the patient's airway (see Chapter 11).

Continuing care intervals should be established with a goal of maintaining or regaining oral health. In the presence of phenytoin-induced gingival enlargement, the interval should be shortened according to the severity of the condition. Frequent maintenance visits, along with excellent oral self-care, have been shown to diminish the drug-induced gingival changes. Calculus and overhanging restorations are irritants and must be removed. It is also imperative that oral hygiene instruction is individualized and reinforced at every appointment. Furthermore, the dental team should be aware that a seizure-predicting or seizure-response service dog may be utilized by the patient during dental appointments. See Box 62.4 regarding ADA compliance and service animals.

DYSFUNCTIONS OF THE PERIPHERAL NERVOUS SYSTEM

Peripheral Neuropathies

Peripheral neuropathies are conditions that develop as a result of damage to the PNS. Normally, the dendrites of peripheral sensory cranial and spinal nerves receive input from the body or external environment, and the axons transmit signals to cells in the CNS. Cells in the CNS process this information and respond via motor, sensory, or autonomic nerves. Peripheral neuropathy is due to damage to the axons or to the myelin sheath around the axon, which distorts the signals between the CNS and the rest of the body.

Motor nerve damage results in muscle weakness, twitching, atrophy, and decreased reflexes. Sensory nerve damage may cause pain, numbness and tingling, paresthesias (prickles or "pins and needles"), or an inability to feel pain (sensory loss). It may also result in temperature sensations (cold or burning), uncoordinated movements, or sensations of imbalance (particularly with eyes closed). Autonomic nerve damage may result in an inability to sweat normally (regulate body temperature), bowel or bladder problems, low blood pressure, malfunction of nerves in the gastrointestinal tract, or malfunction of the nerves involved in eating and swallowing.

Metabolic disorders, particularly diabetes mellitus, are the most common cause of peripheral neuropathy; however, they may also result from autoimmune disorders, infections, genetic disorders, tumors, or conditions that affect the bone marrow. Moreover, peripheral neuropathy may be caused by alcoholism, exposure to poisons, use of specific medications (chemotherapy), injury, and some vitamin deficiencies. It may also be idiopathic.[38,39] Specific symptoms of neuropathic conditions vary depending on the type (or types) of nerves damaged. Some neuropathies are acute in nature and have a sudden onset, a rapid progression, and also slow resolution as the nerves heal. On the other hand, chronic neuropathies develop slowly and progress in a variety of formats that can be described as either episodic, as in reaching a plateau, or as consistently increasing in intensity.[39]

Neuropathic pain is common. It ranges in severity from tingling to burning or stabbing pain. It often affects the ability to participate in daily activities and decreases quality of life. Peripheral neuropathy can

be difficult to treat, but medication, therapy, or surgery may alleviate the pain.[38]

Facial Neuropathy or Bell Palsy

Bell palsy is the most common cause of facial paralysis. It is also known as idiopathic facial paralysis because the exact etiology is unknown. A viral cause is suspected. The onset is acute, usually unilateral, and of temporary duration. Scientists believe that the facial nerve (cranial nerve VII) becomes inflamed due to viral infection. The swelling causes compression that disrupts the flow of blood and oxygen to the nerve cells and leads to facial weakness or paralysis. This disorder can occur at any age, but it is most common in the 15- to 45-year age group and secondarily in the 70 and above age group. Individuals with diabetes, influenza, upper respiratory ailments, or who are pregnant are affected disproportionately. An iatrogenic form of facial neuropathy and paralysis may result from injections of local anesthesia (see Chapter 43) or from oral surgery procedures.[40,41]

Clinical Symptoms

There is no laboratory test and a diagnosis is based on clinical presentation and ruling out other possible causes of facial paralysis. Patients typically describe facial distortion that began suddenly and reached its peak within 48 to 72 hours. The main clinical feature is weakness of the facial muscles on the affected side that ranges from mild to complete paralysis (Fig. 62.10) and may include facial pain. Symptoms that affect the eyes are drooping of eyelids; inability to close the eye completely, which causes dryness; and excessive tearing of the eye. Other symptoms affecting the mouth are drooping of the corner of the mouth, difficulty with eating, food entrapment on the affected side of the mouth, drooling, and altered sensation, including taste. Patients may also experience pain in or behind the ear and increased sensitivity to sound on the affected side of the face.[40,41]

Considerations for Provision of Clinical Dental Hygiene Services and Oral Self-Care Instructions

Approximately 85% of patients experience improvement in symptoms within 3 weeks and most recover completely. Yet, residual symptoms are common when the condition is untreated. Oral corticosteroids are used for their antiinflammatory effects and appear to be of greatest benefit when started within 72 hours of onset of symptoms. Although antiviral agents are sometimes prescribed, there is no evidence to support their use when used alone, and it is unclear whether there are additional benefits when used in conjunction with corticosteroids. Over-the-counter analgesics may alleviate pain; however, their use

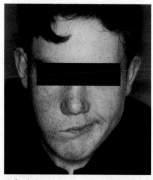

Fig. 62.10 Unilateral facial paralysis in a patient with Bell palsy. In the man's attempt to smile, there is a lack of movement of the entire right face and forehead muscles. (From Little JW, et al. *Dental Management of the Medically Compromised Patient*. Available from: Pageburstls. 9th ed. Elsevier Health Sciences [US]; 2018.)

should be recommended by a physician due to potential adverse drug interactions. Numerous other treatments exist; however, there is either no evidence or only low-quality evidence demonstrating any benefit. These therapies include facial exercises, acupuncture, massage, thermotherapy, electrical stimulation, and surgical treatment.[40,41]

It is essential that patients institute measures to prevent injury to the affected area(s) during convalescence. Eye protection, which may include the use of lubricants, artificial tears, and protective eyewear, is essential if the eye cannot be closed fully.[40,41] Oral trauma, such as cheek biting, is a concern due to both the lack of muscle tone and potential for altered sensation.

Loss of muscle tone in the oral musculature affects the ability to chew and maintain a self-cleansing environment. The retention of food in the vestibule on the affected side increases the risk of periodontal diseases and dental caries. This may be further complicated by xerostomia, glossitis, and candidiasis. The presence of drooling can encourage the development of angular cheilitis.

In the dental setting as well as at home, the patient should wear protective eyewear to prevent foreign material, including aerosols and spatter, from entering the eye. Antifungal medications are prescribed for candidiasis and angular cheilitis. A specific self-care regimen should be implemented. Sensation loss may impede the patient's ability to brush safely and effectively. Establishing a brushing pattern helps the patient avoid missing areas. Interdental care should be chosen based on individual factors. Rinsing with water after eating and using an oral irrigator will help to remove food from the vestibule. The use of a chemotherapeutic mouth rinse without alcohol; a dentifrice containing fluoride, calcium, and phosphate ingredients; and dry mouth products with xylitol is also beneficial.[42]

Trigeminal Neuralgia

Trigeminal neuralgia or tic douloureux is a neuropathy of the trigeminal nerve (cranial nerve V) that results in one of the most painful, chronic disorders of the orofacial region. The condition is seen more often in females, and most cases occur over the age of 50. The cause is thought to be pressure from a blood vessel against the trigeminal nerve as it exits the brainstem. In rare cases, the cause may be pressure from a tumor or a vascular malformation. This pressure can wear away the protective myelin sheath around the nerve, leading to abnormal signals to the brain and resulting in pain. For this reason, it may also be linked to a diagnosis of multiple sclerosis, which is characterized by damage to the myelin sheath, in young adults. Finally, damage to the trigeminal nerve may result from iatrogenic injury during oral or sinus surgery or from facial trauma for some individuals.[43,44]

Clinical Symptoms

Trigeminal neuralgia has two characteristic presentations. Type 1 causes episodes of severe, sudden, burning, or shocking pain that may last for a few seconds or up to 2 minutes and may recur repeatedly within a 2-hour period. Type 2 is a more constant but less intense aching, burning, or stabbing pain.[43] Trigeminal neuralgia can be debilitating, both physically and mentally.[44] Individuals often isolate themselves socially and may benefit from counseling in addition to medical or surgical treatment for their pain.[43]

The symptoms usually occur unilaterally in the areas of the face innervated by the trigeminal nerve, including the cheek, jaw, teeth, gums, and lips. Since the maxillary and mandibular branches are affected more often than the ophthalmic branch, the eye and forehead are less often affected.[45] It can be triggered by even mild vibrations or light contact with the cheek, as may occur in common daily activities such as speaking, eating, shaving, washing the face, applying makeup, brushing teeth, or being exposed to the wind. Attacks are episodic

and periods of remission between attacks may last for months or even years. Eventually, the pain occurs more frequently and lasts longer as periods of remission become fewer and shorter.[43,45]

Diagnosis is difficult and complicated by the large number of other conditions that also cause facial pain. Patient interview and clinical assessment combined with neurological examinations contribute to the differential diagnosis. Moreover, the successful response to a short course of anticonvulsant medication supports a diagnosis of TN1 and low doses of tricyclic antidepressants support the diagnosis of TN2. Patients may also choose to complement pharmacological therapy with a wide variety of other techniques such as yoga/exercise, visualization/meditation, aromatherapy, acupuncture, chiropractic, biofeedback, vitamin or nutritional therapy, or injections of botulinum toxin. Success of these methods varies by individual. Several surgical procedures are available, particularly for TN1, if drug treatment is not tolerated or becomes ineffective as the condition progresses.[43]

Considerations for Provision of Clinical Dental Hygiene Services and Oral Self-Care Instructions

No significant intraoral findings are due to the disease alone. Side effects such as xerostomia may result from medications. The intensity of the pain can cause avoidance of oral self-care based on its potential to trigger an attack. This increases the risk for periodontal and dental diseases. Oral self-care recommendations must be individualized to prevent triggering pain.

Because of the typical location of the pain, dentists are most often contacted initially. The clinician must perform a thorough assessment and consider the patient's report of activities that trigger pain. It is important for dental professionals to be knowledgeable about the characteristic signs and symptoms as reported by individuals who are affected by TN, specifically, "shocking" or "stabbing" facial pain of high intensity and short duration with complete resolution between episodes. Common triggers are also important to recognize, including talking, chewing, or touch.[44]

It is well established that distinguishing trigeminal neuralgia from odontogenic pain is challenging. Several studies report that patients commonly received invasive and possibly unnecessary dental treatment prior to referral to other healthcare professionals.[44,46] Those procedures were primarily tooth extraction and root canal therapy. One retrospective study found that only 21% of dentists made a referral to another healthcare provider. Nearly a quarter of the patients were seen by a neurologist or neurosurgeon within 6 months of symptom onset, but more than 40% took more than 2 years for an evaluation.[46] This emphasizes the need for timely, appropriate referrals and interprofessional collaboration between the dental professional and neurologist or neurosurgeon to determine a correct definitive diagnosis.[44,46]

DISORDERS OF HIGHER CORTICAL FUNCTION

Dementia

Dementia is characterized by a progressive intellectual decline that eventually leads to deterioration of occupational, social, and interpersonal functions. Onset is usually insidious, with memory disturbances frequently attributed to the normal aging process. Even though dementia may occur at all ages, the incidence of most dementias, including Alzheimer disease, rises substantially with increasing age. Dementia differs from the decline of physiologic processes during aging. As patients age, mental processes can slow, but healthy older patients still retain a firm grasp on reality, are oriented, can reason, have good judgment, and can continue to lead an active and self-supporting life. Further characteristics of the normal elderly patient are described in Chapter 47.

All forms of dementia result from the death of nerve cells and/or the loss of communication among these cells. Although genes play a role, a single genetic abnormality has not been associated with the condition. Major risk factors are age and genetics/family history, but risk factors also may include diabetes, Down syndrome, mental illness, hypoxia and anoxia, brain tumor or trauma, toxins, and medications.[47]

Clinical Symptoms

In early stages, individuals often complain of diminished energy and enthusiasm, show less interest in subjects they previously cherished, and may show emotional instability and heightened anxiety levels because of the awareness of failing mental functions. As the disease progresses, other areas of cognition become impaired: orientation, language, perceptions, ability to learn new skills, calculation, abstraction, and judgment. The patient becomes increasingly self-absorbed, anxiety increases, and the recognition of personal failure may lead to depression. At this stage, there may be pronounced mood swings and poor judgment, followed by diminished drive and feeling. As the mental deterioration progresses, anxiety and depression disappear and are replaced by complete flatness of mood. Personal cleanliness deteriorates, and patients will do little, if anything, spontaneously. At this stage, other neurologic dysfunctions, such as hemiparesis (one-sided weakness) and seizures, may develop. Once the patient has reached the point of complete flatness of mood, inability to communicate, and total dependence on others, even treatable dementias are usually irreversible. Consciousness is preserved until terminal stages. Considerations for provision of clinical dental hygiene services and oral self-care instructions for a patient with dementia are discussed further in the next section.

Alzheimer Disease

Alzheimer disease (AD) is a brain degenerative disorder that gradually destroys the ability to remember, reason, learn, and imagine. AD is the most common cause of dementia and is ultimately fatal. It is the seventh leading cause of death in the United States and is the fifth leading cause of death among individuals over age 65. For those over 65, the number of cases is expected to reach 12.7 million by the year 2050.[48] The etiology of AD is similar to that described for dementia, with age as the most significant risk factor. Genetics and family history also are strongly associated with the development of the disease. Other risk factors include smoking and alcohol use, atherosclerosis, Down syndrome, diabetes, mental illness, TBI, and hypertension.[48] The brain lesions of AD are characterized by beta-amyloid plaques—abnormal clumps of beta-amyloid protein and degenerating neurons and other cells—and neurofibrillary or tau tangles, which are irregular knots of cytoskeletal intermediate filaments found within neurons. Both contribute to the decreased activity and progressive destruction of neurons and atrophy of the cerebral cortex, the area of the brain associated with intellectual functions (Fig. 62.11).

Over the past several decades, the relationship between periodontal pathogens and their role in nonoral diseases, such as AD, has been studied extensively. The presence of oral microorganisms, such as *Porphyromonas gingivalis,* and the inflammatory mediators associated with periodontal infection have been identified in the brain tissue, specifically the parts of the brain associated with memory, in patients with AD.[49,50] The existence of *P. gingivalis* in brain tissue may be due in part to the ability of this microbe to secrete proteases called gingipains. Gingipains are specific to *P. gingivalis* and have the ability to break down host tissue and suppress host defenses, specifically the blood-brain barrier in the case of AD. Elevated levels of gingipains have been found in postmortem brain tissue of AD patients.[49] These higher levels of gingipains are associated with tau tangles in the brain that are characteristic

of AD.[50] The relationship between oral microflora and AD is highly complex and not fully understood, and the role of *P. gingivalis* in the pathogenesis of AD continues to be studied. Regardless, it is widely understood that periodontal health and the reduction of the oral bacterial load is beneficial for all patients, especially those with cognitive impairment. While treating patients with AD presents with a unique set of challenges, creating a healthier oral environment is critical to preserving the dentition and maintaining an acceptable quality of life for the patient.

Clinical Symptoms

In the early and middle stages of AD, affected individuals may be painfully aware of their intellectual decline, and it is important to support their emotional and mental health with affection and warmth. In the beginning, there is simple forgetfulness, especially of directions to familiar places or recent events. There also may be personality changes such as restlessness, increased stubbornness, distrust, poor judgment and impulse control, and increased difficulty with activities requiring planning and decision making. Affected individuals may begin to withdraw socially. As the disease progresses, the ability to perform daily living tasks is lost, and there may be trouble recognizing everyone except the person's closest daily companions. Communication becomes difficult as the ability to speak and write declines. In the last stages of the disease, patients with AD become bedridden, have difficulty swallowing and controlling bowel and bladder function, and are unable to recognize themselves or their closest family members.

Currently, the FDA has approved six drugs for the treatment of AD. Donepezil, rivastigmine, galantamine, memantine, and memantine combined with donepezil are used to temporarily treat the symptoms

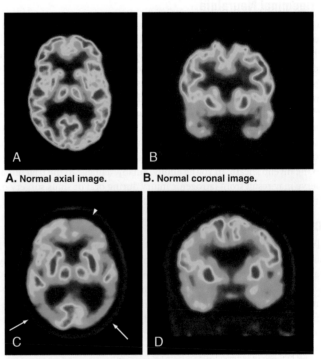

A. Normal axial image.   **B.** Normal coronal image.

C. and D. Reduced activity within temporal and parietal lobes (arrows) and early decreased activity in left frontal lobe consistent with advancing disease (arrowhead).

Fig. 62.11 Fluorodeoxyglucose—positron emission tomography typical pattern for Alzheimer disease. PET scanning using biomarkers for beta-amyloid has allowed researchers to image the presence and distribution of amyloid plaque in AD patients. (From Small BS, Chaves C, Jayashri Srinivasan J. *Netter's Neurology.* Available from: Pageburstls. 3rd ed. Elsevier Limited (UK); 2019.)

of AD in various ways. These drugs may improve the ability to think and remember; however, they do not change the course of the disease and do not alter any of the brain changes associated with AD. Aducanumab, approved through the accelerated approval pathway by the FDA in 2021, works within the brain to reduce the beta-amyloid plaques described above. Aducanumab has only been tested on patients with mild cognitive impairment and mild dementia due to Alzheimer disease and is still being tested by the manufacturer.[48]

In addition to drug therapy, nondrug treatments are also used to support the patient and improve the overall quality of life. Nondrug treatments include cognitive behavior therapy, music therapy, and cognitive stimulation. Because there is no cure for AD, treatment is aimed at slowing progression of the disease and improving quality of life for the patients. The period from the earliest symptoms to death has an average duration of 8 years. Death usually results from a secondary illness such as urinary tract infection or pneumonia.

Considerations for Provision of Clinical Dental Hygiene Services and Oral Self-Care Instructions

Patients with AD have more gingival disease and caries than the normal elderly population, mainly because of poor oral hygiene from significant neglect.[51] Patients forget to brush, forget how to brush, may not want to brush, or may be resistant to a caregiver brushing their teeth. Medications, such as phenytoin to control seizures, may cause gingival enlargement (see Fig. 62.9) and may induce salivary gland dysfunction.

A frightened and frustrated patient may demonstrate uncooperative, even combative, behavior, so patients with AD are managed best with a caring and understanding approach (Box 62.7). Appointments should be scheduled early in the day and preferably when the office is not busy. The office environment should be as free of unnecessary noise, people, and physical clutter as possible. The caregiver should accompany the patient to discuss special patient management issues as well as oral care procedures.

In the early stages of AD, the patient should be encouraged to be self-sufficient. Toothbrushing instructions should be given slowly, step by step, in simple, concrete language. As the disease progresses, the patient becomes more dependent on a caregiver for oral homecare, so the caregiver needs to be familiar with these procedures. Although a power toothbrush may be easier for a caregiver to use on the patient, a manual toothbrush may be necessary if the patient cannot tolerate the noise and vibration from the power toothbrush. Mouth rinses are not usually recommended because the patient may not understand that it would be harmful to swallow. Both the patient and caregiver should be given clear written instructions regarding homecare. Additionally, demonstrating proper oral care techniques and recommending appropriate cleaning aids is a good way to motivate the patient and caregiver and encourage compliance.

CEREBROVASCULAR DISEASE

Cerebrovascular Accident or Stroke

Cerebrovascular accident (CVA) or stroke occurs when there is an abrupt interruption of oxygenated blood circulation to the brain resulting in the death of brain cells and onset of neurologic deficits. This interruption is the consequence of either ischemia or hemorrhage.[52] Strokes are the fifth leading cause of death in the United States.[53] Strokes are also the most common cause of disability in adults, despite the fact that they are preventable and treatable.[52] Risk factors for CVA are listed in Box 62.8.

The major risk factor for CVA is hypertension, which increases the chance of experiencing a stroke by 2 to 4 times. Hypertension is a modifiable risk factor that can be addressed with proper diet, exercise, and prescription medications. Another modifiable risk factor is smoking, which multiplies the chance of having a stroke by two. Nicotine is also known to elevate blood pressure and is a cause of hypertension. Furthermore, hypertension and cigarette smoking are both linked to

---

> **BOX 62.7 Techniques for Communicating With Patients With Alzheimer Disease**
>
> - Greet the patient in a cheerful and reassuring voice. Shake hands with the patient and escort the patient and the caregiver (if present) to the treatment area.
> - Use a calm, soft voice pattern. Speak slowly and clearly, in short sentences; allow ample time for comprehension.
> - The patient's attention span may be short, so schedule extra time for greeting, seating, and handling the patient.
> - Explain procedures before treatment.
> - Repeat instructions and explanations in exactly the same words.
> - Keep everything as simple as possible. Tell patients what you need them to do instead of giving them a choice.
> - Limit use of ultrasonic devices as the water flow may cause the patient to choke or feel overwhelmed by the noise and activity.
> - Distract patients who are uncooperative or argumentative by changing the activity, or take advantage of their forgetfulness by leaving the room for a few minutes and then returning and cheerfully trying the same activity again.
> - Use supportive body posture and facial motion, such as direct eye contact and smiling.

> **BOX 62.8 Risk Factors for Cerebrovascular Accident**
>
> **Modifiable Risk Factors**
> - Hypertension
> - Smoking
> - Heart disease
> - Warning signs or history of TIA or stroke
> - Diabetes
> - Cholesterol imbalance
> - Physical inactivity and obesity
>
> **Nonmodifiable Risk Factors**
> - Age; babies and adults (increases with age)
> - Sex; younger males have higher risk
> - Sex; females have higher lifetime risk (birth control, hormone replacement, pregnancy)
> - Race and ethnicity; African American, Alaska Native, American Indian, Hispanic
> - Family history; genetics
>
> **Other Risk Factors**
> - Anxiety, depression, and high stress levels
> - Exposure to air pollution
> - Other medical conditions; bleeding disorders, sleep apnea, sickle cell disease
> - Medications that can increase bleeding
> - Unhealthy lifestyle habits; poor diet, inactivity, alcohol abuse, drug abuse, too much sleep
> - Overweight and obesity
>
> Source: National Heart, Lung, and Blood Institute; National Institutes of Health; U.S. Department of Health and Human Services. Available at https://www.nhlbi.nih.gov/health/stroke/causes

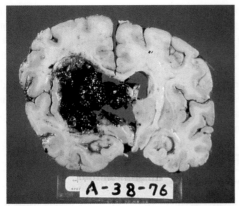

Fig. 62.12 Cerebral infarction in an individual who had chronic hypertension. Blood from the intracerebral hemorrhage has displaced the brain tissue. (From Little JW, et al. *Dental Management of the Medically Compromised Patient.* Available from: Pageburstls. 9th ed. Elsevier Health Sciences [US]; 2018.)

BOX 62.9 Differences Between Right-Sided Brain Damage and Left-Sided Brain Damage

Right-Sided Brain Damage	Left-Sided Brain Damage
• Paralyzed left side	• Paralyzed right side
• Spatial or perceptual deficits	• Language and speech problems
• Impaired thought process	• Decreased auditory memory (cannot remember long instructions)
• Quick, impulsive behavior	
• Patient cannot use a mirror	• Slow, cautious, disorganized behavior
• Difficulty performing tasks (toothbrushing)	
• Memory deficits—for events or people, generalized	• Memory deficits—language-based
• Neglect of left side	• Anxiety

Adapted from Little JW, et al. *Dental Management of the Medically Compromised Patient.* Available from: Pageburstls. 9th ed. Elsevier Health Sciences [US]; 2018.

---

atherosclerosis and narrowing of the arteries.[52] The most important measure in preventing strokes is detection and treatment of hypertension. However, multiple other risk factors may be contributing influences and must be taken into consideration in the development of an effective risk reduction approach that is individualized for each patient.

The most common type of CVA, ischemic stroke, results when a blockage prevents blood flow and adequate circulation of oxygen.[52] The diminished or absent blood flow into the brain tissues may occur in one of three ways: an **embolism** is a blood clot that travels to the brain from another part of the body; **thrombosis** refers to a clot that develops within a blood vessel of the brain or neck; and **stenosis** is a severe narrowing of an artery associated with the brain. The ischemia leads to infarction (necrosis or death) of brain tissue supplied by the affected artery or arteries.[52,54]

The other type of CVA is a hemorrhagic stroke. This type results from the rupture of a brain vessel and leakage of blood into the brain tissue or the space between the brain and skull. The displaced blood exerts pressure on the brain, causing damage. The rupture may be the result of high blood pressure or an **aneurysm**, which is a bulge in an artery due to a weakness in the blood vessel wall (Fig. 62.12).[52,54]

Regardless of the underlying cause of a stroke, an area of brain tissue is deprived of an adequate blood supply for a period of time. The neurons of the brain start to die in minutes.[54] If the oxygenated blood supply is restored to the brain in time, there will be total resolution of the neurologic deficit. A **transient ischemic attack (TIA)** is a transient focal neurologic deficit that persists for less than 24 hours and is followed by complete clinical recovery. Most TIAs last less than 10 minutes as the blockage dissolves on its own and is not in place long enough to cause permanent damage to the brain. TIAs are often referred to as "ministrokes" and more recently as "warning strokes" since 10% to 15% of people will have a major stroke within 3 months of having a TIA.[54] Although a TIA is of shorter duration than a major ischemic stroke, it is still a medical emergency, and the emergency response services (EMS) system should be alerted immediately.[52,54]

Clinical Symptoms

The right and left hemispheres specialize in different functions, and the two sides of the brain are interconnected. Sensory and motor axons cross on their way to or from the cerebral cortex so the left side of the brain controls motor and sensory input for the right side of the body and vice versa. Therefore, the side of the face and body affected is opposite that of the brain injury. Box 62.9 illustrates the differences between right-sided and left-sided brain damage.

CVAs can cause various health complications. Signs and symptoms depend on the brain sites affected, but the following are the more common ones:

- Motor impairments or paralysis. These are the most common deficits and usually involve face, arm, and leg, alone or in combination on the same side. Motor functions affected include cranial nerve functions to muscles of the head and neck, reflexes, gait, balance, and coordination. Often, there is apraxia (the inability to perform purposeful movements), although no muscular paralysis or sensory disturbance is present.
- Language. Difficulty speaking or swallowing (dysphagia) occurs when the muscles of the mouth and throat are affected.
- Cognition. There is often aphasia after a stroke, manifested by disturbances in comprehension and expression. Strokes can cause deficits in thinking, memory, and understanding of concepts.
- Depression. This is the most common affective disturbance after a stroke. Symptoms of depression include lack of interests, energy loss, insomnia, and appetite loss. Stroke patients also may display emotional instability and changes in self-care ability.
- Sensory deficits. Impairments range from loss of primary senses (e.g., vision, pain, temperature, touch) to more complex losses of perception.[55]

Treatment for stroke survivors primarily involves reducing the modifiable risk factors, as listed in Box 62.8, and prescribing anticoagulant or antiplatelet medications to prevent clot formation, antihypertensive agents to reduce blood pressure, and statins to manage cholesterol. A surgical procedure called carotid endarterectomy may be performed to remove plaque buildup from the carotid artery and restore blood flow. Occupational and physical therapy can help the stroke survivor learn new ways of performing activities of daily living, sometimes with the aid of assistive devices such as braces, wheelchairs, and special utensils. Speech therapy may also be indicated.

Considerations for Provision of Clinical Dental Hygiene Services and Oral Self-Care Instructions

The specific oral findings of a CVA survivor depend on the areas of the brain affected and the type of CVA, as well as the resultant dysfunction. Motor dysfunction effects and xerostomic effects of prescribed medications have been described previously. Dental caries and periodontal diseases can be prevalent because of poor oral hygiene. Periodontal disease is associated with the risk of CVA as well as heart disease (see Chapter 21). However, despite periodontal pathogen invasion into the periodontium, which induces bacteremia and a systemic inflammatory response, a causal relationship has not been established.

A positive response to CVA on the health history form should elicit several followup questions, which are listed in Chapter 13. This information, in conjunction with a physician consultation, determines the need for treatment modifications. It is recommended that the CVA survivor not undergo any elective dental care within 6 months of the episode.

A patient who has had a CVA is at a greater risk for having another one, so prevention of a recurrence is of utmost concern. Factors such as pain and anxiety add to the risk and so must be managed by creating a safe and comfortable environment. Efforts should be made to minimize fatigue and optimize energy and patience for clinician and patient.

Blood pressure should be monitored carefully because marked deviations in blood pressure increase the risk for recurrent CVAs. Blood pressure of 180 mm Hg systolic and/or 120 mm Hg diastolic or higher is considered hypertension crisis and warrants immediate medical consultation before any type of dental treatment is initiated. Many CVA and TIA survivors receive anticoagulant therapy, which predisposes them to excessive bleeding. Oral infection presence may cause changes in blood coagulation factors, which may trigger a repeat CVA. The minimum amount of a local anesthetic with vasoconstrictor is recommended.

Identification of a suspected stroke is also critical, and clinicians must be familiar with the signs and symptoms. Watch for sudden numbness or weakness on one side of the face, arm, or leg; confusion or speech difficulties; vision problems; dizziness; or severe headache with no known cause. To identify the signs of a stroke, the acronym FAST has been developed. The letters stand for:

- F—Face drooping on one side
- A—Arm weakness or numbness
- S—Speech difficulty
- T—Time to call 911

Remember to make a note of the time of symptom onset in order to give information to the emergency medical personnel. Transport to the hospital setting, assessment, and diagnosis must be completed as promptly as possible since treatments are most effective when initiated within 3 hours.[54]

During the immediate post-CVA phase, caregivers perform all daily hygiene functions; therefore, they need proper toothbrushing demonstrations and instructions, and/or information about maintenance of any dental prosthesis so that they can perform these tasks until the patient has relearned them. Even during the rehabilitation phase, patients with residual physical deficits may need assistance performing oral hygiene procedures. Special adaptations that foster the CVA survivor's self-sufficiency were described previously and in Chapter 59.

The discomfort from xerostomia can be alleviated by saliva substitutes and associated dry mouth products (see Box 62.3). Fluoride therapy and xylitol gum and mints are beneficial to prevent root caries (see Chapter 19).

APPLICATION TO PRACTICE, SERVICE, OR INTERPROFESSIONAL WORK

Individuals living with disabilities have a higher incidence of oral disease than the general population. Dental hygienists can integrate their knowledge of patients with special needs to make a difference in a population that may not have access to care. Working in public health and partnering with organizations that serve people with disabilities, dental hygienists can provide education to individuals and their caregivers on proper oral self-care, good nutrition, and the importance of maintaining regular preventive care visits. Furthermore, dental hygienists, in collaboration with other healthcare professionals, can provide referrals if necessary to specialty dental or medical providers. Last, dental hygienists can work with other healthcare professionals to improve oral health outcomes and follow best practices.

KEY CONCEPTS

- The provision of effective treatment for the patient with neurologic disabilities presents a potential challenge for the dental team. Poor oral hygiene is often observed in this population for many reasons, which include difficulty performing oral self-care, inability to maintain regular preventive care appointments, and in some cases, caregivers who are overwhelmed. In order to provide an appropriate care plan, dental hygienists must have knowledge of dysfunctions of the motor system, dysfunctions of the central nervous system, peripheral neuropathies, disorders of higher cortical function, and cerebrovascular disease.
- The dental hygienist must understand the etiology, risk factors, pathologic characteristics, clinical symptoms, treatment, and prognosis of neurologic disorders for patient assessment. This will allow the formulation of a customized care plan that outlines treatment and oral self-care recommendations with the goal of optimizing oral and overall health.

ACKNOWLEDGMENT

The authors acknowledge Dorothy J. Rowe, Brenda S. Kunz, Lee E. Wentworth, and Mechee Thomas for their past contributions to this chapter.

REFERENCES

1. Sharma S, Pandey S. Approach to a tremor patient. *Ann Indian Acad Neurol.* 2016;19(4):433–443. https://doi-org.eps.cc.ysu.edu/10.4103/0972 -2327.194409.2. EBSCOhost
2. Louis ED, Ottman R. How many people in the USA have essential tremor? Deriving a population estimate based on epidemiological data. *Tremor and Other Hyperkinetic Movements (New York, N.Y.).* Aug 14, 2014;(259):4. https://doi.org/10.7916/D8TT4P4B.
3. What Is Parkinson's? American Parkinson Disease Assoc. *American Parkinson Disease Association*; 24 Mar. 2022. www.apdaparkinson.org/ what-is-parkinsons/?utm_source=bing. Accessed May 19, 2022.
4. Guo T, Chen L. Gut microbiota and inflammation in Parkinson's disease: pathogenetic and therapeutic insights. *Eur J Inflamm.* 2022:1–15. https://doi-org.eps.cc.ysu.edu/10.1177/1721727X221083763. EBSCOhost
5. Kim JS, Sung HY. Gastrointestinal autonomic dysfunction in patients with Parkinson's disease. *J Mov Disord.* 2015;8(2):76–82. https://doi. org/10.14802/jmd.15008.
6. "Levodopa." Parkinson's Foundation. www.parkinson.org/ UnderstandingParkinsons/Treatment/Prescription-Medications/ Levodopa. Accessed May 31, 2022.
7. Newadkar UR, Khairnar SJ, Dodamani AS, Newadkar RD. Oral health issues and challenges in Parkinson's disease. *Int J Nutr Pharmacol Neurol Dis.* 2017;7:54–59. https://doi.org/10.4103/ijnpnd.ijnpnd_22_17.
8. "What are the risks for cerebral palsy?" Eunice Kennedy Shriver National Institute of Child Health and Human Development, National Institutes of Health, 11 May, 2022, https://www.nichd.nih.gov/health/topics/cerebral-palsy/conditioninfo/risk-factors. Accessed June 2, 2022.
9. Asgarshirazi M, et al. Evaluation of feeding disorders including gastro-esophageal reflux and oropharyngeal dysfunction in children with cerebral palsy. *J Fam Reprod Health.* 2017;11(4):197–201. https://search. ebscohost.com/login.aspx?direct=true&AuthType=ip,uid&db=a9h&AN= 130042486&site=ehost-live&scope=site. EBSCOhost

10. Wasnik M, et al. Dental management of children with cerebral palsy – a review. *Journal of Oral Research & Review*. 2020;12(1):52–58. https://doi-org.eps.cc.ysu.edu/10.4103/jorr.jorr_19_19. EBSCOhost

11. Souza VAF, et al. Factors associated with bruxism in children with developmental disabilities. *Braz Oral Res*. 2015;29:1–5. https://doi.org/10.1590/1807-3107bor-2015.vol29.0009.

12. Jan BM, Jan MM. Dental health of children with cerebral palsy. *Neurosciences*. 2016;21(4):314–318. https://doi.org/10.17712/nsj.2016.4.20150729.

13. Who gets MS? National Multiple Sclerosis Society; 2022. https://www.nationalmssociety.org/What-is-MS/Who-Gets-MS. Accessed July 1, 2022.

14. Mokry LE, et al. Obesity and multiple sclerosis: a mendelian randomization study. *PLoS Med*. 2016;13(6):1–16. EBSCOhost https://doi-org.eps.cc.ysu.edu/10.1371/journal.pmed.1002053.

15. Veronese N, et al. Adherence to a healthy lifestyle and multiple sclerosis: a case-control study from the UK Biobank. *Nutr Neurosci*. 2022;25(6):1231–1239. https://doi.org/10.1080/1028415X.2020.1846357.

16. Bjornevik K, et al. Longitudinal analysis reveals high prevalence of Epstein-Barr virus associated with multiple sclerosis. *Science (New York, N.Y.)*. 2022;375(6578):296–301. https://doi.org/10.1126/science.abj8222.

17. Sexton C, Lalloo R, Stormon N, et al. Oral health and behaviours of people living with Multiple Sclerosis in Australia. *Community Dent Oral Epidemiol*. 2019;47:201–209. https://doi.org/10.1111/cdoe.12445.

18. Amyotrophic Lateral Sclerosis (ALS) Fact Sheet. National Institute of Neurological Disorders and Stroke; April 25, 2022. https://www.ninds.nih.gov/health-information/patient-caregiver-education/fact-sheets/amyotrophic-lateral-sclerosis-als-fact-sheet. Accessed July 1, 2022.

19. "FDA Approved Drugs for Treating ALS." ALS.org., 2022, https://www.als.org/navigating-als/living-with-als/fda-approved-drugs. Accessed July 1, 2022.

20. de Sire A, et al. Functional status and oral health in patients with amyotrophic lateral sclerosis: a cross-sectional study. *Neuro Rehabilitation*. 2021;48(1):49–57. doi:10.3233/NRE-201537 21.

21. "Who is at risk?" Huntington's Disease Society of America, 2022, https://hdsa.org/what-is-hd/history-and-genetics-of-huntingtons-disease/who-is-at-risk/. Accessed July 5, 2022.

22. Munhoz L, et al. The oral manifestations of Huntington's disease: a systematic review of prevalence. *Oral Dis*. Nov 12, 2021. https://doi.org/10.1111/odi.14076.

23. Manley G, et al. Guideline for oral healthcare of adults with Huntington's disease. *Neurodegen. Dis. Manage*. Feb 15, 2012. http://www.ehdn.org/wp-content/uploads/2016/08/Guideline_for_oral_heathcare_of_adults_with_HD.pdf. Accessed July 1, 2022.

24. Saft C, et al. Oral and dental health in Huntington's disease – an observational study. *BMC Neurol*. Sep 3, 2013;(114):13. https://doi.org/10.1186/1471-2377-13-114.

25. van Walsem MR, et al. Health-related quality of life and unmet healthcare needs in Huntington's disease. *Health Qual Life Outcome*. Jan. 7, 2017;15(16). https://doi.org/10.1186/s12955-016-0575-7.

26. Focus on Traumatic Brain Injury Research. National Institute of Neurological Disorders and Stroke, U.S. Department of Health and Human Services; July 6, 2022. https://www.ninds.nih.gov/current-research/focus-disorders/focus-traumatic-brain-injury-research. Accessed July 10, 2022.

27. Alway Y, et al. Factors associated with posttraumatic stress disorder following moderate to severe traumatic brain injury: a prospective study. *Depress Anxiety*. 2016;33:19–26.

28. Centers for Disease Control and Prevention. *Report to Congress on Traumatic Brain Injury in the United States: Epidemiology and Rehabilitation*. Atlanta, GA: National Center for Injury Prevention and Control; Division of Unintentional Injury Prevention; 2015.

29. Centers for Disease Control and Prevention. *Surveillance Report of Traumatic Brain Injury-Related Hospitalizations and Deaths by Age Group, Sex, and Mechanism of Injury—United States, 2016 and 2017*. Centers for Disease Control and Prevention, U.S. Department of Health and Human Services; 2021.

30. Monsour M, et al. A review of the pathology and treatment of TBI and PTSD. *Exp Neurol*. 2022;351:114009. https://doi.org/10.1016/j.expneurol.2022.114009.

31. Post-Traumatic Stress Disorder. National Institute of Mental Health. U.S. Department of Health and Human Services; 2019. https://www.nimh.nih.gov/health/topics/post-traumatic-stress-disorder-ptsd. Accessed July 5, 2022.

32. Developmental Disabilities & Oral Health. National Institute of Dental and Craniofacial Research. U.S. Department of Health and Human Services; 2020. https://www.nidcr.nih.gov/health-info/developmental-disabilities. Accessed July 5, 2022.

33. Spinal Cord Injury. Mayo Clinic, Mayo Foundation for Medical Education and Research; Oct. 2, 2021. https://www.mayoclinic.org/diseases-conditions/spinal-cord-injury/symptoms-causes/syc-20377890. Accessed July 5, 2022.

34. Seizures. Mayo Clinic. Mayo Foundation for Medical Education and Research; Feb. 24, 2021. https://www.mayoclinic.org/diseases-conditions/seizure/symptoms-causes/syc-20365711. Accessed July 5, 2022.

35. Kiriakopoulos E. Understanding Seizures. Epilepsy Foundation. https://www.epilepsy.com/what-is-epilepsy/understanding-seizures. Accessed July 5, 2022.

36. What Is Epilepsy? Epilepsy Foundation; 2022. https://www.epilepsy.com/what-is-epilepsy. Accessed July 5, 2022.

37. Epilepsy Fast Facts. Centers for Disease Control and Prevention; Sept. 30; 2020. https://www.cdc.gov/epilepsy/about/fast-facts.htm. Accessed July 5, 2022.

38. Peripheral Neuropathy. Mayo Clinic. Mayo Foundation for Medical Education and Research; July 3, 2021. https://www.mayoclinic.org/diseases-conditions/peripheral-neuropathy/symptoms-causes/syc-20352061. Accessed July 5, 2022.

39. Peripheral Neuropathy. National Institute of Neurological Disorders and Stroke. U.S. Department of Health and Human Services; May 4, 2022. https://www.ninds.nih.gov/health-information/disorders/peripheral-neuropathy. Accessed July 5, 2022.

40. Bell's Palsy Fact Sheet. National Institute of Neurological Disorders and Stroke. U.S. Department of Health and Human Services; April 25, 2022. https://www.ninds.nih.gov/health-information/patient-caregiver-education/fact-sheets/bells-palsy-fact-sheet. Accessed July 5, 2022.

41. Gagyor I, et al. *Antiviral Treatment for Bell's Palsy (Idiopathic Facial Paralysis)* – Gagyor, I – 2019: Cochrane Library. Cochrane Database of Systematic Reviews. John Wiley & Sons, Ltd; Sept. 5, 2019. https://www.cochranelibrary.com/cdsr/doi/10.1002/14651858.CD001869.pub9. Accessed July 2, 2022.

42. Kandray DP. Treating patients with Bell's palsy. *Dimensions of Dental Hygiene*. 2014;12(3):40–42.

43. Trigeminal Neuralgia Fact Sheet. National Institute of Neurological Disorders and Stroke. U.S. Department of Health and Human Services; Apr. 25, 2022. https://www.ninds.nih.gov/health-information/patient-caregiver-education/fact-sheets/trigeminal-neuralgia-fact-sheet. Accessed July 1, 2022.

44. Porto De Toledo I, et al. Prevalence of trigeminal neuralgia. A systematic review. *JADA (J Am Dent Assoc)*. 2016;147(70):570–576. https://doi.org/10.1016/j.adaj.2016.02.014.

45. Trigeminal Neuralgia. Mayo Clinic. Mayo Foundation for Medical Education and Research; Jan. 26, 2022. https://www.mayoclinic.org/diseases-conditions/trigeminal-neuralgia/symptoms-causes/syc-20353344. Accessed July 5, 2022.

46. Von Eckardstein KL, et al. Unnecessary dental procedures as a consequence of Trigeminal Neuralgia. *Neurosurg Rev*. 2014;38(2):355–360. https://doi.org/10.1007/s10143-014-0591-1.

47. Ranson JM, et al. Modifiable risk factors for dementia and dementia risk profiling. A user manual for brain health services-part 2 of 6. *Alzheimer's Res Ther*. Oct. 11, 2021;13(1):169. https://doi.org/10.1186/s13195-021-00895-4.

48. Alzheimer's Disease Facts and Figures. Alzheimer's Association. *Alzheimers Dement*. 2022;18. https://www.alz.org/media/Documents/alzheimers-facts-and-figures.pdf. Accessed July 10, 2022.

49. Ryder MI, Xenoudi P. Alzheimer disease and the periodontal patient: new insights, connections, and therapies. *Periodontol 2000*. 2021;87(1):32–42. https://doi.org/10.1111/prd.12389.

50. Olsen I, Singhrao SK. Is there a link between genetic defects in the complement cascade and porphyromonas gingivalis in Alzheimer's

disease? *J Oral Microbiol.* 2020;12(1):1–9. https://doi.org/10.1080/2000229 7.2019.1676486. EBSCOhost.

51. Chan AKY, et al. Common medical and dental problems of older adults: a narrative review. *Geriatrics.* Aug. 6, 2021;6(3):76. https://doi.org/10.3390/geriatrics6030076.

52. Brain Basics: Preventing Stroke. National Institute of Neurological Disorders and Stroke. U.S. Department of Health and Human Services; Apr. 7, 2022. https://www.ninds.nih.gov/health information/patient caregiver-education/brain-basics-preventing-stroke. Accessed July 7, 2022.

53. FASTSTATS - Leading Causes of Death. Centers for Disease Control and Prevention; Jan. 13, 2022. https://www.cdc.gov/nchs/fastats/leading-causes-of-death.htm. Accessed July 9, 2022.

54. About Stroke. Centers for Disease Control and Prevention; May 24, 2022. https://www.cdc.gov/stroke/types_of_stroke.htm. Accessed July 5, 2022.

55. Stroke. Mayo Clinic. Mayo Foundation for Medical Education and Research; Jan. 20, 2022. https://www.mayoclinic.org/diseases-conditions/stroke/symptoms-causes/syc-20350113. Accessed July 6, 2022.

63

Professional Development and Job Searching

Elizabeth C. Kornegay

PROFESSIONAL DEVELOPMENT OPPORTUNITIES

Professional development in dental hygiene should be a continual process as professionals assess their careers to adapt to ever-evolving personal characteristics, life changes, and changes within the profession. Analyzing oneself, cultivating and exploring personal and professional interests, learning from mentors, creating professional and personal goals, and organizing those goals in a plan can empower dental hygienists to navigate the profession and offer a path to career satisfaction.

COMPETENCIES

1. Develop a professional career plan by performing a self-assessment, building a network for professional enhancement and a relationship with a mentor, establishing professional career goals, and creating an action plan.
2. Research employment opportunities to identify a desired dental hygiene position.
3. Prepare for a job application by developing a résumé, cover letter, and list of references; prepare for a job interview by creating a list of personal statements, questions, and other considerations. Communicate effectively in a job interview and follow up appropriately afterward.
4. Prioritize employment factors, including compensation, employment rights and evaluation, the expanding scope of dental hygiene, potential sources of burnout or stress, and professionalism on social media websites while balancing your personal and professional values and needs.
5. Describe the importance of leadership in dental hygiene and lifelong learning for career development.

SELF-ASSESSMENT AND PROFESSIONAL GOAL SETTING

Professional development involves identifying one's career goals and learning new knowledge and skills to support one's growth and success in their career. It may lead to a job change, promotion, or improvement in a current job. A successful and fulfilling professional career begins with **self-assessment** and the development of goals and a plan. Engaging in self-assessment is one way to become self-aware by identifying the skills, values, and preferences to help determine professional interests. When people better understand why they are prone to make certain decisions and react to situations in a certain way, they can better understand their behaviors and preferences. The ability to honestly

and routinely self-assess may affect a dental hygienist's desire for career choices and job selection. It is also a solid educational tool for developing critical thinking and problem-solving skills.[1]

Self-awareness is a lifelong process that allows professionals to clearly understand their strengths and opportunities for improvement. Self-awareness allows a dental hygienist to have increased confidence, make sound decisions, and communicate more effectively. This can broaden functions, relationships, and responsibilities within career activities and events, thus enhancing career development and satisfaction.

After professionals understand themselves and what they want in their careers, they should consider what their individual goals are by creating a **career plan**. A career plan is developed by making a list of professional goals that are hoped to be attained during a career, along with actions to take to meet those goals. Goals should be SMART: Specific, Measurable, Achievable, Relevant, and Time-Bound.[2] An example of a SMART goal is: "My goal is to enhance the education I provide to my patients who suffer from diabetes and periodontitis (**Specific**) by taking formal continuing education courses to learn evidence-based information (**Action**) to improve oral health outcomes (**Measurable**) for my patients suffering from both conditions (**Relevant**) by December 31, 2024 (**Time-bound**)."

The plan should be realistic and feasible but not restricted to safe boundaries. It should also be flexible and adjust as life changes occur to ensure job satisfaction throughout a career and include short- and long-term goals. Box 63.1 includes questions to consider when developing a career plan.

Continuing Professional Education

Continuing professional education is formal or informal education for professionals to enhance their learning throughout their careers, help them to stay abreast of new knowledge and skills, maintain and improve competency, and advance a career.[3] Lifelong learning is critical in a career and involves dedicating oneself to learning and treating patients using the most current and research-based care. Dental hygienists can engage in continuing professional education through formal coursework, attending conferences, participating in extracurricular learning environments such as study clubs, maintaining membership in professional associations, and having informal learning opportunities situated in practice.

Many states require continuing education courses for licensure renewal; however, the requirements vary and may be minimal. It is not enough to rely on the information learned during your dental hygiene education. Dental hygienists must continually stay up to date to ensure they are providing appropriate treatment and meeting the current

BOX 63.1 Creating a Career Plan

Section 1: Self-Assessment
What is your passion? What do you enjoy doing and find most rewarding?
What is the relationship between your professional interests and personal desires and needs?
What is your ideal work environment?
What values are important to you?

Section 2: Goal Setting
Goals should be SMART: Specific, Measurable, Attainable, Reliable, and Time-bound
 Short-term goals:
 Mid-term goals:
 Long-term goals:

Section 3: Knowledge, Skills, and Experience
Areas of Strength:
What knowledge and skills do you have that you consider a strength? How do these strengths align with your goals?
What experiences have you had that align with your current position and future goals?

Areas for Growth:
What areas do you need to strengthen?
What knowledge and skills do you need to develop or learn?
What experiences have you not had yet but would be helpful?

Section 4: Development Needs and Skills Required for Current Job and Future Goals
What do you need to do to reach your goals (e.g., completing a master's program, taking an educational methodology course, or volunteering in local dental hygiene programs if you'd like to become a dental hygiene educator in 5 years)?

Section 5: Action Plan
What steps do you plan to take to attain your goals?
What resources will you need for your goals?
What is a reasonable timeline for your goals?

standard of care. Continuing education courses are crucial for disseminating new research and evidence-based recommendations for patient care. Research in dentistry and dental hygiene yields advancements in treatment, instruments, oral health products, and standards of care. Many educational courses also serve as hosts for industries to showcase new and current products, instrument technologies, and resources.

Networks for Professional Enhancement

Networks in dental hygiene are built on professional relationships designed to exchange knowledge and develop a support system for achieving professional goals. A professional network can serve as a career-long resource for job openings, continuing education, leadership opportunities, and reliable references. Professional associations, alumni associations, social media outlets, and community organizations are all places to network and meet other professionals. Networking can build bridges in the professional community and establish personal and professional relationships. Networking can also be a great way to identify a potential mentor.

Building a Relationship With a Mentor

Dental hygienists find it rewarding, personally and professionally, to have one or more mentors throughout their dental hygiene careers. A

mentor is a trusted advisor who serves as a professional resource and provides guidance for career growth, often through mutual engagement over time. Mentors offer support and guidance during career transitions, including from student to clinician, reducing anxiety and improving confidence in clinical practice. Influential mentors can also provide positive differences in protégés' careers and help them to grow professionally; however, both parties in the relationship bear responsibility for success. Good candidates for a mentor include a former professor, a past or present employer or supervisor, close colleagues, or others knowledgeable in a specific area of interest. Dental hygienists may consider seeking mentors by enrolling in advanced education programs or volunteering for professional activities within their national professional organizations, e.g., the Canadian Dental Hygienists Association (CDHA) or the American Dental Hygienists' Association (ADHA), their constituent (state or provincial) organization, local component (area where the dental hygienist resides), and alumni associations, or by collaborating with dental hygienists who have become known in an area of expertise in dental hygiene. Although having a dental hygienist serve as a professional mentor is beneficial in many ways, mentors can also be individuals in other disciplines. By expanding the professional circle, a dental hygienist can help increase opportunities and consider goals from a broader perspective.

DENTAL HYGIENE AS A PROFESSIONAL CAREER

The trajectory for growth in dental hygiene is increasing as the scope of the dental hygienist's role in healthcare expands.[4] According to the Bureau of Labor Statistics, employment of dental hygienists is expected to grow 11% from 2020 to 2030, which is faster than the 8% average for all occupations.[5] This projection is based on population growth, the aging of the current population, growing emphasis on preventive oral healthcare, and research linking oral health and general health. Dental hygienists may work in various settings, including clinical, public health, interprofessional, corporate, research, education, administration, and entrepreneurship (see Table 63.1 for more information about settings).[4]

THE JOB SEARCH

Researching Employment Opportunities

Resources for job searching include professional networks, online job search engines, social media websites, and online classifieds. Word of mouth is also a valuable tool for learning about job opportunities in dentistry, reinforcing the power and importance of strong professional networks. Online resources should be considered for employment searching and as tools to locate a potential employer's website to learn more about the organization, its clients, and its staff, as well as the specific services delivered there. For positions in education, the applicant should visit educational institutions' websites, public health organizations within the state or province of the job seeker's preference, and research facilities or other institutions where research is being conducted. For dental hygiene positions abroad, visit the International Federation of Dental Hygienists (IFDH) (http://www.ifdh.org) or the country's dental hygiene association's website. Box 63.2 identifies sources for locating dental hygiene employment. Before applying, read through the job posting to learn more about the job responsibilities and other information about the job to identify whether it aligns with the applicant's career plan and goals.

Writing a Résumé

The **résumé** is a document highlighting education, experience, skill sets, and achievements that indicate someone's qualifications

TABLE 63.1 **Information on Dental Hygiene Practice Settings and Positions**

Settings	Location(s)	Examples of Roles/Positions
Clinical	General dental office Periodontology office Hospital dental clinics University dental clinics Prison facilities Long-term care facilities Mobile clinics Teledentistry	Clinicians Prevention specialists having a crucial role in oral healthcare and patient health
Public health	Government at the state, local, and federal levels Nonprofit organizations Schools	Clinicians Educators Administrators
Interprofessional	Primary healthcare settings Hospitals Long-term care facilities Community clinics	Clinicians Educators
Corporate	National and international companies Medical device companies Medical technology companies	Sales and marketing positions Product researchers Research assistants Corporate educators Corporate administrators
Research	Universities Private companies Public health departments	Clinical examiner Project manager or planner Academician Interprofessional team member Administrator
Education	Universities Community colleges Corporations	Part-time in a clinical faculty position while continuing in a clinical position Part-time or adjunct faculty member Full-time faculty member Speaker
Administration	Dental offices Universities Community colleges Associations Corporations	Clinical director Educational program director Professional association executive director Research administrator Corporate sales manager
Entrepreneurial	Self-employment	Consultant Nonprofit organizational development Professional speaker and trainer Independent clinical practice owners (as permitted)

BOX 63.2 Sources for Locating Dental Hygiene Employment

- Professional networks (e.g., local professional association, alumni associations, and study clubs)
- Verbal or printed announcements at dental hygiene meetings and continuing education courses
- Public or county health departments
- Dental hygiene education employment opportunities bulletin boards
- Dental hygiene and dental association newsletters and journals
- Professional journals and magazines
- Public employment agencies
- ADHA website: http://www.adha.org/career-center
- Social media websites such as LinkedIn, Facebook, and X, formerly Twitter
- Newspaper and web-based classified advertisements
- Websites for employment opportunities

for a job. Various styles may be used when tailoring a résumé. The functional résumé lists primary skill sets and accomplishments that support a specific job position and reflect ability in individual areas of expertise. Box 63.3 describes the contents of a high-quality résumé.

Honesty and accuracy are the most critical elements of résumé writing. It is important to highlight skills necessary for the desired job and those of a new graduate, such as familiarity with new technologies and treatment modalities. The résumé format should be one to two pages maximum. The résumé must appear polished, neat, and accurate, with correct spelling and grammar. After drafting a résumé, have a mentor or a trusted source review and provide feedback. Sample résumés appear in Figs. 63.1 and 63.2.

Cover Letter

A **cover letter** is an introductory letter designed to introduce the job candidate to a potential employer. The cover letter is the applicant's first

BOX 63.3 Components of a High-Quality Résumé

Personal Identification
- Name
- Address
- Telephone number and email address

Job Objective (Optional)
- Statement of the exact position being sought, giving the résumé focus
- Professional goals

Career Summary
- Skills
- Strengths

Professional Employment Experience
- Summary of any responsibilities not generally encompassed by the normal dental hygiene job description, noting any special awards received; for new licensees, list of special skills or interests from school, jobs in related fields, or academic honors and awards
- Professional experiences with diverse client populations
- Private practice
- Teaching
- Administrative experience
- Research
- Government

Professional Data (Optional)
- Professional affiliations
- Community and professional services
- Publications
- Presentations given
- Continuing education courses attended
- Professional projects
- Leadership roles

References (Optional)
- Write: "References available on request"

contact with a prospective employer and provides a succinct introduction and marketing opportunity spotlighting skills and qualifications. Cover letters should accompany résumés when they are distributed to potential employers. Unless the employer requests an electronic submission, the résumé and cover letter should be typed and printed on high-quality, medium-weight, white or ivory paper. Applicants should hand deliver, mail, or email résumés and cover letters when inquiring about a position. Some businesses are moving to online application portals where application information is submitted through an online intake website (the résumé and cover letter are typically uploaded into the application portal). Job ads typically indicate the method of delivery preferred.

Generally, the format of a cover letter includes an introductory paragraph, a body paragraph, and a closing paragraph. The introductory paragraph should include who the applicant is, why they are writing, and how they learned about the position. The body paragraph is where the applicant summarizes their most vital skills and experiences that are relevant to the position. They should provide specific examples, and this should not be a repeat of the résumé. The closing paragraph should suggest the course of action the applicant

would like to take (e.g., requesting an interview) and information on how to get in contact with them. Fig. 63.3 illustrates a sample cover letter.

Electronic Portfolio

An **electronic portfolio**, also known as an e-portfolio or digital portfolio, is a digital collection of material that provides evidence supporting an applicant's efforts, achievements, and progress gained from education, work, and life experiences. While not typically required, an electronic portfolio can supplement a résumé and allow employers to learn more about an applicant, such as practice principles, community services activities, and notable experiences. A personal website can provide an alternative web presence to social networks, helping build a positive digital identity (see Chapter 8).[6]

References

References are individuals who provide recommendations for a person who is applying for a job. References serve as personal testimonies to the job candidate's competence and character. When identifying potential references, a person should ask if they would be willing to serve as a reference and if they can provide a favorable recommendation. Before distributing the reference list, job seekers should touch base with anyone on their reference list. A friendly phone call periodically keeps the connection current, offers a networking opportunity, and may be a source of job leads. A minimum of three references should be selected and contacted before résumé distribution.

Response and Followup Before the Interview

If no reply has come from the prospective employer, a followup correspondence should be sent at least 1 to 3 weeks after the résumé is sent. Following up avoids any implication of lack of interest or desire for the position and may clarify the status of an application. Fig. 63.4 presents an example of a followup letter.

Preparing for the Job Interview

An employer's initial impression of the applicant may have longstanding implications and determine whether one is hired. Interviews may be intimidating, yet they are vital to understanding whether the office and applicant are a compatible fit. The interview is just as crucial for the applicant as it is for the employer. Both the applicant and office staff need to establish the potential for a positive relationship and synergy.

Before the interview, job applicants should locate important information regarding the practice, university, company, agency, or organization with which they will be interviewing. They should complete an online search to learn about the setting, types of patients seen, mission, values, and philosophy of the office or organization, number and current employees, and any other information (e.g., the administrative department the position is in for a university position). Further, they should refer to the job post for the position description. Reviewing this information can also identify questions to ask during the interview for clarity.

The interview provides an opportunity to ask questions and learn more about the environment to establish whether it may complement the goals of the applicant's career plan. The applicant should prepare questions before the interview regarding the position, job description, practice management, and benefits (vacation time, sick days, holidays, medical and dental insurance, stock options, professional development opportunities, and retirement plan), depending on the setting. Box 63.4 identifies some questions and considerations for job interviews.

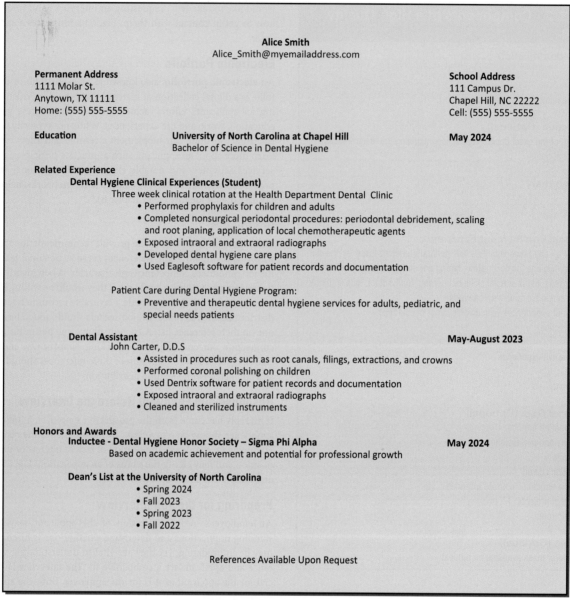

Alice Smith
Alice_Smith@myemailaddress.com

Permanent Address
1111 Molar St.
Anytown, TX 11111
Home: (555) 555-5555

School Address
111 Campus Dr.
Chapel Hill, NC 22222
Cell: (555) 555-5555

Education	University of North Carolina at Chapel Hill	May 2024
	Bachelor of Science in Dental Hygiene	

Related Experience
Dental Hygiene Clinical Experiences (Student)
Three week clinical rotation at the Health Department Dental Clinic
- Performed prophylaxis for children and adults
- Completed nonsurgical periodontal procedures: periodontal debridement, scaling and root planing, application of local chemotherapeutic agents
- Exposed intraoral and extraoral radiographs
- Developed dental hygiene care plans
- Used Eaglesoft software for patient records and documentation

Patient Care during Dental Hygiene Program:
- Preventive and therapeutic dental hygiene services for adults, pediatric, and special needs patients

Dental Assistant   **May-August 2023**
John Carter, D.D.S
- Assisted in procedures such as root canals, filings, extractions, and crowns
- Performed coronal polishing on children
- Used Dentrix software for patient records and documentation
- Exposed intraoral and extraoral radiographs
- Cleaned and sterilized instruments

Honors and Awards
Inductee - Dental Hygiene Honor Society – Sigma Phi Alpha   **May 2024**
Based on academic achievement and potential for professional growth

Dean's List at the University of North Carolina
- Spring 2024
- Fall 2023
- Spring 2023
- Fall 2022

References Available Upon Request

Fig. 63.1 Example of a résumé.

The Interview

Employers frequently outline or discuss the job description, responsibilities, and expectations during the interview. Compatibility is established by linking the candidate's skills and strengths with the job description and needs of the practice. A professional appearance makes a long-standing impression, and applicants should be professional, organized, neat, and clean. Remember that the position is one of a healthcare provider, so it is essential to project professionalism, integrity, and critical thinking skills.

Depending on the time and depth of conversation, some employers may request a second interview. This should include a thorough discussion of the job description, office policies and procedures, work schedule, compensation package of starting wage and benefits, performance evaluation, and frequency and basis of raises. Not all employers use multiple interviews or may discuss these specifics during the interview.

Interview Communication

Professional behavior and effective communication are keys to conducting a successful interview. The applicant should take notes during the interview to reference after the interview. The applicant should listen to each question thoroughly and provide open and honest answers that promote a sense of integrity and self-esteem during the interview. If needing more time to respond to questions or unclear initially about what was asked, one can ask the interviewer to repeat the question or summarize the question to ensure understanding. If there is an unanswerable question, say so instead of faking it. Interview questions should be job related and not used to find out personal information.

Federal and state laws prohibit potential employers from asking certain questions that are not related to the job requirements. Employers should not ask about race, gender, religion, marital status, disabilities, ethnic background, country of origin, sexual preferences,

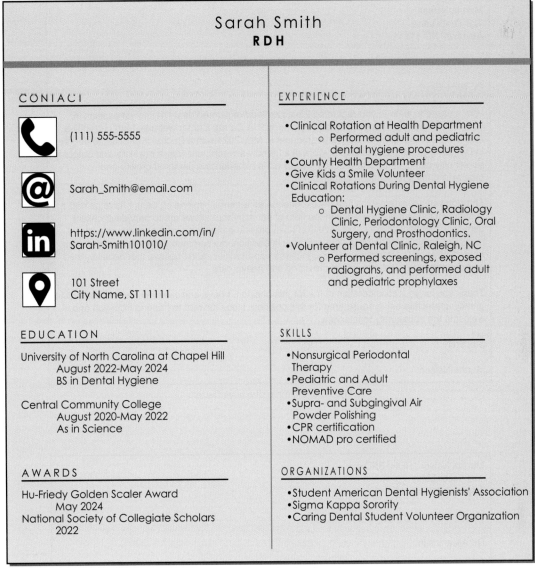

Fig. 63.2 Example of a résumé.

or age because not hiring a candidate based on these factors is discriminatory.[7] If a question seems discriminatory, an applicant does not have to answer and can share that it is against federal and state laws.

When responding to behavioral-based interview questions that warrant providing an example, consider using a structured method such as the STAR method: (1) describe the Situation; (2) explain the Task you had to complete and what your responsibility was in the situation; (3) discuss the specific Actions taken to complete the task; and (4) share the Results of your efforts.[8]

At the end of an interview, employers will hold time for the applicant to ask questions of the employer. Applicants should always have something to ask to show interest, and questions should be specific and provide the information needed to determine if this is a good fit. Box 63.4 lists questions to consider asking during the interview.

Working Interview and Office Observation

Dental hygienists may be asked for or may request a **working interview**, in which they perform the job within the work environment with staff members before being offered the position. This is an excellent opportunity for the applicant and office members to examine their potential working relationship. It also gives the dental hygienist a firsthand view of the interoffice working specificities and their potential to succeed in the environment. The dental hygienist must be licensed in that state to complete a working interview. In addition, if the dental hygienist is performing income-producing procedures, they should be compensated for their work.

If the prospective employee has not completed all licensure procedures or does not wish to complete a working interview, they may ask to observe in an office. Observation will allow the applicant to see how the office functions and better understand the practice's management. Working interviews and observations provide opportunities to gain insight into intraoffice dynamics, including communication between the staff members, management styles, flow of schedule, atmosphere of the working environment, efficiency, teamwork among peers, and client relations. Other important observations may include safety, sanitation, sterilization methods, equipment and instrument quality, and the overall reality of how the office functions.

Martha Nelson
123 Tooth Lane
Anytown, NC 11111

April 20, 2024

Dr. Alice Smith,

I am pleased to write to you regarding the advertised registered dental hygienist position in your office. I heard of the position through the ADHA Career Center website. I am currently a student at the University of ABC and graduate in May 2024 with a Bachelor of Science degree in Dental Hygiene. I am looking for work in a friendly environment where my skills and outgoing personality can contribute to practice growth while experiencing personal growth and broadening my knowledge in dental topics.

Through various externships and my experience as a dental hygiene student, I have gained a substantial amount of knowledge in the field of dentistry that allows me to provide excellent care for patients of all ages. I believe that I can provide a positive dental experience and maintain the high standards of your practice. In addition, my communication skills and patient rapport have been strengthened through these opportunities, and I believe that honesty, trust, and passion are crucial aspects of providing oral health care.

Thank you for your consideration of me for this position. I have enclosed my résumé and would greatly appreciate being considered for this position. I look forward to hearing from you and welcome the opportunity to interview.

Sincerely,

Martha Nelson

Fig. 63.3 Example of a cover letter.

Martha Nelson, RDH, BSDH
123 Tooth Lane
Anytown, NC 11111

May 1, 2024

Dr. Alice Smith,

I recently submitted my cover letter and résumé for the position in your dental practice in Charlotte, North Carolina. I am excited to learn more about this preventive-driven dental practice and the dental hygiene position within it, which was highlighted on the ADHA Career Center website.

My experience working with diverse patent populations at the University of ABC School of Dentistry and external rotations have allowed me to gain fundamental clinical skills, provide patient-centered care, and utilize my Spanish language skills. My experiences with rotations in the clinic and public health, as well as working with special-needs patients using a digital software program, have enhanced my dental technology skills and have trained me to lead in today's dental environment.

I would welcome the opportunity to speak with you further regarding this position. Please feel free to call me during the day at 555-555-5555 or send an email to MarthaNelson@emailaddress.com.

Sincerely,

Martha Nelson, RDH, BSDH

Fig. 63.4 Example of a followup before an interview letter.

BOX 63.4 Questions and Considerations for Job Interviews

General Questions
- How would you describe the work environment?
- What is the management style?
- What are the opportunities for professional growth?
- What are the biggest challenges that someone in this role would face?
- What is the performance review process like?
- What metrics/goals will performance be evaluated against for this position?
- What are the company's/office's/program's most important values? How does the company/office/program uphold its values?
- What do you like most about working at this office/company/program?
- What is the biggest challenge working at this office/company/program?

Questions Specific for Job in a Clinical Setting
Practice Team and Practice Management
- What types of patients/clients and services are provided?
- Are there staff meetings? If so, how often are staff meetings held?

Office Protocols
- What is the practice protocol for medical emergencies, sterilization, antibiotic prophylaxis prior to specific dental hygiene procedures, and restrictions on treating patients with elevated blood pressure?
- Under what circumstances is a patient's physician consulted for advice regarding oral healthcare?
- Does the staff have a practice plan in case of medical emergency?
- Where are the emergency medical kit and oxygen tank located? What do they contain? How frequently are they checked, and by whom?
- How are instruments sterilized? Are the sterilization units monitored?
- Where and how are biohazards disposed of?
- What is the recommended attire? Is protective clothing provided?

Patient Care
- What is the daily schedule for dental hygiene patients?
- What are the appointment lengths for healthy adults, active periodontal therapy care, periodontal maintenance care, new patient care, and/or children?
- Are there days or hours when the dental hygienist will provide patient care in the absence of a dentist (if state supervision laws permit)?
- What are radiographic exposure recommendations for the office?
- How are continued care intervals established for patients?
- What are the elements of nonsurgical periodontal therapy that the practice supports and performs?
- Who discusses risks, benefits, and alternatives to the recommended treatment with the patients?
- Who discusses fees and dental insurance with the patient?
- What products (e.g., antimicrobials, anesthetics, fluorides, and desensitizing agents) are available for patient treatment?
- What products (e.g., toothbrushes, floss, toothpick holders, interproximal devices, fluorides) are available for distribution as samples to patients? What is the process for discussing new products for distribution as samples?
- What methods of pain or dental anxiety control are used and how often?
- What are the recordkeeping and documentation requirements for dental hygiene services?
- What are the additional responsibilities for the dental hygienist?
- What types of instruments are available? What is the instrument maintenance policy? How and when are new instruments ordered?

Closing
- What are the next steps?

Note: Most of these questions are tailored to a clinical dental hygiene position; however, they can be altered to any job setting.

Followup Communications

After the interview, candidates should thank the interviewers in person and in writing. Depending on previous communication, a postinterview thank-you letter (Fig. 63.5) should be mailed or emailed the day after the interview. The letter should be handwritten or typed and signed by the applicant. The letter does not have to be long or detailed. Still, it can show a potential employer a genuine interest and level of respect, making the candidate more memorable to a potential employer. Taking the time to send a thank-you note to the employer can create a positive and lasting impression.

MAINTAINING PROFESSIONALISM ON SOCIAL MEDIA WEBSITES

Although participation in social media (e.g., Facebook and X, formerly Twitter) is common, this can impact decisions for employment. Employers and staff members are likely to search for job candidates' social media sites to learn more about them. Keep these postings professional; remove any potential image-damaging posts and pictures before the job search. Employers and patients have access to social media sites and may view what is public. Potential employers may develop a perception that is misinterpreted or negative.[9] Social media sites should never be used to complain about professional issues or work-related events or comment on patients, patient care, or practice-related issues. Maintaining client privacy and compliance with HIPAA laws is vital for a dental hygiene professional. See Box 63.5 for legal, ethical, and safety issues.

JOB SELECTION CONSIDERATIONS

When considering which position to select, the dental hygienist should compare career goals, needs, and desires with what the potential employer offers. It is also essential to consider the top priorities when selecting a position, such as the overall practice ambiance and atmosphere, practice philosophy and values, practice standards, job responsibilities, general work conditions (e.g., workload, scheduling, equipment), professional growth opportunities, compensation package, job security, location, or practice stability. To guide this process, consider creating a list of five "must-haves" and "can't-haves" in a job to help guide you when job searching and ultimately selecting the appropriate fit for you. Although sometimes challenging, patience and careful job selection are important to identify the best fit. Working with a temporary employment agency before selecting a permanent position is another way to gain clinical experience, create networking opportunities, and identify job opportunities.

Compensation

The methods of compensation for dental hygiene employment are varied and determined by agreement between the employee and employer. Dental hygienists may be paid hourly, daily, salary, or commission. Compensation methods include fixed salary, salary plus commission, salary plus fringe benefits, and commission. Table 63.2 details forms of compensation, and Table 63.3 details types of fringe benefits.

Martha Nelson, RDH, BSDH
123 Tooth Lane
Anytown, NC 11111

May 20, 2024

Dr. Alice Smith,

Thank you for the opportunity to interview for the dental hygiene position in your dental practice. I appreciated meeting you and the team members and learning more about the position.

I am excited about the opportunity to join your team and enjoyed hearing about the team dynamics within the office. You have cultivated an environment focused on providing optimal care for patients efficiently with clear communication and teamwork. As discussed during our meeting, I feel confident that I meet the requirements for this position and can contribute to the positive and charismatic environment.

Please feel free to contact me if I can provide you with any further information. I look forward to hearing from you.

Sincerely,

Martha Nelson, RDH, BSDH

Fig. 63.5 Example of a postinterview thank-you letter.

BOX 63.5 Legal, Ethical, and Safety Issues

- When working in clinical practice settings providing direct access to dental hygiene care without dental supervision, a collaborative practice agreement, or general supervision, the dental hygienist informs patients of any related requirements to see a dentist in addition to the dental hygienist (where laws and regulations specify such requirements).
- It is important to educate all clients, including patients, community groups, legislators and other political leaders, other healthcare providers, and the public on the scope of dental hygiene practice and licensure, especially for the newer expanding roles, including dental therapist (DT), advanced dental therapist (ADT), and advanced dental hygiene practitioner (ADHP).
- Honesty (veracity) and accuracy are the most important elements of résumé writing.
- Dental hygiene employment falls under the Non-Discrimination Act, Title VII of the Civil Rights Act of 1964. The law establishes equal employment opportunity for all during the hiring process and throughout the course of employment.
- Dental practice acts are legislative laws that define the dental hygiene scope of practice. These acts do not apply to the business association between the dentist and the dental hygienist.
- Minimal standards for working conditions are set by each state.
- The Occupational Safety and Health Administration (OSHA) sets minimum federal requirements for workplace health and safety.
- Employment contracts may or may not be legally binding.
- The performance evaluation can be used as a legal supporting document for employee dismissal.
- In the event of dismissal, the dental hygienist must (1) make all attempts to understand clearly the grounds and (2) clarify the severance arrangements.
- Financial arrangements between the dentist and the dental hygienist are solely the concern of those two individuals.
- An independent contractor dental hygienist may hire employees and function as an employer.

Salary Ranges

The job seeker may visit a few helpful websites, including the US Department of Labor's Bureau of Labor Statistics or other salary-aggregating websites, to compare the prospective employer's salary with national, state, or local standards. The dental hygienist also may contact other dental hygienists working in the area, the component dental hygienists' association employment chairperson, or, if possible, a local employment agency specializing in dental office employment to learn about average salary ranges.

EMPLOYMENT AND EVALUATION

Employment Rights

Dental hygiene employment falls under the Non-Discrimination Act, Title VII of the Civil Rights Act of 1964.[10] The law establishes equal employment opportunities for all during the hiring process and throughout employment. Each state sets minimum standards for working conditions. They include guidelines about hours and days of work, minimum wage and reports for pay, employee records, uniforms and equipment, meal periods and eating area, rest periods and rest facilities, and environmental temperature. The Occupational Safety and Health Administration (OSHA) sets minimum federal requirements for industrial safety.

Employment Contracts

An employment contract may be issued to describe the terms of employment agreed on by the dental hygienist and the employer. The contents may include the agreement's administrative terms, settings, employment terms, job description, compensation, probationary period, performance evaluation, and termination procedures (Box 63.6). An employment contract is not a required document and may not be completed.

Performance Evaluation

As a new graduate, gaining feedback from various sources will help to improve skills and build trust with the other office staff members.

TABLE 63.2 Methods of Compensation

Compensation Method	Description
Fixed salary	Guaranteed fixed wage Paid hourly, daily, weekly, or monthly
Salary plus commission	Base salary paid plus an additional percentage of fees charged for dental hygiene services
Salary plus fringe benefits	Fringe benefits or "perks" are special services and items offered in addition to salary (see Table 63.3) Most common fringe benefits: continuing education, free or discounted oral health care, or paid vacations or holidays Fringe benefits paid for by the employer may be tax deductible to the employer
Commission with guaranteed minimum salary	Percentage of fees charged for dental hygiene services is paid, with an assured minimum wage per day, regardless of daily gross production
Commission	Earnings are based on a percentage of fees charged for dental hygiene services and are dependent on productivity
Independent contractor	A dental hygienist may work as an independent contractor, depending on state's scope of practice, with a supervising dentist to provide services to the patients of that dentist by referral prescription Dental hygienist sets and collects all fees and pays overhead costs with the profit fluctuation based on production, collection, and expenses
Profit-sharing bonus	A work incentive is awarded to employees after profit goals are achieved for a specified period May be calculated monthly, quarterly, or annually

TABLE 63.3 Optional Fringe Benefits

Fringe Benefit Category	Type	Description
Paid absences	Sick leave	Salary paid during occasional short-term illnesses May be allowed to accumulate if not used, or unused days are paid at the end of the year as a bonus
	Holidays	Salary paid for usual, nationally observed holidays
	Vacation	Salary paid for vacation time Often varies according to the length of service with the employer
	Educational leave	Salary paid for time off to attend educational programs that are work related
	Emergency personal leave	Paid time off for unexpected events such as a family illness, death, or funeral; jury duty, legal depositions, or court appearances; or extreme weather conditions
	Family leave	Time off, usually without pay but with the guarantee of job protection on return from leave Time limits usually apply
	Extended leave	Leave without pay for a few weeks to several months for the purpose of travel, family, or personal needs The position is held during the absence with an agreed-on time of return
	Sabbatical, developmental, or research leave	Usually involves leave without pay or reduced pay for a few weeks to several months for the purpose of education or research Position is held during the absence with an agreed-on time of return
Employee Assistance Program		Assists employees with personal or work-related problems that may impact job performance, health, or well-being
Retirement		Employer offers retirement plan options for the employee to pay into Employer may match up to a certain percentage Plans may include 401k, 403b, IRAs, profit sharing, or defined benefit (or pension)
Insurance benefits	Health insurance	Employer offers health insurance to employee and employee may pay for all, a portion, or none of the premium
	Dental insurance	Employer offers dental insurance and employee either pays for all, a portion, or none of the premium Employers may elect to provide dental care for their employees instead
	Vision insurance	Employer offers vision insurance and employee either pays for all, a portion, or none of the premium
	Liability (malpractice) insurance	Employer offers and may pay for malpractice insurance Insurance protecting against claims from injuries or damage to other people or property
	Long-term permanent disability insurance	Employer offers disability insurance and employee either pays for all, a portion, or none of the premium Disability insurance pays if employees have an illness or injury leaving them unable to work for a set period of time
	Life insurance	Employer offers life insurance and employee typically elects the amount covered and pays for the premium
Professional expenses	Professional license renewal	Payment or reimbursement for state licensure renewal
	Uniform allowance	Fixed amount of money for scrubs, shoes, and other required work attire or items are provided by employer Typically an annual allowance if provided
	Professional equipment expenses	Designated amount to spend on items necessary to perform work functions (e.g., instruments)
	Professional education assistance	Employer provides a designated amount for continuing education or other means of education associated with work functions
	Professional activities	Employer pays for professional activities such as professional organization membership fees
	Professional journals or texts	Employer pays for subscription for professional journals/texts

Feedback can be gained formally through a performance evaluation or informally. The dental hygienist should be given the opportunity for performance evaluation on a periodic and consistent basis. The **performance evaluation** is a valuable tool that provides a progress report for the employee, recognizes and supports desired behavior, develops strengths, pinpoints weaknesses, and gives specific direction for change. The performance evaluation may assist in determining a salary increase or be used as a legal supporting document for employee dismissal. Ideally, a job evaluation should be performed after the probationary period if the employee is new, then once or twice a year for the duration of employment. Fig. 63.6 provides an example of an employee performance evaluation. Informal feedback generally occurs through day-to-day interactions. Consider asking colleagues in the practice to give feedback on time management or quality of clinical care when patients are shared.

Employee Name: _____ Date: _____
(Registered Dental Hygienist)

Evaluation completed by: _____

	EXCELLENT	ACCEPTABLE	NEEDS IMPROVEMENT
PROFESSIONAL BEHAVIOR:			
1. Attitude	___	___	___
2. Cooperation	___	___	___
3. Responsibility	___	___	___
4. Initiative	___	___	___
5. Communications	___	___	___
6. Contributions to Office	___	___	___
CLIENT MANAGEMENT:			
1. Information and Instruction	___	___	___
2. Assistance in Decision Making	___	___	___
3. Respectful	___	___	___
4. Contribution to Comfort	___	___	___
5. Client Acceptance	___	___	___
RISK MANAGEMENT:			
1. Infection Control	___	___	___
2. Protect Self/Client from Injury	___	___	___
PROCESS OF CARE:			
1. Systematic Approach	___	___	___
2. Performs All Necessary Care	___	___	___
3. Care Procedures (List specific concerns)			

_____
_____
_____
_____

4. Documentation Skills	___	___	___
5. Evaluation Skills	___	___	___
6. Modification of Care	___	___	___
7. Coordination with Other Care	___	___	___

CHANGES/GROWTH SINCE LAST EVALUATION:

_____
_____
_____

GOALS FOR CHANGE/GROWTH:

_____
_____
_____

COMMENTS:

_____
_____
_____
_____

SIGNED:

_____ Date: _____
Supervisor

_____ Date: _____
Employee

Fig. 63.6 Example of an employee performance evaluation.

JOB TERMINATION

Job termination may occur through dismissal by the employer or resignation by the employee. In the event of dismissal, the dental hygienist should make all attempts to understand the reasoning and gain clarification of the reason.

When the dental hygienist resigns from a job, a notice of resignation should be given to the employer as soon as possible, before any coworkers are told. A resignation should allow the employer an adequate and appropriate amount of time to fill the position before departure, and a minimum of 2 weeks' notice should be given to the employer. Maintaining a positive relationship with the employer is essential to assist in future career opportunities by expanding the professional network and potential list of references.

STRESS AND BURNOUT AMONG DENTAL HYGIENISTS

Dental hygienists may experience work-related stress and burnout. Becoming complacent with patient care and losing motivation in efficiency are signs of fatigue and burnout. It is easy to get bored and burned out in a stagnant and unchallenging role or work in an environment with poor staff morale. Sources of stress and burnout in a dental hygiene career may include relationships with staff members and patients; chronic work-related pain; monotonous tasks; and lack of challenges, feeling appreciated, accomplishing goals, or change in responsibilities.

To overcome burnout, dental hygienists can consider sparking a new interest in dental hygiene by attending continuing education courses and implementing the knowledge and skills learned, joining a dental hygiene study club, or becoming active in local or state organizations. They can also take on new roles within a practice and expand their job responsibilities; leading the practice in a community service project or new preventive campaign; working in a different role in another employment setting outside of the typical dental practice; or becoming involved in consumer advocacy at the local or state level to expand the scope of dental hygiene practice, campaign for water fluoridation, or volunteer for community health events. These opportunities can help break up the monotony and create a sense of need and accomplishment. Networking with contacts and mentors may also be a positive influence and resource to identify what may help overcome burnout. See Chapter 66.

DENTAL HYGIENE'S EXPANDING SCOPE

The dental hygiene profession is evolving to accommodate population needs and practice environment changes.[11-12] The development of new technologies, changes in policy at the state and federal levels to address access to care issues, workforce trends, and dental hygienists' professional interests are factors driving advancement within the profession (see Chapter 1).[11]

Laws and regulations governing dental hygiene practice are changing to allow more direct access to dental hygiene services with decreased dentist supervision levels or without supervision, thus offering dental hygienists more opportunities to provide care to those in need. Collaborative practice agreements, general supervision, limited access permits, and public health endorsements give disadvantaged populations more access to preventive and therapeutic dental hygienist care.[11]

As of June 2021, 42 states had permitted direct access to dental hygienists once they had met specific experience and training requirements.[13] **Direct access** to care means that dental hygienists can initiate treatment based on their assessment of patients' needs without a dentist's specific authorization or presence. The administration of local anesthetics and delivery of restorative care by dental hygienists are other areas where the profession has advanced significantly in the past decade. As of July 2021, 46 states plus the District of Columbia permitted dental hygienists to administer local anesthesia.[14] The independent practice of dental hygiene is an option in Canada, with more than 1200 dental hygienists practicing independently in 2021, and the number is increasing.[15] The Canadian Dental Hygienists Association has an independent practice network and a series of professional development courses for dental hygienists to prepare for independent practice available to its members.

Expanding Educational Opportunities

As employment opportunities expand, so does the prospect of advanced education. Positions in education, research, public and community health programs (see Chapter 4), and corporate settings often require educational degrees beyond an associate's degree. To accommodate this need, dental hygiene education programs have created degree completion options designed to allow licensed dental hygienists with an associate's degree to advance their education and earn a baccalaureate degree. As of 2022, there were 58 degree completion programs, many of which offer online coursework and distance education, allowing greater flexibility for completion. Furthermore, as of 2022, there were 18 master of science programs in dental hygiene designed to prepare students to become educators, administrators, and researchers.[11,16]

Beyond traditional education, the establishment of midlevel oral healthcare providers has significantly impacted access to care and dental hygienists' scope of practice. The Advanced Dental Hygiene Practitioner (ADHP) is based on a concept passed by the 2004 ADHA's House of Delegates. The ADHP works as a part of healthcare teams to improve access to oral healthcare for underserved populations through the provision of preventive services currently under the purview of dental hygienists.[17] An ADHP earns a master's degree and serves in a capacity like the nurse practitioner in the medical field. Minnesota was the first state to implement education for licensure of a midlevel provider via the dental therapist (DT) and advanced dental therapist (ADT). The DT may administer services, including extractions and restorative procedures, with the supervision of a dentist. ADTs begin as dental hygienists and may practice as a DT. Still, they have an expanded scope of practice with less limiting restrictions, allowing for evaluation, assessment and treatment plan development, and nonsurgical extractions of permanent teeth. As of June 2022, 13 states had a midlevel oral healthcare workforce model, and other states are pursuing midlevel oral healthcare workforce models.[17] See Chapter 39 for information regarding restorative therapy options and requirements.

LEADERSHIP IN DENTAL HYGIENE

Leadership is paramount for progressive and fundamental change to occur in any profession. Dental hygiene must be supported by leaders who emerge as champions to advocate and support the profession's promotion. Professional leaders must emerge and develop key roles to advocate for themselves, their peers, and the patients they serve. Emerging leaders must possess passion, effective communication, and motivation skills.

Dental hygiene leaders are vital to continue moving dental hygiene with the evolving healthcare models, including integrating interprofessional patient care and increasing access to care through expanded functions and educational opportunities for dental hygienists. Health promotion, improving oral healthcare, and increasing value in the profession are vital goals for leaders in the profession. Dental hygiene leaders may have many roles within private practice, education, research, public health, professional associations, and corporations.[18] They can serve as vital change agents who push for the positive progression of the profession that ultimately impacts the communities in which they serve.

Leadership opportunities in the dental hygiene profession include challenging the way that the profession reacts to conflict and demands; altering traditional practices; advocating for positive, progressive change for patients, communities, and the profession; reforming healthcare and legislation that could influence the scope of practice; and promoting for evidence-based decision making and interprofessional practice. Leaders in dental hygiene may serve to design and implement new models of practice, implement change in educational models, develop doctoral-level educational programs in dental hygiene, enhance interprofessional relationships, collaborate with other professions to improve access to care, and support an evidence-based approach to care.[18]

CAREER SATISFACTION

Evolving in a career is natural, with some realizing early in their career that they need to seek different environments to feel challenged and accomplished. A career is a journey, and as environment and personal life change, so do the desires and needs in the workplace. Excelling in a career involves creating a plan that offers security and confidence and adapting to conform to life changes and personal goals and interests. See the Critical Thinking Exercises to consider this process.

CRITICAL THINKING EXERCISES

1. Answer the following reflection questions:
   - What do you value about yourself as a person?
   - What values are important to you in your career and position at work?
   - What skills and expertise do you have that you can use in your position?
   - What areas do you need to further develop?
2. Write two or three short- (2 years) and long-term (5 to 10 years) professional goals you would like to attain. How do you plan on meeting these goals? What steps will you need to take to achieve these goals? Who can help you obtain these goals?
3. Create a cover letter, résumé, and followup communication letter(s) for your job search. Once you have created these, have someone (e.g., faculty member, mentor, someone within the field) review and provide feedback.
4. Create a table with at least five must-haves and five can't-haves when looking for a position.
5. Develop a list of potential interview questions, pair up with a partner, and pose the questions to each other. Evaluate your answers, body language, and delivery.

CRITICAL THINKING EXERCISES

Discovering opportunities for personal and professional growth may include furthering education, changing your job setting, or expanding your professional responsibilities and practices. Other means to enhance career satisfaction include the following:
- Hold membership and/or leadership roles in professional organizations.
- Contribute to the oral healthcare or interprofessional healthcare team. The dental hygienist must be willing to step in, pick up tasks for other team members, and collaborate to offer superior patient care.
- Continue with lifelong learning and use evidence-based decision making in practice. Dental hygienists must keep abreast of the published research on dental hygiene and dentistry to make relevant evidence-based decisions regarding products, tools, technology, and procedures in practice. The best way of achieving this goal is to conduct literature reviews regularly. Another is to join a study club that can serve as a means for keeping up with research and act as a vehicle for professional networking.

Oral healthcare is a diverse, dynamic profession. Finding a role within it is vital to developing career satisfaction and contributing to the profession. The dental hygienist must seize the opportunity to determine how best to meet both criteria. To begin, complete the questions in Box 63.1 to create a career plan.

KEY CONCEPTS

- A career is a lifelong journey that may evolve to adjust to changes in life.
- The elements of career development include self-assessment, seeking employment, professional development, and career mobility, requiring the dental hygienist's ongoing thoughtful and active participation.
- Dental hygienists need to identify resources, such as mentors and references, for career development and networking.
- Searching for a dental hygiene position begins with writing a résumé, composing a cover letter, preparing a list of questions for an interview, and practicing for the interview.
- Various employment arrangements, terms of employment, and compensation packages are available, depending on the employer and on the dental hygienist's ability to negotiate an agreement with the employer.
- Job performance is determined by a combination of factors, including evaluation of dental hygiene skills and production, adherence to the job description, and contribution to the practice.
- Career satisfaction may be met through continuous self-assessment and adaptation to one's needs and desires.
- The dental hygiene profession is constantly expanding, providing more job opportunities as well as better access to care.

ACKNOWLEDGMENT

The author acknowledges Christine Hovliaras and Jennifer L. Brame for their past contributions to this chapter.

REFERENCES

1. Gadbury-Amyot CC, Woldt JL, Siruta-Austin KJ. Self-assessment: a review of the literature and pedagogical strategies for its promotion in dental education. *J Dent Hyg*. 2015;89(6):357–364.
2. SMART Goals: How to Make Goals Achievable. Mindtools. https://www.mindtools.com/pages/article/smart-goals.htm. Accessed July 18, 2022.
3. Queeney, DS. Continuing professional education. Handbook of adult and continuing education. Wilson AL, Hayes ER, editors. San Francisco: Jossey-Bass; 2000.
4. American Dental Hygienists' Association. Career Center, Career Paths. Available at: http://www.adha.org/professional-roles. Accessed July 18, 2022.

5. Bureau of Labor Statistics, U.S. Department of Labor. Occupational Outlook Handbook, Dental Hygienists. Available at: https://www.bls.gov/ooh/healthcare/dental-hygienists.htm. Accessed June 2, 2022.

6. Parsons KM, Holt ER. Shape your future with an e-portfolio. *Access.* May–June. 2012:19–21.

7. U.S. Equal Employment Opportunity Commission. Employees and Job Applicants. Available at: https://www.eeoc.gov/employees-job-applicants. Accessed June 2, 2022.

8. Boogaard K. *The STAR Method: The Secret to Acing Your Next Job Interview.* The Muse; 2022. Available at: https://www.themuse.com/advice/star-interview-method. Accessed July 18, 2022.

9. Henry RK. Maintaining professionalism in a digital age. *Dimen Dent Hyg.* 2012;10(10):28–30. 32.

10. U.S. Equal Employment Opportunity Commission. Title VII of the Civil Rights Act of 1964. Available at: https://www.eeoc.gov/statutes/title-vii-civil-rights-act-1964. Accessed July 18, 2022.

11. Batrell A, Lynch A, Steinbach P. The American Dental Hygienists' Association leads the profession into 21st century workforce opportunities. *J Evid Based Dent Pract.* 2016;16(suppl 4–suppl 10).

12. Weintraub JS. What should oral health professionals know in 2040: executive summary. *J Dent Educ.* 2017;81(8):1024–1032.

13. American Dental Hygienists' Association (ADHA). *Current Direct Access Map. Chicago, IL;* 2021. Available at: http://www.adha.org/direct-access. Accessed July 20, 2022.

14. American Dental Hygienists' Association (ADHA). Local Anesthesia by State. Available at: http://www.adha.org/scope-of-practice. Accessed July 20, 2022.

15. Spotlight on Independent Dental Hygiene Practice. Canadian Dental Hygienists Association. 2021. Available at: https://www.dentalhygienecanada.ca/pdfs/dhCanada/Independent_Dental_Hygiene_Spotlight_EN.pdf. Accessed July 25, 2022.

16. American Dental Hygienists' Association (ADHA). Education and Careers. Available at: https://www.adha.org/dental-hygiene-programs. Accessed July 19, 2022.

17. American Dental Hygienists' Association (ADHA). Expanding Access to Care through Mid-Level Oral Health Practitioners. Available at: https://www.adha.org/resources-docs/Dental-Therapy-Education-Programs_11-2021.pdf. Accessed July 20, 2022.

18. Wilder RS, Guthmiller JM. Empowerment through mentorship and leadership. *J Evid Base Dent Pract.* 2014;14S:222–226.

64

Practice Management

Haley Dollins

PROFESSIONAL OPPORTUNITIES

Dental hygienists are often tasked with a broad range of duties within both the clinical and nonclinical realms of the dental practice. This skill set may lead to management of a department or an entire dental practice. State-level practice act changes, a global pandemic, and societal needs have required the practice of dental hygiene to expand even further beyond the typical brick-and-mortar business model and have changed the way we communicate with patients. Hygienists must arm themselves with a broad range of management skills and rethink how their role in access and delivery of care, hiring, patient privacy, and communication is approached to help facilitate dental care on a broader spectrum.

COMPETENCIES

1. Describe techniques used for successful practice management.
2. Discuss techniques used for successful patient and record management, including:
   - Listing the elements of a complete case presentation
   - Explaining the risks of relaxed HIPAA policies and procedure enforcement
   - Maintaining detailed records for each patient
   - Discussing quality assurance and the record auditing process
3. List the types of software management systems available as well as their advantages and disadvantages.
4. Discuss time management and scheduling options to create a smooth schedule.
5. Explain economic considerations for a profitable practice, including office overhead, production, and collection.
6. Discuss the marketing of dentistry and dental hygiene, including:
   - Listing the four Ps of marketing
   - Comparing and contrasting types of social media used for marketing
7. Discuss the integral contributions of the dental hygienist to the dental healthcare team.

PRACTICE MANAGEMENT

Participation in management of the dental and/or dental hygiene practice adds a dimension of administrative responsibilities and decision making to the dental hygienist's daily routine and increases the opportunity for professional growth. This role often allows for clinical and nonclinical involvement with the overall dental team and may enhance the team-based environment and individual job satisfaction.

Practice management can be defined as the organization, administration, and direction of the professional practice in a style that facilitates high-quality patient care, efficient use of time and personnel,

reduced stress for staff members and patients, enhanced professional and personal satisfaction for staff, and financial profitability. Those who strive to manage a successful practice must be prepared, organized, and able to act on the goals established for the organization. Dental hygiene managers are strongly recommended to consider professional memberships that support their role (Box 64.1). The practice owner(s) must devise a list of goals and objectives, often as a part of the mission and vision statements. This **mission statement** represents the "what," and the "who" describes what type of business the practice is, and is tied to specific business goals and the philosophies that drive it.[1]

This **vision statement** should be realistic about the current state of the practice, point toward the future, and lay out strategies that will allow the practice to achieve those goals. Consider the vision statement to be the company road map—the "why" and the "how" of the dream.

When writing a vision statement, focus on specifying what makes the practice exceptional and unique to others. Emphasize the specialties of the clinicians, including the key elements of providing quality dentistry, excellent patient service, employee satisfaction, and effective team communication, that contribute to a successful practice. Create and implement a strategic plan that outlines one- to three-year practice goals within your team as a way to identify how the practice will meet or grow the expectations outlined in the vision statement. Consider how all of these elements can be managed successfully by a confident and dedicated leader who is willing to implement them in the practice. While management styles vary, good leaders motivate and inspire coworkers to help advance their field. Team members need to be appreciated and praised, benefits that are often the biggest motivators to many employees.

> *"People ask the difference between a leader and a boss. The leader leads, the boss drives."*
>
> —Theodore Roosevelt

Managers can choose many ways to lead their teams, and the style they choose can easily affect the culture of their practices. An effective leader understands the importance of flexibility and mentorship. As the practice and number of employees continue to grow, so must the goals, strategies, and standards of the practice. Flexibility and good listening skills during communication help to avoid dictatorship and micromanagement and contribute to successful relationships. Frequent communication and appropriate amendments to the office's infrastructure of mission, vision, and strategic plan for the practice and patient care can also greatly enhance colleagues' feelings of inclusion and appreciation. Successes must be rewarded and acknowledged; personnel must also be made aware of shortcomings or deficiencies. Frequently revisiting the practice infrastructure serves as a framework for effective practice growth and supports successful communication during team meetings and quarterly or annual staff reviews. Successful leaders mentor, inspire, and applaud good performance, as well as promote integrity, accountability, and a positive outlook. Leadership is less about power and more about empowerment, as this is what makes a successful team.

> "The quality of a leader is reflected in the standards they set for themselves."
> —Ray Kroc (Founder, McDonald's)

Micromanagement is often viewed as "overmanaging." It creates fatigue for the leaders who choose to manage every detail, is counterproductive for employees, takes overall focus away from patients, and results in loss of team unity, loss of confidence among staff members, and increased staff stress and turnover. Patients also sense a stressful work environment, which may lead to increased anxiety, frustration, and decreased confidence in the team or leader, which may decrease the practice's positive financial growth. An effective leader must understand how to recognize the pitfalls of micromanagement and consistently employ self-management skills to prevent these scenarios.

An undermanaged staff can be just as counterproductive as a micromanaged staff. Poor organization or ineffective leadership may result in employees taking on the attitude of "it's not my job." Poorly managed practices often suffer from decreased employee satisfaction, increased patient frustration and turnover, and loss of financial profitability, resulting in inconsistencies in record keeping and patient care due to high provider and patient turnover.

A **shared leadership** style is often viewed as the best method for successful management. This style involves team empowerment, shared influence, frequent and constructive communication, and, most importantly, flexibility. Shared leadership reduces stress, improves team morale, and maximizes practice profitability and productivity. To develop a shared management approach, the team must start by developing shared goals and answering questions about the future of the practice and enhancements to patient care through the strategic plan. Encouragement of all team members' equal contributions to the office goals helps personnel to become more vested, responsible, and dedicated to carrying out the objectives. A plan may include professional development for employees, as well as individual needs within each department, such as productive use of time, patient needs, current technologies, and treatment modalities. Offices that follow this approach tend to have high financial profitability and patient satisfaction because individual talents are pooled and utilized to the benefit of the whole group.

Standards for Clinical Dental Hygiene Practice

Management styles aside, when devising a framework for quality dental hygiene care provided by the practice, dental professionals should begin with the American Dental Hygienists' Association's Standards for Clinical Dental Hygiene Practice (see Chapter 1).[2] It is imperative that practices consistently revisit this and similar documents and standards to ensure quality delivery of oral healthcare while maintaining provider competency.

Effective Office Collaboration Through Frequent Communication

Collaboration can be defined as working jointly with others in an intellectual endeavor. This type of work is vital to the success of the dental team and encourages high-quality patient care. For collaborative care to exist in a practice, all practitioners must be able to support a diagnosis and deliver the suggested treatment in a respectful manner. Using a collaborative approach requires identifying everyone's knowledge base and areas of expertise and using those attributes to their fullest potential. Team meetings are fundamental to collaboration and often occur in the form of morning huddles as well as weekly or monthly meetings.

Morning huddles are short, as they are intended to identify individual patient needs on a daily basis, resolve any issues identified from the previous day, and enhance management and coordination of procedures planned for that day. These huddles are recommended to last no more than 15 minutes, and typically 5 to 10 minutes, and do not allow time for practice or team development. A creative leader should vary the discussion topics often to avoid monotony and evoke motivation, which may include a quote of the day or word of wisdom. Open discussions and communication are key to a successful and dynamic practice. The leader should never forget or disregard the education and experience of each individual team member. Box 64.2 gives a sample agenda of content to be discussed in a daily huddle.[3]

Because of the ever-changing demands of the profession and patients, a practice manager should schedule different meetings or gatherings to discuss current topics and needs of the practice (Table 64.1). A productive meeting must be well defined, organized, and constructive. Productivity requires advance preparation, including an outline of areas to be addressed; active involvement of others to share concerns; and solutions to instill confidence in one another and effect change. Regular team meetings are most productive when the approach includes shared responsibility, clear standards of patient care, brainstorming, action plans, constructive feedback, empowerment, and praise. Poor meeting planning and communication create frustration for employees. Preparing an effective outline for meetings includes the following three considerations:

1. What is the key motivating issue(s) that should be discussed?
2. What are the topics or issues identified and prioritized by the group?
3. How can successful problem-solving strategies be used during the meeting?

Answering these questions in advance helps meetings flow productively. Assigning a team member to each topic, with a time assigned in the agenda, may prevent deviation or overdiscussion on any matter. If the team cannot conclude an issue, the group may consider tabling the issue for research by the assigned team member and return for review and decision at a specified date. A team member not leading the discussion should be assigned as the timekeeper and another to take notes for documentation of the discussion and decisions made. Posting these notes and subsequent task list in a central employee area such as the break room or a shared file online encourages access, discussion, and brainstorming and helps gain insight into the issues at hand.

Dental hygienists are trained to be critical thinkers through their rigorous dental hygiene education. Though employers or practice managers may be somewhat unfamiliar with their expertise, it is the

BOX 64.2 Daily Huddle Agenda

1. Review the previous day and resolve any open items.
2. Review details of today's schedule.

Administrative:
  a. Changes for today's schedule?
  b. New patients on the schedule?
  c. Significant issues/events regarding any patients on today's schedule (births, birthdays, marriages, deaths, or illnesses)?
  d. Next available open appointments?

Clinical:
Assisting:
  a. Where to place emergencies on the schedule?
  b. All of today's lab cases checked in?
  c. Any stress points on today's schedule?
  d. Any patients overdue for hygiene?
  e. Any photos needed on patients?

Hygiene:
  a. Any patients with emergency dental needs or incomplete prior treatment?
  b. Patient family members due for hygiene to fill openings?
3. Marketing
  a. Referrals asked for
  b. Missed opportunities
  c. Reviews received on website
  d. Referral sources on today's schedule
4. Numbers
  a. Where are we for the day/week/month?
  b. Any collection concerns for today's patients?
  c. Financial arrangements that need to be finalized for today
5. Leadership statement
  a. Can be encouragement, quote of the day, etc., for staff to take with them for the day

Note: This meeting should take no more than 5 to 10 minutes per day unless extended prep time is given prior to patient arrival.

TABLE 64.1 Suggested Meeting Types

1. FYI	Share data, facts, and practice policies or logistics
2. Planning	Create long-range action plans; usually mission oriented
3. Problem solving	Deal with immediate issues related to day-to-day business
4. Decision making	Finalize a process and gain commitment to decisions
5. Monitoring	Review progress of practice or assess team accomplishments
6. Evaluating	Assess the performance of an individual or project
7. Training	Develop skills or knowledge of the team
8. Celebration	Provide social opportunities and reward team performance
9. Marketing	Brainstorm ideas and/or update team on status and successes
10. Patient services	Debrief patient visits and/or plan for future visits or services
11. Team building	Develop a cohesive, congruent, and collaborative team
12. Leadership	Revisit vision, mission, direction, and goals
13. Daily huddle	Review schedule and ensure exceptional patient care
14. Learning moments	Coach and debrief with individuals in training
15. Improving care	Share new educational theories and behaviors that can enhance the patient care experience

BOX 64.3 Steps for Conflict Resolution

1. Explain the current situation as you perceive it. Be brief and to the point, without including your own judgments or feelings.
2. Show that you understand how the other person is feeling and then express your own feelings regarding the matter. Practice active listening.
3. Be respectful of others' opinions and beliefs.
4. Offer a compromise that allows both sides to feel heard and validated.
5. Explain what outcome is likely if all parties can agree.
6. Walk away from the discussion if it escalates to shouting or anger. Collect thoughts, calm down, and appoint another time to meet and discuss the issue.
7. Ask a neutral party to mediate a solution when needed.
8. Be willing to accept the final decision of the situation, whatever it may be.

role of the dental hygienist to educate other healthcare professionals about their vital role in delivering quality oral health services and their expanded abilities to lead in a dental management role.

Conflict Resolution in the Dental and Dental Hygiene Practice

Not all communication among employees is productive and without conflict. Dental professionals often find themselves practicing in close proximity to various individuals and personalities and sometimes experience differences or disagree with one another. A manager or team lead can effectively mediate feelings effectively between employees by following the steps of conflict resolution (Box 64.3). The challenge is to identify an approach that works through differences and find an area of compromise in challenging work environments. Learning and practicing effective communication skills in advance will assist team members when conflict arises.

The first rule of conflict resolution is to understand that people cannot change anyone but themselves. If team members desire a change in a relationship with someone, they must first reflect and understand their own goals, beliefs, and motivations. It may be impractical to think that one team member can work harmoniously with a challenging coworker. Nonetheless, differences do not have to result in constant antagonism and disagreement.

All communication consists of reaction and counterreaction, and altering these interactions can effect change within a team.[4] Exploring how to identify and cope with one's own reactions should preclude any expectation of change in the interactions of another person. Some individuals find it difficult to objectively identify their true feelings or beliefs when reflecting on a situation. It may be helpful for teams to use personality assessments such as Myers-Briggs, DiSC®, Enneagram, or Strengths Finder to identify personality traits and interpersonal reactions from a more scientific standpoint. Discovering each of the team members' character strengths and weaknesses can assist in pinpointing pressure points, as well as which and whose strengths may help to resolve issues. Many dental teams use these assessments upon hiring and revisit them at quarterly team meetings to develop character and increase teamwork before conflict arises. When it does arise, dental professionals must first be introspective and then follow conflict resolution steps to change the situation (see Box 64.3). Respectful behavior among coworkers contributes to a more pleasant workplace for everyone (Figs. 64.1 to 64.3)

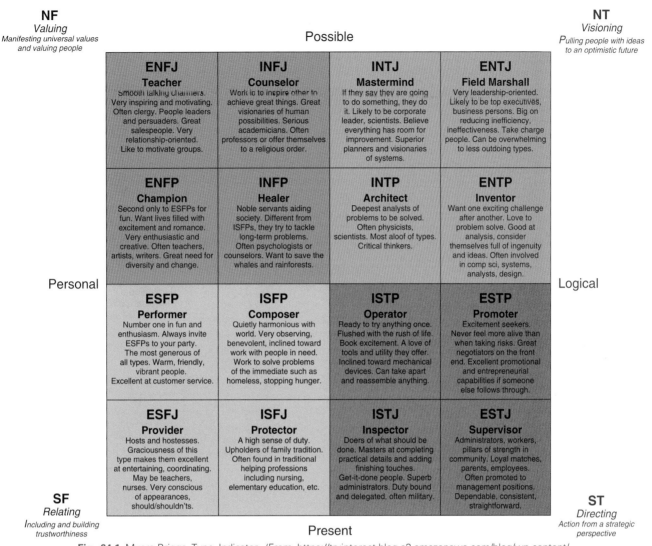

Fig. 64.1 Myers-Briggs Type Indicator. (From https://tryinteract-blog.s3.amazonaws.com/blog/wp-content/uploads/2015/01/personality-types.jpg.)

Personnel Management

Defining specific job descriptions for each team member in the office provides a solid foundation for professional collaboration and teamwork. This allows the employer and employee(s) to recognize and communicate expectations that can reduce workplace stress while increasing productivity and job satisfaction. Job descriptions clarify the role each team member plays and should reflect on their integral role in the bigger picture. Regular review and open discussion about the responsibilities of each contributing team member results in their feeling as though they bring something unique and valued to the team.

A large part of productivity and proficiency in the workplace comes from job satisfaction and the sense of being an appreciated team member. Happy team members are created by allowing each person to work within their own strengths, gifts, and personality. Personality assessments, as previously discussed, may again be applied to understand each team member better, align responsibilities around their characteristics, and foster productivity. Once a personality type is identified, a discussion with that individual employee about their roles, responsibilities, and vision can be used as a means of producing a more tailored job description and result in a feeling of acceptance and flexibility. Placing an optimistic team member in charge of a challenging project may

encourage those working under them, while teaming a detail-oriented person with them may help create structure within the process. Staff members are better prepared to respond appropriately to issues as they arise if they have clear measures of accountability and problem-solving strategies developed to help overcome potential challenges. Finally, creating rubrics that measure success and taking time to reflect on ineffective actions encourages ongoing, positive change as the needs of the practice evolve.

Employees who perceive that they are included, valued, and validated become essential employees. Allowing experienced team members the autonomy to practice using critical thinking skills and evidence-based decision making brings about a feeling of positive impact and value, which is vital to the success of a healthcare team. When every employee in the practice is part of idea generation, each member is more responsive to participating in solutions. Change is difficult, but clear job descriptions and policies, frequent discussions, and employer/employee accountability increase the commitment of everyone involved.

Office Policies

Office policy or procedure manuals should address all areas that are viewed as important to the practice's efficient operation, be

OVERVIEW OF THE DiSC® STYLES

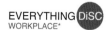

The graphic below provides a snapshot of the four basic DiSC® styles.

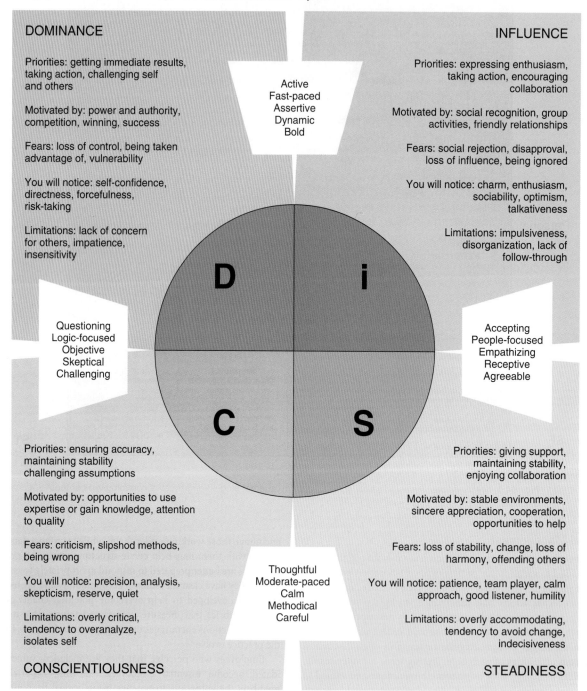

DOMINANCE

Priorities: getting immediate results, taking action, challenging self and others

Motivated by: power and authority, competition, winning, success

Fears: loss of control, being taken advantage of, vulnerability

You will notice: self-confidence, directness, forcefulness, risk-taking

Limitations: lack of concern for others, impatience, insensitivity

INFLUENCE

Priorities: expressing enthusiasm, taking action, encouraging collaboration

Motivated by: social recognition, group activities, friendly relationships

Fears: social rejection, disapproval, loss of influence, being ignored

You will notice: charm, enthusiasm, sociability, optimism, talkativeness

Limitations: impulsiveness, disorganization, lack of follow-through

Active
Fast-paced
Assertive
Dynamic
Bold

Questioning
Logic-focused
Objective
Skeptical
Challenging

Accepting
People-focused
Empathizing
Receptive
Agreeable

D **i**

C **S**

Priorities: ensuring accuracy, maintaining stability challenging assumptions

Motivated by: opportunities to use expertise or gain knowledge, attention to quality

Fears: criticism, slipshod methods, being wrong

You will notice: precision, analysis, skepticism, reserve, quiet

Limitations: overly critical, tendency to overanalyze, isolates self

CONSCIENTIOUSNESS

Thoughtful
Moderate-paced
Calm
Methodical
Careful

Priorities: giving support, maintaining stability, enjoying collaboration

Motivated by: stable environments, sincere appreciation, cooperation, opportunities to help

Fears: loss of stability, change, loss of harmony, offending others

You will notice: patience, team player, calm approach, good listener, humility

Limitations: overly accommodating, tendency to avoid change, indecisiveness

STEADINESS

Fig. 64.2 The DiSC® Styles. (Extracted from the Everything DiSC Workplace® profile, ©2012 by John Wiley & Sons. Everything DiSC, Everything DiSC Workplace, and DiSC are registered trademarks of John Wiley & Sons. All rights reserved. Permission to reprint granted by John Wiley & Sons. For more information on Everything DiSC, please visit www.everythingdisc.com.)

comprehensive, and address a variety of topics essential to management of the practice. They often include information about employee benefits, attendance, hours, dress code, professional expectations and behavior, morning huddles and meetings, inexcusable conduct, penalties for unprofessional actions, career advancement and education opportunities, and patient care. Examples of office policies related to

patient care include infection control, HIPAA, Occupational Safety and Health Administration (OSHA), current CPR/automated external defibrillator (AED) certification, current licensure, continuing education (CE), medical emergency protocols, and patient care approaches.

Office policies often fail to address pressing matters such as conflict resolution among coworkers. It is important to make each employee

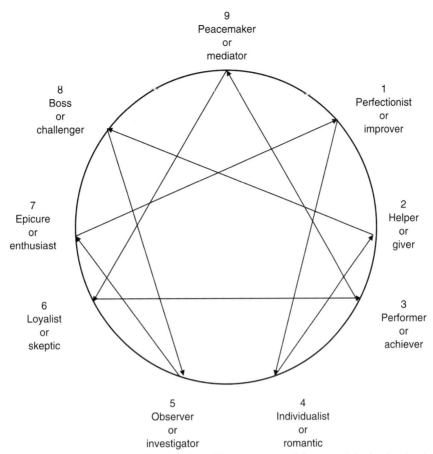

Fig. 64.3 Enneagram Type Indicator. (From Carlson, The enneagram: A framework for faculty development, *J Oral Maxillofac Surg*, Volume 80, Issue 10, 2022, Pages 1583-1586, ISSN 0278-2391.)

aware of the steps to resolve an issue with a coworker and how the office prefers conflicts to be handled. Informing employees of the steps to be taken to resolve conflict in the office can alleviate employee frustrations and lead to quicker resolutions.

As the practice evolves, so should the office policies. A yearly or biyearly review of office policies should be incorporated into leadership or team meetings and reviewed with all team members for clarity. In addition, an employee handbook may also be created and used to explain policies in a detailed manner where necessary to further direct or explain the process.

Periodic performance reviews enhance performance and lower stress levels of the employees because they understand what is expected of them. Job satisfaction results are most positive when each team member knows what is expected and consistent performance evaluation is based objectively on those expectations.

Accountability is the obligation of an individual to account for actions, accept responsibility for them, and report the results in a transparent and respectful manner. Strategies for accountability must be developed to ensure that everyone is acting responsibly and working toward the same goals. Accountability can be just as important as the goal itself. If not enforced, it may encourage laziness, ineffectiveness, and decreased job satisfaction resulting from lack of action on the manager's part. Discussion of circumstances and consequences for failing to perform job responsibilities, collaborate effectively for the achievement of the established goals of the practice, or exhibit productive behaviors and actions is the responsibility of the practice manager. In addition to defining the rights and responsibilities of all office employees, a practice manager must define rights and responsibilities of the patient and ensure that they are available in writing for all patients and team members and fully align.

PATIENT MANAGEMENT AND RECORDS

The patient is the most important member of the oral healthcare team: without patients, there would be no practice. A healthy, functional relationship with the patient must be established early and reinforced often through effective communication regarding treatment needs, individual progress, and education. To be effective at establishing this relationship, the clinician must understand that each patient has basic human needs. Those essential needs, which include safety, belongingness, self-esteem, personal fulfillment, identity, justice, and participation, are sought out simultaneously in relationships and interactions. Human needs are influenced by many factors, such as current and previous experiences and socioethnocultural factors. A clinician who appreciates and understands these needs will be successful at gaining the patient's trust and nurturing the patient-provider bond.

Establishing a healthy relationship starts when the patient makes initial contact with a front-desk employee seeking information or requesting an appointment. Front-desk employees are the first to establish a relationship with the patient and establish the foundation for a successful patient-provider relationship. If front-desk personnel are not welcoming and forthright about office policies and expectations or if they are abrupt or unfriendly, this may cause a negative first impression and may prevent a successful relationship with the patient. This interaction provides an opportunity to showcase the unique qualities of the practice, philosophies, office polices, and/or office expectations for the patient. In recent years, where world events have directly impacted

BOX 64.4 Patient or Client Education Tips

- Provide patients with office expectations and policies (e.g., arriving promptly for scheduled appointments, timely notice if an appointment must be changed).
- Provide practice information about office policies regarding medical precautions and the need for oral radiographs and collaboration with other health professionals.

BOX 64.5 Legal, Ethical, and Safety Issues

Patient autonomy is an important right and ethical principle. Ensure that patients are given all treatment options and a thorough informed consent process is followed.

everyday life, office personnel must take extra care to recognize the unique needs created for each patient and consider these needs with each and every interaction as they may evolve from one appointment or phone call to the next. When office policies change, existing patients should receive those changes in writing. Some practices may ask patients to sign a statement indicating they have been informed and understand the new policies (Boxes 64.4 and 64.5). This update is advised to occur annually as a way to stay on top of communication and create a regular rhythm with patients.

Case Presentation

The dental hygienist is often responsible for presenting or reinforcing a case presentation about dental hygiene care plans and referrals to patients within a general dental or dental hygiene practice (see Chapter 23). To meet the patient's human needs, it is important that the discussion be held in a manner that is informative and nonthreatening to the patient, using common verbiage. Box 64.6 describes the elements of a complete case presentation in detail. Also see Box 64.7.

CRITICAL THINKING EXERCISE

Case presentation: Find a sample patient case with localized severe periodontitis, including a periodontal chart demonstrating deep probing depths. Ensure that the case selected has full-mouth radiographs with evidence of subgingival calculus (potential resource for finding cases: www.dentalcare.com).
a. Role play the case presentation of the dental hygienist presenting findings to the dentist to reach a collaborative dental hygiene care plan.
b. Role play the case presentation as the dental hygienist presenting findings and the recommended dental hygiene treatment plan to the patient. Be certain that the discussion contains all elements, including information about findings, education regarding significance of findings, options for care, choice by the patient, agreement by the patient, and recording of the case presentation in the treatment record.

Patient noncompliance is usually caused by a lack of understanding and results in a lack of patient action after case presentation. Noncompliance may lead to disease progression or increase in systemic health concerns resulting in compromised care, unsatisfactory outcomes for the patient and practitioner, and possible litigation (Box 64.8).

The management of patient nonadherence begins with recognizing when it occurs and documenting it every time. The following list describes the process of documenting patient nonadherence to prescribed care:

BOX 64.6 Elements of a Complete Case Presentation to a Patient

Information
Data collected and assessment findings are shared with the patient using visual aids such as radiographs, photographs, models, or a periodontal chart when appropriate.

Education
An explanation of the significance of the assessment findings is given to the patient, including short- and long-range possibilities and consequences of the condition present. At the same time, the practitioner asks questions and initiates discussion to bring the patient into the conversation so that the patient's level of understanding, priorities, and interest in pursuing care can be determined. Media, research evidence, and other instructional strategies should supplement patient education.

Options
A list of alternative methods of care is given to the patient, including benefits, time involved, treatment risks, risks of not completing treatment, and the cost of each option.

Choice
An informed decision is made by patients based on their understanding of the information presented, priorities, desire for treatment, values, and perceived needs.

Agreement
The patient and professional agree on a course to follow, including sequencing of care and assignment of responsibilities. The dental hygienist, as an advocate, supports the informed decision made by the patient. A written summary of the case presentation should be prepared during the discussion and agreement of care and a copy given to the patient for personal records.

BOX 64.7 Patient or Client Education Tips

Provide written outlines to patients of their assessed needs and sequencing of appointments to help them review and recall verbal case presentations.

- Record recommended care as given to the patient in the record and send copies of the information with the patient.
- Describe all instructions that have not been followed or were partially followed at the recare visit. Include, in quotes, the patient's statement about why the goal was not achieved.
- Describe the patient's nonverbal response when questioned, if noted.
- Document modifications made to recommendations.
- Note any discussion of the consequences of not following recommendations or instructions that occurred between office personnel and the patient.

Patient Records

A complete patient record consists of a comprehensive list of documentation integral to the patient, including both their past and present health findings (Box 64.9).

Patient records serve as a patient's treatment timeline by documenting the patient's dental history with the practice. This record also serves as legal documentation, and it must be completely thorough to accurately verify all experiences shared between office personnel and the patient. Maintaining detailed records for each patient achieves the following:

BOX 64.8 Legal, Ethical, and Safety Issues

In the event of a lawsuit, the judicial decision, outcome, or settlement amount may be altered based on negligence of the practitioner if noncompliance was ignored or not properly documented. The following are examples of noncompliance that may occur during dental hygiene care:

- Routine tardiness or early departure during scheduled appointments resulting in rushed or partial care
- Repeated failed, postponed, or canceled appointments
- Declination of recommended specific procedures, treatment plans, diagnostic tests, or specialist referrals
- Failure to use medications as prescribed or to follow oral hygiene care recommendations

BOX 64.9 Contents of a Patient Record

- Signed HIPAA form
- Current and past health histories
- Intraoral, extraoral, dental, and periodontal charting findings
- Radiographs and findings of other diagnostic tests with corresponding dental and dental hygiene diagnoses
- Informed consents and informed treatment refusals
- Copies of prescriptions, photographs, and study models
- Documented conversations with patients regarding appointments, treatment, and oral hygiene suggestions
- Record of services including all treatment delivered with dates
- Correspondence with other dental or medical specialists

HIPAA, Health Insurance Portability and Accountability Act

- Provides an organized record of all treatment procedures performed
- Includes the patient's oral and health goals related to beliefs, attitudes, and habits
- Provides correlation of dental hygiene care with all other components of the comprehensive care plan
- Aids in evaluating dental hygiene and dental diagnoses
- Serves as a communication tool between all team members and the patient
- Guides consistent, individualized preventive care
- Provides documentation of necessary treatment needs to third-party insurers
- Demonstrates accountability for responsible quality care
- Provides legal protection for oral healthcare providers and serves as documented evidence for defense, if needed

To maintain proper **records management**, treatment entries should be made promptly after any discussion or treatment is performed using clear, concise statements that describe the appointment and are signed by the treating clinician. Clinicians must ensure that a complete and legible name is documented in the chart, as initials are not acceptable for legal documentation, and a provider license number may also be considered for clear identification. Illegible or incomplete written patient records are to blame for numerous incorrect prescriptions, treatments, or diagnoses.

Last, records must be kept on file, even after a patient is no longer an active patient of record. Individual practices must check for state requirements to determine how long this time frame is and what information must be kept.[5]

Patient Satisfaction

To appeal to a broad-based population, practices must offer a comprehensive spectrum of oral health services, including state-of-the-art preventive, therapeutic, maintenance, restorative, cosmetic, nutritional counseling, and reconstruction services, or referrals must be made to specialists who offer such treatments. High-quality care is the key to obtaining patient satisfaction. Displaying a positive professional image and attitude, staying on schedule, adhering to office policies, and building positive provider-patient relationships always reflect positively on the dental hygiene department and the practice. Maintaining current knowledge about oral health conditions, oral hygiene aids and products, clinical and didactic skills, and therapies also increases a patient's confidence in the quality of care. Patients recognize dentists and dental hygienists who are sensitive to human needs, provide consistent technical expertise with an attitude of caring and gentleness, and are respectful of team members and patients.

Correct pronunciation of patients' names can be facilitated by writing them phonetically in the chart. Giving personalized attention, respecting each patient as an individual, listening carefully, thoroughly discussing reported symptoms, and being responsive are methods that help develop special relationships that are appreciated by the patient. As a consumer advocate, the dental hygienist stays abreast of consumer trends and educates patients about oral healthcare changes as new services and products become available. Care plans must be thoroughly explained and alternatives offered, including explanations of all options and the costs of each, with clear recommendations given. Patients need to understand the difference between what treatment is necessary and what treatment is ideal to allow a fully supported and informed decision-making process.

Written, email, text, and/or telephone communications further enhance patient satisfaction. A practice website and brochure should be developed and distributed to describe the philosophy of care, introduce the providers and staff, describe services offered, list office hours plus emergency arrangements, and note special features about the practice for patient convenience. QR codes may also be used in print communications as a quick link to more digital information and further details. Outlines of assessed needs and sequencing of appointments help patients to stay involved with their personal treatment. Sending copies of letters to or from other healthcare professionals concerning needed or ongoing treatment informs the patient of the shared interest in their oral health. Mailing or emailing patients brief personalized notes of appreciation, congratulations, well wishes, and sympathy communicates appreciation and care. Phone or text contact between the dental hygienist and patient should occur after lengthy or complex treatment to check on the patient's comfort or healing.

Patient satisfaction leads to team member satisfaction. The dentist and dental hygienist should recognize one another and all staff members by expressing appreciation for daily cooperation and team spirit, offering congratulations for tasks well done, noting client loyalty, and recognizing referrals received from staff members' marketing efforts.

QUALITY ASSURANCE AND AUDITING OF PATIENT RECORDS

All healthcare providers, including dental and dental hygiene practices, must have a formal written patient care quality assurance plan that includes the following:

- Patient-centered standards of care, focused on comprehensive care, and written in a format that facilitates assessment with measurable criteria
- An ongoing review of a representative sample of patients and patient records to assess the appropriateness, necessity, and quality of the care provided
- Mechanisms to determine the cause of treatment deficiencies

• Patient care review policies, procedures, outcomes, and corrective measures

The practice manager should have a written system and process for regular chart auditing. A valid method of sampling should be created and documented. The review must be consistent and unbiased. Charts may be selected randomly, or a particular area of concern or interest may be audited. For example, a goal of 1% of all monthly records may be set for the practice and every 10th chart may be reviewed until that goal is reached.

A checklist with standards and expectations is helpful for audits. It should have a place to note when policies have not been followed, standards have not been achieved, or treatment deficiencies exist. The record should reflect some commentary or explanation for the deviation. If not, the provider should be asked to comment and to provide needed documentation in the record. Appropriate followup with the patient should also be noted. If not, actions to correct deficiencies must be taken. If multiple providers or team members are responsible for the patient care being audited, a record should be made of standards met and not met for each provider or each procedure being performed. As such, quality assurance involves concurrent review as well as retrospective review of patient records.

Other information examined during record audits as a part of quality assurance includes the distribution and honoring of patient rights. The statement should be delivered to all patients and that fact noted in all records. The practice manager or designee determines if those rights have been granted to all patients and, if not, addresses that concern.

The Association for Healthcare Documentation Integrity has identified best practices for Quality Assessment and Management.[6] They indicate that three types of error can be detected during audits: critical, noncritical, and feedback errors (or educational opportunities). Critical errors affect patient rights, safety, care, or treatment (Box 64.10). Noncritical errors are related to document integrity. Feedback errors do not affect patient care but are minor areas in the system or process needing improvement, commonly typographic or spelling errors that do not affect quality of care.

Some dental software programs can perform patient record audits systematically. The data produced then can be reviewed by the practice manager or designee. Fig. 64.4 presents a sample form used for dental hygiene patient record audits.

Electronic Software and Dental Records

Dental practice software systems have almost entirely replaced the paper dental record with an electronic format. Most state and federal laws now highly encourage or even require digitization. Programs offer a variety of features that encompass day-to-day activities, monthly reporting, and yearly productivity and losses. See Box 64.11.

Electronic health records (EHRs) or electronic dental records (EDRs) are an online combination of information, such as health histories, medical and dental prescriptions, dental and periodontal charting, medical alerts, radiographs, current and future treatment planning, treatment notes, intraoffice communication, oral health education, and other areas that are a part of comprehensive dental care. They also encompass many administrative areas that were formerly completed in a separate system, including appointment scheduling, data management, spreadsheets and e-formatting for billing, e-filing for insurance, pharmacy, specialty referrals, radiograph transfer, and many areas of finance. Networked computers are stationed in each treatment room and administrative workstation so that patient information can be accessed throughout every area of the practice.

Although certain procedures, including dental charting, will always be required, the technology and ability of its systems are continually growing and adapting to meet the needs of the dental industry.

> **BOX 64.10   Example Patient Rights Statement**
>
> **Patient Treatment Rights**
> • Your right to privacy and confidentiality is important to us and will be protected according to all legal and ethical standards.
> • After an assessment has been completed, an explanation of recommended treatment, treatment alternatives, expected outcomes of various treatments, and the risk of no treatment will be explained.
> • Once you understand the information about each procedure, consent for care will be requested. You also have the right to refuse treatment at any time. Before initiating your care, costs will be explained. The provider will strive to complete all treatment that has been discussed and accepted.
> • When treatment is completed, referrals will be made as needed for specialty care that is beyond the scope of practice here.
> • If at any time during or after treatment you wish complete and current information about your care, please contact the front desk and request copies. We also can send information to your other healthcare providers according to the HIPAA statement you signed about privacy of your protected health information.
> • This practice uses strict infection control practices as recommended by the Centers for Disease Control and Prevention and the Occupational Safety and Health Administration. These practices are incorporated to protect you as well as the individuals providing your care.
> • You have the right and are encouraged to be an active participant in your oral healthcare decisions, and your right to individual decisions will be respected. Your treatment outcomes largely depend on your adherence to preventive, self-care, treatment, and followup.
> • We strive to adhere to current standards of care and honor your right to receive such care.
> • We encourage you to inform the practice manager or your care provider if you have any comments, questions, or concerns. They will be addressed to the best of our ability.

Electronic systems aid clinicians in all areas of the assessment, diagnosis, and treatment process. To assist the solo provider and offer a way to provide care without breaching infection control protocols, some software programs coincide with voice-activated applications to record data in all areas of the chart, including periodontal chartings, dental charting, and treatment record notes.

Once patient information is recorded, it then can be compared to past documentation and used for patient educational purposes. Photographs, illustrations, graphs, or spreadsheets illustrate tissue or bone loss and areas of decay in a larger-than-life format that allows the patient to visualize their health status and enhance communication between the provider and patient. Previously documented items, such as the health history or treatment notes, can be easily accessed to review prior to treatment or chairside with the patient.

The EHR format allows patient records to be uniform, understandable, and transferable between providers, while allowing multiple clinicians to view the same records simultaneously, leading to increased communication and quality care for the patient. Many systems are now based in the cloud and allow for easy access both in the office and remotely. The transferability of digital charting allows for confidential and efficient sharing of health information among healthcare providers and addresses interrelated patient needs, increases mobility, enhances image quality, and creates simplified IT tasks with advanced data protection. As an example, the United States Health Insurance Portability and Accountability Act (HIPAA) is a federal law that protects the privacy of health information that can be identified with an

Chart Audit Form

Dental Hygiene Client Chart Audit #: _____   Date: _____

Reviewer: _____   Provider: _____

Note: For each area listed, note yes (Y) or no (N). If no (N) is selected, please give explanation for the deviation in comment section.

Y N   (a) Health history completed, updated, and signed

Y N   (b) Extraoral and intraoral examinations completed

Y N   (c) Periodontal examination completed

Y N   (d) Dental charting completed

Y N   (e) Oral hygiene status/self-care assessed and recorded

Y N   (f) Radiographic surveys and other diagnostic tests completed and evaluated PRN

Y N   (g) Dental hygiene diagnosis, including caries risk assessment and periodontal
           disease classification, completed

Y N   (h) Consultations with other health professionals for diagnoses and care plan, PRN

Y N   (i) Care plan is comprehensive and meets standards

Y N   (j) Consent forms completed and signed, PRN

Y N   (k) Comprehensive care delivered or recommended as appropriate

Y N   (l) Fee payment schedule accurately reflects services provided

Y N   (m) Reevaluation completed or planned appropriately

Y N   (n) Referrals to dentist, specialist, or other healthcare provider, PRN

Y N   (o) Client treatment completed with continued care or periodontal maintenance interval recorded

Y N   (p) Record of services follows documentation guidelines in policy manual

Y N   (q) Other _____

Comments: _____
_____
_____
_____
_____
_____

Followup required: _____

Fig. 64.4 Sample form used for dental hygiene patient record audits. *PRN,* As needed.

BOX 64.11   A Sample of Current Software Systems for the Dental Electronic Health Record

- Patterson Eaglesoft or Fuse
- Dentrix Ascend
- SoftDent
- OpenDental
- MacPractice
- XLDent
- Curve

---

individual patient.[7] The HIPAA Security Rule is an example of national standards for the security of electronic protected health information, and the confidentiality provisions of the Patient Safety Rule permit the sharing of individually identifiable information only as the patient directs or as needed by the patient's healthcare providers for diagnoses and treatment. Dental professionals require the ability to connect with other healthcare professionals to complete their patient's oral/systemic healthcare circle, and a HIPAA-compliant EHR system structure will allow for this communication between various health entities while protecting patient privacy. In addition to the role of HIPAA in the traditional office setting, practice policies and procedures now must be incorporated into virtual appointments to meet these standards on a digital platform (see Chapter 65).

The American Recovery and Reinvestment Act is an example of another federal law that greatly aided the expansion of wireless services and transportability of health records in the United States and required all medical and dental records to be converted to EHR format by 2015. As a result, a task force was established by the American Dental Association (ADA) to put together a dental online database system—the Systematized Nomenclature of Dentistry (SNODENT)—that allowed providers to communicate patient's information to their EHR using a universal method.

Advantages of Electronic Health and Dental Records and Dental Software

Electronic health and dental record software has allowed clinicians to use the totality of a patient's record in an easily accessible way. Electronic records offer many advantages over standard paper files. Electronic files can send alert prompts to remind the provider of patients' needs, such as diagnostic tests, medical history updates, followup visits, and medication refills. Electronic software can assist clinicians in clinical decision making and treatment planning by supporting access to online scientific literature. Dental software allows for remote login and can also provide alerts or notifications for chronic conditions, patient trend tracking, patient treatment preferences, appropriate recare interval reminders/online self-scheduling, pending treatment, past referrals, radiographic needs, allergies, redundant or inconsistent procedures, and reordering needs for supplies. Databases can be linked between dental labs and clinics to check the status of cases and communicate questions between the lab clinician and the provider. Dental software systems may also serve as a safety barrier for the patient and provider by linking with pharmacies to list all current medications or recently filled medications to indicate potential drug interactions or repeat medication prescriptions such as painkillers, including opioids. These electronic reminders can reduce errors in treatment, especially during busy or stressful times or in coordinating between multiple care providers.

At one time or another, almost every patient moves between healthcare settings or experiences out-of-town emergencies, and networked electronic data transfer allows the smooth transfer of information from setting to setting while eliminating time spent scanning, faxing, or copying data or radiographs. Secure internet networks safely transfer patient information through data encryption, the process of transforming data to make them unreadable to anyone except the team member possessing the access key. Encryption is a risky undertaking because the loss of the password results in loss of data; however, it is necessary whenever the security of physical media cannot be ensured. In practice terms, all electronic data must be backed up and properly encrypted before information is sent to an offsite server for safe storage. As previously mentioned, cloud-based systems are completely initiated and used from the cloud. This eliminates the opportunity for loss due to catastrophic events, and because it is entirely Web based, data can be accessed anywhere—there is no need to copy and email data. Information is backed up to the minute, and memory and hardware requirements are reduced because of the cloud-based storage system. Time-consuming backups and external hard drives are no longer necessary. If a power surge or fire destroyed a computer or software, the practice's information would be untouched. See Figs. 64.5 through 64.8.

Upgrading software is also easy with a cloud-based system because it is remote, and the server operates continuously. Failures are possible just as with every other technology, but failures are far less than in most other systems. Date stamping features also add to the level of protection with all electronic files. Each entry is date stamped, documenting when the entry was placed. If changes are made to a previous entry, date stamping documents the newer entry, and security settings can even be changed to limit who in a practice has permission to do so. This feature provides legal protection for all parties involved.

Electronic software increases intraoffice communication. Staff members can inform others that the patient is in the chair, ready for an exam, running late, or has canceled the appointment. Networked programs can be established within a practice for smooth communication between treatment rooms and providers via popup notification or app via monitor or smartwatch, and may even have a specific tone for each provider so that providers know when they are being alerted without degloving. Dropdown features or "auto-notes" can be used and added to clinical entry notes for consistent verbiage and decreased time spent on entry notes. Electronic software eases day-to-day front-desk operations by sending appointment reminders via email, text, or automated phone system regarding upcoming appointments while decreasing time spent scheduling over the phone and returning missed calls to confirm appointments. Patients can schedule or reschedule appointments online and receive online prompts when needed to update their personal medical history in advance, saving time in the office. Insurance coverage also can be autochecked when the patient schedules online to assess or confirm coverage.

Electronic billing is emailed automatically to third-party providers when the clinician submits patient notes and confirms treatments completed during the procedure. Because of reduced paperwork and data entry requirements, administrative personnel have more time for patient education and interaction, allowing for better rapport with office staff. Continued-care prompts can be programmed to appear according to the patient's periodontal status and scheduled while clinicians are entering clinical data, which also assists in communication and accuracy between clinicians and administrative team members. Tracking office and procedure productivity in dental software allows for discussion and treatment improvement within an office team, and the elimination of paper reduces both clutter and environmental footprint.

The implementation of the EHR allows the chairside use of tablets. Because of their size and portability, tablets are ideal for clinical workflow tasks such as entering handwritten notes and signatures into electronic records, generating accurate prescriptions, and sharing information such as radiographic records or intraoral photographs

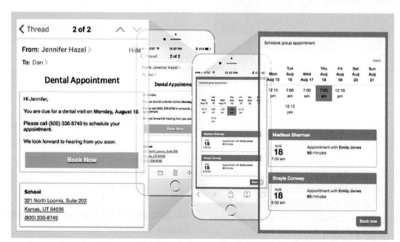

Fig. 64.5 Dentrix Ascend scheduling example for both provider and online patient self-scheduling. (Copyright Henry Schein, Inc. All rights reserved. https://www.dentrixascend.com/features/front-office.)

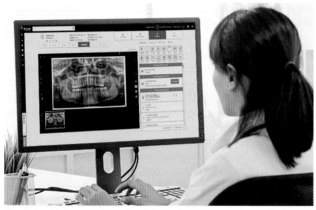

Fig. 64.6 Patterson Fuse cloud–based software radiograph viewer.

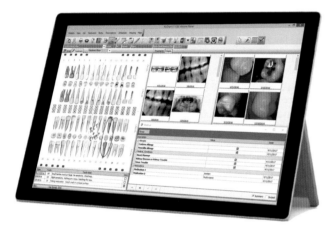

Fig. 64.7 XLDent clinical charting view with Ink Forms sample for tablet-based handwriting. (Courtesy of XLDent.)

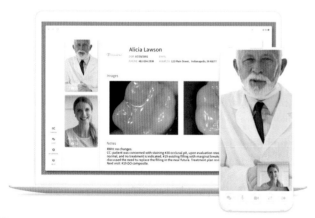

Fig. 64.8 MouthWatch Teledent. (Courtesy of MouthWatch, LLC, https://www.mouthwatch.com/teledent-software/)

with patients for educational purposes. The increased use of teledentistry and collaborative care systems (see Chapters 65 and 9), has also increased the use of these platforms. Teledentistry uses EHRs, programs, and technologies—such as intraoral cameras, live video-feed, and digital radiography—anywhere high-speed internet is available, and it allows providers to diagnose patient needs successfully in remote areas and across the globe. This access allows dental providers in remote sites to collaborate with other dental and healthcare professionals via live feed for the diagnosis of advanced needs, access vital

record information, and provide education in a target language with a click of a button or tap on a screen. See Fig. 64.9.

Electronic files increase communication in the office and between the provider and patient. Some databases allow patients to access their personal records to support the concept that oral conditions are linked to the whole body and affect overall health. Most programs offer features such as "ask a nurse" or "email your provider" to build the relationship between parties. At times, these features also decrease the need for an appointment, saving chair time and the patient's time.

Many software programs feature patient-assisted preventive and disease management services. Online, multimedia oral health education programs can provide patients with valuable information ranging from demonstrations on basic oral hygiene care to detailed explanations of complex dental procedures. Care planning formats, as well as informed consents, can be created while entering data regarding the individual patient. At the same time, patients have an opportunity to increase their awareness and to become active and motivated participants in their personal care plan.

Disadvantages of Electronic Health and Dental Records

Electronic databases and record keeping have many advantages that have revolutionized practice management; however, there are disadvantages with all technologies. Currently, there is not one secure system in which all healthcare entities can share patient records. To this point, there are still no answers to the questions of where the information will be stored or which organization will oversee security and management. Governmental policymakers have not been able to address these concerns.

Small businesses may also find the costs of implementing and maintaining EHRs daunting. These costs include equipment and technology, startup, converting historical medical/dental records to EHRs, ongoing technology upgrades, and ongoing technical support. However, cloud-based systems have helped lower these costs. Practices must comply with HIPAA and revise systems as needed. Those who do not may suffer from loss of accreditation or licensure and lawsuits that may ensue.

CRITICAL THINKING EXERCISE

Visit a local dental or dental hygiene practice to observe the various uses of a patient's electronic record. Report on how each team member, clinical and nonclinical, uses the numerous features of the electronic patient record differently and describe the role each team member plays in ensuring accuracy and documentation in the patient's electronic record.

TIME MANAGEMENT AND SCHEDULING

Appointment scheduling is essential for controlling the flow of an office by allocating appropriate time increments for appointments, lunch breaks, staff meetings, holidays, vacations, and professional meetings or education. Scheduling templates offer a variety of features for practices to track daily, monthly, or yearly office production; pending patient treatment; individual provider productivity; overhead versus production costs; and accounts payable and receivable. Each practice requires and uses various functions, and these systems allow for that tailoring, but most practices use these popular scheduling templates:

- *Unlimited future booking.* This approach allows appointments to be scheduled as far in advance as necessary to accommodate all patients. Most offices use this feature to book the next appointment for patients before they leave the current appointment. Patients appreciate being able to secure a preferred appointment time in advance to best fit their personal schedule. However, this format has some disadvantages. For example, the flexibility to schedule new patients in a timely fashion or the ability to accommodate longer appointments for patients needing periodontal maintenance or scaling and root planing may be lost as an office's schedule may be booked further out and predetermined time frames may conflict with patient availability or time allotted in an autosearch system. Unlimited future booking also requires careful advance planning by the dental hygienist for time away from the practice and may require new office policies to be formed about the advance notice required to request vacation or the use of a temporary staff member to cover time off requests once the schedule has been appointed.

- *Restricted appointment booking.* This approach limits scheduling to a specific period such as 1 to 3 months ahead. Patients who need an appointment but are not scheduled to return in that time frame are placed on a waiting list. Patients who need a continued-care appointment in 4, 6, or 12 months are called or asked to call closer to that date. Often a text, email, or postcard is sent to scheduled patients reminding them of the upcoming appointment or need to schedule. This reminder is helpful for those who travel frequently or have a fluctuating schedule. This restricted format requires less advance planning for needed time off, but it can heavily influence how full the schedule is at any given time.

- *Computer and telephone contact files.* This approach uses a waiting list of patients in need of appointments and their preferred time. Patients who are available on short notice to fill changed or canceled appointments benefit most from these lists. If an office does not participate in this type of booking, it is best to have a list of patients who can be available on short notice and those who need special treatments to be able to fill cancellations. To best use this approach, the ongoing list must include the patient's full name, cell or work phone number and/or email address, treatment and time needed, and availability of the patient by day or time of day to allow for easy scheduling.

- *Production-based booking.* This approach is used to schedule patients based on the type of production or procedure being performed. To use this format, the office first must establish daily production goals. Based on those goals, a format can be tailored to the practice needs. Procedure time blocks are established daily, and patients are scheduled according to the specific procedure block needed. This can provide a more predictable flow to the day and a predictable production goal but can also result in holes in the schedule if the need for that procedure or a patient's availability does not match the schedule.

- *Same-day booking.* There are two avenues, or a hybrid of the two, that offices may take when implementing same-day appointments. The first option may be a dedicated patient column in the schedule that allows for identified times throughout the day when an emergency patient may be appointed for palliative care. This allows the administrative team a clearly identified option for scheduling patients who may contact the office with reported pain. The second option is the addition of a treatment column used specifically for same-day treatment. This column is typically left wide open in structure and scheduled as the day progresses. As a patient is diagnosed through a limited examination, the clinical team decides to capitalize on the patient's need and presence in the office to render same-day treatment. The same-day avenue of scheduling allows for immediate response to patient needs and an increase in production and efficiency on the dental team side, which can create a positive energy in the office through patient gratitude and increased office production.

Dental Hygiene Scheduling

A dental hygienist can provide a variety of services and individualized care to every patient seen in the practice. Full-time dental hygiene work typically involves 32 or more hours a week. While many hygienists have outside influences that may encourage them to work 5 days a week, it is recommended that hygienists listen to their bodies and take the physical toll of dental hygiene into consideration, allowing time for rest. Time away from clinical dental hygiene, as well as varied and core exercise activities, helps to avoid repetitive motion injuries that can affect dental and dental hygiene professionals.

Two typical scheduling approaches for dental hygienists in a general dental practice follow:

- *Traditional dental hygiene booking.* A dental hygienist delivering comprehensive dental hygiene care completes certain procedures at each visit, or series of visits, such as health history review, blood pressure monitoring, preprocedural rinsing, extraoral and intraoral screenings, risk assessments, periodontal charting, dental charting, exposing and interpreting radiographs or other diagnostic tests as needed, scaling and root planing, coronal polishing, pit and fissure sealants, fluoride therapy, restorative functions, patient oral health education, motivational interviewing, and providing recommendations for followup care. For a clinician to provide quality care and comprehensive services for adult patients, a minimum of 1 hour should be allocated per appointment. New patient or periodontal therapy appointments may require additional time. Less time may be needed for pediatric and partially or fully edentulous patients because of reduced charting and treatment requirements. A dental hygiene schedule using a traditional booking format allows the hygienist to treat approximately eight adult patients per day.

- *Assisted/hybrid dental hygiene booking.* Some practices use the support of a hygiene assistant. A dental hygienist and a hygiene assistant work together to increase the number of patients on a given day. Known as Accelerated Dental Hygiene Practice, the use of hygiene assistants allows dental hygienists to work at a faster pace, increasing production and productivity by 50% because assistants are used to the maximum capacity of the scope of practice permitted by law. When the daily production for this team increases, it should reflect an increased salary for the dental provider(s) to help keep momentum and to compensate for the provider who may need to work fewer overall hours as a result of the increased physical workload resulting from the accelerated pace. This scheduling format may become increasingly popular in rural community clinics/settings as a way to increase patient access to care using dental hygienists and advanced practice dental hygiene practitioners, such as dental therapists in combination with a dental assistant.

Continued-Care Systems

The recare, recall, or continued-care system is designed to organize and maintain an appropriate schedule for each patient based on individual needs. When applied to patients with periodontitis who have completed active nonsurgical or surgical periodontal therapy, the term used may be *periodontal maintenance care.* In some practices, the dental hygienist is responsible for establishing and managing the continued care for each patient. The dental clinical team must define and establish office policies and parameters for how continued-care intervals are determined for each patient. Tracking formats provided by dental software programs allow administrative and clinical personnel to schedule patients easily and according to their recare timeline. Online technologies also exist to allow patients to schedule or reschedule their own continued-care appointments online.

Reclamation is a process of electronic periodic purging of all files to identify patients whose care is not complete, who have missed appointments, or who have been absent from the practice and need care. Once identified, patients can be notified of needed treatment and their last appointment at the office. The dental hygienist may be responsible for reviewing charts and managing reclamation protocols.

ECONOMIC CONSIDERATIONS

Practice Overhead

The financial considerations of a practice require determining income and expenditures (e.g., productivity, overhead expenses, collections, and profit). Expenses include the following:

- Employee salaries and fringe benefits
- Rent/lease and utility expenditures
- Lease-hold improvements
- Equipment maintenance and replacement
- Inventory/supplies
- Marketing and advertising
- Accounting and payroll expenses
- Insurance policy payments for the building or personnel

The office overhead, based on these expenses, is a determination of the dollar amount it costs per hour to run the office. Office production is the total fees billed for services performed. Collection and income are the amount of money paid to the office from patients, dental insurance companies, and health agencies. Profit is the amount remaining after all practice operating costs have been paid. Cash flow is the balance between the rate at which money flows into the practice and the rate at which it flows out. Equity is a combination of the practice assets, such as equipment, fittings, and fixtures, and the practice's goodwill.

Financial arrangements must be confirmed with each patient before treatment is performed. The practice's policy statement, presented in writing to new patients, should clearly summarize the financial arrangement options and patient's responsibilities. Financial discussions involving treatment with the patient may involve any individual or combination of members of the dental team. To encourage prompt fee collections, some practices offer a small discount to patients who make payments in full at the time the service is rendered. If the office requires a down payment before extensive services are performed, or if a fee is charged when a patient carries a balance over 30/60/90 days, the patients need to be informed of these policies and any fees that may be added to their account balance. Special long-term financial arrangements by the practice or an outside source such as CareCredit may be offered to assist patients.

Dental insurance assists many patients, including those who otherwise may not be able to afford oral healthcare. Misunderstandings occur when patients do not fully understand their policies and benefit limits or are unfamiliar with how dental insurance coverage is determined. Dental insurance coverage varies greatly from company to company and policy to policy, so it is important to educate patients on their financial responsibilities for services not covered by their dental insurance. Even with the help of the office staff in completing and submitting insurance claims to maximize allowable benefits, it is the patient's responsibility to investigate and understand their individual policy and coverage. Many insurance policies pay a percentage of the "usual and customary" fee for services and require that regular visits be maintained to receive a larger percentage of the service fee. Having a basic understanding of insurance policies and coverage is beneficial for the dental hygienist because many patients will ask the hygienist about dental insurance coverage when specific treatment is recommended. Dental insurance coverage and benefits can vary, depending on the employment model and scope of practice of a dental hygienist. It is important to understand that while many dental hygienists work under a traditional employment setting, there are many scenarios where they may be independently contracted by a program or even self-employed. Theses statuses must be evaluated and managed differently based on the location, scope of practice, and level of supervision.

At this time, it is not legal for a dental hygienist to own and operate a dental practice in most US states and jurisdictions; however, it is legal in some (e.g., Colorado). In several states (e.g., Montana, Oregon, California, Connecticut, and Washington), an independent practice or limited access permit dental hygienist may own a dental hygiene practice. At the time of publication, 19 states allow for direct reimbursement by Medicaid[8] for services rendered, which often allows the dental hygienist to practice outside the four walls of the dental practice, and 42 states allow for some level of direct access to providers.[9] For dental hygienists who choose to own and operate practices, partnerships are made with dental practices to provide patients with dental care as needed, or in some places, a dentist may be hired to work in the practice. These arrangements are unique in that hygienists with collaborative practices or limited access permits work under general supervision or no supervision other than according to a prescription or authorization to provide care. Therefore, the dental hygienist must have knowledge of practice management principles and practices, leadership and managerial roles, and the opportunities to enjoy the rewards of a financially successful practice.

Facility Management

Dental hygiene care rooms and equipment must be cleaned and maintained carefully to ensure the maximum life span of these costly items. To keep overhead costs to a minimum, dental hygienists are expected to perform daily, weekly, or semiannual maintenance (as recommended by manufacturer specifications) to ensure proper equipment function and longevity. Written guidelines are useful to direct personnel in the care of all items. Such guidelines may include information on the following:

- Special cleansing, lubricating, testing, and repairs
- Trained personnel to contact when in need of specialty repair
- Intervals of cleaning/oiling and schedules for changing of O-rings, drains, filters
- Assignment of personnel responsible for equipment resource management

A materials resource inventory file, including Material Safety Data Sheets (MSDSs), is needed for all dental equipment, products, and services. Standards of work provide all dental team members with the information needed to maintain all equipment and products.

Adequate stock should be available, but an excess accumulation of items should be avoided because of shelf life and storage problems. Dental supply companies can supply lists of previous orders, prices, and new items available for purchase; however, if a practice orders from multiple suppliers, a master list should be compiled. An inventory control system can be a paper or electronic system and consists of the following:

- A list of supplies and materials used
- The manufacturer or distributor
- Cost of items
- Quantity and frequency of ordering

Offices should assign to one person the responsibility for ordering supplies and maintaining material and supplies in stock to avoid repeat orders or confusion. Dental hygienists often manage supplies and patient samples for the hygiene department, whereas dental assistants often oversee other materials and supplies needed for the dentist's practice. A specialized budget should be allocated for the dental hygiene department to further break down the budget to allow for the purchase of new instruments, ultrasonic inserts, equipment, consumable products, and technology, in addition to any needed repairs.

Dental Hygiene Revenues

The dental hygiene department is a vital, consistent income source for the dental practice. Without a healthy dental hygiene department, many offices fail to become and/or stay profitable and maximize profitability. Some dentists provide preventive oral health or nonsurgical periodontal therapy services themselves; however, this choice can be counterproductive and costly to production. It is highly recommended that each dental provider work to the highest scope of their practice to allow for the best treatment, increased production, and an efficient overall dental practice. Dental hygienists providing comprehensive care, and especially those with an awareness of practice management, increase the productivity and profits of a practice.

Preventive oral health service fees should be set at a level that validates the education and training of the professional providing the service, and with suitable compensation for the time spent rendering the service. Patients value the quality preventive, nonsurgical, and maintenance care and education provided by the dental hygienist and the relationships that are built through the one-on-one care setting. Additional benefits to the practice are realized when dental hygienists motivate patients to proceed with long-term, comprehensive reconstructive and cosmetic dental treatment, which increases overall profits for the practice.

Some procedures provided directly by the dental hygienist are more productive for the practice and may include radiographs, preventive care and periodontal maintenance, active nonsurgical periodontal therapy, chemotherapeutic drug therapy, periodontal supportive services, dental implant maintenance, emergency periodontal treatment, placement of dental sealants, application of silver diamine fluoride (SDF), cosmetic tooth whitening, and some restorative functions. Protocols and fee structures must be established in the office regarding approaches for each stage of periodontal health and disease. Monitoring of periodontal status is needed at every visit, along with altering or adjusting care plans to address the current status of the patient.

MARKETING DENTISTRY AND DENTAL HYGIENE

Marketing is the business of promoting and selling products or services to the public and may include market research or advertising on many levels. In dentistry, marketing satisfies the needs and wants of the public through an exchange of paid services while obtaining and maintaining the patient base needed for a successful practice—all while building a long-term trusting relationship. To be successful, marketing identifies the "value added" to the focus group the marketer intends to reach. Put simply, a dental practice must create a "product" their focus group of people want, make it available (physically or virtually) in a place those same people visit regularly, price it at a level that matches the value the population feels they will get out of it, and make sure it is available at a time when the buyer is ready to buy. An example of good timing may be marketing tooth-whitening services near the Christmas, graduation, or graduation photo seasons when patients may be interested in gifting this service or buying it for themselves prior to photos.

A "marketing mix" is a combination of factors and strategies launched that can be controlled by a marketer to influence consumers to purchase its products or services. This mix is often defined through the application of the four Ps of marketing, first developed by E.J. White in 1960 and still applied to today's tech-savvy environment:

- Product (or service)
- Price
- Place
- Promotion

Product includes the services provided by the practice as well as the philosophies, objectives, and quality of care provided. Product asks, "What does the customer want, what needs do your product or services satisfy, or what parts might your patient not care about?" *Price* involves the cost of the service, which is based on healthcare financing mechanisms, such as reasonable and customary fees and practice expenses such as materials and staffing. Price asks, "Is the cost versus perceived value to the patient on track, will a small decrease in price gain more market share in sales, will a small increase in an area help gain profit margin where it may be lost in another?" *Place* encompasses the entire location and environment of the practice. Place asks, "Where do patients look for your service or product, can my products be purchased elsewhere, and where or how do I need to try a different avenue of sales?" *Promotion* includes strategies that communicate with target markets and external public groups, such as advertising with a balanced marketing mix of newsletters, television, social media, community events, and all other advertising opportunities. Promotion asks, "What strategies will reach the internal and external client base, when is the best time to promote and with what products or services, what avenues are successful for our competitors, and what avenues have they not tapped that we could?" Brainstorming discussions are an important piece of the marketing puzzle. It is important to ask the "why" and "what if" questions when exploring a new or renewed marketing strategy using the four Ps.

Some practices appoint outside marketing groups to handle all forms of marketing; however, small practices may find these resources unapproachable because of high costs. In a traditional setting, the practice manager is responsible for the marketing relations of the practice. The marketing plan must contain the desired target audience, allotted budget, and mode(s) of advertising selected, as well as evaluation measures, which determine if the marketing is successful for the practice. Within the oral healthcare setting, the entire dental team should be aware of the marketing plan and incorporate it into their daily practice. The most effective marketing is generated by existing patients. Satisfied customers who believe their needs have been met with high-quality oral health services at a reasonable fee and in a caring environment recommend the practice to friends, family, and business associates. Box 64.12 represents marketing strategies that can promote the dental practice. Practice promotion occurs when all team members project the desired professional image and gain public exposure on behalf of the practice. Internal marketing reaps the best results, often in the form of patient referrals. Box 64.13 outlines steps that should be considered for productive internal marketing.[8]

CRITICAL THINKING EXERCISE

Develop a marketing plan to promote the dental hygiene portion of a dental practice.
  a. Include specific activities or behaviors the team members intend to initiate; must identify what each task is intended to accomplish.
  b. Include an overall timeline to complete the project, time frame for each task, labor division outline, outcome evaluation, and budget.

BOX 64.12 Marketing Strategies for Practice Promotion

1. Write or record articles for local newspapers, community websites, area health magazines, X, formerly Twitter, Facebook, Instagram, blogs or vlogs, YouTube, or professional affiliation websites on oral disease and care, dental service updates, emergency dental care, and evaluation of over-the-counter products.
2. Invite local newspaper reports or use social media sites to feature an article on the practice, new technology used, new staff members, or new certification obtained.
3. Participate in broadcast media programming, local radio and television stations with special interest information, talk shows, and community service announcements.
4. Offer lectures to community members regarding oral health and dental diseases to increase awareness.
5. Participate in community wellness fairs that advocate for overall wellness, health, and disease understanding.
6. Sponsor free oral cancer screening days for oral health awareness. Perform oral health screenings at schools, senior centers, health fairs, career days, community and athletic programs, civic groups, and special events.
7. Participate in health coalitions and civic, religious, and fraternal group activities in which the practice professionals meet new people and share common interests, providing business cards and referral slips.
8. Participate in community, cultural, and recreational events in your town, state, or region.
9. Teach health information and cardiopulmonary resuscitation workshops to consumers and other professionals.
10. Teach dental health to local children by sponsoring a "dental day" for oral health month(s) or a "dental hygienist day" for career day events.
11. Sponsor an open house event to welcome neighbors to meet the dental office staff members and learn about services offered.
12. Buy advertising space or time in a telephone book or online Yellow Pages, websites, local paper, radio stations, internet sites, or other community media.
13. Use direct mail methods to distribute practice brochures, oral health education materials, or a newsletter to the patient population or local community. Welcome letters for new community members are also effective, and a community-wide welcome mailer package may also be available to be bundled with other local businesses.
14. Design an SEO-savvy website for the dental practice that can be accessed by the dental consumer through popular search engines and outside websites.

SEO, Search engine optimization.

BOX 64.13 Successful Internal Marketing Tools

1. Train staff to ask patients in good standing for referrals.
2. Remind patients how much your practice appreciates referrals. Place sign(s) in easily seen areas to encourage practice referrals.
3. Use incentives to build a referral system. Examples include tooth whitening, power toothbrushes, a reduced treatment fee, or monthly/seasonal drawings or giveaways.
4. Display posters and/or brochures promoting the dental services offered in the practice.
5. Ask for client testimonials; encourage letters and emails to your office with positive feedback about treatments received from current patients.
6. Build a strong practice website with links to other social media, such as Facebook, Instagram, X, formerly Twitter, YouTube, blogs or vlogs, podcasts, Google Reviews, and LinkedIn.
7. Establish a practice e-newsletter highlighting promotional offerings, events, services, and updates.
8. Consistently survey patients, asking for feedback on how to improve the office.
9. Always provide the best customer service. This leads to satisfied patients, which then leads to patient referrals.
10. Send thank-you notes or emails to patients after each visit, expressing your appreciation for their patronage.
11. Offer various ways to accommodate your patients (e.g., booking an appointment online even if the office is closed).

BOX 64.14 Patient or Client Education Tips

Provide patients with written documentation and practice information through social media, stating the philosophy of care, introducing the staff, describing services offered, listing office hours, and providing suggested websites for continued education, emergency arrangements, and special features of the practice.

Social media is defined as online technologies and applications that people use to create and share content that includes insights, experiences, and opinions via social networking. This may be done on a small platform with a specific group of friends, family, or patients, or it may be done from a large platform to reach a larger audience of acquaintances or the general public. Social media is the newest, trending form of digital advertising and communication; it has revolutionized the marketing world. Social media best lends itself to building relationships and sharing practice updates, feature articles, practice promotion, client referrals, online practice credibility, and advertising. Using social networking shows clients a modern edge to the practice, accessibility to clinicians, and overall approachability. Social media cannot replace all forms of advertising but instead, complements current advertising because large portions of the population access social media on a regular or daily basis, linking print and digital marketing strategies.

Effective websites can showcase a practice or providers' unique talents to set the practice apart and create links to multiple other social media outlets the practice may be using daily to draw in potential new clients (Box 64.14). Website designers or managers must include keyword-rich content and update links constantly, which helps search engines find the practice website and increases viewing—a process called search engine optimization (SEO). The purpose of SEO is to drive traffic to their website and to create pathways that draw visitors to their website from online search engines. This process may draw people to your site(s) based on the location listed, the services offered on your site, or one of multitude of keyword searches a patient may use when searching for a dental practice. In addition, the keywords or phrases used may also affect the place your office has in both page number and listing order when someone searches for a dental office in your area. For example, your office name may show up as number 2 in searches because of the keywords searched and found on your site versus the office down the street, and just because your office name starts with "A" it does not mean you will show up at the top of the list. The rating and frequency of reviews can also affect where your listing appears in a search engine query.

To keep readers stimulated, it is imperative to post beneficial and enlightening articles and video content on a regular basis, to add blog posts frequently, and to update office staff or services along with ongoing management of web-based activity and communication. Social media works well in a budget-minded practice because most forms are free or very inexpensive. Costs for media sites are associated with web design, technologic support, and maintenance, but many offices may choose to place one team member in charge of daily or weekly updates that may incur little to no cost beyond the time spent posting.

Facebook and other such social networking services can feature a practice page, which shows examples of work, patient outcomes, staff, office location(s) and hours, and amenities, and describes services available. This form of social media, along with other media avenues such as Instagram or even Pinterest and Snapchat, allows the client to gain confidence in the practice and feel a sense of comfort from already knowing staff and services before ever setting foot in the practice. These social media outlets can be used to engage clients by posing questions that require input such as, "What do you like about our office?" or posting a team photo or dental-related meme or GIF that says, "Title this." Advertising through this type of social networking also allows a targeted ad campaign based on location, age, gender, education, and interests. These services offer effective and low-cost features that allow communication with existing clients who have the option of encouraging their friends to use the office as well.

X, formerly known as Twitter, is another social media outlet offering a real-time information network that allows members to connect with one another and to receive information of interest in small bursts. These types of sites provide for ongoing conversation and can be used to build a trusting relationship through posts to those with whom one wishes to communicate on a regular basis. These posts can automatically populate on an office's Facebook page at the same time. Sites like these simply require time on the part of the user to post thoughts or ideas on a regular basis.

A blog is a personal online journal meant to be updated frequently and intended for public use. Personal or practice blog sites are easy to implement and can be linked into the practice website. As mentioned earlier, blogs are another resource to be used for search engine marketing, engaging clients in conversations, giving a human voice to the practice, building brand awareness, and generating interest in the practice. Interesting blog posts keep the reader coming back for more, so the topics should be exciting, evoke curiosity, and involve opinions.

YouTube is a form of video marketing that allows a practice or provider to upload and share video advertisements, treatment procedures, and/or educational videos to promote the practice. YouTube allows for great exposure of the upload materials and can expand the practice exponentially. It is important to tag the video or upload with an exciting or descriptive caption for increased interest and viewing. Uploading videos onto YouTube is easy and, best of all, free.

No matter which type of social media the practice decides to use, it is imperative that personal drama and negative opinions be left out at all costs. It is also understandable that sometimes less than flattering reviews may be posted by an unhappy patient. It is best to address any negative reviews openly as soon as possible, with the intention of presenting accurate information for the patient.

INTEGRAL CONTRIBUTIONS OF THE DENTAL HYGIENIST

The dental hygienist is a valuable member of the oral healthcare team and plays an integral role in both drawing patients to a practice and treating them once they are there. The valuable contributions made each day by dental hygienists are not easily measured, but their roles may be recognized. Displaying a positive professional image and attitude, staying on schedule, adhering to office policies, and building positive provider-patient relationships always reflect excellence on the dental hygiene department and the practice. Maintaining current knowledge about oral health conditions, oral hygiene aids and products, clinical and didactic skills, and therapies also increases a patient's confidence in the quality of care. Dental hygienists who speak highly of the practice and the quality of work offered there build confidence in patients that leads to client-to-client referrals.

The clinical role and team leadership role are two of the many hats worn by the dental hygienist. The dental hygienist has the background and knowledge to educate others in the practice as a teammate and mentor, in addition to the role of clinician and patient mentor/educator.

Building a portfolio of contributions to the office, patient outcomes, and overall productivity is a great resource to use when negotiating salary or practice revisions (see Chapter 8). At times, the assets a dental hygienist brings to an office are overlooked and become expected, instead of rewarded. It is the duty of the dental hygienist to record these contributions in measurable terms, using portfolios to highlight these talents.

KEY CONCEPTS

- Practice management refers to the organization, administration, and direction of the professional practice to produce high-quality care, effective use of time and personnel, stress reduction, and satisfaction enhancement.
- The team concept in dental and dental hygiene practice is the interaction and independence of all staff members to promote the unity and efficiency of the group.
- High-quality care and good communication are keys to patient satisfaction.
- Office policies are established to guide expectations and establish consistency.
- Case presentations for dental hygiene therapy explain the examination findings, discuss the treatment options, explain risks and benefits of proposed procedures and refusal of treatment, present an estimate of costs, and make recommendations to guide and motivate the patient in setting goals and choosing a care plan.
- Dental and dental hygiene records serve as a communication, education, assessment, and legal documentation and therefore must be accurate, concise, clear, and thorough.
- Continuing-care and periodontal health maintenance systems are established within dental and dental hygiene practices to ensure regular scheduling of appointments for health maintenance for established patients.
- Economic considerations within a dental and dental hygiene practice include office expenses, production, collection, and profit.
- Marketing a dental and dental hygiene practice involves the planning and management of services that benefit patients at a profit to the practice and involves the participation of all team members.
- Patient satisfaction will do more for practice promotion than any other strategy for marketing.
- Social media should be used to introduce potential patients to the practice as well as showcase the practice's uniqueness, office philosophy, staff, education, services offered, and fees.

ACKNOWLEDGMENT

The author and editors wish to acknowledge Harold Henson, Michelle Sirios, Michele Darby, and Margaret Walsh for their past contributions to this chapter.

REFERENCES

1. Kenny G. Your company's purpose is not its vision, mission, or values. *Harv Bus Rev.* Published September 3, 2014. Available at: https://hbr.org/2014/09/your-companys-purpose-is-not-its-vision-mission-or-values. Accessed August 14, 2022.
2. American Dental Hygienists' Association. Standards for Clinical Dental Hygiene Practice. Available at: https://www.adha.org/resources-docs/2016-Revised-Standards-for-Clinical-Dental-Hygiene-Practice.pdf. Accessed August 23, 2022.

3. Banta L. The a.m. huddle—dentistry's secret weapon for success! *Dent Econ.* Published April 1, 2013. Available at: http://www.dentaleconomics.com/articles/print/volume-103/issue-4/practice/the-am-huddle-dentistrys-secret-weapon-for-success.html. Accessed August 14, 2022.

4. Sharma S. Personnel management: ergonomics and teamwork in dental practice. *Dent Nurs.* 2010;6:12.

5. American Dental Association. *Dental Records—ADA*; 2010. Available at: http://www.vsds.org/docs/librariesprovider50/default-document-library/ada-dental-records-reference-document.pdf?sfvrsn=0. Accessed August 17, 2022.

6. Association of Healthcare Documentation Integrity (AHDI): Healthcare Documentation Quality Assessment and Management Best Practices. Updated July, 2017. Available at: http://www.ahdionline.org/page/qa. Accessed August 17, 2022.

7. Timeline of important events in the history of HIPAA. *HIPAA Journal.* January 2015. Available at: https://www.hipaajournal.com/timeline-of-important-events-history-of-hipaa/. Accessed August 15, 2022.

8. American Dental Hygienists' Association. Reimbursement. Available at: http://www.adha.org/reimbursement. Accessed August 17, 2022.

9. American Dental Hygienists' Association. Direct Access States. Available at: http://www.adha.org/resources-docs/7513_Direct_Access_to_Care_from_DH.pdf. Accessed August 17, 2022.

65

Telehealth

Meghan Wendland and Melanie Simmer-Beck

PROFESSIONAL OPPORTUNITIES

The dental field is experiencing significant innovation in the way oral healthcare services can be delivered due to advances in telehealth technology and the implementation of teledentistry legislation in many states. New models of care that incorporate virtual visits and remote consultations have the potential to decrease barriers to oral healthcare, improve care coordination, and expand the duties of existing oral health professionals. Dental hygienists are educated to complete the assessment and documentation components of the Dental Hygiene Process of Care. Additionally, they are proficient in using electronic health records, taking radiographs and digital images, and communicating their findings. Embracing telehealth provides dental hygienists opportunities to practice to the full extent of their education and credentials, provide oral health services in nontraditional and community-based settings, have a more flexible schedule in traditional settings, and communicate with dental specialists, such as periodontists, more efficiently.

COMPETENCIES

1. Define key terms related to the use of telehealth technology in oral healthcare.
2. Compare and contrast the four telehealth delivery modalities.
3. Describe the four common categories of oral healthcare services delivered via teledentistry.
4. Explain how telehealth technology can be used to decrease barriers to accessing oral healthcare.
5. Summarize how to adapt the dental hygiene process of care using telehealth technology.

INTRODUCTION

Telehealth Defined

Telehealth is defined as "the delivery and facilitation of health and health-related services including medical care, provider and patient education, health information services, and self-care via telecommunications and digital communication technology."[1] Telehealth is a broad category that encompasses all digital healthcare activities and services. Although telehealth and telemedicine are often used synonymously, they are not the same. Telemedicine is defined by the Oxford Dictionary as "medicine practiced with the assistance of telecommunications technology." Therefore, telemedicine is a specific component of telehealth. Like telemedicine, teledentistry is also a specific aspect of telehealth. Telehealth care has been rapidly expanding as the technology and infrastructure (i.e., the internet, computers, smart devices, and electronic health record systems) to support the exchange of data between patients and healthcare providers becomes widely accessible and commonplace.

Telehealth Delivery Modalities

There are four telehealth delivery modalities: **Synchronous (live video)**, **Asynchronous (store-and-forward)**, **Mobile Health (mHealth)**, and **Remote Patient Monitoring (RPM)**. Synchronous and asynchronous are the most common methods to deliver oral healthcare services using telehealth technology (Fig. 65.1).

Direct-to-Consumer Telehealth Services

In telehealth, healthcare services can be divided into three broad categories: direct-to-consumer (DTC), patient-to-provider, and provider-to-provider. Direct-to-consumer means there is no established doctor-patient relationship prior to the encounter. The direct-to-consumer market is experiencing rapid innovation across all four telehealth delivery modalities. DTC telehealth services can be synchronous (e.g., real-time, virtual appointments where a client interacts with a clinician) or asynchronous (e.g., health communication initiated by a client that is sent to a clinician for evaluation or response at a later time). There are also DTC mobile applications (apps) for individuals to access healthcare support services (e.g., health apps that help manage diet and fitness), which are an example of mHealth. Many of these health apps can be linked to biometric monitoring devices, which is a form of RPM telehealth.

Although there are products on the market that provide oral health-related telehealth services directly to consumers, dentistry practiced with the assistance of telecommunications is primarily patient-to-provider and provider-to-provider. The convenience and accessibility make DTC telehealth attractive to the general public, but there are concerns about the lack of regulation and the absence of an established doctor-patient relationship. Therefore, synchronous and asynchronous patient-to-provider and provider-to-provider teledentistry will be the focus of this chapter. Table 65.1 provides examples of direct-to-consumer telehealth services for oral health, along with companies and products that provide the service.

FOUNDATIONS OF TELEDENTISTRY

Teledentistry Defined

Teledentistry is the practice of dentistry with the assistance of telecommunications technology. Teledentistry is not a new dental procedure but a method to deliver oral healthcare virtually or remotely. The same standard of care applies whether the dental encounter is in person or virtual.

Common Forms of Teledentistry

Telehealth is a helpful tool to provide healthcare services virtually, but not all services can be provided via telecommunications. This is especially true in dentistry, where many of the services provided

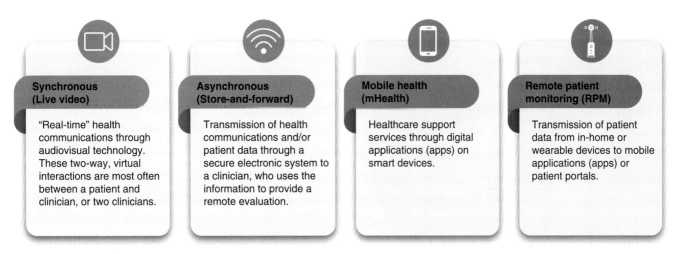

Synchronous (Live video)	Asynchronous (Store-and-forward)	Mobile health (mHealth)	Remote patient monitoring (RPM)
"Real-time" health communications through audiovisual technology. These two-way, virtual interactions are most often between a patient and clinician, or two clinicians.	Transmission of health communications and/or patient data through a secure electronic system to a clinician, who uses the information to provide a remote evaluation.	Healthcare support services through digital applications (apps) on smart devices.	Transmission of patient data from in-home or wearable devices to mobile applications (apps) or patient portals.

Fig. 65.1 The primary delivery modalities used in telehealth. Synchronous (live video) and asynchronous (store-and-forward) are the most common methods used in teledentistry.

TABLE 65.1	Examples of Direct-to-Consumer (DTC) Telehealth Services for Oral Health			
	Synchronous (Live Video)	**Asynchronous (Store-and-Forward)**	**Mobile Health (mHealth)**	**Remote Patient Monitoring (RPM)**
Example	Real-time, virtual consultations for dental questions and concerns	Remote evaluations and treatment plans for orthodontic care	Oral health apps that engage users in their oral healthcare	Smart toothbrushes that collect biometric patient data and provide live coaching through an app
Company/Product	The TeleDentists	Smile Direct Club	Colgate Tooth Fairy	Oral-B iO

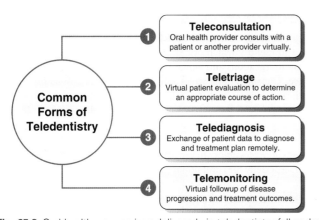

Common Forms of Teledentistry

1. **Teleconsultation** — Oral health provider consults with a patient or another provider virtually.
2. **Teletriage** — Virtual patient evaluation to determine an appropriate course of action.
3. **Telediagnosis** — Exchange of patient data to diagnose and treatment plan remotely.
4. **Telemonitoring** — Virtual followup of disease progression and treatment outcomes.

Fig. 65.2 Oral healthcare services delivered via teledentistry fall under four primary categories. It is important to note that these services are not limited to specific telehealth delivery modalities. How these services are delivered (i.e., synchronous, asynchronous, mHealth, RPM) depends on the needs of the situation.

must be performed in person. There are four common categories of oral healthcare services that can be provided using telehealth technology: **teleconsultation**, **teletriage**, **telediagnosis**, and **telemonitoring** (Fig. 65.2).

The Value of Teledentistry

Innovative oral healthcare delivery models that leverage teledentistry have the potential to achieve the quadruple aim in healthcare, which is to improve health outcomes, enhance the patient experience, reduce costs, and improve provider satisfaction.[2] Studies show that telediagnosis is valid and reliable, and teleconsultation is cost minimizing when compared to in-person evaluations and consultations.[3] Teledentistry is also a tool that can be used to expand opportunities for dental hygienists to practice to the full scope of their education and credentials under the remote supervision of a dentist. Innovative models of dental care delivery provide dental practices an opportunity to adapt to changing landscapes, increase practice capacity without adding operatories, and extend the availability of dental care to patients.

Patient-to-Provider and Provider-to-Provider Teledentistry

Patient-to-provider teledentistry became increasingly popular during the COVID-19 pandemic to provide patients with a way to conveniently access oral healthcare services (i.e., teletriage, teleconsultations, and telemonitoring) on their own schedule from their own device in the safety of their own home. Patient-to-provider dental care is typically delivered synchronously or asynchronously. Videoconferencing software (e.g., Zoom for Healthcare) facilitates virtual visits where the patient can meet with the oral health provider in real time from a computer or smart device. Practice management software or electronic dental records that include a patient portal enable patients to send secure messages to their dental care team with attached images or video to receive professional advice or recommendations at a later time.

Provider-to-provider teledentistry allows oral health professionals to efficiently provide collaborative patient care, like specialist consultations, enhanced referrals, and care coordination. These important aspects of patient care can be accomplished through synchronous (Fig. 65.3) and asynchronous (Fig. 65.4) methods. Advances in technology that facilitate the electronic transfer of patient data from one clinician to another in a fast, easy, safe, and secure manner have accelerated the

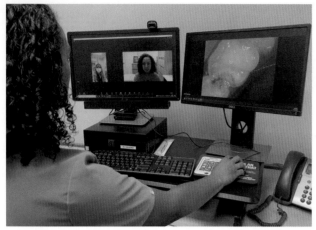

Fig. 65.3 A dental hygienist in the clinic setting communicates with an off-site dentist through live video conferencing. The dentist reviews the patient's clinical data in the electronic health record and is able to provide a consultation in real time using telehealth technology. This is an example of a synchronous provider-to-provider telehealth encounter.

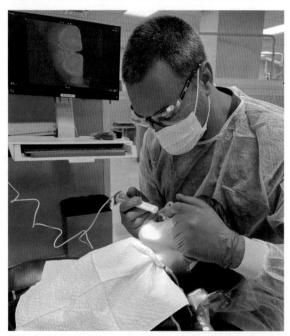

Fig. 65.4 A dental hygienist collects an intraoral video during a pediatric preventive dental visit. The intraoral video, along with radiographs, charting, and detailed documentation in the electronic health record, will allow the supervising dentist to complete the oral evaluation at a later time from any location. This is an example of an asynchronous provider-to-provider telehealth encounter.

adoption of this application of teledentistry. Asynchronous, or store-and-forward, provider-to-provider teledentistry has also been instrumental in hub-and-spoke models of oral healthcare delivery.[4]

If we look at the applications of mHealth and remote patient monitoring in telemedicine, there are opportunities to incorporate these technologies to assist in the delivery of remote oral healthcare. Patient portals that are available as mobile apps provide an mHealth platform for patients to conveniently engage in their oral healthcare. In the future, biometric monitoring devices (e.g., smart toothbrush, glucose monitor, etc.) could be linked to the patient's electronic dental record to provide the dental care team with real-time patient data to assist in

---

BOX 65.1   Critical Thinking Scenario

As a product researcher for a leading corporation in the oral health industry, you use your clinical experience and understanding of the dental field to develop new products. With the rapid growth of teledentistry, you are tasked with launching an innovative smart toothbrush for the Remote Patient Monitoring (RPM) market.
- What patient information (i.e., behaviors, symptoms, biometrics, etc.) would be helpful to track via the smart toothbrush from an oral health perspective?
- How might the smart toothbrush actively engage patients in their oral healthcare and improve their health behaviors?
- How might the smart toothbrush better inform oral health professionals about a patient's oral health status to improve chronic disease management and health outcomes?

the monitoring and treatment of chronic oral diseases. Box 65.1 provides an opportunity to think critically about the future applications of RPM technology in the provision of oral healthcare and health-related services.

It is important to note that there are only two teledentistry Current Dental Terminology (CDT) codes, synchronous and asynchronous, and insurance coverage and reimbursement may vary. Table 65.2 provides examples of patient-to-provider and provider-to-provider teledentistry delivered via the four telehealth modalities, including companies or products that facilitate the delivery of these virtual and remote services.

IMPLEMENTATION CONSIDERATIONS FOR TELEDENTISTRY

When planning to incorporate teledentistry into a practice, the first step is to identify which oral healthcare services will be provided via telecommunications and which modality is most appropriate for each service. Considerations when selecting a delivery modality for oral healthcare services include state laws and regulations, needs of the patients, needs of the practice, access to technology, ease of use for both the provider and the patient, Health Insurance Portability and Accountability Act (HIPAA) compliance, staffing, workflow, and reimbursement. Accessibility to broadband internet can be a major limiting factor, especially for rural populations and community-based settings.

Operations

There are several operational aspects dental hygienists should consider when implementing teledentistry appointments. Items for consideration include:[5]
- What technology, equipment, and teledentistry platforms will be needed for the provider and the client?
- What needs to be communicated to the client?
- What documentation is needed?
- What codes can be used to be reimbursed for services provided? Who can submit these codes?
- What will the workflow look like?

State Policies and Regulations

State statutes and regulations dictate many of the operational aspects of telehealth programs and vary widely from state to state. Teledentistry requirements, permissible practices, and Medicaid and private payer reimbursement should be considered when designing and implementing programs. Although this information is widely available on the

TABLE 65.2 Examples of Patient-to-Provider and Provider-to-Provider Teledentistry

	Synchronous (Live Video)	Asynchronous (Store-and-Forward)	Mobile Health (mHealth)	Remote Patient Monitoring (RPM)
Patient-to-Provider	Real-time virtual consultations for patients of record	Secure messaging to a member of the oral healthcare team through a patient portal	Mobile applications of electronic dental records that allow patients to engage in their care from their smart device	Smart toothbrushes that allow biometric patient data to be sent to their dentist
Company/Product	Zoom for Healthcare	Dentrix Patient Engage	Dentrix Patient Engage	Philips Sonicare FlexCare Platinum Connected
Provider-to-Provider	Real-time virtual consultations among clinicians	Specialist consultations and referrals or remote evaluations and treatment plans through the secure electronic transfer of patient data		
Company/Product	Zoom for Healthcare	Dental practice management software		

internet, the best place to acquire the most up-to-date information is in state dental practice acts. Dental hygienists must be knowledgeable about requirements in the state(s) in which they are delivering teledentistry services. The following questions should be considered when evaluating individual state policies regarding teledentistry:

- Is teledentistry defined?
- Do telehealth laws and regulations include oral health professionals?
- Which telehealth delivery models (i.e., synchronous, asynchronous, mHealth, RPM) are allowed?
- Can out-of-state practitioners provide telehealth visits?
- Is an existing patient-provider relationship required?
- Is informed consent required? If so, how is it obtained and what format is required?
- What specific practices can be delegated to members of the dental team?
- What services are reimbursable through Medicaid or private insurance?

State statutes and regulations should be revisited on a regular basis to make sure teledentistry programs are effectively operating to the full scope of what is permissible and to ascertain continued compliance.[6]

Technology, Equipment, and Platforms

There is no "one size fits all" list of technology, equipment, and platforms needed to implement teledentistry into a dental practice. Listed below are examples of equipment suggested by teledentistry experts. The workflows designed for the particular remote oral health services will dictate what equipment is needed. Table 65.3 lists examples of technology and equipment that can be useful to facilitate teledentistry encounters.[5]

TELEDENTISTRY FOR THE DENTAL HYGIENIST

Teledentistry frameworks and strategies are rapidly evolving as technology improves and state regulations become less restrictive.

Patient Care Services

It is critical for dental hygienists to be innovative and broad minded to identify meaningful ways to utilize teledentistry to increase access to oral healthcare services. Common examples of dental hygiene services that can be provided with the assistance of telecommunications technology are listed in Table 65.4.

TABLE 65.3 Sample Teledentistry Technology and Equipment

For Clients Participating in Synchronous Appointments

Technology for Communications	Smartphone with camera Tablet Computer Webcam Internet Connection

For Oral Health Providers Participating in Synchronous and/or Asynchronous Appointments

Technology for Communications	Smartphone with camera Tablet Computer Webcam Internet Connection
Consent Forms and Client Forms	DocuSign Hello Sign Scannable Apps for creating a fillable online PDF
Electronic Health Record System or Practice Management Software	Epic Dentrix
Digital Imaging	Intraoral Camera (See Chapters 9 and 64) Digital Camera for Extraoral Photos
Portable X-ray Equipment	Nomad (See Chapter 9) Sensors
HIPAA-Compliant Telehealth Service for Videoconference	Zoom for Healthcare Teledentix Epic Mychart Doximity Doxy.Me Google Duo Encrypton software
Other Technology	Dual monitors Green screen

Communication for Virtual Visits

Clear communication with patients is important in all clinical care but especially when new technology is being used to facilitate that

TABLE 65.4 Common Examples of Dental Hygiene Services Provided with the Assistance of Teledentistry

Synchronous	Asynchronous
Virtually interact with clients or other clinicians via live video conferencing	*Store-and-forward patient data to facilitate collaborative care with a supervising dentist*
• Patient assessment/screening • Review health history • Health behavior change interventions • Followup/chronic disease management • Care coordination • Consultations/referrals	• Collect patient data in person to facilitate a remote oral evaluation by a dentist to allow hygienist to provide direct access to hygiene scope of practice • Care coordination • Consultations/referrals

Sample pre-virtual visit communication with patient

Good morning / afternoon [insert patient's name].

You have a virtual visit scheduled with [insert provider's name] on [insert date and time].

To log in for your appointment [insert login instructions].

To prepare for your appointment, find a quiet space with good lighting where your can communicate with your oral health provider. Prior to the appointment, confirm this space has good Wi-Fi and that your technology is working.

Please wash your hands before the appointment in case we ask you to put your fingers in or around your mouth.

If you have photos that you would like to share with us during your virtual visit, please send them to us prior to your appointment so we can review them in advance. [insert instructions on how to send photos].

Providing you a high-quality virtual visit is important to us. Please silence your phones and turn off any other electronic devices during your visit to ensure you do not have any distractions.

Fig. 65.5 Example of what oral health providers may want to include in the preappointment communication for virtual visits.

care. Phone calls, encrypted emails and texts, and secure messages through patient portals are all common methods to communicate directly with patients regarding their oral healthcare. There are many other communication tools available on the market and, as technology evolves, new tools will become available. It is important to ensure that any communication tools are compliant with HIPAA and any additional state and federal regulations regarding the protection of health information in electronic communications.

Prior to a synchronous virtual visit, it is considered good practice to prepare the client by sending them an email about how to best prepare for the appointment (Fig. 65.5). For in-person appointments with a dental hygienist using asynchronous teledentistry, it is best practice to inform the patient prior to the visit that care will include a telehealth component where an on-site dental hygienist will gather diagnostic data, an off-site dentist will review the data remotely, and a comprehensive exam will be completed after the dentist reviews the data. This previsit communication for asynchronous encounters using teledentistry is an important component of informed consent.[5]

Teledentistry Protocols

Practices should establish teledentistry protocols for consistent processes and data collection during an appointment using telecommunications technology. Office policies governing patient privacy, data collection, recordkeeping, and billing may need to be created or modified to support teledentistry appointments. Parents or guardians will still need to be present for visits with minors. Components of the teledentistry protocol will vary depending on your state dental practice act and office policies. For real-time interactions with clients using live video, clients must provide consent to receive care through a telehealth platform. Fig. 65.6 provides an example of how to attain verbal consent for synchronous teledentistry encounters.[5]

Documentation

In accordance with ADHA Standard 6, proper documentation in the patient record is critical for all patient interactions (see Chapter 23). Box 65.2 provides recommendations for documenting the use of teledentistry during a clinical encounter.[5]

Sample verbal consent components

• Good morning / afternoon [insert patient's name]
• My name is [insert your name]. I am a registered dental hygienist at [insert name of practice] *(skip this step if you have already met the patient)*
• Before we begin your telehealth appointment, I need to confirm your identity. Will you please share with me your date of birth? *(skip this step if you have already met the patient and can visually confirm their identity)*
• Before we begin discussing your oral health needs, I need to obtain your consent to receive oral health services through this teledentistry platform [by phone/video]. Do I have your consent? [wait for answer]
• One risk with virtual appointments is that people may hear our conversation, especially if you are in a public area or if other people are around. I am in a private space so that other people will not hear our conversation. Are you also in a private space? [wait for answer]
• Virtual appointments are treated exactly the same as an in-person appointment. Everything we discuss today is confidential and this visit will be recorded in your treatment record for future reference.
• Your virtual appointment today will... [select one option below]
   ○ not be recorded. I ask that you don't record this visit as well.
   ○ be recorded and may be shared with [insert name of supervising dentist or dental referral] to assist with meeting your individual needs.

Fig. 65.6 Example of how to attain verbal consent during a synchronous, virtual visit between a patient and provider.

Coding and Insurance Reimbursement

There are two Current Dental Terminology (CDT) codes for teledentistry: D9995 (synchronous; real-time encounter) and D9996 (asynchronous; information stored and forwarded to dentist for subsequent review). Typically, one of the teledentistry codes is included with the corresponding procedure codes for the oral health services provided during the virtual visit. State regulations will determine which oral

Standards of care must be maintained and consistent with in-person care (see Chapter 7).

REAL-WORLD TELEDENTISTRY APPLICATIONS FOR THE DENTAL HYGIENIST

Synchronous Teledentistry Example
Real-Time Collaboration Among Providers

A dental hygienist works in a pediatric medical office to provide direct access to the full scope of dental hygiene services during well-child visits. The dental hygienist is fully integrated into the medical practice complete with a shared electronic health record system. When questions or concerns arise that require a consultation with a specialist, the dental hygienist is able to connect with a pediatric dentist using live video conferencing. Common equipment needed for this type of teledentistry encounter includes HIPAA-compliant software for live video conferencing, internet, and a camera (extraoral or intraoral). Sample procedure codes to document the services described in this scenario can be found in Table 65.5.

Asynchronous Teledentistry Examples
Portable Preventive Oral Health Services

A dental hygienist brings portable dental and telehealth equipment to a nursing home to provide preventive oral health services under the remote general supervision of a dentist as allowed by the state dental practice act. For each patient, the dental hygienist completes a hygiene assessment, delivers preventive care, and collects necessary clinical and diagnostic data in the electronic dental record (e.g., dental and periodontal charting, radiographs, extraoral and intraoral photographs) for the supervising dentist to complete a remote comprehensive oral evaluation and treatment plan within the timeframe required by the state's teledentistry regulations (e.g., 72 hours). Common equipment needed for this type of teledentistry encounter includes a portable dental operatory, a vehicle to transport the equipment, and the necessary dental supplies to provide the services. Additionally, internet or Wi-Fi, a laptop or tablet, capable software for patient data collection, an intraoral camera, and a handheld x-ray system and digital sensors will be needed. Sample procedure codes to document the services described in this scenario can be found in Table 65.6.

healthcare providers can bill for insurance reimbursement. In many states, these codes will need to be submitted by the dentist who is overseeing the encounter, diagnosing, and treatment planning.

Dental hygienists can play an important role in the provision of virtual and remote oral healthcare. As an integral member of the dental team, whether in person or connected via telehealth, the dental hygienist will continue to be integral to future innovations in oral healthcare delivery. Box 65.3 provides a Critical Thinking Scenario about current access barriers to oral healthcare and the ways in which the dental hygienist can leverage telehealth technology and develop innovative practice models to improve access to care for different populations.

Legal, Ethical, and Safety Issues

Dental hygienists who provide services using teledentistry must be licensed or credentialed in the state where the patient receives services. Barriers to teledentistry include state licensure rules, regulations, and reimbursement policies from Medicaid and private insurers because regulatory oversight varies significantly from state to state. State scope-of-practice requirements may limit the ability of dental hygienists to provide teledentistry services that are reimbursable. Telehealth encounters are subject to HIPAA regulations and standards to ensure patient identifiers and communications are conducted securely. Federal and state regulations regarding privacy and security of protected health information must be followed.[8]

TABLE 65.5   Sample Procedure Codes to Document the Services Described

Hygiene Assessment & Preventive Care Appointment (Originating Site: Pediatric Medical Office)			Pediatric Dentist Remote Evaluation (Distant Site: Pediatric Dental Practice)		
	CDT Code	*Description*		*CDT Code*	*Description*
Diagnostic	D0191	Assessment of patient	*Diagnostic*	D0140	Limited oral evaluation
	D0350	2D photographic image	*Adjunctive*	D9310	Consultation
	D0603	Caries risk assessment—high			
Preventive	D0120	Prophylaxis—child			
	D1206	Fluoride varnish			
	D1310	Nutritional counseling			
	D1330	Oral hygiene instructions			
	D1351	Sealants			
Adjunctive	D9995	Teledentistry—synchronous			
	D9993	Dental case management—motivational interviewing			

TABLE 65.6   Sample Procedure Codes to Document the Services Described

Hygiene Assessment & Preventive Care Appointment (Originating Site: Nursing Home)			Dentist Remote Evaluation (Distant Site: Dental Office)		
	CDT Code	*Description*		*CDT Code*	*Description*
Diagnostic	D0191	Assessment of patient	*Diagnostic*	D0150	Comprehensive oral evaluation
	D0210	Complete series of radiographic images	*Adjunctive*	D9992	Dental case management—care coordination
	D0350	2D photographic image			
	D0603	Caries risk assessment —high			
Preventive	D4346	Scaling in the presence of gingival inflammation			
	D1206	Fluoride application			
	D1310	Nutritional counseling			
	D1330	Oral hygiene instructions			
Adjunctive	D9996	Teledentistry—asynchronous			
	D9993	Dental case management—patient education to improve oral health literacy			

Extended Hygiene Hours in a Private Dental Practice

A small dental practice with one dentist and two dental hygienists is having difficulty meeting the demand for recall exams and preventive care services. The dental team decides to extend the hygiene hours to include evenings and Saturday mornings. The practice will leverage telehealth technology to offer the full scope of hygiene practice allowed under the general supervision of an off-site dentist, who will complete the necessary examinations remotely. Common equipment needed for this type of teledentistry encounter includes a computer with electronic dental record software, internet or Wi-Fi, and a 3D oral scanner. Sample procedure codes to document the services described in this scenario can be found in Table 65.7.

TABLE 65.7 Sample Procedure Codes to Document the Services Described

Hygiene Assessment & Preventive Care Appointment (Originating Site: Dental Practice)			Dentist Remote Evaluation (Distant Site: Dentist's Home)		
	CDT Code	Description		CDT Code	Description
Diagnostic	D0191	Assessment of a patient	Diagnostic	D0120	Periodic oral evaluation
	D0351	3D photographic image	Adjunctive	D9992	Dental case management—care coordination
	D0602	Caries risk assessment—moderate			
Preventive	D4910	Periodontal maintenance			
	D1320	Tobacco cessation counseling			
Adjunctive	D9996	Teledentistry—asynchronous			
	D9993	Dental case management—motivational interviewing			

KEY CONCEPTS

- Telehealth is a broad umbrella term for any health and health-related services delivered through telecommunications technology including but not limited to telemedicine and teledentistry.
- Telehealth services are delivered through four primary methods: live video (synchronous), store and forward (asynchronous), mobile health (mHealth), and Remote Patient Monitoring (RPM).
- Teledentistry is not a new procedure but a method to provide oral healthcare services with the assistance of telecommunications technology.
- Oral healthcare that can be appropriately provided virtually or remotely typically falls under four teledentistry categories: teleconsultation, teletriage, telediagnosis, and telemonitoring.
- The standard of care must be upheld whether the oral healthcare service is provided in person or virtually.

REFERENCES

1. Catalyst NEJM. *What Is Telehealth?*; 2018. Available at: https://catalyst.nejm.org/doi/full/10.1056/CAT.18.0268.
2. Bodenheimer T, Sinsky C. From triple to quadruple aim: care of the patient requires care of the provider. *Ann Fam Med.* 2014;12(6):573–576.
3. Estai M, Kanagasingam Y, Tennant M, et al. A systematic review of the research evidence for the benefits of teledentistry. *J Telemed Telecare.* 2018;24(3):147–156.
4. Glassman P, Harrington M, Namakian M, et al. The virtual dental home: bringing oral health to vulnerable and underserved populations. *J Calif Dent Assoc.* 2012;40(7):569–577.
5. National Network for Oral Health Access (NNOHA). Teledentistry Learning Collaborative: Teledentistry User Guide. Available at: https://www.nnoha.org/news-1/new-resource%3A-teledentistry-user%E2%80%99s-guide.
6. American Dental Education Association. Comparison of State Statutes and Regulations That Address Requirements and Permissible Practices for Teledentistry or Telehealth Conducted by Oral Health Practitioners. Available at: https://adea.org/uploadedFiles/ADEA/Download/ADEA-Teledentistry-Requirements-and-Permissable-Practices-Comparison-Chart.pdf.
7. American Dental Association. D9995 and D9996 – ADA Guide to Understanding and Documenting Teledentistry Events. Available at: https://www.mouthhealthy.org/~/media/ADA/Publications/Files/ADAGuidetoUnderstandingandDocumentingTeledentistryEvents_v3_2021Aug20210804t165513.pdf?la=en.
8. U.S. Department of Health & Human Services. Health Information Privacy. Available at: https://www.hhs.gov/hipaa/index.html.

66

Mental Health and Self Care

Lesley Harbison and Joaquin Borrego

PROFESSIONAL DEVELOPMENT OPPORTUNITIES

With the increase in mental and behavioral health problems such as anxiety and depression, dental hygienists must be equipped with the skills necessary to manage chronic stress in everyday life and in the workplace. Learning stress management skills and self-care will help aid dental hygienists in reducing professional burnout and improve well-being. Additionally, acquiring these skills will improve the overall quality of patient care.

COMPETENCIES

1. Discuss the prevalence of anxiety, depression, and increase in mental disorders.
2. Contrast the relationship between stress and stressors.
3. Compare negative short-term and long-term health outcomes to chronic stress, anxiety, and depression.
4. Analyze the occurrence of professional burnout in the dental hygiene profession and describe factors that influence burnout and time off of work.
5. Correlate the importance of early intervention measures to reduce the occurrence of stress-related chronic conditions and professional burnout.
6. Identify the impact of the practitioner's mental health as it relates to patient care, as well as the role of the practitioner in addressing the overall well-being of the patient.
7. Integrate self-care and stress management strategies.

INTRODUCTION

Life is stressful. Everyone experiences challenges throughout their lifetime. Daily life (e.g., family responsibilities, work pressures, health, and job security) can be a significant source of stress. Even positive life events that make us happy (e.g., birth of a child, getting married, or traveling for fun) can be stressful. Stress is normal. Some stress can be beneficial. Unfortunately, for some, stress can contribute to psychological distress and physical health problems. Stress can also affect the quality of our relationships and social interactions. In general, stress and mental health problems have been reported more frequently in recent years, seemingly coinciding with events such as an increase in civil unrest, wars, and pandemics.

It is important as healthcare providers to prioritize personal mental and behavioral health as well as overall well-being. Providing high-quality care to patients is partially dependent on maintaining a healthy mental state, career enjoyment, and maintaining a work/life balance, among other important aspects. Throughout this chapter, the topic of how mental health problems can directly affect a dental hygienist's personal and professional life, as well as patient care, will be discussed.

Beyond one's own mental health and well-being status, the dental hygienist must also consider the mental health status of their patients. Patients may be dealing with mental and behavioral health problems that have significantly disrupted their daily activities, they may be prescribed medications that affect their oral health, or they may confide in the dental hygienist about stressors they are facing. Understanding the dental hygienist's role in caring for a patient with mental health problems is of vital importance (see Box 66.1). This chapter will detail tools and methods of dealing with work-related stressors as well as how to care for the patient's well-being. This approach to patient care is described as person-centered care, with an emphasis on care that is respectful, compassionate, and responsive to the individual.

RISE IN STRESS-RELATED MENTAL HEALTH PROBLEMS

A survey conducted to research how Americans were feeling during the COVID-19 pandemic found that approximately one-third of respondents reported feeling stressed about the pandemic and found decision making to be difficult.[1] Those who identified as Millennials reported struggling more with daily decision making due to the pandemic as compared to those who identified as older adults (Gen Z, Gen Xers, and Baby Boomers). Millennials also reported experiencing more overall stress than other generational groups. It is understandable that events such as civil unrest and pandemics can contribute to feelings of worry, anxiety, and depression.[1] Worldwide, one out of every eight people is living with a mental health problem, and access to effective mental healthcare is absent in many parts of the world, in both developed and underdeveloped nations.[2] One in five Canadians will experience some mental health problem during any given year.[3] According to the Centers for Disease Control and Prevention, more than one in three high school students expressed persistent feelings of sadness or hopelessness, a 40% increase since 2009.[4] A recent survey found approximately 20% of adults in the United States reported experiencing a mental health illness in 2019.[5]

Dental hygienists will treat many patients during their career, and the probability of treating a patient with a mental health problem is virtually guaranteed. Not only is there a high chance of treating a patient with either an acute or chronic mental health problem, but dental hygienists may also experience times when their own mental health is challenged in one form or another; see Box 66.2. Knowing whom to contact for personal matters as well as understanding what opportunities are available for interprofessional collaboration is a vital piece towards providing patients with the highest quality patient-centered care.

LIFE AND STRESS

Continuous, important, day-to-day decision making can contribute to stress and fatigue and can have a deleterious impact on many. Studies suggest that parenting is significantly impacted by everyday decision making related to work and school.[1] Family responsibility and relationships can be a source of stress in an individual's life, and data reveals parents often feel a lack of emotional support.

Individuals have identified different sources of stress that affect their daily lives (see Fig. 66.1). With regard to personal and family factors, individuals reported personal safety, discrimination, individual, and family health problems, relationships, and responsibilities as sources of stress.[1] Stress related to job stability, money, housing costs, and the economy also rank high. A South African study conducted in 2020 revealed top-ranking concerns to be the economy, childcare and schooling, family health and well-being, and future career possibilities.[6] When several of these common life stressors occur at once and coincide with a significant unforeseen event, a person's potential for developing a mental health issue may increase.

UNDERSTANDING STRESS

Stress is the physiological and psychological *response* to a physical, chemical, or emotional element resulting in tension and may be an aspect of disease causation. People can experience stress either emotionally (e.g., worrying or ruminating thoughts) or physically (e.g., tension headaches or clenched jaw). The element being responded to is referred to as a **stressor** and may be internal (e.g., intrusive thoughts or bodily sensations) or external (e.g., the environment). A stressor can also be an event (e.g., death of a loved one or losing one's job) or a condition (e.g., physical health problems).

As dental hygienists, it is not uncommon to encounter a patient with dental anxiety. It is reported that one out of every six adults experiences dental anxiety, and globally, 1% to 6% experience extreme dental fear.[7] It is important to recognize the signs that a patient with dental anxiety may exhibit. Implementing an in-office stress reduction protocol in order to advance patients through the appointment and accomplish the treatment goals is essential to successful patient outcomes; see Table 66.1. Establishing a stress reduction protocol not only is beneficial to patients who experience dental anxiety but

can also improve the experience of all patients in the dental practice. Patients find it easier to relax and compliance improves once trust is established between the patient and the clinician. Additionally, an anxious patient can lengthen appointment time and disrupt progress, limiting the dental hygienist's ability to efficiently complete treatment goals. When the patient is able to relax, the dental hygienist will feel more relaxed as well. A patient who trusts the practitioner and the process results in the dental hygienist confidently providing excellent care to the patient.[8]

There are many features of the dental environment and aspects of a dental appointment that could induce anxiety. Patients may experience stress from the sounds and smells of the environment or simply from the worry of the financial burdens that come with costly dental treatment. The dental hygiene diagnosis should include application of the dental hygiene human needs conceptual model or the oral health–related quality of life model when identifying issues involving patients' fear and stress (e.g., fear of needles, fear of pain, or financial stress) (see Table 66.2). For more information on dental hygiene diagnosis and the human needs and oral health–related quality of life models, please refer to Chapters 22 and 23.

EFFECTS OF STRESS ON THE BODY

When people experience stress, the body's natural fight or flight response is activated, a self-limiting adaptation to various threats mediated by the sympathetic branch of the autonomic nervous system.[5] An individual may experience dilated pupils, increased heart rate, and a general enhanced state of awareness. The person can also become tense in response to the stressor(s) presented. As noted at the beginning of

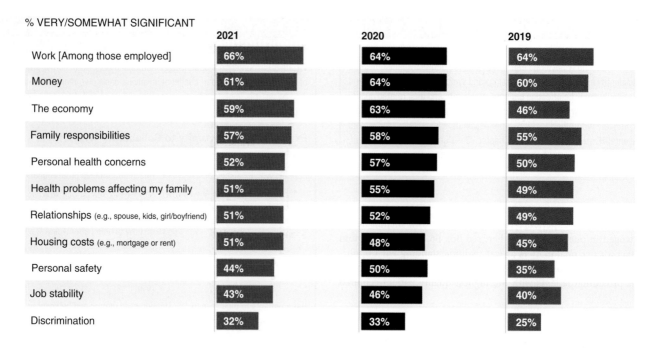

% VERY/SOMEWHAT SIGNIFICANT

	2021	2020	2019
Work [Among those employed]	66%	64%	64%
Money	61%	64%	60%
The economy	59%	63%	46%
Family responsibilities	57%	58%	55%
Personal health concerns	52%	57%	50%
Health problems affecting my family	51%	55%	49%
Relationships (e.g., spouse, kids, girl/boyfriend)	51%	52%	49%
Housing costs (e.g., mortgage or rent)	51%	48%	45%
Personal safety	44%	50%	35%
Job stability	43%	46%	40%
Discrimination	32%	33%	25%

STRESS IN AMERICA™ 2021: STRESS AND DECISION MAKING DURING THE PANDEMIC   © 2021 American Psychological Association

Fig. 66.1 Data from American Psychological Association. Citation: American Psychological Association. *Significant Sources of Stress:2019–2021*. American Psychological Association; 2021. Available at: https://www.apa.org/news/press/releases/stress/2021/october-infographics.

TABLE 66.1	Example of In-Office Stress Reduction Protocol
Patient Concerns	**Office Protocol**
Financial concerns	• Empathetically counsel patients regarding the consequences of postponing treatment (e.g., financial, systemic health, and oral health) • Provide low-interest payment plans • Supply treatment options within various price points
Dental anxiety/phobia	• Regard patient's fears seriously • Provide time to discuss the patient's specific fears • Determine if the patient wants details about procedures or simply the ability to ask questions • Agree on a signal to stop procedure if patient is uncomfortable or just needs a break • Provide a distraction (e.g., headphones, TV, stress ball, or fidget spinner) • Provide information about various mindfulness techniques (e.g., imagery/visualization, breathing technique, or body scanning)
Reviewing medical history	• Ask for a current list of medication at every visit (patients may be hesitant to admit to taking medication for anxiety) • Common medications to include—Selective Serotonin Reuptake Inhibitors (SSRIs), Serotonin and Norepinephrine Reuptake Inhibitors (SNRIs), Tricyclic Antidepressants (TCAs), Benzodiazepines • Xerostomia is a very common side effect with many of the drugs used to treat anxiety and depression • Other conditions or concerns may include bruxism, GERD, xerostomia, poor oral hygiene, poor nutrition, and avoidance of dental care
Patient reveals feelings of depression or being overwhelmed	• Opportunity for interprofessional collaboration • Listen to patients and acknowledge the information that they are sharing • Refer the patient to a healthcare provider • Provide a list of available community mental health resources • Oral health can suffer when life feels overwhelming or symptoms of depression lead to neglect of daily activities such as proper nutrition or oral hygiene

the chapter, we all experience stress, but not everyone experiences the same stressors, nor does everyone respond to those stressors in the same way. Various physical and psychosocial symptoms may result from stressors (Table 66.3). It is important to note that these symptoms are not specific to stress alone; they also present in other clinical conditions such as anxiety, insomnia, and depression.

TYPES OF STRESS

Not all stress that we experience is negative. It is important to differentiate between *eustress* and *distress*. **Eustress** is the stress that people experience due to positive life events (e.g., work promotion or starting your first job after graduation). Eustress can be beneficial as it helps

TABLE 66.2 Dental Hygiene Diagnosis Example

DH Diagnosis—Unmet Human Need	Etiology—due to	Signs and Symptoms—Evidenced by	Client Goal
Freedom from fear/stress	Anxiety about receiving local anesthetic Fear of receiving dental treatment Feeling a lack of control	Reports experiencing a racing heart after receiving local anesthetic in the past Feels tension or tightness in chest during procedures that are "noisy" (e.g., ultrasonic, dental handpiece) Continually postponing needed dental treatment	Be able to receive local anesthetic so that treatment is pain free; feel relaxed during procedures and not feel panicked when there are unfamiliar noises

TABLE 66.3 Possible Physical and Psychological Symptoms of Stress

Physical Symptoms	Psychological Symptoms
• Sleep disturbance (e.g., not able to fall asleep due to being preoccupied) • Muscle tension (e.g., jaw clenching) • Headaches, neck muscle strains • Other bodily sensations (e.g., pit in stomach) • Disruption in eating well (e.g., eating just to eat or eating when stressed) • Fatigue	• Feeling anxious • Feeling overwhelmed • Difficulties concentrating • Constant rumination (continued focus/worry) • Difficulty in making decisions (e.g., not being able to think clearly) • Changes in mood (e.g., irritability) • Inability to make decisions

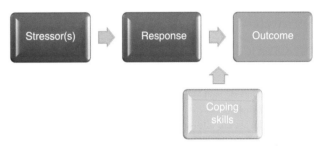

Fig. 66.2 Stress Model. The relationship between stressor(s), stress, and outcome. This diagram displays how coping skills can influence the outcome of a person experiencing a stress response from various stressors.

with such psychological factors such as motivation and focus. Physiologically, the brain releases endorphins when a person experiences eustress. In contrast to eustress, *distress* is a type of stress that can have a deleterious impact on the psychological well-being and physical health of individuals. Psychological *distress* is an outcome of observing or experiencing negative stressors that are severe in nature and/or occur for an extended period. When people experience distress, they may not have the emotional and behavioral capacity to manage the stressors effectively. Physiologically, the brain releases cortisol, a stress hormone, as well as adrenaline, into the body.

Stress can also be characterized with regard to duration. *Acute stress* is usually a one-time occurrence or short-term in nature. Some examples of when people experience acute stress are running late to work due to being stuck in traffic, caring for a child home from school with the flu, or failing an exam. Many individuals with multiple responsibilities or demanding jobs, such as those in healthcare, experience what is known as episodic acute stress.

Contrary to acute stress is *chronic stress*, which is repeated stress that is more long-term in nature. Some examples of chronic stress include being unemployed for an extended period, having a child with a chronic health condition, or repeated exposure to trauma. There is evidence that chronic stress is associated with the development of various diseases such as cardiovascular disease, insulin insensitivity, and cancer.[5] How individuals cope with various stressors will have a significant effect on outcomes and their level of distress (see Fig. 66.2).

In Fig. 66.2, we see a visual of what Brooklyn, in the case study (Box 66.3), is experiencing. Brooklyn is experiencing numerous environmental stressors (the sources of stress) such as job demands, ensuring that her children are involved in extracurricular activities while being a single parent, etc. Brooklyn's response to these stressors is stress in the form of disruption in sleep, feelings of dread, tightness in her stomach, and being short with her children. Brooklyn's coping skills will impact

the short- and long-term outcome of her stress. In one scenario, Brooklyn's healthy coping skills (e.g., practicing mindfulness, exercising, and seeking help) can greatly minimize the negative impact of the stressors she is experiencing. In another scenario, Brooklyn may have less healthy coping skills (e.g., withdrawing, drinking, and stress eating), which may lead to significant distress and increase the probability of developing a psychological disorder such as anxiety or depression.

THE RELATIONSHIP BETWEEN STRESS AND MENTAL AND BEHAVIORAL HEALTH

Decades of research show a clear relationship between stress and mental and behavioral health problems. Psychological distress occurs when the stress that people experience is either too severe, chronic, or a combination of both. Individuals with psychological disorders (e.g., anxiety or depression) report experiencing distress and stress.

Stress and anxiety may be lumped together or thought to be synonymous, but there are differences. As noted earlier, stress is the body's response to stressors. Individuals can often point to stressors that are affecting them and contributing to their stress. However, an individual may experience anxiety in response to stress, or people can experience anxiety in the absence of stressors. With anxiety, a person can feel worry or impending doom, even without an obvious cause. Anxiety is considered more persistent and can lead to significant distress and impairment—just like stress. It is important to note that there are stress-related symptoms (e.g., increased heart rate, irritability, or feeling out of control) that are also found in many anxiety-related disorders such as Panic Disorder, Social Anxiety Disorder, and Generalized Anxiety Disorder. Although the majority of individuals report experiencing stress, fewer report experiencing anxiety-related disorders and major depression (Table 66.4).

According to the National Institute of Mental Health, approximately 31% of the US population will experience an anxiety disorder in their lifetime.[9] On a related note, the prevalence of a major depressive disorder is approximately 8.4% among US adults.[10] The prevalence of a major depressive disorder is higher in females than males and in

BOX 66.3   Case Study

Brooklyn is a 35-year-old female who has been out of school and practicing dental hygiene in a Federally Qualified Health Clinic serving a low-income and diverse population for 5 years. When she first graduated from school, Brooklyn was energized and enthusiastic about serving the community with her newly acquired skills. She thoroughly enjoyed interacting with patients, having her own schedule, and providing therapies that prevented oral disease. Every day was fun. She worked hard and went home exhausted but felt she was compensated fairly for her time.

Since graduating, Brooklyn has worked Monday through Thursday while occasionally picking up an extra Friday through a temping agency. Her typical workday starts at 7:30 AM and often goes past 5 PM. She provides care to roughly one patient per hour and gets 30 to 45 minutes for lunch, depending on how the day is coming together. The practice Brooklyn works for is very busy, and she rarely has a "no show" appointment. She often remarks that once she sets foot in her office, it's "Go time!" and it does not stop until the last patient leaves.

Brooklyn is a single mother with two children at home, ages 10 and 13. She has full custody of her children and transitions from the dental office to "taxi driver" for her kids after work and school. She shuttles them to soccer, taekwondo, and various other activities. Her children want to do it all, and she loves to encourage them. Dinner is often "on the go," and then she wraps up the evening helping her kids finish their homework assignments. Brooklyn is usually mentally and physically exhausted by the end of the day.

Brooklyn loved the fast-paced atmosphere of her job for the first several years, but she has started to notice a subtle shift. Each patient appointment is beginning to feel like a means to an end instead of a unique opportunity to prevent disease and educate individuals. She realizes that she is taking ibuprofen every morning and often in the evening as well. Brooklyn is experiencing sleep disturbances, so her sleep is not as good as it used to be as she wakes up tired most days. She wakes throughout the night and has trouble falling back asleep. She is noticing a growing resentment toward her coworkers, who seem to have more down time during the day. In the morning, on her way to work, she is noticing a tightness in her stomach and almost a feeling of dread. Brooklyn also finds herself snapping at her children and feeling guilty about their constant drive-thru dinners. Finally, Brooklyn finds less satisfaction in her job but feels that she cannot leave her job as she needs the income. All this is contributing to Brooklyn feeling stressed, resentful, and unhappy at work and at home.

Case Study Questions:

What are the stressors in Brooklyn's life contributing to chronic stress?

What are some of the signs Brooklyn is showing of accumulating stress?

How is Brooklyn's work-life balance affecting her overall well-being?

What are some things Brooklyn could do to mitigate the accumulation of stress in her life?

BOX 66.4   Critical Thinking Scenario

Marcus graduated from a baccalaureate dental hygiene program 2 years ago. He has a large amount of student loan debt to pay off. Marcus is eager to please his employer, coworkers, and patients. Recently, Marcus has noticed increased body pain and exhaustion after work.

His manager frequently asks Marcus if he can "squeeze in another patient" into his already busy schedule. Marcus always says "Yes" because he wants his office coworkers to like him and see him as a valuable employee. Marcus is aware that the equipment he uses in his operatory is old and lacks ideal ergonomic function. He also realizes that he seldom has time for bathroom or stretch breaks in between patients, but he rationalizes that he is young and healthy and feels confident that with his positive attitude, he can get through the day.

Critical Thinking Question:

Marcus is a "people pleaser" and relatively new to dental hygiene practice; however, how could he use his leadership role as a dental hygienist to advocate for work policies and ergonomic equipment that benefits not only him but the whole team?

or stress eating) and physical activity (e.g., sitting on the couch). Over time, stress can also negatively affect one's immune system and contribute to increased heart rate and blood pressure.[5]

THE ROLE OF DISTRESS

The *Vulnerability-Stress Model* (also known as the Diathesis-Stress Model) helps explain why individuals exposed to the same stressor or set of stressors respond differently. In being exposed to the same stressors, Person A experiences distress while Person B does not. This model also helps explain why some individuals develop a psychological disorder such as anxiety or depression. In this model, some individuals have a predisposed biological or psychological vulnerability (e.g., genetics or cognitive styles) that *interact* with environmental stressors.[11] Simply stated, some individuals are more susceptible due to a biological predisposition or early life experiences (e.g., childhood trauma) (see Fig. 66.3). Individuals with greater vulnerabilities (e.g., inflexible cognitive styles, poor coping skills) require fewer stress levels and stressors to become distressed (Fig. 66.4). Likewise, individuals with fewer of these biological and psychological vulnerabilities (e.g., flexible cognitive styles, healthy coping skills) may require a greater level or number of stressors to become distressed (see Table 66.6).

PROFESSIONAL BURNOUT

Professional burnout is characterized by emotional and physical exhaustion, detachment from work, and feelings of professional loneliness.[12] Burnout is considered an occupational syndrome with individuals from any profession experiencing symptoms; however, in recent years, burnout has been studied and discussed most earnestly in the healthcare fields.[12,13] Due to the association with risks of mental health challenges such as anxiety and depression, burnout is vital to understand and learn to mitigate. Burnout, like distress, is not an individual mental health diagnosis but rather, an emotional response to chronic stressors.

It is important to understand why some individuals experience burnout. Professional burnout occurs when something has negatively changed within an individual's relationship with their work. Individuals typically start a career with enthusiasm and excitement. Motivation with work is renewed by a desire to perform their skills well, make

young adults aged 18 to 25 years.[10] Symptoms that may appear when an individual has developed anxiety and/or depression will vary in number and may manifest differently in individuals (see Table 66.5). It is important to note that there are specific parameters to being diagnosed with either anxiety or depression, and the symptoms listed here may be a result of some other factors such as duration of symptoms. Additionally, not all symptoms will necessarily manifest themselves in the body. It is important not to try to self-diagnose. Trained professionals (e.g., psychologists, psychiatrists, and other medical professionals) provide diagnosis only after detailed assessments.

Stress can also impact an individual's behavioral (physical) health. Stress can contribute to sleep disturbances (e.g., not being able to sleep or waking up in the middle of the night), headaches, and fatigue.[1] Stress can also contribute to changes in eating (e.g., loss of appetite

TABLE 66.4 Anxiety Related Disorders and Dental Hygiene Treatment Considerations

Condition	Description	DH Treatment Considerations	Resources
Panic Disorder	Regular, sudden attacks of panic or fear. Results in many physical symptoms (e.g., racing heart, feeling faint, choking sensation, dry mouth, or needing to use the bathroom)	Patients with any of these conditions may be prescribed medications to control symptoms. (e.g., antidepressants, antianxiety, or beta-blockers) Antidepressants oral effects: • Xerostomia • Bruxism • Altered taste • Orthostatic hypotension Antianxiety Oral Effects: • Xerostomia • Drowsiness • Double vision • Nausea Beta-Blockers Oral Effects: • Xerostomia (rare) • Altered taste • Orthostatic hypotension Individuals with these disorders are at higher risk of poor oral health due to: • Dental anxiety • Neglecting oral hygiene practices • Nutritional deficiencies • GERD leading to dental erosion • Xerostomia Consider chairside Behavior Guidance such as: • Identify source of anxiety if dentally related • Deep breathing exercises • Communication techniques (e.g., calm voice and distraction) • "Tell-show-do," signaling • N2O Sedation	NHS: https://www.nhs.uk/mental-health/conditions/panic-disorder National Institute of Mental Health: https://www.nimh.nih.gov/health/publications/panic-disorder-when-fear-overwhelms
Social Anxiety Disorder	A persistent fear of being judged or watched by others. Can negatively affect many areas of personal and professional life. Signs and symptoms include: blushing, sweating, rapid heart rate, "mind going blank," feelings of self-consciousness, avoiding eye contact, and changes in posture and voice tone and level.		National Institute of Mental Health: https://www.nimh.nih.gov/health/publications/social-anxiety-disorder-more-than-just-shyness
Generalized Anxiety Disorder	Overall feeling of excessive worry about a variety of topics: resulting in fatigue, inability to focus, sleep disturbance, and feeling on edge.		National Institute of Mental Health: https://www.nimh.nih.gov/health/publications/generalized-anxiety-disorder-gad
Posttraumatic Stress Disorder (PTSD)	May develop when an individual has experienced a shocking, dangerous, or scary event. Can result in feelings of stress and fear, even when there is no danger. Re-experiencing includes bad dreams, flashbacks, and frightening thoughts.		National Institute of Mental Health: https://www.nimh.nih.gov/health/topics/post-traumatic-stress-disorder-ptsd

Data from: National Institute of Mental Health, and Strategies to manage patients with dental anxiety and dental phobia: literature review.

TABLE 66.5 Possible Signs and Symptoms Related to Anxiety and Depression

Examples of Anxiety Symptoms	Examples of Depression Symptoms
• Feeling on edge, restless • Difficulty controlling feelings of worry • Sleep disturbances • Increased heart rate, headaches, or GI disturbances • Irritability • Difficulty concentrating	• Feeling sad, tearful, or hopeless • Decreased energy • Loss of interest in activities • Trouble concentrating, making decisions, and remembering things • Altered appetite and weight change • Feelings of anger and irritability • Disturbances in sleeping and eating

For more information about depression and other mood disorders, please visit: http://www.nimh.nih.gov/health/topics/depression. For more information on anxiety disorders, please visit: http://www.nimh.nih.gov/health/topics/anxiety-disorders.

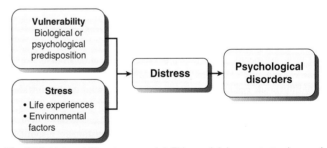

Fig. 66.3 Vulnerability-stress model. This model demonstrates how vulnerabilities within a person coupled with external stress can result in distress and potentially lead to a psychological disorder.

a difference, learn more about their chosen field, and be a valuable member of a team. However, when an individual experiences extensive exposure to chronic stressors, especially those that are work related, burnout may result. Professional burnout can be observed in many professions but has a higher occurrence in professions where individuals work closely together.[12] The dental team is often a small group working closely to care for patients, and this is one factor that puts dental professionals at a higher risk of experiencing burnout.[12] It is important to understand the elements that when combined can contribute to developing professional burnout.

There are many factors that can lead to a dental hygienist experiencing burnout. Each individual is different and will react to various circumstances uniquely; however, there have been numerous studies

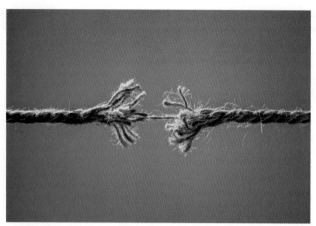

Fig. 66.4 Artistic photo representing how stress may lead to burnout. (iStock.com/BrianAJackson)

TABLE 66.6 **How People Respond to Stressors Differently**	
Possible Stressors Facing Dental Hygienists	**Possible Stressors Facing Patients**
• Limited flexibility in work schedule • Physical pain • Meeting all the needs of your patients • Fast-paced workday/limited breaks	• Fear of pain • Feeling loss of control • Fear of financial burden or not being able to afford dental treatment • Embarrassment over oral health
Factors that increase vulnerability to negative stress responses or lessen a person's ability to handle stress encountered in life	
• Biological factors (e.g., genetics, childhood illness, or viruses) • Past trauma (e.g., abuse, neglect, accident, or loss) • Number and severity of stressors they are coping with at one time	
Protective factors—reduce an individual's vulnerability to biological factors and/or stress factors	
• Healthy coping skills (e.g., communication and problem-solving skills) • Social support from family, friends, and coworkers • Meaning in life (e.g., church membership, volunteer activities, school, or work that brings satisfaction)	

> ### BOX 66.5   Legal, Ethical, and Safety Issues
>
> - Dental hygienists must be aware of the ethical responsibility they have toward their patients for maintaining mental health and well-being. Healthcare providers are at risk of not providing safe, high-quality care when their mental health and well-being suffers.
> - Dental hygienists must recognize their limitations and practice within their scope of practice.
> - Patient behavior, assessment findings, recommendation, and referrals should be recorded in the patient's chart along with treatments as part of the patient's confidential healthcare record.
> - In some states a healthcare provider is required to inform parents or guardians of patients of certain information such as revealed psychological conditions or statements of mental health that could be concerning. Knowledge of state statutes is vital in order to manage confidential information properly.
> - Under the appropriate circumstances (e.g., dental anxiety, medications significantly affecting oral health, or revelation of severe mental health symptoms) and with your patient's consent, contact the patient's primary care physician or mental health professional to work collaboratively.
> - A mental health diagnosis and treatment is not within the dental hygienists' scope of practice, but understanding the signs and symptoms and lifestyle choices that improve resilience to stress is vital for the dental hygienist.

that point to specific, recurrent phenomena. A feeling of detachment from work is one of the leading phenomena correlated with professional burnout. Feeling frustrated with work-related goals, considering leaving the position, or feeling dissatisfied with how their personal needs are being met could lead to a feeling of disengagement or detachment from their job. Emotional and physical exhaustion are also major factors and can stem from numerous sources (e.g., tightly booked schedules or chronic body pain). Other aspects that influence burnout include overall job satisfaction (e.g., acceptable work hours or a fair benefits package). These phenomena—job satisfaction, burnout, and intention to leave—appear to influence each other.[14] Studies demonstrated that individuals who have low job satisfaction and are experiencing burnout are more likely to leave their chosen careers.[13,14]

FACTORS CONTRIBUTING TO PROFESSIONAL BURNOUT

Some individuals may go from loving their chosen career to experiencing burnout, and it is important to understand what leads to this evolution. Each individual is different and will experience various stressors in their life that will inevitably overflow into their work life. How these stressors are managed is a key factor in the development of professional burnout. Major contributing factors that may increase the likelihood of a dental hygienist developing burnout include elements specific to healthcare and dental hygiene in particular.

Dental hygienists are susceptible to musculoskeletal disorders due to the repetitive movements, static positions held for extended periods of time, and vibrating equipment. Musculoskeletal disorders and the chronic pain associated with these disorders place a dental hygienist at a higher risk to experience burnout. Considering the possible need for surgery, a shortened career, or experiencing the need to "recover" from work before enjoying activities such as painting or gardening can affect an individual's mental health and overall job satisfaction. For more information regarding musculoskeletal disorders, please refer to Chapter 12.

The potential stressors of practicing clinical dental hygiene could affect an individual all at once, or they may only face one or two risk factors. Elements that could contribute to burnout such as unsatisfactory pay, a tightly packed patient schedule that results in limited time with each patient, and inadequate time for breaks can all contribute to burnout if endured long enough and without resolution (see Fig. 66.5). An employer may be willing to increase pay but unwilling to lengthen appointment times or schedule breaks between patients. These aspects heavily influence the feeling of being valued and overall job satisfaction, which impacts burnout.

Other factors that can drastically differ, depending on the state in which the dental hygienist is practicing, or the organization for which the dental hygienist is employed, include autonomy and working at the top of your licensure. Several studies have revealed autonomy as a major influence of professional burnout.[12–14] If individuals believe they have no decision-making privileges in regard to their profession, they may begin to feel less valuable and disengaged from their chosen field. When dental hygienists perceive themselves as having autonomy or can clearly identify their professional roles, they experience less professional burnout than those who do not.[12,15] Working at the top of your license means practicing to the full extent of your education and

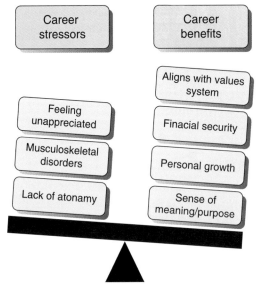

Two areas that have been identified as major stressors in dental hygiene practice are not enough time in work schedule and physical pain.

Fig. 66.5 This figure highlights two major stressors for dental hygienists.

Career stressors

Career benefits

Aligns with values system

Feeling unappreciated

Finacial security

Musculoskeletal disorders

Personal growth

Lack of atonamy

Sense of meaning/purpose

Fig. 66.6 Image demonstrating how it is important to maintain a work-life balance.

training. In this instance, it refers to dental hygienists practicing to the highest extent of their education, training, and experience. An imbalance between the challenges of the working environment and the benefits that are derived from the working environment can also increase the risk of burnout (see Fig. 66.6). This figure depicts the balance a dental hygienist must find between the stress of life and work and the rewards of their career. When the stressors far outweigh the rewards, burnout and/or loss of time at work could occur.

ADVERSE EFFECTS OF BURNOUT

One of the greatest concerns with professional burnout in the health-care field is the possible negative outcome toward patient care. A vast majority of healthcare professionals, dental hygienists included, join the profession because they want to improve the health of individuals and derive great satisfaction in caring for people. However, when burnout occurs and is endured for some time, providers report feeling cynical at work and lose the enthusiasm they once had for their profession. Overall, the result is the provider may not be performing to the best of their ability, which can can significantly affect patient care.

Adverse health outcomes are another concern of unaddressed burnout. One area of particular interest is the relationship between chronic stress and low-grade inflammation, leading to the development of chronic health conditions in the body. Studies have demonstrated the systemic inflammatory response following an acute stressor.[5,16] When the stressor is repeated again and again, those inflammatory markers stay elevated, which is detrimental to the overall health of the individual. Higher work stress is associated with higher inflammatory responses.[5,16]

Understanding the signs of chronic stress and identifying the stressors are important for the dental hygienist entering the healthcare field. Shedding light on the topics of poor mental health and how to improve well-being are not always discussed in sufficient detail. It is vital to recognize that symptoms such as mental fatigue, feeling impatient, frequent headaches, and experiencing anxiety on a regular basis can all contribute to frequent leaves from work and may decrease career longevity.[17] Enduring chronic stress and feelings of burnout may increase the likelihood of having to take a leave from work. Fortunately, dental hygienists can mitigate these risks by addressing the situation early and being proactive with their own mental health and well-being.

SELF-CARE: IMPROVING MENTAL HEALTH AND PREVENTING BURNOUT

As mentioned in the introduction, stress and stressors are inevitable in life. However, **self-care practices**, actions an individual can take through prioritizing personal health and well-being, help to mitigate the negative effects of stress. One of the best ways to protect your body against the effects of chronic stress is through healthy lifestyle choices. Proper nutrition, adequate sleep, water, and exercise are all the first line of defense against the stressors that bombard us in our personal lives and work lives (see Fig. 66.7). There is evidence that brief periods of a mindful activity, such as yoga, can lessen perceived stress and improve an individual's state of mind.[18-20] There are many steps a person can take to reduce the effects of stressors and improve well-being (see Table 66.7).

POSITIVE WORK PRACTICES TO REDUCE BURNOUT

Employers and leadership within companies can reduce the likelihood of burnout among their team by implementing certain policies focused on well-being and consistently checking in with their staff (see Table 66.8). Table 66.7 highlights specific self-care practices that may help to reduce the incidence of burnout among workers. When employers and practitioners learn to recognize chronic stressors, mitigate their effects by mindfully taking time to disconnect from tasks, and remain mindful of their psychological and physical well-being, the team functions at a much higher level.

ACCESSING PROFESSIONAL HELP FOR MENTAL AND BEHAVIORAL HEALTH

Often, feelings of being overwhelmed are dealt with quietly or may manifest themselves in negative ways that affect your psychological well-being, physical health, or relationships with family, friends, and coworkers. Mental health has historically had a stigma that resulted in individuals not reaching out to professionals for help or simply not knowing what to do to relieve their distress. It is important to recognize when you are no longer able to manage your stress (Fig. 66.8).

In today's society, people tend to overextend themselves to the point of exhaustion. This is especially true for healthcare workers who work in fast-paced environments such as dental offices. Although stress is considered a normal part of everyday life and, in some instances, can be positive, people experiencing stress that feels unmanageable or significantly impacts their home, work, or social lives should seek professional help. Individuals are encouraged to not wait until life feels uncontrollable to seek help.

Credentialed mental health professionals can work with you in assessing the severity of your distress, along with identifying an evidence-based treatment that would most benefit you. There are a wide array of mental and behavioral health professionals, including clinical and counseling psychologists, social workers, licensed professional counselors, and marriage

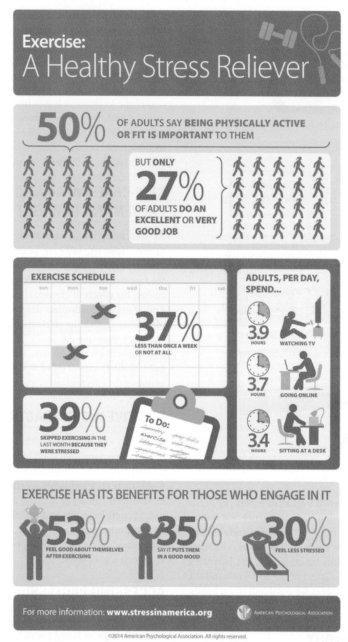

Fig. 66.7 Example of self-care recommendations. Citation: American Psychological Association. *Stress in America 2013: Infographics.* American Psychological Association; 2013. Available at: https://www.apa.org/news/press/releases/stress/2013/infographics.

Question: When should I seek professional help from a healthcare provider?

Answer:

You should seek professional help if you feel overwhelmed and believe your life is out of control and can no longer cope with day-to-day activities. Related: you should seek professional help when the stress is having a significant impact on how you function in your personal, work, and/or social life. You should also seek professional help when you find the symptoms of stress to be distressing.

Fig. 66.8 Knowing when to seek professional help.

and family therapists. When selecting a professional, it is important that the person is licensed and that they offer evidence-based assessments and interventions. There is also a wealth of resources available on the internet for individuals interested in learning about the impact of stress. It is important to ensure the host organization is reputable (e.g., American Psychological Association or National Institute of Health) and avoid the temptation to self-diagnose your difficulties based on information available online. Only a licensed mental health or medical professional can assess and provide an accurate and valid clinical diagnosis.

Mental health and well-being are essential for every individual. This chapter has highlighted the importance of protecting and maintaining personal mental health and well-being in order to provide excellent patient care and enjoy a long and satisfying career. In addition, the

TABLE 66.7 Self-Care Recommendations

Self-care Recommendations	Examples	Importance of self-care	Solutions
Sleep Hygiene	Adults—7 to 9 hours is the recommended minimum • Adult US average is 6.7 hours per night	• Poor sleep leads to feeling sluggish • Feeling irritable • Trouble concentrating • Feelings of stress increase	• Sleep in a dark and cool room • Maintain consistent sleep schedule • Utilize white noise or earplugs if necessary • Avoid large meals or caffeine right before bed • Remove/stop using electronics such as smartphones and television before bed
Physical Activity	Recommendation for adults is 150 minutes of moderate intensity physical activity per week	• Improve mood • Improve sleep quality • Improve cognitive function • Decrease depression and anxiety • Research finds physical activity significantly associated with lower signs of burnout	• Does not have to be high intensity; any accomplished task has psychological benefits (e.g., 15-minute walk, gardening, weightlifting, yoga, etc.)
Healthy Eating Practices	Avoid stress eating • Seek to include predominantly whole foods in your diet and avoid processed food	• Stress eating can lead to feeling of disappointment in yourself • Stress eating may be used as a distraction from the actual cause of the stress • Stress eating may become a habit • Feeling bad about your body • Feeling sluggish or lazy	• Start prepping at least one of your meals during the week (example: meal-prep all lunches for the week) • Cut out one high-sugar or processed food from your diet • Create healthy "snack packs" to grab easily when you are feeling snacky
Staying Hydrated	Water should be your main beverage • Limit diuretics such as alcohol and caffeine	• Important for cells and all body systems function • Mild dehydration can lead to feelings of fatigue • Prevent dry mouth and nasal passages • Dehydration can lead to headaches and sleep disruption	• Eat water-dense foods like watermelon, carrots, cucumbers, and apples • Sip throughout the day instead of chugging large quantities of water at once • Add natural flavor to your water (e.g., fresh cucumber, lemon, or peppermint)
Staying Connected	Reach out for emotional support from friends, family, or a mental health therapist	• Studies reveal an association between reported loneliness and increased inflammatory markers • Increased risk of mortality • Equivalent to smoking 15 cigarettes a day	• Create opportunities to connect with family and community • Make a phone call or an in-person visit instead of sending a text
Schedule Rewarding Activities	Make a point to plan an activity that is rewarding or meaningful in terms of personal value	• Planning activities counteracts feelings of depression and anxiety • Studies show even imagining pleasant activities benefits mood	• Spend time in nature • Schedule quiet time to center thoughts • Do something each week that is extra special or meaningful (e.g., spa treatment, massage, movie night, or scheduling undisturbed time with a good book)
Focus on the Positive	Acknowledge negative feelings but do not dwell on them. Consider what lens you look through. Are you finding deficits in your life, or hope?	• A positive mind is open and neutral • Think more clearly • Connect more • Increase problem-solving skills • More resilient	• Shift focus to things you are grateful for, no matter how small • Practice stating what is true, not just how something feels (e.g., "This is hard, but I can manage it." vs. "I can't stand this!")
Practice Gratitude	Acknowledge the things you are thankful for	Studies show practicing gratitude benefits • Heart health • Better sleep • Improved mood • Less fatigue • Reduced inflammatory biomarkers	• Keep a gratitude journal • Identify at least one thing you are grateful for on a daily basis • Engage in gratitude rituals • Express gratitude towards others • Focus on the positive and the good intent of others

TABLE 66.8   Positive Work Practices to Reduce Burnout

Empower dental team	• Fosters teamwork and communication in quality improvement • Cultivate relationships and use open communication to solve problems • How to build positive culture—regular one-on-one sessions, morning huddles, and group brainstorming
Let employees know they are valued	• Recognize work-life demands • Ensure living competitive wage • Promoting family policies • Considering patient caseload and coverage • Enacting current job hazards policies
Commitment to the health and safety of the dental team	• Highest level of leadership committed to employee well-being (e.g., dentist/owner, office manager, corporate office) • Regularly assess levels of burnout • Ensure workers have time for work breaks and paid leave • Zero-tolerance for violence policy • Commit to safety in the workplace • Prioritizing adequate personal protective equipment

Data from Addressing Health Workers Burnout: The US Surgeons General's Advisory on Building a Thriving Health Workforce.

MENTAL HEALTH RESOURCES

American Dental Association
ADA.org/wellness
Canadian Dental Association
https://www.cda-adc.ca/en/services/essentials/2014/issue5/files/assets/common/downloads/publication.pdf/
The Canadian Dental Hygienists Association
https://www.cdha.ca/cdha/Career_Folder/Healthy_Respectful_Workplace/Psychological_Well-Being/CDHA/Career/Healthy_Workplace/Psychological_Well_Being.aspx

Centers for Disease Control and Prevention
https://www.cdc.gov/mentalhealth
American Psychological Association
https://www.apa.org/
American Psychiatric Association
https://www.psychiatry.org/mental-health

National Institute of Mental Health
https://www.nimh.nih.gov/
National Suicide Prevention Hotline
1-800-272-TALK (8255)
1-888-628-9454 (Spanish)
Crisis Text Line
Text HELLO to 741741

KEY CONCEPTS

- The prevalence of mental health problems has increased in recent years and is a common concern worldwide.
- Dental hygienists will treat many patients with diagnosed mental health problems, dental anxiety, and/or who are experiencing acute episodes of high stress.
- Dental hygienists may experience mental and behavioral health problems during their career.
- Stress is a response to a physical, chemical, or emotional element resulting in tension and may be an aspect of disease causation.
- Stress can be experienced either emotionally or physically.
- The stressor is the element being responded to and may be internal or external.
- Not all stress is bad; eustress is stress people experience due to positive life events such as starting a first job after graduation.
- Distress is a type of stress that can be harmful to overall well-being and physical health, especially when exposure takes place over a long period of time.
- Acute stress is usually a one-time occurrence or short-term in nature.
- Chronic stress is repeated exposures to stressors over a long period of time.
- There is evidence that chronic stress is associated with the development of various diseases such as cardiovascular disease, insulin insensitivity, and cancer.
- Decades of research show a clear relationship between stress and mental and behavioral health problems.
- Psychological distress (anxiety and depression) occurs when the stress that people experience is either too severe, chronic, or a combination of both.

- Stress can have far-reaching effects on psychological health, physical health, sleep disturbance, headaches, fatigue, changes in eating habits, and immune system, among other concerns.
- Professional burnout, an occupational syndrome, is characterized by emotional and physical exhaustion, detachment from work, and feelings of professional loneliness.
- Burnout occurs when an individual experiences extensive exposure to chronic stressors, especially those that are work related.
- Professional burnout has a higher occurrence in professions where individuals work closely together.
- Dental hygienists are susceptible to burnout due to musculoskeletal disorders, demanding schedules, limited time with patients, or limited breaks during the day. Other factors can include pay, benefits, and autonomy.
- Unaddressed burnout may result in time off from work, cynical attitude toward patient care and outcomes, loss of enjoyment with chosen career, or choosing to change careers.
- Self-care practices are actions an individual can take through prioritizing personal health and well-being to help mitigate the negative effects of stress.
- Employers and leadership within companies can reduce the likelihood of burnout among their team by implementing certain policies focused on well-being.
- Employees who recognize chronic stressors can mitigate the negative effects of stress by mindfully taking time to disconnect from tasks and remain mindful of their psychological and physical well-being.
- Only a licensed mental health or medical professional can assess and provide an accurate and valid clinical diagnosis.
- Mental health and well-being are essential for every individual.

effects of stressors and mental health problems and their relationship to oral health are vital for the dental hygienists to understand. With this knowledge, a dental hygienist is well equipped to support their patients through treatments and find enjoyment in a career focused on disease prevention.

REFERENCES

1. American Psychological Association. *Stress in America 2021: Stress and Decision Making During the Pandemic.* American Psychological Association; 2021; 2022.
2. World Health Organization. *Mental Disorders.* World Health Organization; 2022; 2022. https://www.who.int/news-room/fact-sheets/detail/mental-disorders.
3. Canadian Mental Health Association. *Fast Facts about Mental Health and Mental Illness.* Canadian Mental Health Association; 2021; 2022. https://cmha.ca/brochure/fast-facts-about-mental-illness/.
4. Centers for Disease Control and Prevention. *About Mental Health.* Available at: https://www.cdc.gov/mentalhealth/learn/index.htm.
5. Rohleder N. Stress and inflammation – the need to address the gap in the transition between acute and chronic stress effects. *Psychoneuroendocrinology.* 2019;105:164–171. https://doi.org/10.1016/j.psyneuen.2019.02.021.
6. World Federation for Mental Health. *World Mental Health Day 2020. Mental Health for All: Greater Investment-Greater Access.* Available at: https://wfmh.global/img/what-we-do/past-events/2020-wmhd/WMHD2020_v16_resized.pdf.
7. Hauge MS, Stora B, Vassend O, Hoffart A, Willumsen T. Dentist–administered cognitive behavioural therapy versus four habits/midazolam: an RCT study of dental anxiety treatment in primary dental care. *Eur J Oral Sci.* 2021;129(4):e12794-n/a. https://doi.org/10.1111/eos.12794.
8. Appukuttan DP. Strategies to manage patients with dental anxiety and dental phobia: literature review. *Clin Cosmet Investig Dent.* 2016;8:35–50. https://doi.org/10.2147/CCIDE.S63626. Published Mar 10, 2016.
9. National Institute of Mental Health (202a). *Anxiety Disorders*; 2022. https://www.nimh.nih.gov/health/topics/anxiety-disorders.
10. National Institute of Mental Health (202b). *Depression.* Retrieved June 4, 2022. https://www.nimh.nih.gov/health/topics/depression.
11. Zukerman M. *Vulnerability to Psychopathology: A Biosocial Model.* American Psychological Association; 1999.
12. Barnard SJA, Alexander BA, Lockett AK, et al. Mental health and self-care practices among dental hygienists. *J Dent Hyg.* 2020;94(4):22–28.
13. Office of the Surgeon General (OSG). *Addressing Health Worker Burnout: The Surgeon General's Advisory on Building a Thriving Health Workforce.* Office of the Surgeon General; 2022. https://www.hhs.gov/surgeongeneral/priorities/health-worker-burnout/index.html. Accessed July 15, 2022.
14. Patel BM, Boyd LD, Vineyard J, LaSpina L. Job satisfaction, burnout, and intention to leave among dental hygienists in clinical practice. *J Dent Hyg.* 2021;95(2):28–35.
15. Bercasio LV, Rowe DJ, Yansane AI. Factors associated with burnout among dental hygienists in California. *J Dent Hyg.* 2020;94(6):40–48.
16. Dhabhar FS. The short-term stress response – mother nature's mechanism for enhancing protection and performance under conditions of threat, challenge, and opportunity. *Front Neuroendocrinol.* 2018;49:175–192. https://doi.org/10.1016/j.yfrne.2018.03.004.
17. Geisinger ML, Dershewitz JD. Worried sick: anxiety, depression, and the impact on dental health care workers. *J Dent Hyg.* 2022;96(4):6–8.
18. Kanderis Lane CL, Gurenlian JR, Freudenthal J, Denner PR. A 15-minute yoga intervention to reduce entry-level dental hygiene student stress. *J Dent Hyg.* 2021;95(2):63–70.
19. Braun SE, Deeb G, Carrico C, Kinser PA. Brief yoga intervention for dental and dental hygiene students: a feasibility and acceptability study. *J Evid Based Integr Med.* 2019;24:2515690X19855303–2515690X19855303. https://doi.org/10.1177/2515690X19855303.
20. Alire E, Brems C, Bell K, Chiswell A. The role of yoga in treating stress-related symptoms in dental hygiene students. *Int J Yoga.* 2020;13(3):213–222. https://doi.org/10.4103/ijoy.IJOY_5_20.

A | APPENDIX

Dental Charting Symbols and Examples

COMMON CHARTING SYMBOLS

The following matrix and the three different chart examples (anatomical, geometrical, and computer generated [see charts following this box]) of the same patient's clinical chart symbolize dental procedures and conditions.

The matrix is divided into five columns. The first column categorizes **Dental Procedures** according to the categories listed in the book *Current Dental Terminology* (CDT). The second column, **Description,** represents the subcategories of CDT. The third column, **Charting Instructions,** explains how to illustrate the identified dental procedure or condition on the patient's clinical chart. With proper illustration of procedures and conditions and use of correct color coding and symbolization, the dental healthcare team will be able to interpret the patient's clinical chart correctly. The fourth column, **Charting Example,** identifies the tooth number on the charting examples (anatomical, geometrical, and computer generated). Although they differ in design, all charts present the same information. The fifth column, **Black's Classification,** identifies the corresponding classification and tooth surface.

Dental Procedures and Condition	Description	Charting Instructions	Charting Example	Black's Classification
Restorative procedures	Amalgam	Dental caries are outlined and filled in with red.	Tooth #2	Class II MO
		Completed amalgam restorations are colored solid blue or black.	Tooth #18	Class I O
	Resin-based composite	Dental caries are outlined in red.	Tooth #7	Class III M
		Completed restorations are filled with blue or black dots.	Tooth #29	Class II MOD
			Tooth #4	Class V B
	Inlay/onlay Cast metal	Work to be completed is outlined in red and diagonal lines are drawn.	Tooth #31	MOD inlay
		Completed restorations are drawn over in blue or black.		
	Inlay/onlay Resin-based	Work to be completed is outlined in red.	Tooth #14	DOL onlay
		Completed restoration is filled in with blue or black dots.		
	Crown Cast metal	Work to be completed is outlined in red and diagonal lines are drawn.	Tooth #30	
		Completed crown is drawn over with blue or black.		
	Crown Porcelain fused to gold	Work to be completed is outlined in red on the buccal surface or facial surface, and diagonal lines are drawn on the occlusal and lingual surface (posterior teeth) and the lingual surface (anterior teeth).	Tooth #19 Tooth #21 Tooth #15	
		Computer-generated chart draws diagonal lines on all surfaces.		
		Completed crown is drawn over in blue or black.		
	Crown Porcelain or resin-based	Work to be completed is outlined in red.	Tooth #13	
		Completed crown is filled with blue or black dots (computer-generated chart outlined in blue).		
	Stainless steel crown	Work to be completed is identified by writing **SS** in red on the crown of the tooth (computer-generated chart outlined in red).	Tooth #3	
		Completed crown is identified by writing over the SS in blue or black (computer-generated chart outlined in blue).		
	Veneer bonding	Work to be completed is outlined in red on the facial surface only (computer-generated chart filled facial surface in red).	Tooth #8 Tooth #9	
		Completed veneer is filled in with blue or black dots (computer-generated chart filled facial surface in blue).		
	Post and core Buildup	A vertical red line is drawn through the root (approximating the root canal), and a small inverted triangle is drawn in the gingival third of the crown (approximating the pulp chamber of the tooth).	Tooth #30	
		Completed post and core is filled in with blue or black.		
Endodontic procedures	Endodontic therapy (root canal)	When therapy is indicated, a vertical red line is drawn through each root (approximating the root canal).	Tooth #28	
		Completed treatment is drawn over in blue or black.		
	Periapical abscess	A small red circle is drawn at the apex of the root of the infected tooth.	Tooth #27	

From Gaylor LJ. *The Administrative Dental Assistant.* Elsevier; 2021.

COMMON CHARTING SYMBOLS—cont'd

Dental Procedures and Condition	Description	Charting Instructions	Charting Example	Black's Classification
Implant services	Implant	When an implant is indicated, horizontal red lines are drawn across the root of the replaced tooth. When an implant is present, blue or black lines are drawn (computer-generated chart outlined root).	Tooth #13	
Prosthodontics fixed	Fixed bridge	The charting instructions for the type of crown to be used in the construction of the bridge are followed. In addition, connect the teeth involved with two horizontal lines and draw an X through the roots of the missing teeth. When the bridge has been inserted, it is colored over in blue or black.	Tooth #19 Tooth #20 Tooth #21	(Retainer) (Pontic) (Retainer)
Oral surgery	Extraction	A single, angled red line is drawn through the tooth (/) (computer-generated chart draws two lines ‖).	Tooth #1 Tooth #32	
	Extracted or missing tooth	A blue or black X is drawn through the tooth.	Tooth #16	
	Impacted or unerupted tooth	A red circle is drawn around the tooth (crown and root).	Tooth #17	
Other conditions	Rotated tooth	A semicircular red line is placed at the root of the tooth with an arrow pointing in the direction of the rotation.	Tooth #17	
	Drifting tooth	A red line is placed above the crown of the tooth with an arrow indicating the direction of the drift.	Tooth #31	
	Fractured tooth	A red zigzag is placed on the tooth surface where the fracture occurred. If the root is fractured, the zigzag is placed on the root.	Tooth #24	Class IV
	Diastema	When there is more space than normal between two teeth, two vertical red lines are placed between the teeth.	Teeth #8, 9	

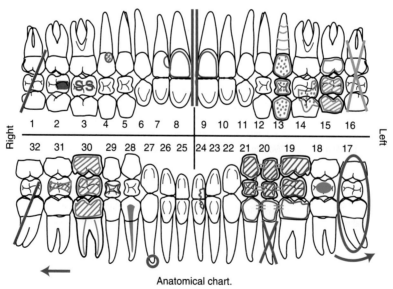

Anatomical chart.

(From Gaylor LJ. *The Administrative Dental Assistant*. Elsevier; 2021.)

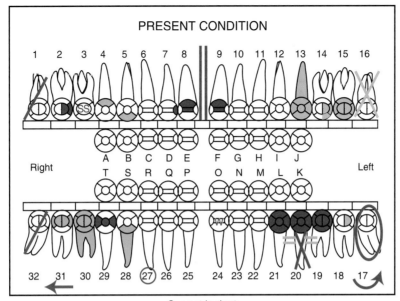

Geometric chart.

(From Gaylor LJ. *The Administrative Dental Assistant.* Elsevier; 2021.)

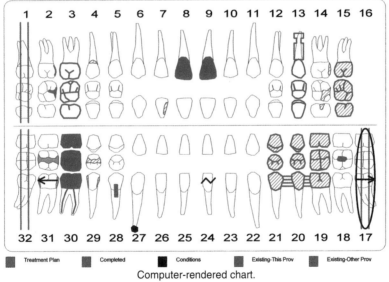

Computer-rendered chart.

(From Gaylor LJ. *The Administrative Dental Assistant.* Elsevier; 2021.)

GLOSSARY

A

Abfractions Noncarious cervical lesions caused by excessive occlusal loading as teeth flex under pressure, resulting in subsequent loss of hard structure at the cementoenamel junction.

Abrasion Pathologic tooth wear caused by a foreign substance.

Abrasive agents Ingredients used to clean and polish teeth to a smooth, lustrous surface.

Abutment Tooth, tooth root, or dental implant that anchors a fixed or removable prosthetic appliance.

Accountability People's ability to answer for their actions.

Acoustic power The rate at which sound power or energy is emitted; produced by the ultrasonic scaler.

Acoustic microstreaming Energy released around ultrasonic devices; commonly occurs around oscillating objects such as cavitation bubbles or the scaler tip. These currents are able to break up colonies of bacteria and disrupt biofilm.

Acquired tooth damage Tooth damage that is caused by any process that results in a loss of the integrity of the tooth.

Acquired immunodeficiency syndrome (AIDS) A set of symptoms and illnesses that develop as a result of advanced HIV infection that has destroyed the immune system.

Acquired pellicle Thin, clear, unstructured organic membrane that forms over exposed tooth surfaces and restorations within minutes after removal by professional and self-polishing techniques.

Active ingredient The specific agent, chemical, or drug component within a particular delivery system that is primarily responsible for the therapeutic effect.

Activities of daily living (ADL) ADLs are those abilities fundamental to independent living, such as bathing, dressing, brushing teeth, toileting, feeding, and continence.

Acute stress Typically a one-time occurrence of stress or short-term in nature; examples can be running late to work due to being stuck in traffic or failing an exam.

Addiction The prolonged and repeated misuse or abuse of any substance—a chronic and compulsive need to use drugs despite causing the user physical and emotional harm.

Adrenal crisis A serious medical condition caused by the body's inability to produce a sufficient amount of cortisol that often follows extreme stress, characterized by sudden dizziness, vomiting, and even loss of consciousness; also called addisonian crisis.

Adrenal insufficiency A disease that occurs when the adrenal glands do not produce enough of the hormone cortisol, and in some cases, the hormone aldosterone; also called Addison disease or chronic adrenal insufficiency.

Adult protective services Services provided by agencies to safeguard vulnerable adults through investigations of reports alleging abuse, neglect, self-neglect or exploitation, and arrangements for the provision of emergency or supportive services necessary to reduce or eliminate risk of harm.

Advanced dental therapist (ADT) Oral healthcare providers, following advanced training and clinical practice, are able to provide all the services that a dental therapist provides plus additional services such as oral evaluation and assessment, treatment plan formulation, non-surgical extraction of certain diseased teeth, and more.

Advocacy Public support for, or championing of, a particular cause or policy.

Aerosols Artificially generated solid or liquid airborne particles less than 50 microns in size.

Air polishing A method of stain and biofilm removal that uses a specially designed device with a handpiece that delivers a spray of warm water and prophy powder under pressure.

Alginate Irreversible, flexible hydrocolloid impression material used primarily for making study casts of a patient's dentition.

Alveolar bone Bone composed of compact or cortical bone and spongy bone that is marked by trabecular spaces seen on radiographs.

Alveolar mucosa Nonkeratinized epithelium characterized by a smooth and shiny surface that covers the vestibule and floor of the mouth and becomes the buccal and labial mucosa.

Alveoli Plural for alveolus, the tooth socket in the alveolar bone, or a sac within the lungs that allows for gases to exchange.

Alzheimer disease A degenerative brain disorder that gradually destroys the ability to remember, reason, learn, and imagine.

Amalgam Alloy of mercury with silver, copper, and tin; used to restore form and function of teeth.

Amide local anesthetics Agents that undergo biotransformation in the liver by microsomal enzymes; metabolic products of amide local anesthetic agents are almost entirely excreted by the kidneys.

Amyotrophic lateral sclerosis (ALS) A progressive neurodegenerative disease that affects nerve cells in the brain and the spinal cord.

Anaerobic Occurring or existing in the absence of free oxygen.

Aneroid manometer A portable and lightweight instrument used to assess blood pressure; it has a glass-enclosed circular gauge containing a needle that registers millimeter calibrations.

Angina pectoris The direct result of inadequate oxygen flow to the myocardium, manifested clinically as a burning, squeezing, or crushing tightness in the chest that radiates to the left arm, neck, and shoulder blade.

Angular cheilitis A manifestation of candidiasis that presents as white and red fissures at the commissures of the mouth.

Ankylosis A disturbance or underdevelopment of the bone on the affected side of a fracture; immobility of a joint resulting from infection, injury, surgery, or disease; fusion of bone to bone or tooth to bone.

Anodontia Congenital absence of teeth. Defects of ectodermal structures are causative effects; also known as *edentia*.

Antimicrobial agents An agent that kills or inhibits the growth of microbes.

Antiseptics Substances or agents that prevent the growth of disease-producing microbes.

Aphthous ulcers A common, painful, shallow lesion, a benign ulcer, that occurs in the soft tissues of the mouth, is well demarcated and round, and usually heals within 10 days.

Apical third The third of the tooth involving the tip or apex of the root.

Apnea Temporary stopping of breathing, especially during sleep.

Approximal (proximal) caries Dental caries between teeth at the point of their proximal contact.

Area-specific curettes Curettes designed for use in specific locations, usually slightly narrower in blade width and longer in terminal shank length than are universal designs (e.g., Gracey curette series).

Arrested caries Dental caries exhibiting recalcified lesions resulting from remineralization that occurs when the caries process halts.

Aspiration pneumonia A pneumonia that occurs when saliva is inhaled into the lungs and an infection results.

Assessment The step in the dental hygiene process of care that involves collecting and analyzing systemic and oral health data with the purpose of identifying a patient or client's needs.

Assessment instruments Instruments, such as the periodontal probe, dental explorer, and mouth mirror, used for taking measurements and for detecting tooth irregularities, restorations, probe depths, soft tissue changes, clinical parameters of oral disease, acquired deposits, and other intra-oral manifestations.

Asthma A chronic inflammatory respiratory disease characterized by an increased responsiveness of the bronchial airways to various stimuli.

Asynchronous (Store-and-Forward) Transmission of patient data through a secure electronic communications system to a health provider who uses the information to evaluate or diagnose a patient's condition and/or update a patient's treatment plan without live interactions.

Atherosclerosis A narrowing of the lumen of the coronary arteries by fibrofatty deposits containing lipids and cholesterol, thereby reducing blood flow volume.

Attached gingiva Portion of the gingiva that is connected firmly to the alveolar bone.

Attrition Tooth-to-tooth wear from opposing tooth contact.

Auscultation Physical assessment technique that uses the clinician's sense of hearing to determine an abnormality; act of listening to and detecting body sounds to determine variations from normal (e.g., listening for clicking sounds in the temporomandibular joint).

Auscultatory gap A period of abnormal silence that occurs between the Korotkoff phases when measuring blood pressure. It can occur in older patients with a wide pulse pressure. This gap usually appears between the first and second systolic sounds.

Autoclave Most common method of heat sterilization in the dental care setting. Uses moist heat and pressure to sterilize instruments and materials that are not sensitive to moist heat.

Autonomy Ethical principle based on the principle of respect for persons. It is the belief that others should not constrain an individual's independent actions and choices.

B

Bacteremia Presence of microorganisms in the bloodstream.

Bacterial plaque biofilm See *Dental plaque; Oral biofilm.*

Bactericidal The ability of a substance to kill microbes, either by killing microbes directly or by negatively affecting the metabolism or reproduction of the microbe.

Bacteriostatic Action by which the metabolism or reproduction of a microbe is negatively affected.

Basic life support (BLS) A level of care provided by certified professionals and individuals to sustain the life of victims of life-threatening illnesses or injuries until they can be given full medical care at a hospital.

Behavior modification Technique used to reinforce desired behaviors and extinguish behaviors considered detrimental via the consistent application of rewards and punishment.

Bell palsy The most common cause of facial paralysis. It is also known as idiopathic facial paralysis because the exact etiology is unknown.

Beneficence Ethical principle that endorses the promotion of benefit, goodness, kindness, and charity and removal of harm.

Bioavailability The extent and amount to which a substance (e.g., fluoride) becomes completely available to its intended biological destination.

Biofilm A complex, three-dimensional arrangement of bacteria living together as a self-sufficient, secure, self-sustaining community that is resistant to conventional antibiotics and antimicrobial agents. Dental plaque is a biofilm; therefore the term *oral biofilm* is often used.

Biologic indicators Commonly referred to as spore tests, a BI is a biological sterility indicator containing nonpathogenic spores that are especially resistant to the sterilization process to test for the killing of all spores, the most resistant microorganisms.

Bitewing radiographs Radiographs that include images of the crown and some of the roots of several teeth in both arches. Bitewing radiographs are standard diagnostic tools for posterior teeth, producing the best image of the tooth crowns, the main area of concern for dental caries and tooth restoration.

Blood dyscrasia A pathologic condition, disease, or disorder that involves abnormal blood material, cells, or platelets.

Body mass index (BMI) A calculation used to estimate body fat calculated by dividing a patient's weight in kilograms by height in meters.

Body mechanics The application of kinesiology, the study of the mechanics of body movement, to daily living activities or exercises to improve stamina, posture, and coordination.

Bone loss (horizontal and vertical) Loss of alveolar bone that normally supports the teeth; the pattern of bone loss may be horizontal when the bone loss is parallel to the cementoenamel junction (CEJ) of adjacent teeth or vertical when the bone loss is oriented diagonally to the CEJ of adjacent teeth.

Bradycardia A slowness of the heartbeat as evidenced by a decline in the pulse rate to less than 60 beats per minute (BPM).

Breach of contract A common concept of liability used in dental malpractice lawsuits (civil law).

Bruxism Stress-induced, involuntary behavior of grinding the teeth together; does not cause bone loss itself but can cause loss of bone secondary to periodontitis, headache, muscle spasm, and facial pain.

Buccal mucosa Tissue that lines the inner cheek; may be glistening pink or pigmented with melanin; frequent areas of cheek-biting lesions.

C

CD4+ T lymphocytes A type of lymphocyte that helps coordinate the immune system's reactions by stimulating the production of various other immune cells that play important roles; also known as T cells.

C-reactive protein A substance produced by the liver in response to inflammation.

Candida albicans The most common causes of fungal infections in humans, often on the skin or mucous membranes; when it occurs under a denture, it is called *denture stomatitis.*

Carcinogenic Cancer causing.

Cardiopulmonary resuscitation An emergency procedure including chest compressions to save the life of a person whose heart stops beating, commonly in a heart attack or near drowning.

Cardiovascular disease (CVD) Alteration of the heart and/or blood vessels that impairs function.

Caries balance Balance between protective factors and pathologic factors to remineralize early carious lesions and/or prevent future caries.

Caries management Care plan to restore and maintain a balance between protective factors and pathologic factors to remineralize early carious lesions and/or prevent future caries, known as the *caries balance.*

Caries risk assessment Process by which the patient is categorized based on the probability of developing dental caries; includes an individual's caries disease indicators, risk factors, and protective factors. The goal of caries risk assessment for individuals 6 years old or older is to assign a caries risk level for developing future caries as the first step in managing the disease process. The level of caries risk (low, moderate, high, or extreme) is based on the presence of caries disease indicators and the balance between pathologic and protective factors.

Career plan A strategy for determining one's own skills and interests, what career best suits the talents identified, and what skills and training are needed for a chosen career or career path.

Carpal tunnel syndrome (CTS) A neurological disorder that occurs when the median nerve that runs from the forearm to the palm of the hand becomes pressed or squeezed at the wrist. Feelings of numbness, weakness, pain in the hand or wrist can occur, and fingers may become swollen and useless.

Case presentation Process of explaining assessment findings to a patient along with options and recommendations for therapy to reach agreement on a care plan and patient goals.

Cavitation Formation and explosive collapse of microscopic bubbles generated by the vibrating ultrasonic tip that aids in debriding biofilm from the tooth surface.

Cavitated lesions Carious lesions on the tooth surfaces that have invaded the dentin that can no longer be repaired by biological means.

Cementoenamel junction (CEJ) Location on a tooth where the cementum and enamel meet; demarcation between the anatomic crown and the anatomic root of the tooth.

Cementum Mineralized bonelike substance that covers the roots of teeth and provides a surface for attachment and anchorage for the periodontal fibers; may be cellular or acellular.

Centric occlusion Relationship between the maxillary and mandibular occlusal surfaces that provides the maximum contact and/or intercuspation.

Centric relation The relation of the mandible to the maxilla when the condyles are in their most posterior and superior positions in the mandibular fossae.

Cephalometric x-ray An x-ray that shows a side view of the head, exposing teeth, jaw, and surrounding structures; used in the assessment of such things as impacted teeth, orthodontic conditions, temporomandibular joint problems, broken teeth or jaws, etc.

Cerebral palsy A chronic, nonprogressive neuromuscular disorder caused by damage to motor areas of the immature brain, affecting primarily the ability to control posture and movement.

Cerebrovascular accident A medical term for a stroke, which occurs when blood flow to a part of the brain is stopped either by a blockage or the rupture of a blood vessel.

Cerebrovascular disease Disease of blood vessels supplying the brain.

Cervical enamel projections Apical extensions of the cementoenamel junction toward the furcation of a molar.

Cetylpyridium chloride A cationic quaternary compound with a broad antimicrobial spectrum, frequently used in mouth rinses and breath sprays.

Chain of infection A process of disease transmission that occurs when an infective agent leaves its reservoir or host, is transported by movement of the pathogen, and enters through a gateway to infect a susceptible host.

Change talk Statements by the client or patient revealing consideration of, motivation for, or commitment to change a behavior, often elicited by motivational interviewing.

Channeling An approach to scaling and peri-odontal debridement that employs continuous, systematic, overlapping working strokes.

Chemotherapeutic agent Chemical agent used to treat a disease or alter host response to the disease.

Chemotherapy Treatment of a disease with a chemical agent that destroys the pathogens caus-ing the disease or alters their ability to replicate; also known as *pharmacotherapy*.

Chief complaint Patient's primary reason for seeking the oral healthcare appointment as verbalized by the patient. The chief complaint is written in the client's own words.

Chlorhexidine gluconate (CHG) A bis-biguanide used as a disinfectant for skin and mucous membranes; an antiplaque and antigingivitis agent. It is used predominantly in prescription mouth rinses, irrigation solutions, and controlled-release products.

Chronic caries A slow, progressive decay process that requires intervention. The carious dentin is firm and often brown to black. In large, open cavi-ties, the decayed dentin can be scooped out in large segments and has the consistency of firm leather.

Chronic obstructive pulmonary disease (COPD) A commonplace, preventable, and treatable disease characterized by persistent respiratory symptoms and airflow restriction due to airway and/or alveolar abnormalities, most often caused by significant exposure to noxious substances.

Chronic stress Stress that is repeated and is more long term in nature; examples might include unemployment for an extended period, or repeated exposure to trauma.

Civil law Includes offenses for violating private or contractual rights; a breach of legal duty against a person. A civil action requires a less strict level of proof called a preponderance of evidence.

Clenching The continuous or intermittent forceful closure of the maxillary teeth against the mandibular teeth.

Client Biologic, psychologic, spiritual, social, cul-tural, and intellectual human being whose behav-ior is motivated by human needs and who has eight human needs related to dental hygiene care; the contemporary healthcare consumer; the term suggests one who is an active participant in oral healthcare and who is responsible for personal choices and the consequences of those choices; may refer to an individual or group; often referred to as a patient in the context of patient care.

Client Self-Care Commitment Model A dental hygiene conceptual model composed of five domains (initiation, assessment, negotiation, commitment and evaluation) that proposes that the relationships among these domains, and the interaction between the client and the dental hygienist can empower clients to make decisions that will enhance their own health through com-mitment and compliance.

Clinical crown Portion of the tooth that is exposed above the epithelial attachment.

Clinical attachment loss (CAL) CAL occurs when the collagen fibers of the periodontal ligament detach from the cementum on the root surface of the tooth, which causes the gingiva to migrate toward the roots of the teeth.

Clinical practice guidelines (CPGs) A second-ary source of evidence at the top of the hierarchy of evidence because it incorporates the best available scientific evidence to support a clinical practice.

Clinical significance A standard used to distin-guish the importance and meaning of the results of a study that is not based on a comparison of numbers, as is statistical significance.

Cochrane Collaboration An international, independent, not-for-profit organization compris-ing over 28,000 contributors from more than 100 countries that produce systematic reviews as a reliable and relevant source of evidence about the effects of healthcare.

Community-acquired pneumonia A type of lung infection that is contracted in a community setting and can cause breathing problems and other symptoms.

Community health A field of public health, it is a discipline concerned with the study and better-ment of the health characteristics of populations in a shared geographic area.

Conceptual model Set of concepts and propo-sitions integrated into a meaningful configuration within the domain of dental hygiene; school of thought. For example the Human Needs Model or the Oral Health-Related Quality of Life Model.

Cone beam computed tomography (CBCT) A special type of x-ray equipment that produces three-dimensional (3D) images of the teeth, soft tissues, nerve pathways, and bone in a single scan.

Concrescence Fusion of two teeth at the root through the cementum only. Originally, teeth are separate but later are joined because of excessive cementum deposition.

Congenital heart disease An abnormality of the heart's structure and function caused by abnormal or disordered heart development before birth. Commonly observed congenital heart malformations are ventricular septal defect, atrial septal defect, and patent ductus arteriosus.

Congestive heart failure A syndrome char-acterized by myocardial dysfunction that leads to diminished cardiac output or abnormal circula-tory congestion.

Conscious sedation Method of pain control that decreases patient's response to pain, anxiety, and stress; client is awake and able to respond, breathe, and cough; also known as *inhalation sedation, nitrous oxide psychosedation,* and *relative analgesia.*

Consistency Degree of firmness or density of the soft tissue; some terms used to define firmness include *spongy, fibrotic,* and *nodular.*

Continued care Preventive care, maintenance care, or periodontal maintenance therapy that occurs at regular intervals after completion of active therapy. Also known as *recare* or *recall.*

Controlled-release drug delivery The use of professionally placed intracrevicular devices that provide local drug delivery for sustained periods of time.

Criminal law Established to prevent harm to society and describes a criminal act and the appropriate punishment. The level of proof for a criminal act is beyond a reasonable doubt.

Critical appraisal The process of systemati-cally assessing the outcome of scientific research (evidence) to judge its dependability, value, and relevance in a specific context.

Critical instruments Infection control term that refers to instruments that penetrate soft tissue or bone. Critical instruments must be heat sterilized between each use or discarded if disposable.

Cross-arch fulcrum Fulcrum established by holding the working end of the instrument and the index finger of the hand holding the instru-ment on separate dental arches.

Cross-contamination Transfer of oral fluids and debris from a client to surfaces, equipment, materials, workers' hands, or another client or person (coworker, family member, or friend).

Cross-hatching An approach to periodontal instrumentation in which the strokes are directed horizontally, vertically, and obliquely to cross hatch the root surface with the blade closed and smooth instrumentation roughness.

Culture A set of guidelines that one can inherit as a member of a particular group or society.

Curette Subgingival scaling instrument designed to enhance access and adaptation on teeth with periodontal pockets. Also spelled curette.

D

Defendant In a legal dispute, the defendant is the person denying the action charged.

Dementia Condition characterized by a progressive intellectual decline that eventually leads to deterioration of occupational, social, and interpersonal functions.

Demographic information Data about the characteristics of a population, such as age, gender, race or ethnicity, education level, and income.

Dental calculus Oral biofilm that has been min-eralized by calcium and phosphate salts within the saliva and can attach to teeth, restorations, and dental appliances; commonly referred to as *tartar*; calcified oral biofilm.

Dental caries An infectious, chronic, bacteria-caused disease characterized by the acid dissolu-tion of enamel and the eventual breakdown of the more organic, inner dental tissues.

Dental charting The graphic representation of the condition of the patient's teeth on a specific date.

Dental hygiene care plan The written blue-print that directs the dental hygienist and patient as they work together to meet the patient's desired oral health outcomes.

Dental hygiene diagnosis The identification of an individual's health behaviors, attitudes, and oral healthcare needs for which a dental hygienist is educationally qualified and licensed to provide. The dental hygiene diagnosis requires evidence-based critical analysis and interpretation of assessments in order to reach conclusions about the patient's dental hygiene treatment needs. The dental hygiene diagnosis provides the basis for the dental hygiene care plan.

Dental hygiene care plan goal The outcome desired to be achieved through specific dental hygiene interventions to satisfy an identified need or problem. The goals are linked to the dental hygiene diagnosis, thus establishing the parameters for measuring the success of the care plan in meeting the needs of the patient.

Dental Hygiene Human Needs Conceptual Model A model based on the premise that human behavior is motivated by fulfillment of human needs; thus it defines the paradigm concepts (client, health/oral health, dental hygiene actions, environment) in terms of human need theory.

Dental hygiene interventions The evidence-based strategies, preventive services, treatment, products, and referrals that when applied, reduce, eliminate, or prevent a diagnosed need or problem. Interventions, like goals, are linked to the dental hygiene diagnosis.

Dental hygiene profession A career requiring specialized education and licensure for healthcare providers that focus on oral health, prevention of oral diseases, and health promotion. Dental hygiene encompasses autonomous, intra- and interprofessional collaboration for shared knowledge and decision making with other healthcare professionals to provide comprehensive patient-centered care. The profession serves clients such as individual patients, families, groups, and communities.

Dental Hygiene Process of Care/ADPIE The process of dental hygiene care involves assessment, dental hygiene diagnosis, care planning, implementation and evaluation, and documentation; evaluation and documentation occurs throughout the process.

Dental hygiene prognosis Evidence-based predictability of the patient's continued health and wellness.

Dental impression Negative imprint taken of the teeth and surrounding tissues so that a diagnostic cast (study model) can be made.

Dental index Quantifiable measure of the amount of oral disease or condition in a population or individual.

Dental plaque Dense, nonmineralized mass of bacterial colonies in a gel-like intermicrobial, enclosed matrix (slime layer) that is attached to a moist environmental surface. Also known as *microbial plaque, oral biofilm, dental biofilm, dental plaque biofilm, bacterial plaque biofilm.*

Dental procedure code A number assigned as a part of a taxonomy defining oral health care services or procedures delivered to patients that frequently is used for billing or insurance reporting purposes, for example, the ADA *CDT Dental Procedure Codes* published annually.

Dentifrice (toothpaste) Substance (gel, paste, or powder) used in conjunction with a toothbrush or interdental cleaner to facilitate bacterial plaque biofilm removal or as a vehicle for transporting therapeutic or cosmetic agents to the tooth and its environment.

Dentinal hypersensitivity A painful condition that occurs when vital dentinal tubules are exposed to the oral environment; fluid movement within the dentinal tubule, caused by a stimulus (thermal, evaporative, tactile, osmotic, or chemical) initiates a pain sensation in the pulp because of dental attrition, dental erosion, gingival recession, and scaling and root planing. Also referred to as *dental hypersensitivity.*

Denture stomatitis Inflammation of the oral mucosa underlying the denture; characterized by redness, pain, and swelling

Developmental disabilities Lifelong severe chronic disabilities that can be cognitive, physical, or both, and present before the age of 21 years.

Diabetes A disease that occurs when blood glucose, also called blood sugar, is too high, commonly because insulin, a hormone made by the pancreas, is insufficient to help food become energy to be used by cells.

Diabetic ketoacidosis A serious complication of diabetes that occurs when the body produces high levels of blood acids, ketones, because the body cannot produce enough insulin.

Diastolic blood pressure A measurement of the minimum pressure occurring against the arterial walls as a result of cardiac ventricular relaxation (diastole) and is the number on the sphygmomanometer when the last heart sound is heard.

Dilaceration A sharp bend in the root surface caused by the displacement of the root during tooth development.

Direct access The ability of dental hygienists to initiate treatment based on their assessment of patients' needs without a dentist's specific authorization or presence during treatment.

Disability A physical or mental condition that limits a person's movements, senses, or activities.

Disability-adjusted life years (DALYs) DALYs referred to the sum of years of potential life lost due to premature mortality and the years of productive life lost due to a disability.

Disclosing agent (disclosant) Liquid concentrate or tablet containing an ingredient that temporarily stains oral deposits and debris so that the patient and clinician can see them.

Disease prevention Specific, population- and individual-based interventions for primary and secondary (early detection) prevention, or stopping diseases from occurring to minimize the burden and associated risk factors.

Disinfected Having sanitized or cleaned (something), especially with a chemical, in order to destroy bacteria.

Distal Situated away from the center of the body. On a tooth, this refers to the tooth surfaces farthest from the midline.

Distant site The location of the healthcare provider while providing remote healthcare services.

Distress A type of stress that can have a deleterious impact on the psychological well-being and physical health of individuals.

Documentation Recording information in dental hygiene records (legal documents) including the complete and accurate recording of all data collected, treatment planned and provided, recommendations, referrals, prescriptions, patient/client comments and related communication, treatment outcomes and patient satisfaction, and other information related to patient care.

Domestic elder abuse An intentional act or failure to act by a caregiver or another person in a relationship involving trust that creates a risk of harm to an older adult, someone age 60 or older.

Drug hypersensitivity Response that occurs when either the medication and/or its metabolites act as immunogens, triggering the immune response (i.e., an allergy).

Drug idiosyncrasy A side effect from a medication that is completely unexpected or qualitatively different from any other known published side effects.

Drug interactions Negative effects that can occur when two or more medications are taken simultaneously.

Drug toxicity Toxin-induced cell damage and/or cell death from a medication.

Dysphagia A medical term for difficulty swallowing accompanied by the sensation of food lodged in the neck or chest.

Dyspnea Difficulty breathing.

E

Early childhood caries (ECC) Severe decay caused by *Streptococcus mutans* and by sugars and acids in a bottle of milk or juice left in contact with a child's primary teeth; causes rapid demineralization of hard tooth structure; affects children ages 0 to 2.

Edentulous Lacking or being without teeth.

Electronic health records (EHRs) An online combination of information, such as health histories, medical and dental prescriptions, dental and periodontal charting, medical alerts, radiographs, current and future treatment planning, treatment notes, intraoffice communication, oral health education, and other areas that are a part of comprehensive dental care.

Electronic nicotine delivery systems (ENDS) An electronic device used to deliver nicotine to the user. Commonly referred to as electronic cigarettes, e-cigarettes, tanks, electronic hookah, or vapor pens.

Electronic portfolio A digital portfolio is a computer-based collection of documents showing performance and accomplishments over time, also called an e-portfolio.

Embrasure space The area immediately under the contact point of adjacent teeth. Size of the embrasure space is important in selecting the correct interdental cleaning aids.

Emphysema Often found in people who smoke or have chronic bronchitis, emphysema is a disorder that results in alveoli (tiny air sacs of the lungs) to become abnormally inflated, damaging the walls and making it harder to breathe; is known as a type of chronic obstructive pulmonary disease (COPD).

End-stage renal disease Kidney failure or when the kidneys stop functioning.

Endogenous stains Stains that originate from within the tooth; examples include tetracycline, pulpal trauma, and developmental conditions such as dentinogenesis and amelogenesis imperfecta.

Endothelium Inner wall of the blood vessels.

Epilepsy A seizure disorder in which the excessive abnormal neuronal discharges from cerebral function disturbances are recurrent and unprovoked.

Ergonomics Study of human performance and workplace design to maximize health, comfort, and efficiency.

Erythema A red area of variable shape and size reflecting tissue inflammation, thinness, and irregularity. The tissue then may be described as erythematous.

Essential oils Volatile oils derived from plants; contain phenolic compounds (e.g., thymol, eucalyptol, menthol, and methyl salicylate) and are used in some commercial mouth rinses.

Ester anesthetics Ester-type local anesthetics (primarily 20% benzocaine) used as topical anesthetic; injectable ester-type local anesthetics are off the market.

Ethics A branch of philosophy that deals with thinking about morality, moral problems, and moral judgments.

Ethical dilemma A situation in which two ethical principles conflict, making it challenging to make a choice.

Eustress A stress that people experience due to positive life events (e.g., work promotion or starting your first job after graduation).

Evidence-based decision making (EBDM) The integration of best research evidence with clinical expertise and the patient's unique values and circumstances.

Exogenous stains Stains that originate from sources outside of the tooth such as food, beverages, tobacco products, or chromogenic (or color-producing) bacteria.

Extraoral fulcrum Fulcrum established outside of the mouth and used predominantly for teeth with deep periodontal pockets; the leverage point may be the patient's jaw or side of the face. Also known as an *external fulcrum.*

Extrinsic motivation Behavior or action initiated from an environmental source. This action is not based on a desire, reason, ability, or need to make a change; it is based on contingencies in the environment.

Extrinsic stains Stains that occur on the tooth surface.

F

Facial The buccal and labial surfaces of teeth and refers to the front of each tooth that is most visible when retracting the lips and cheeks.

Fidelity An ethical principle that involves the obligation to keep implied or explicit promises.

Field block Method of obtaining anesthesia that involves the deposition of solution near large terminal nerve branches.

Filled sealant Sealant composed of a mixture of resins, chemicals, and fillers.

Fluoride Most effective agent and nutrient for the prevention and control of dental caries on smooth surfaces of teeth.

Fluoride-releasing sealant Glass ionomer sealant.

Fremitus The vibration or movement of the teeth when in contacting positions from the patient's own occlusal forces. Used in part to determine occlusal trauma.

Fulcrum Source of stability or leverage on which the finger rests and against which it pushes for the clinician to hold a dental instrument with control during stroke activation.

Furcation Areas between the branching roots of posterior teeth where the root trunk divides into separate roots.

Furcation probe Instrument used to probe or determine the extent and depth of furcation lesions from all sides of the teeth in both arches.

G

Geriatrics The branch of medicine concerned with the illnesses of old age and their treatment.

Gerontology The scientific study of the factors affecting the normal aging process and the effects of aging, especially in relation to quality of life issues.

Gingival abscess A periodontal abscess that is confined to the marginal gingiva and that often occurs in previously healthy gingival areas.

Gingival margin Edge of the marginal gingiva nearest to the incisal or occlusal area of the tooth; marks the opening of the gingival sulcus.

Gingival recession Reduction of the height of the marginal gingiva to a location apical to the cementoenamel junction, resulting in root surface exposure; signifies attachment loss.

Gingival sulcus Space between the marginal gingiva and the tooth. The healthy gingival sulcus measures 0.5 mm to 3 mm from the gingival margin to the base of the sulcus. Also known as a *gingival crevice.*

Gingivitis Inflammation of the gingival tissue with no apical migration of the junctional epithelium beyond the cementoenamel junction; characterized by inflammation and redness of the gingival tissue and bleeding on probing. Gingivitis may also be referred to as dental biofilm-induced gingivitis. See also *Periodontitis.*

Glossodynia Pain in the tongue.

Glycated hemoglobin A1c (HbA1c) A test that measures the amount of blood sugar (glucose) attached to hemoglobin, the part of red blood cells that carries oxygen to the rest of the body.

Gracey curette Unlike the sickle scaler and the universal curette, the Gracey curette is designed to be site specific. The facial surface has only one working blade, angled downward at 70 degrees.

Gravid Pregnant.

H

Halitosis Chronic bad breath that can be caused by volatile sulfur compounds produced by bacteria in the mouth and aggravated by conditions such as dry mouth and dental caries, or caused by systemic problems such as gastric reflux or diabetes.

Health history Assessment of a patient's health status to identify predisposing conditions, current and past treatment experiences, past responses to healthcare, and risk factors that may affect dental hygiene care and outcomes of care. Also known as *medical history.*

Health literacy The degree to which a person has the capacity to obtain, process, and understand basic health information and services needed to make suitable health decisions.

Hematoma Swelling and discoloration of the tissue resulting from the effusion of blood into the extravascular spaces.

Hemodialysis The clinical purification of the patient's blood (a few ounces at a time) by a special filter (called an artificial kidney or a dialyzer), as a substitute for the normal function of the kidney.

Hemorrhage An escape of blood from a ruptured blood vessel, especially when profuse, also called bleeding.

Herpes simplex virus (HSV) A viral infection that causes herpetic lesions.

Hospice A type of care and philosophy of care that focuses on palliation, or comfort, of a chronically ill, terminally ill, or seriously ill patient's pain and symptoms, making them feel better and attending to their emotional and spiritual needs without the intention of curing the illness.

Host defense system A host's natural defense system against invasion by an organism (e.g., the inflammatory process and immune system).

Host immune system Consists of antibodies, lymphocytes, leukocytes, macrophages, and other specialized cells that protect the body from invasion by foreign substances. Specialized cells that fight infectious agents.

Housekeeping surfaces An infection control term that refers to the surfaces such as floors, walls, and sinks. These surfaces may become contaminated during patient care but carry less risk of disease transmission than clinical contact surfaces.

Human immunodeficiency virus (HIV) A virus that attacks cells in the immune system, our body's natural defense against illness. The virus destroys T-helper cells, also called *CD4 cells,* replicates inside these white blood cells, and gradually weakens a person's immune system.

Human need Internal tension that results from an alteration in a state of a person's system. Eight human needs related to dental hygiene practice follow: *Biologically sound and functional dentition:* The need to have intact teeth and restorations that defend against harmful microbes, provide for adequate function, and reflect appropriate nutrition and diet. *Conceptualization and problem solving:* The need to grasp ideas and abstractions in order to make sound decisions about one's oral health. *Freedom from fear and stress:* The need to feel safe and to be free from fear and emotional discomfort in the oral healthcare environment. *Freedom from head and neck pain:* The need to be exempt from physical discomfort in the head and neck area. *Protection from health risks:* The need to avoid medical contraindications to dental hygiene care, including the need to be protected from health risks related to dental hygiene care. *Responsibility for oral health:* The need to be accountable for one's health as a result of interaction among one's motivation, physical capability, and environment. *Skin and mucous membrane integrity of the head and neck:* The need to have an intact and functioning covering of one's head and neck area, including the oral mucous membranes and periodontium, which defend against harmful microbes, resist injurious substances and trauma, and reflect adequate nutrition. *Wholesome facial* *image:* The need to feel satisfied with one's own orofacial features and breath.

Human needs conceptual model Conceptual model of dental hygiene that defines the paradigm concepts of client, environment, health and oral health, and dental hygiene actions in terms of human needs theory.

Human needs theory Theory that explains and predicts human behavior by focusing on human need fulfillment and unmet human needs as motivators.

Human papillomavirus (HPV) A group of more than 150 related viruses. Each HPV virus in this large group is given a number, called its HPV type. HPV can cause warts (papilloma), STDs, cancer, and other diseases or conditions.

Huntington disease A rare, highly complex neurodegenerative disorder resulting from the degeneration of neurons within the basal ganglia (the area deep in the brain that controls movement).

Hydrodynamic theory Most accepted theory today to explain the etiology of dentinal hypersensitivity; this theory proposes that stimuli (e.g., thermal, tactile, chemical) are transmitted to the pulp surface via movement of fluid within the dentinal tubules.

Hypercementosis Excessive formation of cementum in the apical third to half of the tooth after the tooth has erupted.

Hyperglycemia A high blood glucose level resulting from inadequate use or production of insulin, characteristic of diabetes.

Hypertension Condition characterized by a persistent elevation of the systolic and diastolic blood pressures.

Hypertensive crisis A systolic blood pressure greater than 180 mm Hg and/or a diastolic blood pressure greater than 120 mm Hg.

Hypoglycemia A low level of blood glucose that is inadequate to support the body's demand for energy, a symptom of another condition such as diabetes treated by too much insulin.

Hypotension Low blood pressure.

I

Iatrogenic factors Adverse factors caused by the healthcare practitioner that result in a negative outcome for the patient.

Illicit drugs A variety of drugs that are used for nonmedical purposes and are illegal to manufacture, use, or sell.

Immunity The nonsusceptible state of a host to an infectious agent or antigen. In terms of the law, established to protect persons from civil lawsuits and criminal prosecution resulting from filing a report of child abuse and neglect.

Immunization The action of making a person or animal immune to infection, typically by inoculation or vaccination.

Immunosuppression Suppression of the body's natural immune response, measured by a decrease in certain immune system cells.

Implant-supported overdentures Removable complete dentures designed to fit over implant fixtures that are inserted partially or entirely into living bone.

Implementation A step in the dental hygiene process of care, implementation is the act of carrying out the dental hygiene plan of care.

Inactive ingredient (nontherapeutic agent) A product additive that is necessary to make the formulation thick, hold together, clean efficiently, or have a particular color or flavor for consumer appeal.

Incipient caries Carious lesions limited to the enamel surface: if in a pit or fissure, it can be treated with a dental sealant.

Incisal The cutting edges of incisors and canines.

Independent dental hygiene practitioners Dental hygienists licensed to *practice independent dental hygiene* without supervision of a *dentist.*

Indirect illumination Reflecting light off a dental mirror to illuminate or shine light onto a specific area or tooth.

Inflammatory mediators Soluble, diffusible molecules that promote or enhance the process of inflammation and therefore can cause hardand soft tissue destruction observed in periodontal disease. Some examples include endotoxin (LPS), interleukin, tumor necrosis factor-α, and prostaglandins.

Informed consent Written agreement from a mentally competent person that allows an action on the part of the healthcare provider; required before the performance of invasive healthcare procedures or procedures on a minor, and before a person is used as a participant (subject) in research. The agreement may come from a legal guardian or healthcare decision maker in the case of a minor or others who cannot self-determine.

Inhalation sedation Synonym for nitrous oxide and oxygen analgesia; gases are inhaled through the nose, resulting in the reduction in the perception of pain and reduction in anxiety in the patient. Also known as *conscious sedation, psychosedation,* and *relaxation sedation.*

Initial therapy Also known as *phase I periodontal therapy* or *antiinfective therapy,* most of which falls within the scope of dental hygiene practice. Includes client education, diet assessment, tobacco cessation, fluoride therapy, dental sealants, debridement, desensitization, antimicrobial therapy, selective polishing, restorative prosthetic treatment, and occlusal therapy.

Instrument sharpening The use of a stone to produce a sharp cutting edge on a dental hygiene instrument while maintaining the original shape of the instrument.

Intellectual disability A type of developmental disability that must occur before the age of 18 years and be characterized by limitations in adaptive functioning in at least two of the following skill areas: communication, self-care, home living, social or interpersonal skills, use of community resources, self-direction, functional academic skills, work, leisure, health, and safety.

Intrabony periodontal pocket Occurs when the junctional epithelium (JE) has migrated below the crest of the alveolar bone; associated with vertical bone loss.

Interdental papilla Gingival tissue located in the interdental space between two adjacent teeth; the tip and lateral borders are continuous with the marginal gingiva, whereas the center is composed of alveolar gingiva.

Interdisciplinary care providers A team is a group of healthcare practitioners from different fields who work together or toward the same goal to provide the best care or best outcome for a patient or group of patients; also called interprofessional healthcare providers.

Interprofessional collaboration Also known as interprofessional practice, a process which includes communication and decision making among healthcare providers from different disciplines, enabling a synergistic influence of the group's knowledge and skills.

Interproximal or interdental area The proximal surfaces of teeth (mesial and distal surfaces) and the embrasure spaces.

Intraoral fulcrum Traditional fulcrum established inside the mouth against tooth structure.

Intrinsic motivation Behavior that is driven by internal rewards that inspire a person to engage in a behavior because it is naturally satisfying or desirable rather than by external rewards.

Intrinsic stain Internal discoloration of the tooth that may be caused by taking medication (e.g., tetracycline), excessive fluoride ingestion, or genetics during tooth development.

J

Junctional epithelium (JE) Cufflike band of nonkeratinized squamous epithelium that completely encircles and adheres to the tooth surface at the base of the gingival sulcus via hemidesmosomes; histologically the apex, or base of the sulcus, is formed by the JE.

Justice Ethical and legal principle that relies on fairness and equality; people are treated justly when given what they are due, are owed, deserve, or can claim legitimately.

K

Kaposi sarcoma Malignant neoplasm associated with HIV infection and manifesting as brown or purplish tumors on the gingiva near the teeth or on the skin.

Korotkoff sounds The rhythmic, knocking sounds produced when the blood begins to flow intermittently through the brachial artery when the bladder within the occluding cuff is deflated during the blood pressure measurement process.

L

Laser therapy All lasers work by delivering energy in the form of light. When used for surgical and dental procedures, the laser acts as a cutting instrument or a vaporizer of tissue it contacts; in teeth-whitening procedures, the laser acts as a heat source to enhance the effect of tooth-bleaching agents.

Lateral pressure Force used by a dental hygienist to engage the cutting edge of the periodontal scaling instrument against the tooth.

Lavage Therapeutic washing of the periodontal pockets and root surface to remove endotoxins and loose debris with water under pressure.

Legislation Laws or statues enacted by a legislature or other governing body or the process of enacting them.

Leukemia Cancer of the white blood cells, which are produced in the bone marrow to fight infection, so that the bone marrow produces abnormal white blood cells.

Lingual Surface nearest the tongue.

Local anesthesia Loss of sensation in a circumscribed area of the body as a result of the depression of excitation in nerve endings or the inhibition of the conduction process in peripheral nerves; results from use of a local anesthetic agent.

Local delivery Mode of application in which the antimicrobial agent is transported directly to the oral cavity or a specific location within it for topical application.

Local infiltration Injection involving placement of the anesthetic solution close to the smaller terminal endings of the nerve fibers in the immediate area to be treated.

Low birth weight A term used to describe babies who are born weighing less than 5 pounds, 8 ounces (2500 grams).

Low-velocity evacuation tubing (LVE) Tubing that facilitates low level of suctioning to rid the oral cavity of saliva and debris during oral care; also facilitates patient rinsing, operator's ability to see, and oral fluid control during care.

M

Macroglossia A larger than typical tongue; often the result of other conditions such as Down syndrome.

Macrovascular complications Diabetes is a disease of complications, most preventable, including those complications that affect the larger blood vessels, affecting the heart and brain and potentially resulting in heart attack or stroke.

Magnetostrictive Magnetostrictive power scalers, one of two types of ultrasonic devices used in dentistry, operate at an optimal frequency of 20 kHz to 40 kHz, which creates an energy dispersion that allows all sides of the scaler tip to be effective in the removal of biofilm and debris.

Malalignment Malposition of the teeth.

Malocclusion A deviation from the normal relationship between the maxilla and mandible while in centric occlusion.

Materia alba Loosely attached collection of soft oral debris and bacteria seen as a whitish, curdlike mass on the teeth or overlying oral biofilm.

Manual toothbrush An oral hygiene device with brush head holding bristles and a handle, operated by one's hand and arm, not battery or electrically powered.

Mesial A positional term relating to or directed toward the midline of a body. On the tooth, it refers to surfaces closest to the midline.

Metastasize The development of secondary malignant growths at a distance from a primary site of cancer.

Metaanalysis A statistical process often used with systematic reviews; involves combining the data analyses of numerous individual studies into one analysis; considered one of the gold standards for evidence because of strict protocols to reduce bias and to include the findings of only the very best studies.

Metaparadigm A widely accepted view of the discipline which includes paradigm concepts defined by the discipline as its unique perspective. The concepts defined for each discipline differentiate the discipline from others.

Microbiome A collection of microorganisms in a particular environment.

Micrognathia Also known as mandibular hypoplasia, is a condition in which the lower jaw is smaller than usual; may result in breathing or feeding problems in babies.

Microvascular complications Diabetes is a disease of complications, most preventable, including those complications that affect the small blood vessels, potentially causing other health problems or conditions including retinopathy, nephropathy, and neuropathy.

Midlevel oral health practitioner The ADHA defines a midlevel oral health practitioner as a licensed dental hygienist and graduate from an accredited dental hygiene program who is a primary oral healthcare provider of dental hygiene services directly to patients. Midlevel oral health practitioners have an expanded scope of care, as set forth by the appropriate licensing agency or regulatory authority.

Midline An imaginary vertical line that bisects the patient's face.

Minimally invasive dentistry A holistic management philosophy that integrates carious lesion control and minimal operative intervention.

Mitral valve prolapse One of the most frequently occurring valvular heart defects; when the left ventricle pumps blood to the aorta, the mitral valve flops backward (prolapses) into the left atrium.

Mobile Health (mHealth) Health and health-related services supported by mobile applications (apps) on smart devices, such as cell phones and tablet computers.

Mobility Property of a lesion; refers to whether the lesion is free or fixed in relationship to the neighboring tissues; also used to describe the degree of movement of a tooth in a socket infected with periodontitis.

Modified pen grasp Standard grasp used for assessment and treatment instruments.

Monotherapy Treatment with just one drug.

Motivation The incentive or drive to satisfy unmet human needs or human needs in deficit.

Motivational interviewing Form of patient-centered communication to help patients or clients get "unstuck" from the ambivalence that prevents a specific behavior change. The goal is to have the client verbalize arguments for stopping an unhealthy behavior like smoking.

Mouth rinses A liquid mouthwash that can be cosmetic, for a pleasant taste and temporary fresher breath, or therapeutic, with active ingredients to reduce halitosis, plaque, gingivitis, or dental caries.

Mucogingival conditions Conditions that occur when the periodontal disease process extends beyond the attached gingiva and into the alveolar mucosa.

Mucogingival junction Demarcation between the alveolar mucosa and the attached gingiva.

Mucositis A complication of some cancer therapies in which the lining of the digestive system becomes inflamed; often seen as painful sores in the mouth.

Multiple sclerosis (MS) An autoimmune central nervous system disorder in which there is myelin sheath destruction of specific axons, causing multiple neurologic symptoms that accrue over time.

Musculoskeletal disorders (MSDs) Injuries that affect the human body's movement or *musculoskeletal* system (i.e., muscles, tendons, ligaments, nerves, discs, blood vessels, etc.); common MSDs include carpal tunnel syndrome and tendonitis.

Myocardial infarction (MI) A reduction of blood flow through one of the coronary arteries, resulting in an infarct, an area of tissue that undergoes necrosis because of the elimination of blood flow; also known as a *heart attack, coronary occlusion,* and *coronary thrombosis.*

N

Necrotizing ulcerative periodontitis (NUP) A type of periodontal disease characterized by severe pain described as deep jaw pain, fetid odor, bleeding, and loose teeth, with rapid loss of bone and soft tissue.

Neoplasm An abnormal mass of tissue that forms when cells grow and divide more than they should or do not die when they should. Neoplasms may be benign (not cancer) or malignant (cancer).

Nerve block The deposition of anesthetic solution close to a main nerve trunk, often at some distance from the treatment area.

Neuropathy A nerve problem that causes pain, numbness, tingling, swelling, or muscle weakness in different parts of the body; may be caused by cancer/cancer treatment such as chemotherapy; also caused by physical injury, infection, toxic substances, or conditions such as diabetes.

Nicotine replacement therapy (NRT) The most commonly used family of quit smoking medications. NRT reduces withdrawal feelings by supplying a small, controlled amount of nicotine but none of the other dangerous chemicals found in cigarettes.

Nitrous oxide Gas used in combination with oxygen for the control of pain and anxiety during dental and dental hygiene care.

Nodule Elevated solid mass; deeper and firmer than a papule of between 0.5 cm and 2 cm in size.

Nonadherence or noncompliance A lack of client/patient cooperation with recommended oral healthcare.

Noncavitated carious lesions (NCCL) Initial, early, or white spot carious lesions visually confined to the enamel.

Noncritical instruments and devices Infection control term that refers to those items that come into contact only with intact skin.

Nonmaleficence Ethical principle stating that above all, a health professional should do no harm.

Noninvasive debridement Involves removal of any soft deposit, biofilm, plaque, food particles, and pathogens from all areas of the teeth and gums that may cause inflammation and strain on the body's ability to fight infection.

Nonplaque-induced gingivitis Gingival diseases of specific bacterial, viral, or genetic origin; gingival manifestations of systemic conditions such as mucocutaneous disorders and allergic reactions; or traumatic lesions, foreign body reactions, or otherwise nonspecific gingival lesions.

Nonsteroidal antiinflammatory drugs (NSAIDs) Drugs that block enzymes that promote the inflammatory response, thus reducing inflammation.

Nonsurgical periodontal therapy (NSPT) Periodontal scaling and root planing performed with the aim of increasing connective tissue attachment level. Also includes the use of chemotherapeutic agents to control periodontal pathogens.

Nonverbal communication Interactions between two or more persons using body language to communicate a message.

Nosocomial hospital-acquired pneumonia Pneumonia acquired during a hospital stay, exhibiting symptoms within 48 hours after admission.

Nutritional counseling Process used to help patients develop healthful food selection and eating behaviors that promote overall health.

O

Obesity A disorder involving excessive body fat that increases the risk of health problems.

Obstructive sleep apnea A condition that involves the partial or complete collapse of the upper airway while breathing during sleep.

Obturator A removable prosthodontic appliance designed to close a palatal opening as a result of a defect such as an orofacial cleft.

Occlusal Biting or chewing surfaces of posterior teeth.

Occlusion Contact relationship between maxillary and mandibular teeth when the jaws are in a fully closed position.

Occupational exposure Exposure to an infectious agent that occurs in the workplace. A percutaneous injury or contact of mucous membrane or nonintact skin with blood, saliva, tissue, or other body fluids that are potentially infectious. Exposure incidents may pose a risk of hepatitis B virus, hepatitis C virus, or HIV infection and are a matter of medical urgency.

Occupational Safety and Health Administration (OSHA) Federal agency responsible for safety in the workplace.

Opposite-arch fulcrum Intraoral fulcrum established on a tooth surface on the opposing arch from the arch being scaled.

Oral biofilm A biofilm that grows on surfaces within the oral cavity; is a necessary condition for initiation and progression of dental caries and periodontal disease, depending on the pathogens present in the biofilm. See also *Biofilm; Dental plaque.*

Oral biofilm control (plaque control) Regular mechanical or chemical removal of dental plaque from the teeth and adjacent oral tissue or the prevention of its growth and maturation.

Oral candidiasis (thrush) Fungal infection of the oral cavity or oropharynx caused by *Candida albicans;* also known as oral *thrush* on the tongue.

Oral hairy leukoplakia A condition that the Epstein-Barr virus can trigger, most often in people whose immune systems are very weak, for example, people with HIV. The condition causes white lesions or patches on the tongue.

Oral health literacy (OHL) The degree to which a person is able to get, evaluate, understand, and use oral health information and services to make good decisions about health.

Oral Health-Related Quality of Life Conceptual Model (OHRQL) A framework for looking at the complex interrelationship between health and disease, and its biological, psychological, and social consequences, based on the premise that a satisfactory level of oral health, comfort, and function is an integral element of general health. The Health Related Quality of Life (HRQL) domains of Symptom Status, Functional Status, and Health Perceptions are considered in this model.

Oral hygiene Degree to which the oral cavity is kept clean and free of soft and hard deposits by daily oral self-care or, when necessary, oral care provided by a caregiver.

Oral irrigation Method of directing a steady or pulsating stream of water or chemotherapeutic agent over the teeth, over the gingival tissues, or into a periodontal pocket; goal is to remove oral debris, reduce pathogens and their byproducts, or deliver an antimicrobial agent.

Oral malodor (halitosis) Offensive breath odor associated with poor oral hygiene, periodontitis, sinus infection, tonsillitis, lung disease, diabetes, or uremia.

Oral physiotherapy tools Tools used for noninvasive debridement, including brushes for all surfaces (occlusal, buccal, and lingual), floss, stimulators, and tongue cleaners.

Oral rinses Available for both cosmetic and therapeutic use and in prescription and over-the-counter formulations. Therapeutic uses include plaque and gingivitis reduction and caries prevention; cosmetic uses include breath freshening, tartar control, and tooth whitening. Also known as *mouth rinses* and *mouthwashes.*

Orofacial clefts Failure of the lip and palate tissues to close during embryonic development results in orofacial clefts; one of the most common craniofacial anomalies and congenital (birth) defects.

Oropharyngeal Refers to an area consisting of the throat, back third of the tongue, soft palate, and side and back walls of the throat and tonsils.

Oscillation High-frequency vibrations in ultrasonic scaling instruments that cause a forward and backward movement of the tip; this movement produces both mechanical and biophysical forces capable of disrupting and removing deposits from the tooth surface.

Osseointegration Stable and long-term connection of a dental implant placed beneath the mucosa to the supporting bone, which is the apparent direct attachment or connection of osseous tissue to the implant without intervening fibrous connective tissue.

Osteoporosis A disease that thins and weakens the bones, resulting in decreased bone mass and fragile bones that break easily, especially the bones in the hip, spine, and wrist.

Over-the-counter (OTC) drugs Medications and healthcare products that can be purchased without a prescription directly off the store shelf. The American Dental Association Seal of Acceptance includes only OTC products and devices. The Seal is no longer given for prescription drugs.

Oxygen saturation The extent to which hemoglobin in the bloodstream is saturated with oxygen, normally 95% to 100%.

P

Palliative oral care The management and prevention of oral problems caused by a patient's disease or from treatments received by focusing on the patient's immediate comfort and quality of life.

Palpation Act of using the sense of touch to collect patient data; compressing or moving tissue to check for abnormalities during an intraoral and extraoral examination.

Panoramic radiograph Radiograph in which the entire dentition, in addition to the adjacent osseous structures from the orbits of the eyes to the base of the mandible and the temporomandibular joints, is displayed on one rectangular film.

Paradigm A widely accepted worldview of a discipline that shapes the direction and methods of its practitioners, educators, administrators, and researchers.

Parkinson disease A chronic progressive neurodegenerative disorder of the motor system, resulting from the loss of dopamine-producing neurons.

Peri-implant mucositis A reversible inflammatory reaction that resides in the mucosa and does not include loss of supporting bone. In periimplant mucositis, bleeding on probing must be present.

Peri-implantitis Inflammation affecting the soft and hard tissue around a dental implant.

Periapical abscess Localized inflammation that occurs when bacteria or toxins rapidly enter the periradicular tissues, usually from the tooth pulp chamber.

Periapical radiographs Radiographs that include the root apex; may be used to examine anterior and posterior teeth if they are determined to be necessary during the clinical examination.

Pericoronitis Abscess associated with a partially erupted tooth or fully erupted tooth that is covered completely or partially by a flap of tissue (operculum).

Perimylolysis Enamel erosion that is the most common dental finding in a patient who orally purges; also spelled as *perimylosis.*

Periodontal abscess Exacerbated inflammatory reaction occurring usually in a periodontally involved area and caused by a blockage of the area by some foreign body.

Periodontal debridement Removal of subgingival calculus and oral biofilm and its byproducts while preserving as much tooth surface as possible.

Periodontal maintenance (PM) Supportive phase of care initiated after successful completion of active periodontal treatment; also known as *supportive periodontal therapy.*

Periodontal pocket Pathologic deepening of the gingival sulcus from the apical migration of the junctional epithelium and destruction of the periodontium.

Periodontitis Inflammatory disease of the periodontium that results from progression of gingivitis; caused by specific microorganisms; characterized by progressive destruction of the periodontal ligament and alveolar bone, recession, clinical attachment loss, pocket formation, and possible tooth mobility. The four major types are chronic, aggressive, necrotizing, and systemic. See also *Gingivitis*.

Periodontium Supporting structure of tissues that surrounds the teeth; includes the gingiva, periodontal ligament, root cementum, and alveolar bone.

Peritoneal dialysis The clinical purification of the patient's blood (a few ounces at a time) using the patient's own peritoneal lining to filter the blood.

Person-centered care A way of thinking and doing things that sees the people using health and social services as equal partners in planning, developing, and monitoring *care* to make sure it meets their needs. Also referred to as patient-centered care.

Personal protective equipment (PPE) Protective clothing, eye protection, airway protection, and other attire worn with the intent to protect the clinician from blood and body fluid exposure.

PICO The formality of using specific descriptions of the patient, intervention, comparison, and outcomes (PICO) of interest to frame a question that facilitates a computerized literature search by identifying key terms to use.

Piezoelectric Type of ultrasonic scaling device that has a ceramic transducer; alternating currents applied to the transducer create dimensional change that is transmitted to the tip; tip moves in a linear pattern, and only two sides of the tip are activated and applied to the tooth for mechanized instrumentation.

Pit and fissure sealant Thin plastic coating of an organic polymer (resin) placed in the pits and fissures of teeth to act as a physical barrier. Also known as a *dental sealant*.

Plaintiff In a legal dispute, the plaintiff is the person who brings the action or files the suit.

Polydipsia Excessive thirst with an abnormal urge to drink fluids at all times.

Polyphagia Eating of excessive amounts of food.

Polyuria A condition where the body urinates more than usual and passes excessive or abnormally large amount of urine each time a person urinates.

Pontic Artificial tooth or teeth that occupy the edentulous space and replace the missing tooth or teeth.

Population health The outcomes of well-being or disease in a group of individuals, including their distribution within the group.

Posttraumatic stress disorder (PTSD) A disorder that develops in some people who have experienced a shocking, scary, or dangerous event.

Posttreatment instructions Communication and recommendations for self-care of follow-up after healthcare procedures or treatment, usually given verbally and then in writing.

Preeclampsia Pregnancy complication in which the mother experiences high blood pressure—in addition to signs of damage to other organs—often to the kidneys or liver.

Preliminary impression Impressions taken to construct study models for diagnosing,

documenting patients' dental arches as part of permanent records, and enhancing patient education as a visual aid.

Preprocedural rinse A therapeutic oral rinse used before and during professional care to decrease oral microorganisms available to the clinical environment from oral procedures that cause aerosols and spatter.

Preventive sealant Sealant that is placed in caries-free teeth in an effort to prevent dental caries.

Probiotics Supplements and foods with a variety of live microorganisms intended to have health benefits, some of which naturally occur in the body.

Professional burnout A special type of work-related stress that involves a state of physical or emotional exhaustion, including a sense of reduced accomplishment and loss of personal identity.

Professionally applied fluoride Fluoride therapy administered in an oral healthcare setting by a dental hygienist; high-potency, low-frequency fluoride therapy.

Prognosis An evidence-based prediction of the patient's continued health and wellness.

Prophylactic antibiotic premedication Drug therapy administered before invasive dental hygiene instrumentation to patients at the highest risk of a negative outcome from infective endocarditis.

Prosthesis A dental appliance that replaces a missing tooth or covers up tooth defects.

Protective stabilization Any manual method, physical or mechanical device, material, or equipment that immobilizes or reduces the ability of a patient to move arms, legs, body, or head freely.

Proximal contact The contact between teeth (mesial to distal and mesial to mesial at the midline) that stabilizes their position in the dental arch and prevents food impaction between the teeth.

PubMed A computerized scientific database that provides free access to MEDLINE, a database providing citations and abstracts for biomedical literature from around the world.

Public policy A system of laws, regulatory measures, courses of action, and funding priorities concerning a given topic, promulgated by a governmental entity or its representatives.

Pulse The intermittent beat of the heart felt through the walls of an artery, which is an indicator of the integrity of the cardiovascular system.

Pulsus alternans Alternating strong and weak heartbeats, which may indicate ventricular failure.

Pulse oximeter A device that measures your blood oxygen saturation level.

Q

Quadrant Any one of the four quarters of the maxillary and mandibular arches.

R

Rampant caries Rapidly progressive decay that requires urgent intervention to gain control, eliminate the disease, and prevent progression.

Randomized controlled trial (RCT) A type of controlled study using randomization to

provide the strongest evidence for demonstrating cause and effect: that is, the treatment has caused the effect, rather than it occurring by chance.

Recession Reduction of the height of the marginal gingiva to a location apical to the cementoenamel junction, resulting in root surface exposure; signifies clinical attachment loss.

Recurrent caries New caries that occurs under or around a restoration or its margins. These lesions pose a unique threat because they may be difficult to detect and can invade the tissue beneath the restoration.

Reevaluation Appointment that takes place 4 to 6 weeks after completion of nonsurgical periodontal therapy so that a patient's response to active therapy can be determined.

Referral To direct to a source of information or care for a suspected problem, disease, or condition such as child abuse or neglect.

Remineralization Deposition of minerals into previously damaged areas of a tooth; process of replenishing calcium, phosphate, and fluoride ions to damaged tooth structure that has lost minerals; facilitated by fluoride therapy and amorphous calcium phosphate therapy.

Remote Patient Monitoring (RPM) Personal health and medical data collection from an individual in one location via electronic communication technologies, which is transmitted to a provider or data processing service in a different location for use in care and related supportive care.

Removable partial denture Partial denture that can be removed from the mouth by the patient.

Restorative therapy Restoration of damaged tooth structure, defective restorations, a esthetic inconsistencies, and anatomic and physiologic abnormalities.

Rheumatoid arthritis (RA) An autoimmune and inflammatory disease in which the immune system attacks healthy cells by mistake, causing inflammation (painful swelling) in the affected parts of the body. RA often attacks many places at once, affecting joints in the hands, wrists, and knees.

Risk assessment Act of determining the likelihood of a disease occurring in the future based on the balance between risk factors and protective factors.

Risk factors Behaviors and conditions present in the patient/client, child, parent, family, or environment that may contribute to future disease, disability, or abuse and neglect. Conditions, behaviors, lifestyles, or genes that if present will increase the likelihood of a disease occurring.

Root caries Dental caries that involves the tooth root, cementum, or cervical area of the tooth.

Root planing Definitive procedure to remove cementum or surface dentin that is rough, impregnated with calculus, or contaminated with toxins or microorganisms.

Rubber cup polishing Removal of tooth stains after scaling using a low-speed handpiece, prophylaxis angle with rubber cup, and prophylaxis polishing paste; coronal polishing.

S

Salivary gland dysfunction Altered or impaired performance of the glands in the mouth that produce saliva causing dry mouth or xerostomia, most commonly caused by medication usage, radiation therapy, and Sjogren syndrome.

Same-arch fulcrum Intraoral fulcrum established by a finger resting on a tooth surface on the same arch near the area being assessed or treated with a dental hygiene instrument.

Scaling Instrumentation of the crown and root surfaces of the teeth to remove oral biofilm, dental calculus, and extrinsic stains from surfaces without the intentional removal of tooth surface.

Seizure A period of symptoms due to abnormally excessive or synchronous neuronal activity in the brain.

Selective polishing or stain removal Focused polishing on tooth surfaces with visible stains after scaling and debridement is completed, especially when polishing may cause damage or when polishing is contraindicated.

Self-care (home care) A patient's care regimen performed at home daily.

Self-care practices Actions an individual can take through prioritizing personal health and well-being which help to mitigate the negative effects of stress.

Semicritical instruments Infection control term that refers to instruments that are not intended to penetrate soft tissue or bone but contact oral fluids.

Sex steroid hormones Any of a group of hormones that belongs to the class of compounds known as *steroids*, secreted by three "steroid glands"—the adrenal cortex, testes, and ovaries.

Side effects Effects of medication that differ from the intended therapeutic effects resulting from interaction with nontarget tissues. These effects, which are typically undesirable, may be dose related.

Sign Objective condition that can be observed directly.

Single-ended instrument A dental or dental hygiene instrument that has a working end on one end of the handle.

Social determinants of health Conditions in the environment where people live, work, and play that affect health, functioning, and quality of life.

Solid organ transplant A treatment, not a cure, for end-stage *organ* failure of the kidney, liver, pancreas, heart, and lung.

Spasticity A condition associated with damage to the brain or spinal cord in which muscles are continuously contracted, causing stiffness or tightness of the muscles that can interfere with normal movement, speech, and gait.

Special healthcare needs Any physical, developmental, mental, sensory, behavioral, cognitive, or emotional deficiency or limitation that requires medical treatment, *healthcare* intervention, and/ or specialized services.

Sphygmomanometer An instrument to measure blood pressure that consists of a pressure-measuring device called a manometer and an inflatable cuff that wraps around the arm or leg.

Standard of care The degree of care a reasonably prudent professional would exercise under the same or similar circumstances. The standard of care is not defined by the courts but rather is determined by a member of the profession.

Standard oral hygiene care Brushing, flossing, and rinsing are the *standard* way to take **care** of your mouth.

Standard precautions Synthesis of the major features of universal precautions and body substance isolation precautions applied to blood; other body fluids, secretions, and excretions except sweat; nonintact skin; and mucous membranes.

Statistical significance The likelihood that the results were unlikely to have occurred by chance at a specified probability level and that the differences would exist each time the experiment was repeated.

Stem cell transplantation A procedure in which a patient receives healthy blood-forming *cells* (*stem cells*) to replace their own that have been destroyed by disease or by radiation.

Stethoscope An instrument used to amplify sound, consisting of two earpieces, binaurals, plastic or rubber tubing, and a chestpiece. The chestpiece has two sides, the bell and the diaphragm.

Sterilization Destruction of all living organisms, including highly resistant bacterial spores.

Stress reduction protocol Steps taken during a healthcare appointment to reduce the body's cardiovascular and respiratory response to dental anxiety and stress, especially in medically compromised patients.

Stroke A condition that affects the arteries that occurs when a blood vessel that carries oxygen and nutrients to the brain is either blocked by a clot or bursts (or ruptures).

Subgingival calculus Calculus located below the gingival margin and attached to cementum or dentin.

Substance misuse The harmful and often illegal use of substances (like medications, illicit drugs, or alcohol) for a purpose that is not consistent with legal or medical guidelines.

Substance use disorder (SUD) Repeated misuse of substances, including drugs and alcohol.

Substantivity An antimicrobial agent's ability to durably bind with oral tissues and then be released over time, aiding in the agent's effectiveness.

Sulcular epithelium Nonkeratinized epithelial lining of the gingival sulcus.

Suprabony periodontal pocket Occurs when the junctional epithelium (JE) migrates below the cementoenamel junction (CEJ) but remains above the crest of the alveolar bone; commonly associated with horizontal bone loss.

Supragingival calculus Calculus located above the gingival margin; may attach to any hard surface, including enamel, restorative materials, prosthetic appliances, or exposed cementum.

Supraperiosteal injection Deposition of anesthetic solution above the apex of a maxillary tooth, such as the maxillary right central incisor; commonly referred to as a field block.

Symptom Subjective condition reported by the patient.

Synchronous Live, two-way interaction between a patient, or client, and a health provider using audiovisual telecommunications.

Syncope A temporary loss of consciousness due to inadequate blood flow to the brain, also called *fainting*.

Systematic reviews Reviews of published research reports that provide a summary of numerous, high-quality research studies that have investigated the same specific question. Systematic reviews use explicit criteria for retrieval of studies, assessment, and synthesis of evidence from individual randomized clinical trials and other well-controlled methods.

Systemic delivery Mode of application in which the agent (drug) is ingested and then delivered via the bloodstream; agents so delivered include products such as fluoride supplements, fluoridated water, and antibiotic medications.

Systolic blood pressure The maximum pressure occurring in the blood vessels during cardiac ventricular contraction (systole) and is the number on the sphygmomanometer when the first heart sound is heard.

T

Tachycardia Abnormally high heart rate, usually greater than 100 beats per minute (BPM).

Tachypnea Abnormally high breathing rate, usually greater than 20 respirations per minute (RPM).

Tactile sensitivity Ability to distinguish relative degrees of roughness and smoothness on the tooth surface via the vibrations transferred from the instrument's working end, shank, and handle to the clinician's fingers.

Teleconsultation A common form of teledentistry where oral health providers complete remote evaluations and make diagnoses after the review of pertinent patient data.

Teledentistry The practice of dentistry assisted by telecommunications technology.

Telehealth A broad variety of health and health-related services delivered through telecommunications and digital communications technology.

Telemonitoring A common form of teledentistry where oral health conditions are monitored remotely.

Teletriage A common form of teledentistry where oral health providers provide virtual patient evaluations to determine an appropriate course of action.

Temporomandibular joint (TMJ) dysfunction (TMD) Impaired function of the joint characterized by pain, headache, tinnitus, impaired hearing, and pain around the tongue; any one or combination of the following maladies: pain in the area of the TMJ and or muscles of mastication, limitation or deviation in the movement of the mandible, and/or detectable sounds during movement of the mandible. Also known as *temporomandibular dysfunction*.

Teratogen Substances that cause congenital disorders in a developing embryo or fetus; examples include drugs, medicine, chemicals, certain infections, and toxic substances.

Terminal shank The part of a dental or dental hygiene instrument that extends between the blade and the first bend of the *shank*.

Therapeutic communication Process of sending and receiving messages between a patient or client and a healthcare provider that helps the client to make decisions and reach goals related to comfort and health.

Therapeutic effect Interact of medications with their target tissues to produce a desired effect.

Therapeutic sealant Sealant that is placed in teeth with incipient carious lesions in an effort to stop the decay process.

Tobacco and nicotine products Articles or substances that contain tobacco and/or toxins such as nicotine, including cigars, smokeless tobacco, hookah, electronic cigarettes, snuff, snus, and chewing tobacco.

Tobacco cessation Evidence-based intervention for becoming tobacco free.

Tolerance The need to take increased doses of a substance to produce the same response obtained earlier with a smaller dose.

Tooth bleaching (whitening) Use of a chemical oxidizing agent, sometimes in combination with heat, to lighten tooth discoloration.

Topical fluoride Products that are self-applied by patients in a nonprescription form, or professionally applied prescription products that are delivered for variable amounts of time to exposed crown and root surfaces and then expectorated.

Transient bacteremia Temporary presence of bacteria and other microorganisms in the bloodstream.

Transient ischemic attack (TIA) A transient focal neurologic deficit that persists for less than 24 hours and is followed by complete clinical recovery.

Transillumination The passing of a strong beam of light through the teeth for an oral examination using a fiber optic device or a dental mirror.

Trauma Injury that results when the patient inadvertently chews or bites oral tissues while they are still anesthetized. An injury caused by accident or a violent act.

Tremors Involuntary rhythmic repetitions or oscillations of movement at regular intervals.

Trendeleburg A patient position used in the rendering of dental/dental hygiene care where the body lies flat on a 15- to 30-degree incline and the feet are elevated above the head.

Triangular toothpicks A plaque removal device made of a wooden toothpick with a triangle in cross section.

Trigeminal neuralgia A neuropathy of the trigeminal nerve (cranial nerve V) that results in one of the most painful, chronic disorders of the orofacial region; also referred to as tic douloureux.

Trismus Limited ability to open the mouth.

Tuberculosis A contagious disease caused by the bacteria *Mycobacterium tuberculosis*, which usually attacks the lungs but can also damage other parts of the body.

Type 1 diabetes A form of *diabetes* that involves the pancreas making no insulin to regulate blood sugar; formerly called juvenile diabetes.

Type 2 diabetes A form of *diabetes* that is related to the body's inability to use insulin properly to control blood glucose levels; also called insulin resistance.

U

Ulceration Loss of skin surface, with a gray to yellow center surrounded by a red halo; results from destruction of epithelial integrity caused by discrepancy in cell maturation, loss of intracellular attachments, and disruption of the basement membrane.

Ultrasonic scaler Mechanized device that produces vibratory motions of the instrument tip from 18,000 to 50,000 cycles per second; removes all types of supragingival and subgingival deposits from tooth surfaces; includes magnetostrictive and piezoelectric mechanized instruments.

Ultrasonic insert A scaling and debridement instrument designed to fit into an *ultrasonic* scaling unit handpiece, which uses sound waves and water to remove stains, plaque, and calculus.

Unfilled sealant Sealant that does not contain particles and is therefore less resistant to wear; useful in school-based settings when occlusion cannot be adjusted with a finishing burr and dental handpiece.

Universal curette Curette that has two cutting edges on each working end; designed for use in all areas throughout the mouth.

Unmet human needs (human need deficits) Human needs related to oral health, which are in deficit. See also *Human need.*

US Food and Drug Administration (FDA) A federal agency in the United States that is responsible for protecting the public health by ensuring the safety, efficacy, and security of human and veterinary drugs, biological products, and medical devices; and by ensuring the safety of our nation's food supply, cosmetics, and products that emit radiation.

V

Veracity An ethical principle of truth telling, or integrity, that is critical to meaningful communication and relationships between individuals.

Ventilator-acquired pneumonia A lung infection that develops in a person who is on a machine that is used to help a patient breathe by giving oxygen through a tube placed in a patient's mouth or nose, or through a hole in the front of the neck.

Vulnerable adult Anyone over age 18 who has a physical, mental, or emotional disorder that makes self-care difficult; anyone in a hospital, nursing home, transitional care unit, assisted living, housing with services, board and care, foster care, or other licensed care facility; or a person who receives licensed care services.

W

Working end Part of the instrument attached to the shank that determines the general purpose of the instrument.

X

Xerostomia Dry mouth caused by a variety of conditions such as a salivary gland dysfunction, medications, and radiation therapy to the head and neck.

Y

Yokes Devices to hold gas cylinders in contact with the gas machine.

Z

Zones of territory Appropriate distances or personal spaces that are maintained between people in various situations; such zones may be based on the degree of respect, authority, and friendship among the individuals communicating.

INDEX

Page numbers followed by *f* indicate figure, by *t* table, and by *b* box.